# modern NUTRITION in health and disease

EDITORS

# MAURICE E. SHILS, M.D., Sc.D.

Adjunct Professor (Nutrition)
Department of Public Health Sciences
Bowman Gray School of Medicine
Wake Forest University
Winston-Salem, North Carolina
Professor Emeritus of Medicine
Cornell University Medical College
Formerly, Director of Clinical Nutrition
Memorial Sloan-Kettering Cancer Center
New York, New York

# JAMES A. OLSON, Ph.D.

Distinguished Professor of Liberal Arts and Sciences
Department of Biochemistry and Biophysics
Iowa State University
Ames, Iowa

# MOSHE SHIKE, M.D.

Director of Clinical Nutrition
Memorial Sloan-Kettering Cancer Center
Associate Professor of Clinical Medicine
Cornell University Medical College
New York, New York

# modern NUTRITION in health and disease

EIGHTH EDITION

VOLUME 1

Lea & Febiger
PHILADELPHIA · BALTIMORE · HONG KONG
LONDON · MUNICH · SYDNEY · TOKYO
A WAVERLY COMPANY
1994

Lea & Febiger
P.O. Box 3024
200 Chester Field Parkway
Malvern, PA 19355-9725
U.S.A.

Executive Editor—R. Kenneth Bussy
Development Editor—Tanya Lazar
Project Editor—Dorothy DiRienzi
Production Manager—Samuel A. Rondinelli

First Edition, 1955
Second Edition, 1960 Reprinted August, 1961
Third Edition, 1964 Reprinted February, 1966
Four Edition, 1968 Reprinted March, 1970
Reprinted July, 1971
Fifth Edition, 1973 Reprinted September, 1974
Reprinted April, 1975
Reprinted June, 1976
Reprinted November, 1977
Sixth Edition, 1980 Reprinted July, 1980
Reprinted November, 1981
Reprinted August, 1984
Reprinted May, 1986
Seventh Edition, 1988
Eighth Edition, 1994

Library of Congress Cataloging-in-Publication Data

Modern nutrition in health and disease / edited by Maurice E. Shils,
James A. Olson, Moshe Shike.—8th ed.
p. cm.
Includes bibliographical references and index.
ISBN 0-8121-1485-X (set)
1. Nutrition. 2. Diet therapy. I. Shils, Maurice E. (Maurice
Edward), 1914– . II. Olson, James A. III. Shike, Moshe.
[DNLM: 1. Diet Therapy. 2. Nutrition. WB 400 M689]
QP141.M64 1993
613.2—dc20
DNLM/DLC
for Librairy of Congress 92-49855
CIP

NOTE: Although the author(s) and the publisher have taken reasonable steps to ensure the accuracy of the drug information included in this text before publication, drug information may change without notice and readers are advised to consult the manufacturer's packaging inserts before prescribing medications.

Reprints of chapters may be purchased from Lea & Febiger in quantities of 100 or more. Contact Sally Grande in the Sales Department.



PRINTED IN THE UNITED STATES OF AMERICA

Print No. 5 4 3 2 1

# IN MEMORIAM

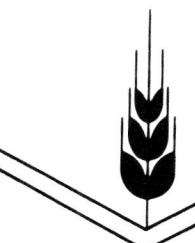

## Robert Stanley Goodhart, M.D.,D.M.S. (1909–1992)

Pioneer in clinical nutrition, ardent supporter of clinical nutrition research and education, founder with Matthew Wohl, M.D. of *Modern Nutrition in Health and Disease* and an editor of its first six editions. He established the standards we strive to emulate.

Maurice E. Shils
James Allen Olson
Moshe Shike

# PREFACE

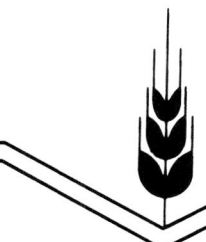

The eighth edition of *Modern Nutrition in Health and Disease* is published 38 years after its first edition appeared. Its new format of two volumes reflects the increasing information in all aspects of its field and the inclusion of many new topics, and will, we hope, permit easier use by the reader.

Its objective remains unchanged: to serve as a major authoritative textbook and reference source in basic and clinical nutrition for students and practitioners in the various aspects of biomedical research and education, medicine, dentistry, osteopathy, dietetics, nursing, pharmacy, and public health. This has been achieved by selecting authors who are authorities in their topic areas in large part as the result of their important personal contributions. These 133 authors of 98 chapters and subsections, representing 10 different countries and many scientific disciplines, are truly the source and strength of this publication.

Approximately one third of the chapters are devoted to energy and specific dietary components. The role of nutrition is then reviewed in relation to integrated biologic systems extending from the cell, to various organ systems, and to intact individuals in situations of physiologic and environmental stresses. Methods of nutritional assessment of the individual are followed by 25 chapters on dietary and nutritional interrelations with diseases, and then by chapters on nutrition support modalities and ethics and by a major section on diet and nutrition in the health of populations.

For the convenience of the reader this edition is in two volumes, each containing a full table of contents, index, and appendices.

When indicated, we have expressed quantitative data both in conventional units and in international system (SI) units. The widespread use of the SI units in major biomedical journals and publications in the United States and other countries makes this dual unitage useful to readers.

We are indebted to members of the Lea & Febiger staff who are identified on the copyright page. Our interactions have been mainly with R. Kenneth Bussy, Senior Executive Editor, and Samuel A. Rondinelli, Production Manager, and we greatly appreciate their cooperation and understanding. Thanks also to Mrs. Holly Lukens, project editor, and her copy editor colleagues for their meticulous work. Maggie Wheelock, Beverly A. Thomas, and Betty Bell Shils have enabled us to manage the enormous amount of communications, record-keeping, and paper work involving the editors, the many authors, the publisher's staff, and the copy editors. To our wives, Betty, Giovanna, and Sherry goes our appreciation for their understanding of the further demands on our time required in the preparation of this book. The senior editor expresses his appreciation to Curt Furberg, M.D., Ph.D. for his support.

*Winston-Salem, North Carolina*
*Ames, Iowa*
*New York, New York*

Maurice E. Shils
James Allen Olson
Moshe Shike

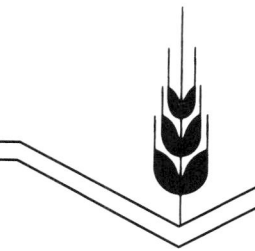

# CONTRIBUTORS

**PHYLLIS B. ACOSTA, Dr. P.H.**
Director, Metabolic Diseases
Ross Laboratories
Columbus, Ohio

**LINDSAY H. ALLEN, Ph.D., R.D.**
Alumni Distinguished Professor of Nutritional Sciences
University of Connecticut
Storrs, Connecticut

**G. HARVEY ANDERSON, Ph.D.**
Acting Dean of Medicine
Professor of Nutritional Sciences, Medical Sciences, and Physiology
Faculty of Medicine
University of Toronto
Toronto, Canada

**JAMES W. ANDERSON, M.D.**
Professor of Medicine and Clinical Nutrition
College of Medicine
University of Kentucky
Chief of Endocrine-Metabolic Section
Veterans Affairs Medical Center
Lexington, Kentucky

**HAROLD M. AUKEMA, Ph.D.**
Research Associate
Department of Animal Science
Texas A&M University
College Station, Texas

**LYNNE M. AUSMAN, D.Sc.**
Scientist I
United States Department of Agriculture
Human Nutrition Research Center on Aging
Tufts University
Boston, Massachusetts

**STEPHEN BARRETT, M.D.**
Instructor of Health Education
Pennsylvania State University
State College, Pennsylvania

**J. CHRISTOPHER BAUERNFEIND, Ph.D.**
Formerly, Director of Agrochemistry and Nutrition and Research Coordinator
Hoffmann-LaRoche
Gainesville, Florida

**GEORGE H. BEATON, Ph.D.**
Professor of Nutritional Sciences
Faculty of Medicine
University of Toronto
Toronto, Canada

**ABBY STOLPER BLOCH, M.S., R.D.**
Coordinator of Clinical Nutrition Research
Memorial Sloan-Kettering Cancer Center
New York, New York

**ALFRED JAY BOLLETT, M.D.**
Clinical Professor of Medicine
School of Medicine
Yale University
New Haven, Connecticut
Vice President for Academic Affairs
Danbury Hospital
Danbury, Connecticut

**IRWIN G. BRODSKY, M.D., M.P.H.**
Research Assistant Professor
Clinical Associate Physician
College of Medicine
University of Vermont
Burlington, Vermont

**HARRY P. BROQUIST, Ph.D.**
Professor of Biochemistry Emeritus
Vanderbilt University
Nashville, Tennessee
Adjunct Professor
Utah State University
Logan, Utah

**RAYMOND F. BURK, M.D.**
Professor of Medicine
Chief of Gastroenterology
School of Medicine
Vanderbilt University
Nashville, Tennessee

**FRANCISCO CHEW, M.D.**
Medical Officer
Division of Nutrition and Health
Instituto de Nutrición de Centro América y Panamá (INCAP)
Gastroenterology Associate
Department of Pediatrics
Hospital Roosevelt
Guatemala City, Guatemala

**ROBERT CHIN, JR., M.D.**
Assistant Professor of Medicine
Section on Pulmonary and Critical Care Medicine
Bowman Gray School of Medicine
Wake Forest University
Winston-Salem, North Carolina

**GRAEME A. CLUGSTON, M.B., D.C.H., Ph.D.**
Nutrition Section
World Health Organization
Geneva, Switzerland

**J. JOSEPH CONNON, M.D.**
Professor of Medicine
Faculty of Medicine
University of Toronto
Physician-in-chief
St. Michael's Hospital
Toronto, Canada

**MARILYN C. CRIM, M.D., Ph.D.**
Assistant Professor
School of Nutrition
Assistant Professor
School of Medicine
Scientist II
United States Department of Agriculture
Human Nutrition Research Center on Aging
Tufts University
Boston, Massachusetts

**KRISHNAMURTI DAKSHINAMURTI, Ph.D.**
Professor of Biochemistry and Molecular Biology
Faculty of Medicine
University of Manitoba
Winnipeg, Manitoba, Canada

**KSHITISH C. DAS, M.D., PhD.**
Professor and Head of Hematology
Faculty of Medicine
Kuwait University
Safat, Kuwait

**EARL B. DAWSON, PhD.**
Associate Professor of Obstetrics and Gynecology
University of Texas Medical Branch
Galveston, Texas

**BESS DAWSON-HUGHES, M.D.**
Chief of Calcium and Bone Metabolism Laboratory
United States Department of Agriculture
Human Nutrition Research Center on Aging
Tufts University
Boston, Massachusetts

**DOMINICK P. DePAOLA, D.D.S., Ph.D.**
President and Dean
Baylor College of Dentistry
Dallas, Texas

**JOHN T. DEVLIN, M.D.**
Associate Professor of Medicine
University of Vermont
Burlington, Vermont
Medical Director, Diabetes Center
Maine Medical Center
Portland, Maine

**PIERRE M. DREYFUS, M.D.**
Professor Emeritus of Neurology and Pediatrics
School of Medicine
University of California
Davis, California

**JOHANNA T. DWYER, D.Sc.**
Professor of Medicine (Nutrition) and Community Health, School of Medicine
Tufts University
Director, Frances Stern Nutrition Center
New England Medical Center Hospitals
Boston, Massachusetts

**LOUIS J. ELSAS, II, M.D.**
Professor and Acting Chairman of Human Genetics
School of Medicine
Emory University
Atlanta, Georgia

**JOHN W. ERDMAN, JR., Ph.D.**
Director of Nutritional Sciences
Professor of Food Science
University of Illinois
Urbana, Illinois

**MARY P. FAINE, M.S., R.D.**
Assistant Professor
Director of Nutrition Education
Department of Prosthodontics
School of Dentistry
University of Washington
Seattle, Washington

**VIRGIL F. FAIRBANKS, M.D.**
Consultant, Mayo Clinic
Professor of Medicine and Laboratory Medicine
Mayo Clinic and Mayo Foundation
Rochester, Minnesota

**MICHAEL D. FALLON, M.D.†**
Formerly, Associate Professor of Pathology
Jefferson Medical College
Thomas Jefferson University
Philadelphia, Pennsylvania

**PHILIP M. FARRELL, M.D., Ph.D.**
Professor and Chairman of Pediatrics
Affiliate Faculty of Nutritional Sciences
University of Wisconsin
Madison, Wisconsin

†Deceased

**LAWRENCE FEINMAN, M.D.**
Chief of Gastroenterology
Veterans Affairs Medical Center
Bronx, New York
Associate Professor of Medicine
Mount Sinai School of Medicine
New York, New York

**ELAINE B. FELDMAN, M.D.**
Professor of Medicine, Physiology, and Endocrinology
Chief of Nutrition
Medical College of Georgia
Augusta, Georgia

**ANN FOGELMAN, R.D., M.P.H.**
Senior Research Associate
Department of Obstetrics and Gynecology
University of Texas Medical Branch
Galveston, Texas

**ALLAN L. FORBES, M.D.**
Medical Consultant (Foods and Nutrition)
Rockville, Maryland
Formerly, Director of Office of Nutrition and Food Sciences
Center for Food Safety and Applied Nutrition
Food and Drug Administration
Washington, D.C.

**GILBERT B. FORBES, M.D.**
Professor of Pediatrics and Biophysics
School of Medicine and Dentistry
University of Rochester
Rochester, New York

**PATTI BAZEL GEIL, M.S., R.D.**
Nutrition Coordinator
Metabolic Research Group
Adjunct Professor of Clinical Nutrition
University of Kentucky
Lexington, Kentucky

**BARRY R. GOLDIN, Ph.D.**
Associate Professor of Community Health
School of Medicine
Tufts University
Boston, Massachusetts

**ELIZABETH J. GONG, M.P.H., M.S., R.D.**
Nutrition Research Associate
Office of the President
University of California
Oakland, California

**ALAN G. GOODRIDGE, Ph.D.**
Professor and Head of Biochemistry
University of Iowa
Iowa City, Iowa

**SHERWOOD L. GORBACH, M.D.**
Professor of Community Health
School of Medicine
Tufts University
Boston, Massachusetts

**HARRY L. GREENE, M.D.**
Director of Nutritional Sciences
Mead Johnson Research Center
Evansville, Indiana

**LOUIS E. GRIVETTI, Ph.D.**
Professor of Geography and Nutrition
University of California
Davis, California

**HERMAN GROSSMAN, M.D.**
Professor of Radiology and Pediatrics
Duke University Medical Center
Durham, North Carolina

**EDWARD H. HAPONIK, M.D.**
Professor of Medicine
Section on Pulmonary and Critical Care Medicine
Bowman Gray School of Medicine
Wake Forest University
Winston-Salem, North Carolina

**ALFRED E. HARPER, Ph.D.**
E. V. McCollum Professor of Nutritional Sciences Emeritus
University of Wisconsin
Madison, Wisconsin

**ROGER C. HARRIS, Ph.D.**
Department of Comparative Physiology
Animal Health Trust
Newmarket, Suffolk, England

**JOHN N. HATHCOCK, Ph.D.**
Chief of Experimental Nutrition Branch
Division of Nutrition
Food and Drug Administration
Washington, D.C.

**KENNETH C. HAYES, D.V.M., Ph.D**
Professor of Biology (Nutrition)
Director of Foster Biomedical Research Laboratory
Brandeis University
Waltham, Massachusetts

**FELIX P. HEALD, M.D.**
Professor of Pediatrics
Director, Division of Adolescent Medicine
School of Medicine
University of Maryland
Baltimore, Maryland

**WILLIAM C. HEIRD, M.D.**
Professor of Pediatrics
Children's Nutrition Research Center
Baylor College of Medicine
Houston, Texas

**VICTOR HERBERT, M.D., J.D.**
Professor of Medicine
Mount Sinai School of Medicine
New York, New York
Chief of Hematology and Nutrition Laboratory
Veterans Affairs Medical Center
Bronx, New York

**BASIL S. HETZEL, M.D.**
Executive Director
International Council of Iodine Deficiency Disorders
Adelaide, Australia

**STEVEN B. HEYMSFIELD, M.D.**
Associate Professor of Medicine
College of Physicians and Surgeons
Columbia University
Director of Human Body Composition Laboratory
Director of Outpatient Obesity Research
Obesity Research Center
St. Luke's-Roosevelt Hospital
New York, New York

**L. JOHN HOFFER, M.D., PH.D.**
Associate Professor of Medicine and Dietetics and Human Nutrition
Associate Director of McGill Nutrition and Food Science Centre
McGill University
Associate Physician
Royal Victoria Hospital
Montreal, Canada

**MICHAEL F. HOLICK, PH.D., M.D.**
Professor of Medicine, Dermatology, and Physiology
School of Medicine
Boston University
Chief of Endocrine Section
Boston City Hospital
Boston, Massachusetts

**BRUCE J. HOLUB, PH.D.**
Professor of Nutritional Sciences
University of Guelph
Guelph, Ontario, Canada

**ERIC HULTMAN, M.D.**
Professor of Clinical Chemistry
Karolinska Institutet
Huddinge, Sweden

**DIANE M. HUSE, R.D., M.S.**
Assistant Professor of Nutrition
Mayo Medical School
Dietician, Clinical Dietetics
Division of Endocrinology, Metabolism, and Internal Medicine
Mayo Clinic and Mayo Foundation
Rochester, Minnesota

**ROBERT A. JACOB, PH.D.**
Research Chemist
United States Department of Agriculture
Western Human Nutrition Research Center
Presidio of San Francisco, California

**KHURSHEED N. JEEJEEBHOY, M.B.B.S., PH.D.**
Professor of Medicine
Faculty of Medicine
Member, Institute of Medical Science
University of Toronto
Staff Gastroenterologist, St. Michael's Hospital
Toronto, Canada

**ALEXANDRA L. JENKINS, R.D.**
Research Associate
Department of Nutritional Sciences
University of Toronto
Senior Research Associate
Clinical Nutritional and Risk Factor Modification Centre
St. Michael's Hospital
Toronto, Canada

**DAVID J.A. JENKINS, M.D., PH.D.**
Professor of Nutritional Sciences and Medicine
Faculty of Medicine
University of Toronto
Staff Physician
Division of Endocrinology and Metabolism
St. Michael's Hospital
Associate Physician
Division of Gastroenterology
Toronto General Hospital
Toronto, Canada

**ERIC JÉQUIER, M.D.**
Professor
Institut de Physiologie
Faculty of Medicine
University of Lausanne
Lausanne, Switzerland

**MORLEY R. KARE, PH.D.**†
Formerly, Director
Monell Chemical Senses Center
Philadelphia, Pennsylvania

†Deceased

**CARL L. KEEN, Ph.D.**
Professor of Nutrition
University of California
Davis, California

**GERALD T. KEUSCH, M.D.**
Professor of Medicine
Division of Geographic Medicine and Infectious Diseases
New England Medical Center Hospitals
Boston, Massachusetts

**JANET C. KING, Ph.D.**
Professor of Nutritional Sciences
University of California
Berkeley, California

**JOEL D. KOPPLE, M.D.**
Professor of Medicine and Public Health
University of California
Los Angeles, California
Chief of Nephrology and Hypertension
Harbor-UCLA Medical Center
Torrance, California

**MARK A. KORSTEN, M.D.**
Associate Professor of Medicine
Mount Sinai School of Medicine
New York, New York
Assistant Chief of Medicine
Veterans Affairs Medical Center
Bronx, New York

**JANE MORLEY KOTCHEN, M.D., M.P.H.**
Professor of Medicine
School of Medicine
West Virginia University
Morgantown, West Virginia

**THEODORE A. KOTCHEN, M.D.**
E. B. Flink Professor and Chairman of Medicine
School of Medicine
West Virginia University
Morgantown, West Virginia

**ELIZABETH A. KRALL, Ph.D.**
Assistant Professor of Nutrition
School of Nutrition
Scientist II
United States Department of Agriculture
Human Nutrition Research Center on Aging
Tufts University
Boston, Massachusetts

**MARIE FANELLI KUCZMARSKI, Ph.D., R.D.**
Associate Professor of Nutrition and Dietetics
College of Human Resources
University of Delaware
Newark, Delaware

**ROBERT J. KUCZMARSKI, Dr.P.H., R.D.**
Nutritionist
United States Department of Health and Human Services
Centers for Disease Control
National Center for Health Statistics
Hyattsville, Maryland

**PAUL A. LACHANCE, Ph.D.**
Professor and Chairman of Food Science
Cook College
Rutgers University
New Brunswick, New Jersey

**JAMES E. LEKLEM, Ph.D.**
Professor of Nutrition and Food Management
Oregon State University
Corvallis, Oregon

**ORVILLE A. LEVANDER, Ph.D.**
Research Chemist
United States Department of Agriculture
Human Nutrition Research Center
Beltsville, Maryland

**ALICE H. LICHTENSTEIN, D.Sc.**
Assistant Professor
United States Department of Agriculture
Human Nutrition Research Center on Aging
Tufts University
Boston, Massachusetts

**CHARLES S. LIEBER, M.D.**
Professor of Medicine and Pathology
Mount Sinai School of Medicine
New York, New York
Director of Alcohol Research Center
Veterans Affairs Medical Center
Bronx, New York

**WILLEM G. LINSCHEER, M.D., Ph.D.**
Professor of Medicine
State University of New York
Chief of Gastroenterology
Veterans Affairs Medical Center
Syracuse, New York

**ALEXANDER R. LUCAS, M.D.**
Professor of Psychiatry
Mayo Medical School
Consultant, Section of Child and Adolescent Psychiatry
Mayo Clinic
Rochester, Minnesota

**DONALD B. McCORMICK, Ph.D.**
Fuller E. Callaway Professor and Chairman of Biochemistry
Emory University
Atlanta, Georgia

**IAN MACDONALD, M.D., D.Sc.**
Emeritus Professor of Applied Physiology
Guy's Hospital
University of London
London, England

**WILLIAM J. McGANITY, M.D.**
Ashbel Smith Professor of Obstetrics and Gynecology
University of Texas Medical Branch
Galveston, Texas

**DONALD S. MCLAREN, M.D., Ph.D.**
Honorary Head of Nutritional Blindness Prevention Programme
Institute of Ophthalmology
London, England

**DONALD J. McNAMARA, Ph.D.**
Professor of Nutrition and Food Science
University of Arizona
Tucson, Arizona

**JOEL B. MASON, M.D.**
Assistant Professor of Clinical Nutrition and Gastroenterology
School of Medicine
Scientist II
United States Department of Agriculture
Human Nutrition Research Center on Aging
Tufts University
Boston, Massachusetts

**RICHARD D. MATTES, M.P.H., Ph.D., R.D.**
Associate Member
Monell Chemical Senses Center
Adjunct Assistant Professor of Nutrition in Medicine
School of Medicine
University of Pennsylvania
Philadelphia, Pennsylvania

**KATHLEEN SHIVE MATTHEWS, Ph.D.**
Wiess Professor of Biochemistry and Cell Biology
Rice University
Houston, Texas

**JAMES H. MEYER, M.D.**
Chief of Gastroenterology
Sepulveda Veterans Affairs Medical Center
Sepulveda, California

**MORTON A. MEYERS, M.D.**
Professor of Radiology
State University of New York
Stony Brook, New York

**J. ROBERTO MORAN, M.D.**
Director of Pediatric Nutrition, Gastroenterology, and Allergy
Mead Johnson Research Center
Evansville, Indiana
Associate Clinical Professor
School of Medicine
Indiana University
Bloomington, Indiana

**HAMISH N. MUNRO, M.D., D.Sc.**
Professor, School of Nutrition
Professor, School of Medicine
Tufts University
Boston, Massachusetts

**QUENTIN N. MYRVIK, Ph.D.**
Vice President and Senior Scientist
Musculoskeletal Sciences Research Institute
Herndon, Virginia
Formerly, Professor of Microbiology and Immunology
Bowman Gray School of Medicine
Wake Forest University
Winston-Salem, North Carolina

**FORREST H. NIELSEN, Ph.D.**
Center Director and Research Nutritionist
United States Department of Agriculture
Grand Forks Human Nutrition Research Center
Grand Forks, North Dakota

**MAN S. OH, M.D.**
Professor of Medicine
Health Science Center at Brooklyn
State University of New York
Brooklyn, New York

**JAMES A. OLSON, Ph.D.**
Distinguished Professor of Liberal Arts and Sciences
Department of Biochemistry and Biophysics
Iowa State University
Ames, Iowa

**ROBERT E. OLSON, M.D.**
Professor of Medicine Emeritus
School of Medicine
Consulting Physician
University Hospital
State University of New York
Stony Brook, New York

**MICHAEL W. PARIZA, Ph.D.**
Director of Food Research Institute
Professor and Chairman of Food Microbiology and Toxicology
University of Wisconsin
Madison, Wisconsin

**F. XAVIER PI-SUNYER, M.D.**
Professor of Medicine
College of Physicians and Surgeons
Columbia University
Director, Division of Endocrinology, Diabetes, and Nutrition
Director of Obesity Research Center
St. Luke's-Roosevelt Hospital
New York, New York

**NORA PLESOFSKY-VIG, PH.D.**
Research Associate
Departments of Genetics and Cell Biology and Plant Biology
University of Minnesota
St. Paul, Minnesota

**ANGELA G. PONEROS-SCHNEIER, M.S.**
Associate Program Coordinator in Food Science
University of Illinois
Urbana, Illinois

**JEANNE I. RADER, PH.D.**
Chief of Nutrient Toxicity Section
Division of Nutrition
Food and Drug Administration
Washington, D.C.

**ROBERT J. ROBERTS, M.D.**
Chairman of Pediatrics
Children's Medical Center
University of Virginia
Charlottesville, Virginia

**DAPHNE A. ROE, M.D.**
Professor of Nutrition
Cornell University
Ithaca, New York

**IRWIN H. ROSENBERG, M.D.**
Professor of Medicine and Nutrition
School of Medicine
Director
United States Department of Agriculture
Human Nutrition Research Center on Aging
Tufts University
Boston, Massachusetts

**ROBERT RUCKER, PH.D.**
Professor of Nutrition and Biological Chemistry
University of California
Davis, California

**ROBERT M. RUSSELL, M.D.**
Professor of Medicine and Nutrition
School of Medicine
Associate Director
United States Department of Agriculture
Human Nutrition Research Center on Aging
Tufts University
Boston, Massachusetts

**HUGH A. SAMPSON, M.D.**
Professor of Pediatrics
School of Medicine
Director of Pediatric Clinical Research Center
Johns Hopkins University
Baltimore, Maryland

**BARBARA O. SCHNEEMAN, PH.D.**
Professor and Chair of Nutrition
University of California
Davis, California

**YVES SCHUTZ, M.P.H., PH.D.**
Institut de Physiologie
Faculty of Medicine
University of Lausanne
Lausanne, Switzerland

**MASUD SEYAL, M.D., PH.D.**
Associate Professor of Neurology
University of California
Davis, California

**MOSHE SHIKE, M.D.**
Director of Clinical Nutrition
Memorial Sloan-Kettering Cancer Center
New York, New York

**MAURICE E. SHILS, M.D., SC.D.**
Adjunct Professor (Nutrition) of Public Health Sciences
Bowman Gray School of Medicine
Wake Forest University
Winston-Salem, North Carolina

**WILEY W. SOUBA, JR., M.D., SC.D.**
Associate Professor of Surgery
Director of Surgical Metabolism
College of Medicine
University of Florida
Gainesville, Florida

**LAWRENCE L. SPRIET, PH.D.**
Assistant Professor of Human Biology
University of Guelph
Guelph, Ontario, Canada

**FRANCENE M. STEINBERG, R.D., PH.D.**
Research Fellow in Nutrition
University of California
Davis, California

**MARIAN E. SWENSEID, PH.D.**
Professor Emerita of Community Health Sciences
School of Public Health
University of California
Los Angeles, California

**VICHAI TANPHAICHITR, M.D., PH.D.**
Professor of Medicine
Director of Research Center
Faculty of Medicine
Ramathibodi Hospital
Bangkok, Thailand

**JAMES A. THOMAS, Ph.D.**
Professor of Biochemistry
Iowa State University
Ames, Iowa

**JANET TIETYEN, M.S., R.D.**
Graduate Research Assistant
Department of Grain Science and Industry
Kansas State University
Manhattan, Kansas

**ANN TIGHE, M.S., R.D.**
Research Dietitian
Obesity Research Center
St. Lukes-Roosevelt Hospital College of Physicians and Surgeons
Columbia University
New York, New York

**BENJAMÍN TORÚN, M.D., Ph.D.**
Senior Scientist and Head
Program of Clinical Nutrition and Metabolism
Instituto de Nutrición de Centro América y Panamá (INCAP)
Professor of Basic and Human Nutrition
University of San Carlos de Guatemala
Guatemala City, Guatemala

**ELKE A. TRAUTWEIN, Ph.D.**
Postdoctoral Fellow in Nutrition
Department of Biology
Foster Biomedical Research Laboratory
Brandeis University
Waltham, Massachusetts

**A. STEWART TRUSWELL, M.D.**
Boden Professor of Human Nutrition
University of Sydney
Sydney, Australia

**JUDITH R. TURNLUND, Ph.D., R.D.**
Research Nutrition Scientist
United States Department of Agriculture
Western Human Nutrition Research Center
Presidio of San Francisco, California

**PENNY S. TURTEL, M.D.**
Special Fellow
Memorial Sloan-Kettering Cancer Center
New York, New York
Clinical Professor
Robert Wood Johnson Medical School
University of Medicine and Dentistry of New Jersey
Piscataway, New Jersey

**ANTOINE J. VERGROESEN, M.D., Ph.D.**
Professor Emeritus of Nutrition
Erasmus University
Rotterdam, The Netherlands

**RICHARD I. VOGEL, D.M.D.**
Professor and Chairperson of Oral Pathology, Biology, and Diagnostic Sciences
New Jersey Dental School
University of Medicine and Dentistry of New Jersey
Newark, New Jersey

**ZI-MIAN WANG, M.S.**
Research Associate
Obesity Research Center
St. Lukes-Roosevelt Hospital
College of Physicians and Surgeons
Columbia University
New York, New York

**ROBIN C. WATSON, M.D.†**
Formerly, Professor of Radiology
Cornell University Medical College
Formerly, Chairman of Medical Imaging
Memorial Sloan-Kettering Cancer Center
New York, New York

**ELSIE M. WIDDOWSON, D.Sc.**
Department of Medicine
Addenbrookes Hospital and Medical Research Council
Cambridge, England

**DOUGLAS W. WILMORE, M.D.**
Frank Sawyer Professor of Surgery
Harvard Medical School
Boston, Massachusetts

**THOMAS M.S. WOLEVER, M.D., Ph.D.**
Associate Professor of Nutritional Sciences
University of Toronto
Toronto, Canada

**RICHARD J. WOOD, Ph.D.**
Scientist I
United States Department of Agriculture
Human Nutrition Research Center on Aging
Tufts University
Boston, Massachusetts

**STEVEN H. ZEISEL, M.D., Ph.D.**
Professor and Chairman of Nutrition
Professor of Pediatrics and Medicine
Schools of Public Health and Medicine
University of North Carolina
Chapel Hill, North Carolina

†Deceased

# CONTENTS

## Volume 1

## part I • SPECIFIC DIETARY COMPONENTS

### A. Major Dietary Constituents and Energy Needs



### B. Minerals

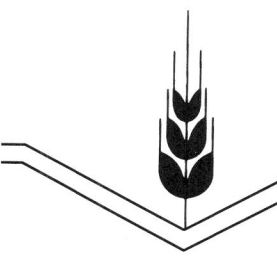

## B. Physiologic and Metabolic Considerations



## C. Nutrition in Growth and Aging

## part III • DIETARY AND NUTRITIONAL ASSESSMENT OF THE INDIVIDUAL



## Volume 2

## part IV • DIET AND NUTRITION IN DISEASE

### A. Dietary and Nutritional Imbalances

## D. Other Diseases, Disorders and Conditions



## E. Systems of Nutritional Support

## D. Food Technology and Toxicology



## E. Nutrition Policy



## APPENDICES



## INDEX

PART I

# Specific Dietary Components

CHAPTER 1

# Proteins and Amino Acids

**Marilyn C. Crim and Hamish N. Munro**



The importance of protein in the diet is primarily as a source of amino acids; some are *essential* (indispensable) dietary constituents because their carbon skeletons are not synthesized in the bodies of animals, whereas others are *nonessential* (dispensable) because they are made within the animal from carbon and nitrogen precursors. A survey of species ranging from protozoa to man shows that all animal species from single-celled organisms onward need some preformed amino acids in their diets.[1] In man, these *essential* amino acids include histidine, isoleucine, leucine, lysine, methionine, phenylalanine, threonine, tryptophan, valine, and possibly arginine (see later in this chapter). In addition, cysteine and tyrosine are synthesized in the body from methionine and phenylalanine, respectively. All these 11 amino acids occur in most proteins. An additional 8 amino acids (alanine, aspartic acid, asparagine, glutamic acid, glutamine, glycine, proline, and serine), also present in proteins, are *nonessential* for man because the body can synthesize them from simple precursors. Other amino acids occur in proteins in nature, but these are made by modifying the side chains of individual amino acids once the protein has been synthesized. Examples are hydroxyproline in collagen made by hydroxylation of certain proline residues in the collagen and 3-methylhistidine in muscle actin and myosin made by methylation of certain histidine residues in these proteins. These derived amino acids are not used again for de novo protein synthesis. When proteins containing them are broken down within the body, they are either metabolized (hydroxyproline) or excreted quantitatively (3-methylhistidine).

Figure 1–1 shows the structural formulas of the 20 amino acids used for protein synthesis. All except glycine have an asymmetric carbon atom and thus can exist as optically active isomers. Only one out of each amino acid isomer pair is used by the body for constructing its proteins. The amino acid isomers used for protein synthesis all have similar structural conformations around the asymmetric carbon atom; the amino group and the carboxyl group occupy the same relative spatial relationship with one another. These amino acids are therefore designated the L-series, whereas those not found in proteins are the D-series, regardless of how they rotate the plane of polarized light. Many metabolic

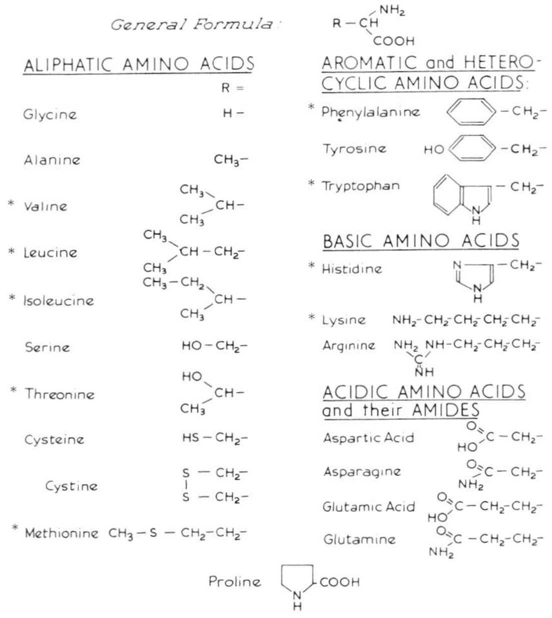
General Formula:
ALIPHATIC AMINO ACIDS
Glycine
Alanine
* Valine
* Leucine
* Isoleucine
Serine
* Threonine
Cysteine
Cystine
* Methionine
AROMATIC and HETERO-CYCLIC AMINO ACIDS:
* Phenylalanine
Tyrosine
* Tryptophan
BASIC AMINO ACIDS
* Histidine
* Lysine
Arginine
ACIDIC AMINO ACIDS and their AMIDES
Aspartic Acid
Asparagine
Glutamic Acid
Glutamine
Proline

**FIGURE 1–1.** Formulas of the 20 common amino acids found in proteins. Essential amino acids are marked with an asterisk(*).

reactions, including those of protein synthesis and transport across cell walls, distinguish L- from D-forms. However, certain reactions (transaminations) can transform the D-form into the L-form and thus make it available to the body. The capacity to use dietary D-amino acids is limited to certain amino acids that vary from species to species.[1] In man, only D-methionine and D-phenylalanine are used. Results of studies with intravenous infusion of D-methionine indicate that it is utilized less efficiently than the L-form.

The structural features of the 20 amino acids show that some are dibasic (arginine, lysine, histidine) and some diacidic (aspartic acid, glutamic acid) (Fig. 1–1). The rest are neutral. These characteristics are important in determining the properties of proteins containing an abundance of dibasic or diacidic amino acids; for example, diacidic amino acids are especially abundant in proteins that are components of membranes. Most amino acids are, however, neutral with an aliphatic or aromatic side chain.

## METABOLISM OF AMINO ACIDS: INTRACELLULAR EVENTS

### FREE AMINO ACID POOLS AND THEIR METABOLIC EFFECTS

Protein consumed in the diet is enzymically hydrolyzed in the alimentary tract and passes into the blood as free amino acids that mingle with amino acids coming from the tissues. Table 1–1 shows the distribution of individual amino acids between the body proteins and the free amino acid pools in the tissues of the young rat. The concentration of protein-bound amino acids in the tissues averages 2 mol/L, whereas the free amino acid pools are about 0.01 mol/L, that is, 0.05% of the concentration of protein-bound amino acids.[2] The tissue concentrations of the free *essential* amino acids are low, whereas those of four of the *nonessential* amino acids (alanine, glutamic acid, glutamine, and glycine) are much higher. On the other hand, the concentrations of all the free amino acids in rat plasma fall within a similar range (Table 1–1).[3,4] This discrepancy occurs because the four nonessential amino acids present in most abundance in the tissues are extensively synthesized within the cells.

Comparison of the concentrations of free essential amino acids in the body with the essential amino acid requirements for the growing rat (Table 1–1) demonstrates that the free amino acid pool must turn over several times daily. The magnitude of the flux of amino acids in the body is increased by recycling of amino acids coming from the breakdown (turnover) of proteins in the tissues.

Transport of free amino acids across cell membranes has been extensively studied, as reviewed by Collarini and Oxender.[5] Several carrier mechanisms have been identified, each common to a number of amino acids. Basic, acidic, and neutral amino acids each enter the tissues by different transport mediators. Within each category, competition for the carrier can be demonstrated between any two amino acids of that class. In addition, within the neutral class more than one transport mechanism has been identified. One system, designated as "A," has high affinity for alanine and for α-aminoisobutyric acid, the latter a synthetic nonprotein amino acid that does not have the complication of being taken up in protein synthesis. This transmembrane carrier is $Na^+$ dependent, is sensitive to respiratory inhibitors, and is affected by hormones. A second major $Na^+$ dependent system for uptake of neutral amino acids is designated as "ASC" from its significance in transportation of alanine, serine, and cysteine. On the other hand, branched-chain and aromatic neutral amino acids are taken up by a different $Na^+$-independent mechanism that is relatively insensitive to respiratory inhibitors. This system, designated "L" for leucine, appears to depend for its driving force on exchange of intracellular neutral amino acids for these extracellular amino acids. In addition to those major categories, some additional subclasses of amino acid transport have also been described. Finally, Meister has proposed a transport mechanism located in the cell membrane and involving glutathione for the actual movement of amino acids into the cells. A review by Meister concludes that this mechanism, the γ-glutamyl cycle, is confined to certain cells, notably those of the kidney tubules.[6]

There has been considerable dispute about whether free intracellular amino acids are the ultimate source for protein synthesis within cells or whether extracellular

**TABLE 1–1.** AMOUNTS OF PROTEIN-BOUND AND FREE AMINO ACIDS IN THE BODY OF A 50-G RAT, AND THE CONCENTRATIONS OF FREE AMINO ACIDS IN RAT PLASMA

| AMINO ACID | TOTAL BODY CONTENT OF AMINO ACIDS (μMOL/100-G RAT) | | FREE AMINO ACIDS IN RAT PLASMA (μMOL/DL) | DAILY AMINO ACID REQUIREMENT (μMOL/100-G RAT) |
|---|---|---|---|---|
| | Protein-Bound | Free | | |
| *Essential* | | | | |
| Arginine | 8,400 | 7 | 16 | — |
| Histidine | 3,600 | 24 | 11 | 140 |
| Isoleucine | 8,400 | 10 | 8 | 400 |
| Leucine | 16,500 | 14 | 16 | 500 |
| Lysine | 8,900 | 15 | 41 | 600 |
| Methionine | 4,050 | 6 | 9 | 350 |
| Phenylalanine | 5,800 | 9 | 9 | 450 |
| Threonine | 7,550 | 20 | 24 | 400 |
| Tryptophan | 980 | 2 | — | 55 |
| Valine | 9,400 | 12 | 18 | 500 |
| *Nonessential* | | | | |
| Alanine | 13,500 | 100 | 32 | — |
| Aspartic acid | 11,300 | 19 | 1 | — |
| Glutamic acid | 17,700 | 132 | 15 | — |
| Glutamine | — | 223 | 55 | — |
| Glycine | 24,700 | 323 | 45 | — |
| Serine | 12,400 | 20 | 23 | — |
| Tyrosine | 3,550 | 8 | 9 | — |

(Adapted from Herbert, J.D., Coulson, R.A., Hernandex, T.: Comp. Biochem. Physiol., *17*:583-598, 1966, in Munro, H.N.: Free amino acid pools and their role in regulation. *In* Mammalian Protein Metabolism. Vol. 4. Edited by H.N. Munro. New York, Academic Press, 1970, pp. 299–386.)

amino acids charge transfer RNA (tRNA) for protein synthesis without entering the cell fluid.[7] Clarification of this mechanism is important in studies of protein synthesis in whole animals because breakdown of tissue protein within cells contributes amino acids that dilute the intracellular free amino acid pool more than the plasma pool. In consequence, isotopically labeled amino acids undergo a greater reduction in specific activity within cells than in the blood, so the rate of synthesis of intracellular proteins computed from the specific activity of the free amino acids in each precursor pool can be quite different. Airhart et al.,[8] who measured the specific activity of liver aminoacyl-tRNA after giving labeled leucine to rats, found that the tRNA had an activity midway between that of free leucine in the plasma and in the liver cells. These investigators concluded that tRNA is charged with amino acids by a pool closely associated with the cell membrane and receives amino acids from both external and intracellular sources. However, by an ingenious use of $^{14}C$-labeled glycine and serine infused into the circulating bloodstream of rats, Fern and Garlick showed that the relative incorporation of these two amino acids into tissue proteins coincided with the ratio of their radioactivities in the intracellular free amino acid pool and not with their relative activities in the plasma.[9]

Amino acids are subjected within the body to a series of metabolic reactions that can be grouped into three categories:

1. Part of the free amino acid pool is incorporated into tissue proteins. Because of protein breakdown (turnover), these amino acids return to the free pool after a variable length of time and thus become available for reutilization in protein synthesis or other reactions.
2. Part of the free amino acid pool undergoes catabolic reactions. This process leads to loss of the carbon skeleton as $CO_2$ or to its deposition as glycogen and fat, whereas the nitrogen is eliminated as urea. Individual pathways of amino acid catabolism are discussed later in this chapter.
3. Some free amino acids are used for synthesis of new nitrogen-containing compounds, such as purine bases, creatine, and epinephrine, which are subsequently degraded without return of end products to the free amino acid pool (e.g., purines are degraded to uric acid, creatine to creatinine, epinephrine to vanillylmandelic acid). In addition, the nonessential amino acids are made in the body using amino groups derived from other amino acids and carbon skeletons formed by reactions common to intermediary metabolism.

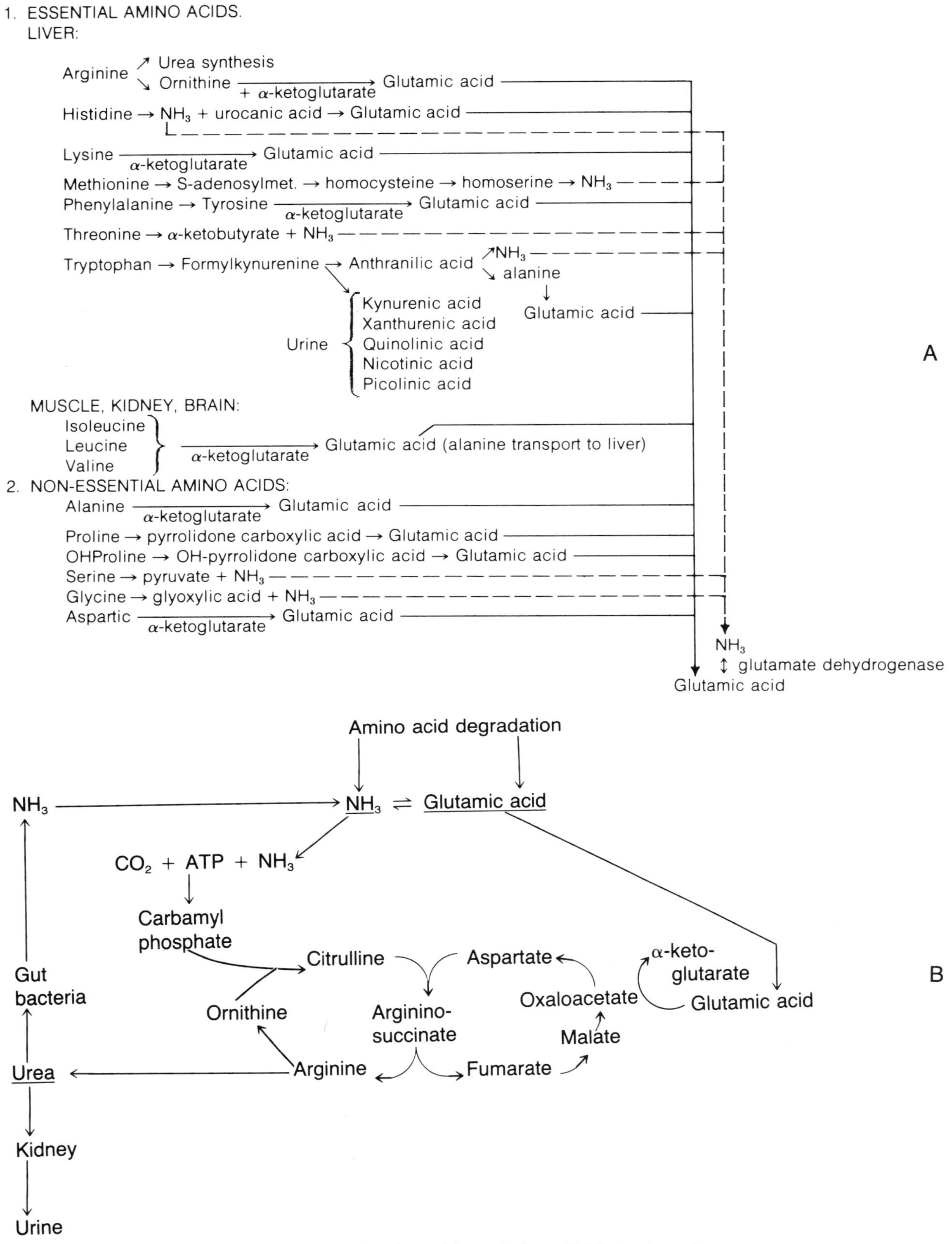
1. ESSENTIAL AMINO ACIDS.
LIVER:
Arginine
Urea synthesis
Ornithine
+ α-ketoglutarate
Glutamic acid
Histidine → NH3 + urocanic acid → Glutamic acid
Lysine
α-ketoglutarate
Glutamic acid
Methionine → S-adenosylmet. → homocysteine → homoserine → NH3
Phenylalanine → Tyrosine
α-ketoglutarate
Glutamic acid
Threonine → α-ketobutyrate + NH3
Tryptophan → Formylkynurenine → Anthranilic acid
NH3
alanine
Glutamic acid
Urine
Kynurenic acid
Xanthurenic acid
Quinolinic acid
Nicotinic acid
Picolinic acid
MUSCLE, KIDNEY, BRAIN:
Isoleucine
Leucine
Valine
α-ketoglutarate
Glutamic acid (alanine transport to liver)
2. NON-ESSENTIAL AMINO ACIDS:
Alanine
α-ketoglutarate
Glutamic acid
Proline → pyrrolidone carboxylic acid → Glutamic acid
OHProline → OH-pyrrolidone carboxylic acid → Glutamic acid
Serine → pyruvate + NH3
Glycine → glyoxylic acid + NH3
Aspartic
α-ketoglutarate
Glutamic acid
NH3
glutamate dehydrogenase
Glutamic acid
A
Amino acid degradation
NH3
NH3
Glutamic acid
CO2 + ATP + NH3
Carbamyl
phosphate
Citrulline
Aspartate
α-keto-
glutarate
Gut
bacteria
Ornithine
ArgInino-
succinate
Oxaloacetate
Glutamic acid
Malate
Urea
Arginine
Fumarate
Kidney
Urine
B

**FIGURE 1–2.** *A*, Degradative pathways of amino acid metabolism. *B*, Mechanism of urea synthesis and recycling. (From Valgeirsdottir, K., Munro, H.N.: Proteins and amino acids. *In* Surgical Nutrition. Edited by J.E. Fisher. Boston, Little, Brown, 1983, pp. 129–164.)

The relative magnitudes of these three pathways in the whole animal are illustrated by studies in which rats were fed by stomach tube with 1-mg doses of uniformly $^{14}C$-labeled L-tyrosine, L-phenylalanine, or L-tryptophan.[10] The proportion of absorbed radioactivity excreted during the first 4 hours in the form of $^{14}CO_2$ or recovered from the liver, gut, and total skeletal musculature in the form of protein-bound activity or nonprotein compounds was determined. At 15 minutes after feeding, 20 to 40% of the absorbed radioactivity of the three amino acids was recovered as acid-soluble compounds in liver, gut, and muscle, a considerable proportion of these compounds being nonaromatic radioactive compounds, indicating rapid breakdown of the free amino acids. Thereafter, acid-soluble $^{14}C$ activity decreased, whereas output as $^{14}CO_2$ rose and eventually accounted for 19 to 40% of the absorbed dose. Protein-bound activity in the three tissues at 4 hours after feeding represented 34 to 51% of the absorbed activity.

## PATHWAYS OF DEGRADATION

Each amino acid is degraded by undergoing a special sequence of chemical reactions (for details see textbooks of biochemistry). In Figure 1–2, the routes of degradation of the essential and nonessential amino acids are summarized to show how $NH_3$ and glutamic acid are made available for excretion as urea. Seven of the ten amino acids essential to the rat are primarily degraded in the liver, whereas the other three (branched-chain amino acids isoleucine, leucine, and valine) are mostly catabolized in muscle, as well as in kidney and brain. Following transamination of the branched-chain amino acids, degradation of the resulting three keto acids involves the enzyme complex dihydrolipoamide acetyltransferase, the activity of which is enhanced by dephosphorylation in response to the influx of these amino acids.[11] The degradative pathways for branched-chain amino acids and their regulation are discussed by Harper et al.[12]

Urea synthesis is performed in the liver[13] (Fig. 1–2 *B*). Ammonia and $CO_2$ first form carbamyl phosphate, which reacts in turn with ornithine to give citrulline, which then acquires another N from aspartic acid to form argininosuccinate. This product splits into arginine and fumarate, the latter returning to the tricarboxylic acid cycle, whereas the arginine is finally split by arginase into urea and ornithine. Ornithine is thus released to participate in another turn of the cycle. Note that glutamic acid contributes N through aspartic acid. Urea is mostly secreted directly into the urine, but some passes into the lumen of the gut, where bacterial urease causes release of ammonia. This ammonia returns via the portal vein to the liver, where it again forms urea. About 20% of the urea formed in the liver is recycled daily in this way.[14]

## OTHER PATHWAYS UTILIZING AMINO ACIDS

### *SYNTHESIS OF NONESSENTIAL AMINO ACIDS*

The division of amino acids into essential and nonessential was originally defined by Rose on the basis of whether they were needed in the diet for optimal growth of rats.[15] Nonessential amino acids could be deleted from the diet without impairing optimal growth. In the case of adults, N balance became negative on withdrawal of essential amino acids. It has since been shown with isotopic labels that nonessential amino acids are made from precursors such as glucose, whereas the carbon skeletons of the essential amino acids do not take up labeled precursors. The pathways of synthesis of the nonessential amino acids are well established (Fig. 1–3).

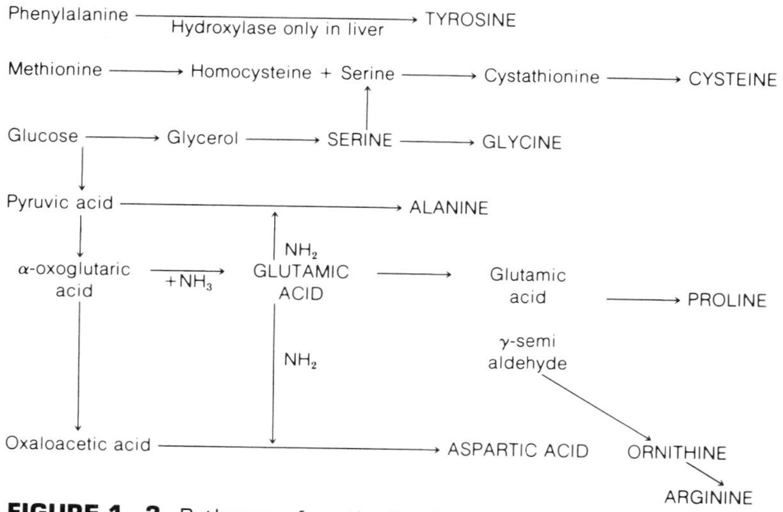
Phenylalanine
Hydroxylase only in liver
TYROSINE
Methionine
Homocysteine + Serine
Cystathionine
CYSTEINE
Glucose
Glycerol
SERINE
GLYCINE
Pyruvic acid
ALANINE
α-oxoglutaric acid
+NH3
NH2
GLUTAMIC ACID
Glutamic acid
PROLINE
γ-semi aldehyde
NH2
Oxaloacetic acid
ASPARTIC ACID
ORNITHINE
ARGININE

**FIGURE 1–3.** Pathways of synthesis of nonessential amino acids. (From Munro, H.N.: Evolution of protein metabolism in mammals. *In* Mammalian Protein Metabolism. Vol. 3. Edited by H.N. Munro. New York, Academic Press, 1969, pp. 133–182.)

These pathways are not always present in all tissues (e.g., tyrosine is formed by hydroxylation of phenylalanine in the liver), and more than one biosynthetic route can exist (e.g., for serine).

## *PURINE AND PYRIMIDINE BIOSYNTHESIS*

Purine and pyrimidine bases are synthesized from simpler carbon and nitrogen precursors including several amino acids (Fig. 1–4).[16] These precursors permit the formation of ribonucleotides of the purines, adenine and guanine, and of the pyrimidines, uracil and cytosine. As high-energy phosphate compounds (di- and triphosphates), all four of these ribonucleotides are involved in many intracellular reactions. The deoxyribonucleotides found in DNA are made by reduction of the ribose in the ribonucleotides.

Biosynthesis of purine nucleotides can occur by two routes: de novo and salvage pathways. In de novo synthesis, glutamine and phosphoribosylpyrophosphate react, followed by a series of reactions, many of which include amino acids, and eventually provide the nucleotide inosine monophosphate (IMP) containing the base hypoxanthine. Adenylic acid (AMP) and guanylic acid (GMP) are then made from this nucleotide by altering substituents on certain carbon atoms of the purine ring. These can be phosphorylated to form the high-energy compounds adenosine diphosphate (ADP), adenosine triphosphate (ATP), guanosine diphosphate (GDP), and guanosine triphosphate (GTP) or can undergo degrada-

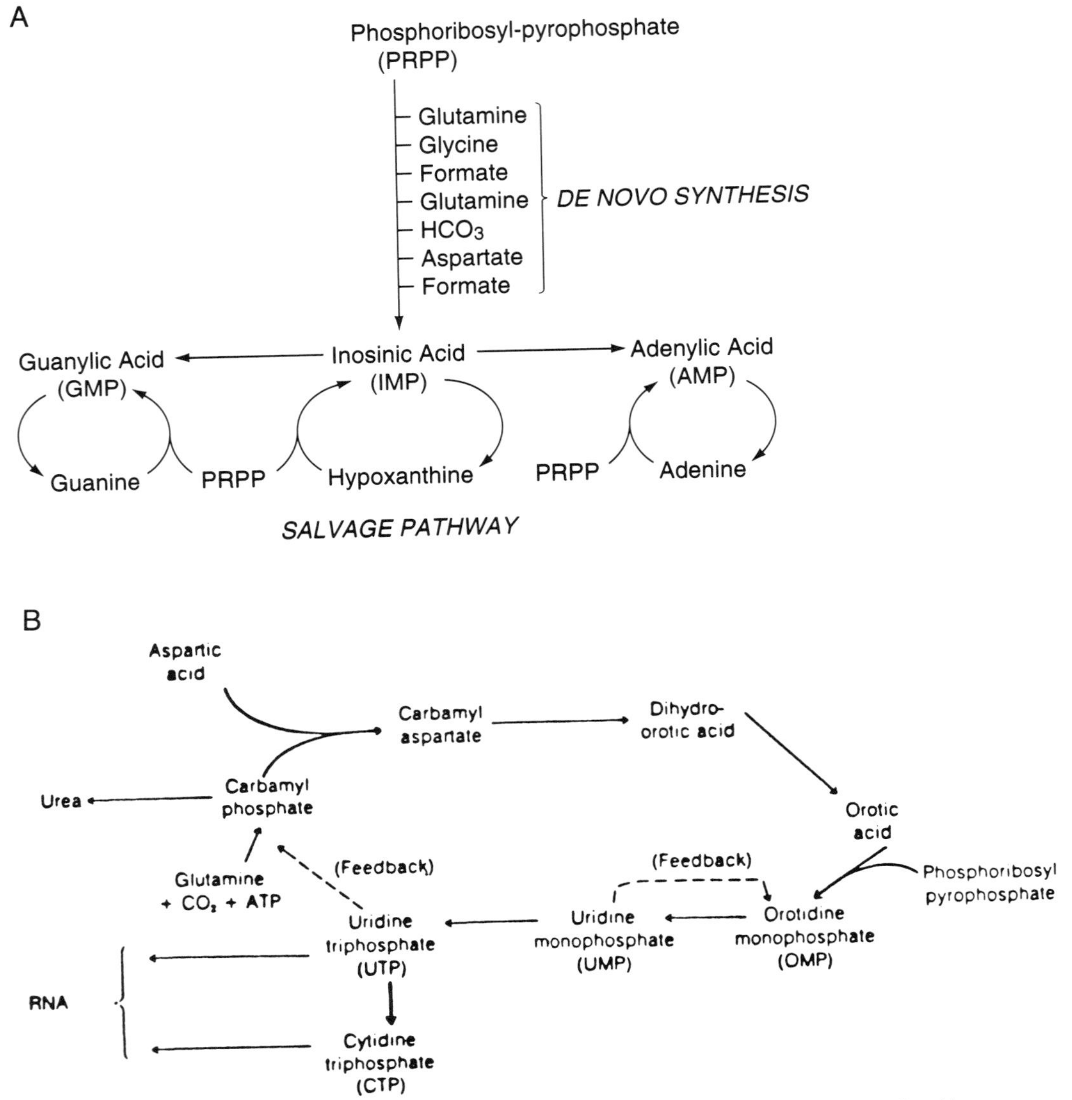
A
Phosphoribosyl-pyrophosphate
(PRPP)
Glutamine
Glycine
Formate
Glutamine
HCO3
Aspartate
Formate
DE NOVO SYNTHESIS
Guanylic Acid
(GMP)
Inosinic Acid
(IMP)
Adenylic Acid
(AMP)
Guanine
PRPP
Hypoxanthine
PRPP
Adenine
SALVAGE PATHWAY
B
Aspartic acid
Carbamyl aspartate
Dihydro-orotic acid
Urea
Carbamyl phosphate
Orotic acid
Glutamine + CO2 + ATP
(Feedback)
(Feedback)
Phosphoribosyl pyrophosphate
Uridine triphosphate (UTP)
Uridine monophosphate (UMP)
Orotidine monophosphate (OMP)
RNA
Cytidine triphosphate (CTP)

**FIGURE 1–4.** *A,* Purine nucleotide synthesis. De novo synthesis of purine nucleotides, nucleotide interchange, the salvage pathways, and purine degradation routes. *B,* Pyrimidine nucleotide synthesis.

tion to adenosine and free adenine or to guanosine and free guanine. In turn, the free bases can then be deaminated to hypoxanthine and xanthine, finally forming uric acid. Although de novo synthesis of AMP and GMP requires many high-energy phosphate bonds, purine nucleotides can also be synthesized by the salvage pathways, in which the free purine bases react with phosphoribosylpyrophosphate to form the mononucleotides.[16]

Synthesis of the pyrimidine bases begins with carbamyl phosphate (Fig. 1–4), which is also a substrate for urea synthesis. Consequently, lack of adequate amounts of arginine to prime the urea synthesis cycle (see Fig. 1–2) can result in diversion of unused carbamyl phosphate to the pyrimidine biosynthetic pathway.[17] This causes overload of the pathway with accumulation of orotic acid and its excretion in the urine (Fig. 1–4). In some species, arginine deficiency can be detected by excessive output of orotic acid in the urine. In some infants of both sexes and in some adult women, mutations involving the enzyme ornithine-carbamoyl transferase result in accumulation of glutamine and ammonia in the blood and diversion of the metabolite carbamoyl phosphate into the pyrimidine synthesis pathway resulting in urinary excretion of orotic acid.[18]

*CREATINE AND CREATININE.*

Most of the creatine of the body is found in skeletal muscle, where it exists both as free creatine and as creatine phosphate. In resting muscle, creatine is present largely in the high-energy phosphate form, whereas in fatigued muscle, creatine phosphate concentration is insignificant.[19] This depletion is the result of the biochemical coupling of the conversion of creatine phosphate to creatine with synthesis of ATP, a reversible reaction mediated by the enzyme ATP-creatine transphosphorylase (also known as creatine phosphokinase).

Creatine is synthesized extramuscularly in a two-reaction sequence (Fig. 1–5). The first is transamidination in the kidney between arginine and glycine, with formation of guanidinoacetic acid and ornithine. Then methylation of guanidinoacetic acid by S-adenosylmethionine in the liver creates creatine, which is transported to the muscle. In muscle, both creatine phosphate and creatine undergo a nonenzymatic irreversible dehydration to form creatinine, the rate being twice as fast for creatine phosphate. Unlike creatine, creatinine is not retained by muscle, but is distributed in total body water and is cleared from the body by the kidney. The rate of creatinine formation by a nonenzymatic reaction from its creatine precursors is remarkably constant, about 1.7% of the total creatine pool per day.

Daily urinary output of creatinine has been used as a measure of total muscle mass in the body, on the assumption that muscle creatine content is fairly constant. Indeed, results of population studies show a good correlation between creatinine output and lean body mass.[20] However, the creatine pool in the muscles of an individual represent a composite of the amount of creatine synthesized and the amount taken in the diet, notably from meat. Crim and colleagues have shown that ingestion of creatine can increase the body pool of creatine appreciably.[21,22] In fact, muscle creatine concentration can vary almost twofold, from 0.3 to 0.5%. The use of urinary creatinine excretion to assess the muscle mass could thus be associated with a considerable error if applied to individuals of populations with different dietary patterns. Clinically, the customary constancy of urinary creatinine output is also used to estimate the adequacy of 24-hour collections of urine. On a short-term basis, such as 1 to 2

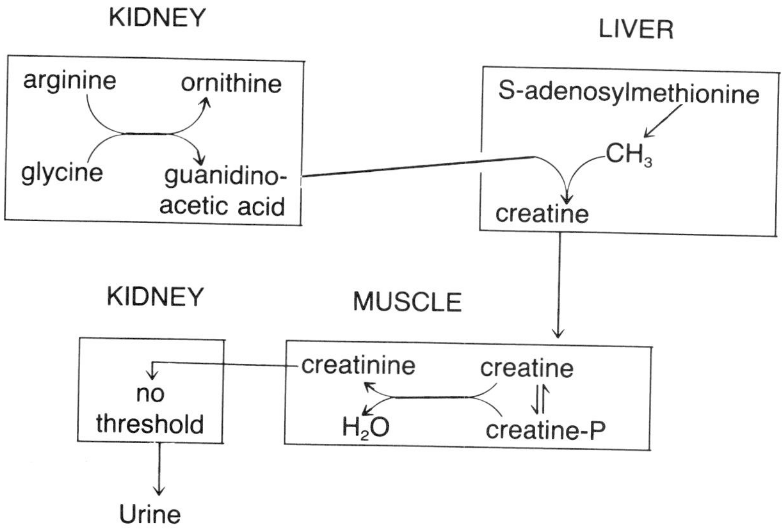
KIDNEY
LIVER
arginine
ornithine
glycine
guanidino-
acetic acid
S-adenosylmethionine
$CH_3$
creatine
KIDNEY
MUSCLE
creatinine
creatine
no
threshold
$H_2O$
creatine-P
Urine

**FIGURE 1–5.** Synthesis of creatine and creatinine. (From Valgeirsdottir, K., Munro, H.N.: Proteins and amino acids. *In* Surgical Nutrition. Edited by J.E. Fisher. Boston, Little, Brown, 1983, pp. 129–164.)

weeks, this estimate is generally accurate, but it assumes that during the collection period there are no significant sources of dietary creatinine, which unlike creatine, is rapidly excreted in the urine.

### *AMMONIA SYNTHESIS IN THE KIDNEY*

An important end product of protein metabolism is urinary ammonia, which increases in amount with acidosis in conditions such as starvation or uncontrolled diabetes mellitus.[23] In such conditions, ammonia formation allows the body to conserve potassium and sodium ions, which would otherwise be used to neutralize the acid excreted. Urinary ammonia is derived from plasma glutamine (Fig. 1–6). In the cells of the proximal convoluted tubule of the kidney, glutaminase causes the amide N of glutamine to form ammonia and glutamate.[24] The latter then yields another $NH_3$, leaving α-ketoglutarate as the other product of the reaction. This product is then available for gluconeogenesis, so in acidosis, the kidney becomes a source of glucose in tandem with $NH_3$ excretion.[25] It has been suggested that the first response to acidosis is the production of glucose by the kidney, to which $NH_3$ formation is secondary.[26]

## UTILIZATION OF DIETARY PROTEIN

In the preceding section, a number of pathways of amino acid metabolism were presented individually. Regulation of protein metabolism in an integrated fashion is necessary to maintain bodily function.

### DIGESTION AND ABSORPTION OF PROTEIN

Digestion of protein begins with pepsin secreted in the gastric juice, followed by proteolytic enzymes from the pancreas and the mucosa of the small intestine.[27,28] These enzymes are mostly made in precursor (zymogen or proenzyme) form and become activated by loss of a small part of their peptide chains through limited proteolysis. The pancreatic proenzymes become activated on meeting the intestinal juice where intestinal enterokinase begins activating trypsinogen to trypsin by limited proteolysis. This is followed by a cascade of activation of the other pancreatic proenzymes through selective proteolysis by active trypsin.

Secretion of proteolytic enzymes by the pancreas appears to be regulated by the presence of dietary protein in the gut contents. Thus, the enzyme trypsin binds to dietary protein in the gut lumen until an excess of the enzyme is present.[29] This excess of free enzyme then operates a feedback regulation system to the pancreatic acinar cells causing inhibition of synthesis of the precursor trypsinogen (Fig. 1–7). Some plants contain inhibitors of proteolytic enzymes, notably soybean trypsin inhibitor. Feeding unheated soybean or its trypsin inhibitor to rats results in hypertrophy of the pancreas,[29] presumably because of tenacious binding of the free trypsin with consequent overstimulation of enzyme formation in the pancreas.

The events occurring in the course of protein digestion are well established.[27] Successive proteolytic enzymes attack peptide bonds selected on the basis of one of the amino acid residues adjacent to the bond. Pepsin has a relatively low specificity, preferentially hydrolyzing bonds adjacent to leucine or the aromatic amino acids, whereas the enzymes of the pancreatic juice show a greater specificity toward bonds adjacent to lysine or arginine (trypsin), to aromatic amino acids (chymotrypsin), or to neutral aliphatic amino acids (elastase). In addition, exopeptidases attack the free ends of the peptide chain. Thus, the carboxyl terminal end loses one amino acid at a time through the action of two carboxypeptidases from the pancreas with different specificities, whereas the intestinal juice contributes aminopeptidases that perform a similar action at the N terminal end of the peptide.

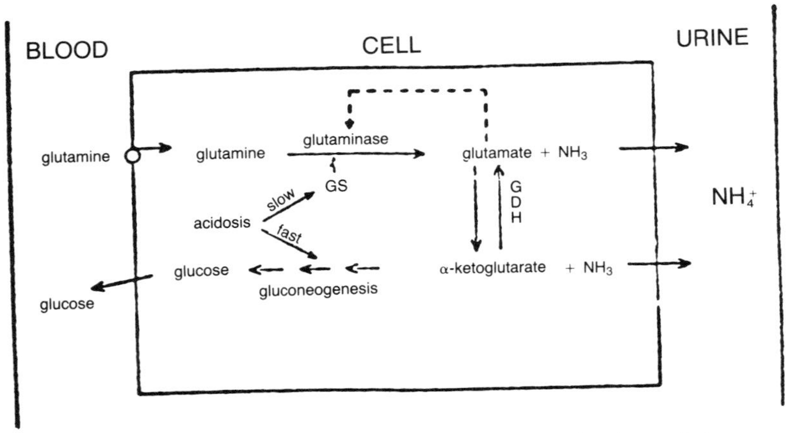
BLOOD
CELL
URINE
glutamine
glutamine
glutaminase
glutamate + NH3
GS
GDH
slow
fast
acidosis
NH4+
glucose
gluconeogenesis
α-ketoglutarate + NH3
glucose

**FIGURE 1–6.** Mechanism for control of ammonia production and gluconeogenesis by the kidney. GS, Glutaminase synthesis; GDH, glutamate dehydrogenase. (From Goldstein, L., Schooler, J.M.: Adv. Enzyme Regul., *5*:71–86, 1967. Copyright by Pergamon Press.)

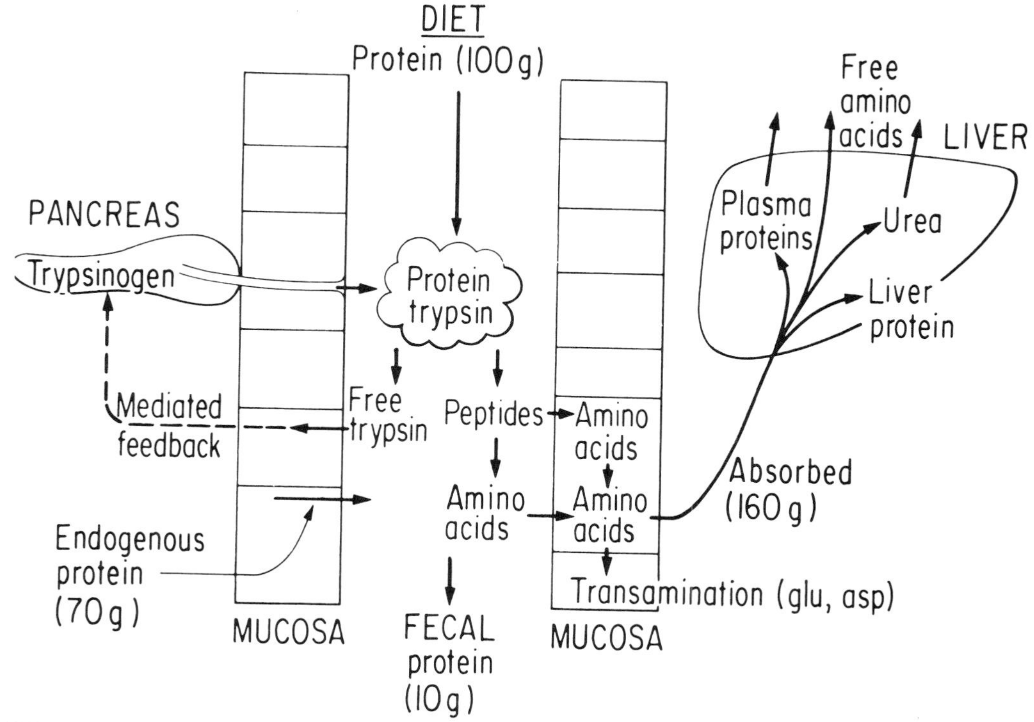

DIET
Protein (100g)
PANCREAS
Trypsinogen
Protein trypsin
Free trypsin
Peptides
Amino acids
Mediated feedback
Endogenous protein (70g)
MUCOSA
FECAL protein (10g)
MUCOSA
Transamination (glu, asp)
Absorbed (160g)
Free amino acids
LIVER
Plasma proteins
Urea
Liver protein


**FIGURE 1–7.** Fate of dietary protein, secretion of endogenous protein, feedback control of pancreatic enzyme secretion, and absorption through the mucosa. (From Crim, M.C., Munro, H.N.: Protein and amino acid requirements and metabolism in relation to defined formula diets. *In* Defined Formula Diets for Medical Purposes. Edited by M.E. Shils. Chicago, American Medical Association, 1977. Reprinted with permission from the American Medical Association.)

The end products of digestion of protein are absorbed through the mucosal cells of the small intestine (Fig. 1–7). Some of the protein in the gut lumen is finally hydrolyzed to free amino acids prior to absorption. Numerous studies confirm that transport of free amino acids into the mucosa involves energy-dependent carriers with some specificity for neutral, basic, and acidic classes of amino acids. However, the absorption of small peptides, notably dipeptides, plays a significant role in assimilation of dietary protein.[30] Because of the presence of peptide hydrolases in the brush border and cytosol of the mucosal cells, these small peptides originating from dietary protein undergo hydrolysis to free amino acids on entering the mucosal cells, so that virtually only free amino acids pass into the portal vein and go to the liver (Fig. 1–7).[31] The transport mechanism for uptake of peptides by mucosal cells differs from the mechanism for free amino acid uptake, notably by the absence of competition for absorption between these two mechanisms. The absorption of peptides is likely to represent a significant major route of amino acid uptake. Thus, although children with Hartnup's disease cannot transport free tryptophan into the mucosal cells, they nevertheless grow almost normally,[32] suggesting that their need for the essential amino acid tryptophan is adequately met by its absorption in peptide form.

It is significant that the mucosal cells can metabolize some incoming amino acids (Fig. 1–7), notably the transamination of glutamic acid to yield alanine. Aspartic acid is also transaminated to alanine by the mucosal cells. Windmueller has demonstrated that glutamic acid and glutamine of dietary origin are extensively converted to alanine,[33] with a smaller yield of ornithine, citrulline, and proline by the pathways shown in Figure 1–3. Similarly, glutamine perfused through the mesenteric vessels going to the gut mucosa is also partly converted to alanine.

Finally, it is necessary to consider endogenous protein added to the gut contents in the form of digestive enzymes and the epithelial cells of the mucosa. Epithelial cells are continuously replaced by mitotic division in the crypts, followed by passage of each cohort of cells up the villus to be sloughed off from its tip.[34] The extent of endogenous protein secretion is controversial, particularly estimates of the contribution of protein from mucosal sloughing. One average estimate is that approximately 70 g of protein (17 g as secreted juices and 50 g as sloughed mucosal cells) is added daily to the intestinal contents (Fig. 1–7). When this amount is added to the 100 g of protein consumed by the average person eating a Western type of diet, a total of 170 g in the gut lumen is available for absorption (Fig. 1–7). Because fecal nitrogen output is equivalent to only 10 g of protein daily, the efficiency of digestion and absorption of both dietary and endogenous protein must be considerable. This turnover of protein in the gut wall is sensitive to nutritional change. Protein deficiency[35] and starvation[36] both reduce the rate of cell division in the mucosa, which correlates with evidence in rats that protein deficiency leads to reduced secretion of endogenous protein into the gut.[37]

## ROLE OF THE LIVER

The absorbed amino acids pass to the liver by way of the portal vein. After a protein-containing meal, the amount and pattern of amino acids change in the portal vein, with a less dramatic increase in amino acid levels in the general circulation. This change occurs because the liver is the main or only site of catabolism for seven of the essential amino acids; the remaining three, the branched-chain amino acids, are degraded mainly in muscle and kidney, a finding first demonstrated by Miller.[38] The liver monitors the absorbed amino acids and adjusts the rate of their metabolism according to bodily needs. Using dogs fed excessive amounts of meat, Elwyn demonstrated that much of this incoming amino acid load was degraded to urea after it entered the liver cells.[39] A small proportion was retained as liver protein, mostly additional enzyme protein, and another small portion was secreted as plasma protein, whereas only about a quarter of the absorbed amino acids passed into the general circulation.

The process of monitoring amino acid intake by the liver regulates the amounts of individual essential amino acids available from the diet to the rest of the body. When the dietary intake of an essential amino acid is progressively increased, induction of liver degradative enzyme activity usually occurs when intake exceeds requirement.[40] This induction (e.g., threonine dehydratase in Figure 1–8) often shows a sudden increase at levels of intake beyond the needs of the body, indicating that the liver accurately monitors intake in relation to the bodily requirements and destroys the excess of essential amino acids. In the case of nonessential amino acids, the levels of degradative enzymes (e.g., glutamic aminotransferase) responsible for their metabolism do not show this inflection, but increase progressively with rising intake (Fig. 1–8). This conservation of essential amino acids is indicated also by studies in which different amounts of lysine were fed to young growing rats.[41] At a daily intake of 100 mg of lysine, gain in body weight was maximal, whereas beyond this intake level, growth was not further stimulated, and $^{14}C$-$CO_2$ production from injected $^{14}C$-lysine rapidly increased, indicating that the liver had begun to destroy the excess lysine.

Finally, synthesis by the liver of degradative and other enzymes of amino acid metabolism is reflected in increased aggregation of polyribosomes after a meal containing protein,[42] a response further augmented by reduced enzyme breakdown caused by substrate stabilization from amino acids derived from the meal. Thus,

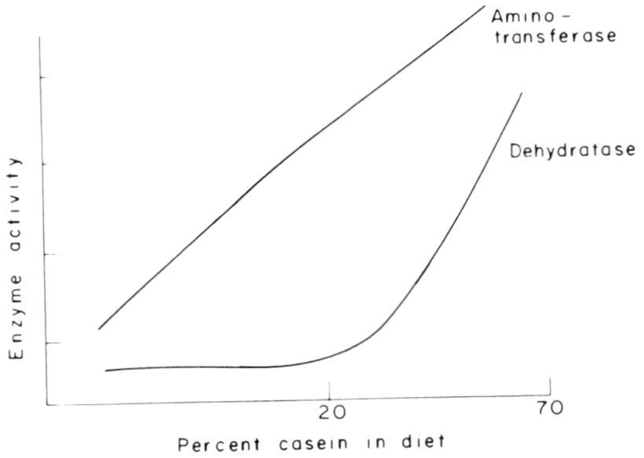

Amino-transferase
Dehydratase
Enzyme activity
20
70
Percent casein in diet


**FIGURE 1–8.** Effect on liver enzymes of increasing the protein content of a diet fed to growing rats. The upper line shows the response of a liver enzyme metabolizing a nonessential amino acid (glutamic acid), while the lower line indicates the response of an enzyme for degradation of an essential amino acid (threonine). (Data from Harper, A.E.: Am. J. Clin. Nutr., *21*:358–366, 1968. Copyright by the American Society for Clinical Nutrition.)

degradative enzymes such as tyrosine aminotransferase[42] and tryptophan pyrrolase[43] show diurnal variations related to protein-containing meal consumption. In addition, other metabolic events in the liver cell are subject to diurnal variations related to protein intake. After a protein-containing meal, levels of liver RNA rise while RNA breakdown decreases, causing a decrease in the free purine nucleotide pool and a stimulation of de novo purine biosynthesis.[44,45] Albumin synthesis does not appear to undergo diurnal rhythm, possibly because hepatic regulation of plasma albumin synthesis is determined by the osmotic pressure of the plasma. On the other hand, $\alpha_{2u}$-globulin made by the liver of the mature male rat and excreted in the urine, shows diurnal responses to protein intake.[46]

## REGULATION OF BLOOD AMINO ACID LEVELS

Although the liver monitors the passage of some amino acids into the peripheral circulation, amino acids may still be presented to peripheral tissues in amounts greater than used for protein synthesis or for other purposes. Consequently, plasma levels of some essential amino acids increase when dietary supply exceeds requirements. The age-dependent response of the plasma tryptophan concentration to different levels of dietary tryptophan is a good example.[47] In one study, as the amount of tryptophan in the diet was increased from less than adequate to more than sufficient for maximal need, at each age, the tryptophan content of the plasma rose after the point of requirement was reached. For rapidly growing rat weanlings, the point of inflection was 0.1% tryptophan in the diet, above which growth was not stimulated and plasma tryptophan started to rise. For mature rats, 0.03% dietary tryptophan was just sufficient to satisfy body weight maintenance; above this level, plasma tryptophan concentration rose. These observations provide the basis for developing a method to determine the dietary intake at which requirements of man for amino acids are met. Figure 1–9 illustrates plasma tryptophan levels at a variety of dietary tryptophan intakes for three age groups.[48] The point of inflection of tryptophan for the young adult (3 mg/kg body weight) agrees with the amount required for N balance.[49] As expected, the point of inflection for children (4 mg/kg body weight) implies a higher requirement, whereas in the case of the elderly the predicted requirement is lower (2 mg/kg). However, other essential amino acids such as lysine have less clear-cut points of inflection, and the use of this criterion as a measure of optimal requirements has been disputed.[50]

The plasma levels of amino acids are also affected by dietary carbohydrate through a mechanism involving insulin secretion. Shortly after an individual consumes carbohydrate, the concentrations of most plasma amino acids decrease because of deposition in muscle through insulin-mediated transport. The effect is maximal for serum levels of branched-chain amino acids, which can fall as much as 40% after a dose of glucose, whereas some amino acids (e.g., tryptophan) are affected only minimally. The alterations in plasma free amino acid patterns caused by protein and carbohydrate components of a meal have significance for the availability of amino acids to the peripheral tissues. In particular, the free tryptophan content of rat brain can be elevated by tryptophan administration, and in consequence this maneuver increases the serotonin content of the brain.[51] Entry of tryptophan into the cells of the brain is also determined by the plasma levels of other competing neutral amino acids, notably the branched-chain amino acids.[51] Consequently, after a meal of carbohydrate, the extensive reduction in plasma levels of branched-chain amino acids results in greater passage of tryptophan into the brain, and more serotonin is synthesized, thus promoting sleepiness.

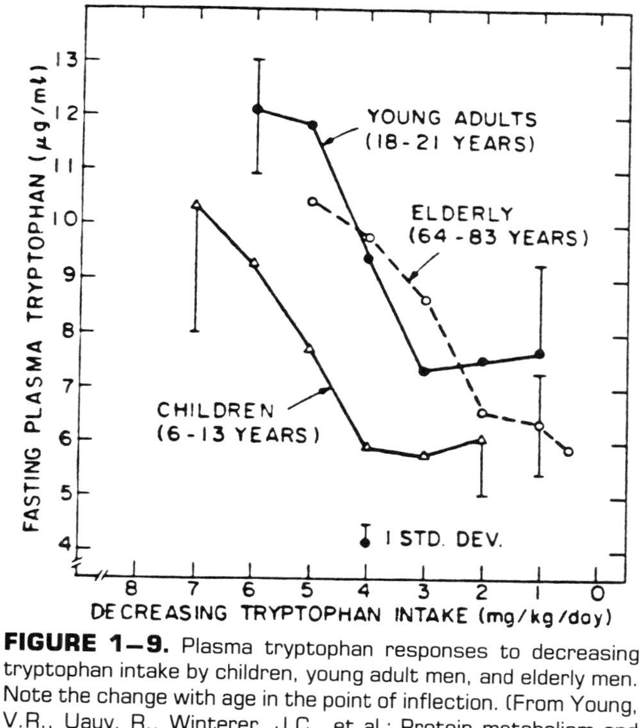
FASTING PLASMA TRYPTOPHAN (µg/ml)
13
12
11
10
9
8
7
6
5
4
YOUNG ADULTS
(18-21 YEARS)
ELDERLY
(64-83 YEARS)
CHILDREN
(6-13 YEARS)
1 STD. DEV.
8
7
6
5
4
3
2
1
0
DECREASING TRYPTOPHAN INTAKE (mg/kg/day)

**FIGURE 1–9.** Plasma tryptophan responses to decreasing tryptophan intake by children, young adult men, and elderly men. Note the change with age in the point of inflection. (From Young, V.R., Uauy, R., Winterer, J.C., et al.: Protein metabolism and needs in elderly people. *In* Nutrition, Longevity, and Aging. Edited by M. Rockstein and M.L. Sussman. New York, Academic Press, 1976, pp. 67–102.)

## ROLE OF SKELETAL MUSCLE IN PROTEIN METABOLISM

Skeletal muscle is the largest tissue in the body. Consequently, metabolism of amino acids in this tissue contributes significantly to overall protein metabolism. Muscle is also the main site of metabolism of the branched-chain amino acids (leucine, isoleucine, and valine). The effects of hormones and of dietary nutrients on muscle protein metabolism have been examined by various techniques. Attempts to assess muscle protein synthesis and degradation in man using stable isotope labeled amino acids have been complicated by methodologic problems.[52–54] These problems include identification of the precursor pool for analysis of isotope concentration, obtaining sufficient isotope concentrations in muscle to permit accurate measurement in small muscle biopsy specimens, isotope recycling, and quantifying the influence of variations in muscle biopsy source, composition, and fiber type.

In man, two additional procedures are used to measure muscle protein metabolism, namely, measurement of the differences in amino acid levels of blood entering and leaving muscle (arteriovenous differences) and measurement of daily urinary excretion of 3-methylhistidine as an index of the rate of myofibrillar protein breakdown. Fasting results in the release of amino acids, primarily glutamine and alanine, equivalent to a loss of 50 g of protein daily from the muscles of a 70-kg man.[55] Alanine is formed by transamination between pyruvate derived from glucose and amino groups transferred from amino acids present in muscle. Thus, alanine becomes a major carrier of nitrogen from muscle to liver, where its carbon skeleton enters the gluconeogenic pathway while its amino group is converted to urea or recycled via transamination. Glutamine, the other major carrier of nitrogen from the muscle, is formed by transamination of glutamic acid in muscle and passes to the intestine, where about half the nitrogen undergoes transamination to alanine, which is carried to the liver by the portal vein for gluconeogenesis. Following hepatic gluconeogenesis, some of the carbon originating in muscle as alanine and glutamine returns to muscle as glucose; this overall exchange between liver and muscle has been named the glucose-alanine cycle. From muscle (about 45% of body weight) a considerable amount of carbon is thus available for metabolism to glucose (and thus energy) during fasting or other emergencies.

Interpretation of arteriovenous difference data is complicated by amino acid recycling within the muscle cell. For example, the diminution of the arteriovenous difference of amino acids after insulin administration could be the result of increased muscle protein synthesis or increased recycling of amino acids within the muscle or decreased muscle protein breakdown.[55] To quantify muscle protein breakdown without involving the confounding effect of amino acid reutilization, urinary 3-methylhistidine can be measured (Fig. 1–10).[56] Methylation of histidine in actin and myosin occurs only after these proteins have been synthesized. When the protein of the myofibril is catabolized, 3-methylhistidine is not reused for protein synthesis but is excreted quantitatively in the urine of several species, thus providing a measure of muscle protein breakdown. Several lines of evidence confirm that 3-methylhistidine in fact fulfills this purpose. First, tRNA and its charging enzymes prepared from rat muscle did not activate 3-methylhistidine,[57] demonstrating that it is not reused for protein synthesis within the muscle cell. Second, analysis of major tissues and organs of the rat shows that skeletal muscle accounts for 75% of the 3-methylhistidine in body proteins. Third, after the administration of $^{14}CH_3$-labeled 3-methylhistidine to rats[57] and to human subjects,[58] essentially all was excreted intact in the urine over a short period.

For those contemplating the use of 3-methylhistidine to measure changes in muscle protein degradation, three limitations should be recognized. First, the human or animal should be consuming a meat-free diet for several days to eliminate 3-methylhistidine from dietary sources. As an alternative, Sjolin et al. have measured output of 1-methylhistidine in the urine.[59] In bovine but not in human muscle, 1-methylhistidine occurs as a

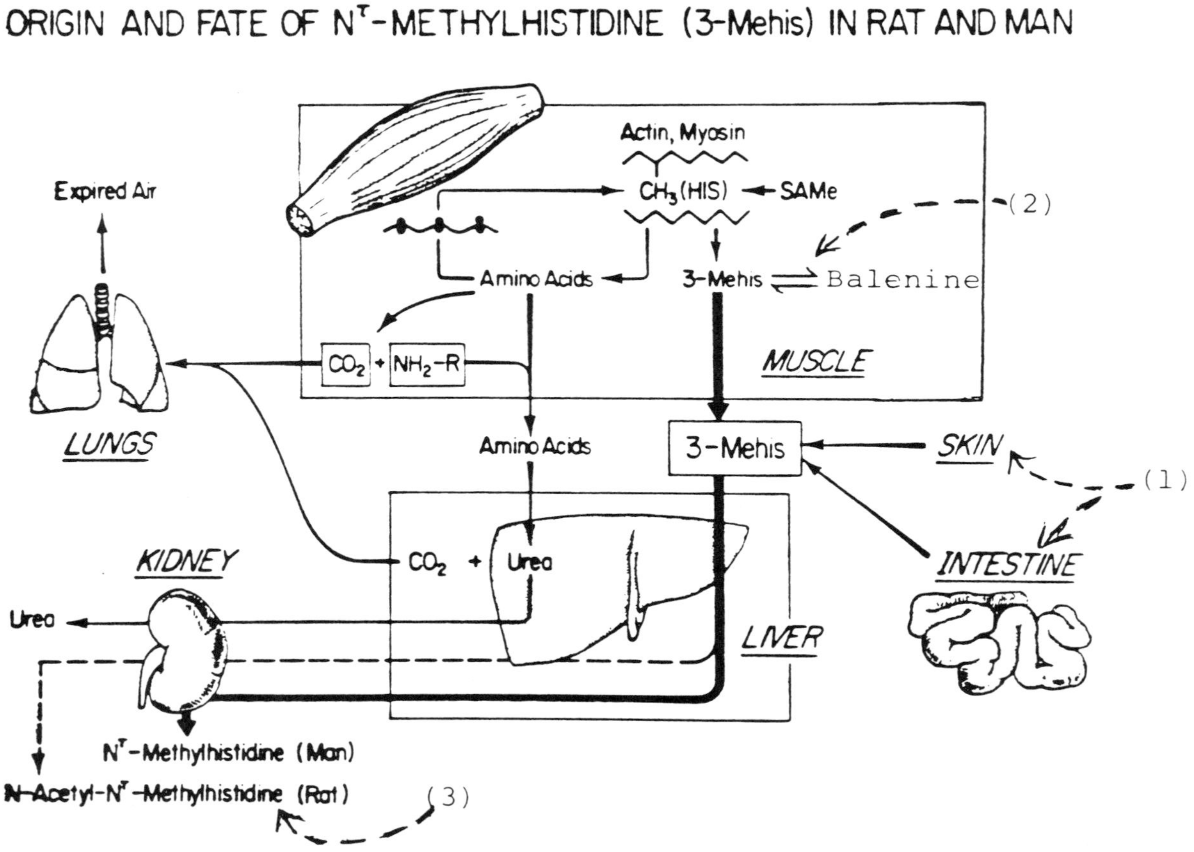
ORIGIN AND FATE OF $N^{\tau}$-METHYLHISTIDINE (3-Mehis) IN RAT AND MAN
Actin, Myosin
$CH_3$(HIS)
SAMe
(2)
Expired Air
Amino Acids
3-Mehis
Balenine
$CO_2$ + $NH_2$-R
MUSCLE
LUNGS
Amino Acids
3-Mehis
SKIN
(1)
INTESTINE
KIDNEY
$CO_2$ + Urea
LIVER
Urea
$N^{\tau}$-Methylhistidine (Man)
N-Acetyl-$N^{\tau}$-Methylhistidine (Rat)
(3)

**FIGURE 1–10.** Pictorial description of the proposed relationship between muscle protein breakdown and urinary output of 3-methylhistidine excretion in the rat and humans. (1), Additional alleged sources of 3-methylhistidine. (2), Exchange of free 3-methylhistidine with the muscle dipeptide balenine (3-methylhistidine-β-alanine). (3), N-acetylation of 3-methylhistidine prior to urinary excretion. (From Munro, H.N., Young V.R.: Use of $N^{\tau}$-methylhistidine excretion as an in vivo measure of myofibrillar protein breakdown. *In* Nitrogen Metabolism in Man. Edited by J.C. Waterlow and J.M.L. Stephen. London, Applied Science, 1981, pp. 495–508.)

peptide, anserine (1-methylhistidine-β-alanine). Thus, the urinary excretion of 1-methylhistidine can provide an estimate of the amount of meat consumed by humans and, in consequence, allows an estimate of this source of urinary 3-methylhistidine. The second limitation is that not all the urinary 3-methylhistidine of endogenous origin comes from skeletal muscle. It has been estimated that about 75% of urinary 3-methylhistidine comes from the skeletal muscle of the rat.[60,61] Afting et al. reported a unique study of a man who had a seemingly total loss of skeletal muscle at the time of his death, but who was still excreting 28% of the normal output of 3-methylhistidine by healthy adults.[62] Thus, 3-methylhistidine must be derived from tissues other than skeletal muscle, such as cardiac and smooth muscle. Nagasawa and Funabiki concluded that skin is a major source of nonmuscular 3-methylhistidine in rats,[60] but Sjolin et al., on the basis of human studies,[63] stated that skin is not a major source of 3-methylhistidine and that the splanchnic area contributes less than 8% of the urinary 3-methylhistidine. The third limitation is that the urinary recovery of injected labeled 3-methylhistidine, although close to 100% within 1 to 2 days in rats, men, adult rabbits, cattle, and adult sheep, is significantly less in lambs, pigs, and growing mice.[64] In the last three groups of animals, the muscles contain large concentrations of the dipeptide *balenine* (3-methylhistidine-β-alanine), which exchanges with labeled 3-methylhistidine and sequesters it. Finally, some of the urinary 3-methylhistidine is excreted in the N-acetyl form, which amounts to 5% in adult man,[58] but is a much larger percentage in the adult rat.[57] This form can be converted to free 3-methylhistidine by acid treatment.

The output of 3-methylhistidine has been used to study the effects of diet on muscle protein breakdown rate.[65] Protein depletion of young, growing rats caused a rapid reduction in output of 3-methylhistidine, which declined steadily to 20% of initial output, whereas output again rose following repletion on a protein-rich diet. In protein-calorie deficiency, however, an initial rise was followed by a gradual fall in 3-methylhistidine output. Thus muscle is conserved in response to protein depletion by reducing breakdown. However, with concurrent calorie deficiency, breakdown at first increases, likely because of the need for carbon for gluconeogenesis, and then diminishes in association with increased use of fat stores for energy.[65] Malnourished children in India showed a low output of 3-methylhistidine per unit of body weight, which rose during repletion.[66] This rise reflects an increase in both muscle mass and protein degradation.

Finally, 3-methylhistidine output is affected by age and by hormonal status. Output per kg body weight is higher in the newborn than in the mature adult,[67] and it declines further in old age, presumably because of the smaller muscle mass of the elderly.[68] Nakhooda et al. observed that the urinary output of 3-methylhistidine increases with the onset of diabetes in a spontaneously diabetic strain of rats and diminishes on treatment with insulin.[69] Output of 3-methylhistidine is increased by thyroxine secretion within the normal range of thyroid activity,[70] but by corticosterone secretion only at plasma levels of this hormone equivalent to severe stress.[71] These variations in 3-methylhistidine output are caused in part by changes in the degradation rate of muscle protein and in part by changes in muscle mass per unit of body weight (e.g., with aging).

## PLASMA PROTEIN METABOLISM

Most major proteins in the plasma are secreted from the liver. Many of these are also glycoproteins, a notable exception being serum albumin. The metabolism of plasma proteins is more conveniently studied than that of most other proteins because plasma proteins are more readily sampled in man. Pool size and turnover rate have been frequently reported for a variety of plasma proteins. These data are obtained by injecting samples of the plasma protein labeled with $^{131}I$ or $^{125}I$ and then measuring the kinetics of the disappearance of the label.[72] Synthesis of plasma proteins can also be measured by administering radioactive $^{14}CO_2$ or, preferably for human studies, the stable isotope $^{13}CO_2$ to label liver arginine in the carbon of the guanido group (see Fig. 1–2). The specific activity of free liver arginine can then be used to correct the rate of incorporation into liver proteins. The rate of plasma protein synthesis can also be calculated from labeled arginine incorporation. In an adaptation of this procedure, $^{15}N$-glycine was fed to human subjects every 3 hours over a 60-hour period to label N in the guanido group of free liver arginine and thus of liver urea.[73]

The rate of synthesis of plasma glycoproteins made in the livers of animals was measured accurately by using a novel method for sampling the specific activity of the hepatic pool of sugars after infusing $^{14}C$-glucose into the blood.[74] As shown in Figure 1–11 uridine diphosphate glucose (UDP-glucose) is in equilibrium with UDP-galactose and UDP-glucuronic acid. The $^{14}C$-activity of hepatic glucuronic acid can be measured by administering a drug (e.g., acetaminophen) that is excreted in the urine as the glucuronide. This specific activity can then be compared with the $^{14}C$ of galactose isolated from a plasma glycoprotein such as $\alpha_1$ acid glycoprotein. From these data, the rate of synthesis of the glycoprotein can be obtained.[75] This procedure can also be adapted to measuring metabolism of other sugars such as galactose.[76]

Table 1–2 shows, for a variety of plasma proteins, the intravascular concentration, the percentage of total body content that is intravascular, the fractional turnover rate, and the mass synthesized per day by human subjects.[77] Nutritional status usually affects these parameters, which have been used to identify protein malnutrition. Rats fed a diet low in protein show a progressive reduction in plasma albumin level because

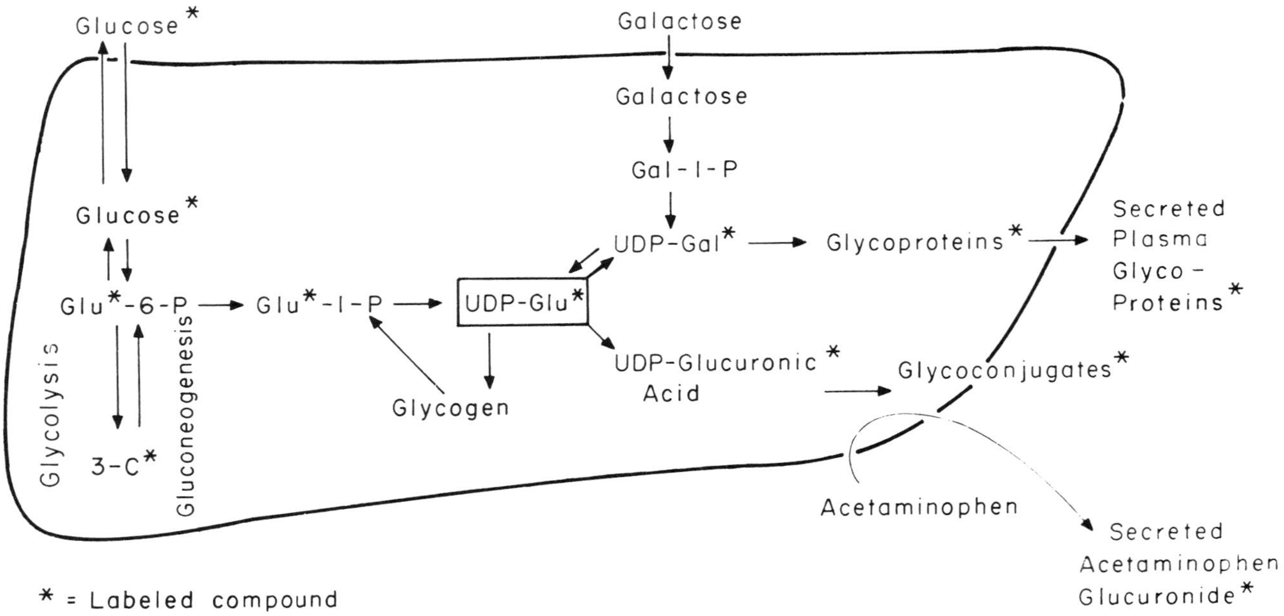
Glucose*
Galactose
Galactose
Gal-1-P
Glucose*
UDP-Gal*
Glycoproteins*
Secreted Plasma Glyco-Proteins*
Glu*-6-P
Glu*-1-P
UDP-Glu*
Glycolysis
Gluconeogenesis
UDP-Glucuronic Acid*
Glycoconjugates*
Glycogen
3-C*
Acetaminophen
Secreted Acetaminophen Glucuronide*
* = Labeled compound

**FIGURE 1–11.** Schematic model of hepatic hexose and uridine diphosphate (UDP)-sugar metabolic pathways. Glu, Glucose; 3-C, trioses. The asterisk shows the pathway of label from labeled glucose. (From Hellerstein, M.K., Greenblatt, D.J., Munro, H.N.: Metabolism, *36*:988–994, 1987.)

**TABLE 1–2.** TURNOVER OF PLASMA PROTEINS IN MAN

| PLASMA PROTEIN | PLASMA CONCENTRATION (G/DL) | INTRAVASCULAR POOL (% TOTAL) | TOTAL PER 70-KG MAN (G) | FRACTIONAL CATABOLIC RATE (% TOTAL MASS/DAY) | AMOUNT SYNTHESIZED (G/DAY) |
|---|---|---|---|---|---|
| Albumin | 4.2 | 45 | 280 | 4 | 11 |
| Transferrin | 0.2 | 49 | 12 | 8 | 1.1 |
| IgG | 1.1 | 58 | 58 | 4 | 2.1 |
| IgM | 0.1 | 74 | 4.5 | 8 | 0.3 |
| Fibrinogen | 0.4 | 84 | 15 | 21 | 2.2 |
| Prealbumin | 0.03 | 40 | 2 | 27 | 0.5 |
| Retinol-binding protein | 0.006 | — | — | 120 | — |

(From Valgeirsdottir, K., Munro, H.N.: Proteins and amino acids. *In* Surgical Nutrition. Edited by J.E. Fisher. Boston, Little, Brown, 1983, pp. 129–164.)

of its reduced synthesis.[78] Feeding of protein then stimulates protein synthesis, slowly followed by restoration of the level of albumin in the plasma. Serum albumin is thus too insensitive to serve as a reliable indicator of subclinical malnutrition. Shetty et al. showed that plasma proteins with more rapid turnover rates than albumin can be more sensitive indicators of protein or calorie depletion and repletion.[79] For example, prealbumin and retinol-binding proteins, which have high rates of turnover, were potentially suitable indicators of changed nutritional status when obese subjects were put on diets restricted in calories and/or protein.

## INTEGRATION OF BODY PROTEIN METABOLISM

### WHOLE-BODY AMINO ACID TURNOVER

From the preceding information, a composite picture of the daily exchange of amino acids in various compartments of the body of an adult man can be assembled.[80] These estimates for a 70-kg man are shown in Figure 1–12. The customary daily protein intake by men in Western countries is about 100 g, augmented by addition of an estimate of about 70 g of protein secreted into the gastrointestinal tract; consequently, the total load

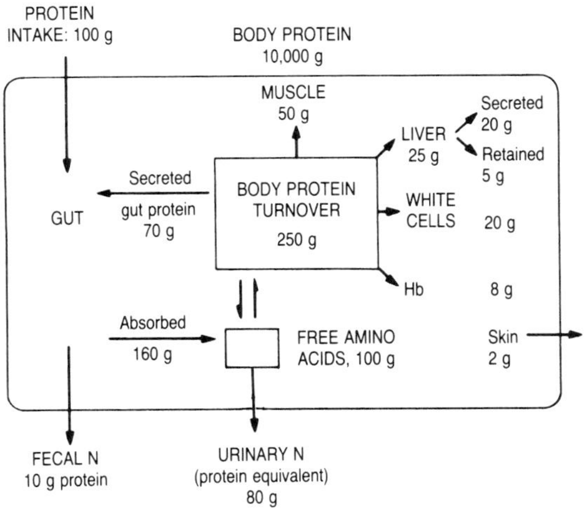
PROTEIN
INTAKE: 100 g
BODY PROTEIN
10,000 g
MUSCLE
50 g
LIVER
25 g
Secreted
20 g
Retained
5 g
Secreted
GUT
gut protein
70 g
BODY PROTEIN
TURNOVER
250 g
WHITE
CELLS
20 g
Hb
8 g
Absorbed
160 g
FREE AMINO
ACIDS, 100 g
Skin
2 g
FECAL N
10 g protein
URINARY N
(protein equivalent)
80 g

**FIGURE 1–12.** Estimated daily turnover of protein in the whole body and some organs of a 70-kg man. (From Hellerstein, M.K., Munro, H.N.: Interaction of liver and muscle in the regulation of metabolism in response to nutritional and other factors. *In* The Liver: Biology and Pathobiology, 2nd Ed. Edited by I.M. Arias, E.B. Jakoby, H. Popper, et al. New York, Raven Press, 1988, pp. 965–983.)

available for absorption is estimated to be 170 g of protein, of which 160 g is calculated to be absorbed as amino acids or small peptides (see Fig. 1–7). Experiments involving amino acids labeled with stable isotopes suggest that 250 to 300 g of protein is synthesized daily in the body of the adult. The difference between the intake of 100 g of protein and the daily synthesis of approximately 300 g indicates extensive reutilization of amino acids in protein metabolism. Some major contributors to this daily protein turnover can be identified, namely, gut, muscle, plasma proteins, white blood cells, and hemoglobin. Note that the free amino acid pool of the body, estimated at 100 g, is primarily made up of nonessential amino acids.

To quantitate whole-body protein synthesis and to identify the effects of changes in protein turnover, the concept of amino acid flux has to be considered (Fig. 1–13).[81] Turnover of protein encompasses synthesis (S) and breakdown (B). When these are equal (S = B), body protein is held constant. When S is less than B, the body is losing protein, whereas when S exceeds B, there is a gain in body protein. To illustrate flux, the remaining 2 items in the equation are the exogenous intake of amino acids as dietary protein (I) and the loss of amino acids by catabolism (C). In Figure 1–13, flux (Q) for a 70-kg man thus consists of I (100 g/day) plus amino acids coming from body protein breakdown B (300 g/day), giving a total amino acid flux of 400 g per day. This is balanced by removal of amino acids from the pool in the form of protein synthesis, S (300 g per day), and amino acid catabolism, C (100 g per day).

Data on the magnitude of protein metabolism in the whole body and its compartments continue to be refined using amino acids labeled with radioactive or stable isotopes of carbon, hydrogen, or nitrogen; stable isotopes are preferred for human studies on grounds of safety. Early studies of whole-body protein and amino acid metabolism were complicated by the use of single-pulse doses of labeled amino acid, often followed by complex kinetic analysis. Garlick and Fern described a study with single doses of $^{15}N$-labeled amino acids and demonstrated that these single doses provide estimates of total daily protein synthesis varying from 100 to 120 g per day (glutamine, alanine) through 250 g (glycine) to 350 g (leucine).[82] These absolute values for total protein synthesis and turnover are subject to large differences incompatible with a single value for protein synthesis. Waterlow and his colleagues used continuous administration of labeled amino acids orally or intravenously to achieve a steady state reflected by a constant concentration of isotopically labeled amino acid in the plasma.[83] Under these conditions, a simple model can be used to derive useful conclusions about the flux of the administered amino acid and the turnover of body protein (Fig. 1–14). By using 1-$^{13}C$-leucine as the amino acid infused intravenously for a few hours,[84] a steady level of $^{13}C$ enrichment can be attained in the free leucine of the plasma that is considered to reflect its level in most tissues. It is therefore accepted as a single metabolic pool from which label is

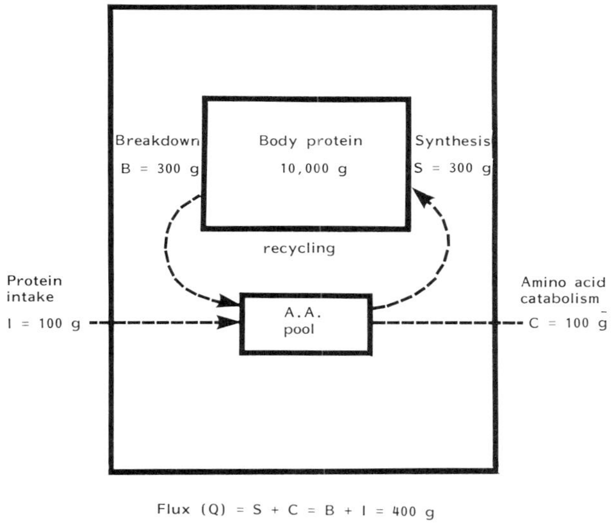
Breakdown
B = 300 g
Body protein
10,000 g
Synthesis
S = 300 g
recycling
Protein
intake
I = 100 g
A.A.
pool
Amino acid
catabolism
C = 100 g

Flux (Q) = S + C = B + I = 400 g

**FIGURE 1–13.** Components of daily whole-body protein turnover for an adult man of 70 kg body weight. The relationships are expressed by the equation Q = B + I = S + C, where Q is total amino acid flux, I is amino acid intake, usually as dietary protein, B is body protein breakdown, S is body protein synthesis, and C is amino acid catabolism. (From Munro, H.N.: Protein nutriture and requirements of the elderly. *In* Human Nutrition: A Comprehensive Treatise. Vol. 6. Edited by H.N. Munro and D.E. Danford. New York, Plenum Press, 1989, pp. 153–181.)

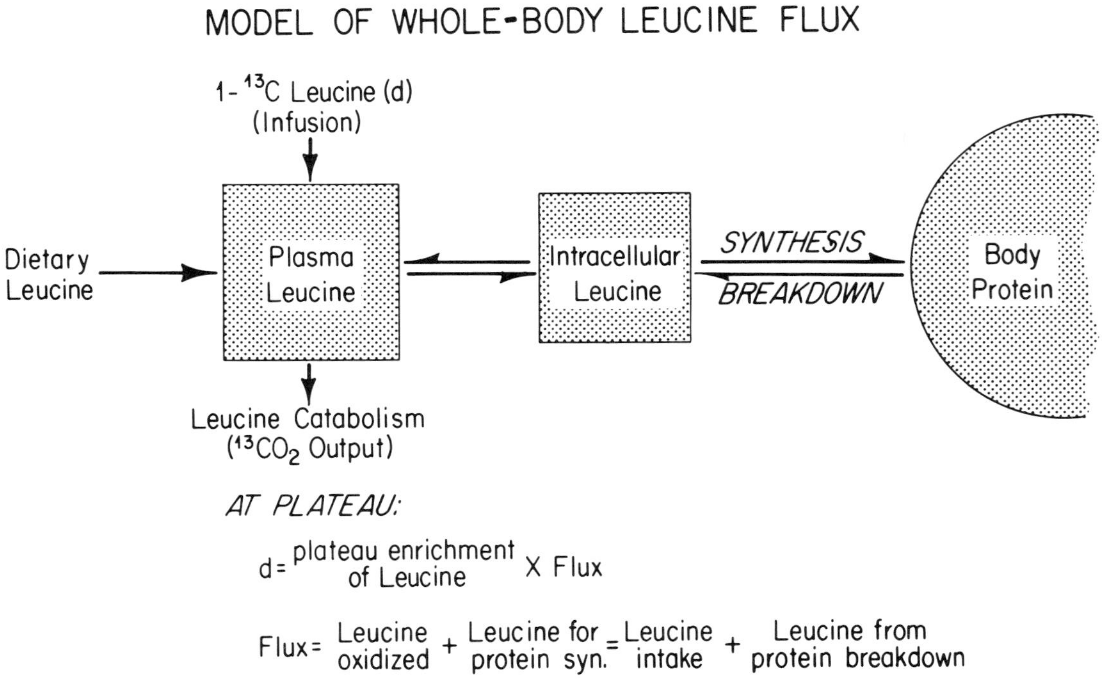
MODEL OF WHOLE-BODY LEUCINE FLUX
1-13C Leucine (d)
(Infusion)
Dietary Leucine
Plasma Leucine
Intracellular Leucine
SYNTHESIS
BREAKDOWN
Body Protein
Leucine Catabolism
(13CO2 Output)
AT PLATEAU:
d= plateau enrichment of Leucine X Flux
Flux= Leucine oxidized + Leucine for protein syn. = Leucine intake + Leucine from protein breakdown

**FIGURE 1–14.** Model of whole-body leucine flux. (Reprinted with permission from Young, V.R., Gersovitz, M., Munro, H.N.: Human aging: protein and amino acid metabolism and implications for protein and amino acid requirements. *In* Nutritional Approaches to Aging Research. Edited by G.B. Moment. Boca Raton, FL, CRC Press, 1981, pp. 47–81.)

**TABLE 1–3.** METABOLISM OF 1-$^{13}$C-LEUCINE IN YOUNG MEN*

| | | PROTEIN SYNTHESIS | | | LEUCINE OXIDATION | | |
|---|---|---|---|---|---|---|---|
| Protein Intake | Nitrogen Balance | Post-Absorptive | Fed | Difference | Post-Absorptive | Fed | Difference |
| g/kg/day | mg/kg/day | | | μmol/kg/h† | | | |
| 0.1 | −42 | 76 | 64 | −8 | 13 | 12 | −1 |
| 0.6 | −21 | 89 | 102 | +13 | 22 | 22 | ±0 |
| 1.5 | +12 | 113 | 113 | ±0 | 18 | 46 | +28 |

*In the postabsorptive and absorptive states at low, marginal, and excess levels of protein intake.
†Expressed as μmoles leucine.
(Adapted from Motil, K.J., Matthews, D.E., Bier, D.M., et al.: Am. J. Physiol., *240:*E712-E721, 1981.)

withdrawn in two directions, namely, for protein synthesis or for catabolism with release of $^{13}CO_2$. Owing to the short time interval of the study, it is assumed that body proteins will not recycle isotope into the metabolic pool. Motil et al. used this concept to study the effect of level of protein intake on the rate of protein synthesis and on leucine oxidation in fasting and fed states.[85] Table 1–3 shows that protein synthesis was increased in both postabsorptive and fed states when protein intake was raised from low through marginal to excess dietary protein, whereas catabolism to $CO_2$ rose sharply only during the absorptive phase after the intake of excess dietary protein.

## METABOLIC INTEGRATION OF ORGANS

From the preceding sections, it is apparent that certain organs play a major cooperative role in ensuring the use of free amino acids.[80,86] This process is seen most convincingly in the response to a meal containing protein, as illustrated in Figure 1–15 for three groups of amino acids: glutamate and glutamine, the aromatic amino acids, and the branched-chain amino acids. The intestinal mucosa responds to an influx of glutamine and glutamic acid from either the diet or the peripheral organs by transamination of a part to pyruvic acid to form alanine. Alanine then passes up the portal vein to

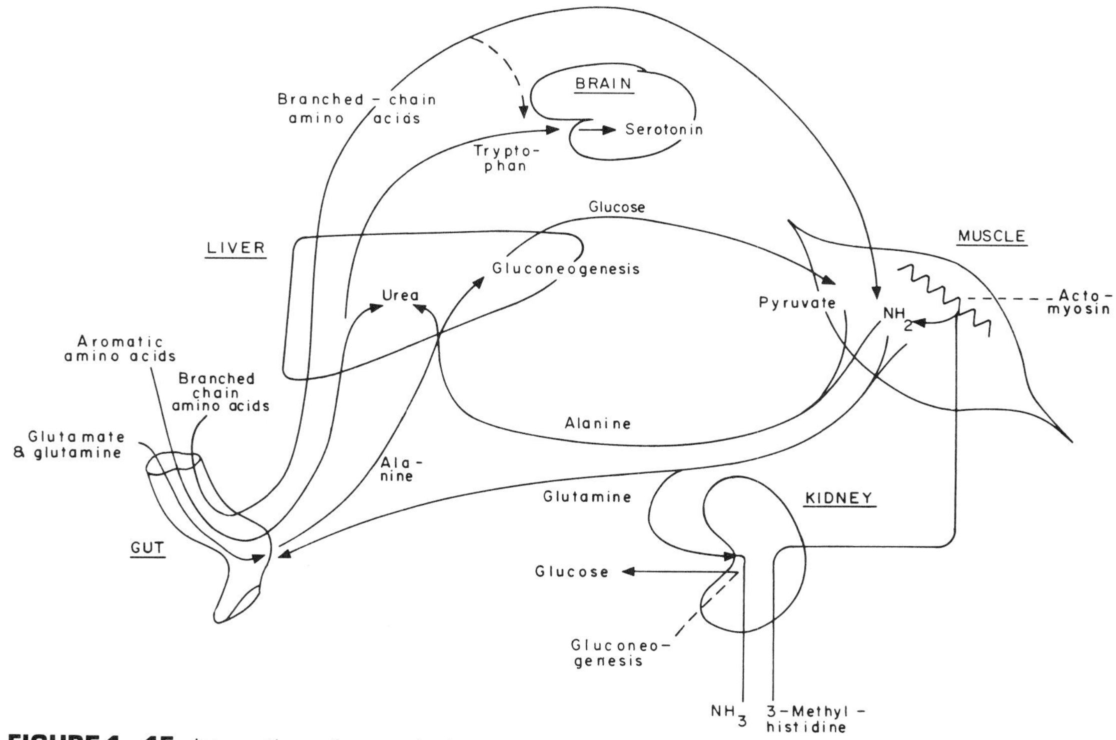
Branched - chain
amino acids
BRAIN
Serotonin
Trypto-
phan
Glucose
LIVER
MUSCLE
Gluconeogenesis
Urea
Pyruvate
Acto-
myosin
$NH_2$
Aromatic
amino acids
Branched
chain
amino acids
Glutamate
& glutamine
Alanine
Ala-
nine
Glutamine
KIDNEY
GUT
Glucose
Gluconeo-
genesis
$NH_3$
3-Methyl-
histidine

**FIGURE 1–15.** Interactions of organs in the metabolism of some major amino acids discussed in the text. (From Hellerstein, M.K., Munro, H.N.: Interaction of liver and muscle in the regulation of metabolism in response to nutritional and other factors. *In* The Liver: Biology and Pathobiology, 2nd Ed. Edited by I.M. Arias, E.B. Jakoby, H. Popper, et al. New York, Raven Press, 1988, pp. 965–983.)

the liver to yield glucose by gluconeogenesis, while the nitrogen becomes urea. In the liver, the rates of catabolism of most incoming essential amino acids are regulated according to the body's needs, as in the case of tryptophan, discussed earlier in this chapter. Such regulation of the rate of hepatic degradation is important because tryptophan is rate limiting for synthesis of the neurotransmitter serotonin in the brain. If the level of plasma tryptophan was not kept within certain limits, the synthesis of serotonin would be uncontrolled.

Branched-chain amino acids are mainly catabolized in the peripheral tissues, notably muscle, adipose tissue, and kidney. DeFronzo and Felig described experiments on human subjects in which the amino acid flux across the splanchnic area (gut and liver) and across the leg were measured by comparing the amounts of each amino acid entering and leaving these body compartments (Fig. 1–16).[87] Following a meal of 250 g of meat, 70% of the amino acids leaving the liver took the form of branched-chain amino acids; this contrasts with their concentration in meat protein (about 20%), thus indicating the selective catabolism by the liver of other entering amino acids. A large percentage of the amino nitrogen taken up by the leg during the absorptive period is similarly accounted for by branched-chain amino acids (Fig. 1–16).

One might expect increased amounts of alanine and glutamine to be released from muscle after a meal because of the transfer of large amounts of branched-chain amino acids to muscle.[88] In contrast, Elia and Livesey showed that, after a meal of meat, glutamine release from a limb is unchanged and alanine output actually decreases.[89] Continuing on this theme, Elia et al. replaced the test meal of meat with a mixed meal containing less protein but including fat and carbohydrate.[90] The response of the plasma amino acid concentrations to the meal was attenuated and so was the uptake of branched-chain amino acids by muscle. In earlier studies in which only protein or amino acids were given, as much as 70% of the administered branched-chain amino acids were taken up by muscle, whereas in the more recent study by Elia et al., muscle uptake over the first 8 hours after the meal accounted for less than 40%. Furthermore, these investigators again identified glutamine as the main vehicle for transporting N from muscle to the viscera and found no large change in output of glutamine from muscle resulting from the meal, whereas release of alanine from muscle was diminished during the period of absorption of the meal. It would thus appear that more studies using meals of normal mixed constituents should be undertaken.

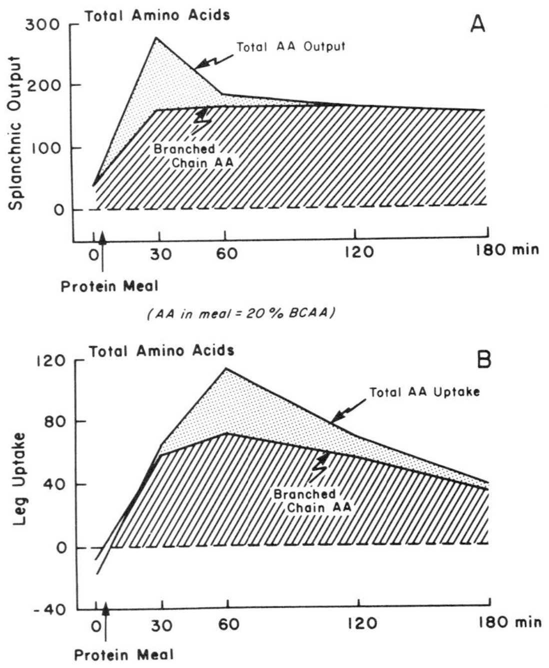

Total Amino Acids
A
Total AA Output
Splanchnic Output
300
200
100
0
Branched Chain AA
0
30
60
120
180 min
Protein Meal
(AA in meal = 20 % BCAA)
Total Amino Acids
B
Total AA Uptake
Leg Uptake
120
80
40
0
-40
Branched Chain AA
0
30
60
120
180 min
Protein Meal


**FIGURE 1–16.** Effect of a meal of protein on splanchnic amino acid release *(A)* and leg uptake of amino acids *(B)*. The exchanges are expressed in µmol/min. (Modified from DeFronzo, R.A., Felig, P.: Am. J. Clin. Nutr., *33*:1378–1386, 1980. Copyright by the American Society for Clinical Nutrition.)

Finally, glutamine is the source of nitrogen for ammonia synthesis by the kidney. The tissues contributing glutamine for this purpose have been elegantly documented in the acidotic rat by Schrock and Goldstein, who used amino acid exchange across the kidney compared with muscle, liver, and gut.[91] Acidosis caused by ammonium chloride ($NH_4Cl$) or hydrochloric acid (HCl) administration resulted in increased ammonia ($NH_3$) output by the kidney, which could be accounted for by release of more glutamine from muscle and liver with gut output remaining unchanged.

To provide a reasonably complete picture of the interaction of metabolites within and between tissues in response to various physiologic conditions, it is necessary to add profiles of interorgan changes in carbohydrate and fat metabolites (Fig. 1–17). The interchange of these among liver, muscle, and adipose tissue is regulated by insulin and glucagon.[80] In the *fasting* state, insulin levels are low and adipose tissue lipase thereby becomes active, releasing large amounts of free fatty acids and glycerol from the fat stores. Coincident with this change, the plasma glucagon level rises and accelerates the utilization of liver glycogen. In the fasting subject, the incoming free fatty acids entering the liver are partly diverted to ketone body formation, whereas in muscle, the free fatty acids, and with more prolonged fasting, the ketone bodies, replace glucose as the major fuel. When the subject is *fed*, the insulin level rises and favors glycogen deposition in liver and in muscle, so carbohydrate becomes the main fuel in both tissues. Insulin also inhibits the action of lipase and thus shuts off the free fatty acids that are the alternative fuel. In muscle, the deposited tissue glycogen provides muscle energy, but under conditions of inadequate oxygen supply, glycogen is metabolized to lactate, which is released into the blood and passes to the liver for gluconeogenesis (Cori cycle).

The interactions of metabolites exchanged between organs are most clearly seen during progressive starvation. As pointed out by Cahill and Aoki, the brain uses large amounts of energy that must be supplied as water-soluble energy substrates, namely, glucose in well-nourished people and ketones during starvation.[92] Figure 1–18 shows metabolic profiles at four stages of the process of starvation. Between meals (interprandial state), blood glucose is maintained for the brain by release of glucose from liver glycogen, while the fall in insulin level allows free fatty acids to be released to provide energy for muscle. At the next stage (overnight fast), liver glycogen is nearly exhausted, and the maintenance of blood sugar now depends on gluconeogenesis from alanine released by muscle and intestine. At the same time, free fatty acids from adipose tissue begin to form ketone bodies in the liver. At the next stage (early starvation), muscle becomes the major source of carbon for glucose released from the liver and utilized by the brain, whereas ketone bodies are the major energy source for muscle. The brain then adapts to using ketone bodies as its major fuel, thus sparing glucose production in the liver. Finally, in prolonged starvation, muscle protein breakdown diminishes, so release of alanine and glutamine from muscle decreases.

The preceding literature analysis presents a picture of cooperation between protein metabolism and energy metabolism. Certain metabolic diseases distort these relationships. These include insulin-dependent diabetes,[87,93] kidney failure,[87] hepatic cirrhosis,[94] fever and sepsis,[95] and cancer.[96–99]

## METABOLIC BODY SIZE AND PROTEIN METABOLISM

It has long been known that among mammals the intensity of energy metabolism decreases as mature body size increases. This general principle of metabolism affects the relative sizes of some organs intimately concerned with metabolic regulation, such as the liver. Table 1–4 is based on regression analysis of data from a wide range of mammals of varying mature size. It shows the results as organ weights or metabolic components per kg body weight for animals weighing 200 g (rat) and 70 kg (man), as predicted by these regression analyses. The proportion of skeletal muscle is constant at 45% of body weight. Blood and heart weights are also maintained at the same weight per kg body weight, but liver and kidney, two organs intimately concerned with metabolism of food, are relatively smaller in man than in

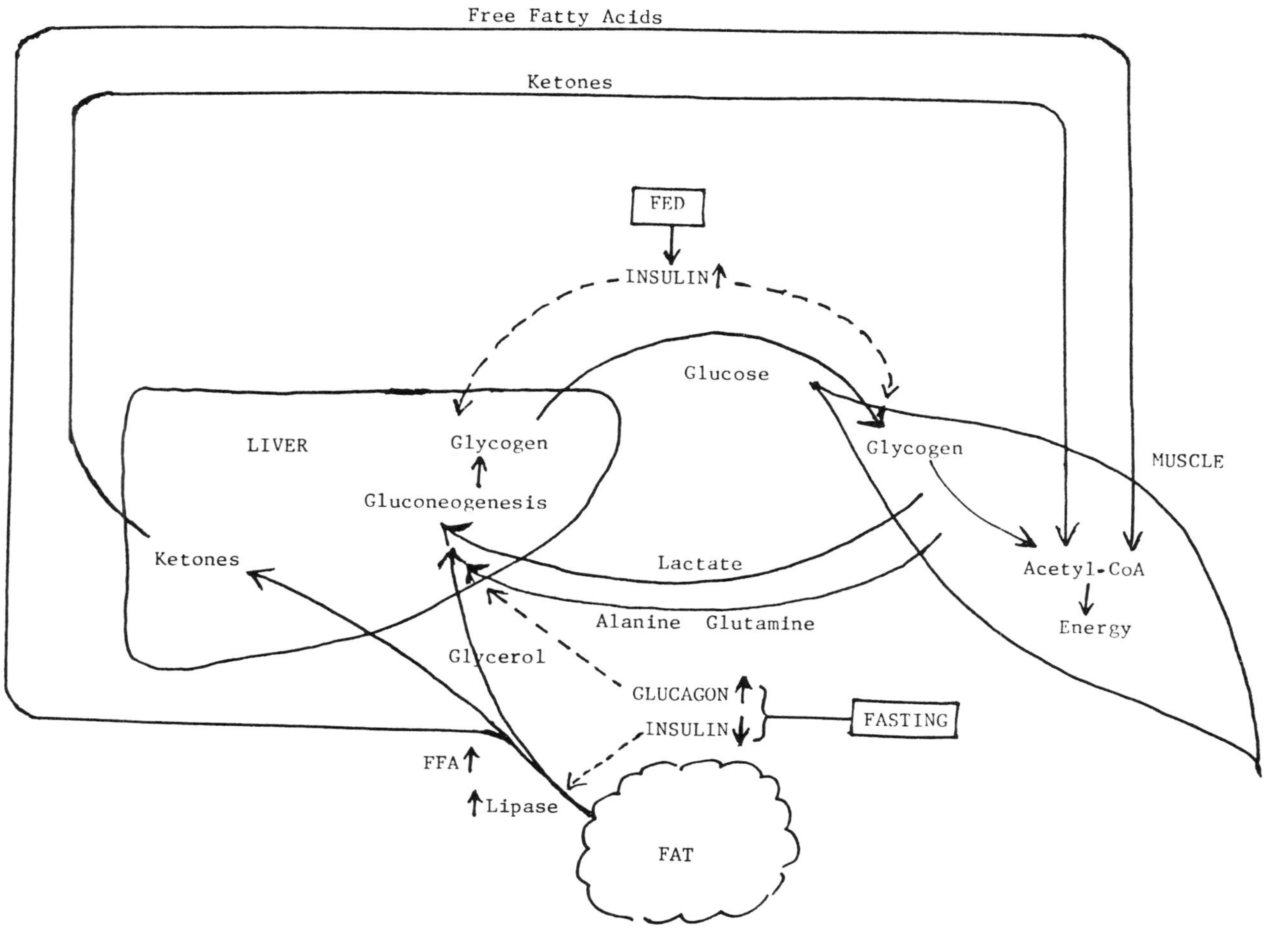
Free Fatty Acids
Ketones
FED
INSULIN↑
Glucose
LIVER
Glycogen
Gluconeogenesis
Glycogen
MUSCLE
Ketones
Lactate
Acetyl-CoA
Energy
Alanine Glutamine
Glycerol
GLUCAGON↑
INSULIN↓
FASTING
FFA↑
↑Lipase
FAT

**FIGURE 1–17.** Role of liver and muscle in the metabolism of carbohydrate and fat in the fed and starved states. (Modified from Hellerstein, M.K., Munro, H.N.: Interaction of liver and muscle in the regulation of metabolism in response to nutritional and other factors. *In* The Liver: Biology and Pathobiology, 2nd Ed. Edited by I.M. Arias, E.B. Jakoby, H. Popper, et al. New York, Raven Press, 1988, pp. 965–983.)

the rat. The endocrine organs (pituitary, adrenal, and thyroid glands) are also smaller relative to body weight. In addition, most metabolic parameters (basal energy metabolism, endogenous urinary N output, requirements for the essential amino acids, total body protein synthesis, and turnover of albumin and ceruloplasmin) are about five times more intense per kg body weight in the rat than in man. However, the daily excretion of creatinine per kg body weight is little affected by the body size of the species, reflecting its relationship with the amount of muscle per kg body weight of rat and man.

## NITROGEN EXCRETION AND NITROGEN BALANCE

The end products of nitrogen (N) metabolism within the body are excreted in the urine, mostly as urea, ammonia, uric acid, and creatinine, whereas unabsorbed protein coming from the diet or protein secreted into the lumen of the intestines and not reabsorbed is lost in the feces. In addition, some nitrogenous materials are lost from the skin both as soluble N (e.g., urea) and as shed epithelial cells. Finally, minor routes of N loss are represented by nasal secretions, hair cuttings, menstrual fluid, and semen.

Each of the major N compounds in urine responds differently to changes in protein intake (Table 1–5).[100] On a diet of normal protein content, urea accounts for more than 80% of urinary N, but this proportion falls when a diet low in protein is consumed. During fasting, the absolute amount and percentage of ammonia N rise in response to the acidosis, despite a decrease in urinary N. On the other hand, creatinine output tends to be independent of dietary protein or calorie intake because it is a product of the pool of creatine in muscle, and this does not alter rapidly with changes in diet.

The overall metabolism of protein in the body is

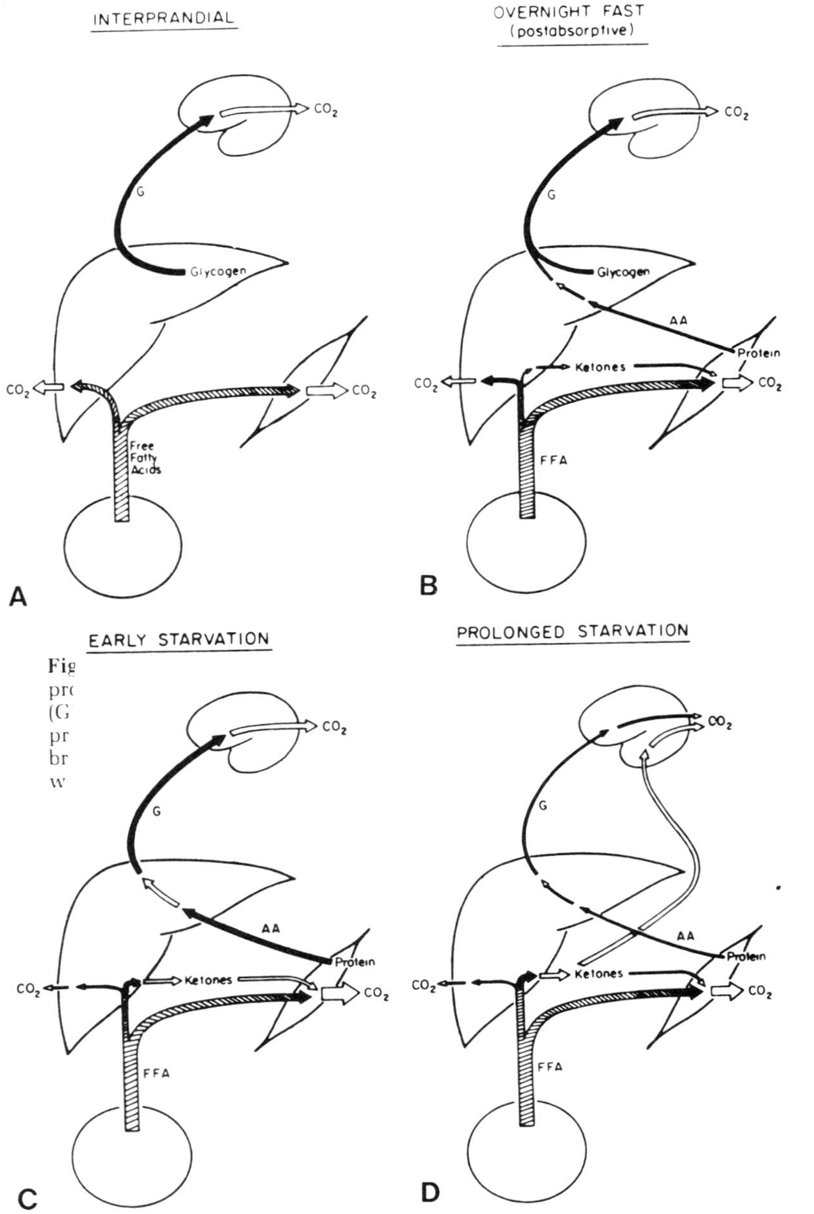
INTERPRANDIAL
OVERNIGHT FAST
(postabsorptive)
$CO_2$
G
Glycogen
Free Fatty Acids
A
AA
Protein
Ketones
FFA
B
EARLY STARVATION
PROLONGED STARVATION
C
D

**FIGURE 1–18.** Sequence of diagrams showing metabolic adaptation of man to starvation. *A,* Man in the interprandial state, with hepatic glycogen providing glucose (G) for brain. *B,* Overnight fasting state, with hepatic gluconeogenesis from muscle-derived amino acids (AA) providing glucose (G) for brain. The remainder of the body is using free fatty acids (FFA). *C,* Early starvation, with muscle providing the major share of gluconeogenic precursor. *D,* Prolonged starvation, with ketoacids mainly rejected by muscle to elevate blood levels to permit their facilitated diffusion into brain. Thus, brain glucose (G) utilization is diminished and, pari passu, muscle proteolysis. (Modified from Cahill, G.F., Aoki, T.T.: Conditions with abnormal energy balance: partial and total starvation. *In* Assessment of Energy Metabolism in Health and Disease. Edited by J.M. Kinney and E. Lense. Columbus, OH, Ross Laboratories, 1980, pp. 129–134. Reprinted with permission of Ross Laboratories, Columbus, OH 43216.)

**TABLE 1–4.** THE INFLUENCE OF BODY SIZE ON THE RELATIVE WEIGHTS OF INDIVIDUAL ORGANS AND ON SEVERAL PARAMETERS OF METABOLISM

| | AMOUNT OF METABOLIC OR BODY COMPONENT/KG BODY WEIGHT | | |
|---|---|---|---|
| Measurement | At 200 g (rat) | At 70 kg (man) | Ratio $\frac{rat}{man}$ |
| Organ weights: | | | |
| Skeletal muscle (g) | 450 | 450 | 1.0 |
| Blood (g) | 52 | 48 | 1.1 |
| Heart (g) | 6.0 | 5.5 | 1.1 |
| Liver (g) | 41 | 19 | 2.1 |
| Kidney (g) | 9.4 | 3.8 | 2.5 |
| Pituitary (mg) | 360 | 80 | 4.5 |
| Adrenal (mg) | 380 | 120 | 3.2 |
| Thyroid (mg) | 150 | 90 | 1.7 |
| Metabolic Parameters: | | | |
| Basal energy metabolism (kcal/day) | 108 | 23 | 4.7 |
| Endogenous urinary N (mg N/day) | 230 | 45 | 5.1 |
| Threonine requirement (mg/day) | 28 | 7 | 4.2 |
| Methionine requirement (mg/day) | 56 | 16 | 3.5 |
| Total body protein synthesis (mg N/day) | 1010 | 218 | 4.6 |
| Creatinine in urine (mg N/day) | 14 | 8 | 1.8 |
| Total body albumin (g) | 4.0 | 4.6 | 0.9 |
| Albumin turnover ($days^{-1}$) | 0.24 | 0.04 | 6.0 |
| Ceruloplasmin turnover ($days^{-1}$) | 0.49 | 0.11 | 4.4 |

(Data from Munro, H.N.: Evolution of protein metabolism in mammals. *In* Mammalian protein Metabolism. Vol. 3. Edited by H.N. Munro. New York, Academic Press, 1969, pp. 133–182.)

**TABLE 1–5.** PARTITION OF URINARY N OUTPUT UNDER DIFFERENT NUTRITIONAL CONDITIONS BY ADULT HUMAN SUBJECTS

| | HIGH-PROTEIN DIET | LOW-PROTEIN DIET | DURING FASTING | |
|---|---|---|---|---|
| | | | Day 1 | Day 2 |
| Urinary N Source | Total daily output (g N) | | | |
| Total N | 16.80 | 3.60 | 10.51 | 8.77 |
| Urea N | 14.70 | 2.20 | 8.96 | 6.62 |
| Ammonia N | 0.49 | 0.42 | 0.40 | 1.05 |
| Uric acid N | 0.18 | 0.09 | 0.12 | 0.17 |
| Creatinine N | 0.58 | 0.60 | 0.44 | 0.39 |
| Undetermined N | 0.85 | 0.27 | 0.59 | 0.54 |
| | Percentage of total N output | | | |
| Urea N | 87.5 | 61.7 | 85.1 | 75.4 |
| Ammonia N | 3.0 | 11.3 | 3.8 | 12.0 |
| Uric acid N | 1.1 | 2.5 | 1.1 | 1.9 |
| Creatinine N | 3.6 | 17.2 | 4.2 | 4.4 |
| Undetermined N | 4.9 | 7.3 | 5.6 | 6.1 |

(From Allison, J.B., Bird, J.C.: Elimination of nitrogen from the body. *In* Mammalian Protein Metabolism. Vol. 1. Edited by H.N. Munro and J.B. Allison. New York Academic Press, 1964, pp. 483–512.)

summarized by N balance, which is the difference between N intake and N output, the difference being positive (N retention, as in active growth), negative (N loss), or zero (N equilibrium). The determination of N balance (B) thus requires a careful estimate of intake (I) and all routes of N loss, namely, urine (U), feces (F), dermal (S), and miscellaneous (M) losses:

$$B = I - (U + F + S + M)$$

The balance obtained is usually a small difference (10 to 15%) between two larger numbers and is subject to the combined errors of these estimates. Furthermore, Wallace pointed out that dietary N intake tends to be overestimated because of unconsumed food, whereas output tends to be underestimated because of unmeasured nitrogen losses.[101] There is thus a built-in bias toward a positive balance. In addition, it is unusual to make direct measurements of dermal losses; the custom is to accept a constant (estimated) correction for dermal N or to ignore this N loss.

Nitrogen balance is also affected by energy intake. Not only does N balance become progressively more negative as energy intake is reduced below the needs of the body, but also it becomes more favorable when energy intake is increased above the subject's requirements for energy.[93,102–104] A direct relationship exists between energy intake and N balance from negative at low-energy levels to positive at excessive intakes of energy. The effect of energy intake on protein requirements is illustrated by the findings of Kishi et al. (Table 1–6), who reported a twofold increase in protein requirements when the energy fed to young Japanese men was decreased from 238 kJ/kg (57 kcal/kg) to 167 kJ/kg (40 kcal/kg).[105] When these data are adjusted to cover 97% of the population (mean + 2SD), the required intake for egg protein varies from 0.5 g protein/kg at 238 kJ/kg (57 kcal/kg) to 1.02 g protein/kg at 167 kJ/kg (40 kcal/kg). (Note that many sedentary individuals require even less energy for weight maintenance.) The improvement of N retention with increased energy does not occur if a limiting amount of dietary protein is available.[93] In conclusion, N balance is clearly the result of both protein intake and energy balance. Studies of factors affecting N balance, such as dietary protein, must therefore be carried out under conditions where the subject's energy intake is carefully defined in relation to individual requirements, a goal not easy to accomplish. New methods for determining total energy expenditure using doubly labeled water may permit more accurate assessments of individual energy needs.[106]

Finally, N balance is influenced by hormones.[107] These can be divided into anabolic (growth hormone, testosterone) and catabolic (corticosteroids, thyroxine). The effects of these hormones are especially pronounced on protein metabolism in muscle. Because skeletal muscle is such a large tissue, anabolic and catabolic changes in muscle tend to determine alterations in N balance, obscuring the effect of these hormones on protein metabolism in other tissues, such as liver.

## REQUIREMENTS OF MAN FOR PROTEIN AND AMINO ACIDS

In contrast to molecular biology, our knowledge of nutritional principles continues to evolve slowly. In the field of protein requirements, a major advance was achieved in 1946 by Block and Mitchell, who showed that various biologic measures of the quality of dietary proteins could be correlated with their content of essential amino acids expressed as a "chemical score," that is, the concentration in least abundance relative to requirements.[108] The emphasis on essential amino acids as an explanation for the need for dietary protein was further

**TABLE 1–6.** EFFECT OF ENERGY INTAKE ON THE AMOUNT OF DIETARY PROTEIN REQUIRED BY ADULT MEN TO ACHIEVE ZERO NITROGEN BALANCE AND ON THE CORRESPONDING SAFE ALLOWANCE OF DIETARY PROTEIN

| ENERGY (KCAL/KG BODY WEIGHT)* | MEAN REQUIREMENT OF DIETARY PROTEIN FOR ZERO N BALANCE (G PROTEIN/KG BODY WEIGHT) | SAFE ALLOWANCE OF PROTEIN (MEAN REQUIREMENT + 2 STANDARD DEVIATIONS) | |
|---|---|---|---|
| | | Grams protein/kg body weight | Grams protein/ 70-kg man |
| 40 | 0.78 | 1.02 | 72 |
| 45 | 0.56 | 0.74 | 52 |
| 48 | 0.51 | 0.62 | 44 |
| 57 | 0.42 | 0.50 | 35 |
| Recommended dietary allowance | | 0.80 | 56 |

*4.18 kcal = 1 kJ.

(Data from Kishi, K., Mitayani, S., Inoue, G.: J. Nutr., *108*:658–669, 1978, in Munro, H.N.: Protein nutriture and requirements of the elderly. *In* Human Nutrition: A Comprehensive Treatise. Vol. 6. Edited by H.N. Munro and D.E. Danford. New York, Plenum Press, 1989, pp. 153–181; and Food and Nutrition Board, National Research Council: Protein and amino acids. *In* Recommended Dietary Allowances. 10th Ed. Washington, D.C., National Academy Press, 1989, pp. 52–77.)

underlined from 1950 to 1960 by a series of quantitative estimates of human requirements for individual amino acids. The protein and amino acid requirements of man have been frequently reviewed, and recommendations have been made in the publications of expert international committees,[109–112] as well as in recommended dietary allowances for the United States.[113] (See Appendix Tables A-2 through A-6 and A-9). The requirements for protein and for individual essential amino acids are considered separately. A detailed analysis of the history of these estimates is provided elsewhere.[114]

## ASSESSMENT OF PROTEIN NEEDS AND ALLOWANCES

The requirement for protein in the diet is usually estimated in one of two ways. The *factorial method* measures all losses of nitrogenous compounds from the body after a period when the diet is protein free and assumes these losses to be obligatory. High-quality dietary protein in amounts sufficient to replace these obligatory N losses ought to provide the adult human with the minimum requirement for protein. This method is therefore based on adding up a series of factors that represent obligatory N losses from the body. The second method for estimating protein requirements is the *nitrogen balance method.* This method determines the minimum amount of dietary protein needed to keep healthy, nonpregnant, nonlactating adults in N balance. Ideally, the two methods should arrive at similar estimates of protein requirements. For infants and children, optimal growth is the criterion used; similarly, additional protein must be provided for pregnancy and lactation.

To determine protein requirements by the factorial method, the magnitudes of the obligatory N losses by each channel listed earlier are required under basal conditions on a protein-free diet. Based on literature surveys by two successive World Health Organization/Food and Agriculture Organization (WHO/FAO) expert committees,[110,111] and confirmed by a recent WHO/FAO/United Nations University (UNU) panel,[112] the minimum *obligatory urinary nitrogen* output has been estimated to be 37 mg N/kg body weight for adult men. On a diet without protein, one still loses N in the feces, representing enzymes and desquamated intestinal cells that have not been fully digested and reabsorbed, amounting to about 12 mg N/kg body weight. Organic nitrogen is also lost from the skin in the form of desquamated cells, hair and nail clippings, and sweat.[115] The cutaneous N loss by adult men eating a normal diet in a temperate environment is in the range of 4 to 8 mg/kg body weight; this amount decreases to 3 mg when a protein-free diet is consumed. In addition to these major routes of N loss are a series of minor routes of N excretion, such as ammonia in the breath, nasal secretions, menstrual flow in the female, and seminal fluid in the male.[115] For all these minor routes, an estimate of 2 mg N/kg body weight for men and 3 mg N/kg for women approximates the average daily loss.

The sum of urinary, fecal, cutaneous, and minor routes of N loss using the factorial approach adds up to 54 mg N/kg body weight for adults. This estimate of obligatory N loss should also be expressed as the amount of body protein that must be replaced daily from dietary sources, using the conversion factor of N $\times$ 6.25 to provide the weight of protein. Thus, the average obligatory N losses would represent a net daily loss of 0.34 g of body protein/kg body weight, if not replaced from the diet and this would therefore become the daily protein requirement of the average adult. The WHO/FAO (1973) report suggests a coefficient of individual variation of 15% for the obligatory N losses in the urine and feces.[111] Consequently, an additional 30% (twice the coefficient of variation of 15%) is added to cover the range of individual losses for 97.5% of the population. The upper limit of the amount of body protein to be replaced thus becomes 0.45 g/kg body weight.

This prediction can be tested by feeding graded amounts of protein and determining the minimum needed to produce zero N balance. However, several investigators have fed diets providing increasing levels of protein in clinical studies and have measured changes in N balance. In general, the addition of increasing amounts of high-quality protein, such as whole-egg protein, has produced a nonlinear response.[116] At low intakes, the improvement in N balance is proportional to the amount of protein added to the diet, but as intake is further increased, the efficiency of utilization decreases. The average amount of protein then needed to achieve zero N equilibrium (i.e., output=intake) is greater than would have been predicted by the factorial method or from the earlier part of the N balance curve. The loss of efficiency as equilibrium is approached has been estimated to add 30% to the amount of whole-egg protein needed for N equilibrium, and therefore the requirement for dietary protein is increased from 0.45 to 0.57 g protein/kg body weight. In addition, if the protein quality of the diet is less than egg protein, the amount needed to replace body protein may need to be correspondingly increased.

These conclusions are less secure than such precise calculations would lead one to believe. As discussed previously, nitrogen balance is influenced by energy intake.[93,105] In the past, not enough attention was paid to ensuring energy equilibrium during N balance experiments; in general, the tendency was to increase energy intake beyond requirements to prevent weight losses on low-protein diets. This approach confounds the N balance data by improving N retention because of the surfeit of calories. Currently energy intake is not used as a factor in determining the protein requirements of various populations.

In addition, it has been suggested that the use of a correction factor of 30% for loss of efficiency of utilization of egg protein may not adequately describê the reduction in utilization of other proteins such as wheat gluten. The correction of 30% was also challenged by the most recent (1985) international committee, who considered that it should be much higher.[112] In addition, Garza et al. concluded that 0.57 g egg protein/kg body weight per day may not be sufficient to provide the optimum protein intake for the average young adult man receiving adequate but not excessive energy intakes.[117] At this intake, serum levels of certain liver enzymes (e.g., transaminases) rose, an effect that disappeared when protein intake was increased. In another study, Garza et al. found that the addition of nonessential amino acids to increase protein intake from 0.57 to 0.8 g/kg allowed young adults to achieve N equilibrium,[118] thus pointing to a requirement for more nonspecific N by the adult in agreement with the evidence of low requirements of adults for essential amino acids (discussed later in this chapter).

## RECOMMENDED DIETARY ALLOWANCES FOR PROTEIN

In 1989, a subcommittee of the United States Food and Nutrition Board issued its updated recommended dietary allowances (RDA) for protein and amino acids[113] (see Appendix Table A–2b). Based largely on the conclusions of the 1985 report of the FAO/WHO/UNU committee,[112] the 1989 RDA recommendations for *safe levels* of protein intake rely more on N balance data than on factorial data. The RDA for protein was established by first estimating the *average requirement* for high-quality, highly digestible protein, so-called reference protein, according to sex, age, and reproductive status. The average requirement was then increased by 2 standard deviations to give the recommended allowance for reference protein (estimated to meet the needs of 97.5% of the population.) Finally, United States protein consumption patterns were reviewed to determine whether essential amino acid composition and protein digestibility were important factors requiring an increase in protein from the reference allowance to the RDA for protein in the United States. Although the RDA subcommittee relied extensively on the information compiled by the international committee, the RDAs are specific to the protein needs of the United States population and are adjusted to fit actual average weights at different ages in the United States.

*For adults,* the *average* daily requirement for reference protein was accepted to be 0.6 g/kg per day, based on extensive published data from long-term and short-term balance studies. This average was then increased by 25% (2SD) to allow for individual variability, and the recommended allowance of reference protein for young men was set at 0.75 g/kg per day. Based on several short-term studies using habitual mixed diets as the source of protein, the RDA subcommittee recommended no increase in protein intake for the adult male in the United States consuming a mixed diet to compensate for protein quality. In contrast, diets with lower digestibility need to be higher in protein. The limited available data for women suggests that their requirement levels, when adjusted for body weight, are similar to those of men. In the final formulation of the RDA for protein, the values are rounded up to the nearest 0.1 g/kg per day resulting in a RDA of 0.8 g/kg per day for young men and women. This value, although derived in a different manner, is the same as the 1980 RDA for this group. The actual grams of protein recommended per day are increased in the 1989 RDA report because of the use of observed *average* body weights for each age and sex group, rather than the lower *reference* weights used previously (Table 1–7).

The RDA for protein for *elderly* adults is also assigned the value of 0.8 g/kg per day. This value is higher relative to lean body mass than in young adults. This occurs because muscle mass decreases significantly with age such that muscle protein turnover, which accounts for 30% of total protein turnover in the young adult, is only 20% of total protein turnover in the elderly.[68] Studies of the protein requirements of elderly men and women are controversial. Two groups found no difference from the needs of young adults.[119,120] In one series, the elderly probably received more energy than they required,[119] whereas those in the second study were evaluated following a period of protein deficiency, which commonly improves the efficiency of use of dietary protein.[120] An additional two studies performed at appropriate levels of energy intake suggest that half the elderly adults find it difficult to achieve zero N balance on 0.8 g protein/kg.[121,122] These findings are of additional interest when one takes into consideration the decrease in muscle mass that occurs with aging and suggest that the efficiency of protein utilization in the elderly is impaired. In addition, the number of chronically ill people who suffer from inadequacy of protein and calories increases with aging. These studies are evaluated elsewhere in more detail.[123]

In *pregnancy,* the RDA for women is increased to provide additional protein for deposition in the maternal (i.e. blood, uterus, breasts), fetal, and placental tissues. The most appropriate method of determining the protein needs of pregnant women is controversial. The factorial method is used to set the RDA for protein requirements for pregnancy. Total protein deposited in pregnancy is estimated to be 925 g, based on maternal weight gain and on infant birth weight at term. The rate of N retention increases during pregnancy; 0.11, 0.52, and 0.92 g N depositions occur daily in the first, second, and third trimesters, respectively. The coefficient of variation in birth weight is 15%, and this variance is used for all components of protein gain in pregnancy. In addition, the efficiency of conversion of dietary protein to fetal, placental, and maternal tissues is assumed to be 70%. These adjustments result in estimates for the requirements for reference protein during the first, second, and third trimester of 1.3, 6.1, and 10.7 g protein per day, respectively. To allow for a maintenance requirement of the added lean tissue and the uncertainty about the rate of tissue deposition, the

**TABLE 1–7.** RECOMMENDED ALLOWANCES OF REFERENCE PROTEIN AND U.S. DIETARY PROTEIN

| CATEGORY | AGE (YEARS) OR CONDITION | WEIGHT (KG) | DERIVED ALLOWANCE OF REFERENCE PROTEIN* (G/KG) | (G/DAY) | RECOMMENDED DIETARY ALLOWANCE (g/kg)† | (g/day) |
|---|---|---|---|---|---|---|
| Both sexes | 0–0.5 | 6 | 2.20‡ | | 2.2 | 13 |
| | 0.5–1 | 9 | 1.56 | | 1.6 | 14 |
| | 1–3 | 13 | 1.14 | | 1.2 | 16 |
| | 4–6 | 20 | 1.03 | | 1.1 | 24 |
| | 7–10 | 28 | 1.00 | | 1.0 | 28 |
| Males | 11–14 | 45 | 0.98 | | 1.0 | 45 |
| | 15–18 | 66 | 0.86 | | 0.9 | 59 |
| | 19–24 | 72 | 0.75 | | 0.8 | 58 |
| | 25–50 | 79 | 0.75 | | 0.8 | 63 |
| | 51+ | 77 | 0.75 | | 0.8 | 63 |
| Females | 11–14 | 46 | 0.94 | | 1.0 | 46 |
| | 15–18 | 55 | 0.81 | | 0.8 | 44 |
| | 19–24 | 58 | 0.75 | | 0.8 | 46 |
| | 25–50 | 63 | 0.75 | | 0.8 | 50 |
| | 51+ | 65 | 0.75 | | 0.8 | 50 |
| Pregnancy | 1st trimester | | | + 1.3 | | +10 |
| | 2nd trimester | | | + 6.1 | | +10 |
| | 3rd trimester | | | +10.7 | | +10 |
| Lactation | 1st 6 months | | | +14.7 | | +15 |
| | 2nd 6 months | | | +11.8 | | +12 |

*Data from WHO/FAO/UNU Report: Energy and Protein Requirements. WHO Technical Report Series No. 724. Geneva, World Health Organization, 1985.

†Amino acid score of typical United States diet is 100 for all age groups, except young infants. Digestibility is equal to reference proteins. Values have been rounded upward to 0.1 g/kg.

‡For infants 0 to 3 months of age, breastfeeding that meets energy needs also meets protein needs. Formula substitutes should have the same amount and amino acid composition as human milk, corrected for digestibility if appropriate.

(Reprinted with permission from Food and Nutrition Board, National Research Council: Protein and amino acids. *In* Recommended Dietary Allowances. 10th Ed. Washington, D.C., National Academy Press, 1989, pp. 52–77. Copyright 1989 by the National Academy of Sciences.)

new RDA for protein during pregnancy provides an additional 10 g per day throughout gestation. Data from animals and humans suggest that protein may be stored early in pregnancy and then mobilized at later stages. Thus, no changes relative to trimester are included in the RDA (Table 1–7). Data from N balance studies during pregnancy indicate that more protein is retained during pregnancy than is calculated by the factorial method, suggesting that protein might be retained at sites other than those used in the calculations, such as skeletal muscle. It is anticipated that such deposition would be adequately covered by the RDA. These recommendations assume the provision of adequate energy throughout pregnancy.

The average protein requirement for *lactation* is estimated from milk composition and the mean volume of milk produced adjusted for 70% efficiency of conversion of dietary protein to milk protein. An additional increase of 25% is added to allow for 2SD variance, resulting in an RDA increment of 15 g of extra protein daily. After 6 months of lactation, the volume of milk produced decreases about 20%, and in consequence the RDA increment for protein is decreased to 12 g per day.

The RDA for protein for *infants and children* are intended to provide adequate protein for a satisfactory rate of growth (Table 1–7). During the first year, an infant increases in weight by about 7 kg and body protein increases by about 3.3 g per day. Infants breast-fed by healthy, well-nourished mothers grow satisfactorily for about 4 months and are usually supplemented with additional foods thereafter. Protein intakes by breast-fed infants vary from 2.43 g/kg per day in the first month to 1.51 g/kg per day in the fourth month. A study of breast-fed infants in the United States demonstrated satisfactory growth at a mean protein intake of 1.68 g/kg per day during the first 3 months. The RDA subcommittee has accepted this as the average human milk protein requirement from birth to 3 months of age. An increase of 25% to include 2SD results in an RDA of 2.2 g/kg per day for infants 0 to 0.5 years of age. For older infants and children, a modified factorial method similar to that used by the 1985 FAO/WHO/UNU committee was used to calculate the protein needs. A protein N increment representing average growth was increased by 50% to allow for variability and then corrected for 70% efficiency of utilization, and this N requirement for growth was added to an estimate of the N maintenance requirement to give the average total N required per day. This estimate was then increased by 25% (2SD) to give the RDA. The protein requirements fall from 1.6 g/kg in the second 6 months of life to 1.0 g/kg for 7 to 14 year olds to 0.8 g/kg for adults (>18 years old).

## OTHER FACTORS INFLUENCING PROTEIN REQUIREMENTS

Although severe psychologic stress increases N output,[124] the ordinary stresses of living are allowed for in the estimates of protein allowances. Although high environmental temperatures cause excessive N loss through sweat, this loss is eventually compensated for by reduced urinary N output. Although heavy work does not seem to affect protein requirements, athletes in training may temporarily need more protein during the period of increase in muscle mass.[125] The effect of the energy content of the diet on protein utilization has been well established, and the necessity for ensuring an adequate but not excessive calorie level during determinations of protein needs has already been emphasized. Illness, which also affects protein requirements, is discussed further later in this chapter.

## ESSENTIAL AMINO ACIDS AND THEIR NEEDS BY MAN

For men, the essential amino acids are isoleucine, leucine, lysine, methionine, phenylalanine, threonine, tryptophan, and valine. Infants also require histidine, and small amounts are also probably needed by adults.[126,127] Arginine is required by the young of most species, but probably not by the human infant.[113] Our ideas on the amino acid needs of adults are based primarily on N balance studies, whereas requirements for infants and children are predicated on the smallest amounts compatible with maximal growth. Irwin and Hegsted reviewed all studies of human amino acid needs published before 1971.[128] Published estimates obtained by N balance measurements show a wide range of estimated needs even within a single study.

To extract useful figures from this literature, the middle of the range of values obtained by Rose and his colleagues has been generally accepted for men on the grounds that requirements for all the essential amino acids were studied by a single investigator under constant conditions. These midrange values, shown in Table 1–8, are expressed per kg body weight for adult men. These values agree closely with data on Japanese men obtained by Inoue et al., who examined the requirement for each amino acid by plotting N balances at several levels of intake and interpolating to zero balance.[129] They also agree with the requirements of women for essential amino acids per kg body weight, as estimated by Hegsted from regression equations obtained by recalculating all available published data on women.[130] These are *average* needs; to compare them with the *allowances* for protein, it would be necessary to increase the estimates by 30% (twice the estimated coefficient of variation) to cover all but the top 2.5% of the population according to a normal distribution. Even so, this adjustment would be based on the assumption that the variability of needs for individual essential amino acids follows that of protein.

The estimates of amino acid needs for young adults have been challenged by Young and colleagues,[131,132] who compute these requirements from estimates of the irreversible loss of essential amino acids by oxidation. Using these data, Young et al. compute by several approaches that the essential amino acid requirements

**TABLE 1–8.** ESSENTIAL AMINO ACID (EAA) REQUIREMENTS IN MG/KG BODY WEIGHT OF HUMAN SUBJECTS OF VARIOUS AGES

| REQUIREMENT | INFANT (HOLT) | CHILD, 10–12 YR. (NAKAGAWA) | MAN (ROSE) | MAN (INOUE) | WOMAN (HEGSTED) |
|---|---|---|---|---|---|
| Histidine | (25) | — | — | — | — |
| Isoleucine | 111 | 28 | 10 | 11 | 10 |
| Leucine | 153 | 49 | 11 | 14 | 13 |
| Lysine | 96 | 59 | 9 | 12 | 10 |
| Methionine and cystine | 50 | 27 | 14 | 11 | 13 |
| Phenylalanine and tyrosine | 90 | 27 | 14 | 14 | 13 |
| Threonine | 66 | 34 | 6 | 6 | 7 |
| Tryptophan | 19 | 4 | 3 | 3 | 3 |
| Valine | 95 | 33 | 14 | 14 | 11 |
| Total EAA (excluding histidine) | 680 | 261 | 81 | 85 | 80 |

(Adapted from Munro, H.N.: Amino acid requirements and metabolism and their relevance to parenteral nutrition. *In* Parenteral Nutrition. Edited by A.W. Wilkinson. London, Churchill Livingstone, 1972, pp. 34–67.)

of the adult are 2 to 3 times greater than those based on N balance. The validity of these estimates generated on a theoretic basis has not been fully tested, and further direct confirmation is necessary.[133]

Regarding amino acid requirements of infants and children, Table 1–8 gives the estimates by Holt and Snyderman of the essential requirements of infants up to 6 months of age who are growing maximally.[134] Although the data were expressed as ranges, we have taken the midpoint of the range of values as the average need. Values of the same order have been obtained by Fomon and Filer from amino acid intakes of infants growing optimally on milk-formula diets.[135] The requirements of older children (10 to 12 years of age) have been estimated by Nakagawa et al.[136]

When expressed per kg body weight, the needs for protein and for each essential amino acid decline progressively with increasing age from infancy (Fig. 1–19). However, the requirements for essential amino acids decrease more extensively than do those for total protein. Consequently, the proportion of total protein needs represented by essential amino acids falls from 43% for infants to 36% for older children and to 19 to 20% for adults. On the basis of this information, it should be possible to dilute egg and other good-quality protein having an overabundance of essential amino acids with nonessential amino acids or with ammonium salts and still maintain N equilibrium. Indeed, some investigators were able to achieve N equilibrium when adult subjects received only 13 to 15% of dietary N in the form of essential amino acids.[137,138] Scrimshaw and co-workers replaced a small part of the nitrogen of egg, beef, and milk with nonessential nitrogen from glycine and diammonium citrate without impairing nutritive value (N balance).[139] At a level of 0.4 g protein/kg body weight, N equilibrium could be maintained with dilution of these proteins up to 25 to 30%. The source of nonessential N may also be important. In contrast to these positive findings, Daniel et al. found that replacement of milk protein with nonessential N significantly reduces the biologic value of the protein for 10- to 11-year-old girls,[140] suggesting that their essential amino acid needs are proportionately higher than those of adults. Snyderman et al., however, observed that nonessential nitrogen added to cow's milk protein to the extent of about 20% stimulated the growth of young infants.[141] The published data on dilution studies are thus too variable to indicate whether proteins can be diluted to a greater extent for adult use than for feeding infants.

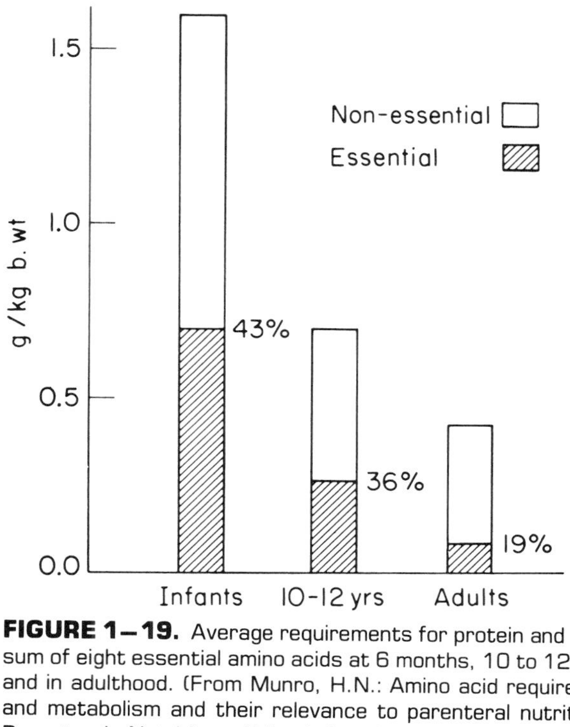
1.5
1.0
0.5
0.0
g / kg b. wt
Non-essential
Essential
43%
36%
19%
Infants
10-12 yrs
Adults

**FIGURE 1–19.** Average requirements for protein and for the sum of eight essential amino acids at 6 months, 10 to 12 years, and in adulthood. (From Munro, H.N.: Amino acid requirements and metabolism and their relevance to parenteral nutrition. *In* Parenteral Nutrition. Edited by A.W. Wilkinson. London, Churchill Livingstone, 1972, pp. 34–67.)

## PROTEIN AND ESSENTIAL AMINO ACID NEEDS IN DISEASE

There are significant difficulties in deciding on protein requirements in disease. Individual diseases affect protein needs to different extents, and each disease process varies in intensity from individual to individual. In some of these conditions (fever, fracture, burns, and surgical trauma), body protein is lost extensively during the acute phase of the disease and needs to be regained during convalescence. The loss of protein during such illness can be appreciable.[142] For example, simple disuse atrophy during a short period of bed rest can cause a loss of 0.3 kg body protein. To this can be added losses related to the particular disease process, such as 0.4 kg body protein after a gastrectomy, 0.7 kg after fracture of a femur, and 1.2 kg after a 35% burn. Opinion is unanimously affirmative on the need to replace such losses during convalescence. Based on animal studies,[143] it is recommended that the essential amino acid pattern for the protein-depleted patient be based on that of the rapidly growing child.[144]

In some diseases, protein intake must be restricted. An example is acute liver failure, in which intake has to be restricted to avoid hepatic coma. In uremia, the capacity to excrete nitrogenous end products is limited and protein intake must also be restricted. In this illness, sufficient protein must be provided to avoid depletion of tissue protein without exceeding the capacity of the patient to deal with the amino acid load. In the dietary management of uremia, an intake of 0.5 g protein/kg body weight allows patients to resist intercurrent infections better than an earlier recommended intake of 0.25 g/kg. To reduce the amount of N to be excreted by uremic patients, N-free analogues of essential amino acids (e.g., keto analogues) are recommended for their ability to provide some of the dietary amino acid supply by transamination to essential amino acids.[145] Finally, evidence suggests that wasting (cachexia) associated with the anorexia of malignant diseases reduces the capacity of the patient to withstand vigorous treatment. Nutritional rehabilitation with amino acids and energy administered parenterally allows the cancer patient better to withstand surgery, chemotherapy, and radiation therapy.[146]

## DIETARY SOURCES OF PROTEIN AND AMINO ACIDS

### FORMS OF DIETARY NITROGEN

In performing N balance studies and similar nutritional experiments using normal diets, it is usually assumed that almost all dietary N takes the form of protein, so dietary N × 6.25 is accepted as a reasonable approximation of the amount of protein in the diet. Natural foods consist mostly of the tissues of plants and animals, so the diet reflects tissue constituents.[147] In animal tissues such as liver and muscle, almost all the N is present in the form of protein, with only a small amount (1 to 2%) as free amino acids or peptides. An equally small amount is in the form of nucleic acids and phospholipid N and, in the case of muscle, as creatine and the dipeptides carnosine, anserine, and balenine. The muscle of fish is richer in nonprotein N (20% or more), however, and contains a greater variety of N compounds. Similarly, about 20% of the N in human milk is nonprotein N, only a third of which is free amino acids.

In plant tissues, the proportion of nonprotein N is variable. Seed N is mostly protein N (95%). In roots, such as the potato and carrot, less than half the total N is protein, and most is present in the form of peptides and free amino acids. Glutamine and asparagine are especially abundant in the potato. In some root crops, such as cassava, the N content leads one to overestimate the already low true protein content of 0.7% as obtained by hydrolysis followed by analysis of individual amino acids. In addition, plant tissues contain an abundance of amino acids that do not occur in proteins. Over 100 have been identified, some of which can be metabolized in the animal body, but many of which are excreted unchanged in the urine. Indeed, a few (e.g., hypoglycin A in the fruit of the West Indian blighia and cyanoalanine in the grain of the East Indian lathyrus) produce serious toxic effects.

In view of these findings, it is reasonable to accept the assumption that the N of Western mixed diets is essentially protein in nature. Use of the conversion factor N × 6.25 implies that the average protein contains 16% N. However, the proteins of individual foods can vary from 15.7% N in milk to 19% in nuts. The use of varying conversion factors from N to protein has, in fact, been used in calculating the protein content of foods assembled in some tables of food composition.

### EVALUATION OF PROTEIN QUALITY

In a preceding section, we pointed out that proteins differ in their capacity to provide amino acids for utilization in the body. As discussed earlier, these differences in protein quality could result in significant changes in the amount of protein needed to meet the needs of certain groups, notably infants. Measures for assessing protein quality have been surveyed in a publication that can be consulted for details.[148] Basically, the evaluation of a protein source begins with N and amino acid analysis and proceeds to biologic tests.

In 1946, Block and Mitchell introduced the concept of assessing the nutritional quality of a protein on the basis of its constituent amino acids.[108] They proposed that the biologic value of a dietary protein would be determined by the essential amino acid present in least concentration relative to the needs of the animal or human. This is therefore the "most limiting amino acid" from which a "chemical score" of protein quality could be calculated. A provisional amino acid pattern for scoring has been provided in the WHO/FAO report on energy and protein requirements.[111] This pattern is based on the essential amino acid needs of the preschool child.

Although amino acid analysis is thus a useful tool in establishing the nutritional potential of a dietary protein, its use has some limitations, including the finding that proteins totally lacking one essential amino acid can still have some biologic value in supporting slow growth. There may also be a problem related to nonavailability of some essential amino acids present in the protein, as discussed later in this chapter. Further information about protein quality can be obtained from biologic tests. Many biologic assays of quality are based on growth of rats in which weight gain or N retention is the criterion of efficiency. In man, growth and N retention have been used for infants and N balance for adults.

The earliest assay used to measure protein quality was the protein efficiency ratio (PER). In this test, young animals (usually rats) are fed the protein source at a standard level (e.g., 9%) for 10 or more days, and the weight gain per g protein eaten over this period provides the PER. For example, in one series of tests, the standard (casein) had a PER of 2.8, soy protein 2.4, and wheat gluten 0.4. This means that the young rat gained 2.8 g for every g of casein eaten, but only 0.4 g for every g of gluten eaten. However, this finding makes gluten appear to be of less value than it really is. If a protein-free diet is fed to young, growing animals, they will lose several grams in weight in a short period. Thus, the grams of weight gain due to gluten are higher when compared with those of animals fed a protein-free diet. In most of the alternative assays described, a control group on zero intake of protein is included.

The classic procedure now used for measuring protein quality by changes in body protein is biologic value. It can be applied to growing or adult animals including man. As originally described, it involves measurement of N intake from the dietary protein and the output of N in the feces and in the urine. Another group is given a protein-free diet to obtain values for excretion of N at zero protein intake. If the output of N in the feces is increased above this basal level, less than 100% of the dietary protein is absorbed. The extent of utilization of this absorbed N is indicated by the proportion excreted in the urine above the basal N output observed with animals or humans fed a protein-free diet. Thus, biologic value is the fraction of absorbed N retained in the body for growth or maintenance.

In animals, a simpler procedure than measurement of biologic value by N balance is to assay the amount of protein N in the body of the animal at the end of the experiment. This amount is compared with the carcass N of a group fed a protein-free diet for the same length of time. The gain in N of the group receiving dietary protein is compared with their N intake, and the proportion retained in their bodies is computed to obtain *net protein utilization* (NPU). Because this index takes no account of digestibility, a poorly digested protein would be recorded as having a low value. The NPU procedure is appealing because of its relative simplicity. It has been widely used with modifications in which the analysis of the carcass N content has been simplified by measuring dry weight or carcass water content. Said and Hegsted modified this procedure by measuring carcass N content at various levels of intake of dietary protein, from which they constructed a dose-response line, the slope of which is determined by the biologic quality of the dietary protein.[149] This procedure is representative of slope ratio assay methods. A problem associated with such dose-response assays is that the line relating protein consumed to growth rate may not be straight.

## AMINO ACID AVAILABILITY FROM THE DIET

In general, the amino acid composition of the protein in a foodstuff is useful in predicting its nutritive value for growing animals and humans, using the chemical score as an index of quality. In certain circumstances, however, amino acid availability can be less than that indicated by chemical analysis. Some raw plants contain inhibitors of proteolytic digestion, the best known being the trypsin inhibitor of the soybean, which is inactivated by cooking.[150] Reduced biologic availability can also occur as a result of heat treatment or of storage under adverse conditions. This second type of underavailability has been extensively studied because of its relevance to food processing procedures.[151]

Four types of damage to amino acids can occur as a result of food processing:

1. Loss of available lysine can occur from mild heat treatment in the presence of reducing sugars, such as during milk processing; in this instance, the sugar lactose reacts with free side chains of lysine residues to render them unavailable. This reaction is called the Maillard or "browning" reaction and may result in a significant loss of lysine at high temperatures. The amount of unavailable lysine can be measured by reacting the available lysine with fluorodinitrobenzene and subtracting the number bound to fluorodinitrobenzene from the total lysine.
2. Under severe heating conditions in the presence of either sugars or oxidized lipids or even without either of these, food proteins can become resistant to digestion, so the availability of all amino acids is reduced.
3. When protein is exposed to severe treatment with alkali, lysine and cysteine residues can react together with the formation of lysinoalanine, which may be toxic.
4. Conditions of oxidation, such as the use of sulfur dioxide, result in a loss of methionine in the protein.

In addition to the loss of essential amino acids from the diet by chemical reactions, their utilization by the recipient can be affected by the presence of excess of other essential or nonessential amino acids.[152] Such disproportionate amounts of amino acids can produce effects on the test animal that are classified into toxicities, antagonisms, and imbalances. These effects have been demonstrated primarily with growing animals that respond to the dietary amino acid excess with a reduction in growth rate and sometimes with other changes. The term *amino acid toxicity* describes adverse effects from intake of large amounts of individual amino acids. Amino acids differ in the level at which such toxic effects occur; the most toxic are methionine and tyrosine, whereas threonine in large excess causes only a moderate reduction in growth rate. *Amino acid antagonism* is the term used when excess of one amino acid in the diet causes depression in growth rate that can be alleviated by the addition of a structurally similar amino acid. The best established example is the antagonism between the branched-chain amino acids leucine, isoleucine, and valine. The term *amino acid imbalance* is used when a change in the proportion of amino acids causes a depression in growth rate that is alleviated by adding more of the most limiting essential amino acid in the diet. The extent to which the normal diet of man can be imbalanced without impairing utilization of essential amino acids is not known. The effects of imbalances are observed in growing animals under special circumstances in which suboptimal intakes of protein are fed. These effects are unlikely to occur in human subjects at normal levels of dietary protein.

## REFERENCES


1. Munro, H.N.: Evolution of protein metabolism in mammals. *In* Mammalian Protein Metabolism. Vol. 3. Edited by H.N. Munro. New York, Academic Press, 1969, pp. 133–182.
2. Christensen, H.N.: Free amino acids and peptides in tissues. *In* Mammalian Protein Metabolism. Vol. 1. Edited by H.N. Munro and J.B. Allison. New York, Academic Press, 1964, pp. 105–124.
3. Munro, H.N.: Free amino acid pools and their role in regulation. *In* Mammalian Protein Metabolism. Vol. 4. Edited by H.N. Munro. New York, Academic Press, 1970, pp. 299–386.
4. Herbert, J.D., Coulson, R.A., Hernandez, T.: Comp. Biochem. Physiol., *17*:583–598, 1966.
5. Collarini, E.T., Oxender, C.L.: Annu. Rev. Nutr., *7*:75–90, 1987.
6. Meister, A.: J. Biol. Chem., *263*:17,205–17,208, 1988.
7. Hider, R.C., Fern, E.B., London, D.R.: Biochem. J., *114*:171–178, 1969.
8. Airhart, J., Vidrich, A., Khairallah, E.A.: Biochem. J., *140*:539–548, 1974.
9. Fern, E.B., Garlick, P.J.: Biochem. J., *142*:413–419, 1971.
10. Dalgleish, C.E., Tabechian, H.: Biochem. J., *62*:625–631, 1956.
11. Reed, L.J., Hackert, M.L.: J. Biol. Chem., *265*:8971–8974, 1990.
12. Harper, A.E., Miller, R.H., Block, K.P.: Annu. Rev. Nutr., *4*:409–454, 1984.
13. Krebs, H.A.: The metabolic fate of amino acids. *In* Mammalian Protein Metabolism. Vol. 1. Edited by H.N. Munro and J.B. Allison. New York, Academic Press, 1964, pp. 125–176.
14. Walser, M.: Urea metabolism. *In* Nitrogen Metabolism in Man. Edited by J.C. Waterlow and J.M.L. Stephen. London, Applied Science, 1981, pp. 229–240.
15. Rose, W.C.: Physiol. Rev., *18*:109–136, 1938.
16. Seegmiller, J.E.: Harvey Lect., *63*:28–51, 1971.
17. Milner, J.A., Visek, W.J.: Nature, *145*:211–212, 1973.
18. Arn, P.H., Hauser, E.R., Thomas, G.H., et al.: N. Engl. J. Med., *322*:1652–1655, 1990.
19. Hultman, E., Bergstrom, J., Nilsson, L.H.: Acta Anaesthesiol. Scand., *(Suppl.) 55*:28–49, 1974.
20. Forbes, G.B., Bruin, G.G.: Am. J. Clin. Nutr., *106*:1359–1366, 1976.
21. Crim, M.C., Calloway, D.H., Margen, S.: J. Nutr., *105*:428–438, 1974.
22. Crim, M.C., Calloway, D.H., Margen, S.: J. Nutr., *106*:371–381, 1975.
23. Cahill, G.F., Owen, O.E.: The role of the kidney in the regulation of protein metabolism. *In* Mammalian Protein Metabolism. Vol. 4. Edited by H.N. Munro. New York, Academic Press, 1970, pp. 539–584.
24. Curtoys, N.P., Lowry, O.H.: J. Biol. Chem., *248*:162–168, 1973.
25. Goldstein, L., Schooler, J.M.: Adv. Enzyme Regul., *5*:71–86, 1967.
26. Simpson, D.P.: J. Clin. Invest., *51*:1969–1978, 1972.
27. Gitler, C.: Protein digestion and absorption in nonruminants. *In* Mammalian Protein Metabolism. Vol. 1. Edited by H.N. Munro and J.B. Allison. New York, Academic Press, 1964, pp. 35–69.
28. Fauconneau, G., Michel, M.C.: The role of the gastrointestinal tract in the regulation of protein metabolism. *In* Mammalian Protein Metabolism. Vol. 4. Edited by H.N. Munro. New York, Academic Press, 1970, pp. 481–522.
29. Green, G.M., Olds, B.A., Matthews, G., et al.: Proc. Soc. Exp. Biol. Med., *142*:1162–1167, 1973.
30. Kim, Y.S., Freeman, H.J.: The digestion and absorption of protein. *In* Clinical Nutrition Update: Amino Acids. Edited by H.L. Greene, M.A. Holliday, and H.N. Munro. Chicago, American Medical Association, 1977, pp. 141–146.
31. Crim, M.C., Munro, H.N.: Protein and amino acid requirements and metabolism in relation to defined formula diets. *In* Defined Formula Diets for Medical Purposes. Edited by M.E. Shils. Chicago, American Medical Association, 1977, pp. 5–15.
32. Asatoor, A.M., Cheng, E., Edwards, K.D., et al.: Clin. Sci., *39*:1P, 1970.
33. Windmueller, H.G.: Adv. Enzymol., *53*:202–237, 1982.
34. Bronstein, A.D., Leleiko, N.S., Munro, H.N.: Biochim. Biophys. Acta, *739*:334–343, 1983.
35. Munro, H.N., Goldberg, D.M.: The effect of protein intake on the protein and nucleic acid metabolism of the intestinal mucosal cell. *In* The role of the Gastrointestinal Tract in Protein Metabolism. Edited by H.N. Munro. Oxford, Blackwell, 1964, pp. 189–196.
36. Ju, J.S., Nasset, E.S.: J. Nutr., *68*:633–645, 1959.
37. Twombley, J., Meyer, J.H.: J. Nutr., *74*:453–460, 1961.
38. Miller, L.L.: The role of the liver and the non-hepatic tissues in the regulation of free amino acid levels in the blood. *In* Amino Acid Pools. Edited by J.T. Holden. New York, Elsevier Science, 1962, pp. 708–721.
39. Elwyn, D.W.: The role of the liver in regulation of amino acid and protein metabolism. *In* Mammalian Protein Metabolism. Vol. 4. Edited by H.N. Munro. New York, Academic Press, 1970, pp. 523–557.
40. Harper, A.E.: Am. J. Clin. Nutr., *21*:358–366, 1968.
41. Brookes, I.M., Owens, F.N., Garrigus, U.S.: J. Nutr., *102*:27–36, 1972.
42. Fishman, B., Wurtman, R.J., Munro, H.N.: Proc. Natl. Acad. Sci. U.S.A., *54*:667–683, 1969.
43. Wurtman, R.J.: Diurnal rhythms in mammalian protein metabolism. *In* Mammalian Protein Metabolism. Vol. 4. Edited by H.N. Munro. New York, Academic Press, 1970, pp. 445–479.
44. Clifford, A.J., Riumallo, J.A., Baliga, B.S., et al.: Biochim. Biophys. Acta, *277*:443–458, 1972.
45. Munro, H.N., Hubert, C., Baliga, B.S.: Regulation of protein synthesis in relation to amino acid supply. *In* Alcohol, Nutrition and Protein Synthesis. Edited by M. Rothschild, M. Oratz, and S.S. Schreiber. New York, Pergamon Press, 1975, pp. 33–66.
46. Driscoll, H., Crim, M.C., Zahringer, J., et al.: J. Nutr., *108*:1691–1701, 1978.
47. Young, V.R., Munro, H.N.: J. Nutr., *103*:1756–1763, 1973.
48. Young, V.R., Uauy, R., Winterer, J.C., et al.: Protein metabolism and needs in elderly people. *In* Nutrition, Longevity, and Aging. Edited by M. Rockstein and M.L. Sussman. New York, Academic Press, 1976, pp. 67–102.

49. Young, V.R., Hussein, M.A., Murray, E., et al.: J. Nutr., *101*:45–50, 1971.
50. Young, V.R., Tontisirin, R.K., Ozalp, I., et al.: J. Nutr., *102*:1159–1170, 1972.
51. Fernstrom, J., Wurtman, R.J.: Science, *178*:414–415, 1972.
52. Waterlow, J.C.: Hum. Nutr.: Clin. Nutr., *38C*:151–154, 1984.
53. Nair, K.S., Halliday, D., Griggs, R.: Am. J. Physiol., *254*:E208–E213, 1988.
54. Garlick, P.J., Wernerman, J., McNurlan, M.A., et al.: Clin. Sci., *77*:329–336, 1989.
55. Pozefsky, T., Felig, P., Tobin, J.D., et al.: J. Clin. Invest., *48*:2273–2282, 1969.
56. Munro, H.N., Young, V.R.: Use of $N^t$-methylhistidine excretion as an in vivo measure of myofibrillar protein breakdown. *In* Nitrogen Metabolism in Man. Edited by J.C. Waterlow and J.M.L. Stephen. London, Applied Science, 1981, pp. 495–508.
57. Young, V.R., Alexis, S.D., Baliga, B.S., et al.: J. Biol. Chem., *247*:3592–3600, 1972.
58. Long, C.L., Haverberg, L., Bilmazes, C., et al.: Metabolism, *24*:929–935, 1975.
59. Sjolin, J., Hjort, G., Friman, G., et al.: Metabolism, *36*:1175–1184, 1987.
60. Nagasawa, T., Funabiki, R.: J. Biochem. (Tokyo), *89*:1155–1161, 1981.
61. Wasner, S.J., Li, J.P.: Am. J. Physiol., *243*:E293–E297, 1982.
62. Afting, E.G., Bernhardt, W., Janzen, W.C., et al.: Biochem. J., *200*:449–452, 1981.
63. Sjolin, J., Stjernstrom, H., Henneberg, S., et al.: Metabolism, *26*:23–29, 1989.
64. Harris, C.I., Milne, G.: Biochem. Soc. Trans., *8*:552, 1980.
65. Haverberg, L., Deckelbaum, L., Bilmazes, C., et al.: Biochem. J., *152*:503–510, 1975.
66. Narasinga Rao, B.S., Nagabushan, V.S.: Life Sci., *12*:205–211, 1973.
67. Munro, H.N., Young, V.R.: Am. J. Clin. Nutr., *31*:1608–1614, 1978.
68. Munro, H.N.: Br. Med. Bull., *37*:83–88, 1981.
69. Nakhooda, A.F., Wei, C.N., Marliss, E.B.: Metabolism, *29*:1272–1277, 1980.
70. Burini, R., Santidrian, S., Moreyra, M., et al.: Metabolism, *30*:679–687, 1981.
71. Tomas, F.M., Munro, H.N., Young, V.R.: Biochem. J., *178*:139–146, 1979.
72. McFarlane, A.S.: Metabolism of plasma proteins. *In* Mammalian Protein Metabolism. Vol. 1. Edited by H.N. Munro and J.B. Allison. New York, Academic Press, 1964, pp. 297–341.
73. Gersovitz, M., Munro, H.N., Udall, J., et al.: Metabolism, *29*:1075–1086, 1980.
74. Hellerstein, M.K., Greenblatt, D.J., Munro, H.N.: Metabolism, *36*:988–994, 1987.
75. Hellerstein, M.K., Munro, H.N.: Metabolism, *36*:995–1000, 1987.
76. Hellerstein, M.K., Munro, H.N.: Metabolism, *37*:312–317, 1988.
77. Valgeirsdottir, K., Munro, H.N.: Proteins and amino acids. *In* Surgical Nutrition. Edited by J.E. Fisher. Boston, Little, Brown, 1983, pp. 129–164.
78. Kirsch, R., Firth, L., Black, E., et al.: Nature, *217*:579, 1968.
79. Shetty, P.S., Jung, R.T., Wastrasiewicz, K.E., et al.: Lancet, *2*:230–232, 1979.
80. Hellerstein, M.K., Munro, H.N.: Interaction of liver and muscle in the regulation of metabolism in response to nutritional and other factors. *In* The Liver: Biology and Pathobiology. 2nd Ed. Edited by I.M. Arias, E.B. Jakoby, H. Popper, et al. New York, Raven Press, 1988, pp. 965–983.
81. Munro, H.N.: Protein nutriture and requirements of the elderly. *In* Human Nutrition: A Comprehensive Treatise. Vol. 6. Edited by H.N. Munro and D.E. Danford. New York, Plenum Press, 1989, pp. 153–181.
82. Garlick, P.J., Fern, E.B.: Whole body protein turnover: theoretical considerations. *In* Substrate and Energy Metabolism. Edited by J.S. Garrow and D. Halliday. London, Libbey, 1985, pp. 7–14.
83. Waterlow, J.C., Garlick, P.J., Millward, D.J.: Protein Turnover in Mammalian Tissues and in the Whole Body. Amsterdam, North-Holland, 1978.
84. Young, V.R., Gersovitz, M., Munro, H.N.: Human aging: protein and amino acid metabolism and implications for protein and amino acid requirements. *In* Nutritional Approaches to Aging Research. Edited by G.B. Moment. Boca Raton, FL, CRC Press, 1981, pp. 47–81.
85. Motil, K.J., Matthews, D.E., Bier, D.M., et al.: Am. J. Physiol., *240*:E712–E721, 1981.
86. Munro, H.N.: J. Parenter. Enteral Nutr., *6*:271–279, 1982.
87. DeFronzo, R.A., Felig, P.: Am. J. Clin. Nutr., *33*:1378–1386, 1980.
88. Felig, P.: Annu. Rev. Biochem., *44*:933–954, 1975.
89. Elia, M., Livesey, G.: Branched-chain amino acid and oxo-acid metabolism in human and rat muscle. *In* Metabolism and Clinical Implications of Branched Chain Amino Acids and Keto Acids. Edited by M. Walser and D.R. Williamson. New York, Elsevier Science, 1981, pp. 257–262.
90. Elia, M., Folmer, P., Schlatmann, A., et al.: Am. J. Clin. Nutr., *49*:1203–1210, 1989.
91. Schrock, H., Goldstein, L.: Am. J. Physiol., *240*:E519–E525, 1981.
92. Cahill, G.F., Aoki, T.T.: Conditions with abnormal energy balance: partial and total starvation. *In* Assessment of Energy Metabolism in Health and Disease. Edited by J.M. Kinney and E. Lense. Columbus, OH, Ross Laboratories, 1980, pp. 129–134.
93. Munro, H.N.: General aspects of the regulation of protein metabolism by diet and by hormones. *In* Mammalian Protein Metabolism. Vol. 1. Edited by H.N. Munro and J.B. Allison. New York, Academic Press, 1964, pp. 381–481.
94. Conn, H.O.: Nutritional management of advanced liver disease. *In* Nutritional Support of the Seriously Ill Patient. Edited by R.W. Winters and H.L. Greene. New York, Academic Press, 1983, pp. 107–132.
95. Beisel, W.R., Wannemacher, R.W., Jr., Neufeld, H.A.: Relation of fever to energy expenditure. *In* Assessment of Energy Metabolism in Health and Disease. Edited by J.M. Kinney and E. Lense. Columbus, OH, Ross Laboratories, 1980, pp. 144–150.
96. Goodlad, G.A.J.: Protein metabolism and tumor growth. *In* Mammalian Protein Metabolism. Vol. 2. Edited by H.N. Munro and J.B. Allison. New York, Academic Press, 1964, pp. 415–444.
97. Munro, H.N.: J. Am. Diet. Assoc., *71*:380–384, 1977.
98. Goodlad, G.A.J., Clark, C.M.: Eur. J. Cancer Clin. Oncol., *16*:1153–1162, 1980.

99. Waterhouse, C., Jeanpetre, N., Keilson, J.: Cancer Res., *39*:1968–1972, 1972.
100. Allison, J.B., Bird, J.C.: Elimination of nitrogen from the body. *In* Mammalian Protein Metabolism. Vol. 1. Edited by H.N. Munro and J.B. Allison. New York, Academic Press, 1964, pp. 483–512.
101. Wallace, W.M.: Fed. Proc., *18*:1125–1130, 1959.
102. Cuthbertson, D.P., Munro, H.N.: Biochem. J., *31*:694, 1937.
103. Munro, H.N.: Physiol. Rev., *31*:488, 1951.
104. Elwyn, D.H., Gump, F.E., Munro, H.N., et al.: Am. J. Clin. Nutr., *32*:1597–1607, 1978.
105. Kishi, K., Mitayani, S., Inoue, G.: J. Nutr., *108*:658–669, 1978.
106. Schoeller, D.A.: J. Nutr., *118*:1278–1289, 1988.
107. Munro, H.N.: A general survey of mechanisms regulating protein metabolism in mammals. *In* Mammalian Protein Metabolism. Vol. 4. Edited by H.N. Munro. New York, Academic Press, 1970, pp. 3–130.
108. Block, R.J., Mitchell, H.H.: Nutr. Abstr. Rev., *16*:249–278, 1946.
109. FAO Report: Protein Requirements. FAO Nutrition Studies No. 16. Rome, Food and Agriculture Organization, 1959.
110. WHO/FAO Report: Protein Requirements. FAO Technical Report Series No. 301. Geneva, World Health Organization, 1965.
111. WHO/FAO Report: Energy and Protein Requirements. WHO Technical Report Series No. 522. Geneva, World Health Organization, 1973.
112. WHO/FAO/UNU Report: Energy and Protein Requirements. WHO Technical Report Series No. 724. Geneva, World Health Organization, 1985.
113. Food and Nutrition Board, National Research Council: Protein and amino acids. *In* Recommended Dietary Allowances. 10th Ed. Washington, D.C., National Academy Press, 1989, pp. 52–77.
114. Munro, H.N.: Historical perspective on protein requirements: objectives for the future. *In* Nutritional Adaptation in Man. Edited by J.C. Blaxter and J. Waterlow. Rank Symposium. London, Libbey, 1985, pp. 155–167.
115. Calloway, D.H., Odell, A.C., Margen, S.: J. Nutr., *101*:775–786, 1971.
116. Calloway, D.H., Margen, S.: J. Nutr., *101*:204–216, 1971.
117. Garza, C., Scrimshaw, N.S., Young, V.R.: J. Nutr., *107*:335–352, 1977.
118. Garza, C., Scrimshaw, N.S., Young, V.R.: J. Nutr., *108*:90–96, 1978.
119. Cheng, A.H.R., Gomez, S., Gergan, J.G., et al.: Am. J. Clin. Nutr., *31*:12–22, 1978.
120. Zanni, E., Calloway, D.H., Zezulka, A.Y.: J. Nutr., *109*:513–524, 1979.
121. Uauy, R., Scrimshaw, N.S., Young, V.R.: Am. J. Clin. Nutr., *31*:779–785, 1978.
122. Gersovitz, M., Motil, K., Munro, H.N., et al.: Am. J. Clin. Nutr., *35*:6–14, 1982.
123. Munro, H.N.: Protein nutriture and requirement in elderly people. *In* Nutritional Problems of the Elderly. Bibliotheca Nutritio et Dieta, No. 33. Edited by J.C. Somogyi and J.F. Fidanza. Basel, Karger, 1983, pp. 61–79.
124. Scrimshaw, N.S., Habicht, J.P., Piche, M.Z., et al.: Am. J. Clin. Nutr., *18*:321–324, 1966.
125. Torun, B., Scrimshaw, N.S., Young, V.R.: Am. J. Clin. Nutr., *30*:1983–1993, 1977.
126. Kopple, J.D., Swendseid, M.E.: J. Nutr., *111*:931–942, 1981.
127. Cho, E.S., Anderson, H.L., Wixom, R.L., et al.: J. Nutr., *114*:369–384, 1989.
128. Irwin, M.I., Hegsted, D.M.: J. Nutr., *101*:539–566, 1971.
129. Inoue, G., Komatsu, T., Kishi, K., et al.: Amino acid requirements of Japanese young men. *In* Amino Acids: Metabolism and Medical Applications. Edited by G.L. Blackburn, J.F. Grant, and V.R. Young. Boston, John Wright, 1983, pp. 55–62.
130. Hegsted, D.M.: Fed. Proc., *22*:1424–1430, 1963.
131. Young, V.R., Nang, R.D., Meredith, C., et al.: Modulation of amino acid metabolism by protein and energy intakes. *In* Amino Acids: Metabolism and Medical Applications. Edited by G.L. Blackburn, J.F. Grant, and V.R. Young. Boston, John Wright, 1983, pp. 13–28.
132. Young, V.R., Bier, D.M., Pellet, P.L.: Am. J. Clin. Nutr., *50*:80–92, 1989.
133. Munro, H.N.: Amino acid requirements and metabolism and their relevance to parenteral nutrition. *In* Parenteral Nutrition. Edited by A.W. Wilkinson. London, Churchill Livingstone, 1972, pp. 34–67.
134. Holt, L.E., Snyderman, E.E.: The amino acid requirements of children. *In* Amino Acid Metabolism and Genetic Variation. Edited by E. Nyhan. New York, McGraw-Hill, 1967, pp. 381–390.
135. Fomon, S., Filer, L.J.: Amino acid requirements for normal growth. *In* Amino Acid Metabolism and Genetic Variation. Edited by E. Nyhan. New York, McGraw-Hill, 1967, pp. 391–401.
136. Nakagawa, I., Takahashi, T., Suzuki, T., et al.: J. Nutr., *83*:115–118, 1964.
137. Kofranyi, E., Jekat, K.: Hoppe Seylers Z. Physiol. Chem., *338*:154–167, 1964.
138. Swenseid, M.E., Feeley, R.J., Harris, E.L., et al.: J. Nutr., *68*:203–211, 1959.
139. Scrimshaw, N.S., Young, V.R., Huang, P.C., et al.: J. Nutr., *98*:9–17, 1969.
140. Daniel, D.A., Doraiswamy, T.R., Swaminathan, M., et al.: Br. J. Nutr., *24*:741–747, 1970.
141. Snyderman, E.E., Holt, L.E., Dancis, J., et al.: J. Nutr., *78*:57–72, 1962.
142. Cuthbertson, D.P.: Protein requirements after injury: quality and quantity. *In* Parenteral Nutrition. Edited by A.W. Wilkinson. London, Churchill Livingstone, 1972, pp. 4–23.
143. Steffee, C.H., Wissler, R.W., Humphreys, E.P., et al.: J. Nutr., *40*:483–497, 1950.
144. Winters, R.W., Hasselmeyer, E.: Intravenous Nutrition in the High Risk Infant. New York, John Wiley & Sons, 1975.
145. Walser, M.: Keto-analogues of essential amino acids. *In* Clinical Nutrition Update: Amino Acids. Edited by H.L. Greene, M.A. Holliday, and H.N. Munro. Chicago, American Medical Association, 1977, pp. 183–191.
146. Copeland, E.M.: The patient with malignancy. *In* Nutritional Support of the Seriously Ill Patient. Edited by R.W. Winters and H.L. Greene. New York, Academic Press, 1983, pp. 231–250.
147. Munro, H.N.: An introduction to nutritional aspects of protein metabolism. *In* Mammalian Protein Metabolism. Vol. 2. Edited by H.N. Munro and J.B. Allison. New York, Academic Press, 1964, pp. 3–39.
148. Pellett, P.L., Young, V.R.: Nutritional Evaluation of Protein Foods. Tokyo, United Nations University, 1980.
149. Said, A.K., Hegsted, D.M.: J. Nutr., *99*:474–480, 1969.

150. Kakade, M.L., Hoffer, D.E., Liener, I.E.: J. Nutr., *103:*1772–1778, 1973.
151. Carpenter, K.: Nutr. Abstr. Rev., *43:*424–451, 1973.
152. Harper, A.E., Benevenga, N.J., Wohlhueter, R.M.: Physiol. Rev., *50:*428–558, 1970.

## SELECTED READINGS

Food and Nutrition Board, National Research Council: Recommended Dietary Allowances. 10th Ed. Washington, D.C., National Academy Press, 1989.

Munro, H.N.: Protein nutriture and requirements of the elderly. *In* Human Nutrition: A Comprehensive Treatise. Vol. 6. Edited by H.N. Munro and D.E. Danford. New York, Plenum Press, 1989, pp. 153–181.

Pellett, P.L.: Protein requirements in humans. Am. J. Clin. Nutr., *51:*723–737, 1990.

Waterlow, J.C., Garlick, P.J., Millward, D.J.: Protein Turnover in Mammalian Tissues and in the Whole Body. Amsterdam, North-Holland, 1978.

WHO/FAO/UNU Report: Energy and Protein Requirements. WHO Technical Report Series No. 724. Geneva, World Health Organization, 1985.

CHAPTER 2

# Carbohydrates

Ian Macdonald



## HISTORY

The earliest record of a carbohydrate is from India in 3000 B.C., when an extraction process for sugar was described. From India sugar cane was brought to Europe, first by Alexander the Great and much later by the returning Crusaders. In 1493 Columbus, on his second voyage, introduced sugar cane to the New World. It was not until 1812 that a Russian chemist named Kirchoff stated that starch, when boiled with dilute acid, was converted to a sugar identical to the sugar of grapes. Seven years later, a similar acid treatment to sawdust, linen, rags, and straw also yielded "grape" sugar.[1] About this time carbohydrates, as they were called by Schmidt in 1844,[2] were found to be composed of atoms of carbon, hydrogen, and oxygen. At the same time, Schmidt showed that sugar was present in blood, though the "honey urine" of the diabetic had been noticed by the Hindus in the sixth century. The presence of starch (glycogen) in the liver of a well-fed animal was discovered by the well-known physiologist Claude Bernard in 1856. He believed it to be formed from food protein.

In more modern times, carbohydrates tended to be dismissed as compounds whose sole role was the provision of energy, but in fact they play an important part in providing satisfactory organoleptic and preservative properties in food. Perhaps because of the desired taste, flavor, and texture of carbohydrates, they have been accused of causing numerous diseases in man, including dental caries, obesity, cardiovascular disease, and diabetes.

## DEFINITIONS

Classically, carbohydrates are substances having the empiric formula $Cn(H_2O)n$. Dietary carbohydrates, however, are usually considered to include those carbohydrates with $n>4$ and the sugar alcohols. This chapter is restricted to the so-called "available" carbohydrates, those that can be digested and/or absorbed in the gut in

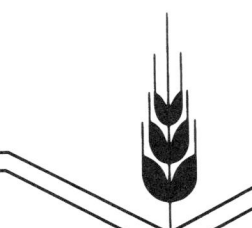

man and metabolized by the body. (For completeness, mention is made of resistant starch). The sugar alcohols, though not consumed in large quantities, do have clinical significance (Table 2–1). The carbohydrates in foods are made up of polysaccharides and sugars, with most foods containing a mixture of both.

### POLYSACCHARIDES

The two main polysaccharides consumed by man are *starch* and *cellulose.* Because it is largely indigestible, cellulose has a minor metabolic role. Starches, found in seeds and roots, are polymers of glucose, with the exception of *inulin* (found in artichokes), which is a polymer of fructose and is also indigestible. Raw starch is difficult to digest because the carbohydrate lies within thin-walled cells, and this makes it difficult for enzymatic attack. However, moist heat causes the starch to swell and burst the confining cell wall, thus becoming readily available for hydrolysis by amylolytic enzymes.

### DISACCHARIDES

Perhaps the most common and best known disaccharide in the diet is *sucrose* (cane sugar, beet sugar), which is made up of a molecule of glucose and a molecule of fructose. Sucrose rotates polarized light to the right, but when hydrolyzed into its constituent molecules, the mixture is often referred to as "invert sugar" because polarized light is now rotated to the left. *Lactose* is a disaccharide of glucose and galactose. Because it is only found in milk, lactose is unique to mammals. *Maltose* consists of two glucose molecules and is formed from the breakdown of starch.

### MONOSACCHARIDES

*Glucose* (grape sugar, dextrose) is the main carbohydrate in the body, although little is consumed in this form. It mainly arises from the hydrolysis of dietary starch. *Fructose* (fruit sugar, levulose) has the same formula as glucose, but the different spatial arrangements of the atoms make polarized light rotate to the left. *Galactose* is also a hexose (six carbon atoms), but is rarely consumed as such.

The pentoses (five carbon atoms) *ribose* and *deoxyribose,* though not consumed in any quantity, are essential components of nucleic acids. The alcohol of glucose, namely, *sorbitol* (glucitol), has a therapeutic value as a replacement carbohydrate in the diet of diabetics and in parenteral feeding. Sorbitol is converted by the liver to fructose.

The alcohol of the pentose xylose is *xylitol,* and it has also been used therapeutically because it has a sweetness similar to that of sucrose. Xylitol is reputed to be less cariogenic and less insulinogenic than sucrose.

## CONSUMPTION PATTERNS

In 1974 the supply of carbohydrates for human consumption was similar in both developed and developing countries (7000 kJ (1680 kcal)/person per day).[3] Although the intake was almost identical, the nature of the carbohydrates eaten and the proportion they contributed to the energy intake were not similar. The carbohydrates from staple foods such as cereals and roots and composed mainly of starch represented 85% of the carbohydrate intake in developing countries, but only 62% in the affluent ones. The difference was largely made up by carbohydrates from fruit and sugar. The proportion of carbohydrate taken as lactose was about 2%. The pro-

**TABLE 2–1.** SUMMARY OF PRINCIPAL DIETARY CARBOHYDRATES

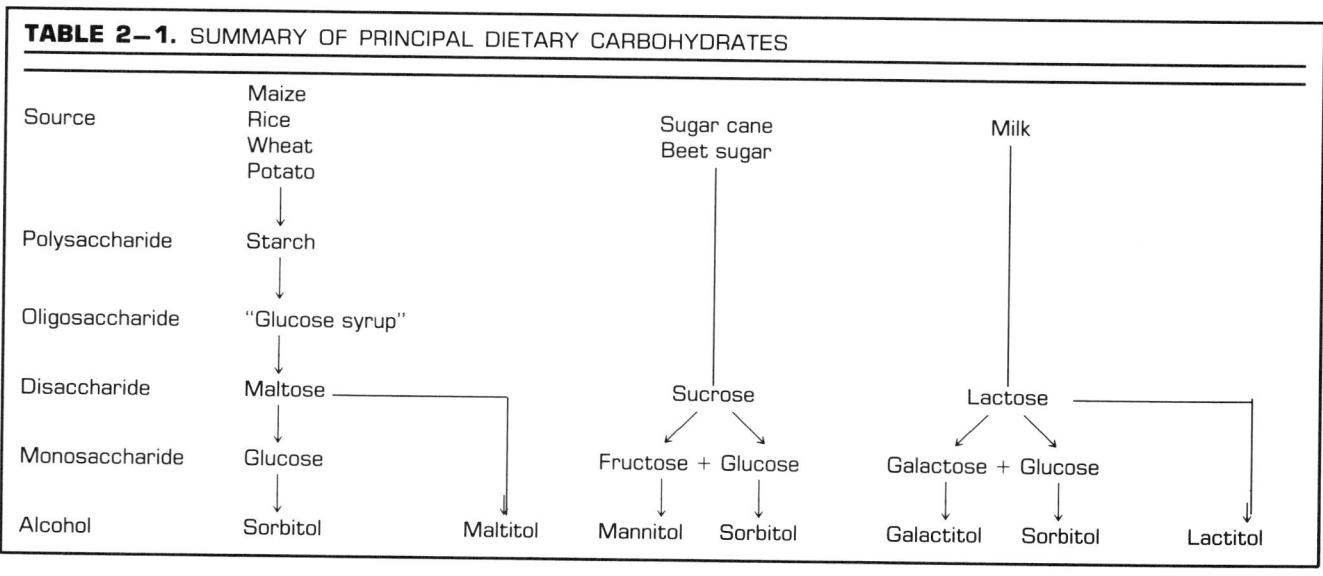

| | | | | | |
|---|---|---|---|---|---|
| Source | Maize<br>Rice<br>Wheat<br>Potato | | Sugar cane<br>Beet sugar | Milk | |
| Polysaccharide | Starch | | | | |
| Oligosaccharide | "Glucose syrup" | | | | |
| Disaccharide | Maltose | | Sucrose | Lactose | |
| Monosaccharide | Glucose | | Fructose + Glucose | Galactose + Glucose | |
| Alcohol | Sorbitol | Maltitol | Mannitol Sorbitol | Galactitol Sorbitol | Lactitol |

portion of energy obtained from carbohydrate falls as income rises.[4]

## CARBOHYDRATE AS AN ENERGY SOURCE

The main function of dietary carbohydrate is to provide energy. Carbohydrates not only contribute to the taste and texture of foods, but they also play a part in determining viscosity, in stabilizing emulsions, and in preserving food. Perhaps their most useful role, apart from nutritional energy, is as sweetening agents.

### DIGESTION

All carbohydrates must be hydrolyzed to their constituent monosaccharides to cross the intestinal wall and be absorbed. After absorption, most of the monosaccharides pass via the portal circulation to the liver, but small quantities are used by the gut wall for maintaining its own viability. Because most of the carbohydrates consumed are not monosaccharides, the alimentary tract has the responsibility to hydrolyze the starches and sugars to monosaccharides. This process commences in the mouth.

### STARCH HYDROLYSIS

Plant starch, which occurs in granules, consists primarily of amylose and amylopectin. Amylose is a straight-chain polymer of glucose linked by α-1,4-glucosidic bonds, whereas amylopectin is a branched-chain polymer of glucose having not only the α-1,4-glucosidic bonds, but also branches of α-1,6-glucosidic bonds approximately every 25 units. The proportion of amylose is approximately 20% and that of amylopectin about 80% in many native starches, with molecular weights of 60,000 d and over 1,000,000 d, respectively. The linkage between glucose molecules is important in view of the specificity of the hydrolyzing enzymes. For example, cellulose is a polysaccharide, but it has a β-1-4 linkage, and because no gut enzyme in man can hydrolyze this linkage,[5] cellulose can theoretically be considered a dietary fiber.

The enzyme that catalyses the hydrolysis of the 1-4-glycosidic bond is an α-amylase present in saliva and in pancreatic juice. The α-amylase splits the starch to maltose, maltotriose, and branched tri-, tetra-, and pentapolysaccharides with only small amounts of glucose. The pancreatic α-amylase, which is the major amylolytic enzyme, probably acts at two sites. One is obviously in the lumen of the jejunum and the other is on the outer surface of the intestinal brush border where pancreatic amylase can be adsorbed. The digestion of starch by this membrane-bound amylase seems to be more efficient than by that in the lumen of the intestine.[6]

The α-1,6 linkages of amylopectin are not affected by α-amylase; hence the branched remnants remain after hydrolysis with α-amylase. These remnants are further split by isomaltase (oligo-1,6-α-glucosidase) present in the brush border of the small intestine.[7]

Among the physical factors that influence the rate of starch hydrolysis is, obviously, the extent of mixing of the digestive juice with the food, for example, as aided by chewing. As in the natural state, starch granules are encased, and failure to remove the outer covering by cooking delays starch hydrolysis. The intestinal discomfort that follows ingestion of large quantities of raw starch is evidence of this fact.

The remaining residues of dietary starch, namely, the oligosaccharides such as maltotriose as well as the remnants of the branched starch (α-limit dextrins with 5 to 10 glucose residues), are hydrolyzed in the brush border of the intestine. Also hydrolyzed by the enzymes in the brush border are the dissacharides lactose and sucrose. The main action sites of these enzymes are the upper and midjejunum. The α-dextrins or branch remnants are split by isomaltose, which removes the α-1-6-glucose stub, and the oligosaccharides are hydrolyzed by maltases (glucosidases), of which there are three. Sucrose is cleaved by sucrase, an enzyme that is also active against maltose and maltotriose. The enzyme lactase (β-glucosidase) is specific for lactose. (Tables 2–2 and 2–3).

The efficiency of these surface enzymes is such that, with the exception of lactase, surface digestion is not rate limiting for absorption and, in fact, a slight excess of

**TABLE 2–2.** HYDROLYSIS OF DIETARY CARBOHYDRATES TO MONOSACCHARIDES

| STARCH | SALIVA AND PANCREATIC JUICE | OLIGOSACCHARIDE | BRUSH BORDER | MONOSACCHARIDE |
|---|---|---|---|---|
| Amylose | Amylase → | Maltotriose | Maltase → | Glucose |
| | | Maltose | Sucrase | |
| Amylopectin | Amylase → | α-Dextrin (branched) | Isomaltase → | Glucose |
| | | Sucrose | Sucrase → | Glucose and fructose |
| | | Lactose | Lactase → | Glucose and galactose |

**TABLE 2–3.** CARBOHYDRATE HYDROLYZING ENZYMES IN HUMAN BRUSH BORDER

| SUBSTRATE | ENZYME | RELATIVE IMPORTANCE FOR SUBSTRATE |
|---|---|---|
| Isomaltose (limit dextrin) | Isomaltase (α-dextrinase) | 95 |
| | Maltase | 5 |
| Maltose and maltotriose | Isomaltase (α-dextrinase) | 50 |
| | Sucrase | 25 |
| | Maltase | 25 |
| Sucrose | Sucrase | 100 |
| Lactose | Lactase | 100 |

monosaccharide is usually found on the luminal side. The splitting of lactose, on the other hand, is a comparatively slow process that releases insufficient glucose and galactose for maximal uptake.[8] If too great a quantity of monosaccharide were released into the gut lumen, the dangers of osmotic efflux of water with subsequent diarrhea and water loss would arise. This problem does not occur because the monosaccharides released probably cause inhibition of the enzymes.

Some vegetables, such as pulses, contain oligosaccharides of the raffinose family such as raffinose itself, stachyose, and verbascose. These oligosaccharides contain α-galactose links. Because these links cannot be hydrolyzed by the gut, the oligosaccharides will, if consumed in large quantities, give rise to flatulence and abdominal discomfort.

The amylolytic enzyme present in the brush border can be influenced by the type of carbohydrate in the diet. When the diet contains large quantities of sucrose, the sucrase and maltase activities are significantly higher after 2 to 5 days than when glucose replaces sucrose, whereas when lactose, maltose, or galactose replaces glucose, no change in sucrase and maltase activity is seen. The clinical interest in the failure of lactose to induce lactase activity lies in the inability to treat subjects with reduced lactase activity by gradually adding lactose to the diet. This finding that the enzyme regulation is not dependent on substrate is reinforced by the finding that fructose is the active principle in sucrose that leads to increased sucrase and maltase activity.

### RESISTANT STARCH

A proportion of dietary starch escapes digestion in the human gastrointestinal tract because (1) it is physically inaccessible to α-amylase (e.g., partly milled grains and seeds), (2) it is in a granular form resistant to enzyme digestion, or (3) it is mainly retrograded amylose formed during the cooling of starch that has been gelatinized by moist heating. This third form of starch, obviously present in many processed foods such as cooled cooked potato, bread, and cornflakes, is both thermally resistant and resistant to α-amylase hydrolysis. It has been estimated that 20% of the carbohydrate from baked beans and 7 to 10% of that from wheat, oats, and potatoes can reach the colon, but only 0.9% of that from rice.[9]

As the resistant starch passes into the large intestine, it is fermented by bacteria. Thus, the energy available to the host is 50 to 80% of that had glucose been the end product of starch digestion. In animal experiments, the digestive energy from resistant starch from peas is 12.2 kJ/g and from maize is 15.5 kJ/g.[10] The end products of fermentation of resistant starch by colonic bacteria are short-chain fatty acids, carbon dioxide, and methane.[11]

## ABSORPTION

Several methods are used, either singly or in combination, to transport monosaccharides across the intestinal mucosa into the splanchnic capillaries. These transport systems include diffusion, facilitated (or carrier-mediated) diffusion, and active transport; the third is distinguished by the need for energy input. Passive diffusion, which applies to the sugar alcohols and to the L-isomers of the monosaccharides glucose and galactose, prevents large quantities from being transported. The water withdrawal these compounds promote while in the gut lumen reduces the steepness of the concentration gradient. The amount that an adult can consume of these passively diffusing sugars and sugar alcohols before symptoms arise is about 50 g at any one time.

In man D-glucose and D-galactose are the only nutritionally significant monosaccharides that are actively absorbed. D-fructose, though not actively absorbed, has a rate of diffusion greater than would be expected by passive diffusion, and its transfer from the lumen is by facilitated diffusion. Although glucose and galactose in the gut lumen can cross the mucosa down a diffusion gradient, the speed of this method is such that water would diffuse in the opposite direction, leading to a lessening in the concentration gradient. When one recalls that the efficiency of diffusion is inversely proportional to the distance, then the advantages of a rapid transport system for glucose and for galactose (in infancy) are obvious.

The cation Na+ is central to the mechanism of active transport of glucose and galactose, where it has been shown that the rate of glucose absorption is related to the flux of Na+ from mucosal to serosal surface,[11] suggesting that Na+ is involved in the carrier mechanism as such, as well as in the system that provides the energy. These and other findings led to the Na+ gradient hypothesis in which the carrier has a binding site for Na+ as well as for the particular sugar,[12] with the suggestion that the carrier has a higher affinity for the sugar when the Na+ site is filled. Inside the cell, a Na+-depleted environment, the Na+ leaves the carrier, the sugar is released, and the free carrier then returns to the surface. Since the Na+ gradient hypothesis was first postulated, it became apparent that not enough energy is available for the sugar transport capability if only the chemical potential for Na+ is considered, based primarily on the finding that K+ replacement of Na+ on the carrier inhibits sugar transport.[13] This finding led to more recent views suggesting that the potential difference across the brush border membrane of the cell may play an important role in the mechanism that concentrates sugar in the cell.

Fructose, which is increasing in the human diet as a result of the advent of high-fructose syrups, comes from the dissacharide sucrose. It is not absorbed actively but by facilitated diffusion, and there does not appear to be any competition from other sugars. The rate of absorption may depend on the concentration of fructose at the brush border because higher plasma concentrations of fructose are found after the ingestion of sucrose than after ingestion of equimolar amounts of glucose and fructose.[14] Clinical confirmation is seen in that, in most adults, 100 g of fructose by mouth will give rise to osmotic diarrhea, whereas more than 250 g of sucrose, which as a dissacharide contains over 100 g of fructose, does not produce any intestinal symptoms.

## INTOLERANCE

Oral tolerance tests using the carbohydrate under investigation are used in the diagnosis of carbohydrate intolerance. Measurements of the appropriate carbohydrate in blood are compared to normal values, and if necessary, an enzyme assay in a mucosal biopsy can be carried out, as can a breath hydrogen examination.

Enzyme or carrier deficiency (and hence dietary carbohydrate intolerance) can be primary or secondary. Primary deficiency has an enzyme or carrier defect; examples include lactase deficiency found in many adults and lactase or sucrase-isomaltase deficiency present at birth. Secondary deficiencies may arise from a disease or disorder of the intestinal tract, and these defects disappear when the disease is resolved. Such diseases include protein deficiency, celiac disease, and intestinal infections.

Adult lactase deficiency is the most common of all enzyme deficiencies; well over half the world's adults are lactose intolerant. Small quantities of lactose can be tolerated, however, and most individuals can tolerate up to 100 ml of milk (5 g lactose) without any symptoms.

## METABOLISM

Glucose is the most common source of energy available to cells. Most cells are able to metabolize glucose to carbon dioxide and water with the release of energy. In this process, the glucose is phosphorylated and converted to trioses before entering the tricarboxylic cycle. However, immediate breakdown to release energy is not the only intracellular fate for glucose. It may be converted to glycogen or to fat for future energy needs. (Although glucose can be converted to fat, fat cannot be converted to glucose.) The other monosaccharides in the diet, fructose and galactose, are metabolized in a comparable fashion.

Although glucose can be utilized by all cells, it is essential in only a few organs, including the brain and red cells. Under normal circumstances the adult brain needs about 140 g glucose/day.[15] During pregnancy and growth, glucose is essential for the formation of cell constituents such as mucopolysaccharides and, of course, for lactose in lactation. Endogenous sources of glucose include some amino acids and the glycerol of glycerides. Glucose is thus ruled out as an essential nutrient in that the body is capable of limited gluconeogenesis.

In the absence of dietary carbohydrate, gluconeogenesis occurs from noncarbohydrate sources up to about 130 g/day. This amount would not meet the needs for glucose were it not that the brain adapts in such a situation and can oxidize ketone bodies.[16] Ketone bodies are formed during the breakdown of fatty acids for energy release and, in the absence of carbohydrate, the final steps in fat breakdown cannot be achieved. About 180 g/day of glucose is needed to complete fat oxidation; the diet should therefore provide about 50 g glucose/day. Thus, one can state a minimum desirable intake of glucose (or its polymer equivalent), but there does not appear to be an ideal level of intake. If dietary recommendations for protein and fat are met, the remainder of the energy needs of the body should be met by dietary carbohydrate.

## STORAGE

The only form of carbohydrate storage in the body is as the polymer of glucose, namely, glycogen. The cost of storing glucose in this way has been calculated as a loss of 5% compared to the direct oxidation of glucose. When glucose is converted to fatty acid, the cost rises to approximately 28%, which makes it a less efficient way of storing energy originating as glucose.[17] Despite the efficiency of glycogen storage, however, the size of the store is small, limited, and negligible compared to the fat store. The size of the store in muscle is about 150 g and can increase about fivefold with training and dietary manipulations, but this amount is still relatively small. Added to this are the following disadvantages: glycogen is not as energy dense as fat, and each gram of deposited glycogen needs about 2.7 g of bound water,[18] making the store even less energy dense compared with triglyceride. The glycogen store in adult liver is about 90 g.

The glycogen in muscle is probably almost entirely derived from circulating glucose because the absence of fructokinase in the muscle cell would prevent fructose metabolism there.[19] In regimen used by athletes, the glycogen store in the muscle can be enlarged for an endurance sporting event.[20]

## CARBOHYDRATE AND ADIPOSE TISSUE

It was first noted in 1852 that dietary carbohydrate could be converted to fat,[21] and this fact is now recognized by all anxious overweight people. Using increases in the respiratory quotient as an indication that carbohydrate was being converted to fat, Benedict and Lee found that the Strasbourg goose force-fed corn had a respiratory quotient of 1.4.[22] It was not clear from this experiment where the fat was formed or deposited, but the three main triglyceride pools are adipose tissue, liver, and plasma.

In adipose tissue, the adipocyte can convert glucose to fatty acid, a process whose rate is variable. Little fructose enters the adipocyte because its transport into the cell is slow compared with that of glucose. Some findings suggest that not all dietary carbohydrates are equal in the extent to which they are converted to fat in adipose tissue, though whether this is a direct or indirect effect is unclear.[22-25]

## CARBOHYDRATE AND LIVER METABOLISM

One assumes that, in a first pass through the liver, much of the glucose that has just been absorbed from the gut is converted by the liver cell to glycogen or to lipid. This simple concept may not be correct, however, and glucose may not be a substrate for liver metabolism. It has been suggested that after absorption glucose is converted to liver glycogen and fat largely through a C3 unit that is formed in tissues other than liver and then recycled to the liver.[26] In normal persons, over two thirds of a glucose load is reported to escape splanchnic removal, and peripheral tissues quantitatively play the dominant role in glucose disposal.[27]

In man most of the fructose absorbed reaches the liver,[28] and little is converted by the intestinal mucosa to glucose, as occurs in rats. Considerable amounts of fructose are removed by the liver because the plasma fructose levels do not rise greatly after fructose ingestion compared to intravenous infusion. The conversion of fructose by the liver can be to glucose, to lipid, or to lactate. The conversion to glucose requires glucose-6-phosphatase. The conversion to lipid can be via glucose, but because the amount of triglyceride formed seems to be greater with fructose than with glucose, another pathway is involved. It has been suggested that fructose, because its breakdown to trioses is not as rate limiting as is that of glucose, forms quantities of glyceraldehyde-P that are then converted to glycerol. This glycerol then forms the basis for attachment of fatty acids.[29]

Fructose also increases the lactate and uric acid levels in the blood, possibly owing to its unlimited rate of breakdown to the trioses.[30] Although these effects may not be important when fructose is given orally, intravenous administration seems to be contraindicated.

Galactose metabolism occurs mainly in the liver, although the kidneys and erythrocytes are involved to a minor extent. Galactose breakdown involves uridine diphosphoglucose and diphosphogalactose before it can be converted to glucose.[31] In milk as well as in gangliosides, cerebrosides, and some phospholipids, galactose is derived from glucose.[32]

The control of carbohydrate metabolism in the liver is hormonal after either short- or long-term ingestion. After long-term ingestion, control is affected by enzyme induction, but in the short term the control is via alterations in inhibitory and/or facilitative factors. Insulin accelerates glycogen formation in keeping with its role as an anabolic hormone. Glucagon has the reverse effect on glycogen in that it accelerates its breakdown, as does circulating epinephrine. Glucagon stimulates insulin release, whereas epinephrine does not; glucagon does not accelerate muscle glycogen breakdown, whereas epinephrine does. Glucocorticoids aid gluconeogenesis.

## CARBOHYDRATE TOLERANCE TESTS

The tolerance test is used clinically to assess the subject's ability to metabolize a given compound or the ability to absorb it. The most common tolerance test is that in which glucose is given by mouth in water and where blood glucose is measured before and at various intervals after ingestion. Any values above normal indicate some inadequate handling of glucose. Details are given in Table 2–4. In view of the ability of insulin to keep blood glucose levels within limits, it is perhaps unwise to assess the extent of glucose absorption from the tolerance curve because varying doses of glucose give similar blood glucose responses.[33] Because insulin can induce liver enzymes, researchers have found that after a period of reduced glucose intake, the serum glucose response to a glucose meal is much greater than if a higher intake of glucose (or its polymers) had preceded the tolerance test.[34]

Galactose tolerance curves are unlike glucose curves in that the maximum galactosemia and the time in which this is achieved are dose related.[35] Because the liver is

**TABLE 2–4.** GLUCOSE CONCENTRATIONS*

| DIABETES MELLITUS | VENOUS BLOOD (MMOL/L) | CAPILLARY BLOOD (MMOL/L) |
|---|---|---|
| Fasting | > 6.7 | > 6.7 |
| After 2 hours | >10.0 | >11.1 |
| IMPAIRED GLUCOSE TOLERANCE | | |
| Fasting | < 6.7 | < 6.7 |
| After 2 hours | 6.7–10.0 | 7.8–11.1 |

*Before and 2 hours after 75 g glucose in 250 to 350 ml water.
(Modified from World Health Organization (WHO): WHO Tech. Rep. Ser., *646*:10, 1980.)

the major site of galactose uptake, galactose tolerance tests have been used to assess liver function. Galactose itself is not insulinogenic.

When glucose accompanies ingested galactose, as in lactose, the serum galactose is modified in that the serum galactose response is decreased by the presence of glucose in the meal, and this decrease is related to the dose of the glucose.[36] Because glucose and galactose share the active absorption system, researchers concluded that the explanation involved competition for active absorption. This cannot be the entire explanation, however, because intravenous glucose given during a galactose tolerance test also reduces the serum galactose response.[37]

The lactose tolerance test may be used to assess lactase deficiency. After ingestion of 50 g of lactose, an increase in the serum glucose concentration of 1.4 mmol/L or more indicates efficient hydrolysis and absorption of lactose.

## CARBOHYDRATE AND SERUM LIPIDS

It has been known since 1961 that dietary carbohydrate can affect the level of lipids in the serum in both the long and the short term.[38,39] Following the short-term ingestion of carbohydrate, the level of serum triglyceride falls. Some researchers consider this effect to be due to an increase in insulin output,[40] but others believe that this explanation may not be entirely correct.[33]

The rise in the level of fasting triglyceride seen after long-term ingestion of a high-carbohydrate diet seems to be short-lived in that, after several weeks, it appears to fall.[41] Furthermore, many people in the world who subsist on a high-carbohydrate diet do not develop hypertriglyceridemia.[42] The increase in the serum triglyceride level varies depending on the type of carbohydrate consumed, with fructose more lipogenic than glucose.[43] All dietary carbohydrates seem to reduce the level of high-density lipoprotein (HDL) cholesterol in the serum[44] and the HDL cholesterol:total cholesterol ratio in the serum is reduced to a greater extent by sucrose than by glucose.[45]

## DIETARY CARBOHYDRATE INTERRELATIONSHIPS

The metabolic response to dietary carbohydrate is not consistent and can be modified by such variables as the other constituents in the food, as well as by, for example, the sex of the consumer.

### CONSISTENCY OF FOOD

The glucose and insulin responses to a carbohydrate are affected by the physical consistency in which it is consumed, as well as by the accompanying fat or "fiber." For example, the glucose and insulin responses to potato are greater than the response to a similar carbohydrate intake given as rice,[46] and ingested ground rice also results in greater serum glucose and insulin response than whole rice.[47] Cooked starch results in a higher insulin response than raw starch, but less than an equivalent amount of glucose.[48]

### ACCOMPANYING CARBOHYDRATES

As already mentioned, fructose seems to be absorbed more rapidly when ingested as sucrose than as an isomolecular mixture of fructose and glucose. In addition, serum galactose levels following galactose ingestion are reduced when accompanied by glucose.

### ACCOMPANYING PROTEIN

When a reducing sugar is heated with a protein, a Maillard reaction reduces the availability of some amino acids, notably lysine.[49] The monosaccharide in the intestinal lumen may influence the rate of uptake of certain amino acids, and fructose seems to accelerate this reaction.[50] Amino acid uptake across the blood-brain barrier is influenced indirectly by serum glucose in that the insulin concentration is directly related to the movement of tryptophan into the brain.[51]

### ACCOMPANYING FAT

Apart from the important role of dietary carbohydrate in preventing ketosis, the type of accompanying ingested carbohydrate modifies the lipid response to carbohydrate. Polyunsaturated fat reduces the rise in fasting serum triglyceride levels seen after a sucrose diet.[52]

### MINERAL BALANCE

It is possible that lactose improves the absorption of calcium from the gut,[53] and carbohydrate intake is associated with sodium retention.[54] The interaction between dietary carbohydrates and mineral absorption and excretion is currently an area of increased interest, though it has been known for at least 20 years that dietary carbohydrates increase calcium and magnesium excretion in the urine. Because amino acids also increase calciuria, insulin is probably not the sole factor.[55]

Fructose seems to enhance, in man, the mineral balance of calcium, copper, zinc, magnesium, and iron.[56] Copper deficiency in rats is exaggerated by sucrose compared to starch,[57] whereas pigs, reputed to be more akin to human beings, do not seem to have any copper:carbohydrate interaction.[58]

In man it has been reported that urinary chromium losses are related to the insulinogenic properties of carbohydrates,[59] and this links with the knowledge that insufficient dietary chromium impairs glucose tolerance.

### ETHANOL

Fructose increases the rate of breakdown of ethanol.[60] In addition, the presence of ethanol slows the metabolism of galactose to carbon dioxide, whereas glucose is unaffected.[61]

### SEX OF THE CONSUMER

After intravenous infusion in primates, males clear fructose more rapidly than females, a difference not seen with glucose.[62] In addition, the fall in plasma triglyceride after intravenous glucose is more marked in men than in women.[63] Apparently, the metabolism of fructose is affected by the sex of the consumer, and premenopausal women fail to show the rise in fasting serum triglycerides seen after ingestion of diets high in fructose (or sucrose).[64] The reason for this difference in response may be that women clear serum triglycerides more rapidly than men.[65]

Glucose tolerance test results vary with the phase of the menstrual cycle; blood glucose levels are highest during ovulation.[65] Estrogens,[67] but not progestogens,[68] impair glucose tolerance. Because these changes are not seen when glucose is given intravenously, they are probably mediated through changes in gastrointestinal motility.[68]

### "SENSITIVITY" OF THE CONSUMER

Those individuals whose fasting serum triglyceride level is raised tend to show a more striking rise in this level when ingesting a high-carbohydrate diet than those with normal levels of fasting serum triglyceride. Presumably, the type IV hyperlipidemic individual is more reactive to dietary carbohydrate, with all its consequences in terms of ensuing disease.

### SPECIES

The absorption of fructose in rats is different from that in man,[69] and the response to dietary carbohydrate can vary with the strain of rat.[70] The metabolism of galactose by the rat[71] and the mouse[72] is dissimilar to that reported in dogs,[73] rabbits,[74] and man.

## CARBOHYDRATE CONSUMPTION AND DISEASE

Concern has been expressed that an excessive intake of dietary carbohydrate, especially sucrose, may play a role in the origin of disease.

### CARIES

The role of carbohydrate in the origin of dental caries varies with the particular carbohydrate as well as with its mode and frequency of intake. Circumstantial evidence suggests a correlation between the amount and especially the frequency of sucrose ingested and the prevalence of caries,[75] but no correlation exists between solubility and caries incidence, although insoluble carbohydrates are noncariogenic.

### OBESITY

Although carbohydrates can be converted into adipose tissue, there is little evidence that they are markedly more efficient in this respect than protein or fat. In fact, with respect to fat, the reverse is true.[76] Differences in the effect on body weight of various carbohydrates are small. Sucrose and fructose in the diet seem to cause a greater weight increase than glucose when rats[23] and baboons[24] are fed isoenergetically. Conversely, weight loss during hypocaloric intake is greater with glucose than sucrose in rats[25] and in man,[77] thereby implying that the energy value of carbohydrates as measured in the laboratory may not be the same as the biologic energy value.

### DIABETES MELLITUS

Evidence associating and relating carbohydrate consumption, and sucrose consumption in particular, to diabetes mellitus is far from conclusive, largely owing to the inability to control variables other than dietary carbohydrate intake.[78,79] There is no evidence that excessive sucrose consumption causes diabetes mellitus.

In the treatment of maturity-onset diabetes (apart from the need to reduce body weight), the consensus is that the amount of carbohydrate in the diet should increase,[80] a view diametrically opposed to that held for many years. Taken as part of a meal, fructose produces a smaller increment in plasma glucose level than does sucrose, glucose, potato starch, or wheat starch. Sucrose, when consumed as part of a meal, does not aggravate postprandial hyperglycemia.[81] The glucose responses to complex carbohydrates are dissimilar and unpredictable, and the use of a glycemic response, which is based on the blood glucose response of a food to that of glucose, has been suggested.[82]

### CARDIOVASCULAR DISEASE

Currently, little evidence suggests that dietary carbohydrates are involved in the origin of cerebrovascular disorders, but they may have a role in ischemic heart disease. Type IV hyperlipidemia is associated with an increased incidence of coronary artery disease. Because in type IV hyperlipidemia the serum lipid, notably the triglyceride, level is dependent on the amount of dietary carbohydrate consumed,[83] it may be deduced that dietary carbohydrate can be of etiologic significance in certain individuals. The type of dietary carbohydrate can alter the level of triglyceridemia in that the effect of dietary sucrose is greater than that of starch, with a fructose:glucose mixture being similar to sucrose.[84]

Several epidemiologic studies and reviews have failed to find sufficient evidence that sucrose is associated with the development of coronary artery disease in the general population.[85–88] With the other variables, such as raised blood pressure and smoking, known to be associated with coronary artery disease, it is not possible to ascribe with any certainty an etiologic role for sucrose or fructose in this condition. Complex carbohydrate intake, however, does not seem to be associated with atherosclerosis in those individuals who subsist on large quantities of these substances.[89]

### CATARACTS

Galactose and glucose can give rise to cataracts because of the further metabolism of these monosaccharides in the lens and subsequent osmotic effects.[90] The glucose cataract is usually seen in diabetics, whose blood glucose levels are raised for a considerable time, whereas the galactose cataract is found in galactosemia[91] or impaired intolerance to galactose.[92]

## INBORN ERRORS AFFECTING DIETARY CARBOHYDRATES

### DIGESTION

When the enzymes concerned with the hydrolysis of carbohydrates are missing or inadequate, the common symptom is osmotic diarrhea. This condition may arise because of a congenital absence of the appropriate enzyme required for the ingestion of lactose,[93] sucrose,[94] or maltose.[95] Inadequacies of these enzymes may also be secondary to gut mucosal damage caused by such conditions as celiac disease or protein deficiency.[96]

### METABOLISM

Genetic errors may occur in the conversion of fructose and galactose with important clinical effects. Absence of the enzyme fructokinase in the liver prevents the breakdown of fructose, which is then excreted in the urine (fructosuria). Diminished activity of fructose-1-phosphate aldolase in the liver results in hypoglycemia and hypophosphatemia with associated vomiting (hereditary fructose intolerance). The hypoglycemia is the result of the inhibition by fructose-1-phosphate of glycogenolysis.[97] These two disorders are inherited as an autosomal recessive trait.[98]

Two clinical forms of galactosemia occur as inborn errors of metabolism and result from enzyme deficiencies. In one condition, the metabolism of galactose is halted at the galactose-1-P step with accumulation of galactose and galactose-1-P, resulting in liver malfunction, cataracts, mental retardation, and failure to thrive. The other deficient enzyme is galactokinase, in which galactose is not phosphorylated.

Certain metabolic errors in the handling of glucose by the body are, strictly speaking, not nutritional in origin. One of these is glucose-6-phosphate dehydrogenase (G6PD) deficiency, which possibly affects over 100 million persons,[99] males more frequently than females. G6PD deficiency is manifested through the red cell and results in an inability to maintain glutathione in a reduced form during exposure to drugs such as sulfonamides, leading to hemolysis and anemia. G6PD deficiency is prevalent in populations subject to malaria and with sickle cell trait.[100]

Rarer metabolic abnormalities affecting carbohydrate metabolism are concerned with gluconeogenesis (G6PD deficiency) or errors in glycogen synthesis and utilization. Glycogen synthesis errors are not common and are of several distinct types.

## REFERENCES


1. Braconnot, H.: Ann. Chim. Phys., *12:*181, 1819.
2. Schmidt, C.: Liebeg's Ann., *51:*30, 1844.
3. Food and Agriculture Organization (FAO): Provisional Food Sheets 1972/74 Average. Rome, FAO, 1977.
4. Perisse, J., Sizaret, F., Francois, P.: FAO Newslett., *7,* 1969.
5. Whelan, W.J.: Biochem. Soc. Symp., *11:*17–26, 1953.
6. Jesuitova, N.N., De Lacey, P., Ugolev. A.M.: Biochim. Biophys. Acta, *86:*205–210, 1964.
7. Dahlqvist, A., Auricchio, A., Semenza, G., et al.: J Clin. Invest., *42:*556–562, 1963.
8. Gray, G.M., Santiago, N.A.: Gastroenterology, *51:*489–498, 1966.
9. Levitt, M.D., Hirsh, P., Fetzer, C.A., et al.: Gastroenterology, *92:*383–389, 1986.
10. Livesey, G.: Am. J. Clin. Nutr., *51:*617–637, 1990.
11. Englyst, H.N., Macfarlane, G.T.: J. Sci. Food Agric., *37:*699–706, 1988.
11. Clarkson, T.W., Rothstein, A.: Am. J. Physiol., *199:*898–906, 1960.
12. Crane, R.K.: A.C.S. Symp. Ser., *15:*2–19, 1975.
13. Crane, R.K., Forstner, G., Eicholz, A.: Biochim. Biophys. Acta, *109:*467–477, 1965.
14. Macdonald, I., Turner, L.J.: Lancet, *1:*841–843, 1968.
15. Cahill, G.F., Owen, O.E., Felig, P.: Physiologist, *11:*97–102, 1968.
16. Owen, D.E., Morgan, A.P., Kemp, H.G., et al.: J. Clin. Invest., *46:*1589–1595, 1967.
17. Horton, E.S.: Am. J. Clin. Nutr., *38:*972–977, 1983.
18. Karlsson, J., Saltin, B.: J. Appl. Physiol., *29:*598–602, 1970.
19. Villar-Palasi, C., Sols, A.: Bull. Soc. Chim. Biol. Paris, *39:*71–75, 1957.
20. Astrand, P.O.: Fed. Proc., *26:*1772–1777, 1967.
21. Lawes, J.B., Gilbert, J.H.: Br. Assoc. Adv. Sci. Rep., *323,* 1852.
22. Benedict, F.G., Lee, R.C.: Carnegie Institute of Washington Publication No. 489, 1937.
23. Allen, R.J.L., Leahy, J.S.: Br. J. Nutr., *20:*339–347, 1966.
24. Brook, M., Noel, P.: Nature, *222:*562–563, 1969.
25. Macdonald, I., Grenby, T.H., Fisher, M.A., et al.: J. Nutr., *111:*1543–1547, 1981.
26. Katz, J., McGarry, J.D.: J. Clin. Invest., *74:*1901–1909, 1984.
27. Katz, L.D., Guckman, G., Rapoport, S., et al.: Diabetes, *32:*675–679, 1983.
28. Cook, G.C.: Clin. Sci., *37:*675–687, 1969.
29. Kupe, I., Lamprecht, W.: Hoppe Seylers Z. Physiol. Chem., *348:*929–935, 1967.
30. Woods, H.F., Alberti, K.: Lancet, *2:*1354–1357, 1972.
31. Leloir, L.F.: Arch. Biochem. Biophys., *33:*186–190, 1951.
32. Kalcka, H.M.: Science, *150:*305–313, 1965.
33. Macdonald, I., Keyser, A., Pacy, D.: Am. J, Clin. Nutr., *31:*1305–1311, 1978.
34. Himsworth, H.P.: Clin. Sci., *1:*1–38, 1933.
35. Williams, C.A., Macdonald, I.: World Rev. Nutr. Diet., *39:*23–52, 1982.
36. Stenstam, T.: Acta Med. Scand., *(Suppl.):*177, 1946.
37. Williams, C.A., Phillips, T., Macdonald, I.: Metabolism, *32:*250–256, 1983.
38. Ahrens, E.H., Hirsch, S., Oettle, K., et al.: Trans. Assoc. Am. Physicians, *74:*134–146, 1961.
39. Havel, R.J.: J. Clin. Invest., *36:*855–859, 1957.
40. Kessler, J.I.: J. Clin. Invest., *42:*362–367, 1963.
41. Antonis, A., Bersohn, I.: Lancet, *1:*3–9, 1961.
42. Schwartz, M.J., Rosenwein, B., Toor, M., et al.: Am. J. Cardiol., *12:*157–168, 1963.
43. Macdonald, I.: Prog. Biochem. Pharmacol., *8:*216–241, 1973.
44. Schonfeld, G., Weidman, S.W., Witztum, J.L., et al.: Metabolism, *25:*261–275, 1976.
45. Macdonald, I: Nutr. Rep. Int., *17:*663–668, 1978.
46. Crapo, P.A., Reaven, G., Olefsky, J.: Diabetes, *26:*1178–1183, 1977.
47. O'Dea, K., Nestel, P.J., Antonoff, L.: Am. J. Clin. Nutr., *33:*760–765, 1980.
48. Collings, P., Williams, C.A. Macdonald, I.: Br. Med. J., *282:*1032, 1981.
49. Landes, D.R., Miller, J.: Cereal Chem., *53:*678–682, 1976.
50. Cooke, G.C.: J. Physiol. (Lond.), *217:*61–70, 1971.
51. Fernstrom, J.D.: Metabolism, *26:*207–223, 1977.
52. Macdonald, I.: Clin. Sci., *43:*265–274, 1972.
53. Condon, J.R., Nassim, J.R., Millard, F.J.C., et al.: Lancet, *1:*1027–1029, 1970.
54. Hoffman, R.S., Martino, J.A., Wahl, G., et al.: Metabolism, *20:*1065–1073, 1971.
55. Holl, M.G., Allen, L.H.: Am. J. Clin. Nutr., *48:*1219–1225, 1988.
56. Holbrook, J.T., Smith, J.C., Reiser, S.: Am. J. Clin. Nutr., *49:*1290–1294, 1989.
57. Fields, M., Ferretti, R.J., Smith, J.C., et al.: Am. J. Clin. Nutr., *39:*289–295, 1984.
58. Schoenemann, H.M., Failla, M.L., Steele, N.C.: Am. J. Clin. Nutr., *52:*147–154, 1990.
59. Anderson, R.A., Bryden, N.A., Polansky, M.M., et al.: Am. J. Clin. Nutr., *51:*864–868, 1990.
60. Brown, SS., Forrest, J.A.N., Roscoe, P.: Lancet, *2:*898–988, 1972.
61. Segal, S., Blair, A.: J. Clin. Invest., *40:*2016–2025, 1961.
62. Jourdan, M.H.: J. Physiol. (Lond.), *201:*27P, 1969.
63. Perry, W.F., Corbett, B.N.: Can. J. Physiol. Pharmacol., *42:*353–356, 1964.
64. Macdonald, I.: Am. J. Clin. Nutr., *18:*369–372, 1966.
65. Kekki, M., Nikkila, E.A.: Metabolism, *20:*878–889, 1971.
66. Macdonald, I., Crossley, J.N.: Diabetes, *19:*450–452, 1970.
67. Buchler, D., Warren, J.C.: Am. J. Obstet. Gynecol., *95:*479–483, 1966.
68. Larsson-Cohn, U. Tengstrom, B., Wide, L.: Acta Endocrinol., *62:*242–250, 1969.
69. Dahlqvist, A., Thompson, D.L.: J. Physiol. (Lond.), *167:*193–209, 1963.
70. Durand, A.M., Fisher, N., Adams, M.: Arch. Pathol., *85:*318–324, 1968.
71. Newstead, G.C.: Proc. Nutr. Soc., *38:*38A, 1979.
72. Williams, C.A., Owens, A.M.: Proc. Nutr. Soc., *43:*58A, 1984.
73. Bollman, J.L., Mann, F.C., Power, M.H.: Am. J. Physiol., *111:*483–491 1935.
74. Roe, J.H., Schwartzmann, A.S.: J. Biol. Chem., *96:*717–735, 1932.
75. Rugg-Gunn, A.J.: Diet and dental caries. *In* Prevention of Dental Disease. 2nd Ed. Edited by J.J. Murray. Oxford, Blackwell Medical Publishers, 1989, pp. 4–114.
76. Wood, J.D., Reid, J.R.: Br. J. Nutr., *34:*15–24, 1975.

77. Macdonald, I., Taylor, J.: Guy's Hosp. Rep., *122*:155–159, 1973.
78. Stare, F.J.: Nutr. Metab., *(Suppl.1)*:133–142, 1975.
79. Kahn, H.A., Herman, J.B., Medalie, J.H., et al.: J. Chronic Dis., *23*:617–629, 1971.
80. American Diabetes Association Report: Diabetes, *20*:633–634, 1971.
81. Bantle, J.P., Laine, D.C., Castle, G.W., et al.: N. Engl. J. Med., *309*:7–12, 1983.
82. Jenkins, D.J.A., Wolever, T.M.S., Taylor, R.H.: Am. J. Clin. Nutr., *34*:362–366, 1981.
83. Nestel, P., Carroll, K.F., Havenstein, N., et al.: Metabolism, *19*:1–18, 1970.
84. Blum, C.B., Levey, R.I., Eisenberg, S., et al.: J. Clin. Invest., *60*:795–807, 1977.
85. M.R.C. Working Party: Lancet, *2*:1265–1271, 1970.
86. Walker, A.R.P.: Atherosclerosis, *14*:137–152, 1971.
87. Keys, A.: Atherosclerosis, *14*:193–202, 1971.
88. Grande, F.: Sugars in cardiovascular disease. *In* Sugars in Nutrition. Edited by H.L. Sipple and K.W. McNutt. New York, Academic Press, 1974, pp. 402–437.
89. Higginson, J., Pepler, W.J.: J. Clin. Invest., *33*:1366, 1953.
90. Van Heyningen, R.: Nature, *184*:194–195, 1959.
91. Rennert, O.M.: Ann. Clin. Lab. Sci., *7*:443–448, 1977.
92. Bhat, K.S., Gopalan, C.: Nutr. Metab., *17*:8, 1974.
93. Dahlqvist, A.: Enzyme deficiency and malabsorption of carbohydrates. *In* Sugars in Nutrition. Edited by H.L. Sipple and K.W. McNutt. New York, Academic Press, 1974, pp. 187–214.
94. Prader, A., Auricchio, S., Murset, G.: Schweiz. Med. Wochenschr., *91*:465–476, 1961.
95. Semenza, G., Auricchio, S., Rubino, A.: Biochim. Biophys. Acta, *96*:487–497, 1965.
96. Bayless, T.M., Christopher, N.L.: Am. J. Clin. Nutr., *22*:181–190, 1969.
97. Nisell, J., Linden, L.: Scand. J. Gastroenterol., *3*:80–82, 1968.
98. Gitzelmann, R., Steinmann, B., Van Der Berghe, G.: Essential fructosuria, hereditary fructose intolerance and fructose-1,6-diphosphate deficiency. *In* Metabolic Basis of Inherited Disease. Edited by J.B. Stanbury et al. New York, McGraw-Hill, 1989, pp. 399–424.
99. Yoshida, A.: Science, *179*:532–537, 1973.
100. Buetler, E., Johnson, C., Powars, D., et al.: N. Engl. J. Med., *290*:826–828, 1974.

## SELECTED READINGS

British Nutrition Foundation: Complex Carbohydrates in Foods. London, Chapman & Hall, 1990.

Dobbing, J. (Ed.): Dietary Starches and Sugars in Man: A Comparison. London, Springer-Verlag, 1990.

Food and Drug Administration Task Force: Evaluation of health aspects of sugars contained in carbohydrate sweeteners. J. Nutr., *116*:11S, 1986.

Reiser, S., Hallfrisch, J.: Metabolic Effects of Dietary Fructose. Boca Raton, FL, CRC Press, 1987.

United Kingdom (UK) Department of Health: Dietary Sugars and Human Disease. London, UK Dept. Of Health Report No. 37, 1989.

Vettorazzi, G., Macdonald, I. (Eds.): Sucrose: Nutritional and Safety Aspects. London, Springer-Verlag, 1988.

CHAPTER 3

# Lipids

Willem G. Linscheer and Antoine J. Vergroesen



## OVERVIEW

Lipids are compounds insoluble in water but soluble in organic solvents, e.g., acetone, ether, and chloroform. Of nutritional interest are triglycerides (TG) (triacylglycerols) sterols, and phospholipids (PL) (diacylglycerophosphatides), consisting mostly of lecithin and sphingolipids (ceramides; glycolipids, such as cerebrosides, gangliosides, and ceramide oligosaccharides; sphingomyelin, the only phosphorylcholine-containing sphingolipid) (see footnote this page). The sources of lipids in food products are of both animal and plant origin, and can be considered of similar nutritional value with a few exceptions. The sterols of plants (phytosterols such as β-sitosterol, stigmasterol) are poorly absorbed, whereas animal tissues contain cholesterol (CH), of which approximately 50% is absorbed. Vegetable food sources may supply a significant amount of "fiber," nonabsorbable carbohydrates, which may interfere with lipid absorption, as well as phytosterols, which inhibit CH absorption. As discussed subsequently, vegetable oils are the sole source of essential fatty acids (EFA) for animals. However, plants synthesize the very long-chain fatty acids (LCFA) (fatty acids with 20 or more carbon atoms) with 3 or

Abbreviations: Acyl-CoA cholesterol acyltransferase (ACAT); adenosine diphosophtase (ADP); adenosine monophosophatase (AMP); adenosine triphosophatase (ATP); β-hydroxy β-methyl glutaryl (HMG); bile salts (BS); cholecystokinin (CCK); cholesterol (CH); cholesterol ester (CE); critical micellar concentration (CMC); cyclic adenosine monophosphate (cAMP); cyclyoxygenase(s) (CO); diglycerides (DG); endoplasmatic reticulum (ER); essential fatty acids (EFA); fatty acids (FA); high-density lipoproteins (HDL); lecithin-cholesterol acyltransferase (LCAT); leukotrienes (LT); lipid transport proteins (LTP); lipoxygenase(s) (LO); long-chain fatty acids (LCFA); long-chain triglycerides (LCT); low-density lipoproteins (LDL); medium-chain fatty acids (MCFA); medium-chain triglycerides (MCT); monoglycerides (MG); 2-monoglycerides (2MG); monounsaturated fatty acids (MUFA); phospholipids (PL); polyunsaturated fatty acids (PUFA); prostaglandin(s) (PG); saturated fatty acids (SAFA); short-chain fatty acids (SCFA); thromboxane (TXA); triglycerides (TG); unstirred water layer (UWL); very low-density lipoproteins (VLDL).

more *cis*-double bonds, which are the EFA typical of animal tissues.

The fat-soluble (pro)vitamins β-carotene, A, D, E, and K, which are also lipids, are discussed in other chapters. It is important to realize that extreme low-fat diets, such as are prevalent in Africa and Asia (or advocated by some food faddists), may lead to deficiencies of these fat-soluble vitamins and EFA. The same deficiencies might occur in patients with a fat-malabsorption syndrome. Because many fatty acids (FA) and sterols have (*cis*-) double bonds in the carbon chain and therefore are prone to oxidation, the presence of natural antioxidants such as vitamin E (α,β,γ,δ tocopherols), and of selenium is important, especially in diets rich in n-3 polyunsaturated fatty acids (PUFA), which induce a significantly higher requirement for these antioxidants.

Cellular lipids are important not only as an energy source but also as structural components of cells. Some are also precursors for steroid hormone synthesis or for other highly active compounds, such as prostaglandins (PG). Phospholipids (PL), which form an interphase between water and other lipids, serve a vital role in cells and blood by binding water-soluble compounds such as protein to a lipid-soluble substance. Furthermore, the PL of the outer cellular membrane can undergo lysis by various phopholipases and release unsaturated fatty acids, e.g., di homo-γ-linolenic and arachidonic acid, the precursor fatty acids for the biosynthesis of various prostaglandins (PG), thromboxanes (TX), and leukotrienes (LT). Phosphatidylcholine may release choline, the precursor for the biosynthesis of acetylcholine.

Dietary lipids consist mainly of triglycerides (TG), a useful and concentrated source of energy (1 g of TG provides approximately 9 kcal (38 kJ) after absorption). Fat maldigestion and malabsorption lead to steatorrhea with an appreciable loss of energy. A fecal fat excretion of 40 g per day, which is common in a patient with severe pancreatitis, represents an energy loss of more than 360 kcal (1500 kJ). An adequate TG supply and efficient intestinal absorption are important for infants and also for adults with a high-energy requirement, such as patients with burns, malignant tumors, or surgical wounds. The alternative energy sources, proteins and carbohydrates, deliver, per gram, 4 kcal or 17 kJ, less than one half the energy density of fats, and require bulky meals to cover high-energy requirements. In practice, the energy density of common sources of proteins and carbohydrates is less because of their fiber and water content.

Triglycerides consist of a molecule of glycerol esterified with 3 fatty acid (FA) molecules. The melting point of a TG is determined by the type of its FA (carbon chain length and the number and *cis* or *trans*-configuration of its double bonds) and the position to which it is esterified with the glycerol molecule (position 1, 2, or 3). The melting point of a TG is important for intestinal absorption and food processing. Varying the chain length of FA, reducing the number of natural *cis*-double bonds, increasing the number of *trans* double bonds, and changing the distribution of FA on the TG molecules results in a range of fats with specific melting behaviors. The FA on position 2 of TG are absorbed easily after digestion as monoglycerides (MG), even if they normally would be absorbed poorly as free FA. This statement is true especially for saturated FA with a chain length of 18 or more and for monounsaturated FA (particularly if the double bond is in the *trans*-configuration) with more than 20 carbon atoms.

The foregoing observations demonstrate why the nutritional characterization of a TG requires more than a FA analysis limited only to chain length and number of double bonds, and why too many nutritional studies on the role of fats can be interpreted only incompletely. Throughout this chapter we use the scientific names of FA determined by the International Union of Chemistry. Most common names and scientific names (Geneva conference) of FA discussed in this chapter are presented in Figure 3–10.

The FA of naturally occurring lipids have even-number carbon atom chains with a typical length of 16 and 18. Notable exceptions are milk fat, coconut oil, and palm kernel oil with a high percentage of short-chain (4–6), medium-chain (6–12), and C14 saturated FA (see Table 3–1). Especially the C12 and C14 saturated FA are responsible for the high atherogenic potential of these common edible fats. On the other side of the range of compositions are 1) peanut oil with 4 to 5% C20:0, C22:0, and C24:0; and 2) fish oils with 5 to 35% C20:1, C22:1, and C24:1; and with 25 to 50% of the polyunsaturated very long FA C20:5 n-3, C22:6 n-3, and C24:6 n-3 all *cis*. The latter compounds are responsible for a range of pathophysiologic effects discussed subsequently. Varieties of rapeseed- and mustard-seed oils are characterized by 35 to 60% of C20:1 n-9 and C22:1 n-9, but new varieties contain less than 1% of these monounsaturated very LCFA. These oils, which are similar to a mixture of soybean and olive oil, do not induce the various specific metabolic changes typical for most of the very LCFA reviewed in the chapter. Some uncommon edible oils are sources of C18:3 n-6,9,12 all *cis* (γ-linolenic acid, not to be confused with the common α-linolenic acid in soybean, linseed and rapeseed oils). Evening primrose and black currant seed oils are cultivated and marketed for presumed health benefits, but as discussed in the section concerning EFA, no evidence exists to justify these specific curative claims. Especially in India, the nutritional value of other sources of edible fats not mentioned in Table 3–1 has been studied, often requiring specific refining techniques to get rid of potentially toxic compounds present in the crude oils (see the last section of this chapter).

Table 3–1 is a review of the more important FA and their natural sources.[1-3] Genetic and climatic differences are responsible for a wide variation in the compositions of vegetable oils. The composition of animal feed determines to a great extent animal fat composition, especially that of nonruminants. For this reason, a fat is insufficiently described by only its source (e.g., safflower

**TABLE 3–1.** AVERAGE TRIGLYCERIDE FATTY ACID COMPOSITION OF IMPORTANT EDIBLE FATS

| FOOD | AVERAGE FAT % | AVERAGE FATTY ACID COMPOSITION | | | | | | |
|---|---|---|---|---|---|---|---|---|
| | | Saturated | | | Mono- and Polyunsaturated | | | |
| | | Total* | 16:0 | 18:0 | 18:1 | 18:2 | 18:3 | 20:4 |
| Milk (cow) | 3.5 | 65* | 25 | 11 | 26 | 1–3 | 2 | tr |
| Butter | 80 | | | | Identical to milk | | | |
| Lard (pig) | 100 | 42 | 28 | 13 | 46 | 6–8 | 2 | 2 |
| Pork | 35 | | | | Approx. as lard | | | |
| Tallow | 100 | 53 | 29 | 20 | 42 | 2 | tr | – |
| Beef | 25 | | | | Approx. as tallow | | | |
| Chicken | 15 | 30 | 25 | 4 | 42 | 21 | – | – |
| Egg | 11 | | | | Identical to chicken | | | |
| Turkey | 20 | | | | Approx. as chicken | | | |
| Groundnut oil | 100 | 19† | 11 | 3 | 40–55† | 20–43† | | |
| Groundnut | 50 | | | | Identical (variable, climate dependent) | | | |
| Sesame oil | 100 | 15 | 9 | 5 | 39 | 40 | 1 | – |
| Sesame seed | 53 | | | | Identical to oil | | | |
| Soybean oil | 100 | 15 | 11 | 4 | 23 | 51 | 7 | – |
| Soybean | 18 | | | | Identical to oil | | | |
| Corn oil | 100 | 13 | 11 | 2 | 25 | 55 | tr | – |
| Corn | 4 | | | | Identical to oil | | | |
| Sunflower seed oil | 100 | 12 | 6 | 4 | 24 | 60–70 | tr | – |
| Olive oil | 100 | 17 | 14 | 3 | 71 | 10 | tr | – |
| Olive | 14 | | | | Identical to oil | | | |
| Cottonseed oil | 100 | 30 | 25 | 3 | 18 | 51 | tr | |
| Safflower seed oil | 100 | 10 | 7 | 3 | 15‡ | 75‡ | tr | |
| Palm oil | 100 | 52 | 45 | 5 | 38 | 10 | – | |
| Coconut oil | 100 | 88* | 8 | 3 | 6 | 2 | – | |
| Palm kernel oil | 100 | 80* | 7 | 2 | 14 | 1 | – | |
| Rapeseed oil (new) | 100 | 7 | 5 | 2 | 53 | 22 | 10 | |
| Rapeseed oil (old) | 100 | 4 | 3 | 1 | 11 | 13 | 9+§ | |
| Mustard seed oil | 100 | 5 | 3 | 1 | 16 | 15 | 10+§ | |
| Cashew nut | 68 | 24 | 14 | 10 | 30 | 35 | tr | |
| Walnut | 63 | 10 | 7 | 2 | 15 | 60 | 10 | |
| Herring[e] (menhaden) | 16–25 | 30 | 19 | 4 | 13 | 1 | 1+‖ | |
| Mackerel[f] | 25 | 25 | 17 | 5 | 18 | 1 | # | |

The figures given are approximations, as climate, species, fodder composition, etc. cause great variations. The data given are compiled from refs. 1,2,3.

*The balance of saturated fatty acids is formed by fatty acids with chain lengths < 12 (butter 14%) and 12 and 14 (butter 16%, coconut and palm kernel 65–70%).

†Circa 4% of C 20:0 and C 22:0, groundnuts from Argentina and Virginia have relatively low C 18:1 and high C 18:2 concentrations.

‡Also safflower seed oil with the reverse C 18:1/18:2 composition is available.

§Contrary to new rapeseed varieties like Canbra and LEAR, old varieties of rapeseed oil and also mustard seed oil have 10% C 20:1 n-9 and 30–50% C 22:1 n-9.

‖Menhaden herring oil has 11% C 20:5 n-3, 9% C 22:6 n-3, but Norwegian herring oil has 13% C 20:1 n-9, 21% C 22:1 n-11, 7% C 20:5 n-3, and 7% C 22:6 n-3.

#Dependent on fishing grounds mackerel oil is similar to Menhaden or to Norwegian/Northsea herring.

seed oil or lard). (See Appendix tables A–19a and b for the average lipid contents of selected foods and oils). The vital importance of the EFA to both man and animals with respect to the adequate composition of the biomembranes and as precursors of the PG, leukotrienes (LT), and various hydroxy FA is discussed later in this chapter. Animals, including man, cannot synthesize EFA; hence, they depend completely on vegetable lipids (directly or indirectly through consumption of herbivores) to meet EFA requirements. Shifting the position of one of the double bonds of the EFA from the n-3, 6, 9 all *cis* or n-6, 9 all *cis* position (biologists prefer to count from the methyl end of the fatty acid), or changing the *cis-* into the *trans-* configuration, as happens during hydrogenation or catalytically by some types of oil processing or by bacteria during fodder digestion in ruminants, results in a complete loss of EFA activity. Even worse PUFA without EFA activity may act as competitive inhibitors of EFA metabolism. For these reasons, careful application of sophisticated analytic methods is crucial in the study of the pathophysiologic effects of EFA and other (poly)unsaturated FA. Edible fats and oils also contain sterols and PL. During the processing of vegetable oils, most of the sterols and PL are removed for technologic reasons as well as because of taste. However, other lipid-containing foods have varying amounts of these compounds, which are integral parts of all animal and plant biomembranes. Man can normally biosynthesize adequate amounts of CH and PL. As discussed in this chapter dietary CH, in contrast to poorly absorbed vegetable sterols, plays an important role in lipoprotein composition and metabolism. Figure 3–1 lists the more important sterols,[4] their main dietary sources, and their molecular differences. Minor differences in structure are responsible for clear differences in absorption, requiring complicated analytic methods for adequate evaluation.

Chemical characterization of sterols is important because plant sterols diminish absorption of CH in mammals and birds; this effect is presumably the result of competition with CH for incorporation into micelles or for transport across the intestinal cell membrane. β-Sitosterol has been used as a therapeutic agent to lower plasma CH-levels, usually in daily doses of 10 to 20 g. However, it has been shown that maximal inhibition of CH absorption—50% reduction—in man is achieved with 3 g of β-sitosterol per day, and no further reduction occurs with higher intakes.[5]

The PL from vegetable sources, although absorbed as well as those from animals, normally have a different FA composition. Oral or intraduodenal administration of soya phosphatidylcholine decreases the absorption of CH; thus, it is a more potent hypocholesterolemic agent in rats[6] and man[7] than TG with a similar FA composition. Furthermore, phosphatidylcholine, given orally, is more efficient in raising blood choline levels than equimolar amounts of free choline,[8,9] which might have significant effects on biosynthesis of acetylcholine in the brain.[10] This finding has interesting therapeutic implications in diseases such as Alzheimer's (pre)senile dementia, tardive dyskinesia, and other conditions probably caused by failing cholinergic activity.

A useful review of the sources of choline and lecithin in the diet has been published.[11] If the preliminary results can be confirmed, the demand will increase for pure phosphatidylcholine (and sphingomyelin). The crude lecithin preparations now available are mixtures of phosphatidylcholine (20 to 25%); phosphatides of serine, ethanolamine, and inositol; nonphosphorus-containing lipids (45 to 50%); and about 10% hydrophilic impurities (sugar and amino compounds). Again, accurate analyses are necessary for a correct evaluation of data; for example, the hypocholesterolemic effects of soya phosphatidylcholine referred to previously could not be confirmed in man by a study in which egg phosphatidylcholine with a different FA composition was used.[12]

Dietary TG, along with carbohydrates, are the main source of digestible energy (consumption of proteins are constant between 10 and 15% of digestible energy

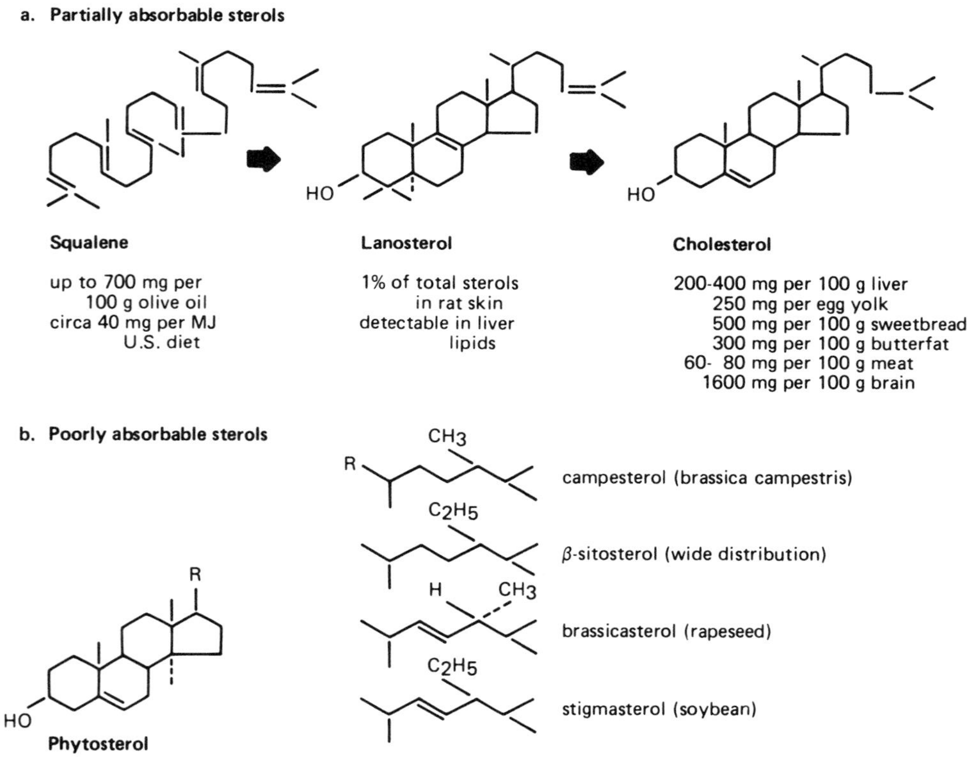
a. Partially absorbable sterols
HO
HO
Squalene
up to 700 mg per 100 g olive oil
circa 40 mg per MJ U.S. diet
Lanosterol
1% of total sterols in rat skin
detectable in liver lipids
Cholesterol
200-400 mg per 100 g liver
250 mg per egg yolk
500 mg per 100 g sweetbread
300 mg per 100 g butterfat
60- 80 mg per 100 g meat
1600 mg per 100 g brain
b. Poorly absorbable sterols
R
HO
Phytosterol
CH3
R
campesterol (brassica campestris)
C2H5
β-sitosterol (wide distribution)
H
CH3
brassicasterol (rapeseed)
C2H5
stigmasterol (soybean)

**FIGURE 3–1.** Molecular structures and average concentrations of the more important sterols in various food components.

[en%]). In most industrialized countries, fat intake is 40 to 45 en%, with a FA composition high in saturated and monounsaturated FA[13] (about 50% and 40% of fat, respectively) and only 2 to 3 en% of EFA. Because this unbalanced composition is considered a causal factor in atherogenesis, modern dietary recommendations emphasize a reduction of total fat intake and a 1 to 1 ratio between saturated FA and EFA.[1,13] A reduction in fat intake results in an increased carbohydrate consumption, accompanied by increased dietary levels of fiber, water-soluble vitamins, and trace elements, assuming that cereals, potatoes, etc. are the main carbohydrate source. However, prosperous population groups in general consider diets high in starch and fiber unattractive and prefer the sweetness of mono- and disaccharides (sucrose, but also, of course, fruits). A healthy diet, however, becomes progressively more difficult with lowering of fat in the diet, because the "hidden" fat in meat and dairy products, bread, pastries, etc. is mainly saturated. Laymen are inclined to limit fat intake by cutting down on "visible" fat intake (oils and spreads), which may be important sources of EFA. Any excess intake of digestible energy (sugar, alcohol, as well as protein) is converted into palmitic and oleic acid and deposited as TG in adipose tissue. In this way, excess food intake contributes to an unphysiologic FA composition of human tissues. The necessity of accurate lipid analysis for human nutrition is not limited to analysis of food lipids, but also applies to analysis of human tissues; blood and subcutaneous fat cells are convenient sources and provide useful information on short- and long-term FA intake, respectively (for reviews, see references 1 to 6). In this context, the consumption of alcohol by adolescents and adults should not be neglected, as it is in many dietary surveys and recommendations. Although reliable figures on actual alcohol intake are difficult to obtain, the average intake in many population groups is certainly more than 10 en%. Therefore, data concerning fat, carbohydrates, and protein consumption and of the vitamins and minerals should be corrected in these studies for energy derived from alcohol.

## DIGESTION AND ABSORPTION

### TRIGLYCERIDES

Although digestion of triglycerides (TG) consists of highly complicated digestive physicochemical reactions and numerous interactions between lipolytic products, PL, bile salts, proteins, and carbohydrates, certain major principles of lipid digestion have been elucidated. Because interactions with carbohydrates and nondigestive proteins have not been clarified and are probably of minor importance, these effects on the intraluminal phase of fat absorption are not discussed. The focus of this discussion is on the main principles of lipid digestion in the gastrointestinal tract, starting with digestion and absorption of TG in the mouth, esophagus, and stomach.

Of the two major groups of ingested lipids, TG and PL, only 2% of the 100 to 140 g of fat ingested daily in the United States and other western countries consists of PL.[14] However, this seemingly small amount of PL plays an important role in the digestion and absorption of TG. Other lipids are either present in such minute quantities that they do not play a role in the absorptive process, or are totally water insoluble and undigestible, such as wax and wax-like compounds, and hence are not absorbable. Being neutral and practically insoluble in water, TG are poorly absorbed and require enzymatic conversion into more water-soluble and polar metabolites for uptake by the gut mucosa. The small amounts of PL present in a normal diet are essential for emulsification of TG into dispersed tiny droplets in the stomach. It creates a large surface area for effective hydrolysis by various digestive lipases. The TG are present inside vegetable cells as small emulsified particles surrounded by a monolayer of PL (mostly lecithin). The PL are, however, removed during oil refining. Emulsifiers are added during manufacturing of soft cheeses, some margarines, and salad sauces. The American diet has changed over the past 10 years in the sense that total fat consumption has decreased and saturated animal lipids have in part been replaced by partly unsaturated vegetable fat. The significance of these modifications is discussed in a subsequent section.

#### *GASTRIC DIGESTION AND ABSORPTION*

The extensive increase of the surface area of ingested TG by emulsification in the stomach has been mediated by a combination of mechanical and physicochemical mechanisms. The mechanical mixing consists of chewing and gastric contractions. Emulsification is enhanced further by dietary PL and simultaneous release of MG and FA from TG by lipase-induced hydrolysis. Chewing furthermore exposes the TG to lingual lipase by disrupting cell walls and mechanical dispersion. The lingual lipase originates from serous glands located on the back of the tongue (Ebner's glands).[15-18] It is the major lipase in the stomach and hydrolyzes, in combination with gastric lipase, approximately 30% of ingested TG during the 2 to 4 hours of gastric emptying after a meal.[19] The two lipases have similar properties, including an acid pH optimum in the range of the physiologic postprandial gastric pH.[20] Both lipases have a preference for cleaving the LCFA at the sn-3 ester linkage. Thus, the postprandial luminal content of the stomach contains TG, diglycerides (DG), and FA.

Milk fat has a different composition; it contains medium-chain TG (MCT, carbon chain length of FA is 6 to 12 carbon atoms). Mother's milk has a high percentage of MCT and also contains lipase, in contrast to cow's milk. These three lipases hydrolyze all FA of the MCT, and part of the medium-chain FA (MCFA) are absorbed by the gastric mucosa because of their hydrophilic properties.

The effects of chewing and gastric fat digestion can be summarized as follows. Ingested long-chain TG (LCT) in vegetable and animal cells are released. All TG are then emulsified and partly hydrolyzed to DG and FA. Emulsification is enhanced by dietary PL and hydrolyzed FA. In emulsified particles, TG and DG are located in the center of the small droplets with a monolayer of PL and FA on the outside. Gastric digestion and intermittent delivery of gastric chyme to the duodenum facilitates further digestion and absorption in the small bowel.[4,13,21-25]

## *INTESTINAL DIGESTION AND ABSORPTION*

Studies by Borgstrom, using a high-fat liquid test meal (75 g of fat) and an intubation technique, demonstrated TG absorption is practically completed in the first 120 cm of the small bowel in healthy volunteers.[26] Gastric chyme, consisting of partly hydrolyzed TG (to 30%, depending on saturation and carbon chain length of FA), is delivered in small quantities to the duodenum by gastric peristalsis and intermittent relaxation of the pyloric musculature. Gastric digestion is limited to incomplete hydrolysis of TG, which results in the formation of oily droplets containing TG, DG, and FA. The LCFA are poorly absorbed in the stomach, because the droplets are too big to diffuse fast through the unstirred water layer (UWL).

Only two hydrolytic products can be absorbed by the intestinal mucosa, 2-MG and FA, and only as free monomers from the aqueous phase at the surface of the luminal membranes of the mucosal cells. From theoretic considerations, one could predict that complete absorption of 75 g fat, as shown by Borgstrom et al.,[26] would require more complete hydrolysis into polar compounds and a solubilizing and delivery system of free monomers (FA and MG) to the UWL at the cell surface. This task could be accomplished only if the following conditions are met. (1) More complete hydrolysis to MG and FA than occurs in the stomach. Because pancreatic lipase has a pH optimum in the alkaline range, acid gastric chyme needs to be neutralized (by pancreatic $NaHCO_3$ and the duodenal mucosa) before lipolysis is maximal. (2) The surface area of TG droplets is enlarged (by detergents) for faster enzymatic hydrolysis. (3) Because MG and FA are poorly soluble in water, a solubilizing transport system (mixed micelles) is required. This system also sustains concentrations of these monomers in this aqueous phase of the UWL at concentrations close to their maximal solubility in water.

On the basis of physicochemical properties of lipids and lipid membranes, one can predict that TG and DG will not permeate the absorptive mucosal membrane and that only 2-MG and mostly protonated (nonionized) FA can pass through the membrane by diffusion as free monomers in the aqueous phase adjacent to the luminal membrane.

**Hydrolysis by Pancreatic Lipase.** The combination of an acid pH and the presence of essential amino acids, FA, and MG in the gastric chyme induces effectively the release of cholecystokinin (CCK) (identical to pancreozymin) and secretin from the duodenal mucosa into the circulation.[27-30] Secretin is the physiologic stimulant for release of most of the pancreatic electrolytes (mostly $NaHCO_3$) and to a minor degree intestinal digestive enzymes; CCK stimulates primarily the synthesis and release of exocrine pancreatic enzymes and, to a lesser degree, the release of electrolytes.[31] The overlapping effect of CCK on pancreatic bicarbonate excretion ensures a more continuous pH adjustment in the duodenum, because secretin release depends primarily on the short episodes of the pH-lowering effect of freshly arrived gastric chyme in the proximal duodenum. Cholecystokinin also induces sustained gallbladder contraction and the synthesis and release of hepatic bile, containing bile salts, PL, and cholesterol. Gastric chyme is effectively "neutralized" by the combined effects of pancreatic $NaHCO_3$ and the buffering properties of the intestinal mucosa. The pH of the bulk phase in the distal duodenum is then sustained at 6.5. In the presence of bile salts, the pH optimum of pancreatic lipase is reduced to 6.[32] Such an excess of lipase is secreted that, under optimal conditions, 100 kg of TG could be hydrolyzed in 24 hours instead of the ingested 100 to 140 g of fat in a normal diet.[33]

In addition to acidic conditions, pancreatic lipase is also inhibited by the simultaneous influx into the proximal duodenum of biliary micelles. The mixed micelles consisting of bile salts (BS), PL, and CH present in bile have a strong affinity for the surface of the emulsified lipid droplets, thereby displacing lipase from its substrate. However, as Borgstrom,[34] Desnuelle,[35] and Morgan and Hoffman[36] have elucidated, lipolysis is effective because a small pancreatic protein, procolipase (10,000 M.W.), is also released by the pancreas simultaneously with lipase (50,000 M.W.) in a ratio of 1:1. Pancreatic trypsin activates procolipase by removing a small group of less than 12 amino acids.[37] In the presence of TG (or FA), colipase then complexes firmly with lipase and also binds to the surface of lipid droplets, thereby supplanting BS and PL molecules. The mixed micelles in bile, consisting of BS, PL, and CH, participate in this complex.[38,39] Thus, colipase gives lipase access to its substrate, and, most likely by its affinity to micelles, it also facilitates micellar uptake of FA and MG. Furthermore, by removing the products of lipolysis, it also increases the effectiveness of lipase (Fig. 3–2). Micellar aggregates, as present in bile, are in fact highly efficient in absorbing from the surface of the TG droplets the 2-MG and FA released by the pancreatic lipase. Because lipolysis is an extremely fast process (the turnover is approximately 400,000 mol/min/mol lipase[40]), the formation of 2-MG

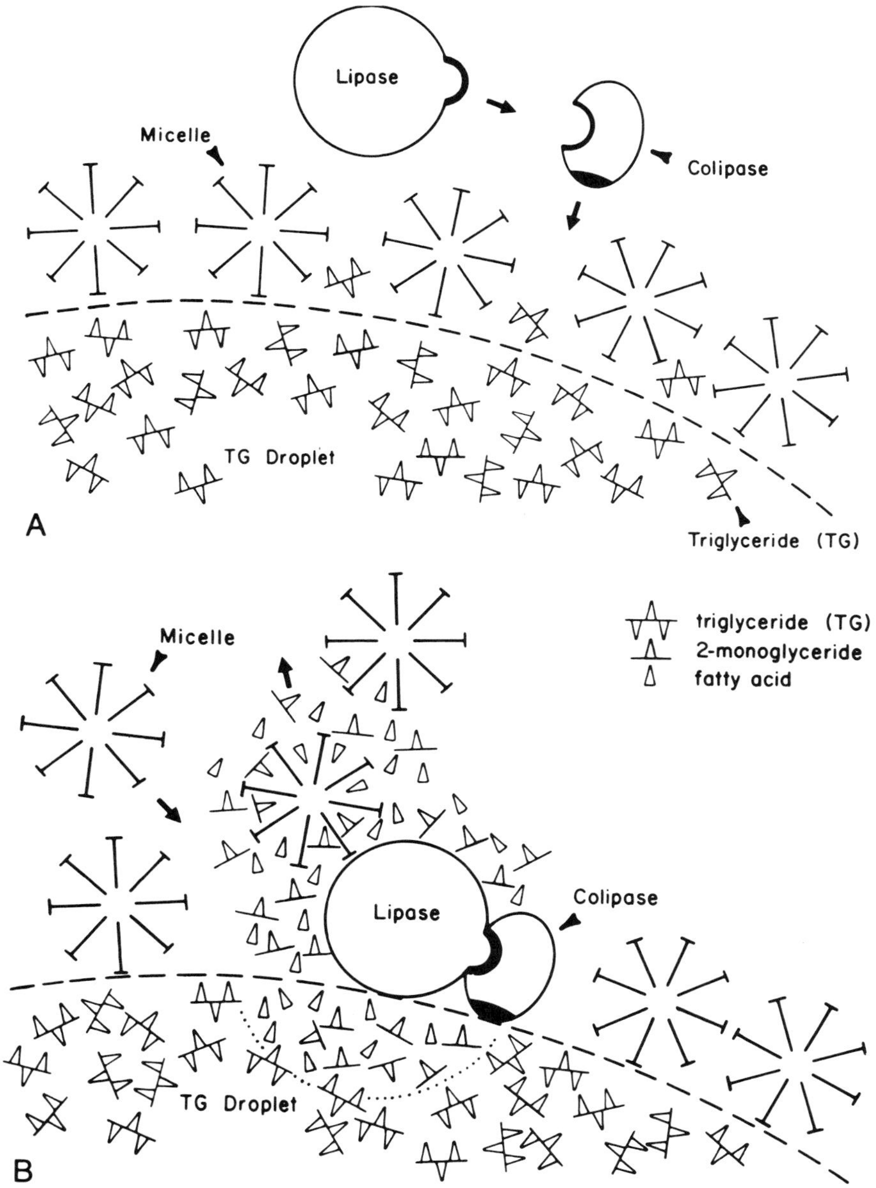
Lipase
Micelle
Colipase
TG Droplet
A
Triglyceride (TG)
triglyceride (TG)
2-monoglyceride
fatty acid
Micelle
Lipase
Colipase
TG Droplet
B

**FIGURE 3–2.** *A*, Bile micelles and their components would prevent access of lipase to its substrate by adhering to the surface of TG droplets. ("Micelle" is the symbol for a bile micelle). *B*, Colipase with a high affinity to TG displaces the micelles and their components and at the same time complexes with the oil phase and the micelles.

and FA takes place at a much higher rate than micellar solubilization. Thus, a new oil phase appears, which consists of droplets of TG, DG in the core, and a rapid increasing fraction of 2-MG and FA on the outside in contact with the aqueous phase.

**Emulsification, Liquid Crystals and Vesicle Formation.** In lipid droplets, an outer layer of emulsifying lipids (MG, FA, biliary PL, and BS) interact with hydrophobic core lipids (TG, DG, CH, and cholesterol ester [CE]). Emulsified particles reach their minimum size when they contain 40% of emulsifying lipids.[38] With further increase in the ratio between emulsifying lipids and core lipids, the emulsifying lipids separate as a coexisting multilamellar liquid-crystalline phase. The latter then change into monolamellar liquid-crystalline vesicles (single bilayered structures, 200 to 600 Å).[38] This process also facilitates hydrolysis by removing the end products of an enzymatic reaction.

As the digestive process proceeds, these vesicles dissolve as their components are incorporated into surrounding micelles. This process is similar to the formation and dissolution of (PL/CH) vesicles in the biliary tract. Formation of these smaller intermediate size particles increases the surface area of the FA- and MG-containing droplets considerably and facilitates incorporation of these compounds into mixed micelles. This relatively new concept has been well supported by in vitro studies of lipid compositions similar to duodenal chyme[38] and studies of duodenal contents obtained from healthy volunteers after administration of a liquid meal.[39]

**Micellar Solubilization.** Pure BS are poor detergents. Mixed bile micelles, however, are efficient detergents because of the presence of PL, which are always secreted simultaneously with BS in relatively fixed molar ratios (1:3). Bile salts are the essential micelle-forming component of the mixed micelles because they are strong amphiphiles.[39] The strong hydrophilic sites are located on one side of the molecule (OH, COOH, $NH_2$) with strongly hydrophobic groups ($CH_2$) on the other side. Their low pKa values (average 3) renders the BS water soluble. The hydrophobic end of the molecule tends to adhere to any hydrophobic surface, and clusters of molecules (micelles) form when the surface is fully covered. The hydrophobic part of the BS is directed toward the core of the aggregate and the hydrophilic sites are located on the outside of the multimolecular sphere.

Micelle formation occurs when a certain concentration of BS has been reached; it is called the critical micellar concentration (CMC). The CMC is different for each BS. The average CMC for the mixture of BS in bile is approximately 2 mmol/L. Physiologic concentrations of BS in intestinal chyme is around 12 mmol/L, but it varies greatly between 2 and 50 mmol/L. Because the highly polar water-soluble BS are poorly absorbed in the proximal small bowel, BS concentrations are sustained in the duodenum and jejunum.

The solubilizing properties of bile micelles for FA and CH are enhanced further by the incorporation of the 2-MG released from the TG by pancreatic lipase. As mentioned, the resistance to hydrolysis of the FA at position 2 by pancreatic lipase actually facilitates micellar solubilization of the lipolytic products. Expanded micelles saturated with MG and FA are still water-soluble macromolecules dispersed throughout the intestinal chyme. Micelles consist of 2 to 40 molecules of BS and can incorporate 2 molecules of mono-olein (less for saturated MG) and 1 molecule of LCFA per mole of BS.[32]

Ionized FA is better solubilized in micelles than protonated FA.[32] The TG and DG are poorly incorporated into the mixed micelles because they have a high partition in the oil phase. The mixed micellar aggregates in bile, consisting of CH, PL, and BS, are in essence macromolecules with a loose, but organized structure determined by attracting and repulsing electromagnetic forces (Van der Waals). The constituents of these aggregates are in continual movement within the micelle and with the aqueous phase. As discussed, these aggregates have the property of incorporating preferentially the two end products of TG lipolysis by pancreatic lipase, 2-MG and FA. Although poorly water soluble, 2-MG and FA can be absorbed as free monomers from the aqueous phase, which is located between the bulk phase and the luminal membrane of the enterocytes (UWL). Uptake thus depends on monomer concentrations in the UWL and on passive diffusion gradients between micelles and cell membranes. No energy-dependent mechanism has been identified.

*Passive Diffusion.* The final step in the digestive phase of absorption, namely, the uptake of free monomers of FA and 2-MG by passive diffusion from a water phase located between micelle and cell membrane, is a rate-limiting step; complicated mechanisms are involved in order to sustain monomer concentrations at the luminal cell surface. To clarify some of these mechanisms, the following discussion includes more details of properties and interactions of the micelles with the oil phase and the cell membrane.

Micelles are called flickering clusters because they are in constant Brownian movement. Their constituents also exchange continuously between the micellar and aqueous phase, thereby sustaining the concentrations of lipid monomers in the intermicellar aqueous phase according to the partition coefficient between the two phases. Because an equilibrium and a fixed ratio exist between the constituents of the micelles and the surrounding aqueous phase, a fast exchange of these constituents between the micelles occurs when micelles move close to each other, thereby changing monomer concentrations in the aqueous phase. Intermicellar concentrations (imc) of monomers of unsaturated micelles are lower than those of the saturated micelles. When the two aggregates come close to each other, monomers move (jump) from the more saturated to the less saturated micelle (through the intermicellar aqueous phase). These movements lead to an equalization of the compositions of the imc and the micelles. Because of their flickering random movements, in combination with the peristaltic movements of the bowel, the intermicellar aqueous phase and the mixed micelles of the intestinal chyme (bulk phase) are saturated with FA and MG because of contact with the different lipid particles saturated with an outer layer of newly formed FA and 2-MG.

Conditions are different in the UWL bordering the mucosal surface. Emulsified oil droplets, because of their large size (25,000 ± 20,000Å), diffuse slowly, compared to the much smaller micelles (30 to 100Å), through the UWL. Micelles, because of their small size and constant movement, migrate into the UWL (thickness 100 to 500 μm in vitro),[41] and, a constant exchange with the micelles in the bulk phase takes place. In contrast to saturation of the intermicellar phase with FA and MG monomers in the bulk phase of the proximal small bowel by the presence of the oil phase of these monomers, no equilibrium phase occurs in the UWL. Almost no oil phase is present, and monomers disappear continually from the aqueous phase across the luminal membrane of the enterocytes. This flow is unidirectional, without back diffusion.[33]

As deduced from the literature and our own observations, we propose the following mechanism for the transport of FA and 2-MG from the surface of their emulsified droplets and other lipid particles in the bulk phase to the cell membrane, as illustrated by Figure 3–3. When imc of monomers decrease, monomers move out of the micelles to establish a new equilibrium according to their partition coefficients. Thus, during absorption, micelles donate their lipid monomers to other micelles and to the cell membrane. Micelles in the UWL, located close to the cell membrane, become partly unsaturated for FA and 2-MG. Depleted micelles are replenished in part by contact with other more saturated micelles and emulsified droplets, creating a kind of chain reaction of monomers jumping from droplets to vesicles, from vesicles to micelles, from micelle to micelle, and from micelle to the cell membrane. As indicated in Figure 3–3, the micelles in the bulk phase are saturated by the presence of excess FA- and MG-containing particles. To date, the rapid exchange of monomers between micelles has been shown,[32] but a chain reaction of monomers jumping from monomer-rich aggregates to less saturated aggregates is difficult to demonstrate. A somewhat similar process, however, has been proposed by Scholander for oxygen transport in hemoglobin solutions when a $pO_2$ gradient is imposed.[42] He postulated that oxygen molecules are handed down from one more saturated hemoglobin molecule to another in a chainlike fashion. Because hemoglobin molecules are large, delivery of oxygen through a shuttle system would be a slower process than a chain reaction of jumping oxygen molecules.

In addition to the transfer of monomers by jumping from micelle to micelle, an exchange of micelles also occurs between the bulk phase and the UWL. This finding led Dietschy to propose a "shuttle system" as the major transport mechanism for lipid monomers.[43] However, micelles move at random and no driving force exists for moving micelles from the bulk phase to the cell membrane or vice versa. Furthermore, the lifetime of a micelle is probably too short for completion of a "shuttle round trip" through the UWL.[44] Dietschy later changed his concept and proposed the possibility of jumping as an additional mechanism of transport, but this concept is difficult to express in a mathematic model.

The most favorable condition for maximal TG absorption by the small bowel mucosa exists in the proximal small bowel, where 2-MG and FA are present in the oil phase as well as in the micellar phase with an aqueous phase practically saturated with monomers.

Although contributing to micellar solubility by expansion of the micelle,[30] PL, mainly lecithin (phosphatidylcholine), inhibit the exchange of monomers between the

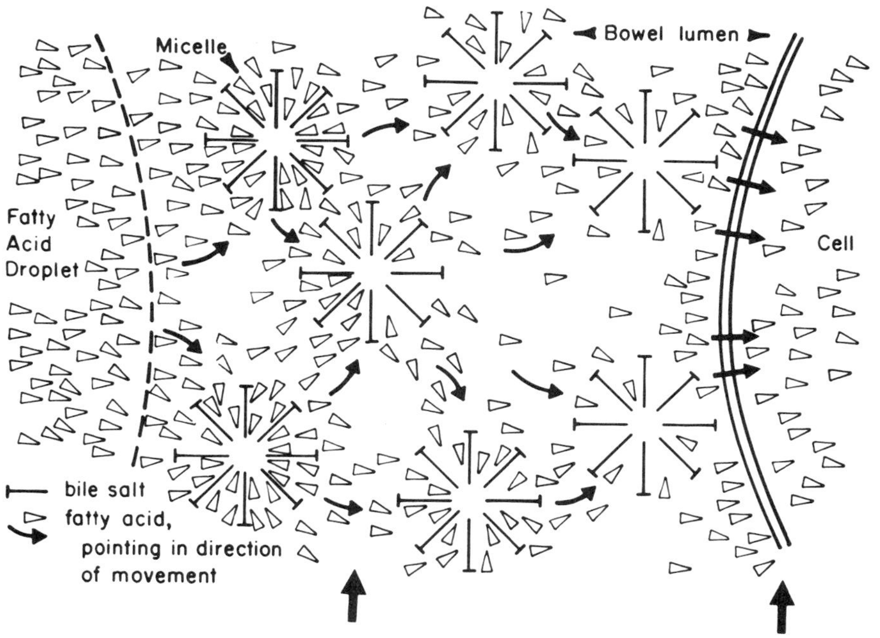
Micelle
Bowel lumen
Fatty Acid Droplet
Cell
bile salt
fatty acid, pointing in direction of movement

**FIGURE 3–3.** Illustration of the transport hypothesis of fatty acids and 2-monoglycerides from the oil droplets to micelles, from the more saturated micelles to the less saturated micelles, and from micelles to cell membrane. The arrows at the base of the figure indicate the unstirred water layer.

micellar and aqueous phase, resulting in decreased monomer activity and FA absorption.[45] However, a phospholipase secreted by the pancreas metabolizes most of the PL to lysoPL (mainly lysolecithin).[46] Lysolecithin does not inhibit monomer activity (monomer activity is an expression of the total amount of protonated FA in solution available for absorption).

From the previous discussion, it is clear that transfer of FA monomers from micelles through the aqueous interface to the cell membrane is optimal when micelles are saturated in the bulk phase. Linscheer demonstrated in the rat that the rate of absorption of oleic acid is proportional to the degree of saturation of micelles with FA[47] (Fig. 3–4). Chijiiwa and Linscheer also demonstrated that the rate of oleic acid absorption from micellar solutions was lower at pH 6.5 than at pH 5.5;[48] more FA could be solubilized at the higher pH than present in the solution, resulting in FA-depleted micelles and decreased monomer activity.[48] These observations have clinical significance, because the pH in the duodenum is lower than in the jejunum. The oil phase also disappears more distally in the jejunum, and micelles become unsaturated for FA and 2-MG. Thus, intraluminal factors are more favorable for lipid absorption in the proximal than in the distal small bowel.

The maximal capability for fat absorption in adults, termed "reserve," is greater than that amount of fat present in an average meal. Relatively independent of the composition of the ingested fat, the average stool fat excretion is 4 to 6 g per day, even when twice the normal amount has been consumed. With an increasing load of fat in adults, absorption is completed somewhat more distally in the small bowel. Newborns, however, have no such reserve, and the source of fat is also important. For infants receiving mother's milk, fat excretion (6% of ingested fat) is similar to that in adults, but infants reared on cow's milk may have, for up to 1 year, a certain degree of fat malabsorption.[49] In contrast to cow's milk, human milk also contains a lipase. This lipase is resistant to gastric acid and pepsin.[21,22]

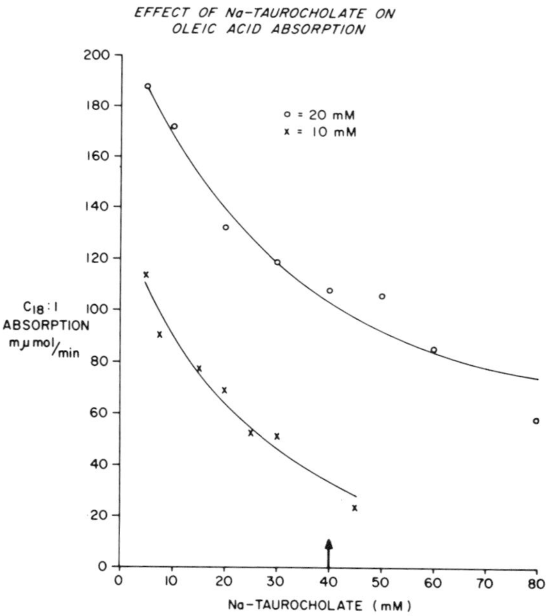
EFFECT OF Na-TAUROCHOLATE ON OLEIC ACID ABSORPTION
o = 20 mM
x = 10 mM
C18:1 ABSORPTION mμmol/min
Na-TAUROCHOLATE (mM)
0
20
40
60
80
100
120
140
160
180
200
10
30
50
70

**FIGURE 3–4.** Rates of absorption by the rat small bowel in vivo (see reference 48 for the technical procedure) at two concentrations of oleic acid (10 mmol (x) and 20 mmol (o) are plotted against increasing concentrations of Na-taurocholate. Micelles become more depleted for fatty acid with increasing concentrations of bile salt.

Babies have a relative deficiency of BS, and the intestinal BS concentration frequently is below the CMC.[50] It is interesting that human milk lipase can hydrolyze the FA from all three positions of the TG. The 2-MG are practically not absorbed without prior micellar solubilization, in contrast to FA the absorption of which is less dependent on micelles.[32] Milk lipase may therefore compensate for the low BS concentrations in the infantile intestinal chyme by completely hydrolyzing TG to FA.

Elderly individuals have a limited capacity for lipid absorption,[51] but because their appetite also decreases, fat intake usually has decreased also. Their reduced fat absorption may manifest clinically as malabsorption of vitamin D; their serum concentrations of vitamin $D_2$ after oral administration of vitamin $D_2$ are lower than in young adults.[51] In addition, the elderly have an increased incidence of achylia gastrica. This condition leads to a higher than normal pH in the proximal duodenum, which further limits the absorption of fat and sterols.[48] This pH effect may also contribute to the mild steatorrhea observed after a partial gastric resection.

## *EFFECTS OF THE NATURE OF TG ON DIGESTION AND ABSORPTION*

**Carbon Chain Length.** The length of the carbon chain of the FA is inversely related to the water solubility and melting point of the TG and their hydrolytic products. Shortening of the chain length increases both the solubility in water and the rate of diffusion in the UWL, thereby increasing the rate of absorption. It also increases the sensitivity of TG to pancreatic lipase, the transfer of hydrolytic products from one particle to the other, and micellar uptake and transport. In addition, rates of hydrolysis are faster and hydrolysis is not limited to the sn-1 and sn-3 position of FA in TG.

A carbon chain length of more than 16 increases the melting point of saturated FA to more than 37°C. Emulsification of solid TG is understandably slower than that of liquid TG. Because FA of various chain length are usually mixed in the diet, total fat absorption is not affected. However, in Australian populations with a high intake of sheep fat, the average 24-hour stool fat is 2 g higher than in the United States.

Practically no short chain FA (SCFA, 2 to 4 carbons) are found in food. The SCFA are formed in the colon of nonruminants, mostly as a result of bacterial metabolism of unabsorbed carbohydrates. Although the small quantities produced have little nutritional value, butyrate can show dramatic effects on cellular differentiation.

**Medium Chain Triglycerides (MCT, C6–C12).** Natural MCT consist of saturated FA with a carbon chain length of 6 to 12 carbon atoms. They occur in milk fat and especially in coconut oil and palm kernel oil. The MCT are fractionated off by margarine manufacturers to increase the melting point of the product. The MCT are retained as a useful byproduct for treatment of patients with fat malabsorption. The advantages of MCT in the intraluminal phase of fat absorption are that they are water soluble, which facilitates emulsification, hydrolysis, and uptake by the intestinal mucosa. The MCFA are also more soluble than LCFA in water, require less BS for solubilization, and diffuse more rapidly through the UWL. Because they are not re-esterified by the enterocyte, they are transported as free FA (bound to albumin) through the portal circulation. The portal flow rate is approximately 250 times faster than lymph flow. Therefore, in comparison with LCT, MCT are digested quickly, require minimal pancreatic lipase activity, and are relatively independent of BS. Because of a different transport mechanism, they are affected only minimally by most metabolic impairments of the enterocytes. They still possess sufficient lipophilic properties for rapid passage through cell membranes. They are not stored in fat depots,[52-55] but rather are largely oxidized to acetic acid. It is therefore not surprising that they can be applied successfully for treatment of most forms of fat maldigestion and malabsorption and in some forms of hyperlipidemia. Side effects related to differences in metabolism are discussed elsewhere.

**Very Long Chain Fatty Acids (C20 and More).** In some parts of the world, edible oils (rapeseed, mustard seed, and fish oils) with a high percentage of very LCFA (C20 and more) are produced and consumed as a natural oil or after (partial) hydrogenation. In addition to di-homo-γ-linolenic acid (C20:3, n-6, 9, 12) and arachidonic acid (C20:4, n-6, 9,12, 15), which occur in TG of animals only in limited amounts (less than 2%), other natural FA with 20 or more carbon atoms and with terminal *cis* double bonds at either the n-3 or the n-9 position can also be present. Peanut oil has a relatively high amount (5 to 10%) of saturated FA with 20 to 24 carbon atoms.

Erucic acid (C22:1 n-9) is present in mustard seed oil (more than 50%) and in many conventional varieties of rapeseed oil (Brassica napus and B. campestris) (20 to 50%), an oil used widely in the margarine industry. Genetic selection of rapeseed oil has led to varieties with less than 1% erucic acid, thereby reducing the risk of potentially harmful side effects. However, in India, Pakistan, and China, rapeseed and other edible cruciferous oils high in C20:1 n-9 and C22:1 n-9 are still being produced. These FA are slowly absorbed and metabolized (see *Metabolism and Transport*).

Marine oils[27] (see Table 3–1) contain up to 50% FA with 20 and more carbon atoms. Many of these oils have 4 to 6 *cis* double bonds starting at n-3 (except some species in such tropical areas as North Australia) and are remarkably high in arachidonic acid, C20:4 n-6. Consumption of fish, seal, and whale oils can lead to high intakes of especially C20:5 n-3 and C22:6 n-3; these are efficiently absorbed, in contrast to saturated and monounsaturated FA of the same chain length, probably because of a lower hydrolysis rate and a higher rate of *trans* esterification to sn-2 MG.[56]

As a side product of the fish meal industry, reasonably large quantities of fish oil are produced (more than $10^6$ tons/year). Fish oil, after partial hydrogenation to improve preservation and melting characteristics, is used in some margarines, shortening, and bakery products.[1,3] Some types of herring, menhaden, and eel oils have about 20% C22:1 n-II, an isomer of C22:1 n-9 (erucic acid). Because of hydrogenation, a whole range of *cis*- and *trans*-isomers with 1 or 2 double bonds is produced, yielding an extremely complicated FA composition.

The very LCFA, and particularly the unsaturated FA, are of great interest because of their extensive use in the margarine industry, differences in absorption and metabolism, and abnormal hydrolysis. These unusual properties can be responsible for a series of interesting pathophysiologic effects, as described subsequently.

**Position of FA on the sn-2 Position.** The MG are better absorbed than FA, and the rates of absorption of FA with a carbon chain length of greater than 18 increase when this FA is located on the sn-2 position. During hydrolysis, FA with more than 20 carbon atoms frequently shift to the sn-2 position, which facilitates their absorption.

**Double Bonds.** Properties of FA are also affected by the presence of double bonds between carbon atoms. Unsaturation lowers the melting point and increases water solubility, which have a similar effect as shortening the carbon chain length. However, TG with C20:5 n-3 and other unsaturated very LCFA are more resistant to pancreatic lipase.[56] The specific effects of unsaturated FA (carbon chain length of 20 or less) on lipid and CH metabolism are discussed elsewhere in this chapter.

## PHOSPHOLIPIDS

Dietary phospholipids (PL) play only a minor role in the digestive process, because the average diet contains approximately only 2 g (mainly from legumes and egg yolk).[11] However, about 12 g are secreted in bile,[38] which plays an essential role in the micellar solubilization of endogenous as well as exogenous CH and solubilizes FA and 2-MG. The role of pancreatic phospholipase A on the absorption of TG has received little attention. The PL, consisting primarily of lecithin, is so efficient in solubilizing 2-MG and FA in the mixed micelles that it inhibits the monomer activity of FA and 2-MG and thereby their rates of absorption.[45] However, pancreatic phospholipase A hydrolyzes PL to lysoPL, which does not inhibit monomer activity or absorption.

In contrast to TG lipase, which hydrolyzes positions 1 and 3 of TG, phospholipase $A_2$ hydrolyzes the FA primarily at position 2. Lysolecithin is an active and potentially toxic molecule, particularly in combination with BS, and it may cause reflux gastritis and pancreatitis when refluxed into the pancreatic duct. Hydrolysis of lecithin is a slower process than hydrolysis of TG. In contrast to lecithin, lysolecithin is well absorbed. It is re-esterified in part after uptake by the enterocyte and used by the cell for chylomicron formation. It is also further hydrolyzed in part by phospholipase $A_1$ (Fig. 3–5).

The PL are secreted in bile in a relatively stable ratio with BS (1:3), and isolated PL deficiencies as a cause of maldigestion are extremely rare. Its main functions in the absorptive process are as follows: (1) emulsifying TG droplets and various mixed lipid particles; (2) solubilizing endogenous and exogenous CH in mixed micelles (preventing gallstone formation and facilitating CH absorption); (3) facilitating micellar solubilization of lipolytic products, steroids, and fat-soluble vitamins; (4) facilitating transport of TG in the intestinal mucosa; and (5) forming vesicles of PL and CH in bile and of PL, MG, and FA in the intestinal lumen. Because secretion of BS and PL by the hepatocyte is always coordinated, biliary BS deficiency is with few exceptions associated with PL deficiency.

## CHOLESTEROL

In contrast to dietary cholesterol (CH), which is dissolved into mixed micelles in the gut, biliary CH is solubilized in part into micelles and in part into PL vesicles (a relatively new concept). Vesicles then dissolve into the mixed micelles. Physiologic malabsorption of CH (50%) is related to its poor micellar solubility.

Like PL, a mixture of exogenous and endogenous CH is absorbed from the intestinal lumen. In contrast to

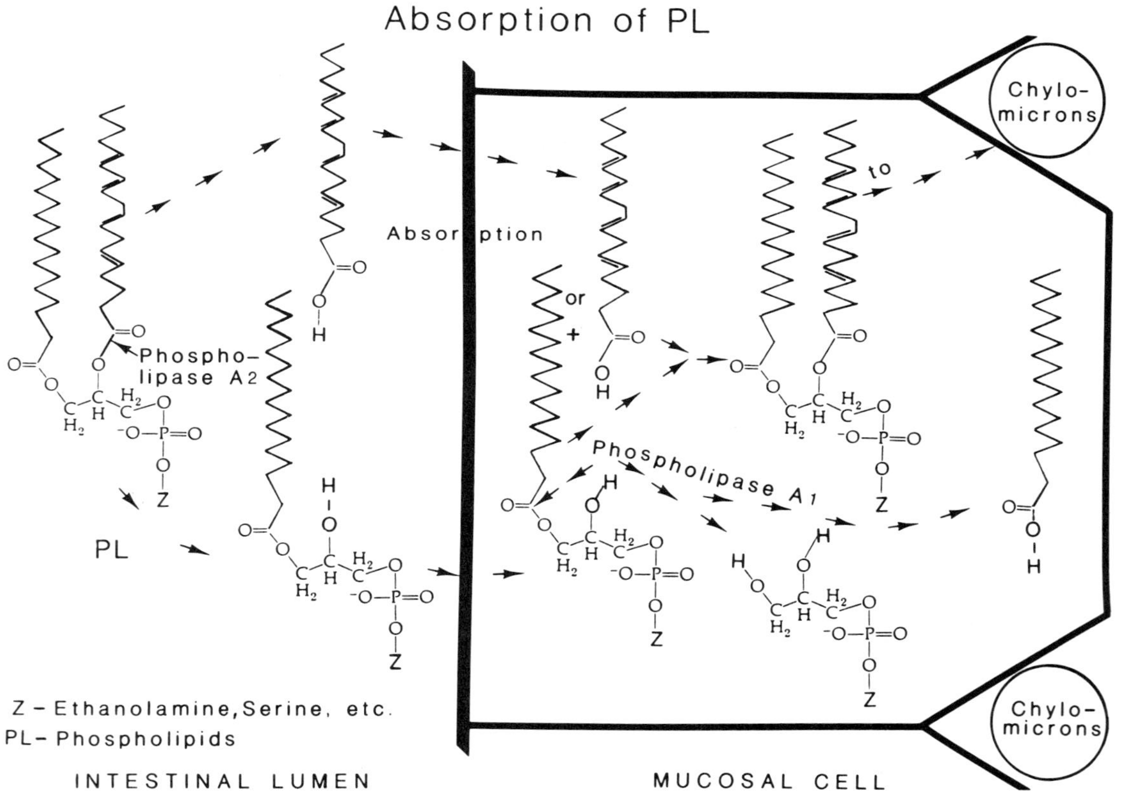
Absorption of PL
Chylo-
microns
to
Absorption
or
+
Phospho-
lipase A2
Phospholipase A1
PL
Z - Ethanolamine, Serine, etc.
PL - Phospholipids
INTESTINAL LUMEN
MUCOSAL CELL
Chylo-
microns

**FIGURE 3–5.** Most of the phospholipids (PL) in the intestinal lumen consist of lecithin (phosphatidyl-choline). Lecithin is poorly absorbed, but pancreatic phospholipase $A_2$ hydrolyzes the unsaturated fatty acid (FA) in the No. 2 position, and the hydrolytic products—lysolecithin and FA—are readily absorbed. Inside the enterocyte the lysolecithin is partly reacylated with an unsaturated FA by lysophosphatidyl choline acyltransferase, the magnitude of which seems to be related to the need for phospholipid for the assembly and transport of chylomicrons. The rest of the absorbed lecithin is further metabolized by hydrolysis of the saturated FA in the No. 1 position by phospholipase $A_1$.

endogenous CH, food CH is esterified in part. Like TG, esterified CH (CE) is not water soluble and cannot be incorporated into micelles. Like TG, it is also hydrolyzed in the intestinal lumen (by an pancreatic esterase), although this process is slower than that for TG. The rate of absorption of CH is also lower than that of FA and MG. In contrast to TG, which are also absorbed in the distal jejunum when a high load is ingested, little absorption of CH takes place in the distal one half of the small bowel. Reasons for the poor absorption of CH are: (1) micellar solubility decreases sharply in the distal jejunum because the lipid oil phase, in which most of the CH is partitioned, disappears; (2) the absorption of FA, MG, and lysolecithin has been completed and pure BS are poor detergents; and (3) CH then precipitates. More CH precipitates when BS are actively absorbed by the distal ileum.

Predictably, exogenous CH absorption depends on the amount of TG in the meal, because it is partitioned in oily emulsions. Because CH is present in all tissues of vertebrates (and some invertebrates, such as the crustaceans crab and shrimp, and higher mollusks, squid), carnivores not surprisingly ingest appreciable quantities of CH (see Fig. 3–1). Not only food but also the bile and, to some extent, the intestine itself (by de novo synthesis of CH and by desquamation of mucosal cells) contribute to the CH available for absorption. The intestinal CH pool is heterogeneous; biliary CH, for example, is absorbed more effectively than dietary CH.[57]

In rats, biliary CH is absorbed primarily in the proximal one half of the small bowel, but dietary CH is absorbed in the distal one half.[58] The absorption and metabolism of CH in the rat is in many respects different from other species. As an example, food has a long transit time in the rat bowel. Although these observations suggest better absorption of endogenous CH, actually only slightly more endogenous than exogenous CH is absorbed. Several investigators, using an isotopic-equilibrium method,[59,60] concluded that in normal human subjects, the maximal capacity for absorbing dietary CH is about 300 to 500 mg per day. Other authors, using combined chemical and isotope balance methods, have shown that 30 to 40% of dietary CH is absorbed in most men over an intake range of 40 mg per day to more than 2 g per day.[61-64] Although disagreement exists about the percentage of CH absorption, all investigators agree that only part of the CH of both origins is absorbed.

The fact that CH is absorbed only by means of micellar solubilization may explain the relatively poor absorption of exogenous CH in healthy subjects, but it does not explain why endogenous CH is also poorly absorbed. Chijiiwa and Linscheer's observation that absorption rates of CH are higher when perfused at the lower pH of the duodenum and proximal jejunum than at the higher pH in the distal part of the small bowel[65] suggests that a high pH may be a contributing factor to CH malabsorption in the distal small bowel. The physiologic malabsorption of CH is essential for the intestinal excretion mechanism of CH. Cholesterol is also the substrate for BS synthesis, but reabsorption of BS is highly efficient and the amount of BS excreted in feces (400 mg) is not the main excretory pathway of CH.

Because no evidence indicates that significant amounts of CH are absorbed from an emulsified oil phase, it seems likely that one of the rate-limiting factors in the absorption of CH is micellar solubilization. The absorption of CH is facilitated by the TG in the diet, because it improves CH uptake by expansion of the biliary micelles.

The intake of CH (0.5 to 1 g per day) accounts for only a small fraction of the total CH transported. Because its contribution to the pool is small, no saturation is apparent for the absorption of dietary CH. Although individual responses of blood CH show variations when animals and men are exposed to increased amounts of dietary CH, and some may even show no clear change,[61] most subjects react with an increase in concentrations of blood (and tissue).[56,60,66,67] Apparently, the augmented absorption is not fully compensated by the reduction of endogenous CH synthesis and by the increased excretion in the bile, because serum CH levels increase in most people by 15% on a high-CH diet.

Another consequence of the limited absorption of a high dietary CH load is the increased concentration of excreted CH and its bacterial degradation products in the colon and rectum, which may have carcinogenic effects. High CH diets are usually low in (vegetable) fibers, however, and are associated with long intestinal transit times and reduced fecal bulk; these factors might well contribute to the (epidemiologically) observed association between high-saturated fat, high-CH, low-fiber diets and colon cancer.

Plant sterols diminish the absorption of CH in animals, presumably because of their competition with CH for incorporation into micelles and for transport across the intestinal mucosa.[5] Absorption of β-sitosterol, a sterol similar in its molecular composition to CH, is less than 5% of a single oral dose in vivo, but its uptake in vitro[68] (inverted sac experiments) is remarkably similar to CH. The enterocytes apparently have an effective selective ability for absorption of sterols in vivo. In some patients with β-sitosterolemia, absorption is increased to about 30%.[69] This rare familial storage disease is characterized by tendon xanthomas, tuberous lesions of the skin, and substantial amounts of plant sterols in plasma, adipose tissue, and erythrocytes, even though plasma concentrations of CH are normal. The accumulation of plant sterols is most likely caused by the loss of normal intestinal selectivity for the absorption of CH rather than by their endogenous synthesis, inasmuch as animal tissue lacks the ability to alkylate the sterol side chain at the C24 position.[4]

Further study of this rare disease might give a better understanding of the development of the more common CH-containing xanthomas at an early age despite near normal concentrations of plasma CH. The intestinal absorption specificity for CH is unlikely to be related to differences in incorporation in micelles, because β-sitosterol and CH have the same partition coefficients between the oil and micellar phases.[64] It is not known whether the specificity is related to the transportation of the sterol into the mucosa, to its intracellular esterification, or to its incorporation into TG-rich lipoproteins (VLDL and chylomicrons). The presence of BS in the bowel lumen seems to be essential for re-esterification inside the enterocytes and for mucosal transport of CH. The poor intestinal absorption of β-sitosterol is used to measure bacterial degradation of sterols in the intestinal tract, which is a necessary step in the combined chemical and isotopic balance studies performed to determine CH absorption in man.[4,57]

Many of the studies reported so far revealed wide variations, intra- and interindividually, with respect to the amount of CH that is degraded; figures of 10 to 500 mg of CH per day have been published.

In summary, approximately one half of the CH in the bowel lumen is of endogenous origin. About 40 to 50% of the CH is absorbed from the bowel lumen. A CH-rich diet increases the CH pool, including higher blood CH levels. Human beings can regulate their blood CH with little variation. Although blood CH increases approximately 15% in response to a high-CH diet, most of the serum CH is of endogenous origin. Thus, the serum CH level is regulated mainly by endogenous synthesis. However, in the long run, a diet low in CH and saturated fats with limited amounts of animal protein leads to significantly lower serum CH levels in a high percentage of the population.[1,2,66]

## MALDIGESTION AND MALABSORPTION

### *FAT ABSORPTION IN THE NEWBORN*

In contrast to adults, newborns have little reserve capacity for lipid absorption. The amount of fecal fat is 4 to 6% of the intake while receiving mother's milk. Infants show a mild fat malabsorption when ingesting cow's milk. Thus, newborns need to cope with some basic physiologic differences as compared to adults. Pancreatic lipase activity and BS secretion are still too low to digest LCT completely. In contrast to human milk, cow's milk does not contain lipase and human milk is richer in MCT.

### *GASTRIC SURGERY*

Gastric resections, particularly the Billroth II resection, interfere with the following physiologic functions of the stomach: (1) reservoir function for hydrolysis by lingual and gastric lipase; (2) portion-wise delivery of gastric chyme to the duodenum, as regulated by pH adjustment in the duodenum; (3) lack of acidification of gastric chyme; (4) reduced duodenal release of CCK and secretin, because the duodenum is bypassed; and (5) acidification of gastric chyme. Patients with a partial gastric resection rarely regain their preoperative body weight and frequently have mild fat malabsorption (approximately 15 g of stool fat per 24 hours instead of 4 to 6 g).[70] Loss of acidity tends to enhance bacterial growth, which interferes with digestion. Low gastric acidity also inhibits, by means of too alkaline a pH, the intestinal absorption of FA and CH. As discussed previously, micellar solutions of FA and CH have higher monomer activity and rate of absorption at a pH of 5.5 than at a pH of 6.5.[48]

### *GASTRIC HYPERACIDITY*

Some gastrin-secreting malignancies (Zollinger-Ellison syndrome) induce hypersecretion of hydrochloric acid by the gastric mucosa, which interferes with neutralization of chyme in the duodenum. As a consequence, lipid hydrolysis is inhibited and micellar solubility is reduced in the proximal small bowel, resulting in steatorrhea and diarrhea.[71]

### *LIPASE DEFICIENCY*

Although lack of lingual lipase activity causes malabsorption in rats,[72] it is unlikely to induce malabsorption in the adult human, because pancreatic lipase is secreted in excessive amounts. Deficiency of pancreatic lipase is of clinical significance only when its secretion is below 10 to 15% of normal levels. Frequently, insufficient pancreatic function interferes also with bicarbonate secretion; hence, gastric chyme will not be adequately neutralized in the proximal small bowel. The abnormally low pH that results interferes with lipase activity. Part of the unabsorbed TG is split by bacterial lipases in the colon,[73] but LCFA are poorly absorbed by the colon.[74] These unsaturated FA, and particularly the hydroxy-FA, change the permeability of the colonic mucosa, resulting in an influx of water into the bowel lumen, causing diarrhea. Steatorrhea caused by pancreatic insufficiency can be treated by fat restriction, oral lipase, with or without alkali, or of inhibitors of gastric acid secretion, or by substitution of LCT by MCT.

### *BILE SALT DEFICIENCY*

Deficiency in BS caused by ileal dysfunction, ileectomy, or liver disease interferes with the transport mechanism of lipolytic products and inhibits lipase activity. Diarrhea caused by fat malabsorption is potentiated by concomitant BS malabsorption (ile-ectomy, nonfunctioning ileum). Dihydroxy BS have an effect similar to FA on the permeability of the colonic mucosa in man.[75]

Deconjugation of BS by bacterial overgrowth in the proximal small bowel also interferes with micellar solubilization of hydrolytic products of lipolysis. The cause of fat maldigestion should be analyzed carefully. Proper treatment, although usually effective, is with a few exceptions only symptomatic; thus, the patient may require lifelong treatment.

Most maldigestion syndromes interfere with, but never totally prevent, fat absorption, primarily because more than one hydrolase is available for digestion and BS rarely are totally absent from the intestinal lumen. Furthermore, although micellar solubilization facilitates absorption, part of the hydrolytic products still reach the intestinal mucosa by diffusion of monomers released from oily emulsions. The slower rate of absorption is thereby compensated for by the excess capacity of the small bowel.

The mucosal malfunction syndromes can be divided into several categories: malfunction of fat uptake (inflammation and mucosal impairment; for example, sprue syndromes and Crohn's disease), decreased surface area (short bowel syndromes), and transport defects (reduced chylomicron formation or bacterial interference with cellular transport, as seen in Whipple's disease). Details about analytic procedures and treatment of these syndromes are discussed in other chapters.

A combination of maldigestion and malabsorption may occur in elderly individuals. However, because so much reserve exists in the digestive system and the intake of fat usually is decreased in older people, clinical fat malabsorption is rare in this population without complicating factors like ischemia of the upper intestine.

## TRANSPORT AND METABOLISM

Absorbed lipids are transported in water-soluble form from the small intestine to other tissues. The FA with chain lengths shorter than 14 C atoms are bound to albumin and preferentially transported directly to the liver by way of the portal vein.

Only a small proportion of the MCFA undergoes a conversion to LCFA and is esterified to TG.[76] Because these FA are not neutralized by re-esterification and are metabolized rapidly, some patients treated with MCT may become acidotic. A small fraction of LCFA is transported by the portal route. This fraction increases when LCT are fed in combination with MCT.

Lipids absorbed from the intestinal lumen consist of FA, 2-MG, lysoPL, some PL, and small amounts of glycerol and CH. Some of these lipid fractions (like LCFA and lysolecithin) are reactive molecules and may lyse cell membranes. The first step in mucosal transport is re-esterification; the second step is synthesis of transport particles, the so-called lipoprotein particles.

### RE-ESTERIFICATION OF TG AND PL

The re-esterification pathways of TG and PL are inter-related. Most TG are resynthesized in the enterocytes by the monoacylglycerol pathway. The FA are activated in the microsomes by fatty acyl: CoA synthase to yield acyl-CoA. Absorbed 2-MG are acylated to form DG and then TG at the endoplasmic reticulum by the action of mono- and diglyceride acyltransferases. The activities of these transacylases is high at the tip of the villi and relatively low in the crypt cells. The second pathway, accounting for 20% of enterocytic TG, is the α-glycerophosphate pathway. α-Glycerophosphate is synthesized de novo from triose phosphate and from absorbed free glycerol. Phosphatidic acid is formed and then dephosphorylated, resulting in a 1,2-diglyceride, which is then esterified to TG. Part of the phosphatidic acid is metabolized into PL, which participate in chylomicron formation. Another minor pathway for the formation of phosphatidic acid is the dihydroxyacetone phosphate pathway.[77] The ratio of TG formed from exogenous sources to that formed from endogenous substrates depends on the amount of exogenous TG present, as discussed elsewhere in this chapter. After ingestion of a high TG meal, more phosphatidic acid is used for PL synthesis because concentrations of PL in the chylomicron are relatively constant (7% in the rat).

### ESTERIFICATION OF CHOLESTEROL

Cholesterol is transported by the chylomicrons in two forms: as free CH, which largely is in the hydrophilic outer layer, and as CE, which mainly resides in the hydrophobic core. Cholesterol is esterified in the mucosa shortly before the chylomicron enters the lymph through the lateral leaky cell membrane of the enterocyte. Esterification is accomplished by incorporation of acyl-CoA into the CH molecule by the microsomal acyl-CoA-cholesterol acyltransferase.

### PRINCIPLES OF INTRAVASCULAR TRANSPORT

Of the three main classes of lipids (TG, PL, and CH), the TG are used primarily as a fuel or are stored in fat depots. The PL and CH are the principal constituents of plasma and biomembranes and also participate in intracellular transport as constituents of micelles and emulsified particles. They are also secreted with BS as mixed micelles into the canicular bile.

Because most of the energy for muscle contractions (including the heart muscle) in the fasting state is supplied by oxidation of FA released by adipose tissue, a continuous uptake of FA from the circulation takes place. In the nonfasting state, FA are derived from chylomicrons and VLDL under the influence of lipoprotein lipase.

Like enterocytes, endothelial cells cannot take in TG, but they do absorb MG and FA. The TG-containing LDL, HDL, and chylomicron remnants, however, can pass through the endothelial gaps and be taken up by pinocytosis. The FA bound to albumin are taken up rapidly by the endothelium. The major source of FA is the TG present in the circulating lipoprotein particles. Although located in the lipid core of the lipoprotein particle, TG are an accessible substrate for lipoprotein lipase present at the surface of the endothelial membrane and also to a hepatic lipase secreted by the liver.

## LYMPHATIC VERSUS PORTAL VENOUS TRANSPORT

Previous studies dating back to the 1950s showed that only 50% of the lipids absorbed from the gut could be recovered in the lymph. Mansbach et al.,[78] in a surprising observation, showed that more than 30% of absorbed LCT was transported by the portal vein, and mostly as TG. Other investigators had reported that only a small percentage of LCFA was transported by the portal route, although this percentage was considerably higher for the unsaturated FA. One of the major contributions of these findings of Mansbach et al. is that absorbed lipids are carried in the portal blood as TG incorporated in lipoprotein particles. Entry of the lipoproteins to blood capillaries is facilitated by an increase of the capillary pores to 300 Å during fat absorption.

Another remarkable finding was the large increase of endogenous TG in portal blood during lipid absorption. Endogenous TG, presumably synthesized in the intestinal endoplasmic reticulum, accounted for most of the increase of lipids in portal blood as compared to concentrations in arterial blood. If the results of these rat experiments can be extrapolated to man, as appears likely, the absorption of dietary fat from the small intestine would stimulate the formation of and release into the circulation of considerable amounts of endogenous fat. It lends credence to the concept that dietary fat restriction has an antiatherogenic effect, even if the ingested fat consists primarily of unsaturated FA, because any ingested TG stimulates synthesis of endogenous FA consisting primarily of saturated FA, like palmitic and stearic acids.

Discovery of these new concepts in the physiology of fat metabolism and transport required accurate measurement of tiny changes in lipid concentrations of portal blood. Although subtle in comparison to lymph, they account for considerable changes in mass movement, because the portal blood flow rate is 250 times faster than lymphatic flow. Modern techniques, like the availability of tiny sonographic probes for measuring flow rates, and better analytic methods contributed greatly to the elucidation of this problem.

## CHYLOMICRONS AND VERY LOW-DENSITY AND LOW-DENSITY LIPOPROTEINS

The long-chain dietary TG are not transported from the intestinal mucosal cells until chylomicrons have been formed. These consist of about 86% TG, 8.5% PL, 3% CH, and CH ester, and 2% protein. Some evidence shows that apo-B proteins in intestinal VLDL and chylomicrons are different from those in liver VLDL. Up to 20% of total VLDL is synthesized in the intestine and carries exogenous lipids, whereas liver VLDL contains only endogenous FA. The apoproteins of the two intestinal lipoproteins are different from liver VLDL in that they contain apo-B 48 instead of apo-B 100 and do not react with the apo-B 100 receptors of peripheral cells. The intestinal VLDL and chylomicrons exchange components with HDL particles during lymphatic transport and blood circulation. The apo-C and E transferred from the high-density lipoproteins (HDL) are essential for the metabolism of the intestinal chylomicron particles, primarily because apo-C is the cofactor for lipoprotein lipase activation, and apo-E, remaining in the chylomicron remnants, is essential for its uptake by the hepatocyte by binding to the apo-E receptors to initiate endocytosis. Lipoprotein lipase not only hydrolyzes TG but also the PL to lysoPL. As illustrated by Figure 3–6, hydrolysis affects particle size. Thus, FA and MG in the circulation originate from exogenous and endogenous sources. Normal individuals have a large reserve of TG in their fat depots and can tolerate prolonged periods of fasting. The constant exchange of surface materials and apolipoproteins, donated by the HDL to chylomicrons and VLDL particles in exchange for PL, induce complicated changes in the properties of the lipoprotein particles and regulate binding to the specific apoprotein binding sites located on the membranes of various cell systems. Transportation of CH and the role of esterification by the lecithin-cholesterol acyltransferase (LCAT) system by transfer of FA from PL is discussed elsewhere.

In short, the principal vehicles for transport of TG from the gut to tissues through lymph and blood circulation to the liver, fat depots, and muscles are the chylomicrons and intestinal VLDL, whereas hepatic VLDL and LDL function primarily as an internal transport mechanism for TG, PL, and CH. Worthy of a more detailed discussion are the interactions among the lipoproteins as affected by exchange or transfer of their constituents, hormones, and enzymes (Fig. 3–7). Alimentary lipemia starts 1 to 2 hours after ingestion of fat, reaches a maximum at 3 to 5 hours, and decreases to reach fasting levels usually by 8 to 10 hours. Hydrolysis of TG in chylomicrons and VLDL is catalyzed by lipoprotein lipase, an enzyme situated in part at the luminal surface of the endothelium, but also present in fat cells. The liver also secretes a lipase into plasma that can hydrolyze lipoprotein TG, but it has different properties from lipoprotein lipase or lipase of endothelial and adipose tissue cells. Lipoprotein lipase activity in blood is affected by many circulating compounds.[79,80] As stated previously, apo-C 2 activates lipoprotein lipase. Because heparin in small doses releases lipoprotein lipase from the surface of endothelial cells into plasma, heparin of endogenous origin may be an important regulating mechanism in the circulation of this enzyme. Furthermore, insulin has a definite stimulating effect on lipoprotein lipase activity, which explains the high incidence of hypertriglyceridemia in uncompensated diabetes mellitus. The earliest effect of insulin on adipose tissue lipoprotein lipase appears to be enhanced

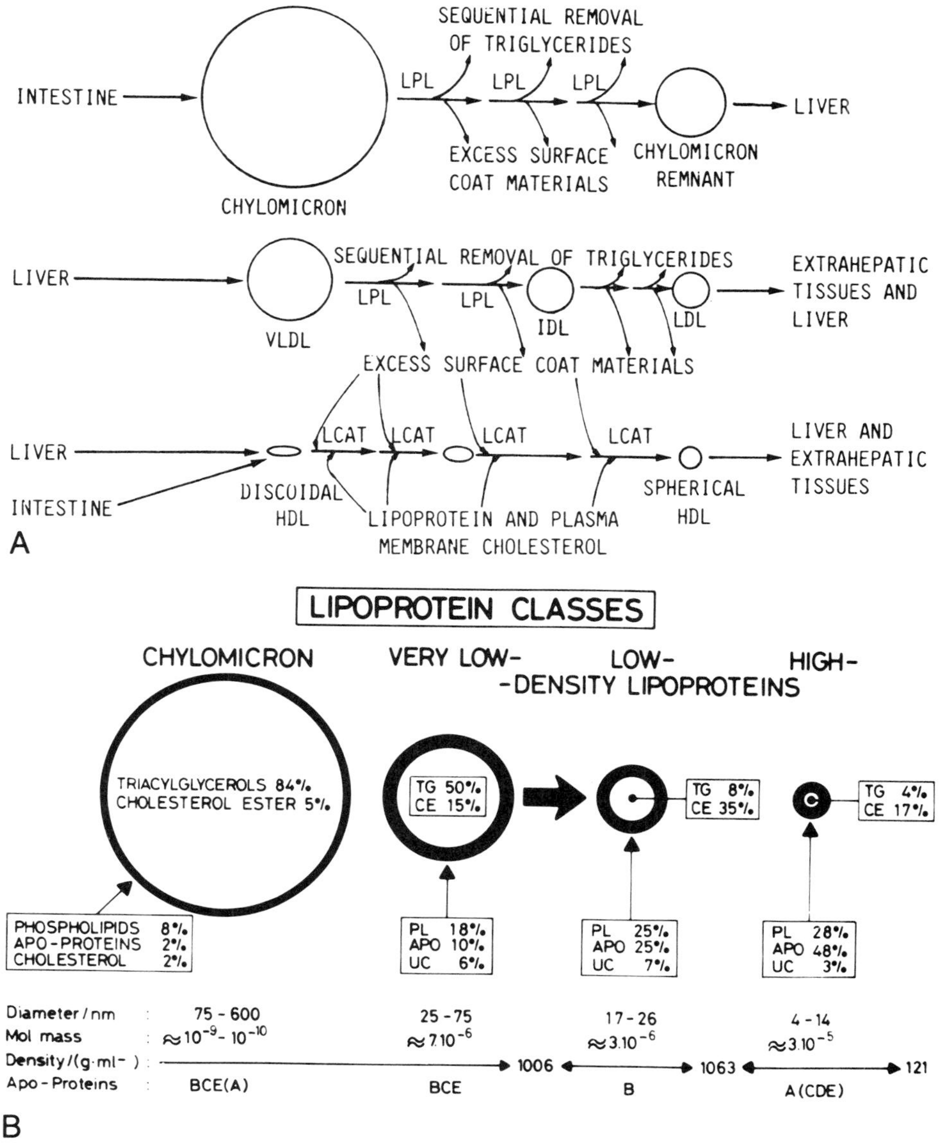
SEQUENTIAL REMOVAL
OF TRIGLYCERIDES
INTESTINE
LPL
LPL
LPL
LIVER
EXCESS SURFACE
COAT MATERIALS
CHYLOMICRON
REMNANT
CHYLOMICRON
LIVER
SEQUENTIAL REMOVAL OF TRIGLYCERIDES
EXTRAHEPATIC
TISSUES AND
LIVER
VLDL
IDL
LDL
EXCESS SURFACE COAT MATERIALS
LIVER
LCAT
LIVER AND
EXTRAHEPATIC
TISSUES
INTESTINE
DISCOIDAL
HDL
SPHERICAL
HDL
LIPOPROTEIN AND PLASMA
MEMBRANE CHOLESTEROL
A
LIPOPROTEIN CLASSES
CHYLOMICRON
VERY LOW-
LOW-
HIGH-
-DENSITY LIPOPROTEINS
TRIACYLGLYCEROLS 84%
CHOLESTEROL ESTER 5%
TG 50%
CE 15%
TG 8%
CE 35%
TG 4%
CE 17%
C
PHOSPHOLIPIDS 8%
APO-PROTEINS 2%
CHOLESTEROL 2%
PL 18%
APO 10%
UC 6%
PL 25%
APO 25%
UC 7%
PL 28%
APO 48%
UC 3%
Diameter/nm : 75 - 600 25 - 75 17 - 26 4 - 14
Mol mass : ≈10^-9 - 10^-10 ≈7.10^-6 ≈3.10^-6 ≈3.10^-5
Density/(g·ml⁻) : 1006 1063 121
Apo-Proteins : BCE(A) BCE B A(CDE)
B

**FIGURE 3–6.** *A*, Schematic representation of lipid transport processes. (From Nishida, T.: *In* Dietary Fats and Health. Edited by E.J. Perkins and W.J. Visek. Champaign, IL, American Oil Chemists' Society, 1983.) *B*, Composition of lipoprotein particles.

secretion of the enzyme by adipocytes.[81] This change leads to increased extracellular activity. Nicotinic acid also activates lipoprotein lipase, but glucagon, adrenocorticotropic hormone, and thyroid stimulating hormone (TSH) inhibit it. In general, its activity is decreased by several hormones with high activity in the fasting state.

The FA of chylomicron and VLDL TG are taken up by extrahepatic tissues and used for: (1) energy production, especially by the heart, red muscle fibers, smooth muscle cells, kidney, and platelets; (2) incorporation into phospholipids of all cellular biomembranes; the FA composition determines to a great extent biomembrane function and integrity, as well as biosynthesis of PG, thromboxanes (TXA), and leukotrienes (LT); and (3) stored energy by its deposition in adipose tissues as TG.

The types of dietary FA determine to a great extent whether they can be used for function 1, 2, or 3. Saturated and monounsaturated FA with chain lengths of 20 carbon atoms or more cannot be used optimally for function 1[82] and MCFA cannot be used for function 3. The FA composition of endogenous TG, transported mainly in VLDL, is nonetheless affected indirectly by dietary composition, because the latter determines adipose tissue composition and the degree of FA biosynthesis from carbohydrates by the liver. Endogenous FA mainly

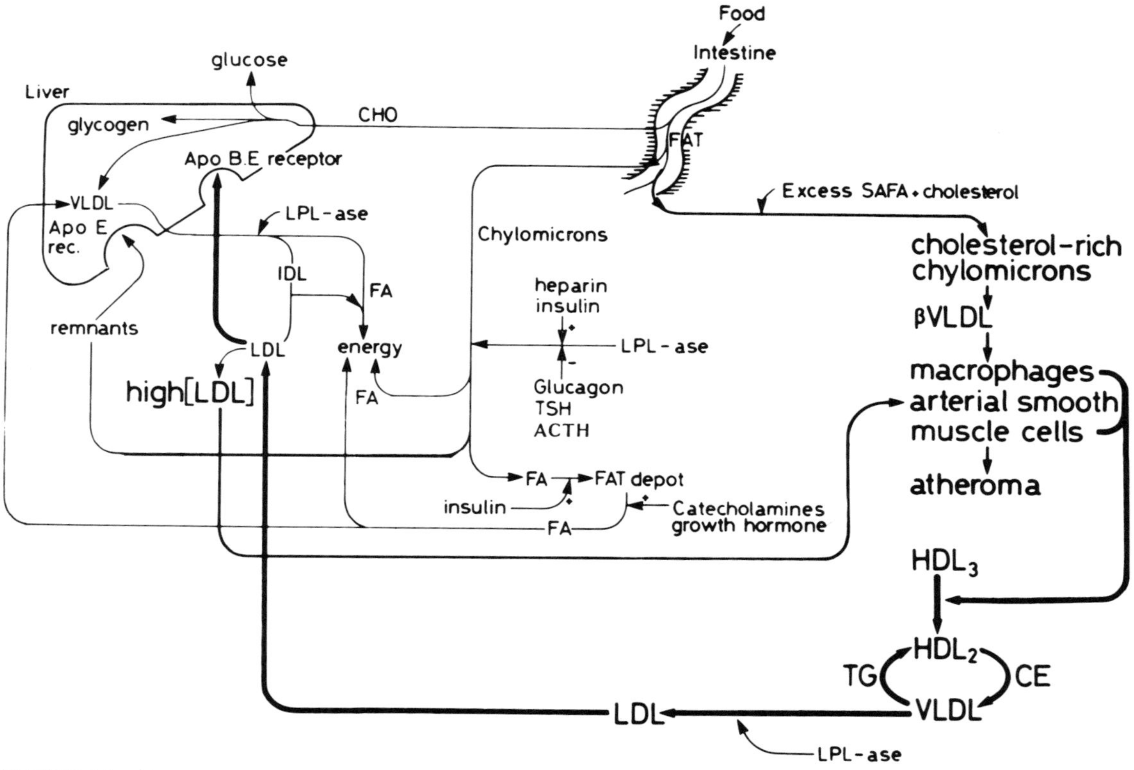
Food
Intestine
glucose
Liver
glycogen
CHO
FAT
Apo B.E receptor
VLDL
Apo E rec.
LPL-ase
Excess SAFA+cholesterol
Chylomicrons
cholesterol-rich chylomicrons
βVLDL
IDL
FA
heparin
insulin
remnants
LDL
energy
LPL-ase
high[LDL]
FA
Glucagon
TSH
ACTH
macrophages
arterial smooth
muscle cells
atheroma
FA
FAT depot
insulin
FA
Catecholamines
growth hormone
HDL3
HDL2
TG
CE
LDL
VLDL
LPL-ase

**FIGURE 3–7.** Simplified scheme of the conversion of absorbed carbohydrates (CHO), fat, and cholesterol to liver VLDL (with apo-B100), chylomicrons (with apo-B48), and β-VLDL. Lipoprotein lipase (LPL-ase) activity is stimulated by heparin and insulin and inhibited by glucagon, thyroid-stimulating hormone (TSH), and adrenocorticotropic hormone (ACTH). Insulin stimulates triglyceride formation in fat depots, and catecholamines and growth hormone stimulate adipose tissue lipase with fatty acids (FA) released as a consequence. Excess VLDL formation in liver by excess dietary CHO or blood FA results in excess formation of LDL and atheroma. The same occurs at too high saturated fat (SAFA) and cholesterol consumption with the consequent formation of the atherogenic β-VLDL. $HDL_3$ is within certain limits capable of removing excess cholesterol from macrophages. The resulting $HDL_2$ particles transport the cholesterol to VLDL and are converted to LDL, which are taken up by liver and peripheral cells. The latter pathway also contributes to atheroma formation, however.

consist of C16:0, C18:0, and C18:1 n-9, contrary to the much greater variety of FA present in normal foods.

The tissue uptake of FA is proportional to its plasma concentration,[83] and probably also depends on FA binding within plasma. Free FA are transported largely in the form of firmly bound but rapidly reversible complexes with plasma albumin, which has two high-affinity binding sites for free FA and four to five weaker sites. Very low concentrations of free FA are present as monomers in solution and, similar to their uptake by enterocytes, are transferred only as free monomers from the aqueous phase into the cells. During fasting, most of the albumin-bound free FA in blood are derived from lipolysis of TG in adipose tissue. In addition, they are released postprandially by hydrolysis of chylomicron and VLDL TG by lipoprotein lipase. Lipolysis of adipose tissue TG increases during fasting to meet the energy requirements of tissues (muscle especially), which depend on FA oxidation for adenosine triphosphate (ATP) synthesis. The capacity of adipose tissue for stored energy is far greater than the available energy from muscle and liver glycogen. It is therefore useful that free FA mobilization increases as a result of stimulation by catecholamine during muscular activity and acute stress. In man, plasma free FA are also increased by growth hormone, glucagon, and thyroxine[83] (see Fig. 3–7). After the FA have entered the cells (particularly adipocyte and muscle cells), they are rapidly re-esterified to TG, if not taken up by mitochondria for oxidation and ATP synthesis. The glycerol-3 phosphate required for re-esterification of FA in extrahepatic tissue is derived from glucose, and therefore TG accumulation depends on insulin concentrations. During TG hydrolysis, glycerol is released. Plasma glycerol concentration is a reliable index of lipolysis because glycerol is not reused for esterification by adipocytes.

The release of free FA depends on the balance between lipolysis and re-esterification. Carbohydrate feeding reduces the concentration of plasma free FA by augmenting insulin concentration. Insulin regulates primarily FA levels in plasma; not only does it have a potent stimulating effect on re-esterification, thereby opposing the effects of catecholamines, growth hormone, and glucagon, but it also inhibits lipolysis. These hormonal interactions are complicated further by locally synthesized prostaglandins $E_1$ and $E_2$, which also inhibit catecholamine-stimulated lipolysis in adipose tissue.[77] Because prostaglandin biosynthesis is stimulated by catecholamines, these observations are compatible with a physiologic role of prostaglandin E in the regulation of lipolysis, possibly by a feedback mechanism.

The intestine and the liver, particularly, take up about 40 to 50% of the free FA leaving plasma in man.[84] In the liver, FA are largely incorporated into TG, and some may be stored there to be used for energy production on subsequent hydrolysis. The major part, however, is incorporated into VLDL and secreted again in the plasma.[85] Increased peripheral lipolysis during prolonged starvation or untreated diabetes results in greater esterification to TG in the liver, thereby producing a fatty liver.[86] Increased synthesis of VLDL also leads to hypertriglyceridemia.[87] The properties of the VLDL secreted by the liver depend to some extent on the load of TG requiring transport, analogous to the situation occurring in the intestinal mucosa. High-carbohydrate feeding in man results in increased production of VLDL with the characteristics of chylomicrons.[83] Diets high in saturated fat and CH also cause major changes in the lipoproteins,[88] including a reduction of typical HDL (without apo-E), an increase of HDL with apo-E (HDLc), and an increase of LDL and of a CH-rich lipoprotein that floats at a density of less than 1.006 g/ml and has β-electrophoretic mobility (β-VLDL).

Important advances in our understanding of the function of apo-E in the metabolism of TG-rich lipoproteins has been derived from mutations of this protein. Three common isoforms of apo-E have now been identified. Two of those (E3 and E4) are associated with normal lipoprotein concentrations. However, E2 is associated with accumulation of chylomicron and VLDL remnants in blood.[79] In rats, the apo-E, together with several C-apoproteins, are added to the surface of chylomicrons from HDL after their secretion from the intestine, mainly in exchange for PL. Until the apo-C is removed from chylomicrons during hydrolysis by lipoprotein lipase, the chylomicron remnants are not taken up by the liver because the liver has predominantly apo-E receptor sites.

As already discussed, two apo-B proteins also play a role in selective hepatic uptake of remnants of VLDL and LDL.[80] HDLc (with apo-E) is formed in plasma or in extracellular space as a result of HDL (without apo-E) accepting CH from peripheral tissue.[89] The free CH is esterified by LCAT. After the HDL enrichment with cholesteryl ester, the apo-E is redistributed from other plasma lipoproteins to HDLc.[88] The HDLc with apo-E interacts with apo-B, E receptors. These receptors are exposed only when the cells lack the required amount of CH for CH homeostasis. The HDL with apo-E not only redistribute CH to other cells that require CH for cell growth and steroid synthesis (e.g., adrenals, testis, and ovary), but redistribute CH also to hepatocytes for biliary secretion or lipoprotein synthesis.

Recent studies have shown that apo-E may serve as the major determinant for lipoprotein recognition by hepatic receptors.[88] In immature dogs and pigs, the liver also possesses typical apo-B,E receptors in addition to the apo-E receptors. The apo-B,E receptor binds LDL and HDL without apo-E. In the liver of adult dogs, the apo-B,E receptor can be induced by treatment with cholestyramine (a drug binding intestinal CH and BS, so that they are no longer available for reabsorption) or by prolonged fasting.[90]

In the immature dog liver, the apo-B,E receptors are blocked by CH feeding, which suggests that the apo-B,E receptors in the immature liver facilitate the increased CH requirement in fast growing tissues in the absence of adequate endogenous CH biosynthesis. Recently, it has been found that a cholesteryl ester transfer protein can transfer cholesteryl esters from HDLc to VLDL and chylomicrons and subsequently transport them to the liver.[91] This pathway will be less effective if the VLDL and chylomicrons are already rich in CH, as is the case in hypercholesterolemia, including those that are diet induced.

Diets high in saturated fats and CH are atherogenic and are associated with a reduction in HDL without apo-E; apparently, the regulating role of HDL in CH metabolism is stressed beyond its capacity in this situation. When the number of other lipoproteins available for CH transport is sufficient, the excess CH is transported to other tissues than the liver and causes atherosclerosis in the arterial walls by accumulation in macrophages and smooth muscle cells in the subendothelial tissue. Especially important in this respect are the β-VLDL that float at a density of less than 1.006 but have a β-electrophoretic mobility and are formed in diet-induced hypercholesterolemia. Species-related differences are apparent in the origin of β-VLDL: in rabbits, these arise as chylomicron remnants,[92] but in dogs and rats, species characterized by a high resistance to atherosclerosis, the β-VLDL appear to be of hepatic origin.[88,93]

Irrespective of their origin, β-VLDL are CH-rich, contain apo-B,E, and interact with a specific high-affinity apo-B,E receptor on the surface of macrophages. Unlike the apo-B,E receptor of fibroblasts or smooth muscle cells, the β-VLDL uptake is not suppressed as the macrophages accumulate CH.[88] Actually β-VLDL seems to be the only naturally occurring lipoprotein that can cause a substantial (20- to 160-fold) increase in the cholesteryl-ester content of macrophages, converting these into foam cells.[94] Because production of β-VLDL can be induced in man by high CH feeding[95,96] and is present in plasma of patients with hyperlipoproteinemia type II, these lipoproteins likely play a role in atherogenesis in man in addition to the well-known atherogenic properties of LDL.[96]

In familial hypercholesterolemia (type II), patients are deficient in apo-B and E receptors in all tissues, or have other defects of receptor-related transport mechanisms; such impairments produce correspondingly high LDL concentrations. This information does not explain, however, how the high LDL concentration can lead to accumulation of cholesteryl ester in subendothelial arterial tissue. Uptake of LDL and its effect on CH metabolism in the hepatocytes is illustrated in Figure 3–8. Diets high in saturated fat (and CH) cause augmented LDL levels in most subjects with the size of these LDL particles being greater than five times that of normal LDL.[88,97,98] In rhesus monkeys, the rise in CH-induced high-molecular weight LDL is correlated with the occurrence and the severity of coronary heart disease.[97] Furthermore, in several animal species, CH feeding leads to a type of LDL containing a variable amount of apo-E next to the normally major apo-B moiety.[88] However, neither the apo-B LDL nor the apo-B,E LDL causes cholesteryl ester accumulation in macrophages. It has been shown that LDL can be modified to an unknown extent, for example, by malondialdehyde released from platelets (malondialdehyde is one of the metabolic end products produced from TXA released during platelet aggregation) or from lipid peroxidation at sites of damaged arterial tissue.[97] This modified LDL appears to be capable of delivering CH to macrophages and might explain the atherogenicity of raised concentrations of LDL. Individual genetically based differences in β-VLDL formation, apo-B,E receptors, and LDL metabolism can explain at least in part the existence of hypo- and hyper-responders to dietary modification in many animal species, including man.[99-102] For a simplified scheme of these pathways, see Figure 3–8.

### HIGH-DENSITY LIPOPROTEINS

Interest in high-density lipoproteins (HDL) was focused primarily on its protective effect against atherosclerosis since attention was drawn to this issue by a review article by Miller and Miller in 1975.[103] Numerous publications have since demonstrated that this particle or better, this group of particles, have many functions, and that reverse transport of CH is only one of the them and is probably the least understood. They originate from the intestinal tract and the liver and can be separated by their differences in apoproteins. These proteins determine some of their functions, but these particles acquire so many other apoproteins from other lipoproteins that it is difficult to determine the role of apo-A1 (intestinal) as opposed to apo-E (liver) proteins in precursor (nascent) HDL. Functions are also determined by their lipid composition, which varies greatly. Their diameter depends on their molecular mass, which may increase from 70 to 100 Å and from 200 to 400 × $10^3$

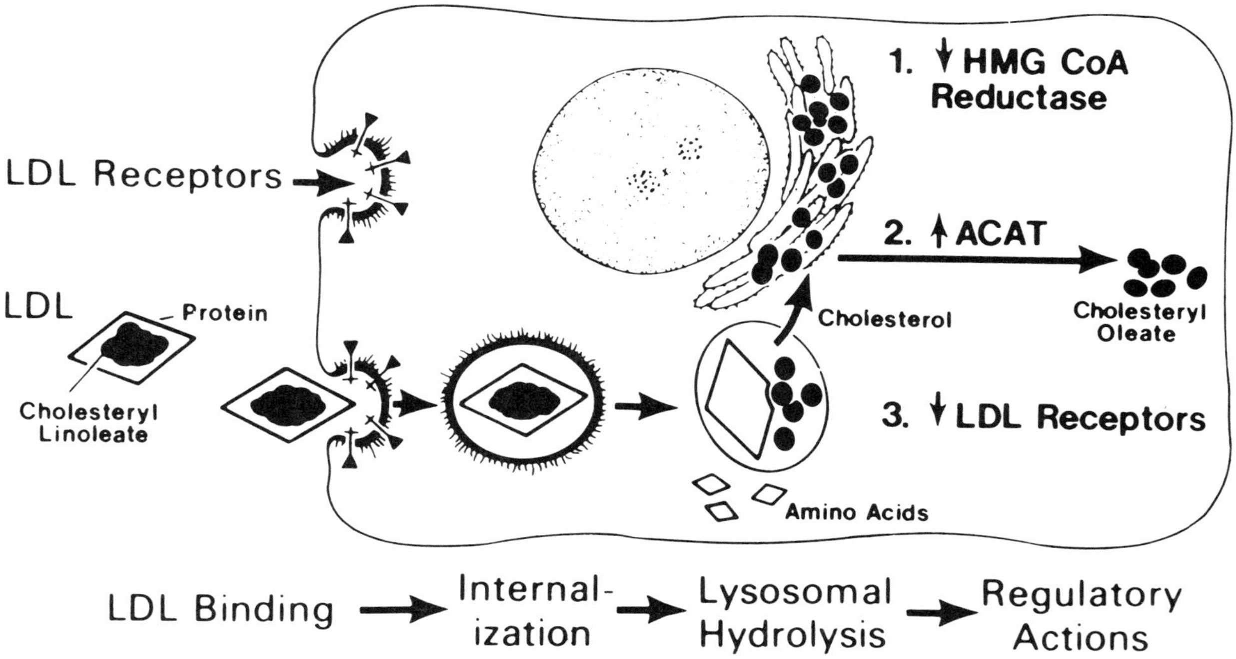
1. ↓ HMG CoA Reductase
LDL Receptors
2. ↑ ACAT
LDL
Protein
Cholesterol
Cholesteryl Oleate
Cholesteryl Linoleate
3. ↓ LDL Receptors
Amino Acids
LDL Binding
Internal-ization
Lysosomal Hydrolysis
Regulatory Actions

**FIGURE 3–8.** Sequential steps in the LDL pathway in cultured mammalian cells. LDL, Low-density lipoprotein; HMG CoA reductase, 3-hydroxy-3-methylglutaryl CoA reductase; ACAT, acyl-CoA: cholesterol acyltransferase. (From Fruchart, Y.C., Shepherd, Y. (Eds.): Human Plasma Proteins. New York, Walter de Gruyter, 1989.)

daltons.[103a] Their concentrations in plasma are lower than the LDL, but in terms of particle numbers, the HDL are the most abundant lipoproteins in circulation. In addition, a greater percentage is distributed in the extravascular space compared to LDL.

All diversified functions of this group of particles have not been identified, but they mostly function as a temporary storage for lipids, CH, and apoproteins. Originating from the liver and the intestinal tract as nascent discoid particles (for a detailed review, see Shepherd and Packard[103a] and Eisenberg[104]), HDL exchange surface lipids and apoproteins with TG-rich transport particles (chylomicrons and VLDL), particularly during lipolysis when these particles decrease in size by losing their TG. The discoid nascent HDL now mature to spherical HDL, at which time they esterify acquired CH to CE by the LCAT system. The LCAT system has a dual action. By transferring CH into CH ester, which moves into the hydrophobic core, more CH can be incorporated in the surface layer of the HDL particle. Lysolecithin is more hydrophilic than lecithin and dissociates readily from the lipoprotein surface into the aqueous environment. The change of composition of HDL facilitates uptake of CH from tissue membranes and transfer of CH and PL from other lipoprotein particles. The effectiveness of HDL as a CH acceptor is enhanced further by the action of a neutral exchange protein, which exchanges TG for CH ester. The TG-enriched HDL becomes susceptible to hydrolysis by circulating lipases and the particle has renewed capacity for CH uptake. The HDL particles function so effectively because they have a relatively large surface area, and because their apoproteins enhance contact with other particles membranes and lipophilic enzymes. The regulation of lipophilic enzymes by HDL is under investigation.

The HDL particles have a long half-life compared to other lipoproteins (10 to 11 hours). Because they have many apoproteins, they are catabolized by several different cell systems. Approximately 25% of HDL is catabolized by the liver. Other organs with a high requirement for CH, such as the adrenals and ovaries, also have a high uptake of HDL.[105]

### LIPID TRANSFER PROTEINS

The exchange of core lipids from lipoprotein particles is mediated not only by incidental collisions or near collisions, similar to the exchange of the constituents of micelles, but also to a major degree by lipid transfer proteins (LTP).[106] These proteins are synthesized by the liver. They are relatively small (60,000 to 70,000 daltons) and they have the unique property to exchange neutral lipids (TG, CE, and PL) from one lipoprotein particle to another.

In regard to the mechanism, formation of a ternary collision complex, consisting of LTP and two different donor/acceptor lipoproteins, has been favored by many investigators over the concept of a shuttle or ping-pong ball mechanism. Most transfer mechanisms of neutral lipids involve enzymatic hydrolysis and re-esterification processes, largely because the lipids must pass through an aqueous phase. This sequence may be different in a complex consisting of two lipoproteins, bridged by a LTP. The role of LTP is minimal in the rat, but it plays a significant role in the exchange of TG from the VLDL for CE donated by the HDL particles in man. LTP is less important for the exchange of these neutral lipids between VLDL and LDL. The CE donated by HDL is returned to the liver when VLDL and LDL are taken up by the hepatocytes. In contrast, the TG incorporated in the HDL particles are hydrolyzed by hepatic lipase secreted into plasma by the liver. Hepatic lipase, which can hydrolyze TG, CE, as well as PL, has a high affinity for HDL and forms a stable complex with HDL. Changes in lipid composition of HDL, and particularly changes in CH, affect their metabolic functions. The implications of these changes have not been determined. Because clearance and uptake of CH and CE by certain cell systems is determined by the interactions among lipoproteins, the role of the LTP in relation to atherosclerosis and energy supply must be analyzed further.

## BIOSYNTHESIS

Given adequate energy uptake, CH and related sterols, phospholipids, sphingo- and glycolipids, and TG can be synthesized by many animal tissues if the requirements for essential minerals, vitamins, essential amino acids, and the EFA are met adequately.

### PHOSPHOLIPIDS

Phospholipids (PL) and CH, which are the principal components of all biomembranes, are both synthesized by the endoplasmic reticulum (ER) of many cell systems, particularly of the liver and intestine. The ER itself consists of a bilayer with PL, being assembled from its components by the synthesizing enzymes located in the ER bilayer. The membranes, consisting of PL, CH, and protein molecules, serve not only as boundaries between individual cells, but also as a means to compartmentalize several major biochemical processes within the cell. The FA composition of the PL contributes significantly to the physical and biochemical properties of the membranes and is influenced directly by the proportion of dietary saturated and mono- and polyunsaturated FA.

The saturated and monounsaturated FA are derived from either diet or de novo synthesis by the condensation of acetate units, eventually followed by direct oxidative desaturation of long chain FA e.g., to oleic acid. In contrast, EFA with *cis* double bonds on the n-3 and/or n-6 position can be derived only from dietary sources (for further details, see the section concerning EFA). Under normal conditions, most tissues have PL in cellular plasma membranes, which are characterized by having predominantly linoleic or arachidonic acid esterified in position 2. On activation of phospholipase $A_2$, the released arachidonic acid is the preferred substrate for both lipoxygenase (LO) and cyclo-oxygenase (CO); this action leads to the instantaneous biosynthesis of various LT, TXA, or PG of the 2-type, as reviewed subsequently.

Continued feeding of an EFA-deficient diet leads to partial replacement of arachidonic acid by C20:3 n-9, 12,15 all *cis*,[107] which is a substrate for LO but not for CO.[108,109] Feeding a diet high in polyunsaturated fats of the n-3 type (linseed and fish oils) results in an enrichment of membrane PL with eicosapentaenoic acid (C20:5 n-3, 6, 9, 12, 15 all *cis*) and docosahexaenoic acid (C22:6 n-3, 3, 6, 9, 12,15, 18 all *cis*)[110]

### *PHOSPHATIDYLCHOLINE*

Phosphatidylcholine is the preferred name for lecithin because the latter term is also used for crude mixtures of various PL, oil, and carbohydrates produced during processing of edible oils. It is a prominent PL in the outer layer of the cell plasma membranes (in platelets, 41%) and in lipoproteins. Dietary phosphatidylcholine is an important contributor to blood and brain choline concentrations,[111] which codetermine the rate of acetylcholine biosynthesis, especially during rapid firing of cholinergic neurons.

Phosphatidylcholine is responsible for the hydrophilic properties of the surface coat of chylomicrons and VLDL. When TG are mobilized from the hydrophobic core by lipoprotein lipase and the particle decreases in size, lecithin is exchanged for apoproteins of the HDL particles. Nascent HDL particles are excellent receptors of free CH from other lipoprotein particles or endothelial membranes. Circulating LCAT, secreted by the liver and activated by apo-A 1 of the HDL surface, synthesizes cholesterol ester through acyltransferase-mediated transfer of the (poly) unsaturated FA located on position 2 of the HDL PL to free CH. The HDL particles have then become spherical (mature) and are partly catabolized by the liver, fibroblasts, and elements of the vascular wall. Lysolecithin can be re-esterified by FA released by lipolysis of TG present in chylomicrons, VLDL, or LDL. LCAT also has lysolecithin-acyltransferase activity.[112]

## REGULATION OF BILIARY PHOSPHOLIPIDS

Synthesis and secretion of biliary PL depends on biliary BS secretion. The BS output is regulated by hepatic uptake of BS from plasma. When plasma BS levels are low during fasting, synthesis and secretion of BS are also at a low level. Plasma concentrations of BS depend on absorption of BS from the intestinal lumen. The release of CCK from the gut mucosa stimulates BS synthesis and induces contraction of the gallbladder. Both actions of CCK result in increased BS levels in blood plasma by absorption from the gut lumen. The composition of the FA of biliary PL is different from that of lipoprotein PL. Secretion rates reach a plateau, and it is most likely that de novo synthesis has a maximum rate of 3 to 4 μmol/min lecithin.[113] Synthesis of PL, which will be incorporated in the hepatic lipoprotein particles, takes place at a slower rate and is independent of BS synthesis.

## STEROLS

Because outstanding reviews of the biosynthesis of CH have been published, only the main points are summarized here.[4,56,83]

Cholesterol can be synthesized in all tissues from acetate. The rate of synthesis is high in the liver and the intestine but low in the adult brain.[114] As early as week 18 of gestation, the fetus is capable of synthesizing CH from small molecules.[115] Incorporation of the carbon of acetate and glucose into CH is higher in the fetus than in the adult; however, it falls sharply at birth and rises again at weaning to a level higher than in adults. The concentrations of β-hydroxy β-methyl glutaryl (HMG)-CoA reductase per milligram of protein in the liver follow a similar growth pattern. Thus, the reduction of HMG-CoA by this enzyme is probably the rate-limiting step in the conversion of acetate into CH in fetal and neonatal life as well as in the adult.[116]

The rate of synthesis not only is different in relation to the stage of development but also varies widely in different tissues and in a given tissue under different conditions. However, the biosynthetic pathway beginning with acetate is similar and has been elucidated.[117,118]

Acetate can be converted into mevalonic acid by a sequence of reactions starting with acetate + ATP + CoA → acetyl-CoA + AMP + PP. However, most of the acetyl CoA used for sterol synthesis is not derived from this reaction but is generated within the mitochondria by the β-oxidation of FA or the oxidative decarboxylation of pyruvate. Pyruvate is converted into citrate, which diffuses into the cytosol and is hydrolyzed to acetyl-CoA and oxaloacetate by citrate-ATP lipase:

$$\text{Citrate} + \text{ATP} + \text{CoA} \rightarrow \text{acetyl-CoA} + \text{oxaloacetate} + \text{ADP} + H_2O$$

The citrate participating in this reaction acts as a carrier to transport acetyl carbon across the mitochondrial membranes, which are impermeable to acetyl-CoA. Subsequently, in the cytosol, acetyl-CoA is converted into mevalonate:

$$2\ \text{acetyl-CoA} \rightarrow \text{acetoacetyl-CoA} + \text{CoA}$$
$$\text{Acetoacetyl-CoA} + \text{acetyl-CoA} + H_2O \rightarrow \text{HMG-CoA} + \text{CoA}$$
$$\text{HMG-CoA} + 2\text{NADPH} + 2H^+ \xrightarrow{\textit{HMG-CoA reductase}} \text{mevalonate} + 2\ \text{NADP}^+ + \text{CoA}$$

HMG-CoA reduction is suppressed by prolonged CH feeding (probably by the increased flux of chylomicron remnants into the liver) and by fasting. A rise in cyclic-AMP concentration also appears to decrease the activity of HMG-CoA reductase.[83] This correlation provides a plausible explanation for the effect of some hormones on HMG-CoA reductase activity, e.g., the stimulatory effect of insulin and the inhibitory effect of glucagon.[119]

Mevalonic acid is phosphorylated, isomerized, and converted to geranyl- and farnesyl-pyrophosphate; which in turn forms squalene. Squalene is then oxidized and cyclized to a steroid ring, lanosterol. In the last steps, lanosterol is converted into CH by the loss of 3 methyl groups, saturation of the side chain, and a shift of the double bond from $\Delta^8$ to $\Delta^5$. During the later stages of CH biosynthesis, the intermediates are bound to a sterol carrier protein. Dietary manipulation, e.g., fat and CH feeding, alters the concentration of this protein and its ability to stimulate later stages in cholesterogenesis in vitro.[120] A similar role in the intact living cell, however, has yet to be demonstrated conclusively.[83]

Suppression of CH synthesis by CH feeding, "feedback inhibition," has been shown to occur in many animal species, including man.[121] In most mammals, the inhibitory effect is confined almost entirely to the liver, although prolonged feeding with CH may also cause some inhibition of sterol synthesis in the intestinal wall and the adrenals. Interruption of the enterohepatic circulation by a bile fistula, an ileal bypass, diets high in β-sitosterol, or therapy with cholestyramine and similar drugs enhances the rate of synthesis of CH in the liver. Part of this effect can probably be explained by a depressing effect of BS, such as taurocholate, on the activity of HMG-CoA reductase in the liver.[122,123]

The effects of various hormones on sterol synthesis in the liver are difficult to interpret because many conflicting data exist.[124] In vivo, the hormones influence the liver not only directly but also indirectly through their actions on other tissues. Of these, adipose tissue plays an important role as a supplier of FA, which are used as a source for the production of acetyl-CoA in the liver. The nutritional state of the subject, for example, influences insulin levels. Because insulin suppresses FA mobilization, the acetyl-CoA pool in the liver is affected by insulin levels, especially in the diabetic state or by prolonged fasting. The regulation of CH synthesis in the small intestine differs from that in the liver. Intestinal synthesis is inhibited only minimally by fasting and is not influenced by CH feeding.[83] However, bile acids in the lumen of the gut do inhibit intestinal synthesis of CH.[125] In rats, guinea pigs, and monkeys, synthesis of CH in other tissues is considerably lower than in the liver and intestinal wall and shows little response to the aforementioned factors influencing synthesis of CH in the liver and intestine.

From these data, the view emerged that the regulation of the amount of CH in the body as a whole is centered in the liver. In several types of human cells, an essential part of this regulatory system is the ability to develop cell surface receptors with high affinity for a specific lipoprotein (LDL).[83] In the presence of LDL receptors, the cell binds LDL and internalizes it; after cholesteryl ester is released from the LDL by hydrolysis, free CH is available for cell growth and maintenance without using the cellular capacity to synthesize its own CH. Thus, free CH inhibits CH synthesis in cells.

In the absence of LDL receptors, as occurs in type IIA hypercholesterolemia, LDL is taken up by a low-affinity process and does not inhibit intracellular synthesis or esterification of CH. The resulting continuous synthesis of CH is responsible for the high levels of CH in familial hypercholesterolemia (type IIA).

Although the lipoprotein particles synthesized by the liver contain mostly CE, the bile contains only free CH. Biliary CH is in part derived from the lipoprotein particles and in part synthesized de novo by the hepatocytes. Synthesis and release of this free CH into the biliary system is regulated by BS-dependent and BS-independent mechanisms. A BS-independent mechanism is the secretion of CH into bile as PL-CH vesicles. The BS-dependent CH secretion varies curvilinearly with BS secretion, but it reaches its maximum rate earlier than PL. However, during fasting, when rates of secretion of BS are low, CH is still secreted by a BS-independent mechanism, which may result in a physiologic or pathologic supersaturation of bile with CH.

Some patients may form CH crystals and eventually CH gallstones. Gallstone formation is related to the duration of the existence of lithogenic bile in the gallbladder and the presence of a nucleating protein. This protein has been isolated, and analysis of its composition is in progress. Supersaturation of bile depends on the micellar solubilization of CH and depends primarily on CH output. As mentioned previously, catabolism of sterols is limited, and elimination of CH depends largely on biliary secretion (600 mg per day) and, to a minor degree, on formation of BS (400 mg per day) from CH. (Fig. 3–9).

The populations of western countries have a diet relatively high in CH, saturated fat, and animal protein. They have a high incidence of CH gallstones (United States, 15%; England, 25%; Sweden, more than 35%). Oriental countries (as is well documented in Japan) and African populations, who ingest low-CH diets, have a low incidence of gallstones. The high incidence of CH gallstones in female American Indians (more than 80%) is related to a genetic disorder, in which the biliary output of BS and PL is low and that of CH is high; to a traditional diet high in CH and animal fat; and to the high incidence of diabetes in this population.

As for the PL, two hepatic CH pools may exist: one based on fast synthesis of biliary free CH for biliary secretion and the other on the slower synthesis of mostly esterified lipoprotein CH, which is secreted by the hepatocytes into the blood. The CH released from absorbed lipoproteins can be used for either the synthesis of new lipoproteins, which will be released into blood plasma, or secretion as biliary CH. Both pools have access to CH absorbed from the small bowel lumen. Only a fraction of CH, secreted by the liver is synthesized de novo.

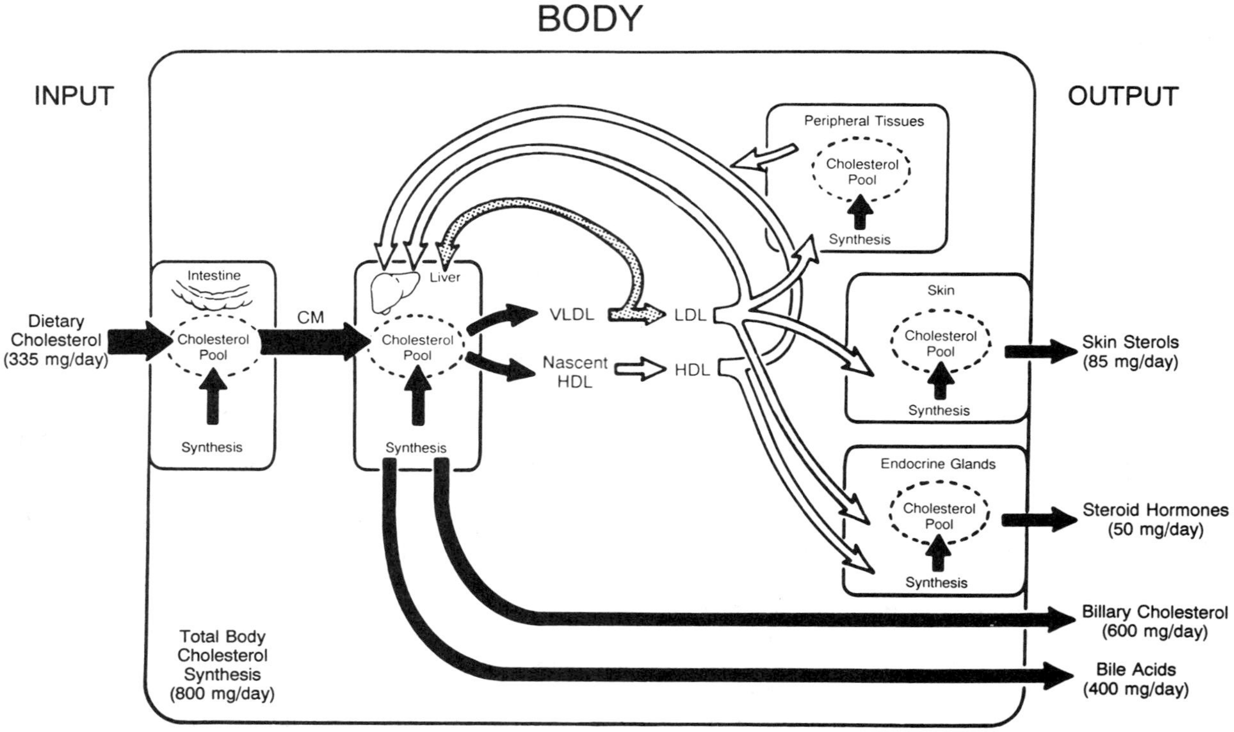
BODY
INPUT
OUTPUT
Peripheral Tissues
Cholesterol Pool
Synthesis
Intestine
Liver
Dietary Cholesterol (335 mg/day)
Cholesterol Pool
CM
Cholesterol Pool
VLDL
LDL
Nascent HDL
HDL
Skin
Cholesterol Pool
Synthesis
Skin Sterols (85 mg/day)
Synthesis
Synthesis
Endocrine Glands
Cholesterol Pool
Steroid Hormones (50 mg/day)
Synthesis
Billary Cholesterol (600 mg/day)
Total Body Cholesterol Synthesis (800 mg/day)
Bile Acids (400 mg/day)

**FIGURE 3–9.** Simplified scheme of the major steps in the transport of cholesterol between the different tissue compartments of the body. Intake of dietary cholesterol is relatively low. Approximately 50% of dietary and biliary cholesterol is not absorbed from the intestine. (From Arias, I.M., Popper, H., Schachter, , et al. (Eds.): The Liver: Biology and Pathology. New York, Raven Press, 1982, p. 477.)

## CHOLESTERYL ESTER

Tissue CH is principally in the free alcohol form, but in blood and adrenals, about two thirds is esterified. In man, the esterification takes place predominantly in the plasma by transfer of the FA from position 2 of plasma PL, under the influence of LCAT, to the 3-β-OH group of CH. Because the FA in position 2 of phospholipids are predominantly polyunsaturated, a high percentage of linoleic acid (more than 55%) is in CH ester circulating in blood plasma, with a low but constant percentage of arachidonic acid (C20:4 n-6 all *cis*)(4 to 6%). Rats and dogs, which are more resistant to developing atherosclerosis, have a higher percentage of C20:4 n-6 all *cis* (about 25%). In contrast, rabbits, which are known to be even more prone to development of atherosclerosis than man, have low C20:4 n-6 concentrations.

The incidence of atherosclerosis in animals seems to be inversely related to the levels of esterified arachidonic acid (see the subsequent section on EFA). In man, arachidonic acid levels do not fluctuate and atherosclerosis is more related to cholesteryl linoleate levels. Man, who regularly consumes diets rich in saturated FA and low in linoleic acid, has lower (35 to 50%) cholesteryl linoleate concentrations with correspondingly higher cholesteryl oleate percentages.[126-128] This condition appears to correlate with a progressively increased risk to develop peripheral vascular disease,[128] and exists also in patients with insulin-independent and insulin-dependent diabetes mellitus, and with a high incidence of diabetic retinopathy and ischemic heart disease.[7,129] LCAT is secreted by the liver and has a high affinity for HDL. It reacts preferentially with the free CH of HDL.[130] As discussed previously, the CE of HDL is subsequently transferred to VLDL.

Several other esterifying enzymes exist. In the mucosa of the small intestine, the absorbed free CH is esterified largely with oleic acid before incorporation into chylomicrons. In the liver, acyl-CoA cholesterol acyltransferase (ACAT), a microsomal enzyme, catalyzes the reaction:

$$\text{Long chain acyl-CoA} + \text{cholesterol} \rightarrow \text{cholesteryl ester} + \text{CoA}$$

ACAT has a marked specificity toward its FA substrate. In the presence of CoA and ATP, C18:1 is the preferred substrate; in the liver of the rat, the order of preference is C18:1>16:0>18:0>18:2. ACAT has been demonstrated in many other tissues, and its activity is increased by an increase in free CH in the cell as a consequence of the uptake of LDL from the medium. The uptake of LDL is mediated by specific LDL receptors, as demonstrated in human skin fibroblasts and aortic smooth muscle cells.

This increase in ACAT activity may have important consequences for the development of atherosclerotic lesions.

## BILE ACIDS

Cholesterol is metabolized mainly by conversion into bile acids and steroid hormones. A small fraction of unabsorbed CH is metabolized by intestinal flora to cholestanol and coprostanol and other poorly absorbed sterols. The catabolism of CH to bile acids accounts for 30 to 60% of the CH lost from the human body, a lower proportion than, for example, in rats (80 to 87% lost as bile acids) (see Fig. 3–9).[4,83] The conversion takes place in the liver and is under negative feedback control by the bile acids reabsorbed from the intestine. The major rate-limiting step in this pathway is the first oxidative step, catalyzed by 7 α-hydroxylase. Subsequently, the 12 α-position is hydroxylated, the 3 β-OH is inverted to the 3 β-position, the 4 double bonds become saturated, and the three terminal carbon atoms of the side chain are removed by a process analogous to β-oxidation. Cholic acid is then formed as cholyl-CoA and is conjugated with glycine or taurine by the formation of a peptide bond between the carboxyl carbon of cholic acid and the amino group of the amino acid.[83]

The pathway for the formation of chenodeoxycholic acid is similar to that for the formation of cholic acid, with the exception that no 12 α-hydroxylation is involved.[131] In man, other pathways also have been found.[83] After their secretion into the intestinal lumen, the conjugated primary bile acids are modified by bacteria in the lower ileum and large intestine; this process results in the formation of deoxycholate, lithocholate, allocholate, and some 20 other bile acid modifications, some of which are reabsorbed. Therefore, human bile contains also deoxycholic, lithocholic, and ursodeoxycholic acids.[83]

About 95% of BS participate in an enterohepatic circulation, which plays an essential role in the absorption of lipids and the regulation of CH metabolism in the liver. If the enterohepatic circulation is interrupted, the rate of synthesis of bile acids increases. This change can occur in Crohn's disease of the distal ileum, after ileal resection, or after a bypass procedure formerly performed for treatment of morbid obesity. Bile acid synthesis increases too by the addition of CH to the diet and by the amount of certain types of fiber added to the food. The latter may be mediated by binding, which inhibits the reabsorption of BS from the intestine.[132] This increase of bile acid synthesis occurs also during therapy with cholestyramine and other anion exchangers that bind bile salts.

## STEROID HORMONES AND VITAMIN D

Cholesterol is an obligatory precursor of the adrenocortical hormones, the sex hormones, and placental hormones. 7-Dehydrocholesterol also serves as the precursor of the vitamin D formed through ultraviolet (UV) irradiation of the skin. In man, the amount of CH converted into steroid hormones is less than that converted into bile acids, but it is by no means negligible (50 mg per day). Because the steroid hormone metabolites principally are excreted in the urine, this loss may be a source of error in the estimation of the overall sterol balance.

## FATTY ACIDS (FIG. 3–10)

With the exception of the n-3 and n-6 PUFA, i.e., the EFA, all other FA can be synthesized by man from any excess of dietary energy. The rate of FA synthesis is strongly linked to the availability of glucose and is depressed by fasting, dietary fat, and insulin deficiency. Glucagon also causes a rapid drop in hepatic lipogenesis, probably mediated by the effect of increased cAMP on a hormone-stimulated protein kinase.[133] The pathway for biosynthesis of saturated FA is basically the same in all organisms examined to date. The universal substrate is acetyl-CoA. Citrate transported from the mitochondria is cleaved to acetyl-CoA and oxaloacetate. This reaction is important in controlling the production of FA.

The first step in the biosynthetic pathway proper is the conversion of acetyl-CoA to malonyl-CoA. This reaction is catalyzed by acetyl-CoA carboxylase, which is rate limiting for FA synthesis.[134] Acetyl-CoA then combines sequentially with a series of malonyl-CoA molecules as follows:

$$\text{Acetyl-CoA} + 7\ \text{malonyl-CoA} + 14\ \text{NADPH} + 14\text{H}^+ \rightarrow \text{C16:0 (palmitic acid)} + 7\ \text{CO}_2 + 8\ \text{CoASH} + 14\ \text{NADP}^+ + 6\ \text{H}_2\text{O}$$

The entire reaction is catalyzed by a group of enzymes known as FA synthetases, which are localized in the cytosol of hepatocytes.

In man, FA synthesis occurs predominantly in the liver; adipose tissue apparently is less active than in many other animal species, such as the rat. In mammals, the product is mainly C16:0, which serves as a substrate for microsomal malonyl-CoA-dependent elongase. Subsequently, $\Delta^9$-oxidative desaturation of C16:0 and C18:0 leads to C16:1 and C18:1 by microsomally bound desaturases with a broad chain length specificity—the $\Delta^9$, $\Delta^6$, $\Delta^5$ and $\Delta^4$ fatty acyl-CoA desaturases.[135] The monoenoic C16:1 n-7 *cis* and C18:1 n-9 *cis* and also linoleic acid (C18:2 n-6, 9 *cis, cis*) and α-linolenic acid (C18:3 n-3, 6, 9 all *cis*) are desaturated by the $\Delta^6$-desaturase, which is the regulatory enzyme in this sequence of reactions and requires the presence of a n-9 *cis* double bond. Consequently, elaidic acid (C18:1 n-9 *trans*, formed by rumen bacteria or by chemical hydrogenation from the natural *cis* type of double bonds) cannot be converted by this enzyme. Newly inserted double bonds are always located between the existing ones and the carboxyl group.

| COMMON NAME | GENEVA NOMENCLATURE | CODE | FORMULA* |
|---|---|---|---|
| Short-chain saturated fatty acids | | | |
| butyric acid | butanoic acid | C4:0 | $CH_3(CH_2)_2COOH$ |
| Medium-chain saturated fatty acids | | | |
| caproic acid | hexanoic acid | C6:0 | $CH_3(CH_2)_4COOH$ |
| caprylic acid | octanoic acid | C8:0 | $CH_3(CH_2)_6COOH$ |
| capric acid | decanoic acid | C10:0 | $CH_3(CH_2)_8COOH$ |
| lauric acid | dodecanoic acid | C12:0 | $CH_3(CH_2)_{10}COOH$ |
| Long-chain fatty acids | | | |
| myristic acid | tetradecanoic acid | C14:0 | $CH_3(CH_2)_{12}COOH$ |
| palmitic acid | hexadecanoic acid | C16:0 | $CH_3(CH_2)_{14}COOH$ |
| stearic acid | octadecanoic acid | C18:0 | $CH_3(CH_2)_{16}COOH$ |
| palmitoleic acid | 9-hexadecaenoic acid | C16:1,n-7 *cis* | $CH_3(CH_2)_5CH{=}\text{©}CH(CH_2)_7COOH$ |
| oleic acid | 9-octadecaenoic acid | C18:1,n-9 *cis* | $CH_3(CH_2)_7CH{=}\text{©}CH(CH_2)_7COOH$ |
| elaidic acid | 9-octadecaenoic acid | C18:1,n-9 *trans* | $CH_3(CH_2)_7CH{=}tCH(CH_2)_7COOH$ |
| linoleic acid | 9,12-octadecadienoic acid | C18:2,n-6,9 all *cis* | $CH_3(CH_2)_4CH{=}\text{©}CHCH_2CH{=}$<br>$\text{©}CH(CH_2)_7COOH$ |
| α-linoleic acid | 9,12,15-octadecatrienoic acid | C18:3,n-3,6,9 all *cis* | $CH_3CH_2CH{=}\text{©}CHCH_2CH{=}$<br>$\text{©}CHCH_2CH{=}\text{©}CH(CH_2)_7COOH$ |
| γ-linoleic acid | 6,9,12-octadecatrienoic acid | C18:3,n-6,9,12 all *cis* | $CH_3(CH_2)_4CH{=}\text{©}CHCH_2CH{=}$<br>$\text{©}CHCH_2CH{=}\text{©}CH(CH_2)_4COOH$ |
| columbinic acid | 5,9,12-octatrienoic acid | C18: n-6, cis,9 *cis*, 13 *trans* | $CH_3(CH_2)_4CH{=}\text{©}CHCH_2CH{=}$<br>$\text{©}CHCH_2CH_2CH{=}$<br>$tCH(CH_2)_3COOH$ |
| Very long-chain fatty acids | | | |
| arachidic acid | eicosanoic acid | C20:0 | $CH_3(CH_2)_{18}COOH$ |
| behenic acid | docosanoic acid | C22:0 | $CH_3(CH_2)_{20}COOH$ |
| eicosenoic acid | 11-eicosenoic acid | C20:1,n-9 *cis* | $CH_3(CH_2)_7CH{=}\text{©}CH(CH_2)_9COOH$ |
| erucic acid | 13-docosaenoic acid | C22:1,n-9 *cis* | $CH_3(CH_2)_7CH{=}\text{©}CH(CH_2)_{11}COOH$ |
| brassidic acid | 13-docosaenoic acid | C22:1,n-9 *trans* | $CH_3(CH_2)_7CH{=}tCH(CH_2)_{11}COOH$ |
| cetoleic acid | 11-docosaenoic acid | C22:1,n-11 *cis* | $CH_3(CH_2)_9CH{=}\text{©}CH(CH_2)_9COOH$ |
| nervonic acid | 15-tetracosaenoic acid | C24:1,n-9 *cis* | $CH_3(CH_2)_7CH{=}\text{©}CH(CH_2)_{13}COOH$ |
| "Mead" acid | 5,8,11-eicosatrienoic acid | C20:3,n-9,12,15 all *cis* | $CH_3(CH_2)_7CH{=}\text{©}CHCH_2CH{=}$<br>$\text{©}CHCH_2CH{=}\text{©}CH(CH_2)_3COOH$ |
| dihomo-γ-linoleic acid | 8,11,14-eicosatrienoic acid | C20:3,n-6,9,12 all *cis* | $CH_3(CH_2)_4CH{=}\text{©}CHCH_2CH{=}$<br>$\text{©}CHCH_2CH{=}\text{©}CH(CH_2)_6COOH$ |
| arachidonic acid | 5,8,11,14-eicosatetraenoic acid | C20:4,n-6,9,12,15 all *cis* | $CH_3(CH_2)_4CH{=}\text{©}CHCH_2CH{=}$<br>$\text{©}CHCH_2CH{=}\text{©}CHCH_2CH{=}$<br>$\text{©}CH(CH_2)_3COOH$ |
| timnodonic acid | 5,8,11,14,17-eicosapentaenoic acid | C20:5,n-3,6,9,12,15 all *cis* | $CH_3(CH_2CH{=}\text{©}CH)_5(CH_2)_3COOH$ |
| clupanodonic acid | 7,10,13,16,19-docosapentaenoic acid | C22:5,n-3,6,9,12,15 all *cis* | $CH_3(CH_2CH{=}\text{©}CH)_5(CH_2)_5COOH$ |
| docosahexaenoic acid | 4,7,10,13,16,19-docosahexaenoic acid | C22:6,n-3,6,9,12,15,18 all *cis* | $CH_3(CH_2CH{=}\text{©}CH)_6(CH_2)_2COOH$ |

*t, *trans* ©, *cis*

**FIGURE 3–10.** Names, codes, and formulas of fatty acids mentioned in this chapter.

In general, the enzymes display highest affinity for the most unsaturated substrate.[136] The order of preference is: α-linolenic acid family (n-3) > linoleic acid family (n-6) > oleic acid family (n-9) > palmitoleic acid family (n-7) > elaidic acid family (n-9, *trans*).[137]

This sequence of preferences has many implications. C20:3 n-9, 12, 15 all *cis* is synthesized from C18:1 n-9 *cis* only in the nearly complete absence of the EFA both of the n-3 and the n-6 types. The presence of C20:3 n-9, 12, 15 in PL instead of C20:4 n-6, 9, 12, 15, C20:5 n-3, 6, 9, 12, 15 and C22:6 n-3, 6, 9, 12, 15, 18 is solid proof for the existence of EFA deficiency.[138,139]

During the catalytic hydrogenation process of vegetable oils (primarily soybean oil) and fish oils for the production of some margarines and shortenings, a variety of geometric (i.e., *trans*) and positional isomers of unsaturated FA are formed in varying amounts. After absorption, these isomers may compete with the EFA and endogenously synthesized FA for desaturation and chain elongation. The biologic effects of *trans* FA have been reviewed.[140] Long-term nutritional evaluation of hydrogenated vegetable oils in mice, rats, and rabbits has shown that no significant differences occur with respect to mortality, life span, growth-rate, organ weights, or histopathology compared to palmitic, stearic, and oleic acids.

Conversion of C18:2 n-6, 9 all *cis* to C20:4 n-6, 9,12,15 all *cis*, however is inhibited by *trans*-9, *trans*-12 octadecadienoic acid (C18:2 n-6, 9 *trans, trans*), a minor component of hydrogenated oils,[140] but only at high concentrations. Furthermore, *trans* FA or their derivatives are not incorporated in position 2 of PL when n-3 or n-6 PUFA. are available. Thus, interference of *trans* FA with the first phase of prostaglandin synthesis, the hydrolysis of biomembrane PL by phospholipase $A_2$, which releases the FA on position 2, seems unlikely.

Dietary PUFA play an important role in controlling the conversion of carbohydrate to storage triacylglycerols by selective inhibition of the lipogenic enzymes.[141,142] Why or how this should be and at what level dietary polyunsaturated FA exert this effect is not known. This phenomenon explains, at least in part, the significant VLDL-lowering effect of linoleic acid-rich diets. As LDL is derived from VLDL, lower VLDL synthesis contributes to the well-known LDL-lowering effects of linoleic acid. In this context, oleic acid may enhance the synthesis of VLDL-CH (whether the oleic acid is from dietary origin or from endogenous synthesis from excess carbohydrates).[143,144] Inhibition by linoleic acid of C18:0-CoA desaturase limits the C18:1 n-9 synthesized and its control of CH synthesis and so may limit VLDL secretion also.

The degradation of LCFA to acetyl CoA by β-oxidation is important for ATP synthesis and energy production, as well as potentially of great importance in regulating the composition of membrane lipids and cholesteryl esters. β-Oxidation normally takes place in mitochondria, and would seem capable of modulating not only the quantity but also, by selective degradation, the variety of FA available for structural lipid synthesis. Unfortunately, little is known regarding the specificity or regulation of β-oxidation. For mitochondrial β-oxidation, the FA have to be transported across the mitochondrial membrane in the form of acyl-carnitine. Two types of carnitine acyltransferase are involved. These transferases are located on the inner and outer surface of the the mitochondrial membrane,[145] which is considered a prime regulatory site for β-oxidation.

Rat liver cells have also peroxisomal β-oxidation activity,[146] a carnitine-independent β-oxidation, which performs for a few β-oxidation cycles.[147] Hereafter, the normal mitochondrial, carnitine-dependent β-oxidation takes care of further metabolism. Although only low peroxisomal activity is found in normal livers, the livers of rats fed clofibrate and its derivatives or oils rich in C20:5 n-3 and C22:6 n-3 contained high levels of peroxisomal activity. Because peroxisomes can produce $H_2O_2$, which is potentially harmful for the cell, the cell needs defense mechanisms against uncontrolled peroxidative reactions.[146] The defense mechanism fails when diets high in n-3 PUFA (α-linolenic acid family) are fed (see subsequent section).

Feeding rapeseed oil (the high C22:1 n-9 *cis* variety) or partially hydrogenated marine oil, rich in *trans* or *cis-trans* mono- and diunsaturated FA with 20, 22, and 24 carbon atoms, causes an acute accumulation of triacyl glycerols (high in C20:1 and C22:1) in the heart and red muscle fibers of many animal species.[82,148] The fat infiltration reaches a peak after approximately 5 days and decreases gradually, but incompletely, on prolonged feeding. This accumulation slowly leads to focal fibrotic changes in the heart. The acute lipidosis can be explained by an inhibition of carnitine acyltransferase by C20:1 and C22:1, resulting in re-esterification of the C20:1 and C22:1 to TG in the cytoplasm.[150] After a few days, increased lipase activity induces FA transport from the heart to the liver,[151] which, contrary to the heart muscle, can metabolize these unusual LCFA, although more slowly than normal.

Fat accumulation in muscle also occurs because C22:1 acyl carnitines are oxidized poorly by mitochondria.[148] In the liver, an adaptive increase in peroxisomal β-oxidation seems to be the most important process explaining the partial adaptation to dietary C20:1 and C22:2.[152] As far as C22:1 FA are concerned, brassidic (C22:1 n-9 *trans*), cetoleic (C22:1, n-11, *cis*), and erucic acid (C22:1 n-9 *cis*) are all oxidized by rat liver peroxisomes at similar rates, corresponding to approximately 20% of the rate obtained with palmitoyl-CoA.[148]

Although peroxisomal β-oxidation of these LCFA is not efficient, it is a process independent of carnitine. In this way, it plays an important role in converting C22:1 FA to SCFA, which can be metabolized by the mitochondria.

It is striking that fats with LCFA ($C_{20}$ or more) have many effects that are similar to the action of drugs like clofibrate. A common feature may be the conversion to CoA esters, which are difficult to metabolize, thus triggering the previously discussed adaptation mechanisms.[153,154] It is therefore not surprising that clofibrate has been found to give partial protection (50%) against C22:1-induced myocardial lipidosis.[155] These data indicate that consumption of oil and fats rich in C20, C22, and C24 monoenoic FA creates some complicated biochemical adaptation processes, which explains the observed growth retardation in experimental animals and functional changes in the heart, adrenals, and the liver (for a complete review, see References 156 and 148).

Very long-chain, C22 PUFA, as present in many marine (fish) oils, can be shortened with concomitant saturation of a double bond (C22:6 n-3 is changed to C22:5 n-3 and to C20:5 n-3[157]). The same pathway is active in converting C22:5 n-6 into C20:4 n-6 (arachidonic acid), and is a peroxisomal process.[158] The partitioning between peroxisomal shortening and complete mitochondrial β-oxidation of C22 FA probably depends on the number and position of double bonds; e.g., isolated rat liver cells oxidize C22:4 n-6 rapidly, whereas the oxidation of C22:6 n-3 is slower and is inhibited more by (+)decanoylcarnitine, an inhibitor of mitochondrial β-oxidation. The feeding state also plays a role; in hepatocytes from fasted rats the mitochondrial β-oxidation of C22:6 n-3 is increased, whereas peroxisomal chain shortening is less affected by fasting and refeeding.[158]

Timnodonic acid (C20:5 n-3), the precursor for the 3-family of prostaglandins (PG), thromboxanes (TXA), leukotrienes (LT) etc. is also present in many fish oils (see the end of this section and Table 3–1). Its metabolism differs from that of arachidonic acid (C20:4 n-6), the precursor of the 2-family of PG, TXA, LT, etc., in the following ways: (1) C20:4 n-6 is biosynthesized efficiently from C18:2 n-6, 9 all *cis* by all animals, including man. However, man, contrary to the rat, has practically no capacity to convert C18:3 n-3, 6, 9 all *cis* into C20:5 n-3.[159] For this reason, man depends on animal sources for C20:5 n-3, but is independent from animal food sources for C20:4 n-6. (2) Arachidonic acid is directed to position 2 of PL, as is C22:6 n-3, but not C20:5 n-3. C20:5 n-3 to some extent is esterified as TG and is oxidized, as observed in rats.[160] (3) C20:4 n-6 is retained more efficiently in the tissues of animals fed a fat-free diet than are C20:5 n-3 and C22:6 n-3. Apparently, important differences exist in the metabolism of both groups of EFA, suggesting that animal tissues try to conserve C20:4 n-6, 9, 12, 15 all *cis* (and probably also the quantitatively less important C20:3 n-6, 9 12 all *cis*). However, these biochemical studies were limited to liver and platelets, while the main biologic activity of the very long-chain n-3 EFA probably is in the retina, testes, and brain, where relatively large quantities of C22:6 n-3 normally are present. Across mammalian species, the levels of C22:6 n-3 in brain and retinal PL are remarkably similar despite wide variations in dietary compositions. The strong affinity of brain lipids for C22:6 n-3 suggests a requirement for n-3 EFA, but this requirement is difficult to study because a n-3 EFA deficiency can develop only under extreme dietary conditions.

## FUNCTIONS OF ESSENTIAL FATTY ACIDS

In studies on essential fatty acids (EFA), the main emphasis has been on C18:2 n-6, 9 all *cis* and C20:4 n-6, 9, 12, 15 all *cis*. The possible dietary importance of C18:3 n-3, 6, 9 all *cis* has not been systematically explored thus far. Serious gaps in our knowledge also exist with regard to the prostaglandins of the 3-series, because most of the research has focused on cyclo-oxygenase products of C20:4 n-6 and less on those of C20:3 n-6 and C20:5 n-3. With respect to the lipoxygenase products of the various EFA, the data are even less complete, although the published results suggest important pathophysiologic functions, especially in inflammatory and thrombotic processes.

Thus, the known functions of the n-3 and n-6 EFA will primarily be considered here in relation to biomembrane structure and the function of various tissues and organs. The emphasis is on their role as precursor FA for the biosynthesis of many PG, TXA, and LT discovered to date. Other products of LO and CO are not discussed because sufficient data are not available. Because a mixture of these products usually is present, it is convenient to use "eicosanoids" (some purists prefer icosanoids) to describe them, unless good reasons emerge to consider the biologic activities of one or more eicosanoids as dominant. However, as reviewed subsequently, the analytic problems in measuring these highly active but short-lived elusive FA derivatives still are too great for the available techniques. Ascribing a certain biologic effect to one or more eicosanoids is therefore always a simplification.

### REQUIREMENTS

Because EFA are necessary for the normal function of all tissues, the list of symptoms of EFA deficiency is long.[107,139,161] Reduced growth rate, abnormal scaliness, increased loss of water by a change of skin permeability, and male and female infertility are the classic signs. To these can be added kidney abnormalities (papillary necrosis, hematuria, and renal hypertension), abnormal liver mitochondria (increased swelling, depressed ATP synthesis), decreased capillary resistance, increased fragility of erythrocytes, increased susceptibility to infections, decreased myocardial contractility, and decreased PG biosynthesis.[161] Convincing evidence has been obtained confirming older data for an essential role for C22:6 n-3 in brain and retinal PL.[162 to 164] One of the most sensitive diagnostic indicators of EFA deficiency is probably an increased triene(n-9)/tetraene (n-6) ratio (greater than 0.1).[107] Feeding diets with 0.1 to 0.5 en% of linoleic acid normalizes an abnormally high triene/tetraene ratio in a few days. Such diets have been accepted in the past as sufficient to cure or to prevent EFA deficiency. However, FA such as C20:5 n-3 and C22:6 n-3 are even more potent in this respect than C18:2 n-6, although they have only a minor effect on the low growth rate and poor skin condition typically associated with EFA deficiency. It is known now that, for optimal function of various tissues, much higher en% of C18:2 n-6 are necessary.

With regard to growth rate, capillary resistance, fragility of erythrocytes, and mitochondrial function of liver and heart, linolenic acid C18:3 n-3 is similar to C18:2 n-6. On the other hand, with regard to skin condition, increased water consumption, and PG biosynthesis, dietary C18:3 n-3 and C20:5 n-3 are inferior to C18:2 n-6 and the other n-6 PUFA. For example, to a greater or lesser extent, a series of synthetic and natural PUFA of variable chain lengths and different degrees of unsaturation can normalize abnormal swelling properties of EFA-deficient rat liver mitochondria. For proper structural function in liver mitochondria, the incorporated FA should have at least 19, but preferably 20, carbon atoms and at least 4 double bonds, two of which should be in the *cis* configuration and in the n-6 and n-9 position; the remaining bonds should be methylene interrupted or farther away from these double bonds.[165] The scaliness of the skin in an EFA-deficient patient has been ascribed to insufficient synthesis of PG,[166] which might be cured by local application of EFA. The efficacy of various EFA of the n-6 type has been confirmed by other authors at low dose levels.[165,167-169]

Columbinic acid (C18:3 n-6, 9, 13 *cis, cis, trans*), present in the seed oil of the columbine, Aquilegia vulgaris, and dihomocolumbinic acid (C20:3 n-6, 9, 13 *cis, cis, trans*) can be used as biochemical tools to differentiate between the structural roles of EFA in various biomembranes and the role of EFA as PG precursor.[167] Columbinic acid, when given to EFA-deficient rats either orally or by topical skin application, efficiently restores their growth rate and normal skin function. Interestingly, dihomocolumbinic acid (C20:3 n-6, 9, 13 *cis, cis, trans*) cured EFA-deficient skin completely, but had disastrous effects on growth rate, liver and heart mitochondria, and kidney function. It cannot be incorporated into membrane PL. The latter occurred only after shortening of the chain to columbinic acid. In severe EFA deficiency, hematuria often is observed because of lesions in the papillary region. This condition was severely aggravated by administration of dihomocolumbinic acid. The abnormal kidney function in EFA deficiency (causing hematuria and hypertension) may be caused by a deficiency of PG biosynthesis. Dihomocolumbinic acid, which cannot be converted to PG, inhibits competitively the conversion of arachidonic acid into PG. Because EFA deficiency results in low concentrations of arachidonic acid, the symptoms of this deficiency are aggravated further. Columbinic acid can prevent the development of infertility in EFA deficiency, which apparently is not caused by low PG biosynthesis. However, when EFA-deficient rats treated with columbinic acid became pregnant, they died of inadequate labor during parturition. Uterine labor depends on normal PG biosynthesis, which was not improved by the addition of columbinic acid.[170]

Until recently, the development of human EFA deficiency was regarded as an extreme rarity. However, with the sensitive triene/tetraene ratio as a diagnostic index,[1,168] the existence of EFA deficiency has been demonstrated in elderly patients with peripheral vascular disease,[171] in patients with fat malabsorption after major intestinal resection,[172,173] during prolonged fat-free intravenous feeding,[170,171] during low-fat, high-protein dietary supplementation for treatment of kwashiorkor,[173a] and after serious accidents and burns.[174] In all these conditions, oral or intravenous feeding of linoleic acid-containing TG rapidly converted not only the abnormal triene/tetraene ratio to normal but also corrected skin abnormalities. Although not tested, the use of PUFA of the n-3 family (e.g., fish oil) would have resulted in persistent dermal lesions that do not respond sufficiently to these FA. The normally low dietary intake of n-6 EFA (in Northwest Europe, North America, Australia, and other countries where the average C18:2 n-6, 9 intake is only 2 to 4 en%) leads to EFA deficiency when a sudden increase of cell regeneration and rapid growth occurs.[172,174] For these reasons, it has been advised [1] that maternal EFA consumption during pregnancy and lactation should be increased from 3 en% to 4.5% and from 5 to 7 en%, respectively, to compensate for losses in the placenta and milk. For example, in human milk, lipid provides 60% of the infant's dietary energy, and 10 to 12% of that is EFA. For the prevention of atherosclerosis, equal amounts of linoleic acid and various saturated FA are recommended.[1] This amount results in 10 to 13 en% of linoleic acid in an American diet.

Lipids are significantly involved in brain development. Most of the EFA in the brain are of the n-3 type, and some authors have postulated that increased intake of EFA of the n-3 type during pregnancy may be advantageous.[168]

Permanent learning defects and alterations in synaptic function in the brain, observed in EFA deficiency, can be prevented by feeding both n-6 or n-6 and n-3 EFA.[162-164] In rats, EFA deficiency cannot be prevented by feeding n-3 PUFA without n-6 EFA, and brain development seemed adequate after feeding diets with high n-6 EFA but free of n-3 PUFA. It was concluded that n-3 PUFA were not essential.[175] The preparation of diets that are really free of n-3 PUFA, however, is technically difficult. In view of the efficiency of incorporation and selectivity of biomembranes for C22:6 n-3, the requisite dietary concentrations of n-3 PUFA unquestionably are extremely low. Whether this conclusion is also applicable to man is questionable. Contrary to rats, man has a limited capacity for chain elongation and desaturation of C18:3 n-3, a common fatty acid in many vegetable oils, to C22:6 n-3,[159] which is not present in vegetable oils.

An impairment in the visual process because of a deficiency in C18:3 n-3 and its metabolites C20:5 n-3 and C22:6 n-3[159] has been demonstrated by a correlation between dietary-induced changes in C22:6 n-3 in the retina and a modification of potentials induced in rod outer segments by light stimulation.[162] Feeding rats fat-free diets from weaning reduced retinal C22:6 n-3 concentrations by only 10-20%; however, feeding 2.5 en% C18:2 n-6-containing diets free of n-3 PUFA decreased C22:6 n-3 concentrations by 60% in the first generation and by more than 87% in the second generation.[164] Female rhesus monkeys were fed during gestation diets with safflower oil (n-6 to n-3 ratio of 255:1) as the sole source of fat. Their offspring that were fed the same diet developed abnormal electroretinogram recordings as compared to the control group consisting of offspring fed soybean oil (n-6 to n-3 ratio of 7). Defects were noted in the rapid phase of retinal dark adaptation and visual acuity thresholds were progressively increased in these infant monkeys. However, learning capacity tested in a spatial reversal learning task was not affected. Apparently, the compensatory increase of n-6 PUFA, especially C22:5, n-6, was sufficient for learning. Retinal n-3 PUFA deficiency could be reversed at the ages of 10 and 24 months by feeding a fish oil rich in 20:5 n-3 and 22:6 n-3.[164] In human nutrition, such extremely high n-6 to n-3 ratios rarely occur because of the wide availability of n-3 PUFA in fish, vegetables, soybean oil, etc., but they may be induced unintentionally by total parenteral nutrition when the sole source of lipid is a safflower oil emulsion. On such a regimen, a 6-year-old child developed peripheral neuropathy and periods of blurred vision.[176] Replacement of this lipid source by a soybean oil emulsion led to a cure of these clinical symptoms.[176]

On the basis of the available evidence, 0.5 to 1 en% of n-3 PUFA in a diet with 5 to 10 en% linoleic acid seems to be an adequate level of EFA intake for humans, which also covers increased EFA requirements during pregnancy, lactation, and infancy. However, the determination of human EFA requirements is complicated because of interactions with other nutrients. Most investigations of interactions have involved only laboratory animals, but the results most likely can be extrapolated to humans. Dietary saturated FA, as evaluated by growth, dermal symptoms, and the triene/tetraene ratio in tissue lipids, increase the EFA requirements. The magnitude of the effect is small, however. Saturated FA in human diets increase significantly the levels of VLDL and LDL CH[177,178] and the thrombotic activity of platelets, which can be counteracted by dietary linoleic acid.[179,180] *Cis*-Monounsaturated FA (mainly C18:1 n-9 *cis* and its product C20:3 n-9, 12, 15 all *cis*) substitute partially for EFA in the lipids of EFA-deficient animals and humans. At high dietary levels of oleic acid, however, metabolism of EFA is suppressed. For example, if the amount of C18:1 n-9 is 10 times higher than that of C18:2 n-6, 9, a triene/tetraene ratio of 1 was observed. This finding is indicative of a frank EFA deficiency.[181]

*Trans*-Monounsaturated FA also have been found to increase the EFA requirement in animals when fed at moderate levels. In man, C18:1 n-9 *trans* (elaidic acid) behaves in respect to blood lipids rather like palmitic acid, if consumed in diets with a moderate CH content.[2,140,156] Finally, an increase of serum CH, induced by high CH feeding, accentuates EFA deficiency in various animal species.

In several human diseases, such as cystic fibrosis,[181] acrodermatitis enteropathica,[181] peripheral vascular disease,[182] and multiple sclerosis,[183] signs of EFA deficiency have been found. In three double-blind trials involving patients with multiple sclerosis who showed minimal disability, treatment with 17 to 23 g of C18:2 n-6 lead to a slower progression of the disease. This result suggests preventive activity. The severe histologic damages in advanced multiple sclerosis exclude the possibility of a curative effect.

Results of several studies suggest that n-6 and n-3 EFA are involved in the regulation of cell-mediated immunity, and that administration of these FA may be beneficial in suppressing pathologic immune responses.[184] In preliminary animal and human studies, fish oil-containing diets also seemed able to modify the course of certain diseases with an inflammatory or immune component.[185] Promising results have been obtained in patients with mild rheumatoid arthritis[186,187] and psoriasis[188,189] using 7 to 70 g of a fish oil concentrate that contained mainly C20:5 n-3 and C22:6 n-3. Such high quantities of n-3 PUFA are not present in normally available food products, however. Further research is needed to find out whether lower amounts might be effective as a preventive measure as demonstrated by long-term studies.

## BIOSYNTHESIS OF EICOSANOIDS

Since the discovery of the biosynthesis of the prostaglandins (PG) $E_2$ and $F_{2a}$ from arachidonic acid (C20:4 n-6, 9, 12, 15 all *cis*) and of $PGE_1$ and $F_{1a}$ from dihomo-γ-linolenic acid (C20:3 n-6, 9, 12, all *cis*) nearly three decades ago,[177,190] our knowledge about the influence of PUFA on the biosynthesis of PG, TXA, LT(s), and hydroxy FA has grown explosively. However, the physiologic significance of the various PG, TXA, LT, and hydroxy FA pathways still requires clarification. The short biologic half-lives, inter- and intraspecies differences, and the synergistic, as well as antagonistic, biologic activities of the various products synthesized by different tissues from the same precursor FA explain why reliable predictions about the influence of changes in dietary PUFA cannot be made (Figs. 3–10 and 3–11). As explained previously, neither linoleic acid (C18:2 n-6, 9 all *cis*) nor α-linolenic acid (C18:3 n-3,6, 9 all *cis*) can be produced by animal organisms. Thus, for adequate biosynthesis of PG through the CO pathway or of LT and hydroxy FA by various LO, man depends on the presence of C18:2 n-6 and C18:3 in the diet. Chain elongation and desaturation of C18:2 n-6 to C20:3 n-6 and C20:4 n-6, which are good substrates for both CO and LO, have been well studied in several animal species[135,191] (Fig. 3–11). The physiologic regulation of chain elongation and desaturation has also been well studied. Effects of insulin, thyroxin, and epinephrine have been demonstrated.[191]

The conversion of 18:3 n-3 to timnodonic acid (20:5 n-3) proceeds efficiently in the rat, but is less effective in man[159] and even less so in rabbits. A variety of lipids rich in certain FA that might serve as precursors of metabolites with desirable effects have been evaluated. Fish oil high in PUFA was fed to obtain an inhibiting effect on the immune mechanism in rheumatoid arthritis.[186,187] Tate et al.,[192] in rat experiments, used a lipid extracted from borage seed, which contains a high concentration of γ-linolenic acid. This FA is a precursor of arachidonic acid. The oil, however, was not chosen to increase the formation of arachidonic acid, but to compete with

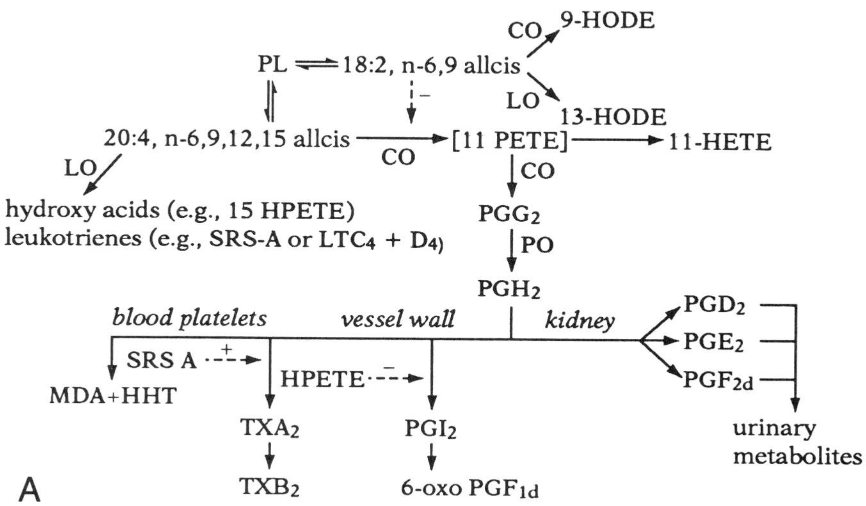
9-HODE
CO
PL
18:2, n-6,9 allcis
LO
13-HODE
20:4, n-6,9,12,15 allcis
CO
[11 PETE]
11-HETE
LO
CO
hydroxy acids (e.g., 15 HPETE)
leukotrienes (e.g., SRS-A or LTC4 + D4)
PGG2
PO
PGH2
blood platelets
vessel wall
kidney
PGD2
PGE2
PGF2d
SRS A
HPETE
MDA+HHT
TXA2
PGI2
urinary metabolites
TXB2
6-oxo PGF1d
A

**FIGURE 3–11.** *A*, Conversion of linoleic acid (C18:2 n-6,9 all *cis*) and arachidonic acid (C20:4 n-6,9,12,15 all *cis*) derived from the 2 position of cell membrane phospholipids (PL) by activation of phospholipase $A_2$ into various hydroperoxy fatty acids, such as 15 HPETE (15 hydroperoxyeicosatetraenoic acid), a product from C20:4 n-6,9,12,15, and hydroxy fatty acids, such as 13 HODE (hydroxyoctadecadienoic acid) by various lipooxygenases (LO). LO also catalyze the formation of leucotrienes (LT-A,B,C,D etc), such as the slow-reacting substance of anaphylaxis (SRS-A, a mixture of $LTC_4$ and $D_4$), $LTA_4$ and $LTB_4$-hydroxyeicosatetra-) (tri-, or penta- if derived from C20:3 n-6,9,12, or C20:5 n-3,6,9,12,15, respectively)enoic acid bound with cysteine, glutathione, and other amino acids. Cyclooxygenase (CO) converts C18:2 n-6,9 all *cis* into 9-HODE and C20:4 n-6,9,12,15 all *cis* via several intermediates into prostaglandins (PG), $PGE_2$, $F_{2a}$, $D_2$ and $I_2$. $PGI_2$ is also known as prostacyclin and $TXA_2$ as thromboxane. The formation of $TXA_2$ by blood platelets is accompanied by the synthesis of malondialdehyde (MDA) and hydroxyheptadecatrienoic acid (HHT). All these compounds have short biochemical half-lifes and are normally measured by bioassays, radioimmunoassays, or chemical analysis of urinary metabolites. Many tissues produce specific types of PG; e.g., kidney produces $D_2$, $E_2$, $F_{2a}$; the ratio is influenced by excess $Na^+$ and availability of C18:2 n-6,9 all *cis*); endothelium produces the vasodilating antithrombotic $PGI_2$, which is inhibited by 15 HPETE; platelets produce, on stimulation by SRS-A, the vasoconstricting, prothrombotic $TXA_2$. HETE, Hydroxyeicosatetraenoic acid.

arachidonic acid as a substrate for oxidative enzyme systems, in order to prevent the formation of inflammatory PG. Although γ-linolenic acid significantly decreased the induction of inflammation in a rat model and a reduction of $PGE_2$ and $LTB_4$ in pouch exudates, its effects were not clearly related to induced changes of the FA composition of the membranes. Unfortunately, this lipid is not available commercially. Evening primrose oil could also have been used for these experiments, but it contains only one half the concentration of γ-linolenic acid. These results are exciting, but such experiments are difficult to perform in a clinical setting. Several studies with fish oil have produced claims of all kinds of beneficial effects and even recommendations for the public. Regrettably, most conclusions are drawn from nonrandomized clinical studies.

Several (nonhydrogenated) fish oils, which are relatively rich in C20:5 n-3 and 22:6 n-3 (cod liver, menhaden, and mackerel), have been selected to evaluate the physiologic effects in man and rabbits of dietary PUFA of the n-3 type in relation to PG and LT biosynthesis. C20:5 n-3 is a poor substrate for CO,[108,193] but a good one for LO.[109]

The PUFA, especially of the n-3 type, are incorporated preferentially at position 2 of most cell membrane PL, and are consequently considered to play an important role in cell membrane integrity and function. Cellular stimulation leads to activation of phospholipase $A_2$ followed by mobilization of the FA on position 2 of cell membrane PL. The types of these FA determine to a great extent the types of CO and LO products. Important in this respect is that C18:2 n-6, C18:3 n-3, C20:3 n-9, and various *cis-trans* isomers show competitive inhibition with C20:3 n-6, C20:4 n-6, and C20:5 n-3, the precursors for the known biologically active PG and LT.[167] Many of the other PUFA are substrates for LO, but insufficient data exist to determine whether these LO products are biologically active.

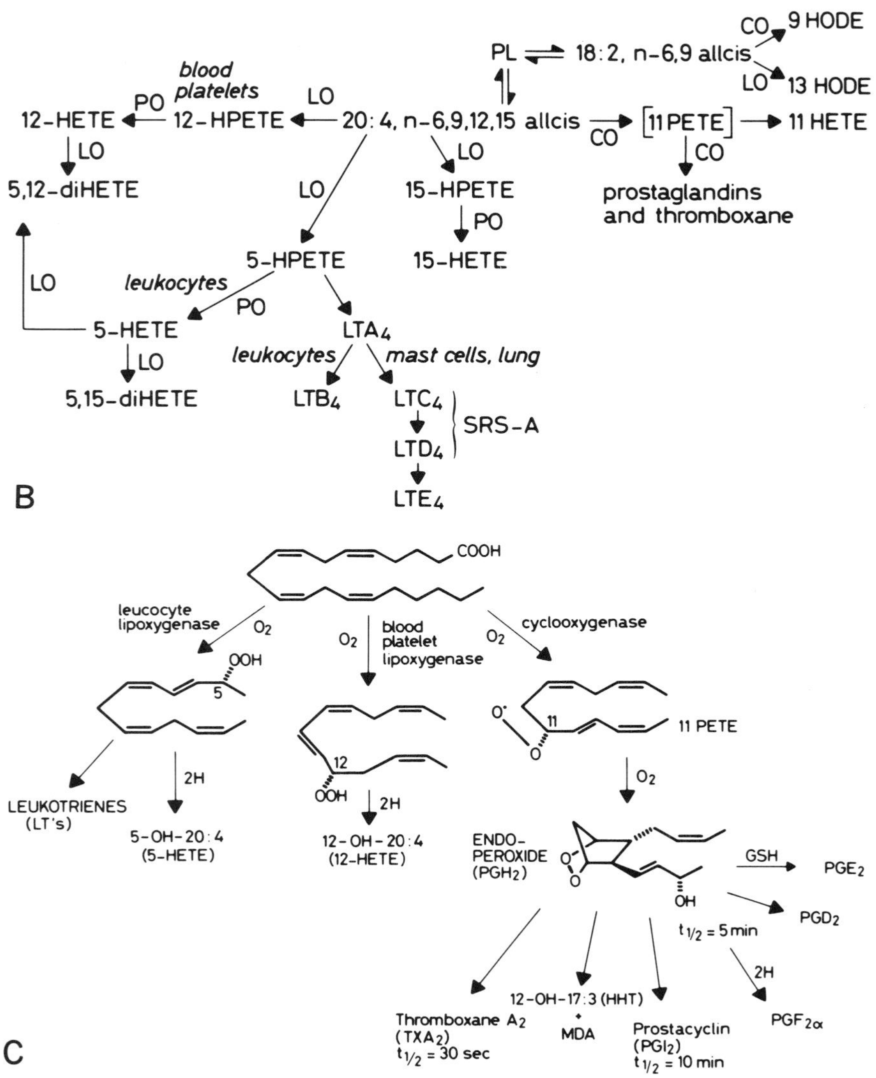

CO
9 HODE
PL
18:2, n-6,9 allcis
LO
13 HODE
blood
platelets
PO
LO
12-HETE
12-HPETE
20:4, n-6,9,12,15 allcis
CO
[11 PETE]
11 HETE
LO
LO
CO
5,12-diHETE
LO
15-HPETE
prostaglandins
and thromboxane
PO
5-HPETE
15-HETE
LO
leukocytes
PO
5-HETE
LTA4
LO
leukocytes
mast cells, lung
5,15-diHETE
LTB4
LTC4
SRS-A
LTD4
B
LTE4
COOH
leucocyte
lipoxygenase
O2
O2
blood
platelet
lipoxygenase
O2
cyclooxygenase
OOH
5
11
11 PETE
12
O2
OOH
2H
2H
LEUKOTRIENES
(LT's)
5-OH-20:4
(5-HETE)
12-OH-20:4
(12-HETE)
ENDO-
PEROXIDE
(PGH2)
GSH
PGE2
OH
PGD2
t1/2 = 5 min
2H
12-OH-17:3 (HHT)
+
MDA
Thromboxane A2
(TXA2)
t1/2 = 30 sec
Prostacyclin
(PGI2)
t1/2 = 10 min
PGF2α
C


**FIGURE 3–11.** continued *B,* Schemes of the various LO and CO products, synthesized from arachidonic acid by different organ systems, emphasizing the various LO catalyzed products. Similar schemes exist for products derived from C20:3 n-6,9,12 all *cis* and C20:5 n-3,6,9,12,15 all *cis.* The latter is a poor substrate for CO, however. *C,* An incomplete, simplified scheme of the molecular changes in C20:4 n-6,9,12,15 all *cis* during the conversion into LT, HETE, PG, and TXA.

For reasons mentioned, the best approach to evaluate the physiologic significance of dietary PUFA and their CO and LO products is through dietary studies in relation to specific organ functions. The existence of relatively specific inhibitors of CO and LO, such as acetylsalicylic acid, indomethacin, eicosatetraenoic acid, and others, facilitates the interpretation of functional changes. The use of dietary EFA of the n-6 or n-3 type in the prevention of atherosclerosis and its complications via the CO and LO pathways (see Fig. 3–11) is briefly discussed in the following section. Needless to say, essential and nonessential PUFA might have other important effects on inflammatory and immunologic processes as well.

## N-6 POLYUNSATURATED FATTY ACIDS AND ATHEROSCLEROSIS

Causally related to the induction and progression of atherosclerosis are the following.

1. Abnormal lipoprotein metabolism leading to increased VLDL and LDL levels. This condition normally is associated with a decreased HDL concentration in blood.

2. Increased tendency of blood platelets to form arterial thrombi. Mural thrombi narrow the lumen directly,

whereas embolizing thrombi are responsible for acute myocardial, cerebral, and renal infarcts. Inasmuch as aggregating platelets also release $TXA_2$, a potent vasoconstrictor, the role of vasospasm cannot be readily differentiated from the reduced blood flow related to the thrombus or embolus itself.

3. Increased arterial blood pressure.
4. Abnormal carbohydrate and insulin metabolism (both insulin-dependent and insulin-independent diabetes mellitus).

Available data support the concept that dietary composition, including the amount and type of FA, CH concentration, and Na− content, in combination with genetically determined predispositions to develop hypercholesterolemia, arterial hypertension, obesity, and diabetes mellitus, determines to a great extent the risk of developing atherosclerosis and its complications. The effects of increased dietary intake of linoleic acid have been studied with respect to the four factors just mentioned and, in general, they have proven beneficial.[1,2]

Measurements of urinary excretion of PG metabolites in rats and man showed clearly that an increase in linoleic acid consumption leads to augmented excretion of PG metabolites.[109,194]

Diets enriched in linoleic acid and reduced in saturated FA significantly lower LDL, VLDL, CH, and TG in man at both 30 and 40 en% of fat levels.[169,178,195] In studies by Iacono et al.,[195] similar diets also lowered moderate age-related hypertension to normal values. The latter results have been confirmed by several other groups[196,197] and are in agreement with epidemiologic data[198] and studies in salt-loaded rats.[199,200] Hornstra concluded from his own studies and the literature[180] that saturated fats, and especially palmitic and stearic acid, are prothrombotic, and that dietary PUFA have an antithrombotic effect in man[179] as well as in rats.[180]

The known pharmacologic effects of PG on kidney function (especially $PGE_2$), platelet aggregation and adhesion ($PGI_1$, $PGE_2$, and $TXA_2$), and blood pressure ($PGE_1$, $E_2$, and $D_2$), and the inhibitory effect of CO inhibitors (aspirin and indomethacin) on the physiologic effects of dietary linoleic acid on blood pressure[200] and platelet function,[109] support the hypothesis that the atherosclerosis-inhibiting action of dietary PUFA is based in part on improved PG biosynthesis. However, in the control of lipoprotein metabolism, no clear role for PG and LT has been identified. Aspirin by its effect on platelet aggregation reduces the incidence of heart attacks and strokes.

The same holds for the observed beneficial effects of increased dietary linoleic acid (40 en% fat, PUFA to saturated FA ratio P/S of about 1) in the prevention of retinopathy and macrovascular complications. Although serum cholesteryl linoleate concentration was increased significantly by the P/S 1 diet, total CH levels during the entire period were similar to those of the control subjects on the P/S 0.3 diet.[127,129] Nevertheless, the incidence of diabetic retinopathy, myocardial infarctions, and mortality resulting from cardiac and cerebral complications was significantly lower with the P/S 1 diet. If results of this important study can be confirmed, the question can be raised whether changes in FA composition of blood lipids (increased linoleic acid at the expense of oleic acid in CE and PL) and cellular membranes might not be more important in diabetes mellitus than the present preoccupation with the possible effects of various lipoprotein concentrations.

## N-3 POLYUNSATURATED FATS, THROMBOSIS, AND ATHEROSCLEROSIS

Eskimos reportedly have a low incidence of myocardial infarction although they consume a diet high in animal protein, fat, and CH.[202] Although this statistic could be expected because of the observed low levels of LDL and VLDL and a high degree of physical activity of Eskimos compared to Danes, another explanation is based on the observed reduced platelet aggregation in vivo, causing the observed prolonged bleeding times typical of Eskimos.[110,202] The diet of Eskimos was (and to some extent still is) characterized by a high intake of C20:5 n-3 and C22:6 n-3. These very long-chain PUFA are incorporated preferentially in plasma and cellular PL at the expense of C18:2 n-6 and C20:4 n-6, the latter being the precursor of the pro-platelet aggregatory $TXA_2$ and of the anti-aggregatory eicosanoids $PGI_2$ and $PGD_2$ (see Fig. 3–11). The increased bleeding times can be explained by a reduced platelet aggregation tendency in vivo owing to a decreased $TXA_2$ biosynthesis. C20:5 n-3 can be converted in vitro into prostanoids of the n-3 series, but with low efficiency. On the other hand, it is a good substrate for various LO, leading to the formation of the other group of eicosanoids, such as LT and hydro (per) oxy fatty acids. The physiologic significance of these compounds has not been studied sufficiently, however. Important species difference appear to exist in regard to the conversion of endogenous C20:5 n-3 into prostanoids of the n-3 series.

Although the conversion of C20:5 n-3 into PG of the n-3 series in vivo is low,[203] the urine of volunteers who consumed fish such as mackerel, or used cod-liver oil, clearly contains significant amounts of the major metabolites of $PGI_3$.[204] However, in the same human study, the amount of the major metabolites of $PGI_2$ (formed from C20:4 n-6) increased even to greater extent, probably because of an increased availability of C20:4 n-6 mobilized from membrane PL caused by substitution by C20:5 n-3 and C22:6 n-3, which have a greater affinity for the position 2 of biomembrane PL. The effect of marine lipids on the synthesis of the 2-series prostanoids may result not only from changes in the availability of C20:4 n-6; but also from alterations in certain properties of lipoproteins. For example, LDL inhibit $PGI_2$ synthesis and promote the formation of $TXA_2$.[205,206] The inhibiting effect of LDL on

$PGI_2$ production, however, is significantly reduced in volunteers who received 6 to 9 g of cod liver oil per day for 2 weeks.[207] Because this effect counteracts the influence of n-3 PUFA on $PG_2$ formation caused by changes in C20:4 n-6 availability, it may, at least in part, explain the inconsistent findings in vivo.

In these studies, only one or two "major" metabolites of a given eicosanoid are analyzed in urine, neglecting the fecal excretion of other metabolites. Furthermore, the "major" metabolite of $PGI_2$ in urine is only 10 to 15% of the total of at least 16 different metabolites.[208]

Apart from prostanoids formed enzymatically, a variety of LO is responsible for the production of hydroxy FA, some of which may have a thromboregulatory role,[209,210] and LT, which are known to affect prostanoid synthesis, asthma, and inflammatory processes.[211] Because the biologic activity of these latter compounds, formed from C20:5 n-3, seems to be less than that of the corresponding products derived from C20:4 n-6, substitution of C20::4 n-6 by C20:5 n-3 can be expected to modulate immunologic and inflammatory reactions.

Animal studies indicate that n-3 PUFA may have important effects on myocardial performance, although contrary to the effects of 18:2 n-6, not always in a beneficial way. In rats fed a diet with 10% (w/w) cod liver oil, the incidence of ST segment elevation in the ECG tested under ether anesthesia was increased, contrary to the response in rats fed palm oil and sunflower seed oil.[212] In rats fed tuna oil (12% w/w) for more than 1 year, tension of isolated papillary muscles developed and the positive inotropic effects of $Ca^{2+}$ were reduced significantly when compared with control animals.[213]

Arrhythmias induced by isoprenaline, however, were reduced to a similar extent after feeding tuna and sunflower seed oils pointing to an antiarrhythmic effect of both n-3 and n-6 PUFA. However, n-3 PUFA might be more active in this respect than n-6 PUFA.[214] Feeding 4.5 to 9.1% w/w mackerel oil (with about 20% C20:5 n-3 + C22:6 n-3) to pigs for 8 to 16 weeks did not detectably affect a series of hemodynamic parameters, measured in vivo, although large changes had been induced in the FA profile of cardiac tissue.[215] Also, recovery of cardiac function after repeated occlusion of the left anterior descending coronary artery was similar to that in control pigs receiving lard instead of mackerel oil. However, the incidence of reperfusion arrhythmias was significantly lower and the reactive hyperemic responses were of longer duration in the mackerel oil-fed animals.[215] On the other hand, the intake of n-3 PUFA from cod-liver oil by rats is associated with a reduced tolerance of the myocardium to stress, induced by repeated intraperitoneal injections of high doses of isoproterenol, and caused more myocardial necrosis and higher mortality than observed in rats fed a control diet low in n-3 PUFA.[216]

Mural thrombus formation has been induced in aortae of rats fed diets deficient in EFA (5 en% hardened coconut oil) or with either 1.5 en% n-3-type PUFA (5 en% cod liver oil) or 3 en% C18:2 n-6 (5 en% sunflower seed oil), using Hornstra's method.[180] Because of the shortage of C20:4 n-6 and consequently a low production of $TXA_2$, thrombus formation is delayed in EFA deficiency. At 2-3 en% C18:2 n-6, biochemical conditions are such that the growth rate of mural thrombus is maximal; this rate decreases again (dose-effect related) at higher dietary C18:2 n-6 concentrations.[180] Because it is claimed that PUFA of the n-3 type reduce arterial thrombus formation because of decreased production of $TXA_2$,[110,202,217] formation of thrombus should have been delayed by the cod liver oil-containing diet, especially because production of both $TXA_2$ and $TXA_3$ was negligible compared to their production in the diet containing 3 en% C18:2, n-6. Thrombus formation in both groups was identical, however, which indicates that, at least in rats, $TXA_2$ production is not well related to in vivo thrombus formation and that n-3 PUFA does not have a specific antithrombotic activity in comparison to n-6 PUFA. Also, at a higher dietary intake (up to 40 en% of either sunflower seed oil or n-3 PUFA-rich fish oils), no significant differences have been observed with regard to the in vivo antithrombotic activities of these oils.[180]

Another animal model of arterial thrombosis is based on the application of an electric current to a coronary artery in dogs, which results in thrombosis. ECG changes were more frequent in control dogs as compared to dogs fed a diet with 25 en% menhaden oil. The average infarct size in most animals in the latter group was smaller, but mortality related to ventricular fibrillation was equal in both groups.[218] Cats fed a diet with 10% menhaden oil developed significantly smaller infarcts, induced by ligating the left middle cerebral artery, in comparison to control animals. As a consequence, the neurologic symptoms caused by the infarct were significantly less severe in the fish-oil-fed cats. In these animal models, the n-3 PUFA-induced reduction of $TXA_2$ is apparently of greater pathophysiologic importance.

Arterial thrombosis and intimal hyperplasia resulting from platelet-stimulated migration of medial smooth muscle cells to the intima are frequent causes of failure of vein grafts used for arterial reconstructions. Antiplatelet aggregation therapy with drugs such as dipyridamole and aspirin has been successful in enhancing graft patency. Cod liver oil in a dose equivalent to 1.8 g of C20: 5 n-3 per day, given to dogs, was more effective than the combination of dipyridamole and aspirin, however, especially if dietary treatment started a few days before the grafts were introduced in the arterial system.[219-221]

In regard to the claimed beneficial effects of n-3 PUFAs on abnormal lipoprotein metabolism, the primary cause of atherosclerosis, the situation is less clear than in regard to arterial thrombosis. In a large series of human intervention studies, high fish- or fish-oil-containing diets always lower plasma TG and VLDL, in comparison to diets with predominantly saturated FA or diets low in total fat and high in carbohydrates. With respect to the biochemical mechanism of the hypotriglyceridemic effect of dietary n-3 PUFA, FA, TG, and VLDL synthesis decreased in the liver and VLDL clearance accelerated [222] (See also the section on biochemistry). Contrary to the well-documented effects of dietary n-3 PUFA on VLDL, the literature on the effect of fish oil on plasma CH and LDL metabolism is confusing. Although in many human studies a moderate lowering effect has been found, in an even greater number of trials, no significant effects were obtained. Indeed, in several instances, a rise in plasma LDL content was reported.[203] These discrepancies are probably related to the initial plasma CH content and lipoprotein profiles, the length of the feeding period, and/or the amount and type of fish (oil) used. Some fish oils have a relatively high content of saturated FA, CH, C and vitamin $D_3$, factors that increase LDL levels.[223] In regard to the influences of fish (oils) on HDL-CH levels, the observed increase can be explained on the basis of its VLDL-lowering activity. In many other studies, however, either no significant effect was found, or a similar increase was observed in the control group.[203] It is distressing that a proper control group was included in only 5 of the 50 studies (published to mid-1989). Another variable affecting LDL levels is the well-documented reduction in the formation of VLDL and their catabolism. Thus, the VLDL to LDL conversion might be enhanced by dietary fish oil, leading to an increased plasma LDL-CH content[224] and, theoretically, to an increased risk for atherosclerosis.

In conclusion, the available data in respect to the effects of n-3 very long-chain PUFA (fish oil) on lipoprotein metabolism do not suggest an antiatherogenic effect similar to the well-documented beneficial effects of n-6 EFA linoleic acid.

The same situation exists with regard to the effects of n-3 PUFA on arterial blood pressure. Contrary to the blood pressure-lowering effect of dietary linoleic acid in NaCl-induced hypertension, the results of fish-oil feeding in 18 human intervention studies are ambiguous.[203,225]

In man, no prospective intervention studies have been reported with respect to the influence of fish (oil) on arterial thrombosis and atherosclerosis, as reflected by statistics on morbidity and mortality of ischemic heart disease (IHD). Such studies are essential before the few, suggestive epidemiologic observations in Eskimos, in Japanese individuals, and in other populations with similar dietary patterns can be evaluated adequately. In the few studies conducted, fish oil treatment did not induce a significant improvement in the clinical condition of patients with angina pectoris or peripheral vascular disease, except in one uncontrolled study involving 12 patients with angina pectoris who observed a dramatic reduction in the requirement for glycerol trinitrate.[203,226]

Because of the small numbers of patients in controlled studies on the preventive effect of diets rich in fish oil on the development of atherosclerosis, several animal studies are of interest. In long-term studies (at least of 2 years duration) with rabbits fed semisynthetic diets without CH but containing the (atherogenic) protein source casein, atherosclerosis of the aorta appeared if the added fat was rich in saturated FA (coconut oil, fully hydrogenated soybean oil). Vegetable oils rich in linoleic acid proved to protect against the development of atherosclerosis,[227] but linseed oil (21% oleic acid, 14% linoleic acid, 53% α-linolenic acid - C18:3 n-3) appeared to be less protective than oils rich in C18:2 n-6.[228,229] This atherosclerosis model was used to compare the effects of fish oil and linseed oil (both rich in n-3 PUFA, but different in content of very long-chain FA) to those of olive oil (mainly C18:1 n-9), palm oil (rich in C16:0), and sunflower seed oil (mainly C18:2 n-6).[230] All diets contained 32% of one of the oils in addition to 8% sunflower seed oil. The latter oil prevented n-6 EFA deficiency in the fish oil-fed group. Protein in the diet consisted of soya protein instead of the more atherogenic casein. Probably because of the use of soya protein, the degrees of atherosclerosis after 90 weeks feeding were only moderate. Nonetheless, more severe lesions developed in the rabbits fed fish oil (P/S ratio 0.7) than in the animals fed palm oil (P/S ratio about 0.2), whereas the linseed oil-fed group (P/S ratio about 5) showed an intermediate effect. Atherosclerosis was not detected in half of the sunflower seed oil-fed animals and to only a minor degree in some of them.[230] Because of the rather large standard deviation in the results, however, no statistical significance was demonstrated between any of the groups. Nevertheless, these findings seriously counteract the claimed antiatherogenic activity of common fish oil (with 20 to 25% C20:5 n-3 and C22:6 n-3) and of linseed oil (with 21% C18:2 n-6 + 53% C18:3 n-3). The P/S ratio, popular since its introduction by Keyes et al. in the early 1960s,[231] has been used to predict the atherogenic potential of a total diet. This use of the P/S ratio clearly is an oversimplification, particularly when n-3 PUFA are simply added to n-6 PUFA in order to calculate the value of P. Similar constraints also exist in calculating the value of S, as Keys et al.[231] demonstrated in 1965. For example, C12:0 and Cl4:0 have a stronger hypercholesterolemic effect than C16:0, which is similar to C18:1 n-9,[232] whereas other saturated FA are rather inactive in this respect.[231]

In a comparable study, rabbits were given a soya protein-containing diet with 1.5% CH added to increase dietary atherogenicity. Administration of a commercial fish oil concentrate "Max EPA," which mainly contains C20:5 n-3 + C22:6 n-3) intragastrically per day for 5 months significantly increased aorta plaque formation.[233] Although this study has been criticized,[234] it demonstrates the limitation of n-3 PUFA to reduce atherogenesis. However, in a hyperlipidemic swine model, 30 ml cod liver oil per day (an excessively high dose, especially when considering the normally high vitamin $D_3$ and A levels in cod liver oil) protected against the development of coronary atherosclerosis induced by balloon abrasion of the coronary arteries.[235] Because mural thrombus formation in this model plays a dominant role in atherogenesis, and because n-3 PUFA have a well-documented antithrombotic effect, these results are in the line of expectation.

These data certainly do not support the widely published assumption that fish oils rich in n-3 FA possess a specific retarding effect on atherogenesis.[110,202,225] In rabbits, at least, they seem to stimulate atherosclerosis. Furthermore, in this study,[230] the rabbits fed fish oil showed dramatically increased levels of serum enzymes, indicative of liver damage (SGOT, SGPT, and alkaline phosphatase). Histopathologic examination confirmed the macroscopically detected liver damage at autopsy. Periportal fibrosis, lipogranulomas filled with lipofuscin, and bile duct hyperplasia were observed. Lipogranulomas were also present in the mesenteric lymph nodes.

Other potentially harmful effects of C20:5 n-3 and C22:6 n-3-rich fish oils are neglected by the advocates of increased human consumption of fish oils. The pathologically increased bleeding times, as observed after aspirin ingestion, also occur in Eskimos on a high-fish-oil diet.[202] Gudbjarnason described in rats a promoting role of C20:5 n-3 and C22:6 n-3 in the development of cardiac necrosis and increased sensitivity to catecholamine stress.[225] Yellow fat disease, as a consequence of feeding n-3 PUFA, has been observed in swine,[236] wild rabbits,[237] Shetland ponies,[238] rats,[239] horses,[240] and mink.[241] Yellow fat disease is a result of vitamin E deficiency, which probably occurs only when oils rich in n-3 PUFA, but low in vitamin E, are present in the food. In piglets, even excess tocopherol cannot prevent yellow fat disease induced by administering mackerel oil.[242] For this reason, long-term studies involving humans ingesting large amounts of n-3 PUFA should be performed with care. On the other hand, the safety of long-term increased consumption of linoleic acid has been amply demonstrated in a variety of animal species, including man.[1,67,128,156,203,232]

## SAFETY ASPECTS OF COMMON AND UNCOMMON EDIBLE LIPIDS

### MEDIUM-CHAIN TRIGLYCERIDES

Medium-chain triglycerides (MCT), used for therapeutic reasons in forms of lipid maldigestion and malabsorption, may have undesirable side effects in some disease entities. When dietary LCT are replaced by MCT, concentrations of MCFA are high in portal blood, as discussed previously. A healthy liver effectively removes MCFA from the circulation and metabolizes them. Patients with cirrhosis of the liver, however, have parenchymal dysfunction and porta-systemic shunts, which cause elevated levels of MCFA in the systemic circulation. These MCFA also cross the blood-brain barrier and may induce encephalopathy and coma in these patients.[243] Although most patients with cirrhosis have a mild fat malabsorption, MCT should not be used for treatment in these patients.

### EFFECTS OF PRODUCTION METHODS ON EDIBLE FATS

Unless the sources of edible fats (seeds, beans, meat) are consumed as such, the fats first must be isolated by crushing, pressing, and/or extraction. In monogastric animals, tissue lipid compositions are similar to dietary fat composition, except that the intestinal absorption of C18:0 and longer chain saturated FA (SAFA) is limited. C22:1 n-9 or n-11 and other very long-chain monounsaturated FA are also somewhat poorly absorbed. In ruminant animals, intestinal bacteria hydrogenate most dietary PUFA before intestinal absorption occurs. As a consequence, ruminant fat has a complex fatty composition, with up to 15% of *trans* and *cis, trans* mono- and diunsaturated FA and with very low EFA levels. A similar mixture results after industrial processing, e.g., partial hydrogenation with Ni- or Cu-based catalysts of initially PUFA-rich oils. Modern food technology has solved the problems of large-scale oil extraction from various common or less common edible fat sources. By applying several techniques (bleaching, deodorizing, steaming at temperatures between 180 and 220°C, and filtration), unwanted and potentially hazardous components and contaminants (pesticides, aflatoxins, polychlorinated biphenyls) are removed.[1] However, if temperatures used for refining are too high (over 220°C), vitamin E activity is lost. Thus, refined oils are often supplemented with desired antioxidants. Considering the wide and undefined range of contaminants present in the raw material after harvesting and storage, well-controlled industrial production of edible oil is preferable to old-fashioned and uneconomic processes, such as cold-pressed "virgin" oils that are preferred by many food faddists.

#### *TRANS FATTY ACIDS*

The long-term biologic effects of *trans* FA, especially those formed during partial hydrogenation of soybean oil, but also from other fat sources, have been studied adequately.[140] Provided that sufficient EFA is present in the diet, no adverse effects have been found. C18:1 n-9 *trans* takes an intermediate position between C18:1 n-9 *cis* and palmitic acid (C16:0), both in its physicochemical and nutritional properties. Columbinic acid (C18:3 n-6, 9, 13 *cis, cis, trans*) is present in high concentrations in the seed oil of *Aquilegia vulgaris*. The interesting effects of this uncommon vegetable oil were discussed in the section on EFA requirements. This oil, although of scientific interest, should not be used for human consumption.

#### *HYDROGENATED FISH OILS AND RAPESEED AND MUSTARD SEED OILS*

These oils are rich in C20, C22, and C24 monoenoic FA. Rapeseed oil is used in many countries as an edible oil and for the production of margarine. As a result of government regulation, the concentration of erucic acid, which is potentially harmful (see *Transport and Metabolism*) has been reduced by genetic selection from 50% to less than 2% in the rapeseed oils of most Western European countries and Canada. In many countries (especially in Asia), however, rapeseed and mustard seed oils still contain a high percentage of C20:1 n-9 and C22:1 n-9 FA.

Fish oils are used primarily in margarine. The *cis* and *trans* very long-chain FA and PUFA present in these oils are responsible for a range of pathophysiologic effects, as discussed previously.

### *USE OF FATS AND OILS FOR FRYING*

Especially during shallow frying, a complex mixture of undesirable polar material, which contains dimeric and polymeric FA, may be produced. The bitter taste and off-flavor of these oxidized fats inhibit the ingestion of large amounts. During deep-frying, the exposure to oxygen is less because of the oil and steam vapor layer covering the surface, but oxidation nonetheless occurs during frequent cooling and reheating cycles, as happens under household and restaurant conditions. Thus, frying oil should be discarded after being used three to five times. It is especially important that the temperature of the oil should not exceed 190° C, which is perfectly adequate for deep frying. With these precautions, deep frying with oils high in C18:2 n-6, 9 and low in n-3 PUFA is perfectly safe.

## UNCOMMON EDIBLE OILS

Table 3–1 provides a list of important edible oils. However, especially in the tropical belt, oils derived from the seeds of trees are often used as well. Furthermore, oils that are produced as byproducts of the rice and cotton industries can be used as edible oils if processed properly.[244] The P/S ratios of most tropical uncommon edible oils (sal, mango-kernel, kokum, pili, etc.), like coconut and palm kernel oil, are low. Oils with an intermediate P/S ratio like palm oil include those of neem, karanja, and mowrah. In contrast, linseed, watermelon seed, cottonseed, rice bran, and ambadi oils have high P/S ratios. The latter oils can therefore be useful in supplying the local population with adequate EFA intakes.

### *COTTONSEED OIL*

This oil is widely consumed in Egypt, India, etc. However, cottonseed oil contains several cyclopropenoid FA, which have unwanted biologic effects as a result of their irreversible binding to SH compounds. For example, they inhibit many dehydrogenases.[245] Furthermore, synergistic activity with aflatoxin and some other chemical carcinogens has been reported. Some varieties of cottonseed oil contain only low concentrations of these FA, however, and "alkali washing" further reduces their content sufficiently for safe usage as an edible oil.

### *RICE BRAN OIL*

This oil is a byproduct of the rice milling industry. Although it is a good edible oil, it contains a lipase that hydrolyzes the oil readily to free FA. If the oil contains less than 10% free FA, it can be refined to an "edible grade" rice bran oil with good nutritional value and without toxic components.[244]

Most of the oils mentioned in this section can be refined for consumption by removing the unsaponifiable colored and bitter substances. However, most of these oils are currently used in a less refined form for soap production. Whether these oils are used for consumption or for other industrial purposes is determined by supply and demand, especially in developing tropical countries.

### *EVENING PRIMROSE AND BORAGE OILS*

These oils are rich in γ-linolenic acid. They are being evaluated for the treatment of rheumatoid arthritis on the hypothesis that this FA competes with arachidonic acid as a substrate for PG formation. In the rat model for inflammatory tissue reactions, administration of borage oil reduced inflammation and the release of these PG.[136] However γ-linolenic acid can also serve as a precursor of arachidonic acid (see Fig. 3–11).

### *AMBADI SEED OIL (HIBERCIES CANNABINICES)*

This oil is used in some areas as an edible oil. Like cottonseed oil, it often contains substantial amounts of cyclopropenoid FA, which should be removed before it is used for animal or human consumption.

### *SAL SEED OIL (SHOREA ROBUSTA)*

Sal forests comprise 10 to 15% of the total forest area of India. The seeds are eaten by cattle but also by poor people when other food is scarce. Currently, 20,000 tons of oil per year is produced, which is only 1% of its potential.[244] Sal fat is rich in C18:0 and C18:1 n-9, a combination that makes it attractive as a cocoa butter substitute and of potential value in confectionery applications. Its refining does not present special problems, and it can be considered safe for human consumption, as shown in long-term animal studies.[243]

In summary, uncommon oils produced mainly in third-world countries may cause toxic side effects, but can be consumed safely after proper refining. However, some of them, like deem (Azadirachta) and karanja seed oil (Pongamit glabra), remain inedible and toxic because of the presence of partially unknown substances not removable by available refining techniques.

## REFERENCES


1. FAO/WHO Expert Consultation: The Role of Dietary Fats and Oils in Human Nutrition. FAO Food and Nutrition Paper 3. Rome, Food and Agriculture Organization, 1978.
2. Vergroesen, A.J., Gottenbos, J.J.: The role of fats in human nutrition: An introduction. *In* The Role of Fats in Human Nutrition. Edited by A.J. Vergroesen. London, Academic Press, 1975, pp. 1–41.
3. Ackman, R.G.: Fatty acid composition in fish oils. *In* Nutritional Evaluation of Long-Chain Fatty Acids in Fish Oils. Edited by S.M. Barlow and M.E. Stansby. London, Academic Press, 1982, pp. 25–88.
4. Myant, N.B.: The Biology of Cholesterol and Related Steroids. 1st Ed. London, William Heinemann Medical Books, 1981.
5. Grundy, S.M., Mok, H.Y.I.: J. Lipid Res., *18:*263–271, 1977.
6. O'Mullane, J.E., Hawthorne. J.N.: Atherosclerosis, *45:*81–90, 1982.
7. Beil, F.U., Grundy, S.M.: J. Lipid Res., *21:*525–536, 1980.
8. Houtsmuller, U.M.T.: Metabolic fate of dietary lecithin. *In* Nutrition and the Brain. Vol. 5. Edited by A. Barbeau, J.H. Growdon, and R.J. Wurtman. New York, Raven Press, 1979, pp. 83–95.
9. Zeisel, S.H., Growdon, J.H., Wurtman, R.I., et al.: Neurology, *30:*1226–1229, 1980.
10. Cohen, E.L., Wurtman, R.J.: Science, *191:*561–562, 1976.
11. Wurtman, J.J.: Sources of choline and lecithin in the diet. *In* Nutrition and the Brain. Vol. 5. Edited by A. Barbeau, J.H. Growdon, and R.J. Wurtman. New York, Raven Press, 1979, pp. 73–83.
12. Simonsson, P., Nilsson, A., Akesson, B.: Am. J. Clin. Nutr., *35:*36–41, 1982.
13. WHO Expert Committee: Prevention of Coronary Heart Disease. WHO Technical Report Series 678, Geneva, World Health Organization, 1982.
14. Borgstrom, B.: Phospholipid absorption. *In* Lipid Absorption: Biochemical and Clinical Aspects. Edited by K. Rommell, H. Goebell, and R. Bohmer. Baltimore, University Park Press, 1976, pp. 65–73.
15. Hamosh, M., Hand, A.R.: Dev. Biol., *65:*100–113, 1978.
16. Hamosh, M., Klaeveman, H.L., Wolf, R.O., et al.: J. Clin. Invest., *55:*908–913, 1975.
17. Hamosh, M., Scow, R.O.: J. Clin. Invest., *52:*88–95, 1973.
18. Hamosh, M., Burns, W.A.: Lab. Invest., *37:*603–608, 1977.
19. Liao, T.H., Hamosh, P., Hamosh, M.: Biochim. Biophys. Acta, *754:*1–9, 1983.
20. Szafran, H., Szafran, S., Popiela, T. et al.: Enzyme, *23:*187–193, 1978.
21. Olivecrona, T., Hernell, O.: Padiatr. Padol., *11:*600–604, 1976.
22. Fredrikzon, B., Hernell, O., Blacksberg, L., et al.: Pediatr. Res., *12:*1048–1052, 1978.
23. Hamosh, M.: Pediatr. Res., *13:*615–622, 1979.
24. Barrowman, J.A., Darnton, S.J.: Gastroenterology, *59:*13–21, 1970.
25. Brockerhoff, H., Jensen, R.G.: Lipolytic Enzymes. New York, Academic Press, 1974.
26. Borgstrom, B., Dahlqvist, A., Lundh, G., et al.: J. Clin. Invest., *36:*1521–1536, 1957.
27. Meyer, J.H.: Release of secretion and cholecystokinin. *In* Gastrointestinal Hormones. Edited by J.C. Thompson. Austin, University of Texas Press, 1975, pp. 475–490.
28. Moore, E.W., Verine, H.I., Grossman, M.I.: Acta Hepatogastroenterol., *26:*30–36, 1979.
29. Malagelada, J., Di Magno, E.P., Summerskill, W.H., et al.: J. Clin. Invest., *58:*493–499, 1976.
30. Ertan, A., Brooks, F.P., Ostrow, Y.D., et al.: Gastroenterology, *61:*686–692, 1971.
31. Grossman, M.I.: Med. Clin. North Am., *52:*1297–1303, 1968.
32. Hofmann, A.F., Mekhijian, H.S.: Bile acids and the intestinal absorption of fat and electrolytes in health and disease. *In* The Bile Acids. Vol. 2. Edited by P.P. Nair and D. Kritchevsky. New York, Plenum Press, 1973.
33. Shiau, Y.: Lipid Digestion and Absorption. *In* Physiology of the Gastrointestinal Tract. Vol. 2. Edited by L.R. Johnson. New York, Raven Press, 1987, pp. 1527–1556.
34. Borgstrom, B.Y.: J. Lipid Res., *16:*411–417, 1975.
35. Desnuelle, P.: The lipases. *In* The Enzymes. Vol. 7. Edited by P.D. Boyer. New York, Academic Press, 1972, pp. 575–616.
36. Morgan, R.G., Hoffman, N.E.: Biochim. Biophys. Acta, *248:*143–148, 1971.
37. Borgstrom, B., Weiloch, T., Erlanson-Albertsson, C.: FEBS Lett., *108:*407–410, 1979.
38. Staggers, J.E., Hernell, O.S., Stafford, R.J., et al.: Biochemistry, *29:*2028–2040, 1990.
39. Hernell, O.S., Staggers, J.E., Martin M.C.: Biochemistry, *29:*2041–2056, 1990.
40. Vandermeers, A., Vandermeers-Piret, M.C., Rathe, J., et al.: Biochim. Biophys. Acta, *370:*257–268, 1974.
41. Dietschy, J.M., Sallee, V.L., Wilson, F.A.: Gastroenterology, *61:*932–934, 1971.
42. Scholander, P.F.: Science, *131:*585–590, 1960.
43. Dietschy, J.M.: Helv. Med. Acta, *37:*89–102, 1973.
44. Aniansson, E.A., Wall, S.N., Almgren, M.: J. Phys. Chem., *80:*905–922, 1976.
45. Saunders, D.R., Sillery, J.: Lipids, *11:*830–832, 1976.
46. Sallee, V.L.: J. Lipid Res., *15:*56–64, 1974.
47. Linscheer, W.G.: Gastroenterology, *62:*777, 1972.
48. Chijiiwa, K., Linscheer, W.G.: Am. J. Physiol., *246:*G492–G499, 1984.
49. Kamer, J.H., van deWeijers, H.A.: Fed. Proc., *20(Suppl. 7):*335–344, 1961.
50. Lavy, U., Silverberg, M., Davidson, M.: Pediatr. Res., *5:*387, 1971.
51. Becker, G.H., Meyer, J., Necheles, H.: Gastroenterology, *14:*80–92, 1950.
52. Senior, J.R.: Introductory remarks by chairman. *In* Medium Chain Triglycerides. Edited by J.R. Senior. Philadelphia, University of Pennsylvania Press, 1968, pp. 3–8.
53. Isselbacher, K.J.: Mechanisms of absorption of long and medium chain triglycerides. *In* Medium Chain Triglycerides. Edited by J.R. Senior. Philadelphia, University of Pennsylvania Press, 1968, pp. 21–34.
54. Scheig, R.: Hepatic metabolism of medium chain fatty acids. *In* Medium Chain Triglycerides. Edited by J.R. Senior. Philadelphia, University of Pennsylvania Press, 1968, pp. 34–50.
55. Hashim, S.A.: Studies of medium chain fatty acid transport in portal blood. *In* Medium Chain Triglycerides.

Edited by J.R. Senior. Philadelphia, University of Pennsylvania Press, 1968, pp. 81–90.
56. Bottino, N.R., Vandenburg, G.A., Reiser R.: Lipids *2*:489–493, 1967.
57. Boyd, G.S.: Cholesterol absorption. *In* The Role of Fats in Human Nutrition. Edited by A.J. Vergroesen. London, Academic Press, 1975, pp. 331–352.
58. Lutton, C., Brot-Laroche, E.: Lipids, *14*:441–446, 1979.
59. Kaplan, J.A., Cox, G.E., Taylor, C.B.: Arch. Pathol. Lab. Med., *76*:359–368, 1963.
60. Wilson, J.D., Lindsey, C.A.: J. Clin. Invest., *44*:1805–1814, 1965.
61. Quintao, E., Grundy, S.M., Ahrens, E.H.: J. Lipid Res., *12*:233–247, 1971.
62. Connor, W.E., Lin, D.S.: J. Clin. Invest., *53*:1062–1070, 1977.
63. Whyte, M., Nestel, P., MacGregor, A.: Eur. J. Clin. Invest., *7*:53–60, 1977.
64. Borgstrom, B.J.: J. Lipid Res., *10*:331–337, 1969.
65. Chijiiwa, K., Linscheer, W.G.: Am. J. Physiol., *252*:G506–G510, 1987.
66. Bronsgeest-Schoute, D.C., Hermus, R.J., Dallinga-Thie, G.M., et al.: Am. J. Clin. Nutr., *32*:2193–2197, 1979.
67. Katan, M.B., Beynen, A.C.: Lancet, *1*:1213, 1983.
68. Treadwell, C.R., Vahouny, G.V.: Cholesterol absorption. *In* Handbook of Physiology. Section 6. Vol. 3. Edited by C.F. Code. Washington, American Physiological Society, 1968, pp. 47–143.
69. Bhattacharyya, A.K., Connor, W.E.: β-Sitosterolemia and xanthomatosis. *In* The Metabolic Basis of Inherited Disease. 4th Ed. Edited by J.B. Stanbury J.B. Wyngaarden, and D.S. Fredrickson. New York, McGraw-Hill, 1978.
70. Gray, J.M.: Maldigestion and malabsorption. *In* Gastrointestinal Disease. Edited by M.H. Sleisenger and J.S. Fordtran. Philadelphia, W.B. Saunders, 1983, pp. 228–256.
71. Shimoda, S.S., Saunders, D.R., Rubin, C.E.: Gastroenterology, *55*:705–723, 1968.
72. Roy, C.C., Roulet, M., Lefebre, D., et al.: Lipids, *14*:811–815, 1979.
73. James, A.T., Webb, J.P., Kellock, T.D.: Biochem. J., *78*:333–339, 1961.
74. Ammon, H.V., Thomas, P.J., Phillips, S.F.: J. Clin. Invest., *53*:374–379, 1974.
75. Mekhjian, H.S., Phillips, S.F., Hofmann, A.F.: Gastroenterology, *62*:783, 1972.
76. Greenberger, N.J., Franks, J.J., Isselbacher, K.J.: Proc. Soc. Exp. Biol. Med., *120*:468–472, 1965.
77. Hajra, A.K., Agranoff, B.W.: J. Biol. Chem., *243*:3458–3465, 1968.
78. Mansbach, C.M., Dowell, R.F., Pritchett, D.: Am. J. Physiol. *26*:G530–539, 1991.
79. Mahley, R.W.: Klin. Wochenschr., *61*:225–232, 1983.
80. Havel, R.J.: Prog. Biochem. Pharmacol., *319*:110–122, 1983.
81. Garfinkel, A.S., Nilsson-Ehle, P., Schotz, M.C.: Biochim. Biophys. Acta, *424*:264, 1976.
82. Vles, R.O.: Nutritional aspects of rapeseed oil. *In* The Role of Fats in Human Nutrition. Edited by A.J. Vergroesen. London, Academic Press, 1975, pp. 434–477.
83. Lewis, B.: The Hyperlipidaemias. Oxford, Blackwell Scientific Publications, 1976.
84. Boberg, J., Carlson, L.A., Freyschuss, U., et al.: Eur. J. Clin. Invest., *2*:454–466, 1972.
85. Havel, R.J.: Metabolism, *10*:1031–1034, 1961.
86. Nestel, P.J., Steinberg, D.: Circulation, *28*:667, 1963 (abstract).
87. Carlson, L.A., Boberg, J., Hogstedt, B.: Some physiological and clinical implications of lipid mobilization from adipose tissue. *In* Handbook of Physiology. Vol. 5. Edited by A.E. Renold and G.F. Cahill. Washington, American Physiological Society, 1965, pp. 625–644.
88. Mahley, R.W.: Med. Clin. North Am., *66*:375–402, 1982.
89. Nestel, P.J., Miller, N.E.: Mobilization of adipose tissue cholesterol in high-density lipoprotein during weight reduction in man. *In* High-Density Lipoproteins and Atherosclerosis. Edited by A.M. Gotto, N.E. Miller, and M.F. Oliver, New York, Elsevier/North Holland Biomedical Press, 1978, pp. 51–54.
90. Mahley, R.W., Hui, D.Y., Innerarity, T.L., et al.: J. Clin. Invest., *68*:1197–1206, 1981.
91. Fielding, P.E., Fielding, C.J.: Proc. Natl. Acad. Sci. USA, *77*:3327–3330, 1980.
92. Ross, A.C., Zilversmit, D.B.: J. Lipid Res., *18*:169–181, 1977.
93. Swift, L.L., Manowitz, N.R., Dunn, G.D., et al.: J. Clin. Invest., *66*:415–425, 1980.
94. Goldstein, J.L., Ho, Y.K., Brown, M.S., et al.: J. Biol. Chem., *255*:1839–1848, 1980.
95. Mistry, P., Nicoll, A., Niehaus, C., et al.: Circulation, 54(Suppl. II):178, 1976.
96. Fredrickson, D.S., Goldstein, J.L., Brown, M.S.: The familial hyperlipoproteinemias. *In* The Metabolic Basis of Inherited Diseases. 4th Ed. Edited by J.B. Stanbury, J.B. Wyngaarden, and D.S. Fredrickson. New York, McGraw-Hill, 1978, pp. 672–712.
97. Rudel, L.L., Shah, R., Greene, D.C.: J. Lipid Res., *20*:55–65, 1979.
98. Tall, A.R., Small, D.M., Atkinson, D., et al.: J. Clin. Invest., *62*:1354–1363, 1978.
99. Lofland, H.B., Jr., Clarkson, T.B., St. Clair, R.W., et al.: J. Lipid Res., *13*:39–47, 1972.
100. Van Zutphen, L.F., Fox, R.R.: Atherosclerosis, *28*:435–446, 1977.
101. Mistry, P., Miller, N.E., Laker, M., et al.: J. Clin. Invest., *67*:493–502, 1981.
102. Katan, M.B., Beynen, A.C.: Lancet, *1*:1213, 1983.
103. Miller, G.J., Miller, N.E.: Lancet, *1*:16–19, 1975.
103a. Shepherd, J., Packard, D.L.: Lipoprotein metabolism. *In* Human Plasma Proteins. Edited by J.C. Fruchart and J. Shepherd. New York, Walter de Gruyter, 1989, pp. 55–78.
104. Eisenberg, S.: High density lipoprotein metabolism: J. Lipid Res. 25:1017–1058, 1984.
105. Andersen, J.M., Dietschy, J.M.: J. Biol. Chem., *252*:3652–3659, 1977.
106. Eisenberg, S., Deckelbaum, R.: Intravascular lipoprotein remodelling: Neutral lipid transfer proteins. *In* Human Plasma Proteins. Edited by J.C. Fruchart and J. Sheperd. New York, Walter de Gruyter, 1989, pp. 153–169.
107. Holman, R.T.: Essential fatty acid deficiency. *In* Progress in the Chemistry of Fats and Other Lipids. Vol. 9. Part 2. Edited by R.T. Holman. New York, Pergamon Press, 1971, pp. 275–348.
108. Lands, W.E.M., LeTellier, P.R., Rome, L.H., et al.: Inhibition of prostaglandin biosynthesis. *In* Advances in the Biosciences 9. Edited by S. Bergstrom. Oxford, Pergamon Press, 1972, pp. 15–28.
109. Vergroesen, A.J., Hoor, F., ten Hornstra, G.: Effects of dietary essential fatty acids on prostaglandin synthesis.

*In* Nutritional Factors: Modulating Effects on Metabolic Processes. Edited by R.F. Beers and E.G. Bassett. New York, Raven Press, 1981, pp. 539–549.

**110.** Dyerberg, J., Bang, H.O., Stoffersen, E., et al.: Lancet, *2:*117–119, 1978.

**111.** Wurtman, R.J.: Precursor control of transmitter synthesis. *In* Nutrition and the Brain. Vol. 5. Edited by A. Barbeau, J.H. Growdon, and R.J. Wurtman. New York, Raven Press, 1979, pp. 1–13.

**112.** Subbaiah, P.V., Albers, J.J., Chen, C.H., et al.: J. Biol. Chem., *235:*9275–9280, 1980.

**113.** Kawamoto, T., Okano, C., Akino, T.: Biochim. Biophys. Acta, *619:*20–34, 1980.

**114.** Waelsch, H., Sperry, W.N., Stoyanoff, V.A.: J. Biol. Chem., *135:*297–302, 1940.

**115.** Solomon, S., Bird, C.E., Ling, W., et al.: Recent Prog. Horm. Res., *23:*297–347, 1967.

**116.** McNamara, D.J., Quackenbush, F.W., Rodwell, V.W.: J. Biol. Chem., *247:*5805–5810, 1972.

**117.** Bloch, K.: Science, *150:*19–28, 1965.

**118.** Cornforth, J.W., Popjak, G.: Meth. Enzymol. *15:*359–393, 1969.

**119.** Ingebritsen, T.S., Lee, H.S., Parker, R.A., et al.: Biochem. Biophys. Res. Commun., *81:*1268–1277, 1978.

**120.** Frnka, J.V., Dempsey, M.E.: Circulation *(Suppl. II):*82, 1975.

**121.** Siperstein, M.D.: Journ. Curr. Top. Cell. Regul., *2:*84–94, 1970.

**122.** Mosbach, E.H.: Arch. Intern. Med., *130:*478–487, 1972.

**123.** Barth, C.A., Hillmar, L.: Eur. J. Biochem., *110:*237–240, 1980.

**124.** Rodwell, V.W., Nordstrom, J.L., Mitschelen, J.J.: Adv. Lipid Res., *14:*1–74, 1976.

**125.** Wilson, J.D.: Arch. Intern. Med., *130:*493–505, 1972.

**126.** Holman, R.T., Johnson, S.: Prog. Lipid Res., *20:*67–73, 1981.

**127.** Houtsmuller, A.J.: The efficacy of linoleic acid in non-insulin dependent diabetes mellitus. *In* The Role of Fats in Human Nutrition. 2nd Ed. Edited by A.J. Vergroesen and M.A. Crawford. London, Academic Press, 1989, pp. 227–361.

**128.** Kingsbury, K.J., Morgan, D.M., Stovold, R.: Postgrad. Med. J., *45:*591–601, 1969.

**129.** Houtsmuller, A.J., Hal-Ferwerda, J., Zahn, K.J., et al.: Prog. Lipid Res., *20:*377–386, 1981.

**130.** Glomset, J.A.: J. Lipid Res., *9:*155–167, 1968.

**131.** Lairon, D., Nalbone, G., Lafont, H., et al.: Biochemistry, *17:*5263–5269, 1978.

**132.** Miettinen, T.A.: Clinical implications of bile acid metabolism in man. *In* The Bile Acids, Chemistry. Physiology and Metabolism. Vol. 2. Physiology and Metabolism. Edited by P.C. Nair and D. Kritchevsky. New York, Plenum Press, 1973.

**133.** Volpe, J.J., Vagelos, P.R.: Physiol. Rev., *56:*339–417, 1976.

**134.** Wakil, S.J.: J. Am. Chem. Soc., *80:*64–65, 1958.

**135.** James, A.T.: Adv. Exp. Med. Biol., *83:*51–74, 1977.

**136.** Mead, J.F., Fulco, A.J.: Metabolism of unsaturated fatty acids. *In* The Unsaturated and Polyunsaturated Fatty Acids in Health and Disease. Edited by N. Kugelmass. Springfield, IL, Charles C Thomas, 1978, p. 77.

**137.** Houtsmuller, U.M.T.: Fette Seifen Anstrichm., *80:*162–180, 1978.

**138.** Holman, R.T.: J. Nutr., *70:*405–410, 1960.

**139.** Holman, R.T.: Biological activities of and requirement for polyunsaturated acids. *In* Progress in the Chemistry of Fats and Other Lipids. Vol. 9. Edited by R.T. Holman. New York, Pergamon Press, 1970, pp. 611–682.

**140.** Gottenbos, J.J.: Biological effects of trans fatty acids. *In* Dietary Fats and Health. Edited by E.G. Perkins, W.J. Visek. Champaign, IL, American Oil Chemists Society, 1983, pp. 375–390.

**141.** Jeffcoat, R., James, A.T.: FEBS Lett., *85:*114–118, 1978.

**142.** Muto, Y., Gibson, D.M.: Biochem. Biophys. Res. Comm., *38:*9–15, 1970.

**143.** Goh, E.H., Heimberg, M.J.: Biochem. Biophys. Res. Commun., *55:*382–388, 1973.

**144.** Goh, E.H., Heimberg, M.: J. Biol. Chem., *252:*2822–2826, 1977.

**145.** Hoppel, C.L.: Carnitine palmitoyltransferase and transport of fatty acids. *In* The Enzyme of Biological Membranes. Vol. 2. Edited by A. Martonosi. New York, Plenum Press, 1976, pp. 119–144.

**146.** Lazarow, P.B.: J. Biol. Chem., *253:*1522–1528, 1978.

**147.** Neat, C.E., Thomassen, M.S., Osmundsen, H.: Biochem. J., *196:*149–159, 1981.

**148.** Christiansen, R.Z., Christophersen, B.O., Bremer, J.: Biochim. Biophys. Acta, *487:*28–36, 1977.

**149.** Beare-Rogers. J.L.: Fortschr. Med., *95:*29–56, 1979.

**150.** Norseth, J.: Biochim. Biophys. Acta, *575:*1–9, 1979.

**151.** Hulsmann, W.C., Stam, H.: Biochem. Biophys. Res. Commun., *82:*53–59, 1978.

**152.** Borrebaek, B., Osmundsen, H., Christiansen, E.N., et al.: FEBS Lett., *121:*23–24, 1980.

**153.** Bronfman, M., Amigo, L., Morales, M.N.: Biochem. J., *239:*781–784, 1986.

**154.** Berge, R.K., Aarsland, A., Osmundsen, H., et al.: The relationship between the levels of long-chain Acyl-CoA and clofibroyl - CoA and the induction of peroxisomal beta-oxidation. *In* Peroxisomes in Biology and Medicine. Edited by H. Fahini and H.D. Sies. Berlin, Springer, 1986, pp. 273–278.

**155.** Christiansen, R.Z., Norseth, J., Christiansen, E.: Lipids, *14:*614–618, 1979.

**156.** Norum, K.R., Christiansen, E.N., Christopherson, B.O., et al.: Metabolic and nutritional aspects of long-chain fatty acids of marine origin. *In* The Role of Fats in Human Nutrition. 2nd Ed. Edited by A.J. Vergroesen and M.A. Crawford. London, Academic Press, 1989, pp. 117–149.

**157.** Schlenk, H., Sand, D.M., Gellerman, J.L.: Biochim Biophys Acta, *187:*201–207, 1969.

**158.** Hagve, T.A., Christophersen, B.O.: Biochim. Biophys. Acta, *875:*165–173, 1986.

**159.** Dyerberg, J.: Nutr. Rev., *44:*125–134, 282, 1986.

**160.** Hagve, T.A., Christophersen, B.O.: Biochim. Biophys. Acta, *796:*205–217, 1984.

**161.** Vergroesen, A.J.: Bibl. Nutr. Dieta, *23:*19–26, 1976.

**162.** Wheeler, T.G., Benolken, R.M., Anderson, R.E.: Science, *188:*1312–1314, 1975.

**163.** Galli, C., Spagnuoli, C., Boricio, E. et al.: Dietary essential fatty acids and prostaglandins. *In* Advances in Prostaglandins and Thromboxane Research. Edited by F. Cocceani and P.M. Olley. New York, Raven Press, 1978, pp. 181–189.

**164.** Neuringer, M., Connor, W.E.: Nutr. Res., *44:*285–294, 1986.

**165.** Houtsmuller, U.M.: Specific biological effects of polyunsaturated fatty acids. *In* The Role of Fats in Human

Nutrition. Edited by A.J. Vergroesen. London, Academic Press, 1975, pp. 331–351.
166. Ziboh, V.A., Hsia, S.L.: J. Lipid Res., *13:*458–467, 1972.
167. Houtsmuller, U.M.: Prog. Lipid Res., *20:*889–896, 1981.
168. Crawford, M.A., Hassam, A.G., Stevens, P.A.: Progr. Lipid Res., *20:*31–40, 1981.
169. Brussaard, J.H., Dallinga-Thie, G., Groot, P., et al., Atherosclerosis, *36:*515–527, 1980.
170. Paulsrud, J.R., Pensler, L., Whitten, C.F., et al.: Am. J. Clin. Nutr., *215:*897–904, 1972.
171. Friedman, Z., Frohlich, J.C.: Pediatr. Res., *13:*932–936, 1979.
172. Collins, F.D., Sinclair, A.J., Royle, J.P., et al.: Nutr. Metab., *13:*150–167, 1971.
173. Shimoyama, T., Kikuchi, H., Press, M., et al.: Gut, *14:*716–722, 1973.
173a. Naismith, D.J.: Br. J. Nutr., *30:*567–576, 1973.
174. Wolfram, G., Eckart, J., Zollner, N.: Klin. Wochenschr., *58:*1327–1337, 1980.
175. Tinoco, J., Williams, M.A., Hincenbergs, J., et al.: J. Nutr., *101:*837–845, 1971.
176. Holman, R.T., Johnson, S.B., Hatch, T.F.: Am. J. Clin. Nutr., *35:*617–623, 1982.
177. Bergstrom, S., Danielsson, H., Samuelsson, B.: Biochim. Biophys. Acta, *90:*207–210, 1964.
178. Lewis, B., Hammett, F., Katan, M., et al.: Lancet, *1:*1310–1313, 1981.
179. Hornstra, G., Chait, A., Karvonen, M.J., et al.: Lancet, *1:*1155–1157, 1973.
180. Hornstra, G.: Effect of type and amount of dietary fats on arterial thrombus formation. *In* Dietary Fats, Prostanoids, and Arterial Thrombosis. The Hague, Martinus Nijhoff, 1982, pp. 1–22.
181. Holman, R.T.: Adv. Exp. Med. Biol., *83:*515–534, 1977.
182. Kingsbury, K.J., Brett, C., Stovold, R., et al.: Postgrad. Med. J., *50:*425–440, 1974.
183. Dworkin, R.H., Bates, D., Millar, J.H., et al.: Neurology, *34:*1441–1445, 1984.
184. Mertin, J., Stackpoole, A.: Cell. Immunol., *62:*293–300, 1981.
185. Taylor, W.A., Hughes, R.A., Lee, T: J. Neuroimmunol., *17:*193–197, 1988.
186. Belch, J.J., Ansell, D., Madhok, R., et al.: Ann. Rheum. Dis., *47:*96–104, 1988.
187. Kremer, J.M., Jubiz, W., Michalek, A., et al.: Ann. Intern. Med., *106:*497–503, 1987.
188. Bittiner, S.B., Tucker, W.F., Cartwright, I.: Lancet, *1:*378–380, 1988.
189. Ziboh, V.A., Cohen, K.A., Ellis, C.N., et al.: Arch. Dermatol., *122:*1277–1282, 1986.
190. van Dorp, D.A., Beerthuis, R.K., Nugteren, D.H., et al.: Biochim. Biophys. Acta, *90:*204–207, 1964.
191. Brenner, R.R.: Factors influencing fatty acid elongation and desaturation. *In* The Role of Fats in Human Nutrition. 2nd Ed. Edited by A.J. Vergroesen and M.A. Crawford. London, Academic Press, 1989, pp. 45–79.
192. Tate, G., Mandell, B., Laposata, M., et al.: J. Rheumatol., *16:*729–733, 1989.
193. Struijck, C.B., Beerthuis, R.K., Pabon, H.J., et al.: Recl. Trav. Chim. Pays Bas, *85:*1233–1250, 1966.
194. Adam, O., Wolfram, G., Zollner, N.: Ann. Nutr. Metab., *26:*315–323, 1982.
195. Iacono, J.M., Judd, J.T., Marshall, M.W., et al.: Prog. Lipid Res., *20:*349–364, 1981.
196. Vergroesen, A.J., Fleischman, A.I., Comberg, H.U., et al.: Acta Biol. Med. Ger., *37:*879–883, 1978.
197. Rao, R.H., Rao, U.B., Srikantia, S.G.: Clin. Exp. Hypertens., *3:*27–38, 1981.
198. Oster, P., Arab, L., Schellenberg, B., et al.: Ernährungsumschau, *27:*143–144, 1980.
199. Triebe, G., Block, H.U., Forster, W.: Acta Biol. Med. Ger., *35:*1223–1224, 1976.
200. Ten Hoor, F., van de Graaf, H.M.: Acta Biol. Med. Ger., *37:*875–877, 1978.
201. Howard-Williams, J., Patel, P., Jelfs, R., et al.: Br. J. Ophthalmol., *69:*15–18, 1985.
202. Dyerberg, J., Jorgensen, K.A.: Prog. Lipid Res., *21:*255–269, 1982.
203. Hornstra, G.: The significance of fish and fish-oil enriched food for prevention and therapy of ischemic cardiovascular disease. *In* The Role of Fats in Human Nutrition. 2nd Ed. Edited by A.J. Vergroesen and M.A. Crawford. London, Academic Press, 1989, pp. 151–235.
204. Fischer, S., Weber, P.C.: Nature, *307:*165–168, 1984.
205. Nordoy, A., Svensson, B., Wiebe, D., et al.: Circ. Res., *43:*527–534, 1978.
206. Beitz, J., Hoffmann, P., Taube, C., et al.: Biomed. Biochim. Acta, *44:*1681–1688, 1985.
207. Beitz, J., Schimke, E., Liebaug, U., et al.: Klin. Wochenschr., *64:*793–799, 1986.
208. Brash, A.R., Jackson, E.K., Lawson, J.A., et al.: Adv. Prostaglandin Thromboxane, Leukotriene Res., *11:*119–122, 1983.
209. Dutilh, C.E., Haddeman, E., Don, J.A., et al.: Prostaglandins Leukot. Essent. Fatty Acids, *6:*111–126, 1981.
210. Croset, M., Sala, A., Folco, G., et al.: Biochem. Pharmacol., *37:*1275–1280, 1988.
211. Lewis, R.A., Austen, K.F.: J. Clin. Invest., *73:*889–897, 1984.
212. Montfoort, A., Van der Werf, L., Hartog, J.M., et al.: Basic Res. Cardiol., *81:*289–302, 1986.
213. McLennan, P., Abeywardena, M.Y., Charnock, J.S.: Prostaglandins Leukot. Essent. Fatty Acids, *27:*183–195, 1987.
214. Gudbjarnason, S.: J. Intern. Med., *225 (Suppl. 1):*117–128, 1989.
215. Hartog, J.M., Lamers, J.M., Achterberg, P.W., et al.: Basic Res. Cardiol., *82 (Suppl. 1):*223–234, 1987.
216. Gudbjarnason, S., Oskarsdottir, G., Duell, B., et al.: Adv. Cardiol., *25:*130–144, 1978.
217. Culp, B.R., Lands, W.E., Lucches, B.R., et al.: Prostaglandins, *20:*1021–1031, 1980.
218. Black, K.L., Culp, B.R., Madison, D., et al.: Prostaglandins Leukot. Essent. Fatty Acids, *3:*257–268, 1979.
219. Cahill, P.D., Sarris, G.E., Cooper, A.D., et al.: J. Vasc. Surg., *7:*108–118, 1988.
220. Casali, R.E., Hale, J.A., LeNarz, L. et al.: J. Surg. Res., *40:*6–12, 1986.
221. Landymore, R.W., MacAuley, M., Sheridan, B., et al.: Ann. Thorac. Surg., *41:*54–57, 1986.
222. Nestel, P., Topping, D., Marsh, Y., et al.: Effects of polyenoic fatty acids (n-3) on lipid and lipoprotein metabolism. *In* Polyunsaturated Fatty Acids and Eicosanoids. Edited by W.E.M. Lands. Champaign, IL, American Oil Chemists Society, 1987, pp. 94–102.
223. Illingworth, D.R., Connor, W.E., Hatcher, L.F.: J. Intern. Med., *225 (Suppl. 1):*91–97, 1989.
224. Hainers, A.P., Sanders, T.A., Imesen, J.D., et al.: Thromb. Res., *43:*643–655, 1986.

225. Knapp, H.R., Whittemore, K.L., Fitzgerald, G.A.: Dietary unsaturates and human vascular function. *In* Polyunsaturated Fatty Acids and Eicosanoids. Edited by W.E.M. Lands. Champaign, IL, American Oil Society, 1987, pp. 41–55.
226. Kristensen, S.D., Schmidt, E.B., Andersen, H.R., et al.: Atherosclerosis, *64:*13–19, 1987.
227. Gottenbos, J.J., Thomasson, H.J.: Coll. Inst. Centr. Nat. Rech. Sci., *99:*221–239, 1961.
228. Kloeze, J., Houtsmuller, U.M., Vles, R.O.: J. Atheroscl. Res., *9:*319–334, 1969.
229. Moore, J.H.: Br. J. Nutr., *23:*125–134, 1969.
230. Hornstra, G., Haddeman, E.: Effect of dietary fatty acid composition on platelet and vascular prostanoid formation. *In* Biology and Pathology of the Vessel Wall. Edited by N. Wolff. Eastbourne, Praeger Scientific, 1983, pp. 119–122.
231. Keys, A., Anderson, J.F., Grande, F.: Metab. Clin. Exp., *14:*776–787, 1965.
232. Bagby, M.O., Smith, C.R., Mikolajeyak, K.L., et al.: Biochemistry, *1:*632–639, 1962.
233. Thiery, J., Seidel, D.: Atherosclerosis, *63:*53–56, 1987.
234. Sanders, T.A.: Atherosclerosis, *67:*91–93, 95, 1987.
235. Weiner, B.H., Olkene, I.S., Levine, P.H., et al.: N. Engl. J. Med., *315:*841–846, 1986.
236. Danse, L.H., Steenbergen-Botterweg, W.A.: Vet. Pathol., *11:*465–476, 1974.
237. Jones, D., Gresham, G.A., Lloyd, H.G., et al.: Nature, *207:*205–206, 1965.
238. Kroneman, J., Wensvoort, P.: Neth. J. Vet. Sci., *1:*42–48, 1968.
239. Danse, L.H., Stolwijk, J., Verschuren, P.M.: Vet. Pathol., *16:*593–603, 1979.
240. Wensvoort, P.: Tijdschr. Diergeneesk, *99:*1060–1066, 1974.
241. Danse, L.H., Steenbergen-Botter-veg, W.A.: Zentralbl. Veterinaermed. (A), *23:*645–660, 1976.
242. Ruiter, A., Jongbloed, A.W., van Gent, C.M., et al.: Am. J. Clin. Nutr., *31:*2159–2166, 1978.
243. Linscheer, W.G.: Replacement of dietary fat by medium chain triglycerides. *In* Medium Chain Triglycerides. Edited by J.R. Senior. Philadelphia, University of Pennsylvania Press, 1968, pp. 165–172.
244. Menon, K.K.G., Mulky, M.J., Mani, V.V.S.: Nutritional and toxicological aspects of uncommon edible oils. *In* The Role of Fats in Human Nutrition. 2nd Ed. Edited by A.J. Vergroesen and M.A. Crawford. London, Academic Press, 1989, pp. 407–440.
245. Allen, E., Johnson, A.R., Fogerty, A.C., et al.: Lipids, *2:*419–423, 1967.

CHAPTER 4

# Dietary Fiber

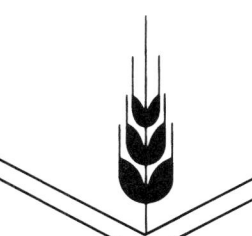

Barbara O. Schneeman & Janet Tietyen



During the last 20 years, dietary fiber has been recognized as an important part of a healthful diet. As a result, numerous clinical trials and animal feeding studies have been conducted with dietary fiber. From 1968 to 1978, the annual number of scientific reports on fiber increased 40-fold.[1] Investigators have evaluated the effects of fiber through use of fiber supplements, meal studies, and high-fiber diets.[2] The unavailable carbohydrate portion of foods is no longer regarded as an inert component with little nutritional value, but rather it is considered important for normal gastrointestinal function. Plants are a unique source of dietary fiber because of the polysaccharide structure of the cell wall, as well as the storage and secretion polysaccharides associated with plant cells and seeds. These polysaccharides cannot be digested by endogenous enzymes secreted in the mammalian small intestine. Within the plant cell wall, dietary fiber components exist in a matrix and are interlinked with other carbohydrates, proteins, fats, and inorganic compounds. This composite structure represents plant fiber as it exists in foods. However, a large body of experimental evidence on the role of fiber in the diet has been gained through feeding of isolated fiber components.

In this chapter, the definitions, chemistry, analysis, and physical properties of dietary fibers as they relate to gastrointestinal function and other physiologic responses are discussed. Data on the food content of total dietary fiber and components are given in Appendix Tables A–18a and A–18b. In other chapters of this book, dietary fiber is discussed with respect to its use in the clinical management of patients with diabetes, hyperlipidemia, and gastrointestinal diseases.

## CHEMISTRY AND CLASSIFICATION

The major fiber components are polysaccharides other than starch and include cellulose, β-glucans, hemicelluloses, pectins, and gums in addition to the nonpolysaccharide component, lignin.[3,4] These polysaccharides are defined by their sugar residues and the linkages between them. Cellulose and β-glucan are glucose polymers with β(1->4) bonds. In the β-glucans the β(1->4) bonds are interspersed with β(1->3) bonds, and this structure makes the molecule less linear than cellulose. Oats and barley are typically rich in β-glucans; however, cellulose is found in all plant tissues. The hemicelluloses are a heterogenous group of polysaccharides with various sugars in the backbone and side chains of the polymers. These polysaccharides are classified based on the predominate sugar residue in their backbone (e.g., xylans, galactans, or mannans) and in their side chains (e.g., arabinose, galactose). In pectins the backbone is predominantly galacturonic acid residues, rhamnose units are inserted at intervals, and side chains contain predominantly arabinose and galactose. Pectins also vary by the degree of methoxyl groups esterified to the uronic acid. Lignin is composed of a mixture of phenolic compounds resulting in a highly complex molecule. Although most foods contain only small amounts of lignin, its presence can greatly affect the digestibility of the cell wall structure, and considerable interest exists in the potential carcinogenic and anticarcinogenic effects of phenolic compounds derived from plant foods.[5] All plant foods contain a mixture of different fiber components that depend on the type of plant tissue and its maturity. Table 4–1 describes some of the predominate fiber components in the major food groups.

Digestion of carbohydrates is based on the linkages between monosaccharides (Table 4–2). In glucose polymers, α -linkages are generally susceptible to digestion by α-amylase secreted in the small intestine, whereas β-linkages are not; however, these bonds can be hydrolyzed by microbial enzymes in the large intestine.[6] The capacity of microbial enzymes to hydrolyze the β-linkage is affected by the linkage sequence of the monosaccharides, as well as polymer structural characteristics such as chain length, degree of branching, and crystallinity.

The most widely accepted definition restricts fiber components to the nonstarch polysaccharides plus lignin. Plant foods also contain compounds such as digestive enzyme inhibitors, cell wall glycoproteins, phenolic esters, or Maillard reaction products that have physiologic activity and may contribute significantly to the properties associated with fiber consumption. These noncarbohydrate constituents, although comprising a small proportion (~5 to 10%) of the dietary fiber complex,[7] may be important in explaining some of the physiologic responses to sources of dietary fiber. For example, glycoproteins contribute to the structural integrity of the cell wall matrix, and Maillard reaction products are nondigestible polymers that provide bulk in the large intestinal contents. Additionally, plant foods can contain ungelatinized or retrograded starch that is resistant to digestion by α-amylase.[8,9] This so-called "resistant starch" can be degraded by the microflora in the large intestine and hence has properties similar to dietary fiber. The amount of resistant starch in a food varies by cooking and holding techniques, maturity of the plant, and the ratio of amylose to amylopectin. Although some controversy has existed as to whether some of the noncarbohydrate compounds as well as resistant starch should be considered part of the dietary fiber, one should not overlook that such components of plant foods have physiologic activities that may contribute to the nutritional importance of foods containing fiber.

Identification and quantification of food components that constitute dietary fiber are difficult because of the diversity of these constituents and their location within the cell wall matrix. In addition to the classification based on carbohydrate units, the components of fiber have been classified based on their dispersion in water. Polysaccharides that readily disperse in water have been described as soluble. Most foods contain a mixture of insoluble and soluble fibers. Anderson and Bridges analyzed the dietary fibers present in major food groups with respect to their solubility and component sugar residues.[10] Soluble fiber content as a percentage of total dietary fiber averaged 32% for cereals, 32% for vegetables, 25% for dried beans, and 38% for fruits. Dried bean, oat, and barley products are relatively concentrated food sources of soluble dietary fiber. Polysaccharide food additives, such as pectin, gums, mucilages, and algal polysaccharides, are additional sources of soluble fiber in the food supply that are consumed at relatively low levels (<2% of fiber intake).[4] These soluble fibers serve functional purposes in food systems by modifying the textural characteristics of foods.

## METHODS OF ANALYSIS

Methods for the determination of fiber in foods have evolved as our knowledge of fiber chemistry and of food analysis has become more complete. The crude fiber method was developed in the 1850s to provide an estimate of the indigestible material in animal feed.[11] This method is not related to any specific carbohydrate fraction of foods, and the losses of fiber components with this procedure can be substantial, resulting in a serious underestimation of fiber content. By recognizing the limitations of the crude fiber method to characterize accurately the fiber content of foods, better analytic

**TABLE 4–1.** MAJOR DIETARY FIBER POLYMERS FOUND IN MAJOR FOOD GROUPS

| FOOD GROUP | POLYMERS PRESENT |
|---|---|
| Cereals | Cellulose, arabinoxylans, β-D-glucans, other noncellulosic polysaccharides, phenolic esters, lignin |
| Vegetables and fruits | Cellulose, pectic substances, xyloglucans, other noncellulosic polysaccharides, lignin, cutin, waxes |
| Seeds | Cellulose, pectic substances, xyloglucans, galactomannans, other noncellulosic polysaccharides |
| Food additives | Gums, algal polysaccharides, alginates, sulfated galactans, cellulose esters and ethers, modified starches |

(Adapted from Selvendran, R.R.: Am. J. Clin. Nutr., *39*:320-337, 1984.)

**TABLE 4–2.** CHARACTERISTICS OF COMMON GLUCOSE POLYMERS

| POLYMER | BOND TYPE | MOLECULE CONFORMATION | PROPERTIES |
|---|---|---|---|
| Starch | | | |
| Amylose | α-(1->4) | Linear | Digestible by α-amylase to glucose |
| Amylopectin | α-(1->4) & α-(1->6) branch points | Branched | Digestible by α-amylase to glucose and limit dextrans |
| Nonstarch | | | |
| Cellulose | β-(1>4) | Linear | Digestible by bacterial enzymes; relatively insoluble |
| Oat or barley β-glucan | β-(1->3) (1->4) | Nonlinear | Digestible by bacterial enzymes; dispersable and viscous in water |

**TABLE 4–3.** METHODS OF ANALYSIS FOR DIETARY FIBER

| METHOD AND REFERENCE | FRACTION ANALYZED |
|---|---|
| Crude Fiber<br>Williams and Olmsted, 1935[11] | Residual following acid and alkali extraction, not related to a specific carbohydrate fraction |
| Neutral Detergent Fiber (NDF)<br>Goering and Van Soest, 1970[13] | NDF includes insoluble polysaccharides and lignin |
| Acid Detergent Fiber (ADF)<br>Van Soest, 1963[12] | ADF includes primarily cellulose and lignin; NDF minus ADF is a rough estimate of hemicellulose content |
| Enzymatic Procedure<br>Prosky et al., 1988[19] | Total dietary fiber (TDF) includes nonstarch polysaccharides plus lignin |
| Southgate, 1976[15] | Unavailable carbohydrates and may include starch; method includes colorimetric determination of carbohydrate fractions |
| Englyst, 1981[17] | Determines nonstarch polysaccharides (NSP); modification of the Southgate procedure to determine carbohydrate fractions with gas-liquid chromatography |
| Theander and Aman, 1981[18] | Determination of hemiculluloses, pectins, cellulose and Klason lignin, and TDF |

schemes have been developed. The major ones in use today are the neutral detergent fiber (NDF) and acid detergent fiber (ADF) methods, the enzymatic procedure (also referred to as total dietary fiber (TDF) and the Prosky method), the Southgate procedure, the Englyst procedure, and the Theander procedure. Published values for fiber content currently use these methods, which are briefly described in this section. The fractions measured by these methods are summarized in Table 4–3.

The NDF and ADF procedures were initially developed for the analysis of animal forages and were modified for application to human foods.[12,13] The NDF procedure estimates insoluble polysaccharides (cellulose, most hemicelluloses) plus lignin, whereas the ADF procedure estimates primarily lignin and cellulose. The difference between NDF and ADF values provides a rough estimate of hemicellulose content. Detergent methods can be used for a simple, rapid estimate of insoluble dietary fiber. The primary limitation of these methods is that they do not estimate the content of soluble polysaccharides and thus underestimate the total fiber content of a food. Because the amount of soluble polysaccharides in foods is variable, no standard conversion factor can be used to convert NDF or ADF values to total dietary fiber content.

The Southgate method, now known to overestimate dietary fiber because of incomplete starch solubilization, was developed to characterize and quantify the unavailable carbohydrate fraction of foods.[14,15] In strong acid solutions, carbohydrates undergo condensation reactions with certain substances to yield products that can be measured colorimetrically. The major disadvantage of colorimetric methods is the lack of an appropriate standard set of monosaccharides. Mutual absorbance interference among groups of sugars and the array of sugars present in a particular food system must be considered in the careful application of colorimetric analysis techniques. More specific gas-chromatographic methods have been developed to characterize neutral sugars, though uronic acid determination remains a colorimetric procedure.[16]

Gas-liquid chromatography (GLC) methods also rely on a set of sugar standards but allow a greater degree of specificity. The original Englyst GLC method was based on that of Southgate, but replaced the colorimetric detection of monosaccharides with chromatographic separation.[17] This method uses a sample size of 1 to 300 mg and has the advantage of being essentially a one-tube procedure. Based on this approach, Southgate and Englyst introduced the concept that this method can be used to quantify the nonstarch polysaccharide (NSP) fraction of foods as a way to quantify dietary fiber.[4] Another chemical analysis approach that is widely used was developed by Theander and Aman.[5,18] The Theander method consists of several analyses of a single sample and provides total, soluble, and insoluble fiber measurements with additional values for hemicelluloses, pectins, cellulose, and Klason lignin. A major difference between these two approaches is the inclusion of Klason lignin by Theander and its exclusion by Englyst.[5] These methods have the advantage of providing more specific information on the carbohydrate fractions in foods, but they are more demanding in terms of analytic skills.

The development of enzymatic methods dates back to the 1930s.[16] Using this approach, the undigested residue following amylolytic and proteolytic enzyme treatment is used for dietary fiber determination. The enzymatic/gravimetric method of Prosky et al. has been tested in interlaboratory studies for the determination of total, soluble, and insoluble dietary fiber.[19] In this procedure, the residue remaining after the enzymatic digestion steps is weighed, corrected for ash and Kjeldahl nitrogen, and used to calculate the percentage of dietary fiber. The Prosky procedure is an official method of the Association of Official Analytical Chemists (AOAC) for total dietary fiber,[19] and it is considered an appropriate method for general food labeling.[20] Another gravimetric method was developed by Mongeau and Brassard.[21] This procedure, which may be more appropriate for cereals, has been adopted by the American Association of Cereal Chemists (AACC).[22] In this AACC method, soluble fibers are precipitated with more concentrated ethanol than in the AOAC method and insoluble fiber is determined by a separate neutral detergent procedure.

In summary, currently available methods to quantify fiber in foods rely on either the weight or monosaccharide profile of the dietary fiber residue. The gravimetric procedures tend to be simpler and more rapid. Table 4–3 summarizes the most widely used methods. Values reported as crude fiber, NDF, or ADF are likely to lead one to underestimate the actual fiber content of a food, whereas the Southgate method typically leads one to overestimate fiber content. The remaining three methods give the best estimate of total dietary fiber content of foods. Both the Theander and the enzymatic procedure include lignin in the total dietary fiber estimate, whereas the Englyst method only includes nonstarch polysaccharides. When using the various food tables available for fiber content, it is important to know the method used in obtaining the values in order to understand what components are included in the estimation. Values of the total dietary fiber content of selected foods and their various constituents are included in the Appendix (Tables A–18a and A–18b). Additional references on the fiber content of foods are articles by Anderson and Bridges[10] and Marlett.[67]

## PHYSICAL PROPERTIES

The chemical composition of dietary fibers as estimated by the monomeric sugar units is not predictive of the physiologic effects of fiber. For example, Table 4–2 lists four polysaccharides that contain glucose units, yet these each vary in their properties. This variation is due in part to the different linkages between the sugar units and polysaccharide chains. These linkages determine the enzymatic digestibility of the polysaccharides as well as their solubility. For this group of polysaccharides, simply knowing the sugar residues would provide little information about the properties of these different polysaccharides when consumed. Similarly, simply characterizing them as soluble or insoluble in water is not sufficient to explain their physiologic effects. Instead, properties such as viscosity, water-holding capacity, bile acid binding ability, particle size, and microbial degradation are better predictors of physiologic function. Table 4–4 summarizes the nutritional implications of properties discussed in this section.

### VISCOSITY

Polysaccharides such as pectins, β-glucans, various gums, and algal polysaccharides are capable of forming highly viscous solutions. The viscosity of individual polysaccharides can be altered by modifying the structure of the polysaccharide. For example, reduction of the molecular weight or methyl ester content of pectins or hydrolysis of the β(1->3) linkages in β-glucans reduces their viscosity. Although it is difficult to use in vitro systems to predict the viscosity in vivo, viscosity within the gastrointestinal contents is increased when these polysaccharides are fed. An increase in viscosity has been associated with slowing the rate of gastric emptying, which slows the delivery of nutrients to the small intestine.[23] Within the small intestine, an increase in viscosity disrupts mixing in the intestinal contents.[24] This effect results in poorer mixing of enzymes and substrates and affects delivery of absorbable nutrients to the mucosal cells. Hence, overall, the presence of highly viscous materials in the stomach and small intestine slows the digestion and absorption of nutrients. Several

**TABLE 4–4.** NUTRITIONAL AND PHYSIOLOGIC IMPORTANCE OF PHYSICOCHEMICAL PROPERTIES OF DIETARY FIBER

| PROPERTY | PHYSIOLOGIC CONSEQUENCES | TYPES OF FIBER | NUTRITIONAL IMPLICATION |
|---|---|---|---|
| Microbial degradation | Breakdown of polysaccharide structure in the large intestine<br>Production of short chain fatty acids (SCFA) and other microbial metabolites<br>Growth of microflora | Polysaccharides<br>Extent of microbial action dependent on solubility | Fecal bulking of fiber dependent on extent of microbial degradation<br>Increase in stool weight due to residual polysaccharides and/or increase in microbial cells<br>Provision of energy by SCFAs to cells and possible metabolic effects<br>Reduction in pH of colon contents |
| Water-holding capacity (WHC) | Swelling with water in the gut contents<br>Increased viscosity of gastrointestinal contents<br>Influence on the microbial breakdown of fiber | Pectins<br>Gums<br>β-glucans<br>Some hemicelluloses | Increased viscosity slowing gastric emptying and the digestion and absorption of nutrients<br>Increased viscosity interfering with mixing in intestinal contents<br>High solubility allowing greater microbial degradation |
| Adsorption/binding of organic molecules | Interaction with bile acids and digestive enzymes in the intestine | Pectins<br>Gums<br>Lignin<br>Nonpurified fiber sources (e.g., cereal brans, legumes) | Increased fecal excretion of bile acids<br>Slower rate of digestion in the small intestine |
| Particle size | Determination of surface area exposed<br>Degree of cell wall disruption due to grinding | Primarily important for nonpurified fiber sources | Increasing surface area and disrupting cell walls enhancing exposure to microbial action and digestive enzymes |

investigators have reported that viscous polysaccharides blunt the appearance of glucose in the plasma when included in a glucose tolerance test,[25] and they can delay the disappearance of starch from the small intestine.[26] These effects of fiber are most likely related to the viscosity of these fiber sources.

## WATER-HOLDING CAPACITY (WHC)

WHC measures the ability of a fiber to hold water and is related to solubility of the polysaccharide. For example, cellulose and lignin are insoluble and have a relatively low WHC. Additionally, a higher crystallinity in the structure of cellulose results in a lower WHC, and modification of the structure of cellulose by making carboxymethylcellulose increases WHC tenfold.[7] In contrast, pectins, gums, β-glucans, and certain hemicelluloses have a high WHC. WHC has an important relationship with several of the physiologic effects of fibers.[27] For a polysaccharide to become viscous in the gut, it must have a high solubility and WHC. Within the large intestine, a high WHC facilitates degradation of the polysaccharides by allowing greater penetration of microbes into the polysaccharide structure.[6] However, WHC can also contribute to fecal bulking of a fiber by holding water in the fecal residue.[27] Consequently, in vitro measures of WHC do not directly predict the fecal bulking ability of a fiber source, and both the ability to retain water in the stool and the relationship between WHC and microbial degradation of the fiber must be considered. When stool weight is increased by increasing fiber intake, the percentage of water in the stool does not necessarily increase because water content of stool is relatively constant at 75 to 80%.[28] Although the WHC of a fiber may not alter the percentage of water in the stool, it can affect the distribution of water in the components of the feces. Water in the stool can be associated with the undegraded residue or incorporated into microbial cells, which are about 80% water. Fibers with high WHC that are degraded by the microflora increase microbial mass to a greater extent than fibers with low WHC; hence more water is associated with microbial cells than with the undigested residue.[29]

## BILE ACID BINDING CAPACITY

Certain fibers are capable of binding bile acids in vitro and in vivo. Wheat bran, guar gum, konjac mannan (a glucomannan), chitosan, and isolated lignin have been shown to bind bile acids in the small intestinal contents.[30,31] In humans, pectin, guar gum, oat bran, and wheat bran have been shown to increase fecal bile acid excretion.[2] Eastwood originally proposed that sources of fiber that bind bile acids and increase their excretion may increase the turnover of cholesterol and contribute to the ability of certain fibers to lower plasma cholesterol. Although this interaction does not appear to be sufficient to explain the hypocholesterolemic effects of fiber completely, it has important consequences for lipid utilization. Within the small intestine, bile acids and phospholipids are required for micelle formation and the subsequent digestion and absorption of lipids.[30] Hence the interaction of certain fibers with bile acids and phospholipids can slow lipid digestion and absorption.

## PARTICLE SIZE

In fiber preparations such as cereal brans, particle size can be varied by grinding. Grinding disrupts the cell wall structure, and typically the degree of disruption increases as a finer particle size is achieved. Several investigators have observed that coarsely ground wheat bran is more effective in increasing stool weight and lowering intracolonic pressure than finely ground wheat bran.[28] This difference reflects that the finely ground structure has an increased surface area that allows greater microbial degradation. Particle size is also important for determining whether the cell wall is left intact in foods or is disrupted by grinding. For example, in finely ground, whole-grain rice, the starch is more digestible than in unground whole grain rice because the bran layers have been disrupted by grinding and hence no longer serve as a barrier to the starch-degrading enzymes.[32]

## MICROBIAL DEGRADATION: SHORT-CHAIN FATTY ACIDS

The polysaccharides associated with dietary fiber are important for the growth and metabolism of the microflora normally present in the human large intestine. This microflora, which is a significant proportion of the fecal weight, has the important function of degrading residual food components and endogenous secretions that enter the large intestine. In healthy subjects consuming a mixed diet, 70 to 80% of the fiber disappears during transit through the gut.[33] Degradation of polysaccharides results in production of carbon dioxide, hydrogen, methane, and short-chain fatty acids (SCFA), of which acetate, butyrate, and propionate are the major anions.

The increase in stool weight attributed to an increase in consumption of fiber from fruits or vegetables is due primarily to an increase in the microbial mass of feces.[29] For example, feeding cabbage fiber increases stool weight about 70%; yet the fiber is degraded and does not survive microbial action to increase stool bulk directly. Thus, the effect of cabbage fiber on stool bulk is indirect because of an increase in microbial growth. On the other hand, wheat bran, which also increases stool weight, survives microbial action to a certain extent. Thus, wheat bran increases stool weight by providing bulk directly as well as by increasing the WHC of the residue. Hence the microbial degradation of fiber is an important determinant of the fecal bulking ability of fiber sources.[34]

### *SHORT-CHAIN FATTY ACIDS*

Cummings estimated that about 200 to 300 mmol of SCFA are produced daily in the colon. These SCFA are absorbed rapidly, and the portal concentration in fed subjects is about 400 μm/L.[35] The potential metabolic importance of SCFA is an active area of current investigation. Colonocytes metabolize SCFAs as an energy source, and butyrate may be the primary energy source for cells in the more distal colon of humans. An exciting area of research concerns the effects of butyrate on chromatin structure in cultured cells. These studies have led to speculation that butyrate may play a role in protecting colon cells from cancer.[36] Propionate enters the portal blood and is cleared by the liver. Propionate may have significant metabolic effects on hepatic lipid or glucose metabolism. Incorporation of labeled acetate into cholesterol is inhibited, but overall cholesterol synthesis, as measured by tritiated water incorporation, is not inhibited in isolated hepatocytes incubated with propionate.[37] Additionally, propionate inhibits incorporation of tritiated water into fatty acids by isolated hepatocytes.[37] Whether this effect of propionate on fatty acid synthesis occurs in intact animals is not known. Acetate, which is the predominate SCFA produced, can be rapidly metabolized to $CO_2$ by peripheral tissues. Two points of importance emerge from the current investigations in this area: (1) SCFAs are a source of energy for the host cells;[38] and (2) these compounds are likely to have metabolic effects that are as yet poorly understood but may be important in explaining the physiologic responses to sources of dietary fiber.

## NUTRITIONAL IMPORTANCE

Several clinical and experimental studies have been conducted in human patients and in animal models to demonstrate the need for fiber in the diet. These studies have shown the potential importance of certain sources of dietary fiber for normal gastrointestinal function, lowering plasma cholesterol, and blunting glycemic response and insulin release.

### GASTROINTESTINAL RESPONSE

In healthy individuals, dietary fiber is clearly important for normal gastrointestinal function, as summarized in Table 4–5. This role is well defined in the large intestine, where dietary fiber provides bulk and the substrates for microbial activity. Several investigators have proposed that the adequacy of fiber intake can be determined by estimating the amount of fiber or nonstarch polysaccharides (NSP) needed to maintain an adequate stool weight and transit time. Using this criterion, the Life Sciences Research Office Expert Panel recommended that a minimum of 20 g of fiber be consumed daily.[2] Spiller estimated that a daily fiber intake of 35 to 45 g was needed to maintain a transit time of less than 2 days and a daily wet stool weight of 160 to 200 g.[39] Data from the United Kingdom also suggest that fiber intake needs to be in this range for adequate stool weight and transit time.[68] In addition, Cummings used data from several clinical studies to estimate the ability of various fiber sources to increase stool weight.[33] The average increase in fecal weight (g) per g fiber fed was 5.7± 0.5, 4.9± 0.9, and 3.9± 1.5 for wheat bran, various fruits and vegetables, and oat products, respectively. Isolated polysaccharides were generally less effective, although some increase in fecal weight was observed. As has been known for over 100 years, coarse wheat bran is clearly effective for increasing fecal weight. Other sources of fiber such as whole-grain cereals, fruits, and vegetables are also effective, however, and may be more acceptable to patients who need to increase fiber intake.[33]

Increased fiber intake has been suggested for disorders involving the large intestine such as constipation, diverticulosis, and irritable bowel syndrome.[27] In all these disorders, numerous factors other than diet can contribute to the development of the disorder. In particular, in irritable bowel syndrome, personality and anxiety as well as dietary factors can be contributing causes. Among identifiable dietary factors, fiber is the only constituent that appears to affect stool weight.[28] Hence, in cases of constipation or irritable bowel syndrome in which a low fiber intake is associated with low stool weight, increasing fiber intake by recommending dietary modifications or by recommending consumption of coarse wheat bran may be beneficial. In symptomatic, uncomplicated diverticulosis, coarse wheat bran consumption has been recommended to increase stool volume and to lower colonic pressure. However, Eastwood pointed out that diverticulosis may be a disease of the very old, and a high-fiber diet cannot necessarily correct the anatomic problems that occur in this population group.[27]

Epidemiologic and experimental evidence has suggested that a diet high in fiber may be associated with a reduced risk of colon cancer. Although several methodologic difficulties have complicated the interpretation of epidemiologic studies, the majority of these studies support the view that fiber-rich diets and consumption of

**TABLE 4–5.** IMPORTANCE OF DIETARY FIBER FOR GASTROINTESTINAL FUNCTION

| GASTROINTESTINAL RESPONSE | PROPERTY OF FIBER | IMPLICATION |
|---|---|---|
| Stomach | | |
| Gastric emptying | Water-holding capacity; viscosity | Slower delivery of nutrients |
| Small intestine | | |
| Lower bile acid reabsorption | Bile acid binding capacity | Bile acid and cholesterol metabolism |
| Digestion and absorption of nutrients | Water-holding capacity; viscosity; binding capacity | Slow fat and carbohydrate absorption |
| Large intestine | | |
| Bulk and transit time | Fermentability of the polysaccharides; water-holding capacity | Stool weight; concentration in stool |
| Microbial growth | Fermentability; water-holding capacity | Short-chain fatty acid production; microbial metabolism |

vegetables are associated with a protective effect against colon cancer. With regard to vegetables, however, one cannot discriminate between effects related to fiber and those related to nonfiber constituents.[40] The incidence of rectal polyps, a benign large bowel dysplasia, were decreased in subjects consuming at least 11 g of wheat bran, suggesting a reduction of risk with an increased fiber consumption.[41] Although these studies support the view that dietary fiber has a protective effect against colon cancer, some animal studies have shown that consumption of highly fermentable polysaccharides, such as gums and pectin, is associated with increased tumor development in animals administered a carcinogen, presumably because of stimulation of mucosal cell growth.[42]

Several plausible mechanisms have been formulated by which fiber may provide protection against colon cancer. These include dilution of contents, adsorption of potential carcinogens, more rapid turnover of contents (decreased transit time), alteration of large intestinal contents by microbial action, and alteration in bile acid metabolism.[34] Our current knowledge indicates that we are still far from establishing a clear cause-and-effect relationship between fiber intake and protection from colon cancer. However, this area of investigation has renewed interest in the nutritional importance of plant-derived foods and has stimulated research activity on the various constituents of plants that may be anticarcinogenic.

In addition to its established role in the large intestine, dietary fiber regulates the rate and site of nutrient absorption in the upper gastrointestinal tract. For example, viscous polysaccharides promote nutrient absorption along a greater length of the small intestine.[43] Although the clinical implications of this effect have not been fully explored, nutrient absorption from the ileum delays gastric emptying, induces satiety, and alters postprandial lipoprotein composition.[44]

## HYPOCHOLESTEROLEMIC EFFECTS OF FIBER

Several long-term epidemiologic studies indicated a positive association between increased fiber intake and a decreased risk of coronary heart disease.[45–47] In most of these studies, this association was no longer significant when controlling for other factors, such as total calorie or fat intake. Thus, evidence for a unique protective role of dietary fiber based on population studies is inconclusive.[48] Nonetheless, this potential association has resulted in many clinical and animal studies conducted to investigate the ability of sources of dietary fiber to lower plasma cholesterol.

In reviewing the large number of clinical and animal studies conducted to test the hypocholesterolemic effects of various sources of dietary fiber, several conclusions can be drawn. Wheat bran and cellulose, both sources of nonviscous, insoluble polysaccharides, do not lower plasma cholesterol levels. In contrast, pectin, guar gum, oat bran, psyllium husk, beans (legumes), and fruits and vegetables have been reported to lower plasma cholesterol and specifically LDL-cholesterol levels.[2,49,50] The extent of the hypocholesterolemic response to sources of fiber is affected by the total amount of fiber fed, by the initial plasma lipid values of the subjects studied, by whether the total diet is self-selected or clinically controlled, and by other dietary variables that influence plasma cholesterol. In studies in which oat products have been added to diets that had already been modified to lower total fat, saturated fatty acids, and cholesterol intake, an additional 3 to 4% reduction in plasma cholesterol level was observed. Thus, dietary fiber's effect on plasma lipids seems to be independent of the effect of dietary fats.[51] In rats, a dose-response relationship exists between consumption of oat products and reduction in plasma cholesterol, again supporting a specific effect of fiber on plasma lipids.[52] Because fiber alone only affects plasma cholesterol to a small extent (e.g., <5%), its effect may not be evident in small clinical trials, in free-living subjects who are not confined to a metabolic unit, or in individuals whose plasma cholesterol is already in the low range (e.g., 4.65 mmol/L <(180 mg/dl)). For example, in free-living subjects a minimum of 40 participants may be needed to detect a difference of 5% in plasma cholesterol levels, given the normal variability that occurs in a population. In evaluating the actions of dietary fiber in therapeutic diets designed to lower plasma lipid levels, it is important to recognize that certain types of fiber, especially those containing soluble, viscous polysaccharides, make a specific contribution to lowering plasma cholesterol. Additionally, foods containing these polysaccharides (e.g., fruits, vegetables, oats, barley, and legumes) are useful in planning diets to lower total fat, saturated fatty acids, and cholesterol intake.

Several mechanisms have been proposed whereby sources of fiber affect cholesterol metabolism. These include increasing the fecal excretion of bile acids, slowing the rate of lipid absorption, and enhancing the production of SCFA by polysaccharide fermentation in the large bowel. Each of these factors undoubtedly contributes to the hypocholesterolemic effects of fiber; however, the relative importance of each is not well understood at this time.

## PLASMA GLUCOSE AND INSULIN RESPONSE

The ability of soluble, viscous polysaccharides to blunt the increase in plasma glucose and insulin following a glucose load has been related to a delay in gastric emptying and an increased viscosity of the gastrointestinal contents. The significance of these effects in the management of diabetic patients is covered in other chapters of this book.

In unrefined foods, the presence of fiber is likely to slow carbohydrate absorption by interfering with the digestion of starch or other saccharides. In unrefined foods, plant cell walls or bran layers in cereal grains can serve as a barrier to the penetration of digestive enzymes. For example, in rice kernels with the bran layer intact, amylase digestion of starch is relatively low, whereas grinding the whole rice kernel to a fine powder increases starch digestion substantially.[32] In evaluating the potential importance of fiber on carbohydrate utilization, it is important to recognize that the presence of fiber may serve as a marker for the structure of plant foods because cell walls are rich in these unavailable polysaccharides. Hence the potential benefit of fiber in slowing carbohydrate utilization may be achieved by consuming foods with intact cell walls, not isolated fiber supplements.

## POTENTIAL PROBLEMS WITH FIBER CONSUMPTION

In many populations of the world, the nutrient quality of the diet is limited because foods high in fiber content and low in available nutrients are the primary foodstuffs. In these populations, consumption of high levels of fiber, along with other compounds in plant foods such as phytates and digestive enzyme inhibitors, an overall low nutrient intake, and the incidence of infections may contribute to potential nutritional problems. In these situations, fiber is not the only nutritional factor that must be examined to improve the overall quality of the diet. Thus, dietary recommendations for populations in North America or the United Kingdom, where excessive consumption of foods high in fat occurs, often at the exclusion of foods high in complex carbohydrates and fiber, may not be applicable to other populations.

Foods containing fiber are known to lower the bioavailability of minerals in part because of the ability of certain fibers to bind minerals and increase their fecal excretion and in part because of the presence of phytates and oxalates, which also bind trace minerals strongly. The decreased mineral absorption associated with high-fiber foods does not necessarily lead to poor mineral status. Generally, mineral intake is increased if foods providing fiber are added to the diet; however, isolated fiber supplements are unlikely to increase mineral intake. Hence mineral status is most likely to be compromised in individuals whose mineral intake is marginal and who consume excessive fiber supplements.

In case studies reported in the clinical literature, individuals have developed intestinal obstructions or bezoars because of dietary fiber.[53,54] Although these reports are rare, they are typically associated with a high level of consumption of a fiber supplement, often in a dry, unhydrated form, or they occur in individuals with a preexisting gastrointestinal problem. Inclusion of foods containing dietary fiber into a varied, balanced diet, as indicated by most of the recommendations in Table 4–6, is unlikely to result in these complications for most individuals.

## CURRENT RECOMMENDATIONS

Twenty years ago, few recommendations were made specifically about dietary fiber intake. The current interest in dietary fiber is largely attributed to the work of Denis Burkitt and Hugh Trowell.[55] Both physicians, who practiced medicine in Africa following World War II, noted the difference in chronic disease patterns between the population of rural Africa and that of their native Britain. Burkitt and Trowell focused on the undigested roughage in the African diet, now known as dietary fiber. Trowell proposed that fiber consumption is a protective factor against certain gastrointestinal and metabolic disorders, such as cardiovascular disease, colonic dysfunction, diabetes, and obesity.[56] Epidemiologic evidence supporting this hypothesis has been collected, though differences in the methods of estimating food consumption patterns and in the analysis of dietary fiber present systematic biases in these types of data.[57] A clear association of fiber intake patterns with the incidence of chronic diseases is difficult to establish because diets that differ in fiber content may also differ greatly in macronutrient composition. Nonetheless, because the data are suggestive, recommendations regarding dietary fiber intake have been issued by governmental and health organizations. These recommendations are directed at a healthy, adult population consuming a typical Western diet. The current dietary fiber intake for the United States population is estimated to be ~1.5 g/1000 kJ. Women typically have a higher fiber intake per 1000 kJ than men.[58–61] Most recommendations would result in increasing fiber intake to 2.4 to 3.6 g/1000 kJ. Table 4–6 summarizes these recommendations, indicating a general consensus on the need to increase fiber intake by consuming foods high in fiber.[62–66]

The 1990 Dietary Guidelines included recommendations on the number of servings of fiber-containing foods for the diet of normal, healthy individuals over the age of 2 years; namely, two or more servings of fruits, three or more servings of vegetables, and six or more servings of grain products.[62] These recommendations are consistent with those of the National Research Council,[48] as well as with the food guide recommended by the United States Department of Agriculture. The selection of this dietary pattern and the choice of higher fiber foods within these categories is probably the best strategy for ensuring the adequacy of fiber intake within a population.

**TABLE 4–6.** DIETARY FIBER RECOMMENDATIONS

| YEAR | TITLE | ORGANIZATION | RECOMMENDATION |
|---|---|---|---|
| 1990 | *Dietary Guidelines for Americans*[62] | U.S. Dept. of Agriculture<br>U.S. Dept. of Health & Human Services | Choose a diet with plenty of vegetables, fruits, and grain products |
| 1987 | *Physiological Effects and Health Consequences of Dietary Fiber*[2] | Life Sciences Research Office, Federation of American Societies for Experimental Biology | Consume a wide variety of whole-grain products, fruits, and vegetables, leading to a dietary fiber intake range of 20 to 35 g/d (10-13 g/1000 kcal) for the healthy, adult population |
| 1988 | "Health implications of dietary fiber"[63] | American Dietetic Association | Daily, consume a high-carbohydrate, low-fat diet containing 20 to 35 g dietary fiber from a variety of food sources for health benefits and to reduce the risk of certain diseases |
| 1988 | *The Surgeon General's Report on Nutrition and Health*[50] | U.S. Dept. of Health and Human Services | Increase consumption of whole-grain foods and cereal products, vegetables (including dried beans and peas), and fruits |
| 1989 | "Dietary fiber and health"[65] | Council of Scientific Affairs, American Medical Association | Obtain an adequate amount of dietary fiber by choosing several servings daily from a variety of fiber-rich foods such as whole-grain breads and cereals, fruits and vegetables, legumes, and nuts |
| 1989 | *Diet and Health*[48] | National Research Council, National Academy of Sciences | Every day eat five or more servings of fruits and vegetables and increase intake of starches and other complex carbohydrates by eating six or more daily servings of a combination of breads, cereals, and legumes |
| 1989 | *Recommended Dietary Allowances, 10th Ed.*[64] | Food and Nutrition Board, National Research Council, National Academy of Sciences | Achieve a desirable fiber intake by consumption of fruits, vegetables, legumes, and whole-grain cereals |
| 1990 | *Nutrition Recommendations*[66] | Health Services Promotion Branch, Dept. of Health and Welfare, Canada | Emphasize cereals, breads, other grain products, vegetables, and fruits |
| 1991 | Dietary Reference Values for Food Energy and Nutrients from the United Kingdom[68] | Department of Health (UK) | Diets should contain an average of 18 g/day (range of 12–24) NSP from a variety of foods whose constituents contain it as a naturally integrated component. |

## REFERENCES


1. Burkitt, D.: Foreword. *In* Dietary Fiber: Basic and Clinical Aspects. Edited by G.V. Vahouny and D. Kritchevsky. New York, Plenum Press, 1986.
2. Pilch, S.M.: Physiological Effects and Health Consequences of Dietary Fiber (FDA 223-84-2059). Bethesda, MD, Federation of American Societies for Experimental Biology, 1987.
3. Selvendran, R.R.: Am. J. Clin. Nutr., *39:*320–337, 1984.
4. Southgate, D.A.T., Englyst, H.: Dietary fibre: chemistry, physical properties and analysis of dietary fibre. *In* Dietary Fibre, Fibre-Depleted Foods and Disease. Edited by H. Trowell, D. Burkitt, and K. Heaton. London, Academic Press, 1985.
5. Marlett, J.A.: Analysis of dietary fiber in human foods. *In* Dietary Fiber: Chemistry, Physiology, and Health Effects. Edited by D. Kritchevsky, C. Bonfield, and J.W. Anderson. New York, Plenum Press, 1990.
6. Salyers, A.: Activities of Polysaccharide-degrading bacteria in the human colon. *In* Dietary Fiber: Chemistry, Physiology, and Health Effects. Edited by D. Kritchevsky, C. Bonfield, and J.W. Anderson. New York, Plenum Press, 1990.
7. Selvendran, R.R., Verne, A.V.F.V.: The chemistry and properties of plant cell walls and dietary fiber. *In* Dietary Fiber: Chemistry, Physiology, and Health Effects. Edited by D. Kritchevsky, C. Bonfield, and J.W. Anderson. New York, Plenum Press, 1990.
8. Englyst, H.N., Macfarlane, G.T.J.: Sci. Food Agric., *37:*699–706, 1986.
9. Dreher, M.L., Berry, J.W., Dreher, C.J.: Crit. Rev. Food Sci. Nutr., *20:*47–71, 1984.
10. Anderson, J.W., Bridges, S.R.: Am. J. Clin. Nutr., *47:*440–447, 1988.
11. Williams, R.D., Olmsted, W.H.J.: Biol. Chem., *108:*653–666, 1935.
12. Van Soest, P.J.J.: Assoc. Off. Anal. Chem., *46:*829–835, 1963.
13. Goering, H.K., Van Soest, P.J.: Forage Fiber Analysis. USDA Handbook 379. Washington, D.C., United States Depart-

ment of Agriculture, United States Government Printing Office, 1970.

14. Southgate, D.A.T.: J. Sci. Food Agric., *20*:331–335, 1969.
15. Southgate, D.A.T.: Determination of Food Carbohydrate. London, Applied Science, 1976.
16. Asp, N.-G., Johansson, C.-G.: Nutr. Abstr. Rev., *54*:736–752, 1984.
17. Englyst, H.: Determination of carbohydrate and its composition in plant materials. *In* The Analysis of Dietary Fiber in Food. Edited by W.P.T. James and O. Theander. New York, Marcel Dekker, 1981.
18. Theander, O., Aman, P.: Analysis of dietary fibers and their main constituents. *In* The Analysis of Dietary Fiber in Food. Edited by W.P.T. James and O. Theander. New York, Marcel Dekker, 1981.
19. Prosky, L., Asp, N.-G., Schweizer, T.F., et al.: J. Assoc. Off. Anal. Chem., *71*:1017–1023, 1988.
20. Schweizer, T.F.: Dietary fiber analysis and nutrition labelling. *In* Dietary Fiber: New Developments. Edited by I. Furda and C. Brine. New York, Plenum Press, 1990.
21. Mongeau, R., Brassard, R.: J. Food Sci., *51*:1333–1336, 1986.
22. American Association of Cereal Chemists: Technical Committee on Dietary Fiber Analysis, Method 32-21, Nashville, TN, 1987.
23. Schwartz, S.E., Levine, R.A., Singh, A., et al.: Gastroenterology, *83*:812–817, 1982.
24. Edwards, C.A.: Physiological effects of fiber. *In* Dietary Fiber: Chemistry, Physiology, and Health Effects. Edited by D. Kritchevsky, C. Bonfield, and J.W. Anderson. New York, Plenum Press, 1990.
25. Jenkins, D.J.A., Wolever, T.M.S., Leeds, A.R., et al.: Br. Med. J., *1*:1392–1394, 1978.
26. Tinker, L., Schneeman, B.O.: J. Nutr., *119*:403–408, 1989.
27. Eastwood, M.: Fiber and gastrointestinal disease. *In* Dietary Fiber: Chemistry, Physiology, and Health Effects. Edited by D. Kritchevsky, C. Bonfield, and J.W. Anderson. New York, Plenum Press, 1990.
28. Eastwood, M., Brydon, W.G.: Physiological effects of dietary fibre on the alimentary tract. *In* Dietary Fibre, Fibre-Depleted Foods and Disease. Edited by H. Trowell, D. Burkitt, and K. Heaton. London, Academic Press, 1985.
29. Stephens, A.: Constipation. *In* Dietary Fibre, Fibre-Depleted Foods and Disease. Edited by H. Trowell, D. Burkitt, and K. Heaton. London, Academic Press, 1985.
30. Gallaher, D., Schneeman, B.O.: Am. J. Physiol., *250*:G420-G426, 1986.
31. Ebihara, K., Schneeman, B.O.: J. Nutr., *119*:1100–1106, 1989.
32. Collier, G., O'Dea, K.: Am. J. Clin. Nutr., *36*:10–14, 1982.
33. Cummings, J.H.: The effect of dietary fiber on fecal weight and composition. *In* CRC Handbook of Dietary Fiber in Human Nutrition. Edited by G.A. Spiller. Boca Raton FL, CRC Press, 1986.
34. Cummings, J.H.: Cancer of the large bowel. *In* Dietary Fibre, Fibre-Depleted Foods and Disease. Edited by H. Trowell, D. Burkitt, and K. Heaton. London, Academic Press, 1985.
35. Cummings, J.H., Pomare, E.W., Branch, W.J., et al.: Gut *28*:1221–1227, 1987.
36. Cummings, J.H., Macfarlane, G.T.: Short chain fatty acid production and metabolism in man. *In* Proceedings of the 14th International Congress of Nutrition. Edited by K.W. Young, L.Y. Cha, L.K. Yull, et al. Seoul, Ewha Women's University, 1990.
37. Nishina, P.M., Freedland, R.A.: J. Nutr., *120*:668–673, 1990.
38. Livesey, G.: The effects of alpha-amylase-resistant carbohydrates on energy utilization and deposition in man and rat. *In* Dietary Fiber: Chemistry, Physiology, and Health Effects. Edited by D. Kritchevsky, C. Bonfield, and J.W. Anderson. New York, Plenum Press, 1990.
39. Spiller, G.A.: Suggestions for a basis on which to determine a desirable intake of dietary fiber. *In* CRC Handbook of Dietary Fiber in Human Nutrition. Edited by G.A. Spiller. Boca Raton FL, CRC Press, 1986.
40. Trock, B., Lanza, E., Greenwald, P.: J. Natl. Cancer Inst., *82*:650–661, 1990.
41. DeCosse, J.J., Miller, H.H., Lesser, M.L.: J. Natl. Cancer Inst., *81*:1290–1297, 1989.
42. Jacobs, L.R.: Influence of soluble fibers on experimental colon carcinogenesis. *In* Dietary Fiber: Chemistry, Physiology, and Health Effects. Edited by D. Kritchevsky, C. Bonfield, and J.W. Anderson. New York, Plenum Press, 1990.
43. Schneeman, B.O.: Macronutrient absorption. *In* Dietary Fiber: Chemistry, Physiology, and Health Effects. Edited by D. Kritchevsky, C. Bonfield, and J.W. Anderson. New York, Plenum Press, 1990.
44. Read, N.W., Sepple, C.P., Brown, N.J.: The ileal brake: is it relevant to the action of viscous polysaccharides? *In* Dietary Fiber: Chemistry, Physiology, and Health Effects. Edited by D. Kritchevsky, C. Bonfield, and J.W. Anderson. New York, Plenum Press, 1990.
45. Kromhout, D., de Lezenne Coulander, C.: Am. J. Epidemiol., *119*:733–741, 1984.
46. Kushi, L.H., Lew, R.A., Stare, F.J., et al.: N. Engl. J. Med., *312*:811–818, 1985.
47. Liu, K., Stamler, J., Trevison, M., et al.: Arteriosclerosis, *2*:221–227, 1982.
48. National Research Council: *In* Diet and Health. Edited by Food and Nutrition Board. Washington, D.C., National Academy Press, 1989.
49. Kris-Etherton, P.M., Krummel, D., Russell, M.E., et al.: J. Am. Diet. Assoc., *88*:1373–1400, 1988.
50. Surgeon General, United States Dept. of Health and Human Services: The Surgeon General's Report on Nutrition and Health. Washington, D.C., U.S. Public Health Service, 1988.
51. Van Horn, L.V., Lui, K., Parker, D., et al.: J. Am. Diet. Assoc., *86*:759–764, 1986.
52. Shinnick, F.L., Ink, S.L., Marlett, J.A.: J. Nutr., *120*:561–568, 1990.
53. Agha, F.P., Nostrant, T.T., Fiddian-Green, R.G.: Am. J. Gastroenterol., *79*:319–321, 1984.
54. Souter, W.A.: Br. Med. J., *1*:166–168, 1965.
55. Trowell, H.C., Burkitt, D.P.: Refined Carbohydrate Foods and Disease. London, Academic Press, 1975.
56. Trowell, H.: Am. J. Clin. Nutr., *29*:417–427, 1976.
57. Bingham, S.: Am. J. Clin. Nutr., *45*:1226–1231, 1987.
58. United States Department of Agriculture: Nationwide Food Consumption Survey Continuing Survey of Food Intakes by Individuals: Men 19-50 Years. Report 85-3. Washington, D.C., Human Nutrition Information Service, 1986.
59. United States Department of Agriculture: Nationwide Food Consumption Survey Continuing Survey of Food Intakes by Individuals: Women 19-50 Years and Their Children 1-5 Years. Report 85-1. Washington, D.C., Human Nutrition Information Service, 1986.
60. Ahrens, E.H.J., Boucher, C.A.: J. Am. Diet. Assoc., *73*:613–620, 1978.
61. Anderson, J.W., Bridges, S.R., Tietyen, J., et al.: Am. J. Clin. Nutr., *49*:352–357, 1989.

62. United States Departments of Agriculture and Health and Human Services: Dietary Guidelines for Americans. No. 232. Washington, D.C., United States Government Printing Office, 1990.
63. American Dietetic Association: J. Am. Diet. Assoc., *88:*216–221, 1988.
64. Food and Nutrition Board, National Research Council: Recommended Dietary Allowance. 10th Ed. Washington, D.C., National Academy Press, 1989.
65. Council of Scientific Affairs: JAMA, *262:*542–546, 1989.
66. Health and Welfare, Canada: Nutrition Recommendations . . . A Call for Action. Ottawa, Minister of Supply and Services of Canada, 1989.
67. Marlett, J.A.: J. Am. Diet. Assoc., *92:*175–186, 1992.
68. Department of Health: Dietary Reference Values for Food Energy and Nutrients for the United Kingdom. London, HMSO, 1991, pp. 61–71.

## SELECTED READINGS

Kritchevsky, D., Bonfield, C., Anderson, J.W., (Eds.): Dietary Fiber: Chemistry, Physiology, and Health Effects. New York, Plenum Press, 1990.

Pilch, S.M. (Ed.): Physiological Effects and Health Consequences of Dietary Fiber. Bethesda, MD, Federation of American Societies for Experimental Biology, 1987.

Schneeman, B.O.: Dietary Fiber: A Scientific Status Summary by the Institute of Food Technologists. Chicago, Institute of Food Technologists, 1989.

Trowell, A., Burkitt, D., Heaton, K. (Eds.): Dietary Fibre, Fibre-Depleted Foods and Disease. London, Academic Press, 1985.

United States Surgeon General: Surgeon General's Report on Nutrition and Health. Washington, D.C., U.S. Department of Health and Human Services, 1988.

CHAPTER 5

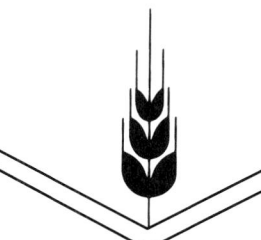

# Energy Needs: Assessment and Requirements

Yves Schutz and Eric Jéquier



To maintain physiologic functions, the human body continuously expends energy by oxidative metabolism. This energy is used to maintain chemical and electrochemical gradients across cellular membranes for the biosynthesis of macromolecules such as proteins, glycogen, and triglycerides, and for muscular contraction. Another part of the energy is lost as heat because of the inefficiency of metabolic transformations. Ultimately all the energy produced by the organism is dissipated as heat.

## MEASUREMENT OF ENERGY EXPENDITURE IN HUMANS

The energy expended by an individual can be assessed by two different techniques: indirect and direct calorimetry. The term indirect calorimetry stems from the fact that the heat released by chemical processes within the body can be indirectly calculated from the rate of oxygen consumption ($\dot{V}O_2$). The main reason for the close relation between energy metabolism and $\dot{V}O_2$ is that the oxidative phosphorylation at the respiratory chain level allows a continuous synthesis of adenosine triphosphate (ATP). The energy expended within the body to maintain electrochemical gradients, support biosynthetic processes, and generate muscular contraction cannot be directly provided from nutrient oxidation. Almost all chemical processes requiring energy depend on ATP hydrolysis. It is the rate of ATP utilization that determines the overall rate of substrate oxidation and therefore $\dot{V}O_2$. With the exception of anaerobic glycolysis, ATP synthesis is coupled with substrate oxidation. The biochemical theory of oxidative phosphorylation considers that 3 mol of ATP are generated per gram-atom of oxygen consumed (i.e., a P:O ratio of 3:1). With the advent of the "chemiosmotic theory" of oxidative phosphorylation, this precise stoichiometry has been questioned, but the concept of a proportionality between $\dot{V}O_2$ and ATP synthesis remains valid.[1]

The energy expenditure per mole of ATP formed should not be calculated from the classic value of 31 kJ for the hydrolysis of 1 mol of ATP under standard conditions (which has no physiologic significance), but from the heat of combustion of 1 mol of substrate, divided by the total number of moles of ATP generated in its oxidation.[2] It is interesting to note that each mole of ATP generated is accompanied by the release of about the same amount of heat (~75 kJ/mol ATP) during the oxidation of carbohydrates, fats, or proteins.[2,3] Because there is a proportionality between $\dot{V}O_2$ and ATP synthesis, and because each mole of ATP synthetized is accompanied by the production of a given amount of heat, one understands the rationale of using $\dot{V}O_2$ measurement to calculate heat production within the body.

There is, however, a slight difference in the heat produced per liter of oxygen consumed when one compares carbohydrate (21.0 kJ/$LO_2$)* and lipid (19.6 kJ/$LO_2$) oxidation (Table 5–1). This is because substrate level phosphorylation in the glycolytic pathway allows the synthesis of 2 mol of ATP without $O_2$ consumption

*1 kJ/$LO_2$ = 5.02 kcal/$LO_2$ (1 kJ = 4.18 kcal)

**TABLE 5–1.** ENERGY YIELDS FROM OXIDATION OF SUBSTRATES

| SUBSTRATES | $O_2$ CONSUMED† | $CO_2$ PRODUCED† | RQ | HEAT RELEASED (PER GRAM) | | ENERGY EQUIVALENT (PER GRAM) | | | |
|---|---|---|---|---|---|---|---|---|---|
| | | | | | | $\dot{V}O_2$ | | $\dot{V}CO_2$ | |
| | | | | kJ | kcal | kJ | kcal | kJ | kcal |
| Starch | 0.829 | 0.829 | 1.00 | 17.6 | 4.20 | 21.2 | 5.06 | 21.2 | 5.06 |
| Saccharose | 0.786 | 0.786 | 1.00 | 16.6 | 3.96 | 21.1 | 5.04 | 21.1 | 5.04 |
| Glucose | 0.746 | 0.746 | 1.00 | 15.6 | 3.74 | 21.0 | 5.01 | 21.0 | 5.01 |
| Lipid | 2.019 | 1.427 | 0.71 | 39.6 | 9.46 | 19.6 | 4.69 | 27.7 | 6.63 |
| Protein | 1.010 | 0.844 | 0.83 | 19.7 | 4.70 | 189.5 | 4.66 | 23.3 | 5.58 |
| Lactic acid | 0.746 | 0.746 | 1.00 | 15.1 | 3.62 | 20.3 | 4.85 | 20.3 | 4.85 |

†In liters per gram of substrate oxidized.
RQ, Respiratory quotient.
(Data from Livesey, G., Marinos, E.: Am. J. Clin. Nutr., *47*:608–628, 1988.)

when 1 mol of glucose is metabolized (compared to 38 mol of ATP synthetized by the complete oxidation of 1 mol of glucose), whereas during fatty acid oxidation, ATP synthesis only occurs by oxydative phosphorylation.

Direct calorimetry consists in the measurement of the heat dissipated by the body by radiation, convection, conduction, and evaporation.[4] Under conditions of thermal equilibrium in a subject at rest and in postabsorptive conditions, heat production, measured by indirect calorimetry, is identical to heat dissipation, measured by direct calorimetry (Fig. 5–1). This is an obvious confirmation of the first law of thermodynamics, which states that the energy released by oxidative processes is ultimately transformed into heat (and external work during exercise). In steady-state conditions, the identity between heat production and heat loss in a resting subject (Fig. 5–1) corroborates the validity (for the whole body) of the method of indirect calorimetry.

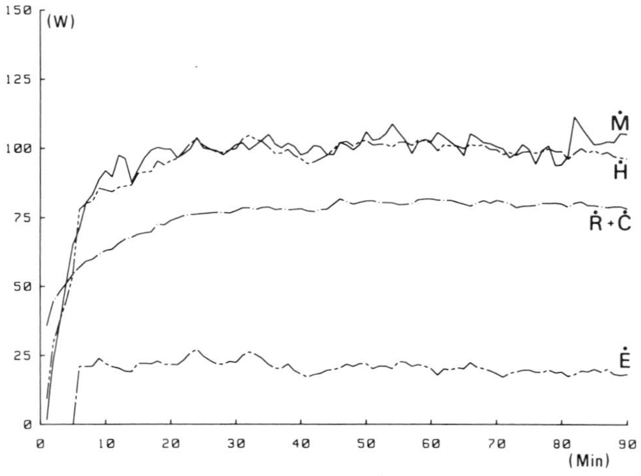
(W)
150
125
100
75
50
25
0
0
10
20
30
40
50
60
70
80
90
(Min)
Ṁ
Ḣ
Ṙ + Ċ
Ė

**FIGURE 5–1.** Metabolic rate (Ṁ), total heat losses (Ḣ), radiative and convective heat losses (Ṙ + Ċ), and evaporative heat losses (Ė) in a male subject, aged 25 years, exposed at 28° C in a direct calorimeter.

## ENERGY METABOLISM AND NUTRIENT UTILIZATION IN HUMANS

The study of energy metabolism and nutrient utilization in humans has recently raised a great interest in the regulation of these processes thanks to advances in the construction of open-circuit ventilated hood indirect calorimeters[5] and comfortable respiration chambers.[6]

With the only measurement of $\dot{V}O_2$ (in liters of $O_2$ STPD (standard temperature (0° C), pressure (760 mm Hg), and dry) per minute), metabolic rate ($\dot{M}$), which corresponds to energy expenditure, can be calculated (in kilojoules per minute) as follows:

$$\dot{M} = 20.3 \times \dot{V}O_2 \quad (1)$$

The number 20.3 is a mean value (in kJ/L) of the energy equivalent for the consumption of 1 L (STPD) of oxygen. The value of the energy equivalent of oxygen depends on the composition of the fuel mixture oxidized (Table 5–1). However, the error in using equation 1 instead of an equation that takes into account the type of fuels oxidized (equations 2 and 3, see below) is no greater than ±1 to 2%.

To take into account the heat released by the oxidation of the three macronutrients (carbohydrates, fats, and proteins), three measurements must be carried out: oxygen consumption ($\dot{V}O_2$), carbon dioxide production ($\dot{V}CO_2$), and urinary nitrogen excretion (N).

Simple equations for computing metabolic rate (or energy expenditure) from these three determinations are written under the following form:

$$\dot{M} = a\,\dot{V}O_2 + b\,\dot{V}CO_2 - cN \quad (2)$$

The factors a, b, and c depend on the respective constants for the amount of $O_2$ used and the amount of $CO_2$ produced during oxidation of the three classes of nutrients (Table 5–1). An example of such a formula (Brouwer's equation) is given below:[7]

$$\dot{M} = 16.18\,\dot{V}O_2 + 5.02\,\dot{V}CO_2 - 5.99\,N \quad (3)$$

where $\dot{M}$ is in kilojoules per unit of time, $\dot{V}O_2$ and $\dot{V}CO_2$

are in liters STPD per unit of time, and N is in grams per unit of time. As an example, if $\dot{V}O_2$ = 600 L per day, $\dot{V}CO_2$ = 500 L per day (respiratory quotient, or RQ, = 0.83), and N = 25 g per day, then $\dot{M}$ = 12,068 kJ per day. With the simpler equation (1) the results give a value of 12,180 kJ per day.

Slightly different factors for the amounts of $O_2$ used and of $CO_2$ produced during oxidation of the nutrients are used by other authors, and the values for the factors a, b, and c are modified accordingly.[8] The difference in energy expenditure calculated by the various formulae is not greater than 3%. Detailed informations about these calculations are described elsewhere.[5,8–9]

Indirect calorimetry also allows computation of the nutrient oxidation rates in the whole body. An index of protein oxidation is obtained from the total amount of nitrogen excreted in the urine during the test period. One approach to calculate the nutrient oxidation rate is based on the oxygen consumption and $CO_2$ production due to the oxidation rates of the three nutrients carbohydrate, fat, and protein respectively.[5] In a subject oxidizing c grams per minute of carbohydrate (as glucose), f grams per minute of fat, and excreting n grams per minute of urinary nitrogen, the following equations, based on Table 5–1, can be used:

$$\dot{V}O_2 = 0.746\ c + 2.02\ f + 6.31\ n \qquad (4)$$

and

$$\dot{V}CO_2 = 0.746\ c + 1.43\ f + 5.27\ n \qquad (5)$$

We can solve equations 4 and 5 for the unknown c and f this way:

$$c = 4.59\ \dot{V}CO_2 - 3.25\ \dot{V}O_2 - 3.68\ n \qquad (6)$$

$$f = 1.69\ \dot{V}O_2 - 1.69\ \dot{V}CO_2 - 1.72\ n \qquad (7)$$

Because 1 g urinary nitrogen arises from approximately 6.25 g protein, the protein oxidation rate (p in grams per minute) is given by the equation

$$p = 6.25\ n \qquad (8)$$

A detailed discussion on the influences of other metabolic processes (such as lipogenesis, gluconeogenesis, and ketogenesis) on the calculated oxidation rates of the nutrients is presented elsewhere.[9] However, intermediate metabolic processes do not influence the results of equations 6 and 7, providing that the intermediate substrate does not accumulate within the body, or is not excreted from the body. When there is accumulation or excretion of an intermediate or end product other than $CO_2$ and $H_2O$, this approach to compute the oxidation rates of nutrients is no longer valid.[9]

## ASSESSMENT OF ENERGY EXPENDITURE IN FREE-LIVING CONDITIONS

Various indirect methods have been used to assess total energy expenditure in humans under natural conditions of life. As shown in Table 5–2, they have been based either on physiologic measurements, human observations and records, kinematic recordings, or more recently isotopic dilution techniques. Although the measurement of energy expenditure using the activity diary has been the object of many studies from the late 1950s, today the two most commonly employed noncalorimetric methods are the heart rate and the doubly-labeled water techniques.

**TABLE 5–2.** NONCALORIMETRIC METHODS FOR ESTIMATING ENERGY EXPENDITURE OR PHYSICAL ACTIVITY IN HUMANS

| |
|---|
| Physiologic measurements |
| Pulmonary ventilation volume |
| Heart rate |
| Electromyography |
| Energy intake/body composition |
| Human observations and records |
| Time and motion studies |
| Activity diary |
| Activity recall (i.e., questionnaire and interview) |
| Kinematic recordings |
| Radar |
| Cine photography |
| Mechanical activity meters (i.e., accelerometers, pedometers) |
| Isotope dilution methods |
| Doubly labeled water ($^2H_2{}^{18}O$) or triply labeled water ($^2H^3H^{18}O$) |

As far back as 1914, the pioneer American investigators Benedict and Talbot suggested that in infants heart rate "may be considered a very fair index of energy metabolism." Briefly, the method involves the establishment of individual regression lines between heart rate and energy expenditure within a range of activities that bracket the habitual heart rate observed in real life. By monitoring heart rate minute-by-minute throughout the day by means of portable small heart-rate integrators, a frequency histogram can be obtained giving the number of minutes spent at each heart rate. By referring this value to the individual regression line, the energy expenditure at a given heart rate can be calculated and integrated during day-time activities. Unfortunately, the relationship between heart rate and energy expenditure is not linear within the sedentary range of measurements. This is primarily due to the confounding effect of variations in stroke volume, which substantially increases in a nonlinear fashion up to about 40% of the maximal aerobic capacity. As a result, the measurement of cardiac output (i.e., heart rate × stroke volume) would predict energy expenditure with more accuracy and precision than heart rate itself, but the noninvasive monitoring of cardiac output in free-living conditions is not possible yet. In addition, a variety of confounding factors (such as eating meals, variation in posture, and cigarette smoking) affects proportionally more heart rate than energy expenditure, so that a transient shift in the regression line occurs with a resultant error of prediction.

The development of respiration chamber from the early 1980s has allowed testing of the validity of the heart rate method for estimating energy expenditure in humans.[6] At the group level, the average accuracy in 4 studies involving 8 to 22 subjects ranged from 1 to 3% in conditions close to energy equilibrium.[10–12] However, the standard deviation of the error is much greater, suggesting that the heart rate method is much less reliable for a given subject than for a group.

More recently, enthusiasm has grown for the stable (nonradioactive) isotope method for estimating energy expenditure using the doubly-labeled water ($^2H_2$ and $^{18}O$). This is the most interesting development in the area of human energy metabolism in recent years and will be briefly discussed. As outlined in Table 5–3, this method has several advantages because it can simultaneously provide an estimation of total body water (and hence body composition) and of water intake (and hence milk intake in studies of infants).

The basis of the method was proposed by Lifson et al. in 1955.[13] Initially, it was the object of extensive studies in small animals; only recently has it been applied to man. The method is based on the difference in the rates of turnover of $^2H_2O$ and $H_2{}^{18}O$ in body water, which is used to estimate $CO_2$ production rate and hence the rate of energy expenditure (Fig. 5–2). Briefly, a subject is given a single oral dose of $^2H_2{}^{18}O$ so that body water is labeled by both isotopes. After an equilibrium is reached, the loss of $^{18}O$ isotope will occur both as $CO^{18}O$ and as water $H_2{}^{18}O$, because the action of carbonic anhydrase causes a rapid exchange of $^{18}O$ between water and carbon dioxide, leading to an isotopic equilibrium of $^{18}O$ in $CO_2$ and body water (Fig. 5–2). The loss of the isotope as water is determined independently by measuring the rate of disappearance of $^2H_2O$. Calculation of $CO_2$ production rate is based on the difference in turnover rates of the oxygen and hydrogen labels (Fig. 5–2).

**TABLE 5–3.** RELATIVE ADVANTAGES AND DISADVANTAGES OF USING THE $^2H_2{}^{18}O$ METHOD TO ASSESS TOTAL ENERGY EXPENDITURE IN HUMANS

Advantages

1. Tracer is a nonradioactive isotope.
2. Long-term energy expenditure determination (2–3 weeks).
3. Simple and convenient technique.
4. Simultaneous assessment of body composition via total body water.
5. Can be used to study a large number of subjects simultaneously.
6. In lactating women, the method provides a simultaneous way of determining breast milk production and estimating the infant's energy expenditure.

Disadvantages

1. Expensive technique (cost of isotope [$^{18}O$] and cost of analysis).
2. Measures $CO_2$ production ($\dot{V}CO_2$) and not $O_2$ consumption ($\dot{V}O_2$); hence there is a five times greater potential error on the energy expenditure calculation by using the caloric equivalent of $\dot{V}CO_2$ than with the caloric equivalent of $\dot{V}O_2$.
3. Needs various correction factors and assumptions (e.g., isotope fractionation factors), which make the magnitude of the error in various situations uncertain.
4. Gives an overall mean value of energy expenditure for a period of 2–3 weeks; it is not possible to measure 24-hour energy expenditure and its components and the day-to-day variability in 24-hour energy expenditure.

(Adapted from Jéquier, E., Acheson, K., Schutz, Y.: Annu. Rev. Nutr., 7:187–208, 1987.)

The disappearance rates can be measured in urine (blood or saliva) for a period equivalent to 2 to 3 biologic half-lives. A theoretical calculation indicates that under normal circumstances the disappearance rate of deuterium (mass 2) and $^{18}O$ (mass 18) is low: assuming a total body water of 45 L and a water input from drink and food of 2.5 L per day, the $^2H_2$ label will be eliminated in an exponential negative fashion at a rate of 6% per day. Because oxygen has an additional route of elimination (expired $CO_2$), the disappearance rate of $^{18}O$ will be greater than that of deuterium.[14]

The assumptions on which the original model is based[13] have been tested in man and will not be described here in detail.[14] The assumption that deuterium is lost only in water, and that $^{18}O$ is lost in water and in $CO_2$ only, may not be entirely correct: under certain circumstances the isotopes may also be sequestrated in body tissues (such as deuterium incorporation into lipids during de-novo lipogenesis) or may be excreted in another form than water, such as in urea or in bicarbonate.

Under controlled conditions, recent studies have compared the energy expenditure obtained by using the doubly-labeled water method with that measured by indirect calorimetry in a respiration chamber or with a hood system. These studies,[15] which involved one to nine subjects, have demonstrated that the error at the group level ranged from 1 to 5%, which corroborates theoretical calculations.[16] However, greater errors are expected for a given individual. In addition, because of the numerous assumptions and correction factors required, the utilization of this method in free-living conditions is more uncertain than in laboratory conditions. Finally, knowledge of the RQ is of primary importance to obtain the energy equivalent of $\dot{V}CO_2$ and to accurately derive energy expenditure (Fig. 5–2). As shown in Table 5–1, the latter substantially varies with the RQ (32% variation from RQ between 0.7 and 1.0).

In subjects of various physiologic and nutritional status (i.e., growing babies, pregnant and lactating women, malnourished individuals in a catabolic phase, or obese individuals under restrictive diets), the $^2H_2{}^{18}O$ method will require additional correction factors because the RQ of the diet (which is commonly used to predict the unknown value) is no longer similar to the metabolic RQ.

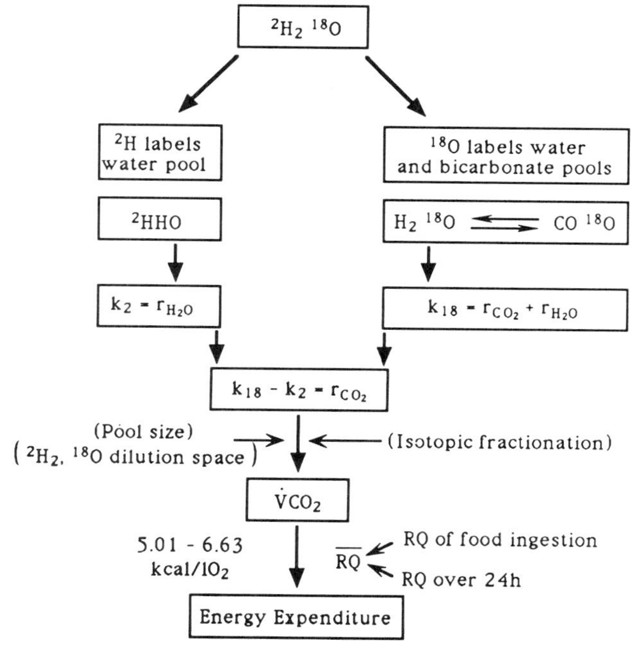
$^2H_2\,^{18}O$
$^2H$ labels water pool
$^{18}O$ labels water and bicarbonate pools
$^2HHO$
$H_2\,^{18}O \rightleftharpoons CO\,^{18}O$
$k_2 = r_{H_2O}$
$k_{18} = r_{CO_2} + r_{H_2O}$
$k_{18} - k_2 = r_{CO_2}$
(Pool size)
($^2H_2$, $^{18}O$ dilution space)
(Isotopic fractionation)
$\dot{V}CO_2$
5.01 - 6.63 kcal/lO$_2$
RQ
RQ of food ingestion
RQ over 24h
Energy Expenditure

**FIGURE 5–2.** Principle of measurement used in the doubly labeled water ($^2H_2{}^{18}O$) technique. Following an oral dose of $^2H_2{}^{18}O$, the difference in the rate of elimination of $H_2{}^{18}O$ ($k_{18}$) versus $^2H_2O$ ($k_2$) in urine, together with a knowledge of the total body water pool and a correction for isotopic effects, provides a measure of the $CO_2$ production rate ($\dot{V}CO_2$). The latter is used to calculate total energy expenditure by means of the energy equivalent of $\dot{V}CO_2$, which varies substantially, from 21.0 to 27.7 kJ/L $CO_2$ at respiratory quotients (RQ) of 1.0 to 0.7, respectively (see Table 5–1). Because the RQ is not measured, it must be estimated from other parameters. The uncertainty because the RQ is unknown could theoretically generate a maximum error of as much as 32%. However, if the dietary intake of the subject is quantitatively measured during the study period and if the subject is in energy equilibrium over the period of measurement, the RQ of the diet can be used to predict the actual RQ of gas exchange, and the error may be reduced to 5 to 10%.

To summarize, the accuracy and precision of the doubly-labeled water method in free-living conditions is probably not constant and depends on the physiologic and nutritional state of the subject as well as the environmental conditions. In future work in the field, it will be necessary to adjust the numerous correction factors and assumptions to specific environmental conditions and to physiologic and nutritional status in order to diminish the uncertainty of the method outside the laboratory.

## ENERGY REQUIREMENTS

The energy requirement of an individual is defined by the World Health Organization (WHO) as "the level of energy intake that will balance energy expenditure when the individual has a body size and composition, and a level of physical activity, consistent with long-term good health. The energy requirement should also allow the maintenance of economically necessary and socially desirable physical activity. In children and pregnant or lactating women, the energy requirement includes the energy needs associated with the deposition of tissues or the secretion of milk at rates consistent with good health."[17] There are two approaches to assess the energy requirement of people of different age, sex, and physical activity:

1. Assessment of food intake followed by the calculation of energy intake
2. Assessment of total energy expenditure

The committee pointed out that (1) the energy needs of a group represent—in contrast to the protein needs—the *average* value of the individuals making up that group, (2) when possible, energy requirement should be based on estimate of energy expenditure rather than on energy intake, and (3) the energy requirement of a typical "reference" man or woman is first established and constitutes a baseline for the assessment of other people with different characteristics. Adjustments for different physiologic states (growth, pregnancy, lactation, and aging) and situations (such as climate) are then made when the group or individual deviates from those reference requirements.

The equation of energy balance can be written as follows:

$$\text{energy intake} = \text{energy expenditure} + \text{changes in stored energy}$$

where energy intake represents the metabolizable energy (either measured or calculated by using Atwater factors) and energy expenditure represents the total energy output. Changes in stored energy are positive when there is an energy gain, and negative when endogenous reserves of energy are used. In an adult individual maintaining weight, changes in stored energy should be close to zero over a few days or weeks, which illustrates the fact that most adult individuals are close to energy balance if one considers it over a prolonged period.

The term "requirements" refers to the "habitual" or "usual" requirements over a certain period. From one day to the next, individuals are not expected to maintain energy balance precisely, and hence energy intake and energy expenditure measurements may not give the same values. The variability of energy intake between subjects is greater than that of energy expenditure (15 to 18% versus 10 to 11% respectively over a 5-day period); this indicates that the habitual requirements can be more adequately obtained from energy expenditure than from energy intake measurements. In addition, it is difficult to measure energy intake accurately without influencing the subject's ingestive behavior.

The energy requirement has been established for maintaining good health, growth, and an "appropriate"

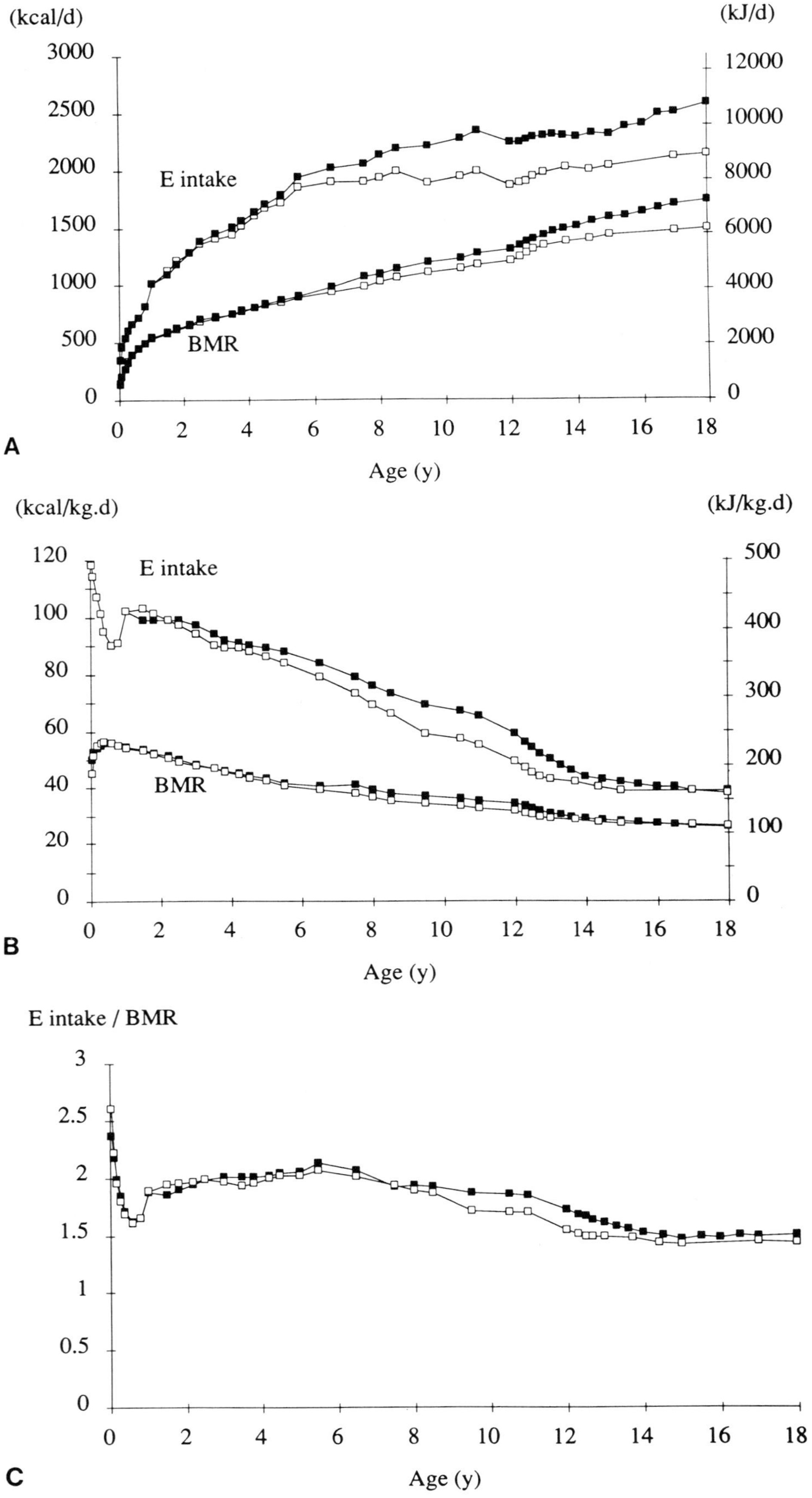

(kcal/d)
(kJ/d)
3000
2500
2000
1500
1000
500
0
12000
10000
8000
6000
4000
2000
0
E intake
BMR
0
2
4
6
8
10
12
14
16
18
A
Age (y)
(kcal/kg.d)
(kJ/kg.d)
120
100
80
60
40
20
0
500
400
300
200
100
0
E intake
BMR
0
2
4
6
8
10
12
14
16
18
B
Age (y)
E intake / BMR
3
2.5
2
1.5
1
0.5
0
0
2
4
6
8
10
12
14
16
18
C
Age (y)


**FIGURE 5–3.** Legend appears on facing page.

**TABLE 5–4.** EVOLUTION OF THE ENERGY REQUIREMENT GIVEN BY VARIOUS JOINT FAO/WHO EXPERT COMMITTEES FROM 1957 TO 1985[17–19]

| FAO/WHO/(UNU) COMMITTEE | REFERENCE INDIVIDUAL (KG) | | EXPRESSION OF REQUIREMENT | PHYSICAL ACTIVITY | ENERGY REQUIREMENT | | | |
|---|---|---|---|---|---|---|---|---|
| | | | | | KCAL/DAY | | KJ/DAY | |
| | MEN | WOMEN | | | MEN | WOMEN | MEN | WOMEN |
| 1957 | 65 | 55 | Per $kg^{3/4}$ | Not categorized | 3200 | 2300 | 13389 | 9823 |
| 1973 | 65 | 55 | Per kg body weight | Moderate activity | 3000 | 2200 | 12552 | 9205 |
| 1985 | 65+ | 55+ | Multiple of BMR | Variable | 2700* | 2100† | 11297 | 8786 |

*No reference individual is considered but the same weight is given for comparison.
†Light activity (1.6 × BMR).

level of physical activity and a satisfactory quality of life. The energy is required to cover the energy needs for basal energy homeostasis (basal metabolic rate), the inefficiency of energy utilization (diet-induced thermogenesis), and the extra cost of physical activity. It cannot be assumed that the observed levels of intake or expenditure are always appropriate for the maintenance of optimal health; actual intakes may be too low in developing countries, whereas the energy expenditure invested for physical activity may be insufficient in affluent societies to maintain optimal cardiovascular functions.

If one examines the evolution of the approach used by expert committee consultation group from the first Food and Agriculture Organization (FAO)/WHO energy meeting[18,19] up to the latest meeting,[17] one can realize the differences in approach used to estimate the energy requirement of individuals (Table 5–4). In addition, it is apparent that the average energy requirement of the individual living in the 1950s was higher than that of today.

## EXPRESSION OF ENERGY REQUIREMENT

The energy requirements can be expressed in absolute values (kJ per day, kcal per day) but they have been commonly expressed in a relative value (Table 5–5) by the different FAO/WHO expert committees: per unit of metabolic body size, i.e., per $kg^{0.75}$,[18] per kilogram body weight,[19] or as a multiple of basal metabolic rate (BMR).[17] An overview of the dynamic changes in energy requirements from birth to adulthood is provided in Figure 5–3, which depicts the evolution of energy intake and BMR when expressed in absolute value, per unit of body weight, or as a multiple of BMR. It is important to remember that the energy expenditure (and hence requirement) per kilogram of body weight is not constant during growth and development: it is much greater in infants and children than in adults (Fig. 5–3). Among adult individuals, the energy requirement per kilogram of body weight will also substantially vary, the highest body weight leading to the lowest value.[17] For example, a young woman of 40 kg will have a predicted BMR of 113 kJ/kg per day (27 kcal/kg per day), whereas a woman of 75 kg will have a value of 90 kJ/kg per day (21.5 kcal/kg per day). This can be explained by two factors: (1) the excess body weight of overweight and obese subjects is mostly composed of adipose tissue of low metabolic activity, and (2) when one derives the energy requirement per unit of body weight, one assumes that the regression line between body weight and energy expenditure has a zero intercept at 0 kg body weight. This is not the case because there is a positive intercept for both basal (Table 5–5) and total energy requirements.[18]

## ESTIMATES OF ENERGY REQUIREMENT

The last consultation groups of FAO/WHO/United Nations University (UNU) (1985)[17] as well as the National Research Council in the United States (1989)[20] have used the same approach to derive total energy requirement of a group of individuals: they use the predicted BMR as a basis. The BMR is predicted from a

**FIGURE 5–3.** Evolution of the basal metabolic rate (BMR), based on Talbot standards,[19] and total energy intakes from birth to 18 years of age, based on tabulated results[17] in male (closed square) and female (open square) individuals. *A*, The absolute value. *B*, Results expressed per unit body weight. *C*, Energy intake expressed as a multiple of BMR. Many important features can be deduced: *B* shows that, per unit body weight, both the BMR and the energy intake vary with age; they are higher in infants and slowly, progressively decrease up to the adulthood. *C* shows that the energy intakes expressed as multiple of BMR has the highest value at birth, substantially decreases during the first year of life, and then takes off again up to 5 years of age (partly because of increased activity at the onset of walking) to finally slowly decrease up to adulthood. Note that this way of expressing the energy requirement considerably flattens the difference between male and female individuals.

**TABLE 5–5.** EQUATIONS FOR PREDICTING BASAL METABOLIC RATE FROM BODY WEIGHT ALONE

| AGE RANGE (YEARS) | KCAL PER DAY | MJ PER DAY |
|---|---|---|
| Males | | |
| 0–3 | 60.9 W − 54 | 0.255 W − 0.226 |
| 3–10 | 22.7 W + 495 | 0.0949 W + 2.07 |
| 10–18 | 17.5 W + 651 | 0.0732 W + 2.72 |
| 18–30 | 15.3 W + 679 | 0.0640 W + 2.84 |
| 30–60 | 11.6 W + 879 | 0.0485 W + 3.67 |
| >60 | 13.5 W + 487 | 0.0565 W + 2.04 |
| Females | | |
| 0–3 | 61.0 W − 51 | 0.255 W − 0.214 |
| 3–10 | 22.5 W + 499 | 0.0941 W + 2.09 |
| 10–18 | 12.2 W + 746 | 0.0510 W + 3.12 |
| 18–30 | 14.7 W + 496 | 0.0615 W + 2.08 |
| 30–60 | 8.7 W + 829 | 0.0364 W + 3.47 |
| >60 | 10.5 W + 596 | 0.0439 W + 2.49 |

W, Body weight expressed in kilograms; MJ, megajoules.
(From WHO: Energy and Protein Requirements. Report of a Joint FAO/WHO/UNU Expert Consultation. Technical Report Series 724. Geneva, World Health Organization, 1985.)

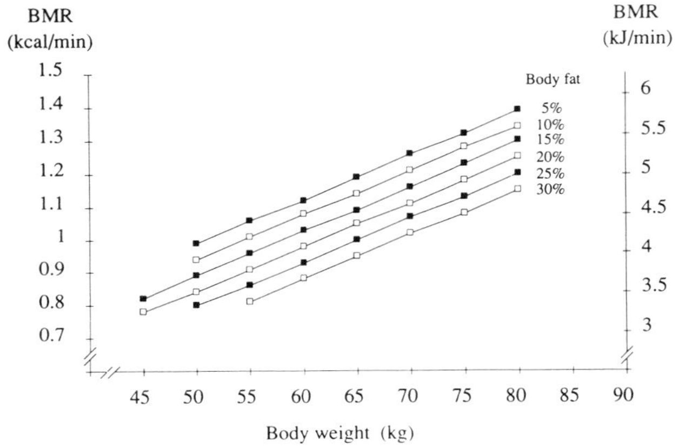
BMR (kcal/min)
BMR (kJ/min)
Body fat
5%
10%
15%
20%
25%
30%
Body weight (kg)
**FIGURE 5–4.** Effect of body composition (% of body fat) on basal (or resting) energy expenditure at different body weight in male (closed square) and female (open square) individuals. The graph clearly shows that, for a given body weight, the lower the percentage of fat, the higher the basal metabolic rate (BMR). In addition, it indicates that the BMR of a 75-kg woman with 30% body fat is not more elevated than the values of a lean man of 60 kg with 10% body fat. (Data from Durnin, J.V.G.A., Passmore, R.: Energy, Work and Leisure. London, Heinemann Educational Books, 1967.)

series of simple linear regression equations (Table 5–5),partitioned into male versus female, and broken down into different age categories (0 to 3, 3 to 10, 10 to 18, 18 to 30, 30 to 60, and >60 years). These equations have been derived from an analysis of the world literature by Schofield et al. (1985).[21] The uncertainty of the prediction is about ±7 to 10% for a single individual, but it is expected to be lower for a group. In individuals of extreme body composition (either very lean or very fat), these equations predicting BMR from body weight are not accurate, because changes in body composition represent an important confounding factor in the prediction of BMR. Figure 5–4, based on tabulated data of Passmore and Durnin,[22] illustrates the influence of body composition on the predicted BMR for individuals with different body fat content (from fat representing 5% of body weight to fat representing 30% of body weight). The figure shows that for a constant body weight, the BMR, in absolute value and expressed per kilogram, decreases with increasing fat content of the body. As a result, fat-free mass is a better predictor of BMR than body weight is. When the body weight is unknown or largely deviates from normality, the median weight, according to age, sex, and height, can be used instead.

Once the BMR is calculated, the factorial approach is used (Fig. 5–5): a BMR factor is defined for the physical activities, which are broken down into occupational activities (work) and discretionary (i.e., desirable) activities. Occupational activities include salaried and nonsalaried chores (such as housework). The energy needs for occupational activities will depend on the type of occupation, the time spent in performing the work, and the physical characteristics of the individuals. These

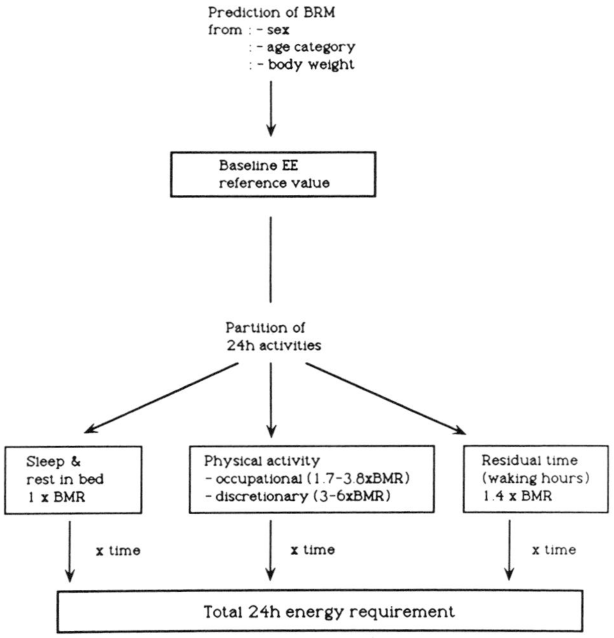
Prediction of BRM
from : - sex
: - age category
: - body weight
Baseline EE
reference value
Partition of
24h activities
Sleep &
rest in bed
1 x BMR
Physical activity
- occupational (1.7-3.8xBMR)
- discretionary (3-6xBMR)
Residual time
(waking hours)
1.4 x BMR
x time
x time
x time
Total 24h energy requirement
**FIGURE 5–5.** Approach used by the FAO/WHO/UNU (1985) consultation group to calculate the energy requirements of adults. BMR, Basal metabolic rate; EE, energy expenditure. (Data from WHO: Energy and Protein Requirements. Report of a Joint FAO/WHO/UNU consultation. Technical Report Series 724. Geneva, WHO, 1985.)

activities are classified into light (1.7 × BMR), moderate (2.2 × BMR for women and 2.7 × BMR for men), and heavy (2.8 × BMR for women and 3.8 × BMR for men). Discretionary activities include socially desirable activities (such as the exploratory activities of children and the participation in tasks implying social improvement), exercise for physical and cardiovascular fitness, and optional household tasks. In addition, the BMR is used to estimate the energy cost of sleeping. Finally, the residual time during which there is no clear definition of activity has been taken as BMR × 1.4.

Once the separate components of energy expenditure (sleep, physical activity, and residual time) have been calculated, the total energy requirement can be calculated by summation. It should be realized that when the energy requirement is calculated *over 24 hours* and categorized into "light," "moderate," and "heavy" work, the value expressed in multiples of BMR is obviously much lower than that calculated during a working task. For example, a group with occupational work classified as "moderate" activity will have an energy requirement calculated over 24 hours of 1.78 × BMR in men and 1.64 × BMR in women because it includes sleeping hours and residual time, whereas during the actual performance of this given task, the energy expended will be 2.7 × BMR for men and 2.2 × BMR for women. The approach used by the expert consultation committee of FAO/WHO/UNU[18] to predict the energy requirements of adults is outlined in Figure 5–5.

Figure 5–6 shows the total energy requirements in an absolute value as a function of body weight and activity level (expressed as a multiple of BMR) in male and female adult subjects. Note that for a given body weight and activity factor, the average energy requirement of a woman (18 to 30 years old) is lower by 12 to 17% than that of a man of the same age category.

Figure 5–7 shows the relative energy cost of walking at different speeds expressed as a multiple of BMR in a 70-kg man and a 70-kg woman. It indicates that, for a given body weight, the factorial approach allows one to estimate the energy requirement of certain activities without considering the gender of the individual.

## ENERGY REQUIREMENTS OF INFANTS, CHILDREN, AND ADOLESCENTS

The FAO/WHO/UNU expert committee has proposed the calculation of energy requirements from birth to 10 years of age from spontaneous energy intake data obtained in healthy children who were growing normally with an arbitrary extra allowance of 5%.[17] The rationale for that was (1) correction for breast milk consumption assessed in the first year of life by the weighing method, and (2) allowance for a desirable level of physical activity in children up to 10 years. After 10 years of age, the energy requirement estimates were based on energy expenditure data using the factorial method, as described above in adults. An extra allowance was made for the energy cost of growth, using a constant value of 21 kJ (5 kcal) per gram of weight gain.

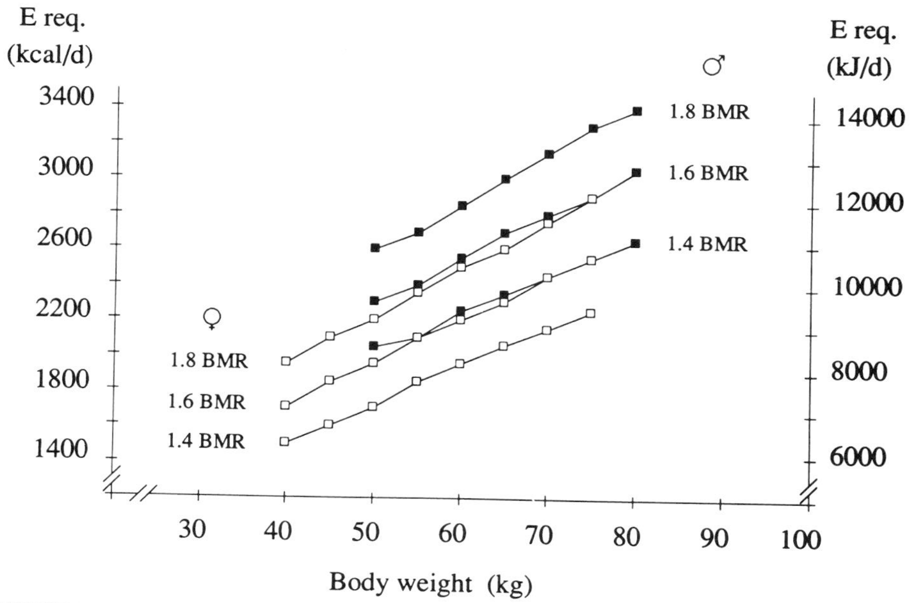
E req. (kcal/d)
3400
3000
2600
2200
1800
1400
E req. (kJ/d)
14000
12000
10000
8000
6000
♂
1.8 BMR
1.6 BMR
1.4 BMR
♀
1.8 BMR
1.6 BMR
1.4 BMR
30
40
50
60
70
80
90
100
Body weight (kg)

**FIGURE 5–6.** Effect of body weight and activity level (expressed as multiple of basal metabolic rate (BMR)) on the daily average energy requirement in a group of male (closed square) and female (open square) adult subjects. (Data from WHO: Energy and Protein Requirements. Report of a Joint FAO/WHO/UNU consultation. Technical Report Series 724. Geneva, WHO, 1985.)

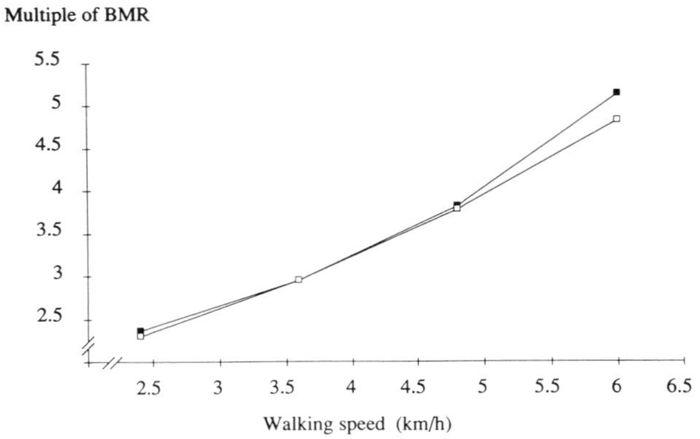
Multiple of BMR
5.5
5
4.5
4
3.5
3
2.5
2.5
3
3.5
4
4.5
5
5.5
6
6.5
Walking speed (km/h)

**FIGURE 5–7.** Gross energy cost of walking on the level (expressed as multiple of basal metabolic rate (BMR)) at various speeds of walking in male (closed square) and female (open square) individuals of 60 kg between 18 and 30 years of age. The increased slope at higher speed is a reflection of the lower work efficiency. (Data from WHO: Energy and Protein Requirements. Report of a joint FAO/WHO/UNU consultation. Technical Report Series 724. Geneva, WHO, 1985.)

## ENERGY REQUIREMENTS DURING PREGNANCY AND LACTATION

The growth of the fetus placenta and the associated maternal tissues during pregnancy requires extra energy. It is well known that the BMR rises during pregnancy, in particular during the last trimester.[23] The increased active tissue mass (fetal, placental, and maternal), the increased cardiovascular and respiratory works, and the metabolic cost of new tissue synthesized explain this rise in BMR. Attempts have been made to estimate the extra energy cost of a full-term pregnancy in healthy women. Classically, a value of 335,000 kJ (80,000 kcal) is given as the total energy cost of pregnancy above prepregnant values, of which about 151,000 kJ (36,000 kcal) are accounted for by maternal lipid storage.[19] The expert FAO/WHO/UNU consultation group advised an average increase of 285 kcal (1190 kJ) per day throughout pregnancy if the woman maintains her level of physical activity throughout pregnancy.

It should be realized that it is difficult to assess accurately the energy needs during pregnancy. On one hand, estimates can be obtained from the factorial method—that is, from the increased BMR observed throughout pregnancy with an allowance for the energy retained in the form of fat and protein in the mother and the baby. However, the extra energy requirement based on BMR alone also depends on the extent to which the mother adapts to the increased energy cost of moving a heavier body (in particular at the third trimester) by spontaneously reducing her rate of physical activity. For example, if a mother gives up her job and leads a sedentary rather than an active life during pregnancy, the increase in energy expenditure observed at rest and the extra energy requirement for tissue storage may be offset by a decrease in activity-related energy expenditure. As a result, the woman may not need an increased amount of food energy as compared to the prepregnant phase. It is more appropriate to assess the changes in total 24-hour energy expenditure in free-living conditions rather than in BMR alone.

Another way to assess the extra energy requirement during pregnancy is to monitor the changes in energy intake during the gestational period. Studies of food intake in well-nourished pregnant European women indicate that a small extra energy intake is necessary to satisfy energy requirement—that is, less than 420 kJ (100 kcal) per day.[24]

Lactation constitutes a major energetic stress in a woman's life because milk production must be sustained continuously over an extended period. The energy cost of lactation depends on two factors: (1) the quantity of milk secreted and (2) the net efficiency of milk synthesis.

The 1985 FAO/WHO/UNU Expert Committee on Energy Requirements estimated the energy cost of lactation by simply adding the computed total cost of milk synthesis (i.e., the sum of the energy content of milk + the net energy cost to synthesize it) to the energy requirement of a nonpregnant, nonlactating woman.[17] The average daily milk secretion during the first 6 months is approximately 750 ml per day,[20] but large variations among individuals are observed. The breast-milk energy content of well-nourished women is on the order of 2.9 kJ/ml (0.70 kcal/ml), so that the energy content of daily milk production amounts to about 2200 kJ per day.

A value of 80% for the efficiency of milk synthesis is currently used for human lactation.[17,20] This value was derived from an average efficiency of human milk production, which was calculated to be 97%; the estimation of 80% results from the most extreme biologic assumptions.[23] As a result, the total cost of milk production is on the order of 2700 kJ per day (2200 ÷ 0.8). However, part of the energy cost of lactation may be sustained by endogenous fat mobilization during pregnancy. Assuming that the extra fat deposited during pregnancy (2 to 4 kg) is mobilized during the first 6 months of lactation, the recommendation of the Expert Committee is an extra 2090 kJ per day throughout lactation.[17,20]

## REFERENCES


1. Flatt, J.P., Pahud, P., Ravussin, E., et al.: Trends Biochem. Sci., *9*:466–468, 1984.
2. Flatt, J.P.: The biochemistry of energy expenditure. *In* Recent Advances in Obesity Research. Vol. 2. Edited by G.A. Bray. London, Newman, 1978, pp. 211–228.
3. Livesey, G., Marinos, E.: Am. J. Clin. Nutr., *47*:608–628, 1988.
4. Jéquier, E.: Direct and indirect calorimetry in man. *In* Substrate and Energy Metabolism. Edited by J.S. Garrow and D. Halliday. London, J. Libbey, 1985, pp. 82–92.
5. Jéquier, E., Acheson, K., Schutz, Y.: Annu. Rev. Nutr, *7*:187–208, 1987.
6. Jéquier, E., Schutz, Y.: Am. J. Clin. Nutr., *38*:989–998, 1983.
7. Brouwer, E.: Eur. Assoc. Anim. Prod. Publ., *11*:441–443, 1965.
8. Brockway, J.M.: Hum. Nutr. Clin. Nutr., *41C*:463–471, 1987.
9. Frayn K.N.: J. Appl. Physiol., *55*:628–634, 1983.
10. Dauncey, M.J., James, W.P.T.: Br. J. Nutr., *42*:1–13, 1979.
11. Spurr, G.B., Prentice, A.M., Murgatroyd, P.R., et al.: Am. J. Clin. Nutr., *48*:552–559, 1988.
12. Ceesay, S.M., Prentice, A.M., Day, K.C., et al.: Br. J. Nutr., *61*:175–186, 1989.
13. Lifson, N., Gordon, G.B., McClintock, R.: J. Appl. Physiol., *7*:704–710, 1955.
14. Schoeller, D.A., Ravussin, E., Schutz, Y., et al.: Am. J. Physiol., *250*:R823–830, 1986.
15. Schoeller, D.A.: J. Nutr., *118*:1278–1289, 1988.
16. Seale, J., Miles, C., Bodwell, C.E.: J. Appl. Physiol., *66*:644–653, 1989.
17. WHO (World Health Organization): Energy and Protein Requirements. Report of a Joint FAO/WHO/UNU Expert Consultation. Technical Report Series 724. Geneva, World Health Organization, 1985.
18. FAO Nutritional Studies No. 15: Calorie Requirements. Report of the Second Committee on Calorie Requirements. Rome, FAO and WHO, 1957.
19. FAO Nutrition Meetings Report Series No. 52 and WHO Technical Report Series No. 522: Energy and Protein Requirements. Geneva, FAO and WHO, 1973.
20. National Research Council: Recommended Dietary Allowances. 10th Ed. Washington, D.C., National Academy Press, 1989.
21. Schofield, W.N., Schofield, E.C., James, W.P.T.: Hum. Nutr. Clin. Nutr., *39C* (Suppl. 1):1–96, 1985.
22. Durnin, J.V.G.A., Passmore, R.: Energy, Work and Leisure. London, Heinemann Educational Books, 1967.
23. Hytten, F., Chamberlain, G.: Clinical Physiology in Obstetrics. Oxford, London, Edinburgh, Boston, Melbourne, Blackwell Scientific Publications, 1980.
24. Durnin, J.V.G.A., McKillop, F.M., Grant, S., et al.: Lancet, *2*:823–825, 1985.

CHAPTER 6

# Water, Electrolyte, and Acid-base Balance

Man S. Oh



## CONTROL OF BODY FLUID VOLUME AND OSMOLALITY

### PRINCIPLES OF CONTROL

The electrolyte compositions of intracellular and extracellular fluid are vastly different, but because cell membranes are freely permeable to water, osmolalities* of intracellular and extracellular fluid are always the same. Any discrepancy in osmolality between intracellular and extracellular fluid causes a rapid shift of water until the two compartments have the same osmolality. A reduction in extracellular osmolality, whether it is caused by retention of water or by loss of solutes, must be followed by a reduction in intracellular osmolality to the same extent, and this is achieved by intracellular shift of water; the result is always an increase in cell volume.

An increase in extracellular osmolality may result from loss of water or gain of solutes. When extracellular osmolality increases by loss of water or by accumulation of a solute that cannot enter the cell freely (e.g., mannitol, sodium, glucose), the osmotic equilibrium occurs by extracellular shift of water reducing cell volume. However, when extracellular osmolality increases by accumulation of a solute that can freely diffuse across the cell membrane (e.g., urea and alcohol), the osmotic equilibrium is achieved by diffusion of the solute into the cells, and no change in cell volume occurs. Osmols that cannot enter the cell freely are effective in causing transcellular shift of water, and hence are called effective osmols, and osmols that can diffuse freely into cells are called ineffective osmols. The plasma osmolality based on effective osmols is effective osmolality. In summary, effective osmolality determines the intracellular volume; the cell volume is increased when effective osmolality is decreased, decreased when effective osmolality is increased, and normal when effective osmolality

*Osmolality refers to concentration of solutes, and is based solely on the number of particles, independent of the size or nature of the solute.

is normal. For example, accumulation of glucose in the extracellular fluid causes shift of water from the cell and thereby reduces serum Na, by a factor of 1.5 mEq/L (1.5 mmol/L)† for each increase of 100 mg/dl in serum glucose. When hyperglycemia is reversed, the reduction in extracellular osmolality causes an intracellular shift of water with serum Na increasing by the same factor.

## BODY FLUID VOLUMES

Using a factor of 2.2 for conversion of kilograms to pounds and a figure of 54% of body weight as the total body water (TBW), we can conveniently estimate the body water (in liters) as: body weight (lb)/4. About 50% of TBW is extracellular volume (ECV), and 50% intracellular volume (ICV). Although most authorities in the field put the normal value of the extracellular volume at 40% of TBW, this figure is based on the space of distribution of sulfate or inulin. When the extracellular volume is measured as the space of distribution of chloride, a larger value (about 50% of TBW) is obtained. Because the space of distribution of chloride is more representative of those of the other major ions of the extracellular fluid such as Na and $HCO_3$, the larger figure (i.e., 50%) seems more physiologically relevant for our discussion.

When a person loses weight acutely, the weight loss can be assumed to be almost entirely that of water. For example, if a person who normally weighs 160 lb (40 L of TBW) develops diarrhea and loses 11 lb of weight in 2 days, the new body water is: 40 L − 5 L (11/2.2) = 35 L. The water content of adipose tissue is only about 10%, and therefore the weight loss resulting from reduction in adipose tissue mass results nearly entirely from the loss of fat; an average-sized person without caloric intake loses about 1/2 lb of body weight daily when fat is the source of calories. However, when protein is the source of energy, weight loss is considerably greater because each gram of protein loss is accompanied by loss of 3 g of tissue water.

## ESTIMATION AND MEASUREMENT OF OSMOLALITY

Plasma osmolality may be measured directly with an osmometer or estimated from the concentrations of the solutes. An osmometer, unable to distinguish between effective and ineffective osmols, only measures total osmolality. Effective osmolality must be estimated, either by adding up all effective osmols or by subtracting ineffective osmolality from total osmolality measured with an osmometer. Because the only significant ineffective osmol in normal plasma is urea, whose concentration is about 5 mosm/L (about 1.5% of total osmolality), the normal plasma osmolality is practically equal to the estimated effective osmolality.

Plasma osmolality can be estimated by multiplying plasma sodium by 2 and then adding up the osmolal concentrations of 2 major nonelectrolyte solutes, urea and glucose:

$$\text{Plasma osmolality} = \text{plasma Na (mEq/L)} \times 2 + \text{glucose (mg/dl)}/18 + \text{urea (mg/dl)}/2.8.$$

Glucose and urea are divided by one tenth of their respective molecular weights, because the volume unit is changed from a deciliter to a liter.

In most instances, osmolality estimated using the above formula is close to the osmolality measured with an osmometer. When the measured osmolality is 10 mosm/L greater than the estimated value, an osmolal gap is said to be present. The osmolal gap suggests the accumulation of nonelectrolyte solutes other than glucose and urea, such as ethanol, methanol, ethylene glycol, and mannitol. Accumulation of anions of acids such as lactate and ketone anions does not lead to an osmolal gap; these anions are balanced by Na, and thus their osmolal contributions are accounted for when plasma Na is doubled.

## MECHANISM OF CELL VOLUME REGULATION

Cell volume is reciprocal to effective osmolality. For certain cells in the body, such as the muscle cells, the reciprocal relationship is maintained in acute as well as in chronic changes in effective osmolality. For certain other cells, such as the brain cells, the cell volume is restored to normal through volume regulatory mechanisms when effective osmolality remains chronically altered. In a *hypo-osmolal* state, the brain cell volume is initially increased, but with a continuing hypo-osmolal state, the volume is normalized over a few days. With subnormal osmolality and normal volume, the solute content of the brain cells is reduced. Thus, sudden normalization of osmolality from a chronic hypo-osmolal state causes a shift of water from the brain into the extracellular fluid (ECF) and hence shrinkage of the brain. Conversely, in a chronic *hyperosmolal* state, when the brain volume is normalized but total solute content of the brain is increased, sudden normalization of osmolality may cause brain edema with intracellular water shift.

## NONRENAL CONTROL OF SALT AND WATER BALANCE

### *CUTANEOUS WATER EXCHANGE*

Water is lost from the skin primarily as a means of eliminating heat. Water loss from the skin without sweat is called insensible perspiration. Sweat contains about 50 mEq/L of sodium and 5 mEq/L of potassium. The

†As indicated here, monovalent ions (e.g., $Na^+$, $K^+$, $Cl^-$, $HCO_3$) have 1 mEq equivalent to 1 mmol; divalent ions have 0.5 mmol/L equivalent to 1 mEq/L.

amount of water loss from the skin is proportionate to the amount of heat generated as is shown by the following formula:

Water loss from the skin = 30 ml per 100 kcal.

### *RESPIRATORY WATER EXCHANGE*

The water content of inspired air is less than that of expired air, and respiratory water loss can be calculated from the ventilatory volume and the difference in partial pressure of water vapor between inspired air and expired air. Because the ventilatory volume is determined by the amount of $CO_2$ production, which in turn depends on the caloric expenditure, the amount of ventilatory water loss in normal environmental conditions depends also on caloric expenditure:

Respiratory water loss
= 13 ml per 100 kcal at normal $PCO_2$.

By pure coincidence, in the absence of fever or hyperventilation, the quantity of water lost from the lung during normal respiration is about equal to the amount produced by metabolism. Respiratory water loss increases with hyperventilation or fever.

### *GASTROINTESTINAL FLUID EXCHANGE*

The net activity of gastrointestinal tract to the duodenum is secretion of water and electrolytes. The net activity from the jejunum to colon is reabsorption. Most of the fluid entering the small intestine is absorbed there, and the remainder is absorbed by the colon, leaving only about 100 ml of water to be excreted daily in the feces. The contents of the gastrointestinal (GI) tract are about isotonic with plasma, and any fluid that enters the GI tract becomes isotonic through secretion and reabsorption. Thus, if water is ingested and vomited, solute is lost from the body.

## ROUTES OF FLUID AND ELECTROLYTE LOSS

### *ABNORMAL LOSSES FROM THE GASTROINTESTINAL TRACT*

Losses of fluid and electrolytes from the GI tract may occur for a variety of reasons: (1) diarrhea, (2) vomiting or gastric drainage, and (3) drainage or fistula from the bile ducts, pancreas, and intestine. Although diarrheal fluid is usually isotonic in terms of the cations (Na and K), diarrhea caused by nonabsorbable solutes such as lactulose, mannitol, sorbitol, or disaccharide (as in a patient with disaccharide malabsorption) causes greater water loss than electrolyte loss.

### *SEQUESTRATION OF FLUID*

Obstruction of bowel may cause transfer of fluid from the extracellular space into the intestinal lumen. Because the composition of the sequestered fluid is similar to that of the ECF, effective arterial volume is reduced without much alteration in composition.

### *SKIN LOSS*

The loss through skin increases with fever, increased metabolism, sweating, and burns. The fluid lost through the skin is hypotonic.

### *LOSS THROUGH VENTILATION*

Only water is lost through the lung with ventilation, and fever and hyperventilation increase water loss through the lung.

### *MISCELLANEOUS LOSSES*

These include drainage from the pleural and peritoneal cavity, seepage from burns, and fluid loss during hemodialysis and peritoneal dialysis.

### *RENAL LOSS*

The kidney may lose sodium and water excessively in a number of situations, which include diuretic therapy, aldosterone deficiency or unresponsiveness to aldosterone, and relief of urinary obstruction.

## PATTERNS OF SALT AND WATER LOSS IN CLINICAL STATES

Depending on the quantity of salt loss in relation to water loss, several types of dehydration are encountered. The net alteration in body composition is determined by the sum of that which has been lost and that which has been added. The net change in dehydration may be (1) isotonic dehydration, (2) hypertonic dehydration, or (3) hypotonic dehydration.

### *ISOTONIC DEHYDRATION*

Salt may be lost isotonically through the GI tract or directly from the ECF by such means as external drainage of pleural effusion and ascites. More often salt is lost with equal or larger water loss, and then the osmolality of the body fluids is subsequently adjusted to isotonicity by oral intake or urinary excretion of water. Because water moves across cell membranes only in response to change in osmolality of the ECF, *isotonic fluid loss is borne completely by the extracellular fluid space.*

### *HYPERTONIC DEHYDRATION*

The primary aberration in hypertonic dehydration is water deficit. Two major mechanisms account for abnormal water deficit: inadequacy of water intake and excessive water loss. Dehydration due to excessive water loss usually develops more rapidly than does dehydration due to reduced water intake. Inadequacy of water intake is always caused by one of the following four conditions: (1) defective thirst mechanism, (2) impaired consciousness, (3) lack of access to water, and (4) inability to drink water.

Water loss may occur excessively through the kidney (e.g., osmotic diuresis and diabetes insipidus) or through the nonrenal routes (e.g., sweating, osmotic diarrhea, vomiting of HCl). Loss of HCl with water is almost equivalent to the loss of pure water, because it leaves behind sodium bicarbonate to replace sodium chloride in the ECF. Even when excessive water loss is the cause of hypertonic dehydration, one of the above conditions limiting water intake must be present in order to maintain hypertonicity. Otherwise, stimulation of thirst by increased osmolality will lead to increased water drinking and correction of hypernatremia.

In hypertonic dehydration total salt content may be normal, increased, or decreased, but it is usually increased because salt administered or ingested in a state of water deficit is retained because of volume depletion.

Water requirement to decrease serum sodium concentration to a desired level can be determined using the following formula:

$$\text{Water requirement} = \left(\frac{\text{actual Na}}{\text{desired Na}}\right) \times \text{TBW in liters} = \Delta\text{Na} \times (\text{TBW/desired Na}),$$

where $\Delta$Na is the difference between actual and normal sodium concentration.

This formula for calculating water requirement is based on the assumption that water is lost without gain or loss of salt. If salt retention is part of the reason for hypernatremia, administration of the total amount of water calculated by the above formula will cause overexpansion of volume. However, if the kidney is functioning normally, the excess salt and water will be excreted. *Rapid correction of hypernatremia to normal levels offers no advantage, and may cause brain edema.* It is advisable to reduce serum sodium at a rate no greater than 0.7 mEq/L per hour, or about 10% of the original value per day except in acute hypernatremia.

### *HYPOTONIC DEHYDRATION*

Fluids lost from the body are almost always either hypotonic or isotonic in relation to sodium concentration, and loss of such fluid cannot cause hypotonicity of body fluid. Hypotonic dehydration occurs usually because the patient loses a sodium-containing solution and replaces it with water or a solution containing fewer cations (sodium + potassium) than the fluid that has been lost.

In the presence of normal renal function, net loss of salt alone is difficult because the hyponatremia would suppress antidiuretic hormone (ADH), resulting in water loss. With severe sodium depletion decreased effective vascular volume causes the release of ADH, which allows retention of water with the development of hyponatremia. Hypo-osmolality of the ECF causes a shift of water into the cells to achieve osmotic equilibrium. *Patients with hypotonic dehydration may therefore present with more evidence of compromised circulation, for a given degree of body water loss, than patients with isotonic or hypertonic dehydration* (Fig. 6–1).

Hypotonic dehydration may be treated by estimating the amount of salt needed to restore the osmolality of the body fluids to normal, administering this amount of salt in the form of hypertonic saline, and adding more normal saline to complete restoration of the ECV. The sodium requirement to increase serum sodium concentration is calculated using the following equation:

$$\text{Na requirement} = (\text{desired} - \text{actual serum Na}) \times \text{TBW (in liters)}$$

Even though the administered sodium would be distributed mainly in the extracellular fluid, TBW is used for this calculation because an increase in serum sodium is accompanied by an exact proportionate increase in

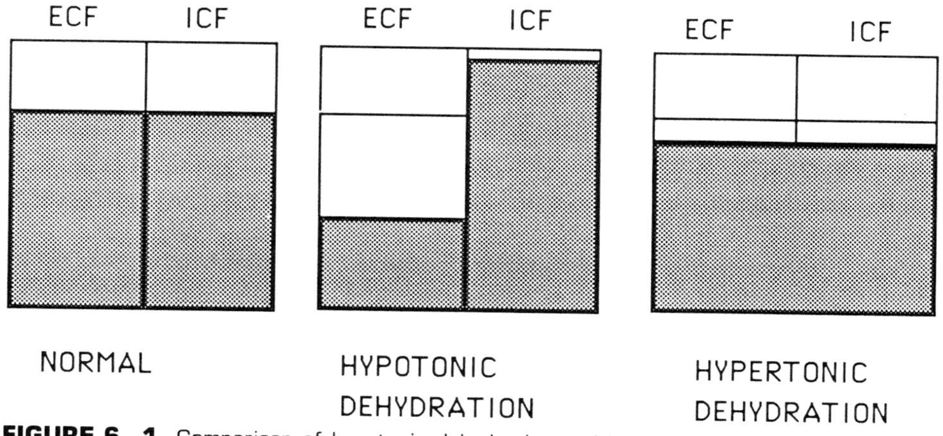
ECF
ICF
ECF
ICF
ECF
ICF
NORMAL
HYPOTONIC DEHYDRATION
HYPERTONIC DEHYDRATION

**FIGURE 6–1.** Comparison of hypotonic dehydration and hypertonic dehydration. For the same amount of total body water loss, the extracellular volume depletion is much greater with hypotonic than with hypertonic dehydration.

serum osmolality (Na × 2 = osmolality). The quantity of solute required to increase serum osmolality is estimated on the basis of TBW, regardless of whether the solute is restricted to the ECF or freely diffusible into cells, because an increase in extracellular osmolality is not possible without an increase in intracellular osmolality to the same extent.

As an alternative therapeutic approach, one can give isotonic saline; as ECF volume increases, ADH will be suppressed, resulting in excretion of free water and restoration of serum sodium to normal. This approach is recommended in patients who suffer mainly from hypovolemia rather than from hypotonicity. In patients with chronic hyponatremia, rapid correction of hyponatremia may be particularly dangerous because of possible occurrence of *central pontine myelinolysis (CPM)*, a demyelinating disease of the central pons and other areas of the brain, which causes a severe motor nerve dysfunction (e.g., quadriplegia). This complication is more likely to occur with rapid treatment of *chronic hyponatremia* than with *acute hyponatremia*. The complication may be avoided by increasing serum sodium more slowly (no faster than 0.5 mEq/L per hour). Although the use of hypertonic saline is the main culprit, administration of isotonic saline may cause sufficiently rapid correction of hyponatremia to cause CPM.

Untreated severe hyponatremia is more serious when it is acute than when it is chronic. Two main dangers of acute hyponatremia are (1) brain edema resulting in herniation of the brain stem and (2) intractable seizure. On the other hand, treatment of acute hyponatremia carries a lower risk of CPM than treatment of chronic hyponatremia does. Hence, hyponatremia may be corrected more rapidly than at 0.5 mEq/L per hour, if the patient has acute symptomatic hyponatremia (e.g., seizure). If the rapidity of the development of hyponatremia is uncertain and the patient is asymptomatic, a conservative approach is indicated.

## PRINCIPLES OF WATER AND ELECTROLYTE THERAPY

### *GOALS OF SALT AND WATER REPLACEMENT*

The goal of therapy is to restore the patient to a state of normal hemodynamics and to restore the body fluid osmolality. There are several components in the program of water and electrolyte therapy: (1) existing deficits must be identified and corrected, (2) daily basal requirements for sodium, potassium, and water must be supplied, and (3) ongoing losses must be quantified and provided for. Short-term parenteral therapy does not require inclusion of calcium, phosphate, and magnesium.

### *BASAL WATER REQUIREMENTS*

The basal requirement for water depends on insensible losses and sensible (urinary) losses of water. Without fever, the amount of water lost from the skin is 30 ml/100 kcal or 8 ml/kg body weight or 3.6 ml/lb. Because, in the absence of fever and hyperventilation, water loss from the lung is about equal to the amount of water produced in metabolism, only the water loss from the skin needs to be included in estimating the basal requirement of water. Urinary loss of water depends on the total amount of solute excreted and urine osmolality. The solute excretion depends mainly on salt ingestion and urea production, the latter being a function of protein intake and catabolism.

### *DAILY WATER REQUIREMENTS*

In the absence of fever and sweating, water loss through the skin is relatively fixed, but the urinary water excretion varies greatly, and depends on the total amount of solute to be excreted and on urine osmolality. For example, for a total solute excretion of 600 mosm per day, the urine volume will be 500 ml at urine osmolality of 1200 mosm/L, and 15 L at 40 mosm/L. For such a person, if the kidney is capable of usual maximal concentration, the minimum water requirement would be 1100 ml (500 ml for urinary water loss plus 600 ml for skin water loss at 2000 cal per day). On the other hand, the maximal allowable water intake would be 15.6 L (600 mosm/40 mosm/L = 15 L) if the kidney can dilute urine to 40 mosm/L. If the kidney can increase the urine osmolality to only 600 mosm/L with the impaired concentration mechanism, the minimum water requirement would be 1.6 L. Similarly, if urine can be diluted to only 300 mosm/L, the maximal allowable water intake would decrease to 2.6 (600/300 + 0.6) L.

Clearly, in the absence of abnormality in urine concentration and dilution, a large variation in water intake will cause neither dehydration nor overhydration. However, underestimation of water need is safer than overestimation for a variety of reasons.

First, the amount of water gained when urine dilution is impaired tends to be greater than the amount of water lost with impaired urine concentration. Second, clinical impairment in urine dilution, as with the *syndrome of inappropriate ADH secretion (SIADH)*, is more common than impairment in urine concentration, as with diabetes insipidus. Finally, in conscious patients thirst is a powerful protection against hypernatremia, whereas patients often lapse into hyponatremic coma without specific complaints.

## CLINICAL PROBLEMS

**1.** A 45-year-old chronic alcoholic was admitted in coma to the emergency room with the following laboratory values: serum Na, 115 mEq/L; serum osmolality, 400 mosm/L; serum glucose, 1000 mg/dl; blood urea nitrogen (BUN), 42 mg/dl; and total serum osmolality, 400 mosm/L.

**i.** The patient's ICV is:

**a.** increased.

b. decreased.
c. normal.
d. not predictable.

ii. When the elevated serum glucose is normalized by metabolism, serum sodium will (assume no change in water content):

a. increase.
b. decrease.
c. remain the same.

iii. When the elevated glucose is normalized by metabolism, extracellular osmolality will (assume no change in water content):

a. increase.
b. decrease.
c. remain the same.

iv. The patient is in coma because of:

a. hyperosmolality.
b. hyponatremia.
c. alcohol intoxication.

2. Which of the following patients has an increased ICV?

a. A diabetic patient with serum sodium of 110 mEq/L and serum glucose of 2000 mg/dl.
b. An alcoholic with serum sodium of 125 mEq/L and serum alcohol of 500 mg/dl.
c. A uremic patient with serum sodium of 150 mEq/L and serum urea nitrogen of 140 mg/dl.
d. A patient with serum sodium of 150 mEq/L accompanied by anasarca.
e. A patient who developed hyponatremia after receiving 200 g of mannitol.

3. A patient has serum sodium of 110 mEq/L and weighs 120 lb. How much sodium is needed to increase serum sodium to 125 mEq/L if TBW is kept constant?

4. A patient with diabetes is admitted to the hospital with serum sodium of 130 mEq/L and serum glucose of 2100 mg/dl. Following treatment with insulin, serum glucose is decreased to 100 mg/dl.

i. What is the new Na concentration (assume no change in TBW and total body Na and K content)?
ii. Is ECV higher or lower after treatment?

5. A patient, who has TBW of 40 L, has serum Na concentration of 180 mEq/L, and you plan to reduce it to 163 mEq/L over the next 24 hours. What is the amount of water required?

6. A 68-year-old woman sustained a stroke and was unattended for 4 days. She was admitted to the hospital with serum sodium concentration of 156 mEq/L. She weighed 120 lb before the stroke. What is the amount of water deficit?

7. A 68-year-old man was admitted to the hospital following 3 days of nausea and vomiting without any water intake. The serum sodium was 152 mEq/L. The patient was hypotensive (blood pressure 70/50 mm Hg), urine volume was 15 ml per hour, and osmolality and sodium concentration were 980 mosm/L and 2 mEq/L, respectively. The patient's body weight before the present illness was 160 lb.

i. How much water did the patient lose, and can you estimate the amount of water loss on the basis of serum Na?
ii. What kind of intravenous fluid would you use to treat this patient?

8. A 48-year-old woman presents with a history of copious diarrhea for 5 days, with water and tea as her only intake. She is very weak, faints on standing; she is nauseated and complains of muscle cramps. Blood pressure in the semirecumbent position is 70/50 mm Hg, pulse rate is 104 beats/min, and hematocrit is 55%. Serum sodium concentration is 120 mEq/L, serum potassium 3.8 mEq/L, serum bicarbonate 16 mEq/L, and chloride 92 mEq/L. The urine volume is 20 ml/h, with an osmolality of 500 mosm/L, and sodium concentration 2 mEq/L. The patient weighs 114.5 lb on admission, and has lost 5.5 lb since the beginning of her illness.

i. What is the ECV loss?
ii. What is the amount of sodium required to bring sodium concentration to normal?
iii. What intravenous solution would you use to treat this patient?

**ANSWERS**

1. *i*, c; intracellular volume is reciprocal with effective osmolality, and in this case effective osmolality is normal.

*ii*, a; serum Na will increase because loss of solute from ECF causes shift of water from ECF into intracellular fluid (ICF).

*iii*, b; loss of glucose will result in a reduction in osmolality.

*iv*, c; hyponatremia causes coma by reducing effective osmolality, but in this patient effective osmolality is normal. A huge osmolal gap (a gap between measured and calculated osmolality) in this patient strongly suggests an accumulation of abnormal osmols such as ethanol.

2. b; the effective osmolality is reduced only in answer b.

3. 15 mEq ($\Delta$Na) $\times$ 30 L (TBW) = 450 mEq.

4. *i*, 160 mEq/L.

*ii,* ECV will decrease as water shifts into the cell. Despite the increase in serum Na, the extracellular effective osmolality is falling with the loss of glucose osmols.

**5.** (17/163) × 40 L = 4.17 L.

**6.** (16/156) × 30 L = 3.1 L.

**7.** *i,* The amount of water loss cannot be estimated on the basis of serum sodium in this patient; water deficit in a hypernatremic patient can be estimated from serum Na only if total body Na and K content has not been altered—that is, when water loss is the sole cause of hypernatremia. If this patient's hypernatremia (Na, 152 mEq/L) had been caused by water loss, the amount of water loss would have been (12/15) × 40 L = 3.1 L. However, the patient's clinical signs of dehydration indicate that the water loss is far greater; the patient must have lost Na as well as water, but water loss was greater than Na loss, resulting in hypernatremia.

*ii,* The patient is suffering mainly from volume depletion, and hypernatremia is only mild. Therefore, isotonic saline would be the best solution to start with; 0.45% saline might also be used.

**8.** *i,* The patient lost 5.5 lbs and therefore 2.5 L of TBW; hence ICV is increased from 15 L (50% of 30 L) to 17.5 L (15 × 280 mosm/L divided by 240 mosm/L = 17.5 L), a gain of 2.5 L. Extracellular volume is therefore reduced by 5 L (2.5 + 2.5 = 5 L).

*ii,* 1100 mEq; 750 mEq of Na is needed to increase serum Na from 120 to 140 mEq/L while maintaining TBW at 37.5 L, and then an additional 350 mEq of Na is needed by adding 2.5 L of isotonic saline (140 mEq/L) to normalize ECV and TBW.

A list of selected readings on this and subsequent topics in this chapter is given at the end of the chapter.

## DISORDERS OF WATER & ANTIDIURETIC HORMONE (ADH) METABOLISM

### REGULATION OF THIRST AND ADH RELEASE

Normal osmolality of body fluids, essential for optimal cell function, is maintained by the interplay of thirst and antidiuretic hormone (ADH; also called vasopressin). A rise in effective osmolality of the ECF (e.g., from reduced water intake) reduces the volume of the cells. The osmoreceptor cells in the hypothalamus respond to the increase in effective osmolality by sending impulses to the cerebral cortex, provoking thirst, and to the supraoptic and paraventricular nuclei, which are the sites of ADH synthesis. The hormone is stored in the posterior pituitary and its stalk, and is released by the impulses coming from the hypothalamic nuclei. Upon its release, ADH is carried by the circulation to the kidney where its antidiuretic effect operates through an increased permeability to water of the collecting duct.

In the normal state, a rise in effective plasma osmolality of as little as 2 to 3% stimulates release of ADH sufficiently for maximal concentration of the urine; a fall in plasma osmolality of as little as 2 to 3% maximally suppresses ADH release. Plasma hypo-osmolality associated with a fall in plasma sodium concentration of 3 mEq/L or more will result in maximal water diuresis, and plasma hyperosmolality caused by a rise in plasma sodium of the similar magnitude will cause maximal antidiuresis (Fig. 6–2). However, hypo-osmolality and severe hyponatremia may be associated with an osmotically concentrated urine because a variety of other factors can also influence ADH release, and these may override the inhibitory effect of hypo-osmolality on ADH release.

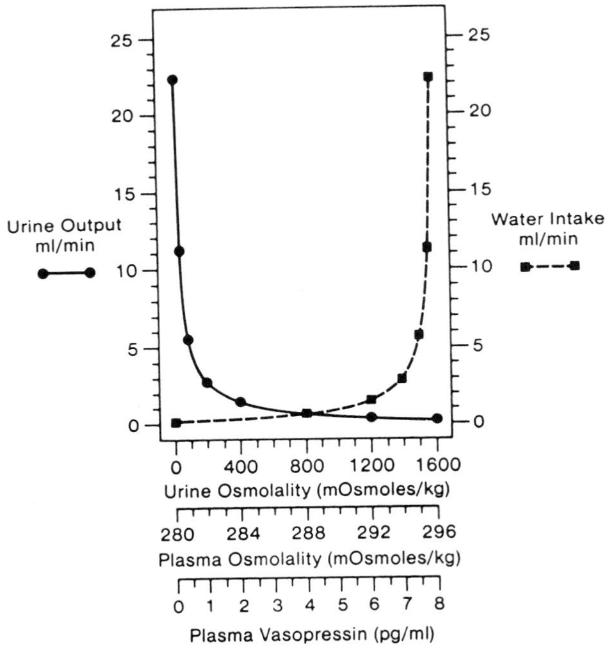

Urine Output ml/min
Water Intake ml/min
0 5 10 15 20 25
0 400 800 1200 1600
Urine Osmolality (mOsmoles/kg)
280 284 288 292 296
Plasma Osmolality (mOsmoles/kg)
0 1 2 3 4 5 6 7 8
Plasma Vasopressin (pg/ml)


**FIGURE 6–2.** The relationship of renal excretion or oral intake of water to urine osmolality, plasma osmolality, and plasma vasopressin in a typical 70-kg human. The line describing urine flow was calculated assuming a solute load of 800 mosm per day. The line describing water intake was obtained by analyzing the relation of water intake to plasma osmolality in 12 healthy adults after infusion of hypertonic saline (unpublished observations of R.L. Zerbe and G.L. Robertson). The contributions of insensible loss and dietary water to total output and intake usually approximate 1.4L per day (1 ml/min). Neither is included in these calculations. (From Robertson, G.L., Berl, T.: Water metabolism. *In* The Kidney. Philadelphia, W.B. Saunders, 1986, p. 389.)

*NONOSMOLAR FACTORS AFFECTING ADH RELEASE AND THIRST*

**Hemodynamic Factors.** Low volume and pressure, operating through baroreceptors, provoke thirst and ADH output; high volume has the reverse effect. Stimulation of thirst and ADH by low volume and pressure is mediated in part through angiotensin II.

**Hormonal Factors.** α Catechols suppress and β catechols enhance ADH output. Prostaglandin inhibits the effect of ADH on the kidney. Angiotensin II stimulates thirst and ADH. Lack of glucocorticoid enhances ADH action on the kidney and may cause increase in plasma ADH.

**Physical and Emotional Stress.** Physical and emotional stress, such as major surgery, enhance ADH output, possibly in part through emetic stimuli.

**Drugs.** Many drugs affect ADH release or action; for example, ethanol inhibits the output of ADH and demeclocycline inhibits the effect of ADH on the kidney. Chlorpropamide increases the action of ADH on the kidney. Some drugs may increase ADH release through emetic stimuli.

**Emetic Stimulus.** Nausea is a potent stimulus for ADH release, and many drugs that are known to cause hyponatremia probably utilize this mechanism.

**Reduced Effective Arterial Volume.** The urine may become osmotically concentrated in the absence of ADH if effective arterial volume (EAV) is very low. The combination of reduced glomerular filtration rate (GFR) and enhanced proximal reabsorption of filtrate reduces the volume of dilute urine formed in Henle's loop. This small volume moves so slowly down the collecting duct that even the limited permeability of the membrane permits withdrawal of a significant fraction of the water from the urine, resulting in urine concentration.

## CLINICAL DISORDERS

There are three main types of clinical disorders of water and ADH metabolism: polyuria, hyperosmolality of the body fluid, and hypo-osmolality of the body fluid.

*POLYURIA*

Polyuria is arbitrarily defined as urine volume in excess of 2.5 L per day, and there are two types: water diuresis and osmotic diuresis. In water diuresis, urine volume is increased with normal total solute excretion. The sine qua non for osmotic diuresis is increased excretion of solute. As a point of reference, solute excretion in excess of 60 mosm/per hour (or 1 mosm/per minute) may be defined as osmotic diuresis.

Water diuresis may result either because of insufficient ADH (central or neurogenic diabetes insipidus) or because of the failure of the kidney to respond to ADH (nephrogenic diabetes insipidus). Insufficient ADH hormone is due either to defective ADH secretion (central, neurogenic, or pituitary diabetes insipidus) or to physiologic suppression resulting from excessive water intake. In pure osmotic diuresis, urine osmolality is usually higher than plasma osmolality because increased plasma osmolality due to water loss leads to increased production of ADH, and a tendency toward antidiuresis. As the osmolal excretion rate increases, urine osmolality falls progressively to approach plasma osmolality but still remains higher than plasma osmolality. Osmotic diuresis is most commonly caused by glucose, salt, or urea.

**Differential Diagnosis.** The diagnosis of osmotic diuresis is confirmed by determining that the rate of solute excretion exceeds 60 mosm/per hour. If urine osmolality is inappropriately low for the degree of osmotic diuresis, a combination of water diuresis and osmotic diuresis should be suspected. Having determined that the patient has osmotic diuresis, one identifies the solute (e.g., glucose, urea, salt).

If water diuresis is diagnosed, the next step is to determine whether the patient's water diuresis is due to primary polydipsia or diabetes insipidus, either central or nephrogenic. Theoretically, diabetes insipidus should be readily distinguishable from primary polydipsia; patients with diabetes insipidus are expected to have a high plasma osmolality, and those with primary polydipsia a low plasma osmolality. However, thirst usually prevents hypernatremia in diabetes insipidus, and rapid renal excretion of water usually prevents hyponatremia in primary polydipsia. Although plasma sodium of patients with diabetes insipidus tends to be higher than that of patients with primary polydipsia, there is much overlap. Therefore a fluid deprivation test, as described below, is usually necessary.

Water is restricted until the serum osmolality is high enough (up to 300 mosm/L) to cause maximal concentration of the urine. If the urine osmolality is maximal (>700 mosm/L) the patient has sufficient ADH production and a normal renal response to ADH; the diagnosis is primary polydipsia. If the urine does not reach maximal concentration with adequate dehydration, the patient has either nephrogenic or central diabetes insipidus. Differentiation between nephrogenic and central diabetes insipidus depends on the response to exogenous ADH. Little or no response to the administered hormone indicates nephrogenic diabetes insipidus.

**Treatment**

*Central Diabetes Insipidus.* Patients with complete deficiency of vasopressin usually need hormonal replacement. Those with partial deficiency may be treated with the hormone or with agents that increase the rate of ADH secretion or end organ responsiveness. In either event, salt restriction and diuretic therapy can help reduce the delivery of salt and hence water to the site where dilute urine is made. Agents used for the treatment of central diabetes insipidus include various ADH analogs, which include desmopressin (dDAVP), lysine-vasopressin (Diapid, Lypressin), and aqueous pitressin, as well as an oral medication, chlorpropamide. The latter increases tubular responsiveness to ADH.

*Nephrogenic Diabetes Insipidus.* The only available treatment is a low-salt diet combined with a thiazide diuretic. The purpose is to increase the proximal tubular reabsorption of salt and hence water, and thereby to reduce distal delivery of urine. A very high dose of desmopressin has been used to overcome tubular unresponsiveness to ADH, but its cost is very high.

*Primary Polydipsia (Dipsogenic Diabetes Insipidus).* There is no satisfactory therapy, because the origin is usually psychogenic. The drugs that interfere with urinary dilution, such as thiazide diuretics, should be avoided. Occasionally, patients with upward reset of the osmostat for thirst may be managed with desmopressin.

*Osmotic Diuresis.* Identify the agent responsible for osmotic diuresis (e.g., urea, glucose, sodium) and treat accordingly.

## *HYPERNATREMIA*

**Causes.** Hypernatremia may be caused either by loss of water or by gain of sodium. In most instances, both causes are present for the following reasons: (1) when hypernatremia is caused by sodium retention, sodium diuresis induced by hypernatremia leads to secondary loss of water; (2) when hypernatremia results from primary water loss, the volume depletion leads to secondary renal retention of sodium. Hypernatremia may be caused by pure water loss with normal body sodium content when water is lost without sodium intake, as in acute diabetes insipidus without sufficient water administration, or when the unattended comatose patient loses water through the skin, lung, and kidney. Sometimes both salt and water are lost but water loss is greater than salt loss, resulting in hypernatremia with decreased body sodium content. Examples include osmotic diuresis, osmotic diarrhea, sweating, and vomiting. Table 6–1 lists causes of hypernatremia.

**Diagnosis.** Hypernatremia may be attributed to one or some combination of three causes: (1) excessive sodium administration, (2) inadequate water intake, and (3) excessive water loss. Whatever the primary defect may be, hypernatremia can be always prevented if water intake is sufficient. In that sense, every patient with hypernatremia may be considered to have inadequate water intake, either absolute or relative. Thus, the evaluation of hypernatremia should always include identification of the causes of inadequate water intake.

Excessive sodium administration as the cause of hypernatremia is usually obvious from the patient's history. Whether hypernatremia is due to insufficient water intake or to excessive water loss can be determined by measurement of urine osmolality and volume. Normal concentration of urine (urine osmolality in excess of 700 mosm/L) suggests that the main problem is insufficient water intake and nonrenal water loss. Urine osmolality between 700 mosm/L and isotonicity suggests partial central diabetes insipidus, osmotic diuresis, diuretic therapy, acquired nephrogenic diabetes insipidus, or renal failure. If urine osmolality is below that of plasma, the findings are consistent with complete central diabetes insipidus and nephrogenic diabetes insipidus, either acquired or congenital.

**Treatment.** Treatment of hypernatremia should be aimed at restoring the normal osmolality and volume. The speed of correction depends on the speed of development and accompanying symptoms. In general, chronic hypernatremia is well tolerated, and therefore

**TABLE 6–1.** CAUSES OF HYPERNATREMIA

**I.** Increased total body sodium content
- **a.** Primary hypodipsia with or without diabetes insipidus
- **b.** Acute diabetes insipidus treated with salt-containing solutions
- **c.** Administration of hypertonic sodium bicarbonate during cardiac arrest or for treatment of lactic acidosis
- **d.** Dialysis accident or accident during hypertonic saline abortion

**II.** Normal total body sodium content
- **a.** Acute diabetes insipidus with inadequate water replacement
- **b.** Unattended comatose patients
- **c.** No access to water or food

**III.** Decreased total body sodium content
- **a.** Osmotic diuresis
- **b.** Sweating
- **c.** Osmotic diarrhea
- **d.** Vomiting

rapid correction offers no advantage and has a disadvantage of possible brain edema. The rate of correction of chronic hypernatremia (of more than 2 days) should not exceed 0.7 mEq/L per hour or about 10% of the serum sodium concentration per day. Hyperacute hypernatremia (less than 12 hours) may be treated rapidly, but it is unlikely that sustained damage, such as intracranial bleeding, will be reversed by rapid treatment. When the patient has hemodynamic alteration due to volume depletion, the initial solution should be isotonic saline; the purpose is to expand the volume without much alteration in osmolality. The amount of water necessary to correct hypernatremia is usually estimated from serum sodium concentration with the assumption that hypernatremia is entirely due to water loss. Although this assumption is unwarranted in most cases of chronic hypernatremia, nevertheless, because volume depletion induced by water loss causes retention of sodium, water requirement to correct hypernatremia still can be estimated from serum sodium concentration on the following basis: (1) if hypernatremia is accompanied by sodium retention, administration of water will cause volume expansion and hence renal excretion of sodium; (2) if urine contains sodium plus potassium at a concentration similar to that of serum sodium, urinary excretion will have little effect on serum sodium concentration.

The amount of water required to reduce serum sodium is then calculated using the following formula:

$$\text{Water requirement (L)} = (\text{actual Na}/\text{desired Na} - 1) \times \text{TBW (L)}.$$

For example, if patient with TBW of 30 L has serum sodium of 180 mEq/L and one intends to reduce serum sodium in the next 24 hours by 18 mEq/L to 162 mEq/L, the amount of water required would be $(180/162 - 1) \times 30 = 3.3$ L.

An easier equation derived from the one above is:

$$\text{Water requirement (L)} = (\Delta\text{Na}/\text{desired Na}) \times \text{TBW (L)},$$

where ΔNa is reduction in serum sodium concentration to be achieved. In the above example, dNa would be 18 mEq/L, and desired Na 162 mEq/L. Hence, water requirement $= (18/162) \times 30 = 3.3$ L. The total water requirement must also include insensible water loss (about 300 to 500 ml per 24 hours).

Urinary electrolyte-free water loss represents the urine water loss in excess of the volume necessary to contain urinary sodium plus potassium at the same concentration as serum sodium. Urinary loss of water affects serum sodium only if the sum of the concentrations of urinary sodium and potassium is different from serum sodium concentration. If the sum is greater than serum sodium concentration, urine output reduces serum sodium; if the sum is less than serum sodium concentration, the effect of urine output is to increase serum sodium. Ideally, the calculation of water requirement should include measurement of electrolyte-free water excretion. If electrolyte-free water excretion is not known, water replacement can proceed with the assumption that the sum of urine Na and K levels is about equal to that in serum. Frequent measurements of serum sodium will detect any error in these assumptions.

### *HYPONATREMIA*

In the absence of abnormal solute accumulation, hyponatremia is associated with low serum osmolality. Occasionally hyponatremia results acutely from shift of water from the cell due to accumulation of solutes restricted to the ECF, such as mannitol or glucose; in this case osmolality is increased. Loss of potassium may also cause hyponatremia as sodium shifts into the cell in exchange for potassium. Most commonly, hyponatremia is caused by either retention of water or loss of sodium.

Normally, a slight reduction in serum sodium concentration, when accompanied by reduction in effective osmolality, results in marked suppression of ADH; this causes excretion of dilute urine until serum sodium is normalized. Persistence of hyponatremia therefore requires an explanation. Four basic mechanisms are responsible for maintenance of hyponatremia: (1) grossly excessive water intake, (2) impairment of renal water excretion despite normal ADH control because of advanced renal failure, (3) impairment of urine dilution by either appropriate or inappropriate ADH secretion, and (4) abnormal urine concentration without participation of ADH because of slow flow of urine in the collecting duct. If low GFR and enhanced proximal reabsorption of salt and water limit delivery of urine to the collecting duct, the fluid may flow so slowly that urine may be concentrated substantially in the presence of little or no ADH.

**Mechanism of Maintenance.** Hyponatremia may be due to excessive water intake or inadequate renal water excretion. Hyponatremia due to excessive water intake is usually obvious from a history of polydipsia and excretion of a large volume of urine. When impaired renal water excretion is the cause, urine volume is not large and urine is inappropriately concentrated. Appropriate urine osmolality in the presence of hyponatremia is defined operationally as a value less than 100 mosm/L. The measurement of urine osmolality in the differential diagnosis of hyponatremia, however, is usually unnecessary because the urine volume is a sufficient clue; in most instances, the volume of appropriately dilute urine (< 100 mosm/L) is fairly large, usually in excess of 10 L a day. Occasionally, however, if daily solute excretion is unusually low, urine volume need not be very great even when the urine is dilute. For example, if a person excretes only 300 mosm of solute in 24 hours, the volume might be only 5 L at an osmolality of 60 mosm/L. A common misconception is that hyponatremia due to impaired urine dilution is always accompanied by very concentrated urine or at least urine osmolality in excess of serum osmolality. However, urine need not be highly concentrated in order to cause or maintain hyponatremia.

Advanced renal failure as a cause of impaired renal water excretion can be easily ruled out by measurement of BUN and serum creatinine. *ADH secretion in the presence of hyponatremia and in the absence of normal to increased effective arterial volume is truly inappropriate, and the term inappropriate secretion of ADH (SIADH) is used.* In contrast, ADH secretion in the presence of hyponatremia is not considered inappropriate if effective arterial volume is reduced.

The vast majority of patients with hypo-osmolality and hyponatremia have either appropriate or inappropriate ADH secretion, and the main distinguishing feature between the two is the status of effective arterial volume. History and physical examination are useful in distinguishing the two, but are often insensitive in detecting subtle alterations in effective arterial volume. The physical signs of volume depletion such as low blood pressure, orthostatic hypotension, and tachycardia are often absent in states of low effective arterial volume, unless volume depletion is severe. Signs such as dry mucous membrane and dry skin and axilla are not as useful in hypotonic dehydration as in hypertonic dehydration. It is known that acute loss of about 10% of blood volume stimulates ADH release through the baroreceptor mechanism, but it is not precisely known what degree of chronic volume depletion is necessary to produce hyponatremia through the distal trickle effect and to stimulate ADH release by the baroreceptor mechanism. If we use diuretic-induced hyponatremia as a guide, the degree of volume depletion necessary to produce hyponatremia need not be very extensive.

The kidney is usually the most sensitive monitor of low effective arterial volume. Low effective arterial volume reduces GFR and enhances tubular reabsorption of sodium, urea, and uric acid, resulting in increases in BUN, serum creatinine, the BUN/creatinine ratio, and serum urate, and a reduction in urinary sodium excretion (usually less than 20 mEq/L). Plasma renin activity and aldosterone tend to be increased.

**Causes.** Hyponatremia caused by hyperlipidemia and hyperproteinemia is called pseudohyponatremia. Symptoms attributable to hyponatremia are absent in pseudohyponatremia because sodium concentration in the extracellular water is normal. This is to be contrasted to hyponatremia caused by accumulation of solutes restricted to ECF (e.g., glucose and mannitol), which is associated with symptoms of hyperosmolality. Some authors also use the term pseudohyponatremia for this latter type of hyponatremia as well, but this usage is incorrect in that situation, because the serum sodium is truly low.

When hyperproteinemia is caused by accumulation of cationic $\gamma$ globulins, as in IgG myeloma, serum sodium is reduced in part because cations of $\gamma$ globulin partly substitute for sodium in balancing extracellular anions. This results in an increase in serum chloride concomitant with a decrease in serum sodium. Because serum osmolality remains unchanged, the increase in serum chloride must equal the reduction in serum sodium (we will ignore the small osmolal contribution of the polyvalent $\gamma$ globulins). At the same time, in order to maintain electrical neutrality, the increase in concentration of cationic charges (in mEq/L) contributed by $\gamma$ globulins must equal the sum of reduction in cationic charge of sodium and increase in anionic charge of chloride. The reduction in sodium concentration (in serum water) by accumulation of cationic $\gamma$ globulin can be estimated by the following equation:

$$\begin{aligned}\text{Reduction in serum Na} &= \text{increase in cationic charge}/2\\ &= \text{change in anion gap}/2.\end{aligned}$$

When a monovalent cation such as lithium or tromethamine (THAM; also called TRIS) accumulates, reduction in serum sodium is equal to the serum concentration of the cation accumulated.

Once the above types of hyponatremia are excluded, usual true hyponatremia, hereafter called hyponatremia, is present. Hyponatremia is associated with normal, increased, or decreased effective arterial volume (Table 6–2).

Patients with hyponatremia accompanied by low effective arterial volume may be dehydrated or edematous; the former are salt-depleted, and the latter have excessive body sodium. With the latter, the kidney retains salt in response to low effective arterial volume, resulting in edema formation.

Low effective arterial volume with salt depletion is caused by either renal or extrarenal salt loss. If the cause of salt loss is renal, renal excretion of salt is inappropriately high (> 20 mEq/L), whereas with extrarenal causes, the kidney would conserve salt. In both dehydrated and edematous subjects, hyponatremia is maintained because water excretion is limited by the enhanced proximal water reabsorption as well as by volume-mediated ADH secretion. The evidence that hyponatremia may result from renal salt wasting due to some unknown humoral substances released in response to cerebral injury is not very conclusive.

Many authors assign myxedema and glucocorticoid deficiency to the category of hyponatremia with apparently normal effective arterial volume, but there is reasonable evidence that effective arterial volume is reduced in both states, as shown by the reduced cardiac output, low GFR, and low renal plasma flow. Thus, the mechanism of hyponatremia is probably the same as that found in edema-forming states and salt-depletion states. Despite low cardiac output and reduced GFR and renal plasma flow, the kidney does not seem to retain sodium in myxedema and glucocorticoid deficiency. On the other hand, in selective glucocorticoid deficiency due to hypopituitarism, the mechanism of hyponatremia appears to be inappropriate secretion of ADH, without evidence of volume depletion.

SIADH causes hyponatremia by excessive and inappropriate retention of water. Expansion of effective arterial volume caused by retention of water stimulates

**TABLE 6–2.** CLINICAL CAUSES OF HYPONATREMIA

- **I.** Pseudohyponatremia: hyperlipidemia, hyperproteinemia
- **II.** True hyponatremia
  - **a.** With increased effective osmolality: hyperglycemia, mannitol
  - **b.** With normal effective osmolality: $\gamma$ globulins, lithium, THAM
  - **c.** With low effective osmolality
    - **1.** Hyponatremia with low EAV
      - **i.** Hyponatremia with edema (sodium excess): congestive heart failure, nephrotic syndrome, cirrhosis of the liver, idiopathic edema
      - **ii.** Hyponatremia with sodium depletion: renal or extrarenal salt wasting
    - **2.** Hyponatremia with normal or expanded EAV
      - **i.** Syndrome of inappropriate ADH secretion
      - **ii.** Water intoxication due to primary polydipsia
      - **iii.** Water overload in advanced renal failure

**TABLE 6–3.** CAUSES OF SYNDROME OF INAPPROPRIATE ADH SECRETION

- **I.** Tumors: cancer of the lung, pancreas, duodenum, ureter, bladder, and prostate; lymphoma, thymoma, mesothelioma, Ewing's sarcoma
- **II.** Intrathoracic causes: virtually any pulmonary lesions
- **III.** CNS abnormalities: virtually any brain lesions
- **IV.** Surgical and emotional stress: emetic?
- **V.** Endocrine causes: glucocorticoid deficiency? and myxedema?
- **VI.** Idiopathic
- **VII.** Drugs
  - **a.** ADH analogues and oxytocin
  - **b.** Drugs that increase ADH release directly: vincristine, vinblastine, cyclophosphamide (?), clofibrate, bromocriptine, carbamazepine, narcotics
  - **c.** Drugs that stimulate ADH possibly through emetic stimulus: tricyclic antidepressants, monoamine oxidase inhibitor, phenothiazines
  - **d.** Drugs that enhance ADH effect on the kidney: chlorpropamide, tolbutamide, diuretics (especially thiazides), acetaminophen, nonsteroidal anti-inflammatory drugs, carbamazepine

various salt-excreting mechanisms, and the kidney excretes salt and water in order to restore the volume to normal. Although salt is excreted, water is retained by the effect of ADH. Volume expansion and hyponatremia attenuate the effect of ADH, and urine tends to become less concentrated for the same amount of ADH, as hyponatremia and volume expansion worsen. Net water retention may slow down eventually or stop despite continuous inappropriately high levels of ADH, and hyponatremia may become fairly stable. Edema does not occur in SIADH despite water retention, because the amount of water retained is small and much of it is retained in the intracellular compartment.

Causes of SIADH are shown in Table 6–3. Virtually any pulmonary disease and any brain lesion may cause SIADH. A vast number of drugs cause SIADH through different mechanisms, but in many instances the exact mechanism is not understood. In some instances, a drug known to cause clinical SIADH may possess the opposite pharmacologic effect in experimental studies. Many of the drugs that have effects on the CNS have anticholinergic effects, which produce dry mouth and increased water ingestion. Many antimetabolites and psychotrophic drugs cause nausea, which is known to stimulate ADH release and cause water retention.

**Clinical Manifestations.** A reduction in serum sodium concentration alone has no direct physiologic effects like those of other electrolyte abnormalities. Hyponatremia causes clinical manifestations only if it is accompanied by cell hypo-osmolality. Cell hypo-osmolality causes muscle cramps, weakness, and fatigue, but the main symptoms are central nervous system (CNS) manifestations such as mental confusion and disorientation. Convulsions and coma may be the outcome of severe and particularly rapidly developing hyponatremia. Coma in hyponatremia frequently follows a seizure. The speed of development and magnitude of hyponatremia are important determinants of clinical symptoms.

**Diagnosis.** Before making the diagnosis of hyponatremia with low effective osmolality, one must exclude pseudohyponatremia and hyponatremia associated with increased effective osmolality. Hyperlipidemia sufficient to cause pseudohyponatremia will be manifested by the lipemic serum, but hyperproteinemia must be confirmed by measurement. Low serum sodium with normal serum osmolality, in the absence of hyperglycemia and azotemia, strongly suggests pseudohyponatremia.

By coincidence, true hyponatremia may be accompanied by accumulation of some other abnormal solutes, such as ethanol, mannitol, ethylene glycol, and methanol; serum osmolality may therefore be normal, giving the impression of pseudohyponatremia. One must be particularly careful not to mistakenly diagnose pseudohyponatremia on the basis of a low serum sodium in the presence of normal osmolality, because substantial ethanol accumulation, which is a frequent event, may be accompanied by true hyponatremia. The true sodium concentration can be confirmed by measuring serum sodium with a sodium-selective electrode without dilution of the sample (direct-reading ion-specific electrode). It is important to note that pseudohyponatremia in the presence of hyperlipidemia or hyperproteinemia is the result of dilution rather than of the technique of sodium measurement. Sodium measurement by an ion-specific electrode with dilution of the sample (indirect-reading ion-specific electrode) will result in the same error as that produced with the flame photometer.

Reduction in serum sodium concentration by displacement of serum water with lipid or protein can also be calculated from the known values of specific gravity of lipid and protein. Each gram per deciliter of triglyceride results in a false reduction in serum sodium by about 1.7 mEq/L, and 1 g/dl of protein falsely reduces serum sodium by about 1 mEq/L. The latter calculation does not include the true reduction in serum sodium that would occur by accumulation of cationic proteins as in multiple myeloma (discussed previously).

Hyponatremia with increased effective osmolality can be diagnosed only if the substances responsible for extracellular shift of water, such as glucose and mannitol, are identified.

**Treatment.** The speed and method of treatment of hyponatremia depend on the severity of symptoms and status of ECV. Treatment for those patients with hyponatremia who suffer from volume depletion should be different from that of patients who suffer mainly from the effects of acute hyponatremia. Treatment of chronic asymptomatic hyponatremia should be different from that of acute symptomatic hyponatremia.

Two well known dangers of severe symptomatic hyponatremia are brain edema leading to herniation and uncontrolled seizure. Both conditions are more likely to occur with acute than with chronic hyponatremia. Until recently, the only potential dangers of rapid correction of hyponatremia were thought to be vascular volume overload and complications of dehydration of the brain (if the brain volume has already been normalized through the volume regulatory mechanisms as described earlier in this chapter). With concomitant use of a diuretic, vascular volume overload can be easily prevented. Apparently, the type of complication that occurs with brain dehydration resulting from acute hypernatremia, such as intracranial bleeding, does not occur with rapid correction of hyponatremia. However, as noted earlier in this chapter, a newly recognized and far more serious danger is central pontine myelinolysis (CPM), a demyelinating disease involving primarily the central pons.

Opinion is widely divided concerning the danger and benefit of rapid correction of hyponatremia. It is my opinion that the danger of CPM resulting from rapid correction is much greater than the danger of complications of sustained hyponatremia resulting from slow treatment. It has been asserted that CPM may develop only if hyponatremia is corrected rapidly to normal or supernormal levels, but that the lesion can be avoided if rapid correction stops at a subnormal level (130 mEq/L). However, there is no dearth of reports of cases of CPM developing after correction of hyponatremia to such subnormal levels. Chronicity of hyponatremia is an important factor for the development of CPM. In the rat, rapid correction of hyponatremia of 3 days' duration resulted in the development of CPM more often and with greater severity than was the case with correction of hyponatremia of 1 day's duration. The vast majority of cases of CPM reported in man followed rapid correction of hyponatremia that had been present for more than 48 hours. However, a few cases of CPM have been reported recently that followed rapid correction of hyponatremia that lasted less than 12 hours. In most reported cases of CPM induced by rapid correction of hyponatremia, the correction was achieved by infusion of hypertonic saline. However, serum sodium may rise very rapidly with administration of isotonic saline also, and, in recent years, the number of cases of CPM that developed following treatment with isotonic saline has been increasing.

In principle, rapid treatment of hyponatremia would be indicated if the danger of untreated or slowly treated hyponatremia is greater than the danger of rapid treatment. Because the danger of CPM with rapid treatment increases with increasing duration of hyponatremia, whereas the danger of untreated hyponatremia diminishes with increasing duration, a rapid increase in serum sodium would be more beneficial and less dangerous in acute hyponatremia than in chronic hyponatremia. Thus, with symptomatic hyponatremia of clearly less than 48 hours' duration, rapid treatment probably would be indicated. Even then, there is no obvious advantage in normalizing serum sodium at once.

In hyponatremia lasting more than 48 hours, which

represents most cases of the so-called acute symptomatic hyponatremia in the hospital, the danger of CPM resulting from rapid treatment probably greatly outweighs the benefit of rapid treatment, and slow treatment is thus recommended.

*Rapid Correction of Hyponatremia.* Rapid removal of water is best accomplished by a loop diuretic, such as furosemide, plus hypertonic saline. The diuretic will remove salt and water, and hypertonic saline returns salt to the body. The net result is removal of water. Administration of hypertonic saline alone would also cause diuresis, but urine usually contains sodium and potassium at high concentrations, partially negating the effect of hypertonic saline. Under the action of furosemide, urine is approximately isotonic. Because the excretion of isotonic urine will have no appreciable effect on serum sodium concentration, the increment in sodium concentration can be estimated with fair accuracy on the basis of the amount of sodium administered.

Some authors have recommended the use of isotonic saline plus furosemide for treatment of acute symptomatic hyponatremia, but the recommendations are illogical. For the same amount of sodium to be administered, isotonic saline contains more water than hypertonic saline does. Administration of isotonic saline instead of hypertonic saline means addition of more water to the body while the therapy is aimed at removing it. The amount of sodium required to increase serum sodium to a desired level is calculated by the following formula:

$$\text{Sodium required (mEq)} = \Delta\text{Na} \times \text{TBW},$$

where ΔNa is defined as desired serum Na − actual serum Na.

However, hypertonic saline contains not only sodium but also water, and the increment in serum sodium concentration for a given amount of hypertonic saline administered is estimated by the following formula:

$$\text{Increment in serum Na} = \frac{(\text{IV Na} - \text{serum Na}) \times \text{IV fluid volume}}{\text{TBW}}$$

We recommend that alternate liters of isotonic saline and half isotonic saline be given to treat hyponatremic dehydration, and that serum sodium be checked at 6-hour intervals. If KCl is administered concomitantly at 30 to 40 mEq/L, then half isotonic saline should be the replacement fluid. Half isotonic saline is about 70% as effective as isotonic saline in expanding ECV if all the administered water and salt are retained. But if all the administered water is excreted while all the sodium is retained, the increment in serum sodium will be only half of that achieved by isotonic saline.

Osmotic diuretics such as mannitol can remove water if renal function is adequate, but the method is not as predictable and convenient as the use of saline plus a loop diuretic is. Administration of urea has also been recommended as a means of treating hyponatremia through osmotic diuresis.

*Slow Correction of Hyponatremia and Maintenance Therapy.* When slow correction of hyponatremia in a volume-expanded subject is desired, water restriction is the best choice. If this is unsuccessful, administer a loop diuretic with increased salt and potassium intake. Furosemide will prevent urine concentration and commit more water to a given amount of solute excreted. Increased intake of salt and potassium increases solute excretion and therefore allows more water to be excreted. Urea has been tried for the same purpose, but offers no theoretic advantage over furosemide plus salt. A number of different agents that interfere with urine concentration at the collecting duct have been tried to manage chronic hyponatremia. Lithium and demeclocycline, which cause nephrogenic diabetes insipidus, have been used with some success, but they are inferior to furosemide because of the side effects. Finally, an ADH antagonist has been used successfully, but its safety is not yet clearly known.

## CLINICAL PROBLEMS

1. A 63-year-old man with a long history of alcoholism and laboratory data suggestive of cirrhosis of the liver was admitted to the hospital complaining of progressive weakness and recent vomiting lasting several days. The patient was lucid and had no neurologic abnormality. His wife described his intake of food as minimal. On examination he had poor skin turgor and no subcutaneous fat; he weighed 120 lb. Blood pressure was 105/70 in the sitting position and fell to 90/– in the upright position. Serum Na concentration was 105 mEq/L and serum K 2.9 mEq/L. The resident made the diagnosis of hypotonic dehydration and treated the patient for 24 hours with 1 L of normal saline every 6 hours (155 mEq/L of Na), each liter containing 40 mEq of K. Within 16 hours the serum Na had risen to 121 mEq/L, and within 24 hours to 128 mEq/L. Three days later the patient was unable to speak or swallow. Computed tomography (CT) scan and magnetic resonance imaging (MRI) of the brain were performed. Which of the following statements is true?
   - **a.** The significant findings on the brain imaging are likely to be in the pons.
   - **b.** The neurologic deterioration is unrelated to the patient's therapy.
   - **c.** The changes in serum Na had no relationship to neurologic manifestations.
   - **d.** The rise in serum Na would have been more rapid had no K been given.

2. A 65-year-old woman was admitted to the hospital because her family felt she was weak and "not quite

herself." She had no complaints and was able to answer questions. Physical examination suggested moderate dehydration; the patient weighted 150 lb, and the resident estimated her fluid loss (correctly, as it turns out) at about 4 L. She had a 10-cm curved scar over the area of the framed frontal lobe of the brain; BUN was 45 mg/dl; creatinine (Cr) 1.3 mg/dl. Serum Na was 182 mEq/L; urine osmolality was 550 mosm/L; urinary Na was 50 mEq/L. Following injection of pitressin the urine osmolality rose to 750 mosm/L. Which of the following statements is true?

  **a.** The patient's hypernatremia is entirely due to water loss.
  **b.** The patient has nephrogenic diabetes insipidus.
  **c.** The patient has a thirst defect.
  **d.** The patient should immediately receive an infusion of pitressin and water sufficient to lower her serum Na to 140 mEq/L within the next 12 to 16 hours.

**3.** A 21-year-old woman was referred from a rheumatology clinic where she was diagnosed as having lupus erythematosus in complete clinical remission on no treatment. The consultant is requested to explain a BUN of 40 mg/dl. Plasma osmolality was 295 mosm/L (normal is about 280). Urinalysis showed normal urinary sediment, and no proteinuria. Urine osmolality was 500 mosm/L. An additional problem noted by the consultant was polyuria and polydipsia, with a 24-hour urine volume of 5 L a day. Blood pressure was 120/80 and pulse rate was 82. Serum creatinine was 0.8 mg/dl and total daily excretion of creatinine was 1.3 g. Which of the following statements is true?

  **a.** She had multiple emboli to the kidneys with loss of renal function and low GFR (glomerular filtration rate).
  **b.** The data given are internally inconsistent: laboratory error.
  **c.** The patient is severely volume depleted and has pre-renal azotemia.
  **d.** The patient was told by a friend to eat a high-protein diet in order to lose weight. She was eating more than 1 kg of beef daily.
  **e.** She had cerebral vasculitis with infarction in the hypothalamus and central diabetes insipidus.

**4.** A 64-year-old man suffering from manic-depressive psychosis was transferred from the psychiatry service with signs of increasing stupor and hypotension. Blood pressure was 110/80 mm Hg in the supine and 80/60 mm Hg in the sitting position. Pulse rate was rapid. Urine volume was 100 ml per hour and its osmolality 240 mosm/L. Serum Na concentration was 165 mEq/L; serum K 4.0 mEq/L; urine Na 3 mEq/L. Which important piece of data has been omitted from the information given?

  **a.** The patient is diabetic and has not taken his insulin.
  **b.** The patient has Addison's disease and has not taken his replacement hormones.
  **c.** The patient is receiving lithium salts for treatment of psychosis.
  **d.** The patient has had severe diarrhea for 4 days.
  **e.** The patient is diabetic and has been taking chlorpropamide.

**5.** A 21-year-old college student is referred to you with complaints of polyuria and polydipsia. Serum Na is 140 mEq/L (normal) and urine osmolality is 120 mosm/L. Urine output is 6.5 L per day. Water is withheld, and urine volume gradually diminishes as urine osmolality rises to 900 mosm/L. Despite continuing water restriction, the urine volume suddenly increases and its osmolality falls to 400 mosm/L. The next step should be:

  **a.** Inject ADH and observe urine osmolality.
  **b.** Begin a program of salt restriction and thiazide diuretics.
  **c.** Treat her with long-acting ADH injections.
  **d.** Explain to her and her family that she has a (neurotic) compulsion to drink water in large amounts and has cheated during the test.
  **e.** Repeat the test under conditions that permit her to be under observation for the entire duration of water deprivation.

## ANSWERS

**1.** a is true. The case is typical of CPM, a complication of rapid correction of hyponatremia. The lesions are seen most often in the central pons but may be seen in the other areas of the brain. A rapid increase in serum sodium following administration of normal saline is mostly due to renal excretion of water with retention of sodium. Simultaneous administration of KCl causes a more-rapid increase in serum Na. As K enters the cell (only a small fraction of K retained in the body remains in the ECF), Na is extruded into the ECF in exchange. When K is excreted in the urine, it will be accompanied by water. Either way, serum Na will rise.

**2.** c. If the hypernatremia were entirely due to water loss, the amount of water loss would be 42 × 40 L (estimated predehydration TBW)/182 = 9.2 L, but the physical examination indicates only modest volume depletion. Hypernatremia therefore must be due to water loss as well as Na retention. Substantial increase in serum Na after exogenous pitressin indicates central diabetes insipidus. The patient would not have allowed serum Na to rise to 182 mEq/L, if thirst was normal. In chronic hypernatremia, the brain cell volume is nearly normal by the volume regulatory mechanisms; rapid correction to normonatremia at this point may lead to brain edema.

3. d is true. High BUN without renal failure and evidence of volume depletion probably indicate increased production of urea, which is due to increased intake of protein. The normal GFR (113 ml per minute) argues against renal failure. In prerenal azotemia, GFR tends to be also reduced. The patient probably has osmotic diuresis, not water diuresis. Urine osmolality of 500 msom/L with 5 L of urine confirms osmotic diuresis. The total daily solute excretion in this case is 5 × 500, or 2500 mosm per day (the upper limit of normal is 1440 mosm per day).

4. c is correct. The patient does not have osmotic diuresis (total daily solute excretion is only 576 mosm per day (240 mosm/L × 2.4 L per day; 100 ml per hour = 2.4 L per day). Urine osmolality of 240 mosm/L in the presence of hypernatremia is grossly inadequate, and suggests diabetes insipidus. Lithium can cause nephrogenic diabetes insipidus. Chlorpropamide causes SIADH, not diabetes insipidus.

5. d is true and e is half true. The patient has primary polydipsia. Normal urine concentration upon water restriction supports the diagnosis. The sudden fall in urine osmolality is probably due to the patient's cheating during the test. Because the diagnosis is certain, a repeat test is unnecessary, but you might want to prove it to the family with another test.

## DISORDERS OF POTASSIUM METABOLISM

### DISTRIBUTION AND FUNCTION

Potassium is the most abundant intracellular cation, with an average concentration of about 150 mEq/L; the extracellular concentration ranges from 3.5 to 5 mEq/L. The average total exchangeable potassium for hospitalized adult males is 42.7 mEq/kg body weight, whereas the figure for women is about 10% less. The normal value of total exchangeable potassium is 8 to 15% less than that of total body potassium.

The two most important physiologic functions of potassium are its effect on transmembrane potential and its role as the major determinant of intracellular ionic strength. The transmembrane electrical potential of most cells is determined by the ratio of intracellular to extracellular potassium concentration; in muscle the transmembrane electrical potential is about 90 mv with the inside of the cell negative to the outside. The membrane potential ($E_m$) is calculated from the Nernst equation:

$$E_m = -60\ K_{in}/K_{ex},$$

where $K_{in}$ and $K_{ex}$ are intracellular and extracellular potassium concentrations, respectively. When the ratio is about 30 to 1, the $E_m$ is normal at $-90$ mv. Because the extracellular potassium concentration is altered more readily in most clinical situations, transmembrane electrical potential is influenced more by the $K_{ex}$ than by the $K_{in}$.

Potassium, being the major intracellular ion, is the main determinant of intracellular ionic strength. Cellular ionic strength greatly influences cellular metabolism as evidenced by the marked clinical abnormalities attributable to cell overhydration or dehydration. In addition, potassium has specific roles in various enzymatic reactions of the cell, such as in protein and glycogen synthesis.

### POTASSIUM BALANCE

The external balance of potassium is determined by intake, renal excretion, and, to a variable extent, extrarenal excretion. Fecal excretion, the most important form of extrarenal excretion, accounts for 5 to 10 mEq per day. Skin losses are normally negligible and need not be accounted for in the calculation of daily balance. Average daily intake of potassium is about 1 mEq/kg body weight, but it varies considerably with diet. The regulation of the $K_{ex}$ is determined mostly by renal excretion, but in the short term transcellular movement plays an important role.

#### *RENAL REGULATION OF POTASSIUM EXCRETION*

Ignoring a small amount of fecal excretion, one can state that urinary K excretion nearly equals K intake. Even with abnormal renal K loss or retention, once a new equilibrium is reached, renal excretion is very close to intake. Potassium is filtered at the glomerulus and most of the filtered potassium is reabsorbed in the proximal tubule and in the loop of Henle. The excreted potassium is derived mostly from tubular secretion by the distal tubule and collecting duct along the electrical potential gradient created by active reabsorption of sodium. The urinary potassium is usually much smaller than the amount secreted by these segments, because some potassium is reabsorbed in the outer medullary collecting duct. The major determinant of urinary potassium excretion is tubular secretion at the distal tubule and cortical collecting duct. At these sites potassium enters the tubular cell in exchange for sodium by the action of the Na-K ATPase, which is stimulated by sodium entry from the lumen and by high potassium concentration at the peritubular side. Entry of sodium from the lumen into the tubular cell is stimulated by aldosterone and inhibited by the diuretics amiloride and triamterene. The following factors increase renal potassium excretion:

1. Increased urine flow to the distal nephron.
2. Increased sodium delivery to the distal nephron.

3. Hormones, such as aldosterone, vasopressin, and $\beta_1$-adrenergic agonists.
4. Poorly reabsorbable anions, such as bicarbonate, sulfate, organic anions, and several antibiotics administered as the sodium salts.
5. High plasma potassium concentration.
6. Acute metabolic and respiratory alkalosis, chronic metabolic and respiratory acidosis, chronic metabolic alkalosis.

## TRANSCELLULAR MOVEMENT OF POTASSIUM

Because potassium concentration is so much greater in the cell than in the ECF, a slight movement of potassium into or out of the cell produces a big change in plasma potassium. When potassium is administered acutely, cellular uptake helps to prevent hyperkalemia, as does renal excretion. The following factors modulate the transcellular movement of potassium.

**1. Insulin.** Insulin causes of shift of potassium into the cell by several mechanisms: (1) by stimulating the Na-K ATPase, (2) by stimulating glycogen synthesis, which causes deposition of about 0.33 mEq of potassium per gram of glycogen, and (3) by increasing phosphorylated intermediary metabolites of glucose to balance potassium.

**2. Blood pH.** It has been considered axiomatic that acidemia shifts potassium out of the cell and alkalemia shifts it into the cell, but the relationship is much more complex. Respiratory acidosis increases serum potassium much less than does metabolic acidosis, and organic acidosis less than inorganic acidosis. The likely explanation is that both bicarbonate anion (in respiratory acidosis) and organic anions enter the cell with proton whereas inorganic anions do not; when an anion and proton enter the cell together, $H^+$-$K^+$ exchange would not be needed. Bicarbonate concentration affects serum potassium independently of pH; an increase in serum bicarbonate decreases serum potassium, and a decrease in serum bicarbonate increases it.

**3. Hyperosmolality.** An increase in body fluid osmolality, as with hypernatremia, hyperglycemia, or mannitol infusion, may cause hyperkalemia by extracellular shift of potassium.

**4. β-Adrenergic Receptors.** Stimulation of the $\beta_2$-adrenergic receptor causes intracellular shift of potassium, and inhibition of the receptor causes the reverse.

## HYPERKALEMIA

Causes and pathogenesis are listed in Table 6–4.

**TABLE 6–4.** CAUSES OF HYPERKALEMIA

- **I.** Pseudohyperkalemia
  - **a.** Thrombocytosis
  - **b.** Marked leucocytosis?
  - **c.** Tourniquet with fist exercise
  - **d.** In-vitro hemolysis
- **II.** Hyperkalemia due to shift from the cells
  - **a.** Acute acidosis
  - **b.** Intravascular hemolysis or rhabdomyolysis
  - **c.** Succinycholine
  - **d.** Cationic amino acids
  - **e.** Hyperosmolality
  - **f.** Familial periodic paralysis
  - **g.** Exercise
- **III.** Hyperkalemia due to impaired renal excretion
  - **a.** Aldosterone deficiency (see **Table 6–5**)
  - **b.** Tubular unresponsiveness to aldosterone
    - **1.** Generalized unresponsiveness to aldosterone: congenital (pseudohypoaldosteronism) and acquired (salt-losing nephropathy, K-sparing diuretics)
    - **2.** Selective potassium secretory defect congenital (type II pseudohypoaldosteronism; Gordon's syndrome?) and acquired (sickle cell disease, systemic lupus, renal transplantation, obstructive uropathy, some case of hyporeninemic hypoaldosteronism)
  - **c.** Advanced renal failure
  - **d.** Severe reduction in distal sodium delivery

*PSEUDOHYPERKALEMIA*

Pseudohyperkalemia refers to hyperkalemia present only in the local blood vessel or in vitro. Thrombocytosis is the most common cause of pseudohyperkalemia. Because hyperkalemia is caused by release of potassium from platelets during blood clotting, the effect is seen in serum but not in plasma, with the increment in serum potassium over the plasma value being about 0.7 mEq/L per million platelets per cubic millimeter. The use of a tourniquet with vigorous fist exercise increases serum and plasma potassium in the local blood vessel by as much as 1 mEq/L as potassium is released by the exercising muscle cells. Hyperkalemia due to in-vitro hemolysis will be accompanied by the reddish tint of serum or plasma. Pseudohyperkalemia due to severe leucocytosis has been reported but the documentation is not very solid.

*HYPERKALEMIA DUE TO SHIFT OF POTASSIUM FROM THE CELL*

**1. Acute Acidosis.** Acute metabolic acidosis of the hyperchloremic type or uremic acidosis can produce hyperkalemia. Organic acidosis also causes hyperkalemia, but less often.

**2. Intravascular Hemolysis or Rhabdomyolysis.** A liter of whole blood contains less than 40 mEq of potassium, and hence even massive hemolysis would not produce hyperkalemia in the absence of concomitant renal impairment. The same is true of rhabdomyolysis.

**3. Administration of Cationic Amino Acids.** Uptake by the cell of cationic amino acids such as arginine, lysine, and ϵ-aminocaproic acid in exchange for potassium can cause hyperkalemia.

**4. Succinylcholine.** The use of this drug in patients with paralyzed muscle is known to cause hyperkalemia, probably because of depolarization of the muscle by the drug.

**5. Familial Periodic Paralysis (Gamstorp's disease; Adynamia Episodica Hereditaria).** This familial disorder with autosomal dominant inheritance is characterized by periodic muscular paralysis associated with hyperkalemia due to shift of potassium out of the muscle cells.

**6. Exercise.** Exercise regularly increases serum potassium, and the effect is magnified during therapy with nonselective β-adrenergic blockers.

*HYPERKALEMIA DUE TO IMPAIRED RENAL EXCRETION*

**1. Aldosterone Deficiency (see Table 6–5).** Aldosterone deficiency may be generalized, as in Addison's disease or by a deficiency of the enzyme 21-hydroxylase, or it may be selective. In the latter situation, glucocorticoid function is normal, and the deficiency can be due to a congenital enzyme defect, to a drug-induced defect of zona glomerulosa function (e.g., heparin), or to lack of renin, which is known as *hyporeninemic hypoaldosteronism,* the most common cause of chronic hyperkalemia. The commonest cause of hyporeninemic hypoaldosteronism is diabetic nephropathy; the other causes include chronic pyelonephritis, gouty nephropathy, obstructive uropathy, hypertensive renal disease, and sickle cell nephropathy.

**2. Tubular Unresponsiveness, Generalized or Selective.**

*Generalized Unresponsiveness to Aldosterone (Type I Pseudohypoaldosteronism).* The defect may be either congenital or acquired. The *congenital* defect becomes manifest during infancy, and is characterized by volume

**TABLE 6–5.** CAUSES OF ALDOSTERONE DEFICIENCY

**I.** Generalized adrenocortical insufficiency
- **a.** Addison's disease
- **b.** 21-Hydroxylase deficiency
- **c.** Hypopituitarism
- **d.** Bilateral adrenalectomy

**II.** Selective aldosterone deficiency
- **a.** Primary defect of the adrenal gland
  - **1.** Corticosterone methyloxidase type I deficiency
  - **2.** Corticosterone methyloxidase type II deficiency
  - **3.** Chronic use of heparin
  - **4.** Idiopathic zona glomerulosa defect
- **b.** Defect in mechanisms that control aldosterone secretion
  - **1.** drugs that affect production of renin and angiotesin II converting enzyme inhibitors, prostaglandin synthesis inhibitors, β-adrenergic blockers
  - **2.** Hyporeninemic hypoaldosteronism

depletion and hyperkalemia with markedly increased levels of plasma renin activity (PRA) and plasma aldosterone. A deficiency of Na-K ATPase has been suggested as the mechanism. *Acquired* resistance to aldosterone is observed in patients with various chronic renal diseases, usually with prominent interstitial involvement. A careful analysis of the literature has revealed that most cases of the so-called salt-losing nephritis are actually caused by tubular resistance to aldosterone. Potassium-sparing diuretics can mimic pseudohypoaldosteronism.

*Selective Defect in K Secretion with Normal Ability to Reabsorb Na (Type II Pseudohypoaldosteronism).* This defect is characterized by tubular resistance to aldosterone without salt wasting. Increased tubular permeability to chloride has been suggested as a mechanism. This would result in increased reabsorption of salt, which would in turn suppress renin and aldosterone secretion, with abolition of the lumen-negative electrical potential.

**3. Severe Renal Dysfunction.** The capacity of the kidney to adapt to increased potassium load is so great that hyperkalemia rarely develops even in moderately severe renal insufficiency. In general, patients with chronic renal failure require maintenance dialysis before hyperkalemia occurs.

**4. Severe Reduction in Distal Sodium Delivery.** Marked reduction in effective arterial volume can impair potassium secretion by reducing delivery of sodium to the distal nephron, and hyperkalemia may develop despite compensatory increase in aldosterone secretion.

### *CLINICAL MANIFESTATIONS*

Clinical manifestations are mainly due to a high $K_{ex}$. Because the increase in potassium in the ECF is proportionately greater than that of the ICF, the membrane potential tends to be reduced. Whether the membrane potential remains reduced in chronic hyperkalemia is uncertain, but the symptoms of hyperkalemia are always more severe with acute hyperkalemia than with chronic hyperkalemia. Hyponatremia and hypocalcemia potentiate the adverse effects of hyperkalemia. Hyperkalemia causes abnormality in rhythm and rate of conduction of cardiac impulse transmission through several mechanisms, associated with various arrhythmias, tall-peaked T waves, low amplitude of the P wave, and widening of the QRS and T wave. As hyperkalemia worsens, the P wave disappears completely and the QRS merges with the T wave, simulating a sine wave. Rapidly ascending neuromuscular weakness or paralysis and cardiac standstill may occur in very severe hyperkalemia.

### *DIAGNOSIS*

1. Repeat the measurement to rule out laboratory error.
2. Measure platelet and white blood cell (WBC) counts; look for red tint in the supernatant. If drawing blood is difficult, repeat the potassium measurement on blood drawn without a tourniquet.
3. Hyperkalemia due to acute acidosis or terminal renal failure will be apparent clinically.
4. Impaired renal excretion as the cause of hyperkalemia is confirmed by demonstrating normal or reduced renal K excretion in the presence of hyperkalemia.
5. The virtual absence of sodium in the urine (less than 5 mEq/L) with other evidence of severe reduction in effective arterial volume suggests reduced distal delivery of sodium as the cause of hyperkalemia.
6. Rule out use of drugs that can precipitate hyperkalemia.

### *TREATMENT*

The measures to be taken for the management of hyperkalemia depend on the urgency of the situation dictated by the level of serum potassium and the electrocardiogram (ECG) findings. *Serum potassium concentration in excess of 7 mEq/L requires immediate treatment,* even if the ECG findings are normal, in order to prevent serious arrhythmias that may suddenly appear. Treatment measures and their rationales follow.

**1. Antagonizing the Action of Potassium on Cell Membrane with Na or Ca Ions.** Hyperkalemia causes a reduction in the resting membrane potential without affecting the threshold potential; this results in slowing of diastolic depolarization. Calcium reduces the threshold potential without affecting the resting membrane potential, and thereby normalizes the speed of diastolic depolarization. The effect of calcium infusion is transient, lasting about 30 minutes. Hyperkalemia reduces the number of sodium channels in the membrane of conducting tissues and consequently reduces conduction velocity. Increase in sodium concentration may reverse this effect of hyperkalemia. Hypertonic sodium may be administered either as the chloride or bicarbonate salt, but the latter is preferred because it will also increase pH and cause intracellular shift of potassium. Calcium salts and sodium bicarbonate should not be mixed; calcium carbonate precipitate will form.

**2. Shift of Potassium into the Cell.** This can be accomplished by the intravenous infusion of glucose and insulin. The usual dose is 25 to 50 g of glucose (50 to 100 ml of 50% solution) with 10 to 20 U of regular insulin over 30 minutes. Sodium bicarbonate, 1 to 2 ampules, can also be given as an intravenous bolus injection to cause intracellular shift of potassium in acidotic patients. Administration of $\beta_2$-agonists has also been used to treat hyperkalemia.

**3. Reduction in Body Potassium Content.** This method may be used when hyperkalemia is less urgent. Potassium content may be reduced by decreased intake, increased renal and fecal excretion, or dialysis. Fecal excretion may be increased by an exchange resin, sodium polystyrene sulfonate (Kayexalate), given with mannitol or sorbitol to prevent constipation. Renal excretion of potassium can be increased by several means. In aldosterone deficiency, the patient may be treated with a liberal salt intake or Florinef (9-α-fluorohydrocortisone) in doses of 0.1 to 0.2 mg per day. In hyporeninemic hypoaldosteronism, Florinef lowers serum potassium but may worsen hypertension, which is common in the syndrome. Ideally, hyporeninemic hypoaldosteronism is treated with administration of loop diuretics or thiazides with liberal salt intake. If acidosis complicates the syndrome, $NaHCO_3$ or sodium citrate (Shohl's solution) may be given. In type II pseudohypoaldosteronism, potassium excretion has been shown to be normalized by nasal insufflation of desmopressin (dDAVP).

**4. Hemodialysis.** This can remove potassium at a rate of about 40 mEq per hour, but the rate is only about 5 mEq per hour with peritoneal dialysis.

## HYPOKALEMIA

The causes and pathogenesis of hypokalemia are listed in Table 6–6.

### *HYPOKALEMIA DUE TO INTRACELLULAR SHIFT*

A sudden shift of potassium into the cell causing hypokalemia is most often due to increased blood pH or to administration of glucose and insulin; occasionally it is due to $\beta_2$ agonists. Intracellular shift of potassium leading to hypokalemia may be caused by increased catecholamine during acute stress such as acute myocardial infarction, delirium tremens, or exogenously administered epinephrine or ritodrine. Barium poisoning causes hypokalemia by inhibiting potassium diffusion out of the cell in the presence of continuous cellular uptake. Hypokalemia observed with hypothermia might have the same mechanism. The mechanism of intracellular potassium shift in familial hypokalemic paralysis is unknown. Intracellular shift may be responsible for hypokalemia observed in patients treated for megaloblastic anemia and in patients with myelogenous leukemia. In the latter, renal potassium wasting due to lysozymuria has also been suggested.

### *HYPOKALEMIA DUE TO POOR INTAKE*

The renal adaptation has evolved towards excellent conservation of sodium but inefficient potassium conservation. Consequently when intake is reduced or curtailed, hypokalemia and potassium depletion can occur. Potassium deficit of about 250 mEq has been attained with potassium intake of 15 to 30 mEq per day for 7 days.

### *HYPOKALEMIA DUE TO GASTROINTESTINAL LOSS*

Vomiting is frequently associated with hypokalemia, but little potassium is contained in the vomitus. The more important mechanism is renal loss due to the secondary metabolic alkalosis. Diarrheal loss of potassium is usually less than 100 mEq per day because potassium concentration in the diarrheal fluid is in-

**TABLE 6–6.** CAUSES OF HYPOKALEMIA

**I.** Intracellular shift
- **a.** Acute increase in blood pH (especially by increase in bicarbonate)
- **b.** Administration of glucose and insulin
- **c.** Familial periodic paralysis
- **d.** Barium poisoning
- **e.** Increase in catecholamine (e.g., acute myocardial infarction, treatment of asthma, $\beta_2$ agonists)
- **f.** Anabolic states or rapid cell growth: treatment of megaloblastic anemia, myelogeneous leukemia, nutritional recovery

**II.** Poor intake or GI loss
- **a.** Diarrhea
- **b.** Poor intake of potassium with high carbohydrate ingestion

**III.** Excessive renal loss
- **a.** Hypermineralocorticoidism (see **Table 6–7**)
- **b.** Increased distal delivery of sodium: diuretics, Bartter's syndrome, metabolic acidosis, metabolic alkalosis
- **c.** Delivery of poorly reabsorbable anions: bicarbonate diuresis, excretion of ketone anions, penicillin, carbenicillin, ampicillin, ticarcillin, nafcillin
- **d.** Unknown mechanisms: magnesium deficiency, potassium-losing nephritis, pseudoaldosteronism (Liddle's syndrome), acute myelogenous leukemia, amphotericin B, para-aminosalicylic acid, rifampin, thallium poisoning, lithium intoxication

**IV.** Skin loss

versely related to the diarrheal volume. When the diarrhea is caused by villous adenoma or by pancreatic cholera (tumor secreting vasoactive intestinal polypeptide, or VIP), considerably greater amounts of potassium can be lost. Abuse of laxatives or enemas is a fairly common cause of hypokalemia.

### *HYPOKALEMIA DUE TO RENAL LOSS*

**1. Hyperaldosteronism and Other States of Mineralocorticoid Excess (Table 6–7).** Increased secretion of mineralocorticoid hormone causes potassium loss only when it is accompanied by adequate distal delivery of sodium, as in primary hyperaldosteronism and hypertensive forms of secondary hyperaldosteronism.

**2. Increased Distal Delivery of Sodium.** Increased distal sodium delivery causes hypokalemia only when plasma aldosterone is normal or increased, as with Bartter's syndrome, diuretic therapy, chronic metabolic acidosis such as renal tubular acidosis.

**3. Delivery of Poorly Reabsorbable Anions to the Distal Nephron.** Poorly reabsorbable anions lead to increased negative charge of the tubular lumen when urine chloride concentration is low, and hence to an increase in potassium secretion. For example, a number of β-lactam antibiotics are sodium salts of poorly reabsorbable anions, and are excreted almost exclusively through the kidney. Excretion of bicarbonate may lead to hypokalemia in respiratory acidosis and metabolic alkalosis, and during therapy with acetazolamide. Excretion of ketone anions contributes to increased renal excretion of potassium in ketoacidosis.

**TABLE 6–7.** CAUSES OF HYPOKALEMIA DUE TO HYPERMINERALOCORTICOIDISM

- **I.** Primary hyperaldosteronism: adenoma or bilateral hyperplasia
- **II.** Secondary hyperaldosteronism with adequate distal sodium delivery
  - **a.** Malignant hypertension
  - **b.** Diuretic therapy
  - **c.** Renal artery stenosis
  - **d.** Reninoma
  - **e.** Bartter's syndrome
  - **f.** Magnesium deficiency
  - **g.** l-DOPA
- **III.** Non-aldosterone hypermineralocorticoidism
  - **a.** 11 β-Hydroxyulase deficiency
  - **b.** 17 α-Hydroxylase deficiency
  - **c.** Cushing's disease
  - **d.** Adrenal cancer or adenoma
  - **e.** Ectopic ACTH-secreting (adrenocorticotropic hormone–secreting) tumor
- **IV.** Mineralocorticoid-like substances: licorice, carbenoxolone

**4. Renal Potassium Wasting of Unknown Cause.** These conditions include magnesium deficiency, Bartter's syndrome, acute myelocytic or acute monocytic leukemia, potassium-losing nephritis, and pseudoaldosteronism (Liddle's syndrome).

**5. Hypokalemia Due to Skin Loss.** Severe potassium depletion has been observed in subjects undergoing intense physical conditioning in a hot climate. Loss of potassium has been attributed to excessive sweating.

### *CLINICAL MANIFESTATIONS*

When hypokalemia and cell potassium depletion occur together, it may be difficult to determine whether both factors contribute to a given manifestation. In hypokalemia without cell potassium depletion, clinical manifestations are limited to neuromuscular and cardiovascular symptoms and signs. When cell potassium depletion is also present, abnormalities in cellular metabolism and structure of various tissues are observed as well.

### *DIAGNOSIS*

1. Repeat the measurement to rule out laboratory error.
2. Hypokalemia due to intracellular shift is transient. History, such as periodic paralysis, and clinical findings, such as acute alkalosis and treatment with β-agonists, will suggest the appropriate cause.
3. Once chronic hypokalemia is documented, measure the 24-hour urine potassium excretion. A value less than 20 mEq per day suggests (1) decreased intake, (2) GI loss, or (3) prior renal potassium loss due to previous diuretic therapy.
4. Urinary potassium greater than 40 mEq per day with serum potassium less than 3 mEq/L suggests renal potassium wasting. Diuretic therapy and hypomagnesemia as the cause of hypokalemia should be ruled out by history and by measuring serum magnesium concentration, respectively. Chronic metabolic acidosis and alkalosis should also be ruled out by blood gas measurements.

### *TREATMENT*

In some instances, the cause of hypokalemia may be directly dealt with, as with removal of a Conn's adenoma or magnesium replacement. In other instances, a potassium supplement is given or measures are taken to reduce urinary potassium excretion.

**1. Administration of Potassium.** If hypokalemia is severe or associated with cardiac arrhythmia, immediate potassium replacement is needed. The route and rate of administration will depend on the severity of hypokalemia and the nature of complications. Because the $K_{ex}$ is a small fraction of the whole body content, hypokalemia due to potassium loss is always accompanied by cellular potassium depletion. Although the serum potassium concentration is an imprecise measure of total body stores, one can use the following rough guide: reduction in serum potassium by 1 mEq/L represents a whole body potassium deficit of about 100 to 200 mEq, and reduction by 2 mEq/L represents the deficit of about 300 to 600 mEq.

A safe rate of intravenous administration of potassium is about 10 mEq per hour. In order to avoid irritation of the vein, the concentration of potassium in the infusate should be kept below 40 mEq/L, but in severe hypokalemia, a higher concentration may be used.

**2. Potassium-Sparing Diuretics.** There are two types of potassium-sparing diuretics. One is spironolactone, a competitive inhibitor of mineralocorticoid hormone, which is effective only when mineralocorticoid activity is present. The other type is effective even without mineralocorticoid excess, and includes amiloride and triamterene.

**3. Low-Salt Diet.** When plasma aldosterone concentration is increased at a fixed level, a high-salt diet increases potassium excretion, and a low-salt diet reduces urinary potassium excretion.

## CLINICAL PROBLEMS

1. A 64-year-old man is admitted to the hospital with severe pneumonia, fever, and bacteremia. The WBC is 28,500. As part of his general evaluation a blood sample is sent for serum electrolyte concentrations. Serum potassium is reported at 6.2 mEq/L. A rapid evaluation of the ECG shows no abnormalities. The patient is not acidotic and renal function is normal. All of the following statements are true except:

   a. The patient should be treated immediately with hemodialysis.
   b. Repeat measurement of potassium concentration in serum and plasma would be useful.
   c. A platelet count might be useful.
   d. This patient may not require treatment for hyperkalemia.
   e. When you draw the blood for repeat measurement you will pay close attention to the technique of obtaining the sample.

2. A 60-year-old woman who has had diabetes mellitus since age 48 is admitted to the hospital because of shortness of breath. Blood pressure is 160/107. She has slight edema. Serum Na is 140, Cl 114, bicarbonate 15, and K 6.5 mEq/L. Blood glucose concentration is 170 mg/dl. She is treated with diuretics and with kayexalate and sorbitol. Serum K the next day is 4.0 mEq/L. Which of the following statements is true?

   a. The odds favor a low plasma cortisol level in this patient.
   b. If plasma cortisol is normal, plasma aldosterone must also be normal.
   c. The patient is likely to have a normal plasma cortisol and low plasma renin activity.
   d. The elevated serum chloride suggests familial renal tubular acidosis.

3. An elderly man is admitted to the emergency room unconscious and breathing rapidly and deeply. He is extremely dehydrated. Catheterization of the bladder reveals no urine. Blood gas determination reveals arterial blood pH to be 7.1; $HCO_3$ is 3 mEq/L; $P_{CO_2}$ is 10 mm Hg. ECG reveals absent P waves, wide QRS, and elevated and peaked T waves. BUN is 280 mg/dl, and glucose is 90 mg/dl. Which of the following would *not* be part of an appropriate therapeutic approach?

   a. Instillation of 50 g of Na polystyrene sulfonate (Kayexalate) into the rectum.
   b. Intravenous administration of 50 g of glucose and 10 U of insulin.
   c. Intravenous administration of calcium chloride.
   d. Intravenous administration of $NaHCO_3^-$.
   e. Simultaneous administration of c and d in one syringe because the patient's condition is critical.

4. A well-known actress in musical comedy complains of severe weakness and is afraid of falling off the stage during dance routines. The only remarkable physical findings are a transient drop in blood pressure upon standing up, sluggish tendon reflexes, and muscle weakness. An ECG shows S-T depression and sagging T waves. An additional complaint is moderate polyuria. Urinary K excretion is 9 mEq in 24 hours. Blood pH is normal. Which of the following statements is true?

   a. The patient ultimately admitted to abuse of laxatives.
   b. The patient has been secretly taking diuretics (and still is).
   c. With fluid restriction, urine osmolality will exceed 1000 mosm/L.
   d. The patient ultimately acknowledged overingestion of licorice.
   e. Treatment calls for intravenous $Ca^{++}$ infusion.

5. A 61-year-old black woman has a blood pressure of 160/104 and serum K of 2.1 mEq/L despite K supplements of 120 mEq per day. Serum Na and Cl are normal, and blood pH is slightly alkaline. She is not diabetic and takes no medication. She is a good historian and seems not to have diarrhea or to have been vomiting. She never eats candy. Twenty-four hour K excretion in the urine is 150 mEq. Plasma renin and plasma aldosterone are both markedly reduced, and plasma cortisol is normal. In response to spironolactone, an inhibitor of mineralocorticoids, there was no change in K excretion. However, in

response to triamterene, blood pressure, serum potassium, plasma renin, and plasma aldosterone all returned to normal. What is your diagnosis?

**6.** A 19-year-old woman is admitted with a diagnosis of severe diabetic ketoacidosis. The blood pH is 7.1, blood glucose is 800 mg/dl, serum Na is 128 mEq/L, serum K is 6.1 mEq/L, BUN is 60 mg/dl (it was 12 mg/dl before this episode), $HCO_3$ is 9 mEq/L, and the anion gap is 27 mEq/L. Treatment with insulin and intravenous NaCl solutions leads to changes in the blood chemistries: blood glucose becomes 200 mg/dl, Na 138 mEq/L, blood pH 7.28, and serum K 2.5 mEq/L. Which of the following statements is true?

**a.** The hyperkalemia on admission means that the patient had an increase in total body potassium.
**b.** Cell potassium may be low while $K_{ex}$ is high.
**c.** Because catecholamines cause K to shift out of cells, the patient's hyperkalemia may be due to the sympathetic stimulation.
**d.** The patient should have received potassium intravenously upon admission in order to avoid hypokalemia.
**e.** If the patient were K-depleted on admission, the ECG would show evidence of K depletion even in the presence of an elevated serum K.

### ANSWERS

**1.** Only a is false. The patient is likely to have pseudohyperkalemia. Because thrombocytosis is the most common cause of pseudohyperkalemia, platelet counts should be measured.

**2.** Only c is true. Blood pressure of 160/107 mm Hg argues against Addison's disease. In hyporeninemic hypoaldosteronism, plasma cortisol is normal, whereas aldosterone is low. In view of the clinical findings this patient is most likely to have type IV renal tubular acidosis (see later section on metabolic acidosis).

**3.** All are true except e; mixing of Ca and $HCO_3$ causes formation and precipitation of $CaCO_3$.

**4.** Only a is true. Low urine K suggests nonrenal loss of K. K depletion causes nephrogenic diabetes insipidus, and therefore urine concentration is impaired. Licorice causes hypokalemia through renal K wasting, and this patient has appropriate renal conservation of potassium. Finally, calcium is used for treatment of hyperkalemia.

**5.** The patient has Liddle's syndrome.

**6.** b is true. Because the high serum potassium is due to transcellular shift, the cell potassium would not be high. Catecholamines cause K to shift into cells, not out of cells. Serum potassium usually drops promptly with treatment of ketosis, but treatment at the beginning is not needed. Because hyperkalemic ECG findings are due to reduced ratio of $K_{in}$ to $K_{ex}$, ECG would not show findings of potassium depletion at the beginning.

## ACID-BASE DISORDERS

### BICARBONATE AND $CO_2$ BUFFERING SYSTEM

pH is customarily expressed as a function of the ratio of $HCO_3$ to $CO_2$, the two major buffers of the body, but all body buffers are in equilibrium with pH. Their relationship to pH is expressed in the equation:

$$pH = pK + \log Buff/HBuff,$$

where Buff/HBuff represents the ratio of a buffer pair. The Henderson-Hasselbalch equation depicts the relationship between pH and the bicarbonate-$CO_2$ buffer pair:

$$pH = 6.1 + \log HCO_3/Pco_2 \times 0.03,$$

where 6.1 is the negative logarithm of the ionization constant (pK) of the $HCO_3$ and $CO_2$ buffer system, and 0.03 is the solubility coefficient of $CO_2$.

The equation is simplified by combining two constants, pK and solubility coefficient of $CO_2$:

$$pH = 6.1 + \log HCO_3/Pco_2 \times 0.03 = 6.1 + \log 1/0.03 + \log HCO_3/Pco_2 = 7.62 + \log HCO_3/Pco_2 = 7.62 - \log Pco_2/HCO_3 = 7.62 + \log HCO_3 - \log Pco_2.$$

When $H^+$ is expressed in nM instead of a negative log value, it can be related to $Pco_2$ and $HCO_3$ in a simple equation:

$$H\ (nM) = 24 \times Pco_2\ (mm\ Hg)/HCO_3\ (mM).$$

According to the Henderson-Hasselbalch equation, pH increases when the $HCO_3/Pco_2$ ratio increases *(alkalosis)*, and pH decreases when the ratio decreases *(acidosis)*. The ratio may be increased by an increase in $HCO_3$ *(metabolic alkalosis)* or by a decrease in $Pco_2$ *(respiratory alkalosis)*. The ratio may be decreased by a decrease in $HCO_3$ *(metabolic acidosis)* or by an increase in $Pco_2$ *(respiratory acidosis)*.

### ACID-BASE BALANCE

On a usual American diet, the daily production of nonvolatile acid is about 90 mEq per day. The main acids are sulfuric acid (about 40 mEq per day), which originates from metabolism of sulfur-containing amino acids, and organic acids (about 50 mEq per day). The total production of organic acid is several thousand milliequivalents per day, but most of these are metabolized to $CO_2$ and water, resulting in regeneration of alkali.

Some of the organic acids cannot be metabolized (e.g., uric acid) or escape metabolism (e.g., citric acid), and their anions are excreted in the urine. Excretion of organic anions represents permanent alkali loss, which amounts to about 50 mEq per day. On a usual diet, a substantial amount of alkali is also absorbed from the GI tract (about 30 mEq per day). Thus, net acid production = (sulfuric acid + organic acid) − alkali absorbed from GI tract. The net alkali absorption from the GI tract can be measured by the convenient new technique utilizing urinary electrolytes. The average net acid production is about 60 mEq per day.

A major function of the kidney in acid-base homeostasis is excretion of acid. Acid is excreted in the form of $NH_4$ and titratable acid (which is measured by titration of urine to the blood pH). The amount of $HCO_3$ generation equals the sum of $NH_4$ and titratable acid. Another important function of the kidney is excretion of $HCO_3$. Renal excretion of $HCO_3$ occurs usually as a compensation for alkalosis, but a small amount of $HCO_3$ excretion occurs normally (about 10 mEq per day). Thus, net renal production of $HCO_3$ can be determined by subtracting $HCO_3$ excretion from acid excretion, and this is called *net acid excretion*. In a condition of acid-base equilibrium, net bicarbonate consumption (measured as net acid production) must equal net renal bicarbonate generation (measured as net acid excretion).

Normally about two-thirds of acid excretion occurs in the form of $NH_4$, and in severe acidosis the excretion rate of ammonia in urine may increase by as much as 10 times. Excretion of titratable acid is limited by the amount of buffer (e.g., phosphate, creatinine, and urate), but the amount may be increased markedly in certain situations, such as β-hydroxybutyrate in diabetic ketoacidosis.

## METABOLIC ACIDOSIS

### *CLASSIFICATION ACCORDING TO NET ACID EXCRETION*

All metabolic acidosis results from reduction in bicarbonate content of the body with two minor and clinically unimportant exceptions: acidosis resulting from dilution of the body fluid by administration of a large amount of saline solution *(dilution acidosis)* and acidosis that results from shift of $H^+$ from the cell. Maintenance of acid-base balance requires that net acid production equal *net acid excretion*. Reduction in bicarbonate occurs when net acid production exceeds net acid excretion. The discrepancy may be due to a primary increase in acid production *(extrarenal acidosis)* or due to a primary reduction in net acid excretion *(renal acidosis)*. In pure extrarenal acidosis, net acid excretion (mostly in the form of $NH_4$) is markedly increased as the kidney compensates for acidosis. On the other hand, in a patient with renal acidosis, net acid excretion may return to normal as acidosis stimulates renal $H^+$ secretion and ammonia production. It is important to note that *the finding of normal net acid excretion in the presence of metabolic acidosis indicates a defect in renal acid excretion and therefore the presence of renal acidosis.*

Renal acidosis is further classified into two types: uremic acidosis and renal tubular acidosis. In *uremic acidosis,* reduced net acid excretion results from reduction in nephron mass (i.e., renal failure), whereas in *renal tubular acidosis (RTA)* reduction in net acid excretion results from a specific tubular dysfunction. Because development of renal acidosis depends on the ability of the kidney to excrete acid as well as the rate of net endogenous acid production, which varies according to diet, the level of renal failure at which uremic acidosis develops is not fixed. On a usual diet, uremic acidosis usually occurs when GFR is less than 20% of normal.

**Renal Tubular Acidosis.** There are three types of RTA. *Type I RTA,* also called classic RTA or distal RTA, is characterized by the inability to reduce urine pH below 5.5. The term distal RTA is actually a misnomer, because acidification of urine to a very low pH occurs at the collecting duct. Furthermore, $H^+$ secretion in the collecting duct is also often impaired in type IV RTA. For these reasons, some authors consider both type I and type IV RTA forms of distal RTA. Still, the terms type I RTA and distal RTA are used synonymously by most authors. In type I RTA, net acid excretion usually remains persistently less than daily acid production, and without alkali therapy, the patients develop progressive severe metabolic acidosis. Type I RTA can develop as a primary disorder or secondary to drug toxicity, tubulointerstitial renal diseases, or other renal diseases.

*Type II RTA,* also called proximal RTA, involves defective renal bicarbonate reabsorption characterized by reduced renal bicarbonate threshold; bicarbonate reabsorption in the proximal tubule is impaired, and severe bicarbonaturia occurs when serum bicarbonate is normal. However, urine can be made free of bicarbonate and acidified normally when serum bicarbonate decreases to a lower level. Most patients with proximal RTA have evidence of generalized proximal tubular dysfunction, which is known as Fanconi's syndrome, and which is manifested by, in addition to reduced renal bicarbonate threshold, aminoaciduria, glucosuria, phosphaturia, and uricosuria. Of these, glucosuria in the presence of normal blood glucose is most useful in diagnosing Fanconi's syndrome. Type II RTA may be a primary disorder or secondary to various genetic or acquired renal dysfunctions. Hypokalemia is a characteristic finding of both type I and type II RTA. A hybrid of type I and II RTA is called *type III RTA.*

*Type IV RTA* is caused by aldosterone deficiency or by tubular unresponsiveness to aldosterone, which leads to impaired potassium secretion in the collecting duct. Although reduction in $H^+$ secretion in the collecting duct plays some role, the major cause of acidosis in type IV RTA is hyperkalemia-induced impairment in ammonia production in the proximal tubule. Type IV RTA is far more common than either type I or type II RTA, and the most common cause of type IV RTA is hyporeninemic hypoaldosteronism (see earlier section on K metabolism).

**Organic Acidosis.** Extrarenal acidosis may result from administration or ingestion of acid, overproduction of endogenous acid, or loss of bicarbonate. Of these, overproduction of endogenous acid is clinically most important, and the two most frequent sources of extrarenal metabolic acidosis are lactic acid and keto acids. Because these acids are normal metabolites of the human body, and the body has a tremendous capacity to metabolize them, only a marked increase in production leads to acidosis. Organic acids are titrated by bicarbonate to form organic anions and $CO_2$. The organic anions may be retained in the body, resulting in increased anion gap, or excreted in the urine. Retention per se of these anions is not responsible for acidosis. These anions are not acid, but their presence provides a clue to the mechanism of a reduced bicarbonate concentration. Removal from the body fluid of such anions by dialysis or by renal excretion would not improve the acidosis. If an organic acid is titrated by bicarbonate, and the resulting organic anion is entirely retained without any urinary loss, alkali would be regained completely by its subsequent metabolism. When some anions are lost in the urine, metabolism of any remaining anions will not restore the alkali content to normal, and acidosis will persist. This is the pathogenetic mechanism of hyperchloremic acidosis during the recovery phase of diabetic ketoacidosis.

*Lactic Acidosis.* Lactic acid is produced from pyruvic acid by the action of the enzyme lactate dehydrogenase (LDH) and a cofactor, NADH (the reduced form of NAD, or nicotinamide-adenine dinucleotide). Metabolism of lactic acid requires its conversion back to pyruvic acid, using the same enzyme and NAD as a cofactor. For this reason, both production and metabolism of lactic acid are influenced by the same factors; increased concentration of pyruvic acid and increased ratio of NADH/NAD increase lactic acid production and at the same time reduce its metabolism. Consequently, most cases of lactic acidosis are caused by increased production as well as reduced metabolism. By far the most common cause of lactic acidosis is tissue hypoxia, which can result from such factors as circulatory shock, severe anemia, severe heart failure, acute pulmonary edema, cardiac arrest, carbon monoxide poisoning, seizures, and vigorous muscular exercise. Normally lactic acid is produced by the extrahepatic tissues and metabolized by the liver, although every organ in the body can produce lactic acid and can utilize it. Acute alcoholism and severe liver disease can cause lactic acidosis by impaired lactic acid utilization in the absence of overproduction.

Lactic acidosis, unless specified otherwise, refers to L-lactic acidosis, because L-lactic acid is the isomer normally produced in the human body. The enzyme LDH, responsible for production of lactic acid in the human body, is an L-isomer. However, several cases of D-lactic acidosis have been reported recently, and the mechanism of acidosis in every case has been the colonic production of D-lactic acid by bacteria. A requirement for overproduction of D-lactic acid is malabsorption syndrome, which allows delivery of nutrients to the colon, where a large number of bacteria normally reside. A second requirement is the colonization in the colon by bacteria producing D-LDH. Treatment of D-lactic acidosis is oral administration of antibiotics.

*Ketoacidosis.* Clinically important keto acids are acetoacetic acid and betahydroxy butyric acid. They are produced in the liver from free fatty acid (FFA), and are metabolized by the extrahepatic tissues. Increased production of keto acid is the main mechanism of ketoacidosis, and requires a high concentration of FFA and its increased conversion to keto acid in the liver. Insulin deficiency is primarily responsible for increased mobilization of FFA from the adipose tissue, and glucagon excess and insulin deficiency cause increased conversion of FFA to keto acids in the liver.

β-hydroxybutyric acid (BB) is produced from acetoacetic acid (AA) by the action of the enzyme β-hydroxybutyrate dehydrogenase, which requires the cofactor NADH. The same enzyme and NAD are required to convert BB to AA. Consequently, the activity of the enzyme does not affect the rate of production of BB or AA. Instead, the ratio of NADH to NAD is the sole determinant of relative production of both acids, and hence the ratio of BB/AA. The clinical diagnosis of ketoacidosis is usually based on the response of the serum to Acetest, which reacts to AA but not to BB. Although BB is the predominant acid in typical ketoacidosis (the usual ratio of BB/AA is about 2.5 to 3), the responses to Acetest can still be used as rough measures of total concentration of keto acids as long as the ratio of BB/AA falls within usual ranges. However, when the ratio of NADH/NAD is abnormally increased, the ratio of BB/AA is also proportionately high; in this setting Acetest may yield negative results despite substantial retention of BB. Such a condition is called *β-hydroxybutyric acidosis,* and this is common in alcoholic ketoacidosis.

### *ANION GAP*

The serum anion gap (AG) is estimated as Serum $Na^+ - (Cl^- + HCO_3^-)$ or $(Na^+ + K^+) - (Cl^- + HCO_3^-)$.

Because serum potassium concentration usually falls within narrow limits, it can be considered nearly constant, and the first of the two equations is more commonly used to estimate the AG, with a normal value of about 12 mEq/L (8 to 16 mEq/L). Some authors subtract the normal AG from the observed AG as I have defined it; calculated thus, the normal anion gap should be zero. The term anion gap implies that there is a gap between cation and anion concentration, but it is emphasized that the concentration of total cations in the serum is exactly equal to the concentration of total anions. Although the total concentration of unmeasured anion (i.e., all anions other than chloride and bicarbonate) is about 23 mEq/L, the AG, $Na^+ - (Cl^- + HCO_3^-)$, is only 12 mEq/L because there are about 11 mEq/L of unmeasured cation (i.e., all cations other than sodium) Fig. 6–3).

The relationship between unmeasured cations and unmeasured anions can be described mathematically in the following manner: total serum cations = total serum anions. Because total serum cations are made up of $Na^+$ and unmeasured cations (UCs) and total serum anions, $Cl^-$, $HCO_3^-$, and unmeasured anions (UAs), $Na^+ + UC = (Cl^- + HCO_3^-) + UA$. Therefore, $Na^+ - (Cl + HCO_3^-) = UA - UC$. Because $Na^+ - (Cl + HCO_3^-) = AG$, $UA - UC = AG$.

The above equation clearly demonstrates that alterations in AG, though measured as $Na^+ - (Cl + HCO_3^-)$, must be accompanied by alterations in UAs or UCs. In fact, experience has shown that an alteration in AG is more easily predicted from changes in UAs or UCs than from changes in Na, Cl, or $HCO_3$. The AG can be increased by increased UAs or decreased UCs, whereas AG can be decreased by decreased UAs or increased UCs. However, the equation also predicts that a change in UAs may not change AG if UCs are also changed in the same direction to the same extent. For example, accumulation of $MgSO_4$ increases both UAs and UCs to the same extent, and AG is therefore unchanged. Clinically a decreased AG is most commonly due to reduction in serum albumin concentration, while an increased AG is most often due to accumulation of anions of acids, such as sulfate, lactate, and ketone anions.

A change in serum Na usually does not cause a change in AG, because chloride usually changes in the same direction. Similarly, a change in bicarbonate concentration may not cause a change in AG if chloride changes in the opposite direction. For example, in metabolic alkalosis bicarbonate concentration increases, but AG is normal because chloride concentration is decreased. When bicarbonate concentration decreases as in metabolic acidosis, a change in chloride concentration depends on whether or not some other anions accumulate to replace bicarbonate. If reduction in bicarbonate concentration is accompanied by retention of another anion to replace bicarbonate, chloride concentration does not increase, resulting in *normochloremic acidosis* with increased AG. Such is the case in organic acidosis and uremic acidosis. On the other hand, when bicarbonate concentration decreases without retention of another anion, maintenance of electrical neutrality requires that chloride concentration increase; AG will be normal and acidosis will be a *hyperchloremic acidosis* (Table 6–8).

Many conditions influence AG but do not cause acidosis, but the presence of these conditions must be known in order to properly interpret AG in the presence of metabolic acidosis. For example, if a patient with a low AG due to hypoalbuminemia develops lactic acidosis, the AG could be normal. Without the knowledge of hypoalbuminemia as a cause of low AG, lactic acidosis in this setting could be overlooked.

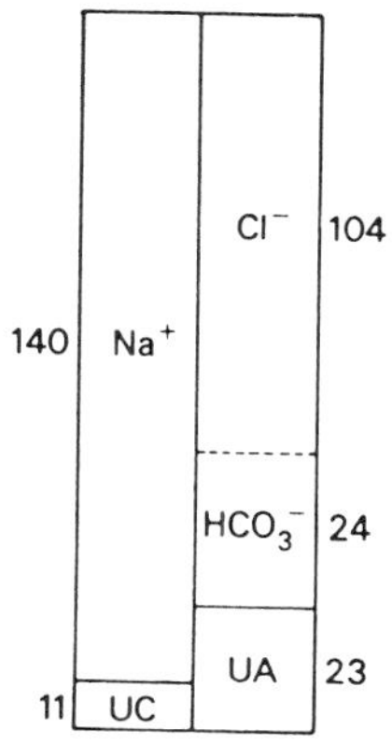
140
Na+
Cl−
104
HCO3−
24
UA
23
11
UC

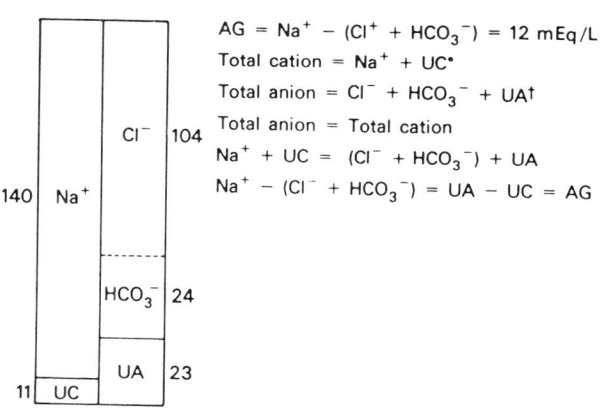

$AG = Na^+ - (Cl^+ + HCO_3^-) = 12$ mEq/L
Total cation = $Na^+$ + UC*
Total anion = $Cl^- + HCO_3^-$ + UA†
Total anion = Total cation
$Na^+ + UC = (Cl^- + HCO_3^-) + UA$
$Na^+ - (Cl^- + HCO_3^-) = UA - UC = AG$

| *UC (Unmeasured cation) | | †UA (Unmeasured anion) | |
|---|---|---|---|
| $K^+$ | 4.5 | Protein | 15 |
| $Ca^{++}$ | 5 | $PO_4^=$ | 2 |
| $Mg^{++}$ | 1.5 | $SO_4^=$ | 1 |
| | | Organic acids | 5 |
| Total UC : 11 mEq/L | | Total UA : 23 mEq/L | |

**FIGURE 6–3.** Anatomy of the anion gap. (From Carroll, H.J., Oh, M.S. (Eds.): Disturbances in acid-base balance. *In* Water, Electrolyte, and Acid-Base Metabolism. Philadelphia, J.B. Lippincott, 1989, p. 242.)

*TREATMENT.*

**Acute Acidosis.** In mild to moderate acidosis, immediate alkali therapy is not indicated. In severe acidosis (pH less than 7.2), the main reason for treatment is to prevent cardiovascular collapse due to arteriolar dilation and decreased cardiac contractility. Older subjects and patients with cardiovascular disease tolerate acidosis poorly. There is no definite level of pH at which treatment with alkali is indicated, but most clinicians would commence alkali therapy when the pH falls below 7.1.

The amount of bicarbonate necessary to increase serum bicarbonate concentration cannot be calculated accurately for several reasons. Rapid correction of severe acidosis with normalization of serum bicarbonate is not only unnecessary but may be harmful for several reasons. When acidosis is corrected with rapid administration of bicarbonate, the corrected blood pH should not exceed 7.2 to 7.3, because rapid increase in pH increases hemoglobin-oxygen affinity, impairing tissue oxygenation without sufficient time to increase the production of red cell 2,3 diphosphoglycerate (DPG). Treatment can be started by administration of 1 or 2 ampules of bicarbonate (44.5 or 50 mEq per ampule) with subsequent dosages decided by blood gas results. The suggestion that treatment of lactic acidosis with sodium

**TABLE 6–8.** CLASSIFICATION OF METABOLIC ACIDOSIS

1. Metabolic acidosis with increased anion gap *(normochloremic acidosis)*
   - Ketoacidosis
   - L-lactic acidosis, D-lactic acidosis
   - β-hydroxybutyric acidosis
   - Uremic acidosis
   - Ingestion of toxins: aspirin (salicylate) ketone, and lactate, methanol (formate), ethylene glycol (glycolate), toluene (hippurate)
2. Metabolic acidosis with normal anion gap *(hyperchloremic acidosis)*
   - Renal tubular acidosis
   - Uremic acidosis (early)
   - Acidosis following respiratory alkalosis
   - Intestinal loss of bicarbonate
   - Administration of chloride-containing acid: HCl, $NH_4Cl$
   - Ketoacidosis during recovery phase

bicarbonate is detrimental has not been thoroughly documented.

**Chronic Acidosis.** In chronic stable metabolic acidosis, the main reasons for alkali therapy are prevention of osteomalacia or rickets, promotion of growth in children, and prevention of nephrocalcinosis and nephrolithiasis. Treatment is indicated in most cases of distal RTA (1 to 3 mEq/kg body weight of alkali per day), because the acidosis is relentless, hypokalemia is severe, and nephrocalcinosis and nephrolithiasis are common. Because patients with distal RTA also need potassium supplement for correction of hypokalemia, agents such as potassium citrate, which contains both potassium and alkali, are preferred. In proximal RTA, on the other hand, treatment is usually not indicated in adults because acidosis is mild and self-limited, complications of acidosis are rare, and correction of acidosis requires a huge amount of bicarbonate. However, when proximal RTA is severe (i.e., serum bicarbonate is below 18 mEq/L) or when it occurs in children, treatment is indicated even for mild acidosis in order to normalize growth. Volume depletion with thiazide diuretics and a low-salt diet enhance tubular bicarbonate reabsorption. Without thiazide or a low-salt diet, bicarbonate requirement usually exceeds 5 to 10 mEq/kg body weight per day.

## METABOLIC ALKALOSIS

### *CAUSES*

At the normal serum bicarbonate concentration, bicarbonate filtered at the glomerulus is virtually completely reabsorbed. As serum bicarbonate concentration rises above the normal level, bicarbonate reabsorption is incomplete and some begins to appear in the urine. As the concentration rises higher, the amount the tubule can reabsorb reaches the maximum level, which is called the tubular maximum for bicarbonate ($Tm_{HCO_3}$). This occurs at plasma bicarbonate concentration of about 27 mEq/L. For example, if a person has normal $Tm_{HCO_3}$ and has plasma bicarbonate concentration of 30 mEq/L, each liter of filtrate will contain 30 mEq of bicarbonate. The tubules will reabsorb 27 mEq for each liter of filtrate and excrete 3 mEq for each liter. At a daily GFR of 200 L, the normal kidney can excrete as much as 600 mEq of bicarbonate when serum bicarbonate concentration reaches a mere 30 mEq/L. In other words, if $Tm_{HCO_3}$ is normal and GFR is normal, about 600 mEq of bicarbonate must be administered daily in order to maintain plasma bicarbonate concentration at 30 mEq/L. Thus, it is nearly impossible to maintain a high plasma bicarbonate in the presence of normal renal threshold unless an enormous amount of bicarbonate is given daily.

For these reasons, development and maintenance of metabolic alkalosis requires not only a mechanism to increase plasma bicarbonate but also a mechanism to keep the concentration increased. Bicarbonate concentration may be increased by administration of alkali, gastric loss of HCl through vomiting or nasogastric suction, or renal generation of bicarbonate. Serum bicarbonate concentration can be maintained at a high level if bicarbonate is not filtered at the glomerulus because of advanced renal failure, or if filtered bicarbonate is absorbed avidly because of increased renal threshold for bicarbonate. The two most common causes for increased renal bicarbonate threshold are *volume depletion* and *K depletion*. Until recently, the mechanism of increased renal threshold for bicarbonate in the presence of volume depletion and K depletion was thought to be enhanced tubular reabsorption, but new evidence suggests that a decrease in GFR plays a significant role.

### *DIAGNOSIS AND TREATMENT*

When volume depletion is responsible for maintenance of metabolic alkalosis and the volume depletion is not caused by renal loss of salt, urinary excretion of Cl is reduced; measurement of urinary Na is an unreliable index of volume depletion in metabolic alkalosis, because excretion of bicarbonate may lead to obligatory loss of Na despite volume depletion. Metabolic alkalosis with reduced urinary chloride is called *chloride-responsive metabolic alkalosis,* and administration of chloride-containing fluid, such as NaCl or KCl solution, ameliorates alkalosis (e.g., vomiting-induced alkalosis). The other type is characterized by normal excretion of chloride in urine, and is called *chloride-resistant metabolic alkalosis,* because administration of Cl does not correct alkalosis (e.g., hypokalemia-induced alkalosis). In edema-forming conditions, administration of Cl may not improve metabolic alkalosis even if the pattern of urinary excretion of Cl suggests chloride-responsive metabolic alkalosis. This is because fluid administration usually does not restore the effective vascular volume to normal in edema-forming states (Table 6–9).

If correction of the underlying cause is not possible, the extracellular bicarbonate concentration can be reduced by renal excretion, chemical buffering, or dialysis. Renal excretion of bicarbonate can be accomplished by correcting abnormal conditions for maintaining high renal bicarbonate threshold; in most instances correction of hypovolemia and hypokalemia, and sometimes treatment of hypercalcemia, will correct metabolic alkalosis. In edema-forming states, metabolic alkalosis may be treated with a carbonic-anhydrase inhibitor, acetazolamide (Diamox), 250 to 500 mg 2 to 4 times a day.

If renal excretion of bicarbonate is not feasible (marked renal impairment or low effective volume that cannot be corrected because of underlying disease), metabolic alkalosis may be treated by direct titration of bicarbonate. For this purpose, ammonium chloride, lysine or arginine chloride, and hydrochloric acid have been used. Removal of bicarbonate by dialysis is effective and predictable, and is particularly useful if the patient has concomitant renal failure.

## RESPIRATORY ALKALOSIS

### *CAUSES*

With the exception of respirator-induced alkalosis and voluntary hyperventilation, respiratory alkalosis is always a result of stimulation of the respiratory center. The two most common causes are hypoxic stimulation of the respiratory center and stimulation through the pulmonary receptors caused by various lung lesions, such as pneumonia, pulmonary congestion, and pulmonary embolism. Certain drugs, such as salicylate and progesterone, stimulate the respiratory center directly. Respiratory alkalosis is common in gram-

**TABLE 6–9.** MECHANISMS FOR GENERATION AND MAINTENANCE OF METABOLIC ALKALOSIS

| CAUSES | MECHANISMS FOR GENERATION | MECHANISMS FOR MAINTENANCE |
|---|---|---|
| Vomiting or gastric suction | **1.** Loss of HCl<br>**2.** Contraction of ECV*<br>**3.** Shift of $H^+$ into cells | **1.** Decreased EAV*<br>**2.** $K^+$ deficiency |
| Contraction alkalosis due to ethacrynic acid | **1.** Contraction of ECV<br>**2.** Shift of $H^+$ into cells<br>**3.** Increased renal $H^+$ excretion | **1.** Decreased EAV<br>**2.** $K^+$ deficiency |
| Congenital chloridorrhea | **1.** Loss of HCl in stool<br>**2.** Increased renal $H^+$ excretion | **1.** Decreased EAV<br>**2.** $K^+$ deficiency |
| Posthypercapnic alkalosis | **1.** Increased renal $H^+$ excretion | **1.** Decreased EAV<br>**2.** $K^+$ deficiency |
| Glucose feeding in fasting | **1.** Shift of $H^+$ into cells | **1.** Decreased EAV?<br>**2.** $K^+$ deficiency |
| Milk-alkali syndrome | **1.** Ingestion of alkali<br>**2.** Increased renal $H^+$ excretion | **1.** Hypercalcemia<br>**2.** Hypoparathyroidism |
| Hypercalcemia of nonparathyroid origin | **1.** Increased renal $H^+$ excretion<br>**2.** Release of bone salts | **1.** Hypercalcemia<br>**2.** Hypoparathyroidism |
| Hypermineralocorticoidism | **1.** Increased renal $H^+$ excretion<br>**2.** Shift of $H^+$ into the cell | **1.** $K^+$ deficiency<br>**2.** Distal $H^+$ secretion |
| Potassium deficiency | **1.** Renal $H^+$ excretion<br>**2.** Shift of $H^+$ into cells. | **1.** $K^+$ deficiency |
| Diuretics | **1.** Increased renal $H^+$ | **1.** Decreased EAV |

*ECV = extracellular volume; EAV = effective arterial volume.

negative sepsis, but the mechanism is unknown (Table 6–10).

*DIAGNOSIS*

Measurements of blood gases will reveal alkaline pH and low $Pco_2$. Chronic respiratory alkalosis with low serum bicarbonate and hyperchloremia will stimulate hyperchloremic metabolic acidosis, but normal or increased blood pH suggests respiratory alkalosis. Once the diagnosis of respiratory alkalosis is confirmed, the most common causes, hypoxemia and pulmonary diseases, should always be ruled out first before considering other causes.

*TREATMENT*

In chronic cases, treatment should only be directed toward removal of causes. In acute symptomatic respiratory alkalosis, rebreathing into a paper bag or breathing of 5% $CO_2$ is effective. In psychogenic hyperventilation, sedatives such as phenobarbital are effective. In severe cases, a mechanical ventilator may be needed after pharmacologic paralysis of the respiratory muscles.

## RESPIRATORY ACIDOSIS

*CAUSES*

The causes are usually apparent. They include diseases of the lung (most common), respiratory muscle, respiratory nerve, thoracic cage, and airways, and suppression of the respiratory center by stroke or by a drug (Table 6–11).

*DIAGNOSIS*

The diagnosis of respiratory acidosis is made from low pH and high $Pco_2$. When $Pco_2$ is mildly increased, pH may be normalized by renal compensation. Metabolic alkalosis might mimic respiratory acidosis because $Pco_2$ will be high with respiratory compensation, but the blood pH in metabolic alkalosis is always high. However, $Pco_2$ in metabolic alkalosis rarely exceeds 60 mm Hg no matter how severe metabolic alkalosis is.

**TABLE 6–10.** CAUSES OF RESPIRATORY ALKALOSIS

1. Hypoxia: living at high altitude and lung diseases
2. Drugs and toxins: salicylate, progesterone
3. Central nervous system disorders: inflammation, tumor, CVA, trauma
4. Psychogenic: anxiety, nervousness, hysteria
5. Reflex stimulation of the lung: any lung disease
6. Rapid recovery from metabolic acidosis
7. Miscellaneous: liver disease, fever, delirium tremens, sepsis, assisted ventilation

*TREATMENT*

The therapeutic effort should be directed at the root cause. Restoration of ventilation by intubation is the key in acute respiratory acidosis of any cause. Administration of sodium bicarbonate will restore the extracellular pH, but the effect on brain pH is delayed because bicarbonate penetrates the blood-brain barrier slowly. Administration of the amine buffer THAM (TRIS) has a theoretical advantage in this particular setting because it increases bicarbonate and decreases $Pco_2$ at the same time: $THAM + H_2CO_3 \rightarrow THAM{-}H^+ + HCO_3^-$.

## MIXED ACID-BASE DISORDERS AND INTERPRETATION OF BLOOD GASES.

The term mixed acid-base disorder refers to a clinical condition in which two or more primary acid-base disorders coexist. The general pattern of presentation of mixed acid-base disturbances is one of obvious disturbance accompanied by an inappropriate (excessive or inadequate) compensation. The "inappropriateness" of the compensation may reflect the effect of a separate primary disorder. There are five possible situations in which two acid-base disorders may be present simultaneously:

1. Respiratory acidosis with metabolic acidosis
2. Respiratory alkalosis with metabolic alkalosis
3. Respiratory alkalosis with metabolic acidosis
4. Respiratory acidosis with metabolic alkalosis
5. Metabolic acidosis with metabolic alkalosis

The combination of respiratory acidosis with respiratory alkalosis cannot occur, because $Pco_2$ cannot be high and low at the same time. However, metabolic acidosis and metabolic alkalosis can coexist, because the terms metabolic acidosis and alkalosis indicate not only a primary decrease or increase in bicarbonate concentration but also the pathophysiologic processes that lead to such changes. For example, an anuric person undergoing continuous gastric suction could have both metabolic acidosis and metabolic alkalosis.

The appropriate degrees of compensation for primary acid-base disorders have been determined by analysis of data from large numbers of patients, and are expressed in the form of equations in Table 6–12. When the two disorders influence the blood pH in opposite directions, the blood pH will be determined by the dominant

**TABLE 6–11.** CAUSES OF RESPIRATORY ACIDOSIS

1. Depression of the respiratory center: general anesthesia, drugs, tumors, CVA, bulbar poliomyelitis, meningitis, pickwickian syndrome, hypothyroidism
2. Defects in nerves and muscles of respiration: poliomyelitis, Guillain-Barré syndrome, spinal cord injury, myasthenia gravis, hypokalemic and hyperkalemic periodic paralysis, severe K depletion
3. Disorders of thoracic cage: Pickwickian syndrome, deformity of the chest, pneumothorax
4. Airway obstruction
5. Pulmonary diseases: chronic obstructive lung disease, severe pneumonia, severe pulmonary congestion, severe bronchial asthma

**TABLE 6–12.** EXTENT OF NORMAL ACID-BASE COMPENSATION FOR VARIOUS DISORDERS

| DISORDER | FORMULA |
|---|---|
| Metabolic acidosis* | $\Delta CO_2 = \Delta HCO_3 \times 1.2 \pm 2.$ |
| Metabolic alkalosis† | $\Delta P_{CO_2} = \Delta HCO_3 \times 0.7 + 5$ |
| Acute respiratory acidosis | $\Delta HCO_3 = \Delta P_{CO_2} \times 0.07 \pm 1.5$ |
| Chronic respiratory acidosis | $\Delta HCO_3 = \Delta P_{CO_2} \times 0.4 \pm 3$ |
| Acute respiratory alkalosis | $\Delta HCO_3 = \Delta P_{CO_2} \times 0.2 \pm 2.5$ |
| Chronic respiratory alkalosis | $\Delta HCO_3 = \Delta P_{CO_2} \times 0.5 \pm 2.5$ |

Note: Δ refers to the difference between normal and actual or expected $P_{CO_2}$ or $HCO_3$.
*$P_{CO_2}$ should be less than 18 mm Hg for pH less than 7.1, and less than 15 mm Hg for pH less than 7.0.
†Compensation may be totally absent. No matter how high serum $HCO_3$, $P_{CO_2}$ rarely rises above 60 mm Hg in metabolic alkalosis.

disorder. If two disorders cancel out each other's effect, blood pH can be normal.

In general, compensation is the best in respiratory alkalosis (pH is often normalized), the next best in respiratory acidosis (pH may become normal), and the third best in metabolic acidosis. Compensation is least effective in metabolic alkalosis, and this is probably because hypoxemia, an inevitable consequence of hypoventilation, prevents hypoventilation.

## CLINICAL PROBLEMS

1. Calculate pH from $P_{CO_2}$ and $HCO_3$.
   a. $P_{CO_2}$, 30 mm Hg, $HCO_3$ 15 mM.
   b. $P_{CO_2}$, 10 mm Hg, $HCO_3$ 2 mM.
   c. $P_{CO_2}$, 80 mm Hg, $HCO_3$ 40 mM.

2. A patient with blood pH 7.32, $P_{CO_2}$ 28 mm Hg, and $HCO_3$ 14 mM has the following urinary values per day: $NH_4$ 60 mEq, titratable acid 20 mEq, and $HCO_3$ 10 mEq. The findings are most consistent with:
   a. respiratory alkalosis.
   b. extrarenal acidosis.
   c. renal acidosis.
   d. metabolic alkalosis.

3. Determine whether serum AG be increased (I), decreased (D), or unchanged (U) with the following:
   a. low serum Na.
   b. low serum Cl.
   c. lithium intoxication.
   d. hypoalbuminemia.
   e. lactic acidosis.
   f. bromide intoxication.
   g. diarrhea-induced metabolic acidosis.
   h. hypermagnesemia due to $MgSO_4$ overdose.

4. A patient with mild renal insufficiency due to diabetic nephropathy has the following laboratory findings: Na 140 mEq/L; K 6.2 mEq/L; $HCO_3$ 16 mEq/L; Cl, 118; serum albumin 2 g/dl; serum creatinine 2.5 mg/dl; and urine pH 5.0. Net acid excretion is 50 mEq per day. The most likely diagnosis is:
   a. type I RTA.
   b. type II RTA.
   c. type IV RTA.
   d. lactic acidosis.
   e. uremic acidosis.

5. A person has normal GFR (180 L per day) and normal renal bicarbonate threshold (i.e., this person will reabsorb $HCO_3$ up to 27 mEq/L of filtrate). If the same subject ingests 720 mEq of $HCO_3$ daily, how high will serum bicarbonate rise? Assume that the net acid production rate from the other sources is zero.

6. Which of the following is the unlikely cause of the following blood gases: pH 7.44, $Pco_2$ 20 mm Hg, $HCO_3$ 14 mM?
   a. Salicylate intoxication.
   b. Progesterone injection.
   c. Pneumocystis carinii pneumonia.
   d. Phenobarbital intoxication.
   e. A trip to Mount Everest.

7. Interpret the following blood gases:

| | *pH* | *$Pco_2$ (mm Hg)* | *$HCO_3$ (mM)* |
|---|---|---|---|
| a. | 7.4 | 20 | 12 |
| b. | 7.14 | 80 | 27 |
| c. | 7.24 | 24 | 10 |
| d. | 7.62 | 30 | 30 |
| e. | 7.62 | 20 | 20 |
| f. | 7.50 | 80 | 60 |
| g. | 7.32 | 30 | 15 |
| h. | 7.02 | 20 | 5 |

## ANSWERS

1. Using the equation pH = 7.62 − log $Pco_2/HCO_3$,
   a. pH = 7.62 − log 30/15 = 7.62 − log 2 − 7.62 − 0.3 = 7.32.
   b. 6.92.
   c. 7.32.

2. c; The blood gas findings are consistent with metabolic acidosis. Net acid excretion of 70 mEq per day is within usual normal range (40 to 100 mEq per day), but it is inappropriately low in the setting of metabolic acidosis; the patient must therefore have renal acidosis.

3. The prediction of AG is best made from the equation Anion Gap = UA − UC.
   a. U; Na is neither UA nor UC; hence AG cannot be predicted.
   b. U; Cl is neither UA or UC.
   c. D; lithium is UC, and high lithium increases UC.
   d. D; albumin is UA, and low albumin decreases UA.
   e. I; lactate is UA.
   f. D; bromide would normally be considered a UA. However, in most clinical laboratories, bromide is measured as chloride, at a falsely higher concentration. Thus, in the presence of high bromide, the total halide (chloride + bromide) concentration is measured higher than normal chloride. The result is pseudohyperchloremia, and AG is reduced.
   g. N.
   h. N; both UA (sulfate) and UC (magnesium) are increased.

4. c; normal net acid excretion despite metabolic acidosis indicates renal acidosis, and argues against lactic acidosis, an extrarenal acidosis. A low AG also argues against lactic acidosis, and the most likely reason for low AG is hypoalbuminemia. Type I RTA is ruled out by urine pH of 5.0. Uremic acidosis is unlikely, because renal function is only mildly impaired, but cannot be entirely ruled out. However, the absence of increased AG does not rule out uremic acidosis because AG is often normal in early uremic acidosis. Type II RTA has not yet been ruled out, but high serum K strongly suggests type IV RTA. High K cannot be explained by this degree of modest renal impairment.

5. Serum bicarbonate will reach a plateau only when the amount ingested equals urinary excretion. When serum bicarbonate is in excess of $Tm_{HCO_3}$, urinary excretion of bicarbonate can be calculated as (serum $HCO_3$ − $Tm_{HCO_3}$) × GFR. At equilibrium, the amount ingested must equal the amount excreted, (serum $HCO_3$ − $Tm_{HCO_3}$) × GFR; 720 = (serum $HCO_3$ − 27) × 180. Hence, serum $HCO_3$ at equilibrium = 720/180 + 27 = 31. To put it differently; when serum $HCO_3$ is 31 mEq/L, each liter of filtrate will contain 31 mEq of $HCO_3$. Because the maximal amount reabsorbed by the tubule is 27 mEq/L (remember $Tm_{HCO3}$ is 27 mEq/L), each liter of filtrate will be accompanied by loss of 4 mEq of bicarbonate in urine. With 180 L of GFR per day, the kidney will excrete 180 × 4 = 720 mEq per day. In other words, serum bicarbonate will gradually rise until it becomes 31 mEq/L, at which point the amount excreted finally equals the intake, and serum bicarbonate becomes stable. The purpose of this exercise is to show you that sustained metabolic alkalosis is possible only when $Tm_{HCO_3}$ is abnormally increased (e.g., by volume deletion or K depletion) or when there is severe renal impairment.

6. d; The blood gas findings are consistent with chronic respiratory alkalosis with compensation. Salicylate intoxication and progesterone injection directly stimulate the respiratory center; Pneumocystis carinii pneumonia causes respiratory alkalosis by hypoxic stimulation as well as by the local reflex (stiffness of the lung due to pneumonia); living in high altitude causes respiratory alkalosis through hypoxemic stimulation; phenobarbital intoxication tends to cause respiratory depression.

7. a. Chronic respiratory alkalosis.
   b. Acute respiratory acidosis.

c. Chronic metabolic acidosis.
d. Mixed respiratory alkalosis and metabolic alkalosis. In this case $P_{CO_2}$ is low and $HCO_3$ is high. When the $P_{CO_2}$ and $HCO_3$ change in opposite directions, the diagnosis of a mixed acid-base disorder is a certainty.
e. Acute respiratory alkalosis.
f. Metabolic alkalosis and respiratory acidosis. The presence of metabolic alkalosis is clear (high pH due to high $HCO_3$), but $P_{CO_2}$ of 80 mm Hg is inappropriately high ($P_{CO_2}$ does not rise in excess of 60 mm Hg no matter how severe the metabolic alkalosis).
g. Chronic metabolic acidosis.
h. Metabolic acidosis with insufficient respiratory compensation (respiratory acidosis).

## SELECTED READINGS

### *CONTROL OF BODY FLUID VOLUME AND OSMOLALITY*

Carroll, H.J., Oh, M.S.: Deficits of salt and water. *In* Water, Electrolyte, and Acid-Base Metabolism. 2nd Ed. Philadelphia, J.B. Lippincott, 1989.

Gennari, F.J.: Current concepts: Serum osmolality: Uses and limitations. N. Engl. J. Med., *310:*102, 1984.

Kinney, J.M.: Influence of intermediary metabolism of nitrogen balance and weight loss: Some considerations basic to an understanding of injury. Metabolism, *8:*809, 1959.

### *DISORDERS OF WATER AND ANTIDIURETIC HORMONE (ADH) METABOLISM*

Carroll, H.J., Oh, M.S.: Water and ADH metabolism. *In* Water, Electrolyte, and Acid-Base Metabolism. 2nd Ed. Philadelphia, J.B. Lippincott, 1989.

Robertson, G.L., Berl, T.: Water metabolism. *In* The Kidney. Edited by B.M. Brenner and F.C. Rector. Philadelphia, W.B. Saunders, 1986.

Sterns, R.H., Riggs, J.E., Schochet, S., Jr.: Osmotic demyelination syndrome following correction of hyponatremia. N. Engl. J. Med., *314:*1529, 1986.

Trachtman, H., Barbour, R., Sturman, J.A., Finberg, L.: Taurine and osmoregulation: Taurine is a cerebral osmoprotective molecule in chronic hypernatremic dehydration. Pediatr. Res., *23:*35–39, 1988.

Weisberg, L.S.: Pseudohyponatremia: A reappraisal. Am. J. Med., *86:*315–318, 1989.

Zerbe, R.L., and Robertson, G.L.: Comparison of plasma ADH measurement with a standard direct test in the differential diagnosis of polyuria. N. Engl. J. Med., *305:*1539, 1981.

### *DISORDERS OF POTASSIUM METABOLISM*

Adrogue, H.J. Madias, N.E.: Changes in plasma potassium concentration during acute acid-base disturbances. Am. J. Med., *71:*456, 1981.

Brown, R.S.: Extrarenal potassium homeostasis. Kidney Int., *30:*116, 1986.

Carroll, H.J., Oh, M.S.: Disorders of potassium metabolism. *In* Water, Electrolyte, and Acid-Base Metabolism. 2nd Ed. Philadelphia, J.B. Lippincott, 1989.

Phelps, K., Lieberman, R.L., Oh, M.S., Carroll, H.J.: The pathophysiology of the syndrome of hyporeninemic hypoaldosteronism. Metabolism, *29:*186, 1980.

Williams, M.E., Rosa, R.M., Epstein, F.H.: Hyperkalemia. Adv. Intern. Med., *31:*265, 291, 1986.

Yasumura, S., Cohn, S.H., Ellis, J.: Measurement of extracellular space by total body neutron activation. Am. J. Physiol., *244:*R40, 1983.

Surawicz, B.: Arrhythmias and electrolyte disturbances. Bull. N.Y. Acad. Med., *43:*1160, 1967.

### *ACID-BASE DISORDERS*

Carroll, H.J., Oh, M.S.: Disturbances in acid-base balance. *In* Water, Electrolyte, and Acid-Base Metabolism. 2nd Ed. Philadelphia, J.B. Lippincott, 1989.

Goldberg, M., et al.: Computer-based instruction and diagnosis of acid-base disorders. JAMA, *223:*269, 1973.

Harrington, J.T.: Metabolic alkalosis. Kidney Int., *26:*88, 1984.

Jacobson, H.R., Seldin, D.W.: On the generation, maintenance, and correction of metabolic alkalosis. Am. J. Physiol, *245:*F425, 1983.

Madias, N.E., Zelma, S.J.: The renal response to chronic mineral acid feeding: A re-examination of the role of systemic pH. Kidney Int., *19:*667, 1986.

Oh, M.S., Carroll, H.J.: The anion gap. N. Engl. J. Med., *297:*814, 1977.

CHAPTER 7

# Calcium and Phosphorus

Lindsay H. Allen and Richard J. Wood



## CALCIUM

The role of calcium as a structural material in bones and teeth has been known for centuries. Prehistoric man suffered from osteoporosis, and although great progress has been made in the last few decades toward quantifying and understanding this disease, much remains to be understood about the importance of dietary calcium intake as a causative, preventative, or therapeutic factor. In addition to calcium's structural role in bone and teeth, it is now recognized that all living cells require calcium to conduct their specialized functions. Intracellular calcium acts as a second messenger and enables cells to respond to stimuli such as hormones or neurotransmitters. Movement of calcium from intracellular compartments to the cytosol initiates events such as cell division, secretion, and movement.

### METABOLISM

Of the approximately 20 mmol (800 mg) consumed daily, about 25 to 50% is absorbed and passes into the exchangeable calcium pool (Fig. 7–1). This pool consists of the small amount of calcium in blood, lymph, and other body fluids, and accounts for 1% of the total body calcium. The remaining 99% is located in bones and teeth. In the adult, the extracellular pool of calcium turns over 20 to 30 times a day, whereas bone turns over every 5 or 6 years. The kidney filters about 216 mmol/per day (8.6 g/per day), almost all of which is reabsorbed so that only 2.5 to 5 mmol/per day (100 to 200 mg) is excreted in urine. Calcium absorption by the intestine, reabsorption by the kidney, and turnover in bone are closely regulated by calcium-regulating hormones: par-

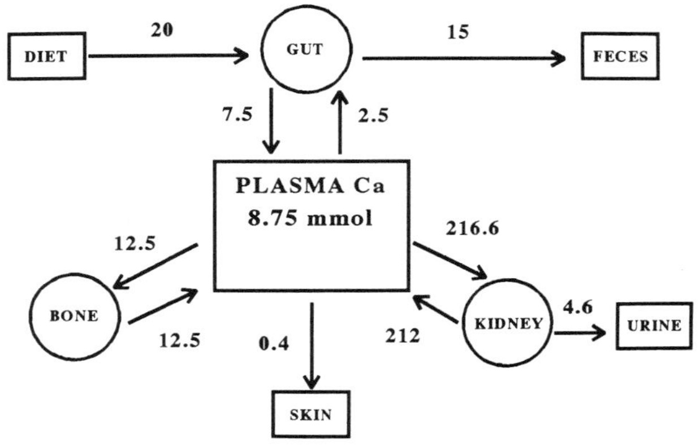
DIET
20
GUT
15
FECES
7.5
2.5
PLASMA Ca
8.75 mmol
12.5
216.6
BONE
12.5
0.4
212
KIDNEY
4.6
URINE
SKIN

**FIGURE 7–1.** Outline of calcium metabolism (mmol/d) under equilibrium conditions (input = output) in adults.

athyroid hormone (PTH), calcitonin, and vitamin D. These hormones act together to maintain calcium homeostasis in the face of variable dietary intakes and changing calcium requirements during growth, pregnancy, and lactation.

Serum total calcium levels are closely regulated at about 2.5 mmol/L (10 mg/dl) to preserve extracellular calcium concentrations and thereby protect normal neuromuscular and hormonal function. The calcium in serum is distributed as follows: ionized 47.5%, protein-bound 46%, calcium citrate 1.7%, $CaHPO_4$ 1.6%, and unidentified complexes 3.2%. Ionized calcium is the functional regulated form, and it equilibrates rapidly with protein-bound serum calcium.

### *ABSORPTION*

The amount of calcium absorbed depends on its interaction with other dietary constituents, and on physiologic factors such as calcium-regulating hormones and stage of the life span.

The solubility of calcium salts is increased in the acid environment of the stomach, but the dissolved ions will to some extent reassociate and precipitate in the jejunum and ileum where the pH is closer to neutral. In the gastrointestinal tract, food constituents are released, such as glucose, fatty acids, phosphorus, and oxalate, that can bind to soluble calcium, resulting in complex luminal interactions. Gastric acidity has little effect on the absorbability of dietary calcium consumed with a meal.[1] In one study achlorhydric subjects absorbed only one-fifth of the calcium from calcium carbonate compared to healthy controls, unless it was ingested with food, in which case absorption was normal.[2] In general the absorption of calcium supplements, and especially those which are less soluble, is substantially better if they are taken with a meal. This may be because the meal stimulates gastric secretion and delays emptying, so that the calcium sources are better dispersed and dissolved.

There are two routes of calcium absorption in the intestine.[3] One is an active, saturable, transcellular process that occurs mainly in the duodenum and proximal jejunum. It is regulated by vitamin D and involves a vitamin D–dependent calcium-binding protein (CaBP or calbindin—see Chapter 17). Ileal absorption may also be affected by vitamin D status.[4] Calcium is pumped out of the enterocyte and into the blood by an adenosine triphosphate (ATP)-dependent pump. Active calcium absorption is affected by the physiology of the host—that is, calcium and vitamin D status, age, pregnancy, and lactation.

The other pathway of calcium absorption is a passive, nonsaturable, paracellular route that is independent of vitamin D regulation and occurs throughout the small intestine. The amount of calcium absorbed in this way depends primarily on its quantity and availability in the diet. Intakes above as little as 3 mmol (120 mg) in a meal will probably be absorbed by this route.[5]

Most calcium absorption occurs in the ileum, where food remains for the longest time. Removal of the ileum has a more devastating effect on human calcium absorption than does removal of the jejunum. Unabsorbed food calcium reaching the terminal ileum is insoluble.

Calcium can also be absorbed by the colon. About 4% of dietary calcium, 200 μmol/per day (8 mg per day), is absorbed by this route; this percentage is higher in individuals who absorb relatively less calcium in the upper intestine.[6] The cecal mucosa of the rat contains vitamin D–dependent calcium-binding protein that increases during dietary calcium deficiency.[7] It remains to be determined whether colonic absorption assumes a more important role in calcium deficiency, or when high-fiber diets are consumed; bacterial fermentation in the colon releases some calcium from its binding to plant constituents such as uronic acids in fiber.

The molecular details of transcellular calcium transport are not fully understood.[8] At the level of the enterocyte, the brush border membrane is the first barrier that calcium must cross to gain access to the cell. The transport of calcium across the brush border membrane is greater in vitamin D–replete compared to vitamin D–depleted animals. Rapid changes in phosphatydlinositol metabolism and membrane lipid composition occur in response to treatment with $1,25(OH)_2D$. For net calcium absorption to occur, calcium must traverse the intracellular environment and reach the basolateral membrane surface for extrusion. The details of intracellular calcium transport are poorly defined. However, it appears that cytosolic calcium-binding protein (calbindin D) is important to facilitate maximal rates of calcium transport. Recently, it has been suggested that at least part of transcellular calcium transport may involve trafficking and compartmentalization by an endosomal-lysosomal pathway or other intracellular organelles. Extrusion of calcium at the basolateral membrane is an energy-dependent process that must move calcium against a significant electrochemical gradient. A component of calcium exit from the cell may also involve a sodium-dependent pathway. A number of hormones, besides $1,25(OH)_2D$, have been shown to affect intestinal calcium absorption; however, our understanding of the mechanism of these effects is rudimentary.

### *STORAGE*

Because more than 99% of the body's calcium is in bone, the skeleton is the major storage site for the maintenance of extracellular fluid (ECF) calcium. In the short term, negative calcium balance involves a harmless mobilization of bone calcium. In the longer term, the chronic removal of skeletal calcium has adverse effects on bone strength.

Release of calcium stored in intracellular locations in cells is an important trigger to many cellular functions, as described in the section on functions.

## HOMEOSTATIC REGULATION

The level of ionized calcium in plasma is controlled by an integrated response of the calcium-regulating hormones that affect calcium transport in the intestine, bone, and kidney. Of these, the most important are PTH, calcitonin, and vitamin D.[9,10]

### *PARATHYROID HORMONE*

The principal mechanism for PTH release is a drop in ECF calcium concentration. The hormone increases the concentration of calcium in ECF by directly stimulating bone resorption and renal tubular reabsorption, and indirectly by increasing intestinal absorption through enhanced formation of $1,25(OH)_2D$ from 25(OH)D in the kidney. High ECF calcium concentrations lead to increased parathyroid cell intracellular calcium, which in turn decreases PTH secretion. PTH is a single-chain polypeptide of 84 amino acids, containing no cysteine. It is biosynthesized on the ribosomes as "preproPTH" containing 31 additional amino acids at the N-terminal, which is rapidly converted to proPTH containing only six additional N-terminal amino acids and then to PTH, which is the form stored in and released from secretory granules. The terminal sequence 1–34 is essential for biologic activity, within which 1–6 is responsible for receptor activation and 26–34 for binding activity. Radioimmunoassays should be directed at the biologically active amino terminal (N-terminal).

PTH interacts with specific receptors on the plasma membrane of bone cells (osteoblasts) and kidney to stimulate the adenylate cyclase system and subsequently cyclic AMP (adenosine monophosphate) production. Cyclic AMP, or cAMP, acts as a second messenger to activate systems such as protein kinase that result in expression of the biologic actions of PTH. No PTH receptors have been identified on osteoclasts: PTH may produce its osteoclastic effect by changing the shape of osteoblasts to make more room for osteoclasts, or through osteoblastic release of a messenger (unidentified) that enhances osteoclastic activity. In the kidney, PTH receptors and PTH-sensitive adenylate cyclase are located in the proximal tubule, and in the granular portion and cortical ascending limb of the distal tubule. It has not been fully clarified how calcium reabsorption is affected.

### *CALCITONIN*

Calcitonin, synthesized by the C cells of the thyroid, is a polypeptide containing 32 amino acids, almost all of which are needed for biologic activity. A rise in serum-calcium is the strongest secretagogue. Calcitonin lowers serum calcium by inhibiting bone resorption and agents that have a resorptive effect on bone. These include PTH, vitamin D metabolites, prostaglandins, and vitamin A. Osteoclasts have calcitonin receptors on the plasma membrane that respond to the hormone with an increase in cAMP production, which in turn mediates the action of calcitonin. The movement of the pseudopod-like extensions of osteoclasts is stopped, and presumably lysosome production is precluded.

### *VITAMIN D*

Vitamin D metabolism is described in detail in Chapter 17. The vitamin enters the circulation after synthesis in the skin or consumption in the diet, and is transported through the body bound to a vitamin D–binding protein. This complex binds to liver cells and permits the vitamin D to enter the cytosol, where it undergoes hydroxylation at carbon 25 by microsomal enzymes similar to the P450 system. The resulting 25(OH)D leaves the liver, is bound again to the binding protein, and enters the kidney where it is further hydroxylated in the mitochondrion to $1,25(OH)_2D_3$, the most active vitamin D metabolite. In calcium deficiency, more $1,25(OH)_2D_3$ is produced, causing enhanced intestinal absorption and renal reabsorption of calcium, and increased bone formation and resorption. There are receptors for $1,25(OH)_2D_3$ on osteoblasts, and it increases the production of osteocalcin (Gla-protein) and other proteins by these cells. How it affects bone turnover and mineralization remains to be determined.

### *OTHER HORMONES*

Although PTH, calcitonin, and vitamin D are the major calcium-regulating hormones, several other hormones affect bone turnover and calcium metabolism.[11] These include glucocorticoids, thyroid hormone, growth hormone, insulin, and estrogen.

Glucocorticoid excess leads to bone loss, especially of trabecular bone, in Cushing's disease or when steroids are used to treat various diseases. The symptoms are delayed growth and skeletal maturation in children, and osteoporosis in adults. The main effect is an inhibition of osteoblastic activity, although osteoclastic activity is also impaired. There is a reduced incorporation of sulfate into cartilage and of amino acids into collagen. Glucocorticoids also impair both the active and passive transport of calcium through intestinal cells, possibly without an effect on vitamin D metabolism.

Thyroid hormones stimulate bone resorption, and both compact and trabecular bone are lost in hyperthyroidism. Hypothyroidism impairs the bone-mobilizing effect of PTH, leading to secondary hyperparathyroidism. The circulating level of $1,25(OH)_2D_3$ tends to be higher, and both the intestinal absorption and renal reabsorption of calcium are increased. Growth hormone stimulates the growth of cartilage and bone throughsomatomedins, growth hormone–dependent polypeptides. It also stimulates the 25(OH)D hydroxylase, increasing serum $1,25(OH)_2D$ levels and the active intestinal transport of calcium. Insulin stimulates the osteoblastic production of collagen and directly reduces the renal reabsorption of calcium and sodium.

Normal serum estrogen levels are essential for the maintenance of normal bone balance. The fall in estrogen levels of postmenopausal women is a major factor in the frequently ensuing bone resorption and osteoporosis. Estrogen receptors have been identified in bone.[12] Estrogen treatment of postmenopausal women reduces bone resorption within weeks without changes in serum PTH, calcitonin, or $1,25(OH)_2D$.[13] However, in the longer term estrogen treatment results in increased PTH and $1,25(OH)_2D$ synthesis, which may explain the observed improvements in the intestinal absorption and renal reabsorption of calcium. Testosterone also inhibits bone resorption,[14] and osteoporosis occurs with hypogonadism in adult men.

## EXCRETION

Calcium is excreted in approximately equal amounts in urine and endogenous intestinal secretions (Fig. 7–1). Calcium loss from the skin is only about 0.4 mmol/per day (15 mg per day), although this will increase substantially with severe sweating.

### *ENDOGENOUS EXCRETION*

Approximately 3.75 mmol per day (150 mg per day) of calcium enter the intestinal lumen in secretions such as succus entericus and bile, but about 30% of this is absorbed so that the minimum endogenous fecal calcium is usually stated to be 2.5 mmol per day (100 mg per day). More recently an endogenous loss closer to 1.1 mmol per day (45 mg per day) has been suggested.[4]

### *URINARY EXCRETION*

Urinary calcium excretion is 2.5 to 6 mmol per day (100 to 240 mg per day) and varies greatly among normal individuals. It accounts for only 0.2% of the calcium filtered by the kidney, because 99.8% is reabsorbed. Renal calcium transport is similar to that in the intestine. Paracellular transport, by which most reabsorption occurs, takes place in the proximal tubule, the thick ascending limb of the loop of Henle, and the connecting and collecting ducts. Active transport is found in the distal convoluted tubule and possibly the proximal tubule, and involves a calcium-binding protein ($CaBP_r$, $calbindin_{28k}$). Within individuals there are large diurnal fluctuations in urinary calcium, due mainly to the calciuretic effect of foods. Approximately 50% of excreted calcium is in the ionized form; the remainder is complexed with sulfate, phosphate, citrate, and oxalate. The amount of calcium in urine is a relatively poor predictor of calcium stone formation.

Urinary calcium excretion increases slightly during childhood, from about 1 to 2 mmol per day (40 to 80 mg per day), and then increases after puberty to approximately 5 mmol per day (200 mg per day) by the age of 20 years. Thus, calcium retention varies with the rate of skeletal growth. Another rise in excretion occurs at menopause, is related to the greater bone resorption, and is treatable by estrogens. This is followed by a decrease after age 65 because of a reduction in glomerular filtration rate and intestinal absorption.

Dietary calcium intake and absorption have a positive but weak relationship with urinary calcium excretion. Metabolizable carbohydrates and protein both produce a calciuretic effect that is linearly related to the intake of these macronutrients, but relatively independent of calcium intake. For each 50-g increment in dietary protein an additional 1.5 mmol (60 mg) of calcium is lost in urine.[15] The relatively high levels of phosphorus in some proteins blunt, but do not eliminate, this calciuretic response. The calciuretic effect of protein involves a reduction of renal calcium reabsorption uncompensated by increased intestinal absorption, so that adults fed high-protein diets are in negative calcium balance. In rats, the calciuretic effect of glucose or arginine infusion is abolished by streptozotocin, suggesting that insulin may be involved in the impairment of renal calcium reabsorption.[16]

There is an inverse relationship between dietary phosphorus intake and urinary calcium. Phosphorus increases PTH synthesis (which reduces urinary calcium) and affects renal tubular calcium transport directly. Changes in urinary calcium are usually accompanied by similar changes in urinary sodium, and vice versa. The two elements share a common reabsorption mechanism in the proximal tubule, but not in the distal tubule where reabsorption is hormonally regulated. The daily addition of 51 mmol (3 g) and 102 mmol (6 g) of sodium chloride to the regular diet of healthy postmenopausal women would mobilize 7.5 and 10%, respectively, of skeletal calcium over 10 years, constituting a potential risk factor for osteoporosis.[17] Caffeine also increases urinary calcium loss.

Infusion of amino acids and glucose to patients receiving total parenteral nutrition (TPN) results in urinary calcium loss and negative calcium balance, which can be ameliorated by the administration of additional phosphorus in the TPN solution.[18]

## FUNCTIONS

Calcium has a structural role in bone and teeth. Bone calcium is relied on to maintain ECF calcium concentrations, which in turn are necessary for normal neuromuscular and other functions. A number of enzymes, including those involved in blood clotting, are calcium-dependent. Changes in intracellular cytosolic calcium trigger events such as contraction, secretion, differentiation, and movement.

*BONES AND TEETH*

The role of calcium in bone is described in more detail in Chapter 89. The chemical structure in bone and teeth is a hydroxyapatite-like crystal, with the general formula $Ca_{10}H(PO_4)_6OH_2$. Bone contains some other calcium salts, especially carbonate. About 80% of bone is dense, cortical bone that has less than 10% soft tissue. By weight trabecular bone is only 25% mineral and is found mostly in the axial skeleton and the ends of long bones. The trabecular type is the one mainly involved in mineral homeostasis and therefore is most depleted during calcium deficiency and osteoporosis. Osteoclasts, bone resorbing cells, respond to PTH, $1,25(OH)_2D$, calcitonin, and prostaglandin $E_2$ by differentiation or osteoblast mediation. They have receptors only for calcitonin[19] and they extrude lysosomal packets containing acid hydrolases that dissolve solid calcium phosphate and help degrade bone matrix. Osteoblasts, which secrete unmineralized collagen and bone matrix, have receptors for PTH, $1,25(OH)_2D$, estrogen, and prostaglandin $E_2$ and regulate the flux of calcium and phosphate in and out of bone. They are unaffected by calcitonin.

The bone calcium pool turns over every 5 to 6 years on average. This varies greatly among specific bones, with the lumbar vertebral bone turning over most rapidly. Dental calcium turnover is negligible. During bone growth and development osteoblastic exceeds osteoclastic activity. Osteoporosis results from a faster rate of bone resorption accompanied by a slower rate of formation.

*INTRACELLULAR REGULATION BY CALCIUM*

Almost all the calcium within cells is bound within organelles such as the endoplasmic reticulum, the nucleus, and vesicles (Fig. 7–2). Consequently the free calcium in cell cytosol is only about $10^{-7}$ mol/L, and there is a 10,000-fold electrochemical gradient for calcium across cell membranes. Very small changes in the release of calcium from intracellular sites, or in its transport across the cell membrane, cause a relatively large increase in cytosol calcium concentration. The changes in cytosol calcium concentrations act as intracellular messengers. In excitable cells such as heart muscle and nerve terminals, channels selective for calcium ions open when the membrane is depolarized; calcium is also released from the internal store (mainly the endoplasmic reticulum). The subsequent rise in cytosolic calcium concentration triggers contraction or secretion.[20] In skeletal muscle calcium is mobilized from the endoplasmic reticulum by an electrical signal, and in other cells inositol trisphosphate ($IP_3$) is the releasing stimulus. The released calcium binds to a calcium-binding protein such as calmodulin, troponin C in muscle, and cytoskeletal proteins. This binding triggers the physiologic event directly or indirectly through phosphorylation of other proteins. Cell recovery involves

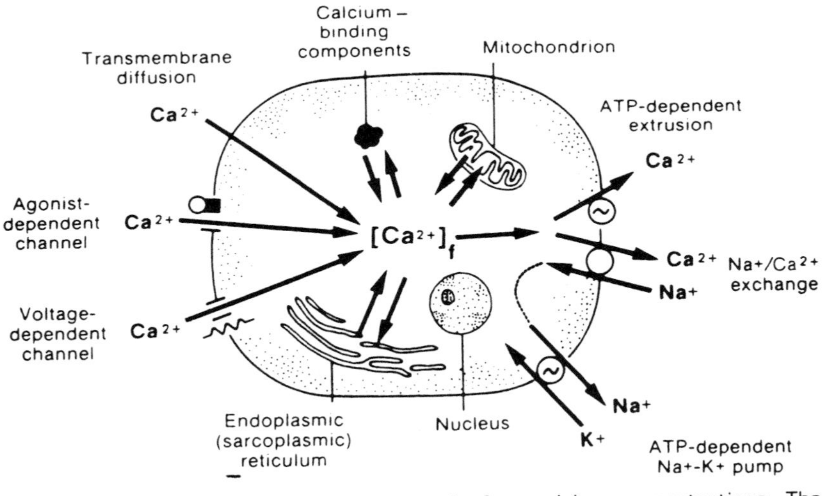
Transmembrane diffusion
Calcium-binding components
Mitochondrion
ATP-dependent extrusion
Agonist-dependent channel
Voltage-dependent channel
Ca2+
[Ca2+]f
Na+/Ca2+ exchange
Na+
K+
Endoplasmic (sarcoplasmic) reticulum
Nucleus
ATP-dependent Na+-K+ pump

**FIGURE 7–2.** Cellular control of cytosolic free calcium concentrations. The cytosolic free calcium concentration $[Ca^{2+}]_f$ is a function of four mechanisms: (1) the rate of influx by diffusion across the plasma membrane; (2) the passage through agonist-dependent and voltage-dependent channels; (3) the rate of efflux by ATP-dependent extrusion (the calcium pump) and $Na^+/Ca^{2+}$ exchange; and (4) the intracellular sequestration by endoplasmic reticulum, mitochondria, or binding components. (From Wasserman, R.H.: *In* Calcium in Human Biology. Edited by B.E.C. Nordin. London, Springer-Verlag, 1988, p. 388.)

pumping calcium out of the cell by a calcium-dependent ATPase and $Na^+/Ca^{2+}$ exchange.

## CHANGES DURING THE LIFE SPAN

Table 7–1 provides an approximation, using values obtained from the literature, of total body calcium, rates of calcium deposition or transfer, and recommended calcium intakes during the life span. The newborn human contains 0.75 mol (30 g) of calcium, which increases to 25 to 30 mmol (1000 to 1200 g) by adulthood. To accumulate this amount, daily retention from the diet is approximately 2.5 to 3.7 mmol (100 to 150 mg) during childhood, peaking at 5 mmol (200 mg) for females to at least 7 mmol (280 mg) per day for males during puberty, and falling to 0.25 to 0.75 mmol per day (10 to 30 mg per day) during early adulthood.[21] Retention tends to become negative in women after menopause, and in men around age 65. Calcium balance is positive during pregnancy and negative during lactation.

### *INFANCY*

In the newborn rat, calcium is probably absorbed by a pinocytotic process because the vitamin D–dependent transcellular route is not operational.[22] A predominantly passive diffusion process has also been suggested to occur in the human infant because calcium intake and absorption are linearly related at least up to intakes of 7.5 mmol/kg per day (300 mg/kg per day).[23] Compared to the equivalent rate of loss in adults, endogenous fecal calcium in premature infants is several times higher, urinary calcium is lower and substantially less than endogenous, and the rate of true absorption is greater.[24] On a daily basis, full-term infants need to absorb about 3.1 mmol (125 mg) to cover a skeletal calcium deposition of 2.5 mmol (100 mg) and a urinary excretion that increases from 0.15 mmol (6 mg) at birth to 0.625 mmol (25 mg) at 1 year.

### *CHILDHOOD AND ADOLESCENCE*

Because bone mass is about 10 mol (400 g) by the end of childhood (10 to 12 years), daily accumulation from birth must average around 2.5 mmol (100 mg). Data are lacking on the absorptive efficiency of younger children. The growth spurt of adolescence involves a peak daily gain of 5 to 10 mmol (200 to 400 mg) or about an average of 6.25 mmol (250 mg) between 12 and 18 years. The total body calcium of boys is about 9 mol (360 g) at 10 years and 22.5 mol (900 g) at 20 years; for girls these values are about 7.2 mol (290 g) and 17.5 mol (700 g), respectively.[25] Isotope studies in teenagers past the growth spurt show an absorptive efficiency of 26% for calcium as carbonate and 41% when given as calcium-citrate-malate,[26] which is similar to the 30% absorbed in adults. Daily urinary losses of adolescents are high, 4.5 to 5.5 mmol (180 to 220 mg), and so a daily calcium intake of 30 mmol (1200 mg) is recommended to cover obligatory losses and optimal retention. Bone mass, which may continue to accumulate up to age 30, may be adversely affected by inade-

**TABLE 7–1.** BODY CONTENT, RATE OF TRANSFER, AND RECOMMENDED DIETARY ALLOWANCES OF CALCIUM DURING THE LIFE SPAN

| GROUP | BODY CALCIUM (G) | RATE OF DEPOSITION OR TRANSFER (MG/D)* | RECOMMENDED INTAKE (MG/D)† |
|---|---|---|---|
| VLBW infant | 8–20 | 100‡ | 160‡ |
| Term infant | 30 | 100 | 400–600 |
| 10 y female | 290 | 100–150 | 800 |
| 10 y male | 360 | 100–150 | 800 |
| Adolescent female§ | 425 | 200 | 1200 |
| Adolescent male§ | 520 | 280–400 | 1200 |
| 18 y female | 630–700 | 50 | 1200 |
| 18 y male | 820–900 | 100 | 1200 |
| Mature female | 920–1000 | 0 | 800 |
| Early postmenopausal female | 920–1000 | −30–−100 | 800 |
| Mature male | 1200 | 0 | 800 |
| 60 y female | 820 | −20 | 800 |
| Midpregnancy | 920–1000 | 50 | 1200 |
| Late pregnancy | 920–1000 | 330 | 1200 |
| Lactation‖ | | 240–300 | 1200 |

VLBW = very low birthweight

*Rate of deposition in bone, or of transfer to fetus (in pregnancy) or milk (lactation).

†Recommended Dietary Allowances, except when noted in table.

‡Units are mg/kg/d.

§Adolescence values are during the period of peak growth rate.

‖May be a temporary bone calcium loss of approximately 50 g.

quate calcium intakes during adolescence and early adulthood.[27]

### *PREGNANCY*

During pregnancy there are changes in maternal calcium-regulating hormones and in the intestinal absorption, renal reabsorption, and bone turnover of calcium.[28,29] Total serum calcium falls gradually during pregnancy, paralleling serum albumin and reflecting hemodilution. Serum ionic calcium changes are negligible. The older literature reported an increase in maternal total PTH, but more recent studies show that levels of intact, biologically active PTH fall to about half of those in nonpregnant women. Calcitonin levels rise early in pregnancy and may afford some protection to the maternal skeleton. Prolactin levels increase 10 to 20 times in pregnancy. This hormone can mobilize bone calcium and may play an as yet unidentified important role in calcium metabolism in human pregnancy. A calcium-mobilizing hormone that is similar to PTH, called PTH-related peptide (PTHRP), has been found in the human mammary gland and stimulates calcium transport in sheep placenta. No role in human pregnancy has yet been identified for PTHRP.

A single study using stable isotopes observed true absorption of calcium to increase from 27% prior to pregnancy, to 54% at 5 to 6 months of gestation and 42% at term.[30] By measuring fetal calcium it can be calculated that daily placental transfer must be about 1.25 mmol (50 mg) at 20 weeks of gestation and 8.3 mmol (330 mg) at 35 weeks. Balance studies show that the increase in maternal calcium retention is insufficient to supply all the calcium transferred to the fetus. The 0.75 mol (30 g) of calcium in the newborn is equivalent to only 2.5% of maternal skeletal calcium, so changes in the latter are difficult to detect. However, a rise in serum osteocalcin and urinary hydroxyproline suggest that some is drawn from maternal bones later in pregnancy.[29] To date there is no evidence that low calcium intakes during pregnancy are harmful to the mother or fetus even after multiple births. Maternal vitamin D deficiency occurs relatively commonly in Europe. This induces maternal osteomalacia, neonatal hypocalcemia and tetany, and tooth enamel hypoplasia. Thus, it appears that the calcium status of the mother and fetus is more affected by maternal vitamin D status than by calcium status.

### *LACTATION*

Maternal calcium intake has no effect on the amount of calcium secreted in breast milk. A woman who produces 750 ml of milk daily for 6 months loses twice as much calcium as in pregnancy—about 1.25 mol (50 g) or 5% of her body calcium. The source of this calcium is unclear. Although intestinal absorption of calcium increases in lactating rats, a single study of women failed to find this increase. Urinary calcium levels are lower. Bone turnover may be higher, as suggested by higher serum osteocalcin levels early in lactation, although serum PTH and calcium are unchanged. Involvement of maternal bone is supported by reports of acute bone demineralization during lactation and recovery post lactation.[31] Although not proven, high prolactin and low estrogen levels in lactation might be responsible for the bone mobilization. The rate of bone loss may be faster in lactating adolescents, in whom it is accompanied by increases in PTH and calcitonin and prevented to some extent by high calcium intakes.[32] The literature is inconclusive concerning the effect of the extent and number of lactations on peak adult bone mass and later risk of osteoporosis.

### *AGING*

There is considerable debate about whether calcium requirements increase with aging in adults. There is frequently a rise in fasting urinary calcium of 20%, reflecting a slight increase in complexed and ultrafiltrable serum calcium. There is some support for the hypothesis that osteoporosis results from the higher urine calcium combined with impaired intestinal absorption.[33]

Several studies have shown that intestinal calcium absorption is decreased in senescent animals and humans. These age-related changes have been explained on the basis of decreased circulating levels of $1,25(OH)_2D$. However, a recent study in healthy women aged 26 to 88 years found that intestinal calcium absorption from the diet did not decrease with age.[34] Moreover, serum $1,25(OH)_2D$ levels increased until about age 65. These data are consistent with a model of intestinal resistance to $1,25(OH)_2D$ and compensatory increases in serum $1,25(OH)_2D$ and PTH to prevent decreases in intestinal calcium absorption. The secondary hyperparathyroidism leads to increased bone turnover and age-related bone loss.

## DIETARY CONSIDERATIONS

The Nationwide Food Consumption Survey of the late 1970s found that calcium intakes were 18.6 mmol (743 mg) daily on average for all people. Approximately 60% of children up to 5 years of age and 40% aged 6 to 11 years had a daily intake below 20 mmol (800 mg). Eighty to 85% of female and 50 to 65% of male adolescents had daily intakes below the recommended level of 30 mmol (1200 mg).[35] Adolescent boys had the highest daily intakes, 29.5 mmol (1179 mg). The lowest daily intakes were 7.3 mmol (530 mg) for women 35 to 50 years of age, with white women consuming more (16 mmol, or 640 mg) than blacks (11.3 mmol or 452 mg), who eat fewer dairy products. No group of women met the Recommended Dietary Allowance (RDA) for calcium on average.

*SOURCES OF DIETARY CALCIUM*

Just over half of the calcium intake of the United States population is from dairy products. Other sources include some green vegetables such as broccoli, nuts, corn tortillas processed with lime, tofu precipitated with calcium, and soft bones of fish. Bioavailability from some nondairy sources is poor. More recently, calcium-fortified foods such as orange juice and flour, and antacids containing calcium, have become important contributors to the intake of some individuals.

*BIOAVAILABILITY*

The absorbability of calcium is mainly determined by the presence of other food constituents (Table 7–2), and the physiologic or nutritional status of the host.[36] Somewhat surprisingly, the solubility of the dominant chemical form of calcium in specific foods, or of calcium supplements, has a negligible effect on calcium absorbability from these sources.[37,38] During the absorption of calcium oxalate there is no tracer exchange, suggesting that absorption occurs without dissociation of the molecule.[39] Likewise, relatively soluble salts such as citrate or citrate-malate bind their calcium tightly, and their solubility is not related to their absorbability. Thus, the form in which the calcium approaches the mucosal brush border and in which it is transported by the paracellular route may be a better predictor of how well it is absorbed. The calcium from most supplements is absorbed as well as calcium in milk is, although absorption from calcium-citrate-malate (CCM) may be superior.

**Food Constituents that Increase Bioavailability.** Lactose enhances the absorption of calcium in animals. It increases the diffusional component of calcium and perhaps of phosphorus, especially in the ileum, and probably acts osmotically to alter the junctions between the epithelial cells.

The lactose in breast milk and formula improves calcium absorption in human infants. In one experiment calcium absorption from formula was 60% compared to 36% from lactose-free formula and 72% from formula treated with lactase.[40] The enhancement of absorption after lactase treatment can be ascribed to the fact that most metabolizable sugars enhance calcium absorption. Beyond infancy it is doubtful whether lactose improves the absorbability of calcium from dairy products. For example, in adults the absorption of calcium from yogurt is the same as that from milk, even though the lactose in yogurt is hydrolyzed in the stomach by lactase originating from the bacteria in the yogurt.[41] The higher prevalence of osteoporosis in lactose-intolerant individuals is more likely related to their low intake of dairy products than to a detrimental effect of lactose on their calcium absorption.

**TABLE 7–2.** DIETARY CONSTITUENTS AFFECTING CALCIUM BIOAVAILABILITY

| EFFECT ON ABSORPTION | DIETARY CONSTITUENT |
|---|---|
| Increase | Lactose (infants) |
| Decrease | Fiber |
| | Phytic acid |
| | Uronic acids |
| | Oxalic acid |
| No effect | Fat (except in steatorrhea) |
| | Protein |
| | Phosphorus |

**Food Constituents that Decrease Bioavailability.** Dietary fiber has such an adverse effect on calcium absorption in humans that it can impair calcium balance significantly.[36] Replacing white flour (22 g fiber per day) with whole wheat flour (53 g fiber per day) in a typical Western diet causes negative calcium balance even with calcium intakes above the RDA. A similar effect is caused by the fiber in fruits and vegetables.

Several constituents of fiber bind calcium. Uronic acids bind calcium strongly in vitro and may explain the inhibition of calcium absorption in humans by hemicellulose. Pectin does not affect calcium absorption in humans, probably because 80% of its uronic acids are methylated and cannot bind calcium. Theoretically a typical vegetarian diet contains sufficient uronic acids to bind 9 mmol (360 mg) calcium, but the majority of these acids are metabolized in the lower intestine so some of the calcium may be absorbable.

Phytic acid is the other major plant constituent that binds calcium. The high phytate content of wheat bran most likely explains its marked adverse effects on calcium absorption.[42] Interestingly, the addition of calcium to wheat dough decreases phytate degradation by 50% during fermentation and baking.[43] Wheat bran impairs calcium absorption to the extent that it has been used therapeutically in absorptive and idiopathic hypercalciurias.

Dark green, leafy vegetables are often relatively high in calcium. Absorption from many of these is expected to be good, if they are low in oxalic acid (e.g., kale, broccoli, turnip and mustard greens, collard). For example, absorption from kale is as good as from milk. The poor absorption of calcium from spinach (5% compared to 27% absorption from milk) has been attributed to its binding to oxalic acid in this plant. However, other factors may also be involved because calcium absorption from calcium oxalate is twice as high as that from spinach.[39] There is no interference of calcium oxalate with the absorption of calcium in milk when the two are consumed together.

**Fat, Protein, and Phosphorus.** Dietary fat has no effect on calcium balance in the healthy adult. Where there is malabsorption of fat (steatorrhea), calcium precipitates with fatty acids to form insoluble soaps in the intestinal lumen. Calcium soap formation in intestinal contents is affected by factors such as pancreatic lipases, the amount of ionized fatty acids, the chain length and saturation of fatty acids, calcium concentration, and monoglycerides.[44] Human infants absorb about 50% of the calcium in formulas based on cow's milk, compared to 65% from breast milk in which fat digestion and absorption are superior.

Although the calciuria induced by high-protein diets causes negative calcium balance in humans that lasts for at least 2 months, this is, surprisingly, not compensated by an increased efficiency of calcium absorption.[45] Neither dietary phosphorus level, nor the calcium/phosphorus ratio, affect calcium absorption in adults[46] or low-birth-weight infants.[47] In contrast, prolonged, continuous feeding of high-phosphorus diets results in hyperparathyroidism and secondary bone resorption.

**Nutrient-Nutrient Interactions.** Because calcium and iron supplements are both commonly recommended for women, interactions between these supplements are of concern. In one study, supplemental calcium carbonate and hydroxyapatite reduced iron absorption by about 50% in postmenopausal women.[48] In another, milk calcium (12.5 mmol, or 500 mg) inhibited the absorption of iron by 30%.[49] When taken with food, supplemental calcium in the form of carbonate, citrate, and phosphate inhibits iron absorption from a ferrous sulphate supplement, from dietary nonheme iron,[50] and from heme iron.[44] However, when taken without food, calcium carbonate does not inhibit the absorption of iron from ferrous sulfate even when supplements contain 15 mmol (600 mg) calcium and 321 μmol (18 mg) iron. Substantial (about 50%) inhibition of iron absorption by calcium citrate and phosphate persists. Thus, taking calcium supplements with meals has a substantial impact on iron absorption. Because the absorption of both heme and nonheme iron is affected, calcium probably affects the intracellular transfer of iron by the enterocyte rather than through a luminal effect. Addition of calcium to wheat dough reduces phytate degradation during fermentation and baking by 50%, reducing iron absorption from the bread.[44]

More recently there has been interest in CCM (a combination of calcium carbonate, citric acid, and malic acid, 5:1:1 mol/mol/mol) as a source of supplemental calcium that is well absorbed. In humans, CCM lowers iron absorption by 30% but not when the CCM is consumed with orange juice.[49] The citric and ascorbic acids in orange juice may be the constituents that alleviate CCM's inhibition of iron absorption, by increasing iron solubility.

Calcium supplements impair the absorption of magnesium by rats, but the results of human studies have been inconsistent. In a recent report, the addition of 22.5 mmol (900 mg) of calcium daily as milk, chloride, or carbonate had no effect on magnesium retention in humans.[5] Daily intakes of calcium above 50 mmol (2000 mg) do not impair zinc absorption or balance.[52]

## CALCIUM DEFICIENCY

When calcium absorbed from the diet is insufficient to balance obligatory fecal and urinary losses, the mineral is drawn from bone to maintain the plasma (ionic) calcium concentration and protect levels of intracellular calcium and the neuromuscular system. While the efficiency of calcium absorption increases when intakes are low, there is a limit to which this can offset body calcium loss. Some balance studies on adult women show that, on average, 13.7 mmol (550 mg) daily is needed to prevent negative calcium balance,[53] whereas other studies suggest this value should be higher. Older individuals may need even higher intakes to stay in balance because their ability to increase their fractional calcium absorption may be impaired.

### *EFFECT ON CALCIUM ABSORPTION*

In general, the efficiency (fractional absorption) of calcium absorption varies inversely with calcium intake. At low daily calcium intakes, below 12.5 mmol (500 mg), absorption is predominantly by active transport.

Chronic dietary calcium restriction is generally believed to increase fractional intestinal calcium absorption by stimulating PTH secretion, which in turn enhances renal $1,25(OH)_2D_3$ synthesis, resulting in increased serum levels of $1,25(OH)_2D_3$. There is also evidence that $1,25(OH)_2D_3$ levels are regulated independently of serum PTH and phosphorus, directly through serum ionized calcium,[54] so that hypocalcemia stimulates $1,25(OH)_2$ synthesis directly.

When calcium intake of human subjects is reduced abruptly from a high or adequate to a low level, within 1 week there is an increase in serum PTH and $1,25(OH)_2D$, an increase in the fractional retention of an oral $^{47}Ca$ dose of about 50%, and a reduction in urinary calcium.[55] Although the early rises in $1,25(OH)_2D$ and calcium retention are probably causally related, the higher levels of the vitamin D metabolite do not persist after 1 week.[55,56] Thus the increased calcium retention, which occurs for at least 2 months after a low-calcium diet is consumed, is independent of $1,25(OH)_2D$-stimulated active transport and may be due to an unidentified factor that stimulates active calcium transport.

In the elderly, the adaptive response to low calcium intake is less dramatic. When subjects were changed from a daily intake of 50 mmol (2000 mg) to 7.5 mmol (300 mg) of calcium intake for 1 to 2 months, absorption increased by 66% in young women (22 to 31 years) but only by 50% in an older group (age 61 to 75).[57] The reasons for this are not understood.

### *EFFECT ON GROWTH*

Severe calcium deficiency limits the growth of rats. Although several epidemiologic studies have suggested associations between children's growth rate and calcium fortification or the consumption of milk, the general conclusion is that growth is not limited by calcium deficiency. The strongest evidence in support of this conclusion is the failure of supplemental calcium and phosphorus to affect the growth rate of calcium- and phosphorus-deficient very-low-birth-weight or premature infants.[58]

### *EFFECT ON PEAK BONE MASS*

Life-long calcium intake may have a significant impact on peak bone mineral density at maturity. Women's reported consumption of calcium during adolescence[27] or since the age of 20 years[59] is a predictor of their peak bone mineral content. In a comparison of regions of low versus adequate calcium intake in Yugoslavia, from at least 30 years of age bone mass of both men and women was related to usual calcium intake.[60]

### *EFFECT ON BONE LOSS OF AGING*

After many years of study, the role of dietary calcium in the causation and treatment of osteoporosis is still the focus of intense debate. Among the reasons for this debate are the complex nature of osteoporosis and, until recently, the low sensitivity with which bone mineral density could be measured. Certainly the rather abrupt changes in bone and calcium metabolism that accompany menopause cannot be attributed to an abrupt decrease in calcium intake or absorption. The question is whether higher intakes before or after menopause can improve peak bone mass or slow the rate of loss with aging. The reader is referred to Chapter 89 on osteoporosis for more detailed information.

A number of investigators have noted a lack of association between current calcium intake and bone mineral density at the mid radius and lumbar spine.[61,62] On the other hand, as discussed above, a significant relationship has been observed between an individual's lifetime history of calcium intake and peak bone mineral content. A higher bone mineral content delays the time at which symptoms of bone loss develop, but does not change the rate of loss.[60]

In designing clinical trials to test the effects of dietary calcium or supplements on bone loss, it is essential to account for factors such as the age, menopausal status, serum estrogen levels, vitamin D status, smoking, parity and lactation history, history of oral contraceptive use, usual calcium intake, and usual level of activity of the participants. Investigations have been inconsistent in the bone sites monitored and the levels of calcium administered.

In spite of these problems, a number of clinical trials—but not all—have found that calcium supplements slow the loss of bone from the appendicular skeleton of postmenopausal women. However, estrogen alone is usually more effective.[63] More recently it has become apparent that calcium carbonate supplements, providing as much as 50 mmol (2000 mg) of calcium per day, slow the rate of loss of cortical bone (such as the proximal forearm) more than that of trabecular bone (lumbar spine).[64,65] Unfortunately most fractures occur in trabecular bone.

Calcium supplements may only protect against bone loss in those women whose usual diet contains relatively low amounts of calcium.[66] Supplements were effective at maintaining skeletal calcium in women more than 6 years after menopause and not receiving estrogen.[67] Calcium-citrate-malate (12.5 mmol, or 500 mg per day) was more beneficial than calcium carbonate, and was even effective in the spine. Neither supplement altered the rate of bone mineral loss in the women who already had reasonable calcium intakes—that is, 10 to 16.25 mmol (400 to 650 mg) per day.

### *OTHER EFFECTS OF DEFICIENCY*

Secondary vitamin D deficiency may result from calcium deprivation. Feeding rats a very-low-calcium diet (0.014%) results in undetectable levels of plasma 25(OH)D.[68] By using low-calcium diets or phytate to reduce the amount of calcium absorbed by rats, inactivation of 25(OH)D in the liver is increased.[69] The mechanism may be mediated by the additional $1,25(OH)_2D_3$ produced in response to secondary hyperparathyroidism. The half-life of the 25(OH)D falls from 15.4 to 9.2 days because of its hepatic conversion to polar inactivation products that are excreted in bile. In one study, a high-fiber diet in humans reduced the 25(OH)D half-life from 27 to 19 days.[70] This may contribute to the vitamin D deficiency that occurs in clinical disorders involving calcium malabsorption, such as gastrointestinal disease.

## ASSESSMENT OF CALCIUM STATUS

In experimental animals severely restricted in dietary calcium, the following effects are consistently observed: hypocalcemia, increased serum levels of PTH and $1,25(OH)_2D_3$, a higher fractional absorption of calcium and phosphate, and lower calcium but higher phosphate in urine. Bone resorption and turnover are stimulated, and decreased bone mineralization ensues. To some extent these deficiency manifestations are found in premature or very low-birth-weight infants whose high calcium (and phosphorus) requirements are not met. In older individuals calcium status is difficult to assess, because the above changes are rarely found before menopause. Serum total and ionic calcium levels are tightly controlled; low levels are usually explainable by low serum albumin to which some calcium is bound, rather than by calcium deficiency.

Abnormal biochemical values are not necessarily proof of a *dietary* calcium deficiency, unless they are normalized by feeding supplemental calcium; vitamin D deficiency, bone diseases, and other hormonal imbalances can produce similar biochemical abnormalities. Urinary hydroxyproline is positively related to bone resorption.

In osteoporotics, the administration of calcium rapidly suppresses urinary hydroxyproline in patients who can absorb calcium, but fails to do so in those who cannot.[33] Urinary nephrogenous cyclic AMP (NCAMP) is increased in response to a higher production of PTH, and calcium supplementation of patients with osteoporosis lowers NCAMP in urine. Although serum osteocalcin (bone gla-protein, BGP) levels are a specific marker for bone formation and turnover, consumption for 1 month of a low (10 mmol or 400 mg per day) calcium diet by young women failed to increase osteocalcin levels in one study.[56]

Calcium balance data provide information on whether the current level of calcium absorption is sufficient to replace calcium excreted in urine, sweat, and endogenous intestinal secretions. If an individual is in negative balance, calcium is being lost from bone. However, balance studies provide no information on the extent to which bone calcium has been lost in the past. Even when calcium balance is positive, as during growth and pregnancy, it may be less than is needed for optimal mineralization. Bone mineral content is a reflection of long-term calcium balance, although the primary problem may or may not be dietary in origin. The sensitivity of techniques for measuring bone loss has improved dramatically in recent years. However, because many factors affect the bone mineral content of an individual, it is usually important to measure changes over time and the effects of supplemental calcium on these changes.

## REQUIREMENTS AND RECOMMENDED DIETARY ALLOWANCES

Recommended intakes are based on the amount of dietary calcium required to replace losses in endogenous intestinal secretions, urine, and sweat, allowing for the efficiency of intestinal absorption.

Breast-fed infants consume on average 6 mmol (240 mg) of calcium per day from 750 ml of breast milk, of which they absorb two thirds. Adding 25% to cover variability in individual requirements means that an average daily intake of 7.5 mmol (300 mg) would be needed, with 5 mmol (200 mg) being absorbed. Absorption of calcium is poorer, closer to 50%, from formulas based on cow's milk, so these are designed to provide 10 mmol (400 mg) per day. The daily RDA for infants is set at 10 mmol (400 mg) for the first 6 months, 15 mmol (600 mg) for 6 to 12 months, and 20 mmol (800 mg) from 1 to 10 years of age.[71]

The RDAs for adolescents and adults are under considerable debate. The 1989 subcommittee took the position that the RDAs for adults should not be revised upward from 20 mmol (800 mg) per day in response to medical concern about the high proportion of postmenopausal women at risk for osteoporosis; persons who have this condition should receive medical attention and their need for supplemental calcium evaluated as part of their treatment. The adult RDA is based on an obligatory loss in urine, sweat, and endogenous daily secretion that averages 5 to 6.4 mmol (200 to 250 mg), and a gastrointestinal absorption of 30 to 40%.

The subcommittee was more convinced that adequate calcium during the period of bone mineralization is important if peak adult bone mass is to be attained. Because peak bone mass does not occur before 25 years of age, recommended daily intakes were increased to 30 mmol (1200 mg) from 11 to 24 years, in both males and females.

The newborn contains about 0.75 mmol (30 g) of calcium, mostly deposited during the third trimester of pregnancy[28] when it is transferred at the rate of 6.25 mmol (250 mg) per day. Calcium secretion in human milk is at most 7.5 mmol (300 mg) per day. Thus, the daily RDA is 30 mmol (1200 mg) during pregnancy and lactation. For women under 25 years of age this represents no increase, but as discussed under the earlier section "Changes During the Life Span," detrimental effects of low-calcium intakes during pregnancy have not yet been demonstrated.

## TOXICITY

No adverse effects have been found with the ingestion of calcium supplements providing as much as 60 mmol (2400 mg) daily, except constipation in some individuals. However, there should be concern about the effect of calcium supplements on iron absorption. Daily intakes above 60 mmol (2400 mg) may impair renal function. Calcium supplementation carries no increased risk for stone formation in normal adults, but may do so in patients with absorptive or renal hypercalciuria, primary hyperparathyroidism, and sarcoidosis. It should also be recognized, however, that the efficiency of absorption from large doses is relatively poor.

## CLINICAL DISORDERS INVOLVING CALCIUM

Clinical disorders involving calcium can be categorized as those in which absorption is excessive or impaired, requirements are high, or supplementation may prevent the onset or symptoms of disease. Osteoporosis is a clinical disorder involving calcium among other factors. This is discussed in detail in Chapter 89.

### *INTESTINAL MALABSORPTION*

A number of intestinal disorders are characterized by calcium malabsorption as well as by vitamin D deficiency and osteomalacia. These include gastrointestinal diseases such as Crohn's and celiac disease, and intestinal resection or bypass. Calcium and vitamin D depletion have been attributed by various investigators to malabsorption, steatorrhea, inadequate oral intake, or a combination of these. A more recent explanation for the low levels of 25(OH)D is the increased hepatic inactivation of this metabolite by the higher levels of $1,25(OH)_2D$ that occur in response to calcium malabsorption.[69]

### IDIOPATHIC HYPERCALCIURIA AND CALCIUM NEPHROLITHIASIS

Most patients with calcium kidney stones have idiopathic hypercalciuria (IH). About 90% of IH cases are characterized by elevated active calcium absorption identifiable by a high urinary calcium-to-creatinine ratio after a calcium load, normal serum calcium and PTH, and elevated serum $1,25(OH)_2D_3$. The vitamin D elevation may be the primary defect, and is associated with a renal phosphate leak.[72] For reasons that are not completely understood, renal stone formers exhibit a lower bone mineral content. Possible explanations are the hypophosphatemia, hypercalciuria, and elevated serum $1,25(OH)_2D_3$ accompanied by a low calcium intake. Unfortunately, maintenance of stone-formers on a low-calcium diet may exacerbate this bone loss.[73] Oral treatment with sodium cellulose phosphate may restore normal absorption, urinary excretion, and calcium balance by binding the mineral in the intestine.

### DISTURBED INTESTINAL ABSORPTION

Excessive intestinal absorption and hypercalcemia occur in sarcoidosis (because of enhanced extrarenal $1,25(OH)_2D_3$ production) and are treatable by adrenocorticosteroid therapy. Elevated $1,25(OH)_2D_3$ also explains hyperabsorption in primary hyperparathyroidism. Impairment of calcium absorption is caused by the reduced synthesis of $1,25(OH)_2D_3$ in chronic renal failure, and hypoparathyroidism.

### PREMATURE AND VERY LOW-BIRTH-WEIGHT INFANTS

Because the daily in utero accretion rates of calcium and phosphorus are 2.5 and 1.9 mmol/kg (100 and 60 mg/kg), respectively, postpartum daily intakes for normal bone mineralization in preterm infants, allowing for absorption, need to be 4 mmol/kg (160 mg/kg) for calcium and 2.4 mmol/kg (75 mg/kg) for phosphorus.[74] For those who are parenterally nourished this amounts to 12.5 to 15 mmol/L (500 to 600 mg/L) of calcium and 12.9 to 14.5 mmol/L (400 to 450 mg/L) of phosphorus, assuming an average daily fluid intake of 120 to 150 ml.[75] The requirements cannot be achieved by feeding breast milk, unless it is fortified with these two minerals or with regular infant formulas. Intakes higher than these lead to calcium and phosphorus solubility problems. Fortification needs to continue even after the infants are discharged to the home.[58] Special preterm formulas are also available that contain high levels of calcium and phosphorus from which up to 85% of the calcium is absorbed.

### HYPERTENSION

A number of population surveys provide correlational evidence that the usual intake of calcium is inversely related to blood pressure. In addition, calcium supplementation can lower blood pressure in both normotensive and hypertensive rats and humans. Patients with essential hypertension and low levels of renin, the renal pressor hormone, demonstrate abnormal calcium metabolism (higher PTH, higher $1,25(OH)_2D$ that is suppressed by oral calcium, low calcitonin and serum ionized calcium) compared to other hypertensives and normal individuals. The low-renin subjects are those who respond consistently to calcium supplements with lowered blood pressure. In addition, only those hypertensives whose blood pressure rises significantly in response to high salt intake show salt-induced increases in $1,25(OH)_2D$ and reductions in serum ionized calcium.[76] Thus low plasma renin, dietary salt sensitivity, and altered calcium metabolism are predictors of a depressor response to supplemental calcium. Other hypertensives may fail to benefit from oral calcium. The renin-aldosterone system and calcium-regulating hormones, particularly $1,25(OH)_2D_3$, may work in a coordinated way to mediate the effects of dietary minerals on blood pressure, through altering the distribution of calcium between intracellular and extracellular compartments.[76] Other mechanisms have been suggested,[77] including a direct effect of calcium-regulating hormones on calcium transport in vascular smooth muscle cells, and a reduced sympathetic outflow from the brain.

### COLON CANCER

Data from a large number of epidemiologic surveys in different countries support the hypothesis that intakes of calcium that meet or slightly exceed the RDA are protective against colon cancer.[78] However, the complexity of human diets precludes confirmation of the correctness of this hypothesis by studying intake of normal foods. For example, higher intakes of calcium from dairy products are usually associated with more fat, protein, vitamin D (where milk is fortified with this vitamin), phosphorus, and riboflavin. Nevertheless, several clinical trials showed a reduction in cell proliferation in the colonic mucosa when calcium supplements were given to subjects at high risk of developing colon cancer.[79] One mechanism by which supplements may be effective is by increasing the concentration of intraluminal calcium ions and calcium phosphate, both of which can precipitate bile acids or fatty acids that can stimulate epithelial cell proliferation in the colon.[80]

## PHOSPHORUS

Phosphorus is an important mineral constituent of the Earth's crust. In soil, phosphorus is commonly found as the inorganic apatite moiety; in water, phosphorus is present as orthophosphate. A small portion of the total phosphorus in water is soluble and available to plants and microorganisms, which incorporate phosphorus into a variety of organic molecules. Organisms higher in the food chain can readily utilize organophosphates obtained from these food sources. In 1862, Hoppe-Seyler noted the striking similarity between the relative amounts of calcium and phosphorus in bone to that of natural mineralogic apatite crystals and hypothesized that bone mineral had a similar apatite-like chemical structure.[81]

## PHOSPHORUS CHEMISTRY AND NOMENCLATURE

Chemically, phosphorus can exist in a variety of oxidation states, ranging from −3 to +5 ($PH_3$ to $P_2O_5$), and can form relatively stable chemical bonds with a wide variety of elements. From the biochemical point of view, however, compounds of phosphorus and oxygen (oxidation state +5) are predominant because of considerations of thermodynamic stability of phosphorus compounds in water.[82] Thus, *phosphate,* rather than phosphorus per se, becomes the center of attention in nutritional biochemistry. Phosphoric acid, $H_3PO_4$, is a strong acid. Monovalent cations, such as sodium, potassium, and ammonium can form highly soluble phosphate salts; whereas, divalent cations, such as calcium and magnesium, form relatively insoluble phosphate compounds.

The general formula for apatite compounds in nature is $M_{10}(RO_4)_6X_2$; where $M_{10}$ can represent a variety of metals, including lead, although in the most abundant natural apatites this metal is usually calcium or magnesium. The $RO_4^{-3}$ group in natural apatites is usually $PO_4^{-3}$. The last radical group ($X_2$) can be $F_2$, $Cl_2$, $Br_2$, $(OH)_2$, or carbonate. The name of the apatite compound is derived from this last radical group; for example, in vertebrate bone the calcium and phosphate containing-apatite form is called hydroxyapatite [$Ca_{10}(PO_4)_6(OH)_2$].

Phosphorus in extracellular fluid accounts for only 1% of the total phosphorus in the body. The majority (70%) of total phosphorus in human plasma is found as a constituent of organic phospholipids. However, the clinically useful fraction in plasma is the total *inorganic* phosphorus concentration. Ten percent of the circulating inorganic phosphorus is bound to protein, 5% is complexed with calcium or magnesium, and the majority of plasma inorganic phosphorus is found as $H_2PO_4^-$ and $HPO_4^{-2}$. These two orthophosphate fractions are found at pH 7.4 in the ratio of 1:4. The fact that plasma inorganic phosphorus is found as both a monovalent and divalent anion can lead to some confusion as to the relationship between various measurement units for plasma phosphorus. The apparent valence of plasma phosphorus at pH 7.4 is negative 1.8, because nine negative charges are associated with 5 mmol of phosphorus. Plasma phosphorus in the amount of 3.1 mg/dl equals 1 mmole/L, but 1.8 mEq/L.[83]

## METABOLISM

The metabolism of phosphorus in the body represents a complex interplay between various factors that can affect the digestion, absorption, distribution, and excretion of this element.

### *DIGESTION*

Insoluble mineral phosphate salts are formed at elevated pH. The acidic milieu of the stomach (pH=2) and most proximal part of the small intestine (pH=5) may play an important role in maintaining the luminal solubility and bioavailability of inorganic phosphorus. In this regard, the potential effects of hypochlorhydria, commonly found in the elderly and in patients on anti-ulcer medications, on the solubility and bioavailability of phosphorus needs further investigation.

In vegetarian diets a large part of the dietary phosphorus may be in the form of phytate. Animals and humans do not possess the enzyme phytase, which is necessary to degrade phytate and liberate phosphorus. However, prokaryotes such as yeasts and bacteria contain phytase. This curiosity of nature is important to human phosphorus nutrition for two reasons; first, the traditional use of yeast in breadmaking liberates some phosphorus from the phytate moiety because of the hydrolytic action of yeast phytases prior to baking[84]; second, intestinal bacteria, which are normally located in the large intestine, can break down some dietary phytate. Germ-free rats and chicks are unable to hydrolyze dietary phytates.[88] Addition of phytase, derived from Aspergillus niger, to chicken and pig rations has a marked positive effect on dietary phosphorus bioavailability from grains.[85] Phytate is poorly digested in the human gastrointestinal tract.[86] Deactivation of endogenous phytase activity in wheat bran results in complete inhibition of phytate digestion in humans who have undergone ileostomy. In contrast, about half the phytate is broken down when the food contained endogenous phytate activity. Soaking grains in water can effectively remove phytate from some foods; for example, 99.6% of the phytate in beans (Phaseolus vulgaris) can be extracted by soaking in water.[87] Milling of grains can remove the outer bran layers, which contain significant amounts of phytate in some cereals. However, these treatments also reduce the phosphorus and mineral content of the food. Prior soaking and germination of sorghum grains, and subsequent fermentation of the flour, can markedly reduce the concentration of pentainositol and hexainositol phosphates[88] and could be important in improving the mineral bioavailability of infant gruels in developing countries and of diets in general. The issue of adaptation to diets high in phytate continues to be raised,[86] but it was recently reported that the inhibitory effects of phytate on iron absorption were still observed in subjects who had been consuming high-phytate diets for many years.[89]

Other organic forms of phosphorus in the diet are primarily derived from typical cellular phosphorus-containing compounds, such as phospholipids and phosphorylated sugars. These compounds are believed to be digested in the intestine to liberate inorganic phosphate, which is transported across the intestinal cell.

*ABSORPTION*

About 60 to 70% of phosphorus is absorbed from a typical mixed diet.[90] Phosphorus absorption in humans has been shown to be linearly related to phosphorus intake over the range of 0.13 to 1 mmol/kg body weight (4 to 30 mg/kg) per day. Physiologic conditions associated with life cycle changes, such as growth, pregnancy, and lactation, are associated with increased phosphorus need and a corresponding increase in phosphorus absorption. In old age changes in phosphorus excretion and adaptation to dietary phosphorus are known to occur.[91] Negative phosphorus balance (2.2 mmol, or 68 mg per day) has been reported in geriatric nursing home patients (65 to 85 years old) even though they were consuming recommended dietary intakes of phosphorus.[92] In this group of subjects, who were not consuming antacids, net fractional phosphorus absorption was 34% and daily urinary phosphorus losses were 10.3 mmol (320 mg).

The cellular and molecular mechanism of intestinal phosphorus absorption is not well understood.[93] Transport of phosphorus across the intestinal cell is by an active, sodium-dependent pathway. Intestinal phosphorus absorption represents the sum of a saturable, carrier-mediated component and a nonsaturable, concentration-dependent component. The apparent affinity ($K_t$) of the saturable phosphorus transport component in the intestine is 2 mmol/L.[94] The kinetics of phosphorus uptake by intestinal brush border vesicle preparations are consistent with the suggestion that phosphorus is transported by a carrier-mediated mechanism.[95] Intracellular phosphorus levels are relatively high and the cell interior is electronegative; thus, it is probable that an active transport process is necessary to get phosphorus into the cell, but that phosphorus may exit the cell by diffusion. A 145-kd polypeptide has been putatively identified as the brush border, sodium-sensitive phosphorus transporter.[96]

Parathyroid hormone does not appear to play a direct role in regulating the absorption of phosphorus across the intestine.[83] Administration of the active metabolite of vitamin D, 1,25$(OH)_2$D, leads to an increase in phosphorus absorption in both normal subjects and uremic patients.[97] Administration of 1,25$(OH)_2$D to rats increases phosphorus absorption in all segments of the small intestine, although the major effect occurs in the jejunum. In contrast, the duodenum is the most responsive site of vitamin D–mediated calcium transport. The steroid-like action of 1,25$(OH)_2$D occurs through a cascade of genome-mediated events.[98] However, 1,25$(OH)_2$D may also have rapid nongenomic effects on some cellular events.[99] Direct in-vitro treatment of isolated rat duodenal enterocytes with 1,25$(OH)_2$D can cause a rapid, cycloheximide-insensitive increase in the rate of phosphorus uptake.[100]

*STORAGE*

Phosphorus is found in all cells and is the sixth most abundant element in the body. The total body content of phosphorus has been assessed by in-vivo neutron activation analysis to be about 16 mol (500 g) in males and 13 mol (400 g) in females.[101] The primary tissue sites of phosphorus storage are in bone hydroxyapatite (85%) and skeletal muscle (14%).

## HOMEOSTATIC REGULATION

Plasma phosphorus reflects the net rate of phosphorus flux between intestine, kidney, bone, and soft tissue. The kidney is the primary regulator of the plasma phosphorus level by altering the rate of phosphorus reabsorption of the filtered phosphorus load. At low renal phosphorus loads essentially all of the filtered phosphorus is reabsorbed and none is excreted in the urine. As the amount of phosphorus in the glomerular filtrate increases the capacity of the renal reabsorptive apparatus is exceeded and phosphorus appears incrementally in the urine. This threshold level, commonly referred to as the TmP/GFR, represents the maximum mass of phosphorus transported (i.e., reabsorbed), or TmP, per unit of filtrate volume, or GFR. The absolute value of TmP/GFR represents the concentration of phosphorus in the reabsorbed fluid that is being returned to the circulation.[83]

Regulation of total body phosphorus over long periods requires the coordinated efforts of the kidney and intestine. Under conditions of low dietary phosphorus intake the intestine must increase its absorptive efficiency to maximize phosphorus absorption and the kidney must increase renal phosphorus transport to minimize urinary phosphorus losses. Hormonally these adaptations result from changes in plasma levels of 1,25$(OH)_2$D and PTH. If these adaptative measures fail to adequately compensate for the lower dietary phosphorus, then bone phosphorus may be initially redistributed to the soft tissues to allow tissue growth to continue. Eventually, however, growth will be limited by the restricted phosphorus supply.

## EXCRETION

Reports of endogenous fecal losses of phosphorus have been variable, ranging between 0.03 and 0.14 mmol/kg (0.9 and 4 mg/kg) per day.[83] The kidneys provide the primary route for phosphorus excretion. The vast majority of the phosphorus in the plasma is filtered at the renal glomerulus, and none is believed to be secreted into the nephron. The fractional excretion of filtered phosphorus can be varied by the kidney from 0.1 to 20%—hence its ability to efficiently regulate plasma phosphorus. About 40% of the total phosphorus reabsorption in the kidney occurs within the first few convolutions of the proximal tubule, and 60 to 70% occurs by the time the ultrafiltrate reaches the last segment of the cortical superficial nephrons. The transport of phosphorus in the renal tubules occurs by two processes. In the proximal tubule an active, sodium-dependent phosphorus transport system has been described. A sodium-independent phosphorus transport system is also found in the kidney. Brush border membranes from proximal tubule cells have a sodium- and pH-dependent, saturable phosphorus transport system. Transport into basolateral membrane vesicles is via passive transport only. The primary regulator of the rate of renal phosphorus reabsorption is the plasma phosphorus concentration. In-vitro studies in porcine and monkey renal cell lines have shown that lowering phosphorus levels in the medium results in a two- to sevenfold increase in phosphorus transport.[102] This autoregulatory phenomenon is probably a widespread process that occurs in most, if not all, cell types, because similar adaptive responses to phosphorus deprivation occur in cardiac and hepatic cell types.

The chief hormonal regulator of renal phosphorus reabsorption is parathyroid hormone, and TmP/GFR is inversely related to plasma PTH and urinary nephrogenous cAMP.[83] Plasma PTH is positively correlated with urinary excretion of phosphorus. PTH affects both the sodium-dependent and sodium-independent transport pathways directly and renal phosphorus handling indirectly by inhibiting proximal and distal bicarbonate reabsorption. The molecular details of PTH action on renal phosphorus transport are not precisely understood. Presumably, the steps involve transmembrane transduction of the cell surface signal and induction of an intracellular second messenger. Some evidence suggests that both high ($K_d=10^{-12}$ mol/L) and low ($K_d=10^{-9}$ mol/L) affinity PTH receptors may be present on renal cell membranes.[103]

The major determinants of urinary phosphorus loss are increases in dietary phosphorus intake, phosphorus absorption, and plasma phosphorus levels. Other important factors that are associated with hyperphosphaturia are hyperparathyroidism, acute respiratory or metabolic acidosis, diuretics, and extracellular volume expansion. Reductions in urinary phosphorus are associated with dietary phosphorus restriction, increases in plasma insulin, thyroid hormone, growth hormone or glucagon, metabolic or respiratory alkalosis, hypokalemia, and extracellular volume contraction.

## FUNCTION AND MECHANISM OF ACTION

The major building blocks of biology are covalent molecules, polymers, proteins, polysaccharides, and nucleic acids. DNA and RNA are polymers based on phosphate ester monomers; the high-energy phosphate bond of ATP is the major energy currency of living organisms; cell membranes are composed largely of phospholipids, and the inorganic constituents of bone are primarily a calcium phosphate salt—that is, amorphorous calcium phosphate and hydroxyapatite. Living matter has a huge demand for phosphorus. A variety of enzymatic activities are controlled by alternate phosphorylation and dephosphorylation of proteins by cellular kinases and phosphatases. The metabolism of all major metabolic substrates depends on the functioning of phosphorus as a cofactor in a variety of enzymes and as the principal reservoir for metabolic energy in the form of ATP, creatine phosphate, and phosphoenolpyruvate. Another important role of phosphorus has to do with the fact that neutral molecules are soluble in lipid and will pass through membranes.[104] Phosphates are ionized at physiologic pH so they may trap phosphorylated molecules within cells. Finally, phosphorus combines with calcium to form hydroxyapatite, the principal inorganic compound found in bone.

## DIETARY CONSIDERATIONS

Any evaluation of dietary phosphorus adequacy should consider not only the quantitative aspects of phosphorus consumption, but also bioavailability of phosphorus from various food sources.

### *FOOD SOURCES*

Phosphorus is found widely distributed in foodstuffs. In the United States, the average daily intake of phosphorus is about 48 mmol (1500 mg) for males and 32 mmol (1000 mg) for females.[71] In general, food sources high in protein (meats, milk, eggs, and cereals) are also high in phosphorus. The relative contribution of the major food groups to the total phosphorus intake is about 60% from milk, meat, poultry, fish, and eggs, 20% from cereals and legumes, and 10% from fruits and fruit juices. Alcoholic beverages on average supply 4% of the phosphorus intake, and other beverages, such as coffee, tea, and regular soft drinks, provide 3%.[105]

### *BIOAVAILABILITY*

Various dietary constituents and the relative amount of other minerals in the diet may inhibit or enhance mineral bioavailability. In general, phosphorus bioavailability is greater from animal products than from plant-based foods.

**Animal Products.** Phosphorus from meat is well absorbed (>70%) by humans.[106] Phosphorus in meat is found mainly as intracellular organic compounds that are mostly hydrolyzed in the gastrointestinal tract, releasing inorganic phosphorus that is available for intestinal absorption. Processed meat also contains various polyphosphates and pyrophosphates as additives.

Inorganic phosphates account for one-third of the phosphorus in milk, 20% occur in ester linkage with amino acids of casein, 40% are in the caseinate micelles, and the remainder are found as water- and lipid-soluble esters.[107] The inorganic phosphate in milk is found mainly as the calcium, magnesium, and potassium phosphate salts. The relative bioavailability of phosphorus in milk has been reported to be 65 to 90% in infants.[71] However, all the phosphorus in milk casein (which represents 20% of the total phosphorus in milk) is recovered in a 5 kd phosphopeptide that is resistant to enzymatic digestion by trypsin and may be of lower bioavailability. The lower casein content of human milk compared to cow's milk may be responsible for the higher bioavailability of phosphorus from human milk.

Most of the phosphorus in eggs is in the form of a 45 kd phosphoprotein called phosvitin, which avidly binds iron. The bioavailability of phosphorus in eggs needs further investigation.

**Plant Products.** Given current public health recommendations to the United States population to increase consumption of cereals, legumes, and vegetables,[108] re-evaluation of the relative bioavailability of phosphorus from plant-based versus animal-based foods is needed. Long ago questions were raised concerning the bioavailability of phosphorus in grains[109] because much phosphorus can be in the form of phytic acid (inositol phosphate), and organophosphate compound used by plants to store phosphorus. In wheat, rice, and maize more than 80% of the total phosphorus is found in phytic acid and 35% is found in mature potato tubers.[87]

**Mineral-Mineral Interactions.** The high levels of phosphorus in formulas fed to support bone growth in premature neonates can decrease magnesium absorption.[110] Phosphorus has been shown to decrease lead absorption in humans.[111]

It has been reported that a diet containing 50 mmol (2 g) of calcium daily does not affect phosphorus absorption.[46] However, high levels of calcium fed with meals inhibit phosphorus absorption in animals[112] and humans, and can be useful therapeutically to ameliorate hyperphosphatemia in patients with chronic renal failure.[113] Ingestion of 25 mmol (1000 mg) of calcium in a meal containing 12 mmol (372 mg) of phosphorus reduces phosphorus absorption from 70 to 31%.[114] The current upsurge of consumer interest in calcium supplementation may have untoward effects on phosphorus balance if supplements are used in excess. The most common mineral-phosphorus interaction results from the ingestion of over-the-counter aluminum- or magnesium-containing antacids. Antacids bind phosphorus in the gastrointestinal tract and reduce phosphorus absorption. Three grams of aluminum hydroxide (25 mmol aluminum) given with a meal reduces phosphorus absorption from 70 to 35%.[115]

## PHOSPHORUS DEFICIENCY

Chronic phosphorus deficiency in animals results in the loss of appetite, development of stiff joints, fragile bones, and a marked increase in susceptibility to infection.[116] An animal deprived of phosphorus will reduce its food consumption and reduce its skeletal mass. Vitamin D–resistant hypophosphatemic rickets was first described in 1937.[117] A mutant mouse breed (Hyp mouse) displays characteristics of hypophosphatemia and low renal phosphorus reabsorption.[118] In normal individuals, phosphorus deficiency is believed to be unlikely to occur because of the widespread availability of phosphorus in the diet.[71] However, premature infants are an exceptional case, as discussed earlier in this chapter, because they are frequently prone to the development of rickets due to an inadequate supply of phosphorus and calcium.[119]

The classic study of phosphorus deficiency in humans was conducted by Lotz et al. in 1968.[120] These investigators induced phosphorus deficiency by feeding normal adults a phosphorus-deficient diet. They found that frank symptoms of phosphorus deficiency, such as anorexia, weakness, debility, and bone pain, did not occur until serum phosphorus levels were lowered to below 0.3 mmol/L (1.0 mg/dl). Administration of phosphorus-binding antacids was necessary to achieve these low serum phosphorus levels. Phosphorus deficiency is accompanied by a reduction in urinary phosphorus excretion and an increase in urinary calcium, magnesium, and potassium excretion. All of the calcium and most of the magnesium is derived from bone. The wide variety of clinical complications that can arise from phosphorus deficiency[121] are illustrated in Figure 7–3.

## ASSESSMENT OF PHOSPHORUS STATUS

The most commonly used index of phosphorus status is the serum phosphorus level. However, this measure of status is inadequate for a variety of reasons. Only 1% of total body phosphorus is in the extracellular fluid, and plasma phosphorus is under physiologic control. Plasma phosphorus is determined by the tubular reabsorptive capacity of the kidney, which in turn is regulated by the level of PTH, growth hormone, and other factors. Moreover, the level of phosphorus in the plasma can be artificially elevated because of muscle and bone catabolism, or acutely decreased because of rapid shifts of phosphorus into the intracellular compartment. Intracellular phosphorus levels in red blood cells, leukocytes, and platelets have been investigated and found to correlate with the circulating phosphorus level; however, intracellular ATP levels are more resistent to change.

Urinary phosphorus levels reflect dietary phosphorus intake under normal conditions. Hypophosphaturia and hypercalciuria occur with phosphate depletion.

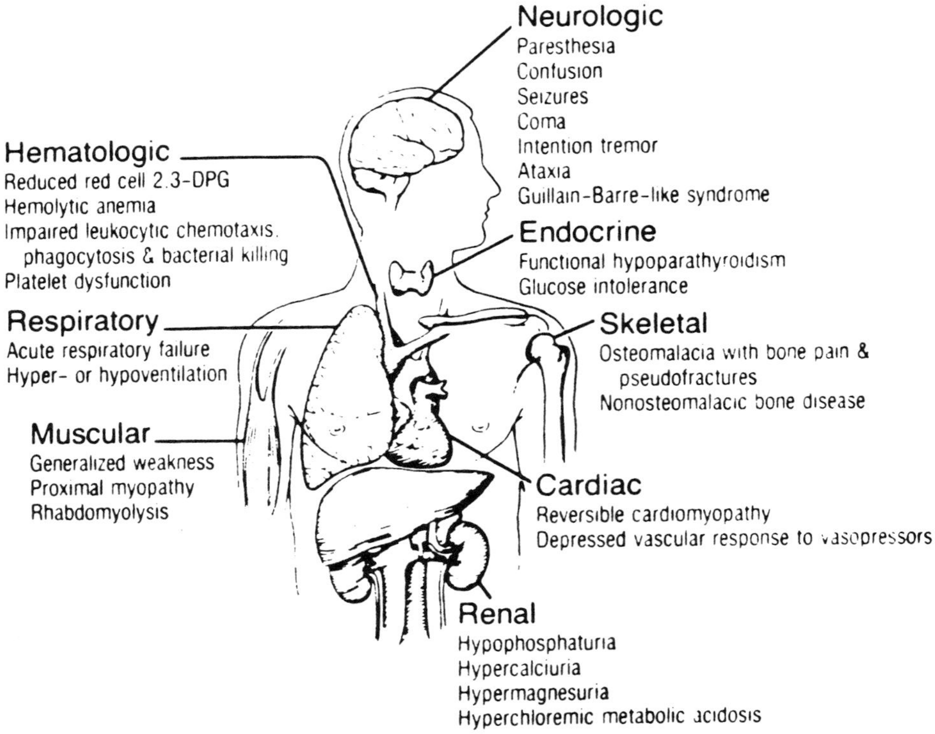
Neurologic
Paresthesia
Confusion
Seizures
Coma
Intention tremor
Ataxia
Guillain-Barre-like syndrome
Hematologic
Reduced red cell 2,3-DPG
Hemolytic anemia
Impaired leukocytic chemotaxis, phagocytosis & bacterial killing
Platelet dysfunction
Endocrine
Functional hypoparathyroidism
Glucose intolerance
Respiratory
Acute respiratory failure
Hyper- or hypoventilation
Skeletal
Osteomalacia with bone pain & pseudofractures
Nonosteomalacic bone disease
Muscular
Generalized weakness
Proximal myopathy
Rhabdomyolysis
Cardiac
Reversible cardiomyopathy
Depressed vascular response to vasopressors
Renal
Hypophosphaturia
Hypercalciuria
Hypermagnesuria
Hyperchloremic metabolic acidosis

**FIGURE 7–3.** The clinical manifestations of severe hypophosphatemia and phosphorus depletion. 2,3-DPG, 2,3-diphosphoglycerate. (From Yu, G.C., Lee, D.B.N.: West. J. Med., *147*:569–576, 1987. Reprinted by permission of the Western Journal of Medicine.)

Likewise, elevated serum alkaline phosphatase and $1,25(OH)_2D$ may be present, but these biochemical changes are not specific enough to accurately predict body phosphorus stores. Newer developments in nuclear magnetic resonance (NMR) techniques offer a powerful research tool to investigate intracellular states of phosphorus under various in-vivo conditions; moreover, whole-body neutron activation analysis can measure total body phosphorus in vivo. However, these expensive and sophisticated methods have limited applicability, and additional approaches to the problem of assessing phosphorus status are needed.

## PHOSPHORUS REQUIREMENTS AND RECOMMENDED INTAKES

The precise requirement for phosphorus is not known. Except in the case of the young infant, the RDA for phosphorus has been set to equal the RDA for calcium. The daily RDA for formula-fed infants from birth to 6 months of age is 9.7 mmol (300 mg) and for infants 6 to 12 months old, 16 mmol (500 mg). The daily RDA for children 1 to 10 years old is 26 mmol (800 mg), 39 mmol (1200 mg) for ages 11 to 24 years, and 26 mmol (800 mg) for ages beyond 24 years.[71]

## DIETARY PHOSPHORUS EXCESS

Hypocalcemia, secondary hyperparathyroidism with excessive resorption and bone loss, has been demonstrated in animals by the long-term feeding of diets containing greater than a 2:1 phosphorus-to-calcium ratio. In infants, high-phosphorus human milk substitutes can cause hypocalcemia and tetany.[71] Phosphorus-to-calcium ratios of typical United States diets frequently exceed a 2:1 ratio; however, these diets are not believed to be harmful.[71]

## CLINICAL DISORDERS AFFECTING PHOSPHORUS BALANCE

Phosphate imbalance can occur for a variety of reasons.[122] The causes of hypophosphatemia can be grouped into three categories based on their respective pathogeneses: rapid shifts of extracellular phosphorus into the intracellular compartment, markedly reduced intestinal absorption or increased intestinal losses, and increased urinary phosphorus losses. Hypophosphatemia is seen clinically associated with nutritional repletion without adequate phosphorus, gastrointestinal malabsorption, starvation, diabetes mellitus, alcoholism, and renal tubular dysfunctions; it is also seen following chronic abuse of phosphate-binding antacids. Nutritional repletion increases intracellular phosphorus demand and can cause rapid shifts of extracellular phosphorus to intracellular sites, particularly in the phosphorus-depleted patient.

Gastrointestinal malabsorption of phosphorus can occur secondary to a decrease of absorptive capacity in diseases that affect large areas of the small intestine, such as Crohn's disease, celiac disease, short bowel syndrome, and radiation enteritis. Other problems associated with gastrointestinal malabsorption include malabsorption of vitamin D and secondary hyperparathyroidism secondary to calcium depletion; these conditions increase the risk of developing negative phosphorus balance. Increased muscle catabolism due to starvation can maintain normal plasma phosphorus levels through phosphorus release from intracellular stores, in spite of underlying phosphorus depletion. Phosphate depletion in alcoholism can occur for several reasons: low dietary phosphorus, malabsorption, increased urinary losses, secondary hyperparathyroidism, hypomagnesemia, and hypokalemia.

Excessive amounts of phosphorus can be lost in the urine of uncontrolled diabetics who have polyuria and acidosis. Plasma phosphorus, however, can be normal or slightly elevated in ketotic patients because of the release of large amounts of phosphorus from intracellular sites. In contrast, fluid and insulin administration in ketotic patients results in a large shift of phosphorus from extracellular to intracellular sites and can quickly precipitate frank hypophosphatemia. Brief periods of experimental acidosis deplete intracellular phosphorus levels; 10 days are required for full repletion of intracellular organic phosphorus. Recovering burn patients are at risk of hypophosphatemia due to massive diuresis. Likewise, excessive urinary phosphorus losses are also seen in patients with dysfunctions of the proximal renal tubule, such as that seen in Franconi's syndrome.

Hyperphosphatemia is usually seen in chronic renal failure, wherein reduced renal function results in increased sensitivity to large dietary phosphorus loads. Hyperphospatemia can also be seen with severe hemolysis, tumor lysis syndrome, rhabdomyolysis, and various endocrine dysfunctions, such as hypoparathyroidism, acromegaly, and severe hyperthyroidism. The clinical sequel of chronic hyperphosphatemia is frequently ectopic calcification, usually when the serum calcium-phosphorus product is greater than 5.65 $mmol/L^2$.[122] Chronic hyperphosphatemia is managed by limiting dietary phosphorus intake where possible and by administering oral phosphate binders containing aluminum, calcium, or magnesium salts. However, prolonged ingestion of high levels of aluminum can induce metabolic bone disease in patients with renal failure, whereas magnesium ingestion can lead to hypermagnesemia or diarrhea.

## REFERENCES


1. Bo-Linn, G.W., Davis, G.R., Buddrus, D.J., et al.: J. Clin. Invest., *70*:640–647, 1984.
2. Recker, R.R.: Calcium absorption and achlorhydria. N. Engl. J. Med., *313*:70–73, 1985.
3. Bronner, F.: Calcif. Tissue Int., *43*:133–137, 1988.
4. Sheikh, M.S., Schiller, L.R., Fordtran, J.S.: Miner. Electrolyte Metab., *16*:130–146, 1990.
5. Sheikh, M.S., Ramirez, A., Emmett, M., et al.: J. Clin. Invest., *81*:126–132, 1988.
6. Barger-Lux, M.J., Heaney, R.P., Recker, R.R.: Calcif. Tissue Int., *44*:308–311, 1989.
7. Petith, M.M., Schedl, H.P.: Gastroenterology, *71*:1039–1042, 1976.
8. Levine, B.S., Walling, M.W., Coburn, J.W.: Intestinal absorption of calcium: Its assessment, normal physiology, and alterations in various disease states. *In* Disorders of Mineral Metabolism, Vol. II. Edited by F. Bronner and J.W. Coburn. New York, Academic Press, 1982.
9. Aurbach, G.D.: Calcium-regulating hormones: Parathyroid hormone and calcitonin. *In* Calcium in Human Biology. Edited by B.E.C. Nordin. London, Springer-Verlag, 1988.
10. Norman, A.: Am. J. Clin. Nutr., *51*:290–300, 1990.
11. Adams, P.H.: Calcium-regulating hormones: General. *In* Calcium in Human Biology. Edited by B.E.C. Nordin. London, Springer-Verlag, 1988.
12. Eriksen, E.F., Colvard, D.S., Berg, N.J., et al.: Science, *241*:84–86, 1988.
13. Stock, J.L., Coderre, J.A., Mallette, L.E.: J. Clin. Endocrinol. Metab., *61*:595–600, 1985.
14. Nordin, B.E.C., Marshall, D.H., Francis, R.M., et al.: J. Steroid Biochem., *15*:171–174, 1981.
15. Kerstetter, J., Allen, L.H.: J. Nutr., *120*:134–136, 1990.
16. Wood, R.J., Allen, L.H.: J. Nutr., *113*:1561–1567, 1983.
17. Zarkadas, M., Gougeon-Reyburn, R., Marliss, E.B., et al.: Am. J. Clin. Nutr., *50*:1088–1094, 1989.
18. Wood, R.J., Sitrin, M.D., Cusson, G.J., et al: JPEN J. Parenter. Enteral Nutr., *10*:188–190, 1986.
19. Bronner, F.: Bone formation and bone resorption. *In* A Basic Science Primer in Orthopaedics. Edited by F. Bronner and R.V. Worrell. Baltimore, Williams & Wilkins, 1991.
20. Campbell, A.K.: Proc. Nutr. Soc., *49*:51–56, 1990.
21. Garn, S.M.: The Earlier Gain and Later Loss of Cortical Bone. Springfield, IL, Charles C Thomas, 1970.
22. Halloran, B.P., DeLuca, H.F.: J. Biol. Chem., *7256*:7338–7342, 1981.
23. Younoszai, M.K.: Development of Intestinal Calcium Transport. *In* Textbook of Gastroenterology and Nutrition in Infancy. Edited by E. Lebenthal. New York, Raven Press, 1981.
24. Moore, L.J., Machlan, L.A., Lim, M.O., et al.: Pediatr. Res., *19*:329–334, 1985.
25. Christiansen C., Rodbro, P., Nielsen, C.T.: Scand. J. Lab. Clin. Invest., *35*:507–510, 1975.

26. Miller, J.Z., Smith, D.L., Floral, L., et al: Clin. Chim. Acta, *183*:107–113, 1989.
27. Halioua, L., Anderson, J.J.B.: Am. J. Clin. Nutr., *49*:534–541, 1989.
28. National Research Council: Nutrition During Pregnancy. Washington, D.C., National Academy Press, 1990.
29. King, J.C., Halloran, B.P., Huq, N., et al.: Calcium metabolism during pregnancy and lactation. *In* Mechanisms Regulating Lactation and Infant Nutrient Utilization. Edited by M.F. Picciano and B. Lonnerdal. In Press.
30. Heaney, R.P., Skillman, T.G.: J. Clin. Endocrinol. Metab., *33*:661–670, 1971.
31. Tylavsky, F.A., Curtis, R.C., Anderson, J.J.B., et al.: J. Bone Mineral Res., *4*:S414, 1989.
32. Chan, G.M., Ronald, M., Slater, P., et al.: Am. J. Clin. Nutr., *46*:319–323, 1987.
33. Nordin, B.E.C.: Nutr. Rev., *47*:65–72, 1989.
34. Eastell, R., Yergey, A.L., Vieira, N.E., et al: J. Bone Min. Res., *6*:125–132, 1991.
35. Morgan, K.J., Stampley, G.L., Zabik, M.E., et al.: J. Am. Coll. Nutr., *4*:195–206, 1985.
36. Allen, L.H.: Am. J. Clin. Nutr., *35*:783–808, 1982.
37. Heaney, R.P., Recker, R.R. Weaver, C.M.: Calcif. Tissue Int., *46*:300–304, 1990.
38. Sheikh, M.S., Santa Ana, C.A., Nicar, M.J., et al.: N. Engl. J. Med., *317*:532–536, 1987.
39. Heaney, R.P., Weaver, C.M.: Am. J. Clin. Nutr., *50*:830–832, 1989.
40. Kabayashi, A., Kawai, S., Ohbe, Y., Nagashima, Y.: Am. J. Clin. Nutr., *28*:681–683, 1975.
41. Smith, T.M., Kolars, J.C., Savaiano, D.A., et al.: Am. J. Clin. Nutr., *42*:1197–1200, 1985.
42. Balasubramanian, R., Johnson, E.J., Marlett, J.A.: J. Am. Coll. Nutr., *6*:199–208, 1987.
43. Hallberg, L., Brune, M., Erlandsson, M., et al.: Am. J. Clin. Nutr., *53*:112–119, 1991.
44. Jandacek, R.J.: Lipids, *26*:250–253, 1991.
45. Allen, L.H., Oddoye, E.A., Margen, S.: Am. J. Clin. Nutr., *32*:741–749, 1979.
46. Spencer, H., Kramer, L., Osis, D., et al.: J. Nutr., *108*:447–457, 1978.
47. Barltrop, D., Mole, R.H., Sutton, A.: Arch. Dis. Child., *52*:41–49, 1977.
48. Dawson-Hughes, B., Seligson, F.H., Hughes, V.A.: Am. J. Clin. Nutr., *44*:83–88, 1986.
49. Deehr, M.S., Dallal, G.E., Smith, K.T., et al.: Am. J. Clin. Nutr., *51*:95–99, 1990.
50. Cook, J.D., Dassenkp, S., Whittaker, P.: Am. J. Clin. Nutr., *53*:106–111, 1991.
51. Lewis, N.M., Marcus, M.S.K., Behling, A.R., et al.: Am. J. Clin. Nutr., *49*:527–533, 1989.
52. Snedeker, S.M., Smith, S.A., Greger, J.L.: J. Nutr., *112*:136–143, 1982.
53. Nordin, B.E.C., Horsman, A., Marshall, D.H., et al.: Clin. Orthop. Relat. Res., *140*:216–239, 1979.
54. Weisinger, J.R., Favus, M.J., Langman, C.B., et al.: J. Bone Min. Res., *4*:929–934, 1989.
55. Dawson-Hughes, B., Stern, D.T., Shipp, C.C., et al.: J. Clin. Endocrinol. Metab., *67*:62–68, 1988.
56. Calvo, M.S., Kumar, R., Heath, R.: J. Clin. Endocrinol. Metab., *70*:1334–1340, 1990.
57. Ireland, P., Fordtran, J.S.: J. Clin. Invest., *52*:2672–2681, 1973.
58. Abrams, S.A., Schanler, R.J., Garza, C.: J. Pediatr., *112*:956–960, 1988.
59. Picard, D., Ste-Marie, L.G., Coutu, D., et al.: Bone Miner., *4*:299–309, 1988.
60. Matkovic, V., Kostial, K., Simonovic, I., et al.: Am. J. Clin. Nutr., *32*:540–549, 1979.
61. Riggs, B.L., Wahner, H.W., Melton, L.J., et al.: J. Clin. Invest., *80*:979–982, 1987.
62. Mazess, R.B., Barden, H.S.: Am. J. Clin. Nutr., *53*:132–142, 1991.
63. Nordin, B.E.C., Horsman, A., Crilly, R.G., et al.: Br. Med. J., *280*:451–453, 1980.
64. Riis, B., Thomsen, K., Christiansen, C.: N. Engl. J. Med., *316*:173–177, 1987.
65. Ettinger, B., Genant, H.K., Cann, C.E.: Ann. Intern. Med., *102*:319–324, 1985.
66. Cummings, R.G.: Calcif. Tissue Int., *47*:194–201, 1990.
67. Dawson-Hughes, B., Dallal, G.E., Krall, E.A., et al.,: N. Engl. J. Med., *323*:878–883, 1990.
68. Vieth, R., Fraser, D., Kooh, S.W.: J. Nutr., *117*:914–918, 1987.
69. Clements, M.R., Johnson, L., Fraser, D.R.: Nature, *325*:62–65, 1987.
70. Batchelor, A.J., Compston, J.E.: Br. J. Nutr., *49*:213–216, 1983.
71. National Research Council: Recommended Dietary Allowances. 10th Ed. Washington, D.C., National Academy Press, 1989.
72. Vosburgh, E., Peters, T.J.: J. R. Soc. Med., *80*:34–37, 1987.
73. Fuss, M., Pepersack, T., Geel, J.V., et al.: Calcif. Tissue Int., *46*:9–13, 1990.
74. Schanler, R.J., Garza, C.: J. Pediatr., *112*:452–456, 1988.
75. Greene, H.L., Hambidge, K.M., Schanler, R., et al.: Am. J. Clin. Nutr., *48*:1324–1342, 1988.
76. Resnick, L.M.: Am. J. Hypertens., *3*:171S–178S, 1990.
77. Luft, F.C.: Am. J. Hypertens., *3*:156S–160S, 1990.
78. Sorenson, A.W., Slattery, M.L., Ford, M.H.: Nutr. Cancer, *11*:135–145, 1988.
79. Wargovich, M.J., Baer, A.R.: Prev. Med., *18*:672–679, 1989.
80. Van der Meer, R., Welberg, J.W.M., Kuipers, F., et al.: Gastroenterology, *99*:1653–1659, 1990.
81. Dallemagne, M.J., Richelle, L.J.: Inorganic chemistry of bone. *In* Biological Mineralization. Edited by I. Zipkin. New York, John Wiley & Sons, 1973.
82. Williams, R.J.P.: Phosphorus biochemistry. Ciba Found. Symp., *57*, 1978.
83. Lee, D.B.N., Brautbar, N., Kleeman, C.R.: Disorders of phosphorus metabolism. *In* Disorders of Mineral Metabolism. Vol III: Pathophysiology of Calcium, Phosphorus, and Magnesium. Edited by F. Bronner and J.W. Coburn. New York, Academic Press, 1981.
84. Le Francois, P., Verel, A., Audidier, Y.: Phytic acid level of white and wholemeal bread doughs: variation with different factors. *In* Nutrient Availability: Chemical & Biological Aspects. Edited by D. Southgate, I. Johnson, and G.R. Fenwick. Cambridge, Royal Society of Chemistry, 1989, pp. 161–163.
85. Simons, P.C.M., Versteegh, H.A.J., Jongbloed, A.W., et al: Br. J. Nutr., *64*:525–540, 1990.
86. Gordon, D.T.: Total dietary fiber and mineral absorption. *In* Dietary Fiber. Edited by D. Kritchevsky, C. Bonfield, and J.W. Anderson. New York, Plenum, 1990.
87. Kratzer, F.H., Vohra, P.: Chelates in Nutrition. Boca Raton, FL, CRC Press, 1986.
88. Svanberg, U., Sandberg, A.S.: Improved iron availability in weaning foods using germination and fermentation. *In* Nutrient Availability: Chemical and Biological Aspects.

Edited by D. Southgate, I. Johnson, and G.R. Fenwick. Cambridge, Royal Society of Chemistry, 1989, pp. 179–181.

89. Brune, M., Rossander, L., Hallberg, L.: Am. J. Clin. Nutr., *49*:542–545, 1989.
90. Avioli, L.: Calcium and phosphorus. *In* Modern Nutrition in Health and Disease. 7th Ed. Edited by R.S. Goodhardt and M.E. Shils. Philadelphia, Lea & Febiger, 1985.
91. Kiebzak, G.M., Sacktor, B.: Age-related phosphaturia and adaptation to phosphorus deprivation in the rat. *In* Homeostatic Function and Aging. Edited by B.B. Davis and W.G. Wood. New York, Raven Press, 1985.
92. Thomas, A.J., Bunker, V.W., Sodha, N., et al: Br. J. Nutr., *62*:211–219, 1989.
93. Favus, M.: Am. J. Physiol., *248*:G147–G157, 1985.
94. Walling, M.W.: Effects of 1,25-dihydroxyvitamin D on active intestinal inorganic phosphate absorption. *In* Vitamin D, Biochemical, Chemical and Clinical Aspects Related to Calcium Metabolism. Edited by A.W. Norman, K. Schaefer, J.W. Coburn, et al. Berlin, de Gruyter, 1977.
95. Berner, W., Kinne, R., Murer, H.: Biochem. J., *160*:467–474, 1976.
96. Peerce, B.E.: Am. J. Physiol., *256*:G645–G652, 1989.
97. Brickman, A.S., Coburn, J.W., Kurokawa, K., et al: N. Engl. J. Med., *289*:495–498, 1973.
98. Norman, A.W., Litwack, G.: Hormones. New York, Academic Press, 1987.
99. de Boland, A.R., Norman, A.W.: Endocrinology, *127*:2475–2480, 1990.
100. Karsenty, G., Lacour, B., Ulmann, A., et al: Am. J. Physiol., *248*:G40–G45, 1985.
101. Aloia, J.F., Vaswani, A., Yeh, J.K., et al.: Miner. Electrolyte Metab., *10*:73–76, 1984.
102. Escoubet, B., Djabali, K., Amiel, C.: Am. J. Physiol., *256*:C322–C328, 1989.
103. Cole, J.A., Eber, S.L., Poelling, R.E., et al.: Am. J. Physiol., *253*:E221–E227, 1987.
104. Westheimer, F.H.: Science, *235*:1173–1178, 1987.
105. Block, G., Dresser, C.M., Hartman, A.M., et al.: Am. J. Epidemiol., *122*:13–26, 1985.
106. Schuette, S., Linkswiler, H.: J. Nutr., *112*:338–349, 1982.
107. Hazell, T.: World Rev. Nutr. Diet., *46*:1–123, 1985.
108. Committee on Diet, Nutrition and Cancer: Diet, Nutrition and Cancer. Washington, D.C., Assembly of Life Sciences, National Research Council, National Academy Press, 1982.
109. Bruce, H.M., Callow, R.K.: Biochem. J., *28*:517–528, 1934.
110. Blake, K.C., Mann, M.: Environ. Res., *30*:188–194, 1983.
111. Giles, M.M., Laing, I.A., Elton, R.A., et al.: J. Pediatr., *117*:147–154, 1990.
112. Lau, K., Chen, S., Eby, B.: Am. J. Physiol., *246*:H324–H331, 1984.
113. Slatopolsky, E., Weerts, C., Lopez-Hiker, S., et al.: N. Engl. J. Med., *315*:157–161, 1986.
114. Schiller, L.R., Santa Ana, C.A., Sheikh, M.S., et al.: N. Engl. J. Med., *320*:1110–1103, 1989.
115. Ramirez, J.A., Emmett, M., White, M.G., et al.: Kidney Int., *30*:753–759, 1986.
116. Knochel, J.P.: Arch. Intern. Med., *137*:203–220, 1977.
117. Albright, F., Butler, A.H., Bloomberg, E.: Am. J. Dis. Child., *59*:529–547, 1937.
118. Eicher, E.M., Southard, J.L., Scriver, C.R., et al.: Proc. Natl. Acad. Sci. U. S. A., *73*:4667–4671.
119. Rowe, J.C., Carey, D.E.: Pediatr. Clin. North Am., *34*:997–1017, 1987.
120. Lotz, M., Zisman, E., Bartter, F.C.: N. Engl. J. Med., *278:*:409–415, 1968.
121. Yu, G.C., Lee, D.B.N.: West. J. Med., *147*:569–576, 1987.
122. Berner, Y.N., Shike, M.: Annu. Rev. Nutr., *8*:121–148, 1988.

## SELECTED READINGS

Allen, L.H.: Calcium bioavailability and absorption: A review. Am. J. Clin. Nutr., *35*:783–808, 1982.

Bronner, F. (ed.): Intracellular Calcium Regulation. New York, Wiley-Liss, 1990.

Bronner, F., Coburn, J.W. (eds.): Disorders of Mineral Metabolism. Vols. II and III. New York, Academic Press, 1981.

Norman, A.W.: Intestinal calcium absorption: A vitamin D-hormone-mediated adaptive response. Am. J. Clin. Nutr., *51*:290–300, 1990.

Nordin, B.E.C. (ed.).: Calcium in Human Biology. London, Springer-Verlag, 1988.

CHAPTER 8

# Magnesium

Maurice E. Shils



Magnesium plays an essential role in a wide range of fundamental cellular reactions. Hence, it is not surprising that deficiency in the organism may lead to serious biochemical and symptomatic changes. McCollum and associates made the first systematic observations of magnesium deficiency in rats and dogs in the early 1930s.[1] The first description of clinical depletion in man was published in 1934 in a small number of patients with various underlying diseases.[2] Flink and associates in the early 1950s initiated their long-term studies documenting depletion of this ion in alcoholics and in patients on magnesium-free intravenous solutions.[3] Although the diets consumed by healthy Americans do not appear to lead to clinically significant hypomagnesemia, an increasing number of clinical disorders have been found to be associated with magnesium depletion. Experimental and clinical observations have revealed important interrelations of this essential ion with other electrolytes, second messengers, hormones and growth factors, their membrane receptors, signal pathways, ion channels, parathyroid hormone secretion and action, vitamin D metabolism, and bone functions.

## BIOCHEMICAL AND PHYSIOLOGIC ROLES

Magnesium is involved in many enzymatic steps in which components of food are metabolized and new products are formed.[4-6] Of magnesium's many known reactions (at least 300), it is sufficient to describe only a small number to emphasize its importance. These include the synthesis of fatty acids, activation of amino acids, protein synthesis, phosphorylation of glucose and its derivatives in the glycolytic pathway, oxidative decarboxylation of citrate, and transketolase reactions. Protein kinases, the enzymes that catalyze the transfer of the $\gamma$ phosphate of magnesium adenosine triphosphate (Mg ATP) to a protein substrate, alone constitute a large and diverse family currently numbering more than 100.[7]

Magnesium is required for the formation of cyclic adenosine monophosphate (cAMP), which was the first "second messenger" identified. It was given this term because it receives messages from outside the cells in the form of hormonal or other stimuli. Binding of a specific hormone at the cell membrane can either stimulate or inhibit activity of the membrane-bound enzyme adenylate cyclase, which forms cAMP and pyrophosphate from ATP. It was then found that a series of proteins (G proteins) in the unstimulated state bind guanosine diphosphate (GDP) in cell membranes; following a stimulation of a specific receptor (e.g., by a $\beta$-adrenergic drug) at the cell surface, GDP dissociates from the $\alpha$ subunit of the particular G protein with its replacement by GTP; activation of adenylate cyclase then releases cAMP (Fig. 8–1). cAMP in turn activates further signals, leading to a biochemical response within the cells (e.g., glycogen breakdown). Discoveries in this field have

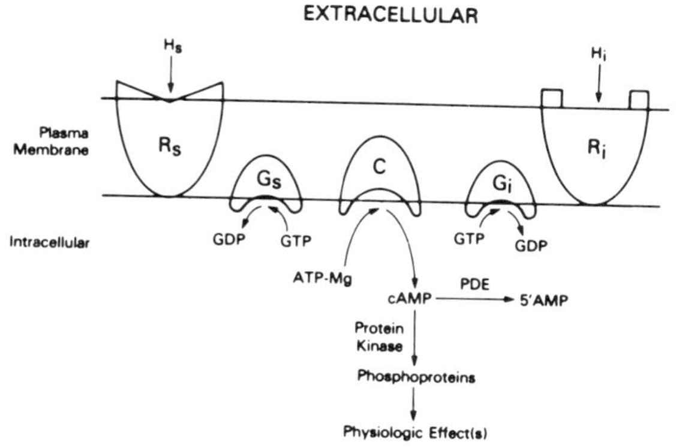
EXTRACELLULAR
Hs
Hi
Plasma Membrane
Rs
Ri
Gs
C
Gi
Intracellular
GDP
GTP
GTP
GDP
ATP-Mg
PDE
cAMP
5'AMP
Protein Kinase
Phosphoproteins
Physiologic Effect(s)

**FIGURE 8–1.** Schematic outline of the adenylate cyclase-cyclic AMP system that involves magnesium. The adenylate cyclase system is a membrane-bound enzyme complex found in virtually every cell; it seems to modulate cAMP through a wide variety of hormones and metabolic agents. Magnesium plays a key role as indicated. $H_s$ and $H_i$ denote stimulatory and inhibitory agents, respectively; $R_s$ and $R_i$ stimulatory and inhibitory receptors; and $G_s$ and $G_i$, the stimulatory and inhibitory guanine nucleotide-binding proteins. C denotes the catalytic unit of adenylate cyclase; PDE indicates phosphodiesterase; cAMP indicates cyclic AMP. (From Spiegel, A.M., Gierschik, P., Levine, M.A., et al.: N. Engl. J. Med., *312*:26–33, 1985.)

multiplied and the original term *adenylate cyclase–cyclic AMP system* has been replaced by the specific designation of one of a number of signal transducer G proteins that control either stimulatory or inhibitory pathways.[8,9] These are derived from a superfamily of genes, are present in all eukaryotic cells, and control metabolic, humoral, neuronal, and developmental functions. More than 100 distinct receptors are coupled by these G proteins to second messengers that in recent years have risen in number from the initial cAMP to include at least 11 others.[9,10]

As noted below, more precise and sensitive methods for determining the concentration of intracellular free $Mg^{2+}$ ($[Mg^{2+}]i$) have lowered earlier estimates. The newer values are in the range at which certain enzymatic systems have their $K_m$ values; hence, variation within the range of 0.5 to 1.0 mmol/L (or lower) would be consistent with its activities as a physiologic modulator.

On the basis of their own work and that of other investigators, White and Hartzell have proposed that $[Mg^{2+}]i$ is carefully regulated and its alterations can have profound effects on cardiac physiology; for example, autonomic control of the heart depends on $[Mg^{2+}]i$ in numerous ways: binding of neurotransmitters to their receptors, coupling of receptors to adenylate cyclase, activation of G proteins and adenylate cyclase, activation of proteins by $Mg^{2+}$-dependent phosphotransferases, rectification of various types of $K^+$ channels, activity of phosphorylated $Ca^{2+}$ channels, voltage-dependent inactivation of $Ca^{2+}$ channels, and optimal activity of mechanisms which maintain $[Ca^{2+}]i$ at resting levels.[11]

The known and postulated mechanisms by which $[Mg^{2+}]i$ regulates ion movements have been reviewed.[12,13] For example, the mechanism in cardiac muscle that allows $K^+$ to move readily into the cell but not out (inwardly rectifying $K^+$ channel) is related to its blocking by intracellular $Mg^{2+}$; the latter ion moves into the aqueous channel pore, thus blocking $K^+$ efflux. The $Mg^{2+}$ cannot pass through the pore because of an outer energy barrier, and it stays until driven intracellularly again at a negative voltage by inward-moving $K^+$. This effect of $[Mg^{2+}]i$ operates in at least four such $K^+$ channels. $Mg^{2+}$ also modulates other channels; in some of these (e.g., calcium, delayed rectifier $K^+$, and $Cl^-$), the channels are markedly potentiated by phosphorylation involving cAMP and are modulated by cytosolic magnesium.[10] Although increased $[Mg^{2+}]_i$ *inhibits* the L-type calcium current in heart cells, rapid increases in the $[MgATP]_i$ result in *enhanced* calcium current.[174]

Magnesium concentration in most cells at resting membrane potential is maintained below electrochemical equilibrium with external ionized magnesium concentrations. Magnesium under these circumstances should slowly accumulate in cells by passive diffusion. This has not been observed, suggesting the existence of magnesium transport systems, some of which must be capable of active magnesium extrusion. Observations on squid axone, barnacle muscle, and red cells from several species indicate that a $Na^+$-dependent magnesium efflux may be the primary mechanism for keeping $[Mg^{2+}]i$ below electrochemical equilibrium. There is also some evidence on the existence of $Na^+$-independent magnesium transport systems.[14] The transport of magnesium across the rat placenta appears to be sodium-dependent.[15] In one study, a calcium-channel blocker inhibited $Mg^{2+}$ influx into magnesium-depleted embryonic chick myocytes.[16] In another study a $Mg^{2+}$-specific current elicited in voltage-clamped paramecium was inhibited when external $Ca^{2+}$ was omitted or when a $Ca^{2+}$ chelator was injected.[17] These observations suggest a role for $Ca^{2+}$ in $Mg^{2+}$ influx.

$[Mg^{2+}]i$ may also play a longer term regulatory role in controlling the set point of a process in cell functions;[18] this action contrasts to the very rapid acute and transient signaling induced by variations in $Ca^{2+}$ movements.

## BODY COMPOSITION

The distribution of magnesium in various compartments of apparently healthy adult individuals is summarized in Table 8–1. Somewhat more than half of the total is in bone with almost all of the rest in soft tissue. Magnesium is the most abundant mineral cation in cells and is second in quantity to potassium.

The greater proportion of intracellular magnesium exists in bound form. Measured by $^{31}P$ magnetic resonance imaging (MRI), frog muscle cells contained magnesium bound to ATP at 5.8 mmol/L, to phosphocreatine

**TABLE 8–1.** DISTRIBUTION AND CONCENTRATIONS OF MAGNESIUM IN A HEALTHY ADULT (TOTAL BODY: 833–1170 MMOL*, OR 20–28 G)

| DISTRIBUTION (PERCENTAGE) | | CONCENTRATION |
|---|---|---|
| Bone | 60–65% | 0.5% of bone ash |
| Muscle | 27% | 3.5–5mmol/kg wet weight |
| Other cells | 6–7% | 3.5–5mmol/kg wet weight |
| Extracellular | <1% | |
| Erythrocytes | | 1.65–2.73§ mmol/L† |
| Serum: | | 0.65–0.88§ mmol/L‡ |
| 55% free $Mg^{2+}$, 13% complexed (citrate, phosphate, etc) | | Ultrafilterable: 0.48–0.66 mmol/L§ <br> Ion electrode—0.53–0.66 mmol/L¶ |
| 32% bound primarily to albumin | | 0.1–0.3 mmol/L |
| Mononuclear blood cells** | | 2.91 ± 0.6 fmol/cell‡ <br> 2.79 ± 0.6 fmol/cell‡‡ <br> 3.00 ± 0.04 fmol/cell§§ |
| Cerebrospinal fluid | | 1.25 mmol/L |
| 55% free $Mg^{2+}$ | | |
| 45% complexed | | |
| Sweat | | 0.3 mmol/L (in hot environment) |
| Secretions (saliva, gastric, bile) | | 0.3–0.7 mmol/L |

*1 mmol = 2 mEq = 24 mg.
†Magnesium falls slowly with aging.
‡Similar at various ages.
§Data from Hosseini, E.: Trace Elem. Med., *5*:47–51, 1988.
¶Data from Altura: Magnesium Trace Elem., *9*:3111, 1990.
**Monocytes and lymphocytes in venous blood.
††Data from Elin, Hossini: Clin. Chem., *31*:377–380, 1985. 1 fmol = 24.3 fg.
‡‡Data from Reinhart, et al.: Clin. Clim. Acta, *167*:187–195, 1987.
§§Data from Yang, et al.: J. Am. Coll. Nutr., *9*:328.1990.

at 1.7 mmol/L, to myosin at 0.3 mmol/L, and to free [$Mg^{2+}$] at 0.6 mmol/L.[19] Magnesium as well as calcium forms complexes with phospholipids of various cell membranes as well as with nucleotides. The ratio of cytosolic magnesium to total magnesium in guinea pig heart was 0.85 in this study.

With relatively limited data available on a few sites in human bone, Wallach has noted in his review that magnesium values cluster about 200 mmol (4.8 g) per kg of bone ash.[20] There appears to be no change with age in the magnesium content of trabecular bone in the iliac crest. Thirty percent of bone is in a surface-limited pool either within the hydration shell or in the crystal surface. In adult men, the large fractional bone magnesium is an integral part of the bone crystal.[21]

## ANALYTIC PROCEDURES

**Methods for Total Magnesium in Blood and Tissue Samples.** The development of analytical methods culminating in the widespread use in clinical chemistry laboratories of atomic absorption spectrophotometry (AAS) has been reviewed.[22] Automated colorimetric methods are also widely used clinically; they are more susceptible to interfering substances but, in experienced hands, compare well with AAS, which is the reference method for serum.[23] For the rapid determination following wet ashing of a number of minerals including magnesium in foods, inductively coupled argon plasma emission spectroscopy is useful.[24]

**Magnetic Resonance Imaging (MRI).** A number of metabolites exist in equilibrium between uncomplexed and complexed $Mg^{2+}$. Because the resonances of such molecules may shift upon $Mg^{2+}$ complexation, MRI spectra can provide information on the level of $Mg^{2+}$ in the cell. ATP is the most useful MRI endogenous indicator because of the presence of $^{31}P$ nuclei and its high concentration and broad distribution in cells. The observed shift difference between $\alpha$ and $\beta$ phosphate resonances is the parameter of choice. Technical issues related to the $^{31}P$ shift of ATP for this measurement have been discussed.[25]

Exogenous MRI indicators have been developed to measure cystolic $Mg^{2+}$; such indicators gain sensitivity and selectivity, for example, by utilizing fluoridated compounds, inasmuch as essentially no fluoride background resonance exists in cells. Mg selective indicators have been developed by modifying EDTA (APTRA chelator) to form $^{19}F$ derivatives of "MRI ophores" with the high sensitivity of $^{19}F$ for MRI detection. Because the dissociation constant for $Ca^{2+}$ is still several hundred times greater than the basal cytosolic Ca level of most cells, $Ca^{2+}$ binding is not a significant interfering problem. (+) Fluorocitrate has been utilized as a magnesium indicator in the form of a membrane permeable ester that is hydrolyzed by intracellular enzymes. Biologic and technical issues with these indicators have been reviewed.[25]

**Fluorescent Indicators.** Recently the modification of the APTRA chelator has resulted in suitable fluorescent magnesium chelators such as FURAPTRA. The presence of $Mg^{2+}$ causes a measurable shift in the excitation spectrum, which allows determination of the ion concentration in cell suspensions and in individual cells by a ratio method. A limitation for this probe is the relatively high affinity for $Ca^{2+}$ by a ratio method. Biologic and technical issues and limitations have been recently reviewed.[25]

**Ion Selective Microelectrodes.** A recently-made-available resin, ETH 5214, apparently overcomes a problem with earlier resins in which $Mg^{2+}$ measurements depended on concentration of $K^+$ and $Na^+$ in the calibration solutions.[26] This and other factors have shifted some $[Mg^{2+}]i$ values closer to 1 mmol.[27]

**[Σ Citrate]/[Σ Isocitrate] Ratio.** The relatively strong $Mg^{2+}$ binding constant of citrate contrasts with the relatively weak binding constants for its metabolic partners, such as oxaloacetate (which are 1 or 2 orders of magnitude lower). Thus, changes in $[Mg^{2+}]$ can have large effects on the equilibrium constants of many of the enzymatic reactions of citrate metabolism.[173]

Free $Mg^{2+}$ concentration in cytoplasm can be measured from the variation in the [Σ citrate]/[Σ isocitrate] ratio in the aconitase reaction because this varies with the $[Mg^{2+}]i$. In the liver of rats starved for 48 hours, this value was 0.61 mM in comparison with that of $^{13}C$ MRI spectrum of citrate in livers of rats starved for 16 hours of 0.46 mM. Using this ratio, the transition from starvation to feeding altered the measured ratio, suggesting the possibility that $[Mg^{2+}]i$ changed from 0.60 to 0.17 mM or less. At the same time, this change was associated with only a small drop in total liver magnesium (8.3 down to 7.6, μmol/kg fresh weight). If the calculation of $[Mg^{2+}]i$ is valid, the changes would imply that, with refeeding, magnesium is moving from the cytosol into some intracellular compartment, most likely the mitochondria.[173]

These newer techniques are enlarging our understanding of the role(s) of free intracellular magnesium, the mechanisms controlling its changes in concentration, and the effect of deficiency.

**Magnesium Isotopes.** These have been used as biologic tracers in following the absorption, distribution in the body, and excretion of this ion. The radioisotope $^{28}Mg$ has been used in human studies[28]; its value is limited by its radioactivity and short half-life of 21.3 hours. Stable magnesium occurs in nature as follows: 78.99% $^{24}Mg$, 10.0% $^{25}Mg$, and 11.01 $^{26}Mg$. The latter has been used for tracer studies,[28] including absorption studies in man,[29] and the $^{25}Mg/^{26}Mg$ ratio has recently been utilized to measure intestinal absorption.[30,31]

## HOMEOSTATIC MECHANISMS

The homeostasis of the individual with respect to mineral balance depends on the amount ingested and the intestinal and renal absorption and excretion and all factors affecting them. A schema for magnesium is given in Figure 8–2.

### DIETARY INTAKE

Magnesium is widely distributed in plant and animal sources but in widely differing concentrations (see Appendix Table A–20).

In considering dietary intake of population groups in the United States, it is noteworthy that data on individual intakes are limited and uncertain because "there is less than 75% analytical data for important sources of the food component."[32] An example of this problem is the comparison of analyzed versus calculated values (using the USDA data base) for the 234 foods in the U.S. FDA Total Dietary Study for eight age-sex groups.[33,34] These foods represent the core items of the U.S. food supply. The analyzed figures were 115 to 124% greater than those of the calculated values (unadjusted for missing values in the data base) among the age groups reported. The sources of magnesium from various food

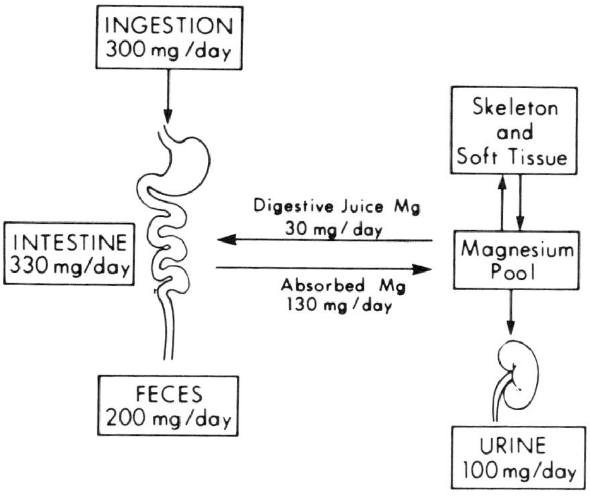
INGESTION
300 mg/day
Skeleton
and
Soft Tissue
Digestive Juice Mg
30 mg/day
INTESTINE
330 mg/day
Magnesium
Pool
Absorbed Mg
130 mg/day
FECES
200 mg/day
URINE
100 mg/day

**FIGURE 8–2.** Magnesium homeostasis in man. A schematic representation of its metabolic economy indicating (a) its relatively poor absorption from the alimentary tract, (b) its distribution into a number of tissue pools with a major distribution into bone, and (c) its dependence on the kidney for excretion. Homeostasis depends upon the integrity of intestinal and renal absorptive processes. (From Slatapolsky, E.: Pathophysiology of Calcium, Magnesium and Phosphorus Metabolism in the Kidney and Body Fluids. Edited by S. Klahr. New York, Plenum Publishing, 1984.

**TABLE 8–2.** CONTRIBUTIONS (AS PERCENTAGE OF DAILY INTAKE) OF VARIOUS FOOD GROUPS TO MAGNESIUM INTAKE (FROM TOTAL DIET STUDY ANALYZED VALUES)

| FOOD GROUP | AGE IN YEARS | | |
|---|---|---|---|
| | 14–16 | 25–30 | 60–65 |
| Dairy | 21 | 13 | 10 |
| Grain | 18 | 16 | 18 |
| Vegetable | 16 | 18 | 18 |
| Animal | 14 | 17 | 15 |
| Fruits | 6 | 6 | 8 |
| Mixed dishes | 11 | 9 | 6 |
| Desserts* | 10 | 6 | 6 |
| Beverages* | 4 | 14 | 15 |
| Fats | 0 | 0 | <1 |

*Not specified.
(From Pennington, J.A.T., Wilson, D.B.: J. Am. Diet. Assoc., *90*:375–381, 1990.)

groups as determined by analysis in the Total Diet Study 1982–1989 are summarized for some of these age groups in Table 8–2. Intake from dairy products and beverages vary with age, inversely or directly, whereas most of the others vary much less.

Magnesium intake data by women aged 20 to 49 years measured from 1985 to 1989 indicate that the amounts consumed vary directly with income and formal education status and that blacks consume less than whites on average.[32] However, the intake differences are not large within given percentile groups based on education status, region, or urbanization.[33]

Per capita availability (i.e., based on disappearance data) of magnesium in the U.S. food supply has been essentially stable at about 14.6 mmol (350 mg) per day since the 1950s with perhaps a small increase in the early 1980s.[32] This figure differs markedly from actual intake data. For example, the mean daily intake from 1985 to 1986 in 4-day surveys using food composition tables by women aged 20 to 49 was 8.62 mmol (207 mg).[33] The mean daily *analyzed* intakes in the Total Diet Study for females 14 to 16, 25 to 30, and 60 to 65 years old was 8.08 mmol (194 mg), 7.88 mmol (189 mg), and 7.79 mmol (187 mg), respectively. For males in the same age groups, the intakes were 12.38 mmol (297 mg), 12.25 mmol (294 mg) and 10.42 mmol (250 mg), respectively.[33]

## ABSORPTION

**Laboratory Animals.** Studies with rats utilizing segment perfusion studies or everted intestinal sacs—many using $^{28}$Mg—have supported, for the most part, the concept that magnesium is often better absorbed in the ileum and colon than in the jejunum (reviewed in reference 35). Magnesium transport by stripped mucosa was measured in the Ussing chamber and found to be secreted across the duodenum[36] but absorbed in the ileum[37] and in the colon.[38] Passive and nonpassive cellular transport processes of magnesium were noted in the ileum and colon.[37,38]

**Human Studies.** The percentage absorption of ingested magnesium by healthy individuals is influenced by its dietary concentration and by the presence of inhibiting or promoting dietary components. Absorptive studies have been conducted in which the amounts of magnesium ingested have varied progressively from very small to very large amounts utilizing the same healthy subjects. $^{28}$Mg has been employed as a tracer to establish fractional absorption.[39,40] In a recent study small amounts of magnesium were fed in the form of a standard meal supplemented by varying amounts of magnesium as the acetate hydrate;[41] fractional absorption was measured over 10 hours using intestinal lavage techniques. Fractional absorption fell progressively from approximately 65 to 70% with intakes of 0.3 to 1.5 mmol (7 to 36 mg) down to 11 to 14% with intakes of 40 mmol (960 to 1000 mg).[40,41] Absorption as a function of intake was curvilinear (Fig. 8–3). The curved portion is compatible with a saturable process (facilitated diffusion or active absorption), and the linear function reflects passive diffusion, as was suggested in children by Milla et al.[42] Estimates of the absorptive fraction related to passive diffusion were 10%[40] and 7%.[41] Using intestinal perfusion techniques in human subjects, magnesium was absorbed in both the jejunum and ileum; it was fully saturable in the ileum but not in the jejunum.[43] If analogous to the rat, human colonic absorption will be significant. The absorption curve of magnesium is compared with that of calcium in Figure 8–4.

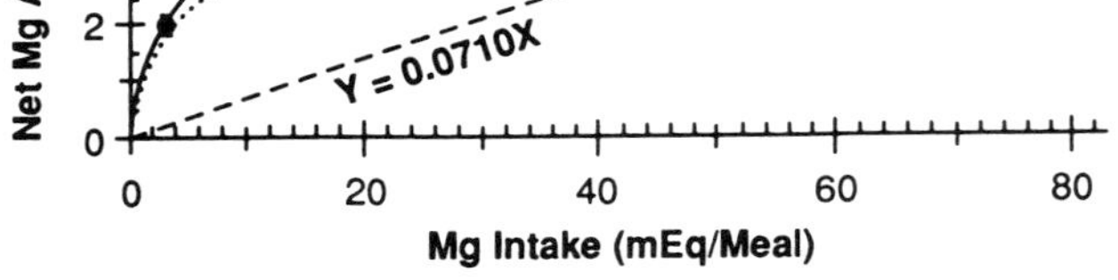
Net Mg Absorption (mEq/10 hours)
Mg Intake (mEq/Meal)
0
2
4
6
8
10
0
20
40
60
80
Y = e^1.286 – 2.889/(X + 1)
Y = 0.0710X

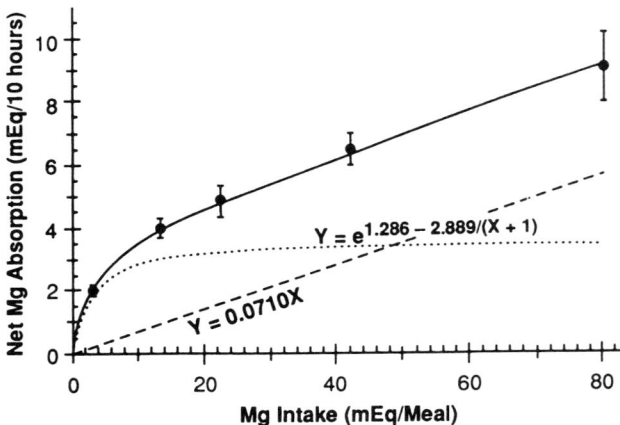

**FIGURE 8–3.** Net magnesium absorption at varying levels of intake of magnesium as derived from linear regression analyses. Experimental conditions are described in the text. The equation for net absorption represents a curved function compatible with a saturable process and a linear function reflecting passive diffusion. (From Fine, K.D., Santa Ana, C.A., Porter, J.L., et al.: J. Clin. Invest., *88*:396–402, 1991, by copyright permission of the American Society for Clinical Investigation.)

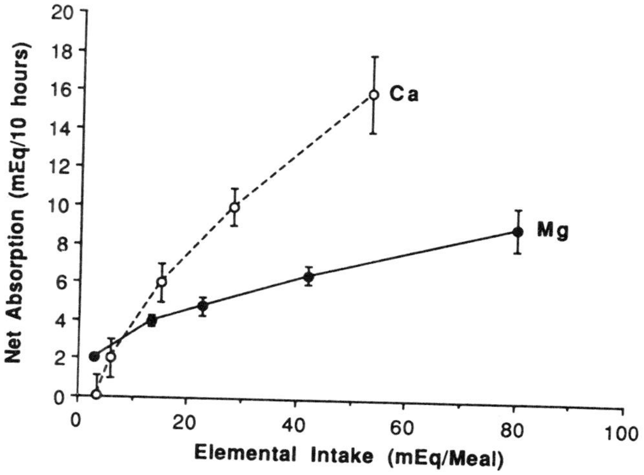
Net Absorption (mEq/10 hours)
Elemental Intake (mEq/Meal)
Ca
Mg
0
2
4
6
8
10
12
14
16
18
20
20
40
60
80
100

**FIGURE 8–4.** Comparison of net magnesium absorption under conditions described in the figure's source reference 41 and in the text with that of calcium measured from meals with and without calcium carbonate. X ± S.E. are indicated by vertical bars. (From Fine, K.D., Santa Ana, C.A., Porter, J.L., et al.: J. Clin. Invest., *88*:396–402, 1991, by copyright permission of the American Society for Clinical Investigation.)

Absorption fractions obtained in older balance studies averaged 50, 60, or 70%. More recent studies have indicated greater variability. With daily magnesium intake of 7.9 to 14.3 mmol (189 to 342 mg), healthy adult males in long-term balance studies excreted 35 to 68% in stool with a fixed daily calcium intake of 5 mmol (200 mg).[44] When free-living adults eating self-selected diets were evaluated periodically over the course of a year, the percentage of absorption of magnesium by men averaged 21%, and by women 27%; their average daily intakes were 13.4 mmol (323 mg) and 9.75 mmol (234 mg), respectively.[45]

**Influence of Other Ions.** A review of long-term balance studies in healthy individuals have, for the major part, indicated that increasing oral calcium intake did not significantly affect magnesium absorption or retention.[46] In those instances when the fractional absorption of magnesium was increased (depending on the calcium source), magnesium retention was not increased because of its increased urinary excretion.[47] With increased oral phosphate, some reports indicated a decrease in magnesium absorption at high levels of phosphate, whereas others found no consistent effect (reviewed in reference 35); when there was decreased absorption of magnesium with high phosphate intake, magnesium balance did not change because of an accompanying decreased urinary magnesium.[48] Increased amounts of magnesium in the diet have been associated with either decreased calcium absorption[35] or no effect.[41] Increased amounts of absorbable oral magnesium have been noted to decrease phosphate absorption,[41,49] perhaps secondary to formation of insoluble magnesium phosphate. Even though increased magnesium intake may have no effect on calcium absorption, renal tubular mechanisms may result in increased calcium excretion.[41] Conversely, decreased absorption of magnesium associated with high phosphate intake did not change magnesium balance because of an associated decreased urinary excretion of magnesium.

**Absorbability of Magnesium Salts in Humans.** The fractional absorption of a salt that is reasonably well absorbed (e.g., magnesium acetate tetrahydrate) will depend on its solubility in intestinal fluids and, as noted above, the amounts given. Five mmol (120 mg) of the acetate in gelatin capsules has been found to be an optimal dose in terms of net absorption.[41] Absorption of Slow-Mg 2 (enteric coated magnesium chloride) was 67% less than the acetate in gelatin capsules.[41] Magnesium citrate has high solubility even in water, whereas magnesium oxide is poorly soluble even in acid solution.[50] The poor solubility of the latter is the basis for the use of magnesium oxide or hydroxide as an osmotic laxative; its excessive ingestion induces diarrhea.[51]

**Magnesium Absorption, Vitamin D, and its Metabolites.** This relationship is considered here in eumagnesemic conditions and below in hypomagnesemic situations. Although reports conflict, the data appear increasingly to favor the concept that, unlike calcium and phosphate, magnesium absorption is not calcitriol-dependent under conditions in which relatively physiologic doses are administered.[52,53] Absorption of magnesium has been noted in individuals having no detectable plasma calcitriol, and there is not a significant correlation between plasma calcitriol and absorption of magnesium.[53,54] Further support for the concept that magnesium and calcium have different intestinal transport processes is the observation that individuals with absorptive hypercalciuria resulting from increased calcium absorption have normal magnesium absorption.[55]

The contradictory results observed in rats were associated with differences in their vitamin D status, calcitriol dosages, and method of study (reviewed in reference 35). When stripped intestinal mucosa of rats was studied under voltage-clamp conditions, calcitriol was without effect in increasing net magnesium absorption in the duodenum (while markedly increasing calcium absorption)[36] or in the ileum[37] or the colon.[38]

**Malabsorption Syndromes.** Intestinal absorption is often reduced in a variety of malabsorption syndromes (Table 8–3). These vary from the more common gastrointestinal disorders associated with steatorrhea and increased intestinal losses to relatively rare situations such as primary idiopathic hypomagnesemia, which is a genetic disorder associated with impairment of facilitated or active absorption.

Serious malabsorption of magnesium may occur because of 1) impaired passage across the disease affected bowel, 2) reduced absorptive surface because of surgical

**TABLE 8–3.** CLINICAL CONDITIONS CONTRIBUTING TO MAGNESIUM DEPLETION

| |
|---|
| *Malabsorption syndromes* |
| Inflammatory bowel disease |
| Gluten enteropathy; sprue |
| Intestinal fistulas, bypass, or resection |
| Bile insufficiency states—e.g., ileal dysfunction with steatorrhea |
| Immune diseases with villous atrophy |
| Radiation enteritis |
| Lymphangiectasia; other fat absorptive defects |
| Primary idiopathic hypomagnesemia |
| Gastrointestinal infections |
| *Renal dysfunction with excessive losses* (see Table 8–4) |
| Tubular diseases |
| Metabolic disorders |
| Hormonal effects |
| Nephrotoxic drugs |
| *Endocrine disorders* (see Table 8–4) |
| Hyperaldosteronism |
| Hyperparathyroidism with hypercalcemia |
| Postparathyroidectomy ("hungry bone" syndrome) |
| Hyperthyroidism |
| *Pediatric genetic and familial disorders* |
| Primary idiopathic hypomagnesemia |
| Renal wasting syndrome (see Table 8–4) |
| Bartter's syndrome (see Table 8–4) |
| Infants born of diabetic or hyperparathyroid mothers |
| Transient neonatal hypomagnesemic hypocalcemia |
| *Inadequate intake, provision, and/or retention of magnesium* |
| Alcoholism |
| Protein-calorie malnutrition (usually with infection) |
| Prolonged infusion or ingestion of magnesium-low nutrient solutions or diets |
| Hypercatabolic states (burns, trauma), usually associated with above entry |
| Excessive lactation |

resection, bowel bypass, or radiation damage, 3) a very rapid transit, or 4) decreased solubility of dietary or secreted magnesium with unabsorbed fatty acids in steatorrhea (Table 8–3); in this case the magnesium (and calcium)–fatty acid complex is lost in the stool.

## RENAL REGULATION

**Filtration and Tubular Absorption.** Magnesium is retained either for tissue growth (including bone) or as turnover replacement; the remainder is excreted in the urine. The kidney plays a critical role in magnesium homeostasis.[56] Approximately 75% of serum magnesium is ultrafilterable in humans at the glomerulus; impaired filtration reduces the amount entering the tubule. Despite compensatory factors in the tubules, serious impairment of glomerular function ultimately causes a rise in serum magnesium unless intake and/or absorption are appropriately decreased. Approximately 15% of the filtered load is absorbed in the proximal convoluted tubule; this is less than half that of sodium and calcium. The proximal straight tubule and descending limb of Henle's loop absorb relatively little, with transport being dependent on luminal magnesium concentration. The thick ascending limb of the loop of Henle appears to be the major site of magnesium reabsorption and the major site of control of excretion, with 50 to 60% of filtered magnesium being reabsorbed between the thin descending limb and the early distal tubule.[57] Changes in concentration of magnesium in the tubular lumen and in the plasma affect renal absorption in this segment. The distal convoluted tubule has limited reabsorption ability (<5% of the filtered load), and the collecting tubules and ducts normally absorbed very little. The healthy kidney with an average intake of magnesium reabsorbs about 95% of the filtered magnesium. Tubular secretion, if it occurs, must be a minor factor.

Studies of overall renal reabsorption of magnesium in various species including humans indicate a maximal transport rate ($T_m$) for this ion.[58] A $T_mMg$ of 0.583 mmol (14 mg) per 100 ml of glomerular filtration per 1.73 $M^2$

for normal subjects was similar to that found in hypoparathyroid and hyperparathyroid (primary) subjects.[58] Any increase in the filtered load was completely excreted. However, observation of segmented reabsorption by micropuncture techniques in thyroparathyroidectomized dogs revealed that the urinary excretory pattern was a summation of the distinct transport properties of the proximal tubule and the loop of Henle; hence, a true $T_m$ was not operative even though the summation resulted in an apparent $T_m$.[59]

**Drug and Hormonal Influences on Renal Regulation.** Magnesium reabsorption in the nephron is influenced by a number of physiologic and metabolic factors as well as by drugs and disease states (Table 8–4). Of particular clinical significance with respect to renal losses are the loop diuretics such as furosemide and ethycrinic acid and certain nephrotoxic drugs. On the other hand, the potassium-sparing diuretics, triamterene and amiloride, also exert a magnesium-sparing effect. The cancer chemotherapeutic agent, cisplatin, may cause serious urinary losses of magnesium because of its tubular toxicity; this may persist for many months after the drug is discontinued. Although a number of hormones in research situations may influence magnesium reabsorption in the rat kidney tubule, their roles and quantitative effects in the normal human kidney are still speculative.

**TABLE 8–4.** METABOLIC, HORMONAL, AND DRUG INFLUENCES ON RENAL MAGNESIUM EXCRETION

| |
|---|
| *Increased excretion* |
| Hypermagnesemia* |
| Hypercalciuria |
| Hyperaldosteronism |
| Hyperparathyroidism† |
| Renal tubular dysfunction |
| Familial renal wasting syndromes |
| Primary magnesuric hypomagnesemia; Bartter's and related syndromes |
| Postrenal obstruction |
| Postrenal transplantation |
| Acute tubulo-interstitial nephritis |
| Nephrotoxic drugs |
| Amphotericin; cisplatin |
| Aminoglycosides; cyclosporin |
| Potassium depletion |
| Alcoholism |
| Increased extracellular fluid volume |
| Phosphate depletion |
| Diuresis |
| Diuretics (thiazides; loop diuretics) |
| Osmotic (diabetes, glucose, mannitol) |
| Acidosis |
| Fasting; diabetic ketoacidosis; $NH_4Cl$ administration |
| Mineralocorticoids‡ |
| Hyperthyroidism |
| *Decreased excretion* |
| Hypomagnesemia |
| Parathyroid hormone |
| Hypocalcemia |
| Alkalosis |
| Hypothyroidism |
| Contracted extracellular fluid volume |
| Antidiuretic hormone |
| Calcitonin |
| Glucagon |
| $K^+$, $Mg^{2+}$ sparing diuretics |

*When associated with excessive magnesium infusion/injection.
†Secondary to hypercalcemia; transient negative balance.
‡Secondary to increased extracellular fluid volume.

**Summary of Homeostatic Factors.** When magnesium intake is severely restricted in human subjects with normal kidney function, magnesium output becomes small (i.e., <0.25 mmol per day) within 5 to 7 days (Fig. 8–5).[56] Supplementing a normal intake increases urinary excretion without altering serum levels provided that renal function is normal and the amounts given do not exceed maximum glomerular filtration. The intestinal and renal conservation and excretory mechanisms in normal individuals permit homeostasis over a wide dietary intake.

## REQUIREMENTS FOR HEALTHY INDIVIDUALS

Data on magnesium intakes in U.S. population subgroups, the issue of adequacy of data on magnesium in foods, and the influences of other dietary factors on absorption were presented earlier. These factors must be taken into account in considering magnesium requirements. The technical issues in conducting metabolic balance studies for magnesium are those that hold for nitrogen and other minerals: namely, completeness and accuracy of intake and excretory values, sufficient time for equilibrium between studies and during collection, adequate numbers of individuals with respect to age and sex to give statistical validity, and systematic gradations of nutrient intake levels that cover the spectrum from negative to positive balances for the subjects. Balance studies that are not based on actual analysis of the magnesium content of the foods actually consumed are unacceptable. This latter point is further emphasized by the variability of magnesium data derived from various microcomputer analysis systems in comparison with the Department of Agriculture's Nutrient Database (which, as pointed out earlier, has some analytic deficiencies of its own).[60] Because of methodologic problems, including those of collection periods and analytic techniques, skepticism is indicated toward the older data[61,62] (reviewed in reference 63). There is considerable variance of data on more recent balance studies.[60,62] The 1989 RDA for adults of both sexes is accepted at 4.5 mg (0.19 mmol)/kg, which is the upper figure for reported magnesium equilibrium among the balance studies reviewed.[62] This translates into RDA values for a 76-kg male and a 62-kg female of 350 mg (14.4 mmol) and 280 mg (11.5

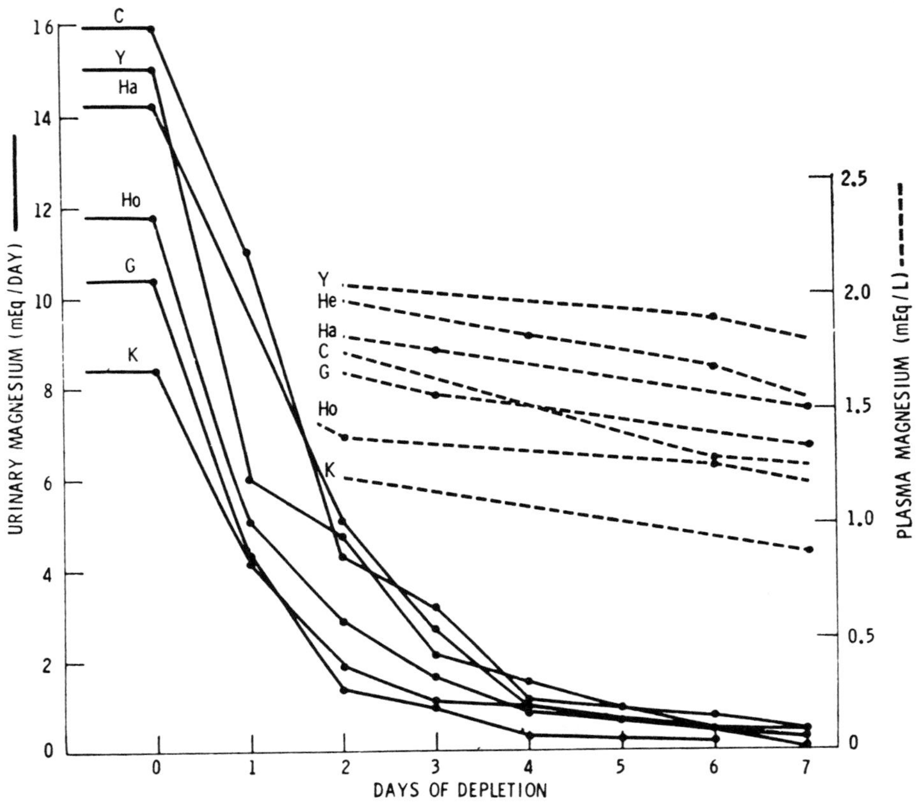

URINARY MAGNESIUM (mEq/DAY)
PLASMA MAGNESIUM (mEq/L)
DAYS OF DEPLETION
C
Y
Ha
Ho
G
K
He
0
1
2
3
4
5
6
7
0.5
1.0
1.5
2.0
2.5
2
4
6
8
10
12
14
16


**FIGURE 8–5.** Plasma and urine magnesium in the week following omission of magnesium from the diet in human experimental deficiency. The rapid decrease in excretion is depicted for 6 subjects. By the tenth day, all plasma values except that of Y were more than 2 standard deviations below the normal mean for the method used. (From Shils, M.E.: Medicine (Baltimore), *48*:61–85, 1969.)

mmol), respectively. The RDA for various groups are given in Appendix Table A–2b.

Serum magnesium levels were determined by atomic absorption spectrophotometry on a U.S. population sample of 15,820 persons between 1971 and 1974 in the NHANES 1 survey.[64] Ninety-five percent of adults aged 18 to 74 had serum levels in the range 0.75 to 0.96 mmol/L (1.50 to 1.92 mEq/L), mean 0.85 mmol/L. The levels of the fifth percentile were at or above the lower levels of normal generally used in clinical laboratories (i.e., 0.70 to 0.73 mmol/L). In my opinion, serum magnesium levels in healthy individuals are a good index of magnesium nutriture; hence, these data indicate that magnesium deficiency in the U.S. population from 1970 to 1974, and presumably now, is uncommon in younger and older adults.

A British study of still older subjects on differing intakes of magnesium indicated plasma levels of magnesium of 0.80 mmol/L (95% confidence limits (C.L.) 0.72 to 8.7) in 21 subjects in a long-term stay unit; six of these in a metabolic study had balances in the range of −1.1 mmol to +0.6 mmol with a mean of −0.2 mmol on a mean daily intake of 5.8 mmol (139 mg) and a mean absorption fraction of 20.7%.[65] Housebound and healthy elderly persons consuming 8.1 mmol (194 mg) and 10.7 mmol (257 mg), respectively, were in metabolic equilibrium. These intakes are below those of the RDA.

As has been consistently noted in various dietary surveys, infants and younger children in the United States consistently ingest magnesium at levels at or above the RDA;[33] even those at ages 1 to 5 years in the lowest fifth percentile achieve intakes of about 90% of the RDA.[32,33]

## MAGNESIUM DEFICIENCY

### SYMPTOMS AND SIGNS

**Laboratory Animals.** Hypomagnesemia is the hallmark of experimental magnesium depletion in many observed species. Although most studied, the rat is not representative of other species with respect to certain of its characteristic deficiency signs, such as hyperemia, repetitive (and usually acutely fatal) tonic-clonic convulsions, and its usually high levels of serum calcium and decreased parathyroid hormone (PTH). Mice on the same diet developed no hyperemia, became hypocalcemic in association with hypomagnesemia, and often died with a single abrupt and massive convulsion.[66] Deficient dogs and monkeys—also on diets of the same composition—developed spasticity, tremors, and occasionally nonfatal convulsions with hypocalcemia; increasing calcium intake did not increase serum calcium or prevent the neuromuscular changes.[67]

Other changes in the rat include reduced growth rate, alopecia, and skin lesions, whereas more chronic deficiency leads to edema, hypertrophic gums, leukocytosis, and splenomegaly. Thymic abnormalities have been noted that have been described by various investigators as malignant lymphosarcoma, disseminated lymphoblastic leukemia, or atrophy; others reported a marked organ enlargement in which normal structure was replaced by cells resembling transformed lymphocytes (reviewed in reference 68). Crystalluria, calcification, and degenerative changes in various organs, especially in the kidney and heart, are prominent in deficient rats and certain other species maintained on low-magnesium diets, particularly when the calcium content is high compared to that of human diets.[69,70]

**Human Magnesium Deficiency.** Symptomatic human deficiency develops in a setting of predisposing and complicating disease states (Table 8–3). These are associated with impaired intake and intestinal or renal tubular malabsorptive conditions.

## EXPERIMENTAL HUMAN DEFICIENCY

In the depletion study in which signs and symptoms occurred, the experimental diet provided about 0.4 mmol (9.6 mg) of magnesium per day; this followed a baseline period with a complete diet including adequate magnesium.[56] Plasma magnesium fell progressively in six subjects to levels that were 10 to 30% those of control periods. Erythrocyte magnesium declined more slowly and to a lesser degree. Urine (Fig. 8–5) and fecal magnesium decreased to extremely low levels within 7 days. Hypomagnesemia, hypocalcemia, and hypokalemia were present in all of the five consistently symptomatic patients. The course of one patient is shown in Figure 8–6. Good intestinal absorption of calcium and low urinary output resulted in positive calcium balance. Serum phosphate values varied among the subjects. Most subjects developed hypokalemia and negative potassium balance resulting from increased urinary losses. Serum sodium remained normal, whereas these subjects were in positive sodium balance. Abnormal neuromus-

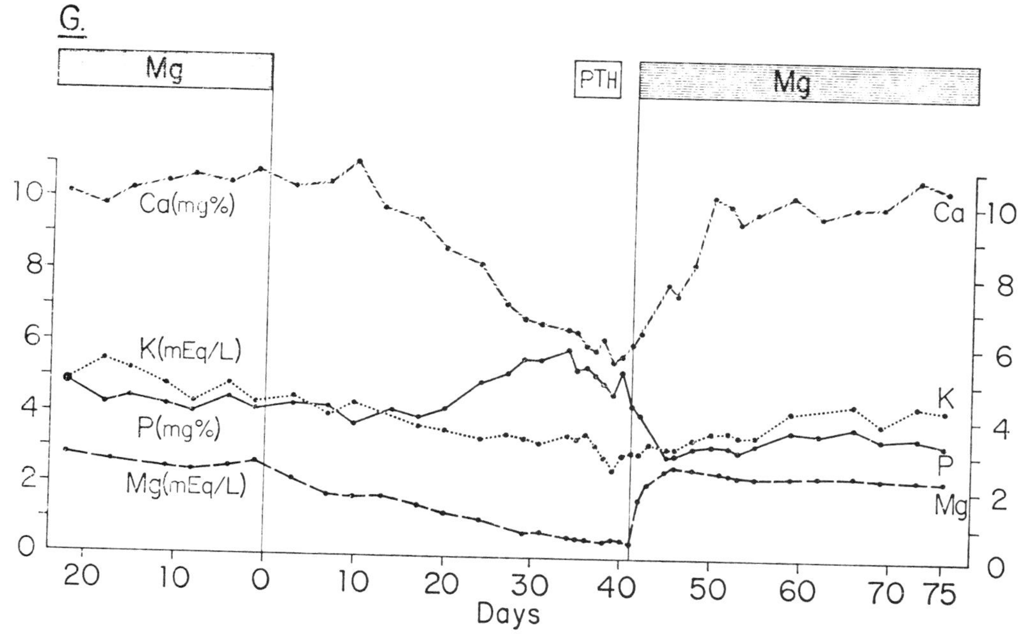
G.
Mg
PTH
Mg
Ca(mg%)
K(mEq/L)
P(mg%)
Mg(mEq/L)
Ca
K
P
Mg
0
2
4
6
8
10
20
10
0
10
20
30
40
50
60
70
75
Days

**FIGURE 8–6.** Blood chemistries in subject on experimental magnesium (Mg) depletion. Mg was omitted after the patient was one month on the control diet. The rise in serum inorganic phosphate (P) with Mg depletion in this patient was unique among the depleted subjects. On depletion day 25, Trousseau's and Chvostek's signs first occurred, and the former became progressively stronger as plasma calcium (Ca), Mg, and potassium (K) continued to decline. On depletion day 35, parathyroid hormone (PTH) was given IM at 50 units t.i.d. for 5 days; this had no effect on plasma Ca but appeared to decrease P. On day 41, anorexia, nausea, paresthesias, and generalized muscle spasticity developed; 17 mEq of Mg IV was then given with rapid improvement. This was followed by similar amounts of Mg IM 12 and 15 hours later. Dietary Mg (40 mEq daily) was resumed on the third repletion day. (From Shils, M.E.: Medicine (Baltimore), *48*: 61–85, 1969.)

cular function occurred in five of the seven subjects after deficiency periods ranging from 25 to 110 days.

All symptoms and signs (including personality changes and gastrointestinal symptoms) reverted to normal with reinstitution of magnesium. A characteristic finding during repletion was the delayed rise in serum calcium and potassium despite the rapid return to normal of serum magnesium; a week or longer passed before they returned to baseline levels. Potassium balances became strongly positive as sodium balances became negative.

**Clinical Deficiency.** The signs and symptoms noted above in experimental deficiency have been described individually or in various combinations in clinical cases of hypomagnesemia. They include Trousseau and Chvostek signs, normal or depressed deep tendon reflexes, muscle fasciculations, tremor, muscle spasm, personality changes, anorexia, nausea, and vomiting. Frank tetany, myoclonic jerks, athetoid movements, convulsions, and coma also have been reported. Convulsions with or without coma occur more frequently in acutely deficient infants than in adults.

The closest disease-related condition to "pure" experimental human magnesium deficiency is an uncommon congenital primary (idiopathic) hypomagnesemia related to a specific defect in intestinal absorption of this ion.[42,71] Hypomagnesemia, hypomagnesuria, hypocalcemia, and hypokalemia with tetany, often with convulsions, were corrected with magnesium supplements. Calcium and vitamin D supplements without magnesium were ineffective in maintaining normocalcemia.

The cellular loss of potassium appears to be secondary to functional impairment of the ATP-dependent Na-K cell membrane dependent pump; as potassium is lost sodium and calcium ions accumulate intracellularly.[72]

## MAGNESIUM DEFICIENCY AND PARATHYROID HORMONE: PHYSIOLOGIC AND BIOCHEMICAL CORRELATES

**PTH Levels in Deficient Humans.** The advent of immunologic assays for circulating PTH has contributed importantly to our understanding of the effect of magnesium depletion on calcium metabolism and has afforded further insight into species differences. The first reported magnesium-depleted patient studied with immunoparathyroid hormone (iPTH) assays had primary hypomagnesemia with undetectable iPTH.[73] When magnesium was given, iPTH levels rose markedly, and this was followed by a good calcemic response. These findings indicated that magnesium depletion was associated with a failure of the parathyroid gland to either manufacture or secrete the hormone. Over the next few years, as more cases with iPTH measurements were reported, it became apparent that the situation was more complex. For example, a survey of data on 36 hypomagnesemic patients from the literature revealed that 10 had iPTH levels that were low or undetectable, 18 had values in the "normal" range (which were, however, inappropriately low for the degree of hypocalcemia present), and 8 had elevated levels.[74] These data suggested that both iPTH secretion and bone reactivity to PTH were involved.

**PTH Levels in Deficient Rats.** The hypercalcemic reaction in magnesium-deficient rats has been noted above. Concentration of PTH in rats, in contrast to humans and other species, responded appropriately to the rising calcium levels induced by the deficiency. In one study plasma iPTH levels exceeded those of controls between deficiency 7 to 14 days and then fell to control levels as plasma calcium continued to increase above that of controls.[75] In another study, as serum magnesium fell and calcium rose, serum iPTH levels rose transiently to twice those of controls during the first 4 days of deficiency; thereafter iPTH fell to levels below those of controls as deficiency progressed with further decline of magnesium and progressive rise in calcium.[76] Severely magnesium-depleted rats were capable of secreting large amounts of iPTH when hypocalcemia was induced by depletion of either calcium or vitamin D.[76]

**Bone Resistance.** As noted, bone resistance to PTH was predicted from the finding of normal or elevated iPTH levels in some hypomagnesemic and hypocalcemic patients and by relative refractoriness of deficient animals and humans to parathyroid extract. Such resistance has been confirmed by observations in dogs with a chronic magnesium depletion.[77] Isolated tibias were perfused with a synthetic bovine PTH (syn b-PTH 1-34); the uptake (i.e., the arteriovenous difference for iPTH across the bones) of control dogs was 37.5% as compared to 10.1% in the depleted animals. This correlated with a significant depression in cAMP production by the deficient dogs. The deficient bones had a histologic picture of skeletal inactivity.

**Impaired PTH Secretion in Severe Human Hypomagnesemia.** Many patients with very low or normal iPTH concentrations developed significant increases in hormone levels following magnesium administration, with the rise in iPTH occurring appreciably earlier than the rise in serum calcium. When iPTH measurements were done serially before and at very short intervals after a rapid bolus intravenous injection of magnesium, serum iPTH rose within 1 minute to very high levels in association with very rapid elevations of serum magnesium but without any detectable rise in serum calcium over the next 30 to 360 minutes. The magnesium-depleted parathyroid gland was capable of producing PTH whereas magnesium supplementation induced rapid secretion.[78,79] The differences in baseline iPTH appear to reflect the severity of the magnesium depletion. Eumagnesemic subjects given magnesium had the expected rise in magnesium with a decline in iPTH.

## SEQUENCE OF CHANGES IN DEFICIENCY AND REPLETION IN HUMANS

**Initiation of Hypocalcemia.** The initiating factor appears to be failure of the normal heterionic exchange of bone calcium for magnesium at the labile bone mineral surface.[80] Impairment of receptor responsiveness to PTH of the osteoclasts follows with reduction of active bone resorption.[77] Hypocalcemia progresses despite increased levels of circulating PTH.[79]

**Perpetuation of Electrolyte, PTH, and Clinical Abnormalities.** As depletion progresses, secretion of PTH diminishes to very low levels despite adequate intraparathyroid gland hormonal reserves.[78,79] The signs of severe magnesium depletion are present at this stage: very low circulating PTH, unresponsive bone, hypocalcemia, hypocalciuria, hypokalemia, sodium retention, and neuromuscular and other clinical signs and symptoms.[56]

**Regression of Magnesium Depletion and Associated Changes.** Following administration of adequate magnesium, serum magnesium rapidly rises presumably with restoration of heterionic calcium exchange but with little or no detectable change in circulating calcium in this early phase. There is an increase in circulating PTH; however, there is a delay in the serum calcium response until receptors to osteoclast PTH regain responsiveness. With a rise in calcium, plasma PTH levels decline appropriately. The delayed rise in serum potassium is presumably secondary to the period required to restore the normal activity of the cellular membrane Na-K pump in various tissues. Clinical signs and symptoms disappear in a matter of hours to a few days.

## OTHER DEFICIENCY MANIFESTATIONS

**Resistance to Vitamin D in Magnesium Deficiency.** The calcemic effect of vitamin D—even in high dose—is blunted in the presence of magnesium depletion in human rickets,[81] in D-deficient laboratory animals,[82] in human malabsorption,[83] and in idiopathic[84] or surgically induced hypoparathyroidism.[85] PTH is necessary for the formation of calcitriol, and calcitriol is necessary for PTH to exert its effect on calcium mobilization from bone;[86] nevertheless, despite low levels of calcitriol in the majority of reported cases with magnesium depletion, serum calcium rose following magnesium repletion.[85,87,88] Magnesium depletion in rats did not affect normal conversion in vivo of calcidiol to calcitriol nor did it modify the in vitro activity of 1, α-hydroxylase in renal mitochondria.[82] It was concluded that vitamin D resistance induced by magnesium depletion is the consequence of impaired skeletal response to calcitriol.

**Urine Citrate Levels.** Magnesium-deficient patients (chronically depleted as the result of intestinal malabsorption or acutely depleted by inadequate magnesium in their TPN solutions) markedly decreased their urinary content of citrate; this was shown to be secondary to increased renal tubular citrate reabsorption.[89] The low urinary citrate is an additional risk factor for renal stone formation.

**Lipids, Lipoproteins, and Prostanoids.** Magnesium deficiency in rats has been associated with increased serum/plasma phospholipids,[90,91] triglycerides,[91] variable total cholesterol,[90,91] low free cholesterol,[91] increased levels of oleic and linoleic acids, and decreased stearic and arachidonic acids.[91] Modifications of lipid and lipoprotein concentrations have also been noted.[91] Some of these may be attributable to reported decreased activity of lipoprotein lipase and lecithin cholesterol acyltransferase.[91]

Plasma prostanoids ($PGE_2$, $PGF_2$-α, 6-keto-$PGF_1$-α, and $TBX_2$) were significantly elevated in both plasma and tissues of deficient rats as compared to controls.[92] Similarly, prostanoids present in the outflow of the vessels of the mesenteric arterial bed were significantly increased in the magnesium deficient rats as compared to controls.[93] It has been hypothesized that magnesium depletion, by inhibiting adenylate cyclase activity and thereby lowering cAMP levels, will permit increased cyclooxygenase activity and stimulation of prostanoid synthesis.[92]

Because of differences in certain biochemical and pathologic changes in the magnesium deficient rat as compared to other species, experimental comparison with other species is necessary before assuming that the lipid and prostanoid changes noted above occur generally.

Lipid alterations have been reported in hypomagnesemic human subjects; however, as discussed below, these are often complicated by factors related to heart and other disease and accompanying medications.

## SOURCES OF MAGNESIUM LOSSES

As noted earlier the normal responses to depletion involve reductions in intestinal and renal excretion, thereby minimizing losses in healthy experimental subjects. Thus, after proportionately large losses of magnesium in urine during the first few days, subsequent daily net losses in four experimental subjects were about 0.35 mmol (8.4 mg).[56] There was no correlation between the extent of net magnesium losses and the time to onset of symptoms. After the first week fecal losses account for one-half to two-thirds of the total. The occurrence of a bout of diarrhea can increase daily stool losses 5 to 7 times the usual daily total net loss.[56]

In an experimental human study of about 3 weeks' duration in which patients became hypomagnesemic (but not symptomatic), there was no decrease in muscle magnesium[94]; presumably, bone was the primary source of magnesium loss.

Wallach has reviewed literature covering 25 years concerning the sources of loss of body magnesium in deficient rats and in humans with various clinical syndromes and associated medications.[95] The human data are variable in terms of estimated muscle and bone losses. In the rat the major loss is from bone with much less lost from muscle; however, the amounts vary depending on age and duration of study. As noted later, the presence of partial starvation, malabsorption, and/or cardiac and renal dysfunction are often associated with chronic acidosis and the use of diuretics. Both may accelerate magnesium and potassium losses as well as other nutrient losses.

## COMPARISON OF EXPERIMENTAL AND CLINICAL DEPLETION

Experimental magnesium depletion in humans and various species of laboratory animals is associated uniformly with an early and progressive fall in serum magnesium. The clinical literature reporting magnesium deficiency is variable in this respect. Such findings include (1) decreased serum and muscle magnesium with normal bone level,[96] (2) decreased serum, variable muscle, and low bone magnesium levels,[97] (3) normal serum and erythrocyte magnesium levels with decreased muscle magnesium and potassium,[98] (4) reduced serum magnesium level with normal muscle content,[99] (5) reduced muscle level in association with normal serum, erythrocyte, and bone magnesium levels and variable muscle potassium,[100] (6) consistently reduced serum magnesium concentrations with variable muscle levels,[101] (7) lack of correlation of reduced, normal, or elevated plasma magnesium with differences in erythrocyte or muscle magnesium,[102] and (8) low serum magnesium with variable muscle magnesium concentration but with a highly significant correlation between serum and bone magnesium levels.[103] Other examples of poor correlations are given later. During magnesium deficiency muscle magnesium varies directly with muscle potassium in humans,[3,103,105] rats,[106] and guinea pigs.[107] These marked variations emphasize the difficulty in ascribing cause and effect to a specific nutrient deficiency in uncontrolled situations in sick individuals. Normal cellular metabolism and homeostasis of cellular composition are critically dependent on an adequate supply of energy and essential nutrients. Significant deficiency of one or more nutrients has an impact on retention of other nutrients; for example, magnesium depletes potassium, whereas potassium depletion reduces the magnesium content of cells.[103,105] Another example concerns the effects of total starvation.[108] Over a 2-month period magnesium was lost from tissue in two ways, firstly, by depletion of lean body mass; in four of six obese subjects a loss of 400 g of nitrogen was calculated to be associated with a loss of approximately 700 mEq of magnesium. Secondly, magnesium was lost by an additional renal loss that appeared to be related, at least in good part, to the degree of acidosis; when 50 to 150 g of glucose were given, urinary magnesium decreased by 55%. Muscle magnesium decreased, but the electrolyte excretion patterns indicated that significant amounts came from bone. Serum magnesium was maintained, presumably by a fairly constant input of magnesium into the blood.

The pattern of increased endogenous loss seen in the starving individual may occur in the sick patient who is eating poorly, is in negative nitrogen balance, and has acidosis, particularly when a serious catabolic state is present (i.e., with trauma, burns, sepsis, and serious inflammatory bowel disease).

It may be useful clinically to distinguish two types of magnesium depletion: (1) that caused by a failure to ingest, absorb, or retain (by the intestine or by renal tubules) sufficient magnesium in an individual who is otherwise reasonably well nourished and with normal glomerular function; this is associated with the characteristic hypomagnesemia and sequelae noted in experimental deficiency; and (2) that associated with concomitant energy and other deficiencies, serious catabolism, potassium depletion, acidosis and/or drugs that result in bone and muscle loss of magnesium. As noted previously, the increased endogenous release of magnesium together with some exogenous magnesium intake may well permit a normal or near-normal serum level, particularly if accompanied by depressed glomerular filtration rate on a prerenal basis (i.e., hypotension, dehydration) or with intrinsic renal dysfunction.

Clinical reports attempting to correlate serum magnesium with tissue levels should provide sufficient clinical, metabolic, and medication data to permit an evaluation of those factors that may affect these levels.

## MAGNESIUM DEPLETION IN VARIOUS DISEASES

**Prevalence.** The list of causes of magnesium depletion (Table 8–3) emphasizes that this condition is not a rare occurrence in acutely or chronically ill patients. Of 2300 patients surveyed in a Veterans Administration hospital 6.9% were hypomagnesemic. Eleven percent of patients having routine magnesium determinations were hypomagnesemic. When patients were hypokalemic, hypomagnesemia occurred in 42%; 29% were hypomagnesemic in the presence of hypophosphatemia, 27% were hypomagnesemic in those with hyponatremia, and 22% in those with hypocalcemia.[109]

Patients in medical and surgical intensive care units (ICUs) have a high prevalence of hypomagnesemia. In a medical ICU, 65% of patients admitted with normal renal function had hypomagnesemia; of these one-third had hypocalcemia corrected with magnesium supplements.[110] Of 193 adult postoperative ICU patients, 117 (63%) were hypomagnesemic and 10 (5%) were hypermagnesemic. Those with serum magnesium <0.5 mmol/L were hypokalemic; the majority had received nephrotoxic agents and they had a higher mortality rate than the others.[111] In 32 pulmonary ICU patients, 9% had low serum magnesium and 47% had low muscle values; there was a significant association between muscle magnesium and muscle potassium concentrations; many of these patients had been treated with steroids, aminoglycosides, diuretics, or digoxin.[112] The frequent associations noted here and below suggest that appropriate estimations of magnesium nutriture should be performed routinely in a variety of clinical conditions.

**Alcoholism.** Magnesium depletion in acute and chronic alcoholism have been documented over many years. Causes include poor intake, increased urinary losses, vomiting, diarrhea, and ketosis.[113]

**Diabetes.** Loss of magnesium in diabetic ketoacidosis has also been known for many years.[114] Ambulatory diabetic patients without renal insufficiency were hypomagnesemic in excess of 30% on a multifactorial basis.[115] A significant negative correlation was noted between serum/plasma magnesium and blood glycohemoglobin in insulin-dependent pregnant women with significant relationships to the rates of spontaneous abortion and malformation.[116] About one-third of infants born to diabetic mothers were hypomagnesemic during the first 3 days of life. Similar negative correlations were noted between plasma and muscle magnesium and glycohemoglobin in adult insulin-dependent diabetes mellitus (IDDM).[117] In one group of children with IDDM, serum magnesium, calcium, PTH, calcitriol, and osteocalcin were lower than in age- and sex-matched controls,[118] whereas in another series magnesium and potassium were low in skeletal muscle.[119] Following oral magnesium supplementation, these values increased significantly. Of interest was the finding of decreased insulin requirement with supplementation.[119]

**Malabsorption.** Serum magnesium is often subnormal in patients with malabsorption syndromes of various causes (Table 8–3). As noted earlier, increased amounts of fatty acids in the intestinal lumen form insoluble soaps with $Mg^{2+}$ leading to loss from both dietary and endogenous sources. In such circumstances, restriction of dietary fat can reduce magnesium losses.[97,120]

**Protein-Energy Malnutrition.** Magnesium depletion occurs in children with inadequate food intakes in association with malabsorption, persistent vomiting and/or diarrhea, and infection. Serum or plasma magnesium was noted to be low in a significant proportion of such children in various studies in Africa,[121] whereas in a study in Central America 50% of serum magnesium values were below 0.65 mmol/L on admission.[122]

**Kidney Disease and Nephrotoxic Drugs.** A number of factors may modify adversely the critical role of the kidney in magnesium homeostasis (Table 8–4). When glomerular filtration is impaired, *hypermagnesemia* is usual. However, *hypomagnesemia* may occur in patients with renal failure because of poor food intake and concomitant losses associated with vomiting, diarrhea, malabsorption, diuretics, nephrotoxic drugs, chronic acidosis, and/or use of magnesium-low dialysate. Increased excretion is also associated with postobstructive nephropathy, chronic glomerulonephritis, acute tubulo-interstitial nephritis, and postrenal transplantation. In congenital urinary magnesium wasting syndromes, the magnesium deficiency is often severe and symptomatic.[123]

**Post Parathyroidectomy Hypomagnesemia.** Symptomatic hypomagnesemia may follow parathyroidectomy for primary hyperparathyroidism in association with the expected hypocalcemia, presumably as part of the "hungry bone" syndrome that occurs as the result of rapid uptake of calcium and magnesium by bone. Symptoms of muscle weakness, tremor, and mental changes can be reversed by magnesium supplementation despite continuing low calcium.[124]

**Congenital Disorders.** Primary hypomagnesemia and congenital renal wasting syndromes reflect deficiencies secondary to malabsorption in the intestine[42] or kidney tubule,[123] respectively. They are differentiated clinically by the finding of a very low urinary output in the former and a relatively high output in the latter. In Barrter's syndrome, hypomagnesemia may occur but is not common. A syndrome similar to that of Barrter's has been described in which there was a normal juxtaglomerular apparatus with severe hypokalemia that responded to large amounts of magnesium.[125]

**Hypertension.** Increased magnesium in vitro relaxes vascular smooth muscle and reduces pressor responses.[126] When 8.3 mmol (200 mg) of $Mg^{2+}$ as the sulfate was infused into normal human subjects over a 3-hour period, serum magnesium was raised from an average of 0.83 mmol/L (1.67 mEq/L) to 1.75 mmol/L (3.5 mEq/L). Systolic and diastolic blood pressures fell by an average of 10 and 8 mm, respectively, and renal blood flow increased significantly.[127] Urinary excretion of 6-keto-$PGF_1$-α (the stable metabolite of prostacyclin) increased markedly, whereas urinary $PGE_2$ did not change. Cyclo-oxygenase inhibition (indomethacin, ibuprofen) completely blocked the magnesium-induced fall in blood pressure, the rise in urinary 6-keto-$PGF_1$-α, and the rise in renal blood flow. The calcium-channel blocker nifedipine also prevented the magnesium-induced rise in 6-keto-$PGF_1$-α and the fall in blood pressure. These findings show that the effect of magnesium was mediated by prostacyclin release, which may be influenced by changes in $Ca^{2+}$ flux.

When magnesium chloride was infused for 90 minutes into healthy subjects to the point of doubling the plasma magnesium, PTH levels fell and those of plasma renin activity and renin increased.[128] Others have found that, when kidneys are perfused with magnesium, renin release is directly related to magnesium concentration.

There are conflicting reports relating serum magnesium levels in hypertensives to those in nonhypertensives— that is, lower in both sexes with hypertension,[129] in men but not in women,[130] or with no difference from controls.[131] Of more relevance are the results of a series of intervention studies. Hypertensive patients on thiazide diuretics were also given magnesium supplements (aspartate-HCl or chloride) with a subsequent drop in blood pressure.[132,133] In contrast, two other studies, also testing magnesium aspartate in comparison with placebo in patients with mild to moderate[134] or mild hypertension,[135] found no decline in blood pressure after 1 month or 3 months, respectively. An 8-month controlled study in subjects with mild hypertension compared either placebo or potassium alone or in combination with magnesium as the chloride; potassium alone or with magnesium caused a significant reduction in blood pressure but magnesium had no added effect to the potassium.[136] The latter three studies were performed in subjects not receiving diuretics who had normal serum magnesium. It is possible that magnesium supplements may lower pressures in those who have become magnesium-depleted as the result of chronic diuretic use.[135]

With the increasing armamentarium of antihypertensive drugs, the state of magnesium nutriture needs to be better evaluated in terms of the effectiveness of the newer drugs. For example, it has been reported that normal or increased levels of magnesium in the diet of spontaneously hypertensive rats did not appear to play an important role in the long-term regulation of blood pressure. However, a response to the calcium-channel blocker nifedipine was most pronounced in the rats on the normal diet and was significantly decreased in those on the magnesium deficient diet.[137]

## CORONARY ARTERY DISEASE

The earlier discussion on the biochemical roles of magnesium has indicated its importance in cardiovascular function. An increasing literature has been concerned with the possible roles of magnesium in various aspects of coronary artery disease (CAD).

**Relation to Magnesium Nutriture.** Some epidemiologic data have suggested a decreased mortality from CAD in populations living in "hard" water areas (i.e., relatively high in calcium, magnesium, and fluoride) as compared to those in "soft" water areas (summarized reference 138). Contrary data from various countries have indicated no association between myocardial disease and mortality and the concentrations of magnesium or calcium in drinking water.[139-141]

The argument has been advanced that the American public has a significant amount of asymptomatic magnesium deficiency, which is a contributing factor to the prevalence of CAD.[138] Data presented earlier contradicts the concept of widespread magnesium deficiency which, together with the continuing decline in age-adjusted death rate from ischemic heart disease in the United States, makes this an unlikely hypothesis.

**Magnesium Status and the Development and Complications of Cardiovascular Disease.** Depressed magnesium status has been implicated to both dysrhythmias and myocardial infarction. Older literature noted low serum/plasma magnesium in individuals complaining of chest pain or with proven myocardial infarction upon admission or soon after hospitalization; most of these reports were either uncontrolled or had inadequate data. More recent studies tend to contradict the suggestion that a prior primary state of magnesium depletion was involved; rather they suggest that other significant events contributed to infarction. A number of factors affect serum and cardiac magnesium concentrations in such patients. These include (1) the time of drawing of blood following onset of chest pain, (2) the prior and often chronic use of diuretics (which may induce magnesium and potassium depletion), (3) postinfarction lipolysis (also induced by ethanol withdrawal, epinephrine, and surgery) causing increased serum fatty acids that lower serum magnesium, and (4) the degree of pain per se (reviewed in reference 61).

In controlled studies in patients with acute infarction or acute ischemic attacks, serum magnesium either fell only slightly and transiently or did not fall at all on admission or over several days (reviewed in references 61 and 142).

Long-term use of diuretics, such as thiazides in high doses or furosemide, is associated with renal loss of both potassium and magnesium; these drugs are associated with depletion of such ions and with an increased prevalence of arrhythmias.[143-145] Further evidence for a role of diuretics in depleting magnesium is the markedly increased retention of a load test of intravenous magnesium chloride by patients with chronic ischemic heart disease (IHD) who had been on long-term diuretics as compared to IHD patients not given diuretics.[146] Patients admitted to the coronary care unit (CCU) who had proven acute infarction had the same magnesium retention as those in whom infarction was ruled out; both had much less retention than the stable chronic IHD patients. However, not all patients with heart disease who take diuretics such as furosemide have low serum or tissue magnesium; conversely, patients can have evidence of low tissue magnesium levels without having received the diuretic.[147]

Magnesium ATP has been reported to be a neurotransmitter released by sympathetic nerves,[148] to decrease the contractile force of atria,[149] and to induce a positive inotropic effect on rat ventricles.[150] More recently, extracellular Mg ATP was noted to induce a transient acidification followed by an alkanization in single rat cardiac cells.[151] The alkanization has been attributed to the activation of a $Na^+/H^+$ antiport,[152] and the decrease in intracellular pH to the activation of a $Cl^-/HCO_3^-$

exchanger.[151] In ischemic conditions, a further fall in pHi could displace intracellular $Ca^{2+}$ ions and open a nonspecific conductance which, in turn, could lead to an arrhythmia.[151]

In the last 8 years, controlled studies have suggested that intravenous magnesium given early after suspected acute myocardial infarction could reduce the frequency of serious arrhythmias and mortality. The results of seven such studies, which included 1301 patients, have been reviewed.[153] A recent editorial in the Lancet briefly noted these reports and considered the mechanisms for reduced mortality because, in its view, "mortality reduction is unlikely to be due to suppression of arrhythmias which cause few deaths in coronary care units."[154] It pointed out that increasing magnesium in serum causes both peripheral and coronary vessel vasodilation, perhaps by competing with calcium at the slow calcium channel of vascular smooth muscle and by stimulation of prostacyclin release from endothelium. The effects of prostacyclin on these circulations are qualitatively similar to those of infused magnesium; magnesium can release prostacyclin with consequent inhibition of platelet adhesion and aggregation. The editorial reported that two large-scale controlled clinical studies testing the effectiveness of magnesium are underway, namely the Leicester Intravenous Magnesium Intervention Trial (LIMIT-2) and the fourth International Study of Infarct Survival (ISIS-4); it suggested caution in the use of intravenous magnesium for this purpose pending the outcome of these studies.*

## ASSESSING MAGNESIUM NUTRITURE

The desirability of having a reliable marker or markers for diagnosing magnesium depletion and the degree of its severity is obvious both in terms of clinical usefulness and in allowing for more precise data on magnesium requirements in healthy individuals. Opportunities exist for improving diagnostic tests.

**Concentrations of Magnesium in Body Fluids, Intact Cells, and Cell Partitions.** As noted earlier, measurement of the level of serum magnesium is often not a reliable indicator of depletion of magnesium in other tissues in various clinical states.

**Total versus Ionized Magnesium.** Protein bound magnesium is subject to variations associated with changes in albumin and acid-base conditions (acidosis decreasing and alkalosis increasing the bonding); hence, the level of ionized or ultrafiltrable magnesium may be more relevant clinically than the level of total magnesium. In a series of 64 patients, 21 had low total serum magnesium but only 5 had low ionized levels. The level of total magnesium was sensitive to ultrafilterable hypomagnesemia but lacked specificity in predicting it.[155] An improved electrode for determining ionized magnesium in whole blood, plasma, and serum has been reported to give good linearity with minimum interference.[156] This approach should give more precision in determining biologically active magnesium but is unlikely to resolve the issue of the discrepancies between serum levels and various tissue levels.

**Free Intracellular $Mg^{2+}$.** The ability to accurately and easily measure changes of $[Mg^{2+}]i$ in various blood and tissue cells together with ions such as $K^+$, $Na^+$, and $Ca^{2+}$ will undoubtedly help in elucidating relationships with magnesium intake and balance, the effects of drugs and disease, and the extent of magnesium depletion. The various techniques for this determination were reviewed earlier. $^{31}P$ NMR spectroscopy is beginning to be applied to erythrocytes in clinical situations.

**Blood Mononuclear Cells.** Magnesium concentrations in human mononuclear cells have been claimed to be a better guide to magnesium nutriture than is the serum level.[157,158] In magnesium deficient rats, however, the percentage of losses of this ion from lymphocytes was similar to that from cardiac and skeletal muscle and very much less than that from serum and erythrocytes.[160] In patients with mild to severe congestive heart failure serum circulating mononuclear cell and skeletal muscle magnesium concentrations were all of little predictive value in assessing the concentration of myocardial magnesium.[147] In experienced hands, the magnesium content of mononuclear blood cells is reproducible (Table 8–1), but variations in the proportion of isolated lymphocytes and monocytes can influence the results.[159]

**Urine Levels of Magnesium.** These measurements are helpful in determining the general cause of hypomagnesemia if the intake of magnesium is known. A low urine magnesium indicates malabsorption, whereas a urine output above intake suggests renal tubular dysfunction.

**Physiologic and Metabolic Measurements: The Magnesium Load Test.** A fairly rapid entry of magnesium into one or more body pools is indicated by the increased retention of magnesium when given previously in an intravenous infusion into magnesium-depleted patients.[146] This semiquantitative load test has been used by certain investigators over the years (see references 157-159); it involves an infusion of a given amount of diluted magnesium salt (which may on occasion cause hypotension), a quantitative urine collection for 12 or more hours, and a magnesium determination. It is an invasive, time-consuming, and expensive test requiring hospitalization for a day and careful urine collection and analysis. It has the advantage of allowing a subject to be his or her own control by repeating the test before and

*The findings of LIMIT-2 indicate a borderline significant reduction with IV magnesium sulfate in mortality (p-0.04) and in the incidence of left ventricular failure (p-0.009) in patients with suspected acute myocardial infarction.[175] There was no evidence of an antiarrhythmic action of magnesium.

after magnesium repletion. It is not standardized in terms of amounts and duration of magnesium infusion and of duration of urine collection.

Despite the numerous *enzymatic* reactions for which $Mg^{2+}$ is essential, there is no diagnostic enzymatic reaction in clinical use for detecting deficiency.

**Classic Balance Studies.** The long-term and expensive metabolic studies used for estimating normal human requirements are not applicable to the study of sick patients. However, estimates of intake (especially by tube or vein) can be done over short periods and, together with urinary and fecal losses, may provide an approximation of the adequacy and needs for magnesium in those circumstances. The results can be correlated with serum and other measurements as guides to need.

**Clinical Observations.** A proper history and physical examination based on the knowledge of the clinical conditions that lead to depletion are important in alerting the physician to incipient or actual magnesium deficiency.

## MANAGEMENT OF DEPLETION

The physician should apply knowledge about predisposing factors in order to anticipate hypomagnesemia and institute early treatments to *prevent* its occurrence or minimize its severity. These include instituting control of underlying disease, minimizing therapeutic insult, and initiating nutritional and dietary changes to minimize magnesium losses in stool and urine.

It is essential to determine the cause of the magnesium depletion. Usually this can be accomplished by a careful history to delineate intestinal and/or renal causes. If the cause is uncertain, a combination of serum and urine determinations is indicated. When the serum magnesium has fallen consistently below the apparent threshold of the normal kidney for several or more days, renal excretion progressively falls. Lower-than-expected urine levels suggest depletion secondary to poor intake, malabsorption, or previous use of medications that enhance magnesium loss. If renal tubular insufficiency is present, urinary magnesium will be appreciably higher, to the point of equaling or exceeding the amount of magnesium absorbed from the intestine or that given parenterally.

The amount, route, and duration of magnesium administration will depend on the severity of depletion and its cause. Symptomatic deficiency (paresthesias, latent or active tetany) is best treated by the intravenous or intramuscular route in conjunction with appropriate therapy for the underlying condition and with correction of other electrolyte and acid-base abnormalities. It is our practice to initiate treatment in symptomatic adolescents and adults with good renal function with 3 g (25 mEq) of 50% magnesium sulfate given intravenously over 2 or 3 hours in saline or dextrose solutions with other nutrients as required. Another 3 or 4 g are then given by continuous infusion over the remaining 24 hours or by periodic intramuscular injections. This regimen is continued for 2 or more days, and the situation is then reassessed. The dosages given must always exceed the daily losses.

Intravenous calcium administration in the treatment of hypocalcemia secondary to magnesium deficiency is usually unnecessary unless incipient or overt tetany is apparent; in this case, a slow calcium infusion is usually necessary only for 1 or 2 days as magnesium replacement takes effect.

The return to the normal range of serum magnesium with the above or higher dosage schedule is relatively rapid. Repletion of magnesium lost from bone and other tissues, however, requires a more prolonged period of magnesium therapy. This treatment should be combined—although at smaller doses or with oral intake if suitable—with periodic evaluation of serum and/or urine magnesium levels as the dosage is reduced to that which achieves a stable and adequate state with normal serum magnesium.

For the asymptomatic patient with serum levels below approximately 0.5 mmol/L (1.0 mEq/L), the dosage prescribed previously is indicated; when the level is higher, half the dosage, given parenterally or orally, should be sufficient unless renal losses are high. In that case, again, the dose must be higher than daily losses.

Where indicated and feasible, supplementary magnesium may be given as gelatin capsules packed with powdered magnesium sulfate (Epsom salts), magnesium chloride, acetate, or other salts with good solubility in enteric fluids. One capsule is given 3 to 6 times per day; multiple doses over the day minimize magnesium-related diarrhea.[51] Improvement of existing steatorrhea will decrease fecal magnesium losses. Treatment of other underlying disease and replacement of potassium deficits are essential.

The need for prolonged magnesium therapy that cannot be met adequately by increased oral intake presents a practical problem. Intramuscular injection of magnesium salts is painful, and chronic injections induce a fibrotic reaction. An alternative is intravenous infusion or the old-fashioned but useful hypodermic clysis. In the latter procedure 50% magnesium sulfate (e.g., 2 g) is diluted in 250 ml of 0.45% saline and infused slowly through a needle of very small bore inserted just under the abdominal skin as frequently as is necessary to meet the patient's magnesium requirement. The intravenous route may be through a peripheral line, a percutaneous catheter into the subclavian vein, or a tunneled central venous catheter. For the patient with serious persistent renal wasting, as may occur with cisplatin toxicity, the latter is useful. The daily requirement for magnesium (together with any other electrolytes that are needed) may be given at home in 2 to 4 hours nightly or less frequently, if indicated. Periodic assessment of serum magnesium levels prior to periodic infusion allows an estimate of needs.

Alternative programs of magnesium replacement in deficient adults have been used, usually with higher doses than advocated here. Flink, for example, recommended 112 to 128 mEq intramuscularly or intravenously over the first day, with smaller doses subsequently.[162] The larger the dose and the faster the rate of administration, the higher the serum level achieved and the greater the amount excreted by the normal kidney.

In the treatment of symptomatic magnesium depletion in infants, the rapid efficacy of relatively small amounts of intravenous or intramuscular magnesium in controlling neuromuscular signs and restoring serum levels is well established. Parenteral administration is recommended at 0.15 to 0.25 mmol(0.3 to 0.5 mEq)/kg body weight as 50% magnesium sulfate over the first several hours followed by an equal amount, either intramuscularly or intravenously, over the remainder of the day. If the child is symptomatic, calcium should also be infused together with potassium and other electrolytes as indicated. Duration, route, and dosage will depend on the severity and cause of the depletion. In cases of chronic malabsorption (e.g., primary hypomagnesemia) 0.5 to 0.75 mmol (1.0 to 1.5 mEq)/kg in multiple divided oral doses should be tested; this dosage schedule raises serum levels to near normal without inducing diarrhea.[163]

## HYPERMAGNESEMIA AND MAGNESIUM TOXICITY

**Hypermagnesemia with Normal Renal Function.** The normal kidney is capable of excreting large amounts of absorbed or injected magnesium ion so rapidly that serum levels usually do not rise to dangerous levels. High-dose parenteral magnesium sulfate is the drug of choice in North America for preventing eclamptic convulsions that may occur with severe hypertension in late pregnancy or during labor.[164] It has also been given in an effort to prevent premature labor.[165] A loading dose is given followed by maintenance doses with the objective of maintaining a high serum level (e.g., 2 to 3 mmol/L (4 to 6 mEq/L)[164] or 2.5 to 4 mmol/L (5 to 8 mEq/L).[165] Patients with normal kidneys are able to excrete 40 to 60 g of magnesium sulfate per day when it is given by persistent infusion.[162] The high doses used clinically rarely cause a degree of hypermagnesemia likely to be associated with serious side effects (see next section) because the patients are closely monitored.

The interdependent and often competitive relations of $Mg^{2+}$ and $Ca^{2+}$ are further demonstrated by the changes in serum $Ca^{2+}$ and circulating PTH levels in patients with therapeutic hypermagnesemia. With the rise in serum magnesium, a fall in PTH may occur with an associated hypocalcemia;[165,166] although some preeclamptic pregnant women had hypocalcemia with little or no change in PTH levels,[167,168] their fetuses at delivery had low calcium and very low PTH levels.[168]

Another example of this $Mg^{2+}-Ca^{2+}$ competition is the observation that magnesium sulfate infusions increased the circulating levels of the vitamin K–dependent, bone-specific protein osteocalcin, presumably as the result of its known inhibition of osteocalcin binding to hydroxyapatite, an effect that can be overcome by calcium.[169] These and many other $Mg^{2+}-Ca^{2+}$ interactions have led to the designation of magnesium as a "mimic weak $Ca^{2+}$ antagonist" and "the mimic/antagonist" of calcium.[170,171] Although this designation holds for many situations, it is also clear that magnesium has independent attributes, some of which have been mentioned earlier.

**Magnesium Toxicity.** In contrast to the planned therapeutic hypermagnesemia noted above, elevated serum levels can occur when magnesium-containing drugs, usually antacids or cathartics, are ingested chronically by individuals with renal insufficiency. Because 20% or more of $Mg^{2+}$ from various salts may be absorbed, the impairment of renal clearance can cause significant elevations of serum magnesium. In acute renal failure with oliguria, especially when accompanied by metabolic acidosis, tissue release in association with magnesium ingestion or parenteral administration may result in some degree of hypermagnesemia.

The many potentially toxic and even lethal effects of magnesium excess are summarized in Figure 8–7.[172] Calcium infusion can counteract magnesium toxicity.[172] Magnesium-containing medications in patients with significant renal disease should be avoided unless there is good reason and the patient is closely monitored. Hypermagnesemia should be suspected in instances of low anion gap in stable patients and a normal anion gap in severely ill acidotic patients.[172]

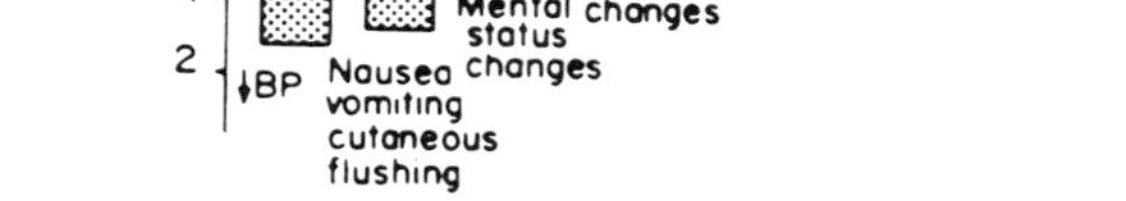

Mg (mEq/L)
16
14
12
10
8
6
4
2
↓BP
Nausea vomiting cutaneous flushing
Mental status changes
ECG changes
↓Reflex
↓Respirations
Coma
Cardiac arrest

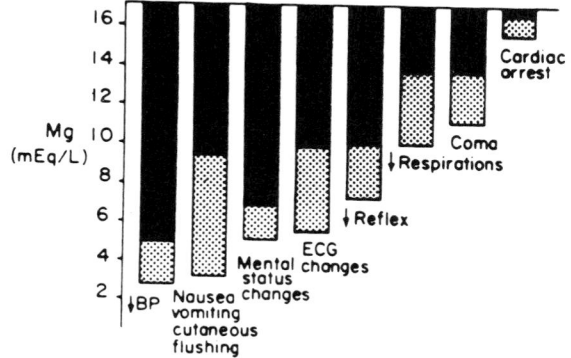


**FIGURE 8–7.** The toxic effects of elevated serum magnesium progress in severity with increasing concentration. Nausea, vomiting and hypotension may occur in the range of 3 to 9 mEq/L; bradycardia and urinary retention also occur in this range. Electrocardiogram changes, hyporeflexia, and secondary central nervous system depression may appear in the 5- to 10-mEq/L range followed at higher concentrations by life-threatening respiratory depression, coma, and asystolic cardiac arrest. (From Mordes, J.P., Wacker, E.C.: Pharmacol. Rev., *29*:274–300, 1978, with permission of the American Society of Pharmacology and Experimental Therapeutics.)

## REFERENCES


1. Kruse, H.D., Orent, E.R., McCollum, E.V.: J. Biol. Chem., *96*:519–536, 1932.
2. Hirschfelder, A.D., Haury, V.G.: JAMA, *102*:1138–1141, 1934.
3. Flink, E.B.: J. Am. Coll. Nutr., *4*:17–31, 1985.
4. Ebel, H., Gunther, T.: J. Clin. Chem. Biochem., *18*:257–270, 1980.
5. Vernon, W.B.: Magnesium, *7*:234–248, 1988.
6. Garfinkel, D., Garfinkel, L.: Magnesium, *7*:249–261, 1988.
7. Knighton, D.R., Zheng, J., Ten Eyck, L.F., et al.: Science, *253*:407–414, 1991.
8. Bernbaumer, L.: FASEB J., *4*:3068–3078, 1990.
9. Seuwen, K., Pouyssegur, J.: Adv. Cancer Res., *58*:75–94, 1992.
10. Simon, M.I., Strathmann, M.P., Gautam, N.: Science, *252*:802–808, 1991.
11. White, R.E., Hartzell, H.C.: Biochem. Pharmacol., *38*:859–867, 1989.
12. Stanfield, P.R.: Trends Neurosci., *11*:475–477, 1988.
13. Agus, Z.S., Morad, M.: Annu. Rev. Physiol., *53*:299–307, 1991.
14. Flatman, P.W.: Annu. Rev. Physiol., *53*:256–271, 1991.
15. Shaw, A.J., Mughal, M.Z., Maresh, M.J.A., et al.: Am. J. Physiol., *261*:R369-R372, 1991.
16. Quamme, G.A., Rabkin, S.W.: Biochem. Biophys. Res. Comm., *167*:1406–1412, 1990.
17. Preston, R.R.: Science, *250*:285–288, 1990.
18. Grubbs, R.D., Maguire, M.D.: Magnesium, *6*:113–127, 1987.
19. Gupta, R.K., Moore, R.D.: J. Biol. Chem., *255*:3987-3993, 1980.
20. Wallach, S.: Magnesium Trace Elem., *9*:1–14, 1990.
21. Alfrey, A.C., Miller, N.L.: J. Clin. Invest., *52*:3019–3027, 1973.
22. Alcock, N.W.: Ann. N.Y. Acad. Sci., *162*:707–716, 1969.
23. Toffaletti, J., Alvarus, B., Bird, C., et al.: Magnesium, *7*:84–90, 1988.
24. Hunt, C.D., Shuler, T.R.: J. Micronutrient Anal., *6*:161–174, 1990.
25. London, R.E.: Annu. Rev. Physiol., *53*:241–58, 1991.z
26. Blatter, L.A.: Pflugers Arch. *416*:238–246, 1990.
27. Murphy, E., Freudenrich, C.C., Lieberman, M.: Annu. Rev. Physiol., *53*:273–287, 1991.
28. Aikawa, J.K., Gordon, G.S., Rhoades, E.L.: J. Appl. Physiol., *15*:503–507, 1960.
29. Schwartz, R.: Fed Proc., *41*:2709–2713, 1982.
30. Lacrosniere, C.S., Cary, E.E., Schwartz, R., et al.: Gastroenterology, *102*:A562, 1992.
31. Schuette, S.A., Ziegler, E.E., Nelson, S.E., et al.: Pediatr. Res., *27*:36–40, 1990.
32. U.S. Dept. H.H.S., Dept. of Agric.: Nutrition Monitoring in the U.S. An Update Report on Nutrition Monitoring. DHHS Publ. No. 89-1255. Hyattsville, MD, Sept., 1989., Washington, D.C., U.S. Govt Print. Off.
33. Pennington, J.A.T., Wilson, D.B.: J. Am. Diet. Assoc., *90*:375–381, 1990.
34. Pennington, J.A.T., Young, B: J. Am. Diet. Assoc., *91*:179–183, 1991.
35. Hardwick, L.L., Jones, M.R., Brautbar, N., et al.: J. Nutr., *121*:13–23, 1991.
36. Karbach, U., Schmitt, A., Hakan Saner, F.: Dig. Dis. Sci., *36*:1611–1618, 1991.
37. Karbach, U., Rummel, W.: Gastroenterology, *98*:985–992, 1990.
38. Karbach, U.: Gastroenterology, *96*:1282–1299, 1989.
39. Graham, L.A., Ceasar, J.J., Burgen, A.S.U.: Metab. Clin. Exper., *9*:646–659, 1960.
40. Roth, P., Werner, E.: Int. J. Appl. Rad. Isot., *30*:523–526, 1979.
41. Fine, K.D., Santa Ana, C.A., Porter, J.L., et al.: J. Clin. Invest., *88*:396–402, 1991.
42. Milla, P.J., Aggett, P.J., Wolff, O.H., et al.: Gut, *20*:1028–1033, 1979.
43. Brennan, P.G., Vergne-Marini, P., Pak, C.Y.C.: J. Clin. Invest., *57*:1412–1418, 1976.
44. Spencer, H., Lesniak, M., Gatza, L.A., et al.: Gastroenterology, *79*:26–34, 1980.
45. Lakshmann, F.L., Rao, R.B., Kim, W.W.: Am. J. Clin. Nutr., *40(Suppl.* 6):1380–1389, 1984.
46. Spencer, H., Osis, D.: Magnesium, *7*:271–280, 1988.
47. Lewis, N.M., Marcus, M.S.K., Behling, A.R., et al.: Am. J. Clin. Nutr., *49*:527–533, 1989.
48. Greger, J.S., Smith, S.A., Snedeker, S.M.: Nutr. Res., *1*:315–325, 1981.
49. Briscoe, A.M., Ragan, C.: Am. J. Clin. Nutr., *19*:296–306, 1966.
50. Lindberg, J.S., Zobitz, M.M., Poindexter, J.R., et al.: J.A.M. Coll. Nutr., *9*:48–55, 1990.
51. Fine, K.D., Santa Ana, C.A., Fordtran, J.S.: N. Engl. J. Med., *324*:1012–1017, 1991.
52. Fox, J., Care, A.D.: *In* Calcified Tissues. Copenhagen, FADL's Forlag, 1976, p. 147.
53. Hodgkinson, A., Marshall, D.H., Nordin, B.E.E.: Clin. Sci., *57*:121–123, 1979.
54. Wilz, D.R., Gary, R.W., Dominguez, J.H., et al.: Am. J. Clin. Nutr., *32*:2052–2060, 1979.
55. Norman, D.A., Fordtran, J.S., Brinkley, L.J., et al.: J. Clin. Invest., *67*:1599–1603, 1981.
56. Shils, M.E.: Medicine (Baltimore) *48*:61–85, 1969.
57. Quamme, G.A., Dirks, J.H.: The physiology of renal magnesium handling. *In* Renal Physiology. Vol. II. Handbook of Physiology. Sect. 8. Edited by E.E. Windhager. New York, American Physiological Society/Oxford University Press, 1992.
58. Rude, R.R., Bethune, J.D., Singer, F.R.: J. Clin. Endocrinol. Metab., *51*:1425–1431, 1980.
59. Wong, N.L., Dirks, J.H., Quamme, G.A.: Am. J. Physiol., *244*:F78-F83, 1983.
60. Nieman, D.C., Butterworth, D.E., Nieman, C.N., et al.: J. Am. Diet. Assoc., *92*:48–56, 1992.
61. Shils, M.E.: Magnesium. In Modern Nutrition in Health and Disease. 7th Ed. Edited by M.E. Shils and V.R. Young. Philadelphia, Lea & Febiger, 1988, pp. 159–192.
62. Food and Nutrition Board, National Research Council: Recommended Dietary Allowances. 10th Ed. Washington, D.C., National Academy Press, 1989.
63. Seelig, M.S.: Am. J. Clin. Nutr., *14*:342–390, 1964.

64. Lowenstein, F.W., Stanton, M.F.: J. Am. Coll. Nutr., *5*:399–414, 1986.
65. Thomas, A.J., Bunker, V.W., Sodha, N., et al.: Br. J. Nutr., *62*:211–219, 1989.
66. Alcock, N.W., Shils, M.E.: Proc. Soc. Exp. Biol. Med., *146*:137–141, 1974.
67. Shils, M.E.: Magnesium deficiency and calcium and parathyroid hormone interrelations. *In* Trace Elements in Human Health and Disease, Vol. 2. Edited by A. Prasad. New York, Academic Press, 1976, pp. 23–46.
68. Alcock, N.W., Shils, M.E., Lieberman, P.H., et al.: Cancer Res., *33*:2196–2204, 1973.
69. Whang, R., Oliver, J., Welt, L.G., et al.: Ann. N.Y. Acad. Sci., *162*:766–774, 1969.
70. Heggtveit, H.A.: Ann. N.Y. Acad. Sci., *162*:758–765, 1969.
71. Yamamoto, T., Kabata, H., Yagi, R., et al.: Magnesium, *4*:153–164, 1985.
72. Whang, R., Whang, D.D.: J. Am. College Nutr., *9*:84–85, 1990.
73. Anast, C.S., Mohs, J.M., Kaplan, S.L., et al.: Science, *177*:606–608, 1972.
74. Shils, M.E.: Ann. N.Y. Acad. Sci., *355*:165–180, 1980.
75. Rayssiguier, Y., Thomaset, M., Garel, J.M.: Horm. Metab. Res., *14*:379–382, 1982.
76. Anast, C.S., Forte, L.F.: Endocrinology, *113*:184–189, 1983.
77. Freitag, J.J., Martin, K.J., Conrades, E., et al.: J. Clin. Invest., *64*:1238–1244, 1979.
78. Anast, C.S., Winnacker, J.L., Forte, L.R. et al.: J. Clin. Endocrinol. Metab., *42*:707–717, 1976.
79. Rude, R.K., Oldham, S.B., Sharp, C.F. Jr., et al.: J. Clin. Endocrinol. Metab., *47*:800–806, 1978.
80. Johannesson, A.J., Raisz, L.G.: Endocrinology, *113*:2294–2298, 1983.
81. Reddy, F., Sivakumar, B.: Lancet, *1*:963–965, 1974.
82. Carpenter, T.O., Carnes, D.L. Jr., Anast, C.S.: Am. J. Physiol., *253*:E106-E113, 1987.
83. Medalle, R., Waterhouse, C., Hahn, T.J.: Am. J. Clin. Nutr., *29*:854–858, 1976.
84. Rosler, A., Rabinowitz, D.: Lancet, *1*:803–804, 1973.
85. Graber, M.L., Schulman, G.: Ann. Intern. Med., *104*:804–805, 1986.
86. Garabedian, M., Tanaka, Y., Holick, M.F., et al.: Endocrinology, *94*:1022–1027, 1974.
87. Rude, R.K., Adams, J.S., Ryzen, E., et al.: J. Clin. Endocrin. Metab., *61*:933–940, 1985.
88. Fuss, M., Cogan, E., Gillet, C., et al.: Clin. Endocrinol., *22*:807–815, 1985.
89. Rudman, D., Dedonis, J.L., Fountain, M.T., et al.: N. Engl. J. Med., *303*:657–661, 1980.
90. Cunnane, S.C., Soma, M., McAdoo, K.R., et al.: J. Nutr., *115*:1498–1503, 1985.
91. Geuex, E., Mazur, A., Cardot, P., et al.: J. Nutr., *121*:1222–1227, 1991.
92. Nigam, S., Averdunk, R., Gunther, T.: Prostagland. Leukotr. Med., *23*:1–10, 1986.
93. Soma, M., Cunnane, S.C., Horrobon, D.F., et al.: Prostaglandins, *36*:431–441, 1988.
94. Dunn, M.J., Walser, M.: Metabolism, *15*:884–895, 1966.
95. Wallach, S.: Magnesium, 7:262–270, 1988.
96. Mac Intyre, I., Hanna, S.S., Booth, C.C., et al.: Clin. Sci., *20*:297–305, 1961.
97. Booth, C.C., Barbouris. N., Hanna, S., et al.: Br. Med. J., *2*:141–144, 1963.
98. Montgomery, R.D.: Lancet, *2*:74–75, 1960.
99. Muldowney, F.P., McKenna, T.J., Kyle, L.H., et al.: N. Engl. J. Med., *281*:61–68, 1970.
100. Lim, P., Jacobs, E.: J. Lab. Clin. Med., *80*:313–321, 1972.
101. Ladefoged, K., Hagen, K.: Clin. Clim. Acta, *177*:157–166, 1988.
102. Stendig-Lindberg, G., Bergstrom, J., Hultman, E.: Acta Med. Scand., *201*:273–280, 1977.
103. Alfrey, A.C., Miller, N., Butrus, D.: J. Lab. Clin. Med., *84*:153–162, 1974.
104. Jones, J.E., Shane, S.R., Jacobs, W.H., et al.: Ann. N.Y. Acad. Sci., *162*:934–946, 1969.
105. Baldwin, D., Robinson, P.K., Zierler, K.L., et al.: J. Clin. Invest., *31*:850–858, 1952.
106. Whang, R., Welt, L.G.: J. Clin. Invest., *42*:305–314, 1963.
107. Grace, N.D., O'Dell, B.L.: J. Nutr., *100*:45–50, 1970.
108. Drenick, E.G., Hunt, J.F., Swendseid, M.E.: J. Clin. Endocrinol., *29*:1341–1348, 1969.
109. Whang, R., Oei, T., Aikawa, J.K., et al.: Arch. Intern. Med., *144*:1794–1796, 1984.
110. Ryzen, E., Wagers, P.W., et al.: Crit. Care Med., *13*:19–21, 1985.
111. Chernow, B., Bamberger, S., Stoiko, M., et al.: Chest, *95*:391–397, 1987.
112. Fiaccadori, E., del Canale, S., Coffrini, E., et al.: Crit. Care Med., *16*:751–760, 1988.
113. Flink, E.B.: Alcoholism, *10*:590–594, 1986.
114. Butler, A.M.: N. Engl. J. Med., *234*:648–656, 1950.
115. Sheehan, J.P.: Magnes. Trace Elem., *9*:320, 1990.
116. Mimouni, F., Miodovnik, R.C., Tsang, J., et al.: Obstet. Gynecol., *70*:85–88, 1987.
117. Sjogren, A., Floren, C.H., Nilsson, A.: Diabetes, *35*:459–463, 1986.
118. Saggese, G., Frederico, G., Beretelloni, S., et al.: J. Pediatr., *118*:220–225, 1991.
119. Sjogren, A., Floren, C.-H., Nilsson, A: Magnesium, *7*:117–122, 1988.
120. Motil, K.J., Altschuler, S.I., Grand, R.J.: J. Pediatr., *107*:473–479, 1985.
121. Rosen, E.U., Campbell, P.G., Moosa, G.M.: J. Pediatr., *77*:709–714, 1970.
122. Nichols, B.L., Alvarado, J., Hazelwood, C.F., et al.: Am. J. Clin. Nutr., *31*:176–188, 1978.
123. Evans, R.A., Carter, J.N., George, C.R.P., et al.: Q. J. Med., *197*:39–52, 1981.
124. Jones, C.T., Sellwood, R.A., Evanson, J.M.: Br. Med. J., *3*:391–392, 1973.
125. Gullner, H.G., Gill, J.R. Jr., Barter, F.C.: Am. J. Med., *71*:578–582, 1981.
126. Altura, B.M., Altura, B.T.: Magnesium Bull., *8*:338–350, 1986.
127. Rude, R., Manoogian, C., Ehrlich, P., et al.: Magnesium, *8*:266–273, 1989.
128. Dechaux, M., Kindermans, C., Laborde, K., et al.: Kidney Intl., *34*:(A-25), S12-S13, 1988.
129. Albert, D.G., Morita, Y., Iseri, T.: Circulation, *17*:761–763, 1958.
130. Bauer, F.K., Martin, H.E., Mickey, M.R.: Proc. Soc. Exp. Biol. Med., *120*:466–468, 1965.
131. Tillman, D.W., Semple, P.F.: Clin. Sci., *75*:395–402, 1988.
132. Dyckner, T., Wester, P.O.: Br. J. Med., *286*:1847–1849, 1983.
133. Reyes, A.J., Leary, W.P., Acosta-Barrios, T.N., et al.: Curr. Ther. Res., *36*:332–340, 1984.

134. Cappucio, F.P., Markandur, N.D., Beymon, G.W., et al.: Br. Med. J., *291*:235–238, 1985.
135. Zemel, P.C., Zemel, M.B., Urberg, M., et al.: Am. J. Clin. Nutr., *51*:665–669, 1990.
136. Patki, P.S., Singh, J., Gokhale, S.V., et al.: Br. Med. J., *301*:521–523, 1990.
137. Overlack, A., Zenzen, J.G., Ressel, C., et al.: Hypertension, *9*:139–143, 1987.
138. Marier, J.R.: Magnesium, *1*:3–15, 1982.
139. Elwood, P.C., Sweetman, P.M., Beasley, W.H., et al.: Lancet, *2*:720–722, 1980.
140. Hammer, D.I., Hayden, S.: JAMA, *243*:2399–2400, 1980.
141. Leoni, V., Fabiani, L., Tichiarelli, L.: Arch. Environ. Health, *40*:274–278, 1985.
142. Rasmussen, H.S.: Magnesium, *8*:316–325, 1989.
143. Dyckner, T., Wester, P.O.: Am. Heart J., *97*:12–18, 1979.
144. Boyd, J.C., Bruns, E.E., Wills, M.R.: Clin. Chem., *29*:178–179, 1983.
145. Whang, R.: Magnesium, *40*:274–278, 1985.
146. Rasmussen, H.S.: Arch. Intern. Med., *148*:329–332, 1988.
147. Ralston, M.A., Murname, M.R., Kelley, R.E., et al.: Circulation, *80*:573–580, 1989.
148. Burnstock, G.: J. Physiol., *313*:1–35, 1981.
149. Burnstock, G., Meghji, P.: Br. J. Pharmacol., *79*:211–218, 1983.
150. Legssyer, A., Poggioli, J., Renard, et al.: J. Physiol., *401*:185–199, 1988.
151. Puceat, M., Clement, O., Vassort, G.: J. Physiol., *444*:241–256, 1991.
152. Wallert, M.A., Frohlich, O.: Am. J. Physiol., *257*:C207–C213, 1989.
153. Teo, K.K., Yusuf, S., Collins, R., et al.: Br. Med. J., *303*:1499–1503, 1991.
154. Editorial: Magnesium for acute myocardial infarction? Lancet, *338*:667–668, 1991.
155. Zaloga, G.P., Wilkens, R., Tourville, J., et al.: Crit. Care Med., *15*:813–816, 1987.
156. Altura, B.T., Altura, B.M.: Mag. Trace Elem., *9*:311, 1990.
157. Reinhart, R.A.: Arch. Intern. Med., *148*:2415–2420, 1988.
158. Ryzen, E.: Magnesium, *8*:201–212, 1989.
159. Yang, X.Y., Hosseini, J.M., Ruddel, M.E., et al.: Magnesium, *8*:100–105, 1989.
160. Ryzen, E., Elbaum, N., Singer, F.R., et al.: Magnesium, *4*:137–147, 1985.
161. Holm, C.N., Jepsen, J.M., Sjogaard, G., et al.: Hum. Nutr. Clin. Nutr., *41C*:301–306, 1987.
162. Flink, E.B.: Ann. N. Y., Acad. Sci., *162*:901–905, 1969.
163. Stromme, J.H., Steen-Johnson, J., Harnaes, K., et al.: Pediatr. Res., *15*:1134–139, 1981.
164. Cunningham, F.G., Lindheimer, M.D.: N. Engl. J. Med., *326*:927–932, 1992.
165. Cholst, I.N., Steinberg, S.F., Tropper, P.J., et al.: N. Engl. J. Med., *310*:1221–1225, 1984.
166. Eisunbud, E., LoBoe, C.L.: Arch. Intern. Med., *136*:688–691, 1976.
167. Cruikshank, D.P., Pitkin, R.M., Reynolds, W.A., et al.: Am. J. Obstet. Gynecol., *134*:243–249, 1979.
168. Donovan, E.F., Tsang, R.C., Steichen, J.J., et al.: J. Pediatr., *96*:305–310, 1980.
169. Wians, F.H. Jr., Strickland, D.M., Hankins, G.D.V., et al.: Magnesium. Trace Elem., *9*:28–35, 1990.
170. Altura, B.M., Altura, B.T.: Fed. Proc., *40*:2672–2679, 1981.
171. Levine, B.S., Coburn, J.W.: N. Engl. J. Med., *310*:1253–1254, 1984.
172. Mordes, J.P., Wacker, E.C.: Pharmacol. Rev., *29*:274–300, 1978.
173. Kwack, H., Veech, L.R.: Curr. Top. Cell. Regul., *33*:185–207, 1992.
174. Rourke, B., Baclex, P.H., Marlan, E.: Science, *257*:245–248, 1992.
175. Woods, K.L., Fletcher, S., Roffe, C., et al.: Lancet, *339*:1553–1558, 1992.


## SELECTED READINGS


Garfinkel, D., Garfinkel, L.: Magnesium and regulation of carbohydrate metabolism at the molecular level. Magnesium, *7*:249–261, 1988.

Hardwick, L.L., Jones, M.R., Brautbar, N., Lee, D.B.N.: Magnesium absorption; Mechanisms and the influence of vitamin D, calcium and phosphate. J. Nutr., *121*:13–23, 1991.

Vernon, W.B.: The role of magnesium in nucleic-acid and protein metabolism. Magnesium, *7*:234–248, 1988.

Wallach, S.: Availability of body magnesium during magnesium deficiency. Magnesium, *7*:262–270, 1988.

Wallach, S.: Effects of magnesium on skeletal metabolism. Magnesium Trace Elem., *9*:1–14, 1990.

White, R.E., Hartzell, H.C.: Magnesium ions in cardiac function. Regulator of ion channels and second messengers. Biochem. Pharmacol., *38*:859–867, 1989.

CHAPTER 9

# Iron in Medicine and Nutrition

Virgil F. Fairbanks



## HISTORY OF IRON IN MEDICINE AND NUTRITION

Iron was a familiar metal in most of the ancient civilizations of the Mediterranean littoral, and was used in numerous tools and weapons. This familiarity with iron may also have led to its early medicinal use. In the earliest extant manuscript, the Ebers papyrus of Egypt, rust was prescribed in an ointment to prevent baldness. In early Greece, a solution of iron in wine was esteemed as a means of restoring male potency. In the seventeenth century of our era, the most important clinical application of iron was discovered: the treatment of chlorosis, a disorder later shown to result from iron deficiency.[1]

Even before the role of iron in nutrition was firmly established, the first clinical description of iron overload disease was reported in 1871.[2] The earliest objective study of iron in human nutrition, performed nearly a century ago and published in 1895, showed that the diets of young women with chlorosis had only enough iron to provide 1 to 3 mg daily, whereas the average iron content of diets of normal persons ranged from 8 to 11 mg daily.[3] Yet it was not until 1932 that a centuries-long controversy concerning the value of iron for treatment of chlorosis was finally resolved beyond doubt.[4] The major aspects of iron metabolism were elucidated before 1960. Thousands of subsequent investigations have filled in important details.

## BIOLOGIC IMPORTANCE

Iron is one of the most abundant metals in the universe and in the earth's crust. It is also one of the most useful, both in technology and in biology, for iron compounds are involved in numerous oxidation-reduction reactions, beginning with the reduction of hydrogen and its incorporation into carbohydrates during photosynthesis in the presence of ferredoxins. Aerobic metabolism depends on iron because of its role in the functional groups of most of the enzymes of the Krebs cycle, as an electron

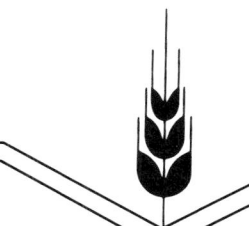

carrier in cytochromes, and as a means of $O_2$ and $CO_2$ transport in hemoglobin.

## AN EXPANDING LITERATURE

The National Library of Medicine lists more than 30,000 articles published just since January 1966 on the subject of iron in biology, medicine, and nutrition. Between 1985 and 1991 approximately 9000 articles on this subject have appeared, at an average rate of about 120 per month. Regrettably, few of these can be cited in this chapter. Many excellent and comprehensive reviews have been published concerning iron metabolism, disorders of iron metabolism, and iron in nutrition, as indicated in the "Selected Reading" list at the end of this chapter. Readers may consult them for additional details.

## IRON METABOLISM

### COMPARTMENTS

In humans, the total quantity of body iron varies with weight, hemoglobin concentration, sex, and size of the storage compartment. Table 9–1 shows approximate normal values for the iron in various compartments. Of these, the largest compartment is the iron in hemoglobin, contained within circulating erythrocytes. The size of this compartment varies considerably according to body weight, sex, and blood hemoglobin concentration. For example, a person weighing 50 kg (110 lb) whose blood hemoglobin concentration is 120 g/L (12.0 g/dL) would have a hemoglobin compartment iron content of 1.1 g. The size of the storage compartment, in which iron is contained in ferritin and hemosiderin, is also markedly influenced by age, sex, body size, and whether there has been excess iron loss as from bleeding or pregnancy, or iron overloading, as in hemochromatosis. Women and children often have little storage iron. The tissue iron pool includes myoglobin and the tiny but essential fraction of iron in enzymes. The "labile pool" is a rapidly recycling component that is defined by iron kinetic studies, but that does not have a definable anatomic or cellular location. The transport compartment is iron bound to transferrin, the iron transport protein in plasma. The transport compartment is small but active; normally 20 to 30 mg cycle through the transport compartment each day. The main metabolic pathways of iron metabolism are illustrated in Figure 9–1.[5] Further details concerning the proteins of the storage and transport compartments are given subsequently. In molar terms, 1 μmol Fe = 55.6 μg and 1 mg Fe = 17.9 μmol.

**TABLE 9–1.** IRON COMPARTMENTS IN NORMAL MAN*

| COMPARTMENT | IRON CONTENT (MG) | TOTAL-BODY IRON (%) |
|---|---|---|
| Hemoglobin iron | 2000 | 67 |
| Storage iron | 1000 | 27 |
| Tissue iron | | |
| Myoglobin iron | 130 | 3.5 |
| Enzyme iron | 8 | 0.2 |
| Labile pool iron | 80 | 2.2 |
| Transport iron | 3 | 0.08 |

*These values represent estimates for an "average" man, that is, 70 kg, 177 cm (70 in.) in height. They are derived from data in several sources. 1 mg Fe = 17.9 μmol.

### *INTAKE*

The average daily intake of iron in North America and Europe is between 10 and 30 mg, about 5 to 7 mg of iron per 1000 calories. A weight-conscious young woman who limits her intake to between 1000 and 1500 calories per day consumes only 6 to 9 mg of food iron. These estimates ignore the iron content of beverages and that added or lost during food preparation. Iron utensils contribute significantly to the iron content of cooked foods. The substitution of aluminum, stainless steel, or plastic-coated pots and pans has certainly had an adverse effect on dietary iron intake.

Failure to consider the iron content of beverages introduces into dietary surveys another source of error that is of varying significance in different areas. Some European ciders and wines may contain 16 mg of iron or more per liter. However, the iron content of American wines and other alcoholic beverages is believed to be negligible. The iron content of city water supplies is usually low, but water from some deep wells or bore holes may contain more than 5 mg of iron per liter.

### *ABSORPTION*

**Mechanisms.** In healthy persons who do not lose iron by bleeding, iron loss is limited. Therefore, normal iron balance is maintained largely by regulation of iron absorption. Ingested inorganic iron is solubilized and ionized by the acid gastric juice, reduced to the ferrous (FeII) form and chelated. Substances that form low-

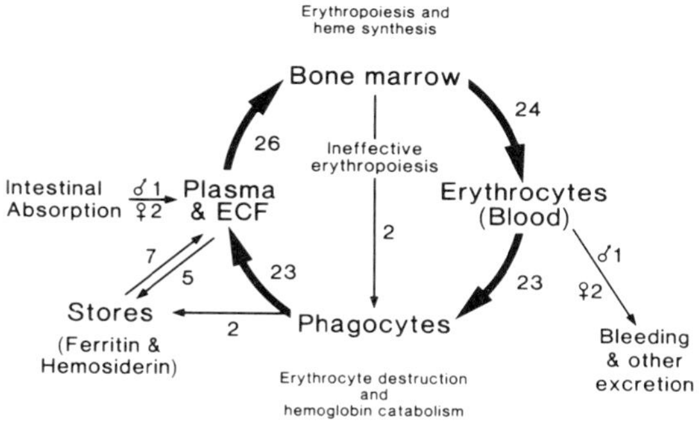
Erythropoiesis and heme synthesis
Bone marrow
24
26
Ineffective erythropoiesis
Intestinal Absorption
♂1
♀2
Plasma & ECF
Erythrocytes (Blood)
2
♂1
7
5
23
23
♀2
Stores
(Ferritin & Hemosiderin)
2
Phagocytes
Bleeding & other excretion
Erythrocyte destruction and hemoglobin catabolism

**FIGURE 9–1.** Pathways of iron metabolism. Iron is tightly conserved in a nearly closed system in which each iron atom cycles repeatedly from plasma and extracellular fluid (ECF) to the bone marrow, where it is incorporated into hemoglobin. Then it travels to the peripheral blood, where within erythrocytes it circulates in the blood for 4 months. It then travels to phagocytes of the reticuloendothelial system, where senescent erythrocytes are engulfed and destroyed, hemoglobin is digested, and iron is released to plasma, where the cycle continues. With each cycle, a small proportion of iron is transferred to storage sites, where it is incorporated into ferritin or hemosiderin, a small proportion of storage iron is released to plasma, a small proportion is lost in urine, sweat, feces, or blood, and an equivalent small amount of iron is absorbed from the intestinal tract. In addition, a small proportion (about 10%) of newly formed erythrocytes normally is destroyed within the bone marrow and its iron released, bypassing the circulating blood part of the cycle (ineffective erythropoiesis). The numbers indicate the approximate amount of iron (in mg) that enters and leaves each of these iron compartments every day in healthy adults who do not have bleeding and other blood disorders. (From Fairbanks, V.F., Klee, G.G.: Biochemical aspects of hematology. *In* Textbook of Clinical Chemistry. Edited by N.W. Tietz. Philadelphia, W.B. Saunders, 1986.)

molecular iron chelates, such as ascorbic acid, sugars, and amino acids, promote iron absorption. Normal gastric secretions contain a stabilizing factor, probably an endogenous chelate, that helps slow the precipitation of ingested iron at the alkaline pH of the small intestine. Impaired iron absorption in achlorhydric or gastrectomized subjects may be related to decreased solubilization and chelation of the ferric iron in food.[6,7]

Absorption may occur at any level of the small intestine, but it is most efficient in the duodenum. Before uptake by the brush border of the mucosal cell, the iron atom must first traverse the mucous layer. The mucus itself has iron-binding properties.[8] The passage of iron through mucus may be facilitated by organic acids[9,10] or taurocholic acid[11] occurring in normal bile, or by polypeptides such as those derived by digestion of meat, fish, or poultry. Whether transferrin in the intestinal lumen may also facilitate passage through the mucin layer is uncertain.

The divalent or Fe(II) form of iron is more readily soluble than the trivalent or Fe(III) form, because of the low solubility of ferric hydroxides and phosphates at the alkaline pH of intestinal fluid. Thus, Fe(II) traverses the mucous layer more readily to reach the brush border of intestinal epithelial cells. There, Fe(II) must be oxidized to Fe(III) before it enters the epithelial cell.

At the cell membrane of the brush border of the epithelial cell, Fe(III) is bound to a receptor protein called membrane iron binding protein (MIBP), which then transfers iron into the cell. This protein has been partially characterized.[12,13] It is a glycoprotein of approximately 160 kilodaltons (kd) that consists of three similar 54 kd monomers. Apotransferrin in the cytosol of intestinal epithelial cells may accelerate iron absorption. The cellular apotransferrin is increased in iron deficiency, and it is plausible that this increase plays a regulatory role by facilitating iron absorption when the body's need for iron is augmented.

Most of the iron that is absorbed from the intestinal lumen passes rapidly through the mucosal cells in the form of small molecules. As the iron enters the plasma, it is oxidized to Fe(III) by ceruloplasmin, which functions as a ferroxidase, and then it is taken up by transferrin. That portion of the cytosolic iron that exceeds the rapid transport capacity combines with apoferritin to form ferritin. Some of the ferritin iron may later be released into the circulation, but most of it remains in the mucosal cells until they are sloughed into the intestinal lumen at the end of their 2- to 3-day life span. Direct entry into lymphatic channels is insignificant.

Heme iron, a major dietary form of iron, is absorbed by a mechanism different from that just described for inorganic and nonheme forms of food iron. Most heme is ingested in the form of hemoglobin or myoglobin. Heme may be absorbed directly by mucosal cells after removal of globin by proteolytic duodenal enzymes, or the protein portion may be removed within the mucosal epithelium.[7-14] In either case, once inside the cells, iron is liberated from heme probably by the enzyme heme-oxygenase.[15] It then traverses the cell to be transferred to plasma as Fe(III). Only a small portion of the heme absorbed by mucosal cells enters the portal blood as heme. Absorption of heme iron is increased in iron deficiency states, but less so than is ingested Fe(II). Absorption of dietary heme iron is not increased by ascorbic acid nor is it depressed by such substances as phytates and desferrioxamine. Its absorption is only slightly inhibited by simultaneous administration of inorganic iron and nonheme iron.[16-18]

**Intraluminal Factors.** Intraluminal factors that decrease absorption include rapid transit time, achylia, malabsorption syndromes, precipitation by alkalinization, phosphates, phytates, and ingested alkaline clays or antacid preparations. Milk proteins, albumin, and soy proteins reduce iron absorption.[19-21] However, ingestion of milk together with cereals neither enhances nor reduces the effect of cereal on iron absorption in humans. Tea and coffee reduce iron absorption substantially, in proportion to the amount of tea or coffee ingested. Iron absorption is reduced about 60% by tea and about 40% by coffee.[22-24] Phytate is inositol hexaphosphate, a substance that normally occurs in the fiber or bran component of wheat, rice, maize, psyllium, walnuts, peanuts, hazelnuts, and plant lignins, and that chelates iron, reducing its absorption.[25–31] As little as 5 to 10 mg of phytate in bread can reduce nonheme iron absorption by 50%.[27] This effect of phytate can be maintained indefinitely.[28] The addition of meat or ascorbic acid to the diet reverses the iron-chelating effect of phytate.[27] Some other plant fibers such as that derived from yod kratin (leaves of the SE Asian lead tree) also reduce iron absorption,[32] but cellulose does not.[33] Beet fiber (beta fiber) also does not appear to inhibit iron absorption.[29] In contrast to the effect of phytate in retarding food iron absorption in humans, both rats and anemic pigs seem to absorb iron equally well from phytate-rich and phytate-poor diets.[34] Concomitant ingestion of zinc and iron salts reduces iron absorption in humans.[35]

As the ingested dose of iron increases, the total amount retained by the body rises steadily, although the percent absorbed decreases. When the logarithm of iron dosage is plotted against the logarithm of iron absorbed, a straight line is obtained.[36] For each 2-fold increment in iron dosage, a 1.6-fold increment in absorption can be anticipated. Uptake is increased by large oral doses of ascorbic acid, by certain weak chelating substances (e.g., citric acid, succinic acid, sugars, and sulfur-containing amino acids) and possibly by the stabilizing gastric factor previously mentioned. Absorption may also be enhanced in the presence of products of digestion of meat from poultry or beef.[37,38] The effects of ethanol ingestion and of deficiency of pancreatic exocrine function on iron absorption have been disputed. Whether ingested or administered parenterally, ethanol has little, if any, direct effect on iron absorption in humans, and may even retard it.[39] In rats, the addition of alcohol to the diet resulted in increased iron absorption.[40] In humans, acute or chronic alcohol consumption does not appear to increase iron absorption.[41]

**Systemic Regulation.** The systemic regulatory mechanisms that influence iron absorption have never been identified in spite of intensive search. They operate to: (1) increase absorption in iron deficiency, in hemochromatosis, during the latter half of pregnancy, and when erythropoiesis is stimulated (including ineffective erythropoiesis), as in anemias or hypoxic states; and (2) decrease absorption in iron overload, in chronic disease such as rheumatoid arthritis, or in other circumstances when erythropoiesis is depressed. With the discovery of MIBP and the demonstration of greater than normal activity of this protein in the hepatocytes and intestinal mucosa of persons with hemochromatosis, the mechanism of systemic regulation of iron absorption may soon be elucidated.

The absorption of iron appears to be modulated by intestinal mucosal cells. The columnar mucosal cells formed in crypts at the base of villi contain a variable amount of transferrin-derived iron. The quantity of intracellular iron regulates, within limits, the quantity of intraluminal iron that enters cells. The iron in intestinal epithelial cells may enter the body according to need, or may remain within these cells to limit absorption and be lost when the cells are sloughed from the tips of villi at the end of their brief life spans. Little iron is incorporated into ferritin in the mucosal cells of iron-deficient subjects, and absorption is enhanced. Conversely, in iron-loaded subjects, the mucosal cells formed are well endowed with iron, but contain little apotransferrin; transport of iron into plasma is limited and the cellular iron is excreted when desquamation occurs.

**Absorption From Foods.** Healthy persons absorb about 5 to 10% of dietary iron, and those who are iron-deficient absorb about 10 to 20%. The maximum amount of iron absorption expected from an average diet in the United States is about 1 to 2 mg in normal adults and 3 to 6 mg in iron-deficient patients.

The earliest measurements of iron absorption were made with balance techniques. The small difference between oral intake and fecal loss is difficult to measure with precision by chemical methods. Furthermore, such methods cannot distinguish excreted iron from iron contained in mucosal epithelial cells that have been desquamated into the intestinal lumen. Such balance studies were done using mixed diets fed over several weeks; the effect of daily variation on results was minimized. Iron absorption, calculated on the basis of positive balance, ranged from 7.3 to 21%.[42]

Since 1950, single foods prepared or grown so as to contain a radionuclide of iron have usually been used to measure the absorption of iron from these foods after they are prepared and fed as in a normal diet. Figure 9–2 presents typical results.[43] The overall absorption in 219 normal subjects approximated 10% and that in 148 iron-deficient patients, 20%. Absorption of iron from food varies widely. It is greatest from meat of mammalian origin, such as beef, less from that of poultry or fish, and least from liver, muscle, eggs, milk, and cereals.[44] It is generally greater in children than in adults.

Figure 9–3 summarizes results obtained in 520 subjects using 7 foods of vegetable origin and 5 of animal origin.[45] Absorption of iron from meat exceeded 10%. Absorption of iron from rice and spinach was poor; it was better from soybeans than from other vegetable sources. Because radioiron-tagged foods were given as a single test dose, daily variations in absorption were not measured, and the effect of possible interactions between specific foods and iron absorption was not determined. For example, ascorbic acid increased, whereas eggs decreased, the uptake of iron from some foods.

Reference has already been made to the effects of polyphenols, such as plant tannins, and of phytate in retarding absorption of food iron. The effects of organic acids, phytates, and polyphenols on absorption of dietary iron were studied by the external tag method in which $^{59}FeSO_4$ is mixed with food before ingestion by human subjects. Iron was poorly absorbed from wheat germ, butter beans, spinach, lentils, and beet greens, all foods

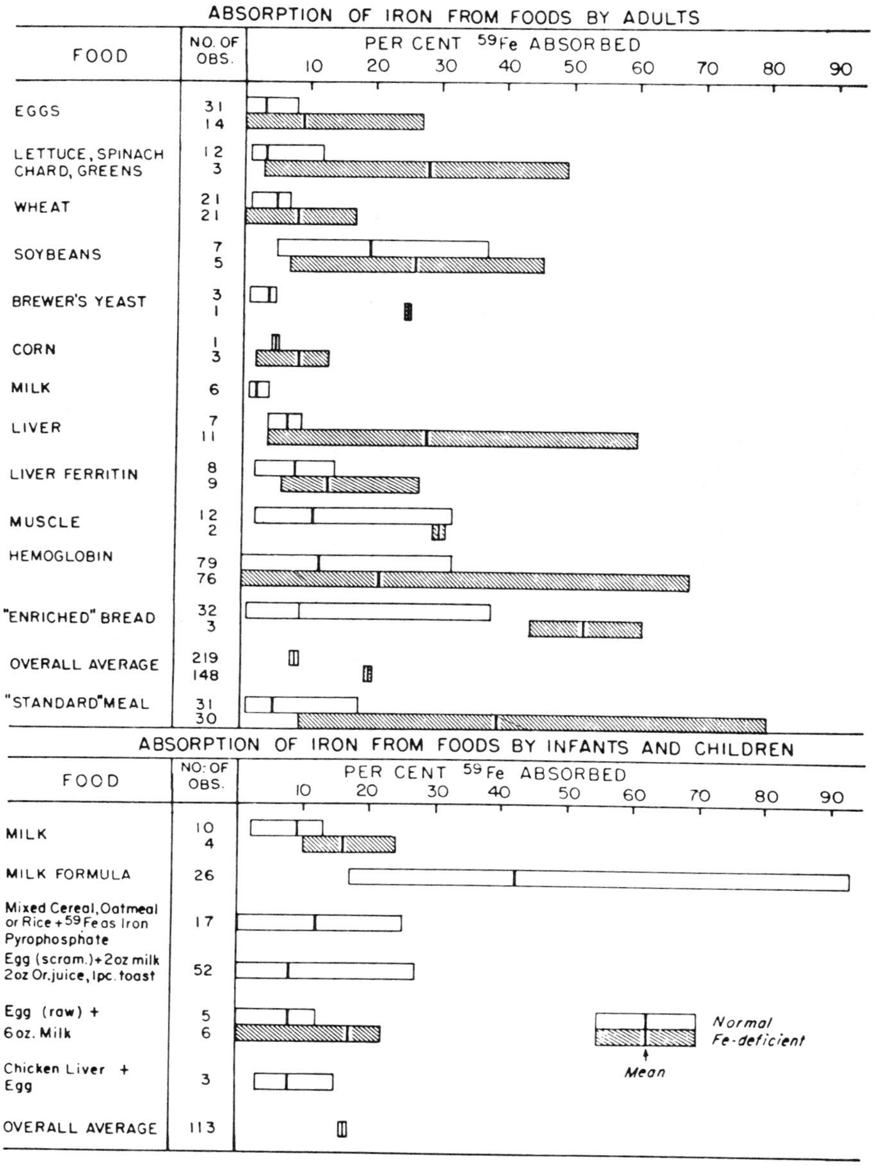
ABSORPTION OF IRON FROM FOODS BY ADULTS
FOOD
NO. OF OBS.
PER CENT 59Fe ABSORBED
10 20 30 40 50 60 70 80 90
EGGS 31 14
LETTUCE, SPINACH CHARD, GREENS 12 3
WHEAT 21 21
SOYBEANS 7 5
BREWER'S YEAST 3 1
CORN 1 3
MILK 6
LIVER 7 11
LIVER FERRITIN 8 9
MUSCLE 12 2
HEMOGLOBIN 79 76
"ENRICHED" BREAD 32 3
OVERALL AVERAGE 219 148
"STANDARD" MEAL 31 30
ABSORPTION OF IRON FROM FOODS BY INFANTS AND CHILDREN
FOOD
NO. OF OBS.
PER CENT 59Fe ABSORBED
10 20 30 40 50 60 70 80 90
MILK 10 4
MILK FORMULA 26
Mixed Cereal, Oatmeal or Rice + 59Fe as Iron Pyrophosphate 17
Egg (scram.) + 2oz milk 2oz Or. juice, 1pc. toast 52
Egg (raw) + 6oz. Milk 5 6
Chicken Liver + Egg 3
OVERALL AVERAGE 113
Normal
Fe-deficient
Mean

**FIGURE 9–2.** Radioiron measurements of the absorption of iron from foods by adults, infants, and children. The length of the bars indicates the variation among different subjects for each food; the heavy vertical lines across each bar indicate the average value. The amount of iron in each feeding varied from 1 to 17 mg. Clear bars indicate normal subjects, whereas crosshatched bars represent iron-deficient patients. (From Moore, C.V.: *In* Symposium on Occurrence, Causes and Prevention of Nutritional Anaemias. Edited by G. Blix. Swedish Nutrition Foundation, Tylösand, 1967, Symposia 6. Uppsala, Almqvist and Wiksells, 1968, pp. 92–103.) 1 mg Fe = 17.9 μmol.

with high phytate content. In contrast, iron absorption was good to moderate from carrots, potatoes, beet roots, pumpkin, broccoli, tomatoes, cauliflower, cabbage, turnips, and sauerkraut, vegetables that contain substantial amounts of malic, citric, or ascorbic acids.[46]

In Western-type whole meals, iron absorption is enhanced by inclusion of beef, poultry, or fish and by ascorbic acid. Meals that included principally pizza or hamburger or spaghetti and cheese result in poor iron absorption, whereas those containing cod, beef, shrimp, or chicken yielded good iron absorption. (It is not clear why iron absorption from the hamburger-based meal is poor; perhaps phytates in the bun or the milk in the milkshake inhibit iron absorption.) In one study, the best

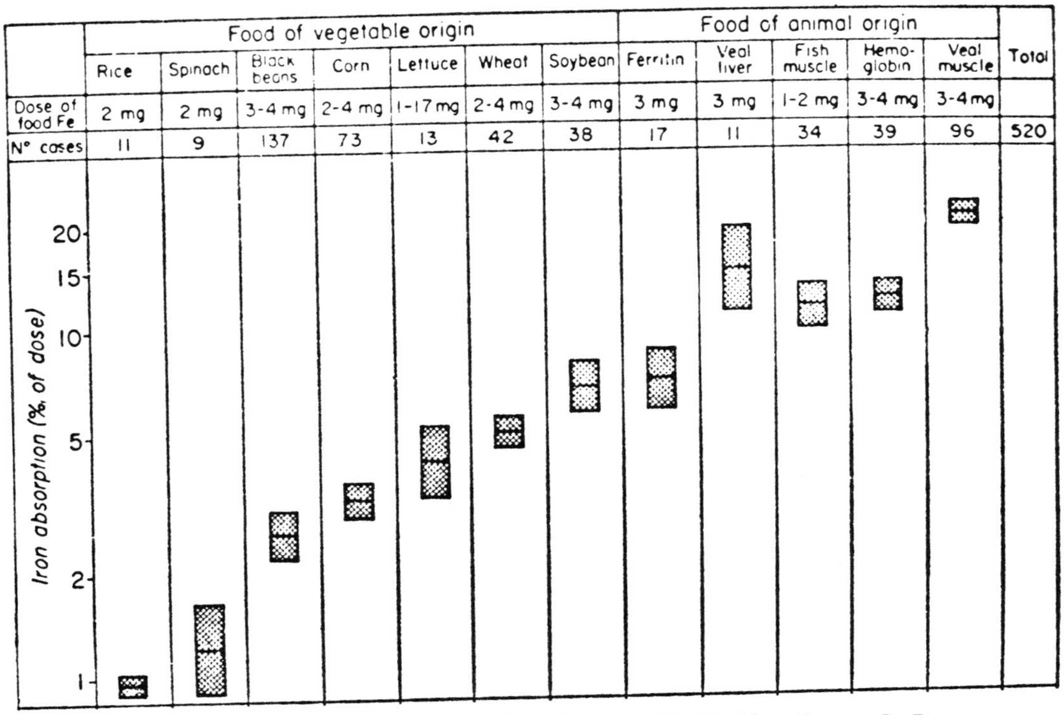
Food of vegetable origin
Food of animal origin
Rice
Spinach
Black beans
Corn
Lettuce
Wheat
Soybean
Ferritin
Veal liver
Fish muscle
Hemo-globin
Veal muscle
Total
Dose of food Fe
2 mg
2 mg
3-4 mg
2-4 mg
1-17 mg
2-4 mg
3-4 mg
3 mg
3 mg
1-2 mg
3-4 mg
3-4 mg
N° cases
11
9
137
73
13
42
38
17
11
34
39
96
520
Iron absorption (%, of dose)
20
15
10
5
2
1

**FIGURE 9–3.** Absorption of iron from foods. (From Layrisse, M., Martinez-Torres, C.: Prog. Hematol., 7:137–160, 1971.)

iron absorption resulted from an Italian meal of antipasto misto, spaghetti, meat, bread, oranges, and wine.[47] In addition to the dietary factors enumerated previously, soy flour proteins have been reported as retarding[48] or enhancing[49] iron absorption, whereas soy sauce enhances iron absorption.[50]

The effects of mixture of foods on iron absorption have also been investigated.[51–53] One vegetable (maize or black beans) and one animal food (fish or veal muscle) tagged with different isotopes ($^{55}Fe$ and $^{59}Fe$) were fed to the same subjects separately and mixed in the same meal. Iron absorption from veal was diminished about 20% when it was combined with vegetable foods; iron absorption from either maize or black beans was almost doubled when these foods were mixed with animal meat. Furthermore, the enhancing effect could be duplicated by substituting amino acids in the same composition as those found in fish muscle; cysteine seemed to be the amino acid primarily responsible for the enhancing effect.

Thus, overall iron absorption from a meal that contains many components cannot be estimated from the percentage of iron absorption that would occur if single foods are fed separately. Therefore, composite data on absorption of iron from a complete diet are of most use, and "standard" or mixed meals to which a tracer dose of inorganic radioiron is added as an external tag are being studied increasingly. Nonheme iron in food appears to be converted into a common pool during cooking and digestion, and absorption of the external tag provides a measure of the iron absorbed from this pool.[44,54,55] In this way, the laborious isotopic labeling of individual foods can be circumvented and the effect of interaction of different foods on absorption can be studied more easily. Radioiron-labeled hemoglobin may be added to food as a means of measuring the absorption of dietary heme iron. Absorption of iron from a complete diet can, therefore, be determined by adding to food both ionic radioiron and hemoglobin-bound radioiron.

## TRANSPORT

In blood or other body fluids, iron is transported by a protein called transferrin. Transferrin binds iron that is either released from intestinal epithelium into the blood or lymph or is secreted from macrophages after the degradation of hemoglobin. Furthermore, transferrin distributes iron throughout the body to wherever it is needed, mostly to erythrocyte precursors in the bone marrow for new hemoglobin synthesis. Transferrin is an elongated protein of approximately 80 kd that has two iron binding sites. One atom of Fe(III) can be bound, together with a bicarbonate ion, at each end of the transferrin molecule. In humans, the two iron-binding sites seem to be functionally equivalent. When no iron is bound to the transferrin molecule, it is designated apotransferrin. Monoferric transferrin has one Fe(III), diferric transferrin has two. When all iron-binding sites are occupied by Fe(III), transferrin is said to be saturated. Normally, plasma transferrin is approximately one-third saturated; it is a mixture of monoferric and diferric transferrin.

The normal concentration of transferrin in plasma is about 2.2 to 3.5 g/L (220 to 350 mg/dl). Because iron is the natural ligand of transferrin, the plasma concentration of transferrin may be measured by the amount of iron that it will bind. This determination is called the total iron binding capacity (TIBC). The normal serum TIBC is about 45 to 80 μmol/L (250 to 450 μg/dl). The amount of iron actually bound to transferrin is measured as the serum iron concentration (SI). The SI ranges from 12 to 31 μmol/L (70 to 175 μg/dl) in males and from 11 to 29μmol/L (60 to 165 μg/dl) in women. Transferrin saturation (Tsat) is calculated as 100 × SI ÷ TIBC. The SI normally exhibits a marked diurnal variation. Highest values occur in midmorning (6 to 10 A.M). Values are about 30% lower in midafternoon, and substantially lower in the evening, with a nadir near midnight. In iron deficiency anemia, SI usually is diminished, TIBC may be increased, and Tsat may be less than 15%. In iron overload disorders, SI is often greater than 40 μmol/L, TIBC is usually normal or diminished, and Tsat may be 100%. In acute diseases, such as acute infections or myocardial infarction, and probably after immunizations, SI is diminished, TIBC is normal, and Tsat is diminished. In chronic disorders such as chronic infections, rheumatoid arthritis, or malignancies, SI is diminished, TIBC often is diminished as well, and Tsat may be normal or low.

When transferrin is 100% saturated, iron that is absorbed by the intestinal mucosa cannot be bound by transferrin: most of this excess iron is deposited in hepatocytes of the liver, the first organ through which flows the blood containing absorbed nutrients including iron. In an extremely rare disorder called congenital atransferrinemia, no transferrin is in plasma to carry the iron. Consequently, absorbed iron is deposited rapidly in hepatocytes of the liver and other organs. In this condition, SI and TIBC are very low and transferrin cannot be measured. Because the normal mechanism for transport of iron to erythrocyte precursors is lacking, severe microcytic anemia develops in addition to iron overload of many organs.

The normal plasma half-time for transferrin is 8 to 10.5 days. However, the transit time of iron through plasma is considerably shorter: the normal plasma iron clearance half-time for transferrin-bound radioiron is about 60 to 90 minutes. As shown in Table 9–1, the total quantity of iron that is transferrin bound at any time is only about 3 mg. Turnover is rapid, however; 25 to 30 mg of iron are transported each day from sites of absorption or release to cells where iron is needed. Normally, 70 to 90% of this iron is taken up by the erythropoietic cells of the bone marrow for formation of hemoglobin. Smaller quantities are delivered to other cells for formation of myoglobin, cytochromes, peroxidases, or other functional iron proteins, and, in pregnant women, to the placenta for fetal needs. A small amount of iron is exchanged with iron released from ferritin and hemosiderin in macrophages.

Transferrin exhibits considerable heterogeneity. At least 19 molecular variants have been recognized. All appear to be functionally identical.

## UPTAKE BY CELLS

Cell membranes contain a protein called transferrin receptor. Early erythrocyte precursors have abundant transferrin receptors on their membranes. The number diminishes as these cells mature and fill with hemoglobin. On the cell membrane, diferric transferrin binds to transferrin receptors, and then the iron-transferrin-transferrin receptor complex is internalized by endocytosis. The binding occurs in pits on the surface of the cell. During endocytosis, the pits become coated vesicles, within which iron is released from transferrin.[56–67]

Most other cells also have transferrin receptors on their membranes. The same mechanism is involved in the internalization of iron in erythrocytes and other cells.

Transferrin receptor is a transmembrane glycoprotein with a molecular weight of approximately 90 kd. It is 760 amino acids in length and consists of two subunits that are linked by disulfide bonds. It is a group II membrane protein; its N terminus is on the cytoplasmic side of the membrane, and its C terminus on the outer surface.[68–71] The transferrin receptor gene is at the end of the long arm of chromosome 3. The gene has been cloned and much of its structure has been elucidated.[72–74]

The cellular regulation of the iron balance appears to depend on the effect of iron, or iron lack, in stimulating the synthesis of ferritin or of transferrin receptors, respectively. This regulatory mechanism involves the effect of iron on iron-responsive elements (IRE) in the untranslated regions of transferrin receptor mRNA and ferritin mRNA. The IRE, which are stem-and-loop structures, have been identified in transferrin receptor mRNA. The loop is the short nucleotide segment CUGUGX on a short stem of nucleotides, where X can be C, A, G, or U. The IRE for transferrin receptor consists of as many as five loops and stems in the 3′ (downstream) untranslated portion of transferrin receptor mRNA.[65–72] Synthesis of transferrin receptor is induced by iron deficiency or, experimentally, by incubation of cells with an iron-chelating agent such as desferrioxamine. Synthesis of transferrin receptor is inhibited by heme, and this inhibition can be blocked by desferrioxamine.[71] Another locus in the 5′ (upstream) untranslated region of transferrin receptor mRNA also appears to contribute to control of transferrin receptor synthesis.[72] As noted subsequently, similar stem-loop IRE are involved in regulation of ferritin biosynthesis.

An iron-responsive element binding protein (IRE-BP) appears to be involved in the activation or repression of ferritin H and L chains and also of the transferrin receptor gene. This IRE-BP, which appears to participate in regulation of iron uptake by the cells, is encoded by a gene in human chromosome 9.[75]

## IRON IN THE ERYTHROBLAST

After endocytosis of the iron-transferrin-transferrin receptor complex in the coated vesicles, iron is released into the cytosol and apotransferrin is returned to extracellular fluid. The release of iron from transferrin is stepwise: one atom may be released by low pH; the other may require mediation by adenosine triphosphate (ATP), hemoglobin, or other substances.[76–81] Within the cytosol of the erythroblast, iron either is transported to mitochondria to be incorporated into heme or is taken up by ferritin within siderosomes. Either transferrin itself or other iron-binding substances[82–84] may participate in iron transport in the cytosol. The mechanism of passage of iron into mitochondria is unknown. In iron deficiency, sideroblasts almost disappear from the marrow. Conversely, in some states of iron overload, they may become more numerous and contain more than the normal number of siderotic granules.

Within the mitochondria, iron is inserted into protoporphyrin, forming heme, a reaction catalyzed by the enzyme heme synthetase (ferrochelatase). Heme inhibits the release of iron from transferrin,[85] an important feedback mechanism for adjusting the supply of iron to the rate of hemoglobin synthesis in the erythroblast.

## IRON UTILIZATION

The amount of iron utilized for hemoglobin synthesis in a normal adult is approximately 20 to 25 mg per day. These values can be calculated as follows. A man with a blood volume of 5000 ml and a hemoglobin level of 150 g/L has 750 g of circulating hemoglobin or 2.55 g of circulating hemoglobin iron (total blood hemoglobin in grams multiplied by 0.34%). Because the normal life span of the red cell is about 120 days, 2.55 g ÷ 120, or 21 mg of iron would be required daily to replace the catabolized hemoglobin. Iron utilization can also be determined after giving a tracer dose of radioiron intravenously. The amount of injected radioactive iron that is used for hemoglobin synthesis and delivered to the peripheral blood in newly formed erythrocytes is then measured. Normally, erythrocyte radioactivity rises for 7 to 14 days and then levels off at 75 to 90% of the injected amount. In iron-deficient persons, utilization typically exceeds 90% of the injected $^{59}Fe$.

Normally functioning bone marrow can effect a sixfold increase in its production of red blood cells and of hemoglobin. Under maximal stimulation, therefore, as much as 100 to 125 mg of iron can be used for hemoglobin synthesis per day. A detailed discussion of iron kinetics measurements is provided by Bothwell and Finch, Finch et al., Fairbanks et al., or Cook et al. (see "Selected Readings").

## REUTILIZATION

The avid manner in which the body conserves and reutilizes iron is an important characteristic of iron metabolism. A normal adult catabolizes enough hemoglobin each day to release 20 to 25 mg of iron, most of which is promptly recycled in the formation of new molecules of hemoglobin. More than 90% of hemoglobin iron is repeatedly recycled. The mechanism for recycling is phagocytosis of old erythrocytes, a process that occurs chiefly in macrophages of liver and spleen.

Digestion of phagocytized red cells proceeds at a rate sufficient to release approximately 20% of the hemoglobin iron within a few hours, and the remainder more slowly. The iron that is released by the action of the monocyte-macrophage system is bound to transferrin and is ultimately redistributed. About 40% of the hemoglobin iron of nonviable erythrocytes reappears in circulating red cells within 12 days. The rate of reutilization varies considerably. In normal persons, 19 to 69% reincorporation occurs in 12 days. The rate of reutilization of iron is more variable in the presence of disease. The remainder of the iron derived from hemoglobin catabolism enters the storage pool as ferritin or hemosiderin and normally turns over slowly: approximately 40% remains in storage after 140 days. When the rate of erythropoiesis increases, however, storage iron may be released more rapidly from the storage pools to plasma transferrin. Conversely, in the presence of chronic disease such as infection or rheumatoid arthritis or malignancy, the storage iron derived from hemoglobin catabolism is reutilized more slowly.

These alterations in the rate of iron reutilization seem to be determined by the rate of iron release from cells of the monocyte-macrophage system to plasma transferrin. Thus, in the presence of chronic disease, the rate of release of iron by macrophages decreases and the storage of iron in the monocyte-macrophage system increases. The effect is a reduced rate of delivery of iron to the developing erythroblast, an accelerated rate of transport to the bone marrow of the iron available in the plasma pool, a reduction in plasma iron concentration, and a reduction in the rate of erythropoiesis. Microcytic erythrocytes may result from the reduced flow of iron from the monocyte-macrophage system to the developing erythroblasts.

In addition to its role in regulating the size of iron stores, the monocyte-macrophage system appears to participate in regulation of the concentration of transferrin. Macrophages of this system have the capacity both to synthesize apotransferrin and to take up and degrade transferrin.

## STORAGE IRON

Iron in excess of need is stored intracellularly as ferritin and hemosiderin, principally in the macrophage ("reticuloendothelial") system of liver, spleen, bone marrow, and other organs. Ferritin is the basic storage for molecule iron; hemosiderin appears to be aggregated ferritin partially stripped of its protein component. A complete ferritin molecule consists of an apoferritin protein shell that is 13 nm in outer diameter and has an internal cavity of 7 nm in diameter.[86–93] Within the internal cavity are one or more crystals of ferric oxyhydroxide, FeOOH, together with trace amounts of phosphate that may occur at imperfections or cleavage planes in the FeOOH crystals (Fig. 9–4).[87] The cavity of each ferritin molecule has the capacity to hold at maximum 4300 iron atoms in the FeOOH crystals, although most ferritin molecules contain 2000 iron atoms.

The apoferritin protein shell is composed of 24 monomers, each with a molecular weight of approximately 20 kd, and each formed, in turn, by 4 long, nearly parallel helical chains of amino acids, 2 short helical segments, and connecting nonhelical segments of amino acids. The monomers are so arranged as to form a nearly spherical structure that is the apoferritin shell, with groups of 4 monomers so aligned that their short helices form pores, altogether 6 in number, that permit ingress and egress of small molecules to the interior of the apoferritin shell. The pores are approximately 0.7 nm diameter, just large enough to permit monosaccharides, flavin mononucleotide, ascorbic acid, and desferrioxamine to enter the interior cavity (Fig. 9–4).[89–91] Furthermore, the pores appear to function as catalytic sites for the binding of Fe(II), its oxidation to FeOOH, and the facilitated passage of the FeOOH so formed to the interior, where it is added to the growing core crystal (Fig. 9–5).[92] Thus, the apoferritin shell not only is an efficient iron trap, but also functions enzymatically.

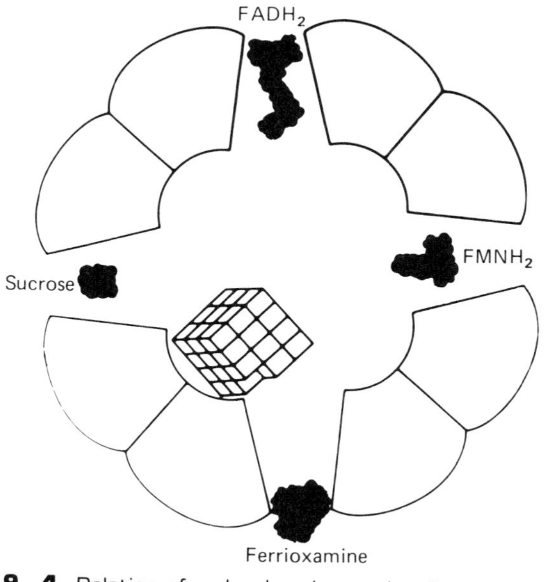
$FADH_2$
$FMNH_2$
Sucrose
Ferrioxamine

**FIGURE 9–4.** Relation of molecular size to the diameter of intermonomeric pores of apoferritin. Small molecules such as sucrose, ascorbate, or flavin adenine nucleotides appear to be capable of diffusing passively through the intermonomeric pores to the internal cavity of ferritin. Desferrioxamine-B may be small enough to enter the internal cavity, but ferrioxamine may be hindered in this passage. $FADH_2$, Reduced flavin adenine dinucleotide; $FMNH_2$, reduced flavin mononucleotide. (From Harrison, P.M.: Semin. Hematol., *14*:557–570, 1977, by permission of Grune and Stratton.)

The oxidation and uptake of iron by apoferritin is rapid. Similarly, the release of iron is rapid.[93] Iron release from ferritin may be mediated by reduced flavin mononucleotide, although an enzymatic mechanism has not been excluded.[91] Human ferritins may exist in multiple isomeric states.[94] H and L monomers differ in molecular weight, the former being about 20 kd and the latter about 18 kd. As many as 25 isoferritins, which vary in the proportion of H and L monomers, may exist. Ferritin that contains mostly H monomers is relatively acidic, contains relatively more iron, and is found predominantly in heart tissue. Ferritin that contains mostly L monomers is relatively basic, contains little iron, and is characteristically found in liver tissue. Ferritin predominantly of the H type is increased in the serum, especially in patients with malignancies such as carcinoma of the breast, embryonal carcinomas, and lymphomas.

Hemosiderin is traditionally differentiated from ferritin by the solubility of the latter in aqueous media and the insolubility of hemosiderin. Chemically, they differ in that hemosiderin contains slightly more iron (about 30% by weight) than does ferritin. Immunologically, they appear to be identical. On electron microscopy, the apoferritin shell of ferritin is not seen, but the electron-dense FeOOH crystalline core appears as a tetrad, because of its octahedral shape. By electron microscopy, hemosiderin contains great numbers of ferritin core crystal tetrads. Thus, a molecular weight cannot be given for hemosiderin. The molecular weight of ferritin depends in part on its iron content, but it usually is stated as 620 kd.

Within cells, apoferritin monomers are synthesized by ribosomes in response to the presence of iron. Regulation of ferritin synthesis depends on an IRE in the ferritin mRNA. An IRE is the nucleotide loop CAGUGX on a short stem of nucleotides. This loop-stem structure that is iron responsive is in the 5′ (upstream) untranslated region of ferritin mRNA. The CAGUGX loop is sensitive to iron or to an iron-induced protein-linked substance that may bind to the IRE stem-and-loop structure. A protein-like "retardation complex" has been described that binds to the IRE and inhibits ferritin synthesis. The presence of iron removes the inhibition of ferritin synthesis.[95] Iron also causes translocation of preformed ferritin messenger RNA to polyribosomes, where synthesis of ferritin occurs.[95–99]

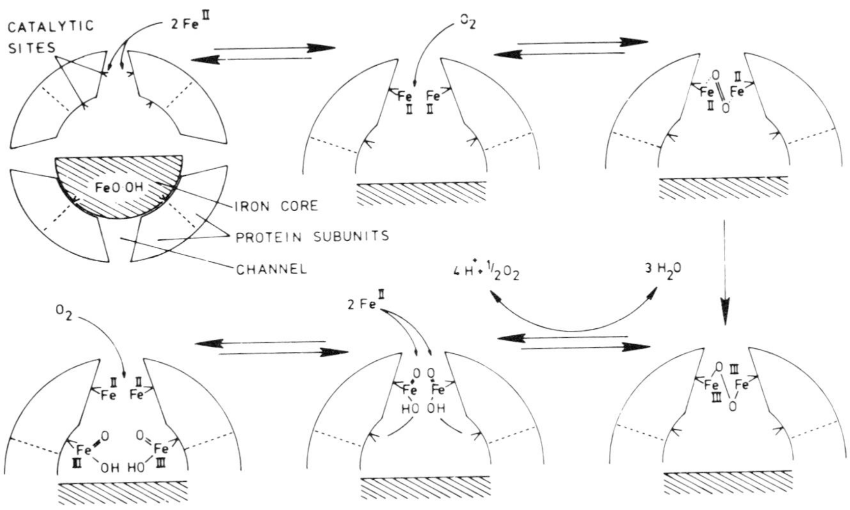
CATALYTIC SITES
2 Fe II
$O_2$
Fe Fe
II II
FeO·OH
IRON CORE
PROTEIN SUBUNITS
CHANNEL
$4H^+ + \frac{1}{2}O_2$
$3 H_2O$
2 Fe II
$O_2$
HO OH
OH HO

**FIGURE 9–5.** Scheme for uptake and deposition of iron by ferritin. Two pairs of iron-binding sites are envisioned in this scheme, and these are located close to the intermonomeric pores of the apoferritin shell. See the text for a more complete explanation of this interesting model. (From Crichton, R.R., Roman, F.: J. Mol. Catalysis, *4*:75–82, 1978, by permission.)

When the IRE is modified, ferritin synthesis does not occur in response to iron.[95]

In the liver and spleen of normal animals, there is a slight preponderance of ferritin over hemosiderin iron. With increasing concentrations of tissue iron, this ratio is reversed, and at high levels, the additional storage iron is deposited as hemosiderin. Both forms are capable of being mobilized for hemoglobin synthesis when the need for iron exists. Such reducing substances as ascorbate, dithionite, and reduced flavin mononucleotide ($FMNH_2$) cause rapid release of iron from ferritin. Thus, $FMNH_2$ might serve as the physiologic mediator of iron release.[91,93]

Quantitative measurement of normal iron stores has proved difficult, but reasonable estimates derived from available data are 300 to 1000 mg for adult women and 500 to 1500 mg for adult men. More individuals appear to fall into the lower half of these ranges than into the upper half, and many healthy women have virtually no iron reserves. Iron is released from ferritin as Fe(II) and as such traverses the cytosol and cell membrane to enter plasma, where it is again oxidized by ceruloplasmin to Fe(III) and taken up by transferrin. An increase in the amount of stored iron may occur as a result of a shift of iron from the red cell mass to the stores. This shift occurs in all anemias except those attributable to iron deficiency. A true increase in the amount of total body iron is found in patients with hemochromatosis, transfusional hemosiderosis or, rarely, after excessive and prolonged iron therapy. The total body burden of storage iron may exceed 30 g. An estimation as to whether iron stores are deficient or excessive may be made from the SI, TIBC, serum ferritin, and stainable iron in bone marrow aspirates.

## ENZYME IRON

At one time, it was almost universally accepted that iron enzymes are "inviolate" in iron deficiency anemia. Extensive studies in animals have shown that iron enzymes are, in fact, sensitive to depletion of iron deficiency. The degree of loss varies from enzyme to enzyme and from tissue to tissue. Cytochrome *c* and aconitase are readily depleted; cytochrome oxidase appears to be less susceptible and catalase is most resistant to depletion. Investigations of human leukocytes and buccal mucosa have shown depletion of cytochrome oxidase, even in relatively mild iron deficiency.[100,101] Iron deficiency in rats is associated with approximately 70% reduction in activity of the iron-sulfur enzymes succinate-ubiquinone oxidoreductase and NADH-ubiquinone oxidoreductase in rat skeletal muscle mitochondria. These important enzymes of the respiratory chain appear to be reduced in quantity rather than impaired in function, because the peptide components as well as the flavin prosthetic groups were reduced.[102] Iron-deficient rats also have hyperphenylalaninemia that is directly proportional to the severity of anemia. The mechanism of this effect is uncertain, as the hepatic activity of the iron-containing enzyme phenylalanine hydroxylase is not reduced. It is suggested that iron deficiency results in metabolism of phenylalanine by an alternative pathway that might generate increased quantities of phenylpyruvic acid and thereby disturb brain function. Treatment of iron deficiency with iron dextran resulted in normal serum concentrations of phenylalanine within 1 week.[103] Poor work performance in iron-deficient rats has been attributed to reduced activity of muscle α-glycerophosphatase dehydrogenase (see "Clinical Manifestations").

Mitochondrial α-glycerophosphate dehydrogenase is a flavoprotein that contains nonheme iron and plays an important electron transport role in aerobic metabolism. That iron deficiency results in impairment of activities of cytochromes and the iron-containing enzymes discussed previously is understandable because iron plays an important role in the function of these enzymes. However, iron deficiency is also associated with reduced activity of many enzymes that do not contain iron. The activity of monoamine oxidase (MAO), a copper-containing enzyme important in the synthesis of neurotransmitters, is diminished in the liver and in platelets of iron-deficient humans.[104–106] MAO activity was normal, however, in the brains of iron-deficient rats.[105]

Some diminution in the activities of other enzymes has been reported in association with iron deficiency in rats. These include hepatic glucose-6-phosphate dehydrogenase,[107] 6-phosphogluconate dehydrogenase,[108] and various transaminases.[109] These alterations appear to be minor and probably are of no physiologic import. Further, it is puzzling that activities of these enzymes should be affected, as none of them contains iron or requires iron as a cofactor.

## IRON LOSS

**Excretion.** The body has a limited capacity to excrete iron. Daily iron loss in adult men is between 0.90 and 1.05 mg or approximately 0.013 mg per kg of body weight irrespective of climate-dependent variation in perspiration.[110,111] The daily external loss is distributed roughly as follows: gastrointestinal blood (hemoglobin), 0.35 mg; gastrointestinal mucosal (ferritin), 0.10 mg; biliary, 0.20 mg; urinary, 0.08 mg; skin, 0.20 mg.

A slight increase in iron excretion, principally fecal, of no more than about 4 mg per day may occur in persons with iron overload, in partial compensation for increased iron stores.[112,113] Urinary iron excretion may be increased significantly in patients with proteinuria, hematuria, hemoglobinuria, and hemosiderinuria; the etiologic role of hemosiderinuria in the iron deficiency associated with cardiac anemia (e.g., implanted artificial heart valves, calcific aortic stenosis) is of considerable clinical importance. The iron excreted in feces is derived from blood lost into the alimentary canal (1.2 ± 0.5 ml whole blood per day),[114] from unabsorbed iron in bile, and from desquamated intestinal mucosal cells.

**Menstruation.** It is difficult to quantitate the "normal" iron loss associated with menstruation or pregnancy. Although the menstrual blood loss for any individual normal woman tends to be constant from month to month, the difference between women is considerable. In studies of Swedish women, the mean menstrual loss was 43 ml, equivalent to an average of about 0.6 to 0.7 mg of iron per day.[115–117] The upper limit of normal menstrual loss was about 80 ml per period. However, women who consider their menses normal may lose more than 100 ml and occasionally more than 200 ml per period. Menstrual blood losses are increased by intrauterine devices and are reduced by contraceptive pills.

**Pregnancy.** The iron "cost" of pregnancy is high. The external loss in urine, feces, and sweat continues and amounts to about 170 mg for the gestational period. About 270 mg (200 to 370 mg) are contributed to the fetus, and another 90 mg (30 to 170 mg) are contained in the placenta and cord. The amount of iron lost in hemorrhage at delivery, underestimated in the past, is now believed to average about 150 mg (90 to 300 mg). Iron is required for the expansion of the red blood cell mass that occurs during the last half of pregnancy, but this amount is recovered in large part when the circulating red blood cell volume returns to normal after delivery. Lactation causes an additional drain of approximately 0.5 to 1 mg of iron per day. The total iron cost of an uncomplicated pregnancy is in the range of 420 to 1030 mg (Table 9–2), or 1 to 2.5 mg per day over the 15 months of pregnancy and lactation. This estimate ignores the loss of iron due to blood lost at delivery because it is approximately equal to the amount of iron conserved by cessation of menses for 1 year. It also ignores the amount of iron needed for the expanded blood volume and increased size of the uterus because most of this iron is conserved and recycled.

**Iron Transfer to the Fetus.** The fetus has a highly effective acceptor system for assimilating iron. Iron from maternal transferrin is transferred to the placental tissue, to the plasma transferrin of the fetus, and then to the fetal tissues, along a unidirectional pathway that operates against increased maternal requirements for iron, even when there is maternal iron deficiency. During the last trimester of pregnancy, 3 to 4 mg of iron are transferred to the fetus each day.

**Bleeding.** Pathologic bleeding from any site constitutes an important form of iron loss: 1 ml of blood with a hemoglobin concentration of 150 g/L contains 0.5 mg of iron. A rough but useful rule of thumb is that 1 ml of packed red cells contains 1 mg of iron. The chronic loss of only a small volume of blood, therefore, may significantly increase iron requirements. For blood donors,

**TABLE 9–2.** IRON "COST" OF A NORMAL PREGNANCY

| | |
|---|---|
| Iron contributed to fetus | 200–370 mg |
| In placenta and cord | 30–170 |
| In blood loss at delivery | 90–310 |
| In milk, lactation 6 months | 100–180 |
| | 420–1030 mg |
| Average per day (pregnancy 9 mo lactation 6 mo) | 1–2.5 |

1 mg Fe = 17.9 μmol.

each 500 ml of blood donated contains between 200 and 250 mg of iron. Spread equally over 1 year, that loss amounts to roughly 0.6 to 0.7 mg per day. A donor who gives blood every 2 months has an increase in the average daily iron loss of 4 mg, and requires at least a fourfold increase in iron intake to avoid becoming anemic. Many women, if they do not receive iron supplementation, cease being blood donors because of anemia. In a controlled study of the effects of iron supplementation for women blood donors, the dropout rate because of anemia was 32% for those not receiving iron supplements and only 4.5% for those given regular oral iron supplement. As little as 39 mg of iron daily (120 mg of ferrous sulfate) in a single dose was sufficient to prevent anemia and allow 96% of adult women to donate blood at 8- to 12-week intervals.[118]

## IRON REQUIREMENTS

### GROWTH

The iron required for growth and its attendant increase in circulating hemoglobin mass depends on the rate of growth, i.e., the rapid growth during infancy and the growth spurt of male adolescents. The basis for estimating iron need is shown in Table 9–3. The average daily iron requirement is 0.35 to 0.7 mg per day for boys and 0.3 to 0.45 mg for girls prior to menarche. Other studies have shown a daily iron requirement of 38 μ/kg of optimal body weight, for both male and female children between ages 4 and 14 years.[119]

### NUTRITIONAL ALLOWANCES

Estimates of the amount of iron required to maintain positive balance are shown in Table 9–4. Recommended dietary intakes of iron in various countries are given in Appendix Tables A–2b, A–3b, A–4d, A–5, A–6, and A–10. Men and nonmenstruating women, in the absence of pathologic bleeding, should have little difficulty obtaining the iron they need from diets customary in the United States (12 to 18 mg per day). The balance may be precarious, however, in many menstruating women and adolescent girls who, because of concern about weight, restrict their diets and frequently have low iron intakes of 10 mg or less per day. The requirements during pregnancy are frequently so large that they are greater than the amount available from diet alone. Particularly in women with depleted stores, supplemental iron therapy is necessary during the latter half of pregnancy and for 2 to 3 months postpartum, to prevent iron deficiency. Full-term neonates do not require iron supplementation for the first 3 months, but should have iron supplementation thereafter as long as they are being formula- or breast-fed. Premature neonates should begin iron supplementation earlier.

## IRON DEFICIENCY AND IRON DEFICIENCY ANEMIA

### PREVALENCE

Iron deficiency is common in infants and nearly always affects the premature infant unless iron supplements are administered. In children over the age of 4 years, anemia has been reported to occur in 0.6 to 7.7%.[117] Relatively advanced iron deficiency anemia was found in 5.5% of poor children aged 5 to 8.[118] For the United States population as a whole, the frequencies of iron deficiency have been estimated as follows: children aged 1 to 2 years, 9.2%; children aged 3 to 10 years, 6.1%; males aged 11 to 14 years, 3.5 to 12.1%; females aged 11 to 14, 6.1%; males older than 14 years, ≤2%; females aged 15 to 44 years, 2.5 to 14.2%; postmenopausal females, 6.1%.[119,120] Thirty-five to 58% of young, healthy women have been found to have some degree of iron deficiency.[121–123] During pregnancy, in the absence of iron supplementation, the incidence is even higher.

In earlier studies of nutritional status of the people of the United States, it appeared that iron deficiency had a high prevalence, especially among the poor and among black people. The methods used for ascertainment of iron deficiency were not very sensitive or very specific. Microcytosis or low blood hemoglobin concentrations have been used as criteria for the prevalence of iron deficiency, on the assumption that other causes are rare. However, because 3% of black Americans have only two

**TABLE 9–3.** ESTIMATES OF AVERAGE DAILY IRON REQUIREMENTS FOR GROWTH

| | | BOYS | GIRLS |
|---|---|---|---|
| Adult wt greater than birth wt by | | 50–100 kg | 45–70 kg |
| Normal body iron per kg | | 50 mg | 35 mg |
| Iron in total wt gained | | 2500–5000 mg | 1575–2450 mg |
| Years of growth | | 20 yr | 15 yr |
| Estimated iron required for growth: | Av per year | 125–250 mg | 100–163 mg |
| | Av per day | 0.35–0.70 mg | 0.3–0.45 mg |

1 mg Fe = 17.9 μmol.

**TABLE 9–4.** RECOMMENDED DAILY INTAKE OF IRON

| CATEGORY | AGE | RECOMMENDED DAILY INTAKE MG |
|---|---|---|
| Infants (full term) | 0–3 mo | — |
| | 3–6 mo | 6.6 |
| | 6–12 mo | 8.8 |
| Children (M and F) | 1–10 yr | 10 |
| Males | 10–18 yr | 12 |
| | 18 yr | 10 |
| Females | > | |
| Nonpregnant | 10–45 yr | 15 |
| Pregnant | | 45 |
| Postmenopausal | | 10 |

(Adapted from Herbert, V.: Am. J. Clin. Nutr., *45*:679–686, 1987). 1 mg Fe = 17.9 μmol.

rather than four α-globin genes, a form of α-thalassemia characterized by microcytosis, and about 1% are β-thalassemia heterozygotes, also with microcytosis, and because the mean hemoglobin concentration of healthy, noniron-deficient black people is slightly lower than that of whites, by about 10 g/L (1.0 g/dL), earlier estimates of the prevalence of iron deficiency in black people are probably overstated. Clearly, however, in tropical regions where helminthiasis is nearly universal and nutrition is poor, and among impoverished people, multiparous women, and premature babies or those breast-fed too long, iron deficiency is a prevalent disorder with adverse consequences. In areas in which intestinal helminthiasis exists in a large proportion of the population, iron deficiency anemia is nearly universal.

Studies of the paleopathology of the ancient inhabitants of the southwestern United States indicate that severe iron deficiency may have been prevalent among sedentary agricultural people of the canyon bottomlands who depended on maize as their nearly sole dietary resource. Maize is poor in iron and also contains phytates that chelate iron, further reducing iron availability. Skeletons excavated in such areas reveal bony deformities and spongy porosity of the skull (porotic hyperostosis), attributed to extreme iron impoverishment.[128,129] Nomadic highland peoples who were hunters appear not to have suffered this deformity. Similarly, the peoples of the Aztec and Mayan cultures of meso-America, where maize was the major food, do not appear to have been afflicted with this disorder, perhaps because they also consumed beans rich in iron.

## ETIOLOGY

Iron deficiency results from one or a combination of the following: inadequate diet, impaired absorption, blood loss, or repeated pregnancies. An iron-poor diet is rarely the primary cause of iron deficiency in adults. Normal excretory loss of iron is so small that once a person has attained adulthood with normal body iron stores, a subsequent iron-poor diet and poor iron absorption depletes iron reserves and leads to anemia only after many years. Thus, the two most common causes of iron deficiency among adults are increased menstrual bleeding and hemorrhage from the alimentary tract. The development of iron deficiency in an adult man or a postmenopausal woman should be assumed to result from blood loss until proved otherwise.

**Defective Absorption.** This problem can be caused by diets that are grossly iron deficient or high in cereal content and low in animal protein. Geophagia interferes in the absorption of iron, probably because the ingested clay either strongly chelates or precipitates iron as insoluble compounds in the lumen of the gut. Clay-eating is practiced particularly by children and adult women. Among the poor, its prevalence is greater than is generally realized. Inadequate uptake of iron occurs in malabsorption syndromes and in chronic diarrhea from any cause. After partial or total gastrectomy, two defects in iron absorption are observed: absorption of food iron is subnormal[130] and the increase in absorption that usually accompanies iron deficiency does not take place.[131,132] When patients with atrophic gastritis and achlorhydria become iron deficient, they also are not able to increase the uptake of iron as much as are comparable individuals with normal gastric function.

**Blood Loss.** Except for pregnancy, large losses of iron are most commonly caused by bleeding. Hemorrhage from wounds, the nose or mouth, genitourinary tract, and hemorrhoids is obvious. Bleeding from the gastrointestinal tract often is occult, and adults may lose as much as 30 ml of blood from the esophagus, stomach, or small bowel without stools being discolored or becoming positive for occult blood by the guaiac test. Hemorrhoidal bleeding is usually obvious, if the patient is observant, but exceptionally fastidious persons may not observe even marked hemorrhoidal bleeding. Occult gastrointestinal bleeding is most commonly related to peptic ulcer, large hiatus hernia, esophageal varices, salicylate ingestion, intestinal diverticula, benign or malignant tumors, intestinal helminthiasis (particularly hookworm disease), regional enteritis, or ulcerative colitis. Occult gastrointestinal blood loss may be detected in nearly 50% of iron-deficient infants; usually no anatomic lesions can be identified. In infants or children, Meckel's diverticulum is one possible cause of occult blood loss that may be particularly difficult to identify.

The effect of normal menstrual blood loss on iron requirements has been discussed. However, women frequently fail to recognize an abnormal flow. Menstrual volume may be excessive if double pads must be worn because one soaks through, duration of periods is greater than 5 days, large clots are passed, and more than 12 pads per period are needed. The use of intrauterine devices increases menstrual bleeding. The admirable and necessary donation of blood for transfusions and the collection of large amounts of blood for diagnostic study are also forms of hemorrhage.

Iron deficiency anemia is common after subtotal gastric resection, particularly when the anastomosis between remaining stomach and small bowel is end-to-side, respectively (e.g., Billroth II). Approximately 45% of patients who have had such an operation ultimately become iron deficient. Sometimes, they have combined iron and vitamin $B_{12}$ or folate deficiency. A few of these patients have low-grade chronic blood loss from lesions around the anastomosis site, not amounting to more than 5 or 10 ml per day.[133] Most such patients, however, appear to have an impaired ability to absorb heme iron.[134] They respond well to the administration of medicinal iron orally, because their absorption of inorganic iron is unimpaired.

Hereditary hemorrhagic telangiectasia is a well-recognized cause of chronic bleeding and iron-deficiency anemia. The diagnosis is usually made early, especially in individuals with a positive family history or typical cutaneous lesions on palms, soles, face, and elsewhere. Similar telangiectases of the gastrointestinal tract in scleroderma or in Turner's syndrome may cause chronic blood loss. The telangiectatic lesions may be widespread in the gastrointestinal tract. A vascular anomaly that is not hereditary, does not have a cutaneous counterpart, and usually is not manifested until middle age is angiodysplasia of the gastrointestinal tract, also called vascular ectasia or arteriovenous anomaly.[135] These tiny telangiectasis-like lesions are most common in the cecum or ascending colon, but may occur at any level of the alimentary canal. They seem to be a relatively frequent cause of occult gastrointestinal blood loss that cannot be diagnosed by traditional radiologic examinations or sigmoidoscopy. Mesenteric angiography, gastroscopy, or colonoscopy usually is required.

Blue rubber bleb nevi usually are hereditary cutaneous hemangiomas that may be associated with similar vascular malformation in the gastrointestinal tract. The latter may bleed and may require surgical excision. The diagnosis may be suspected when the typical skin lesion is found. Diffuse vascular ectasia of the gastric antrum is another uncommon vascular malformation that is associated with gastrointestinal hemorrhage.

Menetrier's disease is gastric mucosal hypertrophy associated with hypersecretion of hydrochloric acid (HCl). Zollinger-Ellison syndrome and pseudo-Zollinger-Ellison syndrome also are characterized by hypersecretion of gastric HCl. Each of these disorders may cause chronic blood loss. Hemocholecyst, or hemorrhage in the gallbladder, is a rare cause of chronic blood loss. It appears to be the result of erosion by gallstones.

Some medications may cause gastrointestinal hemorrhage. Aspirin may cause diffuse hemorrhage gastritis, particularly when ingested together with ethanol. Ingestion of adrenocorticosteroids or nonsteroidal anti-inflammatory agents may also cause gastrointestinal bleeding.

Mild anemia is commonly encountered in elite long-distance runners. The anemia has been characterized as microcytic; plasma hemoglobin concentration is increased and serum iron and ferritin concentrations are decreased. The anemia responds to iron therapy. Significant gastrointestinal blood loss was demonstrated in 20 of 24 long-distance runners, and is postulated as the probable cause of anemia in runners.[136] A similar anemia has been observed in competitive swimmers.[137]

Iron deficiency anemia is a frequent long-term complication of gastric bypass surgery for refractory obesity. In this setting, iron deficiency may be accompanied by vitamin $B_{12}$ deficiency, folate deficiency, or both.[138]

Factitial iron deficiency anemia, also known as the Lasthénie de Ferjol syndrome, may result from self-inflicted blood-letting.[139,140] The condition is rare, and is encountered principally in young women. It is a manifestation of severe psychoneurosis. Diagnosis is difficult; such patients tend to be evasive, denying that the blood loss is self-inflicted, and often are refractory to treatment.

**Iron Sequestration.** In four conditions, the availability of iron for hemoglobin synthesis is reduced despite normal or greater than normal body iron content. These conditions are: (1) idiopathic pulmonary hemosiderosis; (2) paroxysmal nocturnal hemoglobinuria; (3) chronic disease, with inability to mobilize iron from reticuloendothelial cell depots; and (4) the extremely rare disorder congenital atransferrinemia. In these four disorders, increased amounts of iron are found, respectively, in (1) lungs, (2) kidneys, and (3 and 4) the reticuloendothelial system (including liver and bone marrow macrophages), but the amount of iron transported to normoblasts of the bone marrow is reduced. Hence, persons with these disorders may develop iron deficiency anemia. Despite reduced availability of iron from sequestered stores, patients with idiopathic pulmonary hemosiderosis and those with paroxysmal nocturnal hemoglobinuria usually respond to iron therapy with a rise in blood hemoglobin concentration.

Sometimes, the cause of iron deficiency is not found during the course of careful clinical evaluation: the diet seems adequate, no absorptive defect can be recognized, no blood loss can be detected. In all probability, blood loss in such patients goes unrecognized because it is intermittent or small in amount.

## CLINICAL MANIFESTATIONS

It is often assumed that the manifestations of iron deficiency anemia result from reduction of the hemoglobin concentration of the blood. However, three clinical observations contradict this assumption. First, the severity of symptoms is not closely correlated with the degree of anemia. Second, response to treatment often seems to precede any increase in the hemoglobin concentration of the blood. Third, certain clinical manifestations such as koilonychia and esophageal webs cannot be accounted for on the basis of anemia alone. In pernicious anemia, the neurologic symptoms are related to the metabolic effects of vitamin $B_{12}$ deficiency on nonhematopoietic tissues. Similarly, iron deficiency is a systemic disorder in which symptoms do not arise from the anemia alone, and may occur in the absence of anemia.

Iron-deficient rats are unable to exercise normally even if transfused to a normal hemoglobin level, apparently because of an iron deficiency-induced abnormality in muscle metabolism that is attended by lactic acidosis and reduction in α-glycerophosphate dehydrogenase activity.[141,142] Iron-deficient rats also have decreased cold tolerance resulting from failure to increase the blood levels of thyroid hormones, the normal adaptive response of rats to cold.[143]

Many studies in humans have shown effects of iron deficiency similar to those described in rats. Work tolerance is impaired,[144–150] and blood lactate concentration rises more rapidly during work in iron-deficient humans.[151] Iron deficiency anemia may be accompanied by impairment of temperature regulation and a secondary deficiency of thyroid hormone. These abnormalities respond to administration of iron alone.[152]

Iron deficiency in early childhood results in reduction in rates of longitudinal growth and weight gain.[153,154] Much of this growth retardation can be amended by iron supplementation if begun early enough.

Iron deficiency contributes to scholastic underachievement and behavioral disturbances in children,[154–164] possibly through defects in the metabolism of monoamines involved in neural transmission.[155–162] In a study of iron deficiency induced by phlebotomy in seven adult men, disturbance in cognitive function could not be demonstrated with confidence. However, subtle changes in mental function may require a larger series to attain statistical significance. Asymmetries of electroencephalograph recordings in the occipital area were observed and were positively correlated with severity of iron deficiency.[165]

Significant depression of the ST segment of electrocardiograms was observed during treadmill tests in 14 of 55 iron deficiency anemia patients and in only 1 of 55 age- and sex-matched controls. Total dose iron dextran infusion resulted in abolition of the electrocardiographic abnormality in 10 of 11 patients so treated. Because iron replacement corrected the electrocardiographic abnormality before the blood hemoglobin concentration increased, the observed electrocardiographic abnormality may well have been the result of impairment of cytochrome or enzyme function within the cells of the conducting system.[166]

Symptoms of iron deficiency are often so insidious in onset that their duration cannot be dated with accuracy. Patients with iron deficiency anemia may be unaware of being in ill health. However, they commonly experience symptomatic improvement once iron therapy is initiated. In symptomatic patients with moderate to severe degrees of anemia, most of the complaints are common to all anemias: weakness, fatigue, pallor, dyspnea on exertion, palpitation, and a sense of being overly tired. When standardized exercise is carried out on a bicycle ergometer, the time needed to restore cardiorespiratory functions to pre-exercise resting values in iron-deficient subjects is prolonged. Coldness and paresthesias of the hands and feet are noted frequently. Few iron-deficient patients complain of the abnormality causing the anemia, such as hiatus hernia, peptic ulcer, or hemorrhoids.

Manifestations related to the oral cavity and the gastrointestinal tract have attracted attention because of both their frequency and uncertainty as to their pathogenesis. Vague gastrointestinal complaints—capricious appetite, flatulence, epigastric distress, belching, constipation or diarrhea, and nausea—are fairly common. Pica is practiced by some patients with iron deficiency: geophagia, clay-eating, starch-eating, salt-eating, cardboard-eating, and ice-eating. Pica is often but not always corrected by iron therapy. Iron deficiency may cause secondary malabsorption phenomena, possibly related to a decrease in iron-containing or iron-dependent enzymes in intestinal mucosal cells.[167] Glossitis, characterized by varying degrees of papillary atrophy and soreness, is found more often in patients over the age of 40 years and with greater frequency in women than in men. Angular stomatitis occurs in 10 to 15% of patients, particularly among those who are edentulous. Dysphagia, iron deficiency anemia, and postcricoid esophageal stricture, often accompanied by a web at this site, constitute an interesting triad (the Paterson-Kelly or Plummer-Vinson syndrome) found particularly, but not exclusively, in middle-aged women. It has been regarded as a precancerous lesion, but the relationship has been questioned.[168] Gastroscopic examination with gastric biopsy has demonstrated gastritis with varying degrees of glandular damage in about 80% of patients and atrophic gastritis in a few.

Paradoxically, the frequency of glossitis, angular stomatitis, and dysphagia varies greatly among patients in different population groups and seems to be decreasing in communities where iron deficiency remains prevalent. The varying incidence of these epithelial changes plus the fact that they seem to occur more frequently in "low input" (decreased absorption) than in "high output" (blood loss) iron deficiency suggest that they may be caused by associated deficiencies. Hypochlorhydria and achlorhydria occur more commonly than in comparable population groups that are not iron deficient; their incidence varies with the methods used for stimulating gastric secretion, the age of the patient, and the cause of iron deficiency. For instance, achlorhydria is unusual in chronic iron deficiency associated with hookworm disease. Particularly in younger patients with achlorhydria, the secretion of acid may return after treatment with iron. However, it usually does not. The histologic appearance of the gastric mucosa has only rarely been observed to improve. The suggestion that impairment of iron absorption might be the result of iron deficiency as well as its cause was made first many years ago. Iron deficiency may be associated with diminution in the increase in serum iron concentration that normally follows oral iron loading, but such data cannot be interpreted as unequivocally indicating impaired absorption.

The fingernails, and sometimes the toenails as well, may become lusterless, thin, brittle, flattened, and then spoon-shaped (koilonychia). When the blood hemoglobin concentration falls below 60 g/L (6 g/dl), the heart may become dilated and "hemic" murmurs may be heard. Infrequently, the spleen is palpable at the costal margin. Mild degrees of vitiligo and of dependent edema often are noted. Neurologic examination is normal in spite of paresthesias. Rarely, papilledema, visual disturbances, and elevated cerebral spinal fluid pressure, simulating intracranial tumor, may be found in iron-deficient patients; these unusual manifestations are corrected by iron therapy.[6] A complex syndrome occurs among young males in Iran: dwarfism, iron deficiency anemia, hepatosplenomegaly, hypogonadism, and geophagia.[169] A similar syndrome without geophagia has been observed in Egypt; coexistent zinc deficiency may be responsible.

Severe iron deficiency anemia in pregnant rats results in excess embryonic and fetal mortality and increased frequency of microphthalmia or anophthalmia.[170] Iron deficiency may also be associated with impaired hearing in rats. These effects have not been described in humans.

The leukocyte count in severely iron-deficient patients usually is normal, but in 14% of patients, it may be as low as $2.5 \times 10^9$/L. Both neutrophils and lymphocytes are diminished. Thus, the leukocyte differential is normal. Platelet counts may be elevated, but thrombocytopenia also occurs and may be severe.[171]

## DIAGNOSIS

In most disorders, the fully developed disease state is easy to detect, but when its expression is mild, it may be difficult to diagnose. Iron deficiency is no exception. Severe iron deficiency anemia is characterized by hypochromia and microcytosis of the red blood cells. Erythrocytes not only are small and pale when observed on the blood smear, but also they vary greatly in size and shape. The serum iron concentration is diminished, and the TIBC is increased. In consequence, the saturation of the iron-binding protein is reduced; generally, less than 16% of the available iron binding sites are saturated. The free protoporphyrin level of the erythrocytes is increased and the serum ferritin concentration is diminished. Examination of the bone marrow generally reveals a decrease in the amount of storage iron in macrophages.[155,165] Exceptions are patients who have been transfused within the previous few months or who have been given parenteral iron preparations; in such persons, storage iron may be present in bone marrow despite hypochromic, microcytic erythrocytes in blood, low SI, and low serum ferritin concentrations. Such cases are puzzling unless it is recalled that some patients utilize iron dextran poorly. The number of sideroblasts (the normoblasts that contain cytoplasmic granules that stain for iron) is also diminished in the bone marrow of patients with iron deficiency anemia.

The diagnosis of mild iron deficiency anemia, or iron deficiency without anemia, is more difficult to establish than that of the severe form. Mildly anemic patients do not manifest the microcytic hypochromic cells characteristic of the severe iron deficiency state. Neither is the SI invariably diminished nor the TIBC increased. The transferrin saturation may be normal. However, the serum ferritin concentration usually is diminished even in mild iron deficiency, and even after recent administration of exogenous iron such as iron dextran. The free erythrocyte protoporphyrin concentration is increased. With the exception of patients who have received blood transfusions or parenteral iron therapy, the bone marrow iron stores are depleted, even in the mildest degree of iron deficiency.

It is important to differentiate iron deficiency anemia from other anemias, particularly those microcytic anemias that may simulate it. Thalassemias and certain hemoglobinopathies are also characterized by hypochromia and microcytosis of erythrocytes, and are easily misdiagnosed as iron deficiency, sometimes with serious consequences. These disorders are prevalent in North America. α-Thalassemia is particularly common and is often overlooked. Approximately 28% of black Americans lack one of the four normal α-globin genes, and about 3% lack two of these genes. Characteristically, erythrocytes of individuals with only two α-globin genes are slightly smaller than normal and they may have mild hypochromia and slight target cell formation. Those with three normal α-globin genes do not usually exhibit any major blood abnormalities, but for such persons, the median hemoglobin concentration and median mean erythrocyte volume (MCV) are slightly less than the corresponding median values of persons who have four functional α-globin genes.

More than 25% of the Indochinese refugees now living in North America also have forms of α-thalassemia. This population includes persons who lack three of the normal α-globin genes. With only one functioning α-globin gene, they have hemoglobin H disease, characterized by moderate anemia (blood hemoglobin concentration of (80 to 100 g/L (8 to 10 g/dl)) microcytosis, hypochromia, and target erythrocytes. Some have reticulocytosis, elevation in serum bilirubin concentration, and mild splenomegaly. Approximately 10% of the Indochinese refugees have hemoglobin E trait, which is also characterized by mild microcytosis and hypochromia, and may be mistaken for iron deficiency.[172] Indeed, the presence of smaller than normal erythrocytes in the blood of persons from Southeast Asia now residing in North America is more often related to hemoglobin E trait or α-thalassemia than to iron deficiency. β-Thalassemia minor occurs in about 5% of people of Mediterranean, Southern Chinese, or Southeast Asian origin, and in about 1% of black Americans. Thus, it is quite prevalent in North America, and must not be mistaken for iron deficiency, which it may resemble from examination of the blood or blood film. It is characterized by an increase in the hemoglobin $A_2$ content of blood, usually to 4 to 9%. However, when iron deficiency and β-thalassemia minor coexist, the hemoglobin $A_2$ content is often normal, and the correct diagnosis may be overlooked.

δβ-Thalassemia is less common than β-thalassemia. It is characterized by small erythrocytes, hypochromia, and target erythrocytes, and an increase in the hemoglobin F content of blood to 5 to 15% of total hemoglobin. Hemoglobin Lepore trait, once believed rare, is in fact quite common, with a prevalence about one-fortieth that of β-thalassemia minor. It is associated with blood changes like those of β-thalassemia minor, but not with anemia or splenomegaly.

Of these disorders, all but the minor α-thalassemias are easily identified by hemoglobin electrophoresis and the measurement of hemoglobins $A_2$ and F. Identification of the α-thalassemias requires measurement of globin chain synthesis or restriction enzyme-DNA probe studies of the globin genes. These costly tests may not be practical for routine use. Therefore, the diagnosis of α-thalassemias (except hemoglobin H disease) is usually based on exclusion of other known causes of microcytosis: iron deficiency, β-thalassemia, δβ-thalassemia, Hb E disorders, Hb Lepore trait, chronic disease (e.g., infection or malignancy), and sideroblastic anemias. Sometimes, a family history of anemia or microcytosis is a useful clue. Knowledge of the patient's ethnic origin is often helpful, because thalassemias have high prevalence in certain ethnic groups.

Measurement of the SI, TIBC, and Tsat and assay of serum ferritin concentration are sometimes useful in distinguishing iron deficiency from most other disorders that produce microcytic anemias. Except when these conditions coexist with iron deficiency (a common problem), or when there are inflammatory disorders or malignancies (chronic disease), the SI, TIBC, Tsat, and serum ferritin concentration are normal. In early iron deficiency, SI, TIBC, and Tsat often are normal, but the serum ferritin concentration is diminished. In more advanced iron deficiency, the SI, Tsat, and ferritin concentration usually are low and the TIBC may be increased. In chronic disease, on the other hand, the SI and TIBC usually are both diminished, the Tsat is normal, and the ferritin concentration is increased. Unfortunately, exceptions to these generalizations do occur. A particular problem is the interpretation of these tests for iron deficiency in patients who have such disorders as rheumatoid arthritis, chronic renal disease, malignant lymphomas, leukemias, or other malignancies or inflammatory disorders, or in Gaucher's disease. The problem stems from the fact that serum ferritin concentration typically is increased in these conditions, and may reflect the severity of the disease. Thus, an elevated or abnormal serum ferritin concentration in patients with these disorders may cause the physician to assuming erroneously that iron deficiency does not coexist. In such cases, diagnosis requires bone marrow examination with iron stain.

Differentiation of iron deficiency anemia from the sideroblastic anemias is particularly important, because patients with sideroblastic anemia tend to accumulate excess amounts of iron in the tissues. As a result, they frequently develop iron overload disease. In such circumstances, iron therapy not only fails to benefit the patient but hastens the appearance of complications of iron overload disease and may cause earlier death. A dimorphic appearance of erythrocytes in the blood smear is a clue that leads to this diagnosis: erythrocytes seem to be of two distinct populations, some are of normal size and well-filled with hemoglobin, others are microcytic and hypochromic. The serum iron and ferritin concentrations may be elevated. The diagnosis is confirmed by staining a bone marrow specimen by Perls' Prussian blue method and demonstrating the presence of ringed sideroblasts. A discriminative function (DF′) and use of the red cell distribution width (RDW) have been proposed to differentiate iron deficiency from the conditions listed previously.[173–175] Experience has shown these methods are of limited value. Measurement of erythrocyte ferritin concentration may provide information complementary to that of serum ferritin.[176] Furthermore, in chronic disease in which the serum ferritin concentration is elevated, the erythrocyte ferritin concentration may be low. Measurement of both serum and erythrocyte ferritin may help differentiate iron deficiency from chronic disease. Assay for serum transferrin receptor has been proposed as a reliable test for iron deficiency, in which transferrin receptor concentration is increased.[177,178] However, it is too early for a verdict on this new test.

At present, despite the limitations noted, measurement of serum ferritin concentration appears to be the most sensitive, specific, and practical test for diagnosis of uncomplicated iron deficiency. Nonetheless, serum ferritin assay may lead to erroneous diagnosis. Reference (normal) ranges and diagnostic criteria vary from laboratory to laboratory, depending on the method used.

Studies of patients with iron deficiency anemia are never complete until the cause for the deficiency is recognized. The source of any blood loss that may underlie the deficiency state must be identified. Carcinomas of the gastrointestinal tract occasionally are detected in this search long before other manifestations have appeared. At times, it is helpful to tag a sample of the patient's red blood cells with $^{51}Cr$, readminister the blood, and measure the radioactivity of feces: it will be greater than normal if blood is oozing from a gastrointestinal lesion. The same technique may be used to measure menstrual loss.

## TREATMENT

Whereas dietary sources of iron are adequate to maintain normal iron balance in adult males, prevention of iron deficiency anemia during pregnancy or treatment of iron deficiency anemia usually cannot be accomplished by dietary means alone. The amount of iron contained in red meats or liver is simply not enough for this purpose. Iron medication must be administered orally or parenterally. Adequate therapy must not only correct the deficiency, but also treat its cause. Increased menstrual flow, occult loss of blood from the urinary or gastrointestinal tracts, or defective absorption must be detected and corrected, if possible. Appropriate selection of a therapeutic agent requires understanding of the maximum expected hematologic response, the amount of iron required to produce this maximum effect, and the absorption that can be expected from a given iron compound. The physician must observe the patient to make certain that a response is obtained: a satisfactory rise in the hemoglobin level attributable to the iron therapy constitutes final proof of the correctness of the diagnosis.

**Optimal Hematologic Response.** A few days after therapy is initiated, the reticulocyte count begins to rise. It reaches a peak between 7 and 12 days and then falls to normal levels during the next 2 weeks. The height of the reticulocyte peak is inversely proportional to the original hemoglobin value and may exceed 20% in severely anemic patients. The blood hemoglobin concentration begins to increase after about 10 to 14 days. Then, it may increase at a rate of 2 to 3 g/L of blood per day if the anemia is severe and at a rate of 1 to 2 g/L per day if the initial hemoglobin concentration is greater than 75 g/L. As the hemoglobin concentration approaches normal, the rate of increase slows. The anemia is usually half corrected in 3 weeks; normal values usually are attained by 8 weeks of treatment. The response in children is somewhat more rapid than that of adults.

The daily dose of iron ideally should be sufficient to support a maximum hemoglobin increase: 3 g/L (0.3 g/dl) per day or 15 g of new circulating hemoglobin each day, in a patient with a blood volume of 5 L. This rate of increase requires absorption of 50 mg of iron daily. The exact amount obviously varies with the blood volume and with other factors, but 50 mg of absorbed iron is a reasonable average quantity to provide for adults. The comparable figure for children varies with body weight and can be calculated by estimating the blood volume to be 70 ml/kg body weight.

The total amount of iron that must be absorbed or injected to correct the deficiency can also be estimated. If, for example, a woman with severe iron deficiency anemia has a hematocrit of only 0.15, each 1000 ml of blood is deficient by approximately 300 ml of packed red cells. If the patient's blood volume is 4 L, enough iron must be supplied to provide four times as many red cells, i.e., 1200 ml. Because 1 ml of red cells contains about 1 mg of iron, 1.2 g of iron are needed to restore the red cell mass to normal. In addition, 0.5 to 1 g of iron should be provided to replete the stores. The total amount needed to correct the deficiency in this instance, therefore, would be 1.7 to 2.2 g.

**Oral Therapy.** The ideal iron preparation for oral therapy should be well absorbed, well tolerated by the gastrointestinal tract in therapeutic doses, and inexpensive. Because ferrous iron is more efficiently absorbed than the ferric form, simple highly soluble ferrous salts come closest to approaching the ideal. Ferrous sulfate is generally recognized as the standard against which all other compounds must be evaluated. In a comparison of absorption from different iron compounds using a double isotope iron tracer technique, 30 mg of iron as ferrous sulfate and 30 mg as the preparation under study were given on alternate days for a total of 10 days. The two preparations were labeled with two different isotopes of iron so that absorption from the preparation under study could be compared with that from ferrous sulfate (Fig. 9–6). Several compounds were absorbed about as well as ferrous sulfate: ferrous succinate, ferrous lactate, ferrous fumarate, ferrous glycine sulfate, ferrous glutamate, and ferrous gluconate; none was clearly superior. Large amounts of ascorbic acid given with ferrous sulfate increased absorption of iron.[179]

Table 9–5 is a list of many of the commonly available iron pills and provides a comparison of their cost per gram of iron. An iron-deficient patient absorbs approximately 20% of the iron in these tablets. Because the recommended daily dose provides roughly 200 to 240 mg of iron, the desired daily absorption of 40 or 50 mg can be attained. As shown in Table 9–5, both the iron content of commercially available pills and the cost of iron in this form vary enormously: the iron in the more expensive of these pills costs more than 100 times that of the least expensive. Because the price of gold (June, 1991) is \$12.25/g, and the iron in one of these preparations costs the consumer \$44.69/g, at least one pharmaceutical manufacturer has surpassed the ancient alchemists' objective of the transmutation of "baser metals" into gold. Furthermore, it is astonishing that the market price of Simron increased 20% from 1989 to 1991, and the price of Fero-Gradumet increased 46%, whereas the price of some iron preparations declined substantially. These prices must be placed in the context that the commercial

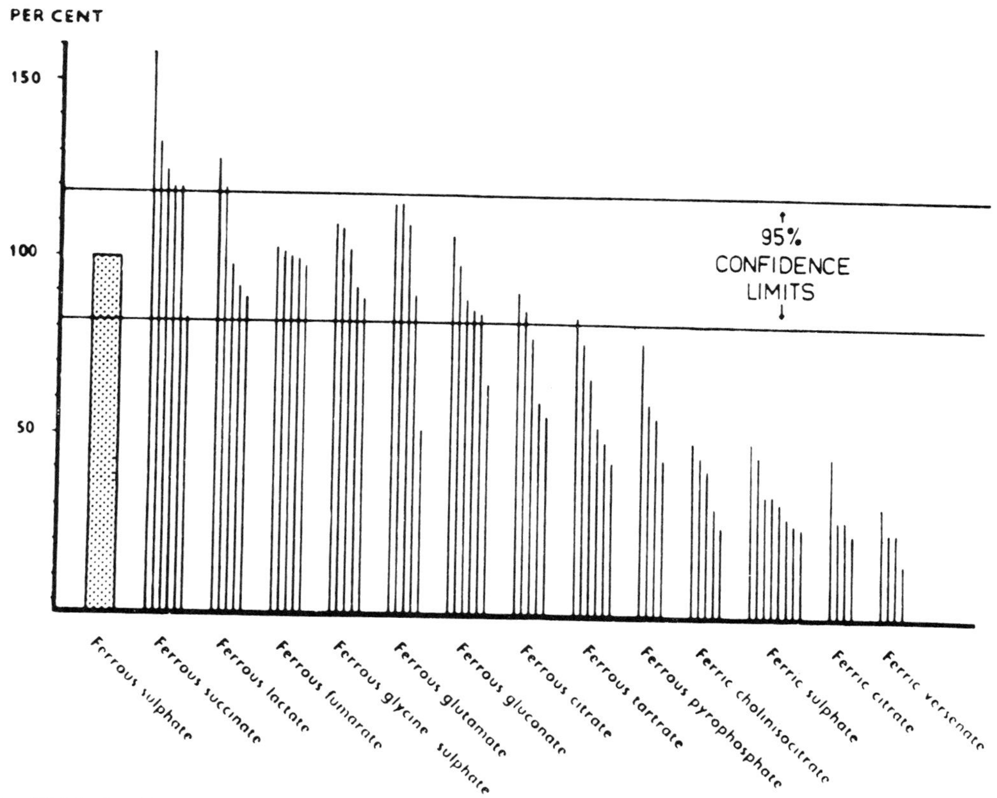
PER CENT
150
100
50
95%
CONFIDENCE
LIMITS
Ferrous sulphate
Ferrous succinate
Ferrous lactate
Ferrous fumarate
Ferrous glycine sulphate
Ferrous glutamate
Ferrous gluconate
Ferrous citrate
Ferrous tartrate
Ferrous pyrophosphate
Ferric cholinisocitrate
Ferric sulphate
Ferric citrate
Ferric versenate

**FIGURE 9–6.** Comparison of the absorption of iron from ferrous sulfate and from various iron compounds. The daily dose is equivalent to 30 mg elemental iron. Ferrous sulfate and other compounds under study were tagged with different isotopes of iron and were given on alternate days for 10 days. (From Brise, H., Hallberg, L., Acta Med. Scand., *376(Suppl.)*:1–73, 1962.) 1 mg Fe = 17.9 μmol.

retail prices of ferrous sulfate and ferrous fumarate, when purchased in bulk as chemicals, are, respectively, 10¢ and 5¢/g of iron. Public concern about the rising cost of medical care must be considered when these extremely overpriced products are prescribed or dispensed.

The gastrointestinally irritating quality of medicinal iron salts has been greatly exaggerated. Iron preparations are better tolerated by patients than is generally believed. In a double-blind study in which iron was given at a slightly lower dosage than that usually employed, no difference could be observed between the effects of placebo and iron.[180] On the other hand, a few patients do have difficulty tolerating iron medication taken in full therapeutic dosage. In those patients who complain of severe epigastric distress, tolerance can frequently be induced by reducing the dose to one tablet per day and then gradually adding one tablet per day until the full therapeutic dose is reached. Alternatively, other preparations may be tried until one is found that can be tolerated. Children tend to have less gastrointestinal distress from iron therapy than do adults. A satisfactory schedule is to give half the adult dose to children who weigh from 15 to 35 kg, and the full dose to those heavier than 35 kg. For smaller children, and those unable to take tablets, liquid preparations are available. Because milk, bread, and other cereals inhibit iron absorption, iron medication should always be taken between meals.

A common error is to discontinue iron therapy after the 2 or 3 months required for correction of the anemia. Replenishment of iron stores occurs slowly when iron is given orally because absorption falls off as the hemoglobin concentration rises toward normal levels. Consequently, oral therapy must be continued for 6 to 12 months if stores are to be repleted. If the chronic bleeding responsible for iron deficiency cannot be corrected or controlled, continuous iron therapy is required.

Iron preparations that contain molybdenum, copper, cobalt, ascorbic acid, various vitamins including folic acid and vitamin $B_{12}$, and liver or bone marrow extracts, are more expensive, no more effective in correcting iron deficiency and, in some instances, have more serious disadvantages. Injections of folic acid and of vitamin $B_{12}$ do not increase the response to iron. Also to be deplored is the prevalent practice of packaging ferrous sulfate in enteric-coated tablets or in capsules containing delayed-release granules. The fraction of iron absorbed from

**TABLE 9–5.** COMPARISON OF IRON CONTENT AND COSTS OF SOME ORAL IRON MEDICATIONS*

| NAME | MANUFACTURER | IRON CONTENT (MG PER TABLET) | COST ($) Per 100 Tablets or Capsules | COST ($) Per Gram of Iron |
|---|---|---|---|---|
| Plain iron tablets or capsules | | | | |
| Ferrous sulfate | | | | |
| Feosol | Manly & James | 66 | 8.50 | 1.28 |
| Generic | Golding† | 66 | 2.29 | 0.35 |
| Ferrous fumarate | | | | |
| Ircon | Kenwood | 66 | 7.26 | 1.10 |
| Generic | Nature-Made | 20 | 3.97 | 1.98 |
| Ferrous gluconate | | | | |
| Fergon | Winthrop-Breon† | 37 | 7.92 | 2.14 |
| Simron | Marion Merrell Dow | 10 | 44.69 | 44.69 |
| Generic | Nature-Made | 37 | 3.97 | 1.07 |
| Enteric-coated tablets | | | | |
| Generic | Goldline | 66 | 3.00 | 0.45 |
| "Delayed-release" capsules | | | | |
| Fero-Gradumet‡ | Abbott | 105 | 30.39 | 2.90 |
| Ferro-sequels | Lederle | 50 | 29.25 | 5.85 |
| Feosol Spansules | Manly & James | 50 | 22.86 | 4.57 |
| Combination tablets or capsules | | | | |
| Geritol | Beecham | 50 | 14.52 | 2.91 |
| Trinsicon | Russ | 90 | 56.70 | 6.29 |
| Unicap Plus Iron | Upjohn | 18 | 9.75 | 5.38 |
| Vitron-C | Fisons | 66 | 10.98 | 1.66 |

*Figures are based on average retail price in the United States in June 1991. Prices vary slightly among pharmacies. Numerous other iron preparations are available and many other manufacturers produce generic iron preparations. Those shown are selected only as examples, and their listing does not imply endorsement.

†Sugar-coated. Potentially dangerous in households with young children.

‡Although the manufacturer represents Fero-Gradumet as a "slow release" form of iron, independent studies indicate that it actually releases iron rapidly, a desirable property. In this regard, it resembles many of the medications listed as "plain iron tablets."

some of these preparations is distinctly less because iron is released more distally in the small intestine or colon, where absorption is less efficient. As a result, the expected response to treatment does not occur or is suboptimal. The failure of the enteric coating to dissolve high in the alimentary tract has been one of the more common explanations for "refractory iron deficiency anemia" in the United States. Good responses may be observed with some so-called delayed-release iron preparations. Fero-Gradumet actually releases iron rapidly and is effective. Another widely used preparation, Feosol Spansule capsules, may be ineffective in some patients.

Oral iron therapy may fail in patients with malabsorption syndromes or with diarrhea, or in those who have had a gastrectomy. In the latter two instances, iron tablets may move so quickly through the small intestine that they reach the cecum before disintegrating.

All iron pills, when taken by a young child in handful amounts, can cause severe and sometimes fatal iron poisoning. Such medications must be kept out of reach of little children. Parents must be warned, and pills must be dispensed in child-proof containers.

**Parenteral Therapy.** Parenteral administration of iron should be reserved for those subjects who are unable to tolerate or absorb orally administered iron, such as the following: (1) patients with ulcerative colitis, regional enteritis, intestinal shunts, colostomy, or ileostomy; (2) patients with malabsorption syndromes; (3) the rare person who is unable or unwilling to cooperate or who has severe intolerance to oral therapy; and (4) patients in whom the rate of blood loss is so rapid that it is desirable both to introduce large amounts of iron into the body quickly and to re-establish iron stores.

The most widely used and most satisfactory parenteral iron preparation is iron dextran (Imferon). It is the only parenteral form of iron (other than transfusion) available in the United States.* This preparation is given intramuscularly or intravenously. The possibility of an anaphylactoid response is slightly greater when iron dextran is given intravenously. Intramuscular administration of iron produces staining of the skin and may also result in local discomfort. Because iron dextran in large doses has the capacity to induce sarcomas in laboratory animals, some concern has been generated about its possible carcinogenecity in humans. Only a few reports cite the appearance of such tumors at injection sites in humans. Nonetheless, the fact that sarcomas have been reported at iron dextran injection sites, both in laboratory animals and in humans, should persuade physicians not to administer iron dextran routinely.

The total dose should be calculated to correct the hemoglobin deficit and to provide at least an additional 1000 mg for storage. An easily remembered formula for estimation of required dose in adults is: one tenth the venous blood hemoglobin deficit (in g/L) times body weight in pounds. To this, add 1000 mg to provide an adequate storage iron reserve. Smaller doses are appropriate for children; the manufacturer's recommendations may be followed.

Intramuscular injections should be given using a "Z-track" technique in which the skin is pulled to one side during the injection. This maneuver helps to minimize unsightly staining of the skin. According to the manufacturer, not more than 5 ml (250 mg) should be injected on any day, whether intramuscularly or intravenously. Systemic reactions are unusual but may be severe: headache, fever, arthralgia, generalized lymphadenopathy, splenomegaly, back pain and, rarely, peripheral vascular collapse, and death. Premedication with adrenocorticosteroids has been used to try to avert this sometimes fatal complication. Neutrophilic leukocytosis of peripheral blood has been reported, as has pleocytosis of the cerebrospinal fluid. Whenever iron dextran is injected, by either parenteral route, a physician should be prepared to treat anaphylactic shock, if it occurs, with epinephrine and other supportive measures. No evidence exists that doses of 2 ml or less are any less likely to cause severe adverse reactions than are larger doses such as total dose infusion by intravenous route. Rates of hemoglobin increase do not differ significantly from those produced by proper oral iron therapy.

Blood transfusions are rarely necessary in the treatment of iron deficiency anemia and should be reserved for patients who have serious complications demanding immediate correction of the anemia: angina, congestive heart failure, or cerebral ischemia. For patients with cardiac failure, transfusions must be given slowly and cautiously. Healthy young adults are able to tolerate levels of hemoglobin as low as 25 or 30 g/L (2.5 or 3.0 g/dl) with remarkably little discomfort or danger. The patient's clinical status, not the numeric value of the blood hemoglobin concentration, should be given primary consideration in reaching a decision regarding the advisability of blood transfusion. Patients with active bleeding who are iron deficient must sometimes be transfused. In these instances, however, the purpose of the transfusion is not primarily to correct the anemia but rather to restore a falling blood volume to normal, thus avoiding the development of hemorrhagic shock.

*Because of recent problems in the manufacture of iron dextran, the product has been withdrawn from the market and was not available in the United States as of April of 1992. The manufacturer has stated that this withdrawal is only temporary, pending approval by the United States Food and Drug Administration of changes in the method of manufacture.

## PROGNOSIS

Recurrence of iron deficiency anemia is common because the precipitating cause is not recognized, continues, or recurs. Patients with chronic severe epithelial changes in the oral cavity may have a slightly higher risk of carcinoma of the upper gastrointestinal tract. In iron-deficient children whose growth and development are retarded, iron therapy frequently produces at least partial correction of the defect.

## SUPPLEMENTS TO PREVENT DEVELOPMENT OF IRON DEFICIENCY

In many countries, the cereal eaten most commonly, wheat flour, usually is fortified with iron. In the United States, flour is enriched with 20 mg iron per pound (460 g): bread baked under commercial conditions contains about 28 mg Fe/kg of wet weight. Thus, gram-for-gram, bread now has an iron content nearly equal to that of beef. That the iron can be absorbed was proved in experiments in which two groups of people were fed bread fortified with radiolabeled iron. Normal subjects absorbed from 1 to 12%, whereas iron-deficient subjects absorbed several times as much. Soluble inorganic iron added to food is absorbed to the same extent as is iron intrinsic to food. However, the usual method for iron fortification of flour in the United States is addition of "reduced iron," which is finely powdered metallic iron. Metallic iron is used because bread that contains added soluble iron (such as ferrous sulfate) rapidly develops an unacceptable flavor. Because absorption of metallic iron is poor, iron fortification of flour has a greater impact on public relations than on nutritional status, e.g., millers are able to list a high percent of the recommended daily allowance. Concern has also been expressed regarding the potential risk of iron fortification of cereal to persons with unrecognized hemochromatosis. However, studies in Sweden, where bread has long been fortified with even larger amounts of iron, have failed to show an adverse effect of this form of iron supplementation on persons who are homozygous for hereditary hemochromatosis.[181]

Because iron in rice and corn is poorly absorbed, these cereals are poor vehicles for fortification. Approximately 10% of the iron is absorbed from iron-fortified cereals prepared for infants.[182] The exact amounts may differ considerably, however, varying not only with the iron compound used but also with the particle size and presumably with method of preparation of the food. Although wheat flour has received the most emphasis as a vehicle for iron supplementation, other foodstuffs may be equally or more suitable, particularly in certain countries. Thus, sugar, fish sauce, salt, and curry powder have each been claimed as suitable vehicles for iron supplementation.

Iron supplementation is recommended for two times in life: infancy and pregnancy. A daily dietary allowance of 1.0 to 1.5 mg dietary iron per kilogram achieves optimal iron nutrition for a substantial majority of the infant population.[183–185] In an infant of average weight, an intake of 6 to 9 mg per day at 3 months of age, gradually increasing to 8 to 12 mg per day at 6 months of age and to 10 to 15 mg per day by 12 months of age will satisfy this requirement. Supplementation by iron-enriched cereals or by iron salts is usually required if an intake of 15 mg per day is to be achieved. In pregnant women, 78 mg of ferrous iron per day for 24 weeks was sufficient to achieve optimal hemoglobin mass and maintain normal iron stores, but 39 mg daily was not.[186] Pregnant women who receive adequate iron supplementation have continually normal values for SI, TIBC, Tsat, ferritin concentration, and free erythrocyte protoporphyrin, although their blood hemoglobin concentration may decline to between 100 and 110 g/L because of expanded plasma volume.

The prevalence of iron deficiency also correlates with age in both sexes. Persons 60 years of age and older have a greater frequency of iron deficiency than younger persons. Males over the age of 60 years are more likely to have hemoglobin concentrations less than 140 g/L and serum iron and ferritin concentrations below normal limits.[187] The low values documented in some studies of elderly individuals probably reflect a higher frequency of occult blood loss or chronic disease in this group.[188] Iron supplementation is not justified for healthy elderly persons who are not iron deficient.

## IRON OVERLOAD

An excessive body burden of iron can be produced by greater than normal absorption from the alimentary canal, by parenteral injection, or by a combination of both mechanisms. The excess iron is deposited largely as hemosiderin in reticuloendothelial cells or in the parenchymal cells of certain tissues. The site of deposition depends in part on the portal of entry. When excess iron is derived from intestinal absorption, it is carried to tissues bound by plasma transferrin and transferred to parenchymal and reticuloendothelial cells as well as to developing erythroblasts. On the other hand, parenterally administered iron, given usually as transfused blood, accumulates largely in reticuloendothelial cells where the transfused erythrocytes are eventually destroyed and their hemoglobin degraded. In iron overload, the SI and Tsat usually are increased, and the TIBC may be depressed. A simple classification based on mechanism of production is:

1. Excessive absorption of iron
   a. Hereditary hemochromatosis
   b. Excessive intake (African or "Bantu" siderosis; prolonged therapeutic administration of iron to subjects not iron deficient)
   c. Chronic alcoholism or chronic liver disease (usually alcoholic cirrhosis) and possibly pancreatic insufficiency
   d. "Shunt hemochromatosis"
   e. Certain types of severe chronic anemia, usually associated with ineffective erythropoiesis and increased hemolysis
2. Transfusional hemosiderosis.

Traditionally, the term hemosiderosis has denoted an increase in iron storage without associated tissue damage; hemochromatosis has indicated that such damage is present, particularly in the liver, that the iron overload is generalized, and that the amount of iron is greatly increased (usually 20 to 40 g). In present usage, however, hemochromatosis has come to mean a severe or potentially severe iron overload disorder with or without evidence of tissue injury.

### HEREDITARY HEMOCHROMATOSIS

Hereditary hemochromatosis (HH) is a relatively common inborn error of metabolism in which the increased intestinal absorption of iron results in slow progressive accumulation of the metal throughout life. It is caused by a recessive gene that is closely linked to the HLA histocompatibility locus on chromosome 6.[189–192] HH is associated with a 5- to 10-fold greater than normal activity of MIBP activity of hepatocytes and intestinal epithelial cells. Thus, MIBP may play a critical role in the development of HH.

Extensive studies of the prevalence of HH indicate that the homozygous condition occurs with a frequency of about 3 in 1000 in Sweden, France, Scotland, Canada (Ontario), the United States (Utah), and Australia. This prevalence rate implies a gene frequency of about 0.04 to 0.09 and a carrier rate of about 10% of whites of northern European derivation. Furthermore, it implies that most cases of hemochromatosis are not correctly diagnosed during life; many are diagnosed as diabetes mellitus, rheumatoid arthritis, or idiopathic cardiomyopathy, without the underlying iron storage disease being recognized. The occasional observation of apparent autosomal dominant inheritance of hemochromatosis now appears to be the result of homozygote-heterozygote matings.

The homozygous state may be manifest any time after puberty in males, but it is unusual before menopause in women, because menstruation functions as a "safety valve."

For some time, controversy arose as to whether HH ought to be regarded as a truly separate nosologic entity or merely an epiphenomenon of alcoholic cirrhosis. However, careful genetic studies have laid to rest the latter hypothesis. In this regard, the close linkage to the HLA locus has been extremely useful. The frequency of the HLA-A3 phenotype in patients with hemochromatosis is about 70%, whereas in the general population the HLA-A3 phenotype has a 28% prevalence. Were hemochromatosis merely an epiphenomenon of alcoholic cirrhosis, the HLA-A3 frequency should also be 70% in the latter group. In fact, it is 28%, as in the general population.[192] Results of these and extensive genetic studies leave no room for doubt that HH and alcoholic cirrhosis are distinct and separate disease entities, although they share some clinical manifestations. Furthermore, both ethanol and iron stimulate collagen biosynthesis. Therefore, the combination of alcohol consumption and iron overload are particularly likely to lead to cirrhosis.

Some physicians may be tempted to use HLA typing as a screening test for hemochromatosis or in the attempt to differentiate it from alcoholic cirrhosis. Either application is illogical, wasteful of resources, and meaningless, because any patient with alcoholic cirrhosis has nearly a 30% likelihood of having the HLA-A3 antigen, and 30% of patients with hemochromatosis do not have HLA-A3. For any person in the United States whose cells have the HLA-A3 antigen, the odds are nearly 100 to 1 that he or she is not homozygous for, and will never develop, hemochromatosis. Furthermore, HLA testing is time-consuming and costly. The procedure has merit, however, for examining the siblings of a patient known to have hemochromatosis, because siblings who are genotypically identical with an affected individual may be presumed also to be homozygous for HH; those who are not genotypically identical may be reassured. In this application, it does not matter what the HLA type is, whether it is A3 or any other type.

The classic "triad" of hemochromatosis—cirrhosis, diabetes, and hyperpigmentation of the skin—are only the most striking clinical features of a far advanced state of this disorder. The other major clinical features of hemochromatosis are fatigue, cardiac arrhythmias, restrictive cardiomyopathy (from iron deposition in heart muscle cells), cardiac failure, arthropathy that may mimic rheumatoid arthritis, hypothyroidism, gonadal failure resulting from reduction in pituitary hormone secretion, and testicular atrophy. Arthritis most often affects the second and third metacarpophalangeal joints, the knee, or hip joint. The diabetes, arthropathy, and sterility usually are irreversible, but cardiac function and hepatic function commonly improve after removal of the excess iron. Patients with hemochromatosis have a substantially increased risk of hepatocellular carcinoma. The frequency of hepatoma is as high as 29% of cases in some series; but overall, about one out of every seven hemochromatosis patients dies of hepatoma. Of patients with liver cirrhosis, approximately 30% develop hepatoma. If cirrhosis is avoided, by timely diagnosis and phlebotomy therapy, the risk of hepatoma becomes minuscule. The risk or progression of hepatoma is not affected by phlebotomy therapy once cirrhosis has developed. Aberrations in mental function may be observed in about one third of patients with hemochromatosis. These aberrations include lethargy, somnolence, confusion, and disorientation.

Patients with HH manifest increased susceptibility to infection. Sudden onset of overwhelming sepsis and shock was once a common cause of death in patients with this disorder. Persons with iron overload of any cause are especially susceptible to septicemia from the marine bacterium Vibrio vulnificus, a microorganism that grows rapidly when iron is readily available.[193–195] The infection usually is acquired by handling or eating raw shellfish, such as oysters. Septicemia is rapidly progressive and is commonly fatal. Cases have also been reported of peritonitis and of septicemia from Yersinia enterocolitica in patients with HH, thalassemia major, or oral iron overdosing. This microorganism appears to be an "opportunistic pathogen," causing severe or fatal infections in persons debilitated from a variety of disorders.

Screening tests for hemochromatosis should include assay of SI, TIBC, Tsat, and ferritin concentration. Taken together, these tests, when abnormal, provide a high level of confidence for identification of persons likely to have hemochromatosis, although a few cases may be missed even with these tests. Persons with SI greater than 32 μmol/L and Tsat greater than 60% on repeated assays (at least twice) must be assumed to be at risk of hemochromatosis until proven otherwise. The observation of persistently elevated SI and Tsat is a hallmark of the homozygous state for HH; these findings may be present for years before elevation of serum ferritin concentration or other clinical or laboratory features of HH are manifest. Elevation in SI and Tsat persist despite vigorous phlebotomy therapy, normalization of iron stores, and serum ferritin concentration.[196] Serum activity of aspartate aminotransferase (AST, SGOT) often is elevated early in the course of HH. Alanine aminotransferase (ALT, SGPT) activity may also be elevated. Serum bilirubin concentration is normal.

Examination of bone marrow iron content is often misleading in HH, because the iron content may be normal. Noninvasive methods for demonstrating iron overload in liver, such as computer assisted tomography (CAT) or magnetic resonance imaging (MRI) scans, have a limited role in diagnosis, for they are insensitive to early iron overload, and they do not document presence or absence of cirrhosis.

The definitive diagnostic test is usually liver biopsy. The specimen should be sectioned and stained with hematoxylin and eosin and with Perl's Prussian blue stain for iron. It is also useful to divide the specimen and chemically assay the iron content. This can also be done using paraffin embedded specimens.

Microscopic examination of iron content generally correlates well with the chemical assay. In normal liver, the iron content is estimated at 0 to 1+ histologically, and less than 50 μmol/g (2.8 mg/g) dry weight. In persons with alcoholic liver disease, the iron content of liver is not more than 0 to 2+ microscopically, and less than 100 μmol/g (5.6 mg/g) dry weight. In hemochromatosis, liver iron content is 3 to 4+ by microscopic estimation, and usually exceeds 100 μmol/g by chemical assay. Most patients with cirrhotic hemochromatosis have liver iron content of at least 200 μmol/g (11 mg/g) dry weight. Because the iron content of liver normally increases slowly with age, a Hepatic Iron Index (HII) can be calculated by dividing hepatic iron content (μmol/g) by age in years.[197,198] Persons who are homozygous for HH have HII values of 2.5 to 10 (mean 6.1). Little overlap in HII values is apparent between some patients homozygous for HH and some heterozygotes, but clear separation exists between these on the one hand and normal controls or alcoholic cirrhotic individuals on the other.[197,198]

Treatment of HH is by a vigorous program of phlebotomy: removal of 500 ml of blood one to three times weekly over the course of 1 to 2 years. Because each 500-ml volume of blood contains 200 to 250 mg of iron, such treatment removes approximately 20 to 40 g of iron. The phlebotomy program must be continued until the iron excess has been removed, the first evidence of which is a falling venous hemoglobin concentration that does not return to 110 g/L (women) or 120 g/L (men) within 1 week. The serum ferritin concentration should be less than 50 μg/L. When this point has been reached, the initial phase of treatment is completed. Thereafter, the patient should have a 500-ml phlebotomy once every 2 to 6 months for the remainder of his or her life, with the objective of not allowing the serum ferritin concentration to exceed 100 μg/L. Measurement of SI, TIBC, and Tsat in phlebotomy-treated patients is not warranted. The SI and Tsat will likely be high.[196] These abnormalities are characteristic of hemochromatosis irrespective of the size of iron stores. SI and Tsat cannot be used as guides to treatment.

The frequency of phlebotomy required varies and must be determined individually. The dramatic improvement in longevity and reduction in complications that attend this treatment have been amply documented. If this program is undertaken before hepatic cirrhosis or diabetes mellitus has developed, survival rates are indistinguishable from those of age- and sex-matched normal subjects.

In addition to iron removal, the endocrine, cardiac, and joint manifestations of HH may require appropriate treatment. Patients with HH must abstain absolutely from alcohol consumption. However, attempts to reduce iron intake by reducing meat or bread consumption are rarely indicated. An ordinary well-balanced diet is recommended.

Such iron chelators as desferrioxamine have no rational place in the treatment of HH. In secondary hemochromatosis, as in transfusion-dependent thalassemia major, however, parenteral administration of iron chelators is essential.

## AFRICAN ("BANTU") SIDEROSIS

Iron overload in black people of South Africa (first recognized in those of the Bantu linguistic stock, although not limited or predetermined by language) results from long-continued exposure to diets containing too much iron, derived largely from cooking pots and from the steel barrels used in the preparation of fermented alcoholic beverages. In adult males, the intake may exceed 100 mg iron per day. The condition frequently manifests in late adolescence, reaches its greatest severity between the ages of 40 and 60 years, and usually is more severe in males, whose alcoholic consumption tends to be greater. The pathologic pattern of the iron overload is one of hepatic and reticuloendothelial involvement. Portal cirrhosis becomes evident in most patients (but not in all) when the hepatic concentration of iron reaches 2 g or more per 100 g of dry weight. Redistribution of iron takes place so that parenchymal deposits of hemosiderin are found in the epithelial cells of many organs, particularly in the pancreas and the myocardium. Approximately 20% of these subjects develop clinical diabetes, but myocardial failure has not been described. To what extent these changes are caused by iron alone, by chronic alcoholism, or by the associated nutritional disturbances is unknown.

## ALCOHOLIC CIRRHOSIS, CHRONIC ALCOHOLISM, AND PANCREATIC INSUFFICIENCY

Patients with alcoholic or nutritional portal cirrhosis of the liver frequently have slightly increased amounts of stainable iron in their livers. The total amount present is rarely greater than 1 g. Clinical similarity to hemochromatosis is accentuated by the occurrence also in alcoholic cirrhosis of increased skin pigmentation, a higher incidence rate of diabetes mellitus than can be ascribed to coincidence, testicular atrophy, and an increased risk of hepatoma. Cardiac failure, when it occurs, can usually be accounted for on other grounds. More males than females are affected and clinical manifestations are most prominent in late middle life.

Several possible explanations for the iron overload have been cited. Patients with hepatic cirrhosis frequently are wine drinkers, and may consume several liters daily. European wines may contain significant quantities of iron (although American wines do not) and several milligrams per day may be derived from that source alone. Patients with chronic liver disease or chronic pancreatitis may have greater than normal intestinal absorption of iron.

Although the controversy over the genetic basis of

"idiopathic" hemochromatosis has been resolved, the issue whether alcoholic cirrhosis per se can lead to serious iron overload remains. Seventy percent of cirrhotic patients with significant iron overload have the HLA A3 allele, a frequency identical with that in hereditary hemochromatosis, whereas the frequency of HLA A3 is 30% in cirrhotic patients without iron overload, a frequency identical within the general population.[192] As noted previously, studies of HLA antigen frequencies in HH and in alcoholic cirrhosis have shown that all or most of the alcoholic cirrhosis patients with iron overload in fact have HH, and that ethanol abuse is additive but not the primary cause.

## SHUNT HEMOCHROMATOSIS

"Shunt hemochromatosis" appears within a few years of the establishment of a shunt between the portal and systemic venous systems. The shunt has usually been created surgically to relieve pressure in esophageal varices, and in most instances, the iron loading has followed end-to-side anastomoses. However, the disorder has also developed spontaneously, presumably from formation of collateral channels between portal and systemic veins. The rate of iron accumulation is astonishingly rapid. The mechanism is unknown. The manifestations are the same as those of hemochromatosis from other causes.

## PROLONGED IRON THERAPY

In a few noniron-deficient patients, the inappropriate administration of iron orally or parenterally, for decades, has led to typical hemochromatosis. Because iron preparations are advertised widely in the United States, are available without prescription, and are consumed in large quantities, it is astonishing that so few cases have been reported. Therefore, the potential of iron preparations to cause iron overload deserves special attention. It is possible to estimate mathematically the amount of iron that might accumulate in the body of normal persons when different amounts of medicinal iron are administered over long periods. These estimates, for which the calculations were shown in the seventh edition of this book, are illustrated in Figure 9–7. As seen from the uppermost curve of this illustration, even at a daily dose of 240 mg of iron (for example, four ferrous sulfate tablets daily), and a total ingested dose of 1.3 kg in 15 years, the increase in body iron content would not approach that commonly encountered in HH. These facts emphasize the remarkable way in which the modulation of iron absorption by the intestinal mucosa tends to protect normal persons from the adverse effects of excessive iron ingestion. The relationships portrayed in Figure 9–7 do not, however, apply to persons who are homozygous for HH. In view of the high prevalence of HH, the widespread use of iron supplements, and the

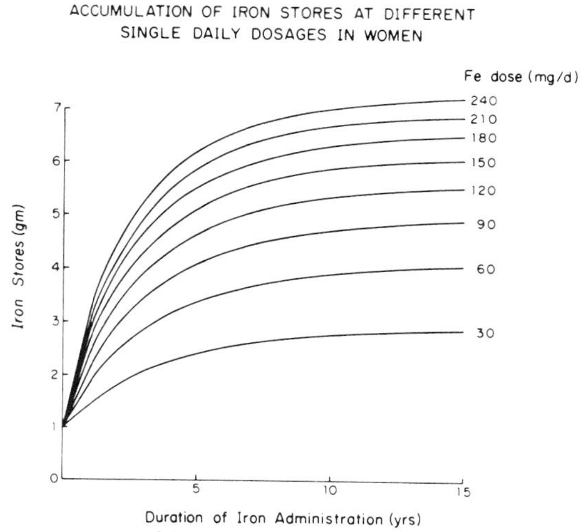
ACCUMULATION OF IRON STORES AT DIFFERENT SINGLE DAILY DOSAGES IN WOMEN
Fe dose (mg/d)
240
210
180
150
120
90
60
30
Iron Stores (gm)
0
1
2
3
4
5
6
7
5
10
15
Duration of Iron Administration (yrs)

**FIGURE 9–7.** The expected accumulation of iron in menstruating women receiving single daily doses that ranged from 30 to 240 mg. These data are based on the assumptions that iron absorption in females is $D^{0.668}$, where D is the dose of iron in g, that iron absorption is modified by stores to the extent of $e^{-0.196(F-1)}$, and that excretion is $.0009\sqrt{F} + .0005$, where F is the iron stores in g. 1 g Fe = 17.9 mmol.

rarity of cases in which hemochromatosis is attributed to chronic ingestion of iron, it is likely that these patients are also homozygous for HH.

Prolonged administration of large doses of iron poses some hazard to persons who are not iron deficient, particularly patients with thalassemia major and other chronic anemias, for whom the ultimate development of hemochromatosis is a serious complication of treatment. For premenopausal women who have normal menses and do not have thalassemia or other chronic anemia, the hazard of serious iron overload resulting from exogenous iron is slight. However, the inappropriate and prolonged administration of iron, orally or parenterally, to adults who are not bleeding and not iron deficient needlessly exposes them to the risk of hemochromatosis with all its serious complications.

## SEVERE CHRONIC ANEMIAS

The amount of iron found in the tissues of patients with refractory anemia, particularly those with hypercellular marrows and ineffective erythropoiesis, is occasionally greater than can be accounted for by the transfusions they have received. In some patients, little blood was given during the course of the illness yet excess iron was present. Some, but not all, of these subjects have been treated inappropriately with iron. Excessive absorption of dietary iron must have occurred, presumably because of the accelerated but ineffective erythropoiesis. Patients at risk include those with sideroblastic anemia, thalassemia major, and paroxysmal nocturnal hemoglobinuria. The cardiac and hepatic complications of hemochromatosis are common causes of death in patients with sideroblastic anemias or β-thalassemia major.

Severe iron overload may occur in patients with congenital dyserythropoietic anemia. Hereditary spherocytosis and thalassemia minor are not usually associated with iron overload, except in those patients in whom the disorder is misdiagnosed as iron deficiency and are given copious amounts of iron over many years. However, in some reports, these disorders coexisted with HH. In view of the high prevalence of the latter disorder in persons of European ancestry, the concurrence of these disorders is hardly surprising. In such patients, large amounts of hemosiderin are found in parenchymal as well as in reticuloendothelial cells.

**Transfusional Hemosiderosis.** Whenever chronic anemia has been treated by numerous transfusions over many years in a patient who does not have chronic bleeding, iron overload is likely to occur. These patients may have the same consequences as described for HH. This complication is found most often in severe thalassemias, such as β-thalassemia major, in some chronic sideroblastic anemias, and in hypoplastic or other refractory anemias. For many of these patients, long-term treatment with the iron-chelating agent desferrioxamine is essential. The desferrioxamine must be administered daily by subcutaneous infusion for 12 to 16 hours each day. This treatment is cumbersome and expensive.

Effective oral iron-chelating agents are in the process of development and may become available within a few years. They will then supplant parenteral desferrioxamine therapy for these patients.

Surprisingly, some patients with marked iron overload resulting from transfusion never manifest severe organ damage. However, some persons with HH and iron overload also do not exhibit evidence of organ damage. These paradoxes may reflect the fact that serious organ injury is more likely to occur in patients subjected to toxic substance(s) or hepatitis in addition to iron excess.

## REFERENCES


1. Fairbanks, V.F., Fahey, J.L., Beutler, E.: History of iron in medicine. *In* Clinical Disorders of Iron Metabolism. 2nd Ed. New York, Grune & Stratton, 1971, pp. 1–41.
2. Troisier, E.: Diabete sucre. Bull. Soc. Anat. (Paris), *46*:231–235, 1871.
3. Stockman, R.: J. Physiol. (Lond.), *18*:484–489, 1895.
4. Heath, C.W., Strauss, M.B., Castle, W.B.: J. Clin. Invest., *11*:1293–1312, 1932.
5. Fairbanks, V.S., Klee, G.G.: Biochemical aspects of hematology. *In* Textbook of Clinical Chemistry. Edited by N. W. Tietz. Philadelphia, W. B. Saunders, 1986.
6. Beutler, E., Fairbanks, V.F., Fahey, J.L.: The metabolism of iron. *In* Clinical Disorders of Iron Metabolism. New York, Grune & Stratton, 1963, p. 39.
7. Conrad, M.E., Schade, S.G.: Gastroenterology, *55*:35–45, 1986.
8. Conrad, M.E., Umbreit, J.N., Moore, E.G.: Gastroenterology, *100*:129–136, 1991.
9. Simpson, R.J., Moore, R., Peters, T.J.: Biochim. Biophys. Acta, *941*:39–47, 1988.
10. Simpson, R.J., Venkatesan, S., Peters, T.J.: Cell Biochem. Funct., *7*:165–171, 1989.
11. Sanyal, A.J., Hirsch, J.I., Moore, E.W.: J. Lab. Clin. Med., *116*:76–86, 1990.
12. Teichmann, R., Stremmel, W.: J. Clin. Invest., *86*:2145–53, 1990.
13. Snape, S., Simpson, R.J., Peters, T.J.: Cell Biochem. Funct., *8*:107–115, 1990.
14. Weintraub, L.R., Weinstein, M.B., Huser, H.J., et al.: J. Clin. Invest., *47*:531–539, 1968.
15. Raffin, S.B., Woo, C.H., Roost, K.T., et al.: J. Clin. Invest., *54*:1344–1352, 1974.
16. Brown, E.B., Hwang, Y.F., Nicol, S., et al.: J. Lab. Clin. Med., *72*:58–64, 1968.
17. Turnbull, A., Cleton, F., Finch, C.A.: J. Clin. Invest., *41*:1897–1907, 1962.
18. Hallberg, L., Sölvell, L.: Acta Med. Scand., *181*:335–354, 1967.
19. Turnlund, J.R., Smith, R.G., Kretsch, M.J., et al.: Am. J. Clin. Nutr., *52*:373–378, 1990.
20. Hurrell, R.F., Lynch, S.R., Trinidad, T.P., et al.: Am. J. Clin. Nutr., *49*:546–552, 1989.
21. MacFarlane, B.J., van der Riet, W.B., Bothwell, T.H., et al.: Am. J. Clin. Nutr., *51*:873–880, 1990.
22. Morck, T.A., Lynch, S.R., Cook, J.D.: Am. J. Clin. Nutr., *37*:416–420, 1983.
23. Munoz, L.M., Lonnerdal, B., Keen, C.L., et al.: Am. J. Clin. Nutr., *48*:645–651, 1988.
24. Fairweather-Tait, S.J., Piper, Z., Fatemi, S.J., et al.: Br. J. Nutr., *65*:61–68, 1991.
25. MacFarlane, B.J., Bezwoda, W.R., Bothwell, T.H., et al.: Am. J. Clin. Nutr., *47*:270–274, 1988.
26. Hallberg, L., Rossander, L., Skonberg, A.-B.: Am. J. Clin. Nutr., *45*:988–996, 1987.
27. Hallberg, L.: Scand. J. Gastroenterol. Suppl., *129*:73–79, 1987.
28. Brune, M., Rossander, L., Hallberg, L.: Am. J. Clin. Nutr., *49*:542-545, 1989.
29. Fairweather-Tait, S.J., Wright, A.J.: Br. J. Nutr., *64*:547–552, 1990.
30. Siegenberg, D., Baynes, R.D., Bothwell, T.H., et al.: Am. J. Clin. Nutr., *53*:537–541, 1991.
31. Fernandez, R., Phillips, S.F.: Am. J. Clin. Nutr., *35*:107–112, 1982.
32. Tuntawiroon, M., Sritongkul, N., Brune, M., et al.: Am. J. Clin. Nutr., *53*:554–557, 1991.
33. Rossander, L.: Scand. J. Gastroenterol. Suppl., *129*:68–72, 1987.

34. Frølich, W., Lys, A.: Am. J. Clin. Nutr., *37*:31–36, 1983.
35. Crofton, R.W., Gvozdanovic, D., Gvozdanovic, S., et al.: Am. J. Clin. Nutr., *50*:141–144, 1989.
36. Beutler, E., Kelly, B.M., Beutler, F.: Am. J. Clin. Nutr., *11*:559–567, 1962.
37. Slatkavitz, C.A., Clydesdale, F.M.: Am. J. Clin. Nutr., *47*:487–495, 1988.
38. Gordon, D.T., Godber, J.S.: J. Nutr., *119*:446–452, 1989.
39. Celada, A., Rudolf, H., Donath, A.: Am. J. Hematol., *5*:225–237, 1978.
40. Mazzanti, R., Srai, K.S., Debnam, E.S., et al.: Alcohol, *22*:47–52, 1987.
41. Chapman, R.W., Morgan, M.Y., Boss, A.M.: Dig. Dis. Sci., *28*:321–327, 1983.
42. Marx, J.J., Gebbink, J.A., Nishisato, T., et al.: Br. J. Haematol., *52*:105–110, 1982.
43. Moore, C.V.: *In* Symposium on Occurrence, Causes and Prevention of Nutritional Anaemias. Edited by G. Blix. Swedish Nutrition Foundation, Tylösand, 1967, Symposia 6. Uppsala, Almqvist and Wiksells, 1968, pp. 92–103.
44. Layrisse, M., Martinez-Torres, C.: Prog. Hematol., *7*:137–160, 1971.
45. Josephs, H.W.: Blood, *13*:1–54, 1958.
46. Gillooly, M., Bothwell, T.H., Torrance, J.D., et al.: Br. J. Nutr., *49*:331–342, 1983.
47. Hallberg, L., Rossander, L.: Scand. J. Gastroenterol., *17*:151–160, 1982.
48. Cook, J.D., Morck, T.A., Lynch, S.R.: Am. J. Clin. Nutr., *34*:2622–2629, 1981.
49. Morris, E.R., Bodwell, C.E., Miles, C.W.: Plant Foods Hum. Nutr., *37*:377–389, 1987.
50. Baynes, R.D., MacFarlane, B.J., Bothwell, T.H., et al.: Eur. J. Clin. Nutr., *44*:419–424, 1990.
51. Layrisse, M., Cook, J.D., Martinez, C., et al.: Blood, *33*:430–443, 1969.
52. Martinez-Torres, C., Layrisse, M.: Blood, *35*:669–682, 1970.
53. Layrisse, M., Martinez-Torres, C., Cook, J.D., et al.: Blood, *41*:333–352, 1973.
54. Pirzio-Biroli, G., Bothwell, T.H., Finch, C.A.: J. Lab. Clin. Med., *51*:37–48, 1958.
55. Cook, J.D., Layrisse, M., Martinez-Torres, C., et al.: J. Clin. Invest., *51*:805–815, 1972.
56. Sly, D.A., Grohlich, D., Bezkorovainy, A.: Biochim. Biophys. Acta, *385*:36–40, 1975.
57. Sullivan, A.L., Grasso, J.A., Weintraub, L.R.: Blood, *47*:133–143, 1976.
58. Hemmaplardh, D., Morgan, E.H.: Biochim. Biophys. Acta, *373*:84–99, 1974.
59. Morgan, E.H., Appleton, T.C.: Nature, *223*:1371–1372, 1969.
60. Martinez-Medellin, J., Schulman, H.M.: Biochim. Biophys. Acta, *264*:272–274, 1972.
61. Cheng, T.P.O.: Cell Tissue Res., *244*:613–619, 1986.
62. Dautry-Varsat, A.: Biochimie, *68*:375–381, 1986.
63. Schneider, C., Williams, J.G.: J. Cell Sci., *3 (Suppl.)*:139–149, 1985.
64. Zerial, M., Melancon, P., Schneider, C., Garoff, H.: EMBO J., *5*:1543–1550, 1986.
65. Cox, T.M., O'Donnell, M.W., Aisen, P., London, I.M.: J. Clin. Invest., *76*:2144–2150, 1985.
66. Morgan, E.H., Baker, E.: Ann. N.Y. Acad. Sci., *526*:65–82, 1988.
67. Ajioka, R.S., Kaplan, J.: Proc. Natl. Acad. Sci. USA, *83*:6445–6449, 1986.
68. Casey, J.L., Di Jeso, B., Rao, K.K., et al.: Nucleic Acids Res., *16*:629–646, 1988.
69. Casey, J.L., Di Jeso, B., Rao, K.K., et al.: Ann. N.Y. Acad. Sci., *526*:54–64, 1988.
70. Müllner, E.W., Kühn, L.C.: Cell, *53*:815–825, 1988.
71. Rouault, T., Rao, K., Harford, J., et al.: J. Biol. Chem., *260*:14,862–14,866, 1985.
72. Casey, J.L., Di Jeso, B., Rao, K., et al.: Proc. Natl. Acad. Sci. USA, *85*:1787–1791, 1988.
73. Enns, C.A., Snomaleinin, H.A., Gebhart, J.E., et al.: Proc. Natl. Acad. Sci. USA, *79*:3241–3245, 1982.
74. Miller, Y.E., Jones, C., Scoggin, C., et al.: Am. J. Hum. Genet., *35*:5783, 1983.
75. Hentze, M.W., Seuanez, H.N., O'Brien, S.J., et al.: Nucleic Acids Res., *11*:6103–6108, 1989.
76. Young, S.P., Roberts, S., Bomford, A.: Biochem. J., *232*:819–823, 1985.
77. Soda, R., Tavassoli, M.: J. Ultrastruct. Res., *88*:18–29, 1984.
78. Bergamaschi, G., Eng, M.J., Huebers, H.A., et al.: Proc. Soc. Exp. Biol. Med., *183*:66–73, 1986.
79. Larrick, J.W., Enns, C., Raubitschek, A., Weintraub, H.: J. Cell. Physiol., *124*:283–287, 1985.
80. Stoorvogel, W., Geuze, H.J., Griffith, J.M., Strous, G.J.: J. Cell Biol., *106*:1821–1829, 1988.
81. Blight, G.D., Morgan, E.H.: Eur. J. Cell Biol., *43*:260–265, 1987.
82. Nunez, M.T., Coles, E.S., Glass, J.: Blood, *55*:1051–1055, 1980.
83. Pollack, S., Campana, T., Weaver, J.: Am. J. Hematol., *19*:75–84, 1985.
84. Funk, F., Lecrenier, C., Lesuisse, E., et al.: Eur. J. Biochem., *157*:303–309, 1986.
85. Ponka, P., Neuwirt, J., Borova, J.: Enzyme, *17*:91–99, 1974.
86. Harrison, P.M., Clegg, G.A., May, K.: Ferritin structure and function. *In* Iron in Biochemistry and Medicine, II. Edited by A. Jacobs and M. Worwood. New York, Academic Press, 1980, pp. 131–171.
87. Harrison, P.M.: Semin. Hematol., *14*:557–570, 1977.
88. Clegg, G.A., Stansfield, R.F.D., Bourne, P.E., et al.: Nature, *288*:298–300, 1980.
89. Harrison, P.M., Treffry, A., Lilley, T.H.: J. Inorg. Biochem., *27*:287–293, 1986.
90. Fischbach, F.A., Gregory, D.W., Harrison, P.M., et al.: J. Ultrastruct. Res., *37*:495–503, 1971.
91. Crichton, R.R., Roman, F., Roland, F., et al.: J. Mol. Catalysis, *7*:267–276, 1980.
92. Crichton, R.R., Roman, F.: J. Mol. Catalysis, *4*:75–82, 1978.
93. Hoy, T.G., Harrison, P.M., Shabbir, M.: Biochem. J., *139*:603–607, 1974.
94. Arosio, P., Adelman, T.G., Drysdale, J.W.: J. Biol. Chem., *253*:4451–4458, 1978.
95. Casey, J.L., Hentze, M.W., Koeller, D.M., et al.: Science, *240*:924–928, 1988.
96. Rogers, J., Munro, H.: Proc. Natl. Acad. Sci. USA, *84*:2277–2281, 1987.
97. Zähringer, J., Baliga, B.S., Munro, H.N.: Proc. Natl. Acad. Sci. USA, *73*:857–861, 1976.
98. Hentze, M.W., Rouault, T.A., Wright-Caughman, S., et al.: Proc. Natl. Acad. Sci. USA, *84*:6730–6734, 1987.
99. Mack, U., Storey, E.L., Powell, L.W., et al.: Biochim. Biophys. Acta, *843*:164–170, 1985.
100. Beutler, E.: Ill. Med. J., *116*:16–19, 1959.
101. Jacobs, A.: Lancet, *2*:1331–1333, 1961.

**102.** Ackrell, B.A.C., Maguire, J.J., Dallman, P.R., et al.: J. Biol. Chem., *259*:10,053–10,059, 1984.
**103.** Mackler, B., Person, R., Miller, L.R., et al.: Pediatr. Res., *13*:1010–1011, 1979.
**104.** Symes, A.L., Sowkes, T.L., Youdim, M.B.H., et al.: Can. J. Biochem., *47*:999–1002, 1969.
**105.** Youdim, M.B.H., Green, A.R.: Ciba Found. Symp., *51*:201–221, 1977.
**106.** Youdim, M.B.H., Green, A.R.: Proc. Nutr. Soc., *37*:173–179, 1978.
**107.** Srivastava, S.K., Zaheer, N., Krishnan, P.S.: Arch. Biochem. Biophys., *105*:446–447, 1964.
**108.** Bailey-Wood, R., Blayney, L.M., Muir, J.R., et al.: Br. J. Exp. Pathol., *56*:193–198, 1975.
**109.** Kyaw, A., Win, T., Pe, U.H.: Biochem. Med. Metab. Biol., *11*:194–197, 1974.
**110.** Green, R., Charlton, R., Seftel, H., et al.: Am. J. Med., *45*:336–353, 1968.
**111.** Bothwell, T.H., Seftel, H., Jacobs, P., et al.: Am. J. Clin. Nutr., *14*:47–51, 1964.
**112.** Finch, C.A.: Physiopathologic mechanisms of iron excretion. *In* Iron Metabolism: An International Symposium. Edited by F. Gross. Berlin, Springer, 1964, pp. 452–465.
**113.** Crosby, W.H., Conrad, M.E. Jr., Wheby, M.S.: Blood, *22*:429–440, 1963.
**114.** Ebaugh, F.G. Jr., Clemens, T. Jr., Rodnan, G., et al.: Am. J. Med., *25*:169–181, 1958.
**115.** Hallberg, L., Nilsson, L.: Acta Obstet. Gynecol. Scand., *43*:352–359, 1964.
**116.** Hallberg, L., Högdahl, A.M., Nilsson, L., et al.: Acta Obstet. Gynecol. Scand., *45*:320–351, 1966.
**117.** Rybo, G.: *In* Iron Deficiency: Pathogenesis, Clinical Aspects, Therapy. Edited by L. Hallberg, H.G. Harwerth, A. Vannotti. New York, Academic Press, 1970.
**118.** Simon, T.L., Hunt, W.C., Garry, P.J.: Transfusion, *24*:469–472, 1984.
**119.** Taylor, P.G., Mendez-Castellano, H., Lopez-Blanco, M.: J. Am. Diet. Assoc., *88*:454–458, 1988.
**120.** Herbert, V.: Am. J. Clin. Nutr., *45*:679–686, 1987.
**121.** Pearson, H.A., Abrams, I., Fernbach, D.J., et al.: Pediatr. Res., *1*:169–172, 1967.
**122.** Karp, R.J., Haaz, W.S., Starko, K., et al.: Am. J. Dis. Child., *128*:18–20, 1974.
**123.** Expert Scientific Working Group: Am. J. Clin. Nutr., *42*:318, 1985.
**124.** Dallman, P.R., Yip, R., Johnson, C.: Am. J. Clin. Nutr., *39*:437–445, 1984.
**125.** Harris, D.C., Aisen, P.: Nature, *257*:821–823, 1975.
**126.** Schlabach, M.R., Bates, G.W.: J. Biol. Chem., *250*:2182–2188, 1975.
**127.** Delaney, T.A., Morgan, W.H., Morgan, E.H.: Biochim. Biophys. Acta, *701*:295–304, 1982.
**128.** El-Najjar, M.Y., Robertson, A.L. Jr.: Science, *193*:141–143, 1976.
**129.** El-Najjar, M.Y., Lozoff, B., Ryan, D.J.: AJR, *125*:918–924, 1975.
**130.** Magnusson, B.E.O.: Scand. J. Haematol. *26 (Suppl.)*,:7–111, 1976.
**131.** Baird, I.M., Wilson, G.M.: Q. J. Med., *28*:35–41, 1959.
**132.** Stevens, A.R. Jr., Pirzio-Biroli, G., Harkins, H.N., et al.: Ann. Surg., *149*:534–538, 1959.
**133.** Kimber, C., Patterson, J.F., Weintraub, L.R.: JAMA, *202*:935–938, 1967.
**134.** Hallberg, L., Sölvell, L., Zederfeldt, B.: Acta Med. Scand., *445 (Suppl. 179)*:269–275, 1966.
**135.** Clouse, R.E., Costigan, D.J., Mills, B.A., et al.: Arch. Intern. Med., *145*:458–461, 1985.
**136.** Stewart, J.G., Ahlquist, D.A., McGill, D.B., et al.: Ann. Intern. Med., *100*:843–845, 1984.
**137.** Selby, G.B., Eichner, E.R.: Am. J. Med., *81*:791–794, 1986.
**138.** Crowley, L.V., Seay, J., Mullin, G.: Am. J. Gastroenterol., *79*:850–860, 1984.
**139.** Bernard, J., Najean, Y., Alby, N., Rain, J.D.: Presse Med., *75*:2087–2090, 1967.
**140.** Fey, M.F., Radvila, A.: Br. Med. J., *296*:1504–1505, 1988.
**141.** Finch, C.A., Mackler, B.: Trans. Assoc. Am. Physicians, *89*:116–119, 1976.
**142.** Finch, C.A., Gollnick, P.D., Hlastala, M.P., et al.: J. Clin. Invest., *64*:129–137, 1979.
**143.** Beard, J., Finch, C.A., Green, W.L.: Life Sci., *30*:691–697, 1982.
**144.** Vellar, O.D., Hermansen, L.: Acta Med. Scand., *522 (Suppl.)*:1–40, 1971.
**145.** Andersen, H.T., Barkve, H.: Scand. J. Clin. Lab. Invest., (Suppl 114) *25*:1–62, 1970.
**146.** Andersen, H.T., Stavem, P.: Nutr. Metab., *14*:129–135, 1972.
**147.** Viteri, F.E., Torun, B.: Clin. Haematol., *3*:609–626, 1974.
**148.** Lieden, G., Adolfsson, L.: Scand. J. Clin. Lab. Invest., *34*:37–42, 1974.
**149.** Gardner, G.W., Edgerton, V.R., Senewiratne, B., et al.: Am. J. Clin. Nutr., *30*:910–917, 1977.
**150.** Charlton, R.W., Derman, D., Skikne, B., et al.: Clin. Sci., *53*:537–541, 1977.
**151.** Ohira, Y., Edgerton, V.R., Gardner, G.W., et al.: J. Nutr. Sci. Vitaminol. (Tokyo), *27*:87–96, 1981.
**152.** Beard, J.L., Borel, M.J., Derr, J.: Am. J. Clin. Nutr., *52*:813–819, 1990.
**153.** Sanstead, H.H., House, F.R., Horton, K.B., et al.: Am. J. Dis. Child., *121*:455–463, 1971.
**154.** Chwang, L.C., Soemantri, A.G., Pollitt, E.: Am. J. Clin. Nutr., *47*:496–501, 1988.
**155.** Pollitt, E., Leibel, R.L.: J. Pediatr., *88*:372–381, 1976.
**156.** Voorhess, M.L., Stuart, M.J., Stockman, J.A., et al.: J. Pediatr., *86*:542–547, 1975.
**157.** Lozoff, B., Brittenham, G.M., Viteri, F.E., et al.: J. Pediatr., *101*:948–952, 1982.
**158.** Oski, F.A., Honig, A.S., Helu, B., et al.: Pediatrics, *71*:877–880, 1983.
**159.** Walter, T., Kovalskys, J., Stekel, A.: J. Pediatr., *102*:519–522, 1983.
**160.** Lozoff, B., Brittenham, G., Viteri, F.E., et al.: *In* Iron Deficiency: Brain Biochemistry and Behavior. Edited by E. Pollitt, R.L. Leibel. New York, Raven Press, 1982, pp. 183–194.
**161.** Pollitt, E., Viteri, F., Saco-Pollitt, C., et al.: *In* Iron Deficiency: Brain Biochemistry and Behavior. Edited by E. Pollitt, R.L. Leibel. New York, Raven Press, 1982, pp. 195–208.
**162.** Youdim, M.B.H., Yehuda, S., Ben-Shachar, D., et al.: *In* Iron Deficiency: Brain Biochemistry and Behavior. Edited by E. Pollitt, R.L. Leibel. New York, Raven Press, 1982, pp. 39–56.
**163.** Walter, T.: Am. J. Clin. Nutr., *50*:655–666, 1989.
**164.** Haas, J.D., Fairchild, M.W.: Am. J. Clin. Nutr., *50*:703–705, 1989.
**165.** Tucker, D.M., Sandstead, H.H., Swenson, R.A., et al.: Physiol. Behav., *29*:737–740, 1982.
**166.** Mehta, B.C., Panjwani, D.D., Jhala, D.A.: Acta Haematol. (Basel), *70*:189–193, 1983.

**167.** Kimber, C., Weintraub, L.R.: N. Engl. J. Med., *279*:453–459, 1968.
**168.** Jacobs, A.: Br. J. Cancer, *15*:736–744, 1961.
**169.** Halsted, J.A., Prasad, A.S., Nadimi, M.: Arch. Intern. Med., *116*:253–256, 1965.
**170.** Shepard, T.H., Mackler, B., Finch, C.A.: Teratology, *22*:329–334, 1980.
**171.** Scher, H., Silber, R.: Ann. Intern. Med., *84*:571–572, 1976.
**172.** Monzon, C.M., Fairbanks, V.F., Burgert, E.O. Jr., et al.: Am. J. Hematol., *19*:27–36, 1985.
**173.** England, J.M., Fraser, P.M.: Lancet, *1*:449–452, 1973.
**174.** Bessman, J.D., Feinstein, D.I.: Blood, *53*:288–293, 1979.
**175.** Bessman, J.D., Gilmer, P.R., Gardner, F.H.: Am. J. Clin. Pathol., *80*:322–326, 1983.
**176.** Peters, S.W., Jacobs, A., Fitzsimmons, E.: Br. J. Haematol., *53*:211–216, 1983.
**177.** Cook, J.D., Dassenko, S., Skikne, B.S.: Br. J. Haematol., *75*:603–609, 1990.
**178.** Skikne, B.S., Flowers, C.H., Cook, J.D.: Blood, *75*:1870–1876, 1990.
**179.** Brise, H., Halling, L.: Acta Med. Scand., *376(Suppl.)*:1–73, 1962.
**180.** Kerr, D.N.S., Davidson, S.: Lancet, *2*:489–492, 1958.
**181.** Olsson, K.S., Safwenberg, J., Ritter, B.: Ann. N.Y. Acad. Sci., *526*:290–300, 1988.
**182.** Schulz, J., Smith, N.J.: Am. J. Dis. Child., *93*:30, 1957.
**183.** Zhan, H., Pollack, S., Weaver, J.: Am. J. Hematol., *31*:203–207, 1989.
**184.** Beutler, E.: Am. J. Med. Sci., *234*:517–527, 1957.
**185.** Moe, P.J.: Acta Paediatr. Scand., *150(Suppl.)*:1–67, 1963.
**186.** De Leeuw, N.K.M., Lowenstein, L., Hsieh, Y.S.: Medicine (Baltimore), *45*:291–315, 1966.
**187.** Singer, J.D., Granahan, P., Goodrich, N.N., et al.: Diet and iron status, a study of relationships: United States, 1971–74. Vital and Health Statistics. Series 11, No 229. DHHS Pub No (PHS) 83–1679. Public Health Service. Washington, U.S. Government Printing Office, December 1982.
**188.** Garry, P.J., Goodwin, J.S., Hunt, W.C.: J. Am. Geriatr. Soc., *31*:389–399, 1983.
**189.** Powell, L.W., Ferluga, J., Halliday, J.W., et al.: Hum. Genet., *77*:55–56, 1987.
**190.** Edwards, C.Q., Griffen, L.M., Dadone, M.M., et al.: Am. J. Hum. Genet., *38*:805–811, 1986.
**191.** Simon, M., Le Mignon, L., Fauchet, R., et al.: Am. J. Hum. Genet., *41*:89–105, 1987.
**192.** Lesage, G.D., Baldus, W.P., Fairbanks, V.F., et al.: Gastroenterology, *84*:1471–1477, 1983.
**193.** Blake, P.A., Merson, M.H., Weaver, R.E., et al.: N. Engl. J. Med., *300*:1–5, 1979.
**194.** Wright, A.C., Simpson, L.M., Oliver, J.D.: Infect. Immun., *34*:503–507, 1981.
**195.** McManus, R.: JAMA, *251*:323–325, 1984.
**196.** Edwards, C.Q., Griffen, L.M., Kaplan, J., Kushner, J.P.: J. Intern. Med., *226*:373–379, 1989.
**197.** Bassett, M.L., Halliday, J.W., Powell, L.W.: Hepatology, *6*:24–29, 1986.
**198.** Adams, P.C.: Dig. Dis. Sci., *35*:690–692, 1990.

## SELECTED READINGS

Bothwell, T.H., Finch, C.A. (eds.): Iron Metabolism. Boston, Little, Brown, 1962.

Conrad, M.E., Barton, J.C., Gams, R.A., et al.: Iron, folic acid and vitamin $B_{12}$. *In* Current Hematology. Vol. 1. Edited by V.F. Fairbanks. New York, John Wiley & Sons, 1981, pp. 123–190.

Cook, J.D., Skikne, B.S.: Iron deficiency: definition and diagnosis. J. Intern. Med., *226*:349–355, 1989.

Edwards, C.Q., Dadone, M.M., Skolnick, M.H., et al.: Hereditary hemochromatosis. Clin. Haematol., *11*:411–435, 1982.

Fairbanks, V.F., Beutler, E.: Iron metabolism. *In* Hematology. 4th Ed. Edited by W.J. Williams, E. Beutler, J. Erslev, et al. New York, McGraw-Hill, 1990, pp. 282–339.

Fairbanks, V.F., Beutler, E.: Iron deficiency. *In* Hematology. 4th Ed. Edited by W.J. Williams, E. Beutler, J. Erslev, et al. New York, McGraw-Hill, 1990, pp. 482–505.

Fairbanks, V.F., Beutler, E.: Congenital atransferrinemia and idiopathic pulmonary hemosiderosis. *In* Hematology. 4th Ed. Edited by W.J. Williams, E. Beutler, J. Erslev, et al. New York, McGraw-Hill, 1990, pp. 506–510.

Fairbanks, V.F., Fahey, J.L., Beutler, E.: Clinical Disorders of Iron Metabolism. 2nd Ed. New York, Grune & Stratton, 1971.

Jacobs, A., Worwood, M. (eds.): Iron in Biochemistry and Medicine. II. London, Academic Press, 1980.

McLaren, G.D.: Iron storage proteins and iron overload. *In* Current Hematology and Oncology. Vol. 6. Edited by V.F. Fairbanks. Chicago, Year Book, 1988, pp. 185–230.

Milder, M.S., Cook, J.D., Stray, S., et al.: Idiopathic hemochromatosis: an interim report. Medicine, *59*:34–49, 1980.

Niederau, C., Fischer, R., Sonnenberg, A., et al.: Survival and causes of death in cirrhotic and non-cirrhotic patients with primary hemochromatosis. N. Engl. J. Med., *313*:1256–1262, 1985.

Schafer, A.I.: Iron overload. *In* Current Hematology. Vol. 1. Edited by V.F. Fairbanks. New York, John Wiley & Sons, 1981, pp. 191–218.

Ward, J.G., Kushner, J.P., Kaplan, J.: Iron metabolism and clinical disorders. *In* Current Hematology and Oncology. Vol. 3. Edited by V.F. Fairbanks. New York, John Wiley & Sons, 1984, pp. 1–50.

Weintraub, L.R., Edwards, C.Q., Krikker, M. (eds.): Hemochromatosis: Proceedings of the First International Conference. Ann. N.Y. Acad. Sci., *526*:141–154, 1988.

Worwood, M.: An overview of iron metabolism at a molecular level. J. Intern. Med., *226*:381–391, 1989.

CHAPTER 10

# Zinc

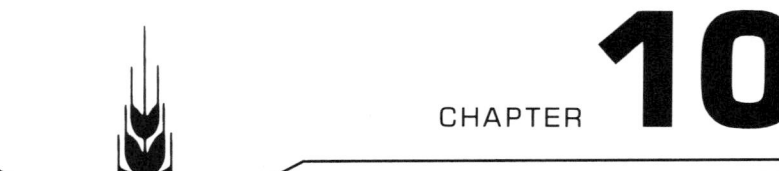

Janet C. King and Carl L. Keen



## HISTORICAL ASPECTS

Zinc (Zn) was recognized as a distinct element in 1509. Evidence of its essentiality was demonstrated in plants in 1869 and in animals in 1934.[1] Because of its wide prevalence in foodstuffs, naturally occurring Zn deficiency was considered unlikely until 1955, when swine parakeratosis was shown to be a Zn-deficiency disease. That humans could suffer from Zn deficiency was suggested by observations that malnourished Chinese patients during World War II had low concentrations of plasma Zn. In 1956, a conditioned Zn-deficiency syndrome in humans was demonstrated. Since 1961, when the endemic hypogonadism and dwarfism of rural Iran was suggested to be derived from Zn deficiency, there has been an increasing appreciation of the magnitude of both the clinical and the public health significance of Zn-deficiency states.[1–3]

## CHEMISTRY

Zn is a IIB element with a completed d subshell and two additional s electrons. Zn has an atomic number of 30, an atomic weight of 65.37 (isotopic mean), and in pure form is a bluish white metal. Zn occurs naturally as five stable isotopes: $^{64}Zn$, 48.89%; $^{66}Zn$, 27.91%; $^{67}Zn$, 4.11%; $^{68}Zn$, 18.57%; and $^{70}Zn$, 0.62%. Six radioisotopes have been identified, of which three, $^{65}Zn$, $^{69m}Zn$, and $^{63}Zn$ are used often in tracer studies (half-lives of 245 days, 13.8 hours, and 38 minutes, respectively). In biologic systems Zn is virtually always in the divalent state. Zn typically forms complexes with a coordination number of 4 with a tetrahedral disposition of ligands around the metal. Zn readily complexes to amino acids, peptides, proteins, and nucleotides. Zn has an affinity for thiol and hydroxy groups and for ligands containing electron-rich nitrogen as a donor. Zn does not exhibit any direct redox chemistry.

## BIOLOGIC ACTIVITY

The net delivery of Zn to an organism is a function of the bioavailability and the total amount of Zn in the diet. Bioavailability is defined as the proportion of Zn, or any other nutrient, in food that is absorbed and utilized. As with most minerals, Zn absorption typically exceeds the amount actually utilized; the excess absorbed is rapidly excreted.

### FOOD SOURCES

Foods differ widely in their Zn content. Zn concentrations range from 0.02 mg/100 g for egg white to 1 mg/100 g for light chicken meat to 75 mg/100 g for oysters. Shellfish, beef, and other red meats are good Zn sources. Whole-grain cereals are relatively rich in total Zn. Most of the Zn is contained in the bran and germ portions, and nearly 80% of the total Zn is lost in the wheat milling process.[2] There is no standard enrichment policy for Zn, but some breakfast cereal manufacturers fortify the Zn content of their product in amounts ranging from 25 to 100% of the United States recommended dietary allowance (RDA). Nuts and legumes are relatively good plant sources of Zn. Plant Zn concentrations may be enhanced if grown in Zn-rich soil or treated with Zn-rich fertilizers.[4]

Total dietary Zn intakes are influenced greatly by food choices. Animal products, especially meat, provide about 70% of the Zn consumed by people in the United States.[5] Cereals are the primary plant source. Frequently, Zn intakes are correlated with protein intake, but the exact relationship is influenced by protein source. Diets consisting primarily of eggs, milk, poultry, and fish have a lower Zn-protein ratio than those composed of shellfish, beef, and other red meats. Similar variations occur in vegetarian diets. Diets with a rich Zn-protein ratio have liberal quantities of legumes, whole grains, nuts, and cheese, whereas those with a low ratio contain primarily fruits and vegetables. Drinking water is typically low in Zn. The mean intake from adult self-selected mixed diets in the United States ranges from 8.6 to 14 mg Zn per day.[2] During the first 6 months of life, Zn intake varies with the mode of feeding. Reported intakes of breast-fed infants range from 0.03 mmol per day (1.9 mg per day) at 1 month of age to 0.04 mmol per day (2.7 mg per day) at 6 months;[6] bottle-fed infants consumed 0.055 and 0.07 mmol per day (3.6 and 4.6 mg per day) at 1 and 6 months, respectively. The Zn content of commercial infant formulas depends on the fortification policy of the manufacturer. Children consume 0.08 to 0.12 mmol per day (5 to 8 mg per day), and adolescent girls report daily intakes of about 0.17 mmol (11 mg); the daily intake of 8 to 13-year-old children is approximately 0.12 to 0.15 mmol (8 to 10 mg), and elderly populations consume 0.11 to 0.15 mmol per day (7 to 10 mg per day).[2,7] Pregnant and lactating women report intakes that fall within a range similar to that of adult mixed diets.[2]

### FACTORS AFFECTING ZINC BIOAVAILABILITY

Absorption of Zn is largely a function of the presence or absence of substances in the food or meal that alter the solubility or availability of Zn compounds at the absorption site. Some dietary components form large, insoluble Zn compounds and thereby inhibit Zn absorption. Other components form soluble, stable compounds that enhance absorption. Competition between Zn and other elements for absorption binding sites can influence absorbability.

Meats, liver, eggs, and seafood are considered to be good sources of Zn because of the relative absence of chemical constituents that inhibit Zn absorption and because of the presence of certain amino acids that improve Zn solubility.

Cysteine and histidine enhance Zn absorbability by forming stable complexes with Zn.[8] Whole-grain cereal products and plant proteins, such as soy protein, contain Zn in a less available form. The phytic acid (inositol polyphosphate) content of plant foods explains, at least in part, the lower availability of Zn from these foods. Fermentation of bread reduces the phytic acid content and significantly improves Zn absorption. Extrusion cooking, which is used for breakfast cereals, seems to inhibit the degradation of phytic acid in the gut and causes less efficient absorption of Zn.[9] Values of the millimolar ratio of phytate to Zn above 10 increases the risk of poor Zn utilization. Removal of phytate from a food such as soy protein can significantly increase the availability of Zn from the product.[10] The effect of other plant and food components such as fiber, tannic acid, and caffeine on Zn utilization by humans is equivocal.[2,9]

### ZINC-NUTRIENT INTERACTIONS

Transport mechanisms into cells for cations are in part determined by their configuration and coordination properties.[11] Thus, elements with similar physicochemical characteristics compete for common pathways. Zn, with a preferred coordination number of 4, competes with copper (Cu) and cadmium (Cd). Mutual affinity for a carrier protein can also result in metal competition. This type of interaction may underlie reported Zn-iron (Fe) interactions.

*ZINC-COPPER*

Large quantities of ingested Zn can interfere with Cu bioavailability.[9] One explanation is that a high intake of Zn induces the synthesis of the Cu-binding ligand, metallothionein, in the mucosal cell. This protein sequesters Cu, making it unavailable for serosal transfer and thus decreases Cu absorption. Relatively low levels of dietary Zn may interfere with Cu absorption. An intake of only 0.28 mmol Zn per day (18.5 mg per day) for 2 weeks reduced apparent Cu retention in a group of young men.[12] Clinical signs of Cu deficiency developed in individuals taking 2.3 mmol Zn per day (150 mg Zn per day) for 2 years. Pharmacologic doses of Zn (3 to 4.6 mmol per day; 200 to 300 mg per day) have been used to treat Wilson's disease, a rare inborn error of Cu metabolism that causes excessive tissue accumulation of Cu.[13] A high intake of Cu does not inhibit Zn absorption.[2]

*ZINC-IRON*

Fe can interfere with Zn absorption when elemental Zn is given in solution, but it has little effect on the utilization of Zn from a complex meal.[14] Using body retention of $^{65}Zn$ as an index of absorption, Valberg et al. found that both inorganic and heme Fe inhibited Zn absorption from a 0.09-mmol (6-mg) dose of Zn as Zn chloride, but had no effect on Zn absorption from an extrinsically labeled turkey test meal.[15] Several human studies have suggested that supplemental Fe may lower plasma Zn concentrations during pregnancy;[2] however, this observation was not made for either pregnant rats or monkeys under controlled conditions.[16,17]

*ZINC-OTHER ELEMENTS*

Although high levels of dietary calcium can impair Zn absorption in animals,[9] the addition of calcium salts to the diets of humans does not typically reduce Zn balance or whole-body retention of $^{65}Zn$. Supplements of 0.4 mmol (50 mg) of tin increased fecal Zn excretion in a human balance study;[18] however, given that the usual intake of dietary tin is <8μmol per day (<1 mg per day), it is unlikely that this element has an adverse effect on Zn absorption in typical diets. Although high levels of dietary Cd can influence the distribution of Zn in the body, Cd does not seem to have a major effect on dietary Zn absorption.

*ZINC-FOLIC ACID*

Hydrolysis of dietary folates to their monoglutamate form requires the Zn-dependent enzyme, pteroylpolyglutamate hydrolase.[19] Administration of an oral dose of pteroylheptaglutamate to a group of Zn-depleted men prevented the usual rise in serum folic acid, whereas the serum response to an oral dose of pteroylmonoglutamate was normal.[20] Folic acid may impair Zn absorption when the dietary Zn intake is low, but not when it is high. Administration of 1.8 μmol (800 μg) of folic acid to a group of adults inhibited Zn absorption when the fractional rate of Zn absorption was higher than 30%.[21] This finding raises concern about pregnant women, who are often given supplemental folic acid to reduce the risk of birth defects.

## METABOLISM

### ZINC IN THE HUMAN BODY

Based on a total body concentration of about 0.3 μmol Zn/g (20 μgZn/g), it is estimated that the newborn contains approximately 0.9 mmol (60 mg) Zn.[22] During growth and maturation, the Zn concentration of the human body increases to approximately 0.46 μmol/g (30 μg/g).[2] The adult total body Zn content ranges from about 2.3 mmol (1.5 g) in women to 3.8 mmol (2.5 g) in men.

Zn is present in all organs, tissues, fluids, and secretions of the body. Zn is primarily an intracellular ion, with well over 95% of the total-body Zn found within cells. Zn is associated with all organelles of the cell, but about 60 to 80% of the cellular Zn is found in the cytosol. The Zn concentration and content of various tissues and the proportion of total body Zn found in them are described in Table 10–1.

### ZINC UPTAKE

*SITES OF ABSORPTION*

Zn is absorbed all along the small intestine; only small amounts are absorbed in the stomach and large intestine. Considering the length and surface area of the various segments of the small bowel, the transit time of digestion, and the endogenous secretion of Zn, most of the element is probably absorbed in the jejunum.[23] After intake of a meal, the intraluminal quantity of Zn increases to about 1.5 to 3 times the amount ingested at the distal duodenum, presumably because of the secretion of Zn-containing digestive juices. The luminal content declines substantially in the jejunum.[24] It was estimated that about 0.05 to 0.08 mmol (3.3 to 5.0 mg) Zn is absorbed from the first 90 cm of the jejunum.

*INTRALUMINAL FACTORS*

During the process of digesting a meal, digestive enzymes release dietary Zn from food matrices and endogenous Zn from various binding ligands. As such, this free Zn is able to form coordination complexes with various exogenous and endogenous ligands, such as amino acids, phosphates, and other organic acids.[9] Histidine and cysteine are the preferred amino acid ligands. Evidence indicates that Zn-histidine complexes are absorbed 30 to 40% more efficiently than Zn sulfate.[8]

**TABLE 10–1.** APPROXIMATE ZINC CONTENT OF MAJOR ORGANS AND TISSUES IN A NORMAL ADULT MAN (70 KG)

| TISSUE | APPROXIMATE Zn CONCENTRATION wet weight μM/g | (μg/g) | TOTAL Zn CONTENT mM | (g) | PERCENTAGE OF BODY Zn (%) |
|---|---|---|---|---|---|
| Skeletal muscle | 0.78 | (51) | 24 | (1.53) | 57 (approx.) |
| Bone | 1.54 | (100) | 12 | (0.77) | 29 |
| Skin | 0.49 | (32) | 2 | (0.16) | 6 |
| Liver | 0.89 | (58) | 2 | (0.13) | 5 |
| Brain | 0.17 | (11) | 0.6 | (0.04) | 1.5 |
| Kidneys | 0.85 | (55) | 0.3 | (0.02) | 0.7 |
| Heart | 0.35 | (23) | 0.15 | (0.01) | 0.4 |
| Hair | 2.30 | (150) | <0.15 | (<0.01) | 0.1 (approx.) |
| Blood plasma | 0.02 | (1) | <0.15 | (<0.01) | 0.1 (approx.) |

(Modified from Mills C. F. (Ed.): Zinc in Human Biology. London, Springer-Verlag, 1989)

Intestinal pH does not appear to influence Zn uptake. As discussed previously, the presence of other divalent metal ions, such as Fe, may compete with Zn for mucosal cell binding sites. Intraluminal prostaglandins seem to influence Zn absorption, with $PGE_2$ enhancing uptake and $PGF_2$ inhibiting.[2,25]

*CELLULAR FACTORS*

The mechanism by which Zn enters mucosal cells is unknown. Presumably, it traverses the unstirred water layer in an exchangeable or diffusible form. Zn uptake across the brush border surface occurs by both a carrier-mediated mechanism and diffusion. At low-normal luminal concentrations of Zn, the carrier mechanism predominates. This mechanism does not require energy. Specific receptor proteins for Zn have not been characterized. Carrier-mediated Zn uptake is stimulated when the dietary supply of Zn is low.[25] The carrier affinity for Zn is not changed with low intake, but the capacity for carrier-mediated transport is considerably greater, thereby suggesting a rise in the number of receptor sites. With high Zn intakes, a nonsaturable mechanism for Zn absorption becomes prominent. This mechanism may involve passive diffusion and/or movement between mucosal cells. The positive, nonspecific effect of lactose and glucose polymers on Zn absorption may represent an increase in pericellular Zn movement.

The disposition of Zn within the cell is diverse. Intercellular Zn may be used by the cell for Zn-dependent processes, become bound firmly to metallothionein and held within the cell, or pass through the cell. Transcellular passage results in a net transport of Zn into the lumen or circulation. Zn trapped within the cell is eventually lost in the feces in the normal course of mucosal cell turnover. Transport of Zn across the serosal membrane is carrier mediated and occurs by an adenosine triphosphate (ATP)-driven mechanism.[26]

*PORTAL TRANSPORT*

Zn is released by the intestinal cells at the basolateral-serosal surface into the mesenteric capillary and is carried by the portal blood to the liver.[26] The absorbed $^{65}Zn$ is initially albumin bound.[26]

*HOMEOSTATIC REGULATION*

Total body Zn content is controlled in part by regulating the efficiency of intestinal absorption and the excretion from endogenous Zn pools. As intraluminal concentrations of Zn rise, the fractional absorption of Zn decreases, but the actual amount of Zn absorbed rises linearly. Thus, at high Zn intakes, regulation of intestinal absorption only provides "coarse control" of total body Zn. An increase in the fecal excretion of endogenous Zn provides the "fine control" needed to balance the net retention of Zn with metabolic needs. Endogenous fecal Zn losses can be increased several fold to maintain Zn homeostasis with high intake of Zn.[27]

The physiologic state of the organism influences the homeostatic regulation of Zn. Experimental Zn deficiency in animals and humans enhances Zn uptake.[28,29] In the rat, a specific increase in the efficiency of Zn absorption is observed in late pregnancy, possibly because of an increase in receptor sites.[30] An enhanced uptake during lactation is also observed, but this is nonspecific and related to mucosal hypertrophy.

The age of the individual influences absorptive capacity. Newborn animals absorb Zn to a higher degree than do older animals, perhaps because of a transport system with a higher affinity for Zn.[31] Zn absorption decreases with age;[32] five healthy men between 65 and 74 years of age absorbed half as much Zn as did five men between 22 and 30 years of age fed the same diet. This reduction in Zn absorption was associated with a decline in endogenous Zn losses, so balance was maintained in the older subjects.

Hormonal influences associated with stress (corticosteroids and select cytokines) can increase the efficiency of Zn absorption.[29] Acute bacterial infection and endotoxemia in the rat significantly increase Zn absorption.[29]

## ZINC TURNOVER AND TRANSPORT

Kinetic modeling using $^{65}$Zn has provided information about Zn pools and their turnover. A two-component model best explains the elimination of absorbed Zn from the body.[2] The initial rapid phase has a half-life in humans of 12.5 days, and a slower turnover phase has a half-life value of about 300 days. The initial rapid half-life primarily represents liver uptake of circulating Zn and its release. The slower turnover rate reflects differing rates of Zn turnover in various tissues other than liver.[2] Zn uptake by the central nervous system and bones is relatively slow; the pancreas, liver, kidney, and spleen have the most rapid rates of accumulation and turnover; uptake and exchange of Zn in red cells and muscle are slower than in the viscera.

Dietary Zn restriction of rats enhanced the retention of $^{65}$Zn in soft tissues and organs, except bone, by a reduction in Zn turnover.[27] These adjustments prevent a measurable decline in tissue Zn concentration. In humans turnover of the slower Zn pool is accelerated by daily loading with 1.54 mmol (100 mg) of Zn.[33]

About 0.05 mmol (3 mg) of Zn is normally circulating in the plasma at any given moment. This Zn is partitioned among α-2-macroglobulin (40%), albumin, 57%, and amino acids, 3%.[34] These loosely bound albumin and amino acid fractions of circulating Zn provide the transport and delivery of Zn to tissues. The amino acid bound fraction determines the amount that is filtered by the kidneys. Because the total amount of Zn present in the major tissues is much larger than the total present in plasma, relatively small variations in the Zn content of tissues, such as the liver, can have dramatic effects on plasma Zn. For example, an increase of liver Zn by 1% caused by enhanced retention of Zn could cause a 40% decline in plasma Zn. Because all absorbed Zn passes through the plasma to the tissues, the flux of Zn through the plasma must be rapid to maintain relatively constant plasma concentrations. Figure 10–1 illustrates the metabolism of Zn.

## STORAGE

There is no specific Zn "store." In all species studied, a marked reduction in dietary Zn intake is quickly followed by the signs of Zn deficiency. Nonetheless, some sources of endogenous Zn are retained preferentially in certain tissues in response to a decrease in dietary Zn. For example, in Zn deficiency, bone uptake and concentration of the element decline, but the rates of bone turnover and release of Zn are not significantly increased. On the other hand, reductions in food intake

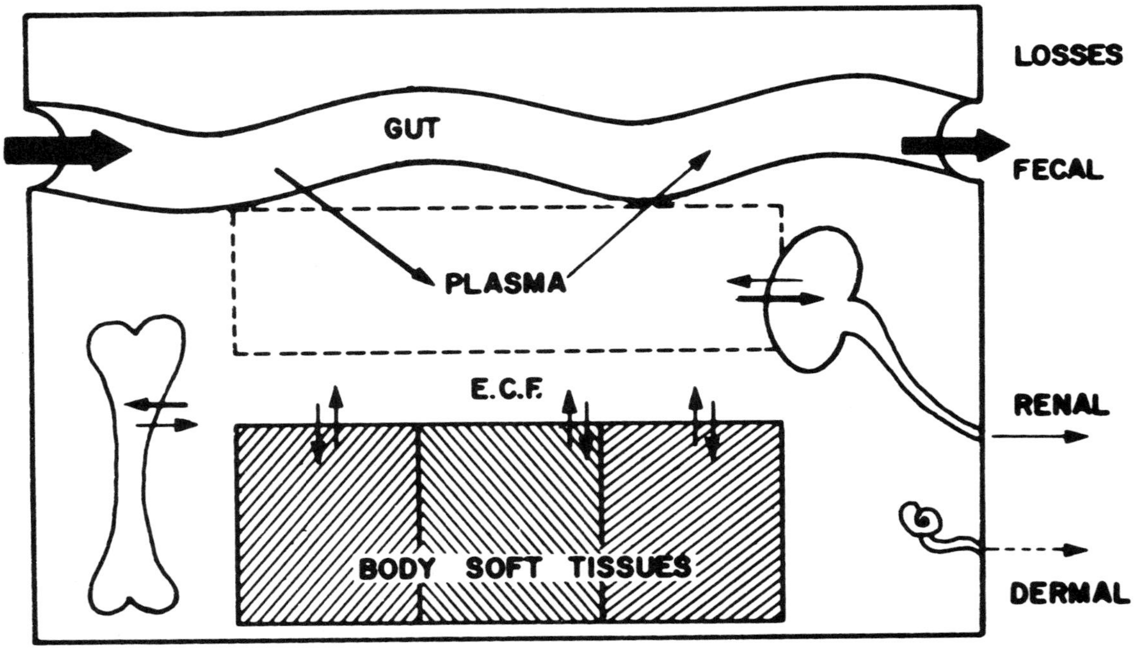
LOSSES
GUT
FECAL
PLASMA
E.C.F.
RENAL
BODY SOFT TISSUES
DERMAL

**FIGURE 10–1.** Schematic representation of the metabolism of zinc in mammals. (From Beisel, W.R., Pekarek, R.S., Wannamacher, R.W., Jr.: Homeostatic mechanisms affecting plasma zinc levels in acute stress. *In* Trace Elements in Human Health and Disease. Vol. 1. New York, Academic Press, 1976.)

associated with Zn deficiency can cause catabolism of muscle tissue and release of Zn into the plasma.[35]

### EXCRETION

The major route for endogenous Zn excretion is into the gastrointestinal tract with ultimate loss in the feces. When tracer doses of Zn are given either orally or intravenously, only about 2 to 10% is recovered in the urine; the remainder is lost in the feces.[2]

Fecal Zn losses are a combination of unabsorbed dietary Zn and endogenous Zn secretions. Pancreatic secretions are a major source of endogenous Zn. Other sources include biliary and gastroduodenal secretions, transepithelial flux of Zn from the mucosal cells, and sloughing of old mucosal cells into the gut.[2] Perfusion studies show that about 0.04 to 0.07 mmol (2.5 to 4.8 mg) Zn is secreted into the duodenum following intake of a meal, presumably as meal-stimulated pancreatic secretions. Much of the Zn secreted into the gut lumen is absorbed and returned to the body. Maintenance of an intact enteropancreatic Zn circulation is important for maintenance of body Zn. The amount of Zn secreted into the gut varies with Zn intake. In humans, endogenous fecal losses may range from <15 μmol/day (1 mg/day) with extremely low intakes to over 80 μmol/day (5 mg/day) with extremely high intakes.[28,36]

Normally, about 6 to 9 μmol (400 to 600 μg) of Zn is excreted daily in the urine. Urinary Zn arises largely from the ultrafilterable portion of the plasma Zn.[2] Dietary Zn only influences urinary losses if the intake is extremely low or extremely high. Under basal conditions, up to 95% of the filtered Zn is reabsorbed in the distal parts of the renal tubule.[37] The amount of Zn excreted in the urine is correlated highly with the rate of urine production (or the urine volume) and creatinine excretion. Catabolic states, such as those resulting from severe burns, major surgery or other trauma, and total starvation, cause clinically significant increases in urinary Zn losses. Chelating agents, such as ethylene diamene tetra-acetic acid (EDTA), also elevate urinary Zn.[2]

Surface losses through desquamation of skin, outgrowth of hair, and sweat contribute up to 15 μmol (1 mg) of Zn daily. A marked reduction or marked increase in dietary Zn intake causes a concomitant change in surface losses.[38] Other sources of loss include the semen and menstrual secretions. An ejaculum of semen contains up to 15 μmol (1 mg) of Zn.[28] Total menstrual losses represent a loss of approximately 1.5 to 8.0 μmol (0.1 to 0.5 mg) per menstrual period.[39]

## BIOCHEMICAL AND PHYSIOLOGIC FUNCTIONS

Zn is recognized to have a multitude of diverse functions, namely, Zn has been identified in numerous enzymes. It is a component of biomembranes, is thought to be necessary for RNA, DNA, and ribosome stabilization, is involved in the binding of a number of transcription factors, stabilizes some hormone-receptor complexes, and may have a regulatory role in tubulin polymerization. Given its multitude of functions, it is not surprising that a deficit of this element can pose serious physiologic challenges. A brief outline of some of the biochemical and physiologic functions of Zn is presented and is followed by a discussion of the signs of Zn deficiency.

### BIOCHEMISTRY

With regard to metalloenzymes, Zn can have a catalytic, structural, or regulatory role. Examples are carbonic anhydrase, Cu, Zn-superoxide dismutase, and fructose bisphosphatase, respectively. Over 200 Zn enzymes have been reported to occur in biologic systems, and Zn enzymes are found in all six International Union of Biochemistry (IUB) classes.[2,40] Because of space constraints, a detailed discussion of all identified Zn enzymes is not feasible here; selected enzymes are discussed in the context of specific physiologic functions and of deficiency signs of Zn. For additional details on Zn enzymes, the reader is directed to several reviews.[2,40,41]

A critical function of Zn is its role in the structure and function of biomembranes. Some investigators have argued that a reduction in the concentration of Zn in biomembranes underlies some of the disorders associated with Zn deficiency,[42] with a loss of Zn from the membrane resulting in an increased susceptibility to oxidative damage, structural strains, and alterations in specific receptor sites and transport systems. The influence of Zn on biomembrane structure and function may be due in part to its ability (1) to stabilize thiol groups and phospholipids, (2) to occupy sites that might otherwise contain transition metals with redox potential (such as Fe), and (3) to be involved in the quenching of free radicals through its association with metallothionein.[43] Biomembrane accumulation of Zn can also result in alterations in membrane structure and function; for example, the release of histamine from mast cells is reduced when Zn masks receptor sites for histamine releasing agents.[44]

In addition to its putative structural role in biomembranes and in many enzymes, Zn helps to stabilize the structures of RNA, DNA, and ribosomes.[2,45] Moreover, several transcription factors have been reported to contain "Zn finger" regions, repeated cysteine- and histidine-containing domains that bind Zn in a tetrahedral configuration. It is currently thought that Zn finger-Zn complex regions are needed for the binding of these transcription factors to DNA; one suggested mechanism of transcription control may involve the binding and release of Zn from these regions in response to meal-associated changes in nuclear Zn content.[46]

Zn may also have a regulatory role in the polymerization of tubulin. Zn has been shown to stabilize neurotubules in vitro, possibly through the formation of Zn mercaptide bridges between the tubulin dimer subunits. The rate of tubulin polymerization is decreased in brain extracts of Zn-deficient rats and pigs; Zn-deficiency-induced reductions in the rate of tubulin polymerization have been postulated to underlie some of the developmental defects associated with Zn deficiency.[47]

### PHYSIOLOGIC FUNCTIONS

To a great extent the appreciation of the physiologic roles of Zn is based on observations of signs of Zn deficiency in experimental animals and in humans. Surprisingly, despite the long list of described Zn enzymes and nonenzymatic Zn-dependent processes, little consensus has been achieved on the precise biochemical lesions underlying the development of the numerous signs of Zn deficiency. In the following sections, we consider some of the signs of Zn deficiency in experimental animals and humans, along with a discussion of some of the potential mechanisms that may underlie their development. At present, however, these mechanisms must be considered speculative. A brief review of the effects of Zn deficiency in experimental animals is presented first, followed by a discussion of the signs of Zn deficiency in humans.

## ZINC DEFICIENCY IN EXPERIMENTAL ANIMALS

A deficiency of Zn develops in a manner *different* from that of most nutrients. Thus, in the case of most nutrients, an insufficient dietary intake causes first a mobilization of stores or functional reserves. Thereafter, tissue concentrations of the nutrient decline, and eventually, one or more specific functions or metabolic pathways dependent on the nutrient deteriorate. Thus, reduction in growth is a *late* manifestation of deficiency. In contrast, when dietary Zn intakes are insufficient, the first responses are a reduction in growth by growing organisms and a decrease in endogenous losses of Zn to conserve tissue Zn. If the dietary deficiency is mild, Zn homeostasis may be reestablished after adjusting the rates of growth and excretion, and no further functional or biochemical changes occur. However, with a markedly deficient diet, the organism cannot reestablish homeostasis through adjustments in endogenous losses and growth, and as a consequence, generalized tissue dysfunction develops quickly. It is thought that the prompt appearance of Zn deficiency signs in animals fed essentially Zn-free diets is associated with the loss of a small, labile pool of Zn located within various tissues.[48]

Zn deficiency can be induced rapidly in some species. For example, within 12 hours of consuming a Zn-deficient meal, plasma Zn concentrations in the rat can be decreased by as much as 50%.[49] That this reduction in plasma Zn can be functionally significant is dramatically illustrated by the observation that the feeding of a Zn-deficient diet to pregnant rats for only a few days during the first trimester is sufficient to cause embryonic abnormalities.[50] Although all species may not respond to a Zn-deficient diet as rapidly as the rat, the lack of any appreciable Zn stores under homeostatic control is a consistent finding for all mammalian species to date.

Early effects of Zn deficiency in many species are anorexia and cyclic feeding. Increased levels of norepinephrine and alterations in its receptor function in the hypothalamus of Zn-deficient animals have been suggested mechanisms underlying the anorexia.[51] Regardless of the biochemical explanation for the anorexia, the cyclic food pattern of Zn-deficient animals may represent an adaptation of the animal to the low Zn diet because, during periods of low food intake, the substantial muscle catabolism and release of Zn into the plasma pool can be used by hepatic and extrahepatic tissues for Zn-dependent processes.[45]

If the period of Zn deficiency is prolonged, additional hallmarks of Zn deficiency are impaired growth, dermatitis, a compromised immune system, and a decreased efficiency of food utilization. Although the lesions underlying the foregoing signs have not been defined, a reduction in cell replication is an early event in Zn deficiency. The reduction in cell division has been related in part to the role of Zn in protein and nucleic acid synthesis, in chromatin decondensation, and in the assembly of the mitotic spindle through its effect on microtubule polymerization.[45]

Associated with Zn-deficiency-induced reduction in cell division is impaired growth, which has been demonstrated for numerous species including humans.[45] It has been suggested that a reduction in growth rate may represent an accommodation of the animal to the Zn deficit, thereby resulting in the availability of more Zn for Zn-dependent metabolic processes. An alternative explanation for the slower rate of growth is that it is secondary to the anorexia and the concomitant reduction in food intake. However, animals fed diets adequate in Zn, in amounts equivalent to those consumed by Zn-deficient animals, gain considerably more weight than the Zn-deficient animals. Thus, the lower weight gain observed with Zn deficiency cannot be ascribed solely to reduced food intake.[51]

In addition to an overall reduction in body size, Zn-deficiency-associated reductions in cell division may also contribute to abnormal bone growth and maturation. Both the number of osteoblasts and the chondrocyte number in epiphyseal cartilage are reduced in Zn deficiency.[52] A reduction in cell division rates may also underlie some of the effects of Zn deficiency on the immune system, in that a deficient animal is often characterized by a small thymus and spleen, with resultant reductions in its capacity for T- and B-lymphocyte production.[53] Zn-deficiency-induced reductions in cell replication rates may also underlie the teratogenicity of embryonic Zn deficiency because an interruption in normal replication rates and patterns could lead to asynchrony in cell and tissue maturation.

As already indicated, a deficiency of Zn during early development can be highly teratogenic. Typical malformations associated with Zn deficiency in experimental animals include brain and eye defects, spina bifida, cleft lip and palate, and numerous malformations of the heart, lung, skeleton, and urogenital system.[50] Biochemical lesions proposed to contribute to the teratogenicity of Zn deficiency include abnormal nucleic acid and protein synthesis, alterations in the differential rates of cellular growth needed for normal morphogenesis, impairment in tubulin polymerization with resultant reductions in cell motility and division, chromosomal defects, excessive cell death in areas adjacent to regions where programmed cell death occurs, and excessive peroxidation of cell membrane lipids.[50] It is evident from the foregoing that the mechanisms leading to Zn-deficiency-associated abnormal development are probably multifactorial in nature. In addition to its impact on the fetus, Zn deficiency during late gestation can result in parturition difficulties with delayed deliveries and excessive bleeding.[50,54] In Zn-deficient rats, the delay in delivery has been linked to a lower-than-normal activity of ovarian 20-α-hydroxysteroid dehydrogenase, an enzyme that catalyzes the degradation of progesterone, which is inhibitory to parturition.[55] The subcellular distribution and metabolism of uterine estrogen-receptor complexes are altered in Zn-deficient rats. A poor response to estrogen priming may contribute to the delivery problems associated with Zn deficiency.

The influence of Zn on the reproductive process is not restricted to females. In Zn-deficient males, the testes are reduced in size with atrophy of the seminiferous epithelium. The resulting testicular dysfunction impairs spermatogenesis and the output of testosterone. It is thought that the primary defect underlying the effect of Zn deficiency on testicular function may involve impaired Leydig cell function with a secondary effect on the pituitary-gonadal axis.[56]

A consequence of Zn deficiency can be marked alterations in several components of the immune system. Immune defects associated with Zn deficiency include reduced thymic hormone production and activity, impaired functions of lymphocytes, natural killer cells and neutrophils, impaired antibody-dependent cell-mediated cytotoxicity, altered immunologic ontogeny, and defective lymphokine production.[53] As discussed previously, Zn-deficient animals can be characterized by thymic atrophy and small spleens. Significantly, Zn deficiency reduces the mass of lymphoid tissues more than that of other tissues. The particular sensitivity of lymphoid tissue to Zn deficiency has not been clarified.[53]

Impaired glucose tolerance has been reported by some investigators to occur in Zn deficiency. The impairment has been related to reduced insulin output, increased insulin degradation by glutathione insulin transhydrogenase, and an increase in peripheral insulin resistance.[2]

Lipid metabolism has also been shown to be affected by Zn deficiency. The reduction in glucose utilization in Zn deficiency has been linked to an overall increased rate of lipid oxidation. Zn-deficient animals can be characterized by hypocholesterolemia (primarily caused by reduction in HDL cholesterol) and by an HDL fraction that is enriched in apo E and low in apo C content.[2,57] Many of the signs of Zn deficiency are similar to those of essential fatty acid deficiency, and tissue arachidonic levels are typically elevated in deficient animals.[58]

In addition to its putative effects on insulin and testosterone, the metabolism of several other hormones has been reported to be influenced by Zn. The synthesis, release, and binding of growth hormone, somatomedin, prolactin, thyroid hormone, corticosterone, luteinizing hormone releasing hormone (LHRH), follicle-stimulating hormone (FSH), and luteinizing hormone (LH) have all been reported to be affected by Zn deficiency, although these findings are not universal.[2,55]

## ZINC DEFICIENCY IN HUMANS

### MILD DEFICIENCY

Although the occurrence of severe Zn deficiency in humans is well documented, whether a physiologically significant mild Zn deficiency exists in humans is controversial. It is inherently unlikely, however, that human Zn deficiency is an "all-or-none" phenomenon. The concept of a graded response to progressive degrees of deficiency is supported by animal studies; for example, when weanling rats were fed graded amounts of dietary Zn ranging from 1 to 12 ppm, the 12-ppm diet supported normal growth, but impairment was increasingly severe with more severe dietary Zn restrictions.[59]

Evidence of mild Zn deficiency in humans is not as straightforward to demonstrate as in experimental animals. If it is accepted that impaired growth velocity is the primary clinical feature of mild Zn deficiency, several studies done in Denver, Colorado, provide convincing evidence.[60,61] Apparently healthy children with low height-for-age percentiles were selected for a double-blind, controlled trial of Zn supplementation. The treatment group received a small (0.08-mmol, 5-mg) Zn supplement. In all studies of these growth-retarded children, Zn supplementation increased the mean height increment and height-for-age percentile increment in comparison to that of placebo controls. Boys frequently had a greater response than girls. In one study, supplemental Zn improved the calculated energy and protein intake.[62] Concurrently with these studies, Zn supplementation in children who were unselected with respect to growth percentiles did not increase their growth velocity.[61]

Mild Zn deficiency may also affect the quality of growth. Zn supplementation of malnourished infants reduced the energy cost of growth, which was probably related to improved synthesis of lean body tissue.[63] Idiopathic dysgeusia was improved in a single-blind trial of Zn therapy, but a subsequent double-blind trial failed to confirm this observation.[64] Other functions that have responded to Zn supplementation include immune function in the elderly,[65] oligospermia,[66] and complications of pregnancy, such as pregnancy-induced hypertension, prematurity, prolonged labor, and intrapartum hemorrhage.[67] In most of the foregoing cases, however, the response was to pharmacologic quantities of Zn, and these findings do not necessarily indicate a Zn deficiency. The response of these conditions to physiologic Zn doses (0.15 to 0.23 mmol per day, 10 to 15 mg per day) needs to be tested using double-blind, controlled designs.

## SEVERE DEFICIENCY

Severe Zn deficiency has been seen in patients with acrodermatitis enteropathica (AE), in patients fed total parenteral nutrition (TPN) solutions lacking Zn, and in experimental human Zn depletion. The clinical features of severe Zn deficiency in the three situations are similar. The expression of Zn deficiency in an individual depends on the severity of the deficiency and other factors.

## CLINICAL MANIFESTATIONS

The primary clinical manifestations of severe Zn deficiency are listed in Table 10–2. In severe deficiencies, growth ceases, whereas a less severe deficiency state causes a decrease in growth velocity. If growth retardation is mild, the response to Zn supplementation is modest. Persons suffering from more severe reduction in growth velocity, as in AE or in Middle Eastern adolescents consuming high-phytate diets, show a greater response to Zn supplementation. The original observations of human Zn deficiency in Persian and Egyptian dwarfs included hypogonadism and delayed sexual maturation.[3] The effect of severe Zn deficiency on hypogonadism among patients with AE is unclear.[68]

**TABLE 10–2.** CLINICAL MANIFESTATIONS OF SEVERE HUMAN ZINC DEFICIENCY*

| |
|---|
| Growth retardation |
| Delayed sexual maturation and impotence |
| Hypogonadism and hypospermia |
| Alopecia |
| Acro-orificial skin lesions |
| Other epithelial lesions, including glossitis, alopecia, and nail dystrophy |
| Immune deficiencies |
| Behavioral disturbances, including impaired hedonic tone |
| Night blindness |
| Impaired taste (hypogeusia) |
| Delayed healing of wounds, burns and decubitus ulcers |
| Impaired appetite and food intake |
| Eye lesions, including photophobia and lack of dark adaptation |

*Features depend on the severity of the deficiency and other factors.

The skin lesions of severe Zn deficiency have a characteristic distribution, primarily at the extremities and adjacent to the body orifices. Lesions may occur elsewhere and can become generalized. Often the rashes are erythematous, vesiculobullous, and pustular.[2,68] Changes in the hair usually become apparent after the onset of dermatitis. The hair may become hypopigmented and acquire a reddish hue.[68] Patchy loss of hair is a common feature.

Diarrhea is a complication of AE and in patients receiving TPN. The mechanism(s) for diarrhea in Zn deficiency is unknown. Decreased mucosal disaccharidase activity and related carbohydrate malabsorption have been suggested,[69] but the diarrhea seen in patients receiving TPN who are not ingesting meals clearly is of a different origin. Other possible explanations include an increase in the synthesis of prostaglandins, especially $PGE_2$, which can cause diarrhea, and a defect in enterocyte transport function.

Consistent with experimental animal data, Zn deficiency in humans alters several aspects of immune function. Thymic hypoplasia has been seen in patients with AE and in individuals suffering from protein-energy malnutrition. Impaired cutaneous responses to mitogens and in vitro lymphoblast responses have been noted as have defects in monocyte and neutrophil chemotaxis.[53]

The cornea, the tissue with the highest Zn concentration in the body, is affected by Zn deficiency. Corneal edema occurs and may progress to corneal clouding and opacities.[68] Healing of more advanced lesions may leave residual scarring, but minor lesions may heal completely. A mild dry conjunctivitis may also occur and may progress to bilateral xerosis and keratomalacia. Vitamin A is ineffective in the treatment of these disorders.

Behavioral changes can occur with Zn deficiency. Irritability, lethargy, and depression are common in children with AE.[68] The administration of large doses of histidine to induce zincuria caused anorexia and dysfunction of smell and of taste in adult subjects.[64] The subjects then became irritable, depressed, easy to anger, lethargic, and sleepy. Some develop a fine tremor, an ataxic gait, and slurred speech. Supplementation with 0.8 mmol (50 mg) of Zn quickly reversed these symptoms.

## BIOCHEMICAL CORRELATES

Although information on the biochemical functions of Zn is extensive, the biochemical correlates of the clinical features of Zn deficiency have not been determined satisfactorily. Disturbances in nucleic acid metabolism and protein synthesis may account for some of the features of Zn deficiency in humans. Elevated blood ammonia and reductions in circulating proteins with short half-lives have been reported in human Zn deficiency.[70] It has been suggested that a relative excess of dietary nitrogen in subjects fed a Zn-deficient diet can cause anorexia.[63]

As in experimental animal models, some of the effects of Zn deficiency in humans appear to be mediated through effects on hormonal function. Hormones reported to be affected by Zn status in humans include growth hormone, the gonadotropins and sex hormones, prolactin, thyroid hormones, corticosteroids, insulin, and the hormone-like substances, prostaglandins.

## CONDITIONS PREDISPOSING TO ZINC DEPLETION

Mild-to-marginal states of Zn deficiency may go undetected because those individuals do not display the specific clinical features of Zn depletion. Individuals at risk include those with decreased absorption, increased losses, or increased needs caused by growth or reproduction, particularly if their dietary Zn intake is also low.

## PRIMARY AND DIETARY-INDUCED ZINC DEFICIENCY

The occurrence of isolated Zn deficiency in normal, healthy free-living adults has not been, and is unlikely to be, documented because of the remarkable ability of individuals to reduce Zn losses and to reestablish homeostasis when the dietary supply is low.[71] However, if Zn need is increased, as in growing infants and children or in pregnant and lactating women, the potential for Zn deficiency may be increased. This is especially true if the dietary supply is inadequate. Although the increase in metabolic requirements for Zn during pregnancy appear to be modest (about 1.5 mmol, 100 mg),[22] certain complications of pregnancy have been linked to poor Zn status, as discussed later in this chapter. Moreover, physiologic Zn supplements have improved growth velocity rates in growth-retarded infants who appeared otherwise healthy.[72] A reliable, sensitive laboratory index of Zn deficiency is needed before the incidence of Zn deficiency in those vulnerable groups can be documented.

Patients receiving TPN have developed the clinical features of Zn deficiency. In many cases, patients who became Zn deficient had conditions that predisposed them to the problem, such as diarrhea, inflammatory bowel disease, or other conditions that caused increased Zn loss. Patients receiving TPN often have increased urinary Zn losses because of release of Zn from catabolized tissues,[73] or because of increased levels of glycosylated amino acid-Zn complexes.[74]

Conditions of semistarvation, such as anorexia and protein-energy malnutrition (PEM), may cause Zn deficiency. Insufficient intake combined with poor digestibility and absorbability caused by the effects of malnutrition on gastrointestinal function are precipitating factors. Poor bioavailability, attributed to high levels of dietary phytate and fiber and geophagia, is the major etiologic factor in adolescent nutritional dwarfism in Egypt and Iran.[75] Other contributory factors include dermal losses caused by excessive sweating and Zn loss through chronic gastrointestinal hemorrhage. Because of high phytate intake, vegetarianism is considered by some to be a risk factor for Zn deficiency, especially in individuals subsisting primarily on cereal-based diets.

## INBORN ERRORS OF ZINC METABOLISM: ACRODERMATITIS ENTEROPATHICA

Acrodermatitis enteropathica (AE) is a rare, inherited, autosomal recessive disease affecting both sexes.[68] The basic defect in AE is an impaired intestinal uptake and transfer of Zn. In young patients with AE, intestinal Zn absorption was reduced, as assessed by whole-body retention of an orally administered dose of $^{65}$Zn.[75] The basic defect in Zn absorption is unknown, but the mucosal mechanism for Zn uptake and transfer at customary luminal concentrations seems to be defective.[68] The beneficial therapeutic effect of large oral doses of Zn may result from a net uptake and transfer of Zn by a less specific mechanism.

The diagnosis of AE is made from the clinical features. Hyperpigmented skin lesions over the acral surfaces of elbows and knees, often also involving the face, buttocks, and other surfaces, are characteristic.[76] The rash usually first occurs in early infancy, but the onset of the disease usually does not appear until solid foods are started or until breast-feeding is completely discontinued. Secondary infection is common. Intestinal disturbances and growth failure are usually present. Psychologic and behavioral abnormalities are prominent, with irritability, lethargy, and depression occurring even during relatively mild stages of the disease.[76] Plasma and serum Zn concentrations are typically less than 6 mmol/L (40 mg/dl).

Oral Zn therapy, which causes a rapid and complete remission of the clinical and biochemical symptoms of AE, has to be continued indefinitely to sustain remission and normal Zn status. The quantity of Zn required is 0.5 to 0.7 mmol per day (30 to 45 mg per day); smaller quantities may be used initially in the very young child or infant.[76]

Another syndrome of altered Zn metabolism is found in lactating women. This condition results from an inability of the mother's mammary gland to secrete normal quantities of Zn into her milk. Apart from low milk Zn concentrations, maternal Zn status is normal. Zn supplementation does not increase milk Zn concentrations.[76] Infants who are entirely breast-fed by these mothers do not develop the clinical features of severe Zn deficiency unless they were born prematurely. Temporary management with Zn supplements is required until breast-feeding is supplemented with other foods.

### SECONDARY ACQUIRED ZINC DEFICIENCY

The major pathophysiologic abnormalities contributing to secondary Zn deficiency are Zn malabsorption and excessive urinary Zn losses. Any disease or condition altering the integrity of the mucosa cell can affect the efficiency of absorption of Zn. Chelating agents and drugs can exacerbate the impact of a disease state on Zn metabolism. Penicillamine in the treatment of Wilson's disease and diethylene triamine penta-acetate (DTPA) in the treatment of the Fe overload of thalassemia patients have caused severe Zn deficiency.[68] Moreover, anticonvulsant drugs, especially sodium valproate, may precipitate Zn deficiency. The antituberculous drug, ethambutol, has chelating properties and has been shown to increase Zn turnover rates in rats.[77]

## EVALUATION OF ZINC STATUS

Despite our knowledge of the biology of Zn and of factors promoting or predisposing persons to Zn depletion, assessment of the incidence of Zn deficiency in humans has been impaired by the lack of sensitive, specific indicators of poor Zn nutriture. Approaches to assessing nutritional status in the laboratory involve the measurement of static indices (e.g., concentration of the nutrient in tissues or fluids or measurement of surrogates for the nutrient, such as metal-containing enzymes and proteins) or functional indices (performance on nutrient-dependent physiologic functions). The problem is that many measurements do not accurately reflect nutritionally available Zn pool sizes.

### STATIC INDICES

Plasma/serum Zn has been denigrated as a measure of Zn status because it does not reflect reductions in dietary Zn intake or changes in whole-body Zn.[48] Both criticisms are valid. Because whole-body Zn content is conserved during Zn deficiency, plasma Zn is not a good marker of Zn status. Moreover, plasma Zn does not fall with changes in Zn intake unless the dietary Zn levels are so low that homeostasis cannot be reestablished. Plasma Zn seems to be a component of a labile, or nutritionally available, total-body Zn pool.[48] Thus, any fall in plasma Zn would suggest a reduction in the size of the labile pool.

Unfortunately, metabolic states other than a change in Zn status alter the labile Zn pool. Stress, infection, food intake, short-term fasting, and the hormonal state all appear to influence the distribution of labile Zn among the tissues and thereby alter the amount in the plasma.[78] Thus, plasma Zn can only be useful for assessment of Zn status if the effect of poor Zn nutriture can be differentiated from these other metabolic conditions. Recent studies suggest that erythrocyte metallothionein concentrations may be useful for diagnosing tissue Zn redistribution.[79]

Other static measures of Zn status hold little promise. Erythrocyte Zn is little affected by Zn deficiency and is not a sensitive index. The response of leukocyte Zn to changes in Zn status is not consistent among laboratories, and the assay is laborious. Hair Zn levels may be depressed in mild Zn-deficiency states, but they tend to remain normal in severe states when hair growth is arrested. Urinary excretion rates are diminished in extremely severe deficiency states, but this measurement is not sensitive to less dramatic changes and is confounded by many clinical disorders that increase urinary Zn losses.

### FUNCTIONAL INDICES

Several different in vitro and in vivo tests of physiologic function have been used to evaluate Zn status. The most definitive index is isotopic measurements of the labile, or nutritionally available, Zn pool size. However, the conditions for making this measurement have not been standardized, and the test is not easily done in a clinical situation. Many of the other functional tests are not routine and lack specificity. For example, measurements of wound healing and nitrogen retention are cumbersome. Dark adaptation requires a high degree of the subject's cooperation and time, and immune function and glucose tolerance tests lack specificity.

## REQUIREMENTS AND RECOMMENDED INTAKES

Human nutrient requirements are generally based on one of the following criteria: (1) the amount required to support balance; (2) the amount required to replace endogenous loss; or (3) the amount needed to maintain normal function. Because a good functional test for Zn status is not available, Zn requirements are generally based on the amount needed to support balance or to replace endogenous losses. Balance studies have not been particularly useful for determining human Zn requirements because both negative and positive balances occurred with daily intakes below 0.08 mmol (5 mg) and above 0.23 mmol (15 mg) in different studies.[71]

The 1989 RDA for Zn are shown in Table 10–3[80] (see also Appendix Table A–2b). The recommendations are based on the intakes required to maintain balance, on measurements of endogenous losses, and on the estimated fractional Zn absorption from typical diets in the United States.

## HIGH-RISK CLINICAL SITUATIONS

### PREGNANCY

Zn is essential for normal growth and development. The requirement for Zn increases during pregnancy. Adverse effects of Zn deficiency have been documented in

**TABLE 10–3.** RECOMMENDED ZINC INTAKES (MG/DAY)

| | AGE (YEARS) | MALES | FEMALES |
|---|---|---|---|
| Infants | 0.0–0.5 | 5 | 5 |
| | 0.5–1.0 | 5 | 5 |
| Children | 1–3 | 10 | 10 |
| | 4–6 | 10 | 10 |
| | 7–10 | 10 | 10 |
| Adolescents | 11–14 | 15 | 12 |
| | 15–18 | 15 | 12 |
| Adults | 19–24 | 15 | 12 |
| | 25–50 | 15 | 12 |
| | 51+ | 15 | 12 |
| Pregnancy | | | 15 |
| Lactation | First 6 months | | 19 |
| | Second 6 months | | 16 |

(From Food and Nutrition Board, National Research Council: Recommended Dietary Allowances. 10th Ed. Washington, D.C., National Academy Press, 1989.)

experimental animals, as discussed earlier in this chapter. Studies of Rhesus monkeys provide information about the effect of a marginal Zn deficiency on outcome in a primate model.[81]

The total incremental Zn need for pregnancy is modest in humans, about 1.5 mmol (100 mg), or an additional demand of 9 μmol (0.6 mg) of Zn per day during late gestation.[22] Women do not appear to increase their Zn intakes during pregnancy. The RDA is 0.23 mmol (15 mg) Zn per day. The average daily intake remains constant at near 0.15 mmol (10 mg). If women do not increase their Zn intakes, adequate delivery of Zn to the developing fetus must be achieved by adjustments in Zn utilization. Studies have failed to show an improvement in Zn absorption in human pregnancy. Endogenous fecal Zn losses have not been measured in pregnant women, but urinary Zn losses increase in late pregnancy after a small decline in the first trimester. By late pregnancy, the concentration of circulating Zn is about 15 to 35% lower in pregnant women than in nonpregnant women.[22] The decline occurs as early as the first gestational month, stabilizes in the second trimester, and then declines further in the third trimester. The fall in plasma Zn may be attributed to expansion of the plasma volume, fetal uptake, and hormonal adjustments in the distribution of labile, or nutritionally available, Zn from the circulation to other tissues, such as the liver.

In 1976 Jameson observed that low maternal serum Zn was associated with congenital malformations, fetal dysmaturity, prematurity, and maternal complications in otherwise healthy women.[82] That report stimulated further research to examine the relationship between Zn status and pregnancy outcome. Several detailed reviews of this topic are available.[22,50,54] Human studies indicate that some pregnant women who deliver infants with congenital abnormalities used Zn differently than women who delivered healthy infants. Several groups reported that mothers of infants with congenital anomalies had lower plasma Zn concentrations than other mothers.[50] Zn deficiency has been implicated specifically in the development of two neural tube defects, anencephaly and spina bifida. The association of plasma Zn with congenital malformations does not imply causation. Perhaps Zn status simply varies with and reflects the real, but unknown, causal factor(s), or perhaps the association between Zn and congenital abnormalities reflects poor or inefficient Zn utilization. Double-blind, supplementation trials of women prior to conception and with sufficient statistical power to detect differences have not been done.

Intrauterine growth retardation has also been associated with a poor Zn status during pregnancy. Infants of low birth weight or those who are small for gestational age have been born to women with low levels of circulating or leukocytic Zn.[83] Other studies show the opposite relationship, however, which is increased plasma Zn and small babies.[84] In such cases, the transfer of Zn from the maternal to the fetal circulation may be inadequate. Many of these studies did not control for other factors that influence birth weight, such as maternal smoking or gestational weight gain.

Maternal morbidity associated with poor Zn status includes prolonged labor, atonic bleeding, and delivery outside of normal term.[22] An increased incidence of pregnancy-induced hypertension also has been associated with a poor maternal Zn status[85] or low Zn intake.[86] The results have not been consistent, however.

## OLD AGE

The mean intake of Zn by the elderly in the United States is less than two thirds of the RDA for Zn.[7] Analysis of the 1977 United States Department of Agriculture (USDA) food consumption survey showed that men and women over 75 years of age consumed 26 and 15%, respectively, less energy daily than did the average young (23 to 34 years of age) man and woman. Moreover, men and women over 75 years of age ate 31 and 17%, respectively, less meat, fish, or poultry than did young adults. These differences in the amount and types of foods consumed probably account for the lower average Zn intakes reported by the elderly. A compilation of 17 different studies indicates that elderly individuals select diets providing 7 to 11 mg of Zn per day, or 47 to 73% of the RDA for men.[7] This does not imply that elderly Americans have insufficient Zn intakes, but they may be at risk of a deficiency if other conditions impairing Zn utilization are present.

Several factors may increase the risk of Zn deficiency in the elderly, namely, a reduced capacity to absorb Zn,[32] the increased likelihood of disease states that alter Zn utilization, the use of drugs such as diuretics that increase urinary Zn excretion, and consumption of fiber, calcium, or Fe supplements that may alter Zn bioavailability.

Assessment of Zn nutriture in the elderly is confounded by the effects of age itself on both functional and static indicators of status. Elderly subjects tend to have lower plasma Zn levels than younger adults.[87] Analysis of the results of the HANES-II survey showed that serum Zn levels of 65- to 74-year-old individuals were lower than those of young adults, and the difference was more obvious among men than women.[7] Generally, the average concentration of Zn in hair samples from elderly subjects is less than that in hair samples from younger adults and adolescents. Nonetheless, only a few elderly subjects had less than 70 μg of Zn/g hair, a concentration often used to define low hair Zn levels.[7]

Several clinical conditions associated with a poor Zn status also are problems commonly reported by the elderly, such as slow wound healing, anorexia, dermatitis, depressed taste acuity, and impaired immune function.[7] Double-blind or single-blind trials of Zn supplementation failed to improve these functions. Moreover, one needs to evaluate physiologic and pharmacologic doses. If Zn absorption is compromised in the elderly, administration of a larger Zn supplement together with a Zn-binding ligand such as histidine may be beneficial.

## MALABSORPTIVE DISORDERS

Diseases of the gastrointestinal tract are frequently complicated by Zn deficiency. Breakdown of integrity of the gastrointestinal tract reduces normal absorption of dietary Zn and disrupts the enteropancreatic Zn circulation. Zn deficiency has developed in the following malabsorptive disorders: Crohn's disease; sprue; short bowel syndrome; and jejunoileal bypass. Crohn's disease, or regional enteritis, is a type of inflammatory bowel disease. Many investigators have reported low serum Zn concentrations in patients with Crohn's disease, and it is not unusual to find depressed urinary Zn excretion.[69] Other clinical features of Zn deficiency have been reported in these patients, such as growth retardation, abnormal taste acuity, delayed sexual maturation, skin lesions, and retinal dysfunction.[88–90] The mechanisms for Zn deficiency and altered Zn metabolism in Crohn's disease are probably multifactorial. Dietary Zn intakes appear to be adequate,[89] but absorption is probably impaired. Using an oral Zn tolerance test, McClain et al. showed that patients with Crohn's disease had a 35% reduction in the area under the serum concentration curve compared to healthy controls.[89] Large gastrointestinal losses may result from the diarrhea common in these patients,[91] and urinary losses may be elevated because of catabolism of skeletal muscle. Plasma Zn concentrations of these patients may be low because of the release of the cytokinin, interleukin-1.

Decreased plasma Zn levels have been reported in patients with celiac sprue.[92] The area under the serum concentration curve for the Zn tolerance test is depressed in untreated sprue patients and improves when a gluten-free diet is fed. This indicates that Zn absorption is impaired. Jones and Peters measured disaccharidase activity in three patients with clinically mild, nonresponsive celiac disease and observed a modest increase in activity of some disaccharidases after Zn therapy.[93] Possibly, a marginal Zn deficiency exacerbates the disease state by further reducing the activity of intestinal disaccharidases.

Patients with short bowel syndrome have a double defect in Zn absorption. First, the absorptive surface of the small bowel is decreased and the transit time is increased. Second, intestinal reabsorption of Zn from the pancreatic juice is impaired if much of the distal bowel is removed.[69] Patients with short bowel syndrome have developed acrodermatitis, abnormal protein metabolism, and impaired immune function. All these problems were corrected with Zn supplementation.

Patients who have had intestinal bypass surgery frequently have depressed serum Zn levels.[69] Dietary Zn intake appears to be adequate in these patients. The capacity to absorb Zn has not been measured in bypass patients, but the oral Zn tolerance test suggests about a two-thirds reduction in the area under the serum concentration curve in postbypass patients in comparison to healthy controls.[94] A poor Zn status may contribute to the frequent incidence of opportunistic infections following jejunoileal bypass surgery.

## ALCOHOLISM

Patients with alcoholic cirrhosis are often characterized by hyperzincuria, hypozincemia, and low liver Zn concentrations compared to controls or to patients without cirrhosis.[95] Potential mechanisms underlying the hyperzincuria include the shifting of Zn in plasma to ligands that are easily excreted and that inhibit tubular reabsorption of Zn.[95,96] Although hypozincemia is most prevalent (70%) in alcoholics with liver disease,[95] it is also observed in some alcoholics (30 to 50%), with no evident liver disease. Consistent with human data, long-term alcohol feeding resulted in lower liver Zn concentrations in monkeys, rats, and pigs.[95,97]

Alcoholism-associated changes in Zn metabolism may well be functionally significant. Several studies have linked Zn deficiency and altered vitamin A metabolism in alcoholism.[95] As discussed previously, Zn deficiency can result in reductions in serum retinol concentrations and elevated liver vitamin A stores, presumably because of a reduction in the synthesis of retinol-binding protein in the liver. Zn deficiency can also result in low retinol-alcohol dehydrogenase activity in the retina. Zn administration to alcoholic patients can improve dark adaptation, a retinol dehydrogenase-dependent function.[96] Zn supplementation of patients with alcoholic cirrhosis has been reported to improve their immune responsivity.[95] Zn supplementation of alcoholics with low plasma Zn levels and hypogonadism can result in a return of normal gonadal function.[98]

Because the teratogenic expression of Zn deficiency is similar to that of fetal alcohol syndrome (FAS), one hypothesis is that the development of FAS is by an alcohol-induced embryonic Zn deficiency. Consistent with this suggestion, plasma and umbilical cord blood Zn concentrations have been reported to be lower in pregnant women who drink compared to controls.[99] Although maternal alcohol feeding in rats is associated with a reduction in placental Zn transfer in the second trimester and with lower than normal fetal liver Zn concentrations, dietary Zn supplementation has not been shown to affect FAS expression in animal models.[100] A direct role for altered Zn metabolism in the development of FAS in humans, however, has not been established. Nonetheless, given the negative effects associated with inadequate Zn delivery to the embryo/fetus, it would seem prudent to monitor closely the Zn status of pregnant alcoholic women and their children.

### DIABETES

Alterations in Zn metabolism have been shown to occur in both diabetic humans and experimental animals. Adult rats with genetically or chemically induced diabetes are characterized by Zn accumulation in the liver and kidney and by hyperzincuria.[101,102] Both type 1 and type 2 diabetic patients can exhibit hyperzincuria, which increases with the severity of the diabetes.[103] It has been postulated that the hyperzincuria can result in a conditioned Zn deficiency in some individuals, and hypozincemia is a relatively common finding in diabetics.[103] Zn supplementation of diabetic patients has been reported to improve their immune function.[53,104] In the rat, diabetes during pregnancy can result in fetal Zn depletion; this deficiency has been linked to the poor reproductive performance associated with diabetes in this model.[102] Whether altered Zn metabolism is also a factor underlying the increased risk of birth defects associated with diabetes in humans remains to be established. The mechanisms underlying altered Zn metabolism in the diabetic have not been firmly identified.

### PATIENTS WITH CHRONIC INFECTIONS AND/OR TRAUMA

As mentioned earlier, tissue-specific hormonal induction of metallothionein can occur during periods of acute disease (infection), stress, and inflammation. One consequence of metallothionein induction is a redistribution of body Zn, with the result that plasma Zn concentrations are often markedly reduced.[26] The long-term implications of low plasma Zn concentrations secondary to recurring acute-phase reactions have not been well defined, although potentially they could lead to Zn deficiency in select extrahepatic tissues. Although it is tempting to suggest that these individuals should be provided with Zn supplements, at present it is not clear whether the reduction in plasma Zn may actually represent a positive response of the patient to some insults. This issue clearly needs clarification.

### AIDS

Because patients with acquired immunodeficiency syndrome (AIDS) often exhibit immunologic abnormalities similar to those associated with Zn deficiency, Zn deficiency has been postulated to underlie the development of some of the disorders associated with AIDS. Although low plasma Zn concentrations have been reported in a number of AIDS patients, individuals with AIDS-related complex (ARC) and asymptomatic human immunodeficiency virus (HIV) positive subjects have been reported to have normal plasma Zn concentrations.[105] Thus, Zn deficiency is not a common contributory factor of HIV infectivity or its clinical expression. However, in the late stages of AIDS, excessive Zn loss from diarrhea, as well as from cytokine-directed redistribution of the element, may be expected to lower plasma Zn concentrations. The effects of chronic hypozincemia secondary to AIDS-related infections have not been delineated.

## ZINC TOXICITY

### ACUTE TOXICITY

Although rare, incidences of acute Zn toxicity in humans resulting from high intakes of Zn have been reported. Isolated outbreaks of Zn toxicity have occurred as a result of the consumption of foods and beverages contaminated with Zn released from galvanized containers. Typical signs of acute Zn toxicosis include epigastric pain, diarrhea, nausea, and vomiting.[106,107] Doses in excess of 200 mg a day are typically emetic. A fatal outcome occurred in a woman who was inadvertently given 1.5 g of Zn intravenously over a 3-day period.[108] Metal fume fever has been reported to occur following the inhalation of Zn oxide fumes. Signs develop within 8 hours and include hyperpnea, profuse sweating, and general weakness.[106] Signs of toxicity disappear 12 to 24 hours after the individual is removed from the Zn-contaminated environment.

### CHRONIC TOXICITY

The major consequence of the long-term ingestion of excessive Zn supplements is the induction of a secondary Cu deficiency caused by the competitive interaction between these elements with regard to intestinal absorption. Levels of Zn supplements as low as 25 mg per day have been reported to induce Cu deficiency. The long-term consumption of Zn supplements in excess of 150 mg per day has also been reported to result in low serum HDL levels, gastric erosion, and depressed immune function.[107]

## REFERENCES


1. Todd, W.R., Elvehjem, C.A., Hart, E.B.: Am. J. Physiol., *107:*146–156, 1934.
2. Hambidge, K.M., Casey, C.E., Krebs, N.F.: Zinc *In* Trace Elements in Human and Animal Nutrition. 5th Ed. Vol. 2. Edited by W. Mertz. Orlando, FL, Academic Press, 1986, pp. 1–137.
3. Prasad, A.S., Halsted, J.A., Nadimi, M.: Am. J. Med., *31:*532–546, 1961.
4. Welch, R.M., House, W.A., Van Campen, D.: J. Nutr., *107:*929–933, 1977.
5. Welsh, S.O., Marston, R.M.: Food Technol., *36:*70–76, 1982.
6. MacDonald, L.D., Gibson, R.S., Miles, J.E.: Acta Paediatr. Scand., *71:*785–789, 1982.
7. Greger, J.L.: Potential for trace mineral deficiencies and toxicities in the elderly. *In* Mineral Homeostasis in the Elderly. Current Topics in Nutrition and Disease. Vol. 21. Edited by C.W. Bales. New York, Marcel Dekker, 1989, pp. 171–200.
8. Schölmerich, J., Freudemann, A., Köttgen, E., et al.: Am. J. Clin. Nutr., *45:*1480–1486. 1987.
9. Sandström, B., Lönnerdal, B.: Promoters and antagonists of zinc absorption. *In* Zinc in Human Biology. Edited by C.F. Mills. London, International Life Sciences Institute, 1989, pp. 57–78.
10. Lönnerdal, B., Bell, J.G., Hendrickx, A.G., et al.: Am. J. Clin. Nutr., *48:*1301–1306, 1988.
11. Hurley, L.S., Keen, C.L., Lönnerdal, B.: Fed. Proc., *42:*1735–1739, 1983.
12. Festa, M.D., Anderson, H.L., Dowdy, R.P., et al.: Am. J. Clin. Nutr., *41:*285–292, 1985.
13. Brewer, G.J., Hill, G.M., Prasad, A.S.: Ann. Intern. Med., *99:*314–320, 1983.
14. Sandström, B., Davidsson, L., Cederblad, A., et al.: J. Nutr., *115:*411–414, 1985.
15. Valberg, L.S., Flanagan, P.R., Chamberlain, M.J.: Am. J. Clin. Nutr., *40:*536–541, 1984.
16. Southon, S., Wright, A.J., Fairweather-Tait, S.J.: Br. J. Nutr., *62:*415–423, 1989.
17. Lönnerdall, B., Keen, C.L., Hendrickx, A.G., et al.: Obstet. Gynecol., *75:*369–374, 1990.
18. Johnson, M.A., Baier, M.J., Greger, J.L.: Am. J. Clin. Nutr., *35:*1332–1338, 1982.
19. Chandler, C.J., Wang, T.T.Y., Halsted, C.H.: J. Biol. Chem., *261:*928–933, 1986.
20. Tamura, T., Shane, B., Baer, M.T., et al.: Am. J. Clin. Nutr., *31:*1984–1987, 1978.
21. Milne, D.B.: J. Trace Elements Exp. Med., *2:*297–304, 1989.
22. Swanson, C.A., King, J.C.: Am. J. Clin. Nutr., *4–6:*763–771, 1987.
23. Weigand, E.: Int. J. Vitam. Nutr., Res. *25(Suppl.):*67–81, 1983.
24. Matseshe, J.W., Phillips, S.F., Malagelada, J.-R., et al.: Am. J. Clin. Nutr., *33:*1946–1953, 1980.
25. Hoadley, J.E., Leinart, A.S., Cousins, R.J.: Am. J. Physiol., *252:*G825–G831, 1987.
26. Cousins, R.J.: Clin. Physiol. Biochem., *4:*20–30, 1986.
27. Coppen, D.E., Davies, N.T.: Br. J. Nutr., *57:*35–44, 1987.
28. Baer, M.T., King, J.C.: Am. J. Clin. Nutr., *39:*556–570, 1984.
29. Cousins, R.J.: Physiol. Rev., *65:*238–309, 1985.
30. Davies, N.T., Williams, R.B.: Br. J. Nutr., *38:*417–423, 1977.
31. Lönnerdal, B.: Intestinal absorption of zinc. *In* Zinc in Human Biology. Edited by C.F. Mills. London, International Life Sciences Institute, 1989, pp. 33–58.
32. Turnlund, J.R., Durkin, N., Costa, F., et al.: J. Nutr., *116:*1239–1247, 1986.
33. Aamodt, R.L., Rumble, W.F., Babcock, A.K., et al.: Metabolism, *31:*326–334, 1982.
34. Harris, W.R., Keen. C.L.: J. Nutr., *119:*1677–1682, 1989.
35. Masters, D.G., Keen, C.L., Lönnerdal, B., et al.: J. Nutr., *113:*905–912, 1983.
36. Jackson, M.J., Jones, D.A., Edwards, R.H.T., et al.: Br. J. Nutr., *51:*199–208, 1984.
37. Victery, W., Smith, J.M., Vander, A.J.: Am. J. Physiol., *241:*F532–F539, 1981.
38. Milne, D.B., Canfield, W.K., Mahalko, J.R., et al.: Am. J. Clin. Nutr., *39:*535–539, 1984.
39. Hess, F.M., King, J.C., Margen, S.: J. Nutr., *107:*1610–1620, 1977.
40. Vallee, B.L.: Zinc in biology and biochemistry. *In* Zinc Enzymes. Edited by T.G. Spiro. New York, John Wiley, 1983, pp. 1–24.
41. Chesters, J.K.: Biochemistry of zinc in cell division and

tissue growth. *In* Zinc in Human Biology. Edited by C.F. Mills. London, International Life Sciences Institute, 1989, pp. 109–118.
42. Bettger, W.J., Fish, T.J., O'Dell, B.L.: Proc. Soc. Exp. Biol. Med., *158:*279–282, 1978.
43. Wilson, R.L.: Zinc and iron in free radical pathology and cellular control. *In* Zinc in Human Biology. Edited by C.F. Mills. London, International Life Sciences Institute, 1989, pp. 147–172.
44. Kazimierczak, W., Adamas, B., Maslinski, C.: Biochem. Pharmacol., *27:*243–249, 1978.
45. Clegg, M.S., Keen, C.L., Hurley, L.S.: Biochemical pathologies of zinc deficiency. *In* Zinc in Human Biology. Edited by C.F. Mills. London, International Life Sciences Institute, 1989, pp. 129–146.
46. Berg, J.M.: J. Biol. Chem., *265:*6513–6516, 1990.
47. Oteiza, P.I., Cuellar, S., Lönnerdal, B., et al.: Teratology, *41:*97–104, 1990.
48. King. J.C.: J. Nutr., *120:*1474–1479, 1990.
49. Hurley, L.S., Gordon, P., Keen, C.L., et al.: Proc. Soc. Exp. Biol. Med., *170:*48–52, 1982.
50. Keen, C.L., Hurley, L.S.: Zinc and reproduction: effects of deficiency on foetal and postnatal development. *In* Zinc in Human Biology. Edited by C.F. Mills. London, International Life Sciences Institute, 1989, pp. 183–220.
51. O'Dell, B.L., Reeves, P.G.: Zinc status and food intake. *In* Zinc in Human Biology. Edited by C.F. Mills. London, International Life Sciences Institute, 1989, pp. 173–182.
52. Bergman, B., Friberg, U., Lohmander S., et al.: Scand. J. Dent. Res., *80:*486–492, 1972.
53. Keen, C.L., Gershwin, M.E.: Annu. Rev. Nutr., *10:*415–431, 1990.
54. Apgar, J.: Annu. Rev. Nutr., *5:*43–68, 1985.
55. Bunce, G.E.: Zinc in endocrine function. *In* Zinc in Human Biology. Edited by C.F. Mills. London, International Life Sciences Institute, 1989, pp. 249–258.
56. McClain, C.J., Gavaler, J.S., VanThiel, D.H.: J. Lab. Clin. Med., *104:*1007, 1984.
57. Koo, S.I., Lee, C.C.: Am. J. Clin. Nutr., *47:*120–127, 1988.
58. Bettger, W.J., Reeves, P.G., Moscatelli, E.A., et al.: J. Nutr., *109:*480–488, 1979.
59. Williams, R.B., Mills, C.F.: Br. J. Nutr., *24:*989–1003. 1970.
60. Walravens, P.A., Hambidge, K.M., Koepfer, D.M.: Pediatrics, *83:*532–538, 1989.
61. Hambidge, K.M., Walravens, P.A., Casey, C.E., et al.: J. Pediatr., *94:*607–608, 1979.
62. Krebs, N.F., Hambidge, K.M., Walravens, P.A.: Am. J. Dis. Child, *138:*270–273, 1984.
63. Golden, M.H.N., Golden, B.E.: Am. J. Clin. Nutr., *34:*900–908, 1981.
64. Henkin, R.I.: Biol. Trace Element Res., *6:*263–280, 1984.
65. Bogden, J.D., Oleske, J.M., Munves, E.M., et al.: Am. J. Clin. Nutr., *45:*101–109, 1987.
66. Abbasi, A.A., Prasad, A.S., Rabbani, P., et al.: J. Lab. Clin. Med., *96:*544–550, 1980.
67. Jameson, S., Burström, M., Hellsing, K.: Tema, 7, 1990.
68. Aggett, P.J.: Severe zinc deficiency. *In* Zinc in Human Biology. Edited by C.F. Mills. London, International Life Sciences Institute, 1989, pp. 259–280.
69. McClain, C.J.: J. Am. Coll. Nutr., *4:*49–64, 1985.
70. Wada, L., King, J.C.: J. Nutr., *116:*1045–1053, 1986.
71. King, J.C.: J. Am. Diet. Assoc., *86:*1523–1527, 1986.
72. Hambidge, K.M.: Mild zinc deficiency in human subjects. *In* Zinc in Human Biology. Edited by C.F. Mills. London, International Life Sciences Institute, 1989, pp. 281–296.
73. Fell, G.S., Cuthbertson, D.P., Morrison, C., et al.: Lancet, *1:*280–282, 1973.
74. Freeman, J.B., Stegink, L.D., May P.D., et al.: J. Surg. Res., *18:*463–469, 1975.
75. Weismann, K., Hoe, S., Nikkelsen, H.I., et al.: Br. J. Dermatol., *101:*573–579, 1979.
76. Hambidge, K.M., Walravens, P.A.: Clin. Gastroenterol., *11:*87–117, 1982.
77. King, A.B., Schwartz, R.: J. Nutr., *117:*704–708, 1987.
78. Cousins, R.J.: Systemic transport of zinc. *In* Zinc in Human Biology. Edited by C.F. Mills. London, International Life Sciences Institute, 1989, pp. 79–94.
79. Grider, A., Bailey, L.B., Cousins, R.J.: Proc. Natl. Acad. Sci. U.S.A., *87:*1259–1262, 1990.
80. Food and Nutrition Board, National Research Council: Recommended Dietary Allowances. 10th Ed. Washington, D.C., National Academy Press, 1989.
81. Keen, C.L., Lönnerdal, B., Golub, M.S., et al.: Pediatr. Res., *26:*470–477, 1989.
82. Jameson, S.: Acta Med. Scand., *593(Suppl.):* 1–89, 1976.
83. Simmer, K., Thompson, R.P.H.: Clin. Sci., *68:*395–399, 1985.
84. McMichael, A.J., Dreosti, I.E., Gibson, G.T., et al.: Early Hum. Dev., *7:*59–69, 1982.
85. Hunt, I.F., Murphy, N.J., Cleaver, A.E., et al.: Am. J. Clin. Nutr., *42:*815–828, 1985.
86. Hunt, I.F., Murphy, N.J., Cleaver, A.E., et al.: Am. J. Clin. Nutr., *40:*508–521, 1984.
87. Chooi, M.K., Todd, J.K., Boyd, N.D.: Nutr. Metab., *20:*135–142, 1976.
88. McClain, C.J., Su, L.-C., Gilbert, H., et al.: Dig. Dis. Sci., *28:*85–87, 1983.
89. McClain, C.J., Soutor, C., Zieve, L.: Gastroenterology, *78:*272–279, 1980.
90. Nishi, Y., Lifshitz, F., Bayne, M.A., et al.: Am. J. Clin. Nutr., *33:*2613–2621, 1980.
91. Sturniolo, G.C., Molokhia, M.M., Shields, R.R., et al.: Gut, *21:*387–391, 1980.
92. Elmes, M., Golden, M.K., Love, A.H.S.: Q. J. Mol. Med., *55:*293–306, 1978.
93. Jones, P.E., Peters, T.J.: Gut, *22:*194–198, 1981.
94. Andersson, K.E., Brat, L., Dencker, H., et al.: Eur. J. Clin. Pharmacol., *9:*423–428, 1976.
95. Halsted, C.H., Keen, C.L.: Eur. J. Gastroenterol. Hepatol., *2:*399–405, 1990.
96. McClain, C.J., Su, L.C.: Alcohol. Clin. Exp. Res., *7:*5–10, 1983.
97. Zidenberg-Cherr, S., Halsted, C.H., Olin, K.L., et al.: J. Nutr., *120:*213–217, 1990.
98. McClain, C.H., Van Thiel, J.H., Parker, S., et al.: Alcohol. Clin. Exp. Res., *3:*135–141, 1979.
99. Flynn, A., Martier, S.S., Sokol, R.J., et al.: Lancet, *1:*572–574, 1981.
100. Zidenberg-Cherr, S., Benak, P.A., Hurley, L.S., et al.: Drug-Nutrient Interact., *5:*257–274, 1988.
101. Failla, M.L., Kiser, R.A.: Am. J. Physiol., *244:*E115–121, 1983.
102. Uriu-Hare, J.Y., Stern, J.S., Keen, C.L.: Diabetes, *38:*1282–1290, 1989.
103. Walter, R.M., Uriu-Hare, J.Y., Olin, K.L., et al.: Diab. Care., *14:*1050–1056, 1991.
104. Niewoehmer, E., Allen, J.I., Boosalis, M., et al.: Am. J. Med., *81:*63–68, 1986.
105. Walter, R.M., Oster, M.H., Lee, T.J., et al.: Life Sci. *46:*1597–1600, 1990.

106. Bertholf, R.L.: Zinc. *In* Handbook on Toxicity of Inorganic Compounds. Edited by H.G. Seiler and H. Sigel. New York, Marcel Dekker, 1988.
107. Fosmire, G.M.: Am. J. Clin. Nutr., *51*:225–227, 1990.
108. Brocks, A., Ried, H., Glazer, G., et al.: Br. Med. J., *1*:1390–1391, 1977.

## SELECTED READINGS

Hambidge, K.M., Casey, C.E., Krebs, N.F.: Zinc. *In* Trace Elements in Human and Animal Nutrition. 5th Ed. Vol. 2. Edited by W. Mertz. Orlando, FL, Academic Press, 1986, pp. 1–137.

Keen, C.L., Gershwin, M.E.: Zinc deficiency and immune function. Annu. Rev. Nutr., *10*:415–431, 1990.

King, J.C.: Assessment of zinc status. J. Nutr., *120*:1474–1479, 1990.

Mills, C.F. (Ed.): Zinc in Human Biology. London, International Life Sciences Institute, 1989.

CHAPTER **11**

# Copper

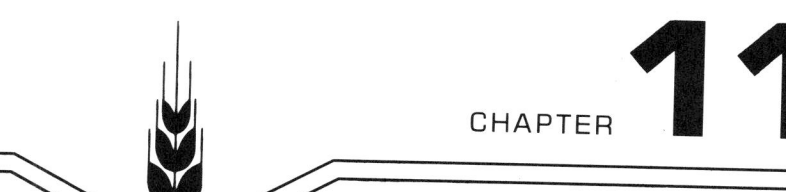

**Judith R. Turnlund**



## HISTORICAL INTRODUCTION

Copper has been used therapeutically since at least 400 B.C., when Hippocrates prescribed copper compounds for pulmonary and other diseases.[1] The use of copper compounds in the treatment of diseases reached its peak in the nineteenth century and subsequently declined when the treatments were not successful.

Copper was identified as a normal constituent of blood and its toxicity was described in the late nineteenth century. By 1900, an anemia that could not be prevented by iron supplements had been observed in animals kept on a whole-milk diet. In 1928, Hart reported that this anemia in rats was responsive to iron only when copper supplements were also given.[2] Experiments in several animal species produced similar results and suggested that copper deficiency anemia occurs in all species. Detailed reviews of the early history of copper have been published.[1,3]

Human disease was first linked to copper metabolism shortly after Wilson's disease was described in 1912, and long before the condition was recognized as an inborn error of metabolism in 1953.[1] As early as 1930, a relationship between anemia in humans and copper deficiency was suspected, but copper supplements only improved hemoglobin synthesis in some instances, so the hypothesis was not well accepted. Conclusive evidence of copper deficiency in humans was not reported until 1964.[4] Menkes' disease, another genetic disorder, was described in 1962 and recognized as a disorder of copper absorption in 1972. Since about 1950, an increasing number of diseases that are not specifically disorders of copper metabolism have been associated with altered, usually increased, levels of copper in blood or other tissues.

An official dietary copper recommendation, an Estimated Safe and Adequate Daily Dietary Intake of 31 to 47 μmol (2 to 3 mg), was first introduced in 1979.[5] The lower end of this range was reduced to 24 μmol (1.5 mg) in 1989.[6]

## CHEMISTRY

Copper, a transition metal with an atomic mass of 63.54 d, has two stable isotopes, $^{63}$Cu and $^{65}$Cu, with natural abundances of 69.2 and 30.8%, respectively. There are a number of radioisotopes of copper, all with relatively short half-lives. The two with the longest half-lives, $^{67}$Cu (61.9 hours) and $^{64}$Cu (12.9 hours), and the stable isotope, $^{65}$Cu, are used as tracers of copper metabolism.

Copper has two oxidation states, $Cu^{+}$ and $Cu^{2+}$, and may shift back and forth between the two during enzyme action. It may occur rarely as $Cu^{3+}$.[7] Only minute quantities of $Cu^{+}$ ions can exist in solution; thus $Cu^{+}$ compounds are highly insoluble and strongly complexed.[8] Copper is most often found in biologic systems as $Cu^{2+}$, each with distinctly different physicochemical properties, are found in copper-containing enzymes. Type 1 is a deep blue protein seen in many copper-containing oxidases. Type 2, present in many multicopper oxidases, is not blue, but is detectable by electron paramagnetic resonance (EPR). Type 3, neither blue nor detectable by EPR, is also found in a number of enzymes. A single protein may contain one or more types of copper.[7,9]

## DIETARY CONSIDERATIONS

Estimates of dietary intake of Americans prior to 1970 were considerably higher than current estimates. This reflects marked improvements in analytical techniques for measuring copper and awareness of the importance of avoiding copper contamination of analytical samples. It was thought that the usual diet contained from 30 to 80 μmol (2 to 5 mg) of copper, but studies, including one study of 132 diet composites, now show that few diets contain over 30 μmol (2 mg) per day.[10] Women consume an average of about 14 μmol (0.9 mg) per day; men, with higher energy intakes, consume about 19 μmol (1.2 mg) per day.[11] As with all nutrients, copper intake can vary widely, depending on food choices. Diets in countries where more whole-grain products, legumes, and organ meats are eaten contain more copper.

### FOOD SOURCES

The richest sources of dietary copper contain from 50 to over 300 nmol/g (0.3 to over 2 mg/100 g). These include shellfish, nuts, seeds (including cocoa powder), legumes, and the bran and germ portions of grains, liver, and organ meats. Most grain products, most products containing chocolate, fruits and vegetables such as dried fruits, mushrooms, tomatoes, bananas, grapes, and potatoes, and most meats have intermediate amounts of copper, from 20 to 50 nmol/g (0.1 to 0.3 mg/100 g). Other fruits and vegetables, chicken, many fish, and dairy products contain relatively low concentrations (less than 20 nmol/g [0.1 mg/100 g]) of copper.[12] Cow's milk is particularly low in copper.

Because information on the copper content of foods is incomplete and data bases often contain missing values, copper intake is underestimated unless missing values are replaced with imputed values. A table of the copper content of foods compiled when much of the available data were from the 1930s and 1940s reported consistently higher copper concentrations[13] than tables that exclude pre-1960 data, suggesting that early values are too high. However, a critical evaluation of the reliability of post-1960 published values for the copper content of foods demonstrated that improvement is still needed.[12]

### BIOAVAILABILITY

Estimates of the bioavailability of dietary copper to humans are usually based on absorption.[14] The amount of copper in the diet appears to influence bioavailability more than the composition of the diet or specific dietary components unless the levels are extremely high or low or when diet composition is unusual. Absorption is discussed under "Metabolism."

### INTERACTIONS WITH OTHER NUTRIENTS

Nutrients known to affect the bioavailability of copper when included in the diet of humans or animals in extreme amounts are iron, zinc, molybdenum, ascorbic acid, and carbohydrates. In addition, high or low levels of dietary copper may affect metabolism of some of these nutrients. Interactions between dietary copper and other nutrients or dietary components have been reviewed.[15,16]

**Iron.** Copper and iron may interact in a number of ways. As discussed under "Copper Deficiency," copper deficiency alters iron metabolism. Anemia, often accompanied by accumulation of iron in the liver, has been reported in all species studied, including humans. An excess of copper has produced anemia in the pig. Excessive iron in the form of inorganic iron salts decreased copper status and, in time, resulted in clinical signs of copper deficiency in several animal species.[16]

**Zinc.** When the diet contains excessive zinc over a sufficient period, the copper status of animals and humans has been impaired and the effect reversed by copper supplements. One explanation for this interaction is that high dietary zinc induces intestinal metallothionein (MT). Copper does not induce MT, but it has a stronger affinity for MT than for zinc. It displaces zinc in intestinal MT and is trapped.[3] Copper depletion was observed in humans when supplements of 280 μmol (50 mg) or more of zinc were given for extended periods. This caused concern that dietary zinc intake slightly above the recommended level might affect copper status, but copper absorption was not affected by 250 μmol (16.5 mg) of zinc per day. High doses of copper have in some cases reduced the effects of zinc deficiency in animals, but these effects were inconsistent.[17] In one study a high-copper diet reduced zinc absorption slightly and increased the excretion of zinc in young men, but did not impair zinc status.[18]

**Molybdenum.** Interactions between copper and molybdenum have been observed frequently in ruminants.[15] Slight excesses of molybdenum in the presence of sulfide produce molybdenum toxicity and secondary copper deficiency. A similar response in rats requires much more molybdenum and is independent of sulphur. One report of a high molybdenum diet in humans increasing urinary copper excretion suggests that a similar interaction could occur in humans. The toxicity of molybdenum in ruminants is ameliorated when dietary copper is increased.

**Ascorbic Acid.** Ascorbic acid supplements have produced copper deficiency in laboratory animals and may affect the copper status of humans. Daily ascorbic acid supplements of 8.5 mmol (1500 mg) given to young men caused ceruloplasmin to decline. Copper absorption was not impaired by 3.4 mmol (600 mg) of ascorbic acid, but ceruloplasmin declined and the results suggested that the oxidase activity of ceruloplasmin may be impaired by excessive ascorbic acid.[15]

**Carbohydrates.** The type of carbohydrate in the diet affects the rate and severity of copper depletion in rats. They are more resistant to copper deficiency when the carbohydrate source is cornstarch than when it is sucrose or fructose. The interaction between carbohydrate source and copper in humans is not clear, because in one study superoxide dismutase (SOD) levels of humans were lower with a high-fructose diet compared to a high-cornstarch diet, but copper retention increased.[19] In addition, research in young pigs, whose cardiovascular and gastrointestinal systems are similar to those in humans, suggests that the interaction observed in rats may not apply to humans.[20]

## METABOLISM

Mammalian copper metabolism is depicted schematically in Figure 11–1. Some copper in the diet is absorbed into the body through the intestinal mucosa, transported via the portal blood to the liver, and incorporated into ceruloplasmin. Ceruloplasmin is released into the blood and delivers copper to tissues throughout the body. Most endogenous copper is secreted into the gastrointestinal tract, where it combines with unabsorbed dietary copper and is eliminated from the body, and a small amount is eliminated through other excretory routes.

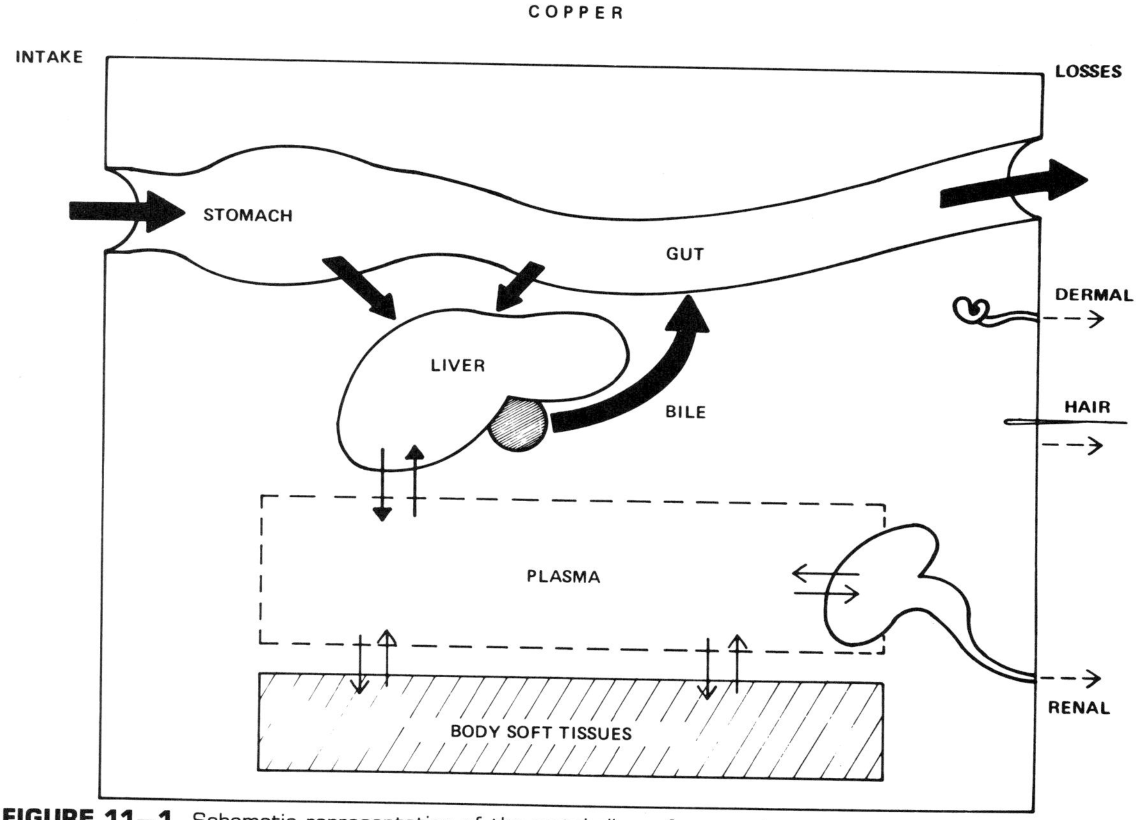
COPPER
INTAKE
LOSSES
STOMACH
GUT
LIVER
BILE
DERMAL
HAIR
PLASMA
RENAL
BODY SOFT TISSUES

**FIGURE 11–1.** Schematic representation of the metabolism of copper in mammals. (From Solomons, N.W.: Zinc and copper. *In* Modern Nutrition in Health and Disease, 7th Ed. Edited by M.E. Shils and V.R. Young. Philadelphia, Lea & Febiger, 1988.)

### ABSORPTION

Studies conducted with laboratory animals have begun to provide some basic information on the mechanism of copper absorption.[3,21] Copper is absorbed primarily in the small intestine, with a small amount absorbed in the stomach. Absorption is probably by a saturable, active transport mechanism at lower levels of dietary copper and, at high levels of dietary copper, passive diffusion plays a role. Absorption may be regulated by the need for copper, with MT in intestinal cells involved in the regulation.

During the past 10 years a stable isotope of copper has made it possible to measure copper absorption in humans more reliably than in the past.[14] Early estimates of copper absorption in humans ranged from 15 to 97%.[1] Estimates of copper absorption varied widely in part because of inadequate methods, and because the level of dietary copper was not known or controlled. A series of stable isotope studies of copper absorption have since demonstrated that the level of copper in the diet strongly influences absorption.[14] As dietary copper increases, the fraction absorbed declines and the amount absorbed increases. Absorption declined from 56% at 13 μmol (0.8 mg) Cu per day to 12% at 120 μmol (7.5 mg) Cu per day, and the amount absorbed increased from 6.9 to 15 μmol (0.44 mg to 0.93 mg), or doubled with a ninefold increase in dietary copper. This suggests that copper homeostasis is maintained in part by regulation of absorption. Another point of regulation appears to be via excretion into the gastrointestinal tract, as discussed under "Excretion."

### STORAGE

The adult human body contains only about 0.79 to 1.9 mmol (50 to 120 mg) of copper,[3] very little compared to other trace elements such as iron and zinc. Animal data suggest that copper is stored in the liver bound to MT-like proteins. Ruminants and a few other animal species can store much more copper in the liver than humans or most animal species. Copper may also be held, at least temporarily, bound to intestinal MT.

### TRANSPORT

Following absorption, copper is transported bound primarily to albumin, and to transcuprein and low-molecular-weight ligands.[21,22] The newly absorbed copper disappears rapidly from the plasma. Most is taken up by the liver and some is taken up by the kidney. Once in the liver, copper is incorporated into ceruloplasmin within hours. Some is incorporated into MT in the liver of animals, particularly when copper intake is high; a role for MT in cellular detoxification has been proposed.[23] A role for copper in the kidney is not known, but copper is probably filtered by the glomerulus and reabsorbed in the tubules,[24] because little copper is excreted in the urine.

Copper is released from the liver into the blood bound to ceruloplasmin and delivered to cells with specific ceruloplasmin receptors on their surface. Ceruloplasmin binds to these receptors; the copper is reduced, dissociates from ceruloplasmin, and is released into the cells.[25]

One suggested sequence leading to excretion of copper in bile is that ceruloplasmin with part of the copper removed may return to the liver, where it is partially degraded[21] and transferred to the bile accompanied by ceruloplasmin fragments. Glutathionine, although not a cuproenzyme, may play a role in the rapid transfer of excessive copper to bile.[26]

### EXCRETION

The primary route of copper excretion is via bile into the gastrointestinal tract. Little of this copper is reabsorbed. It combines with a small amount of copper from intestinal cells and from pancreatic and intestinal fluids, and with unabsorbed dietary copper; it is then eliminated in the feces. The excretion of biliary copper appears to be another point of regulation in the homeostatic control of copper retention. Animals and humans increase endogenous copper excretion when the diet is high in copper and excrete little during copper deficiency or when dietary copper is low.[14,21] The homeostatic regulation of copper absorption and excretion protects against copper deficiency and toxicity over a broad range of dietary intakes.

Other routes of excretion contribute little to total copper losses. Healthy humans excrete only 0.2 to 0.5 μmol (10 to 30 μg) of copper in the urine,[27] but urinary losses can increase markedly in some conditions, such as renal tubular defects.[24] Sweat and integumentary losses are usually less than 0.8 μmol (50 μg) per day.[27]

## FUNCTIONS

### BIOCHEMICAL

Copper functions in vivo as a part of a number of proteins, including many important enzymes. Detailed descriptions of these proteins and their functions have been published.[7,9,21] The copper proteins known to be present in human beings are listed in Table 11–1 and are described briefly in the following paragraphs. Many other copper-containing proteins are found in plants, lower organisms, and some animal species. Some of the better known of these include ascorbate oxidase, carboxypeptidase A, hemocianin, laccase, and uricase.

**TABLE 11–1.** COPPER-CONTAINING PROTEINS IN HUMANS

| |
|---|
| Copper-containing enzymes |
| Amine oxidases |
| Amine oxidase (flavin-containing)[monoamine oxidase, tyramine oxidase](EC 1.4.3.4)* |
| Amine oxidase (copper-containing)[diamine oxidase, histaminase](EC 1.4.3.6) |
| Lysyl oxidase(EC 1.4.3.13) |
| Ferroxidases |
| Ferroxidase I [ceruloplasmin](EC 1.16.3.1) |
| Ferroxidase II |
| Cytochrome *c* oxidase [cytochrome oxidase](EC 1.9.3.1) |
| Dopamine β-monooxygenase [dopamine β-hydroxylase] (EC 1.14.17.1) |
| Superoxide dismutase [hemocuprin, erythrocupin] (EC 1.15.1.1) |
| Extracellular superoxide dismutase |
| Copper/zinc superoxide dismutase |
| Monophenol monooxygenase [tyrosinase](EC 1.14.18.1) |
| Copper-binding proteins |
| Metallothionein |
| Albumin |
| Transcuprein |
| Bood clotting Factor V |
| Low-molecular-weight ligands |
| Amino acids |
| Peptides |

*The recommended names of enzymes are followed by other common names in brackets and by the code numbers assigned by the Nomenclature Committee of the International Union of Biochemistry[46] in parentheses.

## *COPPER-CONTAINING ENZYMES FOUND IN HUMAN BEINGS*

**Amine Oxidases.** Several important amine oxidases are cuproproteins. Relatively small amounts of these enzymes are found circulating in blood plasma, where they inactivate and catabolize physiologically active amines such as histidine, tyramine, and polyamines. They are found in tissues throughout the body. Their activity is elevated in conditions in which connective tissue activation and deposition take place, including liver fibrosis, congestive heart failure, hyperthyroidism, childhood, and senescence.[21]

*Monoamine Oxidase.* Monoamine oxidase is involved in inactivation of catecholamines. It reacts with substances such as serotonin, norepinephrine, tyramine, and dopamine. The enzyme is inhibited by tricyclic antidepressant drugs.

*Diamine Oxidase.* A number of copper-dependent diamine oxidase enzymes are found in cells throughout the body. Diamine oxidase inactivates histamine, acting in the small intestine, where histamine stimulates acid secretion, and in allergic reactions throughout the body, where histamine is released in response to exposure to antigens. It also inactivates polyamines involved in cell proliferation, which suggests that diamine oxidase may play a role in limiting excessive growth. Diamine oxidase activity is highest in the small intestine. Activity is also high in the kidney, where diamine oxidase inactivates diamines filtered from the blood, and in maternal placenta, where it may inactivate amines produced by the fetus.

*Lysyl Oxidase.* Lysyl oxidase, a unique amine oxidase, acts on lysine and hydroxylysine sidechains of collagen and elastin. It deaminates the lysine of newly formed, immature elastin and collagen, after which cross-links are formed. The enzyme functions in the formation of connective tissue, including bone, blood vessels, vasculature, skin, lungs, and teeth. The concentrations are highest during development. Long-term estrogen treatment increases the activity of lysyl oxidase, and malignant transformation decreases activity.

**Ferroxidases**

*Ceruloplasmin.* Ceruloplasmin, also called ferroxidase I, is an $\alpha_2$ glycoprotein with a molecular weight of about 150,000 d. It contains six (possibly seven) atoms of copper per molecule, including $Cu^{2+}$ atoms of all three types described under "Chemistry." Four copper atoms appear to be involved in the oxidation/reduction reactions the enzyme catalyzes. The role of the other atoms is not yet understood. This enzyme catalyzes the oxidation of ferrous iron and plays a role in the transfer of iron from storage to sites of hemoglobin synthesis. Ceruloplasmin also oxidizes aromatic amines and phenols.

Most of the copper in blood plasma is bound to ceruloplasmin. Until 1985, estimates of the ceruloplasmin fraction ranged from 80 to 95%, but recent work suggests that only about 60% of the plasma copper may be in ceruloplasmin.[28] The fraction of plasma copper associated with ceruloplasmin appears to be relatively constant within an individual, but varies considerably among individuals.[27]

*Ferroxidase II.* Ferroxidase II is another enzyme that catalyzes the oxidation of ferrous iron. It accounts for only about 5% of the ferroxidase activity in human plasma, but plays a more important role in some animal species.

**Cytochrome *c* Oxidase.** This enzyme, present in the mitochondria of cells throughout the body, is the terminal link in the electron transport chain. It reduces $O_2$ to form water, and permits the formation of adenosine triphosphate (ATP) in mitochondrial energy production. Cytochrome *c* oxidase is considered the single most important enzyme of the mammalian cell, because it is rate-limiting in electron transport.[22] It contains two or three copper atoms per molecule. The activity of this enzyme is highest in the heart and high in brain, liver, and kidney tissues.

**Dopamine β-Hydroxylase.** This enzyme catalyzes the conversion of dopamine to the neurotransmitter, norepinephrine, in the brain. Estimates of the copper content of dopamine β-hydroxylase range from two to eight atoms per molecule, with the most recent estimates being the higher amount.[29] Dopamine β-hydroxylase concentration is two to three times higher in gray matter of the brain than in white matter, and it is present in the adrenal gland, where it is required for epinephrine production.

**Superoxide Dismutase**

*Extracellular Superoxide Dismutase (EC-SOD).* EC-SOD, a copper-containing enzyme, is present in high amounts in the lungs, thyroid, and uterus and in small amounts in blood plasma. It functions as a scavenger of superoxide radicals and protects against oxidative damage.

*Copper/Zinc Superoxide Dismutase (SOD).* This enzyme, which contains two copper atoms per molecule, is present within most cells of the body, primarily within the cytosol. It protects intracellular components from oxidative damage, converting the superoxide ion to hydrogen peroxide. High concentrations are found in brain, thyroid, liver, pituitary, erythrocytes, and kidney of humans. Erythrocyte levels of SOD are high in alcoholics and individuals with Down's syndrome.

**Tyrosinase.** Tyrosinase catalyzes the conversion of tyrosine to dopamine and the oxidation of dopamine to dopaquinone, steps that take place in the synthesis of melanin. It is present in the melanocytes of the eye and skin and is responsible for the color in hair, skin, and eyes. Deficiency of tyrosinase in skin leads to albinism.

*COPPER-BINDING PROTEINS*

**Metallothionein (MT).** MTs are small, nonenzymatic proteins, rich in cysteine, which is responsible for binding copper. Each molecule can bind 11 or 12 copper atoms, as well as zinc and cadmium. It appears to play a role in metal storage and sequesters excess metal ions, preventing toxicity. The concentration is highest in the liver, where metals accumulate in MT fractions. MT is found in many other human tissues, including small amounts in the blood plasma. The presence in blood plasma has prompted the suggestion that MT also plays a role in copper transport, but if so, the role would be minor.[21]

**Albumin.** Albumin, a protein with a molecular weight of 68,000 d, is the most prevalent protein in blood plasma and interstitial fluids. Albumin binds and transports copper and may also play a role in binding excess copper that would otherwise be toxic. The usual estimate that 5 to 10% of the copper in blood plasma is bound to albumin may be slightly low. A tentative recent estimate is 18%, but this is not yet well established.[21]

**Transcuprein.** Transcuprein, a recently isolated plasma protein with a molecular weight of about 270,000 d, binds copper and is found in human plasma. It has not yet been completely characterized and its functions are not clear, but it may play a role in copper transport. A considerably smaller fraction of serum copper is bound to transcuprein than to albumin.[21]

**Blood Clotting Factor V.** This nonenzymatic component of the blood clotting process has recently been found to contain one atom of copper per molecule.[30] Although this indicates that copper is required for blood clotting, impaired blood clotting is not among the reported manifestations of copper deficiency.

*LOW-MOLECULAR-WEIGHT LIGANDS*

Amino acids and small peptides also carry a small fraction of the copper in the blood plasma. Estimates range from less than 1% to 4%.[21] Histidine, glutamine, threonine, and cystine are examples of amino acids that bind copper in the plasma, and at least one copper peptide complex, glycyl-histidine-lysine, has been isolated from human plasma. The role of these complexes is not known, but the copper carried by low-molecular-weight ligands is thought to exchange with nonceruloplasmin copper in the blood. The ligands may carry copper to cells.[31]

**PHYSIOLOGIC**

Many of the physiologic functions of copper can be deduced from reactions the cuproenzymes catalyze. Others are based on symptoms of copper deficiency. Detailed reviews of the physiologic functions of copper have been published.[1,3,32]

**Connective Tissue Formation.** Copper, through the enzyme lysyl oxidase, is essential for cross-linking of collagen and elastin, which are required for the formation of strong, flexible connective tissue. Thus, it plays a role in bone formation, skeletal mineralization, and the integrity of the connective tissue in the heart and vascular system.

**Iron Metabolism.** Several mechanisms have been proposed for the role of copper in iron metabolism and erythropoiesis.[33] Ceruloplasmin and ferroxidase II oxidize ferrous iron, so it can be transported from the intestinal lumen and storage sites to sites of erythropoiesis. This may explain why anemia develops with copper deficiency, yet iron accumulates in the intestinal lumen and liver. Copper may also be required for the formation of normal bone marrow cells, necessary for the formation of red blood cells.

**Central Nervous System.** Copper plays more than one role in the central nervous system. It is required for the formation or maintenance of myelin, a protective layer covering neurons composed primarily of phospholipids. Phospholipid synthesis depends on cytochrome *c* oxidase activity, which may explain why copper deficiency leads to poor myelination, necrosis of nerve tissue, and neonatal ataxia in copper-deficient animals. The role of cuproenzymes in catecholamine metabolism (the conversion of dopamine to norepinephrine by dopamine β-hydroxylase and the degradation of serotonin, norepinephrine, tyramine, and dopamine by monoamine oxidase) implies a function in normal neurotransmission.

**Melanin Pigment Formation.** The role of copper in the pigmentation of skin, hair, and eyes is related to the requirement for tyrosinase in melanin synthesis. Depigmentation of hair and skin is observed with copper deficiency in several animal species.

**Other Functions.** Other physiologic functions suggested for copper are not as well understood as those described previously. These include roles for copper in thermal regulation, cholesterol metabolism, glucose metabolism, immune function, and cardiac function. Some roles, such as in protection from oxidative damage through superoxide dismutase and in blood clotting through Factor V, are known but have not yet been clearly associated with clinical manifestations of copper deficiency.

## DEFICIENCY IN HUMANS AND ANIMALS

### COPPER DEFICIENCY IN ANIMALS

Copper deficiency has been produced experimentally and observed in areas with copper-deficient soil in rats, mice, guinea pigs, rabbits, chicks, pigs, dogs, cattle, goats, and sheep. Detailed descriptions of deficiency symptoms and comparisons among species have been published.[1,3,24] Animal studies have provided definitive information on the manifestations of copper deficiency. However, the deficiencies produced in animals were more severe than those reported in humans, and species differences make extrapolation to humans difficult.

Anemia, neutropenia, and osteoporosis are observed with copper deficiency in all species. Other well-established manifestations of copper deficiency observed in animal species are skeletal abnormalities, fractures, and spinal deformities; neonatal ataxia; depigmentation of hair and wool; impaired keratinization of hair, fur, and wool; reproductive failure, including low fertility, fetal death, and resorption; cardiovascular disorders including degeneration of myocardium, cardiac hypertrophy and failure, rupture of blood vessels, and electrocardiographic changes; and impaired immune function. Some manifestations of copper deficiency are considered controversial because they have only been observed in one or two species or under specific dietary conditions such as unusually high levels of fructose or zinc.[3] These include changes in lipid and cholesterol metabolism, increased lipid peroxidation, and impaired glucose metabolism.

### COPPER DEFICIENCY IN HUMANS

For years following the discovery of copper deficiency in laboratory animals it was considered unlikely that copper deficiency could occur in humans. Although copper deficiency in humans is relatively rare, it has been reported a number of times since 1964 under special circumstances. Reviews of copper deficiency in humans have been published.[24,33]

Copper deficiency has been clearly documented in infants recovering from malnutrition, in premature and low-birth-weight infants fed milk diets, and in patients receiving prolonged total parenteral nutrition. In established cases, blood was sampled for determination of serum copper and ceruloplasmin prior to administration of copper supplements, and manifestations of copper deficiency were reversed following copper supplementation.

Frank copper deficiency is accompanied by hypocupremia and low ceruloplasmin levels. Levels fall to 30% of normal and below. Serum copper values as low as 0.5 μmol/dl (3 μg/dl) and ceruloplasmin values as low as 35 mg/L (3.5 mg/dl) have been reported.[34] Usual features of copper deficiency are anemia, leukopenia, and neutropenia. The anemia is most often described as normocytic and hypochromic, but is sometimes normochromic and sometimes microcytic. Osteoporosis is often observed when bones are still growing and may be accompanied by flaring of the metaphyses and fractures at the margins of the metaphyses.

The possibility of mild copper deficiency due to marginal copper intake over a long period has been suggested. Possible manifestations, in addition to the features of severe deficiency, are conditions such as arthritis, arterial disease, loss of pigmentation, myocardial disease, and neurologic effects.[24] Diminished glucose tolerance, increased serum cholesterol, and heart beat irregularities have been linked to marginal copper intake.[3] These conditions were not accompanied by the low ceruloplasmin or serum copper levels or other features of severe deficiency, but serum copper levels declined in one individual with these symptoms. Dietary copper intake in these studies was within the range of intakes consumed by a large segment of the population, 13 to 16 μmol (0.8 to 1 mg) per day, and these effects were not produced in other studies at this level of dietary copper.[27] Further research is required to establish whether these conditions are related to copper status or not, but this is complicated by ethical considerations, the possibility that some individuals may have a higher copper requirement than others, and possible nutrient interactions.

## EVALUATION OF COPPER STATUS

Currently used indices of copper status easily detect severe copper deficiency. Serum copper and ceruloplasmin concentrations fall to levels far below the normal range and respond quickly to copper supplementation.[24] Ceruloplasmin has generally been considered the most reliable index of copper status,[35] but some consider red cell superoxide dismutase may be equally or more sensitive.[36] SOD values have not yet been reported in cases of severe copper deficiency in humans, and a level that would indicate copper deficiency has not been established. The normal ranges of these indices vary between laboratories, but are approximately as follows: 10.0 to 24.6 μmol/L (64 to 156 μg/dl) for serum copper; 180 to 400 mg/L (18 to 40 mg/dl) for ceruloplasmin; and 0.47 ± 0.067 mg/g for erythrocyte SOD.[15]

Although serum copper and ceruloplasmin clearly reflect severe deficiency, they may not be sensitive to marginal copper status. In addition, ceruloplasmin is an acute phase reactant and, as a result, serum copper and ceruloplasmin are elevated in a variety of conditions. Serum copper and ceruloplasmin could be within the normal range or even elevated, masking copper deficiency when one of these conditions occurs at the same time.

The search for a reliable index of marginal copper status has been unsuccessful, though a number of possibilities have been suggested.[24] Copper levels in the urine, hair, nails, or saliva do not appear to reflect copper status. Cytochrome oxidase in red cells, or possibly in platelets or white cells,[37] may be sensitive to copper status, but more data are needed. Stable isotope measurements of total body copper, the exchangeable copper pool size, or copper turnover may prove useful in evaluating copper status, but research in this area has just begun.[38]

## REQUIREMENTS AND RECOMMENDED INTAKES

A dietary copper requirement, the lowest dietary level at which copper status can be maintained by most healthy individuals, has not been established. Copper depletion/repletion studies have not been done in healthy humans with a copper intake low enough to produce systematic depletion of copper status. The establishment of a dietary copper requirement has been hampered by concern that marginal copper status may go undetected because of the lack of an index of marginal status. Relatively few cases of frank copper deficiency have been reported, and these have been accompanied by confounding factors such as malnutrition, malabsorption, and excessive gastrointestinal losses, limiting their value in establishing a minimum requirement.

The most relevant example of a diet containing less than the minimum copper requirement may be the following: An enteral diet containing 0.56 pmol/J (15 μg Cu/100 kcal) produced copper deficiency in six out of six severely handicapped patients between the ages of 4 and 24 years after they had consumed the diet for 12 to 66 months. Serum copper values of 1.8 to 7.2 μmol/L (11.7 to 45.7 μg/dl) and ceruloplasmin values of 30 to 125 mg/L (3 to 12.5 mg/dl) were discovered, accompanied by other manifestations of copper deficiency. These values had increased to within the normal range when measured 3 months after copper supplementation.[39] By extrapolation, though it may not be valid to extrapolate from these growing, severely handicapped individuals to healthy adults, copper deficiency could be expected to develop eventually if the diet contained 0.56 pmol/J (15 μg Cu/100 kcal, or 0.44 mg Cu/2900 kcal for men and 0.29 mg Cu/1900 kcal for women).

The above example, combined with a study in which healthy young men maintained copper balance and status at 12 μmol (0.79 mg) per day,[14] suggests the minimum copper requirement of men is somewhere between 7 and 12 μmol (0.44 and 0.79 mg) per day.

The daily dietary copper intake range recommended by the National Research Council of the United States is now 24 to 47 μmol (1.5 to 3.0 mg) for adults. Recommended daily ranges for children are 6 to 9 μmol (0.4 to 0.6 mg) for infants 0 to 6 months of age, increasing to 24 to 39 μmol (1.5 to 2.5 mg) for children over 11 years of age. A daily dietary copper recommendation for adults of below 24 μmol (1.5 mg) is expected in the revised World Health Organization (WHO) publication on Trace Elements on Nutrition.

## TOXICITY IN HUMANS AND ANIMALS

Copper toxicity can occur in all animal species. It has been observed in sheep, cattle, pigs, rats, and poultry, as well as in humans. The effects of copper poisoning and the levels required for deleterious effects to develop have been reviewed.[3]

### COPPER TOXICITY IN ANIMALS

Tolerance to high levels of copper differs greatly from one species to another, with sheep being the most susceptible to copper poisoning and rats having high tolerance to excessive copper. Because of species differences and the effects of the levels of zinc, iron, and molybdenum in the diet, the minimum toxic copper level varies. Deleterious effects were observed in pigs at 4 μmol/g (250 μg Cu/g) diet, but could be avoided by increasing the amount of iron and zinc in the diet. Poultry exhibit slowed growth and egg production at 8 μmol/g (500 μg/g), and fatality can occur at 19 μmol/g (1200 μg/g). Sheep have developed copper toxicosis from diets containing 0.19 μmol/g (12 μg/g), and some breeds of sheep are more susceptible to excess copper than others. Copper chloride is more toxic than copper sulfate; lower levels of copper are toxic when the molybdenum content of the diet is low. Single doses of 0.31 to 1.8 mmol (20 to 100 mg) copper per kilogram of body weight have been toxic. Cattle are susceptible to toxicity when diets contain 3 to 12 times the required level of copper. Ruminants can store more copper in their livers than other animals, and symptoms of toxicity appear when the capacity of the liver to sequester copper has been exceeded. Manifestations of copper toxicity include weakness, tremors, anorexia, and jaundice. Tissue copper levels increase, producing liver, kidney, and brain damage, and hemolytic crisis may follow.

### COPPER TOXICITY IN HUMANS

Acute copper poisoning has been observed to occur in the following ways: accidental consumption by children, ingestion of several grams in suicide attempts, following the application of copper salts to burned skin, drinking water from contaminated water supplies, or consumption of acidic food or beverages that had been stored in copper containers. Excessive copper produces epigastric pain, nausea, vomiting, and diarrhea, which usually prevents the more serious manifestations of copper toxicity. Serious manifestations include coma, oliguria, hepatic necrosis, vascular collapse, and death. Chronic copper toxicosis has been observed in dialysis patients following months of hemodialysis when copper tubing was used and in vineyard workers using copper compounds as pesticides. The amount of oral copper required to produce toxic effects is not well established, but liver damage in two infants may have been related to consuming water with 31 to 47 μmol Cu/L (2 to 3 mg Cu/L) in early infancy.[40] An extremely wide range of oral copper, beginning at 1.1 μmol/kg (0.07 mg/kg) per day, has been associated with gastrointestinal effects. Wilson's disease, a genetic disorder, and certain liver and biliary diseases, described below, are associated with accumulation of toxic levels of copper in the liver and other tissues without excessive intake.

## HIGH-RISK CLINICAL SITUATIONS

### GENETIC DEFECTS IN COPPER METABOLISM

The two best-known defects in copper metabolism in humans are Menkes' disease and Wilson's disease. Several defects in production of cuproenzymes have been identified, including overproduction of SOD in Down's syndrome, absence of tyrosinase in albinism, changes in lysyl oxidase in cutis laxa (Ehlers-Danlos syndrome), and myopathy due to reduction in cytochrome *c* oxidase. Genetic defects in copper metabolism have also been observed in mice and dogs. The reader is referred to a review of genetic diseases of copper metabolism.[41]

**Menkes' Disease.** Menkes' disease is a fatal X-linked disorder characterized by mental retardation, abnormal hair, and maldistribution of copper.[42,43] It occurs in 1 in 50,000 to 100,000 live births and is usually fatal by the age of 3 years. Serum copper and ceruloplasmin levels are low, as are levels in liver and brain, but copper accumulates in intestinal mucosa, muscle, spleen, and kidney. Synthesis of ceruloplasmin, SOD, and cytochrome oxidase is impaired. Abnormalities in connective tissue cross-linking due to dysfunction of lysyl oxidase result in defective arteries in the brain and elsewhere, and in osteoporosis. Progressive nerve degeneration in the brain results in intellectual deterioration, hypotonia, and seizures. Hypothermia is common. Skin and hair are poorly pigmented and hair is characteristically "kinky." The anemia and neutropenia common to nutritional copper deficiency are not found in Menkes' disease, a difference that cannot be explained. Administration of parenteral copper increases serum copper and ceruloplasmin, but does not improve brain function or slow the progressive deterioration.

**Wilson's Disease.** Wilson's disease is an autosomal recessive disease of copper storage. The prevalence of the defect is uncertain, but has been estimated at approximately 1 in 200,000 in the United States. Copper accumulates in the liver, the brain, and the cornea of the eye (Kayser-Fleisher rings). Urinary copper excretion is abnormally high, but ceruloplasmin values are usually low. There appears to be a defect in the catabolism and excretion of ceruloplasmin copper into the bile. If the disease goes untreated, copper accumulation in the liver and brain results in neurologic damage and cirrhosis. Hepatitis, hemolytic crisis, and hepatic failure may ensue. Early diagnosis and treatment can prevent the severe consequences of the disease. Dietary copper restriction was advocated for Wilson's disease at one time, but chelation therapy, usually using D-penicillamine, is much more effective in reducing copper stores.[44] Avoidance of large quantities of foods rich in copper may also be recommended, but diets very low in copper are not necessary. D-penicillamine is an antimetabolite of pyridoxine, so daily pyridoxine supplements of 75 to 150 nmol (12.5 to 25 mg) are recommended. The treatment induces removal of excess copper and prevents reaccumulation through excretion of 16 to 79 μmol (1 to 5 mg) copper daily in the urine. Oral zinc supplements to help avoid copper accumulation have been studied, but cannot be expected to replace chelation therapy.

## CLINICAL CONDITIONS WITH INCREASED RISK OF COPPER DEPLETION

Most severe copper deficiency cases reported to date have been associated with other clinical conditions.[24] Copper deficiency has been documented during total parenteral nutrition, in premature infants fed milk formulas, in infants recovering from malnutrition (usually associated with chronic diarrhea), in infants undergoing chronic peritoneal dialysis, and in severely handicapped patients. Two cases of copper deficiency were observed in full-term infants fed only cow's milk. Increased gastrointestinal losses due to diarrhea or fistulas increase copper losses and the risk of copper depletion. Diseases of malabsorption such as celiac disease and nontropical sprue increase the risk of copper depletion because of both malabsorption and increased losses. Prolonged use of antacids and long-term therapy with very high doses of zinc in treatment of sickle cell anemia have resulted in hypocupremia and some manifestations of copper deficiency.

**Parenteral Nutrition.** The realization that trace element deficiencies sometimes follow prolonged parenteral nutrition prompted recommendations that several trace elements, including copper, be added to the solutions. Guidelines for their preparation and addition were established in 1979, and these elements are now added routinely in the United States. Copper deficiency usually develops after months of parenteral nutrition without added copper; the risk of deficiency developing is increased substantially in individuals with excessive gastrointestinal losses. Free amino acid solutions increase urinary copper losses, adding to the risk. Adults receiving total parenteral nutrition (TPN) who did not have excessive gastrointestinal fluid losses could maintain balance and normal serum and ceruloplasmin levels on only 3.9 μmol (0.25 mg) Cu per day. These values did not increase after supplementation with copper. In contrast, serum copper and ceruloplasmin values declined steadily in others receiving a TPN solution in which copper was not detectable, and these indices increased when oral feeding was resumed. Stable adult patients receiving TPN need about 4.7 μmol (0.3 mg) Cu daily to maintain balance. The requirements are increased to 6 to 8 μmol (0.4 to 0.5 mg) daily with excessive gastrointestinal losses and should be reduced in patients with cholestasis and impaired biliary excretion.[45]

## CLINICAL CONDITIONS ACCOMPANIED BY COPPER ACCUMULATION

Copper can accumulate in the liver in any disease that causes impaired biliary excretion. Wilson's disease was discussed above. Liver copper is extremely elevated in Indian childhood cirrhosis, and very high levels are found in primary biliary cirrhosis and biliary atresia. Copper chelation rather than dietary copper restriction is recommended, and D-penicillamine is effective in reducing the liver copper stores in these diseases.[44]

## CONDITIONS WITH INCREASED SERUM COPPER

Serum copper and ceruloplasmin levels rise progressively during pregnancy, usually reaching twice-normal levels by term. They rise, often to two to three times normal values, in inflammatory conditions, infectious diseases, hematologic diseases, diabetes, coronary and cardiovascular diseases, uremia, and malignant diseases, and following surgery.[1,3] Smoking and some drugs will also increase serum copper concentrations. Ceruloplasmin is an acute-phase reactant, and the rise in ceruloplasmin is probably responsible for the increase in serum copper in the above conditions, because the increases parallel one another. The mechanism for the increase or the role for ceruloplasmin is not understood, but is under investigation in several laboratories.[21]

## REFERENCES


1. Mason, K.E.: J. Nutr., *109*:1979–2066, 1979.
2. Hart, E.B., Steenbock, J., Waddell, J., et al.: J. Biol. Chem., *77*:797–812, 1928.
3. Davis, G.K., Mertz, W.: Copper. *In* Trace Elements in Human and Animal Nutrition, Vol. 1. 5th Ed. Edited by W. Mertz. San Diego, Academic Press, 1987, pp. 301–364.
4. Cordano, A., Baerti, J.M., Graham, G.G.: Pediatrics, *34*:324–336, 1964.
5. Food and Nutrition Board, National Research Council: Recommended Dietary Allowances. 9th Ed. Washington, D.C., National Academy of Sciences, 1980.
6. Food and Nutrition Board, National Research Council: Recommended Dietary Allowances. 10th Ed. Washington, D.C., National Academy Press, 1989.
7. Owen, C.A.: Biochemical Aspects of Copper. Copper Proteins, Ceruloplasmin, and Copper Protein Binding. Park Ridge, NJ, Noyes Publications, 1982.
8. Dyer, F.F., Leddicotte, G.W.: The Radiochemistry of Copper. Washington, D.C., National Academy of Sciences, National Research Council, 1961.
9. Weser, U., Schubotz, L.M., Younes, M.: Chemistry of copper proteins and enzymes. *In* Copper and the Environment. Part II, Health Effects. Edited by J.O. Nriugu. New York, J. Wiley & Sons, 1979, pp. 197–239.
10. Holden, J.M., Wolf, W.R., Mertz, W.: J. Am. Diet. Assoc., *75*:23–28, 1979.
11. Pennington, J.A.T., Wilson, D.B.: J. Am. Diet. Assoc., *90*:375–381, 1990.

12. Lurie, D.G., Holden, J.M., Schubert, A., et al.: J. Food Comp. Anal., *2*:298–316, 1989.
13. Pennington, J.T., Calloway, D.H.: J. Am. Diet. Assoc., *63*:143–153, 1973.
14. Turnlund, J.R., Keyes, W.R., Anderson, H.L., et al.: Am. J. Clin. Nutr., *49*:870–878, 1989.
15. Turnlund, J.R.: J. Am. Diet. Assoc., *88*:303–310, 1988.
16. Gawthorne, J.M.: Copper interactions. *In* Copper in Animals and Man, Vol. 1. Edited by J.M. Howell and J.M. Gawthorne. Boca Raton, FL, CRC Press, 1987, pp. 79–100.
17. Kirchgessner, M.: Interactions of copper with other trace elements. *In* Copper and the Environment, Part II. Health Effects. Edited by J.O. Nriugu. New York, J. Wiley & Sons, 1979, pp. 433–472.
18. Turnlund, J.R., Keyes, W.R., Anderson, H.L.: High dietary copper decreases zinc absorption, as determined with the stable isotope 67Zn. *In* Trace Elements in Man and Animals. Edited by B. Momcilovic. Zagreb, Institute for Medical Research and Occupational Health, University of Zagreb, 1991, pp. 5/13–5/15.
19. Reiser, S., Smith, J.C., Mertz, W., et al.: Am. J. Clin. Nutr., *42*:242–251, 1985.
20. Schoenemann, H.M., Failla, M.L., Steele, N.C.: Am. J. Clin. Nutr., *52*:147–154, 1990.
21. Linder, M.C.: The Biochemistry of Copper. New York, Plenum Press, 1990.
22. Frieden, E.: Clin. Physiol. Biochem., *4*:11–19, 1986.
23. Bremner, I.: J. Nutr., *117*:19–29, 1987.
24. Danks, D.M.: Ann. Rev. Nutr., *8*:235–257, 1988.
25. Harris, E.D., Percival, S.S.: Copper transport: Insights into a ceruloplasmin-based delivery system. *In* Copper Bioavailability and Metabolism. Edited by C. Kies. New York, Plenum Press, 1990, pp. 95–102.
26. Houwen, R., Dijkstra, M., Kuipers, F., et al.: Biochem. Pharmacol., *39*:1039–1044, 1990.
27. Turnlund, J.R., Keen, C.L., Smith, R.G.: Am. J. Clin. Nutr., *51*:658–664, 1990.
28. Wirth, P.L., Linder, M.C.: J. Natl. Cancer Inst., *75*:277–284, 1985.
29. McCracken, J., Desai, P.R., Papadopoulos, N.J., et al.: Biochemistry, *27*:4133–4137, 1988.
30. Mann, K.G., Lawler, C.M., Vehar, G.A., et al.: J. Biol. Chem., *259*:12949–12951, 1984.
31. Neumann, P.Z., Sass-Kortsak, A.: J. Clin. Invest., *46*:646–658, 1967.
32. Solomons, N.W.: J. Am. Coll. Nutr., *4*:83–105, 1985.
33. Williams, D.M.: Semin. Hematol., *20*:118–127, 1983.
34. Fujita, M., Itakura, T., Takagi, Y., et al.: JPEN, *13*:421–425, 1989.
35. Paynter, D.I.: The diagnosis of copper insufficiency. *In* Copper in Animals and Man, Vol. 1. Edited by J.M. Howell and J.M. Gawthorne. Boca Raton, FL, CRC Press, 1987, pp. 101–119.
36. Uauy, R., Castillo-Duran, C., Fisberg, M., et al.: J. Nutr., *115*:1650–1655, 1985.
37. Milne, D.B.: AACC Nutrition Division Newsletter, *8*:1–3, 1990.
38. Turnlund, J.R.: J. Nutr., *119*:7–14, 1989.
39. Higuchi, S., Higashi, A., Nakamura, T., et al.: J. Pediatr. Gastroenterol. Nutr., *7*:583–587, 1988.
40. Muller-Hocker, J., Meyer, U., Wiebecke, B., et al.: Pathol. Res. Pract., *183*:39–45, 1988.
41. Prohaska, J.R.: Clin. Physiol. Biochem., *4*:87–93, 1986.
42. Menkes, J.H.: Brain Dev., *10*:77–79, 1988.
43. Danks, D.M.: Copper deficiency in infants with particular reference to Menkes' disease. *In* Copper in Animals and Man, Vol. 2. Edited by J.M. Howell and J.M. Gawthorne. Boca Raton, FL, CRC Press, 1987.
44. Smithgall, J.M.: J. Am. Diet. Assoc., *85*:609–611, 1985.
45. Fleming, C.R.: Am. J. Clin. Nutr., *49*:573–579, 1989.
46. International Union of Biochemistry: Enzyme Nomenclature. Recommendations (1978) of the Nomenclature Committee of the International Union of Biochemistry. New York, Academic Press, 1979.

## SELECTED READINGS

Davis, G.K., and Mertz, W.: Copper. *In* Trace Elements in Human and Animal Nutrition, Vol. 1. Edited by W. Mertz. San Diego, Academic Press, 1987, pp. 301–364.

Howell, J.M., and Gawthorne, J.M. (eds.): Copper in Animals and Man, Vols. 1 and 2. Boca Raton, FL, CRC Press, 1987.

Kies, C. (ed.): Copper Bioavailability and Metabolism. New York, Plenum Press, 1990.

Linder, M.C.: The Biochemistry of Copper. New York, Plenum Press, 1990.

Mason, K.E.: A conspectus of research on copper metabolism and requirements of man. J. Nutr., *109*:1979–2066, 1979.

CHAPTER 12

# Selenium

Orville A. Levander and Raymond F. Burk



Selenium first attracted practical biologic interest in the 1930s when it was found to cause alkali disease, a chronic poisoning of livestock resulting from the consumption of plants that grow on high-selenium soils.[1] Then, in 1957, Schwarz discovered that traces of selenium prevented liver necrosis in vitamin E–deficient rats.[2] Soon thereafter deficiencies of selenium and vitamin E were shown to be involved in several economically important nutritional diseases in cattle, sheep, swine, and poultry.[3] The first demonstration of a biochemical function for selenium in mammals came in 1973 when it was shown to be a constituent of the enzyme glutathione peroxidase.[4] Reports documenting the importance of selenium in human nutrition appeared in 1979.[5,6] Information about the role of selenium in human nutrition increased rapidly in the 1980s, and a Recommended Dietary Allowance for selenium was established in 1989.[7]

## CHEMICAL FORMS

The chemistry of selenium is similar to that of sulfur, reflecting its position below that element in the oxygen series of the periodic table of elements. Selenium enters the food chain through plants that incorporate it into compounds that usually contain sulfur. This results in plant selenium being in the form of selenomethionine and, to a lesser extent, selenocysteine and other analogs of sulfur amino acids. There is no evidence that plants require selenium for incorporation into a specific molecule that is necessary for their existence.

The predominant form of selenium in animal tissues is selenocysteine.[8] It is synthesized from serine and an unidentified selenium intermediate (Fig. 12–1), and it is incorporated at specific sites in certain proteins known as selenoproteins. Many proteins contain selenium as selenomethionine. Animals appear to metabolize selenomethionine by methionine pathways and thus incorporate it nonspecifically into proteins in place of methionine. These proteins and others that do not contain the element in a fixed stoichiometry are usually referred to as selenium-containing proteins. There is no evidence that animals can synthesize selenomethionine. It is derived exclusively from the diet.

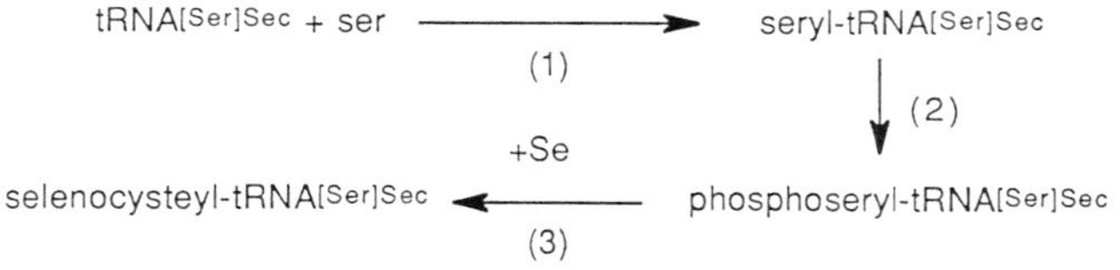
tRNA[Ser]Sec + ser
(1)
seryl-tRNA[Ser]Sec
(2)
phosphoseryl-tRNA[Ser]Sec
+Se
(3)
selenocysteyl-tRNA[Ser]Sec

**FIGURE 12–1.** Synthesis of selenocysteine using tRNA[Ser]Sec as the template. Evidence for this pathway consists of isolation of the intermediates in animal cells[25] and of mutant bacteria with defects at each step.[28] Reaction 1 is carried out by seryl-tRNA synthetase. Reaction 2 is carried out by a kinase in animal cells. Reaction 3 is dependent on a protein thought to be a carrier for reduced selenium.[28]

Some transfer RNAs (tRNAs) contain selenium. The major glutamate isoacceptor in Clostridium sticklandii contains 5-methylaminomethyl-2-selenouridine in the wobble position of the anticodon.[9] Selenium is methylated for excretion,[10] and dimethylselenide is exhaled by animals given a large amount of the element. Trimethylselenonium is a urinary metabolite, but the identity of most of the selenium excreted in the urine is not known.

## DIETARY CONSIDERATIONS

### FOOD SOURCES

Although SI units (Système International d'Unités, or International System of Units) are increasingly used to express concentrations of nutrients in body fluids and tissues, food composition tables primarily express values in micrograms per gram (μg/g). In this regard, 1 μg Se equals 0.0127 μmol Se. The richest food sources of selenium are organ meats and seafoods, 0.4 to 1.5 μg/g fresh weight; followed by muscle meats, 0.1 to 0.4; cereals and grains, <0.1 to >0.8; dairy products, <0.1 to 0.3; and fruits and vegetables, <0.1.[11] The wide variation in the selenium content of cereals and grains is due to differences in the amount of soil selenium available for uptake by plants (phytoavailability). For example, one study showed that the selenium content of corn collected in the People's Republic of China ranged from 0.005 to 8.1 μg/g, depending on whether the samples came from areas with soils that were poor or rich in phytoavailable selenium.[12] Foods from animal sources also vary somewhat in selenium content, but the degree of variation is less because of the tendency toward homeostatic control of selenium under different conditions of exposure. Drinking water generally contributes negligible selenium to the overall intake, except perhaps in some localized highly seleniferous areas.[13]

The Total Diet Study conducted by the United States Food and Drug Administration showed that a typical diet in the United States provided an average daily selenium intake of 100 and 70 μg for adult men and women, respectively, between 1982 and 1986.[14] Lower daily selenium intakes, 30 μg or less, have been reported in countries with selenium-poor soils, such as New Zealand.[15] Since 1985, selenium has been added to fertilizers used on certain crops in Finland such that the daily dietary intake increased from 39 μg in 1984 to 92 μg in 1986.[16] Serum selenium levels in Helsinki also increased from 0.89 ± 0.15 μmol/L (70 ± 12 μg/L) to 1.33 ± 0.11 μmol/L (105 ± 9 μg/L) during this time. Extremely low dietary selenium intakes have been reported in Keshan disease–affected areas of China, from 3 to 22 μg per day.[12] On the other hand, very high dietary intakes (up to 6690 μg per day) have been observed in a region of China with endemic human selenosis.[12] The food in this area had been grown on soil contaminated with selenium leached from a highly seleniferous coal.

### BIOAVAILABILITY

Only a limited number of investigations have been carried out to determine the nutritional bioavailability of selenium in foods consumed by humans. A commonly used procedure to estimate selenium availability has been to follow increases in hepatic glutathione peroxidase activity after feeding various food sources of selenium to selenium-depleted animals. On this basis, selenium fed as mushrooms, tuna, and wheat was 5%, 57%, and 83% as available to rats, respectively, as sodium selenite.[17,18] A human bioavailability trial performed in Finland with men of moderately-low selenium status showed significant differences among various forms of selenium tested (e.g., selenate, wheat, yeast) depending on the criterion of availability used (increase in platelet glutathione peroxidase activity, elevation of plasma or red blood cell selenium content, retention of selenium).[19] This study pointed out the need to consider several variables in such trials including short-term increases in glutathione peroxidase activity, long-term tissue retention of selenium, and metabolic conversion of retained selenium to biologically active forms.

### NUTRIENT-NUTRIENT INTERRELATIONSHIPS

Because of its role in glutathione peroxidase, selenium probably interacts with any nutrient that affects the antioxidant/pro-oxidant balance of the cell. For example, the selenium requirement of chicks is inversely proportional to the dietary vitamin E intake.[20] Selenium also protects against the toxicity of mercury, cadmium, and silver,[21] and a physiologic role for selenium in counteracting heavy metal pollutants has been proposed.[22] The low bioavailability of the selenium in tuna may be due to complexation with mercury, but this issue needs further investigation.[17]

## METABOLISM

Although selenium has chemical similarities to sulfur, its metabolism in animals and bacteria is distinct from that of sulfur. Recent work has begun to elucidate the mechanisms that regulate selenium homeostasis and its incorporation into macromolecules.

### ABSORPTION

Absorption appears to play no role in the homeostatic regulation of selenium. Virtually complete absorption occurs when the element is supplied as selenomethionine,[23] and other forms are generally well absorbed. However, the absorption of inorganic forms varies widely because it is influenced by luminal factors. Thus, selenium absorption is usually in the range of 50 to 100% and is not affected by selenium nutritional status.

### TRANSPORT

Little is known about the transport of selenium. Selenoprotein P and a glycosylated form of glutathione peroxidase are present in plasma, but they both contain selenium as selenocysteine and are unlikely to function in direct transport of the element. Extracellular selenium associated with glutathione, cysteine, and protein thiols has been recognized[24] and might serve a distributive function.

### INCORPORATION INTO PROTEIN

Research using procaryotic systems has outlined the mechanism of selenium incorporation into selenoproteins. Work in animal systems has suggested that they share the basic mechanism with procaryotes, but that some features vary between these systems. Figure 12–1 shows that a unique tRNA, designated $tRNA^{[Ser]Sec}$, participates in the synthesis of selenocysteine. First, $tRNA^{[Ser]Sec}$ is charged with serine. Then the oxygen on the serine side chain is activated. In animals this occurs through phosphorylation.[25] Selenium is then exchanged with the phosphate, yielding selenocysteine. Enzymes are involved at each step of this process. Thus $tRNA^{[Ser]Sec}$ serves as a template for the synthesis of selenocysteine. $tRNA^{[Ser]Sec}$ cannot be charged with selenocysteine directly, so supplying this form of selenium does not improve the efficiency of selenoprotein synthesis. In fact, selenocysteine-beta-lyase catabolizes free L-selenocysteine and presumably keeps its concentration very low.[26] Selenium liberated by this reaction can be utilized to synthesize selenocysteine through the mechanism outlined above.

A second function of $tRNA^{[Ser]Sec}$ is to serve as the transfer RNA for selenocysteine incorporation into selenoproteins. Its anticodon recognizes the messenger RNA (mRNA) codon UGA when it occurs in the proper context. In other contexts this codon serves to terminate protein synthesis. Procaryotes contain a protein translation factor that is necessary for the incorporation of selenocysteine from selenocysteyl-$tRNA^{[Ser]Sec}$ into selenoproteins.[27] This translation factor, which exhibits extensive homology with the elongation factor EF-Tu, might aid in distinguishing between the two functions of the UGA codon.

The selenium used in this process can come from inorganic selenium or from catabolism of selenocysteine or selenomethionine. In procaryotes a protein has been identified that is necessary for the incorporation of selenium to form selenocysteyl-$tRNA^{[Ser]Sec}$ and to form seleno-tRNA.[28] This protein is postulated to be an intracellular carrier for reduced selenium and as such could play a pivotal role in selenium homeostasis. No corresponding protein has yet been found in animal systems.

No other specific mechanisms for the incorporation of selenium into proteins have been described. A number of proteins that contain selenium have been identified, but the form and stoichiometry of the element in them have not been determined. Further work will be necessary to determine whether forms of selenium other than selenocysteine occur stoichiometrically in proteins.

### EXCRETION

Homeostasis of selenium in animals is achieved through regulation of excretion. As dietary intake increases from the deficient into the adequate range, urinary excretion of the element begins to increase.[29] At very high intakes volatile forms of selenium are exhaled. There is no evidence that fecal selenium is regulated. Thus under physiologic conditions, urinary excretion is the primary means whereby body selenium is regulated.

A small percentage of urinary selenium is trimethylselenonium.[30] The remainder has not been identified even though it is regulated. Breath selenium is largely dimethylselenide. The control of excretory metabolite formation may well be linked metabolically with the utilization of selenium for selenoprotein and seleno-tRNA synthesis. However, this relationship has not yet been defined.

## BIOCHEMICAL FUNCTIONS

Approximately 10 selenoproteins are reportedly present in the rat. In addition, a tRNA has been described that contains selenium. Only three animal selenoproteins have been purified and studied in detail. Little is known about the function of other selenoproteins or of seleno-tRNA.

### GLUTATHIONE PEROXIDASE

Glutathione peroxidase uses reducing equivalents from reduced glutathione (GSH) to reduce hydrogen peroxide and nonesterified organic hydroperoxides. It is made up of four identical subunits, each of which contains one selenocysteine in the primary structure.[31] Two forms of this enzyme are known. One is an intracellular form that is found predominantly in cytosolic and mitochondrial compartments. The other is an extracellular form secreted into the plasma by the liver.[32] The extracellular form is glycosylated and has a primary structure that is different from that of the intracellular enzyme.[33] Nonselenium-dependent glutathione peroxidase activity has also been described[34] and is due to the peroxidase activity of several isoforms of glutathione S-transferase.

The function of glutathione peroxidase in vivo is unknown. It cannot metabolize fatty acid hydroperoxides that are esterified in phospholipids[35] and has no protective effect in lipid peroxidation systems. It may serve primarily to metabolize hydrogen peroxide and thus protect against injury. Because the intracellular and extracellular forms of the enzyme are different and are present in compartments with up to 1000-fold differences in GSH concentrations (human plasma is 5 μM in GSH, whereas human liver is 5 to 10 mM in GSH), these forms may have different functions.

Liver and plasma glutathione peroxidase activity can readily be reduced to less than 1% of control activity by feeding rats a selenium-deficient diet.[36] Activities in other tissues decrease also, but to lesser degrees. Measurement of glutathione peroxidase activity can be used to assess selenium nutritional status in humans (see later section on evaluation of nutrient status).

### PHOSPHOLIPID HYDROPEROXIDE GLUTATHIONE PEROXIDASE

A selenium-containing protein has been isolated that inhibits lipid peroxidation in several systems and that can reduce fatty acid hydroperoxides that are esterified in phospholipids.[37] This phospholipid hydroperoxide glutathione peroxidase has a relative molecular mass of 22,000 and is a single polypeptide. Extensive characterization of this protein has not been reported, and routine assays are not yet possible. Nonetheless, this enzyme might be shown to provide some of the antioxidant properties of selenium.

### SELENOPROTEIN P

A second plasma selenoprotein has been purified and characterized that has no glutathione peroxidase activity, is a single polypeptide chain containing seven or more selenocysteine residues, and contains most of the selenium in rat plasma.[38] As measured by specific radioimmunoassay, the serum concentration of this protein falls in selenium deficiency to approximately 10% of control values. However, in one study glutathione peroxidase activity was more sensitive to selenium deficiency than was selenoprotein P.[39] The function of selenoprotein P is not known, but it seems unlikely to be a primary transport protein because all its selenium is covalently bound. Because other selenoproteins serve redox functions, selenoprotein P might also have such an activity. One hypothesis is that it has an antioxidant function.

## BIOLOGIC ACTIVITY

Most micronutrients serve as cofactors for several enzymes and thus have more than one biologic effect. Selenium also has a number of biologic effects, although it is best known as an antioxidant because of its relationship with vitamin E.

Deficiency of selenium leads regularly to marked changes in many biochemical systems. A number of drug-metabolizing enzymes, including the cytochrome P450 system, are affected, some with activities increased and others with activities decreased.[40,41] The underlying causes of these changes have not been established. Glutathione metabolism is also affected by selenium deficiency. In the rat, plasma glutathione concentration is increased two to three times by selenium deficiency.[36] This has been traced to increased synthesis of GSH by the liver and its release into the plasma. Liver, kidney, and lung glutathione S-transferase activities rise in selenium deficiency. Selenium-deficient rodents exhibit changes in glucose metabolism[42] and have alterations in thyroid hormone metabolism.[43] However, their metabolic rate is not affected.[44] This suggests that many of the alterations are compensatory to correct for defects in metabolism that have not been defined.

Pure selenium deficiency does not usually cause clinical illness. Only when animals are raised through several generations on a selenium-deficient regimen do they exhibit any signs (see section below on deficiency). In contrast, first-generation selenium-deficient animals exhibit heightened sensitivity to certain stresses, and that is the basis of most naturally occurring conditions of selenium deficiency. A number of conditions have been described in animals deficient both in selenium and in vitamin E (see section below on deficiency). Thus, vitamin E deficiency is a stress that is poorly tolerated by selenium-deficient animals.

Selenium-deficient animals are more susceptible to injury by certain chemicals. Toxicities of the redox cyclers paraquat, diquat, and nitrofurantoin[45] and of mercury and other heavy metals[46] are increased by selenium deficiency. Not all chemical injuries are aggravated by selenium deficiency. Selenium deficiency protects the rat against acetaminophen and aflatoxin hepatotoxicity, presumably through its effects on GSH metabolism.[45]

## DEFICIENCY IN HUMANS AND ANIMALS

A combined deficiency of both selenium and vitamin E causes liver necrosis in rats and swine, exudative diathesis in chickens, and white muscle disease in sheep and cattle.[3] In animals fed a selenium-deficient diet containing adequate levels of vitamin E, signs attributable to selenium deficiency included hair loss, growth retardation, and reproductive failure in rats fed a deficient diet for two generations[47] and pancreatic degeneration in chicks fed amino acid–based diets severely deficient in selenium.[48] This pancreatic atrophy in the chick, however, can be prevented by feeding high levels of vitamin E or other antioxidants.[49] Pancreatic atrophy can be induced in chicks fed practical rations from a selenium-deficient zone of China, but its severity is less than that seen with the amino acid diet, thereby suggesting the presence of partially protective factors in the practical diet.[50] In one study adult squirrel monkeys fed a low-selenium diet for 9 months lost weight and developed alopecia, myopathy, nephrosis, and hepatic degeneration.[51] However, in another study consistent signs of selenium deficiency proved to be more difficult to produce in rhesus monkeys, even in offspring born to mothers fed a selenium-deficient diet.[52] It was hypothesized that elevated glutathione transferase activity in the tissues of rhesus monkeys may account for their relative resistance to selenium deficiency.

Several lines of evidence suggest that selenium is a nutritionally essential trace element for humans. First of all, selenium is a component of the enzyme glutathione peroxidase, isolated from human red blood cells.[53] Secondly, favorable responses have been obtained after selenium supplementation of depleted patients undergoing long-term total parenteral nutrition (TPN) (see later section on high-risk clinical situations). Finally, selenium has been found to play a role in certain human diseases.

In 1979, Chinese scientists first described in English the relationship of selenium to Keshan disease, an endemic cardiomyopathy affecting children and young women that occurs in a long belt running from northeastern to southwestern China.[6] The acute form is characterized by sudden onset of insufficient heart function, whereas individuals with chronic disease exhibit moderate or severe heart enlargement with varying degrees of heart insufficiency.[54] The histopathologic features include multifocal necrosis, fibrous replacement of the myocardium, and myocytolysis. Keshan disease is related to a low dietary selenium intake and low blood and hair selenium levels.[55] Marginal to deficient vitamin E status has also been observed in subjects residing in endemic areas.[56] A series of intervention trials encompassing more than a million subjects has demonstrated the protective effects of selenium supplements.[57] However, selenium cannot reverse the cardiac failure once it occurs. Because certain features of the disease could not be explained solely on the basis of selenium status (e.g., seasonal variation), a cardiotoxic agent, such as a virus, might also be necessary for the disease to occur.[58] Furthermore, complicating nutritional deficiencies (e.g., protein) may exacerbate the condition.[52] Nonetheless, selenium deficiency appears to be the fundamental underlying condition predisposing individuals to the development of Keshan disease. With the improvement in living conditions in China, the disease is disappearing from several formerly endemic areas.

Another disease that has been associated with poor selenium status in China is Kashin-Beck disease, an endemic osteoarthritis that occurs during preadolescence or adolescence.[59] Necrotic degeneration of the chondrocytes is the most striking pathologic feature of this disease. Dwarfism and joint deformation result from these cartilage abnormalities. Aside from selenium deficiency, a number of other etiologic factors have been suggested for this condition (e.g., mycotoxins in grain, mineral imbalance, organic contaminants in drinking water).[60]

Numerous attempts have been made to associate selenium status with various chronic degenerative human diseases, especially cancer. However, the epidemiologic evidence linking low selenium status and an increased incidence of cancer is conflicting[61] and is often based on small differences in plasma selenium levels between controls and subjects who later developed cancer.[62] Some animal experiments show that high levels of dietary selenium can protect against certain chemically or virally induced cancers, but in some cases selenium itself can stimulate tumorigenesis in rodent models.[63] Thus, any use of selenium as a cancer preventive agent should be approached with caution.

## EVALUATION OF NUTRIENT STATUS

Selenium status can be evaluated by dietary and biochemical means.

### ANALYTICAL EVALUATION

Random urine samples are of little use in assessing selenium status because they are affected by dilution and the selenium content of the previous meal.[64] Blood selenium levels, which vary widely in different countries, are thought to reflect dietary intakes[11] (Fig. 12–2), although a direct relation of dietary selenium to muscle levels or total body selenium content has yet to be established.[64] Average blood selenium levels reported in different areas of the United States range between 2.03 and 3.29 μmol/L,[65] whereas extreme values of 0.10 and 95.0 μmol/L have been reported in areas of China affected by Keshan disease and endemic selenosis, respectively.[12] Plasma selenium levels, which respond to selenium supplementation more rapidly than whole blood levels, are an index of short-term status.[64] Average plasma selenium levels observed in areas with marginally adequate (Maryland) or low (Ohio) levels of soil selenium in the United States were 1.70 and 1.51 μmol/L, respectively.[66,67] Levels less than 0.63 μmol/L are often

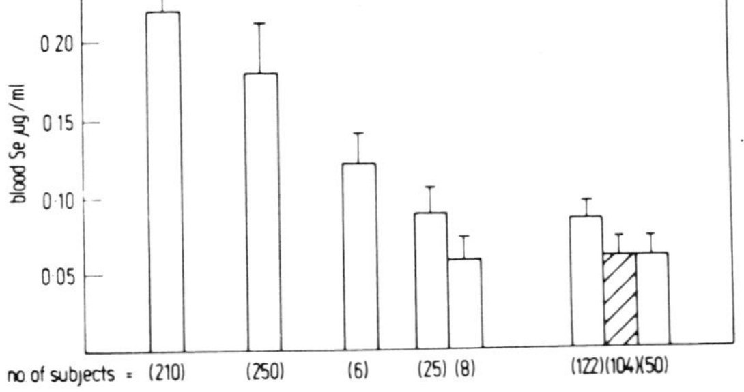
USA
Canada
Sweden
Finland
New Zealand
Auckland
Dunedin
Tapanui
0·25
0·20
0·15
0·10
0·05
blood Se μg/ml
no. of subjects = (210) (250) (6) (25) (8) (122)(104)(50)

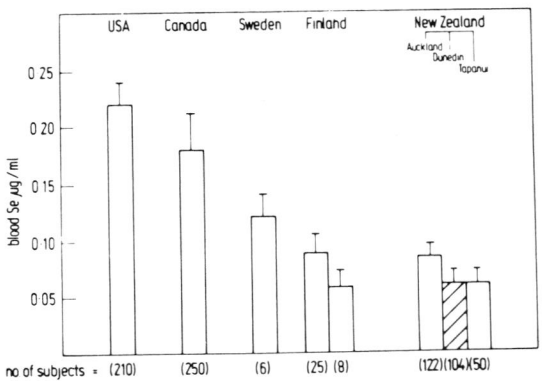

**FIGURE 12–2.** Blood selenium levels reported in healthy adults in various countries. (0.1 μg Se/ml = 1.27 μmol Se/L). (From Thomson, C.D., Robinson, M.F.: Am. J. Clin. Nutr., *33*:303–323, 1980).

seen in healthy residents of the south island of New Zealand.[15] Serum selenium concentrations fall soon after birth and then gradually increase to adult values (Fig. 12–3). Response to selenium supplementation was observed in a New Zealand patient on TPN who had a plasma level of 0.11 μmol/L.[5] Measurement of plasma, serum, or whole blood selenium concentrations has become much easier with the recent introduction of graphite furnace atomic absorption spectrometry with Zeeman background correction.[68] This procedure lends itself to large-scale epidemiologic surveys because no pretreatment of the samples is required other than dilution (i.e., no wet ashing is needed). This method is being used to measure serum selenium concentrations in the Third National Health and Nutrition Examination Survey (NHANES III, 1988–1994) as a way of helping to establish normal selenium ranges in the U.S. population. Determination of total selenium in blood or blood fractions provides no information about the speciation of selenium in blood. The compartmentalization of selenium can influence the interpretation of blood selenium levels (Fig. 12–4). Intake of diets rich in selenomethionine can raise blood selenium concentrations markedly, because this form of selenium is not subject to homeostatic regulation. Also, serum selenium does not reflect the build-up of selenium in the skeletal muscle of animals when high levels of selenomethionine are fed.[70] Hair selenium was used in China to evaluate selenium status,[57] but may not be valid in Western countries where shampoos containing selenium are used. Toenail selenium has been suggested as a convenient noninvasive index of selenium status.[71] However, hair and nail selenium levels, at least in rats, are a function both of the form of selenium fed and of the methionine content of the diet.[70]

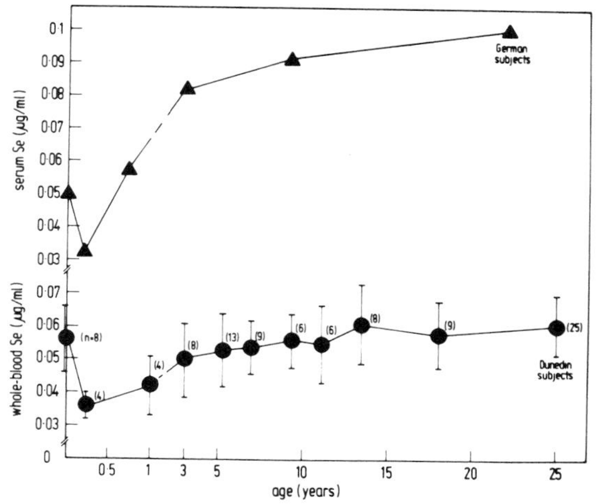
serum Se (μg/ml)
whole-blood Se (μg/ml)
German subjects
Dunedin subjects
age (years)

**FIGURE 12–3.** Serum selenium concentrations in healthy German children and young adults in comparison with whole-blood selenium concentrations in healthy New Zealand children and young adults. (0.1 μg Se/ml = 1.27 μmol Se/L). (From Thomson, C.D., Robinson, M.F.: Am. J. Clin. Nutr., *33*:303–323, 1980.)

Assessment of selenium status by calculating the dietary intake from food composition tables is a risky procedure because of the wide variation in the selenium content of foods. Unless one is certain that the data base used is applicable to the diet in question, the safest approach is direct chemical analysis of the diet. Nonetheless, it is possible to obtain reasonable agreement between calculated and analyzed selenium intakes if the appropriate data base is available.[72]

### BIOCHEMICAL AND CLINICAL EVALUATION

A direct relationship exists between blood glutathione peroxidase activity and blood selenium level up to 1.27 μmol/L.[73] Beyond that point the activity of the enzyme plateaus and cannot be used to evaluate selenium nutriture. Moreover, numerous other factors can affect glutathione peroxidase activity.[74] Nonetheless, glutathione peroxidase activity remains an extremely useful index of selenium status in the nutritional range of dietary intake, and automated enzyme assays suitable for large-scale surveys have been devised.[68] At present, there are no suitable clinical methods for evaluating selenium status.

## REQUIREMENTS AND RECOMMENDED INTAKES

In 1980, the National Research Council established an estimated safe and adequate daily dietary selenium intake for adults of 50 to 200 μg.[75] This recommendation was the first dietary standard for selenium and was based primarily on extrapolation from animal experiments because few human data were available at that time. A nutritionally generous level of selenium for most animals appears to be about 0.1 μg/g of dry diet. If it is assumed that humans consume 500 g of diet (dry basis) daily then, based on the animal results, humans would need 50 μg of selenium per day. Because of uncertainties about the bioavailability of selenium from different diets and possible individual variations in requirements, the dietary recommendation was given as a range.

In the past decade, a number of human studies have been carried out that have greatly increased our understanding of human selenium requirements. Some of the first attempts to delineate human selenium requirements more precisely involved balance studies, but comparison of international balance data revealed that people could maintain selenium balance over a broad range of intake.[62] Therefore, the balance method proved not especially useful in clarifying human selenium requirements. Another approach was to conduct dietary surveys in areas with and without human selenium deficiency—that is, with and without Keshan disease. Such surveys showed that Keshan disease was not present in areas where the selenium intake was at least 19 and 13 μg per day for men and women, respectively.[58] These values can

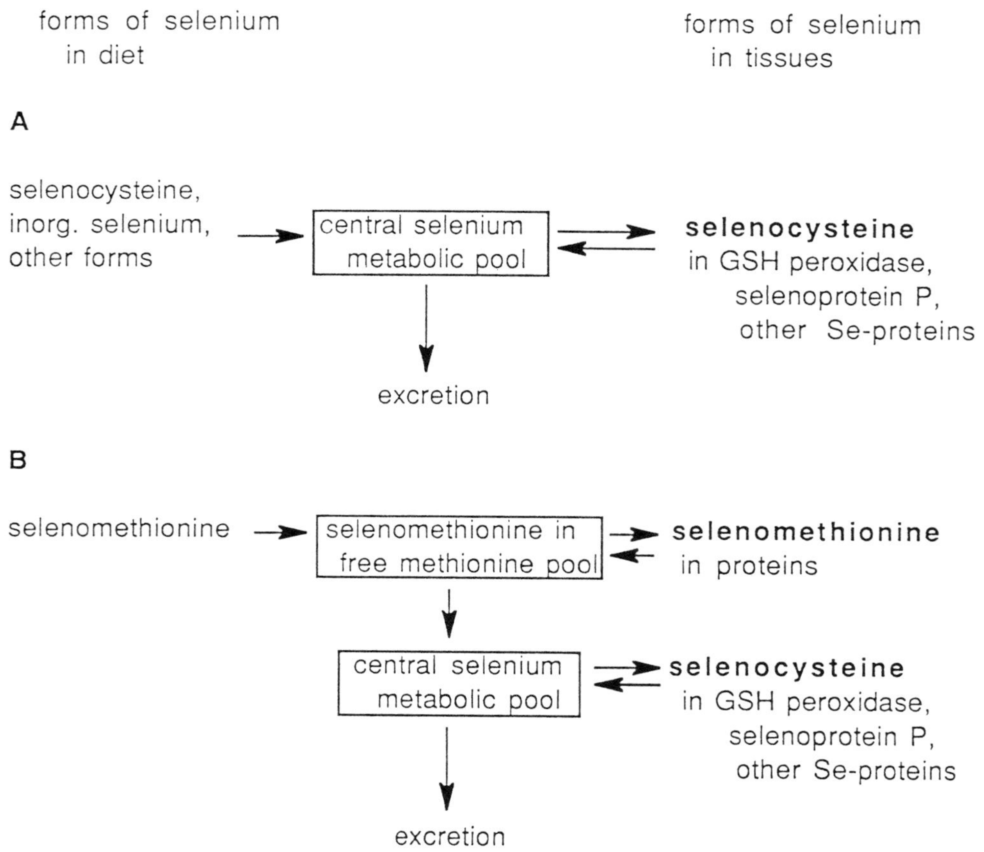
forms of selenium in diet
forms of selenium in tissues
A
selenocysteine, inorg. selenium, other forms
central selenium metabolic pool
selenocysteine in GSH peroxidase, selenoprotein P, other Se-proteins
excretion
B
selenomethionine
selenomethionine in free methionine pool
selenomethionine in proteins
central selenium metabolic pool
selenocysteine in GSH peroxidase, selenoprotein P, other Se-proteins
excretion

**FIGURE 12–4.** Tissue selenium form and concentration as affected by dietary form. Intake of certain forms of selenium restricts the element to the pathways specific to selenium (A). When selenomethionine is ingested, tissue selenium is present in two pools, the methionine pool and the specific selenium pool (B). Its incorporation into the pools can be sequential. This results in higher tissue selenium levels for a certain intake of the element than when it is consumed in the forms given in A. Selenomethionine in proteins serves as an unregulated storage form of selenium (Adapted from Levander, O.A., Burk, R.F.: Selenium. *In* Present Knowledge in Nutrition. 6th Ed. Edited by M.L. Brown. Washington, D.C., International Life Sciences Institute, Nutrition Foundation, 1990, pp. 268–273.)

be considered minimum dietary requirements for selenium.

Human selenium requirements have also been estimated by determining the dietary selenium intake needed to maximize the activity of the selenoenzyme glutathione peroxidase. In these studies, the diets of Chinese men of very low selenium status (residents of an area with Keshan disease) were supplemented with graded doses of selenomethionine.[76] Plasma glutathione peroxidase activity tended to be greatest in those individuals who received 30 μg per day or more of supplemental selenium over a period of several months. That intake plus their habitual dietary intake (11 μg per day) yielded 41 μg per day as the lowest amount tested that caused a plateauing of enzyme activity.

Maximization of plasma glutathione peroxidase activity was accepted by the United States National Research Council as the basis for its Recommended Dietary Allowance (RDA) for selenium in 1989.[7] The Chinese value of 41 μg per day was multiplied by body weight and safety factors to come up with recommendations of 70 and 55 μg per day for adult men and women, respectively. Recommendations for children were extrapolated from the adult values on the basis of body weight. Infant requirements are probably 4 to 7 μg per day, depending on the basis of the estimate.[77] The selenium RDA for infants was set at 10 and 15 μg per day for the first and second 6 months of life, respectively, to allow for growth. Increased allowances for women during pregnancy and lactation were 10 and 20 μg per day, respectively, and were based either on fetal demand or lacteal losses (see Appendix Table A–2b).

Although North Americans should easily achieve the selenium RDA through consumption of a typical mixed U.S. diet, persons living in countries with selenium-poor soils would have difficulty in attaining such intakes (see earlier section on dietary considerations). The Standing Nordic Committee on Food has recommended somewhat lower intakes, 30 to 60 μg per day for teenagers, adults, and pregnant and lactating women, in Scandinavia.[78] The key issue to be resolved is whether or not maximization of glutathione peroxidase activity is necessary for good nutrition. Because the evidence is uncertain, the 1989 RDA for selenium did not take into account any hypothetical role for selenium in the prevention of cancer or other chronic human degenerative diseases (see earlier section on deficiency in humans and animals).

## TOXICITY IN HUMANS AND ANIMALS

The level of dietary selenium needed to cause chronic selenium toxicity in animals is 4 to 5 μg/g.[3] In livestock, chronic selenosis (alkali disease) is characterized by cirrhosis, lameness, hoof malformations, hair loss, and emaciation.[3] Laboratory rats chronically poisoned with selenium exhibit growth depression and cirrhosis. The mechanism of selenium toxicity is not known, and the toxic effects of selenium may be modified by adaptation and certain dietary factors.[11] No sensitive and specific biochemical test is currently available to indicate overexposure to selenium.[79]

Public health surveys carried out in seleniferous areas of the United States failed to establish any symptom specific for selenium poisoning.[80–82] Field studies conducted in Venezuela showed that the incidence of dermatitis, loose hair, and diseased nails was greater in children from a seleniferous area than in those from Caracas,[83] a nonseleniferous area, but no differences were seen in the various biochemical tests performed. A report from China described an outbreak of endemic selenium poisoning in humans.[12] The most common sign of intoxication was loss of hair and nails. In high-incidence areas, lesions of the skin, nervous system, and possibly teeth were observed. Biochemical analyses showed a change in the ratio of plasma selenium to erythrocyte selenium at selenium intakes over 750 μg per day.[84] Signs of selenosis (nail changes) were seen in susceptible patients at intakes of 910 μg per day or more, corresponding to a blood selenium level of 13.3 μmol/L or higher. No signs or symptoms of selenium overexposure were observed among residents of seleniferous ranches in South Dakota or Wyoming whose dietary intake was as high as 724 μg per day.[82] However, an episode of human selenium poisoning was reported in the United States in 1984 involving 13 persons who consumed a "health food" supplement that exceeded the label declaration for selenium by 182 times because of a manufacturing error.[85,86] The total amount of selenium consumed by these victims was thought to have been between 27 and 2387 mg. Signs and symptoms of poisoning included nausea, diarrhea, irritability, fatigue, peripheral neuropathy, hair loss, and nail changes.

## HIGH-RISK CLINICAL SITUATIONS

Subjects who are selenium-deficient as documented by biochemical testing can be considered at risk for developing pathologic conditions. Keshan disease is thought to be such a condition, and Kashin-Beck disease may be another one. Several subjects made selenium-deficient by parenteral nutrition have been reported to have developed a cardiomyopathy similar to Keshan disease.[87,88] Such selenium-deficient subjects might also be sensitive to injury by drugs and chemicals such as nitrofurantoin in the same way animals are.

Total parenteral alimentation leads regularly to selenium deficiency if the element is not administered in the fluids.[89] Semipurified medical diets used to treat conditions such as phenylketonuria are also often low in selenium and can produce selenium deficiency. Thus, subjects eating them might be at risk for conditions related to selenium deficiency. Careful clinical observation will be necessary to document these relationships.

## RECENT DEVELOPMENTS

Since the first draft of this chapter was prepared, remarkable progress has been made regarding various aspects of the molecular biology of selenium, and this topic has been the subject of several excellent reviews.[90-92] A detailed account of the scientific rationale for the 1989 RDA for selenium has also appeared.[93] The recent discovery that the active site of type I iodothyronine deiodinase contains selenocysteine provides yet another example of a selenoprotein with well-defined enzymatic activity.[94,95] Thus, selenium appears to take part in the metabolism of thyroid hormones through its involvement in the deiodination of the prohormone thyroxine to the active hormone $T_3$.[96] Any possible role for selenium in the pathogenesis of endemic cretinism, however, remains to be established. Moreover, serious thyroid failure has been reported in endemic cretins undergoing selenium repletion following iodide loss by the kidney due to increased catabolism of both $T_4$ and $rT_3$.[97] Thus, selenium supplementation of such individuals should only follow iodine supplementation.[98]

## REFERENCES


1. Moxon, A.L., Rhian, M.A.: Physiol. Rev., *23*:305–337, 1943.
2. Schwarz, K., Foltz, C.M.: J. Am. Chem. Soc., *79*:3292–3293, 1957.
3. National Research Council: Selenium in Nutrition. (Revised). Washington, D.C., National Academy of Sciences, 1983.

4. Rotruck, J.T., Pope, A.L., Ganther, H.E., et al.: Science, *179:*588–590, 1973.
5. van Rij, A.M., Thomson, C.D., McKenzie, J.M., et al.: Am. J. Clin. Nutr., *32:*2076–2085, 1979.
6. Keshan Disease Research Group: Chin. Med. J., *92:*471–476, 1979.
7. National Research Council: Recommended Dietary Allowances. 10th Ed. Washington, D.C., National Academy of Sciences, 1989.
8. Hawkes, W.C., Wilhelmsen, E.C., Tappel, A.L.: J. Inorg. Biochem., *23:*77–92, 1985.
9. Ching, W.-M., Alzner-DeWeerd, B., Stadtman, T.C.: Proc. Natl. Acad. Sci. U.S.A., *82:*347–350, 1985.
10. Mozier, N.M., McConnell, K.P., Hoffman, J.L.: J. Biol. Chem., *263:*4527–4531, 1988.
11. International Programme on Chemical Safety: Environmental Health Criteria 58. Selenium. Geneva, World Health Organization, 1987.
12. Yang, G.Q., Wang, S., Zhou, R., et al.: Am. J. Clin. Nutr., *37:*872–881, 1983.
13. National Research Council: The contribution of drinking water to mineral nutrition in humans. *In* Drinking Water and Health, Vol. 3. Washington, D.C., National Academy of Sciences, 1980.
14. Pennington, J.A.T., Young, B.E., Wilson, D.B.: J. Am. Diet. Assoc., *89:*659–664, 1989.
15. Robinson, M.F.: Nutr. Rev., *47:*99–107, 1989.
16. Varo, P., Alfthan, G., Ekholm, P., et al.: Am. J. Clin. Nutr., *48:*324–329, 1988.
17. Levander, O.A.: Fed. Proc., *42:*1721–1725, 1983.
18. Chansler, M.W., Mutanen, M., Morris, V.C., et al.: Nutr. Res., *6:*1419–1428, 1986.
19. Levander, O.A., Alfthan, G., Arvilommi, H., et al.: Am. J. Clin. Nutr., *37:*887–897, 1983.
20. Thompson, J.N., Scott, M.L.: J. Nutr., *97:*335–342, 1969.
21. Levander, O.A., Cheng, L.: Ann. N. Y. Acad. Sci., *355:*1–372, 1980.
22. Parizek, J., Ostadalova, I., Kalouskova, A., et al.: The detoxifying effects of selenium: Interrelations between compounds of selenium and certain metals. *In* Newer Trace Elements in Nutrition. Edited by W. Mertz, and W.E. Cornatzer. New York, Marcel Dekker, 1971, pp. 85–122.
23. Swanson, C.A., Patterson, B.H., Levander, O.A., et al.: Am. J. Clin. Nutr. *54:*917–926, 1991.
24. Vendeland, S.C., Deagen, J.T., Butler, J.A., Whanger, P.D.: FASEB J., *4:*A372, 1990.
25. Lee, B.Y., Worland, P.J., Davis, J.N., et al.: J. Biol. Chem., *264:*9724–9727, 1989.
26. Esaki, N., Nakamura, T., Tanaka, H., Soda, K.: J. Biol. Chem., *257:*4386–4391, 1982.
27. Forchhammer, K., Rucknagel, K.-P., Bock, A.: J. Biol. Chem., *265:*9346–9350, 1990.
28. Leinfelder, W., Forchhammer, K., Veprek, B., et al.: Proc. Natl. Acad. Sci. U.S.A., *87:*543–547, 1990.
29. Burk, R.F., Brown, D.G., Seely, R.J., Scaief, C.C.: J. Nutr., *102:*1049–1055, 1972.
30. Burk, R.F.: Selenium in man. *In* Trace Elements in Human Health and Disease, Vol. II Edited by A. Prasad. New York, Academic Press, 1976, pp. 105–133.
31. Chambers, I., Framptin, J., Goldfarb, P., et al.: EMBO J., *5:*1221–1227, 1986.
32. Avissar, N., Whitin, J.C., Allen, P.Z., et al.: J. Biol. Chem., *264:*15850–15855, 1989.
33. Takahashi, K., Avissar, N., Whitin, J., Cohen, H.J.: Arch. Biochem. Biophys., *256:*677–686, 1987.
34. Burk, R.F., Lawrence, R.A.: Non selenium-dependent glutathione peroxidase. *In* Functions of Glutathione in Liver and Kidney. Proceedings in Life Sciences. Edited by H. Sies and A. Wendel. Berlin, Springer Verlag, 1978, pp. 114–119.
35. Grossmann, A., Wendel, A.: Eur. J. Biochem., *135:*549–552, 1983.
36. Hill, K.E., Burk, R.F., Lane, J.M.: J. Nutr., *117:*99–104, 1987.
37. Ursini, F., Maiorino, M., Valente, M., et al.: Biochim. Biophys. Acta, *710:*197–211, 1982.
38. Read, R., Bellew, T., Yang, J.-G., et al.: J. Biol. Chem., *265:*17899–17905, 1990.
39. Yang, J.-G., Hill, K.E., Burk, R.F.: J. Nutr., *119:*1010–1012, 1989.
40. Burk, R.F., Masters, B.S.S.: Arch. Biochem. Biophys., *170:*124–131, 1975.
41. Reiter, R., Wendel, A.: Biochem. Pharmacol., *32:*3063–3067, 1983.
42. Fischer, W.C., Whanger, P.D.: J. Nutr., *107:*1493–1501, 1977.
43. Beckett, G.J., MacDougall, D.A., Nicol, F., Arthur, J.R.: Biochem. J., *259:*887–892, 1989.
44. Burk, R.F.: Annu. Rev. Nutr., *3:*53–70, 1983.
45. Burk, R.F., Lane, J.M.: Fund. Appl. Toxicol., *3:*218–221, 1983.
46. Parizek, J., Kalouskova, J., Benes, J., Pavlik, L.: Ann. N. Y. Acad. Sci., *355:*347–360, 1980.
47. McCoy, K.E.M., Weswig, P.H.: J. Nutr., *98:*383–389, 1969.
48. Thompson, J.N., Scott, M.L.: J. Nutr., *100:*797–809, 1970.
49. Whitacre, M.E., Combs, G.F., Jr., Combs, S.B., et al.: J. Nutr., *117:*460–467, 1987.
50. Combs, G.F., Jr., Liu, C.H., Lu, Z.H., et al.: J. Nutr., *114:*964–976, 1984.
51. Muth, O.H., Weswig, P.H., Whanger, P.D., et al.: Am. J. Vet. Res., *32:*1603–1605, 1971.
52. Butler, J.A., Whanger, P.D., Patton, N.M.: J. Am. Coll. Nutr., *7:*43–56, 1988.
53. Awasthi, Y.C., Beutler, E., Srivastava, S.K.: J. Biol. Chem., *250:*5144–5149, 1975.
54. Ge, K., Xue, A., Bai, J., et al.: Virchows Arch. [A], *401:*1–15, 1983.
55. Keshan Disease Research Group: Chin. Med. J., *92:*477–482, 1979.
56. Xia, Y., Hill, K.E., Burk, R.F.: J. Nutr., *119:*1318–1326, 1989.
57. Yang, G., Chen, J., Wen, Z., et al.: Adv. Nutr. Res., *6:*203–231, 1984.
58. Yang, G., Ge, K., Chen, J., et al.: World Rev. Nutr. Diet., *55:*98–152, 1988.
59. Mo, D.: Pathology and selenium deficiency in Kashin-Beck disease. *In* Selenium in Biology and Medicine. Edited by G.F. Combs, Jr., J.E. Spallholz, O.A. Levander, and J.E. Oldfield. New York, Van Nostrand Reinhold, 1987, pp. 924–933.
60. Levander, O.A.: Etiological hypotheses concerning Kashin-Beck disease. *In* AIN Symposium Proceedings. Nutrition '87. Edited by O.A. Levander. Bethesda, MD, American Institute of Nutrition, 1987, pp. 67–71.
61. Willett, W.C., Stampfer, M.J.: Br. Med. J., *297:*573–574, 1988.
62. Levander, O.A.: Annu. Rev. Nutr., *7:*227–250, 1987.
63. Birt, D.F., Pour, P.M., Pelling, J.C.: The influence of dietary selenium on colon, pancreas and skin tumorigenesis. *In* Selenium in Biology and Medicine. Edited by A. Wendel. Berlin, Springer-Verlag, 1989, pp. 297–304.

64. Thomson, C.D., Robinson, M.F.: Am. J. Clin. Nutr., *33*:303–323, 1980.
65. Allaway, W.H., Kubota, J., Losee, F., et al.: Arch. Environ. Health, *16*:342–348, 1968.
66. Levander, O.A., Morris, V.C.: Am. J. Clin. Nutr., *39*:809–815, 1984.
67. Snook, J.T., Palmquist, D.L., Moxon, A.L., et al.: Am. J. Clin. Nutr., *38*:620–630, 1983.
68. McMaster, D., Bell, N., Anderson, P., et al.: Clin. Chem., *36*:211–216, 1990.
69. Levander, O.A., Burk, R.F.: Selenium. *In* Present Knowledge in Nutrition. 6th Ed. Edited by M.L. Brown. Washington, D.C., International Life Sciences Institute, Nutrition Foundation, 1990, pp. 268–273.
70. Salbe, A.D., Levander, O.A.: J. Nutr., *120*:200–206, 1990.
71. Morris, J.S., Stampfer, M.J., Willett, W.C.: Biol. Trace Elem. Res., *5*:529–537, 1983.
72. Welsh, S.O., Holden, J.M., Wolf, W.R., et al.: J. Am. Diet. Assoc., *79*:277–285, 1981.
73. Thomson, C.D., Rea, H.M., Doesburg, V.M., et al.: Br. J. Nutr., *37*:457–460, 1977.
74. Ganther, H.E., Hafeman, D.G., Lawrence, R.A., et al.: Selenium and glutathione peroxidase in health and disease—A review. *In* Trace Elements in Human Health and Disease. Vol. 2. Essential and Toxic Elements. Edited by A.S. Prasad. New York, Academic Press, 1976, pp. 165–234.
75. National Research Council: Recommended Dietary Allowances. 9th Ed. Washington, D.C., National Academy of Sciences, 1980.
76. Yang, G.Q., Qian, P.C., Zhu, L.Z., et al.: Human selenium requirements in China. *In* Selenium in Biology and Medicine. Edited by G.F. Combs, Jr., J.E. Spallholz, O.A. Levander, and J.E. Oldfield. New York, Van Nostrand Reinhold, 1987, pp. 589–607.
77. Levander, O.A.: J. Nutr., *119*:1869–1873, 1989.
78. Standing Nordic Committee on Food: Nordic Nutrition Recommendations. 2nd Ed. English version. Copenhagen, Nordic Council of Ministers, 1989.
79. Levander, O.A.: Selenium: Biochemical actions, interactions and some human health implications. *In* Clinical, Biochemical and Nutritional Aspects of Trace Elements. Edited by A.S. Prasad. New York, Alan R. Liss, 1982, pp. 345–368.
80. Smith, M.I., Franke, K.W., Westfall, B.B.: U.S. Public Health Rep., *51*:1496–1505, 1936.
81. Smith, M.I., Westfall, B.B.: U.S. Public Health Rep., *52*:1375–1384, 1937.
82. Longnecker, M.P., Taylor, P.R., Levander, O.A., et al.: Am. J. Clin. Nutr., *53*:1288–1294, 1991.
83. Jaffe, W.G.: Effect of selenium intake in humans and in rats. *In* Proceedings of the Symposium Selenium-Tellurium in the Environment. Pittsburgh, Industrial Health Foundation, 1976, pp. 188–193.
84. Yang, G., Yin, S., Zhou, R., et al.: J. Trace Elem. Electrolytes Health Dis., *3*:123–130, 1989.
85. Jensen, R., Clossen, W., Rothenberg, R.: Morbid. Mortal. Wkly. Rep., *33*:157–158, 1984.
86. Helzlsouer, K., Jacobs, R., Morris, S.: Fed. Proc., *44*:1670, 1985.
87. Johnson, R.A., Baker, S.S., Fallon, J.T., et al.: N. Eng. J. Med., *304*:1210–1212, 1981.
88. Lockitch, G., Taylor, G.P., Wong, L.T.K., et al.: Am. J. Clin. Nutr., *52*:572–577, 1990.
89. Levander, O.A., Burk, R.F.: J. Parenter. Enteral Nutr., *10*:545–549, 1986.
90. Sunde, R.A.: Annu. Rev. Nutr., *10*:451–474, 1990.
91. Bock, A., Forchhammer, K., Heider, J., et al.: Trends Biochem. Sci., *16*:463–467, 1991.
92. Burk, R.F.: FASEB J., *5*:2274–2279, 1991.
93. Levander, O.A.: J. Am. Diet. Assoc., *91*:1572–1576, 1991.
94. Arthur, J.R., Nicol, F., Beckett, G.J.: Biochem. J., *272*:537–540, 1990.
95. Berry, M.J., Banu, L., Larsen, P.R.: Nature, *349*:438–440, 1991.
96. Arthur, J.R.: Can. J. Physiol. Pharmacol., *69*:1648–1652, 1991.
97. Contempre, B., Vanderpas, J., Dumont, J.E.: Mol. Cell. Endocrinol., *81*:C193–C195, 1991.
98. Contempre, B., Dumont, J.E., Bebe, N., et al.: J. Clin. Endocrinol. Metab., *73*:213–215, 1991.

## SELECTED READINGS

Combs, G.F., Combs, S.B.: The Role of Selenium in Nutrition. Orlando, Academic Press, 1986.

Burk, R.F. (ed.): Selenium in Biology and Medicine. Berlin, Springer Verlag, in preparation.

Burk, R.F., Hill, K.E.: Regulation of selenoproteins. Ann. Rev. Nutr., in press.

CHAPTER 13

# Iodine

Graeme A. Clugston and Basil S. Hetzel



## HISTORICAL INTRODUCTION

Iodine is an essential constituent of the thyroid hormones thyroxine 3,5,3′,5′ tetraiodothyronine ($T_4$) and 3,5,3′ triiodothyronine ($T_3$). The major role of iodine in nutrition arises from the importance of thyroid hormones to growth and development.[1–5] The atomic weight of iodine is 126.9 g/atom, and the molecular weights of $T_4$ and $T_3$ are 776.9 and 651.0 g/mol, respectively.

Iodine was discovered by Courtois in 1811 during the course of making gunpowder. Some seaweed ash was being used from which the iodine vaporized as a violet vapor. The element was discovered in the thyroid gland by Baumann in 1895.

The relation of iodine deficiency to enlargement of the thyroid gland, or goiter, was first shown by David Marine, who found that hyperplastic changes occurred regularly in the thyroid when the iodine concentration fell below 0.1%.[3] Subsequently Marine and Kimball (1922) demonstrated in school children in Akron, Ohio that endemic goiter could be both prevented and substantially reduced by administration of small amounts of iodine.[5]

Mass prophylaxis of goiter with iodized salt was first introduced in Switzerland and in Michigan.[5] In Switzerland the widespread occurrence of a severe form of mental deficiency and deaf mutism (endemic cretinism) was a heavy charge on public funds. Following the introduction of iodized salt, however, goiter incidence fell rapidly and new cretins were no longer born. Goiter also disappeared from Army recruits.[5]

A further major development was the administration of injections of iodized oil in Papua New Guinea for people living in inaccessible mountain villages. The successful prevention of goiter and subsequently of cretins was shown in controlled trials over the period 1959 to 1972.[1–5]

More details on the historical aspects will be found elsewhere.[1–5]

## ECOLOGY OF IODINE DEFICIENCY

There is a cycle of iodine in nature. Most of the iodine resides in the ocean. It was present during the primordial development of the earth but large amounts were leached from the surface soil by glaciation, snow, or rain and were carried by wind, rivers, and floods into the sea. Iodine occurs in the deeper layers of the soil and is found in oil-well and natural gas effluents. Water from such deep wells can be a major source of iodine. In general, the older an exposed soil surface, the more likely it is to be leached of iodine.[1,5]

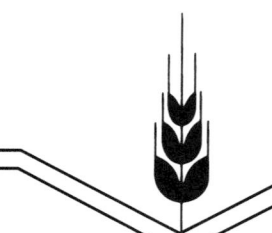

The most likely areas to be leached are the mountainous areas of the world. The most severely deficient areas are those of the Himalayas, the Andes, the European Alps, and the vast mountains of China. But iodine deficiency is likely to occur in all elevated regions subject to glaciation, higher rainfall, and runoff into rivers. It also occurs in flooded river valleys such as the Ganges in India, however.

Iodine occurs in soil and the sea as iodide. Iodide ions are oxidized by sunlight to elemental iodine, which is volatile, so that every year some 400,000 tons of iodine escape from the surface of the sea. The concentration of iodide in the sea water is about 50 to 60 μg/L; in the air it is approximately 0.7 $\mu g/m^3$. The iodine in the atmosphere is returned to the soil by rain, which has concentrations in the range 1.8 to 8.5 μg/L. In this way the cycle is completed.

However, the return of the iodine is slow and small in amount compared to the original loss of iodine, and subsequent repeated flooding ensures the continuity of iodine deficiency in the soil. Hence no "natural correction" can take place, and iodine deficiency persists in the soil indefinitely. All crops grown in these soils will be iodine-deficient. As a result human and animal populations, which are totally dependent on food grown in such soil, become iodine-deficient. The iodine content of plants grown in iodine-deficient soils may be as low as 10 μg/kg, compared to 1 mg/kg dry weight in plants in an iodine-sufficient soil. This accounts for the occurrence of severe iodine deficiency in vast populations in Asia who are living within systems of subsistence agriculture in flooded river valleys (India, Bangladesh, Burma).

An indication of the iodine content of the soil can be given by the local drinking water concentration. In general, iodine-deficient areas have water iodine levels below 2 μg/L as in Nepal and India (0.1 to 1.2 μg/L) compared with levels of 9.0 μg/L in the city of Delhi, which is not iodine-deficient.

Iodine deficiency will persist unless a supplement is provided or diversification of the diet occurs, with increase in iodine intake derived from food sources outside the iodine-deficient area. This has occurred progressively in Europe during the nineteenth century. However, substantial areas of iodine deficiency remain in some countries (Germany, Italy, and Spain), and more-localized areas remain in other countries.

In developing countries more than 1 billion persons are estimated to be at risk of iodine deficiency disorders (IDDs). Most of these persons live in areas where endemic goiter affects at least 10% of the population. Of this large group, 220 million are suffering from goiter, more than 5 million are suffering from mental retardation as gross cretins, and 15 to 25 million suffer from lesser mental defects (Table 13–1).

## PHYSIOLOGY OF IODINE DEFICIENCY

The healthy human adult body contains 15 to 20 mg of iodine, of which about 70 to 80% is in the thyroid gland.[1,2] The thyroid gland, which weighs only 15 to 25 g, possesses a remarkable concentrating power for iodine. The amount of iodine in the gland is closely related to the iodine intake. The content may be reduced to only 1 mg or less in the iodine-deficient enlarged thyroid (goiter).

Iodide is rapidly absorbed through the gut. The normal intake and requirement is 100 to 150 μg per day. Excess iodine is excreted by the kidney. The level of excretion correlates well with the level of intake, so that it can be used to assess the level of iodine intake.

Iodine exists in the thyroid as inorganic iodine; the iodine-containing amino acids, monoiodothyronine (MIT), diiodothyronine (DIT), $T_3$, and $T_4$; polypeptides containing thyroxine; and thyroglobulin. Thyroglobulin is a protein that contains the iodinated amino acids in a peptide linkage. Thyroglobulin is the chief constituent of the colloid that fills the thyroid follicle. It is a glycoprotein (it contains glucose) with a molecular weight of 650,000. It is the storage form of the thyroid hormones and makes up 90% of the total iodine in the gland.

The thyroid has to trap about 60 μg of iodine per day to maintain an adequate supply of thyroxine. This is possible because of the very active iodide-trapping mechanism, which maintains a gradient of 100:1 between the thyroid cell and the extracellular fluid. In iodine deficiency this gradient may exceed 400:1 in order to maintain the output of thyroxine.

This increased trapping of iodine in iodine deficiency can be well demonstrated using radioiodine. In the Argentinean Andes of South America, Stanbury and his

**TABLE 13–1.** PREVALENCE OF IODINE DEFICIENCY DISORDERS IN DEVELOPING COUNTRIES AND NUMBERS OF PERSONS AT RISK (IN MILLIONS)

| GEOGRAPHIC AREA | AT RISK | GOITER | OVERT CRETINISM |
|---|---|---|---|
| Africa | 227 | 39 | 0.5 |
| Latin America | 60 | 30 | 0.3 |
| Southeast Asia | 280 | 100 | 4.0 |
| Asia (other countries including China) | 400 | 30 | 0.9 |
| Eastern Mediterranean | 33 | 12 | — |
| TOTAL | 1000 | 211 | 5.7 |

(From World Health Organization Report to 43rd World Health Assembly. Geneva, World Health Organization, 1990.)

colleagues first showed that urinary radioiodine excretion was inversely related to the severity of iodine deficiency.[5] Concomitantly, the percentage of retention of administered $^{131}I$ was directly related to the severity of iodine deficiency.[5]

The trapping of iodide by the thyroid depends on an active transport mechanism (i.e., it requires energy), which is called the "iodine pump." This mechanism is regulated by the thyroid-stimulating hormone (TSH), which is released from the pituitary to regulate thyroid secretion.

Other ions can compete with iodide, including thiocyanate (SCN-). Thiocyanate is derived from the metabolism of hydrogen cyanide (HCN), which is found in foods such as cassava. Cassava is a dietary staple in Zaire and in many other countries. The occurrence of goiter and severe hypothyroidism in Zaire is associated with the use of cassava, particularly when it is not well cooked.[1,2]

The iodide is released by the thyroid cells into the colloid follicle phase between the cells, and there it is oxidized by hydrogen peroxide from the thyroid peroxidase system (Fig. 13–1).[7] It then combines with tyrosine in the thyroglobulin to form MIT and DIT. The oxidation process then continues with the coupling of MIT and DIT to form the iodotyrosines. This oxidation process can be readily blocked by various drugs including propylthiouracil and carbimazole, which are widely used for the treatment of hyperthyroidism. There may also be a congenital defect in biosynthesis so that iodide cannot be bound to tyrosine; this is a cause of congenital goiter and hypothyroidism, which may run in families. Such a defect does not, however, occur in iodine-deficient goiter. The reason why iodine deficiency causes goiter in some people and not in others is not known.

Finally the iodinated thyroglobulin, including the iodinated amino acids, is absorbed back into the thyroid cells by pinocytosis. It is then exposed to proteolytic enzymes, which break it down to release the $T_4$ and $T_3$ into the blood. The unused iodotyrosines are conserved for incorporation into a subsequent cycle of the biosynthetic process. With states of thyroid stimulation this conservation process may not be able to keep pace with the production of free iodotyrosines, which leak into the circulation but have no biologic effect.

The regulation of thyroid hormones is a complex process involving not only the thyroid, but the pituitary, the brain, and the peripheral tissues.

The thyroid secretion is under the control of the pituitary gland through TSH. TSH is a glycoprotein with a molecular weight of approximately 28,000. There are two subunits: the X subunit has virtually the same structure as other pituitary hormones; the B subunit is specific for TSH but is essentially the same across the different species.

The control of TSH secretion is by a "feedback" mechanism related closely to the level of $T_4$ in the blood. As the blood $T_4$ falls, the pituitary TSH secretion is increased, thereby enhancing both thyroid activity and the output of $T_4$ into the circulation, and so maintaining the necessary level of circulating hormone.

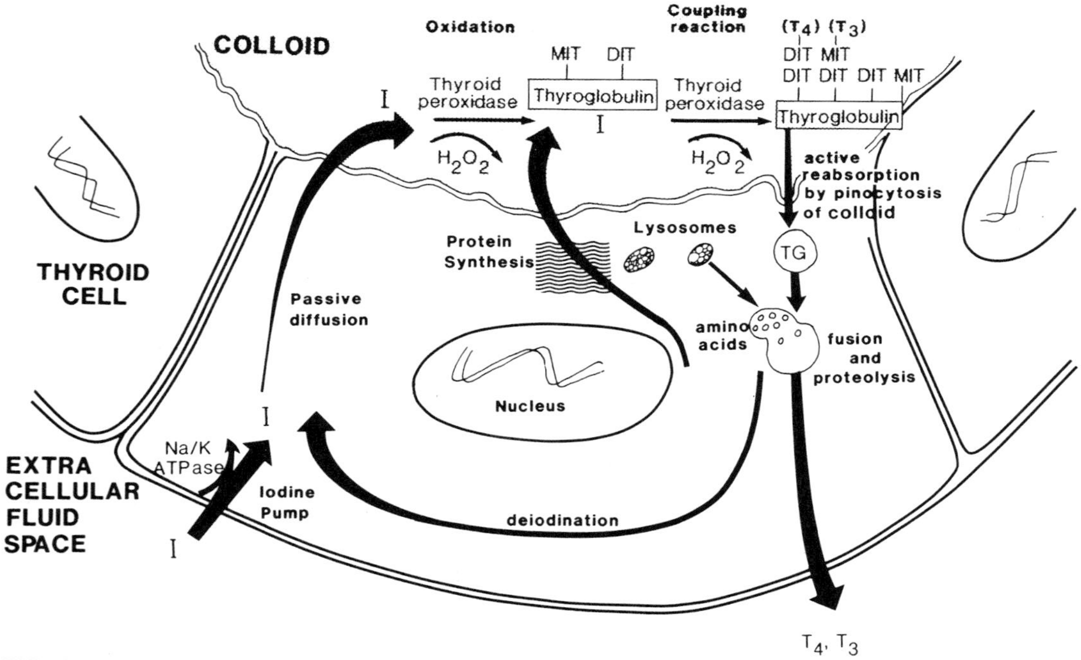
COLLOID
Oxidation
Coupling reaction
(T4) (T3)
MIT DIT
DIT MIT
DIT DIT DIT MIT
I
Thyroid peroxidase
Thyroglobulin
I
Thyroid peroxidase
Thyroglobulin
H2O2
H2O2
active reabsorption by pinocytosis of colloid
Lysosomes
Protein Synthesis
TG
THYROID CELL
Passive diffusion
amino acids
fusion and proteolysis
Nucleus
I
EXTRA CELLULAR FLUID SPACE
Na/K ATPase
Iodine Pump
deiodination
I
T4, T3

**FIGURE 13–1.** Diagram showing pathways of synthesis of thyroid hormones from iodine within the thyroid gland. (From Hetzel, B.S., Maberly, G.F.: Iodine. *In* Trace Elements in Human and Animal Nutrition, 5th Ed. Vol. 2. Edited by W. Mertz. New York, Academic Press, 1986, pp. 139–208.)

If this is not possible because of severe iodine deficiency, then the level of $T_4$ remains lowered and the level of TSH remains elevated. Both these measurements are used for the diagnosis of hypothyroidism due to iodine deficiency at various stages in life but particularly in the neonate.

Levels of blood thyroid hormones and TSH are determined using radioimmunoassay (RIA) when known amounts of radioactively labeled hormones are used and compete with the unknown amount of hormone in the blood in binding to a specific antibody. The technology for these determinations is still advancing, and further improvements are being developed, as discussed later in this chapter.

### DEVELOPMENT OF GOITER

The preceding discussion on the production and regulation of thyroid hormones provides the framework for understanding the production of goiter as a result of iodine deficiency. Although not the only cause, iodine deficiency is the primary cause of goiter. Goitrogens such as thiocyanates that can enhance the effect of iodine deficiency are referred to as secondary factors.[1,2]

The basic effect of iodine deficiency is to interfere with the production of thyroid hormones because iodine is an essential constituent of the $T_4$ and $T_3$ molecules. The lowering of output from the thyroid leads to a fall in the blood levels of $T_4$ but to some increase in $T_3$ (the less iodinated hormone is produced preferentially in iodine deficiency).

The fall in the level of $T_4$ leads to increase in TSH output from the pituitary. TSH increases the uptake of iodide by the thyroid with increased turnover associated with hyperplasia of the cells of the thyroid follicles. The reserves of colloid-containing thyroglobulin are gradually used up so that the gland has a much more cellular appearance than normal. The size of the gland increases with the formation of a goiter. Enlargement is regarded as significant in the human when the size of the lateral lobes is greater than the terminal phalanx of the thumb of the person examined. More-precise measurements can now be made using ultrasonography.[4]

Extensive reviews of the global geographic prevalence of goiter have been published.[1–4]

## IODINE DEFICIENCY DISORDERS (IDD)

The effects of iodine deficiency on growth and development are now denoted by the term iodine deficiency disorders (IDD). These effects are evident at all ages, but particularly in the fetal stage, the neonatal stage, and infancy, which are the periods of rapid growth. The term "goiter" has been used for many years to describe the primary effect of iodine deficiency. Goiter is indeed the most obvious and familiar feature of iodine deficiency. Because knowledge of iodine deficiency has greatly expanded in the last 25 years (Table 13–2), the new term "IDD" was introduced.[3–5]

### FETUS

Iodine deficiency of the fetus is the result of iodine deficiency in the mother. The condition is associated with a greater incidence of stillbirths, abortions, and congenital abnormalities, which can be reduced by iodization (Table 13–2). The effects are similar to those observed with maternal hypothyroidism, which can be reduced by thyroid hormone replacement therapy.[8]

Controlled trials with iodized oil have revealed a significant reduction in recorded fetal and neonatal deaths in the treated group of pregnant women, which is consistent with animal evidence indicating the effect of iodine deficiency on fetal survival.[3–5]

Further data from Papua New Guinea indicates a relationship between the level of maternal thyroxine with the outcome of current and recent past pregnancies, including mortality and the occurrence of cretinism. The rate of perinatal deaths was twice as high among mothers (36.0%) with very low serum concentrations of total thyroxine compared to women (16.4%) with levels above 25 μg/ml.[8,9]

**TABLE 13–2.** THE SPECTRUM OF IODINE DEFICIENCY DISORDERS (IDD)

| | |
|---|---|
| **Fetus** | Abortions |
| | Stillbirths |
| | Congenital anomalies |
| | Increased perinatal mortality |
| | Increased infant mortality |
| | Neurologic cretinism (Mental deficiency, deaf mutism, spastic diplegia, squint) |
| | Myxedematous cretinism (dwarfism, mental deficiency) |
| | Psychomotor defects |
| **Neonate** | Neonatal goiter |
| | Neonatal hypothyroidism |
| **Child and Adolescent** | Goiter |
| | Juvenile hypothyroidism |
| | Impaired mental function |
| | Retarded physical development |
| **Adult** | Goiter with its complications |
| | Hypothyroidism |
| | Impaired mental function |
| | Iodine induced hyperthyroidism |

Data from Hetzel, B.S., Potter, B.J., Dulberg, E.M.: World Rev. Nutr. Diet., *62*:59-119, 1990; and Hetzel, B.S., Dunn, J.T., Stanbury, J.B. (eds.): The Prevention and Control of Iodine Deficiency Disorders. Amsterdam, Elsevier, 1987).

These data, indicating the importance of maternal thyroid function to fetal survival and development, are complemented by extensive animal data.[3]

A major effect of fetal iodine deficiency is the condition of endemic cretinism, which is distinct from the condition of sporadic cretinism.[1–3,9]

Endemic cretinism, which occurs with an iodine intake of below 25 μg per day in contrast to a normal intake of 80 to 150 μg per day, is still widely prevalent, affecting for example up to 10% of the populations living in severely iodine-deficient areas in India, Indonesia, and China.[9,10] In its most common form, it is characterized by mental deficiency, deaf mutism, and spastic diplegia, which is referred to as the "nervous" or neurologic type, in contrast to the less common "myxedematous" type characterized by hypothyroidism with dwarfism.

Apart from its prevalence in Asia and Oceania (Papua New Guinea), cretinism also occurs in Africa (Zaire) and in South America in the Andean region (Ecuador, Peru, Bolivia, and Argentina).[9] In all these situations, with the exception of Zaire, neurologic features are predominant. In Zaire the myxedematous form is more common, probably because of the high intake of cassava.[11] However, there is considerable variation in the clinical manifestations of neurologic cretinism, which include isolated deaf mutism and mental defect of varying degrees. In China the term "cretinoid" is used to describe these individuals.[10]

The apparent spontaneous disappearance of endemic cretinism in Italy and Switzerland raised considerable doubts as to the relation of iodine deficiency to the condition.[1,3,5] However, a controlled trial in the Western Highlands of Papua New Guinea revealed that endemic cretinism could be prevented by correction of iodine deficiency with iodized oil before pregnancy.[1,3,12]

The value of iodized oil injection in the prevention of endemic cretinism has been confirmed in Zaire and in South America. Mass injection programs have been carried out in New Guinea (in 1971 and 1972) and in Zaire, Indonesia, and in China. Recent evaluations of these mass programs in Indonesia and China indicate that endemic cretinism has been prevented where correction of iodine deficiency has been achieved.[2,4,5]

The apparent spontaneous disappearance of the condition is now attributed to increase in iodine intake due to dietary diversification as a result of social and economic development affecting more remote rural areas.

## NEONATE

An increased perinatal mortality rate due to iodine deficiency has been shown in Zaire from the results of a controlled trial of iodized oil injections given in the latter half of pregnancy, alternated with a control injection.[3,4] There is a substantial fall in perinatal and infant mortality with improved birth weight. Low birth weight is generally (whatever the cause) associated with a higher rate of congenital anomalies and higher risk through childhood.

Apart from the question of mortality, the importance of the state of thyroid function in the neonate relates to the fact that at birth the brain of the human infant has only reached about one third of its full size and continues to grow rapidly until the end of the second year.[19] The thyroid hormone, dependent on an adequate supply of iodine, is essential for normal brain development, as has been confirmed by animal studies.[3,14]

Data on iodine nutrition and neonatal thyroid function in Europe confirm that the continuing presence of severe iodine deficiency affects neonatal thyroid function and is hence a threat to early brain development.[15]

There is similar evidence from neonatal observations in Zaire in Africa, where rates of biochemical hypothyroidism of 10% ($T_4$ less than 38.6 nmol/L or 3.0 μg/dl) have been found.[16] In Zaire it has been observed that this hypothyroidism persists into infancy and childhood and, if uncorrected, results in retardation of physical and mental development.

These observations indicate a much greater risk of mental defect in severely iodine-deficient populations than is indicated by the presence of classic cretinism.

## CHILD

Iodine deficiency in children is characteristically associated with goiter. The classification of goiter standardized by the World Health Organization is shown in Table 13–3. The goiter rate increases with age so that it reaches a maximum with adolescence. Girls have a higher prevalence than boys. Goiter rates in 8- to 14-year-old school children are a convenient indicator of iodine deficiency in a community.

School children living in iodine-deficient areas from a number of countries show impaired school performance and lower IQs in comparison with matched groups from areas that are not iodine-deficient. Because many possible causes exist for impaired performance in school or on an IQ test, the interpretation of any differences that might be observed between children living in different areas is difficult. The iodine-deficient area is likely to be more remote, to suffer more social deprivation, to have poorer school facilities, and to be characterized by a lower socioeconomic status and poorer general nutrition. All such factors have to be taken into account, apart from the problem of adapting tests developed in Western countries for use in Third World countries.

The results of a number of studies indicate the significant role of iodine deficiency in intellectual development and in school performance,[17,18] although other factors such as social deprivation and other nutritional factors are also important.

**TABLE 13–3.** DEFINITION OF GOITER STAGES

**A. Definition of goiter**

A normal thyroid gland should have the minimal size compatible with euthyroidism under conditions of normal iodine intake (100 to 150 μg/d). This gland would be nonpalpable or barely palpable. For practical purposes a thyroid gland whose lateral lobes have a volume greater than the terminal phalanges of the thumbs of the person examined is defined as goitrous.

**B. Estimation of thyroid size**

| | |
|---|---|
| Stage 0 | No goiter |
| Stage 1a | Goiter detectable |
| Stage 1b | Goiter palpable and visible only when the neck is fully extended. This stage also includes nodular glands, even if not goitrous; see Section C below. |
| Stage 2 | Goiter visible with the neck in normal position; palpation is not needed for diagnosis. |
| Stage 3 | Very large goiter that can be recognized at a considerable distance. |

In case of doubt between any two of these stages, the lower should be recorded.

The total goiter rate is the prevalence of stages 1 to 3; the visible goiter rate is the prevalence of stages 2 to 3. This classification is appropriate to field surveys for public health purposes. For clinical purposes, more precise information can be obtained by other techniques including scintigraphy and sonography.

**C. Estimation of the consistency of the thyroid by palpation**

The diffuse or nodular consistency of the thyroid should be recorded. Nodules usually occur in areas where marked iodine deficiency has been long-standing. This estimation should be independent of that for the size of the thyroid, with the following exception: when one or more nodules are found in a nongoitrous gland, it will be recorded as Stage 1b because nodularity implies marked modifications in the structure of the gland.

**Definition of IDD as a public health problem**

An area is arbitrarily defined as endemic with respect to goiter if more than 10% of the population or of the children aged 6 to 12 years are found to be goitrous. The figure 10% was chosen because a higher prevalence usually implies an environmental factor, whereas a prevalence of several percent is common even when all known environment factors are controlled.

(From Dunn, J.T., Pretell, E.A., Daza, C.H. (eds.): Towards the Eradication of Endemic Goiter, Cretinism, and Iodine Deficiency. Washington, D.C., Pan American Health Organization, 1986.)

### ADULT

Iodine administration in the form of iodized salt, iodized bread, or iodized oil have all been demonstrated to be effective in the prevention of goiter in adults. Iodine administration may also reduce existing goiter in adults. This is particularly true of iodized oil injections.[1,4,5] This obvious effect leads to ready acceptance of the measure by people living in iodine-deficient communities. A rise in circulating thyroxine can be readily demonstrated in adult subjects following iodization.

The major determinant of brain (and pituitary) $T_3$ is serum thyroxine ($T_4$) and not $T_3$ (as is true of the liver, kidney, and muscle). Low levels of brain $T_3$ have been demonstrated in the iodine-deficient rat in association with reduced levels of serum $T_4$. Both have been restored to normal with correction of iodine deficiency.[19]

These findings provide an explanation for suboptimal brain function in subjects with endemic goiter and lowered serum $T_4$ levels, and for its improvement following correction of iodine deficiency.

In northern India a high degree of apathy has been noted in populations living in iodine-deficient areas. This may even affect domestic animals such as dogs! It is apparent that reduced mental function is widely prevalent in iodine-deficient communities, with effects on their residents' capacity for initiative and decision-making.

Thus, iodine deficiency is a major block to the human and social development of communities living in an iodine-deficient environment. Correction of the iodine deficiency is indicated as a major contribution to development.

## EFFECTS OF IODINE DEFICIENCY IN ANIMALS

Iodine deficiency in farm animals causes reproductive failure and thyroid insufficiency, as reported in the older literature.[7] In areas of iodine deficiency, development of the fetus has been retarded or arrested at some stage in gestation, resulting in resorption, abortion, stillbirth, early death, or the birth of weak, hairless offspring associated with prolonged gestation and parturition and retention of placental membranes. Subnormal thyroid hormone levels in herds of cattle have been accompanied by a high incidence of aborted, stillborn, and weak calves.[7]

An important new dimension has been provided by recent experimental work with animal models.[3,14,19] Severe iodine deficiency has been established prior to and during pregnancy, and then the effects on fetal development have been studied. Iodine deficiency in the sheep (5 to 8 μg per day for sheep weighing 40 kg) is associated with an increased incidence in abortions and stillbirths. At the end of pregnancy the fetus shows a reduced body weight, complete absence of wool growth, deformation of the skull, and retardation of bone development. There is retardation of brain development as indicated by reduced brain weight and a reduced number of cells (as measured by DNA). Similar effects have been observed in the marmoset monkey (0.3 μg per day for a 340-g animal).

In the light of data indicating transfer of $T_4$ across the placenta in the human and in the rat,[20] it may be concluded that the effects of severe iodine deficiency on fetal development are mediated by a combination of maternal and fetal hypothyroidism, the effect of maternal hypothyroidism occurring earlier than the onset of fetal thyroid secretion. This would imply an effect on neuroblast multiplication, which occurs from 40 to 80 days of gestation in the sheep and 11 to 18 weeks in the human.[3,14,21] In the rat (a postnatal brain developer in which neuroblast multiplication occurs in the last third of fetal life), an effect of the maternal thyroid early in pregnancy is indicated by reduced weight and number of embryos, reduced brain weight, and reduced transfer of maternal $T_4$.[3,14,19]

These findings suggest that iodine deficiency has an early effect on neuroblast multiplication; if so, this could be important in the pathogenesis of the neurologic form of endemic cretinism.[3,14,21]

## ASSESSMENT OF IODINE STATUS

The assessment of iodine nutritional status is important in relation to public health programs in which iodine supplementation is carried out. The problem is therefore one of assessment of a population or group living in an area or region that is suspected to be iodine deficient.

The data methods recommended are as follows:

1. *The goiter rate,* including the rate of palpable or visible goiter, classified according to accepted criteria.[22] A classification of goiter severity has been adopted by the World Health Organization.[1,2,22] There are still minor differences in technique between different observers. In general, visible goiter is more readily verified than palpable goiter. Recent observations in Tanzania indicate that palpation of the thyroid overestimates the size of the gland as determined by ultrasonography, particularly in children.[4] However, the assessment of goiter rate in a whole population, although desirable, is time-consuming, costly, and not essential. Limited representative samples of the population sufficient to verify its presence are usually adequate. In adults goiter represents past iodine deficiency. Ultrasonography is going to provide more objective measurements in the future.[4]
2. *The determination of urine iodine excretion.* This can be carried out appropriately on 24-hour samples. However, the difficulties of such collections may be insurmountable. For this reason, as originally suggested by Follis, determinations can be carried out on casual samples from a group of approximately 40 subjects. The iodine levels are expressed as micrograms per 100 ml, and the range is plotted out as a histogram.* This provides a reference point for the level of iodine excretion, which is also a good index of the level of iodine nutrition. The availability of modern automated equipment (auto analyzer) is making the analysis of large numbers of samples feasible. Dry ashing with a muffle furnace or a wet digestion procedure for the conversion of iodine from organic to inorganic form are widely used.[4] Excessive iodine intake can also be conveniently monitored by determination of urine iodine excretion.
3. *The determination of the level of serum thyroxine ($T_4$) or TSH* provides an indirect measure of iodine nutritional status. Various methods and normal levels are shown in Table 13–4. The availability of radioimmunoassay methods with automated equipment has greatly assisted this approach, and TSH is now the preferred method because of better stability under tropical conditions and easier use. Particular attention should be given to levels of TSH in the neonate and pregnant female.

In the developed countries of the world, where iodine deficiency in humans normally does not exist, all babies born are screened to ensure they have adequate thyroid hormone levels. These screening programs use blood from heel pricks of neonates, which is spotted onto filter paper, dried, and sent to a regional laboratory. Blood levels of either $T_4$ or TSH or both are measured by immunoassay techniques. The rate of neonatal hypothyroidism requiring treatment is about 1 per 3500 babies screened. This rate varies little among developed countries.[23]

Neonatal hypothyroid screening has been initiated in several less developed iodine-deficient regions. Severe biochemical hypothyroidism has been reported in up to 10% of neonates in northern India[23] and in Zaire.[4]

*Formerly the level of excretion was expressed in relation to creatinine concentration—that is, micrograms of iodine per gram of creatinine. However, the level of creatinine varies because of nutritional status and introduces an unnecessary additional variable.

**TABLE 13–4.** NORMAL LEVELS FOR SERUM THYROID HORMONES ($T_4$, $T_3$) AND PITUITARY THYROID-STIMULATING HORMONE (TSH)

| HORMONE | ABBREVIATION | MOST COMMON METHOD | REPRESENTATIVE MIDNORMAL VALUES | |
|---|---|---|---|---|
| | | | PRESENT | SI UNITS |
| Thyroxine | $T_4$ | Immunoassay | 8 μg/dl | 100 nmol/L |
| Triiodothyronine (3,5,3′-triiodothyronine) | $T_3$ | Immunoassay | 130 ng/dl | 2.0 nmol/L |
| Thyrotropin (thyroid-stimulating hormone of the pituitary) | TSH | Immunoassay | 2 μU/ml | 2 mU/L |

Abbreviated from Larsen, P.R., Alexander, N.M., Chopra, I.J., et al.: J. Clin. Endocrinol. Metab., *64*:1089-1094, 1987.)

Within an iodine-deficient population, serum $T_4$ levels are lowest at birth and lower in children than in the adult population.[4,11,23] In addition, goitrogens such as cassava seem to be much more potent at reducing serum $T_4$ levels in neonates and children than in adults.

To summarize, the most critical evidence for determining iodine nutritional status comes from measurement of urine excretion of iodine and from the measurement of blood TSH in the neonate or pregnant female. The results of these two determinations indicate the severity of the problem, as indicated in Table 13–5. They can also be used to assess the effectiveness of remedial measures.

## IODINE REQUIREMENTS

In 1989 the Food and Nutrition Board of the National Academy of Sciences National Research Council of the United States confirmed the previous 1980 recommendations for a daily iodine intake of 40 μg for children aged 0 to 6 months, 50 μg from 6 to 12 months, 70 to 120 μg from 1 to 10 years, and 120 to 150 μg from 11 years onward. The recommended rates during pregnancy and lactation were, respectively, 175 and 200 μg. The recommendations applied equally to both sexes[24] (see Appendix Table A-2b).

## IODINE TOXICITY

Iodine toxicity has been critically studied in man, laboratory species, poultry, pigs, and cattle.

Wolff has suggested that daily human intakes of 2000 μg I should be regarded as an excessive or potentially harmful level of intake.[25] Normal diets composed of natural foods are unlikely to supply as much as 2000 μg I per day, and most would supply less than 1000 μg I, except where the diets are exceptionally high in marine fish or seaweed, or where foods are contaminated with iodine from adventitious sources.

Inhabitants of the coastal regions of Hokkaido, the northern island of Japan, whose diets contain large amounts of seaweed, have remarkably high daily iodine intakes amounting to 50,000 to 80,000 μg I.[26] Daily urinary excretion in 5 patients exhibiting clinical signs of iodide goiter exceeded 20 mg I, or about 100 times normal. Similar findings have been reported from two Chinese villages on the Yellow Sea Coast in association with the consumption of large amounts of kelp.[27]

In Japan,[28] it has been shown that:

1. Normal subjects who have not been iodine deficient can maintain normal thyroid function states even when they are taking several milligrams of dietary iodine per day.

**TABLE 13–5.** GRADES OF SEVERITY OF IODINE DEFICIENCY DISORDERS (IDD)

| | MILD IDD | MODERATE IDD | SEVERE IDD |
|---|---|---|---|
| 1. Prevalence of goiter % (total) | 5–19 | 20–29 | >30 |
| 2. Cretinism | 0 | 0 | 0–5 |
| 3. Daily urine I μg/d | 50–100 | 25–49 | <25 |
| Median urine I μg/dl | 3.5–5 | 2–3.4 | 0–1.9 |
| 4. Prevalence of neonatal TSH >50 μU/ml (day 5 of life) | <1% | 1–5% | >5% |

(From WHO/ICCIDD Report of the Consultation on the Assessment and Monitoring of Iodine Deficiency Disorders. Geneva, World Health Organization. In preparation.)

2. Incidence of nontoxic diffuse goiter and toxic nodular goiter are remarkably decreased by high dietary iodine.
3. Incidence of Graves' disease and Hashimoto's disease appears not to be affected by high dietary iodine.
4. However, high dietary iodine may induce hypothyroidism in autoimmune thyroid diseases and may inhibit the effects of thionamide drugs.

Species differences in tolerance to high iodine intakes are significant. In all species studied the tolerance is high relative to normal dietary iodine intakes, pointing to a wide margin of safety for this element.

### IODINE-INDUCED HYPERTHYROIDISM

A mild increase in incidence of hyperthyroidism has now been described following iodized salt programs in Europe and South America and following the use of iodized bread in Holland and Tasmania.[29,30] A few cases have been noted following iodized oil administration in South America. No cases have yet been described in New Guinea, India, or Zaire. This is probably due to the scattered nature of the population into small villages and limited opportunities for observation.[31] Natural remission also occurs. The condition is largely confined to those over 40 years of age; a smaller proportion of the population in developing countries is affected than in developed countries. Detailed observations are available from the island of Tasmania.[30,32]

Joseph et al. reported that daily iodine intakes of less than 0.10 mg pose no risk for patients with autonomous thyroids due to iodine deficiency, but that critical daily intakes are probably between 0.10 and 0.20 mg.[33] The iodation of bread in Tasmania resulted in thyrotoxicosis for some individuals at levels of iodine intake of about 0.20 mg per day.[30,32] Iodated bread in Holland contributed an additional 0.12 to 0.16 mg of iodine per day and increased the incidence of thyrotoxicosis. The spring-summer peak of thyrotoxicosis (related to winter milk) in England occurred with average daily iodine intakes of 0.24 mg for women and 0.32 mg for men.[34] The absence of iodine deficiency in the Japanese population accounts for the absence of iodine-induced thyrotoxicosis.[28]

Thyrotoxicosis is readily controlled with antithyroid drugs or radioiodine. Spontaneous remission also occurs. In general, iodation should be avoided in those over the age of 40 because of the risk of hyperthyroidism,[1,2,4] even with an increase to normal levels of intake, primarily because an autonomous thyroid can develop independently of TSH control, which continues its high rate of secretion in spite of an increase in iodine intake.

However, the correction of iodine deficiency prevents the formation of an autonomous thyroid and so prevents the condition of iodine-induced hyperthyroidism. Hence this condition is included as an "iodine-deficiency disorder" (see Table 13–2).

## CORRECTION OF IODINE DEFICIENCY

### IODIZED SALT

Iodation of salt has been the major method used for the correction of iodine deficiency since the 1920s, when it was first successfully used in Switzerland.[1,4,5] Since then, successful programs have been reported from a number of countries. These include Central and South America (e.g., Guatemala and Colombia), Finland, China, and Taiwan.[5]

The difficulties in producing, monitoring, and distributing iodized salt to the millions that are iodine deficient, especially in Asia, are vividly demonstrated in India, where there has been a breakdown in supply. The difficulties have led to the adoption of a proposal that universal salt iodination for India be achieved by 1992.

In Asia, the cost of iodized salt production and distribution at present is of the order of 3 to 5 cents per person per year.[4] This cost is small in relation to the social benefits that have been described in the previous section. However, there is still the problem of the salt actually reaching the iodine-deficient subject. There may also be a problem with distribution or preservation of the iodine content—salt may be left uncovered or exposed to heat. It should be added after cooking to reduce the loss of iodine.

Finally there is the difficulty of actual consumption of the salt. Although the addition of iodine makes no difference to the taste of the salt, the introduction of a new variety of salt to an area where salt is already available and familiar and much appreciated as a condiment is likely to be resisted. In the Chinese provinces of Sinjiang and Inner Mongolia, the strong preference of the people for desert salt of very low iodine content led to a mass iodized oil injection program to prevent cretinism.[10]

### IODIZED OIL BY INJECTION

The value of iodized oil injection in the prevention of endemic goiter and endemic cretinism was first established in New Guinea with controlled trials involving the use of saline injection as a control. These trials established the value of the oil in the prevention of goiter and the prevention of cretinism.[4,12,35] Experience in South America, Zaire, and China has confirmed the value of the measure. The quantitative correction of severe iodine deficiency by a single intramuscular injection has been demonstrated for a period of over 4 years.[4]

Iodized oil is singularly appropriate for isolated village communities so characteristic of mountainous endemic goiter areas. The striking regression of goiter following iodized oil injection ensures general acceptance of the measure.

In a suitable area the oil (1 ml contains 480 mg) should be administered to all females up to the age of 40 years and all males up to the age of 20 years. A repeat injection would be required in 3 to 5 years, depending on the dose given and the age. In children the need is greater than in adults, and the recommended dose should be repeated in 3 years if severe iodine deficiency persists.[4]

Iodized walnut oil and iodized soya bean oil preparations have been developed in China since 1980.[4]

### IODIZED OIL BY MOUTH

Recent studies in India and China reveal that oral iodized oil lasts only half as long as a similar dose given by injection.[4] A recent review indicates the need for more extensive studies to determine the effectiveness of a massive intervention.[4]

### CHOICE OF INTERVENTION METHODS

There are three grades of severity of IDD in a population, based on the urinary iodine excretion.[4,5] These are as follows:

1. *Mild IDD* with goiter prevalence in the range of 5 to 20% (school children) and with median urine iodine levels in the range 3.5 to 5.0 μg/dl. Mild IDD can be controlled with iodated salt at a concentration of 10 to 25 mg/kg. Mild IDD may disappear with economic development.
2. *Moderate IDD* with goiter prevalence up to 30%, some hypothyroidism, and median urine iodine levels in the range 2.0 to 3.5 μg/dl. Moderate IDD can be controlled with iodinated salt (25 to 40 mg/kg) if the salt can be effectively produced and distributed. Otherwise, iodized oil, given orally or by injection, should be used through the primary health care system.
3. *Severe IDD* with a high prevalence of goiter (30% or more), endemic cretinism (prevalence 1 to 10%), and median urine iodine level below 2.0 μg/dl. Severe IDD requires the use of iodized oil either orally or by injection for the prevention of central nervous system defects.

Iodated salt and iodated oil are the major supplementation measures that have been used on a large scale. More than 20 million injections of iodated oil have been given in Asia with evidence of successful prevention of IDD.

## INTERNATIONAL ACTION

The great gap between our new knowledge of IDD and the application of this knowledge in national IDD control programs, particularly in developing countries, has led to the formation of the International Council for the Control of Iodine Deficiency Disorders (ICCIDD).

The inaugural meeting of this multidisciplinary group of epidemiologists and nutritionists, endocrinologists and chemists, planners and economists was held in Kathmandu, Nepal, in March 1986. A series of papers presented in Kathmandu on all aspects of IDD control programs has been published as a monograph.[4] The ICCIDD has now established a global multidisciplinary network of some 300 people with expertise relevant to IDD and IDD control programs. It works closely with the World Health Organization (WHO), the United Nations International Children's Fund (UNICEF), and the United Nations (UN), as well as with national governments, in the development of national programs.[4,5]

The major concentrations of population are in Asia, where IDD control programs have been established during the last 5 years in India, Indonesia, Nepal, Burma, and Bhutan.[6]

In Latin America earlier efforts have produced a large measure of control in such countries as Argentina, Brazil, Colombia, and Guatemala. Problems have recurred in Colombia and Guatemala that are associated with political and social unrest, however. Major IDD problems have persisted in Ecuador, Peru, and Bolivia, but there has been significant progress in the last 3 years with the combination of national government initiative and support from international agencies.[6]

In Africa there has been a lag in the development of IDD control programs in comparison with the other continents. However, new initiatives have begun following a joint WHO/UNICEF/ICCIDD regional seminar held in Yaounde, Cameroon in March 1987. This seminar set up a joint IDD Task Force, which has now initiated comprehensive planning for the prevention and control of IDD in Africa.[6]

China has also made rapid progress since the passing of the Cultural Revolution in 1976. One-third of the population of China (370 million) is at risk of IDD because of the extensive mountainous areas and the flooded river valleys in that country.[6,10]

The feasibility of substantial progress in the prevention and control of IDD in the next 5 to 10 years was determined in a World Health Assembly Resolution in 1986.[6]

A Global Action Plan designed to achieve the objective of eliminating IDD as a major public health problem (see Table 13–3) by the year 2000 has now been adopted by the UN System,[35] including WHO,[6] UNICEF, and the World Bank.

In September 1990 the World Summit for Children, held at the United Nations in New York, was attended by 71 heads of state and 80 other government representatives. The World Summit signed a Declaration and approved a plan of action that included the elimination of IDD as a public health problem by the year 2000.

This was followed in October 1991 by a Conference entitled "Ending Hidden Hunger." This was a policy and promotional meeting on micronutrients including iodine, vitamin A, and iron. It was attended by multidisciplinary delegations from 55 countries with major IDD problems nominated by heads of state in response to an invitation by the director general of the World Health

Organization (Dr. H. Nakajima) and the executive director of UNICEF (Mr. James Grant). There was a firm commitment at this meeting to the elimination goal for IDD and vitamin A deficiency, with reduction of iron deficiency by one third of 1990 levels.

These objectives were accepted following previous triumphs, as in the eradication of small pox and the success of the expanded program of immunization, which was celebrated at the United Nations in October 1990.

These various developments encourage the hope that significant progress can be made toward the elimination of IDD within the next decade with great benefits to the quality of life of the many millions affected.

## REFERENCES


1. Stanbury, J.B., Hetzel, B.S.: Endemic Goiter and Endemic Cretinism. New York, John Wiley & Sons, 1980.
2. Dunn, J.T., Pretell, E.A., Daza, C.H. (eds.): Towards the Eradication of Endemic Goiter, Cretinism, and Iodine Deficiency. Washington, D.C., Pan American Health Organization, 1986.
3. Hetzel, B.S., Potter, B.J., Dulberg, E.M.: World Rev. Nutr. Diet. *62:*59–119, 1990.
4. Hetzel, B.S., Dunn, J.T., Stanbury, J.B. (eds.): The Prevention and Control of Iodine Deficiency Disorders. Amsterdam, Elsevier, 1987.
5. Hetzel, B.S.: The Story of Iodine Deficiency—An International Challenge in Nutrition. Oxford, Oxford University Press, 1989.
6. World Health Organization Report to 43rd World Health Assembly, Geneva, 1990.
7. Hetzel, B.S., Maberly, G.F. Iodine. *In* Trace Elements in Human and Animal Nutrition. 5th Ed. Edited by W. Mertz. New York, Academic Press, 1986, pp. 139–208.
8. McMichael, A.J., Potter, J.D., Hetzel, B.S.: Iodine deficiency, thyroid function, and reproductive failure. *In* Endemic Goiter and Endemic Cretinism. Edited by J.B. Stanbury and B.S. Hetzel. New York, John Wiley & Sons, 1980, pp. 445–460.
9. Pharoah, P.O.D., Delange, F. Fierro Benitez, R., et al.: Endemic cretinism. *In* Endemic Goiter and Endemic Cretinism. Edited by J.B. Stanbury and B.S. Hetzel. New York, Wiley, 1980, pp. 395–421.
10. Ma, T., Lu, T., Tan, U., et al.: Food Nutr. Bull., *4:*13, 1982.
11. Delange, F., Iteke, F.B., Ermans, A.M. (eds.): Nutritional Factors Involved in the Goitrogenic Action of Cassava. Ottawa, International Development Research Center, 1982.
12. Pharoah, P.O.D., Buttfield, I.H., Hetzel, B.S.: Lancet, *1:*308, 1971.
13. Dobbing, J.: The later development of the brain and its vulnerability. *In* Scientific Foundations of Paediatrics. Edited by J. Davis and J. Dobbing. London, Heinemann Medical, 1974, pp. 565–577.
14. Hetzel, B.S., Chavadej, J., Potter, B.J.: Neuropathol. Appl. Neurobiol., *14:*93–104, 1988.
15. Delange, F., Heidemann, P., Bourdoux, et al.: Biol. Neonate, *49:*322–330, 1986.
16. Ermans, A.M., Moulameko, N.M., Delange, F., Alhuwalia, R. (eds.): Role of Cassava in the Aetiology of Endemic Goiter and Cretinism. Ottawa, International Development Research Center, 1980.
17. Fierro-Benitez, R., Cazar, R., Stanbury, J.B., et al.: Long-term effect of correction of iodine deficiency on psychomotor and intellectual development. *In* Towards the Eradication of Endemic Goiter, Cretinism, and Iodine Deficiency. Edited by J.T. Dunn, E.A. Pretell, C.H. Daza, and F.E. Viteri. Washington, D.C., Pan American Health Organization, 1986, pp. 182–200.
18. Boyages, S.C., Collins, J.K., Maberly, G.F., et al.: Med. J. Aust., *150:*676–679, 1989.
19. Obregon, M.J., Santisteban, P., Rodriguez-Pena, A., et al.: Endocrinology, *115:*614–624, 1984.
20. Vulsma, T., Gons, M.H., DeVijlder, J.J.M., et al.: N. Engl. J. Med., *321:*13–16, 1989.
21. DeLong, R.: Neurological involvement in iodine deficiency disorders. *In* The Prevention and Control of Iodine Deficiency Disorders. Edited by B.S. Hetzel, J.T. Dunn, and J.B. Stanbury. Amsterdam, Elsevier, 1987, pp. 49–63.
22. Thilly, C.H., Delange, F., Stanbury, J.B.: Epidemiologic surveys in endemic goitre and cretinism. *In* Endemic goiter and Endemic Cretinism. Edited by J.B. Stanbury and B.S. Hetzel. New York, John Wiley & Sons, 1980, pp. 157–184.
23. Burrow, G.N. (ed.): Neonatal Thyroid Screening. New York, Raven Press, 1980.
24. Food and Nutrition Board, National Academy of Sciences, National Research Council: Recommended Dietary Allowances. 10th Ed. Washington, D.C., 1989.
25. Wolff, J.: Am. J. Med., *47:*101–124, 1969.
26. Suzuki, H.: Etiology of endemic goiter and iodide excess. *In* Endemic Goiter and Endemic Cretinism. Edited by J.B. Stanbury and B.S. Hetzel. New York, Wiley, 1980, pp. 237–253.
27. Zhu, X.Y., Lu, T.Z., Song, X.K., et al.: The present status of endemic goitre and endemic cretinism in China. *In* Current Problems in Thyroid Research. Edited by N. Ui, K. Torizuka, S. Nagataki, and K. Miyai. Amsterdam, Excerpta Medica, 1983, pp. 13–15.
28. Nagataki, S.: Effects of iodide supplement in thyroid diseases. *In* Recent Progress in Thyroidology. Edited by A. Vichayanrat, W. Nitiyanant, C. Eastman, and S. Nagataki. Bangkok, Crystal House Press, 1987, pp. 31–37.
29. Connolly, R.J., Vidor, G.I., Stewart, J.C.: Lancet, *1:*500–502, 1970.
30. Stewart, J.C., Vidor, G.I., Buttfield, I.H., et al.: Aust. N. Z. J. Med., *3:*203–211, 1971.
31. Larsen, P.R., Silva, J.E., Hetzel, B.S., et al.: Monitoring prophylactic programs; general consideration. *In* Endemic Goiter and Endemic Cretinism. Edited by J.B. Stanbury and B.S. Hetzel. New York, John Wiley & Sons, 1980, pp. 551–566.

32. Vidor, G.I., Stewart, J.C., Wall, J.R., et al.: J. Clin. Endocrinol. Metab., *37*:901–909, 1973.
33. Joseph, K., Mahlstedt, J., Gonnermann, R., et al.: J. Mol. Med., *4*:21–37, 1980.
34. Nelson, M., Phillips, D.I.W.: Hum. Nutr. Appl. Nutr., *39*:213–218, 1985.
35. United Nations Administrative Committee on Coordination/Subcommittee on Nutrition, Paris, 16th Session. Geneva, World Health Organization, 1990.
36. Larsen, P.R., Alexander, N.M., Chopra, I.J., et al.: J. Clin. Endocrinol. Metab., *64*:1089–1094, 1987.

## SELECTED READINGS

*GENERAL*

Hetzel, B.S.: The Story of Iodine Deficiency: An International Challenge in Nutrition. Oxford, Oxford University Press, 1989.

*SCIENTIFIC*

Dunn, J.T., Pretell, E.A., Daza, C.H. (eds.): Towards the Eradication of Endemic Goiter, Cretinism, and Iodine Deficiency. Washington, D.C., Pan American Health Organization, 1986.

*PUBLIC HEALTH*

Hetzel, B.S., Dunn, J.T., Stanbury, J.B. (eds.): The Prevention and Control of Iodine Deficiency Disorders. Amsterdam, Elsevier, 1987.

CHAPTER 14

# Chromium

Forrest H. Nielsen



## HISTORICAL OVERVIEW

By 1948, chromium was recognized as a consistent component of plant and animal tissue. The first suggestion that chromium might have biologic activity appeared in 1954, when it was found that chromium enhanced the synthesis of cholesterol and fatty acids from acetate by rat liver. In 1959, trivalent chromium was identified as the active component of the "glucose tolerance factor," which alleviated the impaired glucose tolerance in rats fed certain diets apparently inadequate in chromium. Between 1964 and 1968, the first reports appeared that indicated chromium could affect glucose tolerance in humans. In these studies, mildly diabetic patients, or subjects with impaired glucose tolerance, received supplements of 2.72 to 3.62 μmol (150 to 200 μg) Cr per day as chromium chloride; the supplementation improved the impaired glucose tolerance of 40 to 50% of these individuals. Subsequently, it was found that the chromium supplementation also decreased serum cholesterol concentrations and normalized the exaggerated insulin responses to glucose loads. Despite these suggestive findings, chromium was not generally accepted as essential for humans until 1977, when chromium deficiency signs in a patient receiving total parenteral nutrition (TPN) were described. Shortly thereafter, other patients receiving TPN were found to exhibit abnormalities of glucose metabolism that were responsive to chromium supplementation.

For citations to original reports that are the basis for the discussion on chromium, the reader is referred to other reviews.[1–18]

## CHEMISTRY

Chromium can occur in oxidation states from 2− to 6+; the most common are 2+, 3+, and 6+. $Cr^{2+}$ is a strong reducing agent and, unless protected by coordination to strong ligands, is readily oxidized to $Cr^{3+}$. $Cr^{6+}$, predominantly combined with oxygen as either chromate ($CrO_4^{2-}$) or dichromate ($Cr_2O_7^{2-}$), is a strong oxidizing agent and is easily reduced to $Cr^{3+}$ in an acid milieu. $Cr^{6+}$ does not form coordination compounds but has been found in biologic materials. $Cr^{6+}$ has an affinity for red blood cells. On in vitro equilibration, or when injected intravenously, $Cr^{6+}$ crosses the erythrocyte membrane and becomes firmly bound to hemoglobin. $Cr^{3+}$ is the most stable oxidation state of chromium and is most likely the form of importance in biologic systems. $Cr^{3+}$ forms many coordination complexes, most of which are hexadentate. In aqueous solutions, $Cr^{3+}$ complexes are characterized by relative kinetic inertness such that ligand-displacement reactions have half-times in the range of several hours. Thus, chromium is unlikely to be involved as the metal catalyst at the active site of enzymes where the rate of exchange needs to be rapid. Such relatively inert chromium complexes, however, may function as structural components; for example, they may bind ligands in the proper orientation for enzymatic catalysis to occur, or be necessary for the tertiary structures of proteins and/or nucleic acids.

The biologically active form of chromium, sometimes called glucose tolerance factor or GTF, has been proposed to be a complex of chromium, nicotinic acid, and possibly the amino acids glycine, cysteine, and glutamic acid. Many attempts have been made to isolate or synthesize the glucose tolerance factor; none have been successful. Thus, the precise structure of this factor and whether or not GTF is the most biologically active form of chromium are points of controversy.

## METABOLISM

$Cr^{6+}$ is absorbed more readily than $Cr^{3+}$. In one study, the $^{51}Cr$ content in blood was three to five times greater when the isotope was fed as $Cr^{6+}$ rather than as $Cr^{3+}$. Inorganic trivalent chromium absorption varies with dietary intake. In one study, human subjects ingesting 181 nmol (10 μg) Cr per day absorbed about 2%. The percentage of chromium absorbed from the diet decreased as the content increased until, at 725 nmol (40 μg) per day, absorption was 0.5%. At dietary intakes from 0.73 to 4.35 μmol (40 to 240 μg) per day, chromium absorption was relatively constant at approximately 0.4%. In another study, two men consuming an average of 667 nmol (36.8 μg) Cr per day exhibited a mean apparent net absorption of 1.8%. Although results of these studies are not in complete accordance, it is apparent that the absorption of trivalent chromium is low, usually less than 2%. Preliminary findings led to the conclusion that biologically active chromium (GTF) is more readily available than inorganic trivalent chromium; however, subsequent studies have indicated that this may not be true. Other evidence suggests that organic chromium may be readily absorbed, but quickly passes through the body unused. An example supporting this concept is that more than 40% of a dose of $^{51}$Cr-*tris* (acetylacetonate) was absorbed from the gastrointestinal tract of rats. As much as 45% of the $^{51}Cr$ appeared in the bile, which suggests a rapid absorption and resecretion.

The mechanism of absorption of chromium from the intestine has not been defined clearly, but based on the preceding findings, it apparently involves processes other than simple diffusion. Numerous dietary factors affect the bioavailability or absorption of chromium. Chromium absorption is increased by oxalate and is higher in iron-deficient than in iron-adequate mice. Also in mice, $^{51}Cr$ absorption from $CrCl_3$ is higher when the dietary carbohydrate is starch than when it is sucrose, fructose, or glucose. In addition to dietary factors, chromium absorption is affected by physiologic factors; for example, it is elevated by chemically induced diabetes and depressed by aging in rats.

Both transferrin and albumin are capable of binding absorbed chromium and transporting it as part of blood serum or plasma. Saturating transferrin with iron reduces the transport and retention of chromium. It has been suggested that transferrin is the main binder of newly absorbed chromium, and albumin assumes the role of chromium acceptor and transporter of chromium if transferrin binding sites are unavailable. Although transferrin and albumin apparently play major roles in chromium transport, other plasma proteins, including α- and β-globulins, and lipoproteins bind chromium and thus may have a role in chromium metabolism.

Chromium is distributed widely throughout the human body in low concentrations without special concentration in any tissue or organ. This statement is tempered by the limited number of studies with adequate analytic and sampling techniques designed to examine the chromium concentrations in human or animal tissues.

Absorbed inorganic trivalent chromium is excreted primarily through the kidney, with small amounts lost in hair, sweat, and bile. As indicated previously, large amounts of some organic forms of chromium may be lost through the bile. The exact mechanisms of metabolism of chromium by the kidney are not known. Most data indicate, however, that renal tubular reabsorption of filtered chromium is high, with a range of 80 to 97% in humans.

## FUNCTIONS AND MODE OF ACTION

Chromium is generally accepted as an essential nutrient that potentiates insulin action and thus influences carbohydrate, lipid, and protein metabolism. The specific biochemical function of chromium, however, has not been clearly defined; that is, the chemical nature of the relationship between chromium and insulin function has not been identified.

As indicated previously, one proposed function of chromium, as GTF, is controversial. It has been suggested that GTF-chromium helps form a complex between insulin and insulin receptors that facilitates the insulin-tissue interaction. Chromium as found in brewer's yeast and in some other naturally occurring and synthetic complexes is more effective in stimulating glucose use than is chromium chloride or the chromium found in torula yeast. This finding, however, may be nothing more than a reflection that some forms of chromium are transported more easily than others to the site of chromium action.

Some patients receiving TPN who exhibited signs of diabetes, including glucose intolerance, were refractory to insulin. After chromium supplementation, however, their diabetic symptoms were alleviated or their need for exogenous insulin was eliminated. This finding supports the concept that chromium has a biochemical function that affects the ability of the insulin receptor to interact with insulin. Although chromium possibly potentiates insulin action through a direct action on insulin or its receptor, another possibility exists. It has been found that in vitro RNA synthesis directed by free DNA is enhanced by the binding of chromium to the template. Furthermore, chromium is concentrated in hepatic nuclei 48 hours after intraperitoneal injection of $CrCl_3$. The chromium is preferentially bound to DNA in chromatin and increases the number of initiation sites, which enhances RNA synthesis. Perhaps chromium, or a biologically active form of chromium, acts similarly to zinc in its "zinc finger" role in regulating gene expression. Thus, chromium possibly regulates the synthesis of a molecule that potentiates insulin action. Some support for this suggestion is the finding that insulin-potentiating substances are often found in materials high in chromium (e.g., brewer's yeast), although the chromium is not necessarily associated with molecules that potentiate insulin action in these materials. Further support is the finding of a 4-hour lag period between the administration of biologically active chromium and its optimal effect on insulin action in vivo.

## DEFICIENCY SIGNS

In 1959, it was reported that chromium-deficient rats exhibit a glucose intolerance similar to that of clinical diabetes mellitus. Since that time, several other deficiency signs have been described for animals, including impaired growth, elevated serum cholesterol and triglyceride concentrations, increased incidence of aortic plaques, corneal lesions, and decreased fertility and sperm count.

Signs of chromium deficiency have been found in three women who were receiving long-term TPN containing low amounts of chromium. One subject who had received TPN for 3½ years exhibited impaired glucose tolerance and glucose use, weight loss, neuropathy, elevated plasma free fatty acid concentrations, depressed respiratory exchange ratio, and abnormalities in nitrogen metabolism. These abnormalities were alleviated by chromium supplementation. Another subject who had received TPN for 5 months developed severe glucose intolerance, weight loss, and a metabolic encephalopathy-like confusional state; all of these abnormalities were reversed by chromium supplementation. Chromium supplementation also reversed the development of an unexplained hyperglycemia and glycosuria in the third subject who had followed a TPN regimen of several months duration.

The three descriptions of human chromium deficiency are not the same. In all three cases, however, the chromium-deficient subjects exhibited impaired glucose tolerance, or hyperglycemia with glycosuria, and a refractoriness to insulin; thus, these should be considered signs of chromium deficiency.

## TOXICOLOGY

Trivalent chromium has such a low order of toxicity that deleterious effects from excessive intake of this form of chromium do not occur readily. Trivalent chromium becomes toxic only at extremely high amounts; chromium then acts as a gastric irritant rather than as a toxic element interfering with essential metabolism or biochemistry. For example, cats tolerated 18.12 mmol (1000 mg) $Cr^{3+}$ per day and rats showed no adverse effects from a diet containing 1.81 mmol (100 mg) $Cr^{3+}$/kg.

Industrial exposure to high amounts of chromium, usually airborne, can cause allergic dermatitis, skin ulcers, and bronchogenic carcinoma. Because chromium is a potent sensitizer, external contacts with chromates, dichromates, and chromic acid in household or industrial materials can induce an allergic eczema in some people. Chromium toxicity through oral ingestion, however, is not a practical concern for humans.

## ASSESSMENT OF STATUS

Chromium concentrations in tissues are 10 to 100 times higher than those in blood. Tissue chromium stores apparently are not in equilibrium with blood chromium stores; thus, a change in fasting plasma or serum chromium concentration is not a good indicator of a mild change in chromium status. The relative content of chromium in plasma was markedly lower in a chromium-deficient woman maintained on TPN for 3½ years, however, than in normal adults. Also, the fasting concentration of serum chromium was depressed in association with impaired glucose tolerance during acute infection. These findings suggest that concentrations of chromium much lower than the normal value of 2.5 to 2.7 pmol (0.14 to 0.15 ng)/ml for serum, or 4.7 to 5.1 pmol (0.26 to 0.28 ng)/ml for plasma might indicate the presence of a severe chromium deficiency.

The serum chromium value may be an indicator of excessive exposure to chromium. Recent findings have shown that serum from tannery workers exposed to trivalent chromium contained a median chromium concentration of 8.9 pmol (0.49 ng)/ml; serum from control subjects contained a median concentration of 2.7 pmol (0.15 ng)/ml. Moreover, workers handling wet hides had significantly higher serum chromium concentrations than those working in other areas of the tannery.

In the late 1970s, the "relative chromium response" (RCR), or 100 times the 1-hour serum chromium concentration after an oral glucose load divided by the fasting serum concentration, was considered an index of chromium status. Recent studies have refuted the RCR, however, as a meaningful indicator of chromium status.

Hair chromium content may reflect endogenous chromium available to hair follicle cells, provided the hair is washed carefully before analysis and is not exposed to dyes, bleach, or other environmental contaminants. Use of hair chromium concentration should be tempered by the fact that it is affected by many variables, including hair growth rate, age, pregnancy, diabetes, and arteriosclerosis. Reported hair chromium concentrations range from less than 3.62 nmol (200 ng)/g to over 16.31 nmol (900 ng)/g. Hair chromium concentrations lower than 3.62 nmol (200 ng)/g might be considered an indication of marginal chromium deficiency in older people.

Because urination is the major excretory route of absorbed chromium, and because urinary chromium may be derived from a biologically active component of plasma chromium, urinary chromium content has been examined closely as a possible index of chromium status. The urinary excretion of chromium by normal healthy adults is low, however, about 3.62 nmol (0.2 μg) per day, which makes the precise measurement of urinary chromium quite difficult. Because of this difficulty, increases, not decreases, in urinary chromium have been examined as an index of chromium status. For example, the possibility that the increase in urinary excretion of chromium after a glucose load might be useful to assess chromium status has been examined. Urinary chromium excretion after a glucose challenge was not predictable, however, and did not indicate chromium status. At present, urinary chromium apparently is useful only as an indicator of exposure to excessive amounts of chromium; for example, median urinary chromium was fourfold higher in tannery workers than in control subjects.

Because the specific biochemical function of chromium has not been identified, the determination of the amount or activity of some substance directly involving chromium cannot be ascertained. Thus, there is no specific biochemical measure of chromium status. Supplementation of chromium, however, has been shown to improve glucose tolerance in children with protein-calorie malnutrition, in some diabetic patients, and in some people with marginally elevated blood glucose concentrations. Thus, an abnormal result of a glucose tolerance test can indicate a low chromium status, and improvement in glucose tolerance after chromium supplementation may be a valid indicator of chromium deficiency.

## DIETARY CONSIDERATIONS

The daily intake of chromium can vary widely depending on the amounts of various foods in the diet. Processed meats, whole grain products including some ready-to-eat bran cereals, and spices are the best sources of chromium. Dairy products, fruits, and vegetables contain low amounts of chromium.

The high dietary intakes of chromium reported generally before 1980 apparently are questionable. Those determinations were flawed by contamination and analytical problems. Recent analyses indicate that many self-selected diets provide less than 906 nmol (50 μg) Cr per day. For example, 22 diets designed by nutritionists to be well balanced contained 241 ± 94 nmol (13.3 ± 5.2 μg; mean ± SD) Cr/1000 kcal. Other reported daily intakes of chromium include 525 nmol (29 μg) in self-selected Finnish diets, 1015 nmol (56 μg) in self-selected Canadian diets, 444 nmol (24.5 μg) in self-selected English diets, and 670 and 507 nmol (37 and 28 μg) for self-selected United States diets.

The current United States estimated safe and adequate daily intakes for chromium[19] (see Appendix Table A-2c) are the following (in nmol or μg): infants aged 0 to 0.5 years, 181 to 725 or 10 to 40, and aged 0.5 to 1 year, 362 to 1087 or 20 to 60; children and adolescents aged 1 to 3 years, 362 to 1450 or 20 to 80, aged 4 to 6 years, 544 to 2174 or 30 to 120, aged 7 to 10 years, 906 to 3624 or 50 to 200, and aged 11 years and older, 906 to 3624 or 50 to 200; and adults, 906 to 3624 or 50 to 200. Some evidence suggests that the lower "adequate" level may be higher than necessary. As indicated previously, the average daily intake of chromium may be well below 906 nmol (50 μg) and may be closer to 453 nmol (25 μg), yet widespread cases of chromium deficiency have not been documented. In addition, supplemental chromium fed to individuals apparently consuming chromium at these low amounts did not show any improvement in glucose tolerance or in plasma insulin, cholesterol, or triglyceride concentrations. Thus, for many people, a daily intake of 453 to 634 nmol (25 to 35 μg) Cr may be adequate. This intake might not be adequate, however, to handle stressors that increase the need for chromium or increase the loss of chromium from the body. These stressors include an elevated intake of simple sugars, strenuous physical exercise or work, infection, and physical trauma. Therefore, the suggested daily intake of 906 nmol (50 μg) Cr probably is valid to ensure good health in most individuals.

## CLINICAL CONSIDERATIONS

Although, as indicated previously, results of some studies do not show a response by healthy humans to chromium supplementation, others do. In one study, significant increases in high density lipoprotein (HDL)-cholesterol values were found in subjects fed 3.62 μmol (200 μg) Cr per day 5 days per week as chromium chloride; no increases in HDL-cholesterol values were seen in subjects fed a placebo. Chromium supplementation also tended to decrease glucose and insulin values. In another double-blind crossover study with 76 subjects, significant improvements in the glucose tolerance in 18 of 20 normal subjects with marginally impaired glucose tolerance were found after they received daily supplements of 3.62 μmol (200 μg) Cr as chromium chloride for 3 months. These findings suggest that chromium nutriture may be of practical concern in developed countries where many refined foods are consumed; appreciable losses of chromium occur in the refining of foods. Moreover, inadequate chromium intake probably is of special concern to people exposed to stressors such as diets high in simple sugars, physical trauma, and infection, which apparently enhance the need for chromium.

Based on current knowledge of chromium function and nutrition, the possibility cannot be ignored that inadequate chromium status may be responsible in part for some cases of impaired glucose tolerance, hyperglycemia, hypoglycemia, glycosuria, and refractoriness to insulin.

## REFERENCES


1. Schwarz, K., Mertz, W.: Fed. Proc., *20* (*Suppl.* 10):111–114, 1961.
2. Schroeder, H.A., Balassa, J.J., Tipton, I.H.: J. Chronic Dis., *15*:941–964, 1962.
3. Mertz, W.: Fed. Proc., *26*:186–193, 1967.
4. Schroeder, H.A.: Am. J. Clin. Nutr., *21*:230–244, 1968.
5. Mertz, W.: Chromium—An overview. *In* Chromium in Nutrition and Metabolism. Edited by D. Shapcott and J. Hubert. Amsterdam, Elsevier/North-Holland Biomedical, 1979, pp. 1–14.
6. Hambidge, K.M.: Chromium. *In* Disorders of Mineral Metabolism. Vol. 1. Edited by F. Bronner and J.W. Coburn. New York, Academic, 1981, pp. 271–294.
7. Borel, J.S., Anderson, R.A.: Chromium. *In* Biochemistry of the Essential Ultratrace Elements. Edited by E. Frieden. New York, Plenum, 1984, pp. 175–199.
8. Anderson, R.A.: Chromium. *In* Trace Elements in Human and Animal Nutrition. Vol. 1. Edited by W. Mertz. San Diego, Academic, 1987, pp. 225–244.
9. Fan, A.M., Harding-Barlow, I.: Chromium. *In* Genotoxic and Carcinogenic Metals: Environmental and Occupational Occurrence and Exposure, Advances in Modern Environmental Toxicology. Vol. XI. Edited by L. Fishbein, A. Furst, and M.A. Mehlman. Princeton, Princeton Scientific Publishing, 1987, pp. 87–125.
10. Offenbacher, E.G., Pi-Sunyer, F.X.: Chromium in human nutrition. *In* Annual Review of Nutrition. Edited by R.E. Olson, E. Beutler, and H.P. Broquist. Palo Alto, CA, Annual Reviews, 1988, pp. 543–563.
11. Anderson, R.A.: Chromium. *In* Trace Minerals in Foods. Edited by K. Smith. New York, Marcel Dekker, 1988, pp. 231–247.
12. Anderson, R.A.: Recent advances in the role of chromium in human health and diseases. *In* Essential and Toxic Trace Elements in Human Health and Disease, Current Topics in Nutrition and Disease. Vol. 18. Edited by A.S. Prasad. New York, Alan R. Liss, 1988, pp. 189–197.
13. Nielsen, F.H.: The ultratrace elements: Arsenic, boron, chromium, nickel, selenium and silicon. *In* Nutritional Status Assessment of the Individual. Edited by G.E. Livingston. Trumbull, CT, Food & Nutrition Press, 1987, pp. 401–415.
14. Anderson, R.A.: Sci. Total Environ., *86*:75–81, 1989.
15. Stoecker, B.J.: Chromium. *In* Present Knowledge in Nutrition. Edited by M.L. Brown. Washington, D.C., International Life Sciences Institute, 1990, pp. 287–293.
16. Saner, G.: Nutr. Int., *2*:213–220, 1986.
17. Mertz, W., Roginski, E.E.: Chromium metabolism: The glucose tolerance factor. *In* Newer Trace Elements in Nutrition. Edited by W. Mertz and W.E. Cornatzer. New York, Marcel Dekker, 1971, pp. 123–153.
18. Anderson, R.A.: Clin. Physiol. Biochem., *4*:31–41, 1986.
19. Food and Nutrition Board, National Research Council: Recommended Dietary Allowances. 10th Ed. Washington, D.C., National Academy Press, 1989.


## SELECTED READINGS


Anderson, R.A.: Chromium. *In* Trace Minerals in Foods. Edited by K. Smith. New York, Marcel Dekker, 1988, pp. 231–247.

Anderson, R.A.: Chromium. *In* Trace Elements in Human and Animal Nutrition. Vol. 1. Edited by W. Mertz. San Diego, Academic, 1987, pp. 225–244.

Borel, J.S., Anderson, R.A.: Chromium. *In* Biochemistry of the Essential Ultratrace Elements. Edited by E. Frieden. New York, Plenum, 1984, pp. 175–199.

Stoecker, B.J.: Chromium. *In* Present Knowledge in Nutrition. Edited by M.L. Brown. Washington, D.C., International Life Sciences Institute, 1990, pp. 287–293.

CHAPTER 15

# Ultratrace Minerals*

Forrest H. Nielsen



Ultratrace minerals have been defined as those elements with estimated dietary requirements usually less than 1 μg/g, and often less than 50 ng/g of diet for laboratory animals.[1] For this chapter, however, the definition has been changed to that of elements for which there is experimental evidence, usually from animal models, suggesting that they are essential for humans, but the nutritional importance has not been established clearly. The reason for the difficulty in establishing importance, apparently, is that they are required in small amounts, meaning 1 mg per day or less. Elements that fit in the ultratrace category are arsenic, boron, bromine, cad-

*The atomic weights (g/mol) of elements discussed in this chapter are: arsenic (74.92), boron (10.81), manganese (54.94), molybdenum (95.94), nickel (58.69), silicon (28.09), vanadium (50.94), bromine (79.90), fluorine (19.00), lead (207.2), and tin (118.7) (see Appendix Table A-1c).

mium, fluorine, lead, lithium, manganese, molybdenum, nickel, silicon, tin, and vanadium.

Since the early 1970s, it has been speculated that the lack of one or more of the ultratrace elements contributed to the occurrence of some human diseases, such as atherosclerosis, osteoporosis, osteoarthritis, and hypertension, with incomplete understanding as to their cause. Convincing evidence that ultratrace element deficiencies result in susceptibility to these chronic disorders, or any human disorder, however, has been elusive. A possible reason for this elusiveness is that experimental approaches used in the past were too simplistic. They usually involved looking for an overt simple or uncomplicated deficiency of a specific ultratrace element that was unlikely because of the powerful homeostatic mechanisms of the human body. When animals and humans are exposed to some form of nutritional, metabolic, hormonal, or physiologic stress, however, some of the ultratrace elements may be of nutritional significance. The insufficient intake of a specific ultratrace element probably becomes obvious only when the body is stressed in some way that enhances the need, or interferes with the use of, that element. Examining the possibility that some of the ultratrace elements are of importance for humans under some form of stress has revealed several candidates of potential nutritional concern; foremost among these is boron. Other ultratrace elements that may be of concern are arsenic, manganese, molybdenum, nickel, silicon, and vanadium.

## ARSENIC

### HISTORICAL OVERVIEW

Since ancient times, arsenicals have been associated with actions benevolent and malevolent. Early in the history of arsenic use, people found that some arsenic compounds were convenient, scentless, and tasteless instruments for homicide. Thus, for about 1100 years, through the nineteenth century, arsenic reigned as the king of poisons. Although arsenic was considered synonymous with poison, its bad reputation did not prevent it from becoming an important pharmaceutic agent. By 1937, the pharmacologic actions of 8000 arsenicals had been recorded. Arsenicals were considered at various times to be specific remedies for the treatment of anorexia and other nutritional disturbances, syphilis, neuralgia, rheumatism, asthma, chorea, malaria, tuberculosis, diabetes, various skin diseases, and numerous hematologic abnormalities. The use of arsenicals for these disorders has either fallen into disrepute or been replaced by more effective alternatives.

Reports describing attempts to produce a nutritional arsenic deficiency first appeared in the 1930s. The first substantial evidence for arsenic essentiality was published in 1975 and 1976. For citations to original reports that are the basis for the discussion on arsenic, the reader is referred to other sources.[1–10]

### CHEMISTRY

Both the trivalent and pentavalent states of arsenic exist in biologic material. The most biochemically important organic arsenic compounds are those that contain methyl groups. The methylation of inorganic oxyarsenic anions occurs in organisms ranging from microbial to mammalian. The methylated end products include arsenocholine, arsenobetaine, dimethylarsinic acid, and methylarsonic acid.

Other arsenic compounds of interest are those possibly formed when arsenate replaces phosphate in biologic molecules. The relatively unstable nature of arsenyl esters apparently is the reason that only indirect evidence exists for compounds such as glucose-6-arsenate and adenosine diphosphate-arsenate. Nonetheless, arsenate ester might be the form of arsenic that performs an essential function.

### METABOLISM

Absorption of inorganic arsenic from the gastrointestinal tract correlates well with the solubility of the compound ingested. In humans and most laboratory animals, more than 90% of inorganic arsenate and arsenite fed in a water solution is absorbed. On the other hand, only 20 to 30% of arsenic in arsenic trioxide or lead arsenate, which are only slightly soluble in water, is absorbed by hamsters, rats, and rabbits.

The form of organic arsenic also determines how well it is absorbed. For example, more than 90% of an oral dose of arsenobetaine was recovered in the urine of hamsters; 70 to 80% of an oral dose of arsenocholine was recovered in the urine of mice, rats, and rabbits; and 45% of an oral dose of dimethylarsinic acid was recovered in the urine of hamsters. In contrast, more than 90% of an oral dose of sodium-*p*-N-glycolylarsanilate was recovered in the feces of rats or humans within 3 days of administration; urinary excretion accounted for only 4 to 5% of the dose.

Arsenate and phosphate, despite structural similarities, do not share a common transport pathway in the duodenum. The absorption of arsenate can be separated into two components. First, arsenate becomes sequestered primarily in or on the mucosal tissue. Eventually, the sites of sequestration become filled with concomitant movement of arsenate to the body. The absorption of arsenate apparently involves a simple movement down a concentration gradient. In rats, some forms of organic arsenic are absorbed at rates directly proportional to their intestinal concentration over a 100-fold range. This finding suggests that organic arsenicals are absorbed mainly by simple diffusion through lipoid regions of the intestinal boundary.

Once absorbed, inorganic arsenic is transferred to the liver, where it is methylated. Thus, blood contains both inorganic, probably protein bound, and methylated forms of arsenic. Before arsenate is methylated, it is reduced to arsenite. Methylation takes place in the liver with S-adenosylmethionine as the methyl donor. In humans, the final product, dimethylarsinic acid, results from the methylation of the monomethylarsenic acid precursor formed from arsenite. The methylation of arsenic can be modified by changing the glutathione, methionine, and choline status of the animal.

The fate of absorbed organic arsenic depends on its form. For example, arsenobetaine passes through the body into the urine without biotransformation. Some orally ingested arsenocholine appears in the urine, and some is incorporated into body phospholipids in a manner similar to choline; however, most is biotransformed to arsenobetaine before being excreted in the urine.

If the ingestion of arsenic is low, no tissue has significant accumulation of arsenic. The highest amounts of arsenic are usually found in skin, hair, and nails, probably the result of arsenite binding to SH-groups of proteins that are relatively plentiful in these tissues.

The excretion of ingested arsenic is rapid, principally in urine. Only minor amounts are removed through sweat, loss of hair and skin, and bile. A reported example of the proportions of the forms of arsenic in human urine after an oral dose of inorganic arsenic is 51% dimethylarsinic acid, 21% monomethylarsonic acid, and 27% inorganic arsenic. The proportions are quite different, however, with the consumption of organic arsenic. For example, an analysis of urine from 102 Japanese students who consumed luxuriant amounts of organic arsenic in seafood revealed 9.4% inorganic arsenic, 3.0% monomethylarsonic acid, 28.9% dimethylarsinic acid, and 58.2% trimethylated arsenic compound.

## FUNCTIONS AND MODE OF ACTION

The metabolic function, or mode of action, of arsenic has not been defined clearly. Recent findings suggest that arsenic has a biochemical role or roles that affect the formation of various metabolites from methionine (e.g., cysteine and taurine), or arginine (e.g., putrescine, spermidine, and spermine), or affects labile methyl-group metabolism. Arsenic deprivation depressed the concentrations of putrescine, spermidine, and spermine in liver of rats fed marginal amounts of methionine, and depressed the taurine concentration in the plasma of hamsters.

Perhaps arsenic has a role in some enzymatic reaction. As an enzyme activator, arsenic as arsenate probably acts as a substitute for phosphate. As an inhibitor, arsenic as arsenite apparently exerts its effects on enzymes by reacting with sulfhydryl groups. It is also possible that arsenic acts in the regulation of gene expression. Arsenite can induce the isolated cell production of certain proteins known as heat shock or stress proteins. The control of production of these proteins in response to arsenite apparently is at the transcriptional level, and may involve changes in the methylation of core histones.

## DEFICIENCY SIGNS

Arsenic deprivation has been induced in chickens, hamsters, goats, miniature pigs, and rats. In the goat, miniature pig, and rat, the most consistent signs of arsenic deprivation were depressed growth and abnormal reproduction characterized by impaired fertility and elevated perinatal mortality. Other notable signs of deprivation in goats were depressed serum triglyceride concentrations and death during lactation. Myocardial damage was also present in lactating goats. The organelle of the myocardium most markedly affected was the mitochondrion at the membrane level. In advanced stages, the membrane actually ruptured. Other signs of arsenic deprivation have been reported. Listing these signs is problematic, because studies with chicks, rats, and hamsters have revealed that the nature and severity of the signs of arsenic deprivation are affected by several dietary manipulations, including variations in the concentrations of zinc, arginine, choline, methionine, taurine, and guanidoacetic acid. In other words, the signs of arsenic deprivation were changed and generally enhanced by nutritional stressors that affected sulfur amino acid or labile methyl-group metabolism.

## TOXICOLOGY

Because of mechanisms for the homeostatic regulation of arsenic, its toxicity through oral intake is relatively low; it is actually less toxic than selenium, an ultratrace element with a well-established nutritional value. Toxic quantities of inorganic arsenic generally are reported in milligrams. For example, the estimated fatal acute dose of arsenic trioxide for humans is 0.35 to 0.91 μmol (70 to 180 mg) or about 10.2 to 26 nmol (0.76 to 1.95 mg) As/kg body weight. The ratio of the toxic to nutritional dose for rats apparently is near 1250. Some forms of organic arsenic are virtually nontoxic; a 56 mmol (10 g)/kg body weight dose of arsenobetaine depressed spontaneous motility and respiration in male mice, but these symptoms disappeared within 1 hour.

Briefly, the signs of subacute and chronic high exposure of arsenic in humans include the development of dermatoses of various types (hyperpigmentation, hyperkeratosis, desquamation, and loss of hair); hematopoietic depression; liver damage characterized by jaundice, portal cirrhosis, and ascites; sensory disturbances; peripheral neuritis; anorexia; and loss of weight.

Results of numerous epidemiologic studies have suggested an association between chronic arsenic overexposure and the incidence of some forms of cancer, although the role of arsenic in carcinogenesis remains controversial. Arsenic does not seem to act as a primary carcinogen, and is either an inactive or extremely weak mitogen.

### DIETARY CONSIDERATIONS

Only data from animal studies are available for estimating the possible arsenic requirement of humans. An arsenic requirement of less than 0.67 nmol (50 ng)/g diet and probably near 0.33 nmol (25 ng)/g diet was suggested for growing chicks and rats fed experimental diets containing about 20% protein, 9% fat, 60% carbohydrate, and 11% fiber, minerals, and vitamins. This regimen translates into an arsenic requirement between 83 and 167 nmol (6.25 and 12.5 μg)/1000 kcal. Based on these calculations, a possible arsenic requirement for humans eating 2000 kcal would be about 160 to 200 nmol (12 to 15 μg) daily. The reported arsenic contents of diets from various parts of the world indicate that the average daily intake of arsenic is in the range of 160 to 534 nmol (12 to 40 μg). Fish, grain, and cereal products contribute the most arsenic to the diet. Clarification of the need for arsenic for optimal health and performance is needed so that a safe and adequate intake of the element can be established.

### CLINICAL CONSIDERATIONS

Until more is known about the biochemical and physiologic functions of arsenic, it is inappropriate to associate specific disorders with deficient arsenic nutriture. At present, it is important to recognize the likelihood that arsenic is essential for humans. Thus, the belief that any form or amount of arsenic is unnecessary, toxic, or carcinogenic is unrealistic, if not potentially harmful.

## BORON

### HISTORICAL OVERVIEW

Between 1939 and 1947, several attempts to induce a boron deficiency in rats were unsuccessful. As a result, boron was generally accepted as essential for plants (suggested in 1910, confirmed in 1923), but not for animals. Since 1981, however, evidence has accumulated that indicates boron is an essential nutrient for animals and humans.

For citations to original reports that are the basis for the discussion on boron, the reader is referred to other reviews.[1,4–7,10–12]

### CHEMISTRY

Boron complexes with organic compounds containing hydroxyl groups; this complexing is best when the groups are adjacent and *cis*. Compounds with more than two hydroxyl groups react more strongly, and the intensity of the reaction increases with the increase in the number of adjacent hydroxyl groups. Thus, boron complexes with many substances of biologic interest, including sugars and polysaccharides, adenosine-5-phosphate, pyridoxine, riboflavin, dehydroascorbic acid, and pyridine nucleotides. To date, two naturally occurring organoboron compounds have been identified. They contain boron bound to four oxy groups. These compounds are aplasmomycin, a novel ionophoric macrolide antibiotic isolated from strain SS-20 of Streptomyces griseus, and boromycin, an antibiotic synthesized by Streptomyces antibioticus.

### METABOLISM

Food boron, sodium borate, and boric acid are rapidly absorbed and excreted largely in the urine. Based on urinary recovery findings, more than 90% of ingested boron is usually absorbed. Without a radioisotope of boron, the study of its metabolism is difficult. Thus, the mechanism by which boron is absorbed from the gastrointestinal tract has not been defined. Boron is distributed throughout the tissues and organs of animals and humans at concentrations mostly between 4.6 and 55.5 nmol (0.05 and 0.6 μg)/g fresh weight. Among the organs that contain the highest amounts of boron are bone, spleen, and thyroid.

### FUNCTIONS AND MODE OF ACTION

Many recent findings support the hypothesis that boron has a function that influences macromineral metabolism. Boron affects steroid hormone metabolism, and vice versa, in humans and animals. Also, the response to boron deprivation seems to be enhanced by nutritional stressors that affect cell membrane function (i.e., calcium, cholecalciferol, magnesium, or potassium deprivation). Thus, boron may have a function at the cell membrane level. Evidence has been reported that is consistent with boron being directly associated with membranes and involved with their functional efficiency in plants. As a result, boron is suspected of having a regulatory role in plants involving such hormones as auxin, gibberellic acid, and cytokinin through controlling a second messenger such as calcium at the cell membrane level.

Boron has been shown to affect the activity of enzymes in vitro and in plants. Boron might be acting in this way when it stimulates RNA synthesis by rat liver and plants. Borate competitively inhibits two classes of enzymes. One class is the pyridine or flavin nucleotide-requiring oxidoreductases, which include aldehyde dehydrogenase, xanthine dehydrogenase, and cytochrome $b_5$ reductase. Borate apparently competes with the enzyme for nicotinamide adenine dinucleotide (NAD) or flavin because of its great affinity for *cis*-hydroxyl groups. The other class of borate-inhibited enzymes are those in which borate and boronic acid derivatives bind to the active enzyme site. These enzymes include chymotrypsin, subtilisin, and glyceraldehyde-3-phosphate dehydrogenase.

## DEFICIENCY SIGNS

Precisely stating the signs of boron deficiency is difficult. The response to boron deprivation is affected by variables that affect macromineral metabolism. For example, signs of boron deficiency in animals vary in nature and severity as the diet varies in its content of calcium, phosphorus, magnesium, potassium, cholecalciferol, aluminum, and methionine. Nonetheless, boron deprivation generally affects variables associated with calcium metabolism in both animals and humans, particularly when they are exposed to stressors altering macromineral metabolism.

### *ANIMAL STUDIES*

Boron deprivation affects the composition, structure, and strength of bone. When compared to animals on a low-boron diet, calcium-deficient rats fed a boron supplement of 0.28, 0.56, or 1.12 μmol (3, 6, or 12 μg)/g diet had vertebrae that were higher in calcium content and required more force to break. A boron supplement of 280 nmol (3 μg)/g to a basal diet containing 43 nmol (0.465 μg) B/g alleviated the cholecalciferol deficiency-induced distortion of marrow sprouts of chick proximal tibial epiphyseal plate, and increased the number of osteoclasts within the marrow sprouts.

Brain composition and function are also affected by boron deprivation. Dietary boron was found systematically to influence brain electrical activity assessed by an electrocorticogram in mature rats; the frequency distribution of the electrical activity was principally affected. In this study, brain copper concentrations were higher in boron-deprived than in boron-supplemented rats. Furthermore, calcium concentrations in total brain and in brain cortex, as well as the phosphorus concentration in the cerebellum, were higher in boron-deprived than in boron-supplemented rats fed a cholecalciferol-deficient diet.

The effect of boron on bone and brain might reflect its known actions on macromineral metabolism. The apparent absorption and balance of calcium, magnesium, and phosphorus were higher in boron-supplemented (250 nmol or 2.72 μg/g diet) than in boron-deprived (14.6 nmol or 0.158 μg B/g diet) rats fed a cholecalciferol-deficient diet. Furthermore, a low-boron diet increased the urinary loss of calcium and magnesium by female rats; the urinary magnesium response was enhanced by feeding a calcium-deficient diet. Supplemental boron also increased the apparent absorption and retention of calcium by sheep.

### *HUMAN STUDIES*

In the first nutritional study with humans, 12 postmenopausal women, who lived in a metabolic unit under close supervision, first were fed a diet that provided 23 μmol (0.25 mg) B/2000 kcal for 119 days, and then were fed the same diet with a daily boron supplement of 280 μmol (3 mg) for 48 days. The boron supplementation reduced the total plasma concentration of calcium and the urinary excretions of calcium and magnesium, and elevated the serum concentrations of 17β-estradiol, testosterone, and ionized calcium.[13]

Subsequently, five men older than age 45 years, five postmenopausal women receiving estrogen therapy, four postmenopausal women not receiving estrogen therapy, and one premenopausal woman were studied.[14] The subjects resided at their homes during the study and were fed a conventional diet that supplied 47.3 mmol (115 mg) magnesium, 176 mmol (706 mg) calcium, 25.2 μmol (1.6 mg) copper, and 21.3 μmol (0.23 mg) boron per 2000 kcal. After an equilibration period of 14 days, during which the subjects were fed the basal-low boron diet (0.021 mmol B) supplemented with 0.28 mmol (3 mg) B per day, there was a depletion period of 63 days, when subjects had only the basal diet. A 49-day repletion period followed, when the basal diet again was supplemented with 0.28 mmol (3 mg) B per day.

When the last 42 days of depletion were compared with the last 35 days of repletion in all 15 subjects, dietary boron affected certain variables associated with calcium and copper metabolism. Plasma ionized calcium, serum calcitonin, 25-hydroxycholecalciferol and enzymatic ceruloplasmin, and erythrocyte superoxide dismutase activity were lower during boron depletion relative to boron repletion, whereas serum creatinine, glucose, and blood urea nitrogen values were higher during boron depletion compared to boron repletion.

Recently, another study with men and postmenopausal women was completed with the same design as the one just described except the diet was adequate in magnesium (129.6 mmol or 315 mg per 2000 kcal) and copper (37.8 μmol or 2.4 mg per 2000 kcal). Alteration of the dietary intake of magnesium and copper apparently determined whether some variables responded to the change in dietary boron. For example, in this study, blood hemoglobin concentration, mean corpuscular hemoglobin concentration, and mean corpuscular hemoglobin were higher, and hematocrit, red blood cell count, and platelet count were lower during boron repletion than during boron depletion; these changes were not noted in the previous study. However, the response to boron deprivation was similar in both studies for many variables including blood urea nitrogen, serum creatinine, and erythrocyte superoxide dismutase.

The last two studies also yielded evidence suggesting that boron can both enhance and mimic some effects of estrogen ingestion in postmenopausal women. When compared to subjects not receiving estrogen therapy, women ingesting estrogen exhibited increased serum

17β-estradiol and plasma copper concentrations; the increases were significantly higher during the high-boron than during the low-boron dietary period. Dietary boron did not affect these variables in the men and women not ingesting estrogen. Estrogen ingestion also apparently increased serum immunoreactive ceruloplasmin, triglycerides, and 25-hydroxycholecalciferol concentrations. Boron supplementation of the low-boron diet also increased these variables in all subjects, not just those ingesting estrogen. These findings support the contention that, if estrogen is beneficial to calcium metabolism, then boron may also be beneficial.

Electroencephalographic (EEG), sensory-motor, and cognitive performance data were also obtained from the second human study. During boron depletion, the subjects displayed impaired performance in tapping, pursuit, search, counting, and encoding tasks. Comparing EEG findings obtained during boron depletion with those from boron repletion indicated that low dietary boron concentrations depressed mental alertness.

## TOXICOLOGY

Boron has a low order of toxicity when administered orally. Toxicity signs in animals generally occur only after the dietary boron concentration exceeds 9.25 μmol (100 μg)/g. When the boron concentration was 13.9 mmol (150 mg)/L in drinking water, rats exhibited depressed growth, continued prepubescent fur, lack of incisor pigmentation, aspermia, and impaired ovarian development. When the boron concentration was raised to 27.8 mmol (300 mg)/L, rats also exhibited depressed values of plasma triglycerides, protein, and alkaline phosphatase, and depressed bone fat and calcium concentrations. Pigs fed 0.74 mmol (8 mg) B/kg body weight per day showed an osteoporosis associated with a reduction in parathyroid activity. Boric acid is the active ingredient in many preparations used to control cockroaches and other crawling household insects.

The low order of toxicity of boron for humans is evidenced by knowledge that, between 1870 and 1920, boron was considered one of the best preservers or extenders of the palatability of foods such as fish, shellfish, meat, sausages, bacon, ham, cream, butter, and margarine. Boron had a vital role as a preservative in preventing food crises during World Wars I and II. In 1904, a study was described in which human volunteers were fed borax and boric acid daily in small doses for extended periods of time or large doses for short periods of time. This report stated that, when doses equivalent to more than 46 mmol (0.5 g) boron daily were consumed, disturbances in appetite, digestion, and health occurred. It was concluded that 46 mmol (0.5 g) boron per day was too much for a normal person to receive regularly, and 370 mmol (4.0 g) boron per day was the limit beyond which a normal person cannot go without harm. More recently, two infants who had their pacifiers dipped into a preparation of borax and honey for several weeks exhibited scanty hair, patchy dry erythema, anemia, and seizure disorders. The seizures stopped and the other abnormalities were alleviated when the use of the borax and honey preparation was discontinued.

In humans, the signs of acute toxicity include nausea, vomiting, diarrhea, dermatitis, and lethargy. In addition, high boron ingestion induces riboflavinuria.

## DIETARY CONSIDERATIONS

For normal development, chicks seem to require about 92.5 nmol (1 μg) B/g diet. As discussed previously, macromineral metabolism is altered in animals ingesting diets usually containing 18.5 to 37.0 nmol (0.2 to 0.4 μg) B/g. In the human studies just described, the subjects responded to a boron supplement after consuming a diet supplying only about 23 μmol (0.25 mg) B/2000 kcal for 63 or 119 days. Thus, humans seem to have a dietary boron requirement above 28 μmol (0.3 mg)/day, and probably closer to 92.5 μmol (1 mg) per day. Overt toxicity signs in animals generally occur only after dietary boron exceeds 9.25 μmol (100 μg)/g. Thus, a conservative upper limit of dietary intake for humans of 925 μmol (10 mg) B per day seems appropriate. In other words, if an intake of 92.5 to 278 μmol (1 to 3 mg) B per day is beneficial to humans, and a daily intake of 925 μmol (10 mg) B, which can be achieved through diet alone, is not harmful, an appropriate suggested safe and adequate daily intake of boron would be 92.5 to 925 μmol (1 to 10 mg).

The daily intake of boron by humans can vary widely depending on the proportions of various food groups in the diet. Foods of plant origin, especially noncitrus fruits, leafy vegetables, nuts, and legumes are rich sources of boron. Wine, cider, and beer are also high in boron. Meat, fish, and dairy products are poor sources of boron. A limited number of surveys indicate that average daily intakes of boron range between 46 and 287 μmol (0.5 and 3.1 mg).

## CLINICAL CONSIDERATIONS

More knowledge about the physiologic or biochemical function(s) of boron is needed before attributing clinical disorders to subnormal boron nutrition. Boron clearly is, however, a biologically dynamic ultratrace element that affects macromineral metabolism in higher animals, including humans. Thus, boron deprivation may have a role in some disorders of unknown cause that exhibit disturbed macromineral metabolism (e.g., osteoporosis, urolithiasis, and abnormal bone associated with long-term total parenteral nutrition (TPN)).

# MANGANESE

## HISTORICAL OVERVIEW

Although manganese was known to be a constituent of animal tissues as early as 1913, it was not until 1931 that manganese deficiency was shown to induce poor growth in mice and abnormal reproduction in rats. Manganese deficiency has since been induced in numerous species of animals, but not in humans, although several well-designed attempts have been made.

For citations to original reports that are the basis for most of the discussion of manganese, the reader is referred to other reviews.[15–18]

## CHEMISTRY

The characteristic oxidative state of manganese in solution, in metal enzyme complexes, and in metalloenzymes is $Mn^{2+}$. $Mn^{3+}$ is important in vivo; it is the oxidative state in the enzyme manganese superoxide dismutase, the form that binds to transferrin, and probably the form that interacts with $Fe^{3+}$. Ingested $Mn^{2+}$ is thought to be converted into $Mn^{3+}$ in the duodenum. $Mn^{2+}$, like $Fe^{3+}$, has a high affinity for imidazole, in contrast to other divalent cations, such as $Zn^{2+}$, $Cu^{2+}$, and $Cd^{2+}$, which have higher affinities for thiol. In manganese-activated biologic reactions, the enzyme-manganese interaction involves either the chelation of the metal ion with a phosphate-containing substrate (particularly adenosine triphosphate) or a direct interaction with the protein. The chemistry of $Mn^{2+}$ is similar to that of $Mg^{2+}$. Therefore, for most enzymatic reactions that are activated by $Mn^{2+}$, the activation is nonspecific, with $Mg^{2+}$ also able to act as the activator.

## METABOLISM

For the adult human, the absorption of manganese from the diet has long been assumed to be near 5%, and to be independent of the body burden or the amount in the diet. This estimate is complicated, however, by the fact that endogenous manganese is almost totally excreted in bile into the intestine. If the body manganese status is adequate, the biliary excretion of absorbed manganese to maintain homeostasis is probably so rapid that it is difficult to determine what portion of fecal manganese was not absorbed from the diet and what portion was excreted in the bile. Thus, the true absorption of manganese by humans probably remains to be determined. In rats, for example, true absorption exceeded apparent absorption because of the endogenous excretion of manganese. Furthermore, the percentage of manganese absorbed from the diet is not constant, but varies with dietary intake. Rats fed diets containing 27, 82, 204, 637, 1183, or 1820 nmol (1.5, 4.5, 11.2, 35, 65, or 100 μg) Mn/g exhibited average true absorption efficiencies of 28.7%, 15.9%, 11.7%, 6.1%, 3.4%, and 2.0%, respectively. Absorption efficiency clearly declined as intake increased. Thus, the often cited hypotheses that manganese homeostasis is regulated mainly by a variable excretion through the digestive tract probably needs to be discarded.

Absorption of manganese apparently occurs equally well throughout the small intestine. In the rat, intestinal manganese absorption is a rapidly saturable process and probably is accomplished through a high-affinity, low-capacity, active transport system. Manganese might well be absorbed by a two-step mechanism; namely, an initial uptake from the lumen followed by transfer across the mucosal cells. The two kinetic processes operate simultaneously, with manganese competing with iron and cobalt for common binding sites in both processes. Thus, one of the metals, if present in a high amount, can exert an inhibitory effect on the absorption of others. In patients with varying iron stores and subjected to duodenal perfusion with manganese, the rate of manganese absorption was higher in iron deficiency and lower in iron-sufficient states. The mechanisms involved in the absorption of manganese apparently are similar to those involved in the absorption of iron.

Absorbed manganese becomes bound to plasma $\alpha_2$-macroglobulin. Hydrated manganese complexes, $Mn^{2+}$ bound to low-molecular weight compounds, and $\alpha_2$-macroglobulin-bound $Mn^{2+}$ in portal blood are removed rapidly by the liver. Like iron, a fraction of the manganese is oxidized to $Mn^{3+}$ and bound to the plasma transport protein transferrin or possibly to a specific transmanganin protein. Transferrin-bound manganese is taken up by extrahepatic tissue.

Within cells, manganese is found predominantly in mitochondria, and thus organs rich in mitochondria, such as liver, kidney, and pancreas, have relatively high manganese concentrations.

As indicated previously, manganese is almost totally excreted in feces; only trace amounts are found in urine. The excretion of absorbed manganese through the bile is rapid and apparently occurs in two waves. The first wave is the result of the clearance of initially absorbed manganese; the second is the result of a combination of initially absorbed manganese and of that arising from the enterohepatic circulation. Several substances, including dopamine, glucagon, and cyclic AMP, reportedly depress the biliary excretion of manganese.

## FUNCTIONS AND MODE OF ACTION

The known biochemical functions of manganese are those of enzyme activation and as a constituent of several metalloenzymes. The enzymes that can be activated by manganese are numerous and include hydrolases, kinases, decarboxylases, and transferases. Most enzymes activated by manganese can also be activated by other metals, especially magnesium. One exception to the nonspecific activation of enzymes by manganese is the manganese-specific activation of glycosyltransferases. Another enzyme that may be specifically activated by manganese is xylosyltransferase. In contrast to the many manganese-activated enzymes, there are only a few manganese metalloenzymes; these include arginase, pyruvate carboxylase, glutamine synthetase, and manganese superoxide dismutase.

## DEFICIENCY SIGNS

Manganese deficiency has been induced in many species of animals. Signs of deficiency include impaired growth, skeletal abnormalities, disturbed or depressed reproductive function, ataxia of the newborn, and defects in lipid and carbohydrate metabolism.

The descriptions of manganese deficiency in humans are not conclusive. A frequently cited case concerns a man who, after consuming a semipurified formula diet for an extended period, developed weight loss, depressed growth of hair and nails, dermatitis, and hypocholesterolemia. Also, his black hair developed a reddish tinge, and his clotting protein response to vitamin K supplementation was abnormal. Subsequent to the appearance of these symptoms, it was realized that manganese had been left out of his diet. The subject responded to a mixed hospital diet. Unfortunately, no supplementation with manganese alone was tried. Thus, although this case is often cited as an example of human manganese deficiency, this isolated evidence is difficult to accept without further verification.

In another study, men were fed a purified diet containing only 2.0 μmol (0.11 mg) Mn per day for 39 days. They exhibited decreased serum cholesterol concentrations and a fleeting dermatitis. Calcium, phosphorus, and alkaline phosphatase activity increased in the blood. Short-term manganese supplementation (10 days), however, did not reverse these changes. Thus, the observed changes cannot be specifically attributed to manganese deprivation.

More recently, 14 young women consumed a conventional diet providing 18.2 μmol (1.0 mg) or 101.8 μmol (5.6 mg) manganese and 14.6 mmol (587 mg) or 33.3 mmol (1336 mg) calcium per day in a 2 by 2 factorially arranged study.[19] Each dietary period was 39 days. Low dietary manganese slightly increased plasma glucose concentration during an intravenous glucose tolerance test (IVGTT). Menstrual losses of manganese, calcium, iron, and total hemoglobin also were increased when the women consumed the low-manganese diet. An interaction between manganese and calcium had small effects on pyruvate kinase activity and the insulin-glucagon ratio during an IVGTT. Because these intriguing findings were not highly significant, they need to be confirmed before conclusively stating that they are signs of manganese deprivation.

Manganese deprivation may contribute to disease processes. A diabetic patient who did not respond to insulin injections responded to oral manganese administration with decreased blood glucose concentrations. Other diabetic patients, however, did not respond to short-term oral administration of manganese. Whole-blood manganese concentrations have been reported to be low in patients with certain types of epilepsy. In rats, manganese deficiency increases the susceptibility to convulsions and results in EEG recordings that are similar to those of epileptic patients. Finally, low serum manganese concentrations, usually in association with low concentrations of copper and zinc, have been found in several persons with weak bones, or impaired bone metabolism; this weakness or impairment was alleviated by supplementation of the diet with manganese, copper, and zinc.

## TOXICOLOGY

Manganese is often considered among the least toxic of the trace elements through oral intake. The major signs of manganese toxicity in animals are depressed growth, depressed appetite, impaired iron metabolism, and altered brain function. Reported cases of human toxicity caused by oral ingestion of high amounts of manganese are essentially nonexistent. The most common form of manganese toxicity in humans occurs as the result of the chronic inhalation of large amounts of airborne manganese as found in mines, steel mills, and some chemical industries. In these cases of toxicity, the principal organ affected is the brain. For example, signs of toxicity were found in Chilean manganese miners; the initial signs were severe psychiatric abnormalities including hyperirritability, violent acts, and hallucinations. These changes were referred to as "manganic madness." With progression of the toxicity, a permanent crippling neurologic disorder of the extrapyramidal system resulted that displayed morphologic lesions similar to those associated with Parkinson's disease.

## DIETARY CONSIDERATIONS

The current United States estimated safe and adequate daily intakes for manganese[20] (see Appendix Table A–2c) are the following (in μmol or mg): infants aged 0 to 0.5 years, 5.5 to 10.9 or 0.3 to 0.6, and aged 0.5 to 1 years, 5.5 to 18.2 or 0.6 to 1.0; children and adolescents aged 1 to 3 years, 18.2 to 27.3 or 1.0 to 1.5, aged 4 to 6 years, 27.3 to 36.4 or 1.5 to 2.0, aged 7 to 10 years, 36.4 to 54.6 or 2.0 to 3.0, and aged 11 years and older, 36.4 to 91.0 or 2.0 to 5.0; adults, 36.4 to 91.0 or 2.0 to 5.0. Few data are available to support these estimates. The values apparently were set mainly through the reasoning that most dietary intakes fall in this range and do not result in deficiency or toxicity signs. Other evidence used was balance data of questionable value. Thus, the estimated safe and adequate intakes of manganese may need some modification as additional data become available. For example, in one study, the calculated minimal requirement for manganese based on obligatory losses in young men consuming a semipurified, manganese-deficient formula diet was 13.5 μmol (0.74 mg) per day. This amount probably did not allow for the storage of manganese for use at times of enhanced need, nor did it allow for the possible inhibition of manganese absorption by dietary substances such as fiber. In another study, five men received varying amounts of manganese in a diet of conventional foods for 105 days. Negative retention of manganese was found at daily dietary intakes of 22.0, 37.5, and 52.6 μmol (1.21, 2.06, and 2.89 mg), but positive retention was found at daily dietary intakes of 48.2 and 69.0 μmol (2.65 and 3.79 mg). By using regression analysis of intake versus balance, a recommended daily intake of 63.7 μmol (3.5 mg) was obtained. This value is difficult to reconcile with the fact that most diets contain a smaller amount of manganese, yet no evidence that manganese deficiency is a problem has appeared. Also, attempts to produce manganese deficiency by feeding diets containing as little as 13.5 or 18.2 μmol (0.74 or 1.0 mg) per day did not result in conclusive or significant effects on the health of adults. Thus, no firm data are available to support changing the lower value of the safe and adequate intake of manganese.

The upper level of acceptable intake probably should be that amount encountered in a diet high in manganese-rich foods and that allows for positive balance if the diet contains high amounts of substances that inhibit manganese absorption. Toxicity does not really enter into the picture in setting this value. Thus, increasing the upper value to 182 μmol (10 mg) per day needs to be considered.

Unrefined cereals, nuts, leafy vegetables, and tea are rich in manganese, whereas refined grains, meats, and diary products contain only small amounts. Thus, Indian diets high in foods of plant origin supply a daily average of 151 μmol (8.3 mg) Mn, whereas highly refined hospital diets in the United States supply less than 6.6 to 32.4 μmol (0.36 to 1.78 mg) Mn per day. Most other reported mean intakes of manganese throughout the world fall between those values.

### CLINICAL CONSIDERATIONS

The importance of manganese in human nutrition needs to be defined before anything can be stated about its clinical importance. Perhaps humans exposed to a stressor that enhances the need for one of the manganoenzymes will be found to be most susceptible to manganese deficiency. For example, ethanol toxicity increases superoxide production, which can be counteracted by manganese superoxide dismutase. Thus, the possibility of becoming manganese-deficient may be enhanced in persons who abuse alcohol.

## MOLYBDENUM

### HISTORICAL OVERVIEW

Evidence for the essentiality of molybdenum first appeared in 1953, when xanthine oxidase was identified as a molybdenum metalloenzyme. Subsequently, attempts to produce molybdenum deficiency signs in rats and chickens were successful only when the diet contained massive amounts of tungsten, an antagonist of molybdenum metabolism. These studies showed that the dietary requirement to maintain normal growth of animals was less than 10.4 nmol (1 μg) molybdenum/g diet, an amount substantially lower than requirements for other trace elements recognized as essential at the time. Thus, molybdenum was not considered of much practical importance in animal and human nutrition. Consequently, over the past 35 years, relatively little effort has been devoted to studying the metabolic and pathologic consequences of molybdenum deficiency in monogastric animals or humans.

For citations to original reports that are the basis for most of the discussion of molybdenum, the reader is referred to other sources.[7,21–24]

### CHEMISTRY

Molybdenum is a transition element that readily changes its oxidation state and can thus act as an electron transfer agent in oxidation-reduction reactions. In the oxidized form of molybdoenzymes, molybdenum is probably present in the 6+ state. Although the enzymes during electron transfer are probably first reduced to the 5+ state, the oxidation state of the completely reduced enzymes is uncertain. Evidence suggests that one or more of the enzymes, in the presence of excess substrate, can have molybdenum present in either the 4+ or 3+ state. The molybdenum apparently is present at the active site of the enzyme in a small nonprotein cofactor containing a pterin nucleus. More than 50% of molybdenum not attached to an enzyme in the liver exists as this cofactor, identified as di-(carboxamidomethyl) molybdopterin, which contains a 5, 6, 7, 8-tetrahydropterin ring and is bound to the mitochondrial outer membrane. This form can be transferred to an apoenzyme of xanthine oxidase or sulfite oxidase, transforming it into an active enzyme molecule.

In addition to the molybdenum cofactor and "enzymatic" molybdenum, the other important form of molybdenum is molybdate. Evidence suggests that molybdenum in blood and urine exists mainly as the molybdate ion ($MoO_4^{2-}$).

## METABOLISM

Molybdenum (except as $MoS_2$) in foods and in the form of soluble complexes is readily absorbed. In humans, between 25 and 80% of ingested molybdenum is absorbed. Molybdenum absorption in rats occurs rapidly in the stomach and throughout the small intestine, the rate of absorption being higher in the proximal than in the distal parts of the small intestine. Whether an active or a passive mechanism is most important in the absorption of molybdenum is uncertain. One study indicated that, at low concentrations, molybdenum absorption is carrier mediated and active. Another study showed that in vivo absorption rates were essentially the same over a 10-fold range of molybdenum concentrations, which suggests that molybdate was absorbed by diffusion only. The possibility exists that molybdate is moved both by diffusion and by active transport, but at high concentrations, the relative contribution of active transport to molybdenum flux is small. The absorption and retention of molybdenum are influenced strongly by interactions between molybdenum and various dietary forms of sulfur.

Molybdate absorbed into the blood is loosely attached to the erythrocytes and tends to bind specifically to $\alpha_2$-macroglobulin. Molybdate in food and water apparently is not chemically changed by absorption and transport in the blood. The organs that retain the highest amounts of molybdenum are the liver and kidney. The molybdenum in liver is entirely present in macromolecular association, partly as known molybdoenzymes and the remainder as molybdenum cofactor.

After absorption, most molybdenum is turned over rapidly and eliminated as molybdate through the kidney; thus, excretion rather than regulated absorption is the major homeostatic mechanism for molybdenum. Significant amounts of this element are excreted in bile.

## FUNCTIONS AND MODE OF ACTION

Molybdenum functions as an enzyme cofactor. Molybdoenzymes catalyze the hydroxylation of various substrates. Aldehyde oxidase oxidizes and detoxifies various pyrimidines, purines, pteridines, and related compounds. Xanthine oxidase/dehydrogenase catalyzes the transformation of hypoxanthine to xanthine, and xanthine to uric acid. Sulfite oxidase catalyzes the transformation of sulfite to sulfate.

Molybdate might also be involved in stabilizing the steroid-binding ability of the unoccupied glucocorticoid receptor. During isolation procedures, molybdate protects steroid hormone receptors, particularly the glucocorticoid receptor, against inactivation. It is hypothesized, however, that molybdate affects the glucocorticoid receptor because it mimics an endogenous compound called "modulator."

## DEFICIENCY SIGNS

Deficiency signs in goats and minipigs are depressed feed consumption and growth, impaired reproduction characterized by increased mortality in both mothers and offspring, and elevated copper concentrations in liver and brain. A molybdenum-responsive syndrome found in hatching chicks is characterized by a high incidence of late embryonic mortality, mandibular distortion, anophthalmia, and defects in leg bone development and feathering. Skeletal lesions, subsequently detected in older birds, include separation of the proximal epiphysis of the femur, osteolytic changes in the femoral shaft, and lesions in the overlying skin that ultimately were attributed to intense irritation in these areas. These apparently dissimilar pathologic changes could possibly be explained by a defect in sulfur metabolism.

Recognition of the role of molybdenum as a component of sulfite oxidase and evidence that sulfite oxidase deficiency deranges cysteine metabolism have resulted in the recognition of human disorders caused by a lack of functioning molybdenum. A lethal inborn error in metabolism that deranges cysteine metabolism has been determined to be a sulfite oxidase deficiency. The disorder is characterized by severe brain damage; mental retardation; dislocation of ocular lenses; increased urinary output of sulfite, S-sulfocysteine, and thiosulfate; and decreased urinary output of sulfate. A patient receiving prolonged total parenteral nutrition (TPN) therapy acquired a syndrome described as "acquired molybdenum deficiency." This syndrome, exacerbated by methionine administration, was characterized by hypermethioninemia, hypouricemia, hyperoxypurinemia, hypouricosuria, and low urinary sulfate excretion. In addition, the patient suffered mental disturbances that progressed to coma. Supplementation with ammonium molybdate improved the clinical condition, reversed the sulfur handling defect, and normalized uric acid production.

## TOXICOLOGY

Large oral doses are necessary to overcome the homeostatic control of molybdenum. Thus, molybdenum is a relatively nontoxic element; in nonruminants, an intake of 1.04 to 52.1 mmol (100 to 5000 mg)/kg of food or water is required to produce clinical symptoms. Ruminants are more susceptible to elevated amounts of dietary molybdenum. The mechanism of molybdenum toxicity is uncertain. Most toxicity signs are similar or identical to those of copper deficiency (i.e., growth depression and anemia). In humans, both occupational and high dietary exposures to molybdenum have been linked through epidemiologic methods to elevated uric acid concentrations in blood and an increased incidence of gout.

### DIETARY CONSIDERATIONS

The current United States estimated safe and adequate daily intakes for molybdenum[20] (see Appendix Table A–2c) are the following (in μmol or μg): infants aged 0 to 0.5 years, 0.16 to 0.31 or 15 to 30, and aged 0.5 to 1.0 years, 0.21 to 0.42 or 20 to 40; children and adolescents aged 1 to 3 years, 0.26 to 0.52 or 25 to 50, aged 4 to 6 years, 0.31 to 0.78 or 30 to 75, aged 7 to 10 years, 0.52 to 1.56 or 50 to 150, and aged 11 years and older, 0.78 to 2.08 or 75 to 200; adults, 0.78 to 2.61 or 75 to 250. Data to support these estimates are scant. These values apparently were set by using balance data, which may be questionable, and through the reasoning that usual dietary intakes are within this range and do not result in signs of deficiency or toxicity.

Recent surveys indicate that the daily intake of molybdenum ranges between 0.52 and 3.65 μmol (50 and 350 μg). Most diets, however, apparently supply about 0.52 to 1.04 μmol (50 to 100 μg) Mo per day; thus, many diets do not meet the minimum level of the suggested safe and adequate intake. The richest food sources of molybdenum include milk and milk products, dried legumes, organ meats (liver and kidney), cereals, and baked goods. The poorest sources of molybdenum include nonleguminous vegetables, fruits, sugars, oils, fats, and fish.

### CLINICAL CONSIDERATIONS

Except for the molybdenum-responsive patient with "acquired molybdenum deficiency" resulting from long-term use of TPN, there is no indication that molybdenum deficiency is of clinical importance. The search for possible molybdenum-responsive syndromes in humans is still warranted, however, especially in those persons treated with TPN or exposed to stressors that enhance the need for the molybdoenzyme sulfite oxidase.

## NICKEL

### HISTORICAL OVERVIEW

The first study of the biologic action of nickel was reported in 1826 when signs of oral nickel toxicity were described in rabbits and dogs. The first reports on the presence of nickel in plant and animal tissues appeared in 1925. Although nickel was first suggested to be nutritionally essential in 1936, strong evidence for essentiality did not appear until 1970. Studies between 1970 and 1975, however, gave inconsistent signs of nickel deprivation, probably because of suboptimal experimental conditions. Since 1975, diets and environments that allow optimal growth and survival of laboratory animals have been used in studies of nickel nutrition and metabolism. Thus, most of the significant biochemical, nutritional, and physiologic studies of nickel have appeared subsequent to 1975.

For citations of original reports that are the basis for the discussion on nickel, the reader is referred to other sources.[1,4–7,10,22–28]

### CHEMISTRY

Monovalent, divalent, and trivalent forms of nickel apparently are important in biochemistry. Like other ions of the first transition series, $Ni^{2+}$ has the ability to complex, chelate, or bind with many substances of biologic interest. The binding of divalent nickel by various ligands, including amino acids and proteins, probably is important in the extracellular transport, intracellular binding, and urinary and biliary excretion of nickel. $Ni^{2+}$, in a tightly bound form, is required for the activity of urease, an enzyme found in plants and microorganisms. In the microbial enzyme, methyl coenzyme M reductase, nickel is present in a chromophore called factor $F_{430}$. Coenzyme M, which is involved in methane formation in anaerobic bacteria, is 2,2′-dithiodiethane sulfonic acid. Factor $F_{430}$ is a tetrapyrrole similar in structure to that in vitamin $B_{12}$. In addition to containing nickel, the formation of factor $F_{430}$ requires the presence of $Ni^{2+}$.

$Ni^{3+}$ apparently is essential for enzymatic hydrogenation, desulfurization, and carboxylation reactions in mostly anaerobic microorganisms. In some of these reactions, the redox action of nickel may involve the 1+ oxidation state, especially in that of methyl-coenzyme M reductase. Nickel also acts as a structural component in some enzymes.

### METABOLISM

When nickel in water is ingested after an overnight fast, or in low quantities, as much as 50%, but usually closer to 20 to 25%, of the dose is absorbed. Certain foodstuffs and simple substances, however, depress this high absorption, including milk, coffee, tea, orange juice, ascorbic acid, and ethylene diamine tetraacetic acid (EDTA). Foods such as those found in a typical Guatemalan meal or in a North American breakfast suppress the absorption of nickel to less than 1%. Thus, nickel is often poorly absorbed (less than 10%) when ingested with typical diets. Nickel absorption is enhanced by iron deficiency, pregnancy, and lactation. Pigs were found to absorb more than 19% of nickel ingested from day 21 of pregnancy until parturition.

A specific nickel carrier mechanism at the brush border membrane of the gut has not been demonstrated; thus, nickel absorption probably depends on the efficiency of mucosal trapping through charge neutralization on the membrane. Thus, nickel seems to cross the basolateral membrane through passive leakage or diffusion, perhaps in the form of a complex with an amino acid or other low-molecular-weight compound.

Nickel is transported in blood principally bound to serum albumin. Small amounts of nickel in serum are associated with the amino acid L-histidine and with $\alpha_2$-macroglobulin. No tissue or organ significantly accumulates orally administered physiologic doses of nickel. In humans, the thyroid and adrenal glands apparently have relatively high nickel concentrations with reported values of 2.40 and 2.25 μmol (141 and 132 μg)/kg dry weight, respectively. Most organs contain less than 0.85 μmol (50 μg) Ni/kg dry weight.

Although fecal nickel excretion (mostly unabsorbed nickel) is 10 to 100 times as great as urinary excretion, most of the small fraction of nickel absorbed is rapidly and efficiently excreted through the kidney as urinary low-molecular-weight complexes. Measurable amounts of nickel are also lost through sweat and bile. The nickel content of sweat is high, which points to active nickel secretion by the sweat glands.

## FUNCTIONS AND MODE OF ACTION

No evidence clearly defines a biochemical function for nickel in higher animals or humans. Nickel might, however, function as a cofactor or structural component in specific metalloenzymes in higher organisms, because such enzymes have been identified in plants and microorganisms. These nickel-containing enzymes include urease, hydrogenase, methylcoenzyme M reductase, and carbon monoxide dehydrogenase.

## DEFICIENCY SIGNS

Signs of nickel deficiency have not been described for humans. The reported signs of nickel deprivation for six animal species—chick, cow, goat, pig, rat, and sheep—are extensive. Unfortunately, many of the reported signs may have been misinterpreted manifestations of pharmacologic actions of nickel. High dietary nickel, used in some experiments may have alleviated an abnormality caused by something other than a nutritional deficiency of nickel (many diets were apparently low in iron). Based on some recent studies with rats and goats, nickel deprivation depresses growth, reproductive performance, and plasma glucose and alters the distribution of other elements in the body, including calcium, iron, and zinc. As with other ultratrace elements, the nature and severity of signs of nickel deprivation are affected by diet composition. For example, vitamin $B_{12}$-deprived, nickel-supplemented rats exhibit abnormalities similar to those exhibited by nickel-deprived rats. The lack of dietary nickel becomes more apparent in rats with an elevated propionic acid metabolism caused by high dietary odd-chain fatty acids; a vitamin $B_{12}$-dependent enzyme, methylmalonyl-CoA mutase, catalyzes the last step in the propionate pathway of odd-chain fatty acid metabolism. Biotin status also affects the response of rats to nickel deprivation.

## TOXICOLOGY

Life-threatening toxicity of nickel through oral intake is unlikely. Because of excellent homeostatic regulation, nickel salts exert their toxic action mainly by gastrointestinal irritation and not by inherent toxicity. Generally, greater than 4.26 μmol (250 μg) Ni/g of diet are required to produce signs of nickel toxicity (such as depressed growth and anemia) in animals; by weight extrapolation, a daily oral dose of 4.26 mmol (250 mg) of soluble nickel should produce toxic symptoms in humans. More moderate doses of nickel, however, may have adverse effects in humans. An oral dose in water as low as 10.2 μmol (0.6 mg) nickel as nickel sulfate, which is well absorbed, given to fasting subjects produced a positive skin reaction in some individuals with nickel allergy. That dose is only a few times higher than the human daily requirement postulated on the basis of results from animal studies.

## DIETARY CONSIDERATIONS

Because nickel is essential for several animals, a reasonable hypothesis is that nickel is required by humans also. Moreover, the nickel requirements of animals should suggest the amount of nickel possibly required by humans. Most monogastric animals have a dietary nickel requirement of less than 3.41 μmol (200 μg)/kg diet. If it is assumed that adult humans consume 500 g of a mixed diet daily (dry basis), then the dietary nickel requirement of humans would be less than 1.70 μmol (100 μg) daily. The finding that an oral dose as low as 10.2 μmol (600 μg) of nickel as nickel sulfate given in water produced a positive reaction in some nickel-sensitive fasting individuals suggests that the threshold level of toxicity can be quite low in some specific situations. Thus, a safe and adequate daily intake of nickel probably is near 1.70 to 5.11 μmol (100 to 300 μg). Total dietary nickel intakes of humans vary greatly with the amounts and proportions of foods of animal (nickel-low) and plant (nickel-high) origin consumed. Rich sources of nickel include chocolate, nuts, dried beans and peas, and grains; diets high in these foods could supply more than 15.33 μmol (900 μg) Ni per day. Conventional diets, however, often provide less than 2.55 μmol (150 μg) daily (some much less than 1.70 μmol (100 μg) daily). Examples of reported intakes are (μmol or μg per day): United Kingdom, 2.38 to 2.55 or 140 to 150; United States, range of 1.18 to 2.76 or 69 to 162; and Denmark, mean of 2.21 or 130 and range of 1.02 to 4.43 or 60 to 260.

## CLINICAL CONSIDERATIONS

Until more is known about the physiologic function of and requirement for nickel, it is inappropriate to suggest specific disorders, other than nickel dermatitis, as wholly or partially attributable to abnormal nickel nutrition.

Because the nickel content in some human diets can be lower than that inducing changes in animals, however, and because the deprivation of nickel in animals can be enhanced by stressors affecting metabolic pathways involving biotin and vitamin $B_{12}$-dependent enzymes, nickel should still be considered a possibly limiting nutrient under specific conditions in humans.

## SILICON

### HISTORICAL OVERVIEW

Silicon was first found in the ash of animals in 1848. In 1901, it was reported that high concentrations of silicon were present in tendons, aponeuroses, and eye tissues. As early as 1911, researchers suggested that silicon might have an antiatheroma action. Until 1972, however, silicon was generally considered nonessential, except in some lower classes of organisms (diatoms, radiolarians, and sponges), in which silica serves a structural role. In that year, the first substantial evidence was published that silicon is an essential element for chickens and rats. Most of the limited studies on the biochemical, nutritional, and physiologic roles of silicon have been published since 1974.

For citations to original reports that are the basis for most of the discussion on silicon, the reader is referred to other sources.[1,4–7,10,29–31]

### CHEMISTRY

The chemistry of silicon is similar to that of carbon, its sister element. Silicon forms silicon-silicon, silicon-hydrogen, silicon-oxygen, silicon-nitrogen, and silicon-carbon bonds. Thus, organosilicon compounds are analogues of organocarbon compounds. The substitution of silicon, however, for carbon, or vice versa, in organocompounds results in molecules with different properties, because silicon is larger and less electronegative than carbon.

In animals, silicon is found both free and bound. Silicic acid probably is the free form. The bound form has never been rigorously identified. Silicon may be present in biologic material as a silanolate, an ether (or ester-like) derivative of silicic acid. $R_1$-O-Si-O-$R_2$ or $R_1$-O-Si-O-Si-O-$R_2$ bridges may play a role in the structural organization of some mucopolysaccharides.

### METABOLISM

Little is known about the metabolism of silicon. Increasing the intake of silicon increases urinary silicon output up to fairly well-defined limits in humans, rats, and guinea pigs. The upper limits of urinary silicon excretion, however, apparently are not set by the excretory ability of the kidney, because urinary excretion can be elevated above these upper limits by peritoneal injections of silicon. Thus, the limits apparently are set by the rate and extent of silicon absorption from the gastrointestinal tract. The form of dietary silicon determines whether it is well absorbed. In one study, humans absorbed only about 1% of a large single dose of an aluminosilicate compound, but absorbed more than 70% of a single dose of methylsilanetriol salicylate, a drug used in the treatment of circulatory ischemias and osteoporosis. Some dietary forms of silicon must be well absorbed, inasmuch as daily urinary silicon excretion in rats and humans can be a high percentage (close to 50%) of daily silicon intake. Silicon absorption is affected in rats by age, sex, and the activity of various endocrine glands. The mechanisms involved in intestinal absorption and in blood transport of silicon are unknown.

Silicon is not protein-bound in plasma; it is believed to exist in plasma almost entirely in the undisassociated monomeric silicic acid form, $Si(OH)_4$. Connective tissues, including aorta, trachea, tendon, bone, and skin, and its appendages contain much of the silicon that is retained in the body. The elimination of absorbed silicon is mainly through the urine, where it probably exists as magnesium orthosilicate.

### FUNCTIONS AND MODE OF ACTION

Both the distribution of silicon in animals and the effect of silicon deficiency on the form and composition of connective tissue support the view that silicon functions as a biologic cross-linking agent that contributes to the architecture and resilience of connective tissue. The connective tissue components in which silicon apparently plays a fundamental role in the cross-linking mechanism are collagen, elastin, and mucopolysaccharide. Silicon is required for maximal bone prolylhydroxylase activity. Silicon also increases the activities of prolyl-4-hydroxylase, galactosyl-hydroxyllysyl glucosyltransferase, and lysyloxidase (three enzymes catalyzing post-translational modifications of collagen) in lungs of rats. These findings suggest that silicon has an important role in bone and cartilage collagen biosynthesis. Recently, it was found that silicon affects gene expression in some diatoms; perhaps a similar role should be examined in higher animals.

Silicon apparently is involved in bone calcification; however, the mechanism of involvement remains unclear. Some findings suggest a catalytic function for silicon. The influence of silicon on collagen and mucopolysaccharide formation and structure may indirectly affect bone calcification. In this regard, the mineralization process is impaired in silicon-deficient animals, although not as much as the formation of organic matrix, whether cartilage or bone.

### DEFICIENCY SIGNS

Most of the signs of silicon deficiency in chickens and rats indicate aberrant metabolism of connective tissue and bone. Chicks fed a semisynthetic, silicon-deficient diet exhibit structural abnormalities of the skull, depressed collagen content in bone, and long-bone abnormalities characterized by small, poorly formed joints and defective endochondral bone growth. Tibias of silicon-deficient chicks exhibit depressed contents of articular cartilage, water, hexosamine, and collagen. Signs of silicon deprivation can be enhanced by low dietary calcium and high dietary aluminum. Rats fed a diet low in calcium and silicon and high in aluminum accumulated high amounts of aluminum in the brain. Silicon supplements prevented the increase in aluminum concentration in the brain. When fed a low-calcium diet, silicon-deprived rats exhibited depressed tibial and skull concentrations of calcium, magnesium, and phosphorus; these changes apparently were less pronounced in silicon-deprived rats fed adequate amounts of calcium.

### TOXICOLOGY

Silicon is essentially nontoxic when taken orally. Magnesium trisilicate, an over-the-counter antacid, has been used by humans for more than 40 years without obvious deleterious effects. Other silicates are food additives used as anticaking or antifoaming agents. Ruminants consuming plants with a high silicon content, however, may develop siliceous renal calculi. Renal calculi in humans may also contain silicates.

### DIETARY CONSIDERATIONS

Although the essentiality of silicon was suggested almost 20 years ago, its minimum requirement has not been ascertained for any animal. Deficiency signs in chickens were prevented by 3.56 to 7.12 μmol (100 to 200 μg) silicon as the silicate/g of diet, or about 0.93 to 1.85 mmol (26 to 52 mg)/1000 kcal. Other silicon compounds, however, apparently are 5 to 10 times as effective per atom of silicon in preventing deficiency signs. Thus, if humans have a requirement for silicon, it probably is in the range of 178 to 712 μmol (5 to 20 mg) per day. Total dietary silicon intake of humans varies greatly with the amounts and proportions of foods of animal (silicon-low) and plant (silicon-high) origin consumed, and with the amounts of refined and processed foods in the diet. The richest sources of silicon are unrefined grains of high fiber content, cereal products, and root vegetables. The average British diet has been estimated to supply 1.10 mmol (31 mg) Si/day. In the United States, the dietary intake of silicon may be in the range of 0.75 to 1.64 mmol (21 to 46 mg) per day.

### CLINICAL CONSIDERATIONS

Although silicon is generally accepted as an essential nutrient, more work is needed to clarify the consequences of silicon deprivation in humans. A severe lack of dietary silicon could have detrimental effects on brain and bone function and composition.

## VANADIUM

### HISTORICAL OVERVIEW

In 1876, Priestley reported on the toxicity of sodium vanadate. It was not until 1912, however, that the first paper on the pharmacologic and toxicologic actions of vanadium appeared. At this time, high vanadium concentrations were discovered in the blood of ascidian worms. The hypothesis that vanadium may play a physiologic role in higher animals has had a long and inconclusive history. In 1950, it was stated that, "we are completely ignorant of the physiological role of vanadium in animals, where its presence is constant."[32] In 1963, after a review of the early studies on vanadium essentiality, Schroeder et al. concluded that, although vanadium behaves like an essential trace metal, final proof of essentiality for mammals was still lacking.[33] Between 1971 and 1974, a number of findings reported by four different research groups led many people to conclude that vanadium is an essential nutrient. Many of these findings, however, may have been the consequence of high vanadium supplements (10 to 100 times the amount normally found in the diet) that induced pharmacologic changes in suboptimally performing animals fed imbalanced diets. The most substantive evidence for vanadium essentiality has appeared only since 1987.

For citations to original reports that are the basis for most of the discussion on vanadium, see other reviews.[1,4–7,10,34–37]

### CHEMISTRY

The chemistry of vanadium is complex because the element can exist in oxidation states from −1 to +5 and can form polymers. In biologic systems, the tetravalent and pentavalent valence states are the most important forms of vanadium. The tetravalent state appears most simply as $VO^{2+}$, or the vanadyl cation, which easily complexes with other substances such as transferrin or hemoglobin, thereby stabilizing it against oxidation. The pentavalent state of vanadium is known as vanadate ($H_2VO_4^-$ or more simply $VO_3^-$). Vanadate forms complexes with other biologic substances, and in particular, with *cis*-diols. Vanadate is reduced easily by ascorbate, glutathione, or NADH.

Three types of behavior can be predicted for vanadium in biologic systems. First, as vanadate, the element competes at the active sites of phosphate-transport proteins, phosphohydrolases, and phosphotransferases. Second, as vanadyl, the element competes with other transition metal ions for binding sites on metalloproteins and for small ligands such as adenosine triphosphate. Third, vanadium participates in redox reactions within the cell, particularly with relatively small molecules that can reduce vanadate nonenzymatically, such as glutathione.

## METABOLISM

Limited information exists about vanadium metabolism at physiologic quantities in animals or humans. Based on the very low concentrations of vanadium normally in urine in comparison with the estimated daily intake and fecal content of vanadium, less than 5% of vanadium ingested is absorbed. A greater percentage (over 30%) of vanadium, however, was found to be absorbed from the intestine of rats under certain conditions. Thus, ingested vanadium may not always be poorly absorbed by the gastrointestinal tract. Dietary vanadium probably occurs mainly as vanadyl or vanadate. Most ingested vanadium probably is transformed in the stomach to vanadyl and remains in this form as it passes into the duodenum. Vanadate, however, is absorbed three to five times more effectively than vanadyl. Thus, the effect of other dietary components on the form of vanadium in the stomach and the speed at which it is transformed into vanadyl apparently affect the percentage of ingested vanadium absorbed. In this regard, a number of substances can ameliorate vanadium toxicity, including ascorbic acid, EDTA, chromium, protein, ferrous iron, chloride, and aluminum hydroxide.

The binding of the vanadyl ion to iron-containing proteins is important in vanadium metabolism. Regardless of its oxidation state on entering the blood, vanadium apparently is converted into vanadyl-transferrin and vanadyl-ferritin complexes in plasma and body fluids. If vanadate appears in the blood, it is quickly converted into vanadyl, most likely in the erythrocytes. It remains to be determined whether ferritin is a storage vehicle for vanadium as well as for iron in the liver, and whether vanadyl-transferrin can transfer vanadium through the transferrin receptor. Little of the absorbed vanadium is retained under normal conditions in the body; most tissues contain less than 196 pmol (10 ng) V/g fresh weight. Urine seems to be the major means of excretion for absorbed vanadium, and bone is a major sink for retained vanadium.

## FUNCTIONS AND MODE OF ACTION

Because vanadium is such an active element in vitro and pharmacologically, numerous biochemical and physiologic functions have been suggested for it. Thus, vanadium has been postulated to play a role in the regulation of (NaK)-ATPase, phosphoryl transferase enzymes, adenylate cyclase, and protein kinases; as an enzyme cofactor in the form of vanadyl; and in hormone, glucose, lipid, bone, and tooth metabolism. No specific biochemical function has been identified for vanadium in higher animals. The recent discovery of enzymes in lower forms of life that require vanadium for activity lends credence to the possibility that vanadium has a similar role in higher animals. These enzymes are nitrogenase in bacteria, which reduces nitrogen gas to ammonia, and iodoperoxidase and bromoperoxidase in algae and lichens, which catalyze the oxidation of halide ions by hydrogen peroxide, thus facilitating the formation of a carbon-halogen bond. The best known haloperoxidase in animals is thyroid peroxidase. Recently, it was shown that vanadium deprivation in rats affected the response of thyroid peroxidase to changing dietary iodine concentration.

## DEFICIENCY SIGNS

Most of the deficiency signs reported for vanadium are questionable. These signs may have been manifestations of pharmacologic actions of vanadium in suboptimally performing animals fed imbalanced diets. The diets used in early vanadium deprivation studies had widely varying contents of protein, sulfur amino acids, ascorbic acid, iron, copper, and perhaps other nutrients that affect, or can be affected by, vanadium. The uncertainty about vanadium deficiency signs has prompted new efforts to characterize a consistent set for animals. In these recent studies, diets apparently contained adequate and balanced amounts of all known nutrients. In these studies, vanadium-deprived goats exhibited an elevated abortion rate and a depressed milk production. About 40% of kids from vanadium-deprived goats died between days 7 and 91 of life with some deaths preceded by convulsions; only 9% of kids from vanadium-supplemented goats died during this time. Serum creatinine and β-lipoprotein concentrations were elevated and that of serum glucose was depressed in the vanadium-deprived goats. Also, skeletal deformations were seen in the forelegs, and forefoot tarsal joints were thickened. In another study, vanadium deprivation increased thyroid weight and thyroid weight to body weight ratio, and decreased growth in rats. This study also showed that stressors that change thyroid status or iodine metabolism enhance the response to vanadium deprivation. Among the findings supporting the interaction between iodine and vanadium were the following: as dietary iodine increased from low to excessive amounts, thyroid peroxidase activity decreased; the decrease was more pronounced in vanadium-supplemented than vanadium-deprived rats. Also, as the amount of dietary iodine increased, the plasma glucose concentration increased in the vanadium-deprived rats, but decreased in vanadium-supplemented rats.

### TOXICOLOGY

Vanadium can be a relatively toxic element. Acute toxicity studies indicate that vanadium is a neurotoxic and a hemorrhagic-endotheliotoxic poison with nephrotoxic, hepatotoxic, and probably leukocytotactic and hematotoxic components. Apparently, this breadth of toxic effects is the reason that a variety of signs of vanadium toxicity for animals have been described that vary among species and with dosage. Some of the more consistent signs include depressed growth, elevated organ vanadium, diarrhea, depressed food intake, and death. Animal data indicate that long-term daily intake over 196 μmol (10 mg) V might lead to toxicologic consequences. Limited studies with humans support this contention. When 12 subjects were given 265 μmol (13.5 mg) V daily for 2 weeks and then 442 μmol (22.5 mg) V daily for 5 months, five patients exhibited gastrointestinal disturbances and five patients exhibited green tongue. In another study, six subjects were fed 88 to 353 μmol (4.5 to 18 mg) V daily for 6 to 10 weeks; green tongue, cramps, and diarrhea were observed at the higher doses. Excessive in vivo amounts of vanadium have been suggested as a factor in manic-depressive illness.

### DIETARY CONSIDERATIONS

If vanadium is essential for humans, its requirement most likely is small. The diets used in animal deprivation studies contained only 39 to 491 pmol (2 to 25 ng) V/g; these often did not markedly affect the animals. Vanadium deficiency has not been identified in humans, yet diets generally supply less than 589 nmol (30 μg) vanadium daily and most supply only 294 nmol (15 μg) daily. Thus, a daily dietary intake of 196 nmol (10 μg) V probably will meet any postulated vanadium requirement. As indicated previously, a daily intake of 196 μmol (10 mg) vanadium produced signs of overt vanadium toxicity. Much lower amounts of vanadium (but still 10 to 100 times the amount normally found in the diet) apparently cause pharmacologic effects in animals and humans. Because these amounts may be toxic under certain situations, daily vanadium intake probably should not exceed 1.96 μmol (100 μg). Thus, a safe and adequate daily intake of vanadium most likely is near 0.196 to 1.96 μmol (10 to 100 μg).

Diets usually supply between 118 and 393 nmol (6 and 20 μg) V per day. Foods rich in vanadium include shellfish, mushrooms, parsley, dill seed, black pepper, and some prepared foods. Beverages, fats and oils, fresh fruits, and fresh vegetables contain the least vanadium.

### CLINICAL CONSIDERATIONS

The clinical importance of vanadium is uncertain. Because vanadium can affect iodine metabolism and thyroid function in animals, vanadium may be of nutritional importance in humans exposed to stressors that cause a subnormal thyroid status. Since 1985, extensive studies have been performed examining the mechanism through which vanadate mimics the action of insulin and prevents the signs of diabetes associated with streptozotocin administration to rats. Because the amounts of vanadium used to induce this action usually result in some toxic manifestations in rats (i.e., depressed growth), it is doubtful that vanadium will be useful in the treatment of diabetic humans. Nonetheless, because vanadium is pharmacologically active, a beneficial pharmaceutical role for this element may be found.

## OTHER ULTRATRACE ELEMENTS

Evidence currently supporting the nutritional importance of ultratrace elements other than those discussed previously is more limited. Recent findings, however, give support to the contention that bromine, fluorine, lead, and tin are essential ultratrace elements.

### BROMINE

In 1988, Anke et al. reported that, when compared to goats fed 250 μmol (20 mg) Br/kg diet, goats fed a diet containing less than 12.5 μmol (less than 1.0 mg) Br/kg diet exhibited depressed growth, conception rate, milk fat production, hemoglobin, and life expectancy.[38] These findings were obtained with a small number of animals; thus, further studies are needed before stating that bromine is an essential element.

### FLUORINE

In 1990, Anke and co-workers reported that, when compared to goats fed 79 to 132 μmol (1.5 to 2.5 mg) F/kg diet, goats fed less than 16 μmol (0.3 mg) F/kg diet exhibited decreased feed efficiency, depressed growth, and reduced life expectancy.[39] These rather general effects suggest, but do not prove, that fluorine is essential. Nonetheless, it is well recognized that fluoride has some beneficial pharmacologic properties that help prevent dental caries and possibly protect against bone fractures associated with osteoporosis. An estimated safe and adequate intake of fluorine for adults is 79 to 210 μmol (1.5 to 4.0 mg)[20] (See Appendix Table A-2c).

### LEAD

Lead deprivation apparently depresses growth, disturbs iron metabolism, and alters the activities of several enzymes and the liver concentrations of several metabolites associated with iron status in rats.[40] In support of the viewpoint that lead is necessary for optimal iron metabolism, lead deprivation was found to elevate iron absorption and retention and to depress iron concentrations in serum and various organs of rats.[41,42] Furthermore, absolute lead retention increased as dietary lead increased from 0.12 to 1.09 nmol (25 to 225 ng)/g diet, decreased as dietary lead increased from 1.09 to 4.95 nmol (225 to 1025 ng)/g diet, and markedly increased as dietary lead increased from 24.15 to 2898.0 nmol (5 to 600 μg)/g diet.[43] These data indicate that homeostatic mechanisms exist for lead and support the concept that lead, at low dietary intakes, is an essential element. In this regard, lead was found to enhance growth and to improve the hematocrits and hemoglobin concentration of iron-deficient rat pups; however, it was suggested that the effects were probably the result of a pharmacologic action of lead.[44] Thus, the mechanism by which lead affects iron metabolism needs to be determined. Nonetheless, the possibility must be considered that lead is an essential element, the need of which may be enhanced by the stressor of suboptimal iron status.

### TIN

In 1990, Yokoi et al. showed that when compared to rats fed 16.9 nmol (2 μg) Sn/g diet, rats fed 0.143 nmol (17 ng) Sn/g diet exhibited poor growth, decreased food efficiency, alopecia, depressed response to sound, and changes in mineral concentrations in various organs.[45] These interesting studies of tin deficiency now need confirmation.

Progress in showing the nutritional significance of the ultratrace elements has been substantial since 1985. Much of this progress has been the result of studies that examined the importance of specific ultratrace elements in organisms exposed to various metabolic, hormonal, physiologic, and nutritional stressors. The findings indicate that situations will be found in which an ultratrace element is of nutritional importance; at present, the prime candidate is boron. Thus, some ultratrace elements are probably more important in human nutrition than is now generally accepted.

## REFERENCES


1. Nielsen, F.H.: Ultratrace elements in nutrition. *In* Annual Review of Nutrition. Vol. 4. Edited by W.J. Darby, H.P. Broquist, and R.E. Olson. Palo Alto, Annual Reviews, 1981, pp. 21–41.
2. Uthus, E.O., Cornatzer, W.E., Nielsen, F.H.: Consequences of arsenic deprivation in laboratory animals. *In* Arsenic: Industrial, Biomedical, Environmental Perspectives. Edited by W.H. Lederer and R.J. Fensterheim. New York, Van Nostrand Reinhold, 1983, pp. 173–189.
3. Nielsen, F.H., Uthus, E.O.: Arsenic. *In* Biochemistry of the Essential Ultratrace Elements. Edited by E. Frieden. New York, Plenum, 1984, pp. 319–340.
4. Nielsen, F.H.: Possible future implications of ultratrace elements in human health and disease. *In* Essential and Toxic Trace Elements in Human Health and Disease, Current Topics in Nutrition and Disease. Vol. 18. Edited by A.S. Prasad. New York, Alan R. Liss, 1988, pp. 277–292.
5. Nielsen, F.H.: The ultratrace elements. *In* Trace Elements in Foods. Edited by K.T. Smith. New York, Marcel Dekker, 1988, pp. 357–428.
6. Nielsen, F.H.: Ultratrace elements: An update. *In* Trace Elements in Clinical Medicine. Edited by H. Tomita. Tokyo, Springer, 1990, pp. 353–360.
7. Nielsen, F.H.: Other trace elements. *In* Present Knowledge in Nutrition. 6th Ed. Edited by M.L. Brown. Washington, D.C., International Life Sciences Institute, 1990, pp. 294–307.
8. Anke, M.: Arsenic. *In* Trace Elements in Human and Animal Nutrition. Vol. 2. Edited by W. Mertz. Orlando, FL, Academic, 1986, pp. 347–372.
9. Vahter, M.: Metabolism of arsenic. *In* Biological and Environmental Effects of Arsenic. Edited by B.A. Fowler. Amsterdam, Elsevier, 1983, pp. 171–198.
10. Nielsen, F.H.: FASEB J, *5*:2661–2667, 1991.
11. Nielsen, F.H.: Other elements: Sb, Ba, B, Br, Cs, Ge, Rb, Ag, Sr, Sn, Ti, Zr, Be, Bi, Ga, Au, In, Nb, Sc, Te, Tl, W. *In* Trace Elements in Human and Animal Nutrition. Vol. 2. Edited by W. Mertz. Orlando, FL, Academic, 1986, pp. 415–463.
12. Nielsen, F.H.: Magnesium, *9*:61–69, 1990.
13. Nielsen, F.H., Hunt, C.D., Mullen, L.M., et al.: FASEB J., *1*:394–397, 1987.
14. Nielsen, F.H., Mullen, L.M., Gallagher, S.K.: J. Trace Elem. Exp. Med., *3*:45–54, 1990.
15. Keen, C.L., Lönnerdal, B., and Hurley, L.S.: Manganese. *In* Biochemistry of the Essential Ultratrace Elements. Edited by E. Frieden. New York, Plenum, 1984, pp. 89–132.
16. Hurley, L.S., Keen, C.L.: Manganese. *In* Trace Elements in Human and Animal Nutrition. Vol. 1. Edited by W. Mertz. San Diego, Academic, 1987, pp. 185–223.
17. Johnson, P.E., Nielsen, F.H.: Copper, manganese, cobalt, and magnesium. *In* Meat and Health, Advances in Meat Research. Vol. 6. Edited by A.M. Pearson and T.R. Dutson. London, Elsevier Applied Science, 1990, pp. 275–299.
18. Keen, C.L.: Manganese. *In* Present Knowledge of Nutrition. 6th Ed. Edited by M.L. Brown. Washington, D.C., International Life Sciences Institute, 1990, pp. 279–286.
19. Johnson, P.E., Lykken, G.I.: J. Trace Elem. Exp. Med., *4*:19–35, 1991.
20. Food and Nutrition Board, National Research Council: Recommended Dietary Allowances. 10th Ed. Washington, D.C., National Academy Press, 1989.
21. Winston, P.W.: Molybdenum. *In* Disorders of Mineral Metabolism. Vol. 1. Edited by F. Bronner and J.W. Coburn. New York, Academic, 1981, pp. 295–315.
22. Rajagopalan, K.V.: Molybdenum. *In* Biochemistry of the Essential Ultratrace Elements. Edited by E. Frieden. New York, Plenum, 1984, pp. 149–174.

23. Mills, C.F., Davis, G.K.: Molybdenum. *In* Trace Elements in Human and Animal Nutrition. Vol. 1. Edited by W. Mertz. San Diego, Academic, 1987, pp 429–463.
24. Rajagopalan, K.V.: Molybdenum: An essential trace element in human nutrition. *In* Annual Review of Nutrition. Vol. 8. Edited by R.E. Olson, E. Beutler, and H.P. Broquist. Palo Alto, Annual Reviews, 1988, pp. 401–427.
25. Nielsen, F.H.: Nickel. *In* Biochemistry of the Essential Ultratrace Elements. Edited by E. Frieden. New York, Plenum, 1984, pp. 293–308.
26. Nielsen, F.H.: Nickel. *In* Trace Elements in Human and Animal Nutrition. Vol. 1. Edited by W. Mertz. San Diego, Academic, 1987, pp. 245–273.
27. Walsh, C.T., Orme-Johnson, W.H.: Biochemistry, *26:*4901–4906, 1987.
28. Anke, M., Groppel, B., Kronemann, H., et al.: Nickel—an essential element. *In* Nickel in the Human Environment. Edited by F.W. Sunderman et al. Lyon, International Agency Research Cancer, 1984, pp. 339–365.
29. Carlisle, E.M.: Silicon. *In* Biochemistry of the Essential Ultratrace Elements. Edited by E. Frieden. New York, Plenum, 1984, pp. 257–291.
30. Carlisle, E.M.: Silicon. *In* Trace Elements in Human and Animal Nutrition. Vol. 2. Edited by W. Mertz. Orlando, FL, Academic, 1986, pp. 373–390.
31. Carlisle, E.M., Curran, M.J.: Alzheimer Dis. Assoc. Disord., *1:*83–89, 1987.
32. Bertrand, D.: Bull. Am. Mus. Nat. His., *94:*403–456, 1950.
33. Schroeder, H.A., Balassa, J.J., Tipton, I.H.: J. Chronic Dis., *16:*1047–1071, 1963.
34. Nielsen, F.H.: J. Nutr., *115:*1239–1247, 1985.
35. Nechay, B.R., Nanninga, L.B., Nechay, P.S.E., et al.: Fed. Proc., *45:*123–132, 1986.
36. Nielsen, F.H.: Vanadium. *In* Trace Elements in Human and Animal Nutrition. Vol. 1. Edited by W. Mertz. San Diego, Academic, 1987, pp. 275–300.
37. Nielsen, F.H., Uthus, E.O.: The essentiality and metabolism of vanadium. *In* Vanadium in Biological Systems. Edited by N.D. Chasteen. Dordrecht, Kluwer Academic, 1990, pp. 51–62.
38. Anke, M., Groppel, B., Arnhold, W., et al.: Essentiality of the trace element bromine. *In* Trace Element Analytical Chemistry in Medicine and Biology. Edited by P. Braetter and P. Schramel. Berlin, Walter de Gruyter, 1988, pp. 618–626.
39. Anke, M., Groppel, B., Krause, U.: Fluorine deficiency in goats. *In* Trace Elements in Man and Animals. Edited by B. Momčilović. Zagreb, IMI, 1991, pp. 26.28–26.29.
40. Kirchgessner, M., Reichlmayr-Lais, A.: Lead deficiency and its effects on growth and metabolism. *In* Trace Element Metabolism in Man and Animals (TEMA 4). Edited by J. McC. Howell, J.M. Gawthorne, and C.L. White. Canberra, Australian Academy of Science, 1981, pp. 390–393.
41. Reichlmayr-Lais, A.M., Kirchgessner, M.: Newer research on lead essentiality. *In* Trace Elements in Man and Animals 5. Edited by C.F. Mills, I. Bremner, and J.K. Chesters. Farnham Royal, Commonwealth Agricultural Bureaux, 1985, pp. 283–286.
42. Reichlmayr-Lais, A.M., Kirchgessner, M.: J. Anim. Physiol. Anim. Nutr., *59:*34–37, 1988.
43. Kirchgessner, M., Reichlmayr-Lais, A.M., Stöckl, K.N.: J. Trace Elem. Electrolytes Health Dis., *2:*149–152, 1988.
44. Uthus, E.O., Nielsen, F.H.: Biol. Trace Elem. Res., *16:*155–163, 1988.
45. Yokoi, K., Kimura, M., Itokawa, Y.: Biol. Trace Elem. Res., *24:*223–231, 1990.

## SELECTED READINGS

Brown, M.L. (ed.): Present Knowledge in Nutrition. Washington, D.C., International Life Sciences Institute, 1990.

Frieden, E. (ed.): Biochemistry of the Essential Ultratrace Elements. New York, Plenum, 1984.

Mertz, W. (ed.): Trace Elements in Human and Animal Nutrition. Vols. 1 and 2. San Diego, Academic, 1987.

CHAPTER 16

# Vitamin A, Retinoids, and Carotenoids

James Allen Olson



## HISTORICAL OVERVIEW

Night blindness was a well-recognized disease in ancient Egypt. The cure, as expressed in the Papyrus Ebers and the London Medical Papyrus, was to apply topically to the eyes juice squeezed from cooked liver. The ancient Greeks, who were familiar with Egyptian medical practice, recommended the ingestion of cooked liver as well as its topical application.[1] Interestingly, this tradition of applying cooked liver oil or juice topically to the eye has persisted in many societies to this day. The active principle of liver oil or juice, of course, is vitamin A.

In the early part of this century, Frederick Gowland Hopkins in England found that a growth-stimulating principle in milk was present in the alcoholic extract rather than in the ash, and soon thereafter Stepp in Germany identified one of these so-called "minimal qualitative factors" as a lipid. In 1913, E.V. McCollum and Marguerite Davis in Wisconsin showed that butter or egg yolk, but not lard, contained an essential growth factor for rats. They termed this factor "fat-soluble A." Concomitantly, Osborn and Mendel in New Haven found a similar fat-soluble growth factor in cod liver oil and butter. Thus, 1913 marks the beginning of the modern nutritional history of vitamin A.

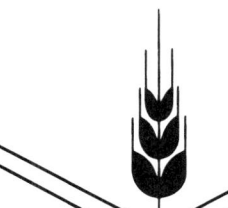

The fact that active fractions from plant tissues were often colored, whereas those from liver and animal tissues were not, puzzled many investigators during the following decade. This problem finally was resolved when Moore in England showed that β-carotene was converted biologically to a colorless form of vitamin A, which was then stored in liver tissue. In 1930, Karrer and his colleagues in Switzerland determined the structures of both vitamin A and β-carotene. Five years later, Wald identified the chromophore of visual pigments as retinene, now termed retinal, thereby defining one of the primary functions of the vitamin. During the 1920s, the marked effects of vitamin A deficiency on appetite, growth, and tissue differentiation were also well noted. These early studies on vitamin A are well reviewed in Moore's elegant treatise.[2]

## CHEMISTRY

Vitamin A and more than 600 carotenoids have been crystallized and fully characterized by a variety of chemical and physical methods. Furthermore, vitamin A and many of its analogues, as well as selected carotenoids, have been synthesized chemically from simple, readily available precursors. Mainly because of the structure of conjugated double bonds that are characteristic of both vitamin A and carotenoids, these substances are sensitive to oxidation.

### NOMENCLATURE

Vitamin A is now considered chemically a subgroup of the retinoids, which are defined as a class of compounds consisting of four isoprenoid units joined in a head-to-tail manner and customarily containing five conjugated double bonds.[3,4] The term vitamin A is used as a generic descriptor for retinoids exhibiting qualitatively the biologic activity of retinol. The numbering system for all-*trans* retinol is depicted in Figure 16–1*A*. Other naturally occurring retinoids of biologic interest, mainly in the all-*trans* form, include retinal (also termed retinaldehyde), retinoic acid, 3-dehydroretinol (vitamin $A_2$), 11-*cis* retinal, 4-oxoretinoic acid, retinyl palmitate, retinyl phosphate, retinoyl β-glucuronide, and retinotaurine (Fig. 16–1*B* to *J*).

The nomenclature of carotenoids primarily is based on β-carotene, or more formally, on β,β-carotene.[4,5] The formulas and numbering system for β-carotene and α-carotene are given in Figure 16–1 *M* and *N*. The term provitamin A carotenoids is used as a generic descriptor for all carotenoids exhibiting qualitatively the biologic activity of vitamin A.

### ISOLATION AND SYNTHESIS

Vitamin A, mainly in the form of esters, was initially prepared commercially by molecular distillation from extracts of fish liver oils.[2] As early as 1937, however, vitamin A was synthesized from β-ionone, although in poor yield. In 1947, a commercially feasible process was developed by Otto Isler in Switzerland, and later another excellent commercial process, using the Wittig reaction, was devised by Pommer.[6] Simple compounds, such as acetone, formaldehyde, isobutylene, acetylene, methanol, hydrogen gas, and acetic acid anhydride, are now used as precursors in the complete synthesis of retinol.

Carotenoids, which contain 40 carbon atoms, are commercially synthesized in the presence of suitable catalysts either from 2 molecules of retinal, a C-20 compound, or from 2 molecules of C-19 aldehyde and acetylene.[6] Most, if not all, of the vitamin A and β-carotene available commercially, whether in concentrated solution, stabilized beadlets, or crystalline form, is of synthetic origin. These synthetic compounds are identical in every way, both chemically and biologically, to the substances isolated from natural sources. Commercially available preparations of vitamin A are almost invariably in the form of fatty acyl esters, i.e., retinyl acetate, propionate, or palmitate, which are more stable than retinol. Stabilized dry forms of vitamin A, which contain an antioxidant in a matrix of gelatin and carbohydrates, are commonly used as supplements in animal feed and can be used as well in humans.

In view of the intense current interest in analogues of vitamin A for the treatment of skin disorders and as possible anticancer agents, many additional retinoids have been synthesized.[7] The formulas of two highly active synthetic retinoids that are *not* found in nature are depicted in Figure 16–1 *K* and *L*. The free acid of Figure 16–1*K*, termed acitretin, rather than the ethyl ester (etretinate), is now used preferentially in therapy.

### PROPERTIES

Vitamin A and carotenoids are soluble in most organic solvents, but not in water. In their extraction from plasma and tissues, therefore, the cell structure must be disrupted, the proteins denatured, and the lipid fraction dissolved in some solvent, such as hexane or dichloromethane, which is immiscible with water. In crystalline form or when dissolved in oil containing an antioxidant, vitamin A is stable for long periods, providing it is kept in a sealed container under a dry nitrogen or argon atmosphere in the dark. Carotenoids, although less stable than retinol, are also preserved well under similar conditions.

Vitamin A and the carotenoids are sensitive to oxidation, isomerization, and polymerization when dissolved in dilute solution under light in the presence of oxygen, particularly at elevated temperatures. The destruction of these compounds is particularly rapid when they are adsorbed as a thin surface film in the presence of light and oxygen.

Vitamin A is stable when stored in frozen liver tissue in the dark at a temperature below −20° C and in frozen serum stored at −70° C in sealed vials under ideal conditions. Carotenoids present in stored frozen serum or tissues tend to be more sensitive than vitamin A to destruction.

Vitamin A has several physical properties that have been used in its analysis: (1) a characteristic ultraviolet (UV) absorption spectrum with an absorption maximum

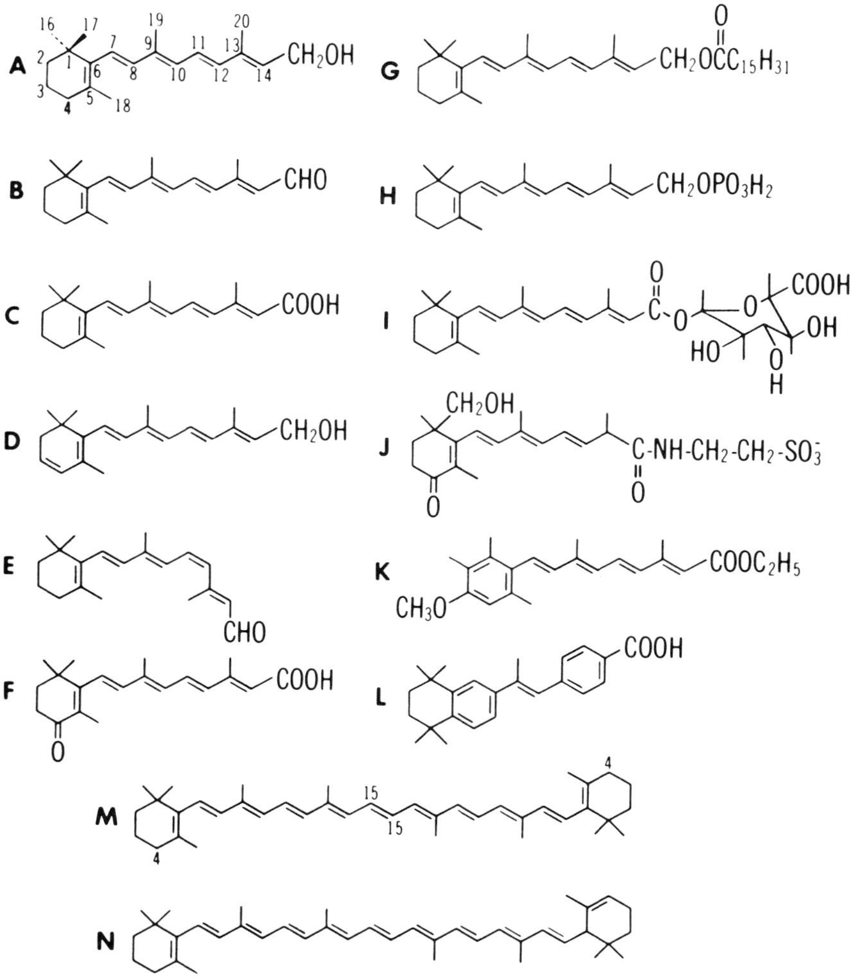

**FIGURE 16–1.** Formulas and numbering systems for retinoids and carotenoids. *A*, All-*trans* retinol; *B*, all-*trans* retinal; *C*, all-*trans* retinoic acid; *D*, 3-dehydroretinol (vitamin $A_2$); *E*, 11-*cis* retinal; *F*, 4-oxoretinoic acid; *G*, retinyl palmitate; *H*, retinyl phosphate; *I*, retinoyl β-glucuronide; *J*, retinotaurine; *K*, trimethylmethoxyphenyl analogue of ethyl retinoate; *L*, tetrahydro, tetramethylnaphthylisopropenylbenzoic acid; *M*, all-*trans* β-carotene; *N*, α-carotene.

(λmax) of 325 nm and a molecular extinction coefficient of 53,000 $cm^{-2}M^{-1}$ ($E^{1\%}_{1cm}$ of 1850) in hexane; (2) greenish fluorescence at 470 nm when excited at 325 nm; and (3) the capability to form a brilliant blue chromophore, albeit transient, with a λmax of 620 nm when exposed to various Lewis acids, such as antimony trichloride, trifluoroacetic acid, and trichloroacetic acid, in anhydrous chloroform.

Carotenoids also show characteristic absorption spectra; β-carotene, for example, has a λmax of 450 nm in hexane with a molecular extinction coefficient of 136,900 $cm^{-2}M^{-1}$ ($E^{1\%}_{1cm}$ of 2550). Under normal laboratory conditions, most carotenoids do not fluoresce to any significant extent. Although carotenoids form colored complexes with Lewis acids, the intensity is much less than those formed with vitamin A.

Most pure retinoids and many individual carotenoids have been well characterized by UV and visible (VIS) absorption spectroscopy, infrared spectroscopy, nuclear magnetic resonance spectroscopy, mass spectrometry, and other physical methods.[7,8]

## BIOLOGIC ACTIVITY

The primary unit of biologic activity for vitamin A is 1 μg of all-*trans* retinol, whether present as the free alcohol or as one of several natural or synthetic fatty acyl esters. Although retinyl esters are more common than retinol in foodstuffs and are almost exclusively present in synthetic preparations of vitamin A, the biologic activity is still calculated in terms of the amount of all-*trans* retinol present.

Whenever appropriate, vitamin A and individual retinoids and carotenoids are preferentially expressed in molar terms in accord with the Système International (SI) (see Appendix Tables A-1a and A-1b). Thus, serum concentrations of retinol are given in micromolar terms (μmol/L) rather than in micrograms per deciliter (μg/dl), and liver concentrations as micromoles per gram, not as micrograms per gram. In this expression, 1 μg retinol is equal to 0.003491 μmol or, conversely, 1 μ mol of retinol equals 286.46 μg of retinol. The use of SI units is less appropriate for expressing the vitamin A content of foodstuffs, which often consists of a mixture of several biologically active forms, often with different bioavailabilities. Recommended dietary intakes are not expressed in SI units for the same reason.

A unit of historical value, which is still extensively used in food composition tables and in labeling of vitamin A supplements, is the International Unit, or IU. One IU equals 0.300 μg of all-*trans* retinol, or a corresponding amount of retinol in ester linkage. Thus, whether the vitamin A in a given solution is present as free retinol, retinyl acetate, or retinyl palmitate, the number of IU will be the same.

Among the 600 or more carotenoids that exist in nature, only about 50 show provitamin A activity. The most active, and often major, provitamin A carotenoid in food is all-*trans* β-carotene. In stimulating the growth of vitamin A-depleted animals, most other provitamin A carotenoids, such as α- and γ-carotene, show biologic activities between 20 and 60%. On the average, other provitamin A carotenoids in foods possess approximately 50% of the growth-promoting action of β-carotene. To express all provitamin A carotenoids as a single unit, the β-carotene equivalent was defined, where 1 μg β-carotene equivalent equals 1 μg of all-*trans* β-carotene or 2 μg of other, largely all-*trans*, provitamin A carotenoids in foods.

To express both preformed vitamin A and β-carotene equivalents as a single nutritive value, the retinol equivalent (RE) was created.[9] One μg RE is equal to 1 μg of all-*trans* retinol in food, or to 6 μg of all-*trans* β-carotene in food, or to 12 μg of other provitamin A carotenoids in foods. Although the ratios are arbitrary, the logic is as follows: In the biologic conversion of β-carotene to vitamin A, one molecule of the former can yield two of the latter. Some β-carotene may also be cleaved in a stepwise manner to yield only one molecule of vitamin A. Not all ingested β-carotene is converted to vitamin A, however, and the absorption efficiency of synthetic β-carotene is poorer than that of vitamin A. Thus, a low dose of ingested vitamin A, on a weight basis, is approximately two to four times as efficacious as a low dose of ingested pure β-carotene.[2,10] Carotenoids in foods are less bioavailable, however, than is preformed vitamin A, and the absorption efficiency of carotenoids, unlike vitamin A, falls with increasing doses or dietary amounts. If the bioavailability of vitamin A in food is presumed to be 1.5 to 3 times greater than that of β-carotene, 1 μg of retinol in food would be equivalent to 6 μg β-carotene. In this nutritional context, 1 μmol retinol equals 3.2 μmol β-carotene. In the absence of carefully controlled studies of this conversion ratio in man under normal dietary conditions, the weight ratio of 1 to 6 is an acceptable, albeit arbitrary, value.

Some confounding factors exist. On the basis of carefully conducted older experiments in animals, 1 IU vitamin A added to a diet was found to be equivalent to approximately 0.6 μg of added β-carotene under optimal conditions of absorption and conversion.[2] Thus, 1 IU β-carotene was defined as 0.6 μg and was presumed to be equal to 1 IU retinol (0.3 μg). Food composition tables have been compiled in large part by simply adding IU from preformed vitamin A and from β-carotene equivalents, although the revision of Handbook 8 expresses values both as total IU and as RE.[161] Confusion exists because the equivalency is different in the two systems: in the RE system, 1 μg retinol equals 6 μg β-carotene, whereas in the IU system, 1 μg retinol equals 2 μg β-carotene. If an IU of retinol is denoted as $IU_a$ and an IU of β-carotene as $IU_c$, where 1 $IU_a$ equals 3 $IU_c$, this impasse might be resolved.[11] Procedures for interconverting various expressions for the biologic activities of vitamin A and carotenoids are given in Appendix Table A1-b.

In vitamin A and all known provitamin A carotenoids, ingested all-*trans* forms are also significantly more active than any of the *cis* isomers. All-*trans* retinal is almost as active as all-*trans* retinol, whereas 3-dehydroretinol shows about 40% as much activity. Retinoic acid is active in growth but ineffective in vision and, depending on the species, in reproduction. The synthetic aromatic retinoid depicted in Figure 16–1*L* is active in growth, but also is highly toxic at elevated doses.[12]

All provitamin A carotenoids possess at least one unsubstituted β-ionone moiety. Carotenoids that are *not* converted into vitamin A still show significant biologic and pharmacologic activity,[13] which is primarily attributed to the physical and chemical properties of their long, highly conjugated systems of double bonds. Thus, biologic activity of carotenoids might be characterized as either nutritional or non-nutritional in nature. Some carotenoids possess both activities, some only one, and some none.[13]

## METABOLISM

The metabolism of vitamin A and carotenoids consists of their digestion and absorption, transport in chylomicra, uptake and storage by the liver, release as holo-retinol-binding protein (holo-RBP), intracellular binding in various tissues, regulation of retinol-binding protein (RBP) expression, biologic transformation, and excretion.[14-16]

## DIGESTION AND ABSORPTION

Preformed vitamin A and carotenoids in the diet are largely released from protein during proteolysis in the stomach. Vitamin A and carotenoids tend to aggregate with lipids into globules, which then pass into the small intestine. The upper intestine is the major site of lipid hydrolysis. Dietary fat, protein, and their hydrolytic products stimulate, through cholecystokinin, the secretion of bile, which first emulsifies lipids and then forms micelles. Bile salts also stimulate pancreatic lipase, which hydrolyzes triglycerides, and other esterases that hydrolyze retinyl esters and cholesteryl esters. Hydrolysis is an important factor in the bioavailability of vitamin A, inasmuch as retinol in a bile salt-containing micelle is well absorbed (70 to 90%) from the small intestine, whereas retinyl esters are poorly utilized. Vitamin A seems to be absorbed by a carrier-mediated process at low concentrations, but mainly by diffusion from the micellar phase at high doses.[14-16]

As already mentioned, carotenoids are not as well absorbed as vitamin A, perhaps in part because of their more fastidious requirements for a suitable micellar suspension.[14-16] Various carotenoids are also absorbed at different rates; ethyl β-apo-8′-carotenoate, for example, is rapidly absorbed from the human intestine without hydrolysis, 4,4′-dimethoxy β-carotene is absorbed less well, and the polar carotenoids, neoxanthin and violaxanthin, are absorbed poorly.[17]

## TRANSPORT IN CHYLOMICRA

Within intestinal cells, newly formed chylomicra contain retinyl ester, cholesteryl ester, some retinol, phospholipids, much triglyceride, and apolipoproteins A-1, A-4, B, and several others. In the complex conversion of the secreted chylomicra into chylomicron remnants in the plasma, the triglyceride content is markedly reduced by the hydrolytic action of lipoprotein lipase, the predominant apolipoproteins on the chylomicron remnant become B and E, and the relative concentration of retinyl ester increases.[15]

## UPTAKE AND STORAGE BY THE LIVER

By interaction with cell surface receptors on liver parenchymal cells for apolipoprotein E, and possibly for apolipoprotein B, chylomicron remnants are internalized by receptor-mediated endocytosis. Retinyl esters are hydrolyzed, combined with cellular retinol-binding protein (CRBP) in the cytosol of the hepatocyte, and then subjected to several possible metabolic routes. In regard to storage, retinol may be directly esterified primarily to retinyl palmitate, which is stored in vitamin A-containing lipid globules in the hepatocyte. Alternatively, retinol may be transferred to stellate cells,[18,19] where retinol is also esterified and stored in vitamin A-containing globules. Stellate cells have also been termed lipocytes, Ito cells, and fat-storing cells.[18,19] Under normal physiologic conditions, stellate cells contain 80 to 90% of the stored vitamin A, hepatocytes 10 to 20% and other liver cells only a few percent.[18-21] The retinyl ester stored in stellate cells and hepatocytes can be readily and completely mobilized and used by the organism.

## RELEASE OF RETINOL INTO PLASMA FROM TISSUES

Within the hepatocyte, a precursor of RBP, preapo-RBP is first formed, which is then proteolytically cleaved, with the loss of a peptide, to apo-RBP.[22] All-*trans* retinol combines with apo-RBP in a specific 1:1 molecular complex to form holo-RBP. The latter is transported through the Golgi apparatus and then is secreted into the plasma. Human RBP, a single polypeptide chain with 182 amino acids in a known sequence,[23] has a molecular weight of 21,230. Within the plasma, holo-RBP combines in a large part with transthyretin (prealbumin), which specifically binds one thyroxine molecule per tetramer.[22]

Retinol might be released into plasma from liver stellate cells by two routes: (1) by its transfer back to parenchymal cells followed by RBP release; or (2) by direct release into the plasma as a RBP complex. Whether one or both of these routes are active is still unclear.[18,19] Route 1 has not been shown experimentally, and whether stellate cells can synthesize RBP,[18,19] or not,[24] is uncertain. Besides the storage of vitamin A, stellate cells synthesize and secrete collagen and proliferate in a fibrotic liver.[19] They are also present in many nonhepatic tissues. Thus, they may well have several physiologic roles.[19]

Although vitamin A is primarily stored in the liver, all tissues contain some vitamin A. Because messenger ribonucleic acid (mRNA) for RBP has been identified in the kidney,[25] lacrimal gland,[26] adipose tissue,[27] and bone marrow as well as in the liver, nonhepatic tissues may well synthesize and secrete RBP. The possible physiologic role of RBP in nonhepatic tissues is not yet clear.

In adults, the total RBP concentration in plasma is 1.9 to 2.4 μmol/L (40 to 50 μg/ml), 80 to 90% of which exists as holo-RBP.[22] In children up to the age of puberty, the total RBP concentration is approximately 50% of the adult level.[28]

Holo-RBP interacts with cell-surface receptors for RBP on target tissue cells, which are mainly epithelial. Retinol is internalized, whereas apo-RBP is modified in conformation and released. This modified apo-RBP no longer binds retinol, no longer interacts with transthyretin, and ultimately is catabolized, primarily by the kidney.[21] Holo-RBP can also be taken up by the liver stellate and parenchymal cells.[18,19]

Retinol bound to RBP can also be transferred to receptor-free lipid membranes at a physiologic rate.[162]

Thus, specific cell surface receptors for holo-RBP are not required for the uptake of retinol by tissues.

## INTRACELLULAR AND INTERSTITIAL BINDING PROTEINS

Cells of most tissues contain a specific binding protein for all-*trans* retinol, cellular retinol-binding protein type I (CRBP-I).[29,30] Most fetal tissues and many adult tissues also contain a binding protein for all-*trans* retinoic acid, cellular retinoic acid-binding protein type I (CRABP-I).[29,30] Müller cells of the retina and pigment epithelial cells of the eye possess a fairly specific binding protein for 11-*cis* retinal, cellular retinaldehyde-binding protein (CRALBP).[30,31] Fetal and adult intestine contains a distinct binding protein for all-*trans* retinol, CRBP type II (CRBP-II),[29,30] and fetal tissues, including the developing chick limb bud, contain CRABP type II (CRABP-II).[30,32] Interphotoreceptor retinol-binding protein (IRBP) is synthesized by photoreceptor cells of the eye and is secreted into the intercellular matrix between the pigment epithelium cells and the photoreceptors.[30,33,34] Other retinoid-binding proteins that are at least partially characterized have been identified in the epididymis, uterus, fetal liver, and Sertoli cells.[18,29,30] The properties of the major retinoid-binding proteins in mammals, including the nuclear retinoid receptors, are summarized in Table 16–1.

Thus, the retinoids clearly are chaperoned by a set of highly specific proteins during their movements in vivo. These proteins seem to function as transport agents, as sequestering entities, as coligands in enzymatic transformations, and as coligands in genetic expression.

Other proteins, such as several fatty acid-binding proteins, serum albumin, and β-lactoglobulin also bind retinoids, and in particular, retinoic acid. These interactions, although relatively nonspecific, may play some physiologic role.

## CONTROL OF EXPRESSION OF RETINOID-BINDING PROTEINS

The synthesis of mRNA for RBP and of RBP by the liver does not seem to be much affected by vitamin A status in vivo,[22] although mRNA for RBP increases in response to both increases and decreases of retinol concentrations in cultured hepatoma cells in vitro.[35] Retinol has little or no direct effect on the steady-state concentrations of retinoid-binding proteins,[36] but retinoic acid increases the synthesis of mRNA for CRBP-I, CRBP-II, CRABP-I, and CRABP-II in several cell types and species.[36-38] Because the genes for most retinoid-binding proteins have been cloned, the site (response element) in the promoter region of the gene for the retinoic acid-receptor complex has been determined in several cases. The mechanisms for controlling the formation of other primarily cytosolic retinoid-binding proteins are less clear.

## METABOLIC TRANSFORMATIONS AND EXCRETION

The major form of vitamin A in the plasma, the retinol-RBP complex (holo-RBP), interacts with a cell-surface receptor for RBP on retinal pigment epithelial

**TABLE 16–1.** PROPERTIES OF MAJOR RETINOID-BINDING PROTEINS

| NAME | ABBREVIATION | APPROXIMATE MOLECULAR WEIGHT (KD) | MAJOR LIGAND |
|---|---|---|---|
| Retinol-binding protein | RBP | 21.2 | all-*trans* retinol |
| Cellular retinol-binding protein, type I | CRBP-I | 15.7 | all-*trans* retinol |
| Cellular retinol-binding protein, type II | CRBP-II | 15.6 | all-*trans* retinol |
| Cellular retinoic acid binding-protein, type I | CRABP-I | 15.5 | all-*trans* retinoic acid |
| Cellular retinoic acid-binding protein, type II | CRABP-II | 15.0 | all-*trans* retinoic acid |
| Cellular retinaldehyde-binding protein | CRALBP | 36.0 | 11-*cis* retinol |
| Interphotoreceptor retinol-binding protein | IRBP | 135 | 11-*cis* and all-*trans* retinal |
| Retinoic acid receptor-α | RARα | 50 | all-*trans* retinoic acid |
| Retinoic acid receptor-β | RARβ | 50 | all-*trans* retinoic acid |
| Retinoic acid receptor-γ | RARγ | 50 | all-*trans* retinoic acid |
| Retinoid X receptor-α | RXRα | 51 | 9-*cis* retinoic acid |
| Retinoid X receptor-β | RXRβ | 51 | 9-*cis* retinoic acid |
| Retinoid X receptor-γ | RXRγ | 51 | 9-*cis* retinoic acid |

cells and is internalized by endocytosis.[39] The cell-surface receptor, which presumably is present on most other cells as well, has a molecular weight of 86 kd and a dissociation constant (Kd) of 31 to 72 nmol/L.[39] Other retinoids in plasma are taken up by cells in other ways, retinoic acid from a complex with serum albumin and the water-soluble retinoid β-glucuronides by diffusion.

The major reactions of vitamin A metabolism, which are summarized in Figure 16–2, are esterification, oxidation at C-15, oxidation at C-4, conjugation, isomerization, other miscellaneous oxidative reactions, and chain cleavage.[14,40] Retinol and retinal, as well as other metabolites reversibly converted to them, all possess significant biologic activity. Retinoic acid and its glucuronide are active in growth but not in vision or, in most species, in reproduction. Except for 14-hydroxy, 4,14-*retro* retinol,[41] more oxidized products, such as 4-hydroxyretinoic acid, 5,6-epoxyretinoic acid, and C-19 metabolites, are largely devoid of biologic activity. Retinoyl β-glucuronide, retinyl β-glucuronide, and retinoic acid are normally present in small amounts (3 to 11 nmol/L, or 1 to 5 μg/L) in human plasma.[42] Retinoyl β-glucuronide is not hydrolyzed in some cells and only slowly in vivo.[43] Retinoic acid can also be covalently bound to proteins,[44,45] possibly by means of a coenzyme A intermediate.[45] The cellular retinoid-binding proteins play a major role in the oxidation/reduction and transesterification of retinol.[30] Intestinal CRBP-II has been particularly closely studied in this regard.[46]

Approximately 5 to 20% of ingested vitamin A and a larger percentage of carotenoids, depending on their nature, bioavailability, and amount, are not absorbed from the intestinal tract and consequently are excreted in the feces. A significant portion (10 to 40%) of *absorbed* vitamin A is oxidized or conjugated in the liver and then is secreted into the bile. Although some of these biliary metabolites, such as retinoyl β-glucuronide, are reabsorbed in the intestine and transported back to the liver, most of the biliary metabolites are excreted in the feces. Vitamin A that is oxidized and chain-shortened in various tissues ultimately is excreted in the urine. Finally, carbon dioxide that is released in the oxidation and cleavage of the side chain in vitamin A is excreted in the respired air. In quantitative terms, of the dietary intake of vitamin A, an average of 10% is not absorbed, 20% appears in the feces through the bile, 17% is excreted in the urine, 3% is released as $CO_2$, and 50% is stored, primarily in the liver.

Most provitamin A carotenoids can be cleaved by a carotenoid 15,15′-dioxygenase in the cytosol of mucosal, hepatic, and some other tissue cells.[47,48] β-Carotene yields two molecules of retinal, which are in large part reduced and esterified to retinyl ester. The cleavage enzyme requires molecular oxygen and apparently contains a metal, possibly iron, at its catalytic site.[47,48] β-Carotene and some other carotenoids can also be cleaved asymmetrically to yield β-apocarotenals that, in turn, are converted to retinal, or possibly directly to retinoic acid.[49,50] At the level of retinal, therefore, which is reversibly reduced to retinol by alcohol dehydrogenases in many tissues, the metabolism of carotenoids and that of preformed vitamin A usually coincide. Much less is known about the metabolism and excretion of carotenoids other than β-carotene.[13] Each carotenoid, however, seems to show a specific pattern of absorption, metabolism, and transport.[17]

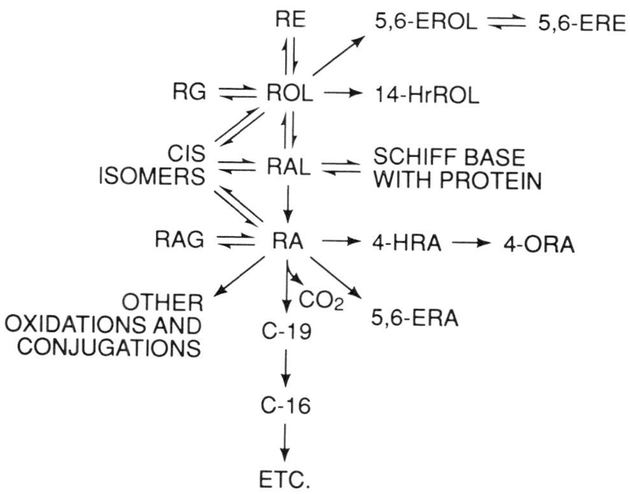
RE
5,6-EROL
5,6-ERE
RG
ROL
14-HrROL
CIS ISOMERS
RAL
SCHIFF BASE WITH PROTEIN
RAG
RA
4-HRA
4-ORA
OTHER OXIDATIONS AND CONJUGATIONS
$CO_2$
C-19
5,6-ERA
C-16
ETC.

**FIGURE 16–2.** Major metabolic transformations of vitamin A. ROL, Retinol; RE, retinyl ester; RAL, retinal; RA, retinoic acid; RG, retinyl β-glucuronide; RAG, retinoyl β-glucuronide; 5, 6-EROL, 5,6-epoxyretinol; 5,6-ERE, 5,6-epoxyretinyl ester; 14-HrROL, 14-hydroxy, 4,14-*retro*-retinol; 4-HRA, 4-hydroxyretinoic acid; 4-ORA, 4-oxoretinoic acid; 5,6-ERA, 5,6-epoxyretinoic acid; C-19 and C-16, chain-shortened, oxidized products with the indicated number of carbon atoms. Double arrows indicate reversible reactions; single arrows denote irreversible changes.

## FUNCTIONS

Functions of vitamin A include vision, cellular differentiation, morphogenesis, and transmembrane transport (in bacteria). Many other complex physiologic processes in animals, such as growth, reproduction, and the immune response, seem to be affected as a result of these cited functions.

### VISION

The role of vitamin A in vision is well defined.[51,52] In the outer segment of rod cells in the retina, 11-*cis* retinal forms a protonated Schiff base with a specific lysine residue of the membrane-bound protein, opsin, to yield rhodopsin, with an absorption maximum of 498 nm. Similar complexes exist in human cone cells to give three specific iodopsins that absorb maximally at 420 nm (blue cones), 534 nm (green cones), and 563 nm (red cones).

When a photon of light strikes the dark-adapted retina, the 11-*cis* bond of retinal in rhodopsin is isomerized to the all-*trans* form. This isomerization destabilizes rhodopsin, which passes through a series of different conformational states and ultimately dissociates into all-*trans* retinal and opsin. Metarhodopsin II and probably other like conformers, but not rhodopsin, may also be phosphorylated by rhodopsin kinase.

All-*trans* retinal may be isomerized back to the 11-*cis* form in the rod outer segment by light in the presence of certain phospholipids. In the dark, however, 11 *cis*-retinol is formed by the action of all-*trans*: 11-*cis* retinyl ester isomerase, a membrane-bound enzyme in retinal pigment epithelial cells.[51] This enzyme might better be called an isomerohydrolase, in that the energy released in the hydrolysis of the retinyl ester bond is directly coupled to the formation of the energy-rich 11-*cis* retinol.[51] The 11-*cis* forms of retinol and retinal are then transported on IRBP to the rod outer segment, whereas all-*trans* retinol is shuttled back on IRBP.[34]

The light-activated transformation of rhodopsin ultimately results in a reduction in the sodium ion current into the rod outer segment, which induces hyperpolarization of the membrane. In the probable sequence of steps in this amplification cascade,[53] summarized in Figure 16–3, light converts rhodopsin to the active intermediate, metarhodopsin II. The latter induces the exchange of guanosine diphosphate (GDP) for guanosine triphosphate (GTP) on a disk protein termed transducin. Transducin contains three subunits, and the complex of GTP with transducin activates phosphodiesterase, which in turn hydrolyzes cyclic guanosine monophosphate (cGMP) to GMP. As the concentration of cGMP falls, the sodium channel closes, leading to membrane hyperpolarization. The cascade is turned off by the time-dependent decay of metarhodopsin II to opsin, by the conversion of metarhodopsin II to an inactive phosphorylated form, and by the hydrolysis of bound GTP by the inherent GTPase activity of transducin.

## CELLULAR DIFFERENTIATION

In vitamin A deficiency, mucus-secreting cells are replaced by keratin-producing cells in many tissues of the body.[36,54] Conversely, the addition of vitamin A to vitamin A-deficient keratinizing cells in tissue culture induces a shift to mucus-producing cells. Retinoids also rapidly induce F-9 teratocarcinoma cells, as well as many other cell lines, to differentiate.[55] In this process, many new proteins appear in the newly differentiated cells. Thus, vitamin A and its analogues, both in vivo and in vitro, markedly influence the way in which cells differentiate.[36,54,55]

The mechanism by which retinoids induce cellular differentiation is becoming clear (Fig. 16–4). Within tissue cells, all-*trans* retinol, in association with CRBP, can be oxidized to all-*trans* retinoic acid and presumably can also be isomerized to 9-*cis* retinol, which in turn can be oxidized to 9-*cis* retinoic acid. All-*trans* or 9-*cis* retinoic acid is transported on CRABP or on other retinoid-binding proteins to the nucleus, where it is tightly bound to one or more of the three (α, β, γ) retinoic acid receptors (RAR) [56-60] or to one or more of the three (α, β, γ) retinoid X receptors (RXR),[61,62] respectively. In the activation of retinoic acid-responsive genes, a heterodimer of RAR and RXR, or in some cases a homodimer of RXR, binds to the response element of the gene to initiate transcription.[63-65] RXR also serves as a coregulator for the expression of genes responsive to triiodothyronine, to calcitriol, and perhaps to other hormones, but not to estrogen.[63-65] In this latter role,

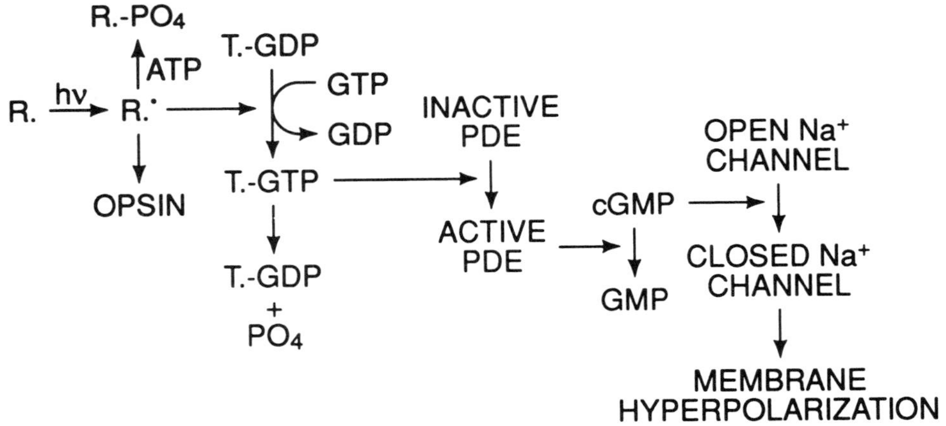
R.-PO4
ATP
T.-GDP
R.
hv
R.·
GTP
GDP
INACTIVE PDE
OPEN Na+ CHANNEL
OPSIN
T.-GTP
cGMP
ACTIVE PDE
T.-GDP
+
PO4
GMP
CLOSED Na+ CHANNEL
MEMBRANE HYPERPOLARIZATION

**FIGURE 16–3.** A possible sequence of steps between the light-induced activation of rhodopsin and hyperpolarization of the rod cell membrane. R., Rhodopsin; R.·, light-activated metarhodopsin II; R-$PO_4$, phosphorylated rhodopsin; ATP, adenosine triphosphate; GTP, guanosine triphosphate; GDP, guanosine diphosphate; cGMP, cyclic 3′, 5′-guanosine monophosphate; GMP, guanosine monophosphate; T., transducin; T.-GDP, a complex of transducin with GDP; T.-GTP, a complex of transducin with GTP; PDE, phosphodiesterase.

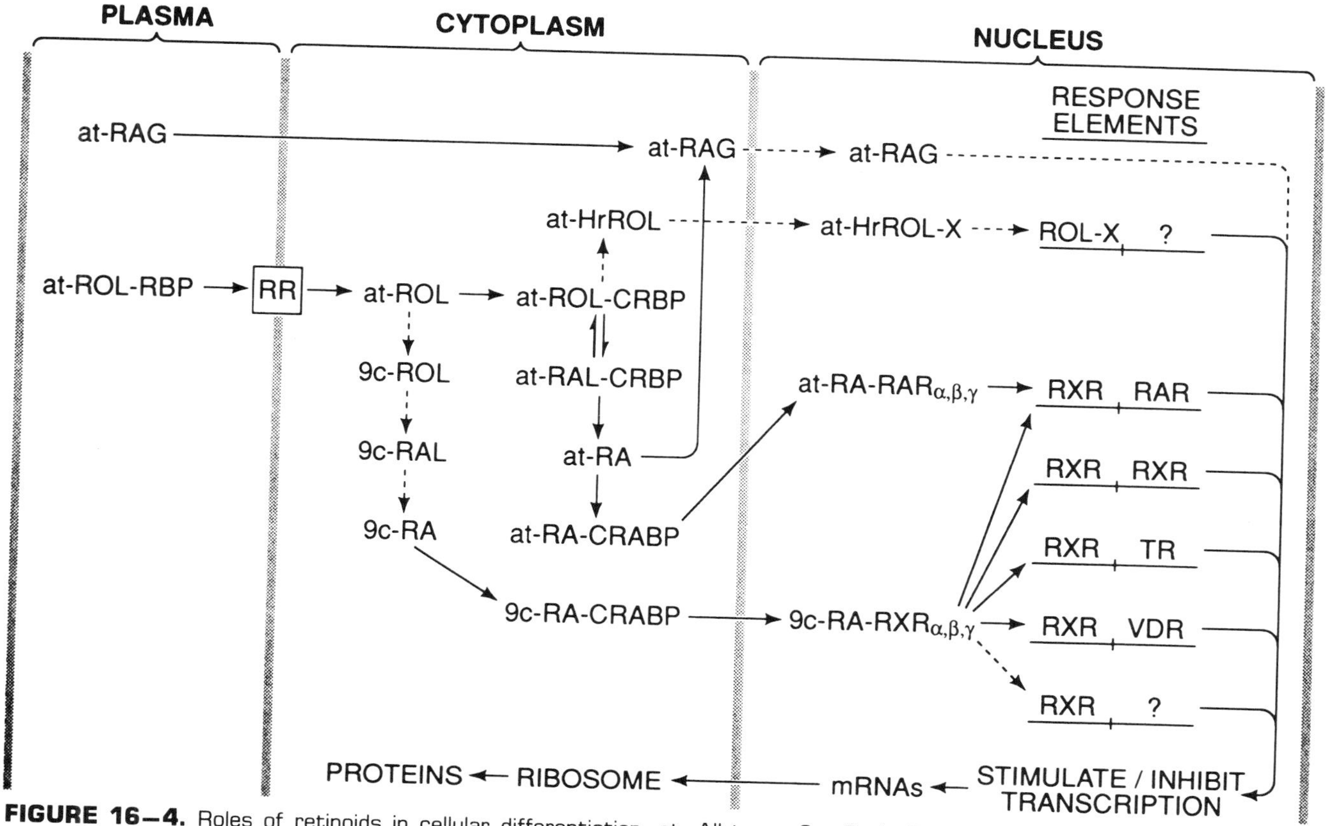
PLASMA
CYTOPLASM
NUCLEUS
RESPONSE ELEMENTS
at-RAG
at-RAG
at-RAG
at-HrROL
at-HrROL-X
ROL-X ?
at-ROL-RBP
RR
at-ROL
at-ROL-CRBP
9c-ROL
at-RAL-CRBP
at-RA-RARα,β,γ
RXR RAR
9c-RAL
at-RA
RXR RXR
9c-RA
at-RA-CRABP
RXR TR
9c-RA-CRABP
9c-RA-RXRα,β,γ
RXR VDR
RXR ?
PROTEINS
RIBOSOME
mRNAs
STIMULATE / INHIBIT TRANSCRIPTION

**FIGURE 16–4.** Roles of retinoids in cellular differentiation. at, All-*trans*; 9c, 9-*cis*; ROL, retinol; HrROL, 14-hydroxy-4,14-*retro*-retinol; RAL, retinal; RA, retinoic acid; RAG, retinoyl β-glucuronide; RR, cell surface receptor for holo-RBP; RBP, plasma retinol-binding protein; CRBP, cellular retinol-binding protein; CRABP, cellular retinoic acid-binding protein; RARα, β, γ, nuclear retinoic acid receptors, forms α, β, and γ; RXRα, β, γ, nuclear 9-*cis* retinoic acid receptors, isoforms α, β, and γ; TR, triiodothyronine bound to the nuclear thyroid receptor; VDR, calcitriol bound to the nuclear vitamin D receptor; X, unknown nuclear receptors; solid arrows, known transformations or effects; dashed arrows, postulated transformations or effects; ?, unknown occupancy.

RXR forms a heterodimer with the appropriate nuclear receptor for other hormones, thereby enhancing its affinity for the response element of the gene. The carboxyl terminal end of these receptors is involved in heterodimer formation.[63-65] Thus, 9-*cis* retinoic acid seems to play a general role in cell differentiation, whereas all-*trans* retinoic acid has more specific effects.

Like the cytosolic retinoid-binding proteins, the nuclear retinoic acid receptors appear in different cells and at different times in development.[58-60] Of particular note is RARγ, which is primarily localized in the skin.[58-60]

Some retinoids may stimulate differentiation by a different pathway; for example, retinoyl β-glucuronide does not bind to CRBP, CRABP, or nuclear RAR, but nonetheless is highly active biologically.[66,67] Similarly, B lymphocytes differentiate in response to 14-hydroxy, 4, 14-*retro*-retinol, but not to all-*trans* retinoic acid.[41] Furthermore, the binding to RAR of various acidic retinoids, both natural and synthetic, relates closely to their invoked cellular responses, but not well to their binding affinities for CRABP, at least in some cellular systems.[68] Finally, single RAR or RXR molecules, or homodimers of them, may activate some genes.[38]

The base sequence in DNA, reading in the 5′ to 3′ direction, at which RAR binds is GGTTCA followed by AGTTCA in the RARβ gene; it is a fourfold repeat of AGGTCA in the CRBP-II gene,[38,59] a direct repeat of GGTCA in the CRBP-I gene,[37,59] and a threefold repeat of TGACC in the laminin B1 gene.[69] The spacing between binding sites, which may well contribute to specificity, usually varies from one to five base pairs. Thus, the DNA binding regions for RAR and RXR are similar.

The RAR and RXR receptors, like other nuclear hormone receptors, possess 6 protein domains with specific functions.[58-60] At the N-terminal end, domains A and B serve as physiologic activators of the receptor; domain C, which is highly conserved, contains zinc-sulfhydryl interactions ("zinc fingers") that bind to DNA; domain D is a hinge region that provides the necessary conformation of the receptor; domain E binds the ligand;

and domain F, at the C-terminal end, enhances dimerization. All nuclear retinoid receptors contain approximately 460 amino acids and have molecular weights of approximately 50 kd.[58,59]

Retinoic acid is known directly to activate the genes for CRBP-I,[37] CRBP-II,[38] RARβ,[69] *Hox*-1.6,[70] laminin B1,[71] and transglutaminase[72,73] in various types of cells. The sequence by which other genes are subsequently activated is not clear. Various isoforms of transforming growth factor β (TGFβ) can be induced or suppressed by retinoic acid, depending on conditions.[74,75] Although most attention has been paid to the activation of gene expression, retinoids can also suppress transcription. Retinoids also show some physiologic effects in enucleated cells.[76] Thus, retinoids seem to play a central role in the development and maintenance of many tissues.

## MORPHOGENESIS

Both a deficiency and an excess of vitamin A and of most other retinoids adversely affect embryogenesis.[2,14] In a more physiologic context, that gradients of vitamin A might normally affect pattern formation in skin was suggested 20 years ago.[77] With the demonstration that an implant containing all-*trans* retinoic acid, when placed in the anterior part of the developing chick limb bud, mimics the activity of the naturally occurring zone of polarizing activity (ZPA) came the hypothesis that all-*trans* retinoic acid might well be one of a presumed host of morphogens that control embryologic development.[78-80]

This interesting concept is supported by: (1) the presence of a higher concentration of all-*trans* retinoic acid, but not of retinol, in the posterior relative to the anterior part of the limb bud;[81] (2) the dependence of digit duplication in the chick limb bud on the concentration of all-*trans* retinoic acid;[82] (3) the observed diffusion of retinoic acid from the implant to nearby cells;[80] (4) the age- and tissue-dependent appearance of CRABP-I, CRABP-II, RARα, RARβ, and RARγ in the embryo,[83] (5) the induction by retinoic acid of several *Hox* genes, which are known to be involved in the development of several species;[84] (6) the presumed "sharpening" effect of the retinoic acid gradient by CRABP;[85] (7) the retinoic acid-induced inversion in limb digit pattern in the absence of a ZPA;[86] (8) similar effects of retinoic acid on other tissues, such as the nervous system, and on other species, such as xenopus;[87] and (9) the conversion of retinoic acid in the chick limb bud to 3,4-didehydroretinoic acid, which is also morphogenically active.[88]

The concept is constrained by the following observations: (1) manyfold higher concentrations of retinoic acid (3 mmol/L) must be present in the implant than occur endogenously (25 nmol/L) in the embryo to produce a morphogenic anomaly; (2) implants transferred from their initial sites into new chick limbs after 12 hours show no biologic activity, although they still contain much retinoic acid;[89] (3) the RARβ receptor, which is strongly induced by retinoic acid, is not increased in the naturally occurring ZPA;[90] (4) some *Hox* genes are not activated as expected by retinoic acid;[91] and (5) the concentrations of retinoic acid required to induce limb duplication are closer to those that produce embryotoxicity and teratogenicity than to those that are endogenously present.[92]

Regardless of these concerns, retinoic acid does affect morphogenesis in specific ways. Thus, defining the mechanisms, regardless of what they might be, underlying its actions will broaden our knowledge of this complex process. Whether retinoic acid serves primarily as an endogenous gradient that signals cells to develop in a specific fashion is much less certain.

## TRANSMEMBRANE TRANSPORT

Bacteriorhodopsin, a light-sensitive, retinal-containing protein similar to rhodopsin, is found in the purple patches on membranes of Halobacterium halobium.[93] In response to light, this protein also undergoes a series of conformational changes that are ultimately linked to the transfer of a proton from the cytosol to the external medium.[93] During this cycle, the 13-*cis* and all-*trans* isomers of retinal are involved, however, rather than the 11-*cis* and all-*trans* forms.

In animals, retinoids do not seem to play similar roles, although they can inhibit some processes involving active transport. On the other hand, all-*trans* retinoic acid and some carotenoids elevate mRNA in cells in vitro for connexin 43, a gap junctional protein involved in intercellular communication.[94]

## IMMUNE RESPONSE

Vitamin A was early termed the "anti-infective" vitamin, based on the increased number of infections noted in vitamin A-deficient animals and humans.[2] In vitamin A deficiency, both specific and nonspecific protective mechanisms are impaired, namely, the humoral response to bacterial, parasitic, and viral infections, cell-mediated immunity, mucosal immunity, natural killer cell activity, and phagocytosis[95,96] (see also Chaps. 41 and 69). Large doses of vitamin A can also serve as an adjuvant.[95] When vitamin A-deficient animals are supplemented with vitamin A, immune responses improve.[95,96] The immune responses to certain antigens in vitamin A-depleted children are also enhanced by vitamin A supplementation.[97] Increased responsiveness in children is less marked than in animals, however, probably because of the presence of multiple nutritional deficiencies in malnourished populations and a poor, but not acutely deficient, vitamin A status.[95]

The activity of T lymphocytes, and in particular of T-helper cells, seems to be mainly affected by vitamin A depletion.[95,96,98] Thus, T-lymphocyte-dependent immune responses are expectedly impaired by vitamin A deficiency. In addition, two classes of T-lymphocyte-independent antigens exist: type 2 and type 1 antigens.

Type 2 antigens, which do not provoke significant responses early in life, require a late-maturing B-cell population, whereas type 1 antigens, which provoke early responses, are less dependent on B-cell maturation and cytokine production.[95] Of these antigens, the humoral response to type 2 antigens, which include many polysaccharide and protein antigens, is depressed in vitamin A depletion, whereas the response to type 1 antigens, which include many lipopolysaccharide antigens, is not.[95] Thus, vitamin A status might well affect resistance to infection by some agents but not by others.

Phagocytosis, particularly the "oxygen burst" following the ingestion of a foreign body, and the secretion of IgA are also depressed in vitamin A deficiency.[95,96] The synthesis of goblet cell mucins is reduced as well by vitamin A depletion, both in the intestinal mucosa and in the conjunctiva of the eye.[95,96] Because protein-energy malnutrition also adversely affects the immune response, children afflicted with both deficiencies are clearly at increased risk of severe infections.

In vitamin A-sufficient animals, carotenoids also enhance the immune response.[95,96] Both nutritionally inactive (canthaxanthin) and nutritionally active (β-carotene) carotenoids have similar effects.[95,99] The mechanism of their action is not known.

### OTHER PROCESSES

Vitamin A is essential, either directly or indirectly, for the proper functioning of most organs of the body. For example, reproductive processes in both males and females and bone development and maintenance are particularly dependent on adequate vitamin A status. Whether these complex physiologic processes have unique needs for vitamin A or are primarily dependent on the action of vitamin A in cellular differentiation is not clear. With increasing indications that vitamin A may influence the synthesis and secretion of various cytokines and growth factors,[74,75] vitamin A might affect complex physiologic processes by means of such factors.

## DEFICIENCY

Most vertebrate species, including man, experimental and farm animals, birds, and fish, suffer from vitamin A deficiency.[2,14] Crustacea and insects also use retinal as a chromophore in their photosensitive pigments. The signs of vitamin A deficiency in most species are similar.

### HUMANS

Vitamin A deficiency is a serious nutritional problem among preschool children in southern and southeastern Asia and in parts of Africa and South America.[100,101] Of an estimated 5 million children who develop xerophthalmia annually, approximately a quarter million become blind and, within 1 year, approximately half those children die.[101] The major signs of vitamin A deficiency in preschool children are a history of night blindness, low serum vitamin A values, and a sequence of abnormalities of increasing severity in the conjunctiva and cornea of the eye, generically termed xerophthalmia. Severe irreversible changes in the cornea, which ultimately perforates with loss of the aqueous humor, is called keratomalacia (see Chap. 55). Another corneal abnormality, punctate keratopathy, is often found, even during the early stages of corneal involvement. These pathologic changes in the conjunctiva and cornea have been well documented.[102]

The conjunctival changes, which include a loss of goblet cells and the development of Bitot's spots overlying keratinized epithelia, are likely caused by a reduced concentration of retinol and of glycoproteins in tear fluid,[103] as well as by slower diffusion of retinol from the plasma to the epithelial layer.[104] The corneal involvement seems to result from proteolytic destruction of collagen and other structural proteins following leukocyte infiltration into the corneal stroma.[104] Viral infections, such as measles, exacerbate the process, and subsequent bacterial infections complicate it. Night blindness results from a reduced concentration of rhodopsin in the rod outer segments because of smaller amounts of vitamin A in the eye. Protein-calorie malnutrition and zinc deficiency, which also lower the rhodopsin content of the eye, exacerbate the condition.[104]

Vitamin A deficiency also produces skin changes in humans, namely, follicular hyperkeratosis and phrynoderma. Because other nutritional deficiencies produce similar skin disorders, these changes are not useful as unique indicators of vitamin A deficiency. Nonetheless, vitamin A is necessary for the maintenance of skin. Normally, vitamin A in the form of holo-RBP diffuses into the dermis and epidermis from capillaries in the skin.[105] On entering cells of the skin, retinol and its oxidation product, retinoic acid, are bound by CRBP and CRABP, respectively. Retinol is also oxidized to 3,4-didehydroretinol, and both alcohols form long-chain fatty acyl esters in all layers of the skin.[106] Under normal conditions, human keratinocytes synthesize keratins with molecular weights of 40,000 and 52,000, as well as many others.[107] When vitamin A is absent, these "small" keratins are replaced by larger keratins (molecular weight ≥67,000) characteristic of the stratum corneum.[107] Retinoids stimulate basal cell proliferation but inhibit the transcription of several epidermal keratins, probably by interacting with RARα or RARγ in the skin.[107,108] TGFα and TGFβ also influence skin development, but in different ways.[107,108] Hair follicles, which are particularly sensitive to vitamin A, become obstructed and enlarged in the deficient condition and are replaced by mucus-secreting glands in vitamin A excess.[109] In all likelihood, vitamin A deficiency sets in motion a large number of changes in skin structure and metabolism that ultimately lead to the observed pathologic signs.

Carotenoids may have favorable effects on health and

may reduce the risk of some chronic diseases. Because carotenoids are not essential nutrients, however, use of the term "carotenoid deficiency" is not warranted.

### OTHER SPECIES

The albino rat has been most extensively studied as a model for vitamin A deficiency. To differentiate between direct effects of vitamin A deficiency and secondary changes resulting from generalized malnutrition, rats have been cycled on retinol-free diets containing retinoic acid for 18 days followed by diets free of both retinol and retinoic acid for 10 days.[110] After five or six cycles, the animals became exquisitely sensitive to removal of retinoic acid from the diet. Three major phases of deficiency are noted: (1) the early period, characterized by reduced food intake and some histologic defects; (2) the midperiod, in which many abnormalities in cellular differentiation, responsiveness to drugs, and metabolism appear; and (3) the late phase, in which neuromuscular defects and other physiologic abnormalities in many tissues and processes become evident. By use of this technique, these signs can be directly attributed to vitamin A deficiency, which clearly can affect nearly all tissues of the body. Similar signs of vitamin A deficiency have been noted in most other affected species by conventional dietary procedures.[2,14]

## EXCESS

In amounts several times higher than the recommended dietary allowances (RDA), preformed vitamin A causes toxicity in man and animals.[111,112] Three toxic syndromes exist: acute, chronic, and teratogenic. Acute toxicity is produced by a single extremely large dose of vitamin A or by several large doses taken during a short period, whereas chronic toxicity is caused by the recurrent ingestion of smaller, but still large, doses. Teratogenic effects, leading to spontaneous abortion, birth defects, and permanent learning disabilities, occur from lower doses, particularly when taken in early pregnancy.[14,112]

Carotenoids, even when taken in extremely large doses for long periods, are generally nontoxic. The only known exception is canthaxanthin, which can induce retinopathy when it is ingested in large amounts for long periods.[113]

### VITAMIN A

#### *HUMANS*

When a single dose of more than 0.7 mmol of vitamin A (>200 mg, or >660,000 $IU_a$) is ingested by adults or when a dose larger than 0.35 mmol (>100 mg or >330,000 $IU_a$) is ingested by children, nausea, vomiting, headache, increased cerebrospinal pressure, vertigo, blurred (double) vision, muscular incoordination, and (in infants) bulging of the fontanelle may occur. Some infants can be adversely affected by single doses of only 0.1 mmol. These signs are generally transient and subside within 1 to 2 days.[111,112] When the dose is extremely large, drowsiness, malaise, inappetence, reduced physical activity, skin exfoliation, itching, particularly around the eyes, and recurrent vomiting soon follow. Finally, when lethal doses are given to young monkeys, which are an excellent model for vitamin A toxicity in the human, the animals have deepening coma, convulsions, and respiratory irregularities, and they finally die of either respiratory failure or convulsions.[114] The median lethal dose ($LD_{50}$ value) of vitamin A injected intramuscularly in a water-miscible form in the young monkey is 0.6 mmol (168 mg) retinol/kg body weight.[114] Extrapolated to a 3-kg child and a 70-kg adult, the total $LD_{50}$ dose would be 1.8 mmol (500 mg) and 41 mmol (11.8 g), respectively. A newborn child, who mistakenly was given 0.09 mmol (25 mg) daily, or 28 μmol/kg for 11 days, died of apparent vitamin A toxicity.[115] The total dose received was 0.31 mmol/kg, similar to the $LD_{50}$ value for young monkeys. Such enormous amounts of vitamin A are present only in high-potency preparations of vitamin A or in large amounts (~500 g) of livers particularly rich in vitamin A (>0.035 mmol/g or >10 mg/g).

Chronic toxicity is induced by the recurrent intake of vitamin A in amounts at least 10 times the RDA, that is, 13 μmol (3.75 mg retinol equivalents or 12,500 $IU_a$) for an infant or 35 μmol (10 mg retinol equivalents or 33,300 $IU_a$) for an adult. A health-food enthusiast who ingested 26 μmol (25,000 $IU_a$) of vitamin A as a supplement daily plus a similar amount in food showed severe signs of toxicity.[112] Approximately 50 signs of chronic toxicity have been reported, of which the most frequent are alopecia, ataxia, bone and muscle pain, cheilitis, conjunctivitis, headache, hepatotoxicity, hyperlipemia, hyperostosis, membrane dryness, pruritus, pseudotumor cerebri, various skin disorders, and visual impairment.[111,112] When the supplemental intake of vitamin A is eliminated, these signs usually disappear over a period of weeks to months, but not always.

In chronic hypervitaminosis A, holo-RBP in the plasma is not elevated, whereas retinyl esters are usually increased markedly.[14] Factors that enhance toxicity include alcohol ingestion, low protein intake, viral hepatitis, other diseases of the liver and kidney, and possibly tetracycline use. Elderly individuals may be more sensitive because of a slower rate of storage in the liver and a reduced plasma clearance of administered vitamin A. Tocopherol, taurine, and zinc are protective in tissue culture cells, but they may or may not be effective in vivo.[112]

Some individuals seem to suffer from vitamin A intolerance, that is, the appearance of signs of toxicity upon routinely ingesting moderate amounts of vitamin

A. This relatively rare condition, which seems to be genetic, mainly affects males.[116]

Both all-*trans* and 13-*cis* retinoic acid, as well as many synthetic retinoids, induce similar toxic states. Indeed, acidic forms of retinoids are usually more toxic than alcoholic forms and some conjugated derivatives.[14] The mechanism of toxicity is ill defined.

Vitamin A and other retinoids are powerful teratogens, both in experimental animals and in women.[14,112,117,118] A single extremely large dose, exposure for as short as a week on high daily doses (0.1 to 0.3 mmol, or 30 to 90 mg), or long-term daily intakes of 26 μmol (25,000 $IU_a$ or 7,500 RE) during early pregnancy can induce spontaneous abortions or major fetal malformations. Common defects are craniofacial abnormalities, including microcephaly, microtia, and harelip, congenital heart disease, kidney defects, thymic abnormalities, and central nervous system disorders. Permanent learning disabilities have been noted in otherwise normal rat pups whose dams received nonteratogenic doses of vitamin A,[14,119] and such effects might occur as well in children exposed to large doses of retinoids early in fetal life. Synergism between vitamin A and other teratogens, such as alcohol and drugs, at nonteratogenic doses of each is probable. Thus, women who are pregnant, or who might become so, should carefully control their intake of vitamin A, both in regard to rich food sources, such as liver, and vitamin A supplements.

Healthy women who routinely ingest diets containing fruits and green leafy vegetables do not require supplements of vitamin A during pregnancy.[14,112] In cases where supplementation is advisable, the total daily intake should not exceed 10 μmol (approximately 3 mg or 10,000 IU) of vitamin A.[14,112] In this regard, vitamin A deficiency, just like its excess, adversely affects the reproductive process.

### *OTHER SPECIES*

Hypervitaminosis A has been described in many domestic animals, including chickens, pigs, and calves.[2,14] The signs of toxicity are similar to those described previously for primates. Although adult rats are particularly resistant to hypervitaminosis A, large doses of retinoids given to the pregnant dam induce many congenital malformations in rat fetuses.

### CAROTENOIDS

Individuals who routinely ingest large amounts of carotenoids, such as found in carrot juice, tomato juice, and red palm oil, may be affected by hypercarotenosis. The condition is characterized by hypercarotenemia and carotenodermia, a yellow, jaundice-like coloration of the skin that is particularly evident in the nasolabial folds, the fat pads of the palms of the hands, and the fatty areas on the soles of the feet. The sclerae of the eyes are clear in hypercarotenosis, but yellow in jaundice. Insofar as is known, the condition is completely benign and slowly disappears upon removing carotenoid-rich foods from the diet. Patients with erythropoietic protoporphyria and related disorders who ingest large daily therapeutic doses of canthaxanthin (0.1 to 0.2 mmol, or 50 to 100 mg) for long periods, however, often show mild retinopathy.[112] A similar condition arises in individuals who use large doses of canthaxanthin to simulate a tan. The retinopathy slowly disappears in most individuals after cessation of treatment.[112]

Hypervitaminosis A does *not* result from the excessive intake of carotenoids, primarily because of the relatively slow rate of conversion of carotenoids into vitamin A and the reduced intestinal absorption efficiency of carotenoids when large amounts are ingested.[14]

## HIGH-RISK CLINICAL SITUATIONS

Newborn infants contain low reserves of vitamin A in the liver. When appropriately nourished, essentially all infants show adequate liver reserves (>0.07 μmol or >20 μg retinol/g) by 1 year of age.[120] Although premature infants show the same median value of liver reserves at birth as term infants, they seem to deteriorate in vitamin A status over the first 2 months of life.[120,121] Because orally administered vitamin A is poorly absorbed in premature infants, this group seems to be at special risk.[122]

Fat malabsorption syndromes, such as cholestasis, cystic fibrosis, sprue, chronic diarrhea, pancreatic insufficiency, and biliary cirrhosis reduce the digestion and absorption of vitamin A and carotenoids and ultimately lead to a state of vitamin A depletion. The effects of these disorders are more marked in young children, who possess limited vitamin A reserves and need vitamin A for growth, than in adults. Nonetheless, adults with chronic malabsorption problems can also be affected, particularly if their diets are low in vitamin A and carotenoids.

Subjects nourished for long periods by means of total parenteral nutrition conventionally receive vitamin A in the infusion fluid. Because variable amounts of the vitamin A present can be adsorbed on the plastic delivery tubing, however, the vitamin A status of these individuals should receive careful attention.[122]

The liver clearly is of primary importance in the storage and utilization of vitamin A. The long-term ingestion of alcohol, even in relatively small amounts, tends to reduce vitamin A storage.[123] In clinical cases of alcoholism, stellate cells tend to disappear, and fibroblasts increase in number. The abnormal dark-adaptation response found in many alcoholic subjects is usually ameliorated by administration of vitamin A. The dosage must be carefully controlled, however, to prevent hepatotoxicity.[123] Other liver poisons, such as halogenated hydrocarbons, and some drugs, such as phenobarbital, also lower liver reserves of vitamin A.[14] Cadmium and other heavy metals, which predominantly affect tubular reabsorption in the kidney, cause a marked excretion of holo-RBP in the urine. Other kidney disorders that cause decreased glomerular and tubular functions give rise to *increased* plasma levels of holo-RBP because of reduced metabolism of RBP in the kidney.[124]

Although estrogens and estrogen-containing contraceptives cause a significant increase in the steady-state concentration of holo-RBP in the plasma, the rate of mobilization of vitamin A from liver reserves is only slightly affected.[14] Thus, in otherwise well-nourished women, the routine use of contraceptive agents does not significantly affect their vitamin A requirement.

Because of the widespread and increasing use of large doses of retinoids, including vitamin A, for the treatment of various skin disorders and some types of cancer, retinoid toxicity will increasingly be encountered. Doses of vitamin A or of other retinoids that have been tolerated by most patients undergoing these treatments are 4.5 to 5.6 μmol (1.3 to 1.6 mg) retinol/kg body weight per day, or approximately 0.21 mmol (200,000 $IU_a$)/$m^2$ per day.[125] Upon lowering the treatment dose, the discomfort lessens.

Because of the teratogenic action of retinoids, fertile women treated with large doses of retinoids should practice rigorous contraception during treatment and for several months, and perhaps for as long as 2 years, after the termination of therapy.[126] Etretinate, because of its long half-life in the body, is particularly hazardous in this regard.[126]

Genetic defects are rare. Nonetheless, a lowered retinol-binding protein concentration, which was accompanied by an enhanced risk of vitamin A deficiency, has been reported in a Japanese family.[127] In some cases of presumed vitamin A intolerance, high plasma retinyl ester concentrations (18 to 87 μmol/L, or 500 to 2500 μg/dl) persisted despite normal intakes of vitamin A.[116,128] The molecular defects, however, have not been clarified.

## PHARMACOLOGIC USES

Retinoids and, to a much smaller extent, carotenoids are extensively used in treating a variety of diseases.

### SKIN

Various retinoids, and particularly 13-*cis* retinoic acid, are used to treat acne and other skin disorders.[129] Although highly effective, retinoic acid is teratogenic at high doses when given orally,[117,118] and it is a skin irritant when applied topically.[130] Although most efficacious retinoids are also toxic, some conjugated forms, such as retinoyl β-glucuronide and hydroxyphenyl retinamide, retain their therapeutic actions with less, if any, toxicity.[131-134] Topical all-*trans* retinoic acid can also reduce wrinkling and hyperpigmentation caused by photoaging.[130,135]

### CANCER

Large doses of vitamin A reduce the recurrence of some forms of skin cancer, including mycosis fungoides, but not melanoma.[136] All-*trans* retinoic acid is effective in treating acute promyelocytic leukemia (APL).[137] In all responsive patients, a specific gene translocation t(15,17) occurs, in which the gene for the retinoic acid receptor RARα is fused with another gene, termed PML, or initially, *myl*.[138] The fusion gene may well produce a gene product with a lower affinity for all-*trans* retinoic acid. Thus, higher concentrations of retinoic acid may be necessary to induce normal promyelocytic differentiation.[137,138] Hydroxyphenyl retinamide reduces mammary cancer in experimental animals,[139] and it is being tested in humans.[140] Many other retinoids have proved effective against a variety of chemically induced and spontaneous cancers in experimental animals and, in a few cases, in humans.[136] Leukoplakia, considered a precancerous condition, responds well to high daily doses of β-carotene in some patients.[141] The dietary intake of carotenoids is associated most closely with a reduced incidence of lung cancer,[142] but also of cancers in other organs.[143,144] Except for the identification of the fusion gene of RARα in APL, the mechanisms of action are not known. Retinoids probably act, however, by stimulating the differentiation of precancerous stem cells, whereas carotenoids probably are involved in a network of antioxidants that include vitamin E, vitamin C, sulfhydryl groups, and a variety of other enzymatic and nonenzymatic processes.[143,144]

### OTHER DISEASES

Whereas retinoids have been most closely associated with protective effects in skin disorders and cancer, carotenoids have been implicated in preventing the oxidation of low-density lipoproteins and consequently reducing the formation of atherosclerotic lesions, in protecting against the development of cortical cataract, and in reducing the oxidative stress induced by smoking.[143,144] Although carotenoids clearly can contribute to antioxidant defenses in cells, their possible importance in such defenses in vivo is still undefined.

## DIETARY CONSIDERATIONS

Vitamin A is *not* a limiting nutrient in healthy individuals who eat an adequate mixed diet, but it is a major nutritional concern among preschool children who ingest highly limited diets in less-industrialized countries.

### FOOD AND OTHER SOURCES

Good dietary sources of preformed vitamin A are liver, other internal organs, whole eggs, dairy products, and whole small fish, whereas good sources of provitamin A carotenoids are carrots, dark green leafy vegetables, yams, spinach, tomatoes, yellow maize, papayas, ripe mangoes, and oranges. The richest sources of preformed vitamin A are the liver oils of marine fish and of marine mammals, whereas those of carotenoids are red palm oil and carrot oil. [14,145](See also Appendix Table A–21 for the vitamin A content of common foods.)

In the United States, multivitamin pills, which usually contain 5.2 to 10.5 μmol (5,000 to 10,000 $IU_a$) of vitamin A, are also a major source of vitamin A for approximately 30% of the adult population.

## REQUIREMENTS AND RECOMMENDED INTAKES

The Food and Agriculture Organization and the World Health Organization (FAO/WHO) recommend both basal and safe levels of vitamin A intake, with the basal level approximately 50% of the safe level.[146] The basal level of intake is sufficient to meet all physiologic needs of the individual without providing for body reserves, whereas the safe level of intake also ensures adequate body reserves to meet needs for approximately 4 months on a diet low in vitamin A and during periods of stress, such as fever or diarrhea. By using a coefficient of variation of 20%, a 40% increment is included in each recommendation to ensure that most (>97%) persons in the given population group receive adequate vitamin A. Thus, the relationships among the mean basal requirement, the basal recommended intake, the mean safe requirement, and the safe recommended intake are 1:1.4:2:2.8, respectively. Single recommendations deal only with the safe recommended intake. In most recommendations, an adequate body reserve is expressed as a liver concentration of 0.07 μmol (20 μg) of vitamin A per gram of wet weight, inasmuch as approximately 90% of the vitamin A in the body is stored in the liver in well-nourished individuals. Recommended dietary intakes (RDI) for vitamin A devised by the FAO/WHO,[146] in the United Kingdom (U.K.),[147] in Japan,[148] and in the United States,[149] where such recommendations are rather oddly called "allowances," are summarized in Table 16–2 (also see Appendix Table A-2 to A-6). In devising these recommendations, expert committees of the FAO/WHO and of the U.K. used modern concepts of vitamin A turnover and replacement, whereas the Food and Nutrition Board of the United States relied on older views of plasma retinol responses to graded doses of vitamin A. The values in all cases are expressed as micrograms retinol equivalents (RE). One microgram RE, which is equal to 3.5 nmol, has been assumed to be nutritionally equivalent to 11 nmol (6 μg) of β-carotene and to 22 nmol (12 μg) of other provitamin A carotenoids.

Mean and median intakes of vitamin A in the United States are approximately 1000 μg RE and 620 μg RE, respectively, of which carotenoids and preformed vitamin A contribute approximately 25% and 75%, respectively.[11,14,145] In one American survey, major ingested food sources of all forms of vitamin A, expressed in RE, were milk and dairy products (31%), vegetables and fruits (22%), the meat group (16%), fats, oils, and fortified margarines (10%), fortified grain (9%), eggs (8%), and miscellaneous foods (4%).[150] Mean and median intakes of vitamin A from foods in the United States have not changed appreciably since 1970, although the use of dietary supplements, particularly among the elderly, has increased.

## NUTRIENT INTERRELATIONSHIPS

Vitamin A status is affected by intakes of protein, fat, iron, zinc, vitamin E, and possibly other nutrients.[14,16,151] Indeed, because of the crucial roles of vitamin A in vision, cellular differentiation, morphogenesis, and most other physiologic processes, *any* nutritional imbalance should adversely affect the functions of vitamin A. *Protein deficiency* reduces carotenoid cleavage and the synthesis of retinoid-binding proteins and receptors. On the other hand, by restraining growth, protein-calorie malnutrition retards the development of acute xerophthalmic signs of vitamin A deficiency. *Fat* is

**TABLE 16—2.** RECOMMENDED DIETARY INTAKES (OR ALLOWANCES) (RDI OR RDA) OF VITAMIN A IN μG RETINOL EQUIVALENTS

| CATEGORY | AGE (YEARS) | FAO/WHO[146] BASAL | FAO/WHO[146] SAFE | UK[147] RNI* | JAPAN[148] | USA[149] RDA |
|---|---|---|---|---|---|---|
| Infants | 0–0.5 | 180 | 350 | 350 | 400 | 375 |
| | 0.5–1.0 | 180 | 350 | 350 | 400 | 375 |
| Children | 1.0–10 | 200–250 | 400 | 400–500 | 400–500 | 400–700 |
| Males | 10–12 | 300 | 500 | 600 | 600 | 1000 |
| | 12–70+ | 300 | 600 | 700 | 600 | 1000 |
| Females | 10–12 | 270 | 500 | 600 | 540 | 800 |
| | 12–70+ | 270 | 500 | 600 | 540 | 800 |
| Pregnancy | | +100 | +100 | +100 | +60 | +0 |
| Lactation | 0–0.5 | +180 | +350 | +350 | +400 | +500 |
| | >0.5 | +180 | +350 | +350 | +400 | +400 |

*RNI, Reference Nutrient Intake, equivalent to the RDI.

required for the efficient intestinal absorption of vitamin A and carotenoids. Although a daily fat intake of only 10 to 20 g is sufficient, the concomitant ingestion of fat and vitamin A is essential. *Iron status*, as indicated by plasma hemoglobin concentrations, is depressed in vitamin A deficiency and enhanced by vitamin A supplements. Although the mechanism is not clear, vitamin A might act on the metabolism and storage of iron or, more probably, on the differentiation of red blood cells in the bone marrow. In *zinc deficiency*, vitamin A in the plasma decreases but that in the liver rises, the synthesis of proteins and nucleic acids is impaired in most organs, including the eye, and night blindness can ensue.[14,151,152] Embryogenesis is impaired by deficiencies of both vitamin A and zinc. Because of the "zinc finger" structure required for the binding of many nuclear transcription factors to deoxyribonucleic acid (DNA), zinc seems to play a general role in gene expression. *Vitamin E* protects vitamin A from oxidation in the gut and presumably in storage globules of the liver and other organs as well. Vitamin E also reduces the rate of hydrolysis of retinyl esters in the liver.[14] Children at high risk of vitamin A deficiency also show low plasma vitamin E levels and low ratios of plasma vitamin E to total lipid.[153] Vitamin A may also interact in various ways with vitamin C, vitamin K, vitamin D, calcium, copper, and iodine.[14,16,151]

## ASSESSMENT OF VITAMIN A STATUS

Vitamin A status can be classified into five categories: (1) deficient; (2) marginal; (3) adequate; (4) excessive; and (5) toxic.[14,154] The deficient and toxic (hypervitaminotic) states are characterized by clinical signs, whereas the other three states are not. In the marginal state, individuals do *not* show clinical signs of deficiency but may have some impaired physiologic responses, such as the immune response, as a result of inadequate concentrations of vitamin A in the liver and in other tissues. In the excessive state, individuals also do *not* show clinical signs of hypervitaminosis A, but such signs may be induced by yet larger vitamin A intakes or by infection, such as viral hepatitis. In a worldwide public health sense, indicators of the deficiency state and of the marginal state are of most importance.

### CLINICAL ASSESSMENT

The most useful clinical sign is the Bitot's spot with conjunctival xerosis, termed X1B by the WHO.[100,102] A public health problem is assumed to exist if the prevalence in preschool age children is greater than 0.5%. Bitot's spots in older children tend not to be responsive to vitamin A treatment; that is, the spots represent permanent lesions caused by earlier episodes of vitamin A deprivation.[102] More serious eye signs, such as corneal xerosis (X2) and corneal ulceration (X3) are specific for vitamin A deficiency, but they are much less prevalent (<0.01%) in children suffering from vitamin A depletion. Corneal scars that occur early in life from inadequate diets rather than from accidents, although also related to vitamin A deficiency, are often difficult to interpret.

### BIOCHEMICAL ASSESSMENT

Vitamin A concentrations in the plasma, milk, or tear fluid are useful indicators of vitamin A status.[154] Plasma vitamin A concentrations lower than 0.35 μmol/L (<10 μg/dl) are indicative of vitamin A deficiency, and those higher than 1.05 μmol/L (>30 μg/dl) are associated with a satisfactory status. Intermediate values, and particularly those between 0.35 and 0.70 μmol/L (10 to 20 μg/dl), are more difficult to interpret, inasmuch as other factors, such as infections and protein-energy malnutrition, lower plasma retinol concentrations.[154] Nonetheless, a frequency distribution curve of plasma retinol values obtained before and after vitamin A supplementation is useful in defining the status of a population.[154] Vitamin A concentrations in breast milk that are lower than 0.35 μmol/L (<10 μg/dl) indicate that the nursing child is at risk of vitamin A deficiency.[14] Values higher than 0.7 μmol/L (>20 μg/dl) should provide adequate vitamin A for growth and development, whereas intermediate concentrations (0.35 to 0.7 μmol/L) should cause concern. Breast milk values higher than 1.4 μmol/L (>40 μg/dl) should allow body reserves to increase. Median vitamin A concentrations of 1.75 nmol/L (0.5 μg/L) were found in the tear fluid of Thai children with marginal vitamin A status, whereas median concentrations in supplemented and well nourished children were 6.3 nmol/L (1.8 μg/L).[154] Vitamin A concentrations in tear fluid have only been measured in one survey, however. Liver vitamin A concentrations associated with deficiency are lower than 17.5 nmol (5 μg)/g, those associated with a marginal status are 17.5 to 70 nmol (5 μg to 20 μg)/g, and those associated with an adequate status are higher than 70 nmol (>20 μg)/g. Although direct measurement is inappropriate in general surveys, analysis of biopsy and autopsy samples, when obtainable, can provide useful information.[14,154]

Three response assays are useful in determining both deficient and marginal vitamin A status.[154] The relative dose response (RDR) assay measures the change in plasma retinol concentration before and 5 hours after the oral administration of 1.6 to 3.5 μmol (450 μg to 1000 μg) retinyl ester in oil. The RDR value, expressed as a percentage, is the increment in plasma retinol observed divided by the concentration at 5 hours. RDR values higher than 50% are characteristic of acute deficiency, values between 20 and 50% indicate marginal status, and values lower than 20% indicate adequate status.[154] A similar procedure has been adapted for use in premature infants, in which the plasma RBP concentration is measured before and after dosing.[154] In the modified relative dose response (MRDR) assay, 3,4-didehydroretinyl acetate (0.35 μmol/kg, or 100 μg/kg body weight) is administered orally in oil, and a single blood sample is taken 5 hours later. A molar ratio of dehydroretinol to retinol in the serum of more than 0.06 is indicative of a marginal or poorer vitamin A status, and a ratio of less than 0.03 is indicative of an adequate status.[154] Intermediate ratios (0.03 to 0.06) are more difficult to interpret.

A large (0.18 mmol) oral dose of deuterated vitamin A in oil, after absorption, will equilibrate with total body reserves of vitamin A within approximately 2 weeks. By measuring the ratio of deuterated to nondeuterated retinol in the plasma, the total body reserves of vitamin A can be estimated.[154,155] A more complete analysis of biochemical indicators is provided in the vitamin A chapter of the previous edition of this book and in a special report.[156,157]

### HISTOLOGIC ASSESSMENT

During vitamin A depletion, goblet cells of the conjunctiva of the eye disappear and epithelial cells become enlarged and keratinized. Conjunctival cells can be adsorbed on a piece of filter paper that is pressed against the eye and then can be stained and examined microscopically. The procedure, termed conjunctival impression cytology (CIC), indicates deficient and marginal status. Four categories are defined: (1) normal; (2) marginal (+); (3) marginal (−); and (4) deficient.[154] Because the interpretation of the two intermediate categories is often difficult, the procedure has primarily been used to detect populations at risk. Although cutoff values have not been set, a population of children in which more than 20% are in the deficient category in both eyes is clearly at risk.[154] Expressed differently, a significant public health problem might well exist if more than 50% are not normal.[154] Skin changes that accompany vitamin A deficiency also occur in many other nutritional deficiencies and can be associated with skin diseases as well. Thus, such changes have not been used as a specific assessment indicator of vitamin A status.

### PHYSIOLOGIC ASSESSMENT

Night blindness, caused by a reduced concentration of rhodopsin in the rod cells of the retina, is a common sign of vitamin A deficiency. A quantitative measurement of dark adaptation requires approximately 30 minutes, uses expensive equipment in a controlled ambient, and is not appropriate for very young children. Thus, for survey procedures, interviews have been conducted with mothers of possibly affected children; the time required for a child to recognize letters or animals under dim light after retinal bleaching, termed the vision-restoration time (VRT), and the time required to sort different colored disks in dim light after bleaching, termed the rapid dark-adaptation time (RDAT), have been determined.[154]

### DIETARY ASSESSMENT

Because the intake of vitamin A-rich foods, such as liver, is infrequent, a 24-hour recall of dietary intake is useful in assessing the vitamin A status of a population but not of an individual.[154] Well-constructed food-frequency questionnaires tend to provide more valid data about an individual's average intake. Because the content of vitamin A and carotenoids can vary greatly in a given food, however, food composition tables provide at best a semiquantitative estimate of vitamin A intake. The actual amounts of vitamin A and carotenoids in ingested foods can be measured, of course, but during the experimental period, individuals usually must be constrained for a significant time in a metabolic ward. Nonetheless, a rapid procedure that is suitable for use in surveys in underdeveloped countries and provides an indication of risk in a preschool population has recently been developed and tested.[154] Dietary data are therefore of greatest value in assessing the food habits of populations at risk of vitamin A deficiency. Such information is essential in devising strategies for improving their nutritional well-being. The appropriate ranges for various indicators of vitamin A status are summarized in Figure 16–5.

## METHODS

Vitamin A and carotenoids are most generally measured by high-pressure liquid chromatography (HPLC).[14,158-160] Straight-phase HPLC is best used for separating *cis-trans* isomers of a given retinoid or carotenoid, whereas reverse-phase HPLC best separates compounds of different polarity. Because both retinoids and carotenoids are easily oxidized and isomerized, biologic samples should be immediately analyzed or stored in the frozen state in the dark, preferably at −70° C. Antioxidants should be present during their extraction by peroxide-free solvents. Laboratories should also be equipped with yellow light to prevent isomerization. Retinoids are usually measured spectrophotometrically at their absorption maximum, such as 325 nm for retinol and retinyl esters and 340 to 360 nm for retinoic acid and its esters. Other detection methods include fluorescence and colorimetric assay after exposure to a Lewis acid or other chromogen.[14,158] Methods used for various specific assays, including enzymatic transformations, have been summarized.[159,160]

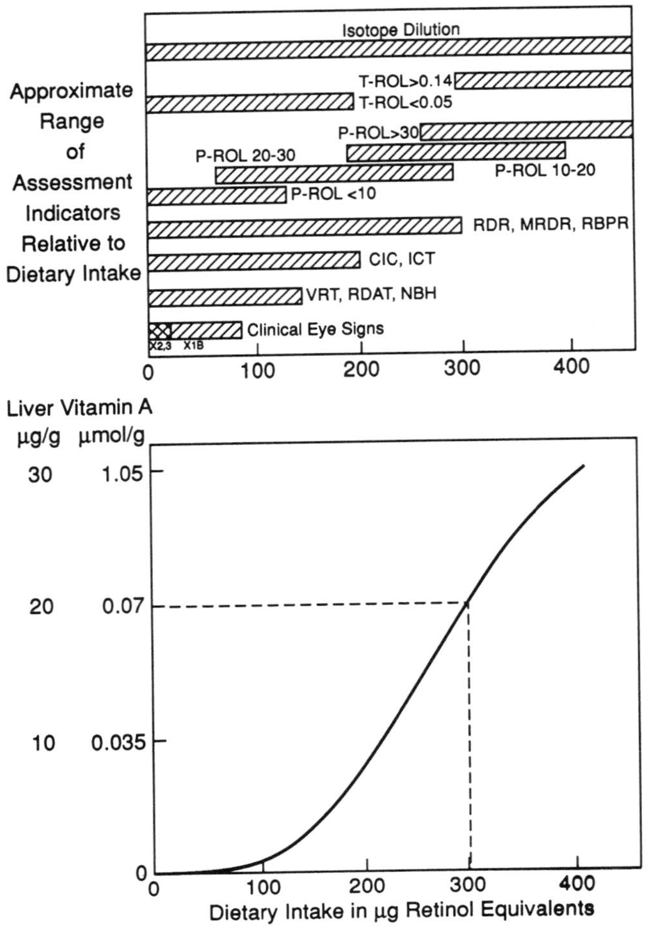
Isotope Dilution
T-ROL>0.14
T-ROL<0.05
P-ROL>30
P-ROL 20-30
P-ROL 10-20
P-ROL <10
RDR, MRDR, RBPR
CIC, ICT
VRT, RDAT, NBH
Clinical Eye Signs
X2,3
X1B
Approximate Range of Assessment Indicators Relative to Dietary Intake
0
100
200
300
400
Liver Vitamin A
μg/g μmol/g
30 1.05
20 0.07
10 0.035
0
0
100
200
300
400
Dietary Intake in μg Retinol Equivalents

**FIGURE 16–5.** An approximate relationship between the average daily dietary intake of vitamin A and provitamin A carotenoids, expressed as micrograms of retinol equivalents, and the vitamin A concentration in the liver of a preschool child. Nonhepatic stores of vitamin A are approximately 10% of the liver reserves when total body stores are high (>30 mg for a 15-kg child), but are proportionally greater (20 to 50%) when body reserves are low (<6 mg for a 15-kg child). A satisfactory liver vitamin A concentration is considered to be 0.07 μmol (20 μg)/g wet weight. The approximate ranges for the responses of various indicators of vitamin A status, relative to dietary intake, are given above the figure. Thus, clinical signs appear when the average daily intake of vitamin A is low, which corresponds to negligible liver reserves. Plasma retinol concentrations <10 μg/dl are usually associated with other signs of vitamin A inadequacy, whereas a plasma retinol concentration in the range of 10 to 20 μg/dl may either be associated with Bitot's spots and other signs of deficiency or be found in a vitamin A-sufficient child, albeit often plagued with infections. Isotope dilution, which involves analysis of the dilution in the plasma of endogenous vitamin A by a dose of deuterated vitamin A, provides information about total body reserves of whatever magnitude. X2, Corneal xerosis; X3, corneal ulceration and keratomalacia; X1B, Bitot's spots with conjunctival xerosis; VRT, vision restoration time; RDAT, rapid dark-adaptation test time; NBH, night blindness by history; CIC, conjunctival impression cytology test; ICT, impression cytology with transfer test; RDR, relative dose response assay; MRDR, modified relative dose response test; RBPR, retinol-binding protein response test; P-ROL, plasma (or serum) retinol concentration; and T-ROL, tear fluid retinol concentration, followed by values expressed in micrograms of retinol per deciliter. Vitamin A equivalencies are: 1 μmol retinol = 286 μg retinol; 1 μg retinol = 1 μg retinol equivalents = 0.0035 μmol retinol. (From Underwood, B.A., Olson, J.A. (Eds.): A Brief Guide to Current Methods of Assessing Vitamin A Status. Washington, D.C., International Vitamin A Consultative Group, International Life Science Institute, Nutrition Foundation. In press.)

## REFERENCES


1. Wolf, G.: Am. J. Clin. Nutr., *31*:290–292, 1978.
2. Moore, T.: Vitamin A. Amsterdam, Elsevier, 1957.
3. IUPAC-IUB Joint Commission on Biochemical Nomenclature: Eur. J. Biochem., *129*:1–5, 1982.
4. Nomenclature Policy: J. Nutr., *120*, 12–19, 1990.
5. IUPAC-IUB Commission on Biochemical Nomenclature: Biochemistry, *10*:4827–4837, 1971.
6. Mayer, H., Isler, O.: Total synthesis. *In* Carotenoids. Edited by O. Isler. Basel, Birkhauser Verlag, 1971, pp. 325–575.
7. Dawson, M.I., Okamura, W.H. (Eds.): Chemistry and Biology of Synthetic Retinoids. Boca Raton, FL, CRC Press, 1990.
8. Frickel, F.: Chemistry and physical properties of retinoids. *In* The Retinoids. Vol. 1. Edited by M.B. Sporn, A.B. Roberts, and D.S. Goodman. New York, Academic Press, 1984, pp. 7–45.
9. World Health Organization: Handbook on Human Nutritional Requirements. Monograph No. 61. Geneva, World Health Organization, 1974.
10. Sauberlich, H.E., Hodges, R.E., Wallace, D.L., et al.: Vitam. Horm., *32*:251–275, 1974.
11. Olson, J.A.: Am. J. Clin. Nutr., *45*:704–716, 1987.
12. Miller, D.A., Stephens-Jarnagin, A., DeLuca, H.F.: Biochem. J., *227*:311–316, 1985.
13. Bendich, A., Olson, J.A.: FASEB J., *3*:1927–1932, 1989.
14. Olson, J.A.: Vitamin A. *In* Handbook of Vitamins. 2nd Ed. Edited by L.J. Machlin. New York, Marcel Dekker, 1990, pp. 1–57.
15. Goodman, D.S.: Biosynthesis, absorption and hepatic metabolism of retinol. *In* The Retinoids. Vol. 2. Edited by M.B. Sporn, A.B. Roberts, and D.S. Goodman. New York, Academic Press, 1984, pp. 1–39.
16. Underwood, B.A.: Vitamin A in animal and human nutrition. *In* The Retinoids. Vol. 1. Edited by M.B. Sporn, A.B. Roberts, and D.S. Goodman. New York, Academic Press, 1984, pp. 281-392.
17. Zeng, S., Furr, H.C., Olson, J.A.: Am. J. Clin. Nutr., *56*:433–439, 1992.
18. Blomhoff, R., Green, M.H., Berg, T., et al.: Science, *250*:399–404, 1990.
19. Blomhoff, R., Wake, K.: FASEB J., *5*:271–277, 1991.
20. Batres, R.O., Olson, J.A.: J. Nutr., *117*:77–82, 1987.

21. Hendriks, H.F.J., Blaner, W.S., Wennekers, M.H., et al.: Eur. J. Biochem., *171*:237–244, 1988.
22. Blaner, W.S.: Endocrinol. Rev., *10*:308–316, 1989.
23. Rask, L., Anundi, H., Peterson, P.A.: FEBS Lett., *104*:55–58, 1979.
24. Yamada, M., Blaner, W.S., Soprano, D.R., et al.: Hepatology, *7*:1224–1229, 1987.
25. Rajan, N., Blaner, W.S., Soprano, D.R., et al.: J. Lipid Res., *31*:821–829, 1990.
26. Lee, S.Y., Ubels, J.L., Soprano, D.R.: Exp. Eye Res. In press.
27. Goodman, D.S., Blaner, W.S., Tsutsumi, C., et al.: Retinol-binding protein (RBP) and its regulation in adipose tissue. *In* Retinoids: Progress in Research and Clinical Applications. Edited by M. Livrea and L. Packer. New York, Marcel Dekker. In press.
28. Vahlquist, A., Rask, L., Peterson, P.A., et al.: Scand. J. Lab. Clin. Invest., *35*:569–574, 1975.
29. Chytil, F., Ong, D.E.: Annu. Rev. Nutr., *7*:321–335, 1987.
30. Wolf, G.: Nutr. Rev., *49*:1–12, 1991.
31. Crabb, J.W., Goldflam, S., Harris, S.E., et al.: J. Biol. Chem., *263*:18,688–18,692, 1988.
32. Bailey, J.S., Siu, C.H.: J. Biol. Chem., *263*:9326–9332, 1988.
33. Bridges, C.D.B., Alvarez, R.A., Fong, S.-L., et al.: Invest. Ophthalmol. Vis. Sci., *28*:613–617, 1987.
34. Chader, G.J.: Invest. Ophthalmol. Vis. Sci., *30*:7-22, 1989.
35. Mourey, M.S., Quadro, L., Panariello, L., et al.: Regulation of retinol-binding protein gene expression by retinoids in cultured hepatoma cells. *In* Retinoids: Progress in Research and Clinical Applications. Edited by M. Livrea and L. Packer. New York, Marcel Dekker. In press.
36. Chytil, F., Haq, R.U.: Crit. Rev. Eukaryotic Gene Expr., *1*:61–73, 1990.
37. Smith, W.C., Nakshatri, H., Leroy, P., et al.: EMBO J., *10*:2223–2230, 1991.
38. Mangelsdorf, D.J., Umesono, K., Kliewer, S.A., et al.: Cell, *66*:555–561, 1991.
39. Bavik, C.O., Eriksson, U., Allen, R.A., et al.: J. Biol. Chem., *266*:14978–14985, 1991.
40. Frolik, C.A.: Metabolism of retinoids. *In* The Retinoids. Vol. 2. Edited by M.B. Sporn, A.B. Roberts, and D.S. Goodman. New York, Academic Press, 1984, pp. 177–208.
41. Buck, J., Derguini, F., Nakanishi, K., et al.: 14-Hydroxy-4, 14-retroretinol mediates intracellular signalling by a pathway distinct from retinoic acid. *In* Retinoids: Progress in Research and Clinical Applications. Edited by M. Livrea and L. Packer. New York, Marcel Dekker. In press.
42. Barua, A.B., Olson, J.A.: Am. J. Clin. Nutr., *43*:481–485, 1986.
43. Barua, A.B., Batres, R.O., Olson, J.A.: Biochem. J., *252*:415–420, 1988.
44. Takahashi, N., Breitman, T.R.: J. Biol. Chem., *264*:5159–5163, 1989.
45. Renstrom, B., DeLuca, H.F.: Biochim. Biophys. Acta, *998*:69–74, 1989.
46. Kakkad, B.P., Ong, D.E.: J. Biol. Chem., *263*:12,916–12,919, 1988.
47. Olson, J.A.: Formation and function of vitamin A. *In* Biosynthesis of Isoprenoid Compounds. Vol. 2. Edited by J.W. Porter and S. L. Spurgeon. New York, Wiley-Interscience, 1983, pp. 371–412.
48. Olson, J.A.: J. Nutr., *119*:105–108, 1989.
49. Napoli, J.L., Race, K.R.: J. Biol. Chem., *263*:17,372–17,377, 1988.
50. Wang, X.D., Tang, G.W., Fox. J.G., et al.: Arch. Biochem. Biophys., *285*:8–16, 1991.
51. Rando, R.R.: Angew. Chem. Int. Ed. Engl., *29*:461–480, 1990.
52. Bridges, C.D.B.: The molecular basis of the visual cycle. *In* Chemistry and Biology of Synthetic Retinoids. Edited by M.I. Dawson and W.H. Okamura. Boca Raton, FL, CRC Press, 1990, pp. 27–50.
53. Stryer, L.: Textbook of Biochemistry. 3rd Ed. New York, H. Freeman, 1988, pp. 1027–1038.
54. Sherman, M.I. (Ed.): Retinoids and Cell Differentiation. Boca Raton, FL, CRC Press, 1986.
55. Jetten, A.M.: Regulation of gene expression by retinoic acid: embryological carcinoma cell differentiation. *In* Mechanisms of Differentiation. Vol. 1. Edited by P.B. Fisher. Boca Raton, FL, CRC press, 1990, pp. 49–74.
56. Petkovich, M., Brand, N.J., Krust, A., et al.: Nature, *330*:444–450, 1987.
57. Giguere, V., Ong, E.S., Segui, P., et al.: Nature, *330*:624–629, 1987.
58. Wolf, G.: J. Nutr. Biochem., *1*:284–289, 1990.
59. DeLuca, L.: FASEB J., *5*:2924–2933, 1991.
60. Wahli, W., Martinez, E.: FASEB J., *5*:2243–2249, 1991.
61. Levin, A.A., Sturzenbecker, L.J., Kazmer, S., et al.: Nature, *355*:359–361, 1992.
62. Heyman, R.A., Mangelsdorf, D.J., Dyck, J.A., et al.: Cell, *68*:397–406, 1992.
63. Yu, V.C., Delsert, C., Andersen, B., et al.: Cell, *67*:1251–1266, 1991.
64. Kliewer, S.A., Umesono, K., Mangelsdorf, D.J., et al.: Nature, *355*:446–449, 1992.
65. Zhang, X.-K., Hoffman, B., Tran, P.B.-V., et al.: Nature, *355*:441–446, 1992.
66. Mehta, R.G., Barua, A.B., Olson, J.A., et al.: Oncology, *48*:505–509, 1991.
67. Sani, B.P., Barua, A.B., Hill, D.L., et al.: Biochem. Pharmacol, *43*:919–922, 1992.
68. Darmon, M., Rocher, M., Cavey, M.T., et al.: Skin Pharmacol., *1*:161–175, 1988.
69. DeThe, H., Vivanco-Ruiz, M., Tiollais, P., et al.: Nature, *343*:177–180, 1990.
70. LaRosa, G.J., Gudas, L.J.: Proc. Natl. Acad. Sci. U.S.A., *85*:329–333, 1988.
71. Vasios, G., Mader, S., Gold, J.D., et al.: EMBO J., *10*:1149–1158, 1990.
72. Davies, P.J.A., Saydak, M.M., Basilion, J.P., et al.: Retinoid receptor-regulated expression of tissue transglutaminase: links to the biochemistry of programmed cell death. *In* Retinoids: Progress in Research and Clinical Applications. Edited by M. Livrea and L. Packer. New York, Marcel Dekker. In press.
73. Denning, M.F., Verma, A.K.: Biochem. Biophys. Res. Commun., *175*:344–350, 1991.
74. Sporn, M.B., Roberts, A.B.: Mol. Endocrinol., *5*:3–7, 1991.
75. Glick, A.B., McCune, B.K., Abdulkarem, N., et al.: Development, *111*:1081–1086, 1991.
76. Bolmer, S.D., Wolf, G.: Proc. Natl. Acad. Sci. U.S.A., *79*:6541–6545, 1982.
77. Olson, J.A.: Isr. J. Med. Sci., *8*:1170–1178, 1972.
78. Tickle, C., Alberts, B., Wolpert, L., et al.: Nature, *296*:564–566, 1982.

79. Summerbell, D.: J. Embryol. Exp. Morphol., *78*:269–289, 1983.
80. Summerbell, D., Maden, M.: Trends Neurosci., *13*:142–147, 1990.
81. Thaller, C., Eichele, G.: Nature, *327*:625–628, 1987.
82. Honig, L.S., Summerbell, D.: J. Embryol. Exp. Morphol., *87*:163–174, 1985.
83. Ruberte, E., Dolle, P., Chambon, P., et al.: Development, *111*:45-60, 1991.
84. Izpisua-Belmont, J.C., Tickle, C., Dolle, P., et al.: Nature, *350*:585–589, 1991.
85. Maden, M., Ong, D.E., Summerbell, D., et al.: Nature, *335*:733–755, 1988.
86. Eichele, G.: Development, *107*:863–867, 1989.
87. Hunter, K., Maden, M., Summerbell, D., et al.: Proc. Natl. Acad. Sci. U.S.A., *88*:3666–3670, 1991.
88. Thaller, C., Eichele, G.: Nature, *345*:815–819, 1990.
89. Summerbell, D., Waterson, N.: Does retinoic acid organize a limb or induce a ZPA? *In* Development Patterns of the Vertebrate Limb. Edited by J.R. Hinchliffe, J.M. Hurle, and D. Summerbell. New York, Plenum, 1991, pp. 151–155.
90. Noji, S., Nohno, T., Koyama, E., et al.: Nature, *350*:83–86, 1991.
91. Brown, R., Brockes, J.P.: Development, *111*:489–496, 1991.
92. Seegmiller, R.E., Harris, C., Luchtel, D.L., et al.: Teratology, *43*:133–150, 1991.
93. Mathies, R.A., Lin, S.W., Ames, J.B., et al.: Annu. Rev. Biophys. Chem., *20*:491–518, 1991.
94. Bertram, J.S.: Retinoids, gap junctional communication and cancer chemoprevention: proposed functional relationship. *In* Retinoids: Progress in Research and Clinical Applications. Edited by M. Livrea and L. Packer. New York, Marcel Dekker. In press.
95. Ross, A.C.: Proc. Soc. Exp. Biol. Med. In press.
96. West, C.E., Rombout, J.H.W.M., Van der Zijpp, A.J., et al.: Proc. Nutr. Soc., *50*:249–260, 1991.
97. Semba, R.D., Muhilal, H., Scott, A.L., et al.: J. Nutr, *122*:101–107, 1992.
98. Carman, J.A., Smith, S.M., Hayes, C.E.: J. Immunol., *142*:388–393, 1989.
99. Bendich, A.: J. Nutr., *119*:112–115, 1989.
100. World Health Organization: Control of Vitamin A Deficiency. Technical Reports Series 672. Geneva, World Health Organization, 1982.
101. Sommer, A.: J. Nutr., *119*:96–100, 1989.
102. Sommer, A.: Field Guide to the Detection and Control of Xerophthalmia. Geneva, World Health Organization, 1982.
103. Ubels, J.L., Macrae, S.M.: Curr. Eye Res.,*3*:815–822, 1984.
104. Olson, J.A. Physiological and metabolic basis of major signs of vitamin A deficiency. *In* Vitamin A Deficiency and Its Control. Edited by J.C. Bauernfeind. Orlando, FL, Academic Press, 1986, pp. 19–67.
105. Törmä, H., Vahlquist, A.: Arch. Dermatol. Res., *275*:324–328, 1983.
106. Törmä, H., Vahlquist, A.: J. Invest. Dermatol., *94*:132–138, 1990.
107. Fuchs, E.: J. Cell Biol., *111*:2807–2814, 1990.
108. Stellmach, V., Leask, A., Fuchs, E.: Proc. Natl. Acad. Sci. U.S.A., *88*:4582–4586, 1991.
109. Hardy, M.H., Dhouailly, D., Törmä, H., et al.: J. Exp. Zool., *256*:279–289, 1990.
110. Lamb, A.J., Apiwatanaporn, P., Olson, J.A.: J. Nutr., *104*:1140–1148, 1974.
111. Bauernfeind, J.C.: The Safe Use of Vitamin A. Washington, D.C., International Vitamin A Consultative Group, Nutrition Foundation, 1980, p. 44.
112. Hathcock, J.N., Hattan, D.G., Jenkins, M.Y., et al.: Am. J. Clin. Nutr., *52*:183–202, 1990.
113. Daicker, B., Schiedt, K., Adnet, J.J., et al.: Graefes Arch. Clin. Exp. Ophthalmol., *225*:189–197, 1987.
114. Macapinlac, M.P., Olson, J.A.: Int. J. Vitam. Nutr. Res., *51*:331–341, 1981.
115. Bush, M.E., Dahms, B.B.: Arch. Pathol. Lab. Med., *108*:838–842, 1984.
116. Olson, J.A.: J. Nutr., *119*:1820–1824, 1989.
117. Lammer, E.J., Chen, D.T., Hoar, R.M., et al.: N. Engl. J. Med., *313*:837–841, 1985.
118. Werler, M.W., Lammer, E.J., Rosenberg, L., et al.: Teratology, *42*:497–503, 1990.
119. Nolan, G.A.: Neurobehav. Toxicol. Teratol., *8*:643–654, 1986.
120. Olson, J.A., Gunning, D.B., Tilton, R.A.: Am. J. Clin. Nutr., *39*:903–910, 1984.
121. Shenai, J.P., Rush, M.G., Stahlman, M.T., et al.: J. Pediatr., *116*:607–614, 1990.
122. Zachman, R.D.: Am. J. Clin. Nutr., *50*:413–424, 1989.
123. Lieber, C.S.: Alcohol Clin. Exp. Res., *15*:573–592, 1991.
124. Shils, M.E., Baker, H., Frank, O.: JPEN J. Parenter. Enterol Nutr., *9*:179–188, 1985.
125. Kligman, A.M., Leyden, J.J., Mills, O., Jr.: Oral vitamin A (retinol) in acne vulgaris. *In* Retinoids: Advances in Basic Research and Therapy. Edited by C.E. Orfanos, O. Braun-Falco, E.M. Farber, et al. Berlin, Springer-Verlag, 1981, pp. 245–253.
126. Kietzmann, H., Schwarze, I., Grote, W., et al.: Dtsch. Med. Wochenschr., *111*:60–62, 1986.
127. Matsuo, T., Matsuo, N., Shiraga, F., et al.: Lancet, *2*:402–403, 1987.
128. Carpenter, T.O., Pettifor, J.M., Russell, R.M., et al.: J. Pediatr., *111*:507–512, 1987.
129. Boyd, A.S.: Am. J. Med., *86*:568–574, 1989.
130. Goldfarb, M.T., Ellis, C.N., Weiss, J.S., et al.: J. Am. Acad. Dermatol., *21*:645–650, 1989.
131. Gunning, D.B., Barua, A.B. Lloyd, R.A.: Unpublished observations.
132. Gunning, D.B., Barua, A.B., Olson, J.A.: FASEB J. *4*:A660, 1990.
133. Biesalski, H.K., Doepner, G., Gerharz, D.D.: Abstract. *In* Proceedings of a Conference on Retinoids: New Trends in Research and Clinical Applications. Palermo, 1991, p. 100.
134. Modiano, M.R., Dalton, W.S., Lippman, S.M., et al.: Invest. New Drugs, *8*:317–319, 1990.
135. Rafal, E.S., Griffiths, C.E.M., Ditre, C.M., et al.: N. Engl. J. Med., *326*:368–374, 1992.
136. Lippman, S.M., Kessler, J.F., Meyskens, F.L, Jr.: Cancer Treat. Rep., *71*:391–405, 493–515, 1987.
137. Degos, L.: All-*trans* retinoic acid in acute promyelocytic leukemia: a model for differentiation therapy of malignancies. *In* Retinoids: New Trends in Research and Clinical Applications. Edited by M. Livrea and L. Packer. New York, Marcel Dekker. In press.
138. Dejean, A., Lavan, C., Chomienne, C., et al.: The t(15,17) translocation of acute promyelocytic leukemia generates a functionally altered retinoic acid receptor. *In* Retinoids: New Trends in Research and Clinical Applications. Edited by M. Livrea and L. Packer. New York, Marcel Dekker. In press.

139. Moon, R.C.: J. Nutr., *119*:127–134, 1989.
140. Costa, A., DePalo, G., Formelli, F., et al.: Breast cancer chemoprevention with retinoids. *In* Retinoids: New Trends in Research and Clinical Applications. Edited by M. Livrea and L. Packer. New York, Marcel Dekker. In press.
141. Garewal, H.S.: Am. J. Clin. Nutr., *53*:294S–297S, 1991.
142. Ziegler, R.G.: Am. J. Clin. Nutr., *53*:265S–269S, 1991.
143. Symposium on Antioxidant Vitamins and β-Carotene in Disease Prevention: Am. J. Clin. Nutr., *53*:1S–396S, 1991.
144. Canfield, L.: Proc. Soc. Exp. Biol. Med, *200*:260–265, 1992.
145. Block, G., Dresser, C.M., Hartman, A.M., et al.: Am. J. Epidemiol., *122*:13–26, 1985.
146. Food and Agriculture Organization/World Health Organization: Requirements for Vitamin A, Iron, Folate, and Vitamin $B_{12}$. Report of a Joint FAO/WHO Expert Committee. Food and Nutrition Series, Report No. 23. Rome, Food and Agriculture Organization, 1988.
147. Dietary Reference Values for Food Energy and Nutrients for the United Kingdom. London, Her Majesty's Stationer's Office (HMSO), 1991.
148. National Institute of Health and Nutrition: Recommended Intake of Nutrients and Energy. Tokyo, Ministry of Health Press, 1985.
149. Food and Nutrition Board, National Research Council: Recommended Dietary Allowances, 10th Ed. Washington, D.C., National Academy Press, 1989.
150. United States Public Health Service: Dietary Source Data, United States 1976–1980. DHHS Publ. No. PHS 83–1681. Hyattsville, MD, United States Department of Health and Human Services, 1983.
151. Mejía, L.A.: Vitamin A-nutrient interrelationships. *In* Vitamin A Deficiency and its Control. Edited by J.C. Bauernfeind. Orlando, FL, Academic Press, 1986, pp. 69–100.
152. Solomons, N.W., Russell, R.M.: Am. J. Clin. Nutr., *33*:2031–2040, 1980.
153. Bergen, H.R., Jr., Natadisastra, G., Muhilal, H., et al.: Am. J. Clin. Nutr., *48*:279–285, 1988.
154. Underwood, B.A., Olson, J.A. (Eds.): A Brief Guide to Current Methods of Assessing Vitamin A Status. Washington, D.C., International Vitamin A Consultative Group, International Life Science Institute, Nutrition Foundation. In press.
155. Furr, H.C., Amedee-Manesme, O., Clifford, A.J., et al.: Am. J. Clin. Nutr., *49*:713–716, 1989.
156. Olson, J.A.: Vitamin A, retinoids, and carotenoids. *In* Modern Nutrition in Health and Disease. 7th Ed. Edited by M.E. Shils and V.R. Young. Philadelphia, Lea & Febiger, 1988, pp. 292–312.
157. Pilch, S.M. (Ed.): Assessment of the Vitamin A Nutritional Status of the U.S. Population Based on Data Collected in Health and Nutrition Examination Surveys. Bethesda, MD, Life Science Research Office, Federation of American Societies for Experimental Biology, 1985.
158. Furr, H.C., Barua, A.B., Olson, J.A.: Retinoids and carotenoids. *In* Modern Chromatographic Analysis of the Vitamins. 2nd Ed. Edited by H.J. Nelis, W.E. Lambert, and A.P. DeLeenheer. New York, Marcel Dekker, 1992, pp. 1–71.
159. Packer, L. (Ed.): Methods Enzymol., *189*:3–536, 1990.
160. Packer, L. (Ed.): Methods Enzymol., *190*:3–448, 1990.
161. Consumer and Food Economics Institute, United States Department of Agriculture: Comparison of Foods. Agricultural Handbook Nos. 8-1 to 8-12. Washington, D.C., United States Government Printing Office, 1976 to 1984.
162. Noy, N., Xu, Z.-J.: Biochemistry *29*:3878–3883, 3883–3888, 1991.


## SELECTED READINGS


Bauernfeind, J.C. (Ed.): Vitamin A Deficiency and its Control. Orlando, FL, Academic Press, 1986.

Dawson, M.I., Okamura, W.H. (Eds.): Chemistry and Biology of Synthetic Retinoids. Boca Raton, FL, CRC Press, 1990.

Furr, H.C., Barua, A.B., Olson, J.A.: Retinoids and carotenoids. *In* Modern Chromatographic Analysis of the Vitamins. 2nd Ed. Edited by H.J. Nelis, W.E. Lambert, and A.P. DeLeenheer. New York, Marcel Dekker, 1992, pp. 1–71.

Livrea, M., Packer, L. (Eds.): Retinoids: New Trends in Research and Clinical Applications. New York, Marcel Dekker. In press.

Olson, J.A.: Vitamin A. *In* Handbook of Vitamins. 2nd Ed. Edited by L.J. Machlin. New York, Marcel Dekker, 1990, pp. 1–57.

Saurat, J.-H. (Ed.): Retinoids: Ten Years On. Basel, Karger, 1991.

Sporn, M.B., Roberts, A.B., Goodman, D.S. (Eds.): The Retinoids. Vols. 1 and 2. New York, Academic Press, 1984.

Underwood, B.A., Olson, J.A. (Eds.): A Brief Guide to Current Methods of Assessing Vitamin A Status. Washington, D.C., International Vitamin A Consultative Group, International Life Science Institute, Nutrition Foundation. In press.

CHAPTER 17

# Vitamin D

Michael F. Holick



Vitamin D has existed on Earth for at least 500 million years. It was first produced in ocean dwelling phytoplankton while they were exposed to sunlight for photosynthesis. Although the physiologic function of vitamin D in these lower life forms is unknown, vitamin D and its precursors may have acted either as a natural sunscreen to absorb high energy ultraviolet radiation, thus protecting ultraviolet sensitive organelles and macromolecules, or as a photochemical signal.[1] For reasons that are not understood, terrestrial vertebrates during evolution became dependent on vitamin D for the development and maintenance of their ossified skeletons. The principal physiologic function of vitamin D in all vertebrates including humans is to maintain serum calcium and phosphorus concentrations in a range that supports cellular processes, neuromuscular function, and bone ossification. Vitamin D accomplishes this goal by enhancing the efficiency of the small intestine to absorb dietary calcium and phosphorus, and by mobilizing calcium and phosphorus stores from bone.

Vitamin D is inherently biologically inactive and requires successive hydroxylations in the liver and kidney to form 1,25-dihydroxyvitamin D ($1,25(OH)_2D$), the biologically active form of vitamin D.[2–4] $1,25(OH)_2D$ interacts with a specific nuclear receptor in its target tissues that results in a biologic response. Recent evidence suggests that $1,25(OH)_2D$ may also have rapid actions on intracellular calcium, phosphatidylinositol metabolism, and cyclic guanosine triphosphate (GTP) metabolism.[2–4]

The identification of vitamin D metabolites led to the development of assays for them. These assays have become valuable diagnostic tools for evaluating patients with hypocalcemic, hypercalcemic, and metabolic bone disorders.

The major target tissues for $1,25(OH)_2D$ are the intestine and bone; however, nuclear receptors for $1,25(OH)_2D$ have been identified in several other tissues and in cultured tumor cells. $1,25(OH)_2D$ inhibits the proliferation and induces terminal differentiation of many tumor and normal cultured cells that possess its receptor.[2–4] These observations have been the impetus for a re-evaluation of the physiologic and pharmacologic actions of $1,25(OH)_2D$.

## HISTORY OF RICKETS

Although historians state that rickets occurred in humans as early as the second century A.D, the disease was not considered a significant health problem until the industrialization of northern Europe. In the seventeenth century, Whistler, DeBoot, and Glissen independently recognized that many of the children who lived in the crowded and polluted cities in northern Europe (Fig. 17–1) developed a severe bone-deforming disease that was characterized by enlargement of the epiphyses of the long bones and rib cage, bowing of the legs, bending of the spine, and weak and toneless muscles (Fig. 17–2).[5] The incidence of this debilitating bone disease increased dramatically in northern Europe and North America during the industrial revolution, and by the latter part of the nineteenth century, autopsy studies done in Leiden, the Netherlands showed evidence that about 90% of the children had rickets.[6] This disease was especially devastating for young women of childbearing age who often had a deformed pelvis, resulting in a high incidence of infant and maternal morbidity and mortality. This high incidence led to the development and widespread use of cesarean sections in Great Britain.

From the earliest recognition of rickets in 1650, scientists and physicians throughout Europe began what would be a 270-year search for the cause and cure of this unfortunate childhood malady. In 1822, Sniadecki observed that children living in Warsaw had a high incidence of rickets, whereas children living in rural areas outside of Warsaw did not.[7] Based on this observation, he advocated the use of exposure to sunlight as a means of curing this disease. Little attention was focused, however, on the environment as the cause of this disorder. In 1889,[8] the British Medical Society conducted an epidemiologic survey and confirmed previous observations that the incidence of rickets was extremely high in the industrialized cities in Great Britain and was less known in rural districts of the British Highlands. This finding was much different from the incidence of rheumatism and malignant disease that was common in all districts in the British Isles.[9] Unfortunately, they were unable to relate the lack of exposure to sunlight with their observations. One year later, however, Palm published an extensive epidemiologic survey and came to the same conclusion as Sniadecki.[10] He collected observations from a number of physicians throughout the British Empire and the Orient. His information revealed that rickets was rare in children living in impoverished cities in China, Japan, and India where people received poor nutrition and lived in squalor, whereas the children of

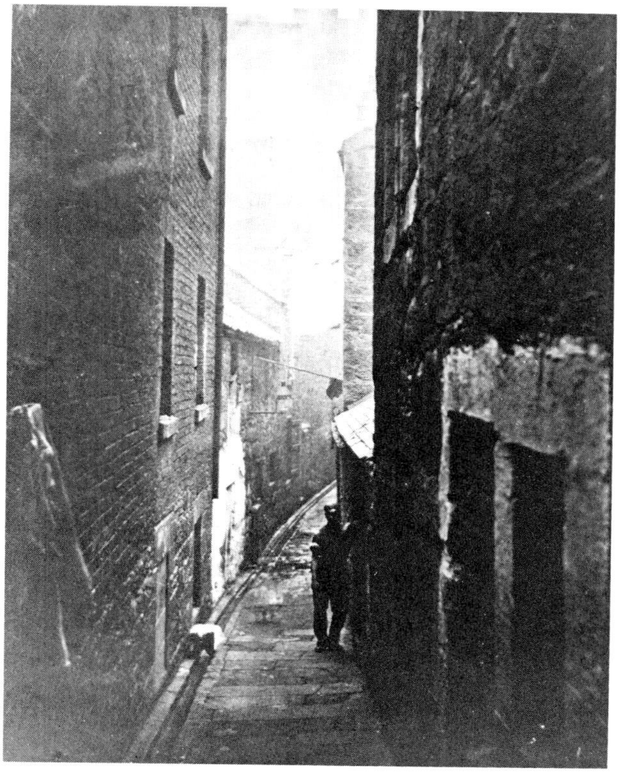

**FIGURE 17–1.** A typical scene in Glasgow in the mid 1800s as captured by this photograph taken by Thomas Annan. (From Thomas Annan's Photographs of the Old Closes and Streets of Glasgow 1868/1877. New York, Dover, 1977.)

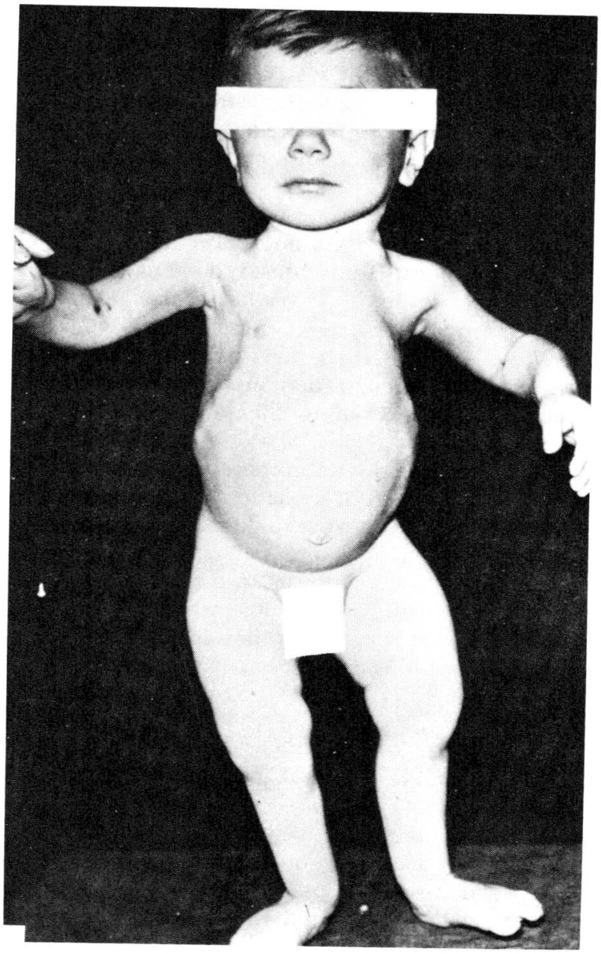

**FIGURE 17–2.** Child with rickets showing rachitic rosary of the rib cage, bowed legs, deformity of the long bones, and muscle weakness. (From Fraser, D., Scriver, C.R.: Hereditary disorders associated with vitamin-D resistance or defective phosphate metabolism. *In* Endocrinology. Vol. 2. Edited by L. DeGroot. New York, Grune and Stratton, 1979.)

middle class and poor who lived in industrialized cities in the British Isles had a high incidence of rickets. Based on this survey, he urged the systematic use of sunbathing as a preventative and therapeutic measure in rickets and other diseases. He also advocated the education of the public to the appreciation of sunshine as a means of health.

Unfortunately, little attention was paid to the insightful observations of Sniadecki and Palm, and another 30 years passed before Huldschinski demonstrated that exposure of rachitic children to radiation from a mercury vapor arc lamp was effective in curing this bone disease.[11] When he exposed one arm of a rachitic child to the ultraviolet radiation, he demonstrated that rickets in the other arm was cured to the same degree as the exposed arm.

He concluded that the phototherapy was not a local effect and speculated that something was made in the skin and could be transported to distal sites to carry out its antirachitic activity. Two years later, Hess and Unger exposed seven rachitic children on a roof of New York City hospital to varying periods of sunshine and reported that radiographic examinations showed improvement of rickets in each child as evidenced by calcification of the epiphyses.[12]

## THE ANTIRACHITIC FACTOR: VITAMIN D

During the eighteenth and nineteenth centuries, cod liver oil was used as a common folklore medicine for the prevention and cure of rickets. As early as 1827, Bretonneau treated acute rickets in a 15-month-old child with cod liver oil and noted the incredible speed with which the patient was cured. His student Trousseau advocated the use of oils from fish and sea mammals accompanied by exposure to sunlight for a rapid cure of rickets.[13] This knowledge prompted an intense investigation to determine what nutritional factor was present in cod liver oil that was responsible for preventing rickets. In 1918, Mellanby reported that he could produce rickets in dogs by feeding them oatmeal and could cure the disease by adding cod liver oil to their diet.[14] Two years later, McCollum et al. examined whether the antirachitic factor in cod liver oil was identical or distinct from vitamin A.[15] Cod liver oil was heated and oxidized in a manner that destroyed all vitamin A activity. When the oil was administered to rachitic rats, it maintained its antirachitic properties. Thus, the antirachitic factor present in cod liver oil clearly was not vitamin A but a new fat-soluble vitamin that was called vitamin D.

Powers et al. showed that exposure to radiation from a mercury arc lamp had the same antirachitic potency as cod liver oil.[16] At the same time, Hess and Weinstock[17] and Steenbock and Black[18] found that exposure of food and a variety of other substances such as rat liver, human serum, cotton, olive and linseed oils, lettuce, growing wheat, and rat chow to ultraviolet radiation resulted in their having antirachitic properties. This concept led Steenbock to patent use of the addition of provitamin D to foods followed by ultraviolet irradiation to impart antirachitic activity. The addition of provitamin $D_2$ to milk followed by ultraviolet irradiation became widely practiced in the United States and Europe in the 1930s. This vitamin D fortification process eradicated rickets as a significant health problem in countries that used this practice. Today, the fortification of milk and infant formula with 400 IU (10 $\mu$g) of vitamin $D_2$ or vitamin $D_3$ has eliminated rickets as a health problem in the United States and Canada. In Europe, vitamin D fortification of milk is prohibited because of severe vitamin D intoxication that resulted from the indiscriminate addition of excessive amounts of vitamin D to infant formulas in the 1940s and 1950s. Today, some foods, including cereals and margarine, are fortified with vitamin D in many European countries.

## PHOTOBIOLOGY

### HISTORY

The first vitamin D that was isolated was a photoproduct from the irradiation of the fungal sterol ergosterol. This vitamin D was known as vitamin $D_1$, until it was realized that it was a combination of substances. As a result, further purification of the irradiation mixture yielded a single compound, which was called ergocalciferol or vitamin $D_2$[19] (Fig. 17–3). At the time of its identification, it was assumed that the vitamin D made in human skin during exposure to sunlight was vitamin $D_2$.[20] In the 1930s, however, it was reported that vitamin D obtained from the irradiation of ergosterol had little antirachitic activity in chickens, whereas the vitamin D that was isolated from the irradiation of cholesterol-like sterol yielded a potent antirachitic substance.[21–24] The confusion as to whether vitamin $D_2$ was identical to the substance produced in human skin was resolved when Windaus and Bock reported the synthesis of a new provitamin D analogue that was similar to ergosterol with the exception that the side chain was that of cholesterol (Fig. 17–3).[25] This provitamin D was called provitamin $D_3$ or 7-dehydrocholesterol, and on irradiation, it gave rise to vitamin $D_3$ (cholecalciferol) (see Fig. 17–3). Vitamin $D_3$, unlike vitamin $D_2$, had equal antirachitic activity in chicks and rats and was identical to the vitamin D found in fish liver oils and mammalian skin. Therefore, it was concluded that 7-dehydrocholesterol rather than ergosterol was the parent compound in the skin and its resulting photoproduct was vitamin $D_3$.

Because of the availability of large quantities of ergosterol, vitamin $D_2$ was the vitamin D used for the fortification of milk in the United States and Canada and for pharmaceutical preparations. During the past two decades, vitamin $D_3$ has also been used to fortify milk and other food substances worldwide.

Originally, it was believed that during exposure to sunlight, provitamin $D_3$ was directly converted to vita-

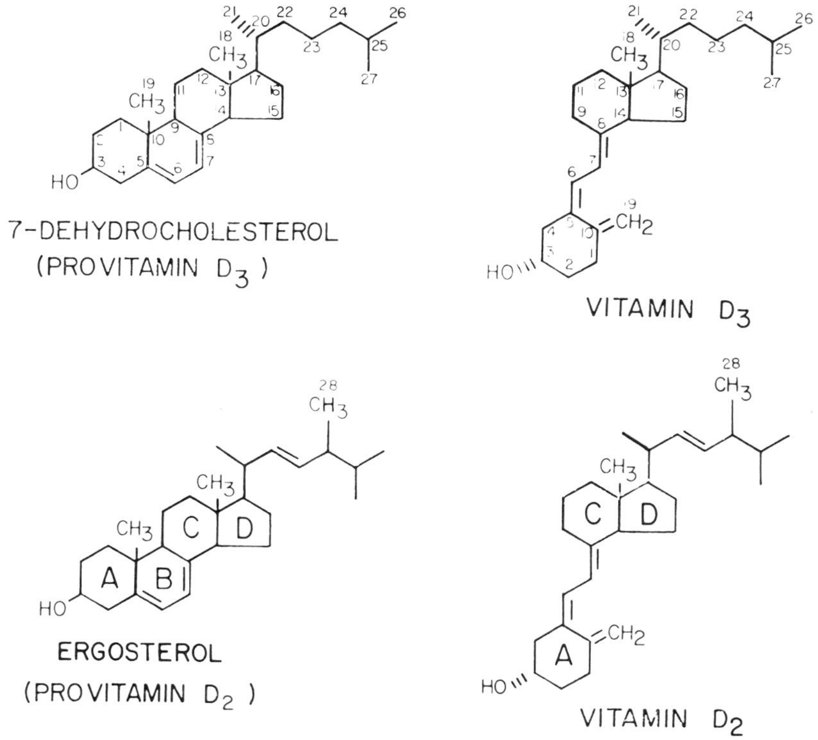
7-DEHYDROCHOLESTEROL
(PROVITAMIN D3)
VITAMIN D3
ERGOSTEROL
(PROVITAMIN D2)
VITAMIN D2

**FIGURE 17–3.** Structure of vitamins $D_3$ and $D_2$ and their respective precursors, 7-dehydrocholesterol and ergosterol. The only structural difference between vitamins $D_2$ and $D_3$ is their side chains; the side chain for vitamin $D_2$ contains a double bond among $C_{22}$, $C_{23}$, and a $C_{24}$ methyl group. (From MacLaughlin, J.A., Holick, M.F.: Mediation of cutaneous vitamin $D_3$ synthesis by UV radiation. *In* Biochemistry and Physiology of the Skin. Edited by L.A. Goldsmith. New York, Oxford University Press, 1983.)

min $D_3$. This concept was then challenged by Velluz et al., who reported that exposure of provitamin $D_3$ in an organic solvent to ultraviolet radiation at 0° C did not yield any vitamin $D_3$.[26] They reported the isolation of a new photoproduct, which they called previtamin $D_3$,[27] that was a thermally labile substance and underwent rearrangement of its double bonds to form vitamin $D_3$ by a temperature-dependent process.

## PHOTOSYNTHESIS OF PREVITAMIN $D_3$ IN HUMAN SKIN

The sun emits a broad spectrum of electromagnetic radiation. The high-energy photons that are most damaging to life on Earth (below 290 nm) are absorbed by the thin layer of ozone that envelops the planet. The small band of radiation between 290 and 315 nm (UV-B radiation) is responsible for the photolysis of provitamin $D_3$ in the epidermis and dermis. During exposure to sunlight, the 5,7-diene of provitamin $D_3$ absorbs radiation with energies between 290 and 315 nm,[28] causing the cleavage of ring B between carbons 9 and 10 (Fig. 17–3) and the formation of a 6,7-*cis* conjugated triene to form a 9,10-seco (seco from the Greek term split) sterol known as previtamin $D_3$ (Fig. 17–4). In adult skin, approximately 60% of the cutaneous stores of provitamin $D_3$ are found in the epidermis, whereas the other 40% resides in the dermis.[29] When white and black adults are exposed to sunlight, approximately 70 to 80% and 95 to 98% of the UV-B photons are absorbed by the epidermis, respectively.[30] Therefore, approximately 80 to 90% of the previtamin $D_3$ that is formed in the skin occurs in the actively growing layers of the epidermis, including the stratum basale and stratum spinosum, and less than 20% occurs in the dermis.[31] In neonates, approximately 50% of the provitamin $D_3$ stores are found in both the epidermis and dermis. Because the thin neonatal epidermis transmits more UV-B photons into the dermis, the dermis is also a major site for previtamin $D_3$ synthesis.

Once previtamin $D_3$ is made in the skin, it immediately begins to thermally equilibrate to vitamin $D_3$ (Fig. 17–4). This thermal equilibration takes approximately 1 to 2 days to reach completion at body temperature (37° C) in humans. Although it is not known how vitamin $D_3$ exits the epidermal cells into the dermal capillary

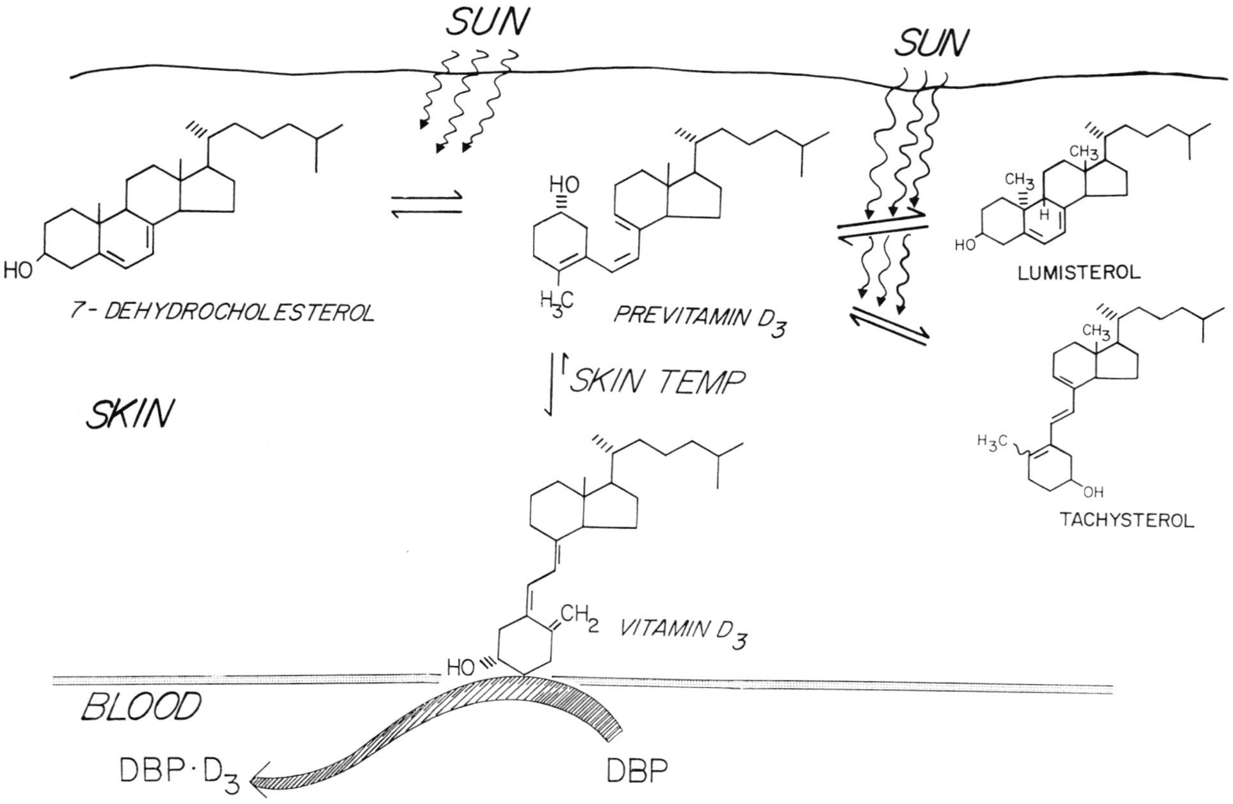
SUN
SUN
7-DEHYDROCHOLESTEROL
PREVITAMIN D3
LUMISTEROL
TACHYSTEROL
SKIN
SKIN TEMP
VITAMIN D3
BLOOD
DBP·D3
DBP

**FIGURE 17–4.** Schematic representation of the formation of previtamin $D_3$ (pre$D_3$) in the skin during exposure to the sun and the thermal isomerization of pre$D_3$ to vitamin $D_3$, which is specifically translocated by the vitamin-D-binding protein (DBP) into the circulation. During the continual exposure to the sun, pre$D_3$ also photoisomerizes to lumisterol$_3$ and tachysterol$_3$, which are photoproducts that are biologically inert (i.e., they do not stimulate intestinal calcium absorption). Because the DBP has no affinity for lumisterol$_3$ but has minimal affinity for tachysterol$_3$, the translocation of these photoisomers into the circulation is negligible, and these photoproducts are sloughed off during the natural turnover of the skin. Because these photoisomers are in a state of quasiphotoequilibrium, as soon as pre$D_3$ stores are depleted (owing to thermal isomerization to vitamin $D_3$), exposure of lumisterol and tachysterol to ultraviolet radiation will provoke these isomers to photoisomerize to pre$D_3$. (From Holick, M.F., MacLaughlin, J.A., Doppelt, S.H.: Science, *211*:590–593, 1981. Copyright 1981 by the American Association for the Advancement of Science.)

bed, some evidence shows that the vitamin D binding protein, which has relatively high affinity for vitamin $D_3$ in comparison to provitamin $D_3$ and previtamin $D_3$, helps to translocate vitamin $D_3$ from the epidermis into the dermal circulation.[31]

## REGULATION OF PREVITAMIN $D_3$ SYNTHESIS IN HUMAN SKIN

### *PHOTOCHEMICAL REGULATION*

Loomis speculated that melanin pigmentation evolved in humans who lived near the equator as a mechanism to prevent sunlight-induced vitamin D intoxication.[32] Although melanin is an excellent natural sunscreen that competes with provitamin $D_3$ for UV-B photons, thereby limiting the cutaneous production of previtamin $D_3$,[29,33] firm evidence exists that sunlight itself is responsible for regulating the total production of vitamin $D_3$ in human skin.[29] Loomis based his theory on the concept that exposure to prolonged intense sunlight would result in an increase in the production of vitamin $D_3$ in the skin. Once previtamin $D_3$ is photosynthesized in the skin, however, either it can thermally isomerize to vitamin $D_3$ or, during exposure to sunlight, it can absorb ultraviolet radiation and isomerize to biologically inert isomers lumisterol and tachysterol (see Fig. 17–4). Thus, if a white individual is exposed to sunlight at the equator, provitamin $D_3$ is rapidly converted to previtamin $D_3$ during the initial few minutes of exposure. Prolonged exposure to sunlight, however, does not increase previtamin $D_3$ production, but rather previtamin $D_3$ is photodegraded to biologically inert isomers (Fig. 17–5).[29]

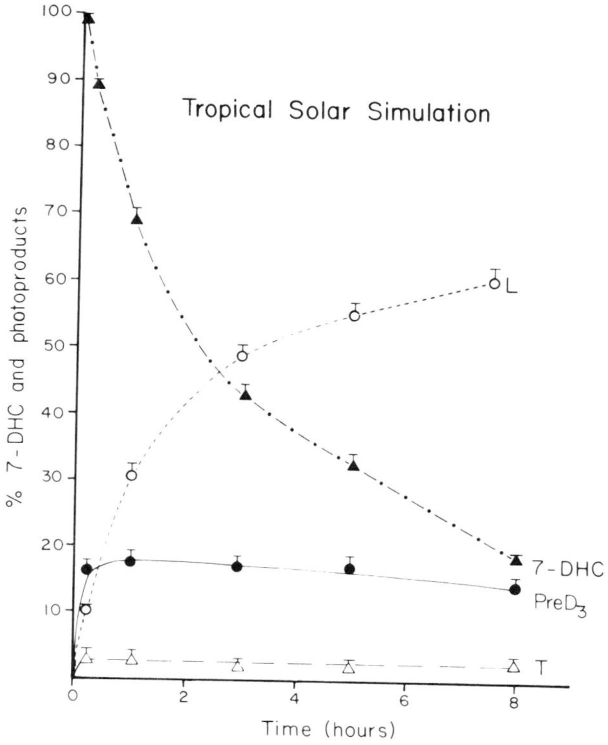
Tropical Solar Simulation
% 7-DHC and photoproducts
Time (hours)
L
7-DHC
PreD3
T

**FIGURE 17–5.** This represents an analysis of the photolysis of 7-dehydrocholesterol (7-DHC) (closed triangles) in the basal cell layer and the appearance of the photoproducts previtamin $D_3$ (pre$D_3$) (closed circles), lumisterol$_3$ (L) (open circles), and tachysterol (T) (open triangles) with increasing exposure time. The bar on the open triangle represents the SEM from three determinations. (From Holick, M.F., MacLaughlin, J.A., Doppelt, S.H.: Science, *211*:590–593, 1981. Copyright 1981 by the American Association for the Advancement of Science.)

Vitamin $D_3$ is exquisitely sensitive to photodegradation when exposed to sunlight (Fig. 17–6). The principal photoisomers that are formed are 5,6-trans-vitamin $D_3$ and supersterols I and II (Fig. 17–6). Thus, once vitamin $D_3$ is made from previtamin $D_3$, it must exit the epidermis into the dermal capillary bed, otherwise it will rapidly be photodegraded during exposure to sunlight.[34]

### *EFFECT OF AGE*

The photoproduction of previtamin $D_3$ in any layer of skin depends on the concentration of provitamin $D_3$, the presence of chromophors that compete with provitamin $D_3$ for UV-B photons, and the quantum of UV-B photons that are able to penetrate the skin and are absorbed by provitamin $D_3$. The average concentration of provitamin $D_3$ in 1 $cm^2$ of young adult skin is approximately 0.8 μg for the epidermis and 0.15 to 0.5 μg for the dermis.[31] An inverse relation exists between the concentrations of provitamin $D_3$ in the epidermis with age (Fig. 17–7).[35] The net effect of this age-related decrease is demonstrated in Figure 17–8. The circulating concentrations of vitamin D were measured in healthy young and elderly subjects who were exposed to the same quantity of whole body ultraviolet radiation. The peak circulating concentrations of vitamin D in the elderly were about 30% of that in young adults.[36]

### *SUNSCREENS*

The awareness that the alarming increase in the incidence of skin cancer is related to chronic exposure to sunlight has led to the recommendation that people should wear sunscreen before going outdoors.[37] The solar radiation that is responsible for causing wrinkles and skin cancer, however, is the same radiation that is responsible for producing previtamin $D_3$ in the skin. Thus, the application of a sunscreen with a sun protection factor of only 8 can completely prevent the cutaneous production of previtamin $D_3$ (Fig. 17–9).[38] The use of sunscreens by children and young adults should not affect their vitamin D status, because it is unlikely that they will always wear a sunscreen before going outdoors. The elderly, however, often are more conscious of their health and apply a sunscreen on their skin before going outdoors. Evidence exists that chronic use of sunscreens by the elderly can decrease circulating concentrations of 25-hydroxyvitamin D (25-OH-D), which is a hallmark for determining vitamin D deficiency. As seen in Figure 17–10, almost one half the subjects who lived in Springfield, Illinois who always wore a sunscreen before going outdoors had overt vitamin D deficiency as determined by low circulating concentrations of 25-OH-D.[39]

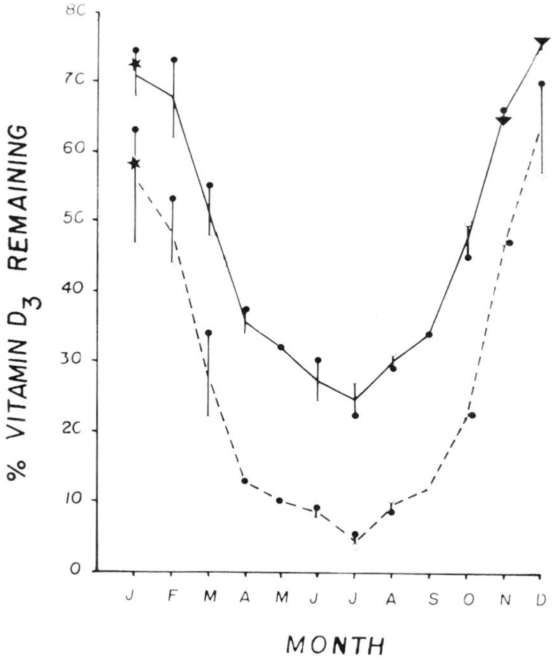
% VITAMIN D3 REMAINING
J F M A M J J A S O N D
MONTH

**FIGURE 17–6.** The percentage of [$^3$H] vitamin $D_3$ remaining after exposure to 1 and 3 h of sunlight in each month of the year. Each point represents the mean ± SE of three determinations. (From Webb, A.R., DeCosta, B.R., Holick, M.F.: J. Clin. Endocrinol. Metab., *68*:822–887, 1989.)

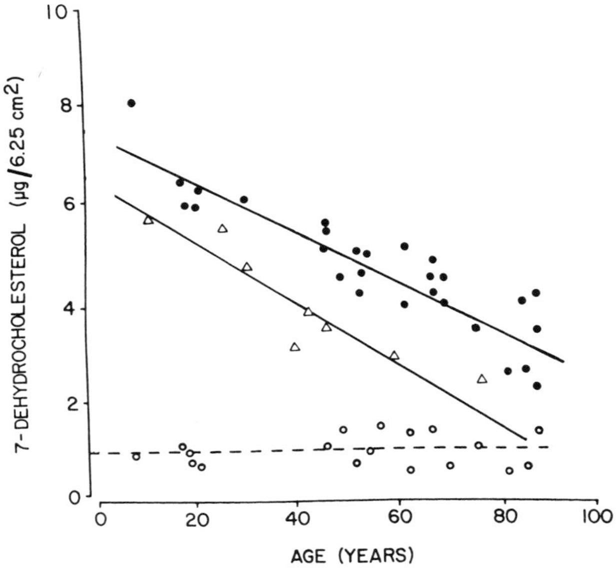
7-DEHYDROCHOLESTEROL (µg/6.25 cm2)
AGE (YEARS)
0
2
4
6
8
10
20
40
60
80
100

**FIGURE 17–7.** Effect of aging on 7-dehydrocholesterol concentrations in human epidermis and dermis. Concentrations of 7-dehydrocholesterol (provitamin $D_3$) per unit area of human epidermis (closed circles), stratum basale (open triangles), and dermis (open circles) were obtained from surgical specimens from donors of various ages. Linear regression analysis gave slopes of −0.05, −0.06, and− 0.0005 for epidermis ($r = -.89$), stratum basale ($r = -.92$), and dermis ($r = -.04$), respectively. The slopes of epidermis and stratum basale are significantly different from the slope of dermis ($P < .001$). (From MacLaughlin, J.A., Holick, M.F.: J. Clin. Invest., *76:*1536–1538, 1985.)

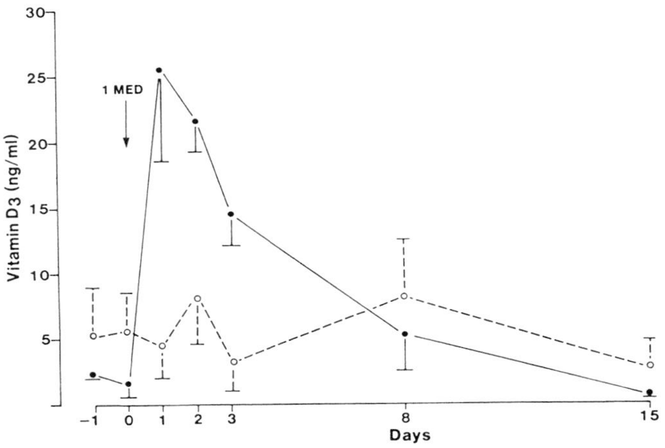
1 MED
Vitamin D3 (ng/ml)
Days
5
10
15
20
25
30
-1
0
1
2
3
8
15

**FIGURE 17–9.** Mean (± SEM) serum vitamin $D_3$ concentrations in eight normal subjects. Four subjects (open circles) applied p-aminobenzoic acid and four applied vehicle (closed circles) to the entire skin before exposure to ultraviolet B (UV-B). On day 0, all subjects underwent total body exposure to 1 MED of UV radiation. To convert nanograms of vitamin D per milliliter to nanomoles per liter, multiply by 2.60. (From Matsuoka, L.Y., Ide, L., Wortsman, J., et al.: J. Clin. Endocrinol. Metab., *64:*1165–1168, 1987.)

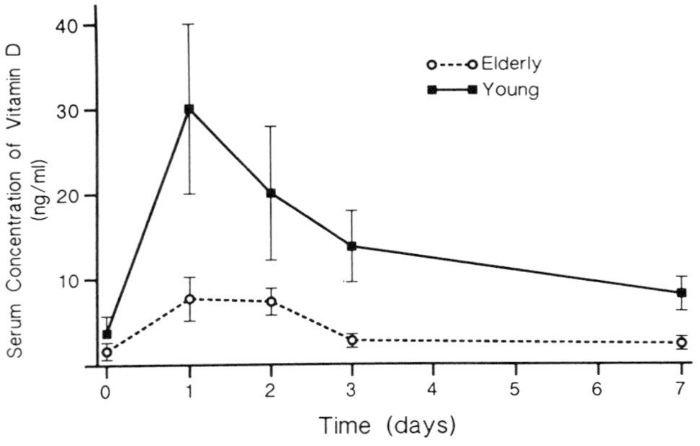
Serum Concentration of Vitamin D (ng/ml)
Elderly
Young
Time (days)
10
20
30
40
0
1
2
3
4
5
6
7

**FIGURE 17–8.** Circulating concentrations of vitamin D in healthy young and elderly volunteers exposed to ultraviolet radiation. To convert nanograms per milliliter to nanomoles per liter, multiply by 2.60. (From Holick, M.F., Matsuoka, L.Y., Wortsman, J.: Lancet, *2:*1104–1105, 1989.)

## *SEASON, LATITUDE, AND TIME OF DAY*

At the turn of the century, a seasonal incidence of rickets was recognized in the industrialized cities of the United States and Europe. Rickets was seen less frequently in children at the end of the summer and more frequently at the end of the winter and early spring.[9] As winter approaches, the solar zenith angle of the sun becomes more oblique. This configuration causes the UV-B photons to be absorbed more efficiently by the stratospheric ozone layer, thereby decreasing the total number of photons that reach the Earth's surface. As a result, the cutaneous synthesis of previtamin $D_3$ is affected by time of day, season of the year, and latitude. As shown in Figure 17–11, exposure to sunlight in Boston (42° N) promoted the cutaneous photosynthesis of previtamin $D_3$ in human skin from March through October. By November, however, the number of 290- to 315-nm photons that penetrated the stratospheric layer into Boston was insufficient to cause significant conversion of provitamin $D_3$ to previtamin $D_3$. Just 10° north in Edmonton (Alberta), Canada, this period was extended between mid-October through mid-March. Further south in Los Angeles (34° N) and Puerto Rico (18° N), the production of previtamin $D_3$ occurred throughout the year (Fig. 17–11).[40]

In Boston in the summer, exposure to sunlight beginning at 5:30 Eastern Standard Time (EST) to 18:30 EST resulted in the cutaneous production of previtamin $D_3$. By October, however, most of the UV-B photons were absorbed by the ozone layer and, as a result, exposure to sunlight before 10:00 EST and after 15:00 EST was

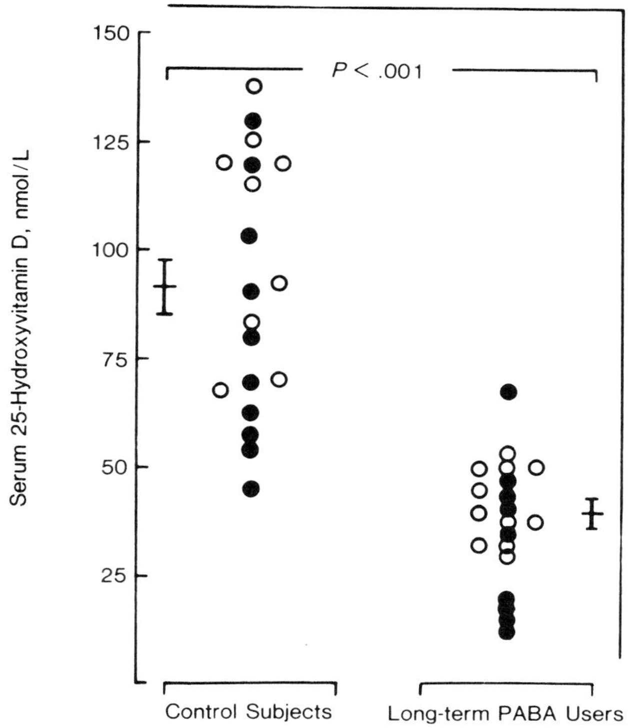
Serum 25-Hydroxyvitamin D, nmol/L
150
125
100
75
50
25
P < .001
Control Subjects
Long-term PABA Users

**FIGURE 17–10.** Serum concentration of 25-hydroxyvitamin D in long-term sunscreen users and in age- and sex-matched controls from same geographic area. Blood samples were obtained simultaneously from patients and controls. The mean serum 25-hydroxyvitamin D level was significantly lower in long-term sunscreen users ($P < .001$). Two long-term sunscreen users had absolute vitamin D deficiency, 25-hydroxyvitamin D level below 20 nmol/L. PABA, p-aminobenzoic acid; open circles, subjects from Philadelphia; closed circles, subjects from Springfield, IL. (From Matsuoka, L.Y., Wortsman, J., Hanifan, N., et al.: Arch. Dermatol., *124:*1802–1804, 1988.)

ineffective in producing previtamin $D_3$ in the skin (Lu and Holick, unpublished results). These observations are beginning to provide guidelines for recommendations regarding the use of sunlight as a means of providing people with their vitamin D requirement. For example, it is reasonable to advise people, especially elderly individuals, that exposure to morning or late afternoon sunlight in the summer is a good source for their vitamin D requirement. At these times, sunlight exposure is less damaging to the skin.

## INTESTINAL ABSORPTION

In nature, only a few foods contain vitamin D: fish liver oils, fatty fish, and egg yolks. Several countries practice the fortification of some foods with vitamin D. In the United States, milk is the principal dietary component that is subject to fortification with either vitamin $D_2$ or vitamin $D_3$. In other countries, some cereals, margarine, and breads have small quantities of vitamin D added to them.

When vitamin D is ingested, this fat-soluble compound is incorporated into the chylomicron fraction and about 80% is absorbed into the lymphatic system.[4] After the ingestion of a single dose of 50,000 IU of vitamin $D_2$, the circulating concentrations of vitamin D begin to increase within hours, peak at 12 hours, and gradually decline to near baseline by 72 hours (Fig. 17–12).[41] This provocative vitamin D absorption test has been useful in determining whether a patient with an intestinal malabsorption syndrome is capable of absorbing this fat-soluble vitamin. A blood sample is drawn just before and 12 or 24 hours after a single oral administration of 50,000 IU of vitamin $D_2$ (see Fig. 17–12). If no elevation in the circulating concentration of vitamin D is observed, complete malabsorption of vitamin D should be suspected; however, any increase in the circulating concen-

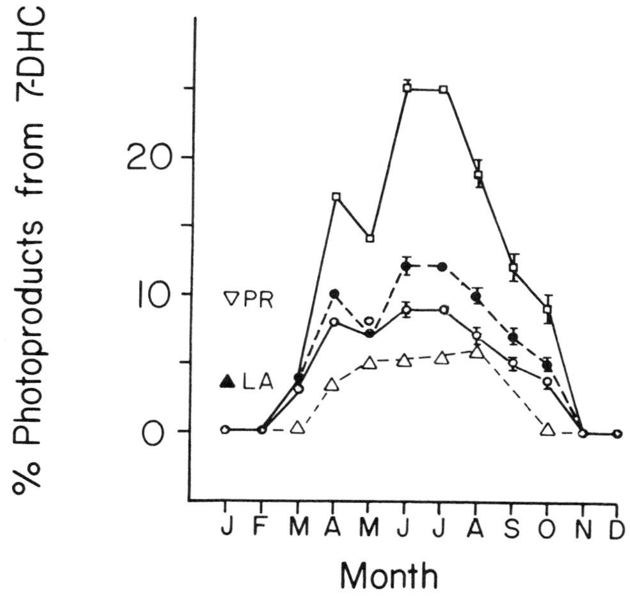
% Photoproducts from 7-DHC
20
10
0
▽PR
▲LA
J F M A M J J A S O N D
Month

**FIGURE 17–11.** [3α-$^3$H] 7-DHC in methanol was exposed to sunlight at different seasons and latitudes. Shown are the mean ± 2 SD (n = 3) annual change in percent conversion of 7-DHC to previtamin $D_3$ after sunlight exposure for 1 h (open circles) and 3 h (closed circles), and total photoproducts (previtamin $D_3$, lumisterol, and tachysterol) after 3 h (open squares) in Boston. The data were collected from November 1985 through 1986 to May 1987, and the figure shows compiled data for the 12 calendar months. For months where data were available for more than 1 yr, the results were the same within the uncertainty of a single point measurement, except for the photosynthesis of previtamin $D_3$ in May, when exposure for 1 and 3 h gave the same result in 1986 (closed circles), and only a 1-h value is available for 1987 (open circles). Also shown is the conversion of 7-DHC to previtamin $D_3$ throughout the year after exposure to 1 h of sunlight in Edmonton (Alberta) Canada, (open triangles) and in January in Los Angeles (LA) and Puerto Rico (PR; single samples accurate to ± 1% photoproduct). (From Webb, A.R., Kline, L., Holick, M.F.: J. Clin. Endocrinol. Metab., *67:*373–378, 1988.)

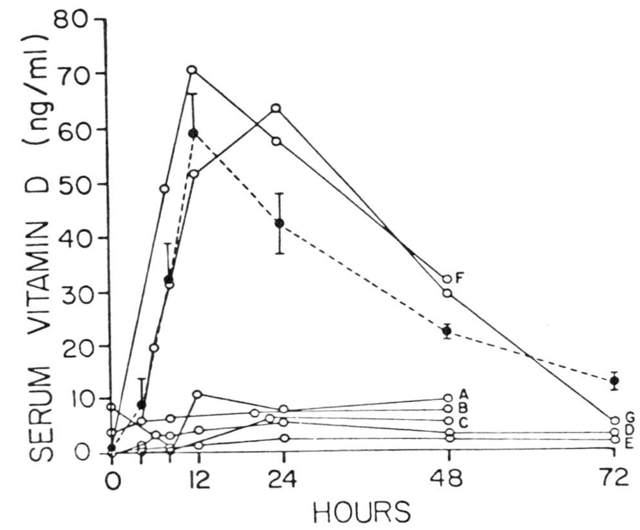
SERUM VITAMIN D (ng/ml)
80
70
60
50
40
30
20
10
0
0
12
24
48
72
HOURS
F
A
B
C
G
D
E

**FIGURE 17–12.** Serum vitamin D concentrations in seven patients with intestinal fat malabsorption syndromes after a single oral dose of 50,000 IU (1.25 mg) of vitamin $D_2$. For comparison, the means and standard errors of vitamin D concentrations measured in seven normal control subjects after a similar dose are indicated by the closed circles and dotted lines. Note that two patients, one with Crohn's ileocolitis (patient F) and one with ulcerative colitis (patient G), had essentially normal absorption curves. Five patients, however, showed a dramatic lack of response, with no values above 25.2 nmol/L (10 ng/ml). (From Lo, C.W., et al.: Am. J. Clin. Nutr., *42*:644–649, 1985.)

tration of vitamin D reflects vitamin D absorption. The dose of vitamin D can, therefore, be tailored accordingly.[4] Thus, patients who suffer from chronic intestinal malabsorption syndromes caused by chronic liver disease, cystic fibrosis, Crohn's disease, Whipple's disease, and sprue are more likely to develop vitamin D deficiency because the small intestine is unable to absorb this fat-soluble vitamin. Diseases that affect the more distal small intestine and large intestine, such as in ileocolitis caused by Crohn's disease and ulcerative colitis, have little effect on absorption of vitamin D (see Fig. 17–12).

## METABOLISM

### VITAMIN D TO 25-HYDROXYVITAMIN D

Once vitamin D (the term vitamin D without a subscript relates to either or both vitamin $D_2$ or vitamin $D_3$ and its metabolites) enters the circulation, it is bound to the group-specific protein commonly known as the vitamin D-binding protein. Vitamin D is transported to the liver, where it undergoes its first hydroxylation on carbon 25, resulting in the formation of the major circulating form of vitamin D, 25-hydroxyvitamin D (25-OH-D) (Fig. 17–13).[2–4,21,42] The production of 25-OH-D by the liver is regulated by a negative feedback mechanism that is controlled by vitamin D, 25-OH-D, and 1,25$(OH)_2$D.[43] This negative feedback control is not regulated tightly in as much as an increase in exposure to sunlight or dietary intake of vitamin D results in an increase in circulating concentrations of 25-OH-D (Fig. 17–14).[44,45] Although the liver is the major site for 25-OH-D production, some extrahepatic sites are capable of this hydroxylation. It is likely that the cholesterol-25-hydroxylase can recognize vitamin D and hydroxylate the side chain on carbon 25 to produce 25-OH-D.[4]

Circulating concentrations of 25-OH-D often are low in patients with severe parenchymal and cholestatic liver disease,[46] in part because of the associated intestinal malabsorption of vitamin D as well as the decrease in the reservoir of the vitamin D-25-hydroxylase in the liver.

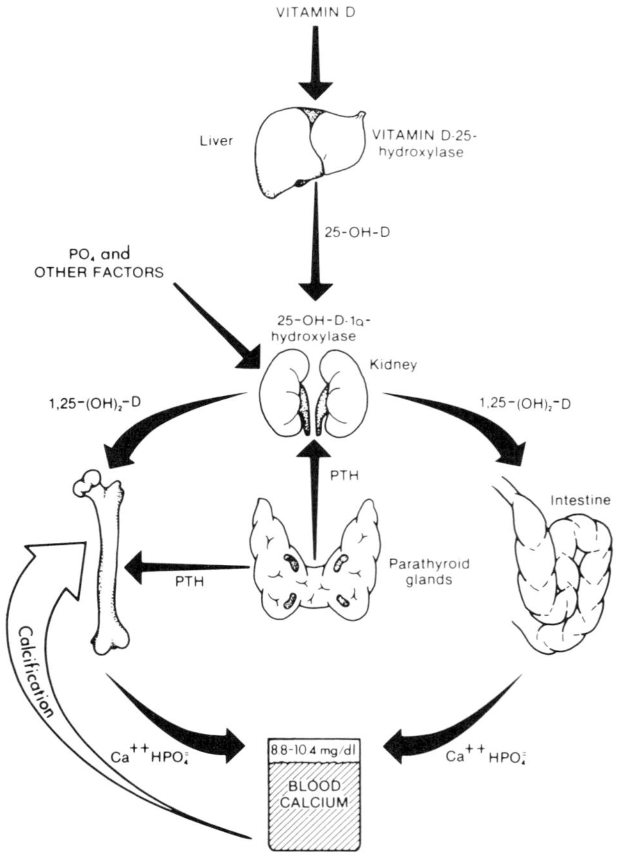
VITAMIN D
Liver
VITAMIN D-25-hydroxylase
25-OH-D
PO4 and OTHER FACTORS
25-OH-D-1α-hydroxylase
Kidney
1,25-(OH)2-D
1,25-(OH)2-D
PTH
Intestine
Parathyroid glands
PTH
Calcification
Ca++ HPO4
8.8-10.4 mg/dl
BLOOD CALCIUM
Ca++ HPO4

**FIGURE 17–13.** Schematic representation of the hormonal control loop for vitamin D metabolism and function. A reduction in the serum calcium below approximately 2.09 mM/L (8.8 mg/ml) prompts a proportional increase in the secretion of parathyroid hormone, which enhances the mobilization of calcium stores from bone. Parathyroid hormone also promotes the synthesis of 1,25$(OH)_2$D in the kidney, which, in turn, stimulates the mobilization of calcium from the bone and intestine. (From Holick, M.F.: Kidney Int., *32*:912–929, 1987.)

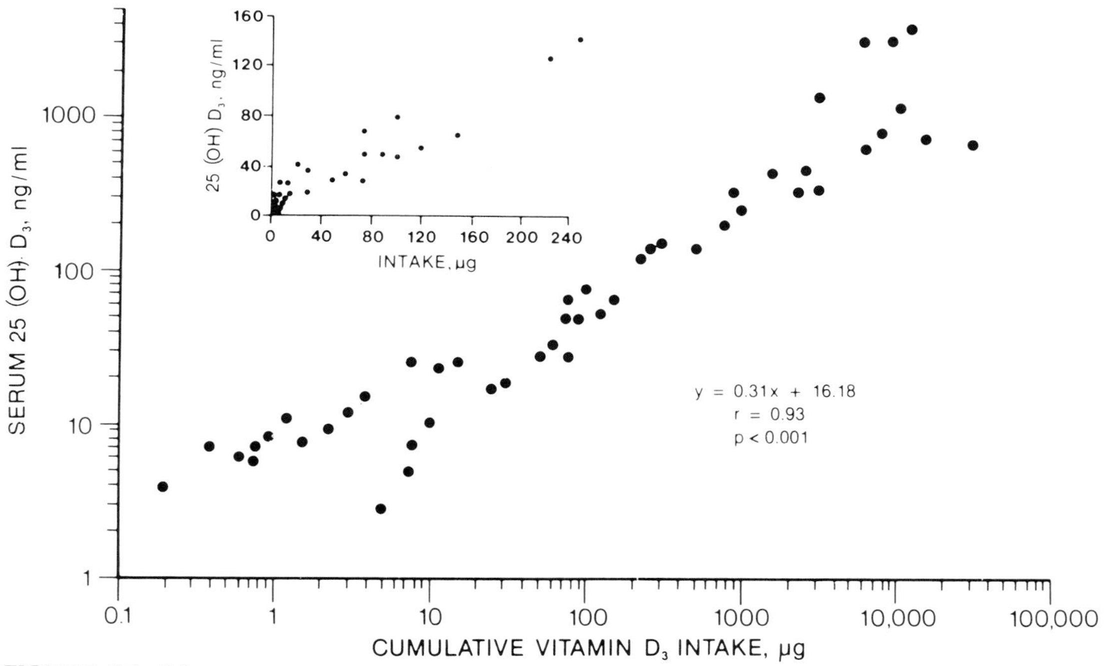
SERUM 25 (OH) $D_3$, ng/ml
1000
100
10
1
0.1
1
10
100
1000
10,000
100,000
CUMULATIVE VITAMIN $D_3$ INTAKE, µg
y = 0.31x + 16.18
r = 0.93
p < 0.001
25 (OH) $D_3$, ng/ml
160
120
80
40
0
0 40 80 120 160 200 240
INTAKE, µg

**FIGURE 17–14.** Serum levels of 25-OH-$D_3$, observed in response to various oral doses of vitamin $D_3$ given to vitamin D-deficient rats. A clear linear correlation extends well into the pharmacologic range for both parameters. To convert nanograms per milliliter to nanomoles per liter, multiply by 2.50. (From Holick, M.F.: Vitamin D: Relevance for Clinical Medicine. Los Angeles, Nichols Institute, 1981.)

Although low circulating concentrations of 25-OH-D can cause vitamin D deficiency bone disease, it is unlikely that these low levels are responsible for the debilitating osteoporosis-like bone disease associated with severe liver failure. Little correlation exists between the severity of osteopenia and fractures in patients with primary biliary cirrhosis and other chronic liver disorders with circulating levels of 25-OH-D. Furthermore, treatment of these patients with 25-OH-D or its metabolites has not provided any significant benefit.[47] Because these patients are more prone to developing vitamin D deficiency as a result of associated fat malabsorption, however, it is prudent to increase their vitamin D intake and monitor circulating concentrations of 25-OH-D.

## 25-HYDROXYVITAMIN D TO 1,25-DIHYDROXYVITAMIN D

Although 25-OH-D is the major circulating form of vitamin D, it is biologically inert at physiologic concentrations. In order for it to become active, it must be hydroxylated on carbon 1 by a specific 25-OH-D-1α-hydroxylase that is present in the kidney (see Fig. 17–13).[1–4,21] Although the kidney is the principal site for the production of 1,25$(OH)_2$D under most circumstances, the placenta also appears to play a role in producing 1,25$(OH)_2$D at a time of increased requirement for calcium by the fetus.[48–50] In a variety of reports, authors cite that there are extrarenal sites for the production of 1,25$(OH)_2$D. Most of these studies were conducted in vitro. Certain cultured cells, such as placental cells, human bone cells, keratinocytes, and stimulated monocytes, also produce 1,25$(OH)_2D_3$.[3,4,51–53] Some people speculate that 1,25$(OH)_2$D may be produced locally in cells to act in an autocrine or paracrine manner. In patients who have had bilateral nephrectomy or have chronic renal failure, the concentrations of 1,25$(OH)_2$D in the circulation usually are low or undetectable. Thus, the kidney is the principal organ responsible for activating vitamin D for the regulation of calcium metabolism.

## ALTERNATIVE METABOLISM OF 25-HYDROXYVITAMIN D

25-OH-D as well as its biologically active metabolite 1,25$(OH)_2$D can act as substrates for a variety of hydroxylases. The principal site of metabolism is the side chain where carbons 23, 24, and 26 undergo hydroxylation and oxidation to yield a plethora of metabolites of 25-OH-D and 1,25$(OH)_2$D.[2–4,21] Although the metabolic importance of these side-chain modifications is uncertain, most likely they are related to the deactivation and rapid clearance of 1,25$(OH)_2$D. This statement is particularly true for the C-23 and C-24 oxidations, which ultimately yield a biologically inactive, water-soluble metabolite 1α-OH-24,25,26,27-tetranor-23-COOH-vitamin $D_3$ (calcitroic acid).[2,54] In addition to the multiple hydroxylations in the side chain, 25-OH-$D_3$ can have its A ring oxidized whereby the C-19 is replaced with a keto group. This reaction occurs in vivo in ruminants and in vitro in chick kidney homogenates, resulting in the conversion of 25-OH-$D_3$ to the *cis* and *trans* isomers of 10-keto-19-nor-25-hydroxyvitamin $D_3$.[2,4,54] Although this keto metabolite is biologically inactive, it is of interest because it co-migrates on many chromatographic systems with 1,25$(OH)_2D_3$ and can be mistaken for 1,25$(OH)_2D_3$. Additional chromatography using methylene chloride as one of the solvents separates these metabolites.[4,55]

To date, more than 25 metabolites of vitamin D have been structurally identified. All of these metabolites are biologically less active on a weight basis when compared to 1,25$(OH)_2$D. At present, many people believe that most of the side-chain and A-ring metabolites exist only in intoxicated states and are not relevant to the physiologic actions of vitamin D.

## REGULATION OF VITAMIN D METABOLISM

The synthesis of vitamin D in the skin and its metabolism to 1,25$(OH)_2D_3$ is regulated carefully by the body. Sunlight regulates the total production of previtamin $D_3$ and vitamin $D_3$ in the skin. Once vitamin D enters the circulation, it can be stored in the fat for later use or metabolized in the liver to 25-OH-D. This hydroxylation step is feedback regulated. The most critical step in the vitamin D metabolism pathway is the production of 1,25$(OH)_2$D by the kidney. During periods of calcium deprivation, circulating ionized calcium concentrations decline. The parathyroid glands immediately detect this decrease and increase the production and secretion of parathyroid hormone.[56] The principal role of parathyroid hormone in calcium metabolism is to increase the tubular reabsorption of calcium from the renal tubular ultrafiltrate and by increasing the renal production of 1,25$(OH)_2$D. 1,25$(OH)_2$D travels to the small intestine where it increases the efficiency of intestinal calcium absorption. 1,25$(OH)_2$D, along with parathyroid hormone act synergistically to induce monocytic stem cells to become mature functioning osteoclasts, which in turn mobilize calcium stores from bone (see Fig. 17–13).

It is generally believed that parathyroid hormone does not directly regulate the renal 25-OH-D-1α-hydroxylase. Evidence suggests that the hypophosphatemic effect of parathyroid hormone is ultimately responsible for enhancing the renal 1α-hydroxylase activity.[57] In healthy men, phosphorus restriction caused an increase in circulating concentrations of 1,25$(OH)_2$D to 80% above control values; this increase was related to an increase in the production rate without any change in the metabolic clearance of this hormone (Fig. 17–15). With phosphorus supplementation, serum concentrations of 1,25$(OH)_2$D decreased abruptly, reaching a nadir within 2 to 4 days. After 10 days of supplementation, the mean concentration of 1,25$(OH)_2$D was 29% lower than the value measured when phosphorus intake was normal (see Fig. 17–15).

Under certain physiologic circumstances, factors other than calcium, phosphorus, and parathyroid hormone may also modulate the activity of 25-OH-D-1-hydroxylase.[4] The efficiency of intestinal calcium transport is enhanced when calcium demands by the body are increased during pregnancy, lactation, and skeletal growth. Because 1,25$(OH)_2$D is the principal hormone responsible for the regulation of calcium absorption in the small intestine, it is not surprising that growth hormone, estrogen, and prolactin can directly or indirectly enhance the renal production of 1,25$(OH)_2$D in various in vitro and in vivo animal models.[58–62] Although estrogen appears to play a significant role in regulating the production of 1,25$(OH)_2$D in the laying hen, estrogen and progesterone likely do not play a significant role in the renal production of 1,25$(OH)_2$D.[63–66] This statement is based on the observation that circulating free concentrations of 1,25$(OH)_2$D do not change in women before, during, and after menopause (Fig. 17–16). Furthermore, circulating concentrations of 1,25$(OH)_2$D were not altered in young women with estrogen deficiency caused by anorexia nervosa.[64] A few authors have suggested that circulating concentrations of 1,25$(OH)_2$D are slightly lower in osteoporotic women compared to age-matched control subjects. Estrogen replacement in postmenopausal women, however, caused only a modest, insignificant elevation in circulating concentrations of 1,25$(OH)_2$D.[67]

It has been demonstrated, however, that the responsiveness of the renal 25-OH-D-1α-hydroxylase to par-

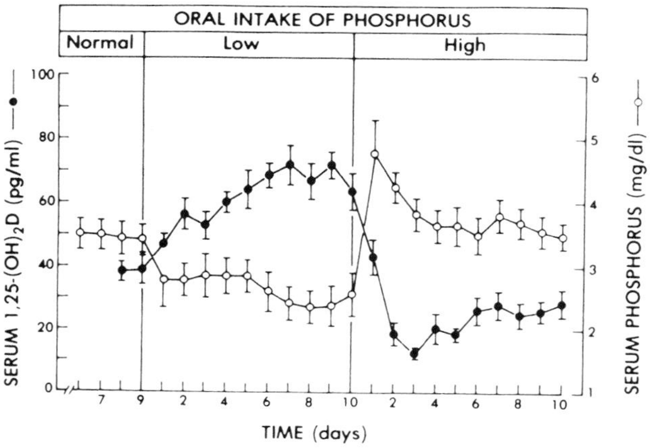
ORAL INTAKE OF PHOSPHORUS
Normal
Low
High
SERUM 1,25-(OH)2D (pg/ml)
SERUM PHOSPHORUS (mg/dl)
100
80
60
40
20
0
6
5
4
3
2
1
7
9
2
4
6
8
10
2
4
6
8
10
TIME (days)

**FIGURE 17–15.** Effect of changes in the oral intake of phosphorus on the fasting serum concentrations of 1,25$(OH)_2$D (to convert pg/ml to pM/L, multiply by 2.40) and phosphorus in six healthy men. The bracketed points depict means values + SEM. (From Portale, A.A., Halloran, B.P., Murphy, M.M., et al.: J. Clin. Invest., *77*:7–12, 1986.)

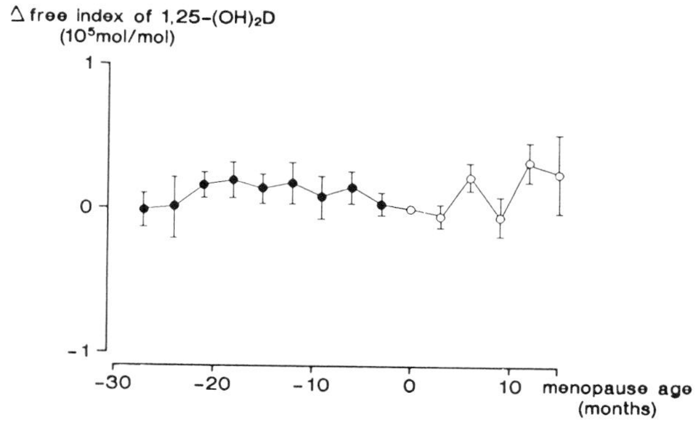
Δ free index of 1,25-(OH)₂D
(10⁵mol/mol)
1
0
-1
-30
-20
-10
0
10
menopause age
(months)

**FIGURE 17–16.** Serum concentrations of free index $1,25(OH)_2D$ in 10 women passing a natural menopause (closed circles, premenopausal; open circles, postmenopausal). Values are the mean ± 1 SEM. (From Hartwell, D., Riis, B.J., Christiansen, C.: J. Clin. Endocrinol. Metab., *71*:127–132, 1990.)

athyroid hormone may be affected by either age or osteoporosis.[67,68] When osteoporotic women were infused with a synthetic fragment of parathyroid hormone, circulating concentrations of $1,25(OH)_2D$ increased twofold within 24 hours in healthy young control subjects, whereas no significant increase was observed in older osteoporotic patients. Whether the moment-to-moment regulation of renal 25-OH-D-1α-hydroxylase in response to parathyroid hormone is altered with aging or osteoporosis, and its role in the disease process, remain to be determined.

## BIOLOGIC FUNCTIONS

### ROLE IN CALCIUM AND PHOSPHORUS METABOLISM

The principal physiologic function of vitamin D in vertebrates including humans is to maintain intracellular and extracellular calcium concentrations within a physiologically acceptable range. Vitamin D accomplishes this goal through the action of $1,25(OH)_2D$ on regulating calcium and phosphorus metabolism in the intestine and bone. $1,25(OH)_2D$ interacts with a specific high affinity receptor in its respective target tissue.[2–4] This rare intracellular protein has been cloned and belongs to the superfamily of the steroid hormone zinc finger receptors.[69] It selectively binds $1,25(OH)_2D_3$ with high affinity, which in turn binds avidly to nuclei and chromatin.[16] This nuclear binding activity likely results in the transcription of hormone-specific mRNA, which in turn govern the translation of several proteins including the calcium-binding protein (Fig. 17–17).[70] This protein is thought to be important in the transcellular transport of calcium in the intestine. The net result is an increase in the absorption of calcium and phosphorus from intestinal contents into the circulation (see Fig. 17–13).

$1,25(OH)_2D$ has a variety of effects on bone cells. In keeping with its principal physiologic function in maintaining serum calcium levels within an acceptable physiologic range for cellular activity, it enhances the mobilization of calcium and phosphorus stores from bone at times of calcium deprivation. $1,25(OH)_2D$ induces stem cell monocytes to become mature osteoclasts.[71] Once mature, osteoclasts lose their nuclear receptors for $1,25(OH)_2D$, and therefore, are no longer responsive to this hormone.[72]

Osteoblasts have nuclear receptors for $1,25(OH)_2D$.[2–4] In vitro studies have suggested that $1,25(OH)_2D$ increases alkaline phosphatase activity and the gene expression for osteocalcin.[73,74] Although vitamin D is regarded as essential for the development and maintenance of a healthy skeleton, evidence is minimal to suggest an active role of $1,25(OH)_2D$ in bone mineralization. Two studies in vitamin D-deficient rats either maintained on a high-calcium, high-phosphorus, vitamin D-deficient diet or infused with calcium and phosphorus to maintain serum calcium and phosphorus concentrations within the normal range showed that they were capable of mineralizing their bones in a similar fashion to groups of rats maintained on a normal-calcium, normal-phosphorus, vitamin-D sufficient diet.[75,76] These data suggest that vitamin D and its metabolites are not absolutely required for the bone ossification process. Instead, vitamin D is responsible for maintaining extracellular calcium and phosphorus concentrations in a supersaturated state that results in the mineralization of bone.[4]

### OTHER BIOLOGIC ACTIONS OF $1,25(OH)_2D$

During the past decade, a considerable amount of effort has been directed toward identifying actions of $1,25(OH)_2D$ that are not directly related to maintenance of calcium and phosphorus homeostasis. The impetus for this search resulted from the observation that a variety of tissues that were not related to calcium metabolism possessed nuclear receptors for $1,25(OH)_2D$ (Table 17–1).[2–4,77] Since these initial observations, careful analysis has shown that these tissues as well as activated B and T lymphocytes[78,79] and several cultured normal and tumor cell lines possess high affinity, low capacity $1,25(OH)_2D$-receptor-like proteins that are quantitatively similar to the intestinal receptor.[2–4]

The first insight into a noncalcemic action of $1,25(OH)_2D_3$ was suggested when promyeloid leukemic cells (line M-1) that had nuclear receptors for $1,25(OH)_2D_3$ responded to this hormone by differentiating into macrophages.[80] $1,25(OH)_2D_3$ induced in a time- and dose-dependent manner phagocytic activity and expression of cell surface antigens including Fc and C3 receptors and lysozyme activity. Similar studies were done in a human promyelocytic leukemic cell line

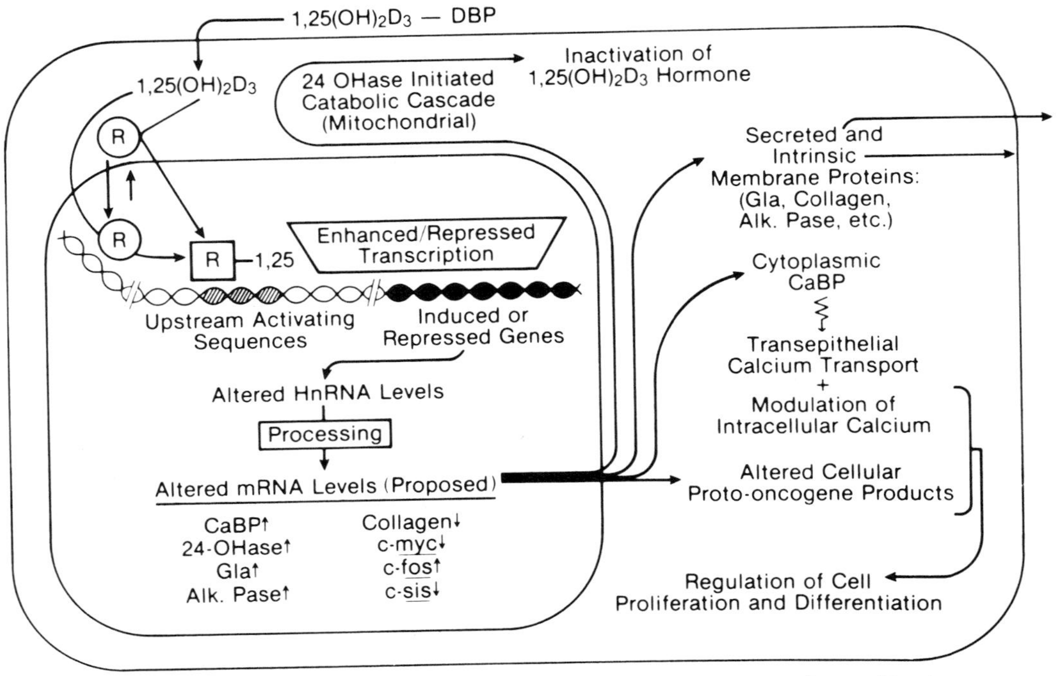

1,25(OH)2D3 — DBP
1,25(OH)2D3
24 OHase Initiated Catabolic Cascade (Mitochondrial)
Inactivation of 1,25(OH)2D3 Hormone
R
R
R
1,25
Enhanced/Repressed Transcription
Secreted and Intrinsic Membrane Proteins: (Gla, Collagen, Alk. Pase, etc.)
Cytoplasmic CaBP
Upstream Activating Sequences
Induced or Repressed Genes
Transepithelial Calcium Transport
+
Modulation of Intracellular Calcium
Altered HnRNA Levels
Processing
Altered mRNA Levels (Proposed)
Altered Cellular Proto-oncogene Products
CaBP↑
24-OHase↑
Gla↑
Alk. Pase↑
Collagen↓
c-myc↓
c-fos↑
c-sis↓
Regulation of Cell Proliferation and Differentiation


**FIGURE 17–17.** Proposed mechanism of action of $1,25(OH)_2D_3$ in target cells resulting in a variety of biologic responses. (From Haussler, M.R., Donaldson, C.A., Kelly, M.A., et al.: Functions and mechanism of action of the 1,25-dihydroxyvitamin $D_3$ receptor. *In* Vitamin D: A Chemical, Biochemical and Clinical Update. Edited by A.W. Norman et al. New York, Walter de Gruyter, 1985.)

**TABLE 17–1.** $1,25(OH)_2D_3$ RECEPTOR DISTRIBUTION AMONG MAMMALIAN TISSUES

| | |
|---|---|
| Intestine | Thymus |
| Kidney | Lymphocytes |
| Bone | Monocytes-macrophages |
| Parathyroid | Testes |
| Brain | Ovary |
| Pituitary | Uterus |
| Parotid | Placenta |
| Pancreas | Breast |
| Stomach | Embryonic liver |
| Skin | Embryonic muscle |

(HL-60). Cell growth was inhibited by as little as $10^{-9}$ M of $1,25(OH)_2D_3$ in a dose-dependent manner.[81] $1,25(OH)_2D_3$ was also found to be an effective antiproliferative agent for cultured tumor cells, such as tumor breast cells and melanoma cells, that possessed its nuclear receptor.[82]

The effect of $1,25(OH)_2D_3$ on leukemia cells is reversible. When clones of HL-60 cells that possessed less than 10% of nuclear binding activity for $1,25(OH)_2D_3$ were incubated with $1,25(OH)_2D_3$, little difference in their proliferative activity was noted.[83]

Of interest was that human epidermal cells had nuclear receptors for $1,25(OH)_2D_3$. $1,25(OH)_2D_3$ inhibited the proliferation and induced terminal differentiation of cultured murine and human keratinocytes in a dose-dependent manner.[84,85] These laboratory observations have been put to practical use by the development of $1,25(OH)_2D_3$ and its analogues as a safe and effective treatment for the hyperproliferative epidermal disorder psoriasis.[86–90]

## USE AND INTERPRETATION OF ASSAYS FOR VITAMIN D AND ITS METABOLITES

### VITAMIN D AND 25-OH-D ASSAYS

The first assays for vitamin D were chick and rat bioassays.[91,92] The rat bioassay, commonly known as the line-test, was used widely to determine the concentration of vitamin D in fortified foods such as milk.[93] The development of specific assays for vitamin D and its biologically important metabolites made these bioassays obsolete.

A specific assay to measure circulating concentrations of vitamin $D_2$ and vitamin $D_3$ has been developed.[94,95] This assay has been of great value in evaluating circulating concentrations of vitamin D after exposure to quantitative doses of UV-B radiation.[44] It has also been useful as a provocative test for determining which patients with intestinal malabsorption syndromes are at risk for developing vitamin D deficiency.[41] Using this assay, the half-life of circulating vitamin D is approximately 24 hours. The serum concentration of vitamin D at any time depends on the most recent ingestion of vitamin D as well as the last exposure to sunlight. The normal range of serum vitamin D is 0 to 310 nmol/L (0 to 120 ng/ml). Consequently, serum vitamin $D_2$ and vitamin $D_3$ concentrations are of little value in determining the vitamin D status of a patient.

Circulating concentrations of 25-OH-D are measured by a specific competitive protein-binding assay using the vitamin D-binding protein.[96–99] Because the half-life of circulating 25-OH-D is approximately 3 weeks, the steady state concentration of 25-OH-D in the circulation summates the concentrations of vitamin D derived from both diet and from photoproduction over several weeks to several months.[91] 25-OH-$D_2$ and 25-OH-$D_3$ can be measured separately.[99,100] Originally, it was thought that 25-OH-$D_2$ was reflective of the dietary component of vitamin D and 25-OH-$D_3$ was reflective of exposure to sunlight. Because milk and multivitamin preparations are now fortified with both forms of the vitamin, however, the separate measurement of these metabolites is of little value.[92]

Measurement of the circulating concentration of 25-OH-D is most valuable for determining the vitamin D status of an individual. The normal circulating concentration of 25-OH-D is usually reported to be between 20 and 150 nmol/L (8 and 60 ng/ml). Serum values below 25 nmol/L (10 ng/ml) are considered to indicate impending or overt vitamin D deficiency. Although most diagnostic laboratories report the upper limit of the normal range for 25-OH-D to be 150 nmol/L (60 ng/mL), a circulating concentration of 250 nmol/L (100 ng/ml) in lifeguards after a full summer of exposure to sunlight is not surprising and is considered normal. Vitamin D intoxication is usually associated with 25-OH-D concentrations above 375 nmol/L (150 ng/ml) with attendant hypercalcemia and hyperphosphatemia.[56,92]

The assay for serum 25-OH-D has clinical utility for determining vitamin D deficiency in patients with intestinal malabsorption syndromes, severe hepatic failure, and the nephrotic syndrome. It is the hallmark assay for determining vitamin D deficiency in very young and elderly individuals.

### 1,25-DIHYDROXYVITAMIN D ASSAYS

Specific assays for 1,25$(OH)_2$D in serum and plasma have been developed with a competitive receptor binding assay using a nuclear/cytosolic receptor for 1,25$(OH)_2$D. After several improvements, the assay now involves the use of a bovine thymus 1,25$(OH)_2$D receptor that recognizes 1,25$(OH)_2D_2$ and 1,25$(OH)_2D_3$ equally well.[91,92,101–103] A bioassay has also been developed using cultured calvaria.[104] This assay, which is tedious to conduct, measures directly the biologic activity of 1,25$(OH)_2$D in serum.

The half-life of circulating 1,25$(OH)_2$D has been estimated to be between 4 and 6 hours. Normal range of serum values is between 38 and 144 pmol/L (16 and 60 pg/ml). As vitamin D deficiency develops, the body responds by increasing the production and secretion of parathyroid hormone (see Fig. 17–13). Parathyroid hormone in turn enhances the 1-hydroxylation of 25-OH-D. Thus, secondary hyperparathyroidism associated with vitamin D deficiency accelerates the conversion of 25-OH-D to 1,25$(OH)_2$D. Because the circulating concentration of 25-OH-D is about three orders of magnitude higher than that of 1,25$(OH)_2$D, even low levels of 25-OH-D in the blood can provide enough substrate for the formation of 1,25$(OH)_2$D. Thus, a patient who is becoming vitamin D deficient will still have enough 25-OH-D substrate for the renal 25-OH-D-1α-hydroxylase. As a result, a patient who has low stores of vitamin D and is becoming vitamin D deficient can have low, normal, or even high circulating concentrations of 1,25$(OH)_2$D.[56] If a patient who is vitamin D deficient enters a hospital and obtains vitamin D either from the short exposure to sunlight while on the way to the hospital or from dietary sources in the hospital, the vitamin D is rapidly metabolized to 25-OH-D and then to 1,25$(OH)_2$D. As a result, circulating levels of 1,25$(OH)_2$D can be elevated to twice normal levels for several months.[44] Thus, serum 1,25$(OH)_2$D concentrations are of little value in evaluating vitamin D deficiency. Needless to say, in an absolute vitamin D deficiency state, circulating concentrations of 1,25$(OH)_2$D are undetectable.

The measurement of circulating concentrations of 1,25$(OH)_2$D has been of great value to clinicians for evaluating patients with inherited and acquired disorders of 25-OH-D metabolism. Patients with chronic renal failure, hyperphosphatemia, hypoparathyroidism, pseudohypoparathyroidism, tumor-induced osteomalacia, hypercalcemia of malignancy (in most cases), or vitamin D-dependent rickets type I (an inborn error reducing the conversion of 25-OH-D to 1,25$(OH)_2$D) often have low circulating concentrations of 1,25$(OH)_2$D.[2–4,56,91,92] Serum concentrations of 1,25$(OH)_2$D are above normal in some patients with primary hyperparathyroidism; vitamin D-dependent rickets type II (an inborn error in which the recognition of 1,25$(OH)_2$D by target tissue receptors is defective); chronic granulomatous disorders such as sarcoidosis, tuberculosis, and silicosis; and lymphoma. It is now recognized that chronic granulomatous disorders and some lymphomas that activate macrophages and lymphoma cells, respectively, can 1α-hydroxylate 25-OH-D, a process that is inhibited by glucocorticoids.[2–4,56,91,92]

## RECOMMENDATIONS

### EXPOSURE TO SUNLIGHT

It is not often appreciated that casual exposure to sunlight during everyday activities provides most humans with their vitamin D requirement.[105] With the increased awareness from scientific and lay press about the causal relationship between long-term exposure to sunlight with skin cancer and skin wrinkling, sunscreen use is more prevalent.[10] Because children and young active adults often are outdoors for short periods of time at least two or three times per week, this casual exposure to sunlight will provide their vitamin D requirement. The elderly population, on the other hand, have a decreased capacity to produce vitamin D in their skin. In addition, they are likely to heed the warnings about the damaging effects of sunlight and use a sunscreen and wear more clothing, thus preventing the cutaneous synthesis of vitamin $D_3$. Because many elderly individuals do not drink milk because of a lactase deficiency or because of their misconception that they no longer need to drink milk (it is only for growing children), their only source of vitamin D is from either a multivitamin pill containing vitamin D or exposure to sunlight. If elderly persons do not take advantage of the beneficial effect of sunlight, they can develop vitamin D deficiency, which can result in secondary hyperparathyroidism. This condition accelerates osteoporosis and can cause a mineralization defect in bones, resulting in adult rickets or osteomalacia. The net effect of this process on bone is likely to weaken bones and increase the risk of fracture.[105–110] Results of several studies indicate that vitamin D deficiency does put elderly individuals at risk for developing hip fractures. A recent epidemiologic survey in a controlled nursing home environment revealed that both free-living and institutionalized elderly persons who took a vitamin supplement or drank two to three glasses of milk per day were vitamin D sufficient. Of those individuals who did not take a vitamin D supplement or drink milk, approximately 80% were overtly to borderline vitamin D deficient by the end of the winter (Fig. 17–18).[111] Thus, especially for elderly people, exposure to sunlight in the morning or late afternoon in the spring, summer, and fall (depending on skin sensitivity to sunlight) will provide the recommended vitamin D requirement and will permit them to store any excess vitamin D in fat for use during the winter months. Elderly individuals need not be exposed to prolonged periods of sunlight, because the amount that they can produce in this period of time should satisfy their body's requirement. Therefore, I recommend for the elderly population in Boston 5 to 30 minutes of exposure (depending on their sensitivity to sunlight) to a suberythemal amount of sunlight. This recommendation is based on our observation that if you take a healthy individual and expose their whole body to one minimal erythemal dose of simulated sunlight, the circulating vitamin D concentrations are comparable to the ingestion of 10,000 IU of vitamin D. After elderly individuals are exposed to sunlight for a short period, they should apply a sunscreen, with a sun protection factor of at least 8, which will protect them from the chronic damaging effects of excessive exposure to sunlight.[10]

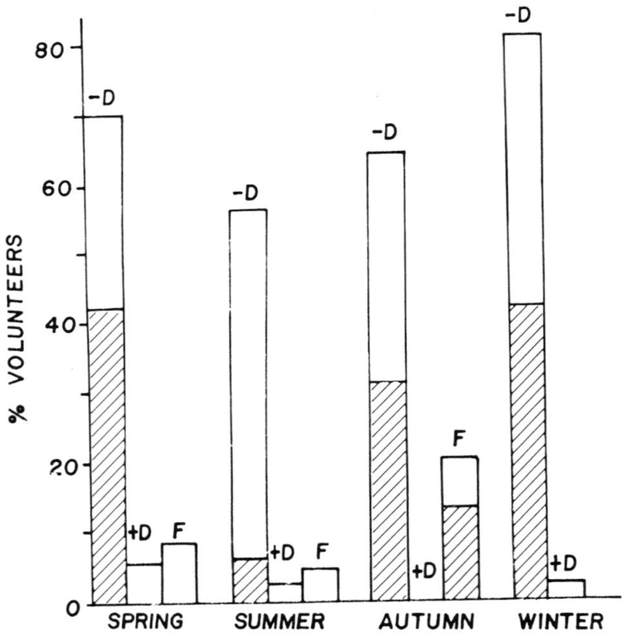
% VOLUNTEERS
80
60
40
20
0
-D
+D
F
SPRING
SUMMER
AUTUMN
WINTER

**FIGURE 17–18.** Seasonal averages of the percentage of volunteers with circulating concentrations of 25(OH)D <37.5 nmol/L (unshaded areas) and 25(OH)D <25.0 nmol (shaded areas). Volunteers are represented as those with (+D) and without (−D) vitamin D supplements and free-living subjects (F), who were without supplements. (From Webb, A.R., Pilbeam, C., Hanafin, N., et al.: J. Clin. Nutr., *51*:1075–1081, 1990.)

## VITAMIN D SUPPLEMENTS

A variety of pharmaceutical preparations are available by prescription. These include a capsule that contains 50,000 IU of vitamin $D_2$ and an oil preparation that contains 100,000 IU/ml. Pharmaceutical preparations containing 50,000 IU of vitamin $D_2$ have been of value in treating vitamin D deficiency in elderly patients and in patients with intestinal malabsorption syndromes, hepatic failure, and nephrotic syndrome. The dose is generally 50,000 IU once per week. Circulating concentrations of 25-OH-D should be evaluated every 2 to 3 months to prevent vitamin D intoxication. Once circulating levels of 25-OH-D are in the mid-normal range, the frequency of administering 50,000 IU of vitamin $D_2$ can be decreased to once or twice per month. For those unable to ingest a capsule containing vitamin D, an alternative source is an oil-based preparation. I usually recommend that patients take 800 IU each day until circulating concentrations of 25-OH-D are in the mid-normal range. Once these concentrations have returned to normal, I recommend an over-the-counter multivitamin containing 400 IU of vitamin D. Because most pharmaceutical companies put in 1.5 to 2 times the amount of vitamin D stated on the label, patients often receive up to 800 IU of vitamin D per day. This amount is usually sufficient to maintain adequate circulating concentrations of 25-OH-D (Fig. 17–19).

## RECOMMENDED DAILY ALLOWANCE OF VITAMIN D FOR HUMANS

Beginning in the 1930s, milk was fortified with 400 IU (10 μg) of vitamin $D_2$ per quart. This fortification process eliminated rickets as a significant health problem in the United States and other countries that used this practice. During World War II, milk was supplemented with up to 2000 IU of vitamin D to compensate for wartime nutritional deprivation that British children had undergone. Manufacturers often put 1.5 to 2 times as much vitamin D in the food preparations to compensate for anticipated vitamin D breakdown during shelf storage. As a result, an epidemic of hypercalcemia in neonates appeared in the 1940s and 1950s.[112] Although the hypercalcemia was easily reversible, many of the infants suffered from hypercalcemia-induced brain damage. As a result, laws were passed in Europe preventing the fortification of milk and infant formulas with vitamin D.

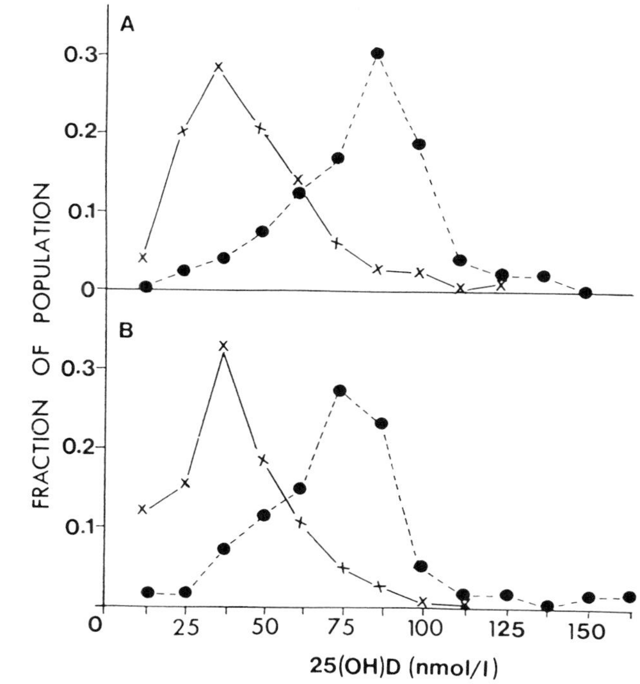
A
B
0.3
0.2
0.1
0
FRACTION OF POPULATION
25
50
75
100
125
150
25(OH)D (nmol/l)

**FIGURE 17–19.** Distribution of circulating concentrations of 25(OH)D for residents with (closed circles) and without (x) vitamin D supplements in September (A) and February (B). Each data point represents n − 10 to n; e.g., 75 represents all samples between 65 and 75.0 nmol/L. (From Webb, A.R., Pilbeam, C., Hanafin, N., et al.: J. Clin. Nutr., *51*:1075–1081, 1990.)

In the United States, infant formula is fortified with 400 IU of vitamin D per quart. It has been estimated that a minimum of 100 IU of vitamin D daily is required to prevent rickets in infants. To provide a margin of safety, the recommended dietary allowance was set at 300 IU for infants from birth to 3 months of age, which is approximately the amount consumed by formula-fed normal infants. Because human milk contains little vitamin D activity, it has been recommended that breast-fed infants receive exposure to sunlight or ingest formula supplemented with vitamin D. The recommended allowance for children older than 3 months has been set at 400 IU to satisfy their requirement during rapid periods of bone growth and mineralization.

In the mid-1960s, studies in infants fed either 300 IU, 350 to 550 IU, or 1380 to 2170 IU daily demonstrated no differences in growth in length or weight or in serum calcium concentrations. Earlier studies, however, suggested that daily ingestion of 2000 to 5000 IU of vitamin D in the diet caused hypercalcemia and all of its clinical features.[112]

Vitamin D deficiency osteomalacia is associated with intakes of less than 100 IU of vitamin D per day. The recommended allowance of 200 IU (5 μg) for adults appears to be reasonable. Because aging does not alter vitamin D absorption,[105] the recommended daily allowance is not increased for elderly adults. Most studies, however, have been conducted in otherwise healthy individuals who received some exposure to sunlight. Thus, the combination of exposure to sunlight with 200 IU of vitamin D is adequate for satisfying the body's requirement for this essential vitamin/prohormone. The exact amount of vitamin D that is required by adults who are not exposed to sunlight is less well understood. A study conducted in young adult submariners who received a vitamin D supplement that contained 600 IU of vitamin $D_2$ for their 3-month mission showed that circulating concentrations of 25-OH-D were maintained at the same levels (Paris, Holick, Bondi, Luria, unpublished results).

Pregnancy increases the demand for vitamin D, especially during the last trimester. As a result, the recommended allowance for vitamin D during pregnancy is increased to 400 IU per day.

## ACKNOWLEDGMENTS

This work was supported in part by the following NIH grants: AG06079, AR36963, DK43690, AG04390.

## REFERENCES


1. Holick, M.F.: Phylogenetic and evolutionary aspects of vitamin D from phytoplankton to humans. *In* Vertebrate Endocrinology: Fundamentals and Biomedical Implications. Vol. 3. Edited by P.K.T. Pang, M.P. Schreibman. Orlando, Academic Press, 1989, pp. 7–43.
2. DeLuca, H.: FASEB J., *2:*224–236, 1988.
3. Reichel, H., Koeffler, H.P., Norman, A.W.: N. Engl. J. Med., *320:*981–991, 1989.
4. Holick, M.F.: Vitamin D: Biosynthesis, metabolism, and mode of action. *In* Endocrinology. Vol. 2. Edited by L.J. DeGroot. New York, Grune and Stratton, 1989, pp. 902–926.
5. Fraser, D., Scriver, C.R.: Hereditary disorders associated with vitamin-D resistance or defective phosphate metabolism. *In* Endocrinology. Vol. 2. Edited by L. DeGroot. New York, Grune and Stratton, 1979.
6. Schmorl, G.: Med. U. Kinderh. IV, 403, 1909.
7. Sniadecki, J. (1840): Cited by W. Mozolowski. Nature, *143:*121, 1939.
8. Owen, I.: Br. Med. J., *1:*113–116, 1889.
9. Holick, M.F.: Vitamin D3: Synthesis and biologic functions in skin. *In* Pharmacology of the Skin. Edited by H. Mukhtar. Boca Raton, FL, CRC Press, 1991, pp. 183–202.
10. Palm, T.A.: Practitioner, *45:*270–279, 321–342, 1890.
11. Huldschinsky, K.: Dtsch. Med. Wochenschr., *45:*712–713, 1919.
12. Hess, A.F., Unger, L.F.: JAMA, *77:*39, 1921.
13. Mayer, J.: Nutr. Rev., *15:*321–323, 1957.
14. Mellanby, T.: J. Physiol., *52:*11–14, 1918.
15. McCollum, E.F., Simmonds, N., Becker, J.E., et al.: J. Biol. Chem., *53:*293–312, 1922.
16. Powers, G.F., Park, E.A., Shipley, P.G., et al.: Proc. Soc. Exp. Biol. Med., *19:*120–121, 1921.
17. Hess, A.F., Weinstock, M.: J. Biol. Chem., *62:*301–313, 1924.
18. Steenbock, H., Black, A.: J. Biol. Chem., *61:*408–422, 1924.
19. Holick, M.F., MacLaughlin, J.A., Parrish, J.A., et al.: The photochemistry and photobiology of vitamin $D_3$. *In* The Science of Photomedicine. Edited by J.D. Regan, J.A. Parrish. New York, Plenum Press, 1982.
20. Fieser, L.D., Fieser, M.: Vitamin D. *In* Steroids. New York, Reinhold, 1959, pp. 90–168.
21. Holick, M.F.: Vitamin D and the skin: Photobiology, physiology and therapeutic efficacy for psoriasis. *In* Bone and Mineral Research. 7th Ed. Edited by J. Heersche, J. Kanis. Amsterdam, Elsevier Science, 1990.
22. Massengale, O.N., Nussmeier, M.: J. Biol. Chem., *87:*423–425, 1930.
23. Steenbock, H., Kletzien, S.W.F.: J. Biol. Chem., *97:*249–264, 1932.
24. Waddell, J.: J. Biol. Chem., *105:*711–739, 1934.
25. Windaus, A., Bock, F.: Hoppe-Seyler's Z. Physiol. Chem., *245:*168, 1937.
26. Velluz, L., Petit, A., Amiard, G.: Bull. Soc. Chim. Fr., *15:*1115–1120, 1948.
27. Velluz, L., Amiard, G., Petit, A.: Bull. Soc. Chim. Fr., *16:*501–508, 1949.
28. MacLaughlin, J.A., Holick, M.F.: Mediation of cutaneous vitamin $D_3$ synthesis by UV radiation. *In* Biochemistry and Physiology of the Skin. Edited by L.A. Goldsmith. Oxford, Oxford University Press, 1983.
29. Holick, M.F., MacLaughlin, J.A., Doppelt, S.H.: Science, *211:*590–593, 1981.
30. Anderson, R.R., Parrish, J.A.: Optical properties of human skin. *In* The Science of Photomedicine. Edited by J.D. Regan, J.A. Parrish. New York, Plenum Press, 1982.
31. Holick, M., MacLaughlin, J., Clark, M., et al.: Science, *210:*203–205, 1980.
32. Loomis, F.: Science, *157:*501–506, 1967.
33. Clemens, T.L., Henderson, S.L., Adams, J.S., Holick, M.F.: Lancet, 74–76, 1982.
34. Webb, A.R., DeCosta, B.R., Holick, M.F.: J. Clin. Endocrinol. Metab., *68:*882–887, 1989.
35. MacLaughlin, J.A., Holick, M.F.: J. Clin. Invest., *76:*1536–1538, 1985.
36. Holick, M.F., Matsuoka, L.Y., Wortsman, J.: Lancet, *2:*1104–1105, 1989.
37. Montagna, W., Carlisle, M.S.: J. Invest. Dermatol., *73:*47–53, 1979.
38. Matsuoka, L.Y., Ide, L., Wortsman, J., et al.: J. Clin. Endocrinol. Metab., *64:*1165–1168, 1987.
39. Matsuoka, L.Y., Wortsman, J., Hanifan, N., et al.: Arch. Dermatol., *124:*1802–1804, 1988.
40. Webb, A.R., Kline, L., Holick, M.F.: J. Clin. Endocrinol. Metab., *67:*373–378, 1988.
41. Lo, C.W., Paris, P.W., Clemens, T.L., et al.: Am. J. Clin. Nutr., *42:*644–649, 1985.
42. Holick, M.F.: Kidney Int., *32:*912–929, 1987.
43. Bell, N.H.: J. Clin. Invest., *76:*1–6, 1985.
44. Adams, J.A., Clemens, T.L., Parrish, J.A., et al.: N. Engl. J. Med., *306:*722–725, 1981.
45. Holick, M.F., Clark, M.B.: Fed. Proc., *37:*2567–2574, 1978.
46. Long, R.G., Skinner, R.K., Meinhard, E., et al.: Gut, *17:*824–827, 1976.
47. Kaplan, M.M., Goldberg, M.J., Matloff, D.S., et al.: Gastroenterology, *81:*681–685, 1981.
48. Gray, T.K., Lester, G.E., Lorenc, R.S.: Science, *204:*1311–1313, 1979.
49. Weisman, Y., Vargas, A., Duckett, G., et al.: Endocrinology, *103:*1992–1996, 1978.
50. Tanaka, Y., Halloran, B., Schnoes, H.K., et al.: Proc. Natl. Acad. Sci. U.S.A., *76:*5033–5035, 1979.
51. Mason, R.S.: Extra-renal production of $1,25(OH)_2D_3$, the metabolism of vitamin D by non-traditional tissues. *In* Vitamin D: A Chemical, Biochemical and Clinical Update. Edited by A.W. Norman. Berlin, Walter de Gruyter, 1985.
52. Howard, G.A., Turner, R.T., Sherrard, D.J., et al.: J. Biol. Chem., *256:*7738–7740, 1981.
53. Bikle, D.D., Nemanic, M.D., Whitney, J.O., et al.: Biochemistry, *25:*1545–1548, 1986.
54. Napoli, J., Horst, R.: Vitamin D metabolism. *In* Vitamin D: Basic and Clinical Aspects. Edited by R. Kumar. Boston, Martinus Nijhoff, 1984.
55. Gray, T.K., Millington, D.S., Maltby, D.A., et al.: Proc. Natl. Acad. Sci. U.S.A., *82:*8218–8221, 1985.
56. Holick, M.F., Potts, J.R., Jr., Krane, S.M.: Calcium, phosphorus and bone metabolism. *In* Harrison's Principles of Internal Medicine, 12th Ed. Edited by J.D. Wilson, E.

Braunwald, K. Isselbacher, et al. New York, McGraw-Hill, 1990.
57. Portale, A.A., Halloran B.P., Murphy, M.M., et al.: J. Clin. Invest., *77:*7–12, 1986.
58. Fraser, D.: Physiol. Rev., *60:*551–663, 1980.
59. Adams, N.D., Garthwite, T.L., Gray, R.W., et al.: J. Clin. Endocrinol. Metab., *49:*628–630, 1979.
60. Kumar, R., Abboud, C.F., Riggs, B.L.: Mayo Clin. Proc., *55:*51–53, 1980.
61. Kumar, R., Merimee, T.J., Silva, P., et al.: The effect of chronic growth hormone excess or deficiency on plasma 1,25-dihydroxy vitamin D levels in man. *In* Vitamin D, Basic Research and Its Clinical Application. Edited by A.W. Norman et al. Berlin, Walter de Gruyter, 1979.
62. Turner, R.T.: 1,25-Dihydroxyvitamin D-1-hydroxylase, measurements and regulation. *In* Vitamin D: Basic and Clinical Aspects. Edited by R. Kumar. Boston, Martinus Nijhoff, 1984.
63. Krabbe, S., Hummer, L., Christiansen, C.: J. Clin. Endocrinol. Metabol., *62:*503–507, 1986.
64. Rigotti, N.A., Nussbaum, S.R., Herzog, D.B., et al.: N. Engl. J. Med., *311:*1601–1606, 1984.
65. Sowers, M.F., Wallace, R.B., Hollis, B.W.: Bone Miner., *10:*139–148, 1990.
66. Hartwell, D., Riis, B.J., Christiansen, C.: J. Clin. Endocrinol. Metab., *71:*127–132, 1990.
67. Riggs, B.L., Gallagher, J.C., DeLuca, H.F., et al.: Mayo Clin. Proc., *53:*701–706, 1978.
68. Slovik, D.M., Adams, J.S., Neer, R.M., et al.: N. Engl. J. Med., *305:*372–374, 1981.
69. Pike, J.W.: Nutr. Rev., *43:*161–168, 1985.
70. Wasserman, R.H., Fullmer, C.S., Shimura, F.: Calcium absorption and the molecular effects of vitamin $D_3$. *In* Vitamin D: Basic, and Clinical Aspects. Edited by R. Kumar. Boston, Martinus Nijhoff, 1984.
71. Bar-Shavit, Z., Teitelbaum, S.L., Reitsma, P., et al.: Proc. Natl. Acad. Sci. USA, *80:*5907–5910, 1983.
72. Merke, J., Klaus, G., Hugel, U., et al.: J. Clin. Invest., *77:*312–314, 1986.
73. Haussler, M.R., Donaldson, C.A., Kelly M.A., et al.: Functions and mechanism of action of the 1,25-dihydroxyvitamin $D_3$ receptor. *In* Vitamin D: A Chemical, Biochemical and Clinical Update. Edited by A.W. Norman et al. New York, Walter de Gruyter, 1985.
74. Demay, M.B., Roth, D.A., Kronenberg, H.M.: J. Biol. Chem., *264:*2279–2282, 1989.
75. DeLuca, H.F.: The metabolism, physiology, and function of vitamin D. *In* Vitamin D: Basic and Clinical Aspects. Edited by R. Kumar. Boston, Martinus Nijhoff, 1984.
76. Holtrop, M.E., Cox, K.A., Carnes, D.L.: Am. J. Physiol., *251:*E20, 1986.
77. Stumpf, W.E., Sar, M., Reid, F.A., et al.: Science, *206:*1188–1190, 1979.
78. Bhalla, A.K., Clemens, T., Amento, E., et al.: J. Clin. Endocrinol. Metab., *57:*1308–1310, 1983.
79. Provvedine, D.M., Tsoukaas, C.D., Deftos, L.J., et al.: Science, *221:*1181, 1983.
80. Abe, E., Miyaura, C., Sakagami, H., et al.: Proc. Natl. Acad. Sci. USA, *78:*4990–4994, 1981.
81. Tanaka, H., Abe, E., Miyaura, C., et al.: Biochem. J., *204:*713–719, 1982.
82. Eisman, J.A.: 1,25-Dihydroxyvitamin D3 receptor and role of 1,25-dihydroxyvitamin D3 in human cancer cells in vitamin D. *In* Vitamin D: Basic and Clinical Aspects. Edited by R. Kumar. Boston, Martinus Nijhoff, 1984.
83. Bar-Shavit, Z., Kahn, A.J., Stone, K.R., et al.: Endocrinology, *118:*679–686, 1986.
84. Hosomi, J., Hosoi, J., Abe, E., et al.: Endocrinology, *113:*1950–1957, 1983.
85. Smith, E.L., Walworth, N.D., Holick, M.F.: J. Invest. Dermatol., *86:*709–714, 1986.
86. Smith, E.L., Pincus, S.H., Donovan, L., et al.: J. Am. Acad. Dermatol., *19:*516–528, 1988.
87. Holick, M.F.: Arch. Dermatol., *125:*1692–1697, 1989.
88. Morimoto, S., Kumahara, Y.: Med. J. Osaka Univ., *35:*51, 1985.
89. Kragballe, K.: Arch. Dermatol., *125:*1642–1652, 1989.
90. Kato, T., Rokugo, M., Terui, T., et al.: Br. J. Dermatol., *115:*431–433, 1986.
91. Holick, M.F., Adams, J.S.: Vitamin D metabolism and biological function. *In* Vitamin D Metabolism and Biological Function. Edited by L.V. Avioli, S. Krane. Orlando, FL, Grune and Stratton, 1990, pp. 155–195.
92. Holick, M.F.: J. Nutr., *120:*1464–1469, 1990.
93. Steenbock, H., Black, A.: J. Biol. Chem., *61:*408–422, 1924.
94. Clemens, T.L., Adams, J.S., Holick, M.F.: Clin. Chim. Acta, *121:*301–308, 1982.
95. Chen, T., Turner, A., Holick, M.F.: J. Nutr. Biochem., *1:*272–276, 1990.
96. Haddad, J.G., Chuy, K.J.: J. Clin. Endocrinol. Metab., *33:*992–995, 1971.
97. Belsey, R., Clark, M.B., Bernat, M., et al.: Am. J. Med., *57:*50–56, 1974.
98. Hollis, B.W., Burton, J.H., Draper, H.H.: Steroids, *30:*285–293, 1977.
99. Chen, T.C., Turner, A.K., Holick, M.F.: J. Nutr. Biochem., *1:*315–319, 1990.
100. Jones, G.: Clin. Chem., *24:*287–298, 1978.
101. Hollis, B.W.: Clin. Chem., *32:*2060–2063, 1986.
102. Horst, R.: Recent advances in the quantitation of vitamin D and vitamin D metabolites. *In* Vitamin D: Basic and Clinical Aspects. Edited by R. Kumar. Boston, Martinus Nijhoff, 1984.
103. Chen, T.C., Turner, A.K., Holick, M.F.: J. Nutr. Biochem., *1:*320–327, 1990.
104. Stern, P.H., Hamstra, A.J., DeLuca, H.F., et al.: J. Clin. Endocrinol. Metab., *46:*891–896, 1978.
105. Holick, M.F.: Clin. Nutr., *5:*121–129, 1986.
106. Krane, S.M., Holick, M.F.: Metabolic bone disease. *In* Harrison's Principles of Internal Medicine. 12th Ed. Edited by J.D. Wilson, E. Braunwald, K.J. Isselbacher, et al. New York, McGraw-Hill, 1990.
107. Chalmers, J., Conacher, D.H., Gardner, D.L., et al.: J. Bone Joint Surg.[ Br.], *49:*403–423, 1967.
108. Doppelt, S.H., Neer, R.M., Daly, M., et al.: Orthop. Trans., *7:*512–513, 1983.
109. Sokoloff, L.: Am. J. Surg. Pathol., *2:*21–30, 1978.
110. Kavookjian, H., Whitelaw, G., Lin, S., et al.: Orthop. Trans., *14:*580, 1990.
111. Webb, A.R., Pilbeam, C., Hanafin, N., et al.: J. Clin. Nutr., *51:*1075–1081, 1990.
112. Chesney, R.W.: J. Clin. Nutr., *119:*1825–1828, 1990.

CHAPTER 18

# Vitamin E

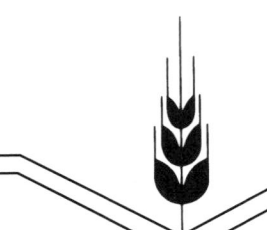

Philip M. Farrell and Robert J. Roberts



During the past decade there have been many developments relating to nutritional and clinical aspects of vitamin E. Methods for assessment of nutritional status have been reexamined critically and improved, particularly with the advent of high performance liquid chromatography (HPLC) to separate the major vitamin E isomers of the tocopherol family.[1-3] Populations of vitamin E deficient patients have been identified and studied with respect to pathologic alterations that might be attributed to the deficiency state.[4] The occurrence of hemolysis in vivo due to tocopherol deficiency has been confirmed and shown to be clinically significant in both infants and older patients with intestinal malabsorption. In addition, it has been demonstrated convincingly in recent years that neurologic dysfunction with degenerative lesions in the spinal cord can develop in chronic vitamin E deficiency.[1] Yet, the vitamin remains an enigma and a continued challenge to both nutritional and clinical scientists. The subcellular role of vitamin E has been particularly difficult to establish, although it clearly functions as a biologic antioxidant. Partly as a result of this gap in knowledge, confusion also persists among medical scientists as to the indications for vitamin E therapy. Although medical benefits of tocopherol pharmacotherapy have been claimed when large doses of dietary supplements were taken by individuals not deficient in vitamin E, the evidence for favorable responses is generally unconvincing.[4-6] The tragic E-Ferol experience using high-dose parenteral vitamin E therapy in newborn premature infants reinforces the risks associated with the trial-and-error approach to clinical problems.[6]

Nevertheless, the essentiality of this vitamin for humans has been well established during the past two decades, and many challenging new concepts have emerged from relevant basic research. The search for clinical disturbances in the human deficiency state has been aided by extensive investigation of the pathobiology of vitamin E deficiency in lower animals. Provocative experimental results in free radical biology have stimulated ever increasing interest during recent years in the antioxidant capability of vitamin E. Thus, review of vitamin E requires comprehensive discussion of current multidisciplinary research, including information on free radical biology and lipid peroxidation.

## HISTORICAL PERSPECTIVE

The early history of vitamin E was reviewed in detail by Mason.[7] Its discovery can be traced to the observation that reproductive failure often occurred in rats fed semipurified diets that contained adequate amounts of vitamins A, B, C, and D and supported good growth and general health. The existence of vitamin E was recognized in 1922 when it became clear that this fat-soluble factor prevented fetal death in animals fed a diet containing rancid lard. By 1925, the term *vitamin E* was accepted as the fifth serial alphabetical designation for vitamins. Subsequently, Evans proposed the word *tocopherol* from the Greek "tos" for childbirth and "phero" meaning to bring forth and "ol" for the alcohol portion of the molecule.

The early years of research were characterized by descriptions of the structural and functional changes of vitamin E deficiency in various animals. Degeneration of the germinal epithelium in the male rat was noted as the underlying problem in testicular atrophy, whereas fetal resorption was identified as the major problem of pregnant females. Paralysis associated with dystrophic muscle and occurrence of encephalomalacia were described in rodents and fowl as reviewed by Nelson.[8] Also, "exudative diathesis" (subcutaneous edema with lipid peroxidation) was described in vitamin E deficient chicks, and an early clue to the nutritional interrelationship with selenium was recognized. In the 1930s, the ferric chloride-dipyridyl method of tocopherol analysis was developed and it became possible to determine the vitamin E content of foods. Lipids with vitamin E activity were isolated from wheat germ oil, and their chemical synthesis was achieved in 1938. Similar methods of chemical synthesis were reported soon thereafter. Nutritional surveys in the 1940s and 1950s revealed that premature infants and patients with malabsorption had low levels of blood tocopherol and abnormal hemolysis of erythrocytes incubated in the presence of hydrogen peroxide.[9-13] Finally, in 1968, vitamin E was recognized formally as an essential nutrient for humans by inclusion in the Recommended Dietary Allowances table of the United States Food and Nutrition Board (National Academy of Sciences).

It is somewhat enigmatic that during the first two decades of vitamin E research the pathologic conditions of the dietary deficiency state in animals were well defined, the chemical nature and biologic properties of the tocopherols were established, and chemical synthesis was achieved, whereas definitive information on subcellular function(s) and the precise role of this vitamin in human health remain to be elucidated. This paradox adds to the challenge of vitamin E research and has stimulated ever increasing scientific interest in tocopherol around the world.

## CHEMISTRY AND NOMENCLATURE

In comparison to the other fat-soluble vitamins, the chemistry of vitamin E is rather complex because there are eight naturally occurring compounds with the characteristic biologic activity. Four vitamers are members of the tocopherol family and four are tocotrienols. Moreover, the stereochemistry of commercially synthesized tocopherols further complicates structural considerations because there are three asymmetric carbon atoms and therefore numerous stereoisomers.

The most abundant and active isomer is α-tocopherol, the structure of which is shown in Figure 18–1. The compound is also referred to as 5,7,8-trimethyl tocol, the latter being 2-methyl-2-(4′,8′,12′-trimethyl-tridecyl)-6-chromanol IX). Natural α-tocopherol as found in foods is [d]-α-tocopherol, whereas chemical synthesis produces a mixture of eight epimers.

In addition to the α vitamer, three other tocopherols with biologic activity are present in foods: β-, γ-, and δ-tocopherols. As illustrated in Figure 18–2, they differ from α-tocopherol only in regard to methyl substitutions on the benzene ring. In particular, β-tocopherol is 5,8-dimethyl-tocol, γ-tocopherol is 7,8-dimethyl tocol, and δ-tocopherol is 8-methyl tocol. The tocotrienols consist of four compounds similar to the corresponding tocopherols but with unsaturated side chains as shown in Figure 18–2. These unsaturated isomers have not been well studied, and only α-tocotrienol appears to have significant vitamin E activity.

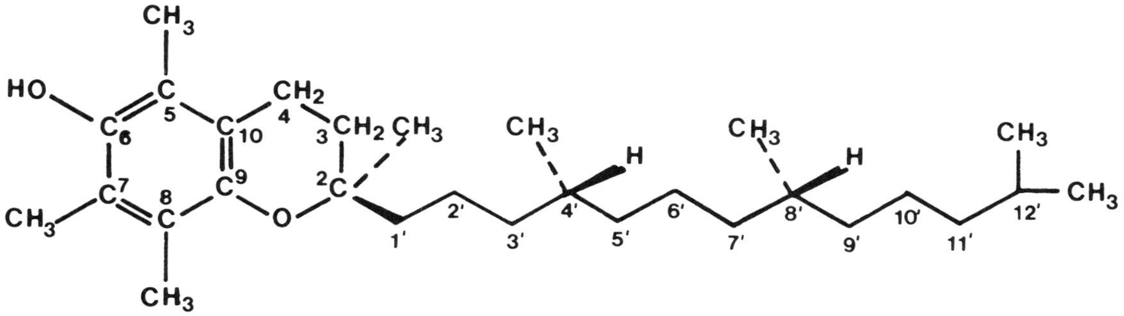

CHEMICAL NAME: 2, 5, 7, 8-Tetramethyl-2-(4′, 8′, 12′-trimethyl tridecyl)-6 chromanol

IUPAC NAME: 2R, 4′R, 8′R-Alpha Tocopherol

TRIVIAL NAME: RRR-Alpha Tocopherol

COMMON NAMES: Natural Vitamin E
Alpha Tocopherol

**FIGURE 18–1.** Structure and nomenclature of the most active vitamin E isomer.

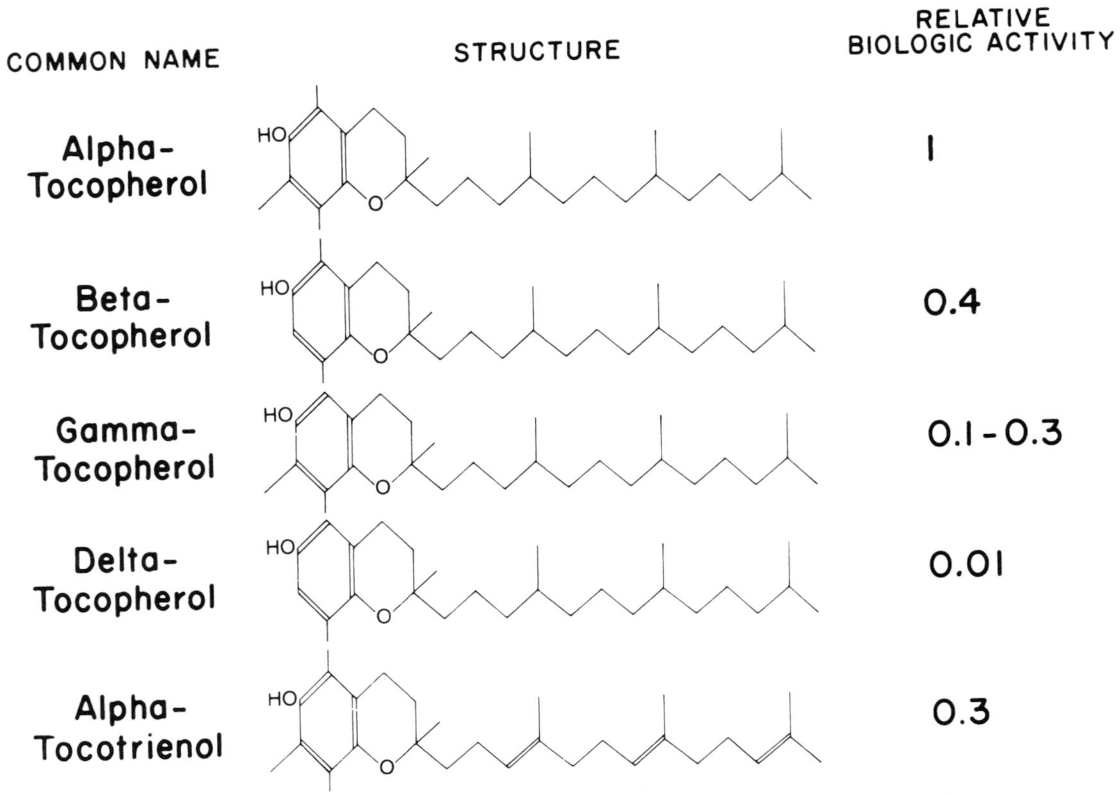
COMMON NAME
STRUCTURE
RELATIVE BIOLOGIC ACTIVITY
Alpha-Tocopherol
HO
O
1
Beta-Tocopherol
HO
O
0.4
Gamma-Tocopherol
HO
O
0.1-0.3
Delta-Tocopherol
HO
O
0.01
Alpha-Tocotrienol
HO
O
0.3

**FIGURE 18–2.** Naturally occurring vitamin E compounds and their biologic activities relative to RRR-α-tocopherol, which is designated officially as having 1.49 IU/mg.

Detailed information on the nomenclature of vitamin E compounds has been published by Kasparek[14] and Bieri and McKenna.[15] In regard to stereoisomers of vitamin E, the International Union of Pure and Applied Chemistry (IUPAC) has recommended that the RS system be used and that the d- and l- prefixes be abandoned.[15] Thus naturally occurring d-α-tocopherol is now designated 2R,4′R, 8′R-α-tocopherol (see Fig. 18–1), synthetic α-tocopherol, made from natural phytol, is 2RS, 4′R,8′R-α-tocopherol, and synthetic all-*rac* α-tocopherol, which contains eight stereoisomers in essentially equal proportions, is denoted 2RS, 4′RS, 8′RS-α-tocopherol. Because different stereoisomers of α-tocopherol show significantly different biologic activities, this rigorous chemical designation is valuable. These facets of nomenclature are included in the policy statement on terminology published by IUPAC and are well described in the nutrition literature.[14,15] On the other hand, inasmuch as the precise mixture of stereoisomers present in blood and tissues usually is not known and because most analytic methods do not distinguish among the stereoisomers, the RS system is generally of less value in nutrition and in clinical medicine. Therefore, in this article, the term *vitamin E* is employed as the generic descriptor for tocol and tocotrienol derivatives with the characteristic biologic activity. In general, α-, β-, δ-, and γ-tocopherol have been used in an unqualified fashion herein to indicate the various vitamers being assessed in human nutrition, and the prefixes d and l have been largely avoided.

Methods for the chemical production of tocopherols have been reviewed by Kasparek.[14] In general, two approaches have been employed, involving either partial synthesis from naturally available compounds or total synthesis. The usual method of complete chemical synthesis depends upon construction of the heterocyclic ring of tocopherols along with the isoprenoid side chain at C-2 using methylated hydroquinones and an aliphatic reactant. Originally, natural phytol was used as the starting material to yield 2RS,4′R,8′R-α-tocopherol. This product contained approximately equimolar amounts of the 2R and 2S stereoisomers and was, therefore, marketed commercially under the designation "[dl]-α-tocopherol," and referred to as "2-ambo-α-tocopherol." Currently, synthetic phytol or isophytol is used to yield a mixture of four racemates or eight stereoisomers which is correctly designated all-*rac*-α-tocopherol. In partial synthetic procedures, methyl groups are introduced into the benzene ring of the lower methyl homolog of 5,7,8-trimethyl tocol. This method yields α-tocopherol from the 5,8-dimethyl, 7,8-dimethyl, and 8-methyl tocol compounds which are naturally present in many sources. In essence, this allows conversion of biologically less active vitamers into the most active RRR-α-tocopherol. The molecular weight of α-tocopherol is 430.66. Thus, 1 mg α-tocopherol/dl of plasma is equivalent to a concentration of 23.22 μmol/L. Although the concentrations of individual compounds of the vitamin E family can be effectively expressed in SI units, the differing biologic activities of various vitamers and of the isomers of each vitamin complicate the utility of such usage. Therefore, international units (IU) and weight measures will be employed in this chapter.

## BIOLOGIC ACTIVITY

There is widespread agreement that vitamin E can function in general as a biologic antioxidant to protect cellular membranes from oxidative destruction. Most of the evidence for this function has been obtained from in vitro experiments, but there are also data from studies of various tissues that tocopherols have antioxidant potential in vivo. Moreover, it has been well established that some manifestations of vitamin E deficiency in chicks and rats can be prevented completely by feeding antioxidants such as ethoxyquin. Many enzyme activities in plasma are altered during severe vitamin E deficiency because tissue necrosis causes release of cellular enzymes.[5,16] Partly as a result of these enzymatic alterations, other functions have been proposed for vitamin E but have not been established. These include regulation of nucleic acid synthesis and gene expression and control of the growth cycle in certain protozoa.[16] The close interaction between vitamin E and selenium also complicates the assignment of specific functions.[17]

McCay and King have reviewed the evidence indicating that α-tocopherol functions as a free radical scavenger in membranes.[18] As illustrated in Figure 18–3, phospholipids in cellular and subcellular membranes contain polyunsaturated fatty acids (PUFA) that are susceptible to peroxidation. Vitamin E is the fat-soluble antioxidant capable of protecting these fatty acids by interrupting free radical reactions that otherwise can cause membrane damage in subcellular organelles. Other antioxidant systems involving enzymes (e.g., glutathione peroxidase and superoxide dismutase) can also function in helping the cell control free radical attacks on peroxidizable fatty acids. Thus, the well-known interrelationship between α-tocopherol and selenium has been explained by the fact that glutathione peroxidase is a selenoenzyme.[17]

The importance of free radicals in cellular metabolism has become apparent because of concurrent investigations in several fields, including studies on the generation of lipid hydroperoxides, on oxidoreductase systems, and on the subcellular role of superoxide dismutase.[18,19] Also, considerable interest has been stimulated in recent years because of concern that adverse effects of environmental toxins are mediated through free radicals, that

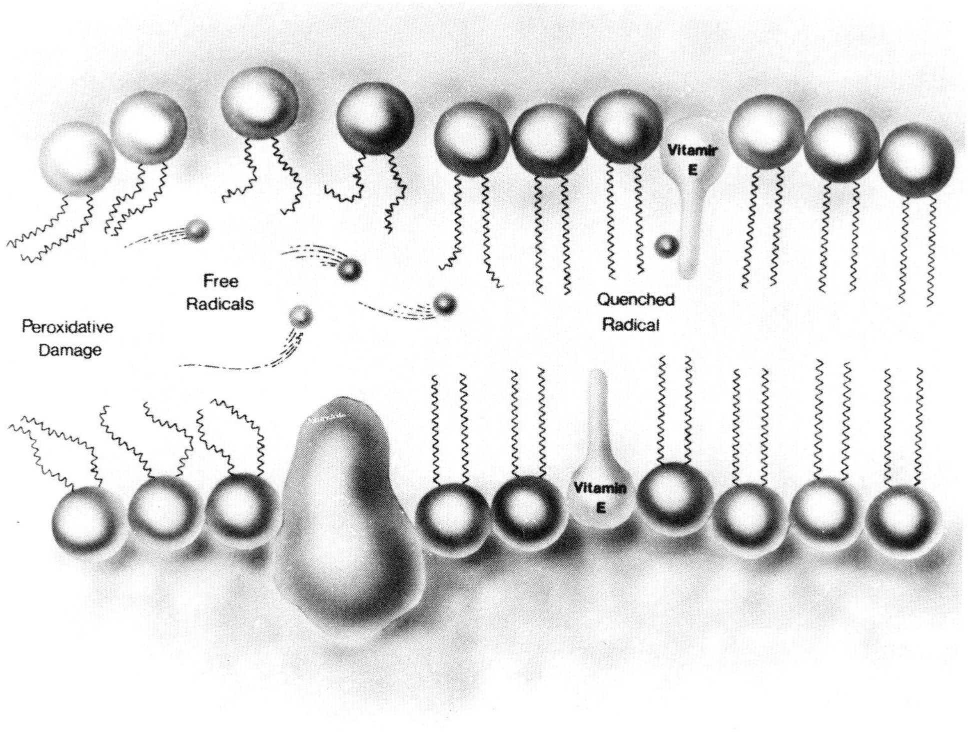
Vitamin E
Free Radicals
Peroxidative Damage
Quenched Radical
Vitamin E

**FIGURE 18–3.** Proposed antioxidant role of vitamin E as a free radical scavenger in biologic membranes halting the chain reaction of polyunsaturated fatty acid peroxidation.

aging is associated with inadequately controlled free radical reactions, and that carcinogenesis can be triggered by peroxidation.[20]

There are several mechanisms for formation of free radicals in biologic systems: (1) cleavage of covalent bonds in organic compounds in which each of the two new molecules retain one electron from the original bonding pair after the splitting; (2) capture of an electron by a receptor molecule such as in the production of the superoxide anion radical when molecular oxygen captures an electron; and (3) self-generation of additional free radicals when reaction occurs with certain compounds such as PUFA molecules. Endogenous production of free radicals can be catalyzed by iron and can also be promoted by inhaled atmospheric pollutants and ingested toxins like carbon tetrachloride.[20] Cellular generation of superoxide and hydrogen peroxide can initiate free radical-mediated lipid peroxidation in exposed membranes. As illustrated in Figure 18–3, a chain reaction can occur during the formation of free radicals because of methylene group reactions of PUFA molecules. It appears that fatty acid radicals formed in this fashion can react spontaneously with oxygen to form a fatty acid peroxy radical; this may propagate the peroxidation of more fatty acid molecules by abstracting hydrogen atoms to form hydroperoxides and new fatty acid radicals. Thus, the self-propagating reaction may lead to oxidation of many fatty acid molecules from production of a single fatty acid radical as the initiating event. As a result of peroxidation of fatty acids, malondialdehyde is produced in tissues subjected to peroxidation of PUFA within phospholipid membranes.[18] Lipid peroxidation can also be detected by analysis of exhaled ethane and pentane.[21]

As envisioned, the major role of vitamin E as an antioxidant is to "neutralize" free radicals, which could otherwise initiate the chain reaction, especially in membranes that contain a large proportion of highly unsaturated fatty acids. To be effective, α-tocopherol must be localized in membrane sites susceptible to free radicals. The chemical reactions involving vitamin E that result in antioxidant activity and the subsequent disposition of vitamin E have not been fully delineated. Degradation products of vitamin E have not been routinely identified or are found only in small quantities, suggesting recycling or regeneration of vitamin E. Recycling or regeneration of vitamin E has been proposed on the basis of experimental evidence showing that both glutathione (GSH) and ascorbic acid can regenerate the tocopheryl radical in a chemical oxidant system.[21] Regeneration of vitamin E would help explain in part the marked discordance between the small amount of vitamin E required relative to PUFA for membrane stabilization (i.e., the ratio of tocopherol molecules to unsaturated fatty acid moieties is surprisingly low in biologic membranes).

In view of the functional relationship between vitamin E and unsaturated fatty acids, it is not surprising that the requirement for α-tocopherol is somewhat dependent upon the amount of PUFA consumed, which can alter membrane fatty acid composition.[5] This relationship appears to be particularly important in young growing animals in which formation of normal membrane structures and maintenance of their integrity are very active biochemical processes.

In addition to the traditional antioxidant activity of vitamin E produced through hydrogen donation, recent studies suggest other cellular protective mechanisms for vitamin E. For example, it has been proposed that vitamin E may protect protein sulfhydryl groups and thereby act as a "sparing agent" during circumstances of increased in vivo oxidative stress. Thus, vitamin E or synthetic phenolic antioxidants may have therapeutic value clinically in circumstances of increased oxidative injury, such as with ischemia reperfusion injury and certain drug-related injury mechanisms. Research is currently underway exploring the role of vitamin E–mediated prevention of cell injury and its relationship to maintenance of protein sulfhydryl groups.[21]

Cellular enzyme antioxidant systems can play a potentially important role in preventing free radical initiation of chain reactions. For instance, glutathione peroxidase is an effective scavenger of hydrogen peroxide because of its high affinity for this substrate. On the other hand, catalase is relatively ineffective at low hydrogen peroxide concentrations.[18] In selenium deficiency, lower glutathione peroxidase activity probably is associated with greater levels of hydrogen peroxide in certain cells; as a result, α-tocopherol might be consumed more rapidly by free radical attacks on unsaturated lipids in the membranes. The enzyme superoxide dismutase appears also to be highly effective in removing superoxide radicals formed by a number of oxido-reductase systems such as microsomal NADPH oxidase.[18] Despite the presence of these antioxidant enzyme systems, tocopherol deficiency in membranes will lead to insufficient protection against hydroxy-radical-induced damage from superoxide formation and hydrogen peroxide in the cell.

An enzyme system that may be extremely important in preserving vitamin E involves the glutathione S-transferases, a group of multifunctional isoenzymes that have remarkably high catalytic activity for lipid aldehydes and have been shown to provide protection against the cytotoxic effects of lipid peroxidation products. Such activity could preserve vitamin E at the expense of intracellular glutathione, which is conjugated to certain lipid peroxidation products by catalytic activity of the glutathione S-transferases.

## STRUCTURAL-FUNCTIONAL RELATIONSHIPS

The biologic antioxidant activity of tocopherol isomers has been measured by using both in vitro and in vivo techniques. It must be recognized that the vitamin E activity of a given isomer will depend not only on the compound's structure, but also on its relative absorption, uptake by target tissues, and turnover rate. Consequently, results of in vitro assay systems do not give the same data as in vivo bioassays. This has lead to controversy over the assignment of relative potencies, an important consideration with respect to dietary allowances. The in vivo bioassay systems used most commonly are based on assessing pathologic changes in rats, chicks, and hamsters. In these bioassays, fetal resorption, production of muscular dystrophy, and occurrence of encephalomalacia may be used to detect relative biologic activity. More recently, quantitative measures of in vivo lipid peroxidation have been used, particularly in rats.[21] Unfortunately, the relative potencies of the vitamers determined by these various in vivo methods can differ substantially, and this fact adds to the controversy.

Table 18–1 summarizes the relative biologic activities of vitamin E compounds according to current consensus.[5,15] The original international standard of vitamin E, synthesized from natural phytol and initially designated "[dl]-α-tocopheryl acetate", was defined as having 1 IU/mg; however, this product is no longer available. The replacement compound (all-rac-α-tocopheryl acetate) is currently being investigated to determine if it has the same biologic activity as the original standard.[22] On the basis of in vivo bioassays, the approximate relative potencies of the other tocopherol isomers compared to α are: β = 40 to 50%; γ = 10 to 30%; δ = about 1%. Thus, the presence and location of methyl groups in the benzene ring is of great importance in determining biologic activity among the tocopherol isomers. As for the stereoisomers, it appears from some data that only the 2-position is significant in influencing biologic antioxidant activity, with the 2R configuration being essential to account for the potency of natural vitamin E.[14,22]

Assessment of γ-tocopherol's relative activity is of special interest because of the high content of this vitamer in the American diet.[23–25] Although 10% of the activity of α-tocopherol has been accepted,[15] recent comparative assessment of lipid peroxidation in vivo by determination of pentane production in iron-loaded rats suggests that γ-tocopherol is 31% as effective as α-tocopherol.[21] In contrast to the in vivo bioassays, the usual in vitro tests indicate that γ-tocopherol in the red blood cell membrane shows 30 to 67% the activity of the α vitamer.[5] Also, measurement of biochemical antioxidant potential in vitro has yielded values as high as 68 to 100% for γ-tocopherol.[23] The difference in γ-tocopherol's level of vitamin E activity has been attributed to a faster turnover rate (compared to that for α-tocopherol) and lesser amounts in the phospholipid membranes where the antioxidant function is needed.[5,24] Because of its uncertain bioavailability, therefore, γ-tocopherol in foods was assigned only 10% the activity of α-tocopherol by the Food and Nutrition Board in the 10th Edition of *Recommended Dietary Allowances.*

Very little information is available on the vitamin E activity of the tocotrienols, but there is evidence that the effects of methyl substitution are similar to those observed with the tocopherol family. Thus, only α-tocotrienol has biologically significant vitamin E activity, approximating 30% that of α-tocopherol.[26]

## DIETARY CONSIDERATIONS

Most of the information on the vitamin E activity in foods has been derived from analysis of tocopherols, rather than tocotrienols. Bauernfeind has presented a list of tocopherol concentrations including the distribution of isomers in various foods.[25] The tocopherol content of diets shows great variation depending upon harvesting, processing, storage, and final food preparation proce-

**TABLE 18–1.** VITAMIN E. ACTIVITIES OF TOCOPHEROL ISOMERS

| COMPOUND | VITAMIN E ACTIVITY |
|---|---|
| [d]-α-tocopherol (RRR-α-tocopherol) | 1.49 IU/mg |
| [d]-α-tocopheryl acetate (RRR-α-tocopheryl-acetate) | 1.36 IU/mg |
| [dl]-α-tocopherol (all *rac*-α-tocopherol) | 1.1 IU/mg* |
| [dl]-α-tocopheryl acetate (all *rac*-α-tocopheryl acetate) | 1.0 IU/mg* |
| "[dl]-α-tocopheryl acetate" ("2-ambo-α-tocopheryl acetate") | 1.0 IU/mg |
| [dl]-β-tocopherol | 0.60 IU/mg† |
| [d]-γ-tocopherol | 0.15–0.45 IU/mg† |
| [d]-δ-tocopherol | 0.015† |

*The original international standard is no longer available, and the activity of the current replacement compound is being investigated to determine if its specific biologic activity is less than 1 IU/mg.[15,22]

†Derived by calculation, since only α vitamers are officially recognized by assigned international units of biologic activity.

(From Bieri, J.G., McKenna, M.C.: Am. J. Clin. Nutr., *34*:289, 1981.)

dures.[25] The major sources of vitamin E consumed by Americans are the vegetable and seed oils, such as corn oil, soybean oil, and safflower oil. Although these common oils, and the less commonly consumed wheat germ, are rich sources of tocopherols, the actual concentration and distribution of vitamin E isomers are quite variable. As shown in Table 18–2, animal products are not good sources. Although butter provides very little α-tocopherol, American margarine contains a range from 3.2 to 32.7 mg/100 g and, therefore, can supply a significant amount of vitamin E in the diet.

The proportion of non-α isomers provided by fats and oils has become a topic of great nutritional interest since corn oil and soybean oil have become major components of the American diet,[5,24] rather than animal fat. Soybean oil has become particularly prevalent and accounted for 74% of oils and fats used in edible United States products according to a USDA survey in 1982/83.[27] Soybeans contain predominantly γ-tocopherol with lesser amounts of δ-tocopherol and only a relatively small amount of α-tocopherol (see Table 18–2). As a result of the rather high content of non-α vitamers, soybean oil provides a disproportionately low amount of vitamin E activity in comparison to its concentration of total tocopherols. Other dietary lipid sources such as coconut and fish oils are low in tocopherols. Except for fish oil, however, the concentration of tocopherols increases in proportion to the amount of PUFA present. (See also Appendix Table A-21 for the vitamin E content of common foods).

In calculating the vitamin E activity of mixed diets, the traditional approach has been to adjust the amount of β-tocopherol by a factor of 0.5, γ-tocopherol by 0.1, and alpha-tocotrienol by 0.3. For instance, the γ-tocopherol content of soybean oil (59.3 mg/100 g) would be multiplied by 0.1 to yield a value of 5.93 mg/100 g and, similarly, the contribution of δ-tocopherol would be reduced from 26 to 0.26 mg/100 g; these concentrations would be added to the 10.1 mg/100 g of α-tocopherol to yield a total "α-tocopherol equivalent" value of 16.29 mg/100 g. For studies of mixed diets in which only RRR-α-tocopherol is reported, the value in milligrams can be increased by 20% to allow for the presence of other vitamin E compounds and thereby estimate "α-tocopherol equivalents."[15]

## INTESTINAL ABSORPTION, TRANSPORT, AND STORAGE

A variety of methods have been used to measure vitamin E absorption and transport as discussed by Bieri et al.[5] Although the data have been obtained almost

**TABLE 18–2.** TOCOPHEROL CONTENT OF REPRESENTATIVE DIETARY COMPONENTS

| | TOCOPHEROLS MEASURED BY VARIOUS TECHNIQUES (mg/100g) | | | |
|---|---|---|---|---|
| DIETARY COMPONENT | α | β | γ | δ |
| Milk | 0.04 | — | — | — |
| Bread—white | 0.04 | 0.02 | 0.24 | 0.1 |
| —whole wheat | 0.16 | 0.15 | 0.38 | 0.2 |
| Beef—steak† | 0.30 | — | — | — |
| —liver† | 0.63 | — | — | — |
| Fish (haddock)† | 0.60 | — | — | — |
| Butter | 1.68 | — | 0.14 | — |
| Lard | 1.20 | — | 0.70 | — |
| Margarine | 11.70* | — | 29.00 | 8.1 |
| Seeds and Nuts | | | | |
| Peanuts | 9.7 | — | 6.60 | — |
| Almonds | 27.4 | 0.30 | 0.90 | — |
| Sunflower seeds | 49.5 | 2.73 | — | — |
| Oils | | | | |
| Corn | 11.2 | 5.00 | 60.20 | 1.8 |
| Cottonseed | 38.9 | — | 38.70 | — |
| Peanut | 13.0 | — | 21.60 | 2.1 |
| Safflower | 38.7 | — | 17.40 | 24.0 |
| Soybean | 10.1 | — | 59.30 | 26.4 |
| Sunflower | 48.7 | — | 5.10 | 0.8 |
| Wheat germ | 133.0 | 71.00 | 26.00 | 27.1 |

*α-tocopherol content varies from 3.2 to 32.7 mg/100 g depending on multiple factors (oil source, processing methods): the average for 27 brands listed by Bauernfeind was 12.0 mg/100 g.

†Values listed are for prepared food (e.g., cooked meat).

(From Bauernfeind, J.: Tocopherols in foods. *In* Vitamin E: A Comprehensive Treatise. Edited by L.J. Machlin. New York, Marcel Dekker, 1980, by courtesy of Marcel Dekker, Inc.)

exclusively in studies of α-tocopherol, it appears that transport processes are similar for the other tocopherol vitamers.[24] On the other hand, tissue storage and turnover are considerably different. The absorption of tocopherols depends upon factors generally important in lipid digestion and intestinal uptake, as discussed elsewhere in the book. Bile salts and pancreatic enzymes are known to be important in the absorption process.[4] In general, the degree of absorption of tocopherols will vary depending upon total lipid absorption.[5] The efficiency of the absorption, however, decreases as large amounts of tocopherol are consumed.[28] Most of the quantitative information has been obtained by administering radioactive α-tocopherol and measuring fecal excretion of radioactivity. The percentage absorption in rats observed by Losowsky et al.[28] decreased from about 60% when 0.04 mg of α-tocopherol was administered (in either arachis oil, a Tween emulsion, or alcohol) to 30% when 20 mg were given. Vitamin E-deficient rats also absorbed about 60% of 0.04 mg of α-tocopherol. In normal humans, an average absorption of at least 50% and perhaps as high as 70% can be assumed for dietary levels of α-tocopherol consumption (e.g., 0.4 to 1 mg);[5,28] however, the efficiency falls to less than 10% with pharmacologic doses such as 200 mg.

The malabsorption of fat seen in patients with various forms of steatorrhea results in a parallel loss of tocopherols. As shown in Figure 18–4, the fecal excretion of radiolabeled tocopherol correlates with the extent of steatorrhea in patients with pancreatic disease, biliary obstruction, celiac disease, postgastrectomy malabsorption, and lymphangiectasia.[29] Children with pancreatic achylia due to cystic fibrosis have been studied extensively with respect to vitamin E status, and their levels of circulating tocopherol have been found to correlate closely with various indices of malabsorption.[30]

Once absorbed, vitamin E isomers are transported with fat predominately by lymphatic vessels to the venous system. Tocopherols are distributed in plasma in association with lipoproteins, but no specific carrier protein has been identified. In general, the concentrations of tocopherol in plasma subfractions vary depending upon the amount of lipid present. A rapid exchange of plasma tocopherol and erythrocyte tocopherol occurs at the red blood cell membrane.[31] α-Tocopherol is taken up by most tissues, including liver, lung, heart, skeletal muscle, and adipose tissue.[32] Contrary to the other

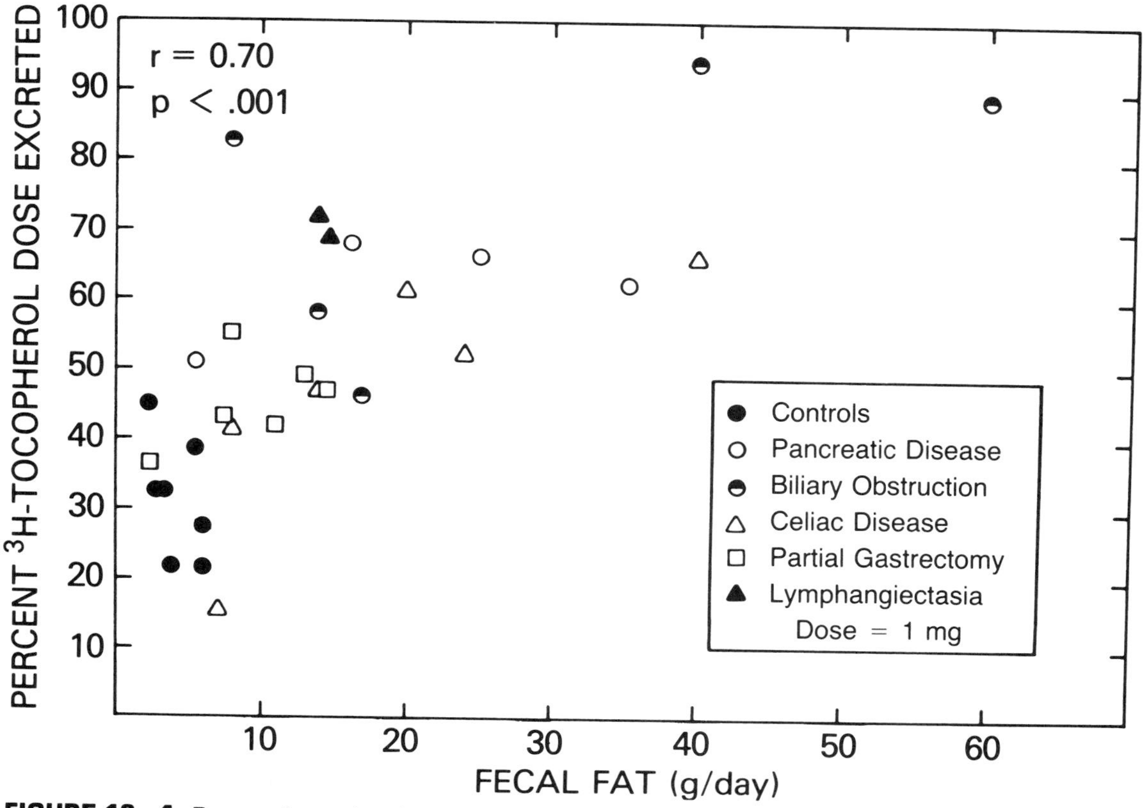
PERCENT ³H-TOCOPHEROL DOSE EXCRETED
100
90
80
70
60
50
40
30
20
10
r = 0.70
p < .001
Controls
Pancreatic Disease
Biliary Obstruction
Celiac Disease
Partial Gastrectomy
Lymphangiectasia
Dose = 1 mg
10
20
30
40
50
60
FECAL FAT (g/day)

**FIGURE 18–4.** Degree of tocopherol malabsorption in patients with various gastrointestinal disorders, as determined by MacMahon and Neal,[29] using 1-mg doses of labeled α-tocopherol. (Reprinted from Farrell, P.M., Machlin, L.J.: *In* Vitamin E: A Comprehensive Treatise. Edited by L.J. Machlin. New York, Marcel Dekker, 1980, pp. 520–620, by courtesy of Marcel Dekker, Inc.)

tissues, fat accumulates α-tocopherol continuously and can sequester the vitamin.[5,32,33] In general, vitamin E compounds are apparently concentrated wherever there is abundant fatty acid, especially in structures of the cell containing phospholipid membranes, such as mitochondria, microsomes, and plasma membranes. When the intake of vitamin E is high, the liver is a major repository, but the total body pool in adipose tissue is much higher. Although adipose tissue is sometimes considered a "store" of vitamin E, it should be recognized that the tocopherol present in adipocytes is not readily available to other tissues.[32]

The concentration of tocopherol present in tissues is related to the amount of vitamin E consumed,[32,34] and the lipid content of the organ in question. The amount of α-tocopherol present in the liver is considered to be an index of dietary intake. Tissues with greater lipid content tend to have more vitamin E. In blood, the amount of lipid present also has a major influence, if not a determining role, on the level of circulating plasma tocopherols.[35] Therefore, vitamin E concentrations in biologic specimens should be expressed both in terms of mg/unit volume or weight and as mg/g lipid.

The metabolism and turnover of α-tocopherol have been investigated only to a limited extent in humans and have not been adequately quantitated in any species. According to the scheme proposed by Gallo-Torres,[36] the chromane ring is hydrolyzed to α-tocopheryl quinone, which may be reduced to the hydroquinone. Further metabolism leads to oxidation of the terminal methyl group in the side chain; the resulting carboxylate may then be shortened, giving rise to tocopheronic acid, which can subsequently be converted to tocopheronolactone. Small amounts of tocopherol metabolites such as tocopheryl quinone and tocopheryl hydroquinone have been found in various tissues. Only traces of tocopherol metabolites are found in urine. Tocopheronolactone has been detected in urine of animals given free tocopherol, but the amount excreted is quite low. The major route of excretion of tocopherol metabolites appears to be fecal elimination, possibly in association with bile secretion.

When a vitamin E-deficient diet is fed to animals, plasma and liver levels of α-tocopherol decrease rapidly. There seem to be two pools present, at least in rats, a rapidly metabolized pool and a component that is retained for longer periods.[32] Depletion of tocopherol from adipose tissue and skeletal muscle is a slow process. Thus, these organs should not be considered physiologic storage sites for vitamin E.

Using both short-term labeling techniques and longer feeding studies, Bieri and Poukka Evarts have assessed γ-tocopherol metabolism in rats in comparison to α-tocopherol.[24] γ-Tocopherol showed similar absorption and initial distribution in plasma lipoproteins. Within 2 hours, however, there was a twofold enrichment of the α-vitamer and by 24 hours a threefold relative increase of α-relative to γ-tocopherol in both chylomicrons and lipoproteins. Tissue deposition was similar for the two isomers at 2 hours, but at 24 hours there was only about half as much labeled γ-tocopherol in liver and spleen. When partially depleted animals were fed for two weeks with a diet providing γ- and α-tocopherols in a 2:1 ratio, an average of only 23% as much γ was deposited in seven tissues. With greater proportions of γ-tocopherol fed longer, relatively more of this isomer was deposited, but never to a level approaching α-tocopherol except in adipose tissue. The results of Bieri and Poukka Evarts indicate that γ-tocopherol disappears from the circulation and tissues much faster than the α vitamer, implying a more rapid turnover rate.[24] Whether this is due simply to the one methyl group difference in structure or to a specific cellular receptor helping to retain α-tocopherol or to some other mechanism remains to be determined.

Quantitative information on γ-tocopherol turnover in humans is lacking. Nevertheless, it is reasonable to conclude that the same faster turnover phenomenon applies to children and adults in view of the low proportion of γ-tocopherol in blood despite higher consumption than that of α-tocopherol. Because depletion of γ-tocopherol from tissues is relatively rapid, one must be careful not to overestimate its contribution to total vitamin E activity in the American diet.

## EVALUATION OF VITAMIN E STATUS

In nutritional surveys and clinical diagnostic studies, assessment of vitamin E status has depended upon biochemical analyses of plasma or serum, erythrocytes, adipose tissue biopsies, and organs obtained at autopsy. In common practice, serum has generally been used for measurement of total tocopherol concentrations. A better assessment, however, is provided by measuring tocopherol isomers either by thin layer chromatography[37] or, preferably, by HPLC.[2,3] The latter will provide precise determination of α-tocopherol concentrations, as well as data on the other isomers. Separation of the β and γ isomers, however, is extremely difficult using either method. As a result, these two vitamers are generally reported together as the β + γ fraction. Although 90% or more of the circulating vitamin E is normally α-tocopherol, large amounts of β + γ-tocopherol and δ-tocopherol can be found in some circumstances. For instance, Gutcher et al. showed that infants on formulas containing corn oil had high levels of circulating γ-tocopherol,[3] and Farrell et al. commented that infants receiving Intralipid (intravenous fat emulsion) had high levels of γ-tocopherol.[38] Also, Horwitt et al. have detected unusually high proportions of β + γ-tocopherol in adults on diets containing a predominance of γ tocopherol (i.e., corn oil supplemented subjects).[39]

In addition to measuring tocopherol concentrations in blood, one finds that the peroxide hemolysis test is helpful in providing an index of antioxidant potential. Although this test is not entirely specific, a normal result [less than 5% hemolysis during 3 hours incubation in 2% $H_2O_2$[30]] can be assumed to rule out vitamin E deficiency. In performing peroxide hemolysis tests, one must be very careful with technical details to avoid artifacts as discussed elsewhere.[30]

Because of the marked influence of plasma lipids on tocopherol concentrations, tocopherol/lipid ratios have been used in some studies as recommended by Horwitt et al.[35] These more recent investigations have demonstrated that although children have significantly lower levels of plasma vitamin E than adults, a tocopherol/total lipid ratio of 0.8 mg/g of total plasma lipids generally indicates adequate nutritional status.[40] Without the concurrent assessment of circulating lipids, it is possible that some individuals with low lipids will be misclassified as vitamin E deficient when they are actually normal. Conversely, some hyperlipidemic subjects can have normal tocopherol concentrations per unit volume of plasma or serum, but in reality may be low in vitamin E.[41]

Most of the previous investigations have utilized colorimetric determination of total plasma or serum tocopherols and have shown that a level above 0.5 mg/dl indicates adequate nutritional status.[5] Although many infants and children have levels less than 0.5 mg/dl because of lower lipid concentrations, they usually do not show other evidence of vitamin E deficiency. This conclusion is based on the finding of normal resistance of erythrocytes to hemolysis in the presence of hydrogen peroxide-promoted membrane peroxidation.[40]

The ideal approach to assessing vitamin E nutritional status, therefore, involves a combination of methods including determination of tocopherol isomers in plasma or serum, measurement of circulating lipids such as the total lipid fraction or cholesterol esters, determination of erythrocyte hemolysis in the presence of 2% hydrogen peroxide, and (if warranted) determination of the tocopherol content of a tissue biopsy.

## PATHOLOGY OF VITAMIN E DEFICIENCY

Table 18–3 summarizes the abnormalities present in animals raised on vitamin E-deficient diets. Perhaps the most notable aspect of vitamin E deficiency in animals is the marked degree of species specificity. Also, there is a great diversity of tissue and organ functions affected by low tocopherol levels. Nelson has reviewed the histopathology of the reproductive organs, skeletal muscles, and nervous system in vitamin E-deficient animals.[8] In general, tissue necrosis is a major feature and is accompanied by accumulation of lipopigments thought to represent peroxidized lipid. In some instances, especially in rapidly growing animals, disorders such as muscular degeneration and encephalomalacia occur over a matter of several days to a few weeks. It must be recognized, however, that young animals that are studied with respect to vitamin E deficiency are typically placed on diets that are virtually devoid of all antioxidants and sometimes contain large amounts of PUFA to further stress vital tissues. It is conceivable that this experimental approach may cause an isolated, severe vitamin E deficiency state in circumstances where other mechanisms involving antioxidants cannot become compensatory.

The search for a clinical correlate of vitamin E deficiency in humans has been based largely on our understanding of the pathologic disturbances in animals on synthetic diets. In humans, rapid development of vitamin E deficiency apparently does not occur except in unusual clinical circumstances. Because of the marked differences in nutritional status between animals investigated comprehensively and human subjects available for clinical investigations, it has become necessary to probe for insidious pathologic processes in humans, possibly leading only to biochemical abnormalities. Yet, extensive research to uncover specific clinical signs of human tocopherol deficiency has met with frustration in

**TABLE 18–3.** VITAMIN E DEFICIENCY*

| CONDITION | TISSUE AFFECTED | SPECIES |
|---|---|---|
| Hemolysis and possible anemia | Erythrocyte | Rat, chick, monkey, premature human, human with malabsorption |
| Neuronal degeneration | Axons† | Rat, monkey, human |
| Nutritional "muscular dystrophy" | Skeletal muscle | Rabbit, fowl, guinea pig, sheep, others |
| Myocardial necrosis and fibrosis | Cardiac muscle | Calf, rat, hamster |
| Reproductive failure | | Rat,‡ mouse,‡ guinea pig,‡ dog, monkey |
| (Fetal death in females)‡ | ?Placenta | |
| (Testicular degeneration in males) | Testicle | |

*Also, encephalomalacia and exudative diathesis in fowl, ceroid pigment deposition in smooth muscle of various species, and possible "disappearance" of mitochondrial and microsomal membranes in ducks and human jejunum.

†Axons of the spinal cord and peripheral nerves degenerate and may accumulate lipopigment.

‡During pregnancy fetal death and resorption have been observed in rats, mice, and guinea pigs.

many instances. This is quite in contrast, of course, to observations on the other fat-soluble vitamins where prominent manifestations of the deficiency state generally develop (e.g., hemorrhage with vitamin K, rickets with vitamin D, and night blindness with vitamin A). It was largely for this reason that vitamin E was not added to the nutrients included on the list of those with a Recommended Dietary Allowance until 1968.

Human vitamin E deficiency can be defined for practical purposes as a low plasma (or serum) tocopherol level (below at least 0.5 mg/dl), accompanied by a low ratio of tocopherol to lipid and/or hemolysis of erythrocytes incubated in 2% hydrogen peroxide. The term *subclinical* or biochemical deficiency may be used to indicate that laboratory evidence of low tocopherol levels in humans is not necessarily equivalent to biologically or clinically evident deficiency. With the exception of the Elgin project described by Horwitt and associates,[42] in which adult male volunteers were placed on special diets low in α-tocopherol, the occurrence of vitamin E deficiency of pure dietary origin is rare in developed countries. On the other hand, there are three categories of patients who have been well established as susceptible to vitamin E deficiency: (1) premature infants, (2) patients with gastrointestinal diseases leading to malabsorption, and (3) individuals with abetalipoproteinemia. Also, children with protein-calorie malnutrition have sometimes been noted to show abnormally low levels of circulating tocopherol. Because the three categories of patients who commonly are low in vitamin E have been reviewed in detail previously,[4] only a brief account has been included herein.

Newborn infants delivered prematurely show evidence of vitamin E deficiency due to several factors, including limited tissue storage at birth, intestinal malabsorption for as long as 8 to 12 weeks,[43] and rapid growth rates that increase nutrient requirements in general. Also, some infant formula preparations have been marginal to low in α-tocopherol content relative to the amount of PUFA and iron present. Although pregnancy is associated with high maternal levels of circulating vitamin E proportional to rising plasma lipids,[35] transplacental delivery of tocopherols to the fetus is limited, resulting in low circulating concentrations in the premature infant. Furthermore, neonatal tissue concentrations are not only low, but a paucity of adipose tissue in premature infants limits their total body vitamin E pool even further.

The possible adverse consequences of vitamin E deficiency in premature infants were first suggested by Owens and Owens in relationship to retrolental fibroplasia (RLF), a tragic disease that nearly caused an epidemic of blindness in premature neonates.[44] This disorder, which is now referred to as retinopathy of prematurity, or ROP, was eventually attributed to oxygen toxicity when hyperoxemia was found to lead to degeneration of retinal arteries. Although the importance of vitamin E deficiency in ROP has been disputed, several investigations of the past decade support the potential benefits of correcting deficiency early in these patients with parenteral or enteral α-tocopheryl acetate.[45,46] On the other hand, there have been well-controlled clinical trials that have yielded negative results— that is, no evidence that vitamin E therapy can prevent or even ameliorate the retinal vascular pathology.[47] Therefore, the prophylactic value of pharmacologic doses of vitamin E remains controversial.[6] The deaths of a number of premature infants treated with an intravenous preparation of vitamin E (E-Ferol) highlights the concern regarding the need to carefully and scientifically elucidate the cause of ROP and the role of pharmacologic treatment with products containing vitamin E.

Hemolytic anemia is another abnormality of premature infants associated with vitamin E deficiency. Oski and Barness were the first to report data indicating that vitamin E deficiency plays a role in the exaggerated anemia that occurs in some premature infants.[48] Although subsequent changes in the composition of infant formula and less use of supplemental iron during the neonatal period have reduced the impact of vitamin E deficiency and raised questions about the reproducibility of the original data,[49] Gross and Melhorn confirmed and extended the original observations with respect to: (1) the pattern of fall in erythrocyte indices, (2) the poor intestinal absorption of vitamin E in premature infants, and (3) the beneficial effects of tocopherol supplementation on hematologic status.[43] In particular, Gross and Melhorn found significantly improved hemoglobin and reticulocyte values in a vitamin E-treated group compared to premature controls (as shown in Figure 18–5).[43] Data on red cell turnover obtained before and after correction of vitamin E deficiency would be helpful in establishing the conclusion concerning hemolysis in vivo. Unfortunately, erythrocyte survival studies involving radioisotope-tagged cells are hazardous to perform in newborns and yield data that are difficult to interpret. Thus, little information is available on erythrocyte kinetics to confirm the clinical observations. Furthermore, current feeding practices seem to have virtually eliminated the hemolytic anemia of prematurity originally described by Oski and Barness.[48] This is probably attributable to the favorable ratio of tocopherol to PUFA in milk formulations used to manage premature infants and the careful use of supplemental iron. Recent studies by Zipursky et al. examined the efficacy of vitamin E supplementation for the *prevention* of anemia in premature infants in a randomized controlled blind trial.[50] They concluded there was no evidence to support the policy of administering vitamin E to premature infants to prevent the anemia of prematurity.

One of the major issues relative to the clinical demonstration of the efficacy of pharmacologic doses of vitamin E relates to the vitamin E status of controls. If control subjects are nutritionally insufficient with respect to vitamin E, then pharmacologic doses of vitamin E will provide sufficiency as well as excess vitamin E levels. On

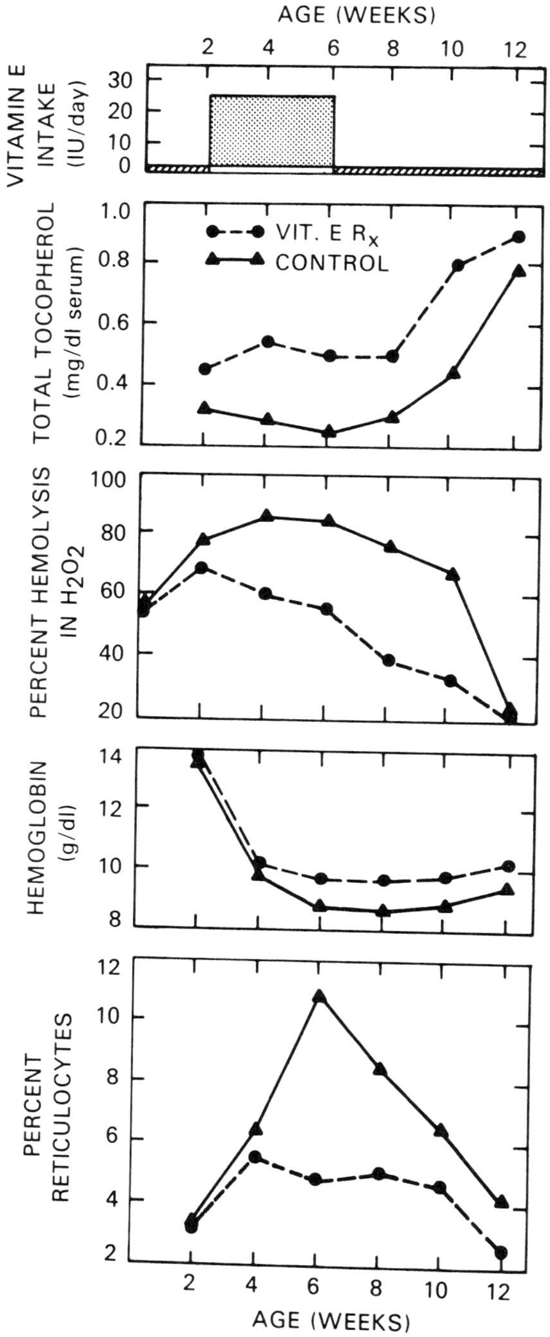
AGE (WEEKS)
2 4 6 8 10 12
VITAMIN E INTAKE (IU/day)
30 20 10 0
TOTAL TOCOPHEROL (mg/dl serum)
1.0 0.8 0.6 0.4 0.2
VIT. E $R_x$
CONTROL
PERCENT HEMOLYSIS IN $H_2O_2$
100 80 60 40 20
HEMOGLOBIN (g/dl)
14 12 10 8
PERCENT RETICULOCYTES
12 10 8 6 4 2
2 4 6 8 10 12
AGE (WEEKS)

**FIGURE 18–5.** Vitamin E and hematologic status of 28- to 32-week-gestation infants studied by Gross and Melhorn. (Reprinted from Farrell, P.M., Machlin, L.J.: *In* Vitamin E: A Comprehensive Treatise. Edited by L.J. Machlin. New York, Marcel Dekker, 1980, pp. 520–620, by courtesy of Marcel Dekker, Inc.)

the other hand, if control subjects are sufficient in vitamin E, then pharmacologic doses will only provide excess vitamin E activity that may lack therapeutic efficacy beyond the vitamin E-sufficient control subjects. Thus, discrepancies in observations in the literature may be explained on the basis of differences between the vitamin E status of control subjects rather than a difference in response to pharmacologic doses of vitamin E. Small but statistically significant differences in hemoglobin values have been demonstrated only in infants with adequate dietary E:PUFA ratios who also received supplementary iron therapy.[51] A review of published randomized trials on the efficacy of vitamin E in retinopathy of prematurity and intracranial hemorrhage concluded that treatment with vitamin E does not result in a significant reduction in either clinical affliction and that possible benefits must be balanced against the potential for serious toxicity.[52]

The second category of human subjects who manifest vitamin deficiency includes a variety of patients with intestinal malabsorption. This is a very heterogeneous group with a common clinical feature, namely steatorrhea. Vitamin E deficiency has been associated with disturbances affecting nearly every component of the gastrointestinal tract, including the stomach (postgastrectomy syndrome), liver (biliary atresia and cirrhosis), pancreas (cystic fibrosis, chronic pancreatitis, and pancreatic carcinoma), and intestinal mucosa (gluten enteropathy and regional enteritis). Although the degree of tocopherol malabsorption varies in these conditions and in individual patients (see Fig. 18–4), it may be concluded in general that if steatorrhea is of sufficient duration and magnitude, vitamin E deficiency is likely to ensue as a consequence of tocopherol malabsorption.

Of those patients with enteropathies leading to chronic steatorrhea, children with cystic fibrosis (CF) have been of particular interest, since they represent a relatively large group of human subjects (1 of 4000 children in the United States) that are readily available for research, and since they manifest a prolonged, permanent digestive defect that cannot be completely corrected by oral pancreatic enzyme replacement therapy. The first report describing vitamin E deficiency in CF patients appeared in 1949 and resulted from a survey of 200 hospitalized patients by Darby et al.[12] Subsequently, Nitowsky and associates showed that low serum tocopherol levels were common in these patients and associated with in vitro hemolysis.[53] Farrell et al. later found that vitamin E deficiency occurred invariably in CF patients with long-term fat malabsorption and that the severity of tocopherol deficiency was proportional to the degree of steatorrhea.[30] Underwood and Denning found that tissue α-tocopherol concentrations were also low,[54] and this was confirmed by others.[30]

Studies on the possible consequences of vitamin E deficiency in patients with cystic fibrosis and other malabsorption syndromes have focused on erythrocyte stability and the neuromuscular system. Although severe anemia is unlikely to occur in patients with malabsorption, significant decreases in the survival of $^{51}Cr$-labeled erythrocytes have been described in CF patients and shown to respond favorably to tocopherol therapy.[4] The average $^{51}Cr$-RBC half-life values observed by Farrell et al. increased significantly in CF patients from 19.0 days to 27.6 days (normal range = 25 to 35 days) before and after supplementation with 100 to 200 IU per day.[30] In a similar experimental design, Leonard and Losowsky found that adults with tocopherol malnutrition due to malabsorption or alcoholism were found to show a similar reduction in the $^{51}Cr$-RBC survival to 19.3 days and an increase to 24.9 days following treatment with vitamin E.[55] It should be noted, however, that the average degree of shortening of erythrocyte survival in tocopherol-deficient patients with malabsorption is not sufficient to produce clinically evident hemolytic anemia. Nevertheless, on the basis of the above studies it is clear that human vitamin E deficiency is associated not only with in vitro hemolysis but also with decreased erythrocyte survival in vivo from diminished antioxidant activity. In addition, a clinical trial of tocopherol supplementation in children with CF (who were initially vitamin E-deficient) demonstrated that hemoglobin values were significantly increased over 18 to 24 months of treatment.[56] This observation confirms the potential hematologic significance of vitamin E deficiency in older individuals with intestinal malabsorption.

Investigation of the neuromuscular system in vitamin E-deficient children with malabsorption has been of interest because of the alterations in lower animals.[8] Some evidence of a primary myopathy has been reported, but the data are unconvincing and not supported by histologic examination of skeletal muscle biopsies.[41] On the other hand, recent investigations of children with chronic cholestasis due to biliary atresia and other etiologies, as well as evaluation of patients with abetalipoproteinemia and cystic fibrosis, suggest that a neurologic disease can develop that is similar to that found in animals.[57–59] These studies were reviewed by Sokol who pointed out the "apparent increased susceptibility of the developing nervous system to injury caused by chronic vitamin E deficiency."[1] The clinical progression of the neurologic disorder in childhood cholestasis includes hyporeflexia at age 18 to 24 months, frank neurologic dysfunction by age 3 to 4 years, and disabling neurologic deficits by 10 years. Sokol further emphasized that the neuropathology of this condition closely resembles the abnormalities found many years ago in animal models of vitamin E deficiency. Histologic abnormalities are especially prominent in the spinal cord where axonal dystrophy leads to degeneration of the posterior columns. Furthermore, published data suggest that the characteristic neurologic symptoms improve with vitamin E treatment and perhaps can be prevented with such therapy in patients with abetalipoproteinemia.[1,57–59]

Several reports suggest that destruction of cellular membranes can occur in patients with vitamin E deficiency such as those with abetalipoproteinemia.[4] Many investigations also indicate that lipopigment (ceroid) will be deposited in human tissues such as small intestine, just as in animals.[8] This deposit is thought to represent accumulation of peroxidized lipid and reflects altered PUFA metabolism.

## NUTRITIONAL REQUIREMENTS

Because of the adequacy of vitamin E nutrition in healthy Americans consuming balanced diets, the recommended daily allowance for this nutrient has been based largely upon dietary analyses. According to a study by Bieri and Evarts in 1972, daily intakes of RRR-α-tocopherol in adults averaged 9 mg (13.5 IU) and ranged from 4.4 to 12.7 mg (6.6 to 19 IU).[60] Witting and Lee found similar values.[61] Because of the dietary contribution of the gamma vitamers, total tocopherol ingestion is generally twofold to threefold higher. Thus, the level of "α-tocopherol equivalents" consumed may range from 6 to 15 mg per day for adults, corresponding to 9 to 22.5 IU per day.[15] Although this is a relatively low level compared to the amounts ingested by young growing animals, there is no indication of deficiency when this amount is ingested. The minimum daily requirement is not known, but the Elgin project revealed that for adult men the level is above 2 mg per day of dietary α-tocopherol.[62]

It has been demonstrated that the requirement for vitamin E in animals is elevated when the intake of PUFA is increased substantially. Horwitt showed that the same applies to humans.[62] Alteration of the fat source in diets consumed by volunteers in the Elgin project elevated the concentration of linoleic acid in adipose tissue markedly and increased the need for dietary tocopherol. Although the consumption of certain oils raises the intake of PUFA, a corresponding increase in vitamin E intake occurs, except in the case of fish oils. When the primary unsaturated fatty acid in the diet is linoleic acid, a ratio of 0.4 mg RRR-α-tocopherol/g of polyunsaturated fatty acid is more than adequate to maintain normal vitamin E status. Bieri and Evarts found that the average α-tocopherol/PUFA ratio in representative American diets was 0.42 mg/g.[60]

In the United States the current recommendations concerning vitamin E allowances reflect the usual dietary intake of Americans. In reaching a conclusion about vitamin E, the committee appointed to develop the tenth edition of *Recommended Dietary Allowances* agreed that 10 mg of α-tocopherol equivalents are satisfactory for young adults [63] (see Appendix Table A-2b). This recommendation is based on assigning γ-tocopherol a vitamin E activity of 0.1 relative to α-tocopherol. The value recommended by the Committee for infants from birth to 3 months of age is 2 mg of α-tocopherol equivalents.[63]

## PHARMACOLOGIC APPLICATIONS AND TOXICITY

The medical uses of vitamin E have been described in detail elsewhere.[4–6] Management of patients with vitamin E deficiency due to malabsorption can generally be achieved by supplementing the diet with water-miscible α-tocopheryl acetate preparations. Although the dose has not been firmly established, experience with CF patients indicates that the following dosages will either correct or prevent vitamin E deficiency: 25 to 50 IU per day for infants; 50 to 100 IU per day for 1 to 10-year-old children; 100 IU per day for 10 to 18-year-olds; and 200 IU per day for those above 18 years of age.[64] Presumably, these same dosages will be effective for other patients with steatorrhea due to pancreatic insufficiency.

On the other hand, patients with biliary atresia and abetalipoproteinemia are extremely difficult to treat and may require parenteral (usually intramuscular) supplementation. An injectable vitamin E preparation has been described and investigated in both infants and adults.[65] Further research, as well as approval of the United States Food and Drug Administration, will be needed before routine intramuscular therapy can be recommended for these two categories of patients.

Premature infants are also difficult to treat adequately using oral supplementation because of the necessity of delayed feedings in critically ill babies, the frequent occurrence of early gastrointestinal intolerance, and the presence of prolonged tocopherol malabsorption. Thus, intramuscular vitamin E is under investigation,[45] and multivitamin mixtures can be given intravenously to provide α-tocopheryl acetate, which is readily hydrolyzed in vivo to α-tocopherol. Gutcher et al. have shown that 3 IU per day rapidly leads to normal plasma tocopherol levels and peroxide hemolysis test results.[66] After a few days, 1 IU/kg per day given intravenously will maintain vitamin E adequacy. When enteral feedings are established, the usual oral dose of water-miscible α-tocopheryl acetate is 25 IU per day.

Pharmacologic use of vitamin E has been recommended in certain disease states that are not accompanied by vitamin E deficiency. This usage constitutes megavitamin therapy and has been reviewed in detail elsewhere.[4] Most of the disorders that have been reported as being responsive to vitamin E supplements, such as ischemic heart disease, intermittent claudication, and pulmonary oxygen toxicity, have not been adequately investigated. Although the most favorable results have been obtained with intermittent claudication, only one controlled study is convincing. This is an ongoing investigation by Haeger that includes objective data on beneficial responses in 158 patients given 300 mg per day.[67]

Because of claims that vitamin E supplementation will lead to great benefits in the quality of one's life, it is not surprising that a large proportion of the American population appears to take vitamin E supplements. The usual doses range from 100 to 800 mg per day, but the amount absorbed is far less. Observational experience over many years and limited studies have indicated no consistent evidence of toxicity when doses of 100 to 800 mg per day are taken orally by adults.[68] It is not appropriate, however, to conclude that long-term self-treatment with large amounts of vitamin E and parenteral tocopherol "therapy" are without risk. Further research is needed in this area, especially in view of the toxicity recently noted in premature infants given parenteral vitamin E[69] and the observation that tocopherol can accumulate continuously in adipose tissue. Indeed, vitamin E toxicity has been demonstrated both in animals and man. In general, doses of vitamin E necessary to elicit toxicity are many times that necessary for nutritional sufficiency. Reported toxic effects in adults have included increased bleeding tendency, impaired immune function, decreased levels of vitamin K-dependent clotting factors, and impairment of leukocyte function.[70] Reports of toxicity in infants include the preparation of E-Ferol previously discussed.[6] The toxicity of this preparation may have been related to non-vitamin E constituents in the formulation.[71] Other reports of vitamin E toxicity include increased risk of sepsis, necrotizing enterocolitis, and hemorrhagic complications. Other studies, however, have failed to identify sepsis, necrotizing enterocolitis, and bleeding disorders as complications associated with vitamin E therapy. The use of plasma or serum of vitamin E determinations to avoid toxicity is problematic because of a lack of reliable correlation with tissue concentrations.[72] Therefore, a cautious approach is recommended, particularly when tocopherol preparations are administered parenterally.

## REFERENCES

1. Sokol, R.J.: Annu. Rev. Nutr., *8:*351–373, 1988.
2. Bieri, J.G., Tolliver, L.J., Catignani, G.L.: Am. J. Clin. Nutr., *32:*2143–2149, 1979.
3. Gutcher, G.R., Lax, A.A., Farrell, P.M.: J.P.E.N., *8:*269–273, 1984.
4. Farrell, P.M., Machlin, L.J.: Human health and disease. *In* Vitamin E, A Comprehensive Treatise. Edited by L.J. Machlin. New York, Marcel Dekker, 1980. pp. 520–620.
5. Bieri, J.G., Corash, L., Hubbard, V.S.: N. Engl. J. Med., *308:*1063–1071, 1983.
6. Martone, W.J., Williams, W.W., Mortensen, M.L., et al.: Pediatrics, *78:*591–600, 1986.

7. Mason, K.E.: The first two decades of vitamin E history. *In Vitamin E, A Comprehensive Treatise. Edited by L.J. Machlin. New York, Marcel Dekker, 1980, pp. 1–6.*
8. Nelson, J.S.: Pathology of vitamin E deficiency. *In* Vitamin E, A Comprehensive Treatise. Edited by L.J. Machlin. New York, Marcel Dekker, 1980, pp. 397–428.
9. Wright, S.W., Filer, L.J. Jr., Mason, K.E.: Pediatrics, *7:*386–393, 1951.
10. Moyer, W.T.: Pediatrics, *6:*893–896, 1950.
11. Gordon, H.H., Nitowsky, Harold M., Cornblath, M.: Am. J. Dis. Child., *90:*669–681, 1955.
12. Darby, C.W., Davidson, A.G.F., Fosbrooke, A.S.: Arch. Dis. Child., *48:*72–75, 1973.
13. Mackenzie, J.B.: Pediatrics, *13:*346–351, 1954.
14. Kasparek, S.: Chemistry of tocopherols and tocotrienols. *In* Vitamin E, A Comprehensive Treatise. Edited by L.J. Machlin. New York, Marcel Dekker, 1980, pp. 7–65.
15. Bieri, J.G., McKenna, M.C.: Am. J. Clin. Nutr., *34:*289–295, 1981.
16. Catignani, G.L.: Role in nucleic acid and protein metabolism. *In* Vitamin E, A Comprehensive Treatise. Edited by L.J. Machlin. New York, Marcel Dekker, 1980, pp. 318–332.
17. Hoekstra, W.G.: Fed. Proc., *34:*2083–2089, 1975.
18. McCay, P.B., King, M.: Biochemical Function. *In* Vitamin E, A Comprehensive Treatise. Edited by L.J. Machlin. New York, Marcel Dekker, 1980, pp. 289–317.
19. McCay, P.B., King, M.M., Poyer, J.L., et al.: Ann. N. Y. Acad. Sci., *393:*23–30, 1982.
20. Pryor, W.A.: Ann. N. Y. Acad. Sci., *393:*1–22, 1982.
21. Pascoe, G.A., Reed, D.J.: Free Radic. Biol. Med., *6:*209–224, 1989.
22. Machlin, L.J., Gabriel, E., Brin, M.: J. Nutr., *112:*1437–1440, 1982.
23. Burton, G.W., Ingold, K.U.: J. Am. Chem. Soc., *103:*6472–6477, 1981.
24. Bieri, J.G., Poukka, R.K., Evarts, R.P.: J. Clin. Nutr., *27:*980–986, 1974.
25. Bauernfeind, J.: Tocopherols in food. *In* Vitamin E, A Comprehensive Treatise. Edited by L.J. Machlin. New York, Marcel Dekker, 1980, pp. 99–167.
26. Bunyan, J., McHale, D., Green, J., Marcinkiewicz, S.: Br. J. Nutr., *15:*253–257, 1961.
27. USDA: Oil Crops—Outlook and Situation Report, May, 1983. Washington, D.C., United States Department of Agriculture, 1983.
28. Losowsky, M.S., Kelleher, J., Walker, B.E.: Ann. N. Y. Acad. Sci., *203:*212–222, 1972.
29. MacMahon, M.T., Neale, G.: Clin. Sci., *38:*197–210, 1970.
30. Farrell, P.M., Bieri, J.G., Fratantoni, J.F., et al.: J. Clin. Invest., *6:*223–241, 1977.
31. Poukka, R.K., Bieri, J.G.: Lipids, *5:*757–761, 1970.
32. Bieri, J.G.: Ann. N. Y. Acad. Sci., *203:*181–191, 1972.
33. Bieri, J.G., Evarts, R.P.: Proc. Soc. Exp. Biol. Med., *149:*500–502, 1975.
34. Wiss, O., Bunnell, R.H., Gloor, U.: Vitam. Horm., *20:*441–455, 1962.
35. Horwitt, M.K., Harvey, C.C., Dahm, C.H., et al.: Ann. N. Y. Acad. Sci., *203:*223–236, 1972.
36. Gallo-Torres, H.E.: Transport and metabolism. *In* Vitamin E, A Comprehensive Treatise. Edited by L.J. Machlin. New York, Marcel Dekker, 1980, pp. 170–267.
37. Bieri, J.G.: Chromatography of tocopherols. *In* Lipid Chromatographic Analysis. Vol. 2. Edited by G.V. Marinetti. New York, Marcel Dekker, 1969, pp. 459–478.
38. Farrell, P.M.: J. Pediatr., *95:*869–872, 1979.
39. Horwitt, M.K., Harvey, C.C., Harmon, E.M.: Vitam. Horm., *26:*487–499, 1968.
40. Farrell, P.M., Levine, S.L., Murphey, M.D., et al.: Am. J. Clin. Nutr., *31:*1720–1726, 1978.
41. Sokol, R.J., Heubi, J.E., Iannaconne, S.T., Bove, K.E., et al.: N. Eng. J. Med., *310:*1209–1212, 1984.
42. Horwitt, M.K.: Vitam. Horm., *20:*541–558, 1962.
43. Gross, S., Melhorn, D.K.: Ann. N. Y. Acad. Sci., *203:*141–162, 1972.
44. Owens, W.C., Owens, E.U.: Am. J. Ophthalmol., *32:*1631–1637, 1949.
45. Johnson, L., Schaffer, D., Boggs, T.R.: Am. J. Clin. Nutr., *27:*1158–1173, 1974.
46. Hittner, H.M., Godio, L.B., Speer, M.E., et al.: Pediatrics, *71:*423–432, 1983.
47. Phelps, D.L., Rosenbaum, A.L., Isenberg, S.J., et al.: Pediatrics, *79:*489–500, 1987.
48. Oski, F.A., Barness, L.A.: J. Pediatr., *70:*211–220, 1967.
49. Goldbloom, R.B., Cameron, D.: Pediatrics, *32:*36–46, 1963.
50. Zipursky, A., Brown, E.J., Watts, J.: Pediatrics, *79:*61–68, 1987.
51. Bell, E.F., Filer, L.J.: Am. J. Clin. Nutr., *34:*414–420, 1981.
52. Phelps, D.L.: Am. J. Clin. Nutr., *46:*187–191, 1987.
53. Nitowsky, H.M., Cornblath, M., Gordon, H.H.: AMA J. Dis. Child., *92:*164–174, 1956.
54. Underwood, B.A., Denning, C.R.: Pediatr. Res., *6:*26–31, 1972.
55. Leonard, P.J., Losowsky, M.S.: Am. J. Clin. Nutr., *24:*388–393, 1971.
56. Kelleher, J., Miller, M.G., Littlewood, J.M., et al.: Int. J. Vitam. Nutr. Res., *57:*253–259, 1987.
57. Guggenheim, M.A., Ringel, S.P., Silverman, A., et al.: Ann. N. Y. Acad. Sci., *393:*84–93, 1982.
58. Muller, D.P.R., Lloyd, J.K.: Ann. N. Y. Acad. Sci., *393:*133–142, 1982.
59. Cynamon, H.A., Milov, D.E., Valenstein, E., et al.: J. Pediatr., *113:*637–640, 1988.
60. Bieri, J.G., Evarts, R.P.: J. Am. Diet. Assoc., *62:*147–151, 1973.
61. Witting, L.A., Lee, L.: Am. J. Clin. Nutr., *28:*571–576, 1975.
62. Horwitt, M.K.: Am. J. Clin. Nutr., *8:*451–461, 1960.
63. Food and Nutrition Board, National Research Council: Recommended Dietary Allowances. 10th Ed. Washington, D.C., National Academy Press, 1989, pp. 99–107.
64. Farrell, P.M., Mischler, E.H., Gutcher, G.R.: Ann. N. Y. Acad. Sci., *393:*96–106, 1982.
65. Newmark, H.L., Pool, W., Bauernfeind, J.C., et al.: J. Pharmacol. Sci., *64:*655–657, 1975.
66. Gutcher, G.R., Farrell, P.M.: J. Pediatr. Gastroenterol. Nutr., *4:*604–609, 1985.
67. Haeger, K.: Ann. N. Y. Acad. Sci., *393:*369–374, 1982.
68. Farrell, P.M., Bieri, J.G.: Am. J. Clin. Nutr., *28:*1381–1386, 1975.
69. Phelps, D.L.: Pediatrics, *74:*1114–1116, 1984.
70. Bell, E.F.: J. Nutr., *119:*1829–1831, 1989.
71. Rivera, A. Jr., Abdo, K.M., Bucher, J.R., et al.: Dev. Pharmacol. Ther., *14:*231–237, 1990.
72. Knight, M.E., Roberts, R.J.: Clin. Perinatol., *14:*843–855, 1987.

## SELECTED READINGS

Bieri, J.G., Corash, L., Hubbard, V.S.: Medical uses of vitamin E. N. Engl. J. Med., *308:*1063–1071, 1983.

Greer, F.R., Zachman, R.D., Farrell, P.M.: Neonatal vitamin metabolism—fat soluble. *In* Principles of Perinatal-Neonatal Metabolism. Edited by R.M. Cowett. New York, Springer-Verlag, 1991, pp. 531–558.

Machlin, L.J. (ed.): Vitamin E, A Comprehensive Treatise. New York, Marcel Dekker, 1980.

Phelps, D.L.: Current perspectives on vitamin E in infant nutrition. Am. J. Clin. Nutr., *46:*187–191, 1987.

Sokol, R.J.: Vitamin E deficiency and neurologic disease. Ann. Rev. Nutr., *8:*351–373, 1988.

CHAPTER 19

# Vitamin K

Robert E. Olson



Long periods of time may elapse between the discovery of a given vitamin deficiency disease, the isolation and determination of the structure of the vitamin, and the final elucidation of its metabolic function. This is true of vitamin K: its deficiency disease, fatal hemorrhage, was discovered in 1929, its isolation and structural determination was accomplished in 1939, and its metabolic function was suspected only after a new amino acid, γ-carboxyglutamic acid (Gla), was discovered in bovine prothrombin in 1974. It is now established that vitamin K is part of a membrane-bound carboxylase system that participates in the posttranslational carboxylation of a number of vitamin K-dependent proteins.

Despite intensive effort in several laboratories over the past 15 years, the vitamin K-dependent γ-glutamylcarboxylase has not yet been isolated and its reaction mechanism is not yet clear, although progress is being made. Furthermore, in this age of molecular biology, the gene that codes for this enzyme has not yet been cloned. What has become clear, however, is that vitamin K is not only associated with coagulation, but also with additional functions in bone, kidney, and possibly other tissues.

## HISTORICAL OVERVIEW

Vitamin K was discovered by Henrik Dam in Copenhagen in 1929 in studies of sterol metabolism in chicks fed fat-free diets.[1] He observed quite unexpectedly that some of the chicks developed hemorrhages under the skin, in muscle, and in other tissues and that blood, occasionally taken for laboratory examinations, showed delayed coagulation. The antihemorrhagic factor was found to be fat soluble. Similar observations were made in 1931 by MacFarlane and his co-workers[2] in Canada and shortly afterward by Holst and Halbrook[3] of the University of California.

In the early 1930s, Dam and co-workers extended their work to show that none of the established vitamins could prevent the hemorrhagic disease and named the new vitamin "K" (for *K*oagulation).[4,5] They demonstrated that vitamin K was distributed in liver, hemp seeds, and green leafy vegetables. In Dam's laboratory Schonheyder discovered in 1936 that the hemorrhagic disease was due to the absence of prothrombin activity in the plasma.[6] About the same time Almquist and Stokstad discovered that fish meal, particularly after putrefaction, was a good source of the vitamin.[7] Efforts were then initiated to isolate the new factor from both alfalfa and putrefied fish meal.

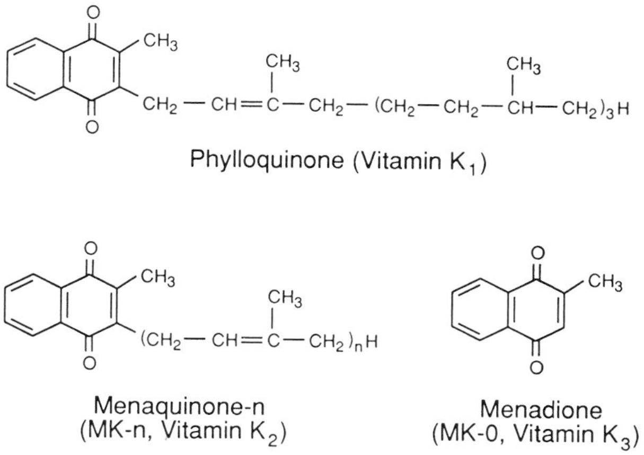
Phylloquinone (Vitamin K1)
Menaquinone-n
(MK-n, Vitamin K2)
Menadione
(MK-0, Vitamin K3)

**FIGURE 19–2.** Structures of vitamin K homologues that are derivatives of 1,4-naphthoquinone. Phylloquinone (vitamin $K_1$), menaquinones (vitamin $K_2$), and menadione (vitamin $K_3$) are shown.

In 1939, Doisy and his colleagues[8] and Dam and his colleagues[9] announced the isolation of vitamin $K_1$ from alfalfa. It was identified as 2-methyl-3-phytyl-1,4-naphthoquinone.[10] In addition, Doisy's group reported the isolation of a related but not identical vitamin K from putrified fish meal, which they named vitamin $K_2$.[11]

In 1941, Campbell and Link discovered[12] that the active agent in spoiled clover that caused a hemorrhagic disease in cattle, first described by Schofield in 1922,[13] was bishydroxycoumarin (dicumarol) and that this compound was antagonistic to vitamin K. The availability of 4-hydroxycoumarin drugs also provided new tools for the investigation of the complexities of blood coagulation. In the next decade three additional vitamin K-dependent coagulation factors were discovered. These were proconvertin (factor VII), Stewart factor (factor X), and Christmas factor (factor IX).[14] During the past 15 years three more coagulation factors dependent on vitamin K (protein C, protein S, and protein Z) have been discovered, of which two (proteins C and S) are anticoagulants.[15]

Studies at the University of Lund by Ganrot and Nilehn in 1968 showed that when the concentration of prothrombin was measured immunochemically in normal and coumarin-anticoagulated human subjects, the antigenic equivalents did not decrease in proportion to the biologic activity as measured by the clotting time.[16] They concluded that coumarin anticoagulant therapy, and by inference vitamin K deficiency, interfered with the normal synthesis of prothrombin and produced an abnormal prothrombin, modified in some way to make it biologically inactive but immunologically reactive.

The study of the chemical properties of bovine prothrombin from normal and anticoagulated cows was then undertaken in several laboratories. In 1974 Stenflo et al. in Sweden,[17] Nelsestuen et al. in the United States,[18] and Magnusson and co-workers in Denmark[19] independently reported that the difference between normal and abnormal prothrombin was the presence of a new amino acid in normal prothrombin, namely, γ-carboxyglutamic acid (Fig. 19–1). This carboxylated glutamic acid was not present in the prothrombin of animals given coumarin drugs or put on vitamin K-deficient diets. It was therefore concluded that vitamin K acts to alter the structure of the vitamin K-dependent proteins post-translationally by facilitating the carboxylation of selected glutamate residues in the primary structure of the protein. This discovery revolutionized ideas about the function of vitamin K and led to studies of the enzymology of the vitamin K-dependent γ-glutamyl carboxylase and related vitamin K enzymes in the microsomes of liver and other tissues. The history of vitamin K research has been extensively reviewed elsewhere.[14,15,20–22]

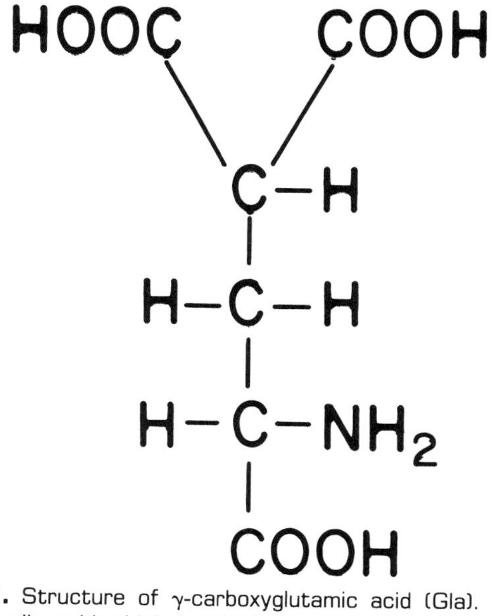
HOOC
COOH
C—H
H—C—H
H—C—NH2
COOH

**FIGURE 19–1.** Structure of γ-carboxyglutamic acid (Gla). Gla is a tricarboxylic acid which is stable in strong base but decomposes with γ-decarboxylation in strong acid. Its isoelectric point is pH 3.0.

## CHEMISTRY

Compounds with vitamin K activity all contain the 2-methyl-1,4-napthoquinone nucleus with a lipophilic side chain at position 3. Vitamin $K_1$, now known as phylloquinone, was identified as 2-methyl-3-phytyl-1,4-naphthoquinone (Fig. 19–2). It is the only homologue of vitamin K synthesized by plants. Vitamin $K_2$, isolated from fish meal, was originally believed to be 2-methyl-3-difarnesyl-1,4-naphthoquinone synthesized by organisms in the fish meal.[23] It has since been shown to have seven isoprene units in the side chain instead of six and is thus called menaquinone-7.[24] The menaquinone family of $K_2$

homologues is a large series of vitamins containing normally unsaturated isoprenyl side chains, which vary in length and are designated MK-n (19–2). Menaquinone-4 (MK-4) is synthesized in animals and birds from the provitamin menadione 2-methyl-1,4-naphthoquinone (formerly known as vitamin $K_3$) by enzymatic alkylation with digeranyl pyrophosphate.[25] The alkylating enzyme has been partially purified and characterized from chick and rat liver microsomes.[26,27] The other menaquinones are products of bacterial biosynthesis and range from menaquinone-7 to menaquinone-13.[28,29] Partially saturated menaquinones, menaquinone-9-H[30] and menaquinone-8-H,[31] are known. The molecular weight of vitamin $K_1$ is 450.68 g/mol.

## FOODS AS A SOURCE OF VITAMIN K

Vitamin K is widely distributed in both animal and vegetable foods and varies from less than 22 nM* (1 μg/100 ml) in milk to over 8.8 μmol/kg (400 μg/100 g) in spinach, kale, and turnip greens. The concentration of vitamin K in the fasting plasma of healthy persons is less than 1 ng/ml (2.2 nM). Liver usually contains a mixture of phylloquinone and menaquinones that totals between 11 and 89 nmol/kg (5 and 40 ng/g). Both biologic and chemical methods have been used to measure vitamin K in foods. Because vitamin K is light sensitive, precautions must be taken to protect the vitamin during analysis.

### BIOLOGIC METHODS

For many years the only satisfactory procedure available for the determination of vitamin K activity of foods was a curative bioassay based on the response of deficient chicks to the added food.[32] In this method, the prothrombin level was measured with Russell's viper venom. The response of unknowns was compared to the dose-response curve using phylloquinone as a standard. The sensitivity of the chick bioassay is 0.22 μmol phylloquinone per kilogram of food (0.1 μg/g) or a total of 4.4 to 6.6 nmol per day (2 to 3 μg per day). Such assays, however, do not yield information about the form of vitamin K present in the material. Furthermore, the various homologues vary in their biologic activity. Matschiner and Doisy found that menaquinone-1 had only 1% of the biologic activity of phylloquinone per os, whereas MK-4, MK-5, and MK-7 were identical to phylloquinone in activity.[32] MK-2 and MK-10 gave 20 to 29% of the activity of phylloquinone and showed that the very short-chain and the very long-chain homologues were less active by mouth than the medium-chain derivatives.

*22 nM is 22 nmol/L

### CHEMICAL METHODS

In more recent times, vitamin K has been determined by chemical methods in which neutral fat solvent extraction of dessicated tissues has been followed by column and thin-layer chromatography, and then by high-pressure liquid chromatography (HPLC), using both direct and reverse phase columns. By using these techniques and HPLC detection by ultraviolet absorption,[33] electrochemical techniques,[34] fluorescence of hydroquinone derivatives,[35] or combined gas chromatography (GC)-mass spectrometry,[36] it's been possible to measure vitamin K homologues in amounts as low as 0.11 pmol/g (50 pg/g) of original material. The molar absorption coefficient for vitamin K homologues at 248 nm is 19,000.

### ANALYTICAL VALUES

The vitamin K content of common foods as determined by a variety of methods is presented in Table 19–1.[37–39] In general, green, leafy vegetables are high in vitamin K (greater than 2.2 μmol/kg, or 100 μg/100 g), fruits and cereals are low (less than 0.33 μmol/kg, or 15 μg/100 g), and meats and dairy products have a wide range (between 0.22 and 1.11 μmol/kg, or 1 and 50 μg/100 g). Human milk contains about 6 nM only (2 to 3 μg/L), whereas cow's milk contains about 18 nM (between 6 and 10 μg/L). It is of interest that tobacco is one of the richest sources of phylloquinone and contains 0.1 mol/kg (5000 μg/100 g). When smoked, a small percentage of vitamin K is volatilized and can be absorbed through the mucous membranes, the nasopharynx, bronchi, and alveoli.[39]

## ABSORPTION, DISTRIBUTION, AND METABOLISM

The absorption of phylloquinone and the menaquinones requires bile and pancreatic juice for maximum effectiveness.[40] Dietary vitamin K is absorbed in the small bowel, is incorporated into chylomicrons, and appears in the lymph.[41] Efficiency of absorption has been measured from 40 to 80%, depending on the vehicle in which the vitamin is administered and the extent of the enterohepatic circulation generally characteristic of isoprenoid lipids. When isotopically labeled phylloquinone was administered to animals[42] and man[43] by mouth in doses ranging from the physiologic to the pharmacologic, the vitamin appeared in the plasma within 20 minutes, peaked at 2 hours, and then declined exponentially to low values over 48 to 72 hours, reaching fasting levels of around 5 nmol (1 to 3 ng/ml). During this period, it appeared to be transferred via the liver from chylomicron remnants to the β-lipoproteins. No specific carrier protein for vitamin K in plasma has been identified. Between 8 and 30% of the administered radioactivity was recovered in polar metabolites in the urine over a

**TABLE 19–1.** AVERAGE VITAMIN K CONTENT OF ORDINARY FOODS.

| FOOD | VITAMIN K* μg/100 g | FOOD | VITAMIN K μg/100 g | FOOD | VITAMIN K μg/100 g | FOOD | VITAMIN K μg/100 g |
|---|---|---|---|---|---|---|---|
| Milk and milk products | | Fats | | Vegetables | | Fruits | |
| Butter | 30 | Beef fat | 15 | Asparagus | 57 | Applesauce | 2 |
| Cheese | 35 | Corn oil | 0 | Beans, green | 46 | Banana | 2 |
| Milk (cow) | 1 | Safflower oil | 10 | Broccoli | 175 | Orange | 1 |
| Milk (human) | 0.2 | Cereal and grain products | | Cabbage | 125 | Peach | 8 |
| Eggs | | Bread | 4 | Kale | 729 | Raisin | 6 |
| Hens (whole) | 11 | Maize | 5 | Lettuce | 129 | Strawberry | 10 |
| Meat and meat products | | Oats | 10 | Peas, green | 29 | Beverages | |
| Bacon | 46 | Rice | 3 | Potato | 1 | Coffee | 38 |
| Beef liver | 92 | Wheat flour | 4 | Pumpkin | 2 | Cola | 2 |
| Chicken liver | 7 | Whole flour | 17 | Spinach | 415 | Tea, black | — |
| Ground beef | 7 | | | Tomato | 6 | Tea, green | 712 |
| Ham | 15 | | | Turnip greens | 650 | Tobacco | |
| Pork liver | 25 | | | Watercress | 80 | Cigarettes | 5000 |
| Pork tenderloin | 11 | | | White turnip | 1 | | |

(Data from Shearer, M.J., Allan, V., Haroon, Y., et al.: *In* Vitamin K Metabolism and Vitamin K-Dependent Proteins. Edited by J.W. Suttie. Baltimore, University Park Press, 1980, pp. 317–327; Dam, H., Glavind, J.: Biochem. J., *32*:485–490, 1938; Matschiner, J.T., Doisy, E.A. Jr.: J. Nutr., *90*:97–100, 1966; and Doisy, E.A. Jr.: Private communication.)

*1 μg vitamin $K_1$ = 2.2 nmol

3-day period in both animals and man, whereas total fecal radioactivity accounted for 45 to 60% of the administered dose over a 5-day period.[43] About one third of this fecal radioactivity was unchanged vitamin $K_1$. The administration of nonabsorbable lipids, such as mineral oil or squalene, greatly reduces the absorption of vitamin K in animals.[44]

Wiss et al.[42] observed that the principal excretory form of vitamin K in rat urine is a metabolite resembling the lactone of vitamin E first described by Simon et al.[45] It was identified as a chain-shortened and oxidized derivative of vitamin K, which forms a γ-lactone and is probably excreted as a glucuronide. Vitamin K-2,3-epoxide has also been identified as a metabolite of vitamin K in animals and is metabolized to a homologous lactone.[46,47] In omnivorous animals both phylloquinone and the higher-molecular-weight menaquinones (MK-7 to MK-13), which are of bacterial origin and probably derived from intestinal flora, are found in the liver.[48–50]

The turnover of vitamin K in the animal body is rapid, and the total body pool is surprisingly small. Bjornsson et al. infused 300 μg of $^3$H-phylloquinone into human volunteers with or without previous drug loading with warfarin or clofibrate.[51] The initial half-time (T½α) for the first exponential phase was 26 ± 8 minutes, and the average terminal half-time (t½β) was 166 ± 9 minutes under all conditions. Shearer et al. found similar results with a 2.2-μmol (1.0-mg) intravenous dose of $^3$H-phylloquinone: T½α equalled 20 to 24 minutes and T½β equalled 120 to 150 minutes.[52] From data on the volume of distribution and clearance rate, Bjornsson et al.[53] calculated the fractional turnover rate to be 0.4/hour, suggesting that the body pool was turning once every 2.5 hours, although more-recent studies by Olson et al.,[54] employing 0.66 nmol (0.3 μg, or 10 μCi) of $^3$H-phylloquinone and longer periods of observation, have suggested that the metabolic turnover time for vitamin $K_1$ is about once per day. From daily intakes of vitamin K of about 0.22 μmol per day (100 μg per day) and the turnover time of 24 hours, the body pool sizes were estimated to be 0.22 μmol (100 μg) or 3.1 nmol/kg (1.5 μg)/kg body weight. This body pool of vitamin K is smaller than that for vitamin $B_{12}$, and exceptionally low for a fat-soluble vitamin.

When menadione (2-methyl-1,4-naphthoquinone) is administered to animals or man, only a small amount (0.05 to 1.0%) is converted to MK-4.[55,56] The principal metabolites of menadione are the sulfate and glucuronide of dihydromenadione.[57,58] As first described by Fieser,[59] menadione also reacts with free sulfhydryl groups, which may account for some of its reported toxicity.[60]

## PHYSIOLOGIC FUNCTION

### REGULATION OF CLOTTING PROTEIN SYNTHESIS

The seven vitamin K-dependent coagulation proteins are proenzymes that are converted to serine hydrolases during coagulation. All require calcium for activation, a phenomenon mediated by their γ-carboxyglutamate residues. The vitamin K-dependent procoagulant factors (II, VII, IX, and X) form the core of the proteolytic cascade leading to fibrin formation in hemostasis as shown in Figure 19–3. This cascade, which accomplishes amplification of proteolytic activity at each stage, has two wings.[61] The intrinsic system, which is operative within the circulation, is activated by surface-mediated reactions involving high-molecular-weight kininogen and prekallikrein. They initiate a series of reactions that result in the activation of factor IX and the conversion of factor X to Xa. The extrinsic system, which is switched on by cell injury via tissue thromboplastin, involves the activation of factor VII, which also converts factor X to Xa. The final common pathway begins with the prothrombinase complex (factor Xa, factor V, $Ca^{++}$, and phospholipid) that converts prothrombin (factor II) to thrombin which, in turn, converts fibrinogen to fibrin.

Protein C is an anticoagulant and serves as a brake on the speed of the intrinsic cascade through a feedback loop involving thrombin. While thrombin is producing fibrin, it is also activating protein C which, in turn, inactivates factors V and VIII, thus slowing its own production. Protein S enhances the activity of protein C in the presence of phospholipid. Antithrombin III, whose cofactor is heparin, also serves as an anticoagulant in plasma by inactivating thrombin and other procoagulant enzymes in the intrinsic system.

Thus the coagulation cascade is tightly regulated by both procoagulants and anticoagulants, some of which are dependent on vitamin K. Because all the vitamin K-dependent coagulation factors are synthesized in the liver, hepatectomy (or severe liver disease) results in lowered plasma levels of these factors and reduced sensitivity of the liver to the administration of vitamin K.

All the genes that code for the seven vitamin K-dependent plasma coagulation factors in human plasma have been cloned, and the complementary DNA (cDNA) sequences have been determined for all but protein Z.[62] The gene for prothrombin is approximately 24 kilobases long and contains 13 introns (which are not translated) and 14 exons. The messenger RNA (mRNA) for prothrombin is about 2000 nucleotides in length and con-

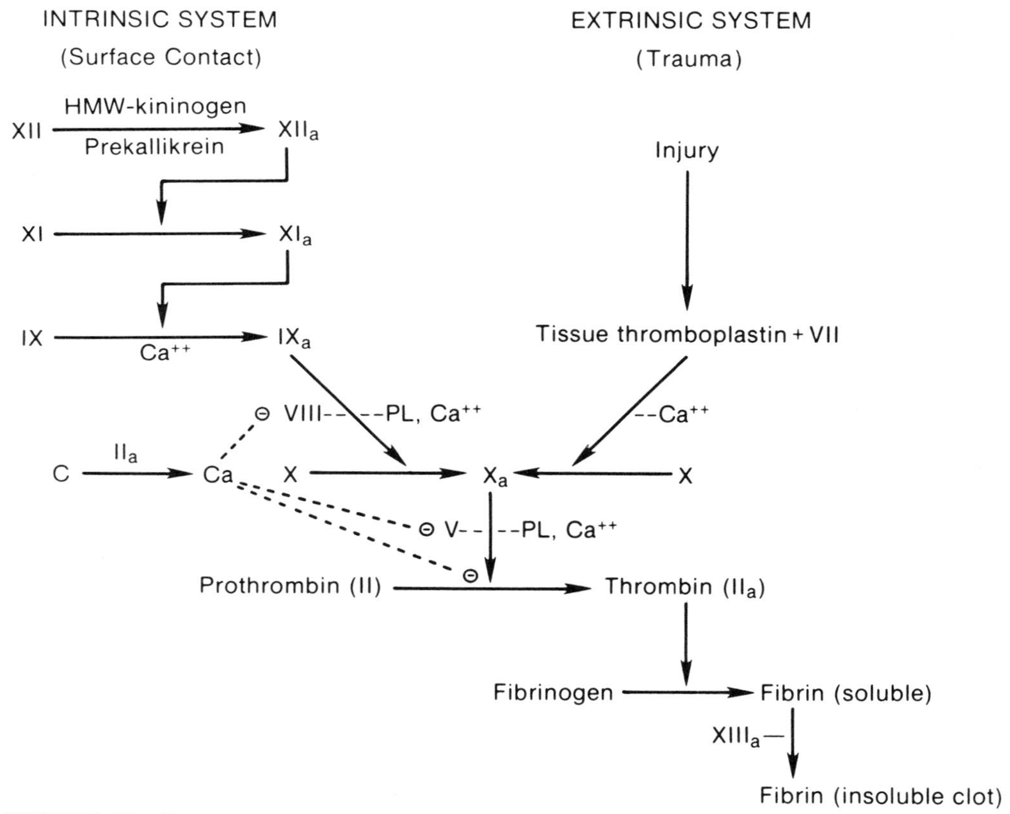
INTRINSIC SYSTEM
(Surface Contact)
EXTRINSIC SYSTEM
(Trauma)
HMW-kininogen
XII
XIIa
Prekallikrein
Injury
XI
XIa
IX
IXa
Ca++
Tissue thromboplastin + VII
⊖ VIII--
--PL, Ca++
--Ca++
IIa
C
Ca
X
Xa
X
⊖ V--
--PL, Ca++
⊖
Prothrombin (II)
Thrombin (IIa)
Fibrinogen
Fibrin (soluble)
XIIIa—
Fibrin (insoluble clot)

**FIGURE 19–3.** The clotting factor cascade. Factors II, VII, IX, and X and proteins C and S contain Gla and are vitamin K dependent. The first four factors occupy the core of the clotting scheme, whereas protein C is an anticoagulant protein that inactivates factors $V_a$ and $VIII_a$. Protein S is a cofactor for protein C and enhances its rate of activation by thrombin. $Ca^{2+}$ is required to activate Gla-containing factors. Factor V (accelerator globulin) and factor VIII (antihemophilic globulin) are cofactors. Factor XIII is a transpeptidase. (Modified from Davie, E.W., Ratnoff, O.D.: Science, *145*:1310–1312, 1964. Copyright 1964 by the American Association for the Advancement of Science.)

tains a noncoding region of 97 base pairs and a poly A tail of 27 base pairs. As shown in Figure 19–4, mature prothrombin contains 579 amino acids and three carbohydrate chains at residues 78, 100, and 373, accounting for 8.2% of the 71,600-kd molecular weight. As synthesized, however, prothrombin has a 43-amino-acid leader sequence containing both signal and propeptide residues. The prosegment, which contains 18 amino acids, is the recognition site for the γ-glutamylcarboxylase.[62]

The prosegment for prothrombin has the following sequence.

*−18*
His-Val-Phe-Leu-Ala-Pro-Gln-Gln-Ala-Arg-Ser-Leu-Leu
-Gln-Arg-Val-Arg-Arg−1

Site-specific mutagenesis has shown that the four amino acids at positions −18 to −15 (His, Val, Phe, and Leu) and the Ala at position −10 are essential for binding of the prothrombin precursor to the γ-glutamylcarboxylase.[63] The enzyme thrombin, which is the proteolytic product of prothrombin, contains two chains linked by a disulfide and contains 308 amino acids.

## VITAMIN K-DEPENDENT γ-GLUTAMYLCARBOXYLASE

The vitamin K-dependent carboxylase system is a membrane-bound component of the endoplasmic reticulum. It has been solubilized[64–66] by various detergents and, in the soluble form, retains most of the properties of the microsomal system. The system requires a Glu-containing peptide substrate, $O_2$, $CO_2$, and either vitamin K plus NADH (the reduced form of nicotinamide-adenine dinucleotide) or a vitamin K hydroquinone. $CO_2$, not $HCO_3^-$, is the active form of carbon dioxide incorporated into the γ-carboxyl group of peptide-bound glutamate ($Gla_p$).[67] Adenosine triphosphate (ATP) is not re-

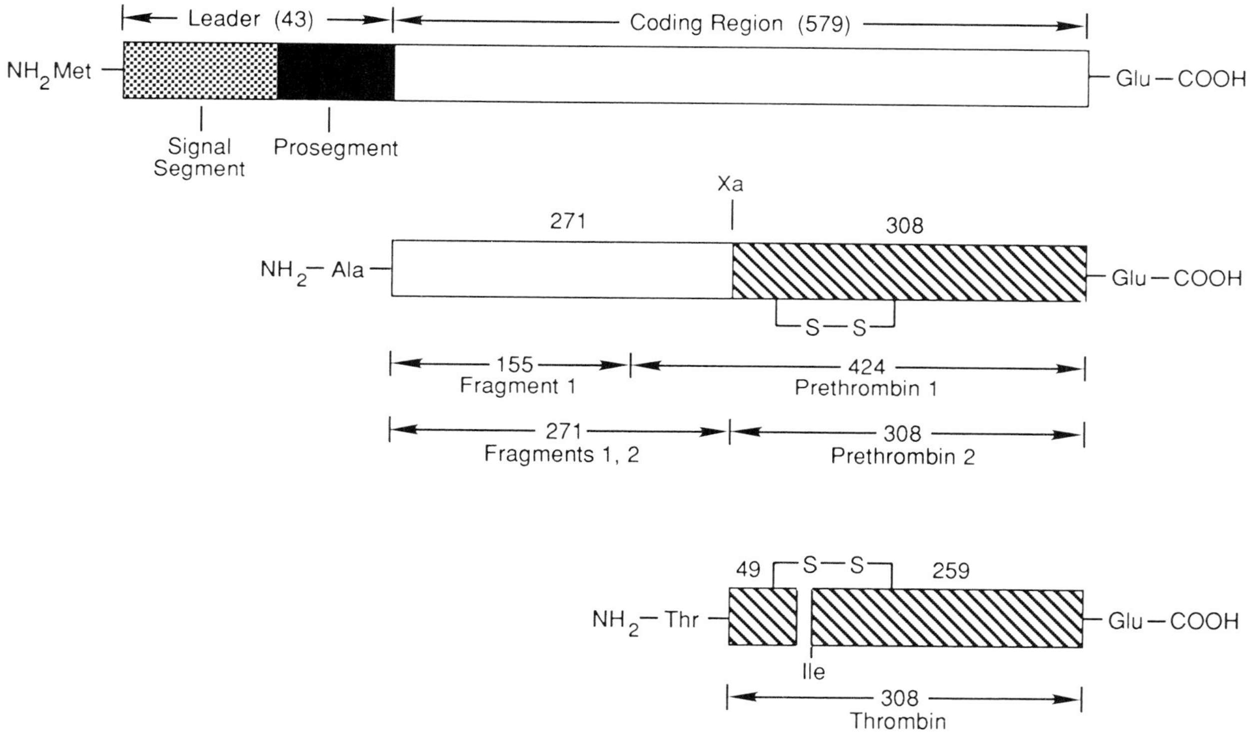
Leader (43)
Coding Region (579)
NH2Met
Glu—COOH
Signal Segment
Prosegment
Xa
271
308
NH2— Ala
Glu—COOH
S—S
155
Fragment 1
424
Prethrombin 1
271
Fragments 1, 2
308
Prethrombin 2
49
S—S
259
NH2— Thr
Glu—COOH
Ile
308
Thrombin

**FIGURE 19–4.** Structure of human prothrombin. A linear model of the nascent peptide is shown at the top. It has three components, a signal segment of 25 amino acids, a basic prosegment of 18 amino acids (in black), and a coding portion of 579 amino acids. The signal segment is cleaved by a signal peptidase on the luminal side of the RER. After carboxylation of 10 N-terminal Gla residues in the mature peptide, the prosegment is cleaved in the Golgi apparatus before secretion. The second linear drawing shows the mature prothrombin secreted into plasma, which has an N-terminal alanine and a C-terminal glutamic acid. The thrombin portion is crosshatched. Prothrombin is split at arginine 271 by activated factor X to generate prethrombin-2, which is converted into an active 2-chain, disulfide-linked thrombin by a second factor $X_a$ clip at arginine 320. The thrombin formed autocatalytically splits prothrombin and fragment 1,2 at arginine 156 to yield prethrombin-1 and fragments 1 and 2. The 10 Gla residues in fragment 1 are at positions 7, 8, 15, 17, 20, 21, 26, 27, 30, and 33 and the carbohydrate moieties are at positions 78, 100, and 373.

quired and biotin is not involved. Reduced vitamin K functions as a cosubstrate in the carboxylation reaction, but also as a cofactor because it is regenerated by two reductases in separate reactions. The overall carboxylation reaction is:

$$KH_2 + O_2 + CO_2 + Glu_p \xrightarrow{Mn^{++}} KO + Gla_p + H_2O$$

Thus the oxidation of $KH_2$ to KO (vitamin K-2,3 epoxide) and $H_2O$ is coupled to the fixation of $CO_2$ in the γ position of peptide-bound glutamate to form $Gla_p$. Artificial substrates imitating partial sequences of prothrombin precursor such as Phe-Leu-Glu-Glu-Leu have proved to be active in this system.[68,69] The rate of carboxylation is conveniently measured by adding $H^{14}CO_3^-$ to the reaction medium and determining the radioactivity incorporated into $Gla_p$.

Despite intense efforts to purify the vitamin K-dependent γ-glutamylcarboxylase over the past 15 years, this enzyme has not yet been purified to homogeneity, although progress has been made.[70] By 1987, the best purification of the carboxylase from liver microsomes was 400 times.[64–66,71–73] In 1989 Hubbard et al. claimed they had purified the vitamin K-dependent carboxylase (M.W. 77,000) to homogeneity (about 10,000 times from bovine microsomes) using synthetic propeptides as affinity columns,[74] but alas, this carboxylase preparation was later shown to be extensively contaminated with a ubiquitous microsomal binding protein (BiP). In 1991 Wu et al. reported the purification of the carboxylase (M.W. 94,000) to near homogeneity, about 70,000 times, from bovine microsomes by affinity chromatography.[75]

The mechanism of the vitamin K-dependent carboxylation is still obscure. A mechanism proposed by Larson and Suttie for the coupling of carboxylation and epoxidation in the vitamin K-dependent carboxylase is shown in Figure 19–5.[76] The reaction is presented as an ordered mechanism with three coupling sites. The first is the combination of the enzyme with $KH_2$ and $O_2$ to yield a ternary enzyme-substrate complex and subsequently KHOOH, the 2-hydroperoxide of vitamin K hydroquinone. This step is inhibited competitively by chlorophylloquinone and tetrachloropyridinol.[77] The second coupling site is between KHOOH and glutamyl peptide activation. The peptide (third substrate) is visualized as binding to the enzyme system after the addition of $KH_2$ and $O_2$. Epoxidation with the formation of KO can occur in the absence of peptide and $CO_2$, but peptide addition stimulates carboxylation and enhances epoxidation.

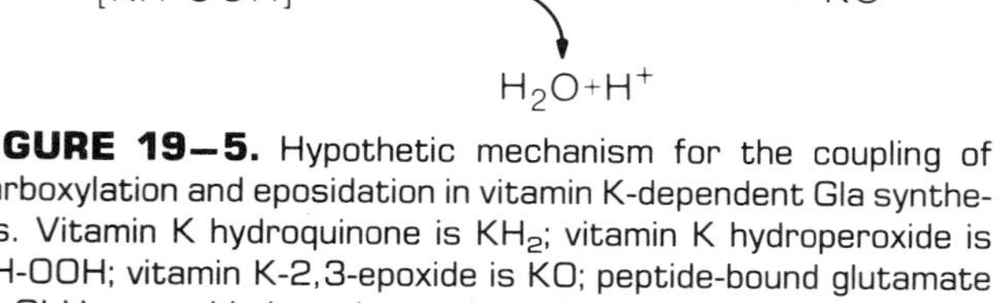
H+
KH2
O2
GLUp
CO2
(-)
GLUp
(-)
GLAp
[KH-OOH]
KO
H2O+H+

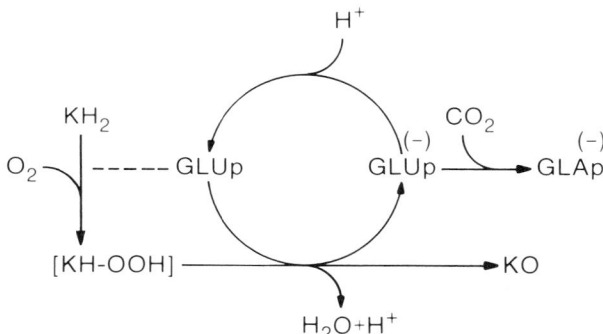

**FIGURE 19–5.** Hypothetic mechanism for the coupling of carboxylation and eposidation in vitamin K-dependent Gla synthesis. Vitamin K hydroquinone is $KH_2$; vitamin K hydroperoxide is KH-OOH; vitamin K-2,3-epoxide is KO; peptide-bound glutamate is GLUp; peptide-bound γ-carboxyglutamate is GLAp. (From Olson, R.E.: Vitamin K. *In* Hemostasis and Thrombosis. Edited by R.W. Coleman, J. Hirsch, V.J. Marder, and E.W. Salzman. Philadelphia, J.B. Lippincott, 1987, pp. 846–860.)

Larson and Suttie proposed that the hypothetical vitamin K-hydroperoxy anion might be sufficiently basic to remove the γ-methylene proton from peptide-bound glutamate.[76] Olson's group, however, argued that the organic hydroperoxy anion was insufficiently basic to remove a proton from the γ-methylene group and suggested an inductive mechanism for the labilization of the γ-methylene proton.[78] Ham and Dowd have suggested, on the basis of the study of a model system, that oxygen addition to reduced vitamin K results in the formation of a very basic epoxy alkoxide anion that can remove a proton from a carbon adjacent to a carboxyl group.[79,80]

The third coupling site is between the activated γ-glutamyl residue and $CO_2$, which appears to be dependent on the $HCO_3^-$ concentration in the medium.[81] The present data favor a nucleophilic attack of the glutamyl carbanion on $CO_2$ to form Gla.

## VITAMIN K CYCLE

The vitamin K cycle is shown in Figure 19–6. In essence it is a salvage pathway for vitamin K, a vitamin present in only nanomolar quantities in liver and other tissues. In this cycle the vitamin K-2,3 epoxide, a product of the carboxylation reaction, is reduced to the quinone by a dithiol-dependent epoxide reductase. The regenerated vitamin K is now reduced to the vitamin K hydroquinone by one of several possible enzymes, at least one driven by a dithiol and several by the reduced form of NAD phosphate (NADPH).[82] The dithiol-dependent reductases for both the epoxide and the quinone are strongly inhibited by warfarin, whereas the NADPH-dependent dehydrogenases are relatively insensitive to warfarin.[83] The net effect of the cycle is the conversion of vitamin K-2,3-epoxide formed in the carboxylation reaction to vitamin K hydroquinone, which becomes available for another round of carboxylation. In this way, vitamin K acts catalytically for Gla synthesis.

## BONE AND KIDNEY PROTEINS CONTAINING γ-CARBOXYGLUTAMATE

Two vitamin K-dependent bone proteins have been discovered in the last 15 years. The first is bone Gla protein (BGP, or osteocalcin) secreted by osteoblasts and

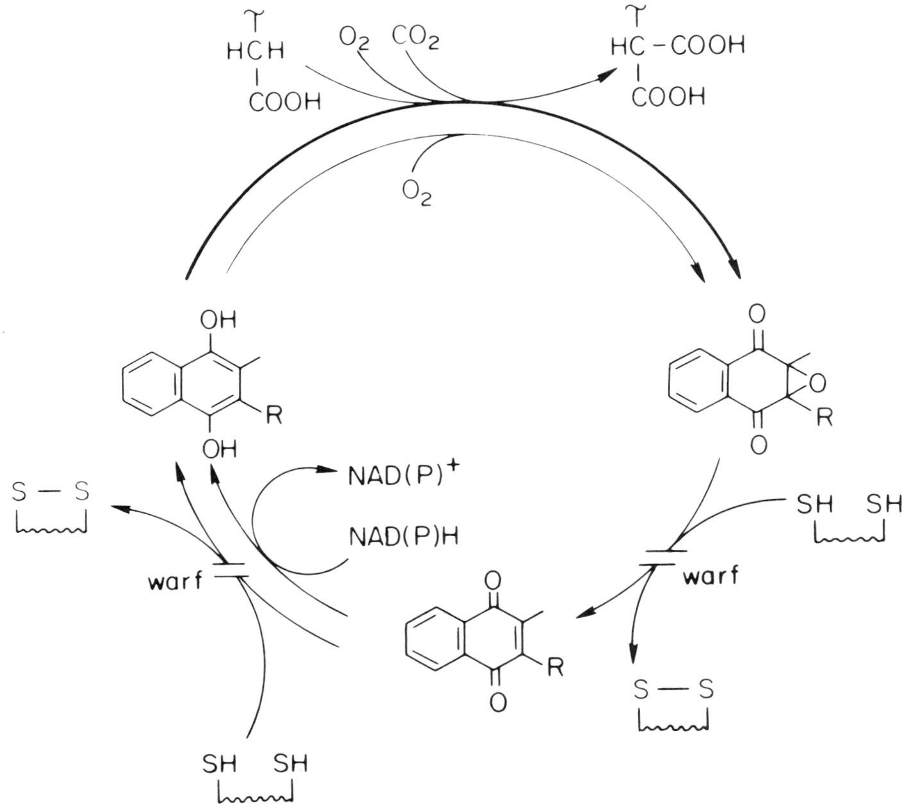
HCH
COOH
$O_2$
$CO_2$
HC-COOH
COOH
$O_2$
OH
R
OH
O
O
R
O
S — S
NAD(P)⁺
NAD(P)H
SH SH
warf
warf
O
R
O
S — S
SH SH

**FIGURE 19–6.** The vitamin K cycle occurs in the hepatic endoplasmic reticulum. The carboxylation and eposidation activities are catalyzed by the same enzyme. The dithiol-dependent reductions of the vitamin K epoxide and of vitamin K are extremely sensitive to the action of coumarin anticoagulants such as warfarin (warf). NADPH-dependent dehydrogenases, however, are not inhibited by warfarin. (From Suttie, J.W., Olson, R.E.: *In* Present Knowledge in Nutrition. 5th Ed. Edited by R.E. Olson. Washington, D.C., International Life Science Institute, 1984, pp. 241–259.)

discovered independently by Hauschka et al. and Price et al. in 1975.[84,85] The second is the matrix Gla protein (MGP) discovered in bone, dentin, and cartilage by Price et al. in 1985.[86]

BGP, which is a water-soluble 49-residue protein with a molecular weight of 5700, contains three Gla residues at positions 17, 21, and 24 and one disulfide bond.[87] BGP is one of the most abundant noncollagenous proteins in bone, accounting for 15 to 20% of noncollagen proteins in most vertebrates. In vitro BGP binds strongly to hydroxyapatite and inhibits its formation. Both properties are lost when the Gla residues are decarboxylated. The nascent peptide of BGP contains a 23-residue leader sequence, a 26-residue propeptide and, as indicated, a 49-residue mature protein that is not homologous with the coagulation proteins. The 26-residue propeptide, however, appears to serve as the recognition site for the γ -glutamylcarboxylase.

MGP, which is a 79-residue protein with a molecular weight of 8700, contains Gla residues at position 2, 37, 41, 48, and 52. It is only 20% homologous with BGP and has different properties, being highly insoluble in neutral salt solutions. It is found in the organic matrix of bone and does not react with hydroxyapatite. The nascent peptide of MGP contains a 19-residue signal sequence but no propeptide. It does, however, have an internal sequence of amino acids in the mature protein from residues 15 to 30 that is homologous with the propeptide in the other vitamin K-dependent proteins. This sequence appears to serve as the recognition site for the γ-glutamylcarboxylase.[88]

Microsomes from embryonic chick bone contain a vitamin K-dependent γ-glutamylcarboxylase that can carboxylate endogenous bone protein and Glu-containing pentapeptides.[89,90] Warfarin inhibits the synthesis of both BGP and MGP. Unlike the coagulation proteins synthesized in the liver, however, vitamin K does not overcome the effect of warfarin on BGP and MGP synthesis.[91] This appears to be the result of the lack of an NADP-linked reductase for vitamin K in bone tissue. This nonresponsiveness of bone tissue to vitamin K in animals on warfarin permitted Price to study the role of the vitamin K-dependent proteins in bone without the risk of a deficiency in vitamin K-dependent coagulation factors.[88]

The synthesis of both BGP and MGP, furthermore, is regulated by 1,25-dihydroxy-vitamin $D_3$ in cultured osteosarcoma cells.[92] This process suggests that BGP and MGP mediate some actions of vitamin D on bone. Although the present data show that a deficiency of BGP does not affect bone structure or fracture repair, plasma BGP is elevated in metabolic bone disease[93] and may stimulate bone remodeling and mobilization of calcium. MGP is associated with the inhibition of growth plate mineralization.

Several cases of the Conradi-Hunermann teratogenic type of chondrodysplasia punctata have been reported in infants born to mothers taking warfarin during the first trimester.[94,95] This defect appears to result from a deficiency of BGP and MGP during embryogenesis.

In 1976, Lian and Prien reported the presence of another Gla-containing protein in the matrix of calcium-containing renal stones in man.[96] It was reported to have a molecular weight of 18,000 and to contain four residues of Gla. It may function to solubilize calcium salts in urine. Hauschka et al. subsequently demonstrated that MK-3 stimulated the synthesis of $^{14}$C-Gla from $^{14}CO_2$ in kidney microsomes from dicoumarol-treated animals.[97] Friedman et al. have localized this synthesis to the tubular cells.[98] Gla biosynthesis has also been demonstrated in a mouse renal adenocarcinoma in tissue culture.[99]

## COUMARIN ANTICOAGULANT DRUGS

The coumarin anticoagulant agents inhibit the biosynthesis of prothrombin and other vitamin K-dependent factors in the liver and thus cause factor deficiencies in the plasma (Fig. 19–7). The 4-hydroxycoumarin drugs do not directly block the vitamin K-dependent carboxylase but block the vitamin K cycle. It is now known that the dithiothreitol (DTT)-driven vitamin KO reductase is not the only reductase blocked by warfarin; a similar DTT-dependent vitamin K reductase also is inhibited.[83] This combined attack by coumarin anticoagulants reduces $KH_2$ to ineffective levels and stops carboxylation. The warfarin receptor, first described by Searcey et al.,[100] has been identified as the vitamin K epoxide reductase.[101] The DTT-driven vitamin K reductase has a very low $K_m$

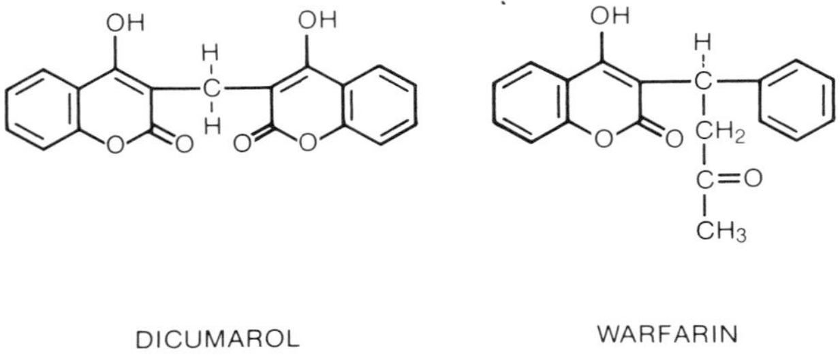

OH
OH
H
C
H
O
O
O
O
OH
H
C
CH2
C=O
CH3
O
O
DICUMAROL
WARFARIN


**FIGURE 19–7.** Structures of two 4-hydroxycoumarin drugs.

when compared to the NADPH-dependent vitamin K reductase. Hence, under physiologic conditions, the DTT-powered warfarin-sensitive enzyme is the pathway used. To overcome a warfarin block, large amounts of vitamin K are necessary. At these high levels, the NADPH quinone reductases, which are relatively insensitive to warfarin, are used to generate $KH_2$.[81]

Overdosage with coumarin drugs can occur in patients who have received these drugs to prevent thrombosis in coronary artery disease or pulmonary embolic disease. The intravenous administration of pharmacologic doses of vitamin $K_1$ in the micromolar range reinitiates prothrombin and other vitamin K-dependent factor synthesis within minutes by bypassing the blocked DTT-dependent vitamin K reductase in the liver. Water-soluble derivatives of menadione (e.g., Synkavite) are largely ineffective against the coumarin anticoagulant drugs because, as previously mentioned, the rate of conversion to MK-4 is so slow that pharmacologically effective levels of the alkylated vitamin are not attained.[26]

## VITAMIN K DEFICIENCY

Primary vitamin K deficiency is uncommon in healthy adults. Several factors protect adults from a lack of vitamin K. These include (1) widespread distribution of vitamin K in plant and animal tissues, (2) the vitamin K cycle, which conserves the vitamin, and (3) the microbiologic flora of the normal gut, which synthesizes menaquinones, which can contribute to the requirement for vitamin K. On the other hand, vitamin K deficiency in the breast-fed newborn remains a major worldwide cause of infant morbidity and mortality.[102,103] The causes of reduced levels of the vitamin K-dependent coagulation factors in adults are largely secondary to disease or drug therapy. The causes of vitamin K deficiency in humans are discussed below.

### HEMORRHAGIC DISEASE OF THE NEWBORN

Newborn infants represent a special case of vitamin K nutrition because (1) the placenta is a relatively poor organ for the transmission of lipids, (2) the neonatal liver is immature with respect to prothrombin synthesis, (3) breast milk is low in vitamin K, and (4) the infant gut is sterile during the first few days of life. As a result a sizable number of infants develop hemorrhagic disease of the newborn (HDN). In normal infants, the plasma prothrombin concentration and that of the other vitamin K-dependent factors are about 20% of adult values at birth and rise slowly to adult values at 3 weeks if the vitamin K intake is adequate. If prothrombin values fall below 10%, hemorrhagic disease of the newborn appears.[102] About 30% of full-term infants have descarboxyprothrombin in their plasma during the first week of life.[91] The level of phylloquinone in the plasma of newborn infants is less than 0.22 nM (0.1 ng/ml).[104] As food is taken, the levels gradually climb to normal adult values over a period of weeks. Some infants, however, who are breast-fed and who have received no prophylactic vitamin K at birth, develop late HDN during the third to the eighth week of life.[103] It is possible that these infants have some abnormality of liver function in addition to low vitamin K levels and that they require intensive vitamin K therapy. Premature infants are even more susceptible to vitamin K deficiency than are full-term ones (Fig. 19–8).[105,106] Because the requirement for vitamin K in the newborn is estimated to be 11.1 nmol per day (5 μg per day), the very low content of vitamin K in human milk 2.2 to 4.4 nM (1 to 2 μg/L)[37] accounts for the greater predisposition of breast-fed infants to develop the hemorrhagic syndrome.[107] Because breast milk is sterile and delays colonization of the gut with bacteria, Seeler and others recommend that babies who are breast-fed receive 2.2 μmol (1 mg) of phylloquinone (Aquamephyton) intramuscularly at birth.[108,109]

Infants of mothers on hydantoin anticonvulsants should have prophylactic vitamin K because diphenylhydantoin is an antagonist to vitamin K.[110] Neonatal complications such as diarrhea, malabsorption, cystic fibrosis, idiopathic cholestasis, atresia of the bile duct, and prolonged parenteral nutrition are all indications for intramuscular or intravenous vitamin K administration to infants.

## DIETARY INADEQUACY

Healthy adult subjects fed low-vitamin K diets (22 to 89 nmol per day, or 10 to 40 μg per day) for several weeks demonstrate a fall in plasma vitamin K levels from 2.2 to 1.1 nM (1.0 ng/ml to 0.5 ng/ml), but no significant change in plasma prothrombin values.[54,111] In two studies of apoplectic patients, intravenous nutrition plus neomycin was required to lower the vitamin K-dependent clotting factors to below 20% of normal in 4 weeks.[112,113] The intravenous administration of vitamin K in various doses (0.07 to 3.3 nmol/kg, or 0.03 to 1.5 μg/kg) to these patients caused a proportional rise in the concentration of prothrombin to normal levels.[113] In unusual cases, self-imposed dietary restriction may induce hypoprothrombinemia with hemorrhage responsive to oral vitamin K.[114,115] Dietary deficiency of vitamin K becomes manifest more quickly in patients following surgery and in debilitated patients with or without antibiotics.[116,117]

In protein-calorie malnutrition, amino acid deprivation may cause hypoprothrombinemia that is not responsive to vitamin K but that does respond to protein feeding.[118]

## TOTAL PARENTERAL NUTRITION

With the advent of subclavian-vein catheterization in 1968 for long-term total parenteral nutrition (TPN) of both surgical and medical patients unable to eat, new

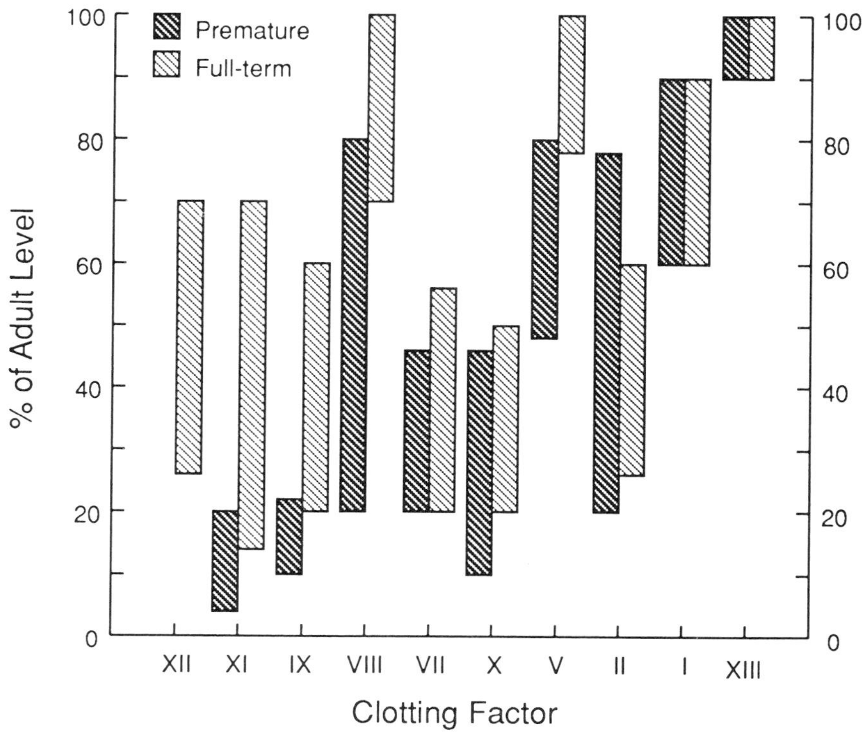
Premature
Full-term
% of Adult Level
0
20
40
60
80
100
XII
XI
IX
VIII
VII
X
V
II
I
XIII
Clotting Factor

**FIGURE 19–8.** Comparison of coagulation factor activities of full-term and premature newborn infants with those of adults. (From Bleyer, W.A., Hakami, N., Shepard, T.H.: J. Pediatr., *79*:838–853, 1971.)

nutritional deficiency syndromes have been reported,[119] among which is hemorrhage due to vitamin K deficiency.[120] It is advisable to give doses of 2.2 μmol (1 mg) of phylloquinone per week (equivalent to about 0.3 μ mol, or 150 μg, of vitamin K per day) to patients on TPN.

## BILIARY OBSTRUCTION

Prior to the discovery of vitamin K and recognition of its deficiency in obstructive jaundice, bleeding commonly occurred after surgical correction of biliary obstruction.[121] Because the secretion of bile salts is essential for the absorption of fats and fat-soluble vitamins, it is not surprising that biliary obstruction was early identified as a cause of vitamin K deficiency. All patients with obstructive jaundice should receive parenteral vitamin $K_1$ (11 μmol per day, or 5 mg per day) for 3 days prior to surgery.

## MALABSORPTION SYNDROME

Depression of the vitamin K-dependent coagulation factors is frequently found in the malabsorption syndromes and in other gastrointestinal disorders (e.g., cystic fibrosis, sprue, celiac disease, ulcerative colitis, regional ileitis, and short bowel syndrome).[122] Severe abnormalities of coagulation with extensive bleeding are not as common in these disorders as in biliary obstruction, but they do occur with sufficient frequency to be a concern of physicians caring for these patients. One of the complications of ileojejunostomy for morbid obesity is hemorrhage due to vitamin K deficiency. Patients with malabsorption should be treated with all the fat-soluble vitamins. Vitamin K should be given orally in doses of 2.2 to 4.4 μmol per day (1 to 2 mg per day) or parenterally in doses of 2.2 to 4.4 μmol per week (1 to 2 mg per week).

## LIVER DISEASE

Patients with parenchymal liver disease may have hypoprothrombinemia and an elevation in plasma descarboxyprothrombin.[123] They are unable to utilize vitamin K in the biosynthesis of vitamin K-dependent clotting factors, usually as a result of destruction of the rough reticulum in the hepatocyte. Patients with liver disease should be challenged with vitamin K to determine the extent of the blockade of prothrombin synthesis. There is no need, however, to give repetitive high doses of vitamin K if the patient is refractory to a single intravenous dose of 22 μmol (10 mg) of vitamin K.[124]

## DRUG THERAPY

Various drugs, including the 4-hydroxycoumarins, salicylates, certain broad-spectrum antibiotics, and vitamins A and E in pharmacologic doses, will antagonize the action of vitamin K.

### *COUMARIN- AND SALICYLATE-INDUCED HEMORRHAGIC DISEASE*

The coumarin anticoagulant drugs can induce serious hypoprothrombinemia and even hemorrhage by blocking the vitamin K epoxide and vitamin K reductases. Some of the contributory causes are reduction in dietary intake of vitamin K, ingestion of interfering drugs, and the inadvertent alteration of the anticoagulant dosage schedule. Coumarin drugs, in rare cases, may cause coumarin skin necrosis. This condition probably occurs because coumarin drugs inhibit the biosynthesis of the anticoagulant protein C before they affect the levels of the procoagulant factors, II, XII, IX, and X. The temporary imbalance may, in fact, stimulate local coagulation in venules with resulting thrombosis.[125] Salicylates in large doses may also depress vitamin K-dependent factors by inhibiting the vitamin K epoxide reductase. When overdosage with or without bleeding occurs, the anticoagulant should be discontinued, 22 μmol (10 mg) of vitamin $K_1$ should be given parenterally, and prothrombin times should be monitored until they are in a satisfactory range.

### *BROAD-SPECTRUM ANTIBIOTICS*

One source of vitamin K in humans is their own intestinal bacteria. Vitamin K, however, is not well absorbed from the colon. The microorganisms synthesizing absorbable menaquinones in the intestine probably reside in the ileum, where absorption of vitamin K is possible.

Sulfaquinoxaline, neomycin, and other broad-spectrum antibiotics are capable of sterilizing the bowel. The classic case is that of a patient who has undergone gastrointestinal surgery preceded by a limited intake of food and bowel-sterilizing antibiotics, who then is treated postoperatively with other antibiotics. The sudden appearance of melena, perhaps with hematemesis, may be the first clue of vitamin K deficiency. Prophylactic vitamin K is effective in preventing this consequence of injury and hospitalization.

Certain broad-spectrum cephalosporin antibiotics (moxalactam, cefamandole) cause vitamin K-reversible hemorrhage in man.[125,126] Lipsky reported that the N-methylthiotetrazole moiety of these antibiotics blocks vitamin K-dependent peptide carboxylation in Triton-solubilized rat liver microsomes in a dose-dependent manner.[127] Shearer et al. concluded that those antibiotics oppose vitamin K by inhibiting hepatic vitamin K epoxide reductase.[128]

*MEGADOSES OF VITAMINS A AND E*

Megadoses of the fat-soluble vitamins A and E are known to antagonize vitamin K. It has been recognized since 1944 that hypervitaminosis A in the rat leads to hypoprothrombinemia that can be prevented by the administration of vitamin K.[129] There is a close relationship above the requirement between the level of dietary retinol (or retinoic acid) and the resulting deficiency of vitamin K as expressed by depressed prothrombin levels in rats.[130] The effect of vitamin A was more severe in males than in females, and retinoic acid was more effective than vitamin A acetate. Because parenterally administered retinoic acid failed to increase the vitamin K requirement, Matschiner et al. concluded that the action of excess vitamin A was to reduce the absorption of vitamin K.[131] Reduced plasma prothrombin levels have been reported in humans intoxicated with vitamin A.[132]

Large amounts of vitamin E antagonize the action of vitamin K in animals.[133] Olson and Jones observed that high dietary intakes of vitamin E in rats increased the vitamin K requirement.[134] Vitamin E does not appear to affect vitamin K uptake or distribution from the gut, nor does vitamin E directly affect the vitamin K-dependent carboxylase in vitro. Bettger et al. found that α-tocopherolquinone is a more potent antagonist of vitamin K activity in the rat than is d-α-tocopherol.[135] Vitamin K deficiency in human subjects taking megadoses of vitamin E has been reported by Corrigan and Marcus.[136] Bleeding was observed in a middle-aged man taking 5 mg of warfarin and 1200 IU of vitamin E each day. Upon discontinuation of megavitamin E therapy, the bleeding tendency disappeared and the prolonged prothrombin time was normalized.

## EVALUATION OF NUTRITIONAL STATUS

The evaluation of individual persons for vitamin K status depends on the proper application of the three classic approaches to patient evaluation, namely, the history, physical examination, and laboratory tests.

### HISTORY

The medical history should include questions about hemorrhage in the mouth or from the nose, from the stomach and intestinal tract (hematemesis and melena), kidney (hematuria), and beneath the skin (ecchymoses). Persons at risk for vitamin K deficiency are newborn infants and adults who are on diets devoid of green, leafy vegetables and animal foods or who have malabsorption or other predisposing conditions. A careful medical history should include questions about these risk factors including coumarin anticoagulant drugs. In addition, the diet history should include a list of foods frequently eaten, a 24-hour recall of foods eaten, and occasionally a 3-day diary.

### PHYSICAL EXAMINATION

Evidence should be sought for a bleeding tendency, which is the cardinal sign of vitamin K deficiency. This can present in one or more of the following ways: bleeding from the nose or mouth; ecchymoses in the groin, around the collar line, or in the legs; splinter hemorrhages under the nails or in the conjunctiva; melena (gross or occult); hematuria; and hematemesis. Pallor may be a sign of previous bleeding. The perifollicular hemorrhages in the skin characteristic of scurvy are not seen in vitamin K deficiency.

### LABORATORY TESTS

A reduction in prothrombin and other vitamin K-dependent factors (X, IX, VII, and protein C) in the plasma is the accepted indicator of vitamin K deficiency. The measurement of plasma phylloquinone, which requires reverse phase high-pressure liquid chromatography, does not correlate too well with vitamin K status.[50] The range of normal is 0.4 to 2.2 nM (0.2 to 1.0 ng/ml), with a mean of 1.1 nM.[137] In individual cases the restriction of vitamin K may lower plasma vitamin K levels about 50%.[54,111] The most sensitive indicator of vitamin K deficiency is the amount of des-γ-carboxyprothrombin (DCP) in the plasma measured by a specific antibody.[138] In healthy persons the DCP concentration is zero, whereas in persons with vitamin K deficiency, liver disease, or both the values can rise to 30% of the total prothrombin (ca. 1.5 μM). Other, more indirect methods measure the ratio of prothrombin activity to total immunochemical equivalents of prothrombin (II:Ag ratio) or the ratio of a thromboplastin activated prothrombin time to that activated by Echis carinatus venom. In vitamin K deficiency these ratios fall.

Finally, urinary Gla can be measured as an index of vitamin K-dependent protein catabolism. A single value of Gla in the urine has little significance, although a given individual may show a fall in urinary Gla when put on a vitamin K-restricted diet.

## NUTRITIONAL REQUIREMENTS

The vitamin K requirement of mammals is met by a combination of dietary intake and microbiologic biosynthesis in the gut. Furthermore, genetic factors influence the vitamin K requirement in both animals and man because males require more vitamin K per kilogram of body weight than females do. In conventional rats, the vitamin K requirement is about 22 nmol/kg (10 μg/kg) of body weight per day, whereas in germ-free rats the requirement is more than doubled, to about 56 nmol/kg (25 μg/kg) per day.[139]

Although vitamin K deficiency depresses the level of the vitamin K-dependent proteins in the plasma, and in some species elevates the level of DCP in plasma, quantitative studies to determine the average requirement of vitamin K in both animals and humans are few, and the extent to which synthesis of menaquinones by intestinal bacteria contributes to the human requirement is unsettled.

Four normal volunteers who were maintained on a purified diet containing about 55 nmol of vitamin $K_1$ per day (25 μg per day) and given antibiotics to suppress intestinal menaquinone syntheses for 5 weeks maintained their prothrombin activity in the range of 70 to 100%.[140] In another study, four healthy young males fed an elemental diet containing 22 nmol per day (10 μg per day) of phylloquinone showed no changes in coagulation factor level or prothrombin antigen activity over an 8-week period. Their plasma phylloquinone values decreased from 2.2 nM (1.0 ng/ml) to 1.1 nM (0.5 ng/ml) over that period.[54] More recently Suttie et al. studied 10 college-aged, nonsmoking males who modified their diets by avoiding vitamin K-rich foods for 3 weeks.[111] Their vitamin K intake dropped from 178 nmol per day (80 μg per day) to about 89 nmol per day (40 μg per day) with a change in plasma phylloquinone from 2.00 ± 0.44 nM (0.90 ± 0.20 ng/ml) to 1.1 ± 0.44 nM (0.50 ± 0.20 ng/ml) during a 3-week period. There was no change in prothrombin time, although there was a 10% change in the Simplastin:Echis clotting ratio and a 20% decrease in Gla excretion. Based on these limited studies it would appear that the requirement of vitamin K in healthy adults is between 0.44 and 1.33 nmol/kg per day (0.2 and 0.6 μg/kg per day), or an average daily requirement of about 66 nmol per day (30 μg per day).

Of the vitamin K homologues stored in human liver, 50% are derived from long-chain menaquinones (reflecting microbiologic synthesis in the gut). It is not clear, however, that this hepatic store reflects bioavailability for prothrombin synthesis.[50] Menaquinones are not found in the plasma of Americans unless they are severely hyperlipemic. Because these more recent data preclude the assumption that the hepatic menaquinones are mobilized for vitamin K-dependent protein synthesis in proportion to their concentration, it is not possible to calculate the contribution of menaquinones to the vitamin K requirement in man.[47,141] An educated guess is that they may contribute from 10 to 30% of the daily requirement.

From the dietary information presented in Table 19–1, it can be calculated that the range of diets common in the United States will contain between 0.3 and 1.1 μmol (150 and 500 μg) of phylloquinone per day, an amount more than adequate to supply the dietary requirement.

## NUTRITIONAL ALLOWANCES

The recommended dietary allowances (RDA) for vitamin K were set by the Food and Nutrition Board for children and adult men and women for the first time in the tenth edition of the RDA (1989)[142] (see Appendix Table A–2b). RDA are defined as the levels of intake of essential nutrients that, on the basis of current scientific knowledge, are judged to be adequate to meet the needs of all healthy persons.

Because the data base for setting requirements for vitamin K in man is slim, and because the RDA should be at least two standard deviations above the mean requirement, the values presented in Table 19–2 are considerably higher than the estimated requirements. This is appropriate because the data available do not include information about the requirements for bone and kidney metabolism, and none of the studies on human requirements have employed the specific antibodies of Blanchard et al. to measure DCP,[138] which is the most sensitive indicator of vitamin K deficiency.

## TOXICITY

There are no reports of toxic effects of phylloquinone at 500 times its RDA. Although this lack of toxicity is true for phylloquinone, it is not true of the vitamin precursor, menadione (2-methyl-1,4-naphthoquinone), unsubstituted in the 3 position, and its water-soluble derivatives such as Synkavite. Menadione can combine with sulfydryl groups in membranes and cause hemolytic anemia, hyperbilirubinemia, and kernicterus in infants.[143] Menadione should not be employed any longer as a therapeutic form of vitamin K.

## RECENT DEVELOPMENTS

After this review was prepared, a paper appeared that reported that the gene for the vitamin K-dependent γ-glutamylcarboxylase had been cloned.[144]

Starting with a nucleotide coding for a 37-amino acid sequence from the bovine γ-glutamyl carboxylase, these investigators screened a cDNA library from bovine liver and found 3 partial clones. An Eco RI-cDNA fragment of 280 bp from the bovine library was then used to screen a human erythroleukemia (HEL) cDNA library, and 1 clone of the gene for the human carobxylase with an internal Eco RI site was obtained.

Several observations indicate that the entire coding sequence is probably contained within this cDNA. These are: (1) the methionine identified as the first amino acid is the only in-frame methionine between a stop codon 27 nucleotides upstream and the first tryptic peptide 195 nucleotides downstream; (2) the open reading frame codes for 758 amino acids and predicts a molecular weight of 87,542, which, if one takes into account that the

**TABLE 19–2.** FOOD AND NUTRITION BOARD (NAS/NRC) RECOMMENDED DIETARY ALLOWANCES FOR VITAMIN K (1989).

| CATEGORY | AGE (YEARS) OR CONDITION | WEIGHT (kg) | VITAMIN K* (μg) |
|---|---|---|---|
| Infants | 0.0–0.5 | 6 | 5 |
| | 0.5–1.0 | 9 | 10 |
| Children | 1–3 | 13 | 15 |
| | 4–6 | 20 | 20 |
| | 7–10 | 28 | 30 |
| Males | 11–14 | 45 | 45 |
| | 15–18 | 66 | 65 |
| | 19–24 | 72 | 70 |
| | 25–50 | 79 | 80 |
| | 51+ | 77 | 80 |
| Females | 11–14 | 46 | 45 |
| | 15–18 | 55 | 55 |
| | 19–24 | 58 | 60 |
| | 25–50 | 63 | 65 |
| | 51+ | 65 | 65 |
| Pregnant | | | 65 |
| Lactating | 1st 6 months | | 65 |
| | 2nd 6 months | | 65 |

*1 μg Vitamin $K_1$ =2.2 nmol

protein is glycosylated, agrees with the weight of 94 kd estimated by mobility in SDS-polyacrylaminde gel electrophoresis; and (3) the cDNA codes for functional carboxylase in mammalian cells.

The enzyme activity coded by the human cDNA was expressed in human kidney 293 cells using the vector pCMV5 with/without the enzyme cDNA. Forty-eight hours after transfection, cells were harvested, microsomes prepared, and γ-glutamyl carboxylase activity determined by standard techniques using $^{14}CO_2$ and FLEEL as substrates. Under all conditions, including activation by $(NH_4)_2SO_4$ and a 19-residue peptide from profactor IX, the microsomes programmed by enzyme cDNA resulted in an increase in activity of 9- to 27-fold over the mock-transfected cells.

## REFERENCES

1. Dam, H.: Biochem. Z., *215*:475–492, 1929.
2. McFarland, W.D., Graham, W.R., Richardson, F.: Biochem. J., *25*:358–366, 1931.
3. Holst, W.F., Halbrook, E.R.: Science, *77*:354–355, 1933.
4. Dam, H., Schonheyder, F.: Biochem. J., *28*:1355–1359, 1934.
5. Dam, H.: Biochem. J., *29*:1273–1285, 1935.
6. Schonheyder, F.: Biochem. J., *30*:890–896, 1936.
7. Almquist, H.J., Stokstad, E.L.R.: J. Nutr., *12*:329–335, 1936.
8. Binkley, S.B., MacCorquodale, D., Thayer, S.A., et al.: J. Biol. Chem., *130*:219–234, 1939.
9. Dam. H., Geiger, A., Glavind, J., et al.: Helv. Chim. Acta, *22*:310, 1939.
10. MacCorquodale, D.W., Cheney, L.C., Binkley, S.B., et al.: J. Biol. Chem., *131*:357–370, 1939.
11. McKee, R.W., Binkley, S., Thayer, S.A., et al.: J. Biol. Chem., *131*:327–344, 1939.
12. Campbell, H.A., Link, K.P.: J. Biol. Chem., *138*:21–33, 1941.
13. Schofield, F.W.: Can. Vet. Rec., *3*:74–79, 1922.
14. Olson, R.E., Suttie, J.W.: Vitam. Horm., *35*:59–108, 1977.
15. Olson, R.E.: Ann. Rev. Nutr., *4*:281–337, 1984.
16. Ganrot, P.O., Nilehn, J.E.: Scand. J. Clin. Lab. Invest., *22*:23–28, 1968.
17. Stenflo, J., Fernkind, P., Eagan, W., et al.: Proc. Natl. Acad. Sci. U.S.A., *71*:2730–2733, 1974.
18. Nelsestuen, G.L., Zytokovicz, T.H., Howard, J.B.: J. Biol. Chem., *249*:6347–6350, 1974.
19. Magnusson, S., Sottrup-Jensen, L., Peterson, T.E., et al.: FEBS Lett., *44*:189–193, 1974.
20. Doisy, E.A., Binkley, S.B., Thayer, S.A.: Chem. Rev., *28*:477–517, 1941.
21. Dam, H., Sondegaard, E., Olson, R.E.: Vitamin K. *In* Vitamins in Medicine. Edited by B.M. Baker and D.H. Bender. London, William Heinemann, 1982, pp. 92–113.

22. Suttie, J.W.: Vitamin K. *In* Fat-Soluble Vitamins. Edited by A.T. Diplock, Lancaster, PA, Technomic Publishing Co., 1985, pp. 225–311.
23. Binkley, S.B., McKee, R.W., Thayer, S.A., et al.: J. Biol. Chem., *133*:721–729, 1940.
24. Isler, O., Ruegg, R. Chopard-dit-Jean Lilt, et al.: Helv. Chim. Acta, *41*:786–807, 1958.
25. Martius, C., Esser, H.O.: Bioch. Zeit., *331*:1–9, 1958.
26. Dialameh, G.H., Yekundi, K.G., Olson, R.E.: Biochim. Biophys. Acta, *223*:332–338, 1970.
27. Lee, F.C., Olson, R.E.: Biochim. Biophys. Acta, *799*:166–170, 1984.
28. Matschiner, J.T., Taggart, W.V., Amelotti, J.M.: Biochemistry, *6*:1243–1248, 1967.
29. Pennock, J.F.: Vitam. Horm., *24*:307–329, 1966.
30. Gale, P.H., Arison, B.H., Trenner, N.R., et al.: Biochemistry, *2*:196–200, 1963.
31. Scholes, P.B., King, H.K.: Biochem. J., *97*:766–768, 1965.
32. Matschiner, J.T., Doisy, E.A. Jr.: J. Nutr., *90*:97–100, 1966.
33. Shearer, M.J.: Adv. Chromatogr., *21*:243–300, 1983.
34. Ueno, T., Suttie, J.W.: Anal. Biochem., *133*:62–67, 1983.
35. Haroon, Y., Bacon, D.S., Sadowski, J.A.: Clin. Chem., *32*:1925–1929, 1986.
36. DiMari, S.J., Supple, J.H., Rapaport, H.: J. Am. Chem. Soc., *88*:1226–1232, 1966.
37. Shearer, M.J., Allan, V., Haroon, Y., et al.: Nutritional aspects of vitamin K in man. *In* Vitamin K Metabolism and Vitamin K–Dependent Proteins. Edited by J.W. Suttie. Baltimore, University Park Press, 1980, pp. 317–327.
38. Dam, H., Glavind, J.: Biochem. J., *32*: 485–490, 1938.
39. Doisy, E.A. Jr.: Private communication.
40. Mann, J.D., Mann, F.D., Bollman, J.L.: Am. J. Physiol., *158*:311–314, 1949.
41. Blomstrand, R., Forsgren, L.: Int. Z. Vitaminforsch., *38*:328–344, 1968.
42. Wiss, O., Gloor, H.: Vitam. Horm., *24*:575–586, 1966.
43. Shearer, M.J., Barkham, P., Webster, G.R.: Br. J. Haematol., *18*:297–308, 1970.
44. Matschiner, J.T., Hsia, S.L., Doisy, E.A. Jr.: J. Nutr., *91*:299–306, 1967.
45. Simon, E.J., Gross, C.S., Milhorat, A.T.: J. Biol. Chem., *221*:797–805, 1956.
46. Matschiner, J.T., Bell, R.G., Amelotti, J.M., et al.: Biochim. Biophys. Acta, *201*:309–315, 1970.
47. Olson, R.E.: Vitamin K. *In* Hemostasis and Thrombosis. 2nd Ed. Edited by R.W. Coleman, J. Hirsch, V.J. Marder, and E.W. Salzman, Philadelphia, J.B. Lippincott, 1987, pp. 846–860.
48. Matschiner, J.T., Amelotti, J.M.: J. Lipid Res., *9*:176–179, 1968.
49. Rietz, P., Gloor, U., Wiss, O.: Int. Z. Vitamforsch, *40*:351–362, 1970.
50. Shearer, M.J., McCarthy, P.T., Crampton, O.E., et al.: The assessment of human vitamin K status from tissue measurements. *In* Current Advances in Vitamin K Research. Edited by J.W. Suttie. New York, Elsevier, 1987, pp. 437–452.
51. Bjornsson, T.D., Meffin, P.J., Swezey, S.E., et al.: Disposition and turnover of vitamin K in man. *In* Vitamin K Metabolism and Vitamin K-Dependent Proteins. Edited by J.W. Suttie. Baltimore, University Park Press, 1980, pp. 328–332.
52. Shearer, M.J., McBurney, A., Barkhan, P.: Vitam. Horm., *32*:513–542, 1974.
53. Bjornsson, T.D., Meffin, P.J., Swezey, S.E., et al.: Pharmacol. Exp. Ther., *210*:322–326, 1979.
54. Olson, R.E., Meyer, R.G., Chao, J., et al.: Circulation, *70*:97, 1984.
55. Billeter, M., Bolliger, W., Martius, C.: Biochem. Z., *340*:290–303, 1964.
56. Taggart, W.V., Matschiner, J.T.: Biochem. J., *8*:1141–1146, 1969.
57. Dialameh, G.H., Taggart, W.V., Matschiner, J.T., et al.: Int. J. Vitam. Nutr. Res., *41*:391–400, 1971.
58. Losito, R., Owen, C.A. Jr., Flock, E.V.: Biochemistry, *6*:62–68, 1967.
59. Fieser, L.F., Turner, R.B.: J. Am. Chem. Soc., *69*:2335–2338, 1947.
60. Mezick, J.A., Cornwell, D.G.: Biochim. Biophys. Acta, *219*:361–364, 1970.
61. Davie, E.W., Ratnoff, O.D.: Science, *145*:1310–1312, 1964.
62. Davie, E.W.: The blood coagulation factors: their cDNAs, genes, and expression. *In* Hemostasis and Thrombosis. 2nd Ed. Edited by R.W. Coleman, J. Hirsch, V.J. Marder, and E.W. Salzman. Philadelphia, J.B. Lippincott, 1987, pp. 242–267.
63. Furie, B., Furie, B.C.: Blood, *75*:1753–1762, 1990.
64. Giradot, J.-M.: J. Biol. Chem., *257*:15008–15011, 1982.
65. Olson, R.E., Hall, A.L., Lee, F.C., et al.: Vitamin K–dependent carboxylase. *In* Post-Translational Covalent Modifications of Proteins. Edited by B.C. Johnson. New York, Academic Press, 1983, pp. 295–319.
66. Larson, A.E., Suttie, J.W.: FEBS Lett., *118*:95–98, 1980.
67. Jones, J.P., Gardner, E.J., Cooper, T.G., et al.: J. Biol. Chem., *252*:7738–7742, 1977.
68. Suttie, J.W., Hagemen, J.M., Lehrman, S.R., et al.: J. Biol. Chem., *251*:5827–5830, 1976.
69. Houser, R.M., Carey, D.J., Dus, K., et al.: FEBS Lett., *75*:226–230, 1977.
70. Suttie, J.W.: Ann. Rev. Biochem., *54*:459–477, 1985.
71. Wallin, R., Suttie, J.W.: Arch. Biochem. Biophys., *214*:155–163, 1982.
72. DeMetz, M., Vermeer, C., Soute, B.A.M., et al.: FEBS Lett., *123*:215–218, 1981.
73. Olson, R.E., Hall, A.L., Lee, F.C., et al.: Chemica Scripta, *27A*:187–192, 1987.
74. Hubbard, B.R., Ulrich, M.M.W., Jacobs, M., et al.: Proc. Natl. Acad. Sci. U.S.A., *86*:6893–6897, 1989.
75. Wu, S.-M., Morris, D.P., Stafford, D.W.: Proc. Natl. Acad. Sci. U.S.A., *88*:2236–2240, 1991.
76. Larson, A.E., Suttie, J.W.: Proc. Natl. Acad. Sci. U.S.A., *75*:5413–5416, 1978.
77. Willingham, A.K., Laliberte, R.E., Bell, R.G., et al.: Biochem. Pharmacol., *25*:1063–1066, 1976.
78. Hall, A.L., Kloepper, R., Zee-Cheng, R. K.-Y., et al.: Arch. Biochem. Biophys., *214*:45–50, 1982.
79. Ham, S.W., Dowd, P.: J. Am. Chem. Soc., *112*:1660–1661, 1990.
80. Dowd, P., Ham, S.W., Geib, S.J.: J. Am. Chem. Soc., *113*:7734–7743, 1991.
81. Larson, A.E., Friedman, P.A., Suttie, J.W.: J. Biol. Chem., *256*:11032–11035, 1981.
82. Wallin, R.: Biochem. J., *236*:685–693, 1986.
83. Fasco, M.J., Hildebrandt, E.F., Suttie, J.W.: J. Biol. Chem., *257*:11210–11212, 1982.

84. Hauschka, P.V., Lian, J.B., Gallop, P.M.: Proc. Natl. Acad. Sci. U.S.A., *72:*3925–3929, 1975.
85. Price, P.A., Otsuka, A.S., Poser, J.W., et al.: Proc. Natl. Acad. Sci. U.S.A., *73:*1447–1451, 1976.
86. Price, P.A. Urist, M.R., Otawara, Y.: Biochem. Biophys. Res. Commun., *117:*765–771, 1983.
87. Price, P.A., Poser, J.W., Raman, N.: Proc. Natl. Acad, Sci. U.S.A., *73:*3374–3375, 1976.
88. Price, P.A.: Ann. Rev. Nutr., *8:*565–583, 1988.
89. Lian, J.B., Friedman, P.S.: J. Biol. Chem., *253:*6623–6626, 1978.
90. Gallop, P.M., Lian, J.B., Hauschka, P.V.: N. Engl. J. Med., *302:*1460–1466, 1980.
91. Motohara, K., Endo, F., Matsuda, I.: Lancet, *2:*242–244, 1985.
92. Price, P.A., Baukol, S.A.: J. Biol. Chem., *255:*11660–11663, 1980.
93. Price, P.A., Parthemore, J.G., Deflos, L.J.: J. Clin. Invest., *66:*878–893, 1980.
94. Warkany, J.: Am. J. Dis. Child., *129:*287–288, 1975.
95. Fourie, D.T., Hay, I.T.: S. Afr. Med. J., *49:*2081–2083, 1975.
96. Lian, J.B., Prien, E.L. Jr.: Fed. Proc., *35:*1763, 1976.
97. Hauschka, P.V., Friedman, P.A., Traverso, H.P., et al.: Biochem. Biophys. Res. Commun., *71:*1207–1213, 1976.
98. Friedman, P.A., Mitch, W.E., Silva, P.: J. Biol. Chem., *257:*11037–11040, 1982.
99. Traverso, H.P., Hauschka, P.V., Gallup, P.M.: Calcif. Tissue Int., *30:*73–76, 1980.
100. Searcey, M.T., Graves, C.B., Olson, R.E.: J. Biol. Chem., *252:*6260–6267, 1977.
101. Thijssen, H.A.W., Baars, L.G.M.: J. Pharm. Exp. Ther., *243:*1082–1088, 1987.
102. Brinkhous, K.M., Smith, H.P., Warner, E.D.: Am. J. Med. Sci., *193:*475–480, 1937.
103. Lane, P.A., Hathaway, W.E.: J. Pediatr., *106:*351–359, 1985.
104. Shearer, M.J., Rahim, S., Barkhan, P., et al.: Lancet, *2:*460–463, 1982.
105. Hellman, L.M., Shettles, L.B.: Bull. Johns Hopkins Hosp., *65:*138–141, 1939.
106. Bleyer, W.A., Hakami, N, Shepard, T.H.: J. Pediatr., *79:*838–853, 1971.
107. Sutherland, J.M., Glueck, H.I., Gleser, G.: Am. J. Dis. Child., *113:*524–533, 1967.
108. Seeler, R.A.: Ill. Med. J., *147:*59–61, 1975.
109. Shearer, M.J.: Br. J. Haematol., *75:*156–162, 1990.
110. Evans, A.R., Forrester, R.M., Discombe, C.: Lancet, *1:*517–518, 1970.
111. Suttie, J.W., Mummah-Schendel, D.V., Shah, B.J., et al.: Am. J. Clin. Nutr., *47:*475–480, 1988.
112. Udall, J.A.: JAMA, *194:*107–109, 1965.
113. Frick, P.G., Riedler, G., Brogli, H.: J. Appl. Physiol., *23:*387–389, 1967.
114. Kark, R., Lozner, E.L.: Lancet, *2:*1162–1164, 1939.
115. Aggeler, P.M., Lucia, S.P., Fishbon, H.M.: Am. J. Dig. Dis., *9:*227–229, 1942.
116. Ansell, J.E., Kumar, R., Deykin, D.: JAMA, *238:*40–42, 1977.
117. Pineo, G.F., Gallus, A.S., Hirsh, J.: Can. Med. Assoc. J., *109:*880–883, 1973.
118. Damrongsak, D.: Fat-soluble vitamins. *In* Protein-Calorie Malnutrition. Edited by R.E. Olson. New York, Academic Press, 1975, pp. 195–197.
119. Dudrick, S.J., Wilmore, D.W., Vars, H.M., et al.: Surgery, *64:*134–142, 1968.
120. Ryan, J.A. Jr.: Complications of total parenteral nutrition. *In* Total Parenteral Nutrition. Edited by E. Fischer. Boston, Little, Brown, 1976, pp. 55–100.
121. Boland, E.W.: Proc. Mayo Clin., *13:*70–72, 1938.
122. Savage, D., Lindenbaum, J. Clinical and experimental human vitamin K deficiency. *In* Nutrition in Hematology. Edited by J. Lindenbaum. New York, Churchill Livingstone, 1983, pp. 271–319.
123. Blanchard, R.A., Furie, B.C., Jorgenson, M., et al.: N. Engl. J. Med., *305:*242–248, 1981.
124. Mehta, R., Reilley, J.J., Olson, R.E.: JPEN J. Parenter. Enteral Nutr., *15:*350–353, 1991.
125. McGehee, W.G., Klotz, T.A., Epstein, D.J.: Ann. Intern. Med., *101:*59–60, 1984.
126. Hooper, C.A., Harvey, B.B., Stone, H.H.: Lancet, *1:*39–40, 1980.
127. Lipsky, J.J.: Lancet, *2:*192–193, 1983.
128. Shearer, M.J., Bechtold, H., Andrassy, K., et al.: J. Clin. Pharmacol., *25:*88–95, 1988.
129. Light, R.F., Alsher, R.P., Frey, C.N.: Science, *100:*225–230, 1940.
130. Matschiner, J.T., Doisy, E.A. Jr.: Proc. Soc. Exp. Biol. Med., *109:*139–142, 1962.
131. Matshiner, J.T., Amelotti, J.M., Doisy, E.A. Jr.: J. Nutr., *91:*303–306, 1967.
132. Smith, F.R., Goodman, D.W.: N. Engl. J. Med., *294:*805–808, 1976.
133. March, B.E., Wong, E., Seier, L., et al.: J. Nutr., *103:*371–377, 1973.
134. Olson, R.E., Jones, J.P.: Fed. Proc., *38:*2542, 1979.
135. Bettger, W.J., Jones, J.P., Olson, R.E.: Fed. Proc., *41:*344, 1982.
136. Corrigan, J.J., Marcus, F.I.: JAMA, *230:*1300–1301, 1974.
137. Sadowski, J.A., Hood, S.J., Dallal, G.E., et al.: Am. J. Clin. Nutr., *50:*100–108, 1989.
138. Blanchard, R.A., Furie, B.C., Kruger, S.F., et al.: J. Lab. Clin. Med., *101:*242–255, 1983.
139. Gustafsson, B.E., Daft, F.S., McDaniel, et al.: J. Nutr., *78:*461–468, 1962.
140. O'Reilley, R.A.: Am. J. Physiol., *221:*1327–1330, 1971.
141. Olson, R.E.: Vitamin K. *In* Modern Nutrition in Health and Disease. Edited by M. Shils and V. Young. Philadelphia, Lea & Febiger, 1988, pp. 328–339.
142. Food and Nutrition Board, National Research Council: Recommended Dietary Allowances. 10th Ed. Washington, D.C., National Academy Press, 1989.
143. DiPalma, J.R., Ritchie, D.M.: Annu. Rev. Pharmacol. Toxicol., *17:*133–148, 1977.
144. Wu, S.M., Cheung, W.F., Frazier, D., et al.: Science, *254:*1634–1638, 1991.

## SELECTED READINGS

Olson, R.E.: The function and metabolism of vitamin K. Annu. Rev. Nutr., *4*:281–337, 1984.

Suttie, J.W.: Vitamin K. *In* Present Knowledge of Nutrition. 6th Ed. Edited by M. Brown. Washington, D.C., Int. Life Science Institute, 1990, pp. 122–131.

Shearer, M.J.: Annotation: Vitamin K and vitamin K–dependent proteins. Br. J. Haematol., *75*:156–162, 1990.

CHAPTER 20

# Thiamin

Vichai Tanphaichitr



## HISTORICAL LANDMARKS

Although Neiching, the Chinese medical book, mentioned beriberi in 2697 B.C., it was not known for centuries that this illness was due to thiamin deficiency. In 1884, Takaki, a surgeon general of the Japanese navy, concluded that beriberi was caused by a lack of nitrogenous food components in association with excessive intake of non-nitrogenous food. In 1911, Funk, a chemist working at the Lister Institute in London, was convinced that he had isolated the antiberiberi principle possessing an amine function from rice bran extracts. He named it "vitamine." His crystalline substance was shown later to have little antineuritic activity. In 1926, Jansen and Donath, Dutch chemists working in Java, succeeded in isolating and crystallizing antiberiberi factor from rice bran extracts. By 1934 Williams, a U.S. chemist, had isolated a sufficient quantity of thiamin so that its structure could be determined. Its synthesis was accomplished in 1936. In 1937, Lohman and Schuster discovered that the active coenzyme form of thiamin was thiamin pyrophosphate (TPP, also known as cocarboxylase).[1-4]

## CHEMISTRY

The chemical name of thiamin, formerly known as vitamin $B_1$, vitamin F, aneurine, or thiamine, is 3-(4-amino-2-methylpyrimidin-5-ylmethyl)-5-(2-hydroxyethyl)-4-methylthiazolium (Fig. 20–1).[5] The free vitamin is a base. It is isolated or synthesized and handled as a solid thiazolium salt—that is, as thiamin hydrochloride or thiamin mononitrate. The synthesis of thiamin is accomplished by either the pyrimidine and thiazole rings being prepared separately and condensed via the bromide, or the pyrimidine ring being synthesized and the thiazole ring formed in situ on it.[2] The molecular weight of thiamin hydrochloride is 337.28 g/mol.

Thiamin hydrochloride is a white crystalline substance. It is readily soluble in water, only partly soluble in alcohol and acetone, and insoluble in other fat solvents. In the dry form it is stable at 100° C. Thiamin in aqueous solutions is stable below pH 5.0 to heat and to oxidation; above pH 5.0 it is destroyed relatively rapidly by autoclaving and at pH 7.0 or above by boiling.

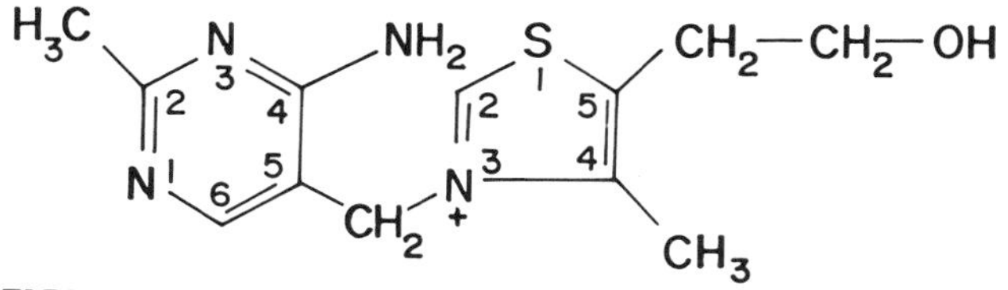

H3C
N
NH2
S
CH2—CH2—OH
N
CH2
N+
CH3


**FIGURE 20–1.** Structural formula of thiamin.

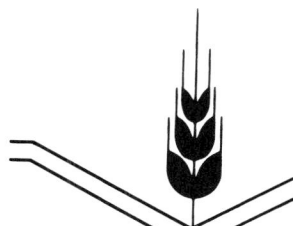

Thiamin can be readily cleaved at the methylene bridge into 2-methyl-4-amino-5-methyl-pyrimidylsulfonate and 4-methyl-5-(2-hydroxyethyl)thiazole by sulfite treatment at pH ≧6.0. At pH ≧8.0, thiamin turns yellow and is destroyed by a complex series of irreversible reactions. In strong alkaline solution in the presence of oxidizing agents, such as potassium ferricyanide, thiamin is converted to thiochrome, which is fluorescent and is used to determine thiamin content. Thiamin is precipitated by iron and ammonium citrate, tannin, and various alkaloids. Thiamin forms esters at the hydroxyethyl side chain with various acids. The most important ones are thiamin monophosphate (TMP), TPP, and thiamin triphosphate (TTP).[2,4]

## MOLECULAR STRUCTURE AND BIOLOGIC ACTIVITY

Both pyrimidine and thiazole moieties are needed for its vitaminic activity, which is maximal when only one methylene group bridges the two moieties. In the thiazole portion, the quaternary nitrogen and a hydroxyethyl group at carbon 5 are needed, as is the amino group at carbon 4 in the pyrimidine portion.[2,4] Several thiamin antagonists are synthesized to produce thiamin deficiency in animals, including oxythiamin, pyrithiamin, and amprolium.[2,4]

## DIETARY CONSIDERATIONS

Thiamin status is affected by the diet and by a variety of other factors.

### FOOD SOURCES

Thiamin, although found in a large variety of animal and vegetable products, is abundant only in a few foods. Excellent sources of thiamin are yeast, lean pork, and legumes, which contain 22.6 to 90.5, 2.7 to 3.9, and 2.0 to 3.8 μmol (6 to 24, 0.72 to 1.04, and 0.53 to 1.00 mg) of thiamin per 100 g of edible portion, respectively. In cereal grains, thiamin is low in the endosperm but high in the germ. The thiamin contents in rice bran, home-pounded rice, and milled rice are 7.5 to 15.1, 0.3 to 0.5, and 0.1 to 0.15 μmol/100 g (2 to 4, 0.08 to 0.14, and 0.02 to 0.04 mg/100 g), respectively. Thiamin is absent from fats, oils, and refined sugars. Milk and milk products, seafoods, fruits, and vegetables are not good sources.[2,6,7] (See also Appendix Table A–21 for the thiamin content of common foods.)

### FACTORS AFFECTING THIAMIN STATUS

Thiamin status depends on its bioavailability in food products, ethanol consumption, the presence of antithiamin factors (ATF) in the diet, and folate and protein status.[2,7,8]

**Thiamin Losses Resulting from Food Processing.** Thiamin is rapidly destroyed above pH 8. Thus, the addition of sodium bicarbonate to green beans and peas to retain their green color or to dried beans to soften their skins inactivates thiamin.[2]

Thiamin is also destroyed at high temperature. Thiamin losses during the cooking and canning of meats, baking of bread, and cooking of vegetables are 25 to 85%, 5 to 35%, and 0 to 60%, respectively. In pasteurization, sterilization, spray-drying, roller-drying, and the condensation of milk, thiamin losses are 9 to 20%, 30 to 50%, 10%, 15%, and 40%, respectively. Freezing does not affect the thiamin content of foods. Processing foods at higher temperature and under alkaline conditions in the presence of oxygen or other oxidants leads to the formation of thiamin sulfides and disulfides, thiochrome, and other oxidation products. Only thiamin sulfides and disulfides still retain the biologic activity of thiamin.[2]

Because thiamin is highly water-soluble, significant amounts are lost in discarded cooking water.[7,8] Thiamin is also destroyed by x rays, γ rays, ultraviolet irradiation, and sulfites that form in treating dehydrated fruits with $SO_2$.[2]

**Ethanol Ingestion.** Thiamin deficiency in chronic alcoholics is caused by multiple factors, which include a low thiamin intake, impaired intestinal absorption, defective phosphorylation, and an apotransketolase deficiency. Ethanol given orally or intravenously also inhibits intestinal thiamin uptake.[2,9]

**ATF.** Two types of ATF exist: thermolabile and thermostable.

The thermolabile ATF include thiaminases I (EC 2.5.1.2) and II (EC 3.5.99.2). Thiaminase I is found in the viscera of freshwater fish, in shellfish, in ferns, in a limited number of sea fish and plants, and in several microorganisms, including Bacillus thiaminolyticus and Clostridium thiaminolyticus. Thiaminase I cleaves thiamin by an exchange reaction with an organic base or a sulfhydryl compound via a nucleophilic displacement on the methylene group of the pyrimidine moiety of thiamin. Thiaminase II is found in several microorganisms, including Bacillus aneurinolyticus, Candida aneurinolytica, Trichosporon, and Oospora. It hydrolyzes thiamin to 2-methyl-4-amino-5-hydroxymethyl pyrimidine and 4-methyl-5-(2-hydroxyethyl)thiazole. Thiamin is accessible to thiaminases when tissues are broken up at pH 4 to 8 or when excreted from cells. Thiaminases act during food storage or preparation prior to ingestion or during passage through the gastrointestinal tract. Thus, habitual intakes of raw freshwater fish with or without fermentation, raw shellfish, and ferns are risk factors for the development of thiamin deficiency.[7,8,10,11]

Thermostable ATF have been demonstrated in ferns, tea, betel nut, some vegetables, other plants, and even in some animal tissues. In animal tissues, myoglobin, hemoglobin, and hemin may be involved. The ATF found in plants and vegetables are related to ortho- and para-polyphenolic compounds such as caffeic acid (3,4-

dihydroxycinnamic acid), chlorogenic acid [3-(3,4-dihydroxycinnamoyl) quinic acid] and tannic acid (tannin).[2,7] The antithiamin activity of polyphenols requires a pH ≧6.5 and oxygen. At high pH polyphenols ionize and the thiazole moiety of thiamin is ruptured at carbon 2 to yield the SH form of thiamin. In the presence of oxygen, polyphenols oxidize and polymerize to yield active quinones and relatively less active polymerized products. Quinones interact with the SH form of thiamin to give thiamin disulfide. Further hydrolysis and oxidation yield inactive products. Ascorbic acid and other reducing agents prevent the formation of quinones and thiamin disulfide. Divalent cations, such as $Ca^{++}$ and $Mg^{++}$, augment the precipitation of thiamin by tannin, thereby making thiamin less bioavailable. Consequently, ascorbic, tartaric, and citric acids present in many fruits and vegetables protect thiamin, presumably by sequestering the divalent cations. The drinking of tea, coffee, or decaffeinated coffee and the chewing of tea leaves or betel nut deplete thiamin in humans. Ascorbic acid intake improves thiamin status of the subjects.[11,12]

**Folate and Protein Status.** Thiamin is poorly absorbed in subjects with folate or protein deficiency.[9]

## METABOLISM

Ingested thiamin is fairly well absorbed, rapidly converted to phosphorylated forms, stored poorly, and excreted in the urine in a variety of hydrolyzed and oxidized products.

### ABSORPTION

The small intestine absorbs thiamin by two mechanisms: active transport (<2 μmol/L) and passive diffusion (>2 μmol/L). A specific sodium- and energy-dependent carrier seems to exist. In this regard, a specific thiamin-binding protein is associated with thiamin transport across the cell membrane of Escherichia coli. Active thiamin absorption is greatest in the jejunum and ileum.[2,7,13,14] Thiamin exit from the mucosal cell on the serosal side depends on $Na^{+}$ and on the adenosine triphosphatase (ATPase) at the serosal pole of the cell.[2,7]

### TRANSPORT

Thiamin is carried by the portal blood to the liver. Most of thiamin in plasma is mainly bound to albumin. The transport of thiamin into erythrocytes seems to be a facilitated diffusion process, whereas its entry into other cells is an active process.[2,14]

### TISSUE DISTRIBUTION AND STORAGE

The total amount of thiamin in the normal adult is approximately 0.11 mmol (30 mg). High concentrations are found in the skeletal muscles, the heart, the liver, the kidneys, and the brain. About 50% of the total thiamin is present in muscle. The biologic half-life of $^{14}C$-thiamin in the body is 9 to 18 days. Because thiamin is not stored in large amounts in any tissue, a continuous supply of thiamin is necessary.[2,7]

### METABOLIC MODIFICATION

Of the total thiamin in the body, about 80% is TPP, 10% is TTP, and the remainder is TMP and thiamin. The three tissue enzymes known to participate in the formation of the phosphate esters are thiamin pyrophosphokinase, which catalyzes the formation of TPP from thiamin and ATP; TPP-ATP phosphoryl transferase, which catalyzes the formation of TTP from TPP and adenosine triphosphate (ATP); and thiamin pyrophosphatase, which hydrolyzes TPP to form TMP. Out of 25 to 30 urinary metabolites of thiamin in rats and men, pyrimidine carboxylic acid, thiazole acetic acid, and thiamin acetic acid predominate.[2,4]

### EXCRETION

Thiamin and its metabolites are mainly excreted in the urine. Very little thiamin is excreted in the bile. Early milk contains a low thiamin level. Thiamin administered by oral or parenteral routes is rapidly converted to TPP and TTP in the tissues. Thiamin much in excess of tissue needs is rapidly excreted in the urine.[2,4]

## FUNCTIONS

Thiamin mainly acts in α-keto acid decarboxylation, in transketolation, and possibly in nerve conduction.

### BIOCHEMICAL FUNCTIONS

In mammalian systems, TPP functions as a $Mg^{++}$-coordinated coenzyme for active aldehyde transfers, which include the oxidative decarboxylation of α-keto acids and the transketolase reaction.[2,4,7,14] The key feature of TPP is that the carbon atom between the nitrogen and sulfur atoms in the thiazole ring is much more acidic than most CH groups. It ionizes to form a carbanion, which readily adds to the carbonyl group of α-keto acids or ketoses. The positively charged ring nitrogen of TPP then acts as an electron sink to stabilize the formation of a negative charge, which is necessary for decarboxylation. Protonation then gives hydroxyethyl TPP.[15]

*OXIDATIVE DECARBOXYLATION OF α-KETO ACIDS*

Pyruvate, α-ketoglutarate, and branched-chain α-keto acids undergo oxidative decarboxylation. The net reaction of the oxidative decarboxylation of pyruvate catalyzed by the pyruvate dehydrogenase complex is:

$$\text{Pyruvate} + \text{CoA} + \text{NAD}^+ \rightarrow \text{AcetylCoA} + CO_2 + \text{NADH} + H^+$$

In addition to CoA and $NAD^+$, TPP, lipoic acid, and flavin adenine dinucleotide (FAD) also serve as coenzymes. The pyruvate dehydrogenase complex, which is an organized assembly of three enzymes localized in the mitochondria, sequentially catalyzes the conversion of pyruvate into acetyl CoA.[2,4,7,15]

The net reaction in the oxidative decarboxylation of α-ketoglutarate, which takes place in the tricarboxylic acid cycle and is catalyzed by the α-ketoglutarate dehydrogenase complex, is:

$$\alpha\text{-ketoglutarate} + \text{CoA} + \text{NAD}^+ \rightarrow \text{SuccinylCoA} + CO_2 + \text{NADH} + H^+$$

The coenzyme requirements and the steps in the formation of succinyl CoA are analogous to the oxidative decarboxylation of pyruvate.[2,4,7,15]

The oxidative decarboxylation of the three branched-chain α-keto acids (α-ketoisocaproate, α-keto, β-methylvalerate, and α-ketoisovalerate) yield isovaleryl CoA, α-methylbutyryl CoA, and isobutyryl CoA, respectively. These reactions are catalyzed by a branched-chain α-keto acid dehydrogenase complex, which is analogous to those for pyruvate and α-ketoglutarate.[2,4,7,15]

*TRANSKETOLASE REACTION*

A TPP-dependent transketolase found in the cytosol catalyzes the reversible transfer of a glycolaldehyde moiety from the first two carbons of a donor ketose phosphate to the aldehyde carbon of an aldose phosphate in the pentose phosphate pathway. These reactions are:

$$\text{Xylulose-5-phosphate} + \text{Ribose-5-phosphate} \rightleftharpoons \text{Glyceraldehyde-3-phosphate} + \text{Sedoheptulose-7-phosphate}$$

$$\text{Xylulose-5-phosphate} + \text{Erythrose-4-phosphate} \rightleftharpoons \text{Glyceraldehyde 3-phosphate} + \text{Fructose-7-phosphate}$$

### BIOCHEMICAL ABNORMALITIES IN THIAMIN DEFICIENCY

Although the precise biochemical defect responsible for the pathophysiologic manifestations of thiamin deficiency is not established, thiamin may well play three major roles at the cellular level. The first relates to energy metabolism—namely, a reduction in the oxidative decarboxylation of α-keto acids leads to a failure of ATP synthesis. The second concerns abnormal carbohydrate metabolism resulting from a lower transketolase activity. The third deals with the function of membranes and nerve conduction.[7]

### OTHER PHYSIOLOGIC FUNCTIONS

The work of Von Muralt[16] and Cooper et al.[17] has suggested that thiamin plays a special role in neurophysiology that is independent of its coenzyme function. TTP (or TPP) may occupy a site on the membrane that is either in a sodium channel or proximal to it. The suggested mechanism is that initiation of a nerve impulse induces the dephosphorylation of thiamin phosphate, thereby causing a displacement of thiamin so that $Na^+$ can freely cross the membrane.[7,17]

## DEFICIENCY

Thiamin deficiency in animals and humans affects the cardiovascular, muscular, nervous, and gastrointestinal systems.[7]

### HIGH-RISK SITUATIONS

Populations vulnerable to the development of beriberi include breast-fed infants whose nursing mothers are thiamin-deficient; adults who have high carbohydrate intake derived mainly from milled rice, with or without ATF consumption; and chronic alcoholics. Dietary factors are major causes of thiamin deficiency in Asia, whereas alcoholism is of greatest concern in the West. An increase in thiamin requirement due to strenuous physical exertion, fever, pregnancy, lactation, or adolescence will precipitate clinical manifestations in marginally nourished persons. Other persons at risk are renal patients on dialysis, patients on parenteral nutrition, and hypermetabolic patients.[8,18–21]

### CLINICAL MANIFESTATIONS

The clinical manifestations of beriberi vary with age and with the systems involved. The disease is divided into infantile and adult beriberi.[8,18,19]

**Infantile Beriberi.** The disease is most commonly found between the age of 2 and 3 months. Infants may present with the cardiac (acute fulminating), aphonic, or pseudomeningitic form, or with a combination of these conditions. Infants with cardiac beriberi usually experience an acute attack, which includes a loud piercing cry, cyanosis, dyspnea, vomiting, tachycardia, and cardiomegaly; death may occur within a few hours of the onset unless thiamin is administered. The striking feature in aphonic beriberi is the tone of the child's cry, which varies from hoarseness to complete aphonia. Infants with pseudomeningitic beriberi exhibit vomiting, nystagmus, purposeless movement of the extremities, and convulsions that are accompanied by a "normal" cerebrospinal fluid.[7,8,18]

**Adult Beriberi.** Children and adults may present with the dry (paralytic or nervous), wet (cardiac), cerebral, or subclinical form.

The predominant features in dry beriberi are peripheral neuropathy, which is characterized by a symmetric impairment of sensory, motor, and reflex functions affecting the distal segments of limbs more severely than the proximal ones, calf muscle tenderness, and difficulty in rising from a squatting position.[8,18,19]

In addition to peripheral neuropathy, common signs found in wet beriberi include edema, tachycardia, wide pulse pressure, cardiomegaly, and congestive heart failure. Some patients have abnormal electrocardiograms. Typical hemodynamic findings in wet beriberi include high cardiac output and low peripheral and pulmonary vascular resistance. However, low cardiac output does not exclude the diagnosis of wet beriberi. In some patients there is sudden onset of a cardiac manifestation known as acute fulminant or "shoshin" beriberi. The predominant features are tachycardia, dyspnea, cyanosis, cardiac enlargement, and circulatory collapse.[8,18,19]

Neuropathologic studies of Wernicke-Korsakoff syndrome (cerebral beriberi) suggest that the distribution of the brain lesions in Wernicke's disease and in Korsakoff's psychosis are similar. Wernicke's disease is characterized by nystagmus, ophthalmoplegia, ataxia of gait, and mental confusion. Korsakoff's psychosis refers to a unique mental disorder in which retentive memory is impaired out of all proportion to other cognitive functions in an otherwise alert and responsive patient. A diagnosis of Wernicke-Korsakoff syndrome should be reserved for patients having combined manifestations of Wernicke's disease and a persistent or enduring defect in learning and memory. Though Wernicke's disease and Korsakoff's psychosis are mainly found in alcoholics, both disorders have been observed in other conditions associated with thiamin deficiency. An abnormal transketolase in fibroblasts from some patients with Wernicke's disease suggests that this genetic aberration may play a role in the susceptibility of some alcoholic patients to Wernicke's disease.[3,7,20,21]

Persons with subclinical thiamin deficiency often show some psychologic disturbances including irritability, frequent headaches, and unusual fatigue.[3]

### TREATMENT

Thiamin should be promptly administered to beriberi patients. The daily dosage usually ranges from 0.19 to 0.38 mmol (50 to 100 mg) given intravenously or intramuscularly for 7 to 14 days, after which 0.04 mmol (10 mg) per day should be administered orally until the patients fully recover. To prevent the recurrence of beriberi, patients should be advised to change their dietary habits and to stop drinking alcohol.[8,18]

Several thiamin derivatives, such as thiamin propyl disulfide (TPD) and thiamin tetrahydrofurfural disulfide (TTFD), have also been used for treating thiamin deficiency.[14] These derivatives are barely soluble in water and are only minimally decomposed by thiaminase. Even when given orally they produce a significantly higher thiamin level in the blood, the tissues, and the cerebrospinal fluid than does thiamin hydrochloride, because the intestinal transport of these compounds is not rate-limited. In alcoholics, oral TPD is effective in correcting laboratory and clinical evidence of thiamin depletion refractory to oral thiamin hydrochloride administration. In studies of subacute necrotizing encephalomyelopathy (SNE), TPD and TTFD were more efficacious than thiamin hydrochloride in raising the thiamin level in the cerebrospinal fluid.[2,14]

### RESPONSE TO THIAMIN ADMINISTRATION

In wet beriberi, improvement is characterized within 6 to 24 hours after thiamin administration by reduced restlessness; the disappearance of cyanosis; reduction in heart rate, respiratory rate, and cardiac size; and clearing of pulmonary congestion. In dry beriberi, more time elapses before improvement is observed.[8,18,19] In Wernicke's disease, ophthalmoplegia and gaze palsies often begin to resolve during the first day. Nystagmus, ataxia, and confusion may improve within days to weeks. Recognizable improvement in Korsakoff's psychosis may take 1 to 3 months.[7,20,21]

## EVALUATION

Various biochemical tests based on thiamin metabolism or the biochemical functions of TPP have been developed to detect thiamin deficiency and to establish thiamin adequacy in man. These include the measurement of blood thiamin, pyruvate, α-ketoglutarate, lactate, and glyoxylate, and of urinary thiamin, thiamin metabolites, and methylglyoxal. A thiamin-loading test has also been devised. At present the most reliable and feasible method of evaluating human thiamin adequacy is the measurement of erythrocyte transketolase activity (ETKA) and its percentage of enhancement resulting from added TPP, which is known as the thiamin pyrophosphate effect (TPPE). The diagnostic criteria for assessing human thiamin inadequacy consist of low ETKA, usually accompanied by a TPPE of 16% and above. However, in chronic thiamin deficiency, the TPP added in vitro cannot restore ETKA fully; under such a condition TPPE may be in the normal range of 0 to 15%.[8,18,19,22]

## REQUIREMENTS AND RECOMMENDED INTAKES

Because thiamin is essential for the metabolism of carbohydrates and branched-chain amino acids, the recommended thiamin intake is expressed in terms of total caloric intake. The current recommended thiamin allowances in the United States are 1.9 μmol/4184 kJ (0.5 mg/1000 kcal) for children, adolescents, and adults, and 1.5 μmol/4184 kJ (0.4 mg/1000 kcal) for infants (see Appendix Table A–2b). These recommendations are based on assessing the effects of varying levels of dietary thiamin on the occurrence of deficiency signs, on the excretion of thiamin or its metabolites, and on ETKA. A minimal thiamin intake of 3.8 μmol per day (1.0 mg per day) is recommended for adults, even though they consume less than 8368 kJ (2000 kcal) daily. An additional thiamin intake of 1.5 μmol per day (0.4 mg per day) is recommended throughout pregnancy to accommodate maternal and fetal growth and increased maternal caloric intake. To account for both thiamin secretion in milk and increased energy consumption during lactation, an increment of 1.9 μmol per day (0.5 mg per day) is recommended throughout lactation.[23] The 1989 recommended thiamin allowances in Thailand also agree with values in the United States.

Patients with thiamin deficiency can be treated with physiologic doses of thiamin. However, patients with thiamin dependency only respond to pharmacologic doses of thiamin. These disorders include thiamin-responsive megaloblastic anemia, thiamin-responsive lactic acidosis, thiamin-responsive branched-chain ketoaciduria, and SNE.[7,14]

## TOXICITY

Excessive amounts of ingested thiamin are rapidly cleared by the kidneys. No evidence exists of thiamin toxicity by oral administration.[4,23]

## REFERENCES


1. Williams, R.R.: Toward the Conquest of Beriberi. Cambridge, MA, Harvard University Press, 1961.
2. Gubler, C.J.: Thiamin. *In* Handbook of Vitamins: Nutritional, Biochemical, and Clinical Aspects. Edited by L.J. Machlin. New York, Marcel Dekker, 1984, pp. 245–297.
3. Haas, R.H.: Annu. Rev. Nutr., *8:*483–515, 1988.
4. McCormick, D.B.: Thiamin. *In* Modern Nutrition in Health and Disease. 7th Ed. Edited by M.E. Shils and V.R. Young. Philadelphia, Lea & Febiger, 1988, pp. 355–361.
5. International Union of Nutritional Sciences Committee on Nomenclature: J. Nutr., *117:*7–15, 1987.
6. Davidson, S., Passmore, R., Brock, J.F., Truswell, A.S.: Human Nutrition and Dietetics. 6th Ed. Edinburgh, Churchill Livingstone, 1975.
7. Tanphaichitr, V., Wood, B.: Thiamin. *In* Present Knowledge in Nutrition. 5th Ed. Edited by R.E. Olson, H.P. Broquist, C.O. Chichester, et al. Washington, D.C., Nutrition Foundation, 1984, pp. 273–284.
8. Tanphaichitr, V.: Epidemiology and clinical assessment of vitamin deficiencies in Thai children. *In* Child Health in the Tropics. Edited by R.E. Eeckels, O. Ransome-Kuti, and C.C. Kroonenberg. Dordrecht, Martinus Nijhoff Publishers, 1985, pp. 157–166.
9. Leevy, C.M.: Ann. N. Y. Acad. Sci., *378:*316–326, 1982.
10. Murata, K.: Ann. N. Y. Acad. Sci., *378:*146–155, 1982.
11. Vimokesant, S., Kunjara, S., Rungruangsak, K., et al.: Ann. N. Y. Acad. Sci., *378:*123–136, 1982.
12. Hilker, D.M., Somogyi, J.C.: Ann. N. Y. Acad. Sci., *378:*137–144, 1982.
13. Itokawa, Y., Kimura, M., Nishino, K.: Ann. N. Y. Acad. Sci., *378:*327–336, 1982.
14. Davis, R.E., Icke, G.: Adv. Clin. Chem., *23:*93–140, 1983.
15. Stryer, L.: Biochemistry. 3rd Ed. New York, W.H. Freeman and Co., 1988.
16. Von Muralt, A.: Ann. N. Y. Acad. Sci., *98:*499–507, 1962.
17. Cooper, J.R., Pincus, J.H.: Neurochem. Res., *4:*223–239, 1982.
18. Chaithiraphan, S., Tanphaichitr, V., Cheng, T.O.: Nutritional heart disease. *In* The International Textbook of Cardiology. Edited by T.O. Cheng. New York, Pergamon Press, 1986, pp. 864–870.
19. Tanphaichitr, V., Vimokesant, S.L., Dhanamitta, S., et al.: Am. J. Clin. Nutr., *23:*1017–1026, 1970.
20. Blass, J.P.: Thiamin and the Wernicke-Korsakoff syndrome. *In* Vitamins in Human Biology and Medicine. Edited by M.H. Briggs. Boca Raton, CRC Press, 1981, pp. 107–135.
21. Adams, R., and Victor, M.: Principles of Neurology. 4th Ed. New York, McGraw-Hill, 1989.
22. Tanphaichitr, V., Lerdvuthisopon, N., Dhanamitta, S., et al.: Intern. Med., *6:*43–46, 1990.
23. Food and Nutrition Board, National Research Council: Recommended Dietary Allowances. 10th Ed. Washington, D.C., National Academy Press, 1989.

## SELECTED READINGS


Brown, M.L.: Thiamin. *In* Present Knowledge in Nutrition. 6th Ed. Edited by M.L. Brown. Washington, D.C., ILSI-Nutrition Foundation, 1990, pp. 142–145.

Chaithiraphan, S., Tanphaichitr, V., Cheng, T.O.: Nutritional heart disease. *In* The International Textbook of Cardiology. Edited by T.O. Cheng. New York, Pergamon Press, 1986, pp. 864–870.

Gubler, C.J.: Thiamin. *In* Handbook of Vitamins: Nutritional, Biochemical, and Clinical Aspects. Edited by L.J. Machlin. New York, Marcel Dekker, 1984, pp. 245–297.

Haas, R.H.: Thiamin and the brain. Annu. Rev. Nutr., *8*:483–515, 1988.

Tanphaichitr, V., Wood, B.: Thiamin. *In* Present Knowledge in Nutrition. 5th Ed. Edited by R.E. Olson, H.P. Broquist, C.O. Chichester, et al. Washington, D.C., Nutrition Foundation, 1984, pp. 273–284.

CHAPTER 21

# Riboflavin

Donald B. McCormick



The "water-soluble B" fraction, reported by McCollum and Kennedy in 1916 to contain an antiberiberi substance,[1] was subsequently shown by Emmett and Luros (1920)[2] and Smith and Hendrick (1926)[3] to contain at least a second more heat-stable antipellagra factor, which was termed $B_2$. It soon became apparent that this $B_2$ fraction was a complex containing a yellow growth factor called riboflavin in England and vitamin G in the United States, as well as the subsequently identified pellagra-preventive factor (niacin) and the rat antidermatitis factor (vitamin $B_6$). Although a water-soluble, yellow fluorescent compound was known in the latter part of the nineteenth century (Blyth, 1879)[4] to occur in such natural materials as whey, association of the pigment with vitaminic properties was not secured until its isolation in 1933 by several groups.[5–7] Terms applied to riboflavin indicated the origin (e.g., lactoflavin (milk), ovoflavin (egg), hepatoflavin (liver), and uroflavin (urine). Warburg and Christian in Germany had meanwhile isolated by 1932 a yellow respiratory ferment (now called "Old Yellow Enzyme") from yeast.[8] This flavoprotein was soon dissociated into a protein apoenzyme and a yellow prosthetic coenzyme that was clearly similar to riboflavin.[9] Stern and Holiday (1934) found that the coenzyme was an alloxazine derivative,[10] and Theorell (1934) demonstrated that it was a phosphate ester.[11]

By 1935, the groups of Kuhn at Heidelburg[12,13] and Karrer in Zurich[14,15] had achieved synthesis of the vitamin. Theorell, in 1937, secured the structure of the simpler coenzyme as riboflavin 5′-phosphate (flavin mononucleotide, or FMN).[16] By 1938, Warburg and Christian had isolated and characterized the more abundant but complex prosthetic group, flavin-adenine dinucleotide (FAD), and showed its participation as the coenzyme of D-amino oxidase.[17–20] In more recent years, it has become known that there are diverse natural flavins that have alterations in the side chain or ring system of the basic flavin structures.[21] No less than four 8α-modified forms of FAD occur covalently attached to important flavoproteins in the mammal: the N(3)-histidyl-linked cases of succinate and sarcosine dehydrogenases of the inner mitochondrial membrane, S-cysteinyl-linked monoamine oxidase of the outer mitochondrial membrane, and the N(1)-histidyl-linked L-gluconolactone oxidase of the liver microsomal fraction.

## CHEMISTRY, INCLUDING PRINCIPAL ANALOGUES

Riboflavin (vitamin $B_2$) was chemically specified as 6,7-dimethyl-9-(1′-D-ribityl)isoalloxazine, but with evolution of systematic nomenclature is now correctly given as 7,8-dimethyl-10-(1′-D-ribityl)isoalloxazine. The free vitamin is a weak base normally isolated or synthesized as a yellowish-orange amorphous solid. The 5′-hydroxymethyl terminus of the ribityl side chain in the vitamin is reacted to become an orthophosphate ester in the simpler coenzyme, FMN, which can be further enlarged to the more complex and frequently encountered FAD with a pyrophosphate-bridged adenylate moiety (Fig. 21–1). The molecular weight of riboflavin is 376.4; thus, 1 mg riboflavin = 2.66 μmol.

There are some biosynthetic variations on the parent vitaminic structure, such as the 8-dimethylamino group of roseoflavin produced by Streptomycetes davawensis[22] and 5′-glycosides of riboflavin, which can be formed by plant and fungal species.[23] Several natural variants of the coenzyme forms are listed in Table 21–1.

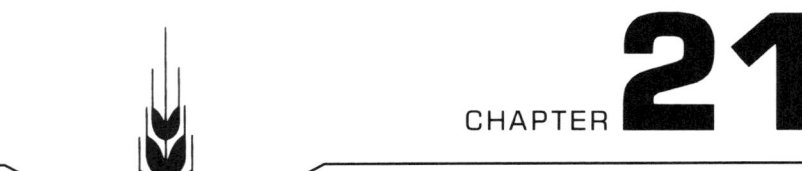

Chemical syntheses of riboflavin and similar isoallox-

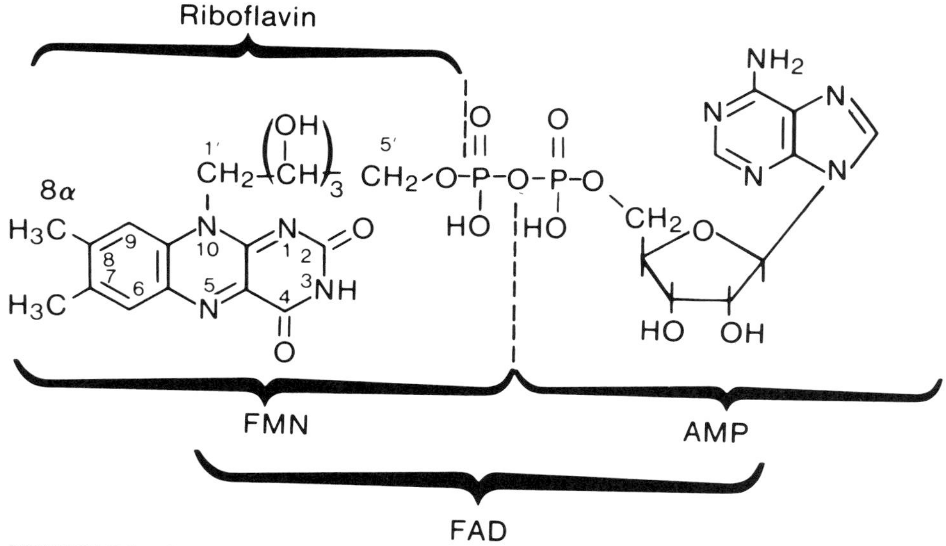
Riboflavin
FMN
AMP
FAD

**FIGURE 21–1.** Riboflavin and flavin mononucleotide (FMN) as components of flavin-adenine dinucleotide (FAD).

azines have been accomplished by several routes,[24] most of which have been adapted from the earlier procedures of Kuhn and Karrer and more recently from modifications introduced by Tishler and his associates.[25]

Riboflavin is only modestly soluble in aqueous solutions, though strong acid flavinium salts formed at low pH ($<1$) and flavin anion formed at alkaline pH ($>10$) are considerably more soluble. Neutral and slightly alkaline solutions are yellow with a long-wavelength absorption band near 450 nm. Strongly acidic flavin solutions are paler, because their primary absorbance shifts with intensification to about 385 nm. Solutions of the neutral oxidized (quinoid) form of the vitamin are strongly fluorescent with an emission wavelength at 525 nm. Riboflavin also has phosphorescent character reflecting triplet state reactivity following light excitation. One consequence of flavin photochemistry is the photolability of the side chain. Riboflavin is photodegraded ultimately to yield vitaminically inactive lumiflavin (7,8,10-trimethylisoalloxazine) under alkaline conditions and lumichrome (7,8-dimethylalloxazine) at all pH values, especially in neutral to acidic solutions. Flavins are chemically and biologically reduced, often through the radical (semiquinone) forms, to the nearly colorless, nonfluorescent 1,5-dihydro forms that rapidly reoxidize upon exposure to air (oxygen).

Chemical syntheses of flavocoenzymes involve phosphorylation of riboflavin,[26] commonly with chlorophosphoric acid, to form crude FMN, which is purified chromatographically. Conversion of FMN to FAD usually involves condensation of activated AMP, such as adenosine 5′-phosphoromorpholidate, with an FMN salt.[27,28] Extension of these techniques has been useful to form coenzyme analogues.[29]

## BIOLOGIC ACTIVITY RELATING TO STRUCTURE

Numerous analogues of riboflavin and the coenzyme derivatives have been tested in whole organisms[30] and with apoflavoproteins,[21,31] respectively. In general, the full D-ribityl side chain is needed, though weak vitaminic activity has been found with the D-arabo configuration. D-galactoflavin is an antagonist. In addition to a normal pyrimidinoid portion, both 7- and 8-methyl substituents are required for optimal vitaminic activity, though sparing with corresponding monoethyl analogues has been reported. The 7,8-dihaloflavins are inhibitors, as is isoriboflavin with a 6,7-dimethyl structure. The 5′-phosphate, commonly occurring as the dianionic ester, is needed for binding in FMN-dependent systems, and an additional 5′-AMP moiety is needed with FAD-dependent enzymes.

## ABSORPTION, TRANSPORT, METABOLISM, AND EXCRETION

The processes by which riboflavin and lesser amounts of natural derivatives are released by digestion of complexes with food proteins and then absorbed, transported, and metabolically altered has been reviewed in a fairly comprehensive manner.[21] Salient features are that coenzyme forms of the vitamin (mainly FAD and less FMN) are released from noncovalent attachment to proteins as a consequence of gastric acidification. Nonspecific action of pyrophosphatase and phosphatase on the coenzyme forms occurs in the upper gut. Several percent of 8α-(amino acid)riboflavins originally in cova-

**TABLE 21–1.** NATURALLY OCCURRING VARIANTS OF FLAVIN MONONUCLEOTIDE (FMN) AND FLAVIN-ADENINE DINUCLEOTIDE (FAD)

| NAME | SOURCES |
|---|---|
| 6-S-Cysteinyl(peptide)-FMN | Trimethylamine dehydrogenase (bacterium W3A1, Hyphomicrobium X) |
| 8α-S-Cysteinyl(peptide)-FAD | Monoamine oxidase (outer mitochrondrial membrane) |
| | Cytochromes c-532 and c-533 (Chromatium strain D, Chlorobium thiosulfatophilum) |
| 8α-O-Tyrosyl(peptide)-FAD | p-Cresol methylhydroxylase (Pseudomonas putida) |
| 8α-N(1)-Histidyl(peptide)-FAD | L-Glucono-γ-lactone oxidase (rat liver microsomes) |
| | L-Galactonolactone oxidase (Saccharomyces cerevisiae) |
| | Cholesterol oxidase (Schizophyllum commune, Gleocystidium chrysocreas) |
| | β-Cyclopiazonate oxidocyclase (Penicillium cyclopium) |
| | Thiamin dehydrogenase (soil bacterium ATCC 25589) |
| 8α-N(3)-Histidyl(peptide)-FAD | Succinate dehydrogenase (inner mitochrondrial membrane) |
| | Sarcosine dehydrogenase (Pseudomonas, mitochondria) |
| | D-6-Hydroxynicotine oxidase (Arthrobacter oxidans) |
| | Fumarate reductase (Escherichia coli) |
| | Choline oxidase (Alcaligenes spp., Arthrobacter globiformis) |
| | D-Gluconate dehydrogenase (Pseudomonas aeuginosa, P. fluorescens) |
| Coenzyme $F_{420}$ (5-deaza-5-carba-7,8-didemethyl-8-hydroxy; 5′-phospholactyldiglutamyl | Methane synthetase (Methanobacterium) |

(Updated from Merrill, A.H., Jr., Lambeth, J.D., Edmondson, D.E., et al.: Annu. Rev. Nutr., *1*:281–317, 1981.

lent attachment to certain enzymes, such as mitochondrial succinate dehydrogenase or monoamine oxidase, and traces of other ring and side-chain substituted flavins are also released by these actions following proteolysis. The vitamin is primarily absorbed in the human in the proximal small intestine by a saturable transport system that is rapid and proportional to dose before leveling off at 66.5 μmol (25 mg) of riboflavin. Bile salts appear to facilitate the uptake, and a modest amount of the vitamin circulates via the enterohepatic system. Active transport at lower levels of intake may be $Na^+$-dependent and involve phosphorylation. An active transport process dependent on $Na^+$ has been indicated from studies on riboflavin uptake in rat intestine in vivo[32] and in vitro.[33,34] In the human, some of the riboflavin circulating in blood plasma is loosely associated with albumin, though significant amounts complex with other proteins. A subfraction of IgG has been found to bind avidly to a small portion of the total free flavin in blood,[35] and several immunoglobulins contribute significantly to the circulatory transport of the vitamin.[36] As found earlier in other mammals, such as the cow,[37] pregnancy increases the level of a riboflavin carrier protein in humans as well.[38] In this connection, there are differential rates of uptake for the vitamin at the maternal and fetal surfaces of the placenta.[39] The entry of riboflavin into mammalian cells appears to be carrier-mediated (facilitated) at physiologic concentrations, but diffusion contributes to entry at higher levels.[40,41] Uptake exhibits relative specificity, and a riboflavin-binding protein has been found in the plasma membrane of rat liver cells.[42] The nonepithelial hepatocyte does not depend on $Na^+$ for riboflavin import,[43] as do bipolar epithelial types such as the enterocyte[33,34] or renal proximal tubular cell.[44] In all cases, metabolic trapping dependent on cytosolic flavokinase follows passage of the vitamin through the plasma membrane, which also contains nonspecific alkaline phosphatase that can catalyze release of vitamin from its internal phosphate ester.[40]

Metabolic interconversions of flavins at the cellular level are outlined in Figure 21–2. Conversion of riboflavin to coenzymes occurs within the cellular cytoplasm of most tissues, but particularly in the small intestine, liver, heart, and kidney.[21,40,45] The obligatory first step is the adenosine triphosphate (ATP)-dependent phosphorylation of the vitamin catalyzed by flavokinase. The FMN product can be complexed with specific apoenzymes to form several functional flavoproteins, but the larger quantity is further converted to FAD in a second ATP-dependent reaction catalyzed by FAD synthetase (pyrophosphorylase). It seems likely that the biosynthesis of flavocoenzymes is tightly regulated and dependent on riboflavin status.[46] Thyroxine and triiodothyroxine stimulate FMN and FAD synthesis in mammalian systems.[47,48] This seems to involve a hormone-mediated increase in an active form of flavokinase.[49] As a product of the synthetase, FAD is also an effective inhibitor at this step and may regulate its own formation.[50] FAD is the predominant flavocoenzyme present in tissues where it is mainly complexed with numerous flavoprotein dehydrogenases and oxidases. Less than 10% of the FAD can also become covalently attached to specific amino acid residues of a few important apoenzymes. Examples include the 8α-N(3)-histidyl FAD within succinate dehydrogenase and 8α-S-cysteinyl FAD within monoamine oxidase, both of mitochondrial localization. Turnover of covalently attached flavocoenzymes requires intracellular proteolysis, and further degradation of the coenzymes involves nonspecific pyrophosphatase cleavage of FAD to adenosine monophosphate (AMP) and FMN and action by nonspecific phosphatases on FMN. A 5′-nucleotidase recently purified from human placenta has been shown to possess specific FAD pyrophosphatase when stimulated with cobalt.[51]

Because there is little storage of riboflavin as such, the urinary excretion reflects dietary intake and catabolic and photodegradative events.[40] The diverse flavin-related products identified in the urine of humans and other mammals are shown in Figure 21–3. Both 7- and 8-hydroxymethylflavins appear in urine from the human and rat and are the result of microsomal mixed-function oxidases.[52] Smaller amounts of side-chain degradation products, such as lumichrome, 10-formylmethylflavin, and 10-(2′-hydroxyethyl)flavin, are also excreted and may largely result from intestinal microorganisms.[21,53–55] Traces of 8α-flavin peptides and catabolites are found in urine and feces.[55,56] A recently identified 5′-riboflavinyl peptide ester also occurs in human urine.[57] For normal adults eating varied diets, riboflavin accounts for 60 to 70% of urinary flavin, 7-hydroxymethylriboflavin accounts for 10 to 15%, 8α-sulfonylriboflavin accounts for 5 to 10%, 8-hydroxymethylriboflavin accounts for 4 to 7%, riboflavinyl peptide ester accounts for 5%, and 10-hydroxyethylflavin accounts for 1 to 3%, with traces of lumiflavin and varyingly the 10-formylmethylflavins and carboxymethylflavins.[40]

Secretion of flavin into milk, an early recognized source[4] that came to be called lactoflavin, has been reexamined on the bases of better techniques for separation and identification. For milk from both cows[58] and humans,[59] the flavin in highest concentration other than the free vitamin is FAD, which can account for over a third of total flavin. Much of this is hydrolyzed to FMN during pasteurization. Fairly significant quantities of the 10-(2′-hydroxyethyl)flavin are notable, because this catabolite has antivitaminic activities as reflected in competitive inhibition both of cellular uptake[43] and subsequent flavokinase-catalyzed phosphorylation of riboflavin.[60] Hence, this catabolite, which may reach 10 to 12% of flavin in cows milk, subtracts from the biologic activity of the food. Several percent of both 7- and 8-hydroxymethylriboflavins are also present, with more of the former. Smaller amounts of other catabolites, including the 10-formylmethylflavin and lumichrome, account for most of the rest.

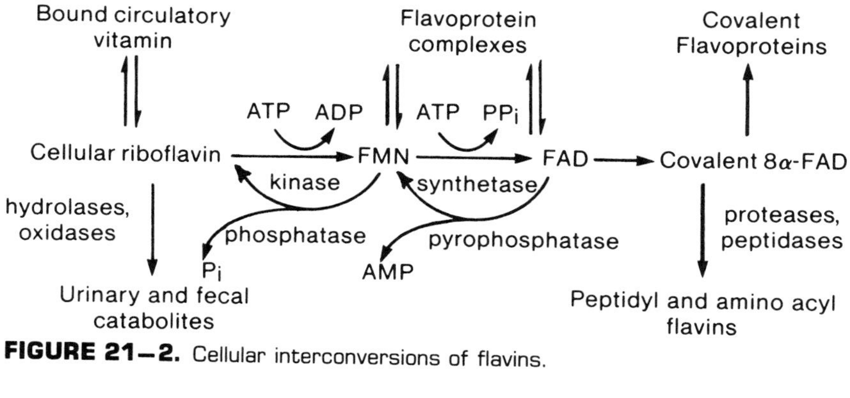
Bound circulatory vitamin
Flavoprotein complexes
Covalent Flavoproteins
ATP
ADP
ATP
PPi
Cellular riboflavin
FMN
FAD
Covalent 8α-FAD
kinase
synthetase
hydrolases, oxidases
phosphatase
pyrophosphatase
proteases, peptidases
Pi
AMP
Urinary and fecal catabolites
Peptidyl and amino acyl flavins

**FIGURE 21–2.** Cellular interconversions of flavins.

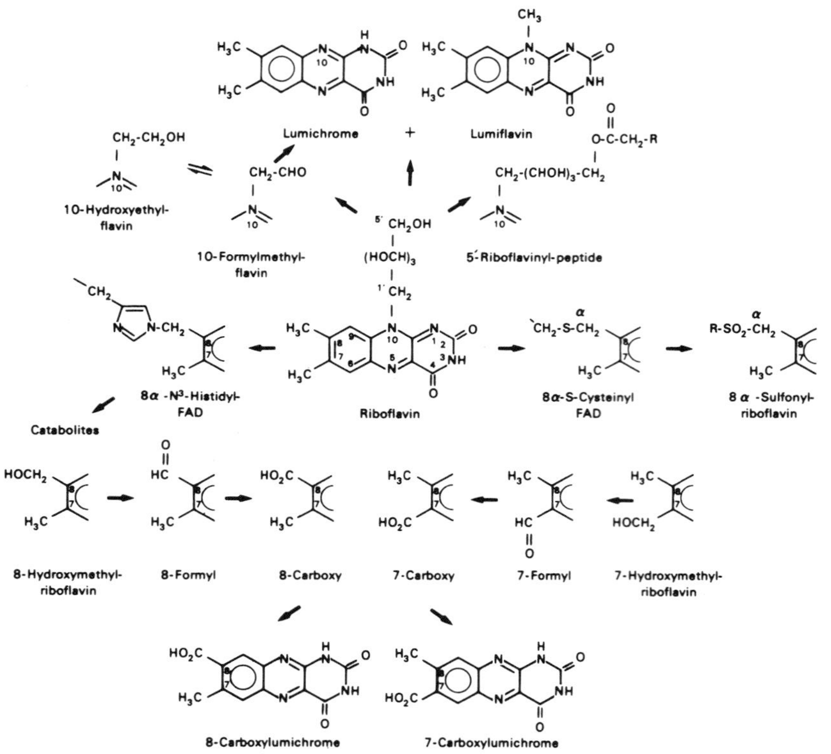

**FIGURE 21–3.** Urinary flavins and products related to riboflavin and 8α-flavocoenzymes.

## BIOCHEMICAL AND PHYSIOLOGIC FUNCTIONS

In bound coenzymic form, riboflavin participates in oxidation-reduction reactions in numerous metabolic pathways and in energy production via the respiratory chain. A variety of chemical reactions are catalyzed by flavoproteins.[21,45,61] The redox functions of a flavocoenzyme, illustrated in Figure 21–4, include one-electron transfers, during which the biologically encountered, neutral, oxidized quinone level of flavin is half reduced to the radical semiquinone, which can exist within natural pH ranges as neutral or anionic species. A further electron transfer can lead to a fully reduced hydroquinone. Additionally, a single-step two-electron transfer from substrate to flavin can occur with hydride ion transfer, as from reduced pyridine nucleotide or by base abstraction of a substrate proton together with carbanion addition.[21]

There are flavoprotein-catalyzed dehydrogenations that are both pyridine nucleotide-dependent and -independent, reactions with sulfur-containing compounds, hydroxylations, oxidative decarboxylations, dioxygenations, and reduction of $O_2$ to hydrogen peroxide. The intrinsic abilities of flavins to be varyingly potentiated as redox carriers upon differential binding to proteins, to participate in both one- and two-electron transfers, and in reduced (1,5-dihydro) form to react rapidly with oxygen permits wide scope in their operation.

## DEFICIENCY AND EXCESS

Though riboflavin has a wide distribution in foodstuffs, many people live for long periods on low intakes; consequently, minor signs of deficiency are common in many parts of the world.[62] Moreover, such deficiency as is encountered almost invariably occurs in combination with deficiency of other water-soluble vitamins.[40] Clinical deficiency of riboflavin has been induced by feeding a riboflavin-deficient diet, by the administration of an antagonist such as galactoflavin, or both. The deficiency syndrome is characterized by sore throat, hyperemia and edema of the pharyngeal and oral mucous membranes, cheilosis, angular stomatitis, glossitis (magenta tongue), seborrheic dermatitis, and normochromic, normocytic anemia associated with pure red cell cytoplasia of the bone marrow.[63] As noted previously, however, some of these symptoms, such as glossitis and dermatitis, when encountered in the field may have resulted from other complicating deficiencies. Severe riboflavin deficiency can also affect the conversion of vitamin $B_6$ to its coenzyme and even curtail conversion of tryptophan to niacin.[40]

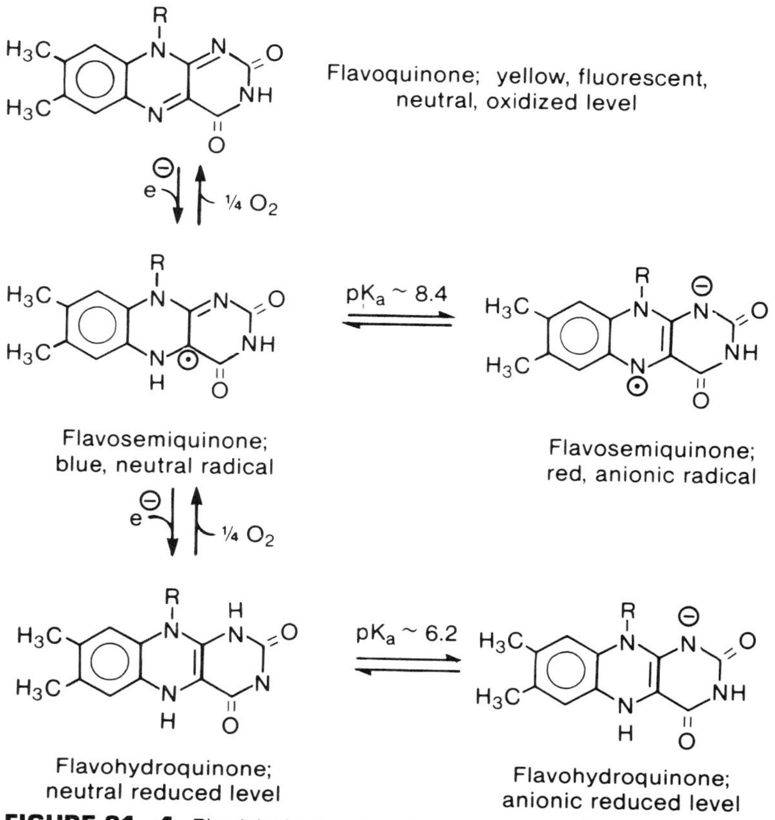
Flavoquinone; yellow, fluorescent, neutral, oxidized level
¼ O2
pKa ~ 8.4
Flavosemiquinone; blue, neutral radical
Flavosemiquinone; red, anionic radical
¼ O2
pKa ~ 6.2
Flavohydroquinone; neutral reduced level
Flavohydroquinone; anionic reduced level

**FIGURE 21–4.** Physiologically relevant redox states of flavocoenzymes.

Toxicity from ingestion of excess riboflavin by experimental animals or humans is doubtful. The capacity of the human gastrointestinal tract to absorb orally administered riboflavin may be less than 20 mg in a single dose.[64,65] The limited solubility and absorptivity of this vitamin as encountered in multivitamin preparations and in natural foodstuffs and its ready excretion (which is typical of water-soluble vitamins) normally precludes a health risk. There is one report of electroencephologram (EEG) abnormalities in two patients during long-term treatment with riboflavin and niacin.[66]

## CAUSES OF DEFICIENCY

Pure, uncomplicated riboflavin deficiency is probably never encountered in patients, but is accompanied by multiple nutrient deficiencies. Ariboflavinosis can result from such primary and secondary factors as commonly affect supply or utilization of other nutrients as well.[67] Inadequate dietary intake most commonly related to limited availability of food, but sometimes exacerbated by poor storage or processing, remains the major cause. Additionally, anorexic persons rarely ingest adequate amounts of riboflavin and other nutrients.

Decreased assimilation results from abnormal digestion, absorption, or both. Lactose intolerance as a result of lactase insufficiency, mostly encountered among blacks and Asians, argues against such afflicted persons' consuming milk, which is a good source of the vitamin. Malabsorption can occur as a result of tropical sprue, celiac disease, malignancy and resection of the small bowel, and gastrointestinal and biliary obstruction. Poor absorption also results from disorders that increase motility and decrease gastrointestinal passage time, such as diarrhea, infectious enteritis, and irritable bowel syndrome.

Rarely encountered, but usually significantly improved by therapeutic treatment with riboflavin, are certain inborn errors in which the genetic defect is in the formation of a normal flavoprotein. Cases in this category include fatty acid desaturases in which specific defects have been found for the mitochondrial FAD-dependent dehydrogenases for short-chain,[68] long-chain,[69] and multichain acyl-CoAs.[70] The young patients have a lipid storage myopathy, often accompanied by carnitine insufficiency, and exhibit glutaric aciduria.[71–75] A low-FMN-dependent pyridoxine 5′-phosphate oxidase activity due to an erythrocyte deficiency of FMN, confirmed by response to oral riboflavin, was reported in the majority of subjects with D-glucose-6-phosphate dehydrogenase deficiency in two studies.[76,77]

Such cases seem to involve an accelerated conversion of FMN to FAD so that glutathione reductase is saturated. This contrasts with heterozygous β-thalassemia, in which there is an inherited slow erythrocyte conversion of riboflavin to FMN, a decrease in subsequent FAD, and a high stimulation of the erythrocyte glutathione reductase by extraneous FAD.[76,78,79]

Defective utilization can result from disturbances in hormonal production, certainly as relates to thyroid hormone,[47,48] but less likely as may be affected by oral contraceptives.[75] Phenothiazine derivatives appear to impair use of riboflavin.[81]

Increased destruction of riboflavin occurs during treatment of neonatal jaundice with phototherapy.[82,83] In this case, the side chain of the vitamin is photochemically destroyed as it is involved in the photosensitized oxidation of bilirubin to more polar excretable compounds.[84,85]

The finding that phenobarbital induces microsomal oxidation of the 7-methyl function of the vitamin[52] lends credence to the belief that long-time use of barbiturates may jeopardize flavin status.

Enhanced excretion of riboflavin occurs in catabolic patients undergoing nitrogen loss. The relationship of the vitamin to protein status has long been recognized. Also, certain antibiotics and phenothiazine drugs increase excretion of riboflavin.[86,87]

Increased requirements can, of course, be the consequence of one or more of the previously mentioned factors. For example, protein-calorie malnutrition commonly accompanies a diminution in both absorption and utilization of riboflavin. Systemic infections even without gastrointestinal involvement sometimes lead to increased requirements that can result from decreased intake, defective absorption, poor utilization, and increased excretion.

## DIETARY CONSIDERATIONS

The requirement levels for riboflavin, in contrast to those for thiamin, are not raised when energy utilization is increased.[88] Because of the interdependence of protein, energy intake, and metabolic body size, however, recommended dietary allowances (RDA) calculated on these three bases do not differ significantly. Because RDA values are given in milligrams,[88] this mass unit has been used here. Nonetheless, 1 μmol riboflavin equals 0.376 mg, or inversely, 1 mg riboflavin equals 2.66 μmol. Thus, 0.4, 0.6, 1.2, and 1.7 mg riboflavin can be expressed as 1.06, 1.6, 3.2, and 4.5 mol, respectively. Clinical signs of deficiency in adults can be prevented with intakes of riboflavin above 0.4 mg/1000 kcal, but over 0.5 mg/1000 kcal may be required to maintain tissue reserves in adults and children as reflected in urinary excretion, red cell riboflavin, and erythrocyte glutathione reductase. From these considerations, the riboflavin allowances are now computed as 0.6 mg/1000 kcal for people of all ages. This leads to RDA ranging from 0.4 mg per day for early infants to 1.7 mg per day for young adult males (see Appendix Table A–2b). However, for elderly people and others whose daily calorie intake may be less than 2000 kcal, a minimum of 1.2 mg per day is recommended. Because pregnancy imposes extra demands, as reflected by decreased excretion and an elevated FAD stimulation of erythrocyte glutathione activity, an additional 0.3 mg per day is recommended. The lactating woman secretes approximately 35 μg/100 ml of milk for an output of about 0.26 mg per day (750 ml) during the first 6 months and 0.21 mg per day (600 ml) during the second 6 months. Because the utilization of the additional riboflavin for milk production is assumed to be 70%, an additional intake of 0.5 mg is recommended for the first 6 months and 0.4 mg for the second.

Small amounts of riboflavin, occurring largely as digestible coenzymes, are present in most plant and animal tissue. Especially good sources are eggs, lean meats, milk, broccoli, and enriched breads and cereals.[89] Such losses as occur during cooking are largely attributable to leaching of the heat-stable but light-sensitive flavins into water. (See Appendix Table A–21 for the riboflavin content of common foods).

When supplementation or therapy with riboflavin is warranted, oral administration of 5 to 10 times the RDA usually is satisfactory.[86]

## METHODS FOR ASSAY AND STATUS DETERMINATION

Numerous biochemical methods are aimed at the separation and quantitation of the diverse natural flavins.[90,91] Among the more sensitive are those that invoke specific binding, such as riboflavin with egg white riboflavin-binding protein, FMN with apoflavodoxin, and FAD with apoproteins for D-amino acid oxidase or glucose oxidase. However, nutritional status is commonly assessed by measuring urinary excretion of the vitamin in fasting, random, or 24-hour specimens, or by load return tests, measurement of erythrocyte riboflavin concentration, and determination of the erythrocyte glutathione reductase activity coefficient.[67,92]

Urinary riboflavin can be measured by fluorometric as well as by microbiologic procedures. Under conditions of adequate intake, the amount excreted per day is more than 0.32 μmol (120 μg), or at least 0.21 μmol (80 μg) are excreted per gram of creatinine. The rate of excretion expressed as μg/g creatinine is greater for children than for adults who normally have ≧80 μg/g but fall to <27 μg/g when deficient. Conditions causing negative nitrogen balance and the administration of antibiotics and certain psychotropic drugs (phenothiazine) increase urinary riboflavin as a consequence of tissue depletion and displacement, respectively. A load return test augments the applicability to a given case. Only high-performance liquid chromatography (HPLC) of suitable extracts followed by specific identification of each flavin is able to distinguish the natural vitamin from other urinary flavins.[55]

Erythrocyte riboflavin can also be determined by either fluorometric or microbiologic means. Because changes observed are rather small, there is some problem with sensitivity and interpretation of results. Nevertheless, it is clear that values below 27 nmol (10 μg)/dl cells should be considered to be reflecting a deficient status, as compared to ≧40 nmol to (≧15 μg)/dl for an acceptable status. Again, HPLC has been used to monitor more exactly the riboflavin composition of human blood.[93]

The most commonly used current method for assessing riboflavin status utilizes the determination of FAD-dependent glutathione reductase activity in freshly lysed red cells as detailed for routine clinical use[94] from the procedure described by Sauberlich et al.[95] Activities of holo and apo forms of glutathione reductase in erythrocyte hemolysates are measured before and after addition of FAD, respectively, by spectrophotometric determinations of NADPH (the reduced form of nicotinamide-adenine dinucleotide phosphate) oxidation. Values obtained are expressed in terms of "activity coefficients," or AC, (AC $=\Delta A_{340}$ with FAD/$\Delta A_{340}$ without FAD), which represent the degree of stimulation of apoenzyme resulting from addition of FAD in vitro. An AC of 1.0 would indicate no stimulation and only the presence of holoenzyme as a result of excess FAD (and riboflavin) in the original erythrocytes. Guidelines suggested for such coefficients are <1.2, acceptable; 1.2 to 1.4, low; >1.4, deficient. Though it is currently the biochemical method of choice for assessing riboflavin status, the erythrocyte glutathione reductase assay has some drawbacks.[67] The test cannot be used in persons with glucose 6-phosphate deficiency because of an increased avidity in the reductase for FAD in this disease, which is about 10% among black Americans. In vitro treatment of blood with inosine and adenine leads to elevated activity coefficients.[96]

## REFERENCES


1. McCollum, E.V., Kennedy, C.: J. Biol. Chem., *24:*491–502, 1916.
2. Emmett, A.D., Luros, G.O.: J. Biol. Chem., *43:*265–286, 1920.
3. Smith, M.I., Hendrick, E.G.: U.S. Public Health Rep., *41:*201–207, 1926.
4. Blyth, A.W.: J. Chem. Soc., *35:*530–539, 1879.
5. Kuhn, R., Gyorgy, P., Wagner-Jauregg, T.: Ber. Dtsch. Chem. Gesellsch., *66B:*317, 576–580, 1034–1038, 1933.
6. Ellinger, P., Koschara, W.: Ber. Dtsch. Chem. Gesellsch., *66B:*315–317, 1933.
7. Booher, L.E.: J. Biol. Chem., *102:*39–46, 1933.
8. Warburg, O., Christian, W.: Biochem. Z., *254:*438–458, 1932.
9. Warburg, O., Christian, W.: Biochem. Z., *266:*377–411, 1933.
10. Stern, K.G., Holiday, E.R.: Ber. Dtsch. Chem. Gesellsch., *67:*1104–1106, 1442–1452, 1934.
11. Theorell, H.: Biochem. Z., *272:*155–156, 1934.
12. Kuhn, R., Reinemund, K., Kaltschmitt, H., et al.: Naturwissenschaften, *23:*260, 1935.
13. Kuhn, R., Reinemund, K., Weygand, F., et al.: Chem. Ber., *68:*1765–1774, 1935.
14. Karrer, P., Schöpp, K., Benz, F.: Helv. Chim. Acta, *18:*426–429, 1935.
15. Karrer, P., Salomon, H., Schöpp, K., et al.: Helv. Chim. Acta, *18:*1143–1146, 1935.
16. Theorell, H.: Biochem. Z., *290:*293–303, 1937.
17. Warburg, O., Christian, W.: Biochem. Z., *295:*261, 1938.
18. Warburg, O., Christian, W.: Biochem. Z., *296:*294, 1938.
19. Warburg, O., Christian, W., Griese, A.: Biochem. Z., *297:*417, 1938.
20. Warburg, O., Christian, W.: Biochem. Z., *298:*150–168, 1938.
21. Merrill, A.H., Jr., Lambeth, J.D., Edmondson, D.E., et al.: Annu. Rev. Nutr., *1:*281–317, 1981.
22. Otani, S.: Studies on roseoflavin: Isolation, physical, chemical, and biological properties. *In* Flavins and Flavoproteins. Edited by T.P. Singer. Amsterdam, Elsevier, 1976, pp. 323–327.
23. Whitby, L.G.: Glycosides of riboflavin. *In* Vitamins and Coenzymes. Methods in Enzymology. Vol. 18, part B. Edited by D.B. McCormick and L.D. Wright. New York, Academic Press, 1971, pp. 404–413.
24. Lambooy, J.P.: The alloxazines and isoalloxazines. *In* Heterocyclic Compounds. Vol. 9. Edited by R.C. Elderfield. New York, Wiley, 1967, pp. 118–223.
25. Tishler, M., Pfister, K., Babson, R.D., et al.: J. Am. Chem. Soc., *69:*1487–1492, 1947.
26. Flexer, L.A., Farkas, W.G.: XIIth International Congress Pure Applied Chemistry, New York, Sept. 1951, Abstracts p. 71.
27. Moffatt, J.G., Khorana, H.G.: J. Am. Chem. Soc., *80:*3756–3761, 1958.
28. Moffatt, J.G., Khorana, H.G.: J. Am. Chem. Soc., *83:*649–658, 1961.
29. Föry, W., McCormick, D.B.: Chemical synthesis of flavin coenzymes. *In* Vitamins and Coenzymes. Methods in Enzymology. Vol. 18. Part B. Edited by D.B. McCormick and L.D. Wright. New York, Academic Press, 1971, pp. 458–464.
30. McCormick, D.B., N. Y. State J. Med., *62:*2842–2844, 1962.
31. McCormick, D.B.: Metabolism of riboflavin. *In* Riboflavin. Edited by R.S. Rivlin. New York, Plenum Press, 1975, pp. 153–198.
32. Rivier, D.A.: Experientia, *29:*1443–1446, 1973.
33. Meinen, M., Aeppli, R., Rehner, G.: Nutr. Metab., *21(Suppl. 1):*264–266, 1977.

34. Daniel, H., Wille, U., Rehner, G.: J. Nutr., *113*:636–643, 1982.
35. Merrill, A.H., Jr., Froehlich, J.A., McCormick, D.B.: Biochem. Med., *25*:198–206, 1981.
36. Innis, W.S.A., McCormick, D.B., Merrill, A.H., Jr.: Biochem. Med., *34*:151–165, 1985.
37. Merrill, A.H., Jr., Froehlich, J.A., McCormick, D.B.: J. Biol. Chem., *254*:9362–9364, 1979.
38. Natraj, U., George, S., Kadam, P.: J. Reprod. Immunol., *13*:1–16, 1988.
39. Dancis, J., Lehanka, J., Levitz, M.: Am. J. Obstet. Gynecol., *158*:204–210, 1988.
40. McCormick, D.B.: Physiol. Rev., *69*:1170–1198, 1989.
41. Bowman, B.B., McCormick, D.B., Rosenberg, I.H.: Annu. Rev. Nutr., *9*:187–199, 1989.
42. Nokubo, M., Ohta, M., Kitani, K., et al.: Biochim. Biophys. Acta, *981*:303–308, 1989.
43. Aw, T.-Y., Jones, D.P., McCormick, D.B.: J. Nutr., *113*:1249–1254, 1983.
44. Bowers-Komro, D.M., McCormick, D.B.: Riboflavin uptake by rat kidney cells. *In* Flavins and Flavoproteins. Edited by D.E. Edmondson and D.B. McCormick. New York, Walter de Gruyter, 1988, pp. 449–453.
45. McCormick, D.B.: Riboflavin. *In* Present Knowledge in Nutrition. 6th Ed. Edited by M.L. Brown. Washington, D.C., International Life Sciences Institute Nutrition Foundation, 1990, pp. 146–154.
46. Lee, S.S., McCormick, D.B.: J. Nutr., *113*:2274–2279, 1983.
47. Rivlin, R.S. (Ed.): Riboflavin. New York, Plenum Press, 1975.
48. Rivlin, R.S.: Nutr. Rev., *37*:241–245, 1979.
49. Lee, S.S., McCormick, D.B.: Arch. Biochem. Biophys., *237*:197–201, 1985.
50. Yamada, Y., Merrill, A.H., Jr., McCormick, D.B.: Arch. Biochem. Biophys., *278*:125–130, 1990.
51. Lee, R.S., Ford, H.C.: J. Biol. Chem., *263*:14878–14883, 1988.
52. Ohkawa, H., Ohishi, N., Yagi, K.: J. Biol. Chem., *258*:5623–5628, 5629, 1983.
53. Oka, M., McCormick, D.B.: J. Nutr., *115*:496–499, 1985.
54. Chastain, J.L., McCormick, D.B.: J. Nutr., *117*:468–475, 1987.
55. Chastain, J.L., McCormick, D.B.: Am. J. Clin. Nutr., *46*:830–834, 1987.
56. Chia, C.P., Addison, R., McCormick, D.B.: J. Nutr., *108*:373–381, 1978.
57. Chastain, J.L., McCormick, D.B.: Biochim. Biophys. Acta, *967*:131–134, 1988.
58. Roughead, Z., McCormick, D.B.: J. Nutr., *120*:382–388, 1990.
59. Roughead, Z., McCormick, D.B.: Am. J. Clin. Nutr., *52*:854–857, 1990.
60. McCormick, D.B.: J. Biol. Chem., *237*:959–962, 1962.
61. Edmondson, D.E., McCormick, D.B. (eds.): Flavins and Flavoproteins. New York, Walter de Gruyter, 1987.
62. Bates, C.J.: World Rev. Nutr. Diet., *50*:215–267, 1987.
63. Wilson, J.A.: Disorders of vitamins-deficiency, excess and errors of metabolism. *In* Harrison's Principles of Internal Medicine. 10th Ed. Edited by R.G. Petersdorf et al. New York, McGraw-Hill, 1982, pp. 461–470.
64. Stripp, B.: Acta Pharmacol. Toxicol., *22*:353–362, 1965.
65. Mayersohn, M., Feldman, S., Gibaldi, M.: J. Nutr., *98*:288–296, 1969.
66. Santanelli, P., Gobbi, G., Albani, F., et al.: Neurophysiol. Clin., *18*:549–553, 1988.
67. Nichoalds, G.E.: Riboflavin. Symposium in laboratory medicine. *In* Clinics in Laboratory Medicine. Vol. 1. No. 4. Philadelphia, W.B. Saunders, 1981, pp. 685–698.
68. DiDonato, S., Gellera, C., Peluchetti, D., et al.: Ann. Neurol., *25*:479–484, 1989.
69. Amendt, B.A., Moon, A., Teel, L., et al.: Pediatr. Res., *23*:603–605, 1988.
70. Gilkeson, G.S., Caldwell, D.S.: Arthritis Rheum., *31*:695–696, 1988.
71. Iafolla, A.K., Kahler, S.G.: J. Pediatr., *114*:1004–1006, 1989.
72. Mandel, H., Africk, D., Blitzer, M., et al.: J. Inherited Metab. Dis., *11*:397–402, 1988.
73. Turnbull, D.M., Bartlett, K., Eyre, J.A., et al.: Dev. Med. Child Neurol., *30*:667–672, 1988.
74. Turnbull, D.M., Shepherd, I.M., Ashworth, B., et al.: Brain, *111*:815–828, 1988.
75. Lipkin, P.H., Roe, C.R., Goodman, S.I., et al.: J. Pediatr., *112*:62–65, 1988.
76. Anderson, B.B., Clements, J.E., Perry, G.M., et al.: Eur. J. Haematol., *38*:12–20, 1987.
77. Powers, H.J., Bates, C.J.: Hum. Nutr. Clin. Nutr., *39*:107–115, 1985.
78. Anderson, B.B., Perry, G.M., Clements, J.E.: Br. J. Haematol., *57*:711–714, 1984.
79. Anderson, B.B., Perry, G.M., Clements, J.E., et al.: Eur. J. Haematol., *42*:354–360, 1989.
80. Roe, D.A., Boguzz, S., Sheu, J., et al.: Am. J. Clin. Nutr., *35*:495–501, 1982.
81. Horvath, C., Szonyi, L., Mold, K.: Teratology, *14*:167–170, 1976.
82. Rublatelli, F.F., Allegri, G., Costa, C., et al.: J. Pediatr., *85*:865–867, 1974.
83. Gromisch, D.S., Lopez, R., Cole, H.S., et al.: J. Pediatr., *90*:118–122, 1977.
84. Knobloch, E., Mandys, F., Hodr, R.: J. Chromatogr., *428*:255–263, 1988.
85. Knobloch, E., Hodr, R.: Czech. Med., *12*:134–144, 1989.
86. Goldsmith, G.A.: Prog. Food Nutr. Sci., *1*:559–609, 1975.
87. Pinto, J., Huang, Y.P., Rivlin, R.S.: Clin. Res., *27*:444A, 1979.
88. Food and Nutrition Board, National Research Council: Riboflavin. *In* Recommended Dietary Allowances. 10th Ed. Washington, D.C., National Academy Press, 1989, pp. 132–137.
89. Watt, B.K., Merrill, A.L.: Composition of food: Raw processed, prepared. *In* Agriculture Handbook No. 8. Washington, D.C., U.S. Department of Agriculture, 1963.
90. McCormick, D.B., Wright, L.D. (Eds.): Vitamins and Coenzymes. Methods in Enzymology. Vol. 18, Part B. New York, Academic Press, 1971.
91. McCormick, D.B., Wright, L.D. (Eds.): Vitamins and Coenzymes. Methods in Enzymology. Vol. 66. Part E. New York, Academic Press, 1980.
92. Briggs, M. (Ed.): Vitamins in Human Biology and Medicine. Boca Raton, FL, CRC Press, 1981.
93. Ishida, T., Horiike, K.: Nippon Rinsho, *48*:589–591, 1989.
94. McCormick, D.B.: Vitamins. *In* Textbook of Clinical Chemistry. Edited by N.W. Tietz. Philadelphia, W.B. Saunders, 1986, pp. 927–964.
95. Sauberlich, H.E., Judd, J.H., Jr., Nichoalds, G.E., et al.: Am. J. Clin. Nutr., *25*:756–762, 1972.
96. Trout, G.E.: Proc. Soc. Exp. Biol. Med., *191*:12–17, 1989.

## SELECTED READINGS

McCormick, D.B.: Riboflavin. *In* Present Knowledge in Nutrition. 6th Ed. Edited by M.L. Brown. Washington, D.C., International Life Sciences Institute Nutrition Foundation, 1990, pp. 146–154.

McCormick, D.B.: Two interconnected B vitamins: riboflavin and pyridoxine. Physiol. Rev., *69:*1170–1198, 1989.

CHAPTER 22

# Niacin

Marian E. Swendseid and Robert A. Jacob



The search for the cause of pellagra, the classic disease now associated with niacin deficiency, is one of the most fascinating episodes in medical science.[1] First recognized in 1735 by the Spanish physician, Casals, pellagra was rampant among many maize-eating populations throughout the world for the next two centuries. In the early 1900s the disease became an epidemic in the southeastern United States, and it was there that Goldberger established that pellagra was not an infectious disease but was caused by an unknown dietary deficiency.[1] In 1937 Elvehjem et al.[2] found that nicotinic acid was effective in treating pellagrous lesions in dogs and, within the year, nicotinic acid was reported to cure pellagra in humans.[3]

In 1945 the amino acid tryptophan (Trp) was shown to replace niacin in improving the growth of rats fed a high-corn diet.[1] Trp was firmly established as a niacin precursor by a series of studies demonstrating that Trp supplements increased the excretion of niacin metabolites and that labeled niacin could be isolated from an incubation mixture of liver tissue and labeled Trp. Trp also proved to be a niacin precursor in humans and could at least partially replace the requirement for preformed niacin in the diet. The recognition that Trp was a precursor of niacin explained the connection between corn-containing diets and pellagra because corn has a low content of both niacin and Trp. Questions still remain about the cause of the pellagra epidemics, however, and deficiencies of other vitamins such as riboflavin may have been contributing factors.[4] The underlying biochemical defects that lead to the symptoms of pellagra are also not understood.[1]

## CHEMISTRY AND ANALYTIC METHODS

Niacin is a generic term that includes both nicotinic acid (pyridine-3-carboxylic acid) and nicotinamide. The structures of these vitamers are shown in Figure 22–1 together with the two coenzymes that are the metabolically active forms of niacin, the pyridine nucleotides, nicotinamide adenine dinucleotide (NAD), and NAD phosphate (NADP). Free forms of the vitamin are white stable crystalline solids, with nicotinamide being more soluble in water, alcohol, and ether than nicotinic acid. Many analogues of niacin have been synthesized, some of which have antivitamin activity. Analogues that have an antivitamin effect in animals include 3-acetylpyridine, 6-aminonicotinamide, and 2 amino-1,3,4,thiazole.[5] In developing chicks, 6-aminonicotinamide and 3-acetylpyridine are teratogens causing abnormal limb formation. 6-Amino-nicotinamide and 2-amino 1,3,4 thiazole and its derivatives have marked antitumor activity in animal models.[5]

The acid or amide form of niacin can be determined by a chemical reaction with cyanogen bromide,[6] by microbiologic assays using bacteria requiring niacin for growth,[6] or by high-pressure liquid chromatography (HPLC).[7] The coenzymes of niacin, NAD and NADP, are measured by enzyme-cycling spectrophotometric or HPLC procedures.[8,9] The metabolites of niacin, such as the methylated derivative, $N^1$-methylnicotinamide (NMN), are measured by HPLC techniques.[7,10] NMN can also be determined by fluorescence based on the reaction of ketones with NMN in alkaline solution to form a fluorescent product.[11]

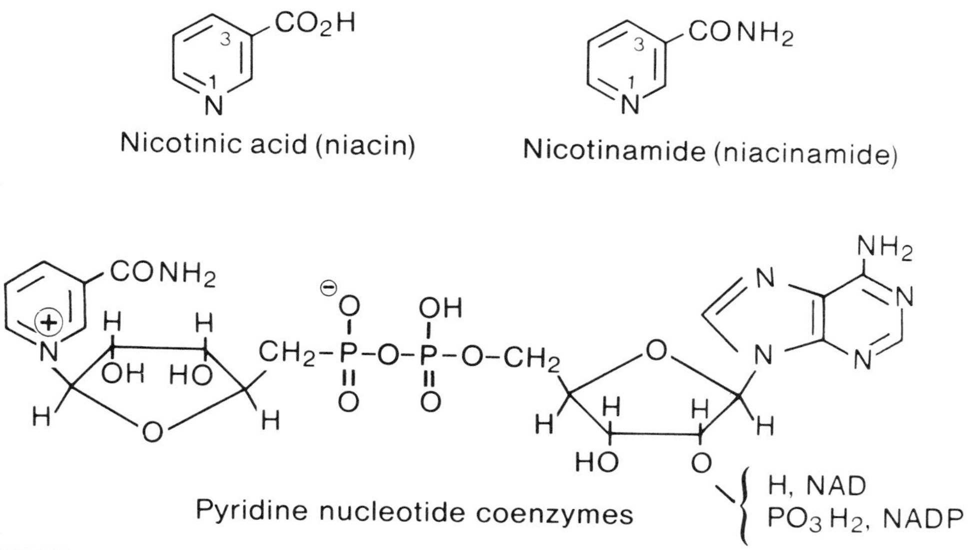
Nicotinic acid (niacin)
Nicotinamide (niacinamide)
Pyridine nucleotide coenzymes
H, NAD
PO3H2, NADP

**FIGURE 22–1.** Structures of vitamins and the two coenzyme forms containing the nicotinamide moiety. (From McCormick, D.B. Niacin. *In* Modern Nutrition in Health and Disease, 7th Ed. Edited by M.E. Shils and V.R. Young. Philadelphia, Lea & Febiger, 1988, p. 371.)

## DIETARY CONSIDERATIONS

Only small amounts of the free forms of niacin occur in nature. Most of the niacin in food is present as a component of NAD or NADP and is relatively stable during cooking and storage. In many foods, particularly cereals, niacin is of low biologic availability because it is bound to macromolecules of either complex carbohydrates (niacytin) or peptides (niacinogens). Good sources of niacin include meats (especially liver), fish, legumes, some nuts such as peanuts, and some cereals. Coffee and tea also contain the vitamin in appreciable amounts. The roasting of green coffee beans converts trigonelline (1-methyl nicotinic acid) to nicotinic acid. The bioavailability of niacin in corn is increased by pretreatment with alkali (lime water), a procedure used in Central America and Mexico in the preparation of tortillas. New varieties of corn such as Opaque-2 contain more niacin and also more tryptophan than conventional sources. Government policies on enrichment of flour have made foods such as bread good sources of niacin. (See Appendix Table A–21 for the niacin content of common foods).

Niacin is unique among the B vitamins in that a precursor can contribute substantially to meeting the dietary niacin requirements. An intake of 290 μmol (60 mg) of the niacin precursor, the essential amino acid Trp is estimated to provide an average of 8.2 μmol (1 mg) niacin or 1 mg niacin equivalent (NE); therefore recommended dietary allowances (RDA) for niacin are given in terms of milligrams of NE rather than in milligrams of niacin.[12] Because most proteins contain approximately 1% Trp, it is theoretically possible that a diet containing >100 g of protein and no preformed niacin could meet the RDA for niacin. Under most conditions studied, Trp appears to be used first for maintenance of protein and amino acid homeostasis, and then for the synthesis of niacin.[13]

## METABOLISM AND FUNCTION

Niacin, in its active metabolic forms, has a pervasive role in metabolism functioning in catabolic reactions, particularly in energy-related pathways and also in biosynthetic processes.

### ABSORPTION AND TRANSPORT

NAD and NADP, the chief dietary forms of niacin, are hydrolyzed by enzymes in the intestinal mucosa to yield nicotinamide as the major end product.[14] Intestinal bacteria can convert nicotinamide to nicotinic acid. Both vitamers are absorbed by facilitated diffusion at low concentrations and by passive diffusion at higher concentrations, and both appear in blood plasma.[14] Even large doses (24.6 mmol (3g) or more) of niacin are efficiently absorbed from the intestine.

Niacin is rapidly removed from blood plasma by the tissues, particularly the liver and red cells; in the postabsorption state only small amounts remain in plasma. Although most tissue cells absorb niacin by passive diffusion, facilitated diffusion also takes place in some cells such as those of the kidney and the erythrocyte.[14]

## STORAGE AND EXCRETION

Once niacin enters the cell it is converted to its coenzyme forms. In addition to NAD bound to enzymes, NAD not attached to an apoenzyme may also be present. This free NAD is sometimes designated as "storage" NAD.[15] In the rat, high concentrations of NAD are found in heart, liver, kidney, and muscle tissues.[16] In the rat, higher hepatic NADP levels were found in one study when Trp rather than preformed niacin was administered, suggesting a limitation on the utilization of niacin for NADP synthesis.[17] The NAD in body tissue appears to have a relatively high turnover rate. One study showed that in human subjects ingesting approximately half the RDA for niacin (49 to 82 μmol (6 to 10 mg NE) per day), NAD levels in red cells fell by 70% in 36 days.[18] In the same study the pool of available niacin was found to be reduced both in size and in rate of turnover as determined by isotope enrichment of NMN excreted following test doses of ring-labeled [$^2H_4$] nicotinamide.[19] In experimental studies with human subjects, clinical signs of pellagra developed in 50 to 60 days after the initiation of a corn diet containing approximately 66 μmol (8 mg) NE per day.[20]

In the liver, any excess of free niacin that accumulates is methylated to NMN by N-methyl transferase. NMN is the major niacin metabolite excreted in urine. Other metabolites found in urine include the oxidized derivatives of NMN, 2- and 4-methyl pyridone, and nicotinuric acid, the conjugate of nicotinic acid and glycine. The oxide and hydroxyl forms of niacin are also excreted in small amounts.[21]

## BIOSYNTHESIS AND REGULATION OF NAD AND NADP

The biosynthesis of NAD and NADP from Trp occurs in all organisms studied, with the formation of quinolinate as the key intermediate. In mammals, in liver and kidney, quinolinic acid is converted to nicotinic acid ribonucleotide, from which the coenzymes NAD and NADP are synthesized, as depicted in Figure 22–2. The efficiency of formation of these coenzymes is affected by both nutritional and hormonal factors. Deficiencies of vitamin $B_6$ or riboflavin slow the conversion because these vitamins are co-factors for enzymes acting in the Trp metabolic pathway. Activities of several of these enzymes, including Trp oxygenase, quinolinate phosphoribosyl transferase, and picolinate carboxylase, are also modulated by protein, energy, and niacin intakes. Although large individual differences in the conversion efficiency of Trp to niacin have been reported, an average conversion ratio is estimated to be 60 mg Trp to 1 mg niacin (or 35 μmol Trp to 1 μmol niacin).[22] In the third trimester of pregnancy, however, the efficiency of this conversion increases threefold,[23] possibly because of the stimulating effect of estrogen on Trp oxygenase, the putative rate-limiting enzyme in the conversion pathway.[24]

NAD can also be synthesized from nicotinic acid and nicotinamide. The biosynthesis of NAD from nicotinic acid involves the amidation of nicotinic acid adenine dinucleotide, a process that is essentially irreversible, as shown in Figure 22–2. The biosynthesis of NAD from nicotinamide occurs in all tissues and appears to be regulated by the concentration of extracellular nicotinamide, which in turn is under hepatic and hormonal control.

The hydrolysis of hepatic NAD stores to nicotinamide and adenosine diphosphate ribose (ADPR) is of particular importance in niacin metabolism because it allows the release of nicotinamide for transport to and absorption by tissues needing niacin. The hydrolysis of NAD (and NADP) in the liver and other tissues is catalyzed by two classes of enzymes, the NAD glycohydrolases and the poly (ADPR) polymerases. The activity of these enzymes appears to account in large measure for the rapid cellular turnover of the pyridine nucleotides. Some bound forms of NAD, however, are relatively immune to glycohydrolase action. The NAD of glyceraldehyde 3-phosphate dehydrogenase is one example thus ensuring that the glycolysis pathway will be spared to some extent in niacin deficiency states.[15]

## FUNCTION

At least 200 enzymes are known to be dependent on NAD and NADP with the nicotinamide moiety acting as electron acceptor or hydrogen donor. Most of the NAD-dependent enzymes are involved in catabolic reactions, such as the oxidation of fuel molecules as shown in Figure 22–3, whereas NADP more commonly functions in reductive biosyntheses of such compounds as fatty acids and steroids. A small number of dehydrogenases can use both coenzymes. Because of their involvement in hydrogen-transfer reactions, the pyridine nucleotides function in the synthesis and degradation of all the macronutrients: carbohydrates, fatty acids, and amino acids.

NAD also has an important nonredox function, in that it serves as a substrate for glycohydrolases catalyzing the transfer of one or more ADPR moieties to protein acceptor molecules (M) and regenerating nicotinamide:

$$\text{ADPR-nicotinamide}(\text{NAD}^+) + \text{M} \rightarrow \text{ADPR-M} + \text{nicotinamide} + \text{H}^+.$$

Examples of mono ADPR transfer products in prokaryotes are diphtheria toxin, which inhibits protein synthesis, and cholera toxin, which regulates adenylate cyclase activity. Poly (ADPR) polymerase, found in nuclei of eukaryotic cells, catalyzes the transfer of many ADPR moieties to acceptor proteins such as the histones. These poly ADP-ribosylated proteins appear to function in DNA repair, DNA replication, and cell differentiation. When a

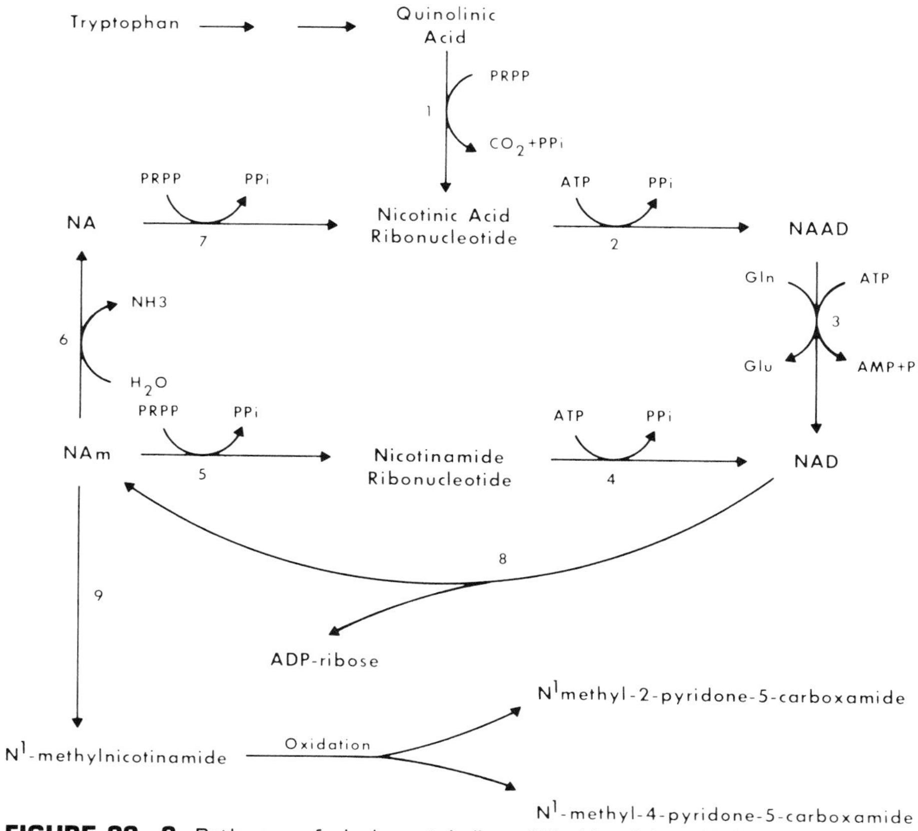
Tryptophan
Quinolinic Acid
PRPP
1
$CO_2$+PPi
PRPP
PPi
NA
7
Nicotinic Acid Ribonucleotide
ATP
PPi
2
NAAD
Gln
ATP
3
Glu
AMP+PPi
NH3
6
$H_2O$
PRPP
PPi
NAm
5
Nicotinamide Ribonucleotide
ATP
PPi
4
NAD
8
9
ADP-ribose
$N^1$methyl-2-pyridone-5-carboxamide
$N^1$-methylnicotinamide
Oxidation
$N^1$-methyl-4-pyridone-5-carboxamide

**FIGURE 22–2.** Pathways of niacin metabolism. NA, Nicotinic acid; NAm, nicotinamide; NAAD, nicotinic acid adenine dinucleotide; PRPP, phosphoribosyl pyrophosphate. 1, Quinolinate phosphoribosyltransferase; 2 and 4, adenyltransferases; 3, NAD synthetase; 5, nicotinamide phosphorbosyltransferase; 6, nicotinamidase, 7, nicotinate phosphoribosyltransferase; 8, poly (ADP-ribose) synthetase or NAD glycohydrolase; 9, $N^1$-methyltransferase. (From Jacob, R.A., Swendseid, M.E.: *In* Present Knowledge of Nutrition. 6th Ed. Edited by M.L. Brown. Washington, International Life Sciences Institute-Nutrition Foundation, 1990, p. 165.)

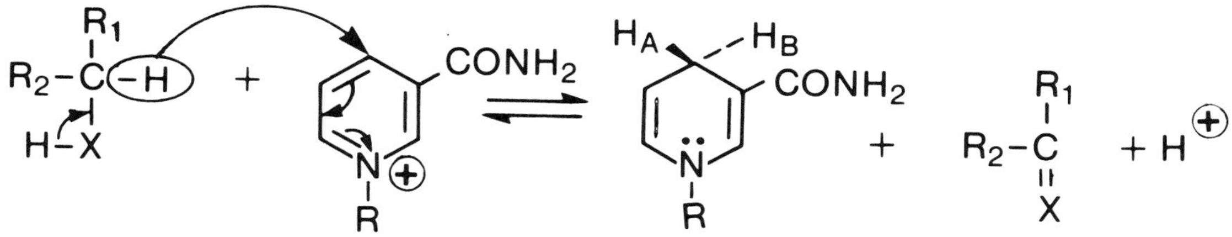
$R_1$
$R_2$-C-H
H-X
+
$CONH_2$
N
R
$H_A$
$H_B$
$CONH_2$
N
R
+
$R_1$
$R_2$-C
X
+ $H^+$

**FIGURE 22–3.** Mechanism of operation for nicotinamide adenine dinucleotide in substrate oxidation. (From McCormick, D.B.: Niacin. *In* Modern Nutrition in Health and Disease. 7th Ed. Edited by M.E. Shils and V.R. Young. Philadelphia, Lea & Febiger, 1988, p. 373.)

niacin supplement was given to rats, hepatic levels of NAD and ADP-ribosyl residues bound to proteins were both increased, suggesting that niacin status influences the extent of ADP ribosylation of proteins.[25] Quiescent human peripheral blood lymphocytes in culture continually produce NAD and utilize it for poly ADP ribosylation.[26] Oxidant or DNA strand-break stressors cause depletion of the NAD pools accompanied by increased poly ADPR polymerase activity in a variety of cultured cells including lymphocytes, endothelial cells, and murine macrophages.[27,28] Under some conditions adenosine triphosphate (ATP) levels also are reduced. There are many reports of low levels of NAD in tumor cells accompanied by elevated ADPR polymerase activity.[15,29]

If a tissue has only a limited capacity to resynthesize NAD from the nicotinamide produced by the polymerase reaction, increased polymerase activity may lead to tissue-specific niacin deficiency states.

Niacin may also have biologic functions independent of its role as a pyridine nucleotide. Nicotinic acid is a component of the glucose tolerance factor, an organo-chromium complex isolated from yeast that potentiates the insulin response.[30] This effect is not produced by free niacin forms.

### INTERACTIONS WITH OTHER NUTRIENTS

Because of its pervasive role in redox reactions, niacin interacts with all nutrients involved in oxidation of fuel molecules either as substrates or as coenzymes. Many of the metallodehydrogenases also are NADP-dependent, an example of niacin and trace element interactions. The first step in many redox reactions is a reduction of a flavoprotein by the reduced form of NADP, or NADPH, which indicates the close metabolic relationship between riboflavin and niacin. In the synthesis of niacin from Trp, riboflavin and vitamin $B_6$ are essential cofactors. Conversely, niacin participates in the biosynthesis of active forms of these two vitamins and of other vitamins as well, such as folic acid.

Excess leucine in the diet has been postulated as the cause of pellagra found in populations consuming a millet, jowar, with a high leucine content.[31] In experimental animals excess leucine was reported to increase hepatic NAD glycohydrolase activity, and 2-oxoisocaproate, an analogue of leucine, depressed NAD biosynthesis from Trp and nicotinic acid in isolated rat hepatocytes. Whether excess leucine influences niacin status in vivo is still uncertain, however, because in several studies in rats[32] and humans[18,22,33] excess leucine had no effect on niacin metabolism or status.

## BIOCHEMICAL ASSESSMENT OF NIACIN STATUS

Measurement of the urinary excretion of the two major methylated metabolites, NMN and 2-pyridone, has been used to determine niacin status. The Interdepartmental Committee on Nutrition for National Defense published criteria suggesting that urinary levels of <5.8 μmol per day (0.8 mg per day) of NMN is an indicator of niacin deficiency.[34] The ratio of 2-pyridone to NMN was proposed as a niacin deficiency marker because it is independent of age and of creatinine excretion and can be used on casual urine samples. In rats, however, this ratio strongly depends on the level of protein intake; thus, the ratio may primarily measure protein status rather than niacin status.[35] In a study of experimental niacin deficiency in adult males,[18] the ratio of 2-pyridone to NMN was not sensitive to a marginal niacin intake of 82 μmol (10 mg) NE per day and was not totally reliable for evaluating an intake of 49 μmol (6 mg) NE per day when protein intakes were adequate and constant. In the same study, urinary excretion of <8.8 μmol per day (1.2 mg per day) of either NMN or 2-pyridone reliably identified subjects receiving the lowest niacin intake of 49 μmol (6 mg) NE per day.

The concentrations of niacin derivatives in blood have not been generally used as markers of niacin status. Although blood pyridine nucleotide concentrations in subjects fed a niacin-deficient diet decreased approximately 40% in one study,[15] the effects of pellagra or experimental niacin deficiency on blood pyridine nucleotides in other studies have been inconsistent. As earlier indicated,[18] red cell NAD levels decreased by about 70% when adult males were fed low-niacin diets containing either 49 or 82 μmol (6 or 10 mg) NE per day for 36 days. In contrast, red cell NADP levels remained unchanged.[33] The red cell NAD concentration may thus be a sensitive indicator of niacin depletion, and a decreased ratio of red cell NAD/NADP may identify subjects at risk of developing niacin deficiency. Plasma Trp levels remained normal in subjects receiving 82 μmol (10 mg) NE per day but fell by about 45% in those receiving 49 μmol (6 mg) NE per day.[33] Thus, reduced red cell NAD levels together with low plasma Trp levels may represent a more severe niacin deficiency than one in which only red cell NAD levels are reduced.

## REQUIREMENTS

The RDA for adults,[12] based on the conversion factor of 290 μmol (60 mg) Trp to 8.2 μmol (1 mg) niacin, range from 123 to 148 μmol (15 to 20 mg) NE for males and 107 to 123 μmol (13 to 15 mg) NE for females (see Appendix Table A–2b). In terms of energy, recommendations are for 54 μmol (6.6 mg) NE/4200 kJ (1000 kcal), but the total niacin intake should not be less than 107 μmol (13 mg) per day for adults of all ages. Most of the evidence for these allowances was derived from studies of adult men and women conducted during the 1950s. There are no data on niacin requirements of children through adolescence. Because milk from well-nourished mothers appears to be adequate to meet niacin needs of infants, however, the RDA for infants up to 6 months of age is set at 65.6 μmol (8 mg) NE/4200 kJ (1000 kcal), which is the average content of niacin in human milk. Direct evidence also does not exist for the niacin requirements of women during pregnancy and lactation. Because the energy requirement is increased by 1260 kJ (300 kcal) per day in pregnancy, the RDA was increased by 16.4 μmol (2 mg) NE per day for pregnant women. The RDA for lactating women includes an additional allowance of 41 μmol (5 mg) NE per day, which is based on the calculated content of 750 ml breast milk (8.2 to 10.7 μmol or 1.0 to 1.3 mg) plus the energy increment required to support lactation.

The calculated average daily reported intakes of niacin in the United States are 221 μmol (27 mg) NE for women and 336 μmol (41 mg) for men.[36] The corresponding values for preformed niacin are 131 and 197 μmol (16 and 24 mg).

## DEFICIENCY STATES

Although pellagra has almost disappeared from industrialized countries except for its occurrence in alcoholics, it is still endemic in India and in parts of China and Africa. Clinical signs of pellagra are commonly referred to as the 3 Ds: diarrhea, dementia, and dermatitis. The most characteristic sign is a pigmented rash that develops symmetrically in areas of the skin exposed to sunlight. The color of the rash is similar to a sunburn, although in chronic cases a darker color may develop. Changes in the digestive tract are associated with vomiting or diarrhea, and the tongue becomes bright red. Neurologic symptoms include anxiety and insomnia and, in more severe cases, disorientation and delusions.

Reports of pellagra-like syndromes have been described in the absence of a dietary niacin deficiency. In such cases, pellagra results from a disturbance in Trp metabolism, which causes a reduction in the conversion of Trp to niacin. Pellagra is sometimes associated with the carcinoid syndrome, where the conversion of Trp to 5-0H Trp and serotonin becomes the major catabolic pathway of Trp. As a consequence, the amount of Trp that is converted to niacin is reduced. Prolonged treatment with the drug isoniazid may also lead to niacin deficiency secondary to depletion by the drug of pyridoxal phosphate, a coenzyme required in the Trp-to-niacin pathway. Patients with Hartnup's disease, an autosomal recessive disorder, develop pellagra because of a defect in the absorption of Trp in the intestine and kidney. Treatment with large doses of nicotinamide 0.3 to 2 mmol (40 to 250 mg) per day results in marked improvement in skin and neurologic abnormalities.

Niacin deficiency has been produced in dogs, pigs, monkeys, chickens, rats, and trout. Pigs, which are particularly sensitive to niacin deficiency, exhibit a scaly dermatitis. Skin lesions, however, do not occur in all species as, for example, in young monkeys. Niacin-deficient animals generally experience a lack of appetite, poor growth, and inflammation of the mouth and tongue mucosa. In dogs this latter condition is referred to as "black tongue" disease.

## PHARMACOLOGIC EFFECTS AND TOXICITY

It was first reported in 1955 that large doses of nicotinic acid reduced serum cholesterol concentrations human subjects.[37] Subsequently, in patients participating in the Coronary Drug Project, the administration of nicotinic acid was associated with a reduction in recurrent myocardial infarctions and in long-term total mortality from heart disease.[38] It is now well established that nicotinic acid given as a drug in doses of 12.3 to 24.6 mmol (1.5 to 3 g) per day can result in decreased total and low-density lipoprotein cholesterol levels and increased high-density lipoprotein cholesterol levels in plasma. Side effects from the administration of these large amounts of nicotinic acid include flushing of the skin, hyperuricemia, abnormalities in liver function, and occasionally hyperglycemia. These effects are reversed if the drug is reduced in amount or discontinued. Although the lipid-decreasing effect of nicotinic acid has been extensively investigated, its mechanism of action is not known. It does not appear to be related to any vitamin or coenzyme function because nicotinamide does not have a similar effect.

The toxicity of high concentrations of nicotinamide is documented in intact animals, regenerating tissues, and cells in culture. The oral median lethal dose ($LD_{50}$) for the rat is 28.7 mmol (3.5 g)/kg for nicotinamide and 28.9 to 42.6 mmol (4.5 to 5.2 g)/kg for nicotinic acid. Nicotinamide fed at concentrations of 1 to 2% of the diet inhibits growth in young rats. Growth retardation may result from the increased synthesis of NAD, which in turn reduces ATP and other substances required for RNA and DNA synthesis.[39] Metabolic effects of high nicotinamide doses in animals include phosphaturia due to an increase in the concentration of NAD, an inhibitor of the $Na^+$-dependent transport of phosphate through the kidney tubule membrane.[40] In adult rats large doses of nicotinamide were shown to increase activities of drug-metabolizing enzymes, including components of the hepatic microsomal mixed-function oxidase system and uridine diphosphoglucuronyl transferase.[41] Long-term administration of large doses of nicotinamide to rats caused increased lipid and decreased choline concentrations in liver, presumably because of depletion of methyl groups that are used for methylation of niacin metabolites.[42]

## REFERENCES


1. Jukes, T.H., Sebrell, W.H., Roe, D., et al.: Fed. Proc., *40*:1519–1537, 1980.
2. Elvehjem, C.A., Madden, R.J., Strong, F.M., et al.: J. Biol. Chem., *123*:137–149, 1938.
3. Spies, T.D., Cooper, C., Blankenhorn, M.A.: JAMA, *110*:622–627, 1938.
4. Carpenter, K.J., Lewin, W.J.: J. Nutr., *115*:543–552, 1985.
5. Weiner, M., Van Eys, J.: Nicotinic acid: Nutrient-cofactor-drug. *In* Clinical Pharmacology. Vol. 1. Edited by M. Weiner. New York, Marcel Dekker, 1983, pp. 109–131.
6. Eitenmiller, R.R., De Souse, S.: Niacin. *In* Methods of Vitamin Assay. 4th Ed. Edited by The Association of Vitamin Chemists. New York, John Wiley & Sons, 1985, pp. 385–398.

7. McKee, R.W., Kang-Lee, Y.A., Panaqua, M., et al.: J. Chromatogr., *230:*309–318, 1982.
8. Nisselbaum, J.S., Green, S.: Anal. Biochem., *27:*212–217, 1969.
9. Stocchii, V., Cucchiarini, L., Canestrari F., et al.: Anal. Biochem., *167:*181–190, 1987.
10. Shibata, K., Kawada, T., Iwai, K.: J. Chromatogr., *424:*23–28, 1988.
11. Clark, B.R.: Methods Enzymol., *66:*5–8, 1980.
12. Food and Nutrition Board, National Research Council: Recommended Dietary Allowances. 10th Ed. Washington, D.C., National Academy Press, 1989, pp. 137–142.
13. Vivian, V.M., Chaloupka, M.M., Reynolds, M.S.: J. Nutr., *66:*587–598, 1958.
14. Henderson, L.M.: Annu. Rev. Nutr., *3:*289–307, 1983.
15. Bernofsky, C.: Mol. Cell. Biochem., *33:*135–141, 1980.
16. Shibata, K., Murata, K.: Nutr. Internat., *2:*177–181, 1986.
17. McCreanor, J.M., Bender, D.A.: Br. J. Nutr., *56:*577–586, 1986.
18. Jacob, R.A., Swendseid, M.E., McKee, R.W., et al.: J. Nutr., *119:*591–598, 1989.
19. Jenden, D.J., Rice, K.M., Jacob, R.A., et al.: Fed. Proc., *46:*1086, 1987.
20. Goldsmith, G.A., Sarett, H.P., Register, U.D., et al.: J. Clin. Invest., *31:*533–542, 1952.
21. Mrocheck, J.E., Jolley, R.L., Young, D.S., et al.: Clin. Chem., *22:*1821–1827, 1976.
22. Patterson, J.I., Brown, R.R., Linkswiler, H., et al.: Am. J. Clin. Nutr., *33:*2157–2167, 1980.
23. Wertz, A.W., Lojkin, M.E., Bouchard, B.S., et al.: J. Nutr., *64:*339–353, 1958.
24. Rose, D.P., Braidman, I.P.: Am. J. Clin. Nutr., *24:*673–683, 1971.
25. Bredehorst, R., Lengyel, H., Hilz, H., et al.: Hoppe-Seylers Z. Physiol. Chem., *361:*559–562, 1980.
26. Carson, D.A., Seto, S., Wasson, D.B.: J. Immunol., *138:*1904–1907, 1987.
27. Schraufstatter, I.U., Hinshaw, D.B., Hyslop, P.A., et al.: J. Clin. Invest., *777:*1312–1320, 1986.
28. Junod, A.J., Jornot, L., Petersen, H.: J. Cell. Physiol., *140:*177–185, 1989.
29. Wenner, C.E., Weinhouse, S.: Cancer Res., *13:*21–26, 1953.
30. Mertz, W.: Nutr. Rev., *33:*129–135, 1975.
31. Gopalan, C., Rao, K., S.J.: Vitam. Horm., *33:*505–528, 1975.
32. Cook, N.E., Carpenter, K.J.: J. Nutr., *117:*519–526, 1987.
33. Fu, C.S., Swendseid, M.E., Jacob, R.A., et al.: J. Nutr., *119:*1949–1955, 1989.
34. Sauberlich, H.E., Dowdy, R.P., Skala, J.H.: Laboratory Tests for the Assessment of Nutritional Status. Boca Raton, FL, CRC Press, 1974, pp. 70–74.
35. Shibata, K., Matsuo, H.: J. Nutr., *119:*896–901, 1989.
36. United States Department of Agriculture. Nationwide Food Consumption Survey. Nutrient Intakes: Individuals in 48 States. Year 1977–78. Report No. 1–2, Consumer Nutrition Division, Human Nutrition Information Service. Hyattsville, MD, U.S. Dept. of Agriculture, 1984.
37. Altschul, Z., Hoffer, A., Stephen, J.D.: Arch. Biochem. Biophys., *54:*588–559, 1955.
38. Canner, P.L., Berge, K.G., Wenger, N.K., et al.: J. Am. Coll. Cardiol., *8:*1245–1255, 1986.
39. Ravel, M., Mandel, P.: Cancer Res., *22:*456–462, 1962.
40. Kempson, S.A., Colon-Otera, G., Ou, S.Y.L., et al.: J. Clin. Invest., *67:*1347, 1981.
41. Nomura, K., Shui, M., Sano, K., et al.: Int. J. Vitam. Nutr. Res., *53:*35–43, 1983.
42. Kang-Lee, Y.A., McKee, R.W., Wright, S.M., et al.: J. Nutr., *113:*215–221, 1982.

## SELECTED READINGS

Berger, N.A.: Poly(ADP-ribose) in the cellular response to DNA damage. Radiat. Res., *101:*4–15, 1985.
Bernofsky, C.: Physiologic aspects of pyridine nucleotide regulation in mammals. Mol. Cell. Biochem., *33:*135–143, 1980.
Henderson, L.M.: Niacin. Annu. Rev. Nutr., *3:*289–307, 1983.
Jukes, T.H., Sebrell, W.H., Roc, D.A., et al.: The conquest of pellagra. Fed. Proc. *40:*1519–1537, 1980.
Weiner, M., Van Eys, J.: Nicotinic acid: Nutrient-cofactor-drug. *In* Clinical Pharmacology. Vol. 1. Edited by M. Weiner. New York, Marcel Dekker, 1983.

CHAPTER 23

# Vitamin $B_6$

James E. Leklem



Since the discovery and identification of the structure of vitamin $B_6$ some 50 years ago, there have been significant advances in our knowledge of the functions of vitamin $B_6$ and the quantitative need for this vitamin.[1] Gyorgy and Lepkovsky were among the first to isolate vitamin $B_6$ in crystalline form. In the subsequent decade Snell and co-workers were instrumental in elucidating the various forms of vitamin $B_6$ and developing microbiologic analytic techniques for measuring these forms in biologic systems.[1,2]

## CHEMISTRY

Vitamin $B_6$ is the name for derivatives of 3-hydroxy-5-hydroxymethyl-2 methyl pyridine.[3] The 4 position can be found as the methyl hydroxy (pyridoxine), the aldehyde (pyridoxal), or the methylamine (pyridoxamine). Each of these forms can also be phosphorylated at the 5 position (Fig. 23–1). Pyridoxal 5′-phosphate (PLP) and pyridoxamine 5′-phosphate (PMP) are the active coenzyme forms, with PLP being the primary form of biologic interest.

The free forms of vitamin $B_6$ are considered relatively labile, with the degree of lability influenced by pH. All three forms are relatively heat stable in an acid medium, but they are heat labile under alkaline conditions.[4] The hydrochloride and base forms are readily soluble in water and are only minimally soluble in common organic solvents. In aqueous solution the forms are light sensitive, but this sensitivity is also pH-dependent. Pyridoxine hydrochloride is the form of vitamin $B_6$ that is most commonly found in vitamin pills and used in the fortification of foods.

The coenzyme forms of vitamin $B_6$ are PLP and PMP. The PLP form is found covalently bound to enzymes via a Schiff base with the ϵ-amino group of lysine. In the formation of the Schiff base the strong electron-attracting character of the pyridine ring and the subsequent withdrawal of electrons from one of the three substituents (R group, hydrogen, or carboxyl group) attached to the α-carbon of the amino acid substrate are key features in the majority of enzymatic reactions.[5] Nearly 100 enzymatic reactions have been reported in which PLP plays a coenzyme role.[6] Although transamination reactions are one of the types of reactions, there are several other classes of reactions involving the α-, β-, or γ-carbon of amino acids.

## FOOD SOURCES AND FORMS

An understanding of the various forms and the quantities of these forms in foods is important in the evaluation of the bioavailability and metabolism of vitamin $B_6$. The methods used for determining the amount of vitamin include microbiologic[7] and high-performance liquid chromatography[8] techniques.

The relative proportion of each of the three forms in

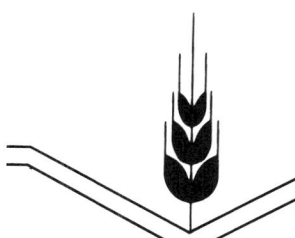

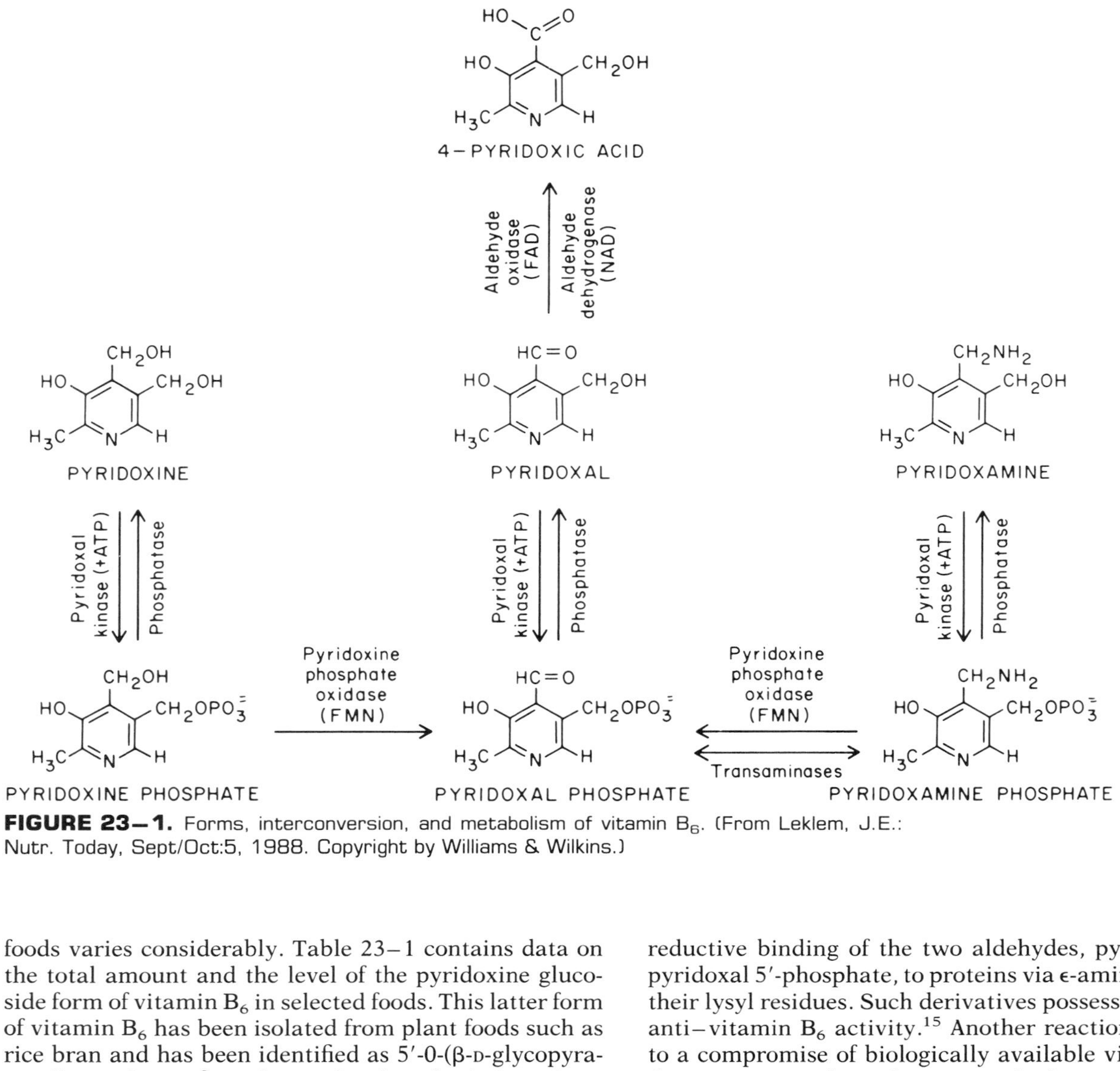
4-PYRIDOXIC ACID
Aldehyde oxidase (FAD)
Aldehyde dehydrogenase (NAD)
PYRIDOXINE
PYRIDOXAL
PYRIDOXAMINE
Pyridoxal kinase (+ATP)
Phosphatase
Pyridoxine phosphate oxidase (FMN)
Transaminases
PYRIDOXINE PHOSPHATE
PYRIDOXAL PHOSPHATE
PYRIDOXAMINE PHOSPHATE

**FIGURE 23–1.** Forms, interconversion, and metabolism of vitamin $B_6$. (From Leklem, J.E.: Nutr. Today, Sept/Oct:5, 1988. Copyright by Williams & Wilkins.)

foods varies considerably. Table 23–1 contains data on the total amount and the level of the pyridoxine glucoside form of vitamin $B_6$ in selected foods. This latter form of vitamin $B_6$ has been isolated from plant foods such as rice bran and has been identified as 5′-0-(β-D-glycopyranosyl) pyridoxine.[9] To date only plant foods have been found to contain this interesting form of vitamin $B_6$.[10] The absence of the glucoside form in animal products suggests that it does not have a biologic function. In plants it may serve as a storage form of vitamin $B_6$. Generally speaking, plant foods contain predominately pyridoxine, whereas animal products contain primarily pyridoxal and pyridoxamine (mainly as the phosphorylated forms[4]). (See also Appendix Table A–21 for the vitamin $B_6$ content of common foods).

Food processing and storage may affect the vitamin content of foods.[11,12] Losses of 10 to 50% have been reported for a wide variety of foods and processing techniques. The forms of vitamin $B_6$ may also change as was observed in heat-sterilized milk in which pyridoxal was converted to pyridoxamine.[12] Pyridoxine added to flour and baked into bread is stable.[13] Thermal processing[14] and low-moisture storage of certain foods results in reductive binding of the two aldehydes, pyridoxal and pyridoxal 5′-phosphate, to proteins via ε-amino groups of their lysyl residues. Such derivatives possess low or even anti–vitamin $B_6$ activity.[15] Another reaction that leads to a compromise of biologically available vitamin $B_6$ is the conversion of pyridoxine to 6-hydroxypyridoxine in the presence of ascorbic acid.[16]

## ABSORPTION

Proper assessment of the requirement of vitamin $B_6$ requires an understanding of how much vitamin $B_6$ is biologically available (i.e., absorbed and utilizable). Absorption of the several forms of vitamin $B_6$ has been examined primarily in animals[17] and to a limited extent in humans.[18] The three primary forms of vitamin $B_6$ are absorbed to a major extent by a nonsaturable passive process,[19] mainly in the jejunum.[20] After hydrolysis of the phosphorylated forms by alkaline phosphatase and uptake into the intestine of the three forms, each can be phosphorylated and thus retained (a process referred to

**TABLE 23–1.** VITAMIN $B_6$ AND PYRIDOXINE GLUCOSIDE (PNG) CONTENT OF COMMONLY CONSUMED FOODS

| FOOD | VITAMIN $B_6$ (mg/100 g) | PNG (mg/100 g) |
|---|---|---|
| Vegetables | | |
| Carrots, raw | 0.170 | 0.087 |
| Cauliflower, frozen | 0.084 | 0.069 |
| Broccoli, frozen | 0.119 | 0.078 |
| Spinach, frozen | 0.208 | 0.104 |
| Cabbage, raw | 0.140 | 0.065 |
| Sprouts, alfalfa | 0.250 | 0.105 |
| Potatoes, cooked | 0.394 | 0.165 |
| Beans/Legumes | | |
| Soybeans, cooked | 0.627 | 0.357 |
| Beans, navy, cooked | 0.381 | 0.159 |
| Beans, lima, frozen | 0.106 | 0.039 |
| Peas, frozen | 0.122 | 0.018 |
| Peanut butter | 0.302 | 0.054 |
| Beans, garbanzo | 0.653 | 0.111 |
| Lentils | 0.289 | 0.134 |
| Animal products | | |
| Beef, ground, cooked | 0.263 | n.d. |
| Tuna, canned | 0.316 | n.d. |
| Chicken breast, raw | 0.700 | n.d. |
| Milk, skim | 0.005 | n.d. |
| Nuts/Seeds | | |
| Walnuts | 0.535 | 0.038 |
| Cashews, raw | 0.351 | 0.046 |
| Sunflower seeds | 0.997 | 0.046 |
| Almonds | 0.086 | –0– |
| Fruits | | |
| Orange juice, fresh | 0.043 | 0.016 |
| Tomato juice, canned | 0.097 | 0.045 |
| Blueberries, frozen | 0.046 | 0.019 |
| Banana | 0.313 | 0.010 |
| Pineapple, canned | 0.079 | 0.017 |
| Peaches, canned | 0.009 | 0.002 |
| Avocado | 0.443 | 0.015 |
| Raisins, seedless | 0.230 | 0.154 |
| Cereals/Grains | | |
| Wheat bran | 0.903 | 0.326 |
| Shredded wheat, cereal | 0.313 | 0.087 |
| Rice, brown | 0.237 | 0.055 |

n.d. = none detected
All values given as milligrams of pyridoxine per 100 g of food. 1 mg $B_6$ = 5.91 μmol.

as metabolic trapping). However, forms of vitamin $B_6$ exit from the basolateral membrane side of the intestine mainly as the nonphosphorylated vitamers.

## BIOAVAILABILITY

Studies in both animals and humans[21,22] have provided information on the relative availability of vitamin $B_6$. A summary of the studies in humans is given in Table 23–2. Generally the availability of vitamin $B_6$ is greater than 75% in most foods studied.[21] In some of the studies there appears to be an inverse relationship between the amount of pyridoxine glucoside (PNG) in a food and the bioavailability of vitamin $B_6$. However, PNG is absorbed and partially converted to 4-pyridoxic acid. Other factors that may limit availability are food processing (formation of ε-pyridoxylysine), the amount of fiber (incomplete digestion), and the presence of other forms of vitamin $B_6$ (6-hydroxypyridoxine).

**TABLE 23–2.** STUDIES IN WHICH BIOAVAILABILITY OF VITAMIN $B_6$ FROM FOODS HAS BEEN ASSESSED IN HUMANS

| FOOD | ESTIMATED BIOAVAILABILITY |
|---|---|
| Whole wheat bread | >85% |
| Cooked wheat bran | >85% |
| Wheat, rice, corn brans | 60–65% |
| Peanut butter | 63%, compared to tuna |
| Bananas | 98%, compared to tuna |
| Hazelnuts | 96%, compared to tuna |
| Soybeans | 41%, compared to tuna |
| Orange juice | 50%, compared to pyridoxine |

(From Leklem, J.E.: Vitamin $B_6$. *In* Handbook of Vitamins, 2nd Ed. Edited by L.J. Machlin. New York, Marcel Dekker, 1991, pp. 341–392.)

## TRANSPORT AND METABOLISM

Vitamin $B_6$ is transported in the blood both in the plasma and in red cells. PLP and pyridoxal (PL) are both bound to albumin,[23] with the PLP binding more tightly. In the red cell, both PLP and PL are bound to hemoglobin.[24,25] The extent of the role the red cell plays in vitamin $B_6$ transport, however, remains to be determined.[26]

The liver is the primary organ responsible for metabolism of $B_6$ vitamers.[23,27] As a result, the liver supplies the active form of vitamin $B_6$, PLP, to the circulation and other tissues. Figure 23–1 depicts the interconversion of the $B_6$ vitamers and the enzymes involved. The three nonphosphorylated forms are converted to the respective phosphorylated forms by pyridoxine kinase. Zinc and adenosine triphosphate (ATP) are cofactors for this kinase.[28] Pyridoxamine 5′-phosphate and pyridoxine 5′-phosphate can then be converted to PLP via a flavin mononucleotide (FMN) oxidase.[29]

Phosphorylated forms can be hydrolyzed by alkaline phosphatases.[27,28] The pyridoxal that results from this dephosphorylation, as well as that which is present from dietary sources, can then be converted to 4-pyridoxic acid (4-PA) in a nonreversible reaction that involves flavin adenine dinucleotide (FAD) and an aldehyde oxidase.[28] This reaction occurs in human liver, but the extent to which the reaction occurs in other tissues is not known. Because of the role riboflavin coenzymes play in the metabolism of vitamin $B_6$, one would expect riboflavin status to affect vitamin $B_6$ status. Whole blood PLP concentrations in persons with oral lesions (presumably deficient in riboflavin) were normal in one study, however, and supplemental riboflavin had no effect on these levels.[30] In-vitro studies utilizing erythrocytes indicate that riboflavin increases the rate of conversion of pyridoxine (PN) to PLP.[31]

Because PLP is a highly reactive molecule and readily forms a Schiff base with proteins, high cellular concentrations of PLP may be detrimental. The activity of the aldehyde (pyridoxal) oxidase in human liver appears to be sufficient, however, to convert excess PL to 4-PA and thus prevent high levels of PLP from accumulating.[28]

In the circulating plasma, PLP and PL account for nearly 75 to 80% of the total vitamin $B_6$.[4,32,33] PN is the next most common form, and although PN is taken up into tissues and can be converted to PNP, many tissues lack sufficient oxidase activity to convert PNP to PLP.[34] For example, in muscle tissue PN is not converted to PLP, and thus PL is the only form that serves as a source of PLP.

There are several body pools of vitamin $B_6$.[35] The major pool is in the muscle, where most of the vitamin $B_6$ is present as PLP bound to glycogen phosphorylase.[36] The total body pool of vitamin $B_6$ is estimated to be 1000 μmol, of which 800 to 900 μmol are present in muscle.[37] Turnover of the various pools will vary depending on the metabolic state and nutritional well-being of the organism.[4] Turnover of PLP in the plasma has been associated with a two-compartment model,[4,38] and the turnover of the slowly-turning-over pool is estimated to be 25 to 33 days.

## FUNCTIONS

The numerous functions of vitamin $B_6$ in humans are complex, multifaceted, and interrelated. Because of the reactivity of PLP with amino acids and several nitrogen-containing compounds, the biochemical functions of vitamin $B_6$ center around these molecules.[39] In the case of glycogen phosphorylase it is probably the phosphate group of PLP that is involved in the coenzyme role.[40] The role of PLP can be viewed from a systems/cellular perspective. These systems/cellular processes are listed in Table 23–3. A brief description and other highlights of each of these follows.

**TABLE 23–3.** SYSTEMS OR CELLULAR PROCESSES IN WHICH PYRIDOXAL 5′-PHOSPHATE FUNCTIONS

| CELLULAR PROCESS OR ENZYME SYSTEM | SYSTEM/FUNCTION |
|---|---|
| 1-Carbon metabolism, steroid modulation | Immune |
| Transaminases, glycogen phosphorylase | Gluconeogenesis |
| Tryptophan metabolism | Niacin formation |
| Heme synthesis, $O_2$ affinity, transaminases | Red cell metabolism |
| Lipid and neurotransmitter synthesis | Nervous system |
| Binding of PLP to lysine of steroid receptor | Steroid (hormone) function |

(Data from Leklem, J.E.: Vitamin $B_6$. *In* Handbook of Vitamins, 2nd Ed. Edited by L.J. Machlin. New York, Marcel Dekker, 1991, pp. 341–392.)

## GLUCONEOGENESIS

PLP is involved in gluconeogenesis via its role in transamination reactions[39] and in the action of glycogen phosphorylase.[36,40] However, in one study a low intake of 1.2 μmol vitamin $B_6$ (0.2 mg) per day in humans as compared to a "normal" intake of 10.6 μmol (1.8 mg) per day for 4 weeks did not adversely affect fasting plasma glucose but did result in impaired glucose tolerance.[41] Glycogen phosphorylase activities in liver and muscle are reduced in vitamin $B_6$–deficient rats,[36,42] but a deficiency of the vitamin per se does not result in mobilization of the vitamin $B_6$ (PLP) stored in muscle.[43] However, in rats a caloric deficit does lead to decreased muscle phosphorylase content.[44] Thus, the reservoir of vitamin $B_6$ in muscle seems to be utilized only when gluconeogenesis increases.[45]

## NIACIN FORMATION

The direct conversion of tryptophan to niacin involves a PLP-requiring enzyme, kynureninase. After 4 weeks of feeding women a diet containing 1.2 μmol (0.2 mg) of vitamin $B_6$ per day and after a tryptophan level of 2 g, the total urinary excretion of the two major niacin metabolites, N′-methyl-2-pyridone-5-carboxamide and N′-methylnicotinamide, was moderately less than that excreted when 10.6 μmol (1.8 mg) of vitamin $B_6$ was fed.[39,45] Thus, a low intake <6.0 μmol (<1.0 mg) per day of vitamin $B_6$ had only a slight effect on the conversion of tryptophan to niacin.

## LIPID METABOLISM

The role of vitamin $B_6$ in lipid metabolism remains controversial. Animals that were fed diets deficient in either fatty acids or vitamin $B_6$ showed similar visual signs and symptoms.[46] Vitamin $B_6$–deficient rats fed high-protein (70%) diets have also been found to have fatty livers in some studies,[47] but not in others. Increased levels of linoleic and γ-linolenic acid, and decreased arachidonic acid in liver phospholipids have been observed in vitamin $B_6$–deficient rats.[48,49] The changes in fatty acid levels may be related to altered phospholipid levels due to high levels of S-adenosylmethionine inhibiting methylation of phosphoethanolamine.[50] This latter effect would tie together altered amino acid metabolism (homocysteine) and the changes in phospholipids and associated fatty acids.

The relationship between vitamin $B_6$ and cholesterol also remains controversial.[51] In humans a deficiency of vitamin $B_6$ is not associated with a significant change in serum cholesterol.[4] Although supplemental intakes of vitamins in general or of vitamin $B_6$ per se alter serum cholesterol levels (they either decrease or prevent an increase),[4] there are no definitive studies on the effect of supplemental vitamin $B_6$ on serum cholesterol level. Nonetheless, plasma PLP levels are positively correlated with plasma high-density lipoprotein (HDL) cholesterol levels and negatively correlated with total cholesterol and low-density lipoprotein (LDL) cholesterol levels in monkeys.[52]

## ERYTHROCYTE METABOLISM AND FUNCTION

In the erythrocyte PLP serves as a coenzyme for transaminases. Both PLP and PL bind to hemoglobin. PL binds to the α chain of hemoglobin and increases $O_2$ binding affinity, whereas PLP binds tightly to the β chain and lowers $O_2$ binding affinity, a situation that may be important in sickle cell anemia.[53] A severe chronic deficiency of vitamin $B_6$ can lead to hypochromic, microcytic anemia. In addition, some patients with sideroblastic anemia and other anemias do respond favorably to pyridoxine therapy.[54,55]

### NERVOUS SYSTEM

Several in-depth reviews on the vitamin $B_6$ and nervous system function are available.[56–58] PLP is a coenzyme for enzymatic reactions that lead to the synthesis of several neurotransmitters, including serotonin (from tryptophan), taurine, dopamine, norepinephrine, histamine and γ-aminobutyric acid. Neurologic abnormalities in human infants[59] and animals[56] deficient in vitamin $B_6$ have also been seen.

Infants who were fed a formula in which the vitamin $B_6$ was destroyed during processing showed abnormal electroencephalogram (EEG) tracings and convulsions.[59] Treatment with 591 μmol (100 mg) of vitamin $B_6$ corrected the EEG abnormalities. Pyridoxine-dependent seizures, an autosomal recessive disorder, are also associated with abnormal EEG patterns, and both these and the convulsions are corrected by 178 to 591 μmol (30 to 100 mg) of pyridoxine per day. Adults fed a diet low in vitamin $B_6$ and high in protein also have been observed to have abnormal EEG findings,[60] whereas those fed similar diets for a shorter period (21 days) had no abnormal EEGs.

Extensive studies in animals fed varying intakes of vitamin $B_6$ showed that the progeny of dams had altered fatty acid levels in the cerebellum and cerebrum regions of the brain.[58,61] Other changes in nerve cells, including reduced γ-aminobutyric acid levels[62] and altered amino acid levels, have been observed. These findings point to a need for an adequate amount of vitamin $B_6$ during nervous system development.

### HORMONE MODULATION

Litwack and colleagues have demonstrated that PLP binds to steroid receptors.[63] PLP also binds to a second site on the steroid receptor and inhibits the binding of the steroid receptor to DNA.[63] This results in a decreased action of the steroid. Reactions between PLP and receptors for estrogen, androgen, progesterone, and glucocorticoid at physiologic concentrations of PLP suggest that the vitamin $B_6$ status of an individual may have significance in endocrine-mediated diseases.

## VITAMIN $B_6$ STATUS

Determination of the vitamin $B_6$ status of an individual is of paramount importance in understanding the relationship between health and nutrient intake, factors that influence the requirement for vitamin $B_6$, and factors that affect overall metabolism of vitamin $B_6$. Assessment of vitamin $B_6$ status can be grouped into three categories: direct, indirect, and dietary intake.[65] Table 23–4 lists several indices used to evaluate vitamin $B_6$ status and suggested values for adequate status.

### DIRECT METHODS

Direct measures are those which reflect one or more of the metabolites of the $B_6$ vitamers. Currently, the most frequently used direct measure is plasma PLP concentration. Support for the use of this comes from both animal models[66] and human studies.[4] Proper evaluation of plasma PLP concentration requires an understanding of factors that influence this level. Table 23–5 lists several such factors and the qualitative change that has been observed.[4] Ideally one would prefer to measure PLP in tissues. Recent work has suggested the erythrocyte PLP level may be useful as an index.[67] Until methodologic problems are resolved and further data are available, the use of this procedure as an index of vitamin $B_6$ is open to

**TABLE 23–4.** INDICES USED TO ASSESS VITAMIN $B_6$ STATUS AND SUGGESTED MINIMAL VALUES FOR ADEQUATE STATUS

| INDEX | ADEQUATE STATUS |
|---|---|
| Direct | |
| Plasma pyridoxal 5′-phosphate | >30 nmol/L |
| Plasma total vitamin $B_6$ | >40 nmol/L |
| Urinary 4-pyridoxic acid | >3.0 μmol/d |
| Urinary total vitamin $B_6$ | >0.5 μmol/d |
| Indirect | |
| Erythrocyte alanine transaminase index | <1.25 |
| Erythrocyte aspartic transaminase index | <1.80 |
| 2 g L-Tryptophan load; urinary xanthurenic acid | <65 μmol/d |
| 3 g L-Methionine load; urinary cystathionine | <350 μmol/d |
| Diet intake | |
| Vitamin $B_6$ intake; weekly average | >1.2–1.5 mg/d |
| Vitamin $B_6$:protein ratio (mg/g) | ≥0.016 |

(From Leklem, J.E.: J. Nutr., *120*:1503–1507, 1990.) 1 mg $B_6$ = 5.91 μmol.

**TABLE 23–5.** FACTORS INFLUENCING PLASMA PLP CONCENTRATION

| FACTOR | EFFECT ON PLASMA PLP |
|---|---|
| Diet | |
| ↑ Vitamin $B_6$ | ↑ |
| ↑ Protein | ↓ |
| ↑ Glucose | ↓, acute |
| ↓ Bioavailability | ↓ |
| Physiologic | |
| ↑ Exercise, aerobic | ↑, acute |
| ↑ Age | ↓ |
| Pregnancy | ↓ |
| ↑ Alkaline phosphatase activity | ↓ |
| Smoking, chronic | ↓ |

(From Leklem, J.E.: J. Nutr., *120*:1503–1507, 1990.)

question. Plasma total vitamin $B_6$ and plasma PL concentrations are additional direct measures that are useful. Because PL is the form that crosses into the cell, measurement of PL may be more relevant than measurement of PLP.

Urinary direct measures include the major metabolic product 4-PA and total vitamin $B_6$ (the sum of the nonphosphorylated and phosphorylated forms). Under normal conditions, 40 to 60% of the daily vitamin $B_6$ intake is excreted as 4-PA.[68] Similarly, urinary $B_6$ vitamers represent 8 to 10% of the daily intake.[18] Urinary 4-PA excretion is considered a short-term indicator of status. Excretion is reflective of and influenced by vitamin $B_6$ intake over a 1- to 4-day period. To utilize properly urinary total vitamin $B_6$ as an indicator of status, several 24-hour urine collections over 1 to 3 weeks are needed. Our knowledge of the factors (dietary and physiologic) that affect urinary 4-PA and total vitamin $B_6$ is limited primarily to the effect of protein intake,[69] with only 4-PA being significantly affected (inverse relation) by protein intake.[4]

## INDIRECT METHODS

The indirect measures of vitamin $B_6$ status currently employed are based on products of metabolic pathways or specific enzymes that require PLP. Thus, they indirectly reflect PLP levels in certain tissues. They are therefore not necessarily reflective of the total vitamin $B_6$ in tissues, nor are they always reflective of circulating levels of PLP or $B_6$ vitamers. The most common indirect measures that have been used are urinary metabolites of the tryptophan pathway or methionine pathway, and erythrocyte transaminase activity and stimulation.[65] Other less common tests are urinary oxalate excretion and EEG patterns.

### *TRYPTOPHAN AND METHIONINE LOAD TESTS*

The tryptophan load test has been one of the most widely used indices of vitamin $B_6$ status[70] and is based on the fact that several steps in the major catabolic pathway of tryptophan are PLP-dependent. The sensitivity of each of these reactions to a vitamin $B_6$ deficiency varies, and cellular compartmentalization of some of the enzymes also affects this test. A 2-g oral load of L-tryptophan is administered and the urinary excretion of metabolites such as xanthurenic acid and kynurenic acid is determined. The sensitivity of the test to intakes of vitamin $B_6$ between 5.9 and 14.8 μmol (1.0 and 2.5 mg) (common intakes in adults) is not known. Thus, this test may have limited utility as an index of vitamin $B_6$ status except in situations in which the intake is low (less than 4.7 μmol (0.8 mg) per day)). Brown has questioned the use of this test because of an adverse effect on the metabolism of tryptophan of factors independent of vitamin $B_6$ intake.[71]

The methionine load test has also been used as an indirect measure of vitamin $B_6$ status. As is true for the tryptophan load test, this test is considered primarily reflective of the liver levels of vitamin $B_6$. In the methionine pathway there are four PLP-dependent steps. The step catalyzed by cystathionase, in which cystathionine is cleaved to form homoserine and cysteine, appears to be especially sensitive to a vitamin $B_6$ deficiency. Indeed, cystathionine is excreted in elevated amounts following a 3-g methionine load.[72] The urinary excretion of cystathionine in subjects fed diets deficient in vitamin $B_6$ is elevated more in men than in women, possibly because men ingested more protein. Thus, there appears to be a protein effect similar to that seen for vitamin $B_6$ metabolism[69] and tryptophan metabolism.[60,73]

### *ERYTHROCYTE TRANSAMINASE (AMINOTRANSFERASES)*

Measurement of erythrocyte alanine aminotransferase (EALT, or EGPT) and aspartic acid aminotransferase (EAST, or EGOT) transaminase activity and/or stimulation is one of the more commonly employed indirect indices of vitamin $B_6$ status. They are considered long-term measures of vitamin $B_6$ status because of the life span of erythrocytes.[65] Activities of the respective transaminases are measured in vitro in the presence and absence of excess PLP.[74] From this the percentage of stimulation (stim) is calculated:

$$\%\ \text{Stim} = \frac{\text{stim activity} - \text{unstim activity}}{\text{unstim activity}} \times 100\%$$

According to studies in women EALT activity (index and percentage of stimulation) is more sensitive than EAST activity to vitamin $B_6$ intake.[75] However, the relative activity of EALT is only one twentieth that of EAST. The EALT enzyme is also more prone to loss of activity when erythrocytes are frozen. Because there have been no long-term studies (longer than 6 weeks) in which different levels of vitamin $B_6$ have been fed and transaminase activities have been measured, the utility of transaminase activity measures as an index of a specific vitamin $B_6$ intake is unknown. Also, there is a limited understanding of the temporal relationship between enzyme activity measurement and intake of vitamin $B_6$. A further consideration in using transaminase data to indicate status is the finding of three phenotypes of EALT.[76]

### DIETARY INTAKE OF VITAMIN $B_6$ AND PROTEIN

A proper assessment of vitamin $B_6$ status and interpretation of blood or urinary measures requires that both vitamin $B_6$ and protein intakes be determined. Because of the possible role carbohydrate may have, this should also be documented.[65] These intakes should be determined at intervals over several weeks, or a detailed diet history should be obtained.

Assessment of vitamin $B_6$ status in a healthy population is best made using a direct measure, an indirect measure, and the appropriate dietary information. Although these measures may be useful in certain clinical conditions, the numerous factors that can influence metabolism of vitamin $B_6$ can preclude proper assessment.[77] In clinical situations a measure of tissue levels of PLP or a functional test would be preferable.

## VITAMIN $B_6$ DEFICIENCY

The assessment of any vitamin deficiency can be made on outward clinical signs or via biochemical/functional tests. The clinical signs accompanying vitamin $B_6$ deficiency usually occur in the latter stages of deficiency and are often those seen with other water-soluble vitamins. Table 23–6 provides a listing of the signs commonly seen with severe and chronic vitamin $B_6$ deficiency.[4] Those signs seen in infants were first observed because of an error in food processing of formula that was subsequently fed to infants.[59] In the earlier stages of vitamin $B_6$ deficiency, direct measures of vitamin $B_6$ status would be expected to become lower, and indirect measures would be expected to become abnormal. The changes in EAST and EALT activity (and percentage of stimulation) do change in vitamin $B_6$ deficiency,[75] but only with a chronic deficiency.

## REQUIREMENTS

With the many areas of metabolism and physiologic functions in which vitamin $B_6$ is involved, the establishment of proper and adequate requirements is imperative. Numerous factors can influence vitamin $B_6$ requirements.[4] For a majority of these we do not have adequate information on the quantitative effect on vitamin $B_6$ requirement. The 1989 recommended dietary allowances (RDA) for vitamin $B_6$ for various age groups are summarized in Table 23–7[77] (see Appendix Table A–2b). These RDA are generally lower than prior RDA for vitamin $B_6$ (i.e., the 1974 and 1980 versions), especially for adult men and women.

Of the factors affecting vitamin $B_6$ need, the effect of protein has been studied in greatest detail. Protein intake is inversely correlated with plasma PLP concentration and urinary 4-PA excretion.[69] Under conditions of low intakes of vitamin $B_6$, protein intake is directly correlated with excretion of tryptophan metabolites.[73] Specific studies directed toward the quantitative effect of bioavailability on vitamin $B_6$ requirement have not been conducted. Because the vitamin $B_6$ content of human milk has been determined[4] and found to be influenced by intake,[78] an assessment of the vitamin $B_6$ needs of infants can be made. Current RDA for infants up to 6 months old is set at 1.8 μmol (0.3 mg), an amount which would require an intake of 1.5 to 2 L of milk (assuming a vitamin $B_6$ content of 0.75 to 1.0 μmol/L).

The effect of sex and age on vitamin $B_6$ requirements has received only minimal attention.[4] In studies of vitamin $B_6$ metabolism in males and females, there is a tendency for plasma PLP levels to be lower in females than in males. Several studies suggest that vitamin $B_6$ status decreases with age,[4,79] especially plasma PLP levels. However, the application of such findings to

**TABLE 23–6.** CLINICAL SIGNS OF VITAMIN $B_6$ DEFICIENCY

| SIGNS OCCURRING PRIMARILY IN INFANTS | SIGNS OCCURRING PRIMARILY IN ADULTS |
|---|---|
| Abnormal electroencephalogram pattern | Stomatitis |
| Convulsions | Cheilosis |
| | Glossitis |
| | Irritability |
| | Depression and confusion |

(Adapted from Leklem, J.E.: Vitamin $B_6$ metabolism and function in humans. *In* Clinical and Physiological Applications of Vitamin $B_6$. Edited by J.E. Leklem and R.D. Reynolds. New York, A.R. Liss, 1988, pp. 3–28.)

**TABLE 23–7.** RECOMMENDED DIETARY ALLOWANCES (1989)[77] FOR VITAMIN $B_6$ AND ASSOCIATED VITAMIN $B_6$ TO PROTEIN RATIOS*

| AGE GROUP (IN YEARS) OR CONDITION | VITAMIN $B_6$ (mg/day) | | VITAMIN $B_6$:PROTEIN (mg/g) | |
|---|---|---|---|---|
| Infants 0.0–0.5 | 0.3 | | 0.023 | |
| 0.5–1.0 | 0.6 | | 0.043 | |
| Children 1–3 | 1.0 | | 0.063 | |
| 4–6 | 1.1 | | 0.046 | |
| 7–10 | 1.4 | | 0.050 | |
| | Males | Females | Males | Females |
| Adults 11–14 | 1.7 | 1.4 | 0.038 | 0.030 |
| 15–18 | 2.0 | 1.5 | 0.034 | 0.030 |
| 19–24 | 2.0 | 1.6 | 0.034 | 0.035 |
| 25–50 | 2.0 | 1.6 | 0.032 | 0.032 |
| 51+ | 2.0 | 1.6 | 0.032 | 0.032 |
| Pregnant | | 2.2 | | 0.036 |
| Lactating 1–6 months | | 2.1 | | 0.032 |
| 2nd 6 months | | 2.1 | | 0.034 |

*This ratio was derived by dividing the RDA for vitamin $B_6$ by the RDA for protein for the respective age group. The RDA for vitamin $B_6$ for adults was established by using twice the RDA for protein (126 g/day for males and 100 g/day for females) and a vitamin $B_6$/protein ratio of 0.016 mg/g. 1 mg $B_6$ = 5.91 μmol.

(From Food and Nutrition Board, National Research Council: Recommended Dietary Allowances. 10th Ed. Washington, D.C., National Academy Press, 1989.)

requirements is not known. The vitamin $B_6$ RDAs for adult males and females are based on metabolic studies, vitamin $B_6$ intake data, and protein intakes of populations.[77] Establishment of the current RDA is based primarily on the protein–vitamin $B_6$ interrelationship. For adults a value of 0.095 μmol (0.016 mg) of vitamin $B_6$ per gram of protein has been set.

## CLINICAL CONDITIONS

Several reviews have examined the relationship between vitamin $B_6$ nutrition and disease states.[80–82] In a number of disease states there is an apparent alteration of vitamin $B_6$ metabolism as reflected in altered tryptophan metabolism or decreased plasma PLP concentration. Disease states in which tryptophan metabolism has been found to be altered include asthma,[83] diabetes,[84] breast and bladder cancer,[71] and rheumatoid arthritis.[85] Conditions in which plasma PLP concentration has been found to be decreased include asthma,[86] renal disease,[87] alcoholism,[88] coronary heart disease,[89] breast cancer,[90] Hodgkin's disease,[91] sickle cell anemia,[53] diabetes,[92] and smoking.[93] In many of these studies only one measure of vitamin $B_6$ status was determined; thus the extent to which true status is compromised is unknown.

Vitamin $B_6$ (as pyridoxine hydrochloride) has been used as a preventive agent or as a therapeutic agent to treat several diseases. Papers from recent conferences on this aspect of vitamin $B_6$ are available.[82,95] Disorders that have been treated with PN include Down's syndrome, autism, hyperoxaluria, gestational diabetes, carpal tunnel syndrome, depression, and diabetic neuropathy.[82] In nearly every case, there has been limited therapeutic benefit. However, the dose of pyridoxine and length of administration has varied from study to study; thereby making evaluation of efficacy difficult.

## DRUG–VITAMIN $B_6$ INTERACTION AND TOXICITY

With the widespread use of clinical drugs in our society, the need to understand the effect of drug use on vitamin $B_6$ metabolism is needed. Table 23–8, taken in part from a review by Bhagavan,[95] lists several drugs that have an effect on vitamin $B_6$ metabolism. In many cases the drugs either react with PLP, induce PLP-dependent enzymes, or interfere with vitamin $B_6$ metabolism.[96] In most cases, administration of pyridoxine corrects the altered metabolism of vitamin $B_6$. The possible effects of excess vitamin $B_6$ (>10 mg per day) on drug efficacy should be considered in those cases in which the drug reacts directly with PLP.

The use of high doses of pyridoxine to treat certain disorders such as premenstrual syndrome and other neurologic diseases has resulted in a small number of cases of neurotoxicity[97] and photosensitivity.[4] These symptoms are rarely if ever seen with doses of 11.8 to 1479 μmol (2 to 250 mg) and usually are seen only with chronic use.[98]

**TABLE 23–8.** DRUG-VITAMIN $B_6$ INTERACTIONS

| DRUG | EFFECT ON VITAMIN $B_6$ METABOLISM/FUNCTION |
|---|---|
| Iproniazid (hydrazines) | Reacts with PL and PLP |
| Cycloserine | Reacts with PLP, forms oxime |
| L-3,4-dihydroxyphenylalanine | Reacts with PLP, forms tetrahydroquinoline derivative |
| Penicillamine | Reacts with PLP, forms thiazolidine |
| Ethinylestradiol, mestranol | Increased enzyme levels and retention of PLP in tissue |
| Ethanol | Increased catabolism of PLP |
| Theophylline, caffeine | Inhibition of pyridoxal kinase |

(Data from Bhagavan, H.N.: Interaction between vitamin $B_6$ and drugs. *In* Vitamin $B_6$: Its Role in Health and Disease. Edited by R.D. Reynolds and J.E. Leklem. New York, A.R. Liss, 1985; and Ubbink, J.B., Bissbort, S., Vermaak, W.J.H., et al.: Enzyme, *43*:72–79, 1990.)

## REFERENCES


1. Leklem, J.E., Reynolds, R.D. (eds.): Methods in Vitamin $B_6$ Nutrition. New York, Plenum Press, 1981.
2. Snell, E.E.: Vitamin $B_6$ analysis: Some historical aspects. *In* Methods in Vitamin $B_6$ Nutrition. Edited by J.E. Leklem and R.D. Reynolds. New York, Plenum Press, 1981, pp. 1–19.
3. IUPAC-IUB Commission on Biochemical Nomenclature. Eur. J. Biochem., *40*:325–327, 1973.
4. Leklem, J.E.: Vitamin $B_6$. *In* Handbook of Vitamins. 2nd Ed. Edited by L.J. Machlin. New York, Marcel Dekker, 1991, pp. 341–392.
5. Leussing, D.L.: Model reactions. *In* Coenzymes and Cofactors. Vol 1. Vitamin $B_6$ Pyridoxal Phosphate. Edited by D. Dolphin, R. Poulson, and O. Avramovic. New York, John Wiley & Sons, 1986, pp. 69–115.
6. Sauberlich, H.E.: Interaction of vitamin $B_6$ with other nutrients. *In* Vitamin $B_6$: Its Role in Health and Disease. Edited by R.D. Reynolds and J.E. Leklem, New York, A.R. Liss, 1985, pp. 193–217.
7. Polansky, M.: Microbiological assay of vitamin $B_6$ in foods. *In* Methods in Vitamin Nutrition. Edited by J.E. Leklem and R.D. Reynolds. New York, Plenum Press, 1981, pp. 31–44.
8. Gregory, J.F.: J. Food. Comp. Analysis, *1*:105–123, 1988.
9. Yasumoto, K., Tsuji, H., Iwami, K., et al.: Agric. Biol. Chem., *41*:1061–1067, 1977.
10. Kabir, H., Leklem, J.E., Miller, L.T.: J. Food Sci., *48*:1422–1425, 1983.
11. Richardson, L.R., Wilkes, S., Ritchey, S.J.: J. Nutr., *73*:363–368, 1961.
12. Woodring, M.J., Storvick, C.A.: J. Assoc. Off. Agric. Chem., *43*:63–80, 1960.
13. Perera, A.D., Leklem, J.E., Miller, L.T.: Cereal Chem., *56*:577–580, 1979.
14. Gregory, J.F., Kirk, J.R.: J. Food Sci., *42*:1554–1561, 1977.
15. Gregory, J.F.: J. Nutr., *110*:995–1005, 1980.
16. Tadera, K., Arima, M., Yoshino, F., et al.: J. Nutr. Sci. Vitaminol., *32*:267–277, 1986.
17. Henderson, L.M.: Intestinal absorption of $B_6$ vitamers. *In* Vitamin $B_6$: Its Role in Health and Disease. Edited by R.D. Reynolds and J.E. Leklem. New York, A.R. Liss, 1985, pp. 11–53.
18. Wozenski, J.R., Leklem, J.E., Miller, L.T.: J. Nutr., *110*:275–285, 1980.
19. Roth-Maier, D.A., Zinner, P.M., Kirchgessner, M.: Int. J. Vitam. Nutr. Res., *52*:272–279, 1982.
20. Middleton, H.M.: J. Nutr., *115*:1079–1088, 1985.
21. Leklem, J.E.: Food Technol., October, 194–196, 1988.
22. Gregory, J.F., Kirk, J.R.: The bioavailability of vitamin $B_6$ in foods. *In* Vitamin $B_6$: Its Role in Health and Disease. Edited by R.D. Reynolds and J.E. Leklem. New York, A.R. Liss, 1985, pp. 3–23.
23. Lumeng, L., Brashear, R.E., Li, T-K.: J. Lab. Clin. Med., *84*:334–343, 1974.
24. Mehansho, H., Henderson, M.: J. Biol. Chem., *255*:11901–11907, 1980.
25. Benesch, R.E., Yung, S., Suzuki, T., et al.: Proc. Natl. Acad. Sci. U.S.A., *70*:2595–2599, 1973.
26. Anderson, B.B., Perry, G.M., Clements, J.E., et al.: Am. J. Clin. Nutr., *50*:1059–1063, 1989.
27. Lumeng, L., Li, T-K.: Mammalian vitamin $B_6$ metabolism: Regulatory role of protein-binding and the hydrolysis of pyridoxal 5′-phosphate in storage and transport. *In* Vitamin $B_6$ Metabolism and Role in Growth. Edited by G.P. Tryfiates. Westport, CT, Food and Nutrition Press, 1980, pp. 27–51.
28. Merrill, A.H., Henderson, J.M., Wang, E., et al.: J. Nutr., *114*:1664–1674, 1984.
29. Wada, H., Snell, E.E.: J. Biol. Chem., *236*:2089–2095, 1961.
30. Lakshmi, A.V., Bamji, B.S.: Br. J. Nutr., *32*:249–255, 1974.
31. Perry, G.M., Anderson, B.B., Dodd, N.: Biomedicine, *33*:36–38, 1980.
32. Coburn, S.P., Mahuren, J.D.: Anal. Biochem., *129*:310–317, 1983.
33. Hollins, B., Henderson, J.M.: J. Chromatogr., *380*:67–75, 1986.
34. Pogell, B.M.: J. Biol. Chem., *232*:761–766, 1958.
35. Coburn, S.P.: Ann. N. Y. Acad. Sci., *585*:76–85, 1990.
36. Krebs, E.G., Fischer, E.H.: Vitam. Horm., *22*:399–410, 1964.

37. Coburn, S.P., Lewis, D.L., Fink, W.J., et al.: Am. J. Clin. Nutr., *48*:291–294, 1988.
38. Shane, B.: Vitamin $B_6$ and blood. *In* Human Vitamin $B_6$ Requirements. Washington, D.C., National Academy Press, 1978, pp. 111–128.
39. Leklem, J.E.: Vitamin $B_6$ metabolism and function in humans. *In* Clinical and Physiological Applications of Vitamin $B_6$. Edited by J.E. Leklem and R.D. Reynolds. New York, A.R. Liss, 1988, pp. 3–28.
40. Helmreich, E.J.M., Klein, H.W.: Angew. Chem. (Engl.), *19*:441–455, 1980.
41. Rose, D.P., Leklem, J.E., Brown, R.R., et al.: Am. J. Clin. Nutr., *28*:872–878, 1975.
42. Angel, J.F., Mellor, R.M.: Nutr. Rep. Int., *9*:97–107, 1974.
43. Black, A.L., Guirard, B.M., Snell, E.E.: J. Nutr., *107*:1962–1968, 1977.
44. Black, A.L., Guirard, B.M., Snell, E.E.: J. Nutr., *108*:670–677, 1978.
45. Leklem, J.E., Brown, R.R., Rose, D.P., et al.: Am. J. Clin. Nutr., *28*:146–156, 1975.
46. Birch, T.W.: J. Biol. Chem., *124*:775–793, 1938.
47. Abe, M., Kishino, Y.: J. Nutr., *112*:205–210, 1982.
48. Cunnane, S.C., Manku, M.S., Horrobin, D.F.: J. Nutr., *114*:1754–1761, 1984.
49. Delrome, C.B., Lupien, P.J.: J. Nutr., *106*:169–180, 1976.
50. Loo, G., Smith, J.T.: Lipids, *21*:409–412, 1986.
51. Chi, M.S.: Nutr. Res., *4*:359–362, 1984.
52. Fincham, J.E., Faber, M., Weight, M.J., et al.: Atherosclerosis, *66*:191–203, 1987.
53. Reynolds, R.D., Natta, C.L.: Vitamin $B_6$ and sickle cell anemia. *In* Vitamin $B_6$: Its Role in Health and Disease. Edited by R.D. Reynolds and J.E. Leklem. New York, A.R. Liss, 1985, pp. 301–306.
54. Bottomley, S.S.: Iron and vitamin $B_6$ in the sideroblastic anemias. *In* Nutrition in Hematology. Edited by J. Lindenbaum. New York, Churchill Livingstone, 1983, pp. 203–223.
55. Horrigan, D.L., Harris, J.W.: Vitam. Horm., *26*:549–568, 1968.
56. Dakshinamurti, K.: Adv. Nutr. Res., *4*:143–179, 1982.
57. Bender, D.A.: J. Neurochem., *18*:2407–2416, 1971.
58. Kirksey, A., Morre, D.M., Wasynczuk, A.Z.: Ann. N.Y. Acad. Sci., *585*:202–218, 1990.
59. Coursin, D.B.: JAMA, *154*:406–408, 1954.
60. Canham, J.E., Baker, E.M., Harding, R.S., et al.: Ann. N.Y. Acad. Sci., *166*:16–29, 1969.
61. Thomas, M.R., Kirksey, A.: J. Nutr., *106*:1415–1420, 1976.
62. Wasynczuk, A., Kirksey, A., Morre, D.M.: J. Nutr., *113*:746–754, 1983.
63. Litwack, G., Miller-Diener, A., DiSorbo, D.M., et al.: Vitamin $B_6$ and the glucocorticoid receptor. *In* Vitamin $B_6$: Its Role in Health and Disease. Edited by R.D. Reynolds and J.E. Leklem. New York, A.R. Liss, 1985, pp. 177–191.
64. Bender, D.A.: World Rev. Nutr. Diet, *51*:140–188, 1987.
65. Leklem, J.E.: J. Nutr., *120*:1503–1507, 1990.
66. Lumeng, L., Ryan, M., Li, T-K.: J. Nutr., *108*:545–554, 1978.
67. Leklem, J.E., Reynolds, R.D.: Challenges and directions in the search for clinical applications of vitamin $B_6$. *In* Clinical and Physiological Applications of Vitamin $B_6$. Edited by J.E. Leklem and R.D. Reynolds. New York, A.R. Liss, 1988, pp. 437–454.
68. Shultz, T.D, Leklem, J.E.: Urinary 4-pyridoxic acid, urinary vitamin $B_6$ and plasma pyridoxal phosphate as measures of vitamin $B_6$ status and dietary intake in adults. *In* Methods in Vitamin $B_6$ Nutrition. Edited by J.E. Leklem and R.D. Reynolds. New York, Plenum Press, 1981, pp. 389–392.
69. Miller, L.T., Leklem, J.E., Shultz, T.D.: J. Nutr., *115*:1663–1672, 1985.
70. Brown, R.R.: The tryptophan load test as an index of vitamin $B_6$ nutrition. *In* Methods in Vitamin $B_6$ Nutrition. Edited by J.E. Leklem and R.D. Reynolds. New York, Plenum Press, 1981, pp. 321–340.
71. Brown, R.R.: Possible role for vitamin $B_6$ in cancer prevention and treatment. *In* Clinical and Physiological Applications of Vitamin $B_6$. Edited by J.E. Leklem and R.D. Reynolds. New York, A.R. Liss, 1988, pp. 279–302.
72. Linkswiler, H.M.: Methionine metabolite excretion as affected by a vitamin $B_6$ deficiency. *In* Methods in Vitamin $B_6$ Nutrition. Edited by J.E. Leklem and R.D. Reynolds. New York, Plenum Press, 1981, pp. 373–381.
73. Miller, L.T., Linkswiler, H.: J. Nutr., *93*:53–67, 1967.
74. Woodring, M.J., Storvick, C.A.: Am. J. Clin. Nutr., *23*:1385–1395, 1970.
75. Brown, R.R., Rose, D.P., Leklem, J.E., et al.: Am. J. Clin. Nutr., *28*:10–19, 1975.
76. Ubbink, J.B., Bissbort, S., van den Berg, I., et al.: Am. J. Clin. Nutr., *50*:1420–1428, 1989.
77. Food and Nutrition Board, National Research Council: Recommended Dietary Allowances. 10th Ed. Washington, D.C., National Academy Press, 1989.
78. Styslinger, L., Kirksey, A.: Am. J. Clin. Nutr., *41*:21–31, 1985.
79. Lee, C.M., Leklem, J.E.: Am. J. Clin. Nutr., *42*:226–234, 1985.
80. Reynolds, R.D., Leklem, J.E. (eds.): Vitamin $B_6$: Its Role in Health and Disease. New York, A.R. Liss, 1985.
81. Merrill, A.H. Jr., Henderson, J.M.: Annu. Rev. Nutr., *7*:137–156, 1987.
82. Leklem, J.E., Reynolds, R.D. (eds.): Clinical and Physiological Applications of Vitamin $B_6$. New York, A.R. Liss, 1988.
83. Collip, P.J., Goldzier, S., Weiss, N.: Ann. Allergy, *35*:93–97, 1975.
84. Musajo, L., Benassi, C.A.: Adv. Clin. Chem., *7*:63–135, 1964.
85. Flinn, J.H., Price, J.M., Yess, N., et al.: Arthritis Rheum., *7*:201–210, 1964.
86. Reynolds, R.D., Natta, C.L.: Am. J. Clin. Nutr., *41*:684–688, 1985.
87. Stone, W.J., Warnock, L.G., Wagner, C.: Am. J. Clin. Nutr., *28*:950–957, 1975.
88. Lumeng, L., Li, T-K.: J. Clin. Invest., *53*:693–704, 1974.
89. Serfontein, W.J., Ubbink, J.B., DeVilliers, L.S.: Atherosclerosis, *55*:357–361, 1985.
90. Potera, C., Rose, D.P., Brown, R.R.: Am. J. Clin. Nutr., *30*:1677–1679, 1977.
91. Devita, V.T., Chabner, B.A., Livingston, D.M., et al.: Am. J. Clin. Nutr., *24*:835–840, 1971.
92. Hollenbeck, C.B., Leklem, J.E., Riddle, M.C., et al.: Am. J. Clin. Nutr., *38*:41–51, 1983.
93. Serfontein, W.J., Ubbink, J.B., DeVilliers, L.S., et al.: Atherosclerosis, *59*:341–346, 1986.
94. Dakshinamurti, K. (ed.): Ann. N. Y. Acad. Sci., *585*, 1990.
95. Bhagavan, H.N.: Interaction between vitamin $B_6$ and drugs. *In* Vitamin $B_6$: Its Role in Health and Disease. Edited by R.D. Reynolds and J.E. Leklem. New York, A.R. Liss, 1985, pp. 401–415.
96. Ubbink, J.B., Bissbort, S., Vermaak, W.J.H., et al.: Enzyme, *43*:72–79, 1990.
97. Schaumburg, H., Kaplan, J., Windebank, A., et al.: N. Engl. J. Med., *309*:445–448, 1983.
98. Cohen, M., Bendich, A.: Toxicol. Lett., *34*:129–139, 1986.

## SELECTED READINGS

Dakshinamurti, K. (ed.): Vitamin $B_6$. Ann. N.Y. Acad. Sci., *585*, 1990.

Leklem, J.E., Reynolds, R.D. (eds.): Clinical and Physiological Applications of Vitamin $B_6$. New York, A.R. Liss, 1988.

Leklem, J.E., Reynolds, R.D. (eds.): Methods in Vitamin $B_6$ Nutrition. New York, Plenum Press, 1981.

Merrill, A.H. Jr., Henderson, J.M.: Diseases associated with defects in vitamin $B_6$ metabolism or utilization. Annu. Rev. Nutr., 7:137–156, 1987.

Reynolds, R.D., Leklem, J.E. (eds.): Vitamin $B_6$: Its Role in Health and Disease. New York, A.R. Liss, 1985.

CHAPTER **24**

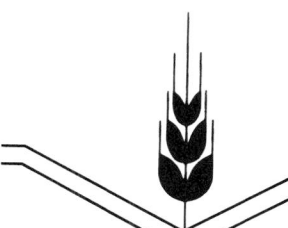

# Pantothenic Acid and Coenzyme A

**Nora Plesofsky-Vig**



## HISTORICAL OVERVIEW

Independent research paths led to the isolation and characterization of pantothenic acid.[1,2] The vitamin $B_2$ complex derived from liver was separated into its individual components, which were tested for their effects on specific animal disorders. In one of the last steps, pantothenic acid was separated from vitamin $B_6$ by adsorption chromatography; pyridoxol and its derivatives (vitamin $B_6$) adsorbed to fuller's earth, while pantothenic acid remained in the filtrate. Vitamin $B_6$ cured rats of the dermatitis produced by vitamin $B_2$ deficiency, but dermatitis in chicks was cured only by the filtrate component that became known as the "chick antidermatitis factor." Biochemical and physiologic tests showed that this factor was identical to the pantothenic acid shown earlier by R. J. Williams to be essential for the growth of yeast. Derivatives of the same factor were found independently to be essential for the growth of lactic acid bacteria.

In 1940, R. J. Williams and R. T. Major successfully synthesized pantothenic acid.[2] Not until 1947, however, was its biologically functional form demonstrated by F. Lipmann and his colleagues to be within coenzyme A (CoA),[3] which they showed was an essential cofactor for such biologic acetylation reactions as the acetylation of sulfonamide in the liver and of choline in the brain. Pantothenate-containing CoA has since been shown to be essential to the respiratory tricarboxylic acid cycle, fatty acid synthesis and degradation, and many other metabolic and regulatory processes. The accepted biochemical structure of CoA was first published in 1953.[4]

## CHEMISTRY

Pantothenic acid [1,2,5] consists of pantoic acid in amide linkage to β-alanine (Fig. 24–1). Pantetheine is formed by the addition of β-mercaptoethylamine, which provides the reactive sulfhydryl group, to pantothenic acid. Pantetheine is an essential growth factor for the yogurt-producing bacterium Lactobacillus bulgaricus. The 4′-phosphopantetheine in CoA is linked by an anhydride bond to the nucleotide adenosine monophosphate, which additionally is modified by a 3′-hydroxyl phosphate. The active sulfhydryl group exposed at the tip of pantetheine is commonly esterified either to acetate or to longer chain acyl groups.

Although pantothenate is found most frequently within CoA, 4′-phosphopantetheine is linked in a few cases directly to a protein.[6] This type of linkage is central to fatty acid synthesis. The acyl carrier protein of bacteria is modified by 4′-phosphopantetheine in phosphodiester linkage to a serine residue; eukaryotes have a larger multifunctional fatty acid synthetase that is similarly modified. Other proteins that contain phosphopantetheine include the citrate lyase of anaerobic bacteria and enzymes involved in synthesis of peptide antibiotics, such as tyrocidine and gramicidin S.

CoA and other pantothenate derivatives participate in two basic types of reactions.[5] One type involves nucleophilic addition to the carbonyl group that is thioesterified to CoA, leading to formation of a new ester bond and displacement of CoA. As a leaving group, CoA facilitates the transfer of acetyl or acyl groups. In the second type of reaction, the α-carbon of the acyl group is acidified by its

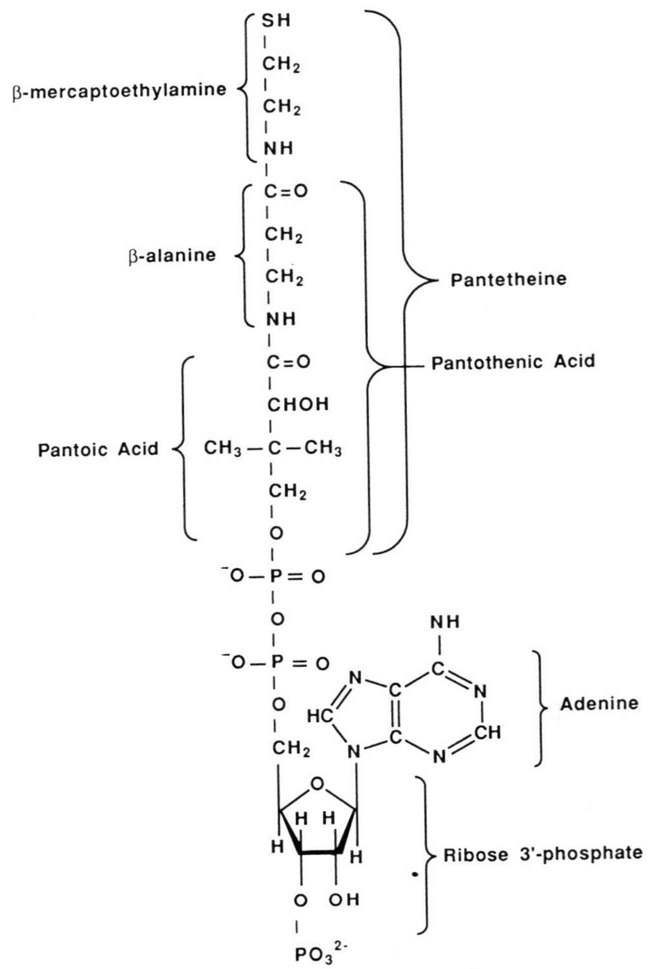
β-mercaptoethylamine
β-alanine
Pantoic Acid
Pantetheine
Pantothenic Acid
Adenine
Ribose 3'-phosphate

**FIGURE 24–1.** Coenzyme A and intermediates.

proximity to the thioester with CoA and it attaches to an electrophilic center, leading to condensation reactions and carbon-carbon bond formation or cleavage. Both of these reactions are used during fatty acid synthesis;[7] acetate groups are transferred from CoA to an enzyme sulfhydryl group, and a malonyl group is donated by CoA to the enzyme-linked phosphopantetheine. After these acyl-transferase reactions, the introduced acetate condenses with the malonate or growing fatty acid chain linked to pantetheine. During respiratory metabolism, acetyl-CoA (derived from pyruvate) condenses with oxaloacetic acid to form citric acid. In this first step of the tricarboxylic acid cycle, only the condensation reaction of CoA occurs.

## FUNCTIONS IN CELLULAR METABOLISM

Bound pantothenate performs multiple roles in cellular metabolism and regulation.[5,8] Esterified CoA is essential to the synthesis of fatty acids and to their incorporation into membrane phospholipids. It is also required for the synthesis of cholesterol, steroid hormones, dolichol, vitamin A, vitamin D, and all compounds formed from isoprenoid units;[9] the isoprenoid precursor mevalonic acid is the condensation product of three molecules of acetyl-CoA. Pantothenate also contributes to the synthesis of amino acids, such as leucine, arginine, and methionine. Through succinyl-CoA, it is essential to the synthesis of δ-aminolevulinic acid, the precursor of the corrin ring in vitamin $B_{12}$ and the porphyrin rings of hemoglobin and the electron-carrying cytochromes. The degradation of fatty acids through β-oxidation and the oxidative degradation of amino acids also depend on CoA, which then makes the products of catabolism available for energy extraction through the tricarboxylic acid cycle. Plants and microorganisms also use acetyl-CoA to build sugars in the glyoxylate cycle. Other molecules to which CoA contributes an essential acetyl group are the neurotransmitter acetylcholine and the sugars *N*-acetylglucosamine, *N*-acetylgalactosamine, and *N*-acetylneuraminic acid, important components of glycoproteins and glycolipids.

## FUNCTIONS IN PROTEIN MODIFICATION

CoA plays a central role in the modification of cellular proteins with acetyl and fatty acyl groups,[6] modifications that strongly affect the activity, structure, and localization of proteins.

### AMINO TERMINAL ACETYLATION

The most common modification is cotranslational acetylation of the amino terminal residue of proteins. Depending on the organism, 50 to 90% of all eukaryotic proteins are N-terminally acetylated.[10] The terminal methionine may become acetylated or, more commonly, it is cleaved and the second amino acid, usually alanine or serine, becomes acetylated.[6] A proposed function of N-terminal acetylation is to protect cellular proteins from degradation. In support of this proposal, certain acetylated proteins were resistant in vitro to ubiquitin-dependent proteolysis, whereas their unacetylated counterparts were degraded.[11] Recent studies show, however, that in a more complete assay mixture, N-acetylated proteins were also subject to ubiquitin-dependent degradation.[12] The importance of peptide acetylation is shown by a yeast mutant that is defective in N-terminal acetyltransferase activity. Several cellular processes were disrupted in the mutant, including cell cycle progression and sexual development.[13] None of the approximately 20 proteins whose block in acetylation was detectable, however, appeared to be dramatically destabilized, which gives little support to the proposed stabilizing function of protein acetylation. Evidence exists that N-terminal acetylation may influence protein structure, because acetylation of the calcium-binding protein calpactin I both increases the α-helical content near its amino terminus and is required for the protein to assemble with the small regulatory subunit of this complex.[14]

N-terminal acetylation also occurs during the processing of mammalian peptide hormones from their polyprotein precursors,[6] and this post-translational addition of acetyl groups strongly affects hormone activity. The presence or absence of acetylation depends on the tissue examined. The precursor pro-opiomelanocortin gives rise both to α-melanocyte-stimulating hormone (MSH) and to the opioid β-endorphin.[15] Although both of these hormones become N-terminally acetylated in the intermediate pituitary, neither becomes acetylated in the anterior lobe of the pituitary gland, and β-endorphin is not acetylated in brain. Acetylation has different effects on the activities of these two hormones,[16] stimulating α-MSH activity but inactivating β-endorphin, which is rendered unable to bind to the opioid receptors. Acetylation may provide a mechanism for differentially activating these two products of a single precursor.

## INTERNAL ACETYLATION

Microtubules, composed of polymerized dimers of α- and β-tubulin, are an important component of the cellular cytoskeleton that affects cell shape and motility. A subset of the α-tubulin within these structures becomes acetylated on the ϵ-amino group of an internal lysine residue,[17] and the acetylated α-tubulin is detected in cells by specific antibodies.[18] Acetylation appears to stabilize microtubule structure,[6] because microtubules containing the modified α-tubulin are resistant to depolymerizing agents such as colchicine. In turn, drugs that stabilize microtubules, like taxol, induce α-tubulin acetylation. Acetylation occurs after microtubule assembly, and isolated acetylase activity was more active with the microtubule than with the tubulin dimer as substrate.[19]

Acetylated microtubules are not distributed randomly in cells.[6] They are excluded from the leading edge microtubules of migrating human 3T3 cells, and in rat cerebellum, acetylated α-tubulin is concentrated in axons compared with dendrites. In chick muscle fibers, acetylated microtubules underlie motor endplates,[20] where they participate in vesicle and organelle transport; the unacetylated cytoplasmic microtubules, in contrast, contribute to the flexible alteration of cell shape. In developing mouse embryos, the nonrandom distribution of acetylated microtubules is associated with cell differentiation.[21] Progeny cells inherit distinct patterns of microtubules, and the subpopulations of microtubules became redistributed during the subsequent process of cell polarization.

Another major group of proteins that undergo selective acetylation includes the histones and certain other DNA-binding proteins.[6,22] Like α-tubulin, the histones become modified on the ϵ-amino group of internal lysines. All four of the core histones—H4, H3, H2A, and H2B—which are encircled with nucleosomal DNA, become acetylated within their amino terminal regions; only the internucleosomal histone H1 has no internal acetylation sites. Histones H4 and H3 each have four possible sites for acetylation. Histone acetylation is thought to weaken interactions between nucleosomes that depend on the N-terminal tails of histones, resulting in the destabilization of chromatin structure. Several types of evidence indicate that chromatin unfolds as a result of hyperacetylation of histones.[6,22] This evidence includes the increased susceptibility of DNA to nucleases, the increased solubility of chromatin,[23] and the decrease in the number of negative supercoils within a nucleosome.[24]

Hyperacetylated histones tend to be associated with newly synthesized DNA or with transcriptionally active DNA. The functions of histone acetylation in relation to DNA replication versus gene transcription have been dissected in the ciliated protozoan Tetrahymena thermophila.[25] The advantage of this organism is that it contains two kinds of nuclei, both of which are active in DNA replication, but only one of which (the macronucleus) is transcriptionally active. Acetyl groups were linked only transiently to newly synthesized histones that participate in chromatin assembly, whereas acetate was added continually to histones in transcriptionally active chromatin. Different sites within the histones become acetylated during these two activities,[26] and distinct enzyme systems appear to be involved.[27] Direct evidence for a connection between histone acetylation and gene transcription was provided by an antibody against the ϵ-acetyl lysine of histones.[28] The chromatin fraction from chick embryo erythrocytes that bound to this antibody was strongly enriched in the transcriptionally active α-D-globin gene sequences. Mutation of the reversibly acetylated lysines in yeast histone H4 provides genetic evidence that histone acetylation strongly enhances gene transcription. Replacement of all four lysines in H4 strongly inhibited transcription of specific genes.[29]

## ACYLATION WITH FATTY ACIDS

A widespread type of peptide modification that is mediated by CoA is the attachment of long chain fatty acyl groups to cellular and viral proteins.[6,30–32] In several cases, this modification affects the protein's ability to participate in regulatory steps that mediate signal transduction.[32] The fatty acids that are most commonly attached to proteins are myristic acid, which is a 14-carbon saturated fatty acid, and palmitic acid, a 16-carbon saturated fatty acid. These two fatty acids are linked to proteins at mutually exclusive sites, and they affect peptide localization or activity in distinct ways.

### *MYRISTIC ACID*

Myristate, a rare fatty acid, usually forms an amide bond to the free α-amino group of the exposed N-terminal amino acid of a protein. Stringent sequence requirements for this attachment reflect the substrate specificity of the isolated enzyme that catalyzes myristate addition.[33] An N-terminal glycine is absolutely critical for myristoylation; in addition, small uncharged residues in the subterminal position and in the fifth position, where serine is especially favorable, are important. The enzyme shows a strong preference for myristoyl-CoA as donor over other acyl-CoA. This type of myristate addition occurs cotranslationally and turnover on the protein has not been reported. Myristoylated proteins are located in the cytoplasm and at various intracellular membranes, including the plasma membrane, the endoplasmic reticulum, and the nucleus. Myristoylation may enhance other localization signals within proteins and it may affect protein interactions.

A cell-transforming viral protein and its cellular counterpart are the best studied myristoylated proteins. The mature $pp60^{src}$ protein, which is a tyrosine kinase, associates with the cytoplasmic face of the plasma membrane. This membrane location depends on the addition of myristic acid to the N-terminal glycine residue of $pp60^{src}$, and nonmyristoylated proteins that lack the requisite glycine remain free in the cytoplasm.[34] The nonmyristoylated forms of viral $pp60^{src}$ are unable to transform cells, probably because of the changed intracellular location of the protein. The $pp60^{src}$ mutation results in decreased tyrosine phosphorylation of a small group of membrane-associated proteins that may, therefore, be involved in cell transformation.[35] An analogue of myristic acid with reduced hydrophobicity also blocked the association of viral $pp60^{src}$ with membranes, presenting the possibility of its use as an antitumor agent.[36]

Several other viral proteins become N-terminally myristoylated,[6,30,31] including the gag polyprotein capsid precursors of mammalian retroviruses and the capsid protein of papovaviruses, VP2, and of picornaviruses, VP4. Acylation of these structural proteins is required for the formation of mature virus particles. Cellular proteins that are modified with myristate[6,30–32] include constitutive proteins such as NADH-cytochrome $b_5$ reductase, and regulatory proteins that participate in signal transmission, such as cyclic adenosine monophosphate (cAMP)-dependent protein kinase and the B subunit of calcineurin, a calmodulin-dependent protein phosphatase. The α-subunits of G proteins,[32] a large family of guanosine triphosphate (GTP)-binding proteins involved in transmembrane signaling, are also modified with myristate. The interrelationship of myristoylation and other types of regulatory modifications is demonstrated by a 68,000-dalton macrophage protein that is a major substrate for protein kinase C.[37] Myristoylation enhances the phosphorylation of this protein by bringing substrate and kinase together at the plasma membrane, but phosphorylation leads to dissociation of the 68,000-dalton protein from the membrane.

The importance of this cotranslational peptide modification for cell viability and growth has been demonstrated genetically in yeast.[38] Disruption of the structural gene for *N*-myristoyl transferase, the enzyme that catalyzes transfer of myristate from CoA to the N-terminal glycine of peptides, was recessively lethal for cells. Nonterminal myristoylation sites have been identified less frequently within proteins. The immunoglobulin heavy chain in B lymphocytes is post-translationally myristoylated on the side chain of an amino acid, probably lysine, as the protein is transported through the Golgi complex to the cell surface.[39] In addition, mitochondria from mammalian cells contain an enzyme activity that adds myristate to certain imported proteins.[40,41]

### *PALMITIC ACID*

Transfer of palmitate, a common fatty acid, from acyl-CoA to viral and cellular proteins[6,30–32] is more widespread than myristoylation. Unlike myristate, palmitate forms an ester bond with amino acid side chains, and it turns over on the protein, being added post-translationally. The enzymes that transfer palmitate are relatively nonspecific for acyl substrate, and they transfer other fatty acids in vitro at lower efficiency. At least two different cellular activities palmitoylate proteins, one in the Golgi complex and the other in the cytoplasm. Proteins that are palmitoylated generally associate with the plasma membrane.

The best studied of the palmitoylated proteins is the viral and cellular ras protein. The ras protein binds guanine nucleotides and hydrolyzes GTP, and in yeast, it modulates adenylate cyclase activity.[42] Viral members of the ras family that are deficient in GTPase activity are oncogenic, including the ras proteins of Harvey murine and Kirsten sarcoma viruses. The ras protein undergoes several types of modification.[43] The addition of farnesol, an isoprenoid intermediate in cholesterol biosynthesis, causes the ras protein to associate weakly with plasma membranes, and palmitoylation further strengthens this membrane binding and is required for strong transforming activity. A similar pattern of modification is shown by several related cellular proteins. Other proteins involved in GTP binding are also farnesylated, such as the γ subunit of transducin. Farnesylation of this subunit appears to be necessary for GTP binding by the peptide complex, which transduces the effect of light on photoreceptors in rod outer segments. This isoprenyl modification is suggested to enhance transducin subunit association in a membrane-independent manner.[44]

Other viral proteins that are palmitoylated are the structural glycoproteins of vesicular stomatitis virus and Sindbis virus and the large tumor antigen of simian virus 40. The hemagglutinins of several influenza viruses are esterified to fatty acids, and this modification contributes to the fusogenic properties of the proteins.[45] Among cellular proteins, the modification is found on cytoplasmic domains of several transmembrane receptors, including the iron-transferrin receptor, the photoreceptor rhodopsin, the insulin receptor, the nicotinic acetylcholine receptor, and the $\beta_2$-adrenergic receptor. An essential role in signal transduction is suggested for fatty acylation of the human $\beta_2$-adrenergic receptor.[46] A receptor protein that was unacylated because it lacked the requisite cysteine residue showed a strongly reduced ability to activate adenylate cyclase in response to stimulation. Fatty acylation may play a similar role in other G protein-coupled receptors that have a similarly located cysteine. Other palmitoylated proteins structurally link plasma membrane components to intracellular or extracellular proteins. These include gap junction proteins of heart and eye lens[47] and platelet glycoproteins that mediate cell adhesion to the subendothelium.[48] The importance of palmitoylation for interactions with other proteins is demonstrated by the lymphoma transmembrane glycoprotein, GP85, which requires palmitate modification to bind with high affinity to erythrocyte ankyrin.[49] Vinculin and ankyrin are palmitoylated proteins that are linked to intracellular, cytoskeletal proteins.

A general requirement for palmitoyl-CoA has been demonstrated for vesicular transport through the Golgi complex. The addition of palmitoyl-CoA to Golgi membranes stimulated in vitro transport of a glycoprotein; a nonhydrolyzable analogue of palmitoyl-CoA inhibited transport.[50] Specific steps in transport that depend on fatty acyl-CoA were identified as the budding of vesicles from donor Golgi[50] and the fusion of these vesicles with acceptor Golgi cisternae.[51] This acyl group requirement may reflect the importance of reversible palmitoylation of resident proteins for regulating vesicular transport through the Golgi complex.

Several highly differentiated cells contain characteristic proteins that are esterified to palmitic acid. The transglutaminase of keratinocytes requires palmitoylation for its anchorage in the membrane where it cross-links peptides into an envelope that contributes to cell cohesiveness.[52] One of the major peptide components of pulmonary surfactant, SP-C, contains two esterified palmitate groups.[53] The glycoprotein in gastric mucus is fatty acylated, with a highly acylated protease-resistant fraction (20 mol fatty acid/mol glycoprotein).[54] The mucus glycoprotein of cystic fibrosis patients is still more highly acylated, and its strongly protease-resistant fraction has 66 mol fatty acid/mol glycoprotein, probably contributing to the insoluble mucous secretions of these patients.[55] In developing brains, there is fatty acylation of GAP-34,[56] a major component of growth cone membranes of elongating axons. Furthermore, the proteolipid subunit of brain myelin was one of the first proteins observed to be covalently modified with palmitic acid.

## DEFICIENCY AND EXCESS

Pantothenic acid deficiency notably affects the adrenal cortex, the nervous system, skin, and hair. Rats deficient in pantothenate develop hypertrophy of the adrenal cortex, followed by hemorrhage and necrosis;[2,57] the competitive inhibitor ω-methylpantothenic acid reduced corticosterone production by adrenal glands.[57] Impaired antibody formation, inflammation of the respiratory tract, anemia, loss of hair pigmentation, and reproductive failure have also been reported.[2] Surprisingly, pantothenate deficiency increased the resistance of rats to certain viral infections.[2] Pantothenate-deficient chicks show dermatitis, poor feathering, and axon and myelin degeneration within the spinal cord.[1,2] Deficiency in dogs produces hypoglycemia, gastrointestinal symptoms, rapid respiration and heart beat, and convulsions.[1,2] Most of these symptoms were reversed by the administration of pantothenic acid; the use of pantothenate supplementation to restore hair color in humans, however, proved a failure.[2] Pantothenic acid deficiency in humans is rare, but its induction is associated with fatigue and depression.[1] High doses of orally administered calcium pantothenate were not toxic to rats, dogs, rabbits, or humans. The toxic oral dose for mice (LD 50), however, was 42 mmol (10 g)/kg, and it led to death by respiratory failure.[2]

## EVALUATION OF PANTOTHENATE STATUS, REQUIREMENTS, AND DIETARY CONSIDERATIONS

Assays for pantothenic acid in biologic sources other than urine involve the use of enzymes to release the pantothenate component of CoA. Pantothenic acid content of blood, urine, and tissues has been determined by microbiologic assays with yeast and lactobacilli.[58] The exchange of radioactive β-alanine with that in preexisting pantothenic acid, catalyzed by pantothase, has been used to measure pantothenate concentration in food sources,[59] and a radioimmunoassay has also been used for quantitation.[60]

Pantothenic acid is distributed widely in cells and tissues. Rich dietary sources of the vitamin are liver, kidney, yeast, egg yolk, and fresh vegetables. Especially high levels of pantothenate are found in royal jelly of bees and in the ovaries of tuna fish and cod.[2] At human parturition, the level of pantothenic acid is five times lower in the mother's serum compared with that of the infant,[57] and within the first 4 days after parturition, human milk shows a fivefold increase in its pantothenate content, from 2.2 to 11.2 μmol/L (48 μg to 245 μg/dl).[2] Although pantothenic acid is relatively stable at neutral pH, cooking is reported to destroy 15 to 50% of the vitamin present in raw meat.[2] It has been estimated that 46 μmol (10 mg) pantothenic acid are provided daily by a 2500-calorie diet from plant and animal sources.[1] The recommended daily intake of pantothenic acid is 18 to 32 μmol (4 to 7 mg) for adults, but it is lower for younger age groups, ranging from 9 μmol (2 mg) daily for infants to 18 to 23 μmol (4 to 5 mg) daily for children 7 to 10 years of age[61] (see Appendix Table A–2c). Synthetic D-pantothenate, the active enantiomer, is available as a calcium or sodium salt, but the alcohol derivative panthenol, which is converted by humans to pantothenic acid, is used widely in multivitamin preparations because of its greater stability.[58]

## METABOLISM

The main route of synthesis of CoA from pantothenic acid[8] is through phosphorylation of the free acid to form 4′-phosphopantothenic acid, which subsequently condenses with cysteine. The resulting 4′-phosphopantothenoylcysteine is decarboxylated to yield 4′-phosphopantetheine, and CoA is formed by sequential steps of transfer of adenosine monophosphate and phosphate from adenosine triphosphate. Among the hydrolytic reactions that subsequently liberate pantothenic acid from CoA is the unique and final reaction in which pantetheine is hydrolyzed to pantothenate and cysteamine.[62] Free pantothenic acid is excreted in urine.

## REFERENCES


1. Wagner, A.F., Folkers, K.: Vitamins and Coenzymes. New York, John Wiley & Sons, 1964.
2. Robinson, F.A.: The Vitamin Co-Factors of Enzyme Systems. Oxford, Pergamon Press, 1966.
3. Lipmann, F., Kaplan, N.O., Novelli, G.D., et al.: J. Biol. Chem., *167:*869–870, 1947.
4. Baddiley, J., Thain, E.M., Novelli, G.D., et al.: Nature, *171:*76, 1953.
5. Metzler, D.E.: Biochemistry. New York, Academic Press, 1977.
6. Plesofsky-Vig, N., Brambl, R.: Annu. Rev. Nutr., *8:*461–482, 1988.
7. Wakil, S.J., Stoops, J.K., Joshi, V.C.: Annu. Rev. Biochem., *52:*537–579, 1983.
8. Lehninger, A. L.: Biochemistry. 2nd Ed. New York, Worth Publishers, 1975.
9. Goldstein, J.L., Brown, M.S.: Nature, *343:*425–430, 1990.
10. Driessen, H.P.C., de Jong, W.W., Tesser, G.I., et al.: CRC Crit. Rev. Biochem., *18:*281–306, 1985.
11. Hershko, A., Heller, H., Eytan, E., et al.: Proc. Natl. Acad. Sci. U.S.A., *81:*7021–7025, 1984.
12. Mayer, A., Siegel, N.R., Schwartz, A.L., et al.: Science, *244:*1480–1483, 1989.
13. Mullen, J.R., Kayne, P.S., Moerschell, R.P., et al.: EMBO J., *8:*2067–2075, 1989.
14. Johnsson, N., Marriott, G., Weber, K.: EMBO J., *7:*2435–2442, 1988.
15. Herbert, E., Uhler, M.: Cell, *30:*1–2, 1982.
16. O'Donohue, T.L., Handelmann, G.E., Miller, R.L., et al.: Science *215:*1125–1127, 1982.
17. LeDizet, M., Piperno, G.: Proc. Natl. Acad. Sci. U.S.A., *84:*5720–5724, 1987.
18. Piperno, G., Fuller, M.T.: J. Cell Biol., *101:*2085–2094, 1985.
19. Maruta, H., Greer, K., Rosenbaum, J.L.: J. Cell Biol., *103:*571–579, 1986.
20. Jasmin, B.J., Changeux, J.-P., Cartaud, J.: Nature, *344:*673–675, 1990.
21. Houliston, E., Maro, B.: J. Cell Biol., *108:*543–551, 1989.
22. Csordas, A.: Biochem. J., *265:*23–38, 1990.
23. Ridsdale, J.A., Hendzel, M.J., Delcuve, G.P., et al.: J. Biol. Chem., *265:*5150–5156, 1990.
24. Norton, V.G., Imai, B.S., Yau, P., et al.: Cell, *57:*449–457, 1989.
25. Allis, C.D., Chicoine, L.G., Richman, R., et al.: Proc. Natl. Acad. Sci. U.S.A., *82:*8048–8052, 1985.
26. Chicoine, L.G., Richman, R., Cook, R.G., et al.: J. Cell Biol., *150:*127–135, 1987.
27. Richman, R., Chicoine, L.G., Collini, M.P., et al.: J. Cell Biol., *106:*1017–1026, 1988.
28. Hebbes, T.R., Thorne, A.W., Crane-Robinson, C.: EMBO J., *7:*1395–1402, 1988.
29. Durrin, L.K., Mann, R.K., Kayne, P.S., et al.: Cell, *65:*1023–1031, 1991.
30. Towler, D.A., Gordon, J.I., Adams, S.P., et al.: Annu. Rev. Biochem., *57:*69–99, 1988.
31. Schultz, A.M., Henderson, L.E., Oroszlan, S.: Annu. Rev. Cell Biol., *4:*611–647, 1988.
32. James, G., Olson, E.N.: Biochemistry, *29:*2623–2634, 1990.
33. Towler, D.A., Adams, S.P., Eubanks, S.R., et al.: Proc. Natl. Acad. Sci. U.S.A., *84:*2708–2712, 1987.
34. Pellman, D., Garber, E.A., Cross, F., et al.: Proc. Natl. Acad. Sci. U.S.A., *82:*1623–1627, 1985.
35. Linder, M.E., Burr, J.G.: Proc. Natl. Acad. Sci. U.S.A., *85:*2608–2612, 1988.
36. Heuckeroth, R.O., Gordon, J.I.: Proc. Natl. Acad. Sci. U.S.A., *86:*5262–5266, 1989.
37. Aderem, A.A., Albert, K.A., Keum, M.M.: Nature, *332:*362–364, 1988.
38. Duronio, R.J., Towler, D.A., Heuckeroth, R.O., et al.: Science, *243:*796–800, 1989.
39. Pillai, S., Baltimore, D.: Proc. Natl. Acad. Sci. U.S.A., *84:*7654–7658, 1987.
40. Vijayasarathy, C., Bhat, N.R., Avadhani, N.G.: J. Biol. Chem., *264:*7772–7775, 1989.
41. Stucki, J.W., Lehmann, L.H., Siegel, E.: J. Biol. Chem., *264:*6376–6380, 1989.

42. Fujiyama, A., Tamanoi, F.: Proc. Natl. Acad. Sci. U.S.A., *83:*1266–1270, 1986.
43. Hancock, J.F., Magee, A.I., Childs, J.E., et al.: Cell, *57:*1167–1177, 1989.
44. Fukada, Y., Takao, T. Ohguro, H., et al.: Nature, *346:*658–660, 1990.
45. Lambrecht, B., Schmidt. M.F.G.: FEBS Lett., *202:*127–132, 1986.
46. O'Dowd, B.F., Hnatowich, M., Caron, M.G., et al.: J. Biol. Chem., *264:*7564–7569, 1989.
47. Manenti, S., Dunia, I., Benedetti, E.L.: FEBS Lett., *262:*356–358, 1990.
48. Muszbek, L., Laposata, M.: J. Biol. Chem., *264:*9716–9719, 1989.
49. Bourguignon, L.Y.W., Kalomiris, E.L., Lokeshwar, V.B.: J. Biol. Chem., *266:*11761–11765, 1991.
50. Pfanner, N., Orci, L., Glick, B.S., et al.: Cell, *59:*95–102, 1989.
51. Pfanner, N., Glick, B.S., Arden, S.R., et al.: J. Cell Biol., *110:*955–961, 1990.
52. Chakravarty, R., Rice, R.H.: J. Biol. Chem., *264:*625–629, 1989.
53. Curstedt, T., Johansson, J., Persson, P., et al.: Proc. Natl. Acad. Sci. U.S.A., *87:*2985–2989, 1990.
54. Slomiany, A., Jozwiak, Z., Takagi, A., et al.: Arch. Biochem. Biophys., *229:*560–567, 1984.
55. Slomiany, A., Witas, H., Aono, M., et al.: J. Biol. Chem., *258:*8535–8538, 1983.
56. Skene, J.H.P., Virag, I.: J. Cell Biol., *108:*613–624, 1989.
57. Baker, H., Frank, O.: Clinical Vitaminology. New York, Interscience Publishers, John Wiley & Sons, 1968.
58. Bird, O.D., Thompson, R.Q.: Pantothenic acid. *In* The Vitamins. Vol. 7. 2nd Ed. Edited by P. Gyorgy, W.N. Pearson. New York, Academic Press, 1967.
59. Airas, R.K.: Methods Enzymol., *122:*33–35, 1986.
60. Wittwer, C., Wyse, B., Hansen, R.G.: Anal. Biochem., *122:*213–222, 1982.
61. Food and Nutrition Board, National Research Council: Recommended Dietary Allowances. 10th Ed. Washington, D.C., National Academy Press, 1989.
62. Wittwer, C.T., Wyse, B.W., Hansen, R.G.: Methods Enzymol., *122:*36–43, 1986.

## SELECTED READINGS

Csordas, A.: On the biological role of histone acetylation. Biochem. J., *265:*23–38, 1990.

Goldstein, J.L., Brown, M.S.: Regulation of the mevalonate pathway. Nature, *343:*425–430, 1990.

James, G., Olson, E.N.: Fatty acylated proteins as components of intracellular signaling pathways. Biochemistry, *29:*2623–2634, 1990.

Olson, R.E.: Pantothenic Acid. *In* Present Knowledge in Nutrition. 6th Ed. Edited by M.L. Brown. Washington, D.C., International Life Science Institute Nutrition Foundation, 1990, pp. 208–211.

Plesofsky-Vig, N., Brambl, R.: Pantothenic acid and coenzyme A in cellular modification of proteins. Annu. Rev. Nutr., *8:*461–482, 1988.

Towler, D.A., Gordon, J.I., Adams, S.P., et al.: The biology and enzymology of eukaryotic protein acylation. Annu. Rev. Biochem., *57:*69–99, 1988.

CHAPTER 25

# Folic Acid and Vitamin $B_{12}$

Victor Herbert and Kshitish C. Das



## HISTORY

The unraveling of the relation of vitamin $B_{12}$ and folic acid to anemia traces back almost two centuries.[1-4] In 1822, the physician Combe reported in Edinburgh on the "history of a case of anemia" that he surmised was due to "some disorder of the digestive and assimilative organs."[5] Thus was launched the study of pernicious anemia in particular and megaloblastic anemia in general, after restimulation by physician Thomas Addison's description, in 1849 and 1855,[6] of what his contemporaries evidently recognized as pernicious anemia. The nutritional basis of pernicious anemia was suspected by the American physician Austin Flint in 1860, when he stated that "in these cases there exists degenerative disease of the glandular tubuli of the stomach."[7]

Another two-thirds of a century had passed when the classic work of physician William Castle and his associates demonstrated that normal human gastric juice contains an "intrinsic factor" (i.e., within the body) that combines with an "extrinsic factor: (i.e., outside the body—in food) contained in animal protein to result in absorption of the "antipernicious anemia principle."[8] Vitamin $B_{12}$ was finally reported as isolated in 1948 in the United States,[9] and three weeks later, entirely independently, in England.[10] Berk and his associates showed that this vitamin was "extrinsic factor" and "antipernicious anemia principle."[11]

Early reports of disease now recognizable as probable folate deficiency include those of Channing,[12] Barclay,[13] and Osler.[14] A decade later Wills and her associates described in Hindu women in Bombay a macrocytic anemia, usually associated with pregnancy,[15] that responded to therapy with a commercial preparation of autolyzed yeast called Marmite; these workers produced in monkeys a similar macrocytic anemia that responded to a "Wills factor" present in crude but not in purified liver extracts.

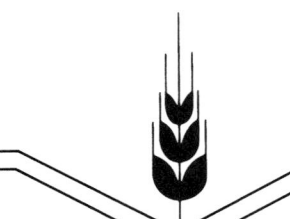

The more purified liver extract was found to be a fairly pure solution of vitamin $B_{12}$, whereas the "Wills factor" from the crude liver extract was found to be folic acid. This was clarified by advances in knowledge of folic acid (e.g., the purification of pteroylglutamic acid in 1943,[16]

its crystallization in the same year,[17] and its synthesis and structural identification in 1946[18]) and by the isolation of vitamin $B_{12}$ in crystalline form in 1948. The rapid isolation of the vitamin was greatly aided by a microbiologic assay based on Shorb's discovery that the growth factor required by Lactobacillus lactis Dorner was the "animal protein factor" necessary for animals fed an all-vegetable diet.[19] The amounts of vitamin $B_{12}$ present in liver extracts closely paralleled their potency in the treatment of pernicious anemia.

Folic acid has proved to be the same as the Wills factor; "vitamin M" contained in dried brewer's yeast that corrected the deficiency anemia, leukopenia, diarrhea, and gingivitis of monkeys[21]; "vitamin Bc" contained in yeast that corrected the deficiency syndrome in chicks characterized by anemia and growth failure; and the Norite eluate factor of liver, essential to the growth of Lactobacillus casei[22] (and therefore also called the "L. casei factor").[23,24] Sulfanilamide was shown to act by competitive inhibition of a bacterial metabolite, *para*-aminobenzoic acid. This metabolite was later found to be an essential component of L. casei factor.[24,25]

The term folic acid was coined in 1941 by Mitchell and co-workers because they found this material in a leafy vegetable (spinach).[26] At that time, it was not recognized that vitamin $B_{12}$, and not folic acid, was the active ingredient in the oral liver therapy that Minot and Murphy reported in 1926 as successful in treating pernicious anemia (for which work they received the Nobel Prize in Medicine in 1934).[27] Considerable progress has since been made in our understanding of the metabolic role of folic acid in health and disease, and of the use of folate antimetabolites in the treatment of some infectious diseases and cancers.

## CHEMISTRY

Neither cyanocobalamin nor pteroylglutamic acid, the common pharmaceutical forms of Vitamin $B_{12}$ and folic acid, is present *as such* in significant quantity in either the human body or the various foods from which these agents were isolated. They are present in various reduced metabolically active coenzyme forms, often conjugated in peptide linkage. During the extraction procedures, these labile active forms are either destroyed by oxidation (particularly folates) or oxidized and converted to cyanocobalamin or pteroylglutamic acid, which are the stable forms of the respective vitamins. Not until they are reduced by metabolic systems present within gut and other tissue cells do these stable forms become metabolically active cobalamins or folates.

### VITAMIN $B_{12}$

Figure 25–1 shows the structural formula of vitamin $B_{12}$ (cyanocobalamin): Delineation of this structure,

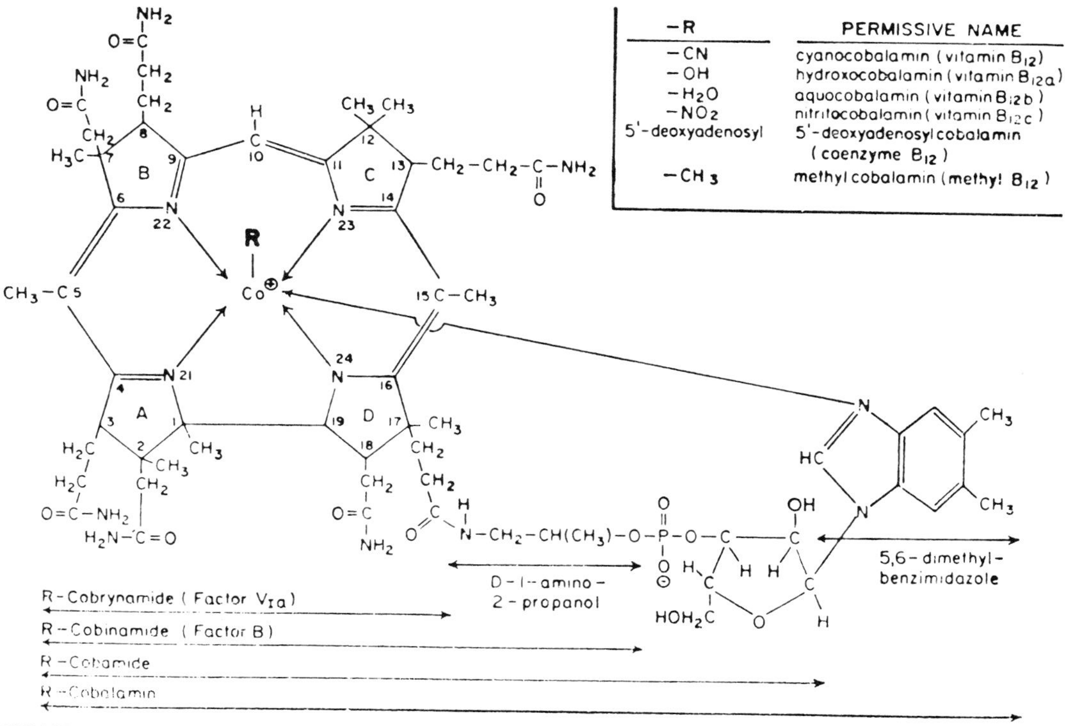

-R
PERMISSIVE NAME
-CN
cyanocobalamin (vitamin B12)
-OH
hydroxocobalamin (vitamin B12a)
-H2O
aquocobalamin (vitamin B12b)
-NO2
nitritocobalamin (vitamin B12c)
5'-deoxyadenosyl
5'-deoxyadenosylcobalamin (coenzyme B12)
-CH3
methylcobalamin (methyl B12)
R
Co
D-1-amino-2-propanol
5,6-dimethyl-benzimidazole
R-Cobrynamide (Factor VIa)
R-Cobinamide (Factor B)
R-Cobamide
R-Cobalamin


**FIGURE 25–1.** Structural formula of vitamin $B_{12}$ (cyanocobalamin). The numbering system for the corrin nucleus is made to correspond to that of the porphin nucleus by omitting the number 20. (Modified from Brown and Reynolds: Annu. Rev. Biochem., *32*:419, 1963.)

using x-ray crystallography, by Hodgkin and her coworkers was partly responsible for her winning the 1964 Nobel Prize in Chemistry. The chemistry of the vitamin has been reviewed in detail.[28] The two major portions of the molecule are the corrin nucleus (a planar group) and a "nucleotide" lying in a plane nearly at right angles to the corrin nucleus and linked to it by D-1-amino-2-propanol. The nucleotide (5-6-dimethylbenzimidazole) is attached to ribose by an α-glycoside linkage. A second bond between the two major parts of the molecule is the coordinate linkage of the cobalt atom to one of the nitrogen atoms of the nucleotide.

In cyanocobalamin, the anionic (-R) group in coordinate linkage with the cobalt is cyanide. The original isolation of $B_{12}$ from liver yielded a stable product, cyanocobalamin, because the unstable linkage of the 5′-deoxyadenosyl anionic group to the rest of the molecule in coenzyme $B_{12}$ (the form naturally dominant in liver) was ruptured and replaced by cyanide, which leached from the charcoal columns used in the isolation procedure.

Cyanocobalamin crystals (M.W. 1355.42) are dark red, and the substance absorbs water (the USP product contains 12% absorbed moisture). Cobalamins are destroyed by heavy metals and strong oxidizing or reducing agents, but not by autoclaving for short periods at 121° C. Ascorbate and other nutrients that are strong reducing agents, when placed in solution with cobalamins, destroy cobalamins by converting them to various analogues,[29] some of which may actually block cobalamin metabolism (i.e., function as antimetabolites).[30] Aqueous solutions are neutral with maximum stability at pH 4.5 to 5.0.

Coenzyme $B_{12}$ (5-deoxyadenosylcobalamin) and methylcobalamin (methyl-$B_{12}$) are the two vitamin $B_{12}$ coenzymes known to be metabolically active in mammalian tissues. Both are unstable in light and undergo photolysis with formation of aquocobalamin or, in the presence of potassium cyanide, cyanocobalamin. Under the rules of the International Union of Pure and Applied Chemistry (IUPAC) Commission on Biochemical Nomenclature,[31] cyanocobalamin is a permissive (semisystematic) name for vitamin $B_{12}$, and the term vitamin $B_{12}$ without qualification means cyanocobalamin exclusively. However, the term is also entrenched in the literature as a generic term for all the cobalamins active in man. The permissive term cobalamin (or vitamin $B_{12}$ ) is used to describe the vitamin $B_{12}$ molecule minus the cyanide group, and is prefixed by the designation of the anionic R group (Fig. 25–1) attached to the cobalt. The terms coenzyme $B_{12}$ and vitamin $B_{12}$ coenzyme are not interchangeable; the former means 5′-deoxyadenosylcobalamin exclusively, and the latter applies to any coenzyme form of $B_{12}$.

Coenzyme $B_{12}$ is more potent therapeutically than cyanocobalamin.[32] All forms of $B_{12}$ appear equipotent when used in greater than minimal daily doses (0.08 mmol = 0.1 μg).

## FOLIC ACID

Figure 25–2 presents the structural formula of folic acid (pteroylglutamic acid, PteGlu or $PteGlu_1$), the reference compound of the folate vitamin forms. The major subunits of the molecule are the pteridine moiety linked by a methylene bridge to para-aminobenzoic acid, which is joined by peptide linkage to glutamic acid.

Crystalline folic acid is yellow (M.W. 441.4). The free acid is almost insoluble in cold water, but the disodium salt is more soluble—about 1.5 g/dl (34.0 nmol/L). Injectable solutions are prepared by dissolving folic acid in isotonic sodium bicarbonate solution, or by using the disodium salt. Folic acid is destroyed at a pH below 4, but is relatively stable above pH 5, with no destruction in 1 hour at 100° C. The molecule usually splits into pteridine and *para*-aminobenzoyl glutamate.

Recommendations of an advisory panel to several Commissions on Nomenclature are as follows: "Folate and folic acid are the preferred synonyms for pteroylglutamate and pteroylglutamic acid, respectively. . . . The term folates may also be used in a generic sense to designate any member of the family of pteroylglutamates, or mixtures of them, having various levels of reduction of the pteridine ring, one-carbon substitutions, and numbers of glutamate residues."[31] The term "folacin" is no longer to be used.

Pteroylglutamic acid, an oxidized compound, is not normally found as such in foods or in the human body in significant concentrations. The forms that are found in such sources are the reduced forms indicated in Figure 25–3. They differ from the parent compound by virtue of one to three structural modifications. First, all are reduced folates and, except for 7,8-dihydrofolate, all are 5,6,7,8-tetrahydrofolates (THF). Second, as indicated in Figure 25–3, various one-carbon adducts may be linked to THF at the N-5, N-10, or N-5, 10 position, conferring on folates their role as one-carbon carriers. N5-formyl

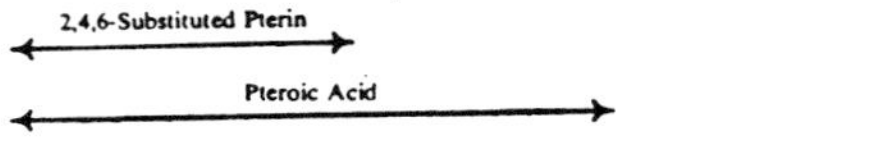
Para-aminobenzoic Acid (PABA)
Glutamic Acid
Para-aminobenzoylglutamic Acid
2,4,6-Substituted Pterin
Pteroic Acid

*Site of attachment of extra glutamate residue(s) of pteroyl di-, tri-, or hepta-glutamate.

Folic Acid (Pteroylmonoglutamic Acid)

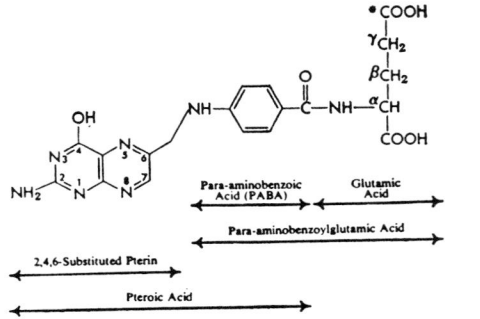

**FIGURE 25–2.** Structural formula of folic acid (pteroylglutamic acid). (From Herbert, V.: Drugs effective in megaloblastic anemia: vitamin $B_{12}$ and folic acid. *In* The Pharmacologic Basis of Therapeutics. 5th Ed. Edited by L.S. Goodman and A. Gilman. New York, Macmillan, 1975, pp. 1324–1349, with permission of Macmillan Publishing.)

| | R | OXIDATION STATE |
|---|---|---|
| $N^5$ formyl THFA | —CHO | formate |
| $N^{10}$ formyl THFA | —CHO | formate |
| $N^5$ formimino THFA | —CH=NH | formate |
| $N^{5,10}$ methenyl THFA | ⋗CH | formate |
| $N^{5,10}$ methylene THFA | >$CH_2$ | formaldehyde |
| $N^5$ methyl THFA | —$CH_3$ | methanol |

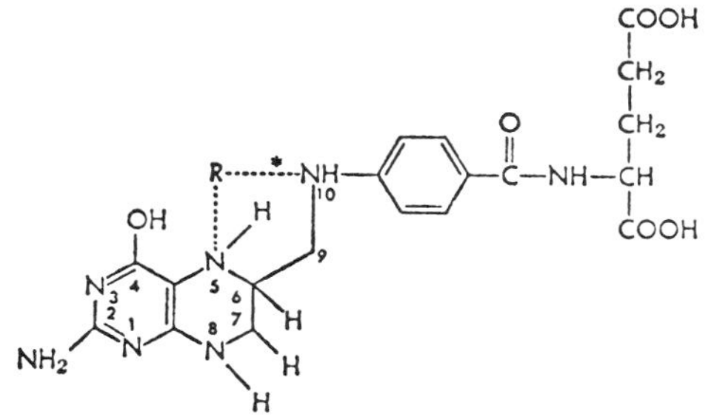
COOH
$CH_2$
$CH_2$
O
R
NH
10
C—NH—CH
COOH
OH
H
9
N
5
6
N
3
4
2
1
8
7
H
$NH_2$
N
N
H
H

*Broken lines indicate the $N^5$ and/or $N^{10}$ site of attachment of various 1-carbon units for which THFA acts as a carrier.

5,6,7,8-Tetrahydrofolic Acid (THFA)($FH_4$)(R=—H)

**FIGURE 25–3.** Structures and nomenclature in the folate field. The table above the formula lists some of the possible one-carbon adducts formed with THFA. (From Herbert V.: Drugs effective in megaloblastic anemia: vitamin $B_{12}$ and folic acid. *In* The Pharmacologic Basis of Therapeutics. 5th Ed. Edited by L.S. Goodman and A. Gilman. New York, Macmillan, 1975, pp. 1324–1349, with permission of Macmillan Publishing.)

THF (folinic acid, citrovorum factor) represents nonenzymatic conversion of folate during processing of natural materials.[33] Third, the number of glutamate residues may vary from one to seven, and sometimes up to 11, each linked by peptide bonds between its amino group and the γ-carboxyl group of the preceding glutamate (see Fig. 25–2).

## UNITS OF MEASUREMENT AND METHODS OF ASSAY

### VITAMIN $B_{12}$

Human serum levels of vitamin $B_{12}$ are measured in picograms (pg = $10^{-12}$ g; also called micromicrograms, or μμg) per ml of serum. Normal values range from 200 to 900 pg/ml (146.6 to 659.7 μmol/L); that below 80 pg/ml (58.64 μmol/L) represents unequivocal $B_{12}$ deficiency according to the World Health Organization (WHO) Scientific Group on Nutritional Anemias.[34] However, the analyzed level below which an unequivocal deficiency actually exists will vary from laboratory to laboratory, depending on the microbiologic or radioassay method used; there is no "gold standard" method for assay.[34,35] In fact, as vitamin $B_{12}$ deficiency develops, $B_{12}$ analogue levels may rise, making assays that measure total corrinoids instead of cobalamins alone unreliable.

The tiny quantity of vitamin $B_{12}$ activity in human serum may be measured only microbiologically or by radioassay. There are many microbiologic assays for vitamin $B_{12}$. Radioassay has several advantages over microbiologic assay: (1) false low results do not occur if serum contains antibiotics or other substances that inhibit growth of microorganisms, and (2) one can perform differential radioassay to separate cobalamins from other corrinoids,[36,37] which cannot be adequately done by differential microbiologic assay. Radioassay for vitamin $B_{12}$ was first described by Herbert in 1958.[38] The most widely employed assay uses coated charcoal to separate free from bound vitamin $B_{12}$,[39] but many other satisfactory separation methods exist.[34,35]

Human serum and tissues contain not only biologically active "true $B_{12}$" (i.e., cobalamins), but also analogues (i.e., noncobalamin corrinoids) of varying to no activity; some may even be antimetabolites.[40] Radioassays that use pure intrinsic factor measure true $B_{12}$. Those that do not use pure intrinsic factor or that use it without its blocking nonintrinsic component by an analoge measure "total $B_{12}$" ("total corrinoids"—i.e., cobalamins plus noncobalamin analogues) rather than true $B_{12}$. Thus such assays may not detect early vitamin $B_{12}$ deficiency, because in early deficiency only that portion of total $B_{12}$ that is true $B_{12}$ may fall, and analogues may still be in the normal range [41] or may even rise. In addition, heat plus the presence of large amounts of vitamin C or other nutrients with strong reducing activity may destroy vitamin $B_{12}$ unless the $B_{12}$ is protected by cyanide, -S, or another protective mechanism.[29,30]

Differential radioassay is necessary to distinguish cobalamin from noncobalamin corrinoids in human serum, erythrocytes, liver, nervous system, and bile. Exposure of $B_{12}$ to vitamin C converts vitamin $B_{12}$ to noncobalamin corrinoids that nondifferential microbiologic assays and radioassays are unable to distinguish from true $B_{12}$.[42]

Larger quantities of vitamin $B_{12}$ than those present in human serum may be assayed calorimetrically, spectroscopically, fluorometrically, or chemically. A serum standard has been proposed.[43] The USP assay for vitamin $B_{12}$ in pharmaceutical preparations is spectrophotometric. A preparation from of liver extract for injection was deleted from the USP in 1960; however, such largely obsolete often allergenic products may still be in use. Differential radioassay demonstrate that 10 to 30% of such "$B_{12}$" in multivitamin-mineral pills may be such analogues.

### FOLIC ACID

Normal human serum contains 5 to 16 ng (1 ng = $10^{-9}$ g) which is the same as 1 millimicrogram, (or 1 mμg), or 11.33 to 36.25 nmol/L of folic acid activity (i.e., PteGlu equivalents) per ml. These tiny quantities could be measured only microbiologically, as originally described in 1959,[44] until a radioisotopic assay was described in the 1970s.[45,46] The dominant form of folate in serum and red cells is 5-methyltetrahydrofolate (Fig. 25–3); folate assays must therefore be capable of measuring this derivative. The only microbiologic assay that adequately measures serum and red cell folate uses L. casei. Similarly, the only radioassays that accurately measure serum folate are those that measure 5-methyltetrahydrofolate. Simultaneous radioisotope determinations of serum vitamin $B_{12}$ and folate can be done in the same sample.[47] The results correlate well with those of other radioassays.

Because serum folate is labile, false low values for serum folate activity occur if the serum has not been protected against oxidative destruction before assay. Such protection is brought about by storing the serum frozen, storing it in the presence of a reducing agent such as ascorbate, or both. However, ascorbate may destroy $B_{12}$ in storage. Larger quantities of folate activity than those normally present in human serum may be measured chemically, fluorometrically, by paper and thin-layer chromatography, enzymatically, or by animal assay.[40]

## ABSORPTION

### VITAMIN $B_{12}$

There are two separate and distinct mechanisms for the absorption of vitamin $B_{12}$. The physiologic mechanism operates as follows: (1) Ingested vitamin $B_{12}$ is freed from its polypeptide linkages in food by gastric acid and by gastric and intestinal enzymes. (2) The free vitamin $B_{12}$ attaches to salivary R binder polypeptide in preference to the gastric intrinsic factor (IF) of Castle. (3) The R binder is destroyed in the small intestine by pancreatic trypsin, thereby releasing $B_{12}$. Free $B_{12}$ then combines with IF; this is a glycoprotein with a molecular weight of about 50,000 that is, produced by normal gastric parietal cells, which dimerizes on combination with vitamin $B_{12}$ so that a complex is formed containing two molecules of vitamin $B_{12}$. (4) The $B_{12}$-IF complex is carried down to the ileum, where it attaches to receptors for $B_{12}$-IF on the brush border of the ileal mucosal cells in the presence of ionic calcium and a pH above 6. (5) The vitamin $B_{12}$-IF complex is taken up by the ileal enterocyte (epithelial cell). (6) The vitamin then diffuses, or is transported across the enterocyte via transcobalamin (TC) II into the portal venous blood, at which point it is attached to serum vitamin $B_{12}$-binding proteins.

Pancreatic bicarbonate and trypsin facilitate this mechanism by selectively destroying R binders.[48] Pancreatic enzymes also effect transfer of biliary cobalamin from R binder to intrinsic factor, creating much of the enterohepatic cobalamin circulation[49] that is so important to the vitamin $B_{12}$ economy of the vegetarian. TC II preferentially binds cobalamins and delivers them to all tissues that need them. TC II is to cobalamin economy what transferrin is to iron economy. Holo-TC III is more a reflection of cobalamin stores.

The pharmacologic mechanism appears to be diffusion. It accounts for the absorption along the entire length of the small intestine of approximately 1% of any quantity of free vitamin $B_{12}$ in the small bowel. This mechanism makes possible oral (rather than parenteral) therapy for vitamin $B_{12}$ deficiency caused by vitamin $B_{12}$ malabsorption. However, such therapy is less reliable than parenteral therapy.[4]

### FOLATE

Food folate is absorbed primarily from the proximal third of the small intestine, although it can be absorbed from the entire length of the small bowel.[50] Folate in food is present primarily in polyglutamate form. Before absorption, the "excess" glutamates must be split off the side chain of the vitamin molecule by enzyme conjugases (pteroylpolyglutamate hydrolase). The products of conjugase action are detectable in the intestinal lumen before absorption, and are due to a surface-active brush border conjugase functionally and chromatographically distinguishable from intracellular conjugase. The bioavailability of ingested folate monoglutamates (PteGlu) is significantly greater than that of folate polyglytamate ($PteGlu_n$) in humans presumably because of the requirement for hydrolysis of the latter.[50] The folate hydrolase (conjugase) present in the brush border of small intestinal enterocytes, though much less abundant than intracellular folate hydrolase, is more than adequate for digestion of the recommended dietary allowance (RDA) of 3 μg (6.8 nmol) folate/kg body weight. Conjugase action may be specifically inhibited by food factors described in yeast and beans and may be nonspecifically impaired at acid pH. The altered activity of the brush border folate hydrolase in certain diseases and following exposure to drugs such as salicylazosulfapyridine, alcohol, and diphenylhydantoin appears to play a significant role in causing malabsorption and deficiency of folate.[50]

Impaired mucosal transport of monoglutamyl folates after deconjugation probably accounts for most instances of folate malabsorption. Active mucosal transport is accelerated by glucose and galactose and impaired by unidentified factors present in many foods. However, studies using mild folate binder (see later) suggest that folate uptake in the gut is facilitated by prior binding. It is probable that a small but relatively unchanging percentage of ingested folate is absorbed by passive diffusion after deconjugation, as is the case with vitamin $B_{12}$.

Folic acid absorbed from the intestine at physiologic concentrations is largely converted to reduced forms and then methylated or formylated, whereas at higher concentrations, it is transported through the enterocytes without such modifications.[51] However, transfer of folate from the intestine to the circulation occurs faster with reduced and formylated or methylated forms than with folic acid.[52] The mechanism by which folate is transported from the enterocytes to the lamine propria of the villi or the circulation is poorly understood; a carrier-mediated system has been postulated.[53]

## TRANSPORT, DISTRIBUTION, STORAGE, AND EXCRETION

### VITAMIN $B_{12}$ (FIG. 25–4*A*)

**Binding Proteins.** Vitamin $B_{12}$ in human serum is bound to three different vitamin $B_{12}$-binding proteins: transcobalamins I, II, and III (TCI, TCII, and TCIII). The normal total $B_{12}$-binding capacity (TBBC) of serum ranges from about 1000 to 1800 pg/ml (700 to 1260 pmol/L), and the unsaturated vitamin $B_{12}$-binding capacity (UBBC) ranges from 600 to 1400 pg/ml (420 to 980 pmol/L), largely due to TCII (450 to 1000 pg/ml, or 315 to 700 pmol/L).[51] TCI and TCIII are glycoproteins that are synthesized mainly in granulocytes,[54] but possibly also in salivary glands, gastric mucosa, and some hepatomas.[55] They have a molecular weight of about 60,000, and appear to have largely a storage function, although TCIII may be involved in redelivery of vitamin $B_{12}$ to the liver, to which TCIII may attach via a terminal galactose. The amounts of unsaturated TCI and TCIII in serum range from 30 to 110 pg/ml (21 to 77 pmol/L) and 120 to 3000 pg/ml (84 to 210 pmol/L), respectively.[56] These glycoproteins are referred to by some as cobalophilins or haptocorrin (R proteins). They are microheterogenous mixtures of various isoproteins in different proportions.[57]

TBBC, UBBC, and serum vitamin $B_{12}$ levels all tend to be elevated in any situation in which the total body neutrophil pool is increased (as in myeloproliferative disorders). This elevation is caused by an increase in the amounts of unsaturated TCI and TCIII.[58] These glycoproteins, however, do not appear to deliver vitamin $B_{12}$ to the bone marrow or nerve tissue.[54,59]

**Transport In and From Blood.** TCII, unlike the cobalophilins (TCI and TCIII), is not glycosylated. It has an apparent molecular weight of 38,000,[57] is synthesized largely in the liver,[60] is a β-globulin, and is chiefly responsible for transport and delivery of the vitamin. Relatively little vitamin $B_{12}$ is attached to it in vivo because of the rapidity with which it is degraded as it delivers $B_{12}$ to tissues. When a sample of blood is drawn, only 10 to 20% of plasma vitamin $B_{12}$ (which is mainly methyl-$B_{12}$) is bound to TCII; the rest is bound to cobalophilin, largely TCI (which is 80 to 100% saturated with $B_{12}$). The plasma survival time of TCIII is very short (minutes) compared to TCII, which in turn is short (hours) compared to TCI (days) and to the cobalophilins in chronic myelogenous leukemia and hepatoma.[55]

Vitamin $B_{12}$, upon entering the blood, is bound by TCs in proportion to their binding capacity and delivered by TCII to liver, bone marrow cells, reticulocytes, lymphoblasts, fibroblasts, and tumor cells via a mechanism similar to that by which intrinsic factor delivers the vitamin to ileal mucosal cells. Bone marrow cells, reticulocytes, and many other cells contain on their surfaces "receptor sites" for the TCII-$B_{12}$ complex. These sites will take up the complex only in the presence of ionic calcium and a pH greater than 6;[61] liver cells may also contain receptor sites for TCIII.[54,55] Thus, delivery of $B_{12}$ to the gut enterocyte and the immature erythrocytes both require (1) a transport protein, (2) pH above 6, (3) ionic calcium, and (4) a receptor site for the protein–vitamin $B_{12}$ complex on the surface of the cell.

The importance of TCII in the absorption, transport, and delivery of vitamin $B_{12}$ to the tissues is emphasized by the finding of individuals with congenital absence of TCII who have defective vitamin $B_{12}$ delivery and therefore require treatment with large frequent parent-

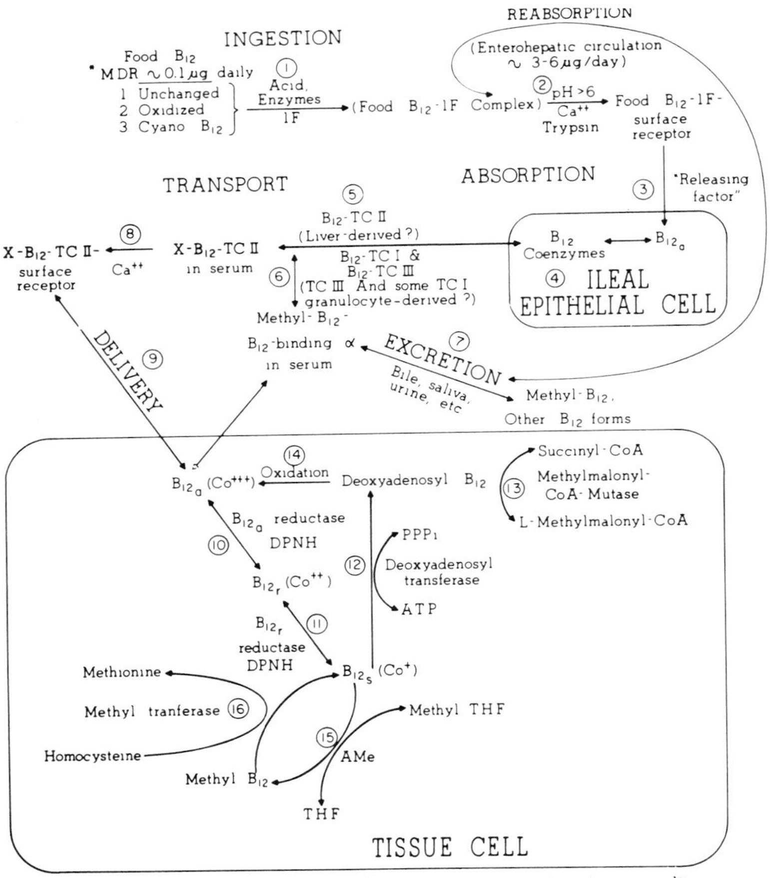
INGESTION
Food B12
*MDR ~0.1 μg daily
1 Unchanged
2 Oxidized
3 Cyano B12
Acid, Enzymes
IF
(Food B12-IF Complex)
REABSORPTION
(Enterohepatic circulation ~ 3-6 μg/day)
pH >6
Ca++
Trypsin
Food B12-IF-surface receptor
"Releasing factor"
ABSORPTION
TRANSPORT
B12-TC II (Liver-derived ?)
B12-TC I & B12-TC III (TC III And some TC I granulocyte-derived ?)
Methyl-B12-
B12-binding α in serum
X-B12-TC II-surface receptor
Ca++
X-B12-TC II in serum
B12 Coenzymes
B12a
ILEAL EPITHELIAL CELL
DELIVERY
EXCRETION
Bile, saliva, urine, etc
Methyl-B12, Other B12 forms
Oxidation
B12a (Co+++)
Deoxyadenosyl B12
Succinyl-CoA
Methylmalonyl-CoA-Mutase
L-Methylmalonyl-CoA
B12a reductase DPNH
PPPi
Deoxyadenosyl transferase
ATP
B12r (Co++)
B12r reductase DPNH
B12s (Co+)
Methionine
Methyl tranferase
Homocysteine
Methyl B12
Methyl THF
AMe
THF
TISSUE CELL

*MDR = Adult minimum daily requirement from exogenous sources to sustain normality

**FIGURE 25–4.** *A*, Cobalamin ($B_{12}$) metabolism in man. *B*, Flow chart of folate metabolism in man. Circled numbers identify individual steps in folate metabolism. In mammals, the same enzyme catalyzes reactions 12, 14, and 19, and another single enzyme catalyzes both steps 16 and 21. THF, Tetrahydrofolate; DHF, dihydrofolate. *In* Textbook of Medicine. 14th Ed. Edited by P.B. Beeson and W. McDermott. Philadelphia, W.B. Saunders, 1975.)

eral doses of the vitamin.[62] The possible "acute phase reactant" status of TCII may be important, including its elevated level in autoimmune disease.[63]

**Storage.** "Normal" stores of vitamin $B_{12}$ range between 1 and 10 mg (0.75 to 7.5 μmol),[64] with the liver containing 50 to 90% of the total stored vitamin (averaging 1 μg $B_{12}$, or 0.8 nmol/g of liver). Some of the stores are not cobalamins but rather noncobalamin analogues. Average vitamin $B_{12}$ stores range between 2 and 5 mg (1.5 to 3.75 μmol). There is little evidence for significant catabolism of vitamin $B_{12}$ by man, and it is probable that loss occurs only by excretion, mainly in the bile. The noncobalamin analogues do not appear to derive mainly by catabolism, but seem to be absorbed across the ileum. The whole-body turnover of vitamin $B_{12}$ is between 0.1 and 0.2% daily, regardless of whether body stores are normal or reduced. Coenzyme $B_{12}$ appears to be the main storage form, and methyl-$B_{12}$ appears to be the main serum transport form.[31]

**Excretion.** The normal enterohepatic circulation of vitamin $B_{12}$ may account for approximately 0.6 to 6 μg (0.45 to 4.5 nmol) of the vitamin excreted daily in the bile and reabsorbed in the ileum.[4] This almost total conservation of vitamin $B_{12}$ explains why pure vegetarians, who eat almost no vitamin $B_{12}$, take decades to develop deficiency of the vitamin. It is only when the reabsorption phase of the enterohepatic circulation of the vitamin is damaged, by damage to the stomach, ileum, or pancreas, that vitamin $B_{12}$ deficiency disease develops more rapidly (i.e., in 3 to 6 years).[65]

The effect of the enterohepatic circulation is to remove noncobalamin vitamin $B_{12}$ analogues from the body,

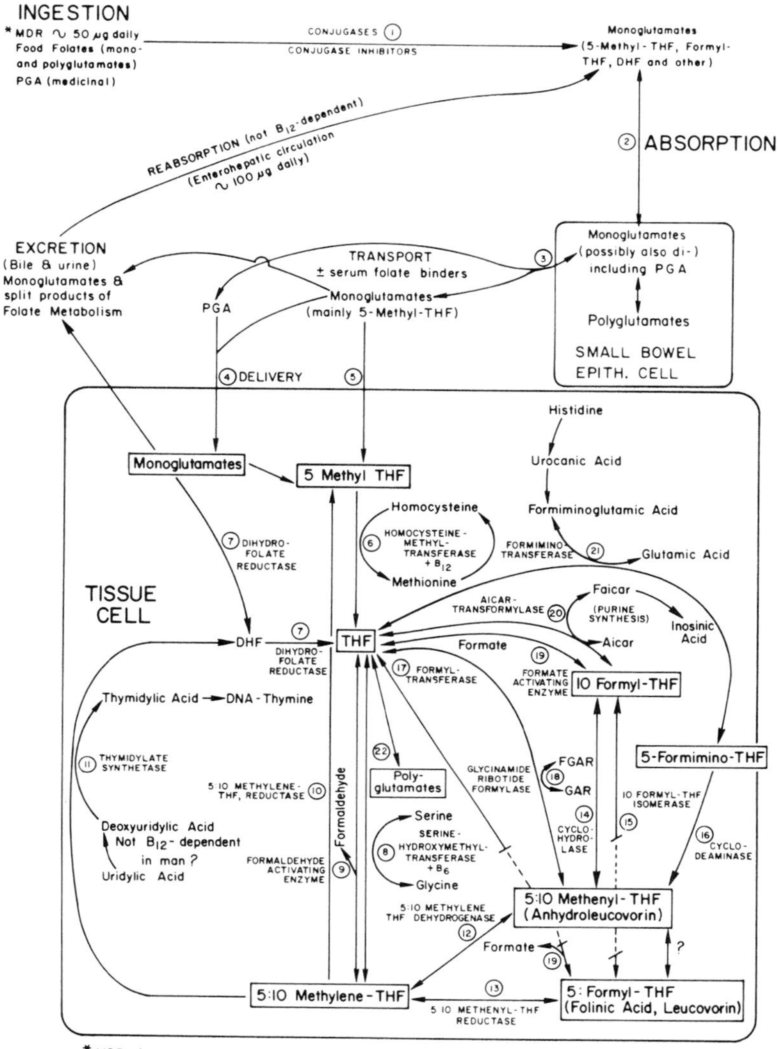
INGESTION
* MDR ∿ 50 μg daily
Food Folates (mono- and polyglutamates)
PGA (medicinal)
CONJUGASES ①
CONJUGASE INHIBITORS
Monoglutamates (5-Methyl-THF, Formyl-THF, DHF and other)
REABSORPTION (not B12-dependent)
(Enterohepatic circulation ∿ 100 μg daily)
② ABSORPTION
EXCRETION
(Bile & urine)
Monoglutamates & split products of Folate Metabolism
TRANSPORT
± serum folate binders
③
Monoglutamates (possibly also di-) including PGA
Polyglutamates
SMALL BOWEL EPITH. CELL
PGA
Monoglutamates (mainly 5-Methyl-THF)
④ DELIVERY
⑤
TISSUE CELL
Monoglutamates
5 Methyl THF
Histidine
Urocanic Acid
Formiminoglutamic Acid
Homocysteine
⑥ HOMOCYSTEINE-METHYL-TRANSFERASE + B12
Methionine
FORMIMINO-TRANSFERASE ㉑
Glutamic Acid
⑦ DIHYDRO-FOLATE REDUCTASE
AICAR-TRANSFORMYLASE ⑳
Faicar
(PURINE SYNTHESIS)
Inosinic Acid
Aicar
DHF
⑦ DIHYDRO-FOLATE REDUCTASE
THF
Formate
⑲
⑰ FORMYL-TRANSFERASE
FORMATE ACTIVATING ENZYME
10 Formyl-THF
Thymidylic Acid → DNA-Thymine
⑪ THYMIDYLATE SYNTHETASE
5·10 METHYLENE-THF, REDUCTASE ⑩
Formaldehyde
㉒
Poly-glutamates
GLYCINAMIDE RIBOTIDE FORMYLASE
FGAR
⑱
GAR
5-Formimino-THF
10 FORMYL-THF ISOMERASE
⑭ CYCLO-HYDRO-LASE
⑮
⑯ CYCLO-DEAMINASE
Deoxyuridylic Acid
Not B12-dependent in man?
Uridylic Acid
Serine
⑧ SERINE-HYDROXYMETHYL-TRANSFERASE + B6
Glycine
FORMALDEHYDE ACTIVATING ENZYME ⑨
5·10 METHYLENE THF DEHYDROGENASE
⑫
5:10 Methenyl-THF (Anhydroleucovorin)
Formate
⑲
?
5:10 Methylene-THF
⑬
5·10 METHENYL-THF REDUCTASE
5: Formyl-THF (Folinic Acid, Leucovorin)

* MDR = Adult minimum daily requirement from exogenous sources to sustain normality

**FIGURE 25–4.** *(continued)*

because about 60% of the corrinoids excreted in bile are analogues,[66] and cobalamin is normally preferentially reabsorbed over analogues.[67] The role of noncobalamin vitamin $B_{12}$ analogues in human vitamin $B_{12}$ economy is unknown, but some may act as antivitamins and could prove harmful.[37] Although noncobalamin carrinoids in humans may primarily derive from vitamin supplements fed to livestock and subsequently ingested by humans, analogue levels of Americans are similar to those in Kalahari Bushmen never exposed to supplements.

## FOLATE (FIG. 25–4*B*)

**Binding Proteins and Transport.** Transport of folate is much less clearly elucidated than that of vitamin $B_{12}$. Folate in plasma appears to be distributed in three fractions; free folate and that loosely bound to low-affinity binders are similar in magnitude, with much less being bound to high-affinity binders. Low-affinity binding is a nonspecific property of many different plasma proteins, including albumin, and is similar to nonspecific binding of bilirubin and various drugs. It was detected many years ago using ultrafiltration, equilibrium dialysis, and gel filtration. The potential binding capacity is several hundred times greater than the amount of folate in serum. Early data showing failure to half-saturate these binders at high concentrations of free folate indicate that the affinity constant of the system is less than 104 L/mol, which might be compared to the 106 L/mol affinity constant of the carrier-mediated cell transport system for folate.[66]

Study of the high-affinity serum folate binders was initiated by the discovery of such binders in chronic myeloid leukemia cells, and in the serum of the same patients.[67] They are demonstrable in granulocytes of a proportion of nonleukemic subjects, and are released into the serum by these cells. Although their release has not yet been detected in most normal subjects, all human (and animal) serum contains these binders, which more often than not are largely saturated.[68]

Only one class of high-affinity serum folate binders are thought to exist. These binders are glycoproteins with a molecular weight of about 40,000; they are probably synthesized in and released from granulocytes, but are modified in liver and perhaps in kidney.[68] They have binding constants (Kd) of approximately $10^{-10}$ mol/L folic acid and of the order of $10^{-8}$ mol/L 5-methyltetrahydrofolate, the main forms of folate present in serum. Although these affinities indicate that binder would only be half saturated at usual serum methyltetrahydrofolate concentrations, they normally average 67% saturation. This higher-than-expected saturation may be due to the binding of small quantities of nonmethyl unsubstituted folates on binders. Because of their low concentration in plasma, these binders carry less than 5% of serum folate.

Their physiologic function has not yet been demonstrated, but they may play a role in (1) folate delivery to liver, similar to the role of transcobalamin I in vitamin $B_{12}$ transport, (2) controlling folate distribution, breakdown, and excretion in deficient states, and (3) transporting oxidized folates from cerebrospinal fluid to blood. They are also present in milk, where they may enhance folate absorption from gut, and they may be related to a membrane protein-mediated uptake of folate. High-affinity folate binding protein found in human serum appears to have a higher affinity for folic acid (PteGlu) than for reduced folate.[69] Folate-binding proteins in several tissues closely resemble the serum binders.[66]

Folate is delivered to bone marrow cells, reticulocytes, liver, cerebrospinal fluid, and renal tubular cells against a concentration gradient in a manner that suggests energy-dependent carrier-mediated transport.[70] The transport constant (Km) of these systems is about $10^{-6}$ M. Methyltetrahydrofolate, which accounts for almost all serum folate, appears to be transported more efficiently than folic acid across the intestinal cells and into the cells of the body. A red cell membrane protein that binds folates (including methyltetrahydrofolate) and is immunologically cross-reactive with folate binders in placenta, milk, and serum increases in quantity when cells are grown in low-folate medium. This phenomenon suggests that it may be important in cellular folate transport.

**Storage.** Normal total-body folate stores range from 5 to 10 mg (11.3 to 22.6 mmol), of which approximately half is in the liver. It has been suggested that the enterohepatic circulation, which transports about 0.1 mg (0.226 mmol) of biologically active folate daily, is important in the maintenance of serum folate levels.

Most stored folate is present as polyglutamates,[33] which have far greater molecular size and charge than monoglutamates. Transport across cell walls probably requires hydrolysis to monoglutamates, and the enzymes responsible for polyglutamate systhesis and hydrolysis are thus thought to play a major role in folate storage. These enzymes, which have been incompletely characterized, are known respectively as polyglutamate synthetase and conjugase (pteroylpolyglutamate hydrolase; γ-glutamylcarboxypeptidase). Conjugase, which has been more fully studied than the synthetase, is present in almost all mammalian tissue and is under partial hormonal control. Some of the folate-dependent reactions shown in Figure 25–4*B* are altered by varying glutamyl chain lengths. Folate polyglutamate synthetase has been purified from human liver and organs of other mammals; the enzyme is relatively unstable and is found in low quantity. The folate monoglutamates are the circulating and transport forms, whereas polyglutamates are the main intracellular storage forms of this vitamin. Recent evidences indicate that folate polyglutamates are the preferred substrates and active coenzyme forms in various 1-carbon metabolism and thereby regulate these metabolic processes.[66]

**Excretion.** Folate is excreted in urine and bile in metabolically active and inactive forms. Urinary excretion of the biologically active material occurs after glomerular filtration of the free fraction and reabsorption of some filtered folate by active transport across the tubular cell wall. The principal breakdown product of folate in urine, acetamidobenzoylglutamate, suggests that the principal route of folate catabolism occurs through oxidative cleavage of the folate molecule at the 9–10 bond, with acetylation of the *para*-aminobenzyl moiety in the liver before excretion.[71] Some workers believe that scorbutic patients may lose large amounts of folate through irreversible oxidation of 10-formylfolate and excretion of the latter in the urine.[72]

As mention previously, about 100 μg of biologically active folate is excreted in the bile daily. Studies with radioactive tracer folates indicate that a large proportion of injected radioactivity is excreted in the bile as a biologically inactive compound that is not a product of 9–10 cleavage, but that has not been well characterized. Alcohol interferes with the folate enterohepatic cycle. In chronic alcoholics, all six major causes of folate deficiency, as defined earlier, may occur simultaneously.[73] For these reasons, nearly all alcoholics are in negative balance, and the majority are clinically folate-deficient.

## NUTRITIONAL REQUIREMENTS IN HEALTH

The term *minimal daily requirement* (MDR), as used in this chapter, means the minimum *from exogenous sources* required to sustain normality, with normality defined as the absence of any biochemical hypofunction that is correctable by addition of greater quantities of the vitamin. By this definition, the MDR for vitamin $B_{12}$ of a normal subject would be only 0.1 μg (0.075 nmol), because this quantity will sustain normality in a normal subject.[74] The MDR for vitamin $B_{12}$ of a patient with gastric or ileal structural or functional damage would be greater because such damage eliminates not only the normal absorption of vitamin $B_{12}$ from exogenous (food) sources, but also the normal daily reabsorption from the ileum of almost all the vitamin $B_{12}$ normally excreted each day in bile.

The MDR can be reduced to a formula: MDR (units/day) = UBS (units ÷ D (days), where MDR = minimal daily requirement of nutrient from exogenous sources, UBS = utilizable body stores of nutrient, and D = number of days required to develop tissue deficiency after cessation of absorption from exogeneous sources of nutrient (with appropriate correction for incomplete cessation of absorption).[75] Utilization rate is constant in the normal person, but first-order as negative balance progresses. As suggested previously, one can predict the time it would take any given nutrient deficiency to develop in any given person after reduction or cessation of absorption of the nutrient if one knows (or can reasonably estimate) the MDR for the nutrient and the utilizable body stores thereof.

The RDA for folate and $B_{12}$ is intentionally substantially greater than the MDR in order to produce some measurable amount of body stores to allow for normal variation in utilization and transient increased requirements (see Appendix Table A–2b). There is a tendency to err on the side of larger body stores when information is incomplete. Small storage surpluses of nutrients are rarely detrimental, whereas small deficits may result in deficiency over a long period of subtle negative balance.

## VITAMIN $B_{12}$

These requirements have been estimated from three different types of studies: (1) those designed to determine the minimal amount needed to prevent or to cure megaloblastic anemia resulting from vitamin $B_{12}$ deficiency, (2) those correlating the relationship between the levels of vitamin $B_{12}$ in serum and in liver in deficient and healthy subjects, and (3) those correlating body stores and turnover rates of vitamin $B_{12}$.

The results of such studies [34] demonstrated the following: (1) The minimum quantity of vitamin $B_{12}$ required to produce a hematologic response in patients with uncomplicated vitamin $B_{12}$ deficiency was approximately 0.1 μg (0.075 nmol) daily; 0.5 to 1 μg (0.375 to 0.75 nmol) of the vitamin daily produced maximum hematologic responses, with similar amounts maintaining a normal picture. (2) Patients with moderate vitamin $B_{12}$ deficiency resulting from $B_{12}$ malabsorption had an average liver vitamin $B_{12}$ content of 0.16 μg (0.12 nmol)/g wet weight of liver, associated with serum vitamin $B_{12}$ levels ranging from 80 to 130 pg/ml (60 to 97.5 pmol/L) and an average total body $B_{12}$ of approximately 250 μg (0.186 μmol). A second group of individuals who were also suffering from vitamin $B_{12}$ malabsorption, but who had not yet developed morphologic evidence of blood damage due to vitamin $B_{12}$ deficiency, all had serum levels between 130 and 200 pg/ml (97.5 to 150 pmol/L), associated with approximately 0.28 μg (0.21 nmol) of vitamin $B_{12}$/g wet weight of liver and an average total body vitamin $B_{12}$ content of approximately 525 μg (0.394 μmol). (3) The daily whole-body turnover of vitamin $B_{12}$ measured with tracer doses of radioactive vitamin indicated a radioactivity turnover of between 0.1 and 0.2% daily, regardless of whether the body vitamin $B_{12}$ stores are normal or reduced.

Loss of 0.1 to 0.2% of radioactive vitamin $B_{12}$ daily means less than that quantity of vitamin is lost from the body stores daily because the radioactive $B_{12}$ excreted in the bile mixes with nonradioactive $B_{12}$ in the diet, and some of the radioactive $B_{12}$ that would otherwise be reabsorbed in the ileum is replaced by absorbed nonradioactive vitamin. The net result is a gradual reduction in the radioactivity of the body vitamin $B_{12}$ stores, but a much lesser reduction in the actual vitamin $B_{12}$ content of those stores.

The 1989 RDA for vitamin $B_{12}$ is 2 μg (1.5 nmol) per day for adolescents and normal adults [74] (see Appendix Table A–2b). This figure is less than that of the 1980 RDA revision, but the same as that recommended by the "aborted" NAS 1980–1985 RDA Committee.[65] The Joint FAO/WHO Expert Group recommended in 1987 a daily intake of 1 μg (0.75 nmol) vitamin $B_{12}$ for the normal adult (see Appendix Table A–10) and 2 μg (1.5 nmol) for those with achlorhydria.[34] The 1 μg is based not only on radioactivity turnover studies, but also on studies of minimal amounts needed to prevent or to cure megaloblastic anemia resulting from vitamin $B_{12}$ deficiency, and on studies of the relationship between the levels of vitamin $B_{12}$ in serum and in liver in deficient and in healthy subjects. The 1989 RDA of 2 μg (1.5 nmol) for adults carries a greater margin above normal physiologic requirements for absorption of the vitamin by the nonachlorhydric adult than does the FAO/WHO recommendation, resulting in larger tissue stores. There is no clear evidence that these larger stores constitute a benefit (or a harm).

Vitamin $B_{12}$ deficiency does not occur in normal children on adequate calorie and animal protein intakes. The Joint FAO/WHO Expert Group calculated desirable intakes of vitamin $B_{12}$ for children as 0.04 μg (0.03 nmol)/kg body weight per day to a maximum of 1 μg (0.75 nmol) per day.[34] The 1989 RDA figures are 0.3 and 0.5 μg (0.23 and .38 nmol) for infants up to 6 and 12 months old, respectively, progressing to 1.0 μg (.75 nmol) for children 7 to 10 years old.[74]

Pregnancy produces an increased requirement for vitamin $B_{12}$ owing to the fetal drain on maternal stores. The fetus removes approximately 0.2 μg (0.15 nmol) of vitamin $B_{12}$ daily from the maternal stores in the latter half of pregnancy. The Joint FAO/WHO Expert Group calculated the desirable daily intake of vitamin $B_{12}$ in pregnancy to be the adult 1 μg (0.75 nmol) plus an additional 0.4 μg (0.3 nmol), and in lactation an additional 0.3 μg (0.225 nmol) on top of the adult 1 μg (0.75 nmol).[34] The 1989 RDA adds an additional 0.2 μg (0.15 nmol) daily for pregnancy and 0.6 μg (0.45 nmol) per day of lactation[74] (see Appendix Table A–2b).

Vitamin $B_{12}$ deficiency does not occur in breast-fed infants unless their mothers are deficient in the vitamin. Infants showing such deficiency respond hematologically to 0.2 μg (0.15 nmol) vitamin $B_{12}$ orally.[75] In economically advanced countries, breast milk with a content of about 0.4 μg (0.3 nmol)/L supplies about 0.3 μg (0.225 nmol) of vitamin $B_{12}$ daily, which is clearly adequate as manifested by the lack of evidence of any deficiency in the infant. Available evidence suggests that the milk from mothers whose serum contains vitamin $B_{12}$ concentrations close to the lower limit of normality (i.e., 200 pg/ml (150 pmol/L)) is also adequate, whereas the milk of vegetarian mothers who have still lower serum levels is not adequate when it falls to 0.07 μg (0.053 nmol/L of breast milk or less. The Joint FAO/WHO Expert Group therefore recommended a daily intake of 0.1 μg (0.075 nmol) of vitamin $B_{12}$ in breast milk as adequate for infants.[34] The 1989 RDA recommended 2.6 μg for lactating women.[74]

The natural source of this vitamin in nature is synthesis by microorganisms; hence it is not found in plants except when they are contaminated by microorganisms. Fruits, vegetables, and grains and grain products are usually devoid of vitamin $B_{12}$. Small amounts of vitamin $B_{12}$ in legumes, which contain microorganisms, and in contaminated food may provide the only dietary source of vitamin $B_{12}$ for strict vegetarians. Rich sources of vitamin $B_{12}$—greater than 10 μg (7.5 nmol)/100 g of wet weight—are organ meats such as lamb and beef liver, kidney, and heart, and bivalves (clams, oysters) that siphon large quantities of vitamin $B_{12}$–synthesizing microorganisms from the sea (See Appendix Table A–21a). Moderately high amounts—3 to 10 μg (2.25 to 7.5 nmol)/100 g of wet weight—are present in nonfat dry milk, some seafood (crabs, rock fish, salmon, sardines), and egg yolk. Moderate amounts—1 to 3 μg (0.75 to 2.25 nmol)/100 g of wet weight—are found in fluid milk products, cream, cheddar cheese, and cottage cheese. Bacteria in the knobby growth of some seaweeds make the vitamin.

The vitamin $B_{12}$ molecule is resistant to heat unless exposed in an alkaline medium to temperatures in excess of 100° C. Boiling muscle meat at 170° C for 45 minutes results in a loss of 30% of the vitamin from the meat. Milk pasteurized for 2 to 3 seconds loses 7% of its available vitamin $B_{12}$; when boiled for 2 to 5 minutes, it loses 30%. Sterilization in a bottle for 13 minutes at 119 to 120° C causes a loss of 77%; rapid sterilization (3 to 4 seconds) with superheated steam at 143° C destroys only about 10% of vitamin.[64] In the presence of ascorbic acid, vitamin $B_{12}$ is less heat-stable, and substantial amounts in food may be destroyed by 0.5 g of ascorbic acid.[41]

The enzymatically active forms of vitamin $B_{12}$ (coenzyme $B_{12}$) and methylcobalamin) are the dominant forms in foodstuffs, in which they are generally attached to polypeptides. Cyanocobalamin per se is probably not present to a significant extent in any natural source, but may result from the action of cyanide (from tobacco smoke) on natural vitamin $B_{12}$ coenzymes.

## FOLIC ACID

The MDR for folate is approximately 50 μg (113.3 nmol) for adults. The FAO/WHO Expert Group in 1987 recommended a daily dietary intake for adults of 3.1 μg (2.3 nmol)/kg of body weight, to equal a daily intake of 200 μg (453.33 nmol) for a 65-kg man and 170 μg (128 nmol) for a 55-kg woman[34] (Appendix Table A–10). This amount will provide stores sufficient to prevent deficiency for 3 to 4 months of zero intake. To meet the added needs of pregnant women, WHO/FAO recommends a supplement of 200 to 300 μg (453.33 to 680.0 nmol) daily, so that the daily folate intake is no less than 350 μg (793.33 nmol) (or 7 μg/kg body weight), and a supplement of 100 μg (226.67 nmol) per day during lactation (i.e., a total of 5 μg, or 11.33 nmol, per kg body weight). The 1989 RDA (see Appendix Table A–2b) ranges from 25 μg (56.7 nmol) for young infants, 35 μg for those 6 to 12 months old, and 50, 75, and 100 μg (227 nmol) for those 1 to 3, 4 to 6, and 7 to 10 years old, respectively. Males of 11 to 14 years of age should receive 150 μg, and thereafter 200 μg; females 11 to 14 years old should receive 150 μg, and thereafter 180 μg. Pregnant women should receive 400 μg, and lactating women should receive 280 μg for the first 6 months and 260 μg for the second 6 months.[74] On the basis of percentage, these values are appreciably lower than those of the 1980 RDA.

The daily folate requirement is increased by factors that increase metabolic rate (such as infection and hyperthyroidism) and by those that increase cell turnover (such as hemolytic anemia, rapid tissue growth in the fetus, and malignant tumors). Folate consumption by individual cells is proportional to their rate of one-carbon-unit transfer. As noted earlier, alcohol interferes with folate utilization, and thereby increases folate requirement.

**Natural Sources of Folate.** Unlike vitamin $B_{12}$, which is present only in animal protein, folates are ubiquitous in nature, being present in nearly all natural foods (see Appendix Table A–21a) . Again unlike vitamin $B_{12}$, folate is highly susceptible to oxidative destruction: 50 to 95% of the folate content of foods may be destroyed by protracted cooking or other processing, such as canning, and all folate is lost from refined foods such as hard liquor and hard candies. Foods with the highest folate content per unit of dry weight include yeast, liver and other organ meats, fresh green vegetables, and some fresh fruits.

The naturally occurring folates are active metabolic forms, usually in polyglutamate linkage[33] (with pteroylheptaglytamates dominant in yeast). Conjugases present in vegetable and mammalian tissues[76] (including human intestine) liberate pteroyldiglutamates and pteroylmonoglutamates from the conjugates, thereby making the folate available for absorption. As mentioned earlier, about 90% of the monoglutamate is absorbed by humans when ingested alone, but this percentage is markedly decreased in the presence of many foods, irrespective of whether the folate was derived from or added to the food.[77]

The pharmaceutic product pteroylglutamic acid (PGA), like the pharmaceutic product cyanocobalamin, is not usually found as such in natural sources. Its isolation from natural sources, like the isolation of cyanocobalamin, was the result of oxidation and deconjugation of the naturally occurring conjugated forms to a stable form.

## CAUSES OF NUTRITIONAL DEFICIENCY

In the final analysis, nutritional deficiency means that the amount of a biologically active nutrient in one or more intracellular systems is inadequate to sustain normal biochemical functions. Such inadequate use falls in one or more of six basic categories: inadequate ingestion, inadequate absorption, inadequate utilization, increased requirement, increased excretion, and increased destruction. Any one or combination of these three inadequacies and three excesses may result in nutritional deficiency. Table 25–1 presents the currently known possible etiologic factors in each of these six categories that may produce a nutritional deficiency of vitamin $B_{12}$ or folic acid. The ensuing sections will discuss in more detail mechanisms of inadequate absorption and utilization of these two vitamins.

## VITAMIN $B_{12}$ DEPLETION: PROGRESSION AND DETECTION

From normality to deficiency is an overlapping continuum of two stages of progressive depletion followed by two of progressive deficiency.[78] The sequence of events in developing vitamin $B_{12}$ deficiency is delineated in Figure 25–5 and involves the concept of four stages of depletion for vitamins using vitamin $B_{12}$[78] and folate [73] as models. In the first stage, negative vitamin $B_{12}$ balance begins when vitamin $B_{12}$ absorption falls low enough to deplete the amount of vitamin $B_{12}$ on its primary delivery protein, TCII, resulting in a low holo-TCII level, even though total vitamin $B_{12}$ level remains within normal limits. For any laboratory test, because of individual variability, deviation from the value normal for the individual often precedes deviation from the range of normal for the laboratory. A decrease in holo-TC level may be the earliest detectable sign of developing vitamin $B_{12}$ deficiency.[78]

The serum cobalamin level has been generally considered a sensitive index for the detection of clinical disorders caused by cobalamin deficiency. However, normal serum cobalamin level is found in a significant minority of patients with typical or atypical clinical features of this vitamin deficiency; on the other hand, many patients with low serum cobalamin concentrations, particularly vegetarians and vegans, do not show significant clinical evidence of deficiency.[79-81] Elevated levels of methylmalonic acid and total homocysteine in serum, measured by recently improved techniques of gas chromatography–mass spectrometry are found in over 90% of cases of cobalamin deficiency.[80,81]

The deoxyuridine (dU) suppression tests in bone marrow cells and PHA-stimulated lymphocytes (microculture of whole-blood lymphocytes) are highly sensitive tests for the detection of early, subtle, or occult deficiency of vitamin $B_{12}$ or folate and of deficiency masked by concomitant iron deficiency or thalassemia.[82] Recent studies on patients with acquired immunodeficiency syndrome (AIDS) who developed cobalamin deficiency have shown that the earliest serum marker of subnormal vitamin $B_{12}$ absorption, and therefore of negative vitamin $B_{12}$ balance, is a fall in serum holoTCII, even when serum homocysteine level and classic Schilling test (oral free radio $B_{12}$) are both normal[78]; an abnormal food Schilling test (oral protein–bound radio-$B_{12}$) may indicate subnormal vitamin $B_{12}$ absorption in these patients. This may correlate well with the development of an abnormal dU suppression test. This may explain why about 10% of Hindu Indian vegetarians with early cobalamin deficiency did not yet have an elevated mean corpuscular volume (MCV) (particularly with their frequent iron deficiency) or anemia.

## FOLATE DEPLETION: PROGRESSION AND DETECTION

The sequence of events in developing folate deficiency in man is depicted in Figures 25–6 and 25–7. The stages are as follows[73]:

*Stage 1:* Early negative nutrient balance characterized by a fall in serum folate to below 3 ng/ml (6.8 nmol). The state of body folate stores as indicated by a red cell folate level >200 ng/ml (453.3 nmol/L) is not detectably affected.

*Stage 2:* Folate depletion as indicated by a low serum folate, and characteristically by a fall in erythrocyte folate below 160 ng/ml (362.67 nmol/L) (and pari passu by a fall in hepatic folate content).

*Stage 3:* Folate deficient erythropoiesis. This condition is indicated by defective DNA synthesis, an abnormal diagnostic deoxyuridine (dU) suppression test correctable in vitro by folates, and granulocyte nuclear hypersegmentation.

*Stage 4:* Clinical folate deficiency as manifested by gross macro-ovalocytosis, elevated mean corpuscular volume (MCV), and anemia.

More than half of folate-depleted individuals who have not yet reached the stage of anemia will be missed by

**TABLE 25–1.** CAUSES OF VITAMIN $B_{12}$ DEFICIENCY

**I.** Inadequate ingestion
  **A.** Poor diet (lacking microorganisms and animal foods, which are the sole $B_{12}$ sources)
    **1.** Strict vegetarianism (eating no meat, fowl, seafood, eggs, milk, or any products thereof)
    **2.** Chronic alcoholism (no $B_{12}$ or folate in hard liquor: folate deficiency occurs first, and is more common, partly because body stores of $B_{12}$ last much longer than those of folate)
    **3.** Poverty, religious tenets (Hinduism, Seventh-Day Adventism,* certain Catholic orders), dietary faddism
**II.** Inadequate absorption
  **A.** Gastric disorder, producing inadequate or absent secretion by gastric parietal cells of intrinsic factor
    **1.** Addisonian pernicious anemia (PA—that form of $B_{12}$ deficiency disease due to inadequate intrinsic factor secretion of uncertain cause)
      a) Hereditary absence of normal intrinsic factor secretion: absent secretion at birth (circulating antibody to intrinsic factor never present) supports theory that antibody only occurs when antigenic stimulus is produced by intrinsic factor, which enters blood from damaged parietal cells and is recognized as foreign by the immunologic surveillance system); rare
      b) Congenital production of defective intrinsic factor molecule (three published cases)
      c) Autoimmunity-associated gastric atrophy. These patients usually have nondiagnostic-for-PA circulating parietal cell antibody, which is an index only of past or present gastric damage and not of amount of intrinsic factor secretion (circulating diagnostic-for-PA antibody to intrinsic factor is always present under age 21; there is a gradual decrease in measurable antibody, so that by age 65 only two-thirds of patients present with measurable circulating antibody to intrinsic factor)
        1) Juvenile pernicious anemia (usually presents between ages 3 and 14)
        2) Hereditarily determined degenerative gastric atrophy (gradually progressing with increasing age; almost half of all adult PA cases fall into this category)
        3) Acquired gastric atrophy as the end-result of superficial inflammatory gastritis; superficail gastritis with atrophy (almost half of all adult PA cases fall into this category, which includes acquired gastric damage related to iron deficiency or alcohol)
        4) Endocrine disorders (hypothyroidism, polyendocrinopinopathy) associated with gastric damage
    **2.** Gastrectomy
      a) Total
      b) Subtotal (approximately 20% develop PA within 10 years after surgery, associated with atrophy of remaining parietal cells)
        1) Proximal
        2) Distal
        3) Lesions that destroy the gastric mucosa (ingested corrosives, linitis plastica)
        4) Intrinsic factor inhibitor in gastric section
      c) Antibody to intrinsic factor (in saliva or gastric juice)
        1) "Blocking" antibody (attaches to intrinsic factor to block ability of intrinsic factor to take up $B_{12}$
        2) "Binding" antibody (attaches to intrinsic factor at site distal to site of $B_{12}$ attachment)
      d) Small intestinal disorder (affecting ileum, which is the main site of $B_{12}$ absorption)
        1) Gluten-induced enteropathy (childhood and adult celiac disease); idiopathic steatorrhea; nontropical sprue
        2) Tropical sprue ($B_{12}$ is often the first nutrient to be subnormally absorbed and the last to return to normal absorption)
        3) Regional enteritis
        4) Strictures or anastomoses of the small bowel, other "stagnant bowel" syndromes
        5) Intestinal resection
        6) Cancers and granulomatous lesions involving the small intestine
        7) Other conditions characterized by chronically disturbed intestinal function

screening tests that do not recognize that folate depletion may precede anemia by months.

## METABOLIC FUNCTIONS AND INTERRELATIONSHIPS

### DNA SYNTHESIS

As illustrated in Figure 25–8, both vitamin $B_{12}$ and folic acid are required for synthesis of thymidylate and, therefore, of DNA. A vitamin $B_{12}$–containing enzyme removes a methyl group from methyl folate and delivers it to homocysteine, thereby converting homocysteine to methionine (methyl-homocysteine) and regenerating tetrahydrofolic acid (THFA) from which the 5,10-methylene THFA involved in thymidylate synthesis is made. Methyl folate is the dominant form of folate in human serum and liver, and probably also in other body storage depots for folate. Because methyl folate may only return to the body's folate pool via a vitamin $B_{12}$–dependent step, a patient with vitamin $B_{12}$ deficiency has much of his folate "trapped" as methyl folate, which is metabolically inactive. This "folate trap" hypothesis helps explain the

**TABLE 25–1.** *(continued)*

8) Drugs damaging $B_{12}$ absorption
i. Para-aminosalicylic (PAS)
ii. Colchicine
iii. Neomycin
iv. Ethanol
v. Metformin (and other biguanide antidiabetic agents?)
vi. Oral contraceptive agents (suggested, but no sound evidence for it)
9) Specific malabsorption for vitamin $B_{12}$
i. Long-term ingestion of calcium-chelating agents
10) Due to inadquately alkaline pH in ileum (Zollinger-Ellison syndrome, pancreatic disease)
11) Unknown causes (lack of intestinal receptors for $B_{12}$-intrinsic factor complex? Absence of "releasing factor"?)
i. Congenital (Imerslund-Grasbeck syndrome: receptors probably functioning)
ii. Acquired (forme fruste of sprue; receptors absent or nonfunctional?)
e) Competition for vitamin $B_{12}$ by intestinal parasites or bacteria
1) Fish tapeworm (Diphyllobothrium latum)
2) Bacteria: the blind loop syndrome
f) Pancreatic disease (normal pancreatic exocrine secretion of trypsin and bicarbonate required for normal $B_{12}$ absorption)
g) HIV infection (AIDS) leading to gastrointestinal dysfunction and malabsorption

**III.** Inadequate utilization
**A.** Vitamin $B_{12}$ antagonists
1. Substituted $B_{12}$ amides and anilides (experimental agents)
2. Cobaloximes (experimental agents)
3. Anti-$B_{12}$ analogues?
**B.** Congenital or acquired enzyme deficiency or deletion
1. Methylmalonyl-CoA mutase
2. Methyltetrahydrofolate-homocysteine methyltransferase
3. $B_{12}$a reductase,
4. $B_{12}$r reductase,
5. Deoxyadenoxyltransferase
6. Other enzyme reduction or deletion
**C.** Abnormal $B_{12}$-binding protein in serum, irreversibly binding $B_{12}$ and making it unavailable to tissues
1. Increased TC1 or TCIII glycoprotein (myeloproliferative disorders—"granulocyte-related" $B_{12}$ binders)
2. Increased TCII protein (liver disease; "liver-related" $B_{12}$ binders)
3. Other abnormal $B_{12}$ binding (a glycoprotein in some cases of hepatoma)
**D.** Inadequate serum $B_{12}$-binding protein (congenital or acquired)
1. TCII protein (lack produces megaloblastic anemia; it delivers $B_{12}$ to blood cells, as transferrin delivers iron)
2. TCI glycoprotein (lack not known to produce megaloblastic anemia; it is mainly a storage protein for $B_{12}$, somewhat akin to ceruloplasmin for copper)
3. TCIII (larger amounts produced in vitro by granulocytes)

**IV.** Increased requirement (normal adult daily requirement for exogenous sources is 0.1 μg (0.073 nmol)
**A.** Hyperthyroidism
**B.** Increased hematopoiesis?
**C.** Infancy
**D.** Parasitization
1. By fetus
2. By malignant tissue?

**V.** Increased excretion
**A.** Inadequate $B_{12}$-binding protein in serum
**B.** Liver disease (inadequate storage capacity for $B_{12}$)
**C.** Renal disease?

**VI.** Increased destruction by antioxidants
**A.** Pharmacologic doses of ascorbic acid

*Only 1–2% of Seventh Day Adventists eat no animal foods

hematologic damage of vitamin $B_{12}$ deficiency that is not clinically distinguishable from that of folate deficiency.[37] In both instances, the hematologic defect results from lack of adequate 5,10-methylene THFA, which delivers its methyl group to deoxyuridylate to convert that substance to thymidylate, and thus makes DNA during the S (synthesis) phase. In either deficiency, lack of adequate DNA synthesis causes many hematopoietic

**SEQUENTIAL STAGES OF VITAMIN B12 STATUS**

Biochemical and hematological sequence of events as negative vitamin B12 balance progresses.

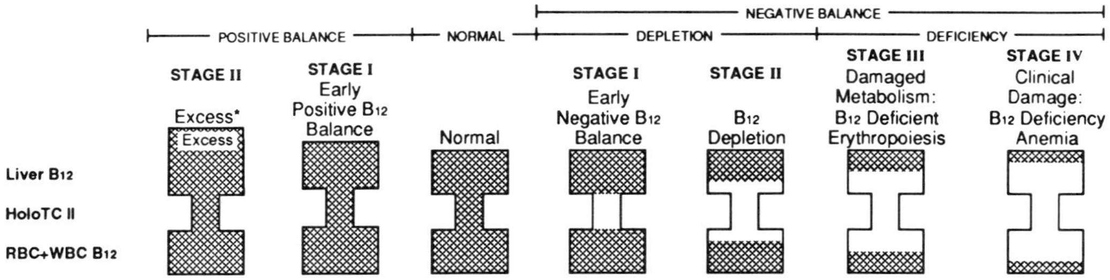
NEGATIVE BALANCE
POSITIVE BALANCE
NORMAL
DEPLETION
DEFICIENCY
Excess
Liver B12
HoloTC II
RBC+WBC B12

| | STAGE II Excess* | STAGE I Early Positive B12 Balance | Normal | STAGE I Early Negative B12 Balance | STAGE II B12 Depletion | STAGE III Damaged Metabolism: B12 Deficient Erythropoiesis | STAGE IV Clinical Damage: B12 Deficiency Anemia |
|---|---|---|---|---|---|---|---|
| HoloTC II (pg/ml) | >100 | >100 | >50 | <40 | <40 | <40 | <40 |
| TC II % sat. | >5% | >5% | >5% | <4% | <4% | <4% | <4% |
| Holohap (pg/ml) | >500 | >400 | >180 | >180 | <150 ¥ | <100 | <100 |
| dU Suppression | Normal | Normal | Normal | Normal | Normal | Abnormal | Abnormal |
| Hypersegmentation | No | No | No | No | No | Yes | Yes |
| TBBC† % sat. | >50% | >40 | >15% | >15% | >15% | <15% | <10% |
| Hap % sat. | >50% | >40 | >20% | >20% | >20% | <20% | <10% |
| RBC Folate (ng/ml) | >160 | >160 | >160 | >160 | >160 | <140 | <100 |
| Erythrocytes | Normal | Normal | Normal | Normal | Normal | Normal | Macroovalocytic |
| MCV | Normal | Normal | Normal | Normal | Normal | Normal | Elevated |
| Hemoglobin | Normal | Normal | Normal | Normal | Normal | Normal | Low |
| TC II | Normal | Normal | Normal | Normal | Normal | Elevated | Elevated |
| Methylmalonate ↑ ≠ | No | No | No | No | No | ? | Yes |
| Myelin Damage | No* | No | No | No | No | ? | Frequent |

* Cyanocobalamin excesses (injected or intranasal) produce transient rise in B12 analogues on B12 delivery protein (TC II); the significance of such rises is unknown (Herbert et al, 1987). Cyanocobalamin acts as an anti-B12 in a rare congenital defect in B12 metabolism.
≠ In serum and urine.
† TBBC= Total B12 binding capacity.
¥ Low holohaptocorrin correlates with liver cell B12 depletion. There may be hematopoietic cell and glial cell B12 depletion prior to liver cell depletion, and those cells may be in STAGE III or IV negative B12 balance while liver cells are still in STAGE II.

**FIGURE 25–5.** Biochemical and hematologic sequences of events as negative vitamin $B_{12}$ balance progresses. Earliest abnormalities in each stage are boxed.

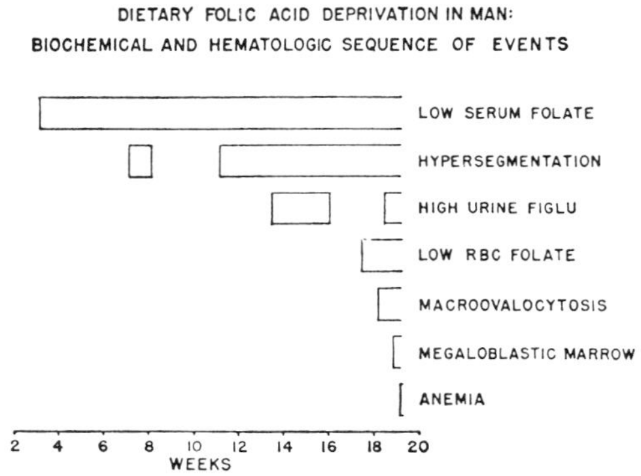
DIETARY FOLIC ACID DEPRIVATION IN MAN:
BIOCHEMICAL AND HEMATOLOGIC SEQUENCE OF EVENTS
LOW SERUM FOLATE
HYPERSEGMENTATION
HIGH URINE FIGLU
LOW RBC FOLATE
MACROOVALOCYTOSIS
MEGALOBLASTIC MARROW
ANEMIA
2 4 6 8 10 12 14 16 18 20
WEEKS

**FIGURE 25–6.** Biochemical and hematologic sequence of events in developing dietary folate deficiency in man. (From Herbert, V.: Trans. Assoc. Am. Physicians, *75*:307, 1962.)

cells to die in the bone marrow, possibly without ever completing the S phase of cell replication (i.e., a form of "ineffective erythropoiesis").

Megaloblastosis (the presence of giant germ cells) is the end product of deranged DNA synthesis of any cause. The finely stippled sieve-like open chromatin in megaloblasts suggest a defect in nuclear maturation. The precise molecular basis of megaloblastic maturation is obscure. Poor thymidylate synthesis (due to folate and/or vitamin $B_{12}$ deficiency) may fail to promote elongation of DNA chains in the presence of a relatively normal capacity to initiate DNA synthesis. This process occurs, presumably, because the lowered thymidylate concentrations remain adequate to serve as substrate for "initiating" but not for "elongating" the DNA chain by polymerase.[83] Alternatively, the mechanism of the defect may be "illicit" incorporation of thymidylate precursors (such as deoxyuridylate) into DNA, with subsequent cleavage of the DNA containing the illicit nucleotide.[84] Decreased synthesis and methylation of arginine-rich nuclear histone may contribute to megaloblastic maturation in pernicious anemia.

Morphologic changes are most striking in bone marrow cells, with the "ineffective hematopoiesis" resulting in peripheral blood pancytopenia (anemia, leukopenia, and thrombopenia).[85] However, megaloblastosis is also present in all other duplicating cells of the body[86] and may be strikingly noted in the epithelial cells of the entire alimentary tract, producing glossitis and variable degrees of megaloblastosis along the entire alimentary tract epithelium. It is not yet clear why gut changes associated with vitamin $B_{12}$ deficiency are often related to constipation, whereas those associated with folate deficiency are more commonly related to diarrhea. These differences may be connected to phenomena other than the nutrient deficiency per se.

SEQUENTIAL STAGES OF FOLATE STATUS

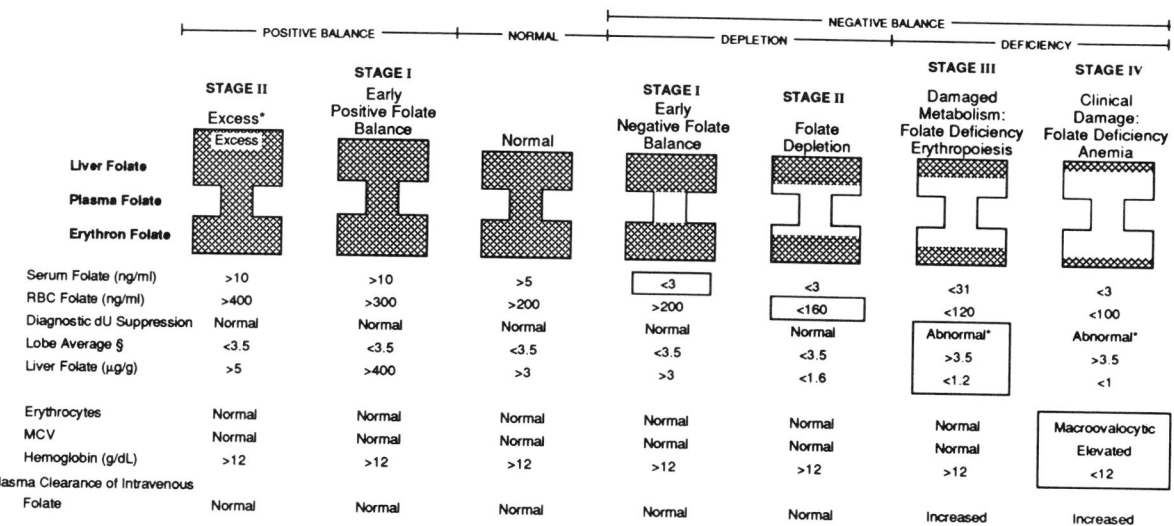

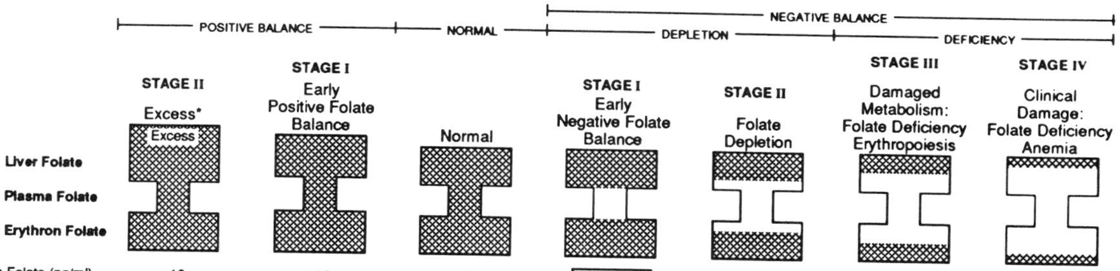
POSITIVE BALANCE
NORMAL
NEGATIVE BALANCE
DEPLETION
DEFICIENCY
STAGE II
Excess*
Excess
STAGE I
Early
Positive Folate
Balance
Normal
STAGE I
Early
Negative Folate
Balance
STAGE II
Folate
Depletion
STAGE III
Damaged
Metabolism:
Folate Deficiency
Erythropoiesis
STAGE IV
Clinical
Damage:
Folate Deficiency
Anemia
Liver Folate
Plasma Folate
Erythron Folate

| | Positive Balance: Stage II Excess* | Positive Balance: Stage I Early Positive Folate Balance | Normal | Negative Balance (Depletion): Stage I Early Negative Folate Balance | Negative Balance (Depletion): Stage II Folate Depletion | Negative Balance (Deficiency): Stage III Damaged Metabolism: Folate Deficiency Erythropoiesis | Negative Balance (Deficiency): Stage IV Clinical Damage: Folate Deficiency Anemia |
|---|---|---|---|---|---|---|---|
| Serum Folate (ng/ml) | >10 | >10 | >5 | <3 | <3 | <31 | <3 |
| RBC Folate (ng/ml) | >400 | >300 | >200 | >200 | <160 | <120 | <100 |
| Diagnostic dU Suppression | Normal | Normal | Normal | Normal | Normal | Abnormal* | Abnormal* |
| Lobe Average § | <3.5 | <3.5 | <3.5 | <3.5 | <3.5 | >3.5 | >3.5 |
| Liver Folate (µg/g) | >5 | >400 | >3 | >3 | <1.6 | <1.2 | <1 |
| Erythrocytes | Normal | Normal | Normal | Normal | Normal | Normal | Macroovalocytic |
| MCV | Normal | Normal | Normal | Normal | Normal | Normal | Elevated |
| Hemoglobin (g/dL) | >12 | >12 | >12 | >12 | >12 | >12 | <12 |
| Plasma Clearance of Intravenous Folate | Normal | Normal | Normal | Normal | Normal | Increased | Increased |

* Dietary excess of folate reduces zinc absorption.

Due to hormonal effects (on receptors?), there may be folate deficiency (i.e. Stage III-IV negative balance) in cervical epithelial cells (a reversible lesion) (possibly precancerous?) when there is only early negative balance (i.e. Stage I-II negative balance) in the erythron (Ran et al, Blood, November 1990).

**FIGURE 25–7.** Sequence of events in developing folate deficiency. Earliest abnormalities in each stage are boxed.

## "PACKAGING" FOLATE IN CELLS

Another important interrelationship of these two vitamins is the involvement of vitamin $B_{12}$ in the transport and storage of folate in cells. In vitamin $B_{12}$ deficiency, transport of methyltetrahydrofolate into bone marrow cells and into transformed lymphocytes is impaired, a defect that is corrected by the addition of vitamin $B_{12}$.[87] Similarly, humans and experimental animals with vitamin $B_{12}$ deficiency have low erythrocyte folate and decreased liver folate stores. These defects are probably attributable to failure of vitamin $B_{12}$–dependent homocysteine:methionine transmethylation. Failure to remove the methyl group from folate, which causes an intracellular "methyl trap," may interfere with dissociation of the carrier-folate complex at the inner cell wall and may impair transport into the cell. It does impair folate storage because tetrahydrofolate is preferred over methyltetrahydrofolate as a substrate for polyglutamate synthetase.[88,89]

## NERVE DAMAGE

**Vitamin $B_{12}$.** Inadequate myelin synthesis with resultant neurologic damage results from vitamin $B_{12}$ deficiency but not from folate deficiency.[86] The biochemical basis for this defective myelin synthesis is unknown. Because myelin is a lipoprotein, vitamin $B_{12}$ must have some as yet undetermined role in synthesis of either the lipid or the protein component of myelin. The hypothesis that the neurologic damage relates to the $B_{12}$ requirement for the propionate-methylmalonate conversion is probably not correct because infants born without the apoenzyme for this conversion do not have damaged myelin, and the abnormalities reported in fatty acids in myelin of vitamin $B_{12}$–deficient subjects[90] may well relate to plasmalogen[91] rather than to $B_{12}$ deficiency. The nervous system damage caused by vitamin $B_{12}$ deficiency involves, in addition to myelinated peripheral nerves, the myelinated posterior and lateral cords of the spinal column.[86] Therefore, nervous system damage from this deficiency has been variously termed subacute combined degeneration, combined system disease, posterolateral sclerosis, and funicular degeneration. However, the disease usually starts insidiously and not subacutely. Combined lesions are often absent, and lesions of the peripheral nerves occur more frequently and earlier than lesions of the central nervous system. For these reasons, the nervous system changes are more accurately described by direct reference to the actual involvement (i.e., peripheral nerve, spinal cord, or cerebral damage).

The various neurologic symptoms and signs resulting from the inadequate myelin synthesis caused by vitamin $B_{12}$ deficiency include paresthesia, especially numbness and tingling in the hands and feet, diminution of vibration sense and/or position sense (usually but not always occurring first in the ankles and feet), unsteadiness, poor muscular coordination with ataxia, moodiness, mental slowness, poor memory, confusion, agitation, depression, and central scotomata (sometimes with dim vision due to optic atrophy and tobacco amblyopia). Delusions, hallucinations, and even overt psychosis (usually with paranoid ideas) may occur. The wide variety of sensory and motor changes tend to be symmetric, expecially if present for weeks or months.

Early subtle nerve damage (inability to sense position in index toes, inability to perceive the vibrations of a 256-vps tuning fork) precedes by months grosser nerve damage (inability to sense position in great toes, inability to perceive the vibrations of a 128-vps tuning fork).[86] Correction by vitamin $B_{12}$ therapy confirms that the damage is due to vitamin $B_{12}$ deficiency rather than to the normal process of aging.

In comparing "private" with "ward" patients in large hospital populations, it was observed that economically advantaged people with vitamin $B_{12}$ deficiency tend to have relatively severe neurologic damage and relatively mild hematologic damage, whereas economically deprived people with vitamin $B_{12}$ deficiency tend to have neurologic and hematologic damage of approximately equal severity.[86] An explanation for the variable degree of hematologic damage with fixed amount of neurologic damage in vitamin $B_{12}$ deficiency is the quantity of folate in the diet. Well-to-do people tend to eat better diets, richer in high-folate foods such as fresh fruits, vegetables, and meats. The folate retards development of hematologic damage while allowing neurologic damage to progress.

Cerebration may improve rapidly when vitamin $B_{12}$ deficiency is appropriately treated, but the neurologic damage resulting from inadequate myelin synthesis heals slowly. Because the nerve damage is related to deterioration of the axon underneath the deteriorated myelin, healing is related to the speed of regeneration of damaged axons; this regeneration creeps peripherally from the nerve head at the rate of 0.1 mm per day.

**Folate.** Folate deficiency does not damage myelin, but is associated with a high frequency of irritability, forgetfulness, and often hostility and paranoid behavior. These phenomena often strikingly improve within 24 hours of the start of therapy with folic acid. Other neurologic sequelae attributed by some to folate deficiency have been reviewed elsewhere,[92] but the association has not been convincingly demonstrated.

## SELECTIVE NUTRIENT DEFICIENCY

An important area of nutrition research concerns selective nutrient deficiency in one cell line or one tissue but not another in the same patient. This condition can result from one tissue obtaining food folate first, as do intestine cells when food folate is decreased. Another cause may be the presence of a more effective mechanism for folate uptake and a less effective one for folate rejection and loss in relation to one cell line as compared to another. Selective folate deficiency can occur, for example, in white cells but not in red cells.[93] Therefore, lymphocytes (which in their resting form in the human blood appear impervious to vitamin $B_{12}$ and folic acid, and to other nutrients such as nicotinamide can be used to measure past nutrient deficiency up to 2 months after therapy; they can also reveal covert folate deficiency in patients who lack macro-ovalocytosis because of coincident iron deficiency or hemoglobinopathy.[94] Only when lymphocytes are making DNA do they appear to be pervious to nutrients.[92]

## VITAMIN $B_{12}$ IN NUTRIENT METABOLISM

### FATS AND CARBOHYDRATES

Because coenzyme $B_{12}$ is required for the hydrogen transfer and isomerization whereby methylmalonate is converted to succinate,[95] $B_{12}$ is involved in both fat and carbohydrate metabolism. There is not yet evidence to associate this metabolic defect with neurologic damage of vitamin $B_{12}$ deficiency in man. Researchers have also shown that rat glial cells in vitamin $B_{12}$–deficient media produce two odd-chain fatty acids that are not found when the cells are grown in the presence of vitamin $B_{12}$ deficiency.[96] Further, nerve biopsies from subjects with vitamin $B_{12}$ deficiency incubated in $^{14}C$-labeled propionate produced $^{14}C$-labeled fatty acids.[97] The explanation for this finding and its relationship to the functional and histologic changes have not yet been elucidated.

Recently, it has been suggested that defective methionine synthesis (lack of transferable methyl group) reduces the supply of adenosylmethionine (AdoMet), which is required for essential methylation in the nervous system.[98] This attractive theory deserves to be examined in the human. Cobalamin neuropathy in the fruit bat is not the result of impaired methylation, but rather the result of impaired conversion of methylmalonate to succinate, because the neuropathy is delayed by supplementation with valine or isoleucine.[99] However, the possibility remains that homocysteine, which piles up in cobalamin deficiency, may be a neurotoxin involved in the rapid onset of cognitive dysfunction; this dysfunction was noted recently in cases in which transcobalamin II has no cobalamin to deliver to the nervous system.[78] A comprehensive delineation of the neuropsychiatry of cobalamin deficiency has been published.[100]

### PROTEIN AND FAT

As noted earlier, vitamin $B_{12}$ is involved in protein synthesis through its role in the synthesis of the amino acid methionine, and possibly in other ways as well. Because methionine is involved in making available more of the lipotropic substances choline and betaine, this is another area where cobalamin may play a role in lipid metabolism.

### AS A REDUCING AGENT

Vitamin $B_{12}$ appears to be involved in maintenance of sulfhydryl (SH) groups in the reduced form necessary for function of many SH-activated enzyme systems. Vitamin $B_{12}$ deficiency is characterized by a decrease in reduced glutathione (which is changed from reduced glutathione (GSH) to oxidized glutathione (GSSG) of erythrocytes and liver. This condition may be corrected by administration of vitamin $B_{12}$. In vitro, vitamin $B_{12}$ derivatives catalyze the nonenzymatic oxidation of sulfhydryl derivatives.

## FOLATE IN ONE-CARBON-UNIT TRANSFERS

Folate coenzymes are concerned with mammalian metabolic systems involving transfer of a 1-carbon unit (Fig. 25–4*B*). These reactions include (1) de novo purine synthesis (formylation of glycinamide ribonucleotide (GAR) and 5-amino-4-imidazole carboxamide ribonucleotide (AICAR), (2) pyrimidine nucleotide biosynthesis (methylatin of deoxyuridylic acid to thymidylic acid), (3) three-amino-acid conversions—the interconversion of serine and glycine (which also requires vitamin $B_6$), catabolism of histidine to glutamic acid, and conversion of homocysteine to methionine (which also requires vitamin $B_{12}$), (4) generation of formate into the formate pool (and utilization of formate), and (5) methylation of small amounts of transfer RNA. Folate is not involved in the physiologic methylation of biogenic amines.[101]

There is no evidence that ascorbate plays any role in the reduction of pteroylglutamic acid to tetrahydrofolic acid, a reaction mediated by folate reductases, but it may protect THFA against further oxidative destruction.

## ROLES IN THERAPY

The only established therapeutic use of vitamin $B_{12}$ or folic acid is in treating deficiency of the respective vitamins. Claims made for nutritional value of either of these vitamins in clinical situations in which deficiency of the vitamin does not exist are without foundation.

When the deficiency is of vitamin $B_{12}$, only this vitamin should be used for therapy; conversely, when the deficiency is of folate, only that vitamin should be used for therapy. The use of folic acid in the treatment of a patient whose deficiency is of vitamin $B_{12}$ often produces temporary hematologic improvement, but allows the neurologic damage of the underlying vitamin $B_{12}$ deficiency to progress, often to an irreversible state. Because preparations of liver extract (deleted from the USP in 1960) contain hematopoietic materials other than vitamin $B_{12}$ (e.g., folic acid, folinic acid), they constitute "shotgun therapy," like many other multi-ingredient therapies, and such use is to be avoided.

The signs and symptoms of deficiency of vitamin $B_{12}$ or folate in humans are listed in Table 25–2.

### CRITICALLY ILL PATIENTS

It is rarely necessary to institute immediately therapy before determining the cause of megaloblastic anemia. Major indications for *emergency* therapy include severe thrombocytopenia (platelet count less than 50,000/mm$^3$) associated with bleeding, severe leukopenia (white cell count less than 3000/mm$^3$) associated with infection, infection itself, coma, severe disorientation, marked neurologic damage, severe hepatic disease, uremia, or other debilitating illness complicating the anemia. The anemia itself is not a problem because the dyspnea and occasional angina that may accompany a hematocrit of less than 15 volumes % are relieved by a transfusion of one to two units of packed erythrocytes. Transfusion is unwarranted in the absence of *symptoms* of anemia. When venous pressure is elevated, transfusion of packed erythrocytes should be accompanied by withdrawal of equivalent or slightly smaller quantities of whole blood, which will reduce rather than raise the venous pressure. Transfusion of whole blood without withdrawal of blood has been responsible for acute rises in venous pressure with resultant irreversible congestive failure in elderly patients with megaloblastic anemia and unrecognized elevated venous pressure. Ideally, venous pressure should be determined before transfusion and monitored during both the transfusion of packed cells and the simultaneous withdrawal of whole blood. An alternative to exchange transfusion is to precede the administration of blood by the parenteral injection of a diuretic.

When, for one of the reasons discussed previously, immediate vitamin therapy is necessary before etiologic diagnosis, 100 μg (76.0 nmol) of cyanocobalamin and 15 mg (34 μmol) of folic acid are given intramuscularly, followed by 5 mg (11.3 μmol) of folic acid by mouth and 100 μg (75.0 nmol) of vitamin $B_{12}$ intramuscularly daily, for a week. Such treatment produces excellent hematologic response except in patients in whom hematopoiesis is suppressed by infection, uremia, chloramphenicol administration, or some other factor.

### VITAMIN $B_{12}$ DEFICIENCY

Vitamin $B_{12}$ deficiency in man is nearly always the result of inadequate ingestion and/or inadequate absorption, and therapy is guided by adequate etiologic diagnosis (see Tables 25–1 and 25–2).

Inadequate ingestion of vitamin $B_{12}$ is corrected by adding to the daily diet any food containing vitamin $B_{12}$ (i.e., animal products, including meat, milk, fish, shellfish, or poultry). If the patient, because of poverty, cannot afford animal products or, for religious or other reasons, is a strict vegetarian, adequate treatment consists of 1 μg

**TABLE 25–2.** CAUSES OF FOLIC ACID DEFICIENCY

**I.** Inadequate ingestion
- **A.** Poor diet (lacking unprocessed fresh, uncooked, or slightly cooked food or fruit juices—folates are heat-labile)
  - **1.** Nutritional megaloblastic anemia.
    - a) Tropical
    - b) Nontropical
    - c) Scurvy (diets low in vitamin C are low in folate)
  - **2.** Chronic alcoholism with or without cirrhosis

**II.** Inadequate absorption (affecting upper third of small intestine, which is the main site of folate absorption; because most food folates are in polyglutamate forms, biliary and intestinal $\gamma$-glutamyl conjugates are necessary to split off excess glutamates to make folates absorbable)
- **A.** Malabsorption syndromes
  - **1.** Gluten-induced enteropathy (childhood and adult celiac disease; idiopathic steatorrhea, nontropical sprue; coincident $B_{12}$ malabsorption rare)
  - **2.** Any other chronic functional or structural disorder involving the upper small intestine
    - a) Tropical sprue (coincident $B_{12}$ malabsorption almost invariably present)
    - b) Associated with herpetic and other skin disorders
  - **3.** Drugs
    - a) Anticonvulsants (e.g., phenytoin, primidone)
    - b) Barbituates
    - c) Cycloserine
    - d) Ethanol
    - e) Metformin
    - f) Amino acid excess (glycine or methionine)
    - g) Nitrofurantoin ? (antimicrobial)
    - h) Glutethimide ? (sedative)
    - i) Cholestyramine
    - j) Salicylazosulfapyridine (Azulfidine)
- **B.** Specific malabsorption for folate
  - 1. Congenital nonconjugase defects (four cases published)
  - 2. Acquired nonconjugase defects
  - 3. Inadequate biliary or intestinal conjugates
  - 4. Conjugase inhibitors (such as contained in some beans)
- **C.** Blind loop syndrome (more commonly, bacteria make folate and actually raise serum folate level of host)

**III.** Inadequate utilization (metabolic block)
- **A.** Folic acid antagonists (dihydrofolate reductase inhibitors)
  - 1. 4-Amino-4-deoxyfolates i.e., methotrexate—(Chemotherapy, immunosuppression, psoriasis)
  - 2. 2,4 Diaminopyrimidine e.g., pyrimethamine, trimethoprim—(malaria, toxoplasmosis; antibacterial)
  - 3. Triamterene (diuretic)
  - 4. Diamidine compounds i.e., pentamidine, isothionate—(Pneumocystis carinii, protozocidal)

(0.75 nmol) of vitamin $B_{12}$ orally supplied daily as a liquid or tablet of $B_{12}$-containing food supplement.

When the vitamin $B_{12}$ deficiency is the result of inadequate absorption, 1 $\mu$g (0.75 nmol) of vitamin $B_{12}$ parenterally (subcutaneously or intramuscularly) daily constitutes adequate therapy. A single injection of 100 $\mu$g (75.0 nmol) or more of vitamin $B_{12}$ produces a complete therapeutic remission in any patient whose deficiency is not complicated by unrelated systemic disease or other factors. The remission is sustained for life by monthly injections of 100 $\mu$g (75.0 nmol) of vitamin $B_{12}$. It is important to inform the patient who has permanent gastric or ileal damage that monthly injections of vitamin $B_{12}$ must be continued for life.

For simultaneous differential diagnosis and therapy, patients should be treated with an injection of 1 $\mu$g (0.75 nmol) of vitamin $B_{12}$ daily for 10 days after a control period of a few days to establish the constancy of the reticulocyte level, and the elimination of dietary sources of vitamin $B_{12}$ and folic acid (by provision of a diet consisting exclusively of well-cooked finely particulate grains or vegetables, such as rice and beans, and beverages devoid of vitamin $B_{12}$ and folate, such as tea, coffee, and soft drinks).[102]

Initial therapy with doses of vitamin $B_{12}$ greater than 1 $\mu$g (0.75 $\mu$mol) daily is desirable when the vitamin $B_{12}$ deficiency is complicated by other debilitating illness such as infection, hepatic disease, uremia, coma, severe disorientation, or marked neurologic damage. In such patients, 30 $\mu$g (22.5 nmol) or more of vitamin $B_{12}$ is given daily parenterally for 5 to 10 days. Daily parenteral doses larger than 30 $\mu$g (22.5 nmol) have no proven therapeutic advantage, and much of the excess is rapidly excreted in the urine.[103]

Vitamin $B_{12}$ can also be administrated in a nasal gel, facilitating self-administration. Preliminary data indicate that nasal $B_{12}$ is more effectively absorbed than oral $B_{12}$ in normal individuals, that it is effective in counter-

**TABLE 25–2.** *(continued)*

- **B.** Diphenylhydantoin and possibly other anticonvulsant (possibly block cell uptake or use of folate)
- **C.** Enzyme deficiency
  - **1.** Congenital
    - a) Formiminotransferase
    - b) Dihydrofolate reductase
    - c) Methyltetrahydrofolate transmethylase
    - d) Other enzymes (some secondarily affect folate)
  - **2.** Acquired
    - a) Liver disease
      - i. Formimotransferase
      - ii. Other enzymes
- **D.** Vitamin $B_{12}$ deficiency (reduced folate uptake and retention)
- **E.** Alcohol (both specific and nonspecific damage)
- **F.** Ascorbic acid deficiency
- **G.** Dietary amino acid excess (glycine, methionine)

**IV.** Increased requirement
- **A.** Extra tissue demand
  - 1. By fetus
  - 2. By malignant tissue (especially lymphoroliferative disorders)
  - 3. By breastfed infant
- **B.** Infancy
- **C.** increased hematopoiesis
- **D.** increased metabolic activity
- **E.** Lesch-Nyhan syndrome
- **F.** Drugs (L-Dopa?)

**V.** Increased excretion
- **A.** Vitamin $B_{12}$ deficiency (? of obligatory excretion of folate in urine and bile; possible inability to reabsorb methylfolate excreted in bile because $B_{12}$ is required for it)
- **B.** Liver disease?
- **C.** Kidney dialysis
- **D.** Chronic exfoliative dermatitis

**VI.** Increased destruction
- **A.** Oxidant in diet?

acting intestinal $B_{12}$ malabsorption, and that it can be used to treat $B_{12}$-deficient patients.[104]

Hydroxocobalamin and other depot preparations of vitamin $B_{12}$ may be retained longer at the site of injection and in serum, but this possible slight therapeutic advantage over cyanocobalamin does not warrant their greater cost; they also may have undesirable side effects. More detailed discussion of vitamin $B_{12}$ preparations, routes of administration, dosage, and therapeutic responses may be found elsewhere.[4]

## FOLATE DEFICIENCY

For combined differential diagnosis and therapy, the patient is treated with 100 μg (226.67 nmol) of folic acid orally daily (if the suspected diagnosis is folate malabsorption). This dosage produces a maximal hematologic response in patients with folate deficiency, but does not produce hematologic response in patients with vitamin $B_{12}$ deficiency.[102] As in treated vitamin $B_{12}$ deficiency, treatment of folate deficiency returns subnormal leukocyte and platelet levels to normal within a week of the start of therapy, at approximately the time of the reticulocyte peak.

Therapy with doses of folic acid larger than 0.1 mg (226.67 nmol) daily is desirable when the folate deficiency state is complicated by conditions that may suppress hematopoiesis (such as unrelated systemic disease), conditions that increase folate requirement (pregnancy, hypermetabolic states, alcoholism, hemolytic anemia), and conditions that reduce folate absorption. Therapy should then consist of 0.5 to 1 mg (1.33 to 2.266 μmol) daily. There is no evidence that doses greater than 1 mg (2.266 μmol) daily have any greater efficacy; additionally, loss of folate in the urine becomes roughly logarithmic as the amount administered exceeds 1 mg (2.266 μmol).

Maintenance therapy is normally 0.1 mg (226.67 nmol) of folic acid daily for 1 to 4 months, which then should be discontinued only if the diet contains at least one fresh fruit or fresh vegetable daily. If the daily folate requirement is increased owing to an increased metabolic or cell-turnover rate, the maintenance dose should be 0.2 to 0.5 mg (0.453 to 1.133 μmol) daily.

Ideal nutritional therapy for dietary folate deficiency is the ingestion of one fresh fruit or one fresh vegetable daily. Such a diet would probably eliminate nutritional folate deficiency from the earth.[104] At present, nutritional folate deficiency probably affects approximately a third of all the pregnant women in the world.[64]

## PREVENTION OF FOLATE DEFICIENCY

Pregnant women should receive folate supplements, which have also been recommended in clinical disorders that increase the risk of folate deficiency. However, major problems have been encountered in the delivery of such supplements to patients. Because of resultant gastrointestinal upsets, significant numbers of pregnant women do not ingest iron tablets given to them. Tablets containing both iron and folate may be better tolerated, inasmuch as the adverse gastrointestinal effects of iron ingestion may be decreased when folic acid is simultaneously ingested.[105] However, the iron in the mixed supplement should not exceed the 30 mg (0.54 mmol) iron daily pregnancy supplement. The largest component of the problem is that antenatal care is not available for, or taken advantage of by, large numbers of pregnant women, particularly in populations in which folate deficiency is common.

As an alternative approach to the alleviation of the problem, a series of studies was devised to determine the feasibility of fortifying staple foods with folic acid. When the data generated in these studies were judged against criteria delineated by an Expert Committee of the World Health Organization (WHO) and Food and Agricultural Organization (FAO),[106] such fortification appeared feasible, inexpensive, effective, and safe in populations with a demonstrable need for increased dietary levels of folic acid. Although fortification might increase the incidence and/or severity of neurologic damage in subjects with pernicious anemia, little published data exist to support this view. The WHO and other bodies have recommended that authorities concerned with populations in which folate deficiency is common should initiate trials to determine the feasibility and effectiveness of food fortification with folate in those populations.[107]

## TOXICITY

Vitamin $B_{12}$ and folic acid, when ingested in their human-active forms, are nontoxic in man not only in small doses but also in doses that exceed the minimal daily adult human requirement by 10,000 times for vitamin $B_{12}$ and several hundred times for folic acid. Being water-soluble, excesses of these vitamins tend to be excreted in the urine rather than, like fat-soluble vitamins, being stored in tissues. Vitamin $B_{12}$ and folic acid both appear to require binding to polypeptides as a precondition of storage: excesses above the limited binding capacity in serum and tissues tend to be excreted rather than retained.

A rare allergic reaction has been reported, possibly due to impurities in a rare preparation of crystalline cyanocobalamin. Hydroxocobalamin injections and injections of various depot preparations of cyanocobalamin have been associated with the appearance of antibody to plasma vitamin $B_{12}$-binding protein.[108] Although the significance of this antibody is not yet clear, such preparations offer no clear advantage over cyanocobalamin to warrant their use, especially in view of their greater cost and the pain on injection of some of the depot preparations. The pharmaceutical preparation cyanocobalamin is not metabolically active in humans. Tissue enzymes remove the cyanide to make the cobalamin active. The rare infant who is born with a congenital lack of this cyanide-removing mechanism can, of course, be harmed by cyanocobalamin, which serves in that case as an antimetabolite of vitamin $B_{12}$.[109]

The efficacy and safety of the vitamin $B_{12}$ analogues created by nutrient-nutrient interaction in vitamin-mineral supplements is unknown.

Daily doses of up to 15 mg (43 μmol) in healthy humans without convulsive disorders are without known toxic effects: this daily dose is well below that which could lead to precipitation of crystalline folic acid in the kidneys (such precipitation produces renal toxicity in rats given massive doses of folic acid). One questionable instance of an allergic reaction to folic acid has been reported in man.[3] Very large amounts of folic acid in its pharmaceutical oxidized form (pteroylglutamic acid) may be noxious to the nervous system and can reverse the anti-epileptic effects of phenobarbital, phenytoin, and primidone, and have provoked seizures in patients otherwise under control on anticonvulsant therapy.[92,110]

Although no such effect has been observed in controlled studies using oral doses of 15 mg (34 μmol) folic acid daily, experimental and clinical evidence suggests that very high concentrations of folic acid can have a convulsant effect.[91] The convulsant dose in normal rats was shown in one study to be 45 to 125 mg (102 to 283.3 μmol) if administered intravenously and 15 to 30 mg (34 to 68 nmol) if preceded by the induction of a focal cortical lesions. Convulsions have been reported in one of eight epileptics given parenteral folic acid under electroencephalographic monitoring. This reaction occurred after the rapid intravenous infusion of 14.4 mg (32.64 μmol) folic acid, which presumably elevated serum folate concentration in the cerebral vessels several times higher than would be the case after folic acid ingestion.[92] Anticonvulsant drugs and folic acid compete with each other for absorption across the intestinal epithelial cells, and probably also compete at the brain cell wall.[110] However, despite evidence in uncontrolled studies suggesting increased fit frequency in epileptics given oral therapeutic doses of folic acid, no such effect of oral folic acid has so far been demonstrated in carefully conducted controlled trials.

Oral folic acid supplements of 350 μg (793.3 μmol) daily reduce zinc absorption and may be a problem where maternal zinc depletion and intrauterine growth retardation are common.[65]

**TABLE 25–3.** CLINICAL PICTURE OF THE MEGALOBLASTIC ANEMIAS

1. Symptoms
   - Weakness, tiredness
   - Dyspnea
   - Sore tongue
   - Paresthesia ($B_{12}$ deficiency only)
   - Diarrhea (especially folate deficiency)
   - Constipation (especially $B_{12}$ deficiency)
   - Irritability and forgetfulness (especially folate deficiency)
   - Anorexia
   - Syncope
   - Headache
   - Palpitation
2. Signs
   - Megaloblastic bone marrow (orthochromatic megaloblasts, giant metamyelocytes)
   - Anemia, leukopenia, thrombocytopenia, with macro-ovalocytes (normal MVC = 87 ± 5 $\mu m^3$) and "hypersegmented polys" (normal Arneth count 2 lobes = 20 to 40%, 3 lobes = 40 to 50%, 4 lobes = 15 to 25%, 5 lobes = 0 to 5%, 6 lobes = 0 to 0.1%, more than 6 lobes = 0) (normal "lobe average" = 3.17 = 0.25). (Rule of fives: When 100 neutrophils are counted, the presence of more than 5% containing 5 or more lobes means hypersegmentation.)
   - Morphologic red herrings: congenital hypersegmentation (approximately 1% of population), hypersegmentation with renal disease; twinning deformities; macrocytes of pyruvate kinase deficiency, aplastic anemia, reticulocytosis, hypothyroidism, neoplasia.
   - Fever
   - Icterus plus pallor (lemon-yellow skin)
   - Glossitis
     - Acute
     - Chronic atrophic
   - Neurologic damage (only proven in $B_{12}$ deficiency, which damages myelin)
     - Vibration sense diminished
     - Position sense diminished, ataxia, "combined systems disease"
     - Impaired mentation, paranoid ideation (seen in both deficiencies)
   - Malabsorption
   - Achylia gastrica (primary with $B_{12}$ deficiency, secondary with folate deficiency) (reduced/intrinsic factor)
   - Splenomegaly (in approximately one-third of cases, if looked for radiologically)
   - Weight loss (especially folate deficiency)
   - Pigmentation: vitiligo
   - Postural hypotension (especially $B_{12}$ deficiency)
   - Low serum vitamin $B_{12}$ or folate level
   - Low or absent vitamin $B_{12}$ in TCII
   - Low red cell $B_{12}$ or folate level: low lymphocyte $B_{12}$ or folate
   - Elevated serum lactic dehydrogenase (LDH)
   - Elevated urine formiminoglutamate
   - Methylmalonic aciduria ($B_{12}$ deficiency only)
   - High serum iron, increased saturation of iron-binding capacity of serum, increased bone marrow iron stores, normal free erythrocyte protoporphyrin (findings that may obscure occult Fe deficiency)
   - Low red cell folate is present in either deficiency
   - Circulating antibody to intrinsic factor in two thirds of pernicious anemia patients
   - Circulating antibody to gastric parietal cells in most patients with gastric damage, regardless of cause
   - Abnormal "dU suppression test" (corrected by adding vitamin in vitro)
   - Abnormal liver function tests
   - Subnormal intestinal absorption

## REFERENCES


1. Castle, W.B.: Trans. Am. Clin. Climatol. Assoc., *73*:54–80, 1961.
2. Kass, L.: Pernicious Anemia. Philadelphia, W.B. Saunders Co., 1976.
3. Chanarin, I.: The Megaloblastic Anaemias. Oxford, Blackwell Scientific Publications, 1979.
4. Herbert, V.: Drugs effective in megaloblastic anemia: vitamin $B_{12}$ and folic acid. *In* The Pharmacological Basis of Therapeutics. 5th Ed. Edited by L.S. Goodman and A. Gilman. New York, Macmillan, 1975, pp. 1324–1349.
5. Combe, J.S.: Trans R. Med. Chir. Soc. Edinb., *7*:194–198, 1824.
6. Addison, T.: On the Constitutional and Local Effects of Disease of the Suprarenal Capsules. London, S. Highley, 1855.
7. Flint, A.: Am. Med. Times, *7*:181–184, 1960.
8. Castle, W.B.: Am. J. Med. Sci., *178*:748–764, 1929.
9. Rickes, E.L., Brink, N.G., Koniuszy, F.R., et al.: Science, *107*:396–398, 1948.
10. Smith, E.L., Parker, L.F.J.: Biochem. J., *43*:8A, 1948.
11. Berk, L., Castle, W.B., Welch, A.D., et al.: N. Engl. J. Med., *39*:911–915, 1948.
12. Channing, W.: N. Engl. Q. J. Med. Surg., *1*:157–180, 1824.
13. Barclay, A.W.: Quoted by Castle.[1]
14. Osler, W.: Br. Med. J., *1*:1–4, 1919.
15. Wills, L., Clutterbuch, P., Evans, B.D.F.: Biochem. J., *31*:2136–2147, 1937.
16. Stokstad, E.L.R.: J. Biol. Chem., *149*:573–574, 1943.
17. Pfiffner, J.J., Binkley, S.B., Bloom, E.S., et al.: Science, *97*:404–405, 1943.
18. Angier, R.B., Boothe, J.H., Hutchings, B.L., et al.: J. Am. Chem. Soc., *103*:667–672, 1946.
19. Shorb, M.S.: Science, *107*:397–398, 1948.
20. This reference has been deleted.
21. Day, P.L., Mims, V., Totter, J.R., et al.: J. Biol. Chem., *157*:423–424, 1945.
22. Snell, E.E., Peterson, W.H.: J. Bacteriol., *39*:273–280, 1940.
23. Stokstad, E.L.R., Hutchings, B.L., Subba Row, Y.: J. Am. Chem. Soc., *70*:3–8, 1948.
24. Woods, D.D.: Br. J. Exp. Pathol., *21*:74–83, 1940.
25. Rubbo, S.D., Gillespie, J.M.: Nature, *146*:838–839, 1940.
26. Mitchell, H.K., Snell, E.E., Williams, R.J.: J. Am. Chem. Soc., *63*:2284–2290, 1941.
27. Minot, G.R., Murphy, W.P.: JAMA, *87*:470–476, 1926.
28. Dolphin, D. (ed.): $B_{12}$. Vols. 1 and 2. New York, John Wiley & Sons, 1982.
29. Herbert, V., Drivas, G., Foscaldi, R., et al.: N. Engl. J. Med., *307*:225–256, 1982.
30. Kondo, H., Binder, M.J., Kolhouse, J.F., et al.: J. Clin. Invest., *70*:899–898, 1982.
31. IUPAC-IUB Commission on Biochemical Nomenclature: Nomenclature of vitamins, coenzymes and related compounds. Tentative rules. *In* Folates and Pterins. Vol. I: Chemistry and Biochemistry of Folates. Edited by R.L. Blakley and S.J. Benkovic. New York, John Wiley & Sons, 1984, p. 29.
32. Sullivan, L.W., Herbert, V.: N. Engl. J. Med., *272*:340–346, 1965.
33. Herbert, V.: Am. J. Clin. Nutr., *21*:743–752, 1968.
34. FAO/WHO Expert Group: Requirements of Vitamin A, Iron, Folate and Vitamin $B_{12}$. Geneva, FAO/WHO, 1987.
35. Herbert, V., Colman, N., Palat, D., et al.: J. Lab. Clin. Med., *104*:829–841, 1984.
36. Kolhouse, J.F., Kondo, H., Allen, R.H., et al.: N. Engl. J. Med., *299*:785–792, 1978.
37. Herbert, V.: Lab. Invest., *52*:3–19, 1985.
38. Herbert, V.: Am. J. Clin. Nutr., *7*:433–437, 1959.
39. Herbert, V.: Vitamin $B_{12}$ and folate metabolism. *In* $B_{12}$ and Folate Analysis with Radionuclides in Hematopoietic and Gastrointestinal Investigations with Radionuclides. Edited by A.J. Gilson, W.M. Smoak, and M.B. Weinstein. Springfield, IL, Charles C Thomas, 1972, pp. 8–20.
40. Herbert, V., Colman, C.: Vitamin $B_{12}$ and folacin radioassays in blood serum. *In* Methods of Vitamin Assays. 4th Ed. Edited by J. Augustin, B.P. Klein, and D. Becker et al. New York, John Wiley & Sons, 1985, pp. 515–534.
41. Donaldson, R.M.: N. Engl. J. Med., *299*:827–828, 1978.
42. Kanazawa, S., Herbert, V., Herzlich, B., et al: Lancet, *1*:707–708, 1983.
43. Internat. Comm. Stds. Haematol. (ICSH): Br. J. Haematol., *64*:809–811, 1986.
44. Herbert, V., Wasserman, L.R., Frank, O., et al.: Fed. Proc., *18*:246, 1959.
45. Waxman, S., Schreiber, C., Herbert, V.: Blood, *36*:228–235, 1960.
46. Rothenberg, S.P., da Costa, M., Rosenberg, Z.: N. Engl. J. Med., *286*:1335–1339, 1971.

46a. Longo, D.L., Herbert, V.: J. Lab. Clin. Med., *87*:138–151, 1976.

47. Gutcho, S., Mansbach, L.: Clin. Chem., *23*:1609–1614, 1977.
48. Allen, R.H., Seetharm, B., Allen, N.C., et al.: J. Clin. Invest., *61*:1628–1634, 1978.
49. Kanazawa, S., Herzlich, B., Herbert, V.: Am. J. Gastroenterol., *80*:964–969, 1985.
50. Halsted, C.H.: Intestinal absorption of dietary folates. *In* Folic Acid Metabolism in Health and Disease. Edited by M.F., Picciano, E.L.R. Stokstad, and J.F. Gregory III. New York, Wiley-Liss, 1990, pp. 23–45.
51. Strum, W.B.: Biochim. Biophys. Acta, *554*:249–257, 1979.
52. Darcy-Villon, B., Selhub, J., Rosenberg, H.: Am. J. Physiol., *255*:361–366, 1988.
53. Said, H.M., Redha, R.: Biochem. J., *247*:141–146, 1987.
54. Carmel, R., Herbert, V.: Blood, *40*:542–549, 1972.
55. Allen, R.H.: Prog. Hematol., *9*:57–84, 1975.
56. Jacob, E., Wong, K.-T. J., Herbert, V.: J. Lab. Clin. Med., *89*:1145–1152, 1977.
57. Jacob, E., Baker, S.J., Herbert, V.: Physiol. Rev., *60*:918–960, 1980.
58. Begley, J.A., Hall, C.A.: Blood, *45*:287–293, 1975.
59. Corcino, J., Zalusky, R., Greenberg, M., et al.: Br. J. Haematol., *20*:511–520, 1971.
60. Cooksley, W.G.E., England, J.M., Louis, L., et al.: Clin. Sci. Mol. Med., *47*:531–545, 1974.

60a. Savage, C.R., Jr., Green, P.D.: Fed. Proc., *34*:905, 1975.

61. Retief, F.P., Gottlieb, C., Herbert, V.: J. Clin. Invest., *45*:1907–1914, 1966.

61a. Hakami, N., Neiman, P.E., Cannelos, G.P., et al.: N. Engl. J. Med., *285*:1163–1170, 1971.

**62.** Scott, C.R., Hakami, N., Teng, C.C., et al.: J. Pediatr., *81:*1106–1111, 1972.

**63.** Sattar, M.A., Das, K.C.: Med. Lab. Sci., *48:*36–42, 1991.

**64.** Herbert, V.: Public issues and nutrition research opportunities. *In* Food and Agricultural Research Opportunities to Improve Human Nutrition for the 21st Century. Edited by A.R. Doberenz, J.A. Milner, and B.S. Schweigert. Newark, DE, University of Delaware College of Human Resources Press, 1986, pp. 1313–1322.

**65.** Herbert, V.: Am. J. Clin. Nutr., *45:*671–678, 1987.

**66.** Ratnam, M., Freisheim, J.H.: Proteins involved in the transport of folates and antifolates by normal and neoplastic cells. *In* Folic Acid Metabolism in Health and Disease. Edited by M.F. Picciano, E.R.L. Stokstad, and J.F. Gregory III. New York, Wiley-Liss, 1990, pp. 91–120.

**67.** Rothenberg, S.P.: Proc. Soc., Ex. Biol. Med., *133:*428–432, 1970.

**68.** Colman, N., Herbert, V.: Blood, *48:* 911–921, 1976.

**69.** Colman, N., Herbert, V.: Ann. Rev. Med., *31:*433–439, 1980.

**70.** Goldman, I.D.: Ann. N.Y. Acad. Sci., *186:*400, 1971.

**71.** Murphy, M., Keating, M., Boyle, P., et al: Biochem. Biophys. Res. Commun., *71:*1017–1021, 1976.

**72.** Stokes, P.L., Melikian, V., Leeming, R.L., et al.: Am. J. Clin. Nutr., *28:*126–129, 1975.

**73.** Herbert, V.: Development of human folate deficiency. *In* Folic Acid Metabolism in Health and Disease. Edited by M.F. Picciano, and E.L.R. Stokstad. New York, Wiley-Liss, 1990, pp. 195–210.

**74.** Food and Nutrition Board, National Research Council: Recommended Dietary Allowances. 10th Ed. Washington, D.C., National Academy Press, 1989.

**75.** Jadhav, M., Webb, J.K.G., Vaishava, S., et al.: Lancet., *2:*903–907, 1962.

**76.** Reed, B., Weir, D.G., Scott, J.M.: Am. J. Clin. Nutr., *29:*1393–1396, 1976.

**77.** Colman, N., Green, R., Metz, J.: Am. J. Clin. Nutr., *28:*459–464, 1975.

**78.** Herbert, V., Fong, W., Gulle, V., et al.: Am. J. Hematol., *34:*132–139, 1990.

**79.** Herbert, V., Jacob, E.: JAMA, *230:*241–242, 1974.

**80.** Allen, R.H., Stabler, S.P., Savage, D.G., et al.: Am. J. Hematol., *34:*90–98, 1990.

**81.** Lindenbaum, J., Savage, D.G., Stabler, S.P., et al.: Am. J. Hematol., *34:*99–107, 1990.

**82.** Das, K.C., Herbert, V.: Am. J. Hematol., *31:*11–20, 1989.

**83.** Hoffbrand, A.V., Ganeshaguru, K., Hooton, J.W.L., et al.: Clin. Haematol., *5:*727–745, 1976.

**84.** Luzzatto, L., Falusi, A.O., Joju, E.A.: N. Engl. J. Med., *299:*1156–1157, 1981.

**85.** Sarode, R., Garewal, G., Marwah, N., et al.: Trop. Geogr. Med., *41:*331–336, 1989.

**86.** Herbert, V.: The Megaloblastic Anemias. New York, Grune & Stratton, 1959.

**87.** Tisman, G., Herbert, V.: Blood, *41:*465–469, 1973.

**88.** Allen, R.H.: Prog. Hematol., *9:*57–84, 1975.

**89.** Pearson, A.G., Turner, A.J.: Nature, *258:*173–174, 1975.

**90.** Frenkel, E.P.: J. Clin. Invest., *50:*33A, 1971.

**91.** Marcus, A., Ullman, H.L., Safier, L.B., et al.: J. Clin. Invest., *41:*2198–2203, 1962.

**92.** Colman, N., Herbert, V.: Folate metabolism in brain. *In* Biochemistry of Brain. Edited by S. Kumar. Oxford, Pergamon Press, 1979, pp. 127–142.

**93.** Das, K.C., Herbert, V.: Br. J. Haematol., *38:*219–233, 1978.

**94.** Green, R., Kuhl, W., Jacobsen, R., et al.: N. Engl. J. Med., *307:*1322–1325, 1982.

**95.** Arnstein, H.R.V., Wrighton, R.J. (eds.): The Cobalamins. London, Churchill Livingstone, 1971.

**96.** Barcley, F.W., Sato, G.H., Abeles, R.H.: J. Biol. Chem., *247:*4270–4276, 1972.

**97.** Frenkel, E.P.: J. Clin. Invest., *52:*1237–1245, 1973.

**98.** Weir, D.G., Keating, S., Molley, A., et al.: J. Neurochem., *51:*1949–1952, 1988.

**98a.** Herbert V.: Am. J. Clin. Nutr., *46:*387–402, 1987.

**99.** Viera-Makings, E., Metz, J., Van der Westhayzen, J., et al.: Biochem. J., *226:*707–711, 1990.

**100.** Healton, E., Savage, D., Brust, J.C.M., et al.: Medicine, *40:*229–245, 1991.

**101.** Meller, E., Rosengarten, H., Friedhoff, A., et al.: Science, *187:*171–173, 1975.

**102.** Herbert, V.: N. Engl. J. Med., *268:*201, 368, 1963.

**103.** Herbert, V.: Semin. Hematol., *7:*2–8, 1970.

**104.** Colman, N., Demartino, L., McAleer, E.: Blood, *68:*45A, 1986.

**105.** Sood, S.K., Ramachandran, K., Mathur, M., et al: Q. J. Med., *44:*241–250, 1975.

**106.** FAO/WHO: WHO Tech. Rep. Ser. No. 477. Geneva, 1971.

**107.** WHO: WHO Tech. Rep. Ser. No. 580. Geneva, 1975.

**109.** Fenton, W.A., Rosenberg, L.: Inherited disorders of cobalamin transport and metabolism. *In* Metabolic Basis of Inherited Disease. 6th Ed. Edited by J.B. Stanbury, J.B. Wyngaarden, D.S., Fredrickson, et al. New York, McGraw-Hill, 1989, pp. 2065–2082.

**110.** Colman, N., Herbert, V.: Folates and the nervous system. *In* Folates and Pterins. Vol. 3. Edited by R.L. Blakley. New York, John Wiley & Sons, 1986, pp. 339–358.

**111.** Herbert, V.: *In* Textbook of Medicine. 14th Ed. Edited by P.B. Beeson and W. McDermott. Philadelphia, W.B. Saunders, 1975.


## SELECTED READINGS


Fenton, W.A., Rosenberg, L.E.: Inherited disorders of cobalamin transport and metabolism. *In* The Metabolic Basis of Inherited Diseases. 6th Ed. Edited by C.R. Scriver, A.L. Beaudet, and D. Valle. New York, McGraw-Hill, 1989, pp. 2065–2082.

Herbert, V.: Nutrition science as a continually unfolding story: The folate, vitamin $B_{12}$ paradigm. The 1986 Herman Award Lecture. Am. J. Clin. Nutr., *46:*387–402, 1987.

Picciano, M.R., Stokstad, E.L.R., Gregory, J.F., III (eds.): Folic Acid Metabolism in Health and Disease. New York, Wiley-Liss, 1990, pp. 1–277.

Rosenblatt, D.S.: Inherited disorders of folate transport and metabolism. *In* The Metabolic Basis of Inherited Diseases. 6th Ed. Edited by C.R. Scriver, A.L. Beaudet, and D. Valle. New York, McGraw-Hill, 1989, pp. 2049–2064.

Woodson, R.D. (ed.): Symposium on new frontiers in vitamin $B_{12}$ metabolism. Am. J. Hematol., *34:*81–128, 1990.

CHAPTER 26

# Biotin

Krishnamurti Dakshinamurti



## HISTORY

Biotin is a water-soluble vitamin. Kogl and Tonnis isolated crystalline biotin in 1936. Du Vigneaud determined its chemical structure in 1942. The chemical synthesis of biotin was achieved by Harris in 1943. Further significant advances involved the identification of biotin as the prosthetic group of the biotin-containing carboxylases, understanding the molecular mechanism of the action of biotin in biotin enzymes[1,2] and clarifying the regulatory features of biotin enzymes.[3] The recognition of biotin-responsive multiple carboxylase deficiency syndromes and the hypothesis of nonprosthetic group function for biotin are among recent developments.

## CHEMISTRY

Biotin has a bicyclic structure consisting of a ureido ring fused with a tetrahydrothiophene ring with a valeric acid substituent, which was shown to be *cis*-hexahydro-2-oxo-1H-thieno [3,4] imidazole-4-valeric acid (Fig. 26–1). Only the (+) stereoisomer of biotin has significant biologic activity. Biotin is soluble in water (0.82 mmol/L at 25° C). It is more soluble in hot water and in dilute alkali and four times more so in 95% ethanol than in cold water. It is not soluble in other organic solvents. Various biotin derivatives, analogues, and antagonists are known. Dethiobiotin, a sulfur-free analogue of biotin is the direct precursor of biotin in microorganisms. Biocytin (biotinyl lysine, Fig. 26–1) is released on proteolytic digestion of biotin-containing proteins. The molecular weight of biotin is 244.31 g/mol.

## DISTRIBUTION

Numerous microorganisms, algae, and plant species synthesize biotin and are food sources for animals. Biotin is distributed in a variety of foods.[13] The best sources of biotin are liver (about 100 μg/100 g), egg yolk (about 50 μg/100 g), soybeans (about 60 μg/100 g), and yeast (about 100 μg/100 g). Cereals, legumes, and nuts are moderate sources (10 to 40 μg/100 g). The biotin content of legumes increases on germination. Vegetables, fruits, and meats are poor sources of biotin, the exceptions being cauliflower and mushrooms (about 17 μg/100 g). The biotin content of human and cow's milk is in the range of 12.3 to 20.5 nmol/L. Most of the biotin of natural products is protein bound. Biotin consumption in the United States has been reported to be 28 to 42 μg per day and that in western Europe is 50 to 100 μg per day.

## ABSORPTION AND EXCRETION

It is often stated that enteric synthesis of biotin by bacteria is a source of biotin for humans, based on observations that the total biotin excreted in urine and feces exceeds the dietary intake. Biotin absorbed in

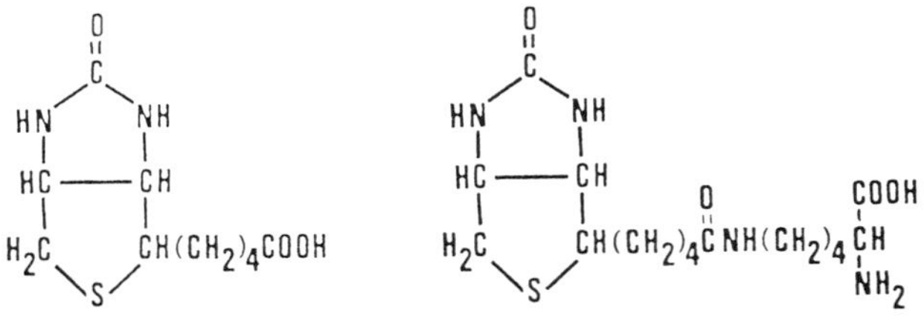

Biotin Biocytin

**FIGURE 26–1.** Structures of biotin and biocytin.

excess of requirement and storage capacity of tissues, along with its metabolites such as bisnorbiotin and biotin sulfoxide, is excreted in urine. Unabsorbed biotin and biotin synthesized by bacteria, essentially in the large intestines, are excreted in feces. The absorption of biotin is higher in the jejunum than in the ileum and is minimal in the colon. Biotin is absorbed better when given orally than when instilled directly into the colon.[4] Because of this fact and the observation that urinary excretion varies with dietary intake whereas fecal excretion is independent of dietary intake, enterically synthesized biotin may be less important for the nutrition of the host than previously thought.

Proteolytic digestion of biotin-containing proteins in the gastrointestinal tract releases biocytin rather than free biotin. It is cleaved further by biotinidase (EC 3.5.1.12) into biotin and lysine before biotin can be absorbed (Fig. 26–2). The absorption of biotin in the rat intestine was thought to occur solely by passive diffusion. Later work with cells in culture[5] and with rat jejunal segments[6,7] showed that at physiologic concentrations of biotin, a saturable process using a biotin-binding carrier is involved in its transport. Thus, the transport of biotin in the rat small intestine is biphasic. At a biotin concentration in the gut below 50 nmol/L (50 nM), the saturable uptake mechanism operates to make enough biotin available to the animal. Such a biphasic system is advantageous in the context of fluctuating biotin intake, borne out by the rarity of primary biotin deficiency in healthy humans. Patients with late-onset multiple carboxylase deficiency who have a deficiency of biotinidase lack the system for absorbing biotin in the nanomolar range, although they respond to pharmacologic doses of biotin. Because biotin-binding activity and biotinidase activity coincide in fractions of human serum, biotinidase might well be a biotin-carrier protein in human serum.[8] A decreased level of plasma biotin has been reported in biotinidase-deficient patients. Significantly, low levels of plasma biotin are also observed in epileptic patients receiving long-term anticonvulsant therapy. These anticonvulsant agents compete with biotin for the biotin-binding activity of biotinidase.[8]

## METABOLISM AND ASSAY

The valerate side chain of biotin can be degraded oxidatively by mammals to form bisnorbiotin, a carboxylic acid that is two carbons shorter than biotin. Most biotin excreted in urine, however, is in the form of free biotin, with only a small amount as metabolites. Biotin in biologic material can be measured based on the biotin-dependent growth of microorganisms such as Lactobacillus plantarum (ATCC 8014), L casei (ATCC 7469), Saccharomyces cerevisiae (ATCC 7754), and the protozoa Ochromonas danica. Variants of an isotope dilution assay for biotin are also used to measure biotin.[9] Biotin levels in human plasma are in the range 0.82 to 2.87 nmol/L, with the mean value around 1.6 nmol/L. Values below 1.02 nmol/L are indicative of a deficient condition.

## REQUIREMENT

No definitive studies on human biotin requirements have been conducted. Hence, there is no specific recommendation regarding dietary allowance.[10] In adults receiving total parenteral nutrition, daily administration of 60 μg prevented the appearance of signs of deficiency. In view of the incomplete knowledge of the bioavailability of biotin in foods, a range of daily intake of 30 to 100 μg has been recommended for adults (see Appendix Table A–2c). Although blood biotin levels fall progressively throughout gestation, such low biotin values are not associated with low-birth-weight infants. Hence, no increment for pregnancy and lactation has been recommended. Based on the biotin content of human milk, which is all in the free, available form, and assuming a daily milk consumption of 750 ml by the infant, the daily biotin intake of breast-fed infants would be in the range 2 to 15 μg per day. For formula-fed infants, an intake of 10 to 15 μg biotin per day has been recommended during the first year. Recommended intakes for children and adolescents are gradually increased to adult levels by the age of 11 years.

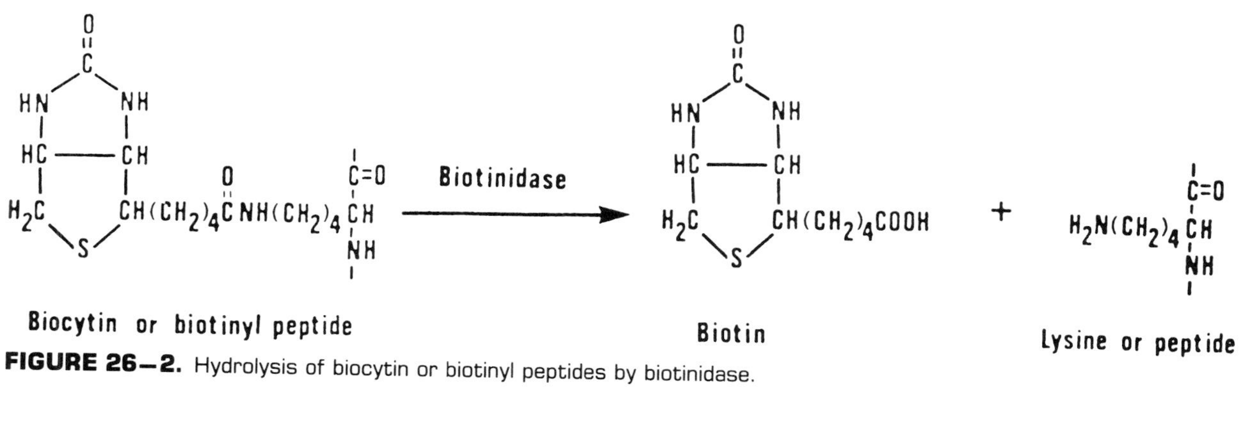
Biotinidase
Biocytin or biotinyl peptide
Biotin
Lysine or peptide

**FIGURE 26–2.** Hydrolysis of biocytin or biotinyl peptides by biotinidase.

## FUNCTIONS

The essential requirement for biotin by higher organisms arises from its obligatory involvement in carbohydrate and lipid metabolism and in the further use of the deaminated residues of certain amino acids. The four biotin enzymes in mammalian tissues are acetyl CoA carboxylase (ACC), pyruvate carboxylase (PC), propionyl CoA carboxylase (PCC), and β-methylcrotonyl CoA carboxylase (MCC). Each of the biotin-dependent carboxylases catalyzes an adenosine triphosphate (ATP)-dependent $CO_2$ fixation reaction and biotin functions as a $CO_2$ carrier on the surface of the enzyme.

**Prosthetic Group Functions.** The best known and understood role of biotin is as the prosthetic group of several biotin-containing enzymes. One phase of all biotin-dependent carboxylation reactions involves the transfer of $CO_2$ from carboxybiotin to substrate. The carboxylations carried out by these enzymes proceed with the intermediate participation of a substrate carbanion. In the ATP-dependent carboxylases, bicarbonate is phosphorylated to form carbonyl phosphate, which is electrophilic and attacks the sterically less-hindered nitrogen of the nucleophilic isourea-like tautomer of the biotinyl moiety of the enzymes. The resulting *N'*-carboxybiotinyl enzyme can then exchange the carboxylate function with a reactive carbon or nitrogen center in the substrate.

Acetyl CoA carboxylase is a cytosolic enzyme, whereas the other three biotin enzymes, PC, PCC, and MCC, are mitochondrial enzymes. The role of biotin enzymes in intermediary metabolism is shown in Figure 26–3. Biotin enzymes are involved in the metabolism of carbohydrates and lipids as well as in the metabolism of some amino acid residues.

ACC (EC 6.4.1.2) catalyzes the ATP-dependent carboxylation of acetyl-CoA leading to the formation of malonyl CoA. ACC is recognized as the major regulatory enzyme of lipogenesis. PC (EC 6.4.1.1) is a key regulatory enzyme of gluconeogenesis in the liver and kidney, where it catalyzes the first step in the synthesis of glucose from pyruvate. It is also present in lipogenic tissues (liver, adipose, lactating mammary gland, and adrenal) and participates in fatty acid synthesis by transporting acetyl groups through citrate, and reducing groups through malate, from mitochondria to cytosol. In all tissues, it has an anaplerotic role in the formation of oxaloacetate. PCC (EC 6.4.1.3) is a key enzyme in the catabolic pathway of isoleucine, threonine, methionine, and valine and also of odd-chain fatty acids. The enzyme catalyzes the conversion of propionyl CoA to methylmalonyl CoA, which enters the tricarboxylic acid cycle by way of succinyl CoA. MCC (EC 6.4.1.4) catalyzes the conversion of β-methylcrontonyl-CoA to β-methylglutaconyl-CoA, a key reaction in the degradative pathway of leucine.

Biotin is covalently linked to the ϵ-amino group of lysine in all carboxylases. The amino acid sequences near the biotin-binding site of PC from sheep, chicken, and turkey livers; of transcarboxylase of Propionibacterium shermanii; and ACC of E. coli show a great deal of homology. In all cases, an Ala-Met-Bct-Met (Bct for biocytin) sequence occurs. Of the four mammalian biotin

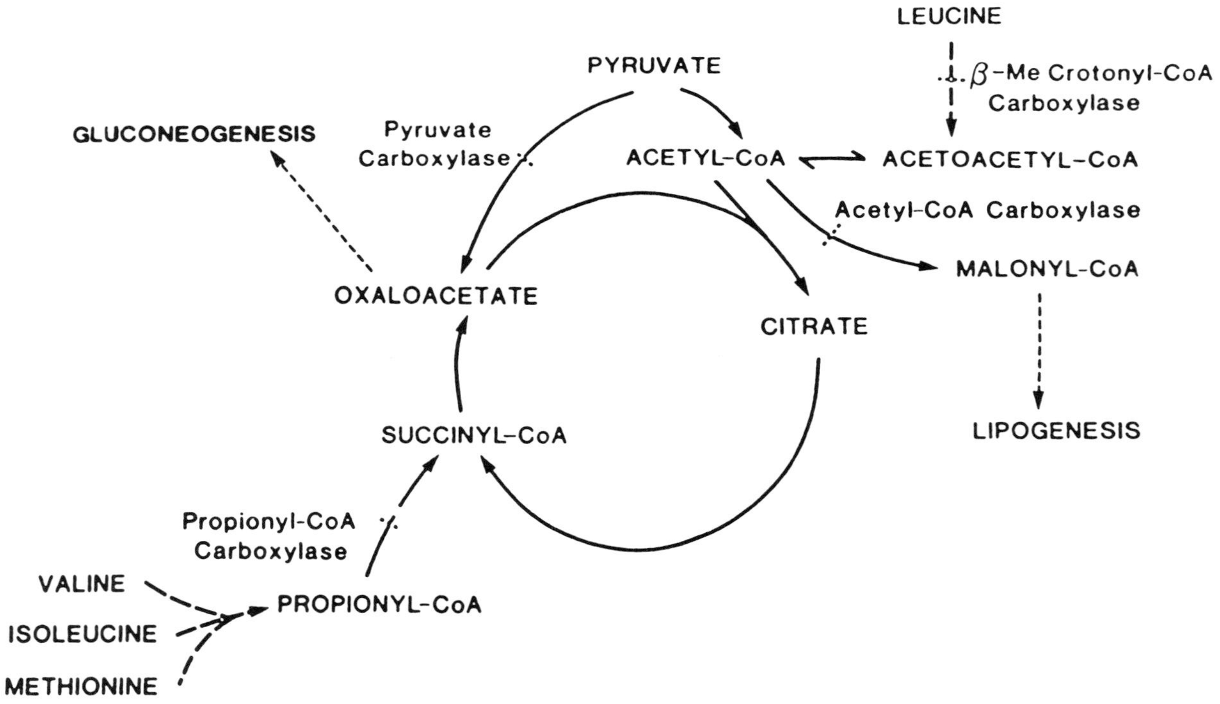
LEUCINE
PYRUVATE
β-Me Crotonyl-CoA
Carboxylase
GLUCONEOGENESIS
Pyruvate
Carboxylase
ACETYL-CoA
ACETOACETYL-CoA
Acetyl-CoA Carboxylase
MALONYL-CoA
OXALOACETATE
CITRATE
SUCCINYL-CoA
LIPOGENESIS
Propionyl-CoA
Carboxylase
VALINE
PROPIONYL-CoA
ISOLEUCINE
METHIONINE

**FIGURE 26–3.** Biotin carboxylases in cellular metabolism.

enzymes, only ACC and PC have regulatory features. Short- and long-term modulations of both enzyme activity and the amount of the enzyme protein by dietary factors and hormonal status are known to occur.[3]

**Nonprosthetic Group Functions.** A requirement for biotin by cells in culture has been established. Cells multiply continuously in basal medium supplemented with delipidized serum and serum lipid extract, but not in basal medium supplemented with serum lipid extract alone. Various reports indicate that cell growth depends on some biotin-mediated activity, the level of which decreases when cells are grown in a biotin-deficient medium.[7] The addition of biotin to the culture medium of cells results in enhanced protein synthesis, DNA synthesis, and cell growth.[11–13] The stimulation of testicular protein synthesis by testosterone also requires normal biotin status.[14] Apart from these effects, the only protein shown to be specifically induced by biotin is glucokinase. Biotin enhances the amount of translatable mRNA coding for glucokinase.[15]

## BIOTIN DEFICIENCY

Human biotin deficiency was first demonstrated by feeding volunteers a biotin-deficient diet.[16] After 5 weeks, all subjects showed prominent symptoms of deficiency; namely, changes in mental status, myalgia, hyperesthesia, localized paresthesia, and anorexia accompanied by nausea. After 7 weeks, maculosquamous dermatitis of the extremities was also prominent. Within 3 to 5 days of daily injections of 150 μg biotin, all symptoms of biotin deficiency disappeared. Acquired biotin deficiency has been described in other reports. A similar syndrome was noted in an 11-year-old boy with hyperuricemia and mental retardation who developed alopecia totalis and generalized erythematous scaly dermatitis.[17] Examination of urinary organic acid excretion revealed intermediates indicating deficiencies of MCC and PCC (Fig. 26–4). In all instances of reported dietary biotin deficiency, raw eggs were a significant component of the patient's diet. Raw egg white contains the protein avidin, which binds biotin almost irreversibly. The dissociation constant (kd) of $10^{-15}$ mol/L is the strongest noncovalent binding between two biologic molecules thus far reported. The avidin-biotin complex is not broken down during proteolytic digestion in the gut. Several cases of biotin deficiency accompanying total parenteral nutrition have been reported.[18,19] Some clinicians suggest, therefore, that biotin be included at a dose of 20 μg per day in such infusions.

The visible pathologic changes in biotin-deficient animals and humans are scaly, seborrheic dermatoses, often accompanied by alopecia. These symptoms are also common to a deficiency of essential fatty acids. Thus, combined defects, such as the decrease in the synthesis of long-chain fatty acids, in tissue linoleic acid, and in the conversion of linoleic acid to eicosatrienoic and eicosatetraenoic acids in the biotin-deficient animal, could contribute to a defective composition of stratum corneum lipids, resulting in impaired epidermal barrier function. The immune system is also impaired in the biotin-deficient animal. Immunodeficiency is noted in

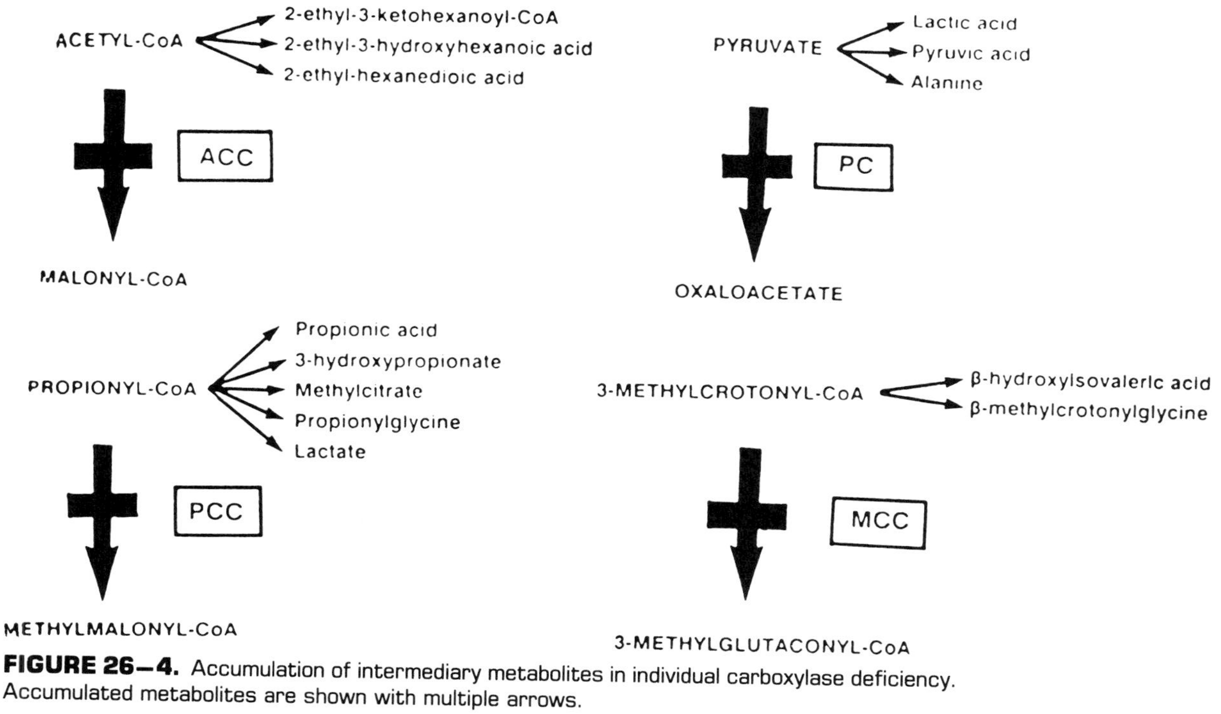
ACETYL-CoA
2-ethyl-3-ketohexanoyl-CoA
2-ethyl-3-hydroxyhexanoic acid
2-ethyl-hexanedioic acid
ACC
MALONYL-CoA
PYRUVATE
Lactic acid
Pyruvic acid
Alanine
PC
OXALOACETATE
PROPIONYL-CoA
Propionic acid
3-hydroxypropionate
Methylcitrate
Propionylglycine
Lactate
PCC
METHYLMALONYL-CoA
3-METHYLCROTONYL-CoA
β-hydroxylsovaleric acid
β-methylcrotonylglycine
MCC
3-METHYLGLUTACONYL-CoA

**FIGURE 26–4.** Accumulation of intermediary metabolites in individual carboxylase deficiency. Accumulated metabolites are shown with multiple arrows.

patients with the biotin-dependent multiple carboxylase deficiency syndrome (MCD).[20] The mechanism leading to immunodeficiency in animals and man still remains to be investigated. Neurologic disorders, including seizures and developmental delay, have been reported in children with MCD or who were receiving total parenteral nutrition. The neurologic symptoms of biotin deficiency are similar to those seen in other conditions of lactic acidosis, including Leigh's subacute necrotizing encephalomyelopathy. The rapid response of neurologic abnormalities to biotin treatment indicates that the defect is a reversible metabolic condition, perhaps related to impaired pyruvate carboxylation. Congenital malformations have been reported in chick embryos of domestic fowl maintained on a biotin-deficient diet. The teratogenic effects of biotin deficiency seem to be species-specific, with severe effects in mice.[21] Because a drastic deficiency of biotin would be incompatible with life, the rate of fetal resorption in the biotin-deficient dams is high.

## INHERITED BIOTIN DEFICIENCY

Since 1976, the incidence in infants of organic acidemia has been investigated with newer techniques; many of these disorders have been characterized as occurring in association with the lack of one or more of the biotin carboxylases. Inherited disorders of individual carboxylases are distinct from the biotin-responsive MCD in as much as patients with inherited disorders do not respond even to pharmacologic doses of biotin. In MCD, all three mitochondrial carboxylases are deficient. Two distinct types of MCD have been recognized based on the nature of the clinical presentation and also on the serum biotin concentration of the patient. The neonatal form is recognized during the first week of life by vomiting, lethargy, and hypotonia.[22] Metabolic ketoacidosis in the infant is associated with excretion of metabolites characteristic of MCD (see Fig. 26–4). The infant could die in an overwhelming acidotic episode before development of cutaneous eruptions, although skin lesions usually are a component of the clinical picture. Carboxylase activities of blood leukocytes are low before treatment with biotin, but return to normal levels after biotin administration. Nevertheless, serum concentration and urinary excretion of biotin by the untreated infant is normal. When skin fibroblasts from the patient are cultured in a medium containing physiologic concentrations of biotin, the carboxylase activities are below normal levels. When the fibroblasts are cultured in a medium containing a high concentration of biotin, however, the carboxylase activities increase to normal levels. A deficiency of biotin holocarboxylase synthetase, the enzyme that covalently adds the biotin prosthetic group to the apobiotin carboxylase (Fig. 26–5), is regarded the primary biochemical lesion in the neonatal type of MCD. The beneficial response of the affected infant to pharmacologic doses of biotin administered prenatally suggests a defective holocarboxylase synthetase with a Michaelis constant (Km) for biotin about 60 times greater than the normal Km of 8 μmol/L (8 μM).[22] An autosomal recessive mode of inheritance for this disorder is indicated.

ATP + Biotin + [Holocarboxylase] Synthetase ⟶
Biotinyl-5'-AMP Synthetase + PPi

Biotinyl -5'-Amp Synthetase + Apo biotin carboxylase ⟶
Biotin carboxvlase + Synthetase + AMP

**FIGURE 26–5.** Biotin holocarboxylase synthetase.

The clinical presentation of patients with the late-onset type of biotin-responsive MCD is similar to that of patients with the neonatal form.[23] The disorder remains undetected until severe clinical abnormalities occur, usually around 3 to 6 months of age. Clinical expression is variable, with a dermatologic picture suggesting acrodermatitis enteropathica and neurologic symptoms such as seizures, ataxia, and myocloni combined with muscular hypotonia. Metabolic acidosis and organic aciduria are inconsistent findings, making it difficult to rely on these signs for diagnosis. Blood levels of biotin and its urinary excretion are low, in contrast to the normal levels seen in the neonatal variant of MCD. Leukocytes isolated from patients before treatment have low levels of carboxylase activities, which increase to normal after treatment with pharmacologic amounts of biotin. The carboxylase activities of skin fibroblasts from the patient are normal, regardless of the biotin concentration of the culture medium. The late-onset (or juvenile) form of MCD is associated with defective biotin absorption, presumably the result of deficiency of biotinidase. Biotinidase specifically cleaves biocytin in the gut before absorption of biotin. It is also implicated in the transport of biotin[8] and in the renal resorption of biotin.

Although dietary biotin deficiency in humans is encountered only rarely, better diagnostic procedures have led to the recognition that MCD syndrome in infants and children is more prevalent than anticipated. An incidence of biotinidase deficiency between 1 in 17,500 and 1 in 340,000 births (95% confidence limits) has been calculated, which would be in the same order of magnitude as for other metabolic disorders.[24] For both neonatal and late-onset variants of MCD, prenatal diagnosis is possible by direct analysis of amniotic fluid for methylcitric acid or 3-hydroxyisovaleric acid. The most dramatic approach to treatment has been the prenatal treatment of high risk pregnancy.[25] The results were unequivocal. In the first such report, a mother at high risk was given biotin orally (10 mg per day) starting from week 34 of gestation. After initiation of oral biotin therapy, the mother's urinary excretion of biotin increased over 100-fold. Nonidentical healthy twins were delivered by cesarean section at 38 weeks of gestation.

Assay of biotin-dependent carboxylases in cultures of fibroblasts established from the foreskins of both twins established MCD in one of the twins, whereas the other was normal. This finding was confirmed by genetic complementation studies. The affected twin has since shown normal physical and mental development on a daily intake of 10 mg biotin. Thus, residual developmental delay and neurologic impairment seen in some postnatally treated MCD patients can be avoided. The excellent maternal tolerance, the benign nature of high levels of biotin in the unaffected twin, and the therapeutic efficacy in the affected twin justify, in retrospect, this approach. Biotin is relatively nontoxic. Doses as high as 60 mg per day over 6 months have been given to children without adverse effects. Even the 10-mg per day dose can be adjusted down depending on the patient's response.

## REFERENCES


1. Utter, M.F., Bardeen, R.E., Taylor, B.L.: Adv. Enzymol., *42*:1–72, 1975.
2. Wood, H.G., Bardeen, R.E.: Annu. Rev. Biochem., *66*:385–413, 1977.
3. Dakshinamurti, K., Chauhan, J.: Annu. Rev. Nutr., *8*:211–233, 1988.
4. Bowman, B.B., Selhub, J., Rosenberg, D.E.: J. Nutr., *116*:1266–1271, 1986.
5. Dakshinamurti, K., Chalifour, L.E.: J. Cell Physiol., *107*:427–438, 1981.
6. Said, S.M., Redha, R.: Am. J. Physiol., *252*:G52–G55, 1987.
7. Dakshinamurti, K., Chauhan, J., Ebrahim, H.: Biosci. Rep., *7*:667–673, 1987.
8. Chauhan, J., Dakshinamurti, K.: Biochem. J., *256*:265–270, 1988.
9. Dakshinamurti, K., Landman, A.D., Ramamurti, L., et al.: Anal. Biochem., *61*:225–231, 1974.
10. Food and Nutrition Board, National Research Council: Recommended Dietary Allowances. 10th Ed. Washington, D.C., National Academy Press, 1989, pp. 165–169.
11. Bhullar, R.P., Dakshinamurti, K.: J. Cell Physiol., *122*:425–430, 1985.
12. Cheng, D.K.S., Moskowitz, M.: J. Cell Physiol., *113*:487–493, 1982.
13. Cohen, D.C., Gospodarowicz, D.: J. Cell Physiol.: *124*:96–106, 1985.
14. Paulose, C.S., Thliveris, J., Dakshinamurti, K.: Horm. Metab. Res., *21*:661–665, 1989.
15. Chauhan, J., Dakshinamurti, K.: J. Biol. Chem., *266*:10035–10038, 1991.
16. Sydenstricker, V.P., Singal, S.A., Briggs, A.P., et al.: JAMA, *118*:1199–1200, 1942.
17. Sweetman, L., Surh, L., Baker, H., et al.: Pediatrics, *68*:553–558, 1981.
18. Innis, S.M., Allardyco, D.B.: Am. J. Clin. Nutr., *37*:185–187, 1983.
19. Mock, D.M., de Lorrimer, A.A., Liebman, W.M., et al.: N. Engl. J. Med., *304*:820–823, 1981.
20. Saunders, J.E., Malamud, N., Cowan, M.J., et al.: Ann. Neurol., *8*:544–547, 1980.
21. Watanabe, T.: J. Nutr., *113*:574–581, 1983.
22. Burri, B.J., Sweetman, L., Nyhan, W.L.: J. Clin. Invest., *68*:1491–1495, 1981.
23. Wolf, B., Feldman, G.L.: Am. J. Hum. Genet., *34*:699–716, 1982.
24. Wolf, B., Heard, G.S., Jefferson, L.G., et al.: J. Inherited Metab. Dis., *9 (Suppl. 2)*:303–306, 1986.
25. Roth, K.S., Yang, W., Allan, L., et al.: Pediatr. Res., *16*:126–129, 1982.


## SELECTED READINGS


Dakshinamurti, K., Bhagavan, H.N. (eds): Biotin, Annals of New York Academy of Sciences. Vol. 447. New York, New York Academy of Sciences, 1985.

Dakshinamurti, K., Chauhan, J.: Biotin. Vitam. Horm., *45*:337–384, 1989.

Sweetman, L., Nyhan, W.L.: Inheritable biotin-treatable disorders and their associated phenomena. Annu. Rev. Nutr., *6*:317–343, 1986.

CHAPTER **27**

# Vitamin C

**Robert A. Jacob**



## HISTORY

Among specific nutritional deficiency diseases, scurvy has ranked with the highest in its toll of human suffering and death. The symptoms are rather characteristic and appear to be described as far back as the ancient civilizations of the Egyptians, Greeks, and Romans. The disease was rampant in the sea explorers of the sixteenth to eighteenth centuries, A.D. , in whom typical physical symptoms of bleeding and rotting gums, swollen and inflamed joints, dark blotches on the skin, and muscle weakness occurred within months of departure. Throughout this period, the British expeditions suffered greatly because of scurvy. Of Admiral Anson's six ships circling the globe in 1740 to 1744, only the flagship returned, and 1051 men died. The carnage prompted the British Admiralty to seek the cure for scurvy, and in 1747, the Scottish surgeon James Lind performed an early clinical nutrition experiment on board ship, whereby six different diet supplements given to six pairs of scorbutic sailors demonstrated the efficacy of oranges and lemons (and to a lesser extent apple cider) in curing scurvy. Yet Lind is credited erroneously with the discovery that citrus fruits can cure scurvy, which had been noted in many earlier accounts. In his famous 1753 *Treatise of The Scurvy,* Lind reasoned that scurvy resulted from blocked perspiration resulting from damp salty sea air, resulting in "putrid humors" that had poisonous and noxious qualities when retained in the body. Captain James Cook in voyages from 1768 to 1775 first proved that long sea voyages did not necessarily result in scurvy. Throughout these voyages, he required that the crew eat local greens and grasses at every opportunity, maintain cleanliness, and practice fastidious personal hygiene. The British Admiralty were beset by inconsistent and conflicting accounts of scurvy cures, and it was not until 48 years after Lind's experiment that lemon or lime juice was made a part of routine British naval provisions.

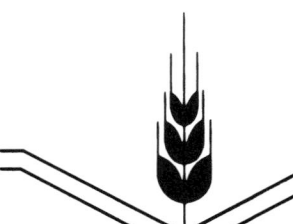

The lessons of the Renaissance explorers were poorly learned by succeeding generations, however. Scurvy beseiged nineteenth century populations on land, including much of Europe during the Great Potato Famine, armies of the Crimean and United States Civil war, arctic explorers, and California gold rush communities. In 1907, scurvy was produced experimentally in the guinea pig, and from 1928 to 1930, Albert Szent-Györgi and Glen King independently published their isolation of vitamin C or "hexuronic acid."[1,2] This pure substance alone was shown to prevent and cure scurvy in guinea pigs. It was later named ascorbic acid for its antiscorbutic properties. The molecular structure was determined and an effective laboratory synthesis was developed in 1933. The history of scurvy and vitamin C has been summarized in a well-annotated volume.[3]

## CHEMISTRY AND ANALYSIS

Ascorbic acid (AA) is the enolic form of an α-ketolactone. The molecular structure (Fig. 27–1) contains two ionizable enolic hydrogen atoms that give the compound its acidic character ($pKa_1$ at carbon 3 =4.17; $pKa_2$ at carbon 2 =11.57). The asymmetric carbon 5 atom allows two enantiomeric forms, of which the L form is naturally occurring. Ascorbic acid is a stable, odorless white solid, formula $C_6H_8O_6$(176.13 g/mol), which is soluble in water, slightly soluble in alcohol, and insoluble in organic solvents. In aqueous solution, the compound is easily oxidized to the diketo form, dehydroascorbic acid (DHAA), and further to diketogulonic, oxalic, and threonic acids, as well as to other minor products (Fig. 27–1). The oxidation of AA to DHAA is reversible, but oxidation beyond DHAA is irreversible and is enhanced by alkaline pH and metals, especially copper and iron. Hence, procedures for stabilizing the vitamin in biologic specimens involve acidification with the addition of a reducing agent and a metal chelator. Because DHAA is readily reduced in vivo, it possesses vitamin C (antiscorbutic) activity, whereas diketogulonic acid has no activity.

The chemical name for AA is 2, 3-didehydro-L-threo-hexano-1, 4-lactone; other terms have included hexuronic acid, cevitamic acid, L-xyloascorbic acid, and vitamin C. Currently, vitamin C is used as the generic descriptor for all compounds exhibiting qualitatively the biologic activity of ascorbic acid. Therefore, this term refers to either or both of the common biologically active forms, AA and DHAA. Its use as a generic descriptor such as vitamin C "activity" or "nutriture", is preferred, rather than a synonym of AA.

A variety of analytic procedures for determining the amount of vitamin C in biologic specimens, foods, and pharmaceutical products have been described in which colorimetric, fluorometric, chromatographic, and electrochemical techniques are used.[4–9] Total vitamin C, AA, or DHAA can be determined depending on the particular assay technique. For example, AA may be determined by colorimetric techniques based on its ability to reduce chromogens such as 2, 6-dichloroindophenol or an α, α-dipyridyl-iron complex. Methods that measure the total amount of vitamin C (AA + DHAA) involve oxidation of AA to DHAA and/or diketogulonic acid with copper, iodine, or ascorbate oxidase, followed by derivatization to form colored (e.g., hydrazones with 2, 4-dinitrophenylhydrazine) or fluorescent (o-phenylenediamine) products. Total vitamin C content has also been determined (as AA) after reduction of sample DHAA with dithiothreitol or homocysteine. Ascorbic acid or DHAA can be determined by the difference after measurements with and without sample pretreatment with exogenous oxidizing or reducing agents. Ascorbic acid and DHAA

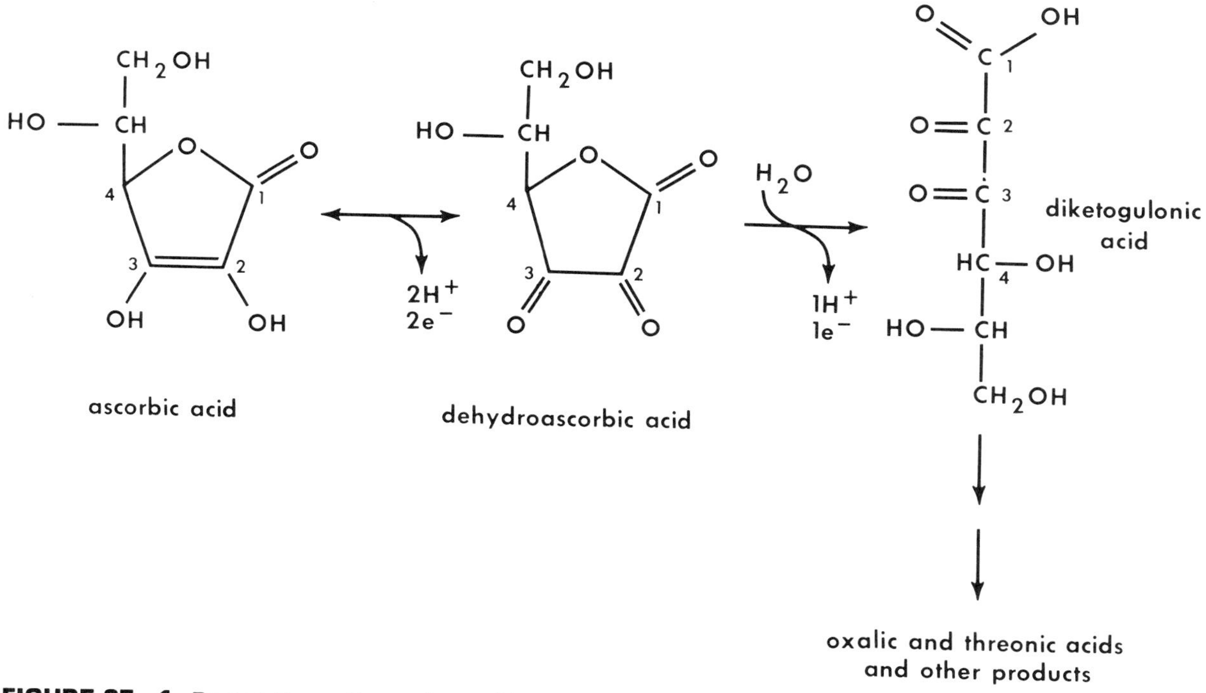
ascorbic acid
2H+
2e−
dehydroascorbic acid
H2O
1H+
1e−
diketogulonic acid
oxalic and threonic acids and other products

**FIGURE 27–1.** Degradation pathway of ascorbic acid.

have been determined simultaneously in a variety of samples by high performance liquid chromatography (HPLC) using post-column derivatization with dimethyl-o-phenylenediamine, or by using dual ultraviolet (UV) detectors.[5]

Although colorimetric methods are convenient and generally reliable, the newer HPLC methods provide improved specificity and sensitivity. A variety of chromatographic conditions have been used, and AA or DHAA can be determined by the use of electrochemical or fluorescent detection modes.[5,7] Isoascorbic (erythorbic) acid, the epimer of L-ascorbic acid, can also be determined by HPLC. Sauberlich et al. caution that its presence in the diet (added as an antioxidant) may result in erroneously high AA values determined by some non-HPLC analytic methods.[10]

Ascorbic acid is easily oxidized to DHAA, and further to the inactive diketogulonic acid at neutral or alkaline pH. The preservative for AA that is added to the sample depends on the selected analytic method. Acidic preservatives, such as trichloroacetic acid and perchloric acid, are suitable for methods that measure total vitamin C, because the acidity prevents the conversion of DHAA to diketogulonate. However, methods that measure the reduced form (AA) specifically must incorporate a reducing agent such as metaphosphoric acid or dithiothreitol as preservative. In the latter case, a metal chelating agent such as ethylene diamine tetraacetic acid (EDTA) is often added to sequester catalytic metals like copper and iron.

**TABLE 27–1.** RANGE OF REPORTED VITAMIN C CONTENTS OF SELECTED FOODS[11–13]

| FOOD | mg/100 g* |
|---|---|
| Black currants | 200 |
| Broccoli | 70–163 |
| Brussels sprouts | 90–150 |
| Cauliflower | 50–90 |
| Strawberries | 40–90 |
| Lemons | 50–80 |
| Cabbage | 31–83 |
| Oranges | 40–78 |
| Spinach, fresh | 6–70 |
| Spinach, frozen | 5–44 |
| Grapefruit | 28–48 |
| Pineapple | 20–40 |
| Turnips | 15–40 |
| Liver, kidney | 10–40 |
| Potatoes | 10–30 |
| Tomatoes | 9–30 |
| Peaches | 5–25 |
| Beans | 10–22 |
| Bananas | 7–19 |
| Peas | 10–15 |
| Cucumber | to 14 |
| Apples | 5–10 |
| Lettuce | 1–7 |
| Cow's milk | 1–2 |
| Apple juice | Up to 2 |
| Meat, beef, and pork | Up to 2 |

*mg/100 g × 56.8 = μmol/kg.

## BIOLOGIC ACTIVITY AND DIETARY INTAKE

Ascorbic acid and DHAA provide biologic vitamin C activity (antiscorbutic), whereas their immediate oxidation product diketogulonic acid and the AA epimer isoascorbic (erythorbic) acid do not. Erythorbic acid, however, is used widely as a food preservative because it possesses antioxidant properties similar to L-ascorbic acid. In this sense, the presence of erythorbic acid in biologic tissues or fluids provides some vitamin C-like activity, analogous to the role of AA as a biologic antioxidant.

More than 80% of the vitamin C in Western diets comes from foods of vegetable origin, chiefly citrus fruits, green vegetables, peppers, tomatoes, berries, and potatoes (Table 27–1).[11–13] A minor portion comes from enriched or fortified products, meat, fish, poultry, eggs, and dairy products, and essentially none from grains. In the United States, the average per capita intake of vitamin C from the food supply in 1985 was 109 mg for adult men, 77 mg for adult women, and 84 mg for children aged 1 to 5 years.[14] The mean total vitamin C intake may be considerably higher because of AA added in some processed foods for its antioxidant properties, and, moreover, because of the consumption of vitamin C supplements. Vitamin C is the nutrient taken most frequently as a supplement, particularly among the elderly population. For example, among elderly healthy Boston area residents, 35% of men and 44% of women used vitamin C supplements, with median supplemental intakes of 300 mg per day.[15]

Values for vitamin C content of food items listed in tables of food composition may represent either AA or total vitamin C, depending on the particular analytic method used. Results to date suggest that the percent of total vitamin C content in fresh fruits and vegetables that is DHAA is on the order of 5 to 10%, whereas storage and/or processing may increase the proportion to 30% or greater.[12] As shown in Table 27–1, the AA content of fresh fruits and vegetables may vary appreciably, even among different samples of the same item.[11–13] The amount of available vitamin C in foods may be significantly reduced because of destruction that occurs during cooking and loss in cooking water. (See also Appendix Table A–21 for the vitamin C content of common foods.)

## METABOLISM

### ABSORPTION AND BIOAVAILABILITY

Ascorbic acid is absorbed in the human intestine through an energy-dependent active process that is saturable and dose dependent. The intestinal absorption of AA and its entry into cells may be facilitated by conversion into DHAA, which penetrates membranes better than the reduced form at physiologic pH. After its entry into the intestinal epithelium or tissue cells, DHAA can readily be reduced back to AA. At low doses (less than 30 mg per day), AA is nearly completely absorbed, and 70 to 90% of the usual dietary intake of AA (30 to 180 mg per day) is absorbed.[16,17] However, absorption falls to 50% with a dose of 1.5 g and to 16% with a 12-g dose.[16] Single AA doses greater than 200 mg that contained $^{14}C$-labeled AA resulted in postabsorptive degradation of AA in the intestine to carbon dioxide, which was expired in the breath.[18] The amount of label recovered increased from 1 to 30% with increasing amounts of AA carrier dose, indicating greater postabsorptive AA degradation with the larger doses. The presence of large amounts of unabsorbed AA in the intestine accounts for the osmotic diarrhea and intestinal discomforts often reported by persons ingesting large doses of AA. Maximal AA absorption is attained by the ingestion of several spaced doses of less than 1 g throughout the day rather than ingestion of a single megadose. The saturable absorption mechanism probably explains the greater bioavailability sometimes seen after healthy subjects ingest AA in sustained release forms compared to equivalent pure doses. In such cases, the bioavailability increases from 121 to 165%, based on measurement of increases in blood AA levels.[19]

Results of comparisons of the bioavailability of pure synthetic AA versus natural forms have not been consistent.[20–22] Overall, the bulk of the data suggest the bioavailability is not significantly different, although the question is not resolved unequivocally.

**TABLE 27–2.** VITAMIN C CONTENT OF HUMAN TISSUES AND FLUIDS

| SPECIMEN | VITAMIN C (μmol/100 g wet*) |
|---|---|
| Pituitary gland | 227–284 |
| Adrenal glands | 170–227 |
| Eye lens | 142–176 |
| Brain | 74–85 |
| Liver | 57–91 |
| Spleen and pancreas | 57–85 |
| Kidneys | 28–85 |
| Heart muscle | 28–85 |
| Semen (whole) | 20–60 |
| Lungs | 40 |
| Skeletal muscle | 17 |
| Testes | 17 |
| Thyroid | 11 |
| Plasma | 1.7–8.5 |
| Saliva | 0.01–0.5 |

*μmol/100 g wet × 0.176 = mg/100 g wet.

## DISTRIBUTION AND TRANSPORT

As seen in Table 27–2, vitamin C content in body tissues varies widely, with the highest levels in pituitary, adrenals, leukocytes, eye lens, and brain, and the lowest levels in plasma and saliva.[23] Vitamin C concentrations also vary widely in different blood cell types.[24–29]

The total AA body pool in adults has been determined experimentally by feeding isotopically ($^{13}C$, $^{14}C$, $^{3}H$) labeled AA as a tracer.[30–32] Kallner et al. used pharmacokinetic calculations to determine AA body pool and turnover in healthy men given doses of 1-$^{14}C$-labeled AA along with steady state AA intakes of 30 to 180 mg per day.[30] They found that the body half-life of AA was inversely related to the AA intake, and that the total body pool of AA increased to a maximum value of about 20 mg/kg body weight or about 1500 mg for an average size man. The maximum body pool was reached at a plasma AA concentration of 57 μmol/L (1.0 mg/dl), attained by 95% of the male population with an AA intake of 100 mg per day.[30] Baker et al. calculated body AA pool sizes of 1486 to 1542 mg in healthy male prisoners consuming 75 mg AA per day along with labeled vitamin during experimental vitamin C depletion and repletion.[32] Clinical symptoms of scurvy appeared at a total body AA pool below 300 mg per day, and disappeared when larger body pools were present.[32] In other studies, which did not involve the use of direct isotopic techniques, the estimated AA body pool was 22 mg/kg body weight and 32 to 34 mg/kg fat-free weight.[33] A calculation of the maximum AA body pool based on vitamin contents of human tissues gives a value of 5 g/70 kg body weight, estimated as attainable by an AA intake of 200 mg/day.[34]

The high concentrations of intracellular AA relative to the blood suggest an energy-driven cellular transport process. The vitamin is actively transported into human leukocytes by a saturable, temperature-dependent process that exhibits stereospecific preference for L- over D-form epimers and shows different transport kinetics depending on the cell type.[35] Evidence suggests that DHAA is the form of the vitamin that actually crosses the membranes of intestinal epithelial cells and leukocytes, after which it is reduced intracellularly to the active reduced form.[33,36] More than one DHAA reductase enzyme, which uses reduced glutathione and/or reduced nicotinamide adenine dinucleotide phosphate (NADPH) to catalyze reduction of DHAA intracellularly, seems to be involved.[37] Accumulation of AA into isolated human neutrophils is mediated by both high and low affinity transporters and is almost entirely in the reduced form intracellularly, and its localization to the cytosol suggests a protective antioxidant function.[36] In the plasma of healthy men and women, vitamin C exists in the free (nonprotein-bound) and reduced form.[38]

## HOMEOSTASIS

The dose-dependent intestinal absorption of AA discussed previously provides a mechanism whereby whole body status of AA is regulated. A second important mechanism involves renal action to conserve or to excrete unmetabolized AA. The amount of AA excreted depends on the amount of AA cleared by glomerular filtration and the amount subsequently resorbed by the renal tubules. The amount of AA cleared by glomerular filtration depends on the plasma AA level and the glomerular filtration rate. As this amount increases, the ability of the renal tubules to reabsorb AA reaches a maximum and the unresorbed excess AA is excreted in the urine. This point, called the renal threshold, occurs in humans at plasma AA levels of about 68 μmol/L (1.2 mg/dl). Renal clearance of AA was found to depend directly on plasma concentrations in a linear fashion between plasma AA of 57 and 227 μmol/L (1.0 and 4.0 mg/dl),[39] and sigmoidally over a larger range. Hence, renal regulation of AA operates to conserve body AA stores during low AA intakes through renal tubular reabsorption, and to limit plasma AA levels by excretion of excess AA loads that exceed the renal threshold. Melethil et al. showed that plasma AA concentration-time profiles are similar for subjects ingesting AA doses of 0.5, 1.0, or 2.0 g per day for 1 week, and that the percent of the dose recovered in the urine decreased significantly with the increasing dosage, indicating that both renal tubular resorption and gastrointestinal absorption of AA are saturable processes.[39]

The dependence of intestinal absorption and renal reabsorption on the external AA load provides an effective systemic regulation of AA status. In addition, homeostatic regulation of AA metabolism may also operate at the cellular level. Some cells or body tissues, including lymphocytes,[29] the brain,[40] and the aqueous humor of the eye,[41] are resistant to AA loading, possibly because of regulation by the AA transport system. The enzymatic regeneration of cellular AA (the active form) from DHAA (the oxidized form) may represent a cellular mechanism to regulate conservation and use of the vitamin.[37]

### TURNOVER AND CATABOLISM

The average half-life of AA in the adult human is about 16 to 20 days. In healthy nonsmoking men ingesting steady-state AA intakes of 30 to 180 mg per day, however, the half-life of radioisotope-labeled AA was inversely related to the dosage. The half-life of AA decreased from 40 to 8 days with increasing steady-state AA intakes from 30 to 180 mg per day, along with increased total AA turnover (14 to 134 mg per day) and AA body pool (11 to 22 mg/kg body weight).[30] The whole body turnover of vitamin C, or catabolic rate, was shown in experimental studies to depend on the AA body pool size.[32] In healthy prisoners depleted of AA, the catabolic rate decreased from 45 mg per day at an initial body pool of 1500 mg, to 9 mg per day at a pool size of 300 mg, a point below which frank symptoms of scurvy appeared in all subjects. Overall, the body turnover of AA amounted to about 3% of the existing body pool per day.[32] At very low or zero intakes of AA, essentially no unmetabolized AA is excreted, yet an obligatory metabolic loss of several milligrams per day occurs. Intake of 8 to 10 mg per day of the vitamin is sufficient to compensate for obligatory catabolism and provide enough AA to satisfy critical functions and prevent overt scurvy symptoms.

In humans, AA is catabolized through oxidation to DHAA, hydrolysis of DHAA to diketogulonate, and decomposition of the latter compound to a variety of compounds including oxalic and threonic acids, L-xylose, and ascorbate-2-sulfate (see Fig. 27–1). The principal route of AA elimination is through urinary excretion, with unmetabolized AA and all of the above named metabolites being eliminated. The initial oxidation of AA to DHAA proceeds through a partially oxidized free radical intermediate, monodehydroascorbate, which is unstable but has been detected by electron paramagnetic resonance spectroscopy. A large amount of ingested AA is metabolized to exhaled $CO_2$ in rats (20 to 30% of intake) and guinea pigs (60 to 70%). This pathway, however, is a minor route of AA catabolism in humans consuming normal dietary intakes of the vitamin.[18] Negligible amounts of AA or its metabolites are excreted in feces. The percentage of unmetabolized AA excreted in urine relative to catabolic products increases greatly with increasing dietary intake of AA. Oxalic acid constitutes a minor fraction (5 to 10%) of AA metabolites, but it seems to be an obligatory product in that it is found even at very low dietary AA intakes. With increasing AA intakes, however, conversion of AA to oxalate is limited.[13,42]

## BIOCHEMICAL FUNCTIONS

The functions of AA are based primarily on its properties as a reversible biologic reductant. As such, it provides reducing equivalents for a variety of biochemical reactions, is essential as a cofactor for reactions requiring a reduced metal ion ($Fe^{+2}$, $Cu^{+1}$), and serves as a protective antioxidant that operates in the aqueous phase and can be regenerated in vivo when oxidized. Few of the roles of AA have been established on a definitive molecular basis. The roles in metal catalyzed hydroxylations that use molecular oxygen are best defined (Fig. 27–2). In such cases, AA is believed to act to reduce the metal catalyst, allowing reactivation of the metal-enzyme complex, and/or as a cosubstrate involved in the reduction of molecular oxygen. The biochemical roles of AA have been reviewed.[33,43]

### COLLAGEN FORMATION

One of the best established roles of AA is as a reductive cofactor for post-translational hydroxylation of peptide-bound proline and lysine residues during formation of collagen.[43,44] The hydroxyproline and hydroxylysine units allow cross-linking to stabilize the triple helical structure of tropocollagen, an essential subunit of procollagen. The reaction occurs in the endoplasmic reticulum of the fibroblast before excretion of procollagen from the cell. The enzyme involved in proline hydroxylation,

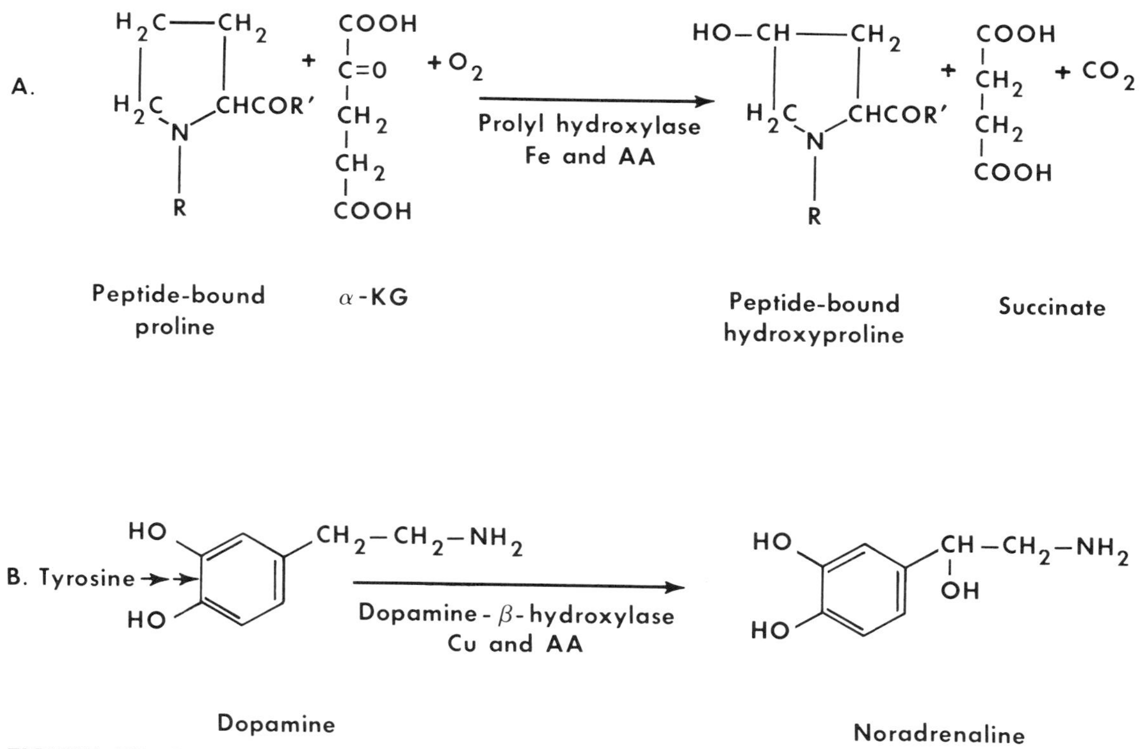
A.
Prolyl hydroxylase
Fe and AA
Peptide-bound proline
α-KG
Peptide-bound hydroxyproline
Succinate
B. Tyrosine
Dopamine-β-hydroxylase
Cu and AA
Dopamine
Noradrenaline

**FIGURE 27–2.** Reactions that require ascorbic acid as a cofactor with metals for hydroxylations of proline *(A)* and dopamine *(B)*. AA, Ascorbic acid; α-KG, α-ketoglutarate; noradrenaline, norepinephrine.

prolyl hydroxylase, requires molecular oxygen, AA, iron, and α-ketoglutarate (Fig. 27–2*A*). During the hydroxylation reaction, the enzyme-bound iron is oxidized to $Fe^{+3}$ and the AA is involved in reactivating the enzyme by reduction of iron back to the ferrous state. In an analogous reaction, AA participates as a cofactor in the hydroxylation of lysine residues catalyzed by copper-dependent lysyl hydroxylase. Prolyl and lysyl hydroxylases are also called dioxygenases, referring to the ability of the enzymes to provide two oxygen atoms to the same or separate substrates.

Ascorbic acid may also serve as a reductant for diverse metal-dependent polymerization and cross-linking reactions of connective tissue, and as carrier for sulfate groups needed for production of glycosaminoglycans (e.g., chondroitin and dermatan sulfate). Although not all details of the processes are clearly resolved, the absolute requirement for AA in the formation of mature connective tissue explains the primary physical manifestations of AA deficiency, the connective tissue disorders associated with scurvy.

## CARNITINE BIOSYNTHESIS

Carnitine is required as a transporter of long chain fatty acids across the mitochondrial membrane wherein β-oxidation provides energy to cells, especially for cardiac and skeletal muscle. Esterification with carnitine appears to provide a mechanism for transport, storage, and excretion of long chain fatty acid acyl groups. Humans obtain carnitine from the diet (primarily from animal products) and also biosynthesize carnitine as do animals. The biosynthesis involves the methylation of lysine with methionine as methyl donor, and requires AA, iron, and vitamins $B_6$ and niacin as cofactors for various enzymes of the pathway.[45] Ascorbate is required along with iron at two steps in the pathway involving mitochondrial and cytosolic hydroxylases, in reactions similar to the hydroxylation of proline and lysine during collagen formation. In AA-depleted guinea pigs, carnitine levels are significantly reduced in muscle, but not in brain or serum.[46–48] Studies with perfused guinea pig livers indicate that during AA deficiency, the rate-limiting enzyme for carnitine synthesis is γ-butyrobetaine, 2-oxo-glutarate-dioxygenase.[48]

The loss of fatty acid-based energy production because of limited carnitine biosynthesis may explain the fatigue and muscle weakness observed in human AA deficiency,[49] although such a connection has not been established definitively.

## NEUROTRANSMITTER SYNTHESIS

Ascorbic acid is required as a cofactor for the copper-containing dopamine-β-mono-oxygenase enzyme that catalyzes hydroxylation of the dopamine side chain to form norepinephrine (Fig. 27–2*B*). Ascorbic acid provides electrons for reduction of molecular oxygen, transferred by copper to dopamine, and hydrogen atoms to reduce the other oxygen atom to water. Hence, the mechanism for dopamine hydroxylation is different from that of prolyl and lysyl hydroxylations, which involve dioxygenase enzymes and reactivate the enzyme-metal complex by reduction of the metal. In guinea pigs, synthesis of biogenic amines has been shown to be AA-dependent. Ascorbic acid appears also to be involved in the hydroxylation of tryptophan to form serotonin in the brain, and in degradation of tyrosine by p-hydroxyphenylpyruvate hydroxylase, although in the latter reaction, it acts as a nonessential reducing agent. The important role of AA in neurotransmitter synthesis and metabolism likely underlies the high concentrations of AA found in adrenal and brain tissue (even during low plasma AA levels) and the relative resistance of these organs to AA depletion.[33,43]

## MIXED-FUNCTION OXYGENASE SYSTEM

The microsomal drug-metabolizing system operates in liver microsomes and reticuloendothelial tissues to inactivate and metabolize a wide variety of substrates, such as endogenous hormones or xenobiotics (e.g., drugs and carcinogens). Modifications such as hydroxylation or demethylation of lipophilic substrates increase their aqueous solubility and excretion in urine. The systems operate with oxygenase enzymes, flavoproteins, cytochrome P450 protein, oxygen, and reducing agents such as NAD(P)H. The activity of the system often seems to depend on AA, although a role for the vitamin has not been elucidated.[33] Results of animal studies indicate that AA depletion reduces the activity of system enzymes and the integrity of cytochrome P-450 electron transport. Studies in animals and humans show that drug-metabolizing activity is reduced during AA deficiency, and that stress (from steroid hormone activation) and/or use of drugs may alter AA metabolism and lower AA body status. Users of oral contraceptives have been shown to have reduced levels of plasma and leukocyte AA. Exposure of rats to polychlorinated biphenyls significantly increases their requirement for AA.

Vitamin C is also involved in the hepatic microsomal hydroxylation of cholesterol in the excretion of cholesterol as bile acids. The first step, 7α-hydroxylation of the steroid nucleus, requires cytochrome P-450-dependent mixed-function oxygenase activity. Studies with guinea pigs have shown that marginal AA depletion reduces the activity of this rate-limiting step in cholesterol degradation. Results from animal studies have been inconsistent, some indicating no direct effect of increased AA intake on the mixed-function oxygenase activity,[33] whereas another reporting increased rate of cholesterol conversion and decreased blood and liver lipid levels as ascorbate dose increased.[34]

## IRON ABSORPTION

Ascorbic acid enhances the intestinal absorption of nonheme iron.[50,51] Generally, the enhancement of iron absorption is proportional to the amount of AA in a meal, although observed differences in the effect of AA may result from varying amounts of substances in the foods that promote or inhibit iron absorption. The mechanism of action is believed to involve the ability of AA to reduce intraluminal iron to the more absorbable ferrous state and/or to form soluble iron complexes at the alkaline pH in the duodenum. The vitamin seems especially effective in counteracting food components such as phytates and tannins, which inhibit iron absorption by forming insoluble complexes. Although the effect of AA in enhancing iron absorption has been demonstrated rather convincingly by using a variety of techniques, results of studies in humans have not always shown improvement in iron status with addition of AA to meals.[33,50] The noneffects of AA on iron status observed in some human studies are likely attributable to experimental conditions such as type of diets, level of AA and iron content, iron status, and length of response period.

## OTHER FUNCTIONS

**Reductive Protection of Folic Acid and Vitamin E.** The reducing property of AA may also improve the stability and use of folic acid and vitamin E (α-tocopherol). The reduced forms of folic acid, dihydro- and tetrahydrofolates, may be stabilized by AA, thus preventing their excretion in urine.[33] Vitamins C and E act as radical scavenging antioxidants in the aqueous and lipid (cell membrane) phases, respectively. Mixed results and conclusions have been reported from studies of AA-tocopherol interactions.[42] In in vitro electron paramagnetic resonance spectroscopy studies, Niki showed that AA spares membrane-bound α-tocopherol by reducing the tocopheroxyl radical back to the active tocopherol form at the membrane interface.[52] On the other hand, no tocopherol sparing by AA was seen in guinea pigs receiving deuterium-labeled tocopherol acetate as an isotope dilution marker.[53] In this study, no significant effects of three levels of AA intake were seen on tocopherol blood or tissue status, or on body pool and turnover of tocopherol at either of two tocopherol intake levels.[53] Hence, whether or not AA significantly affects the use of tocopherol in vivo has not been established.

**Cyclic Nucleotides.** Ascorbic acid may increase cellular levels of cyclic adenosine monophosphate and cyclic guanosine monophosphate (cAMP and cGMP) by increasing their synthesis and/or decreasing their enzymatic degradation rate.[33,43] For example, AA-induced changes in histamine release and dopamine stimulative effects have been interpreted as evidence for this interaction. Although AA has been shown to be related to cyclic nucleotide levels in some studies, the notion that AA directly affects those levels, or that such an effect has physiologic significance, is not established.

**Miscellaneous Functions.** Vitamin C, as ascorbate-2-sulfate, has been suggested to serve as a sulfating agent, of cholesterol as part of its catabolism, and of mucopolysaccharides during formation of connective tissue. The apparent stimulation by AA of prostaglandin synthesis in isolated cells has been hypothesized as a means to explain some of the functions of the vitamin. Evidence relating AA to immunocompetence, antioxidant defense, and other clinical benefits covers the range from AA deficiency to megadose intakes. These effects are discussed in *Clinical Aspects.*

## DEFICIENCY

### MANIFESTATIONS

Humans, along with monkeys and guinea pigs, are among the few species of animals unable to synthesize AA from glucose. Lack of the enzyme required to convert L-gulonolactone to 2-keto-L-gulonolactone is believed to be the key missing element in man. When dietary intake of AA is insufficient, a set of reproducible conditions is observed in humans that is termed scurvy. The scurvy symptoms listed in Table 27–3 have been observed in naturally occurring as well as in experimentally induced scurvy.[8,32] The mesenchymal symptoms result primarily from defects in connective tissue formation. A variety of hemorrhagic manifestations occur, including bleeding into joints, the peritoneal cavity and/or pericardial sac, and the adrenals in severe cases. A decrease in the ability of the gingiva to resist inflammation and bleeding seems to be an early physical sign of AA deficiency. Standardized bleeding indices taken in healthy adult men undergoing controlled experimental AA depletion and repletion are shown in Figure 27–3.[54] During periods of AA depletion (AA intake of 5 mg per day), the men were nonscorbutic, but were in a state of biochemical AA deficiency (as judged by plasma and leukocyte AA levels); the propensity of the gingiva to bleed or to become inflamed was inversely related to AA intake. The mechanism responsible for the hemorrhagic manifestations of AA deficiency has not been elucidated. No specific defects of the blood clotting mechanism have been identified. Presumably, a defect in vascular integrity related to the role of the vitamin in connective tissue formation is the important factor, but no specific histologic defect has been identified. The weakness and fatigue associated with scurvy are analogous to symptoms of human carnitine deficiency and may be related to a defect in carnitine biosynthesis. Psychologic symptoms are likely related to altered neurotransmitter synthesis and metabolism.

**TABLE 27–3.** CLINICAL MANIFESTATIONS OF VITAMIN C DEFICIENCY

| |
|---|
| Mesenchymal |
| Petechiae |
| Ecchymoses |
| Coiled hairs |
| Perifollicular hemorrhages |
| Inflamed and bleeding gums |
| Hyperkeratosis |
| Sjögren's syndrome |
| Dyspnea |
| Joint effusions |
| Arthralgia |
| Edema |
| Impaired wound healing |
| Systemic |
| Weakness |
| Fatigue |
| Lassitude |
| Psychologic and Neurologic |
| Depression |
| Hysteria |
| Hypochondriasis |
| Vasomotor instability |

In infants, AA deficiency manifests with bone abnormalities, including impaired bone growth and disturbed ossification.[8] Hemorrhagic symptoms may occur, such as retrobulbar and subperiosteal hemorrhages, epistaxis, hematuria, purpura, and resultant hypochromic anemia because of blood loss. The affected infants often are irritable because of tender extremities and pseudoparalysis.

Some historically reported symptoms of scurvy may be attributable to coexisting nutrient deficiencies such as of thiamine, "wet beriberi" (edema), vitamin A (night blindness), vitamin D (rickets), and folic acid (megaloblastic anemia).

### PREVALENCE

Clinical scurvy is rare in modern Western societies, and usually occurs in individuals with exceptionally poor diets, such as in alcoholism and drug abuse, or that have a near total lack of AA-containing foods. Most often, it is noted in elderly men who live alone and eat a diet frequently low in fruits and vegetables. Because breast milk provides adequate AA, infantile scurvy is seen most often after weaning, between 6 and 12 months. Modern infant formulas are fortified with sufficient AA such that infantile scurvy is now almost nonexistent.

A greater proportion of low blood AA levels is observed in the elderly population, especially those people that are institutionalized, homebound or chronically sick.[55,56] However, active, healthy elderly persons show adequate vitamin C status, with blood AA levels no different than younger adults when adjusted for AA intakes.[15,28] Vitamin C pharmacokinetics were found to be affected by AA status but not by age when healthy elderly men were compared with young men in vitamin-depleted and

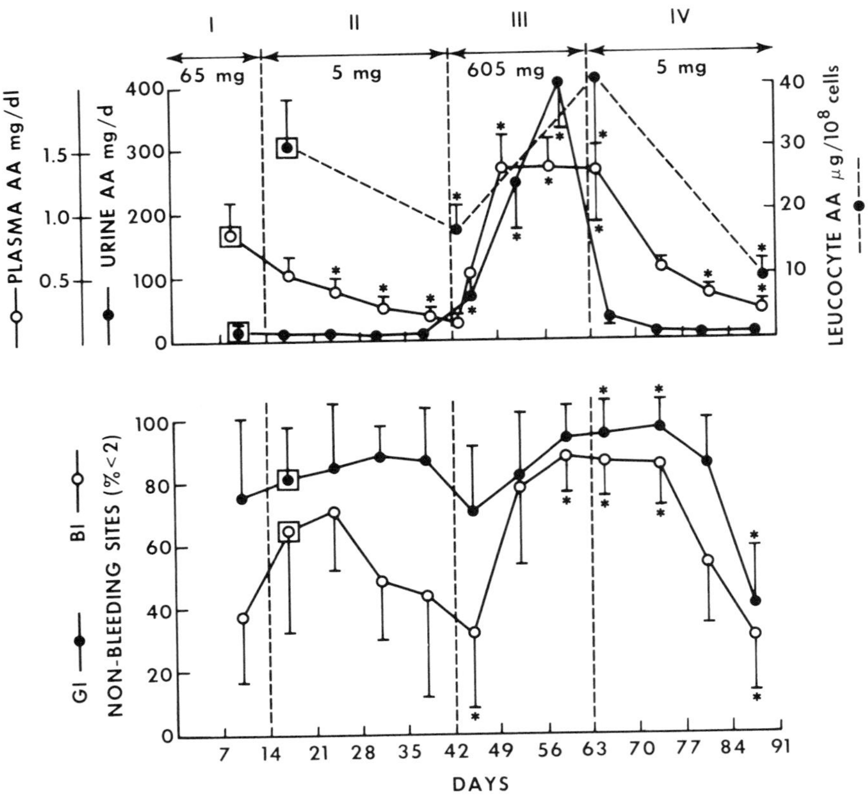

I
II
III
IV
65 mg
5 mg
605 mg
5 mg
PLASMA AA mg/dl
URINE AA mg/d
LEUCOCYTE AA µg/10^8 cells
GI
BI
NON-BLEEDING SITES (%<2)
DAYS


**FIGURE 27–3.** Blood and urine ascorbic acid levels and gingival bleeding indices in 11 healthy adult men receiving various ascorbic acid intakes between 5 and 605 mg per day as shown at top. GI, Gingival index; BI, bleeding index (mg/dl × 56.8 = µmol/L). (From Leggott, P.J., Robertson, P.B., Rothman, D.L., et al.: J. Periodontol., *57*:480–485, 1986.)

supplemented states.[57] No definitive relationship between age and vitamin C status has been established. The trend to lower plasma and leukocyte AA levels observed in the aged seems most likely attributable to decreased dietary AA intake and a lower lean body mass.[58] Many factors related to aging have been postulated to explain lower AA levels in elderly individuals, including decreased intestinal absorption and/or renal tubular reabsorption, increased use because of sickness or drug therapy, and increased turnover, possibly related to lower levels of the DHAA reductase that regenerates the active AA form. Convincing evidence that any of these factors results in deficient AA status in this group or increases their AA requirement has not been reported.

## STATUS ASSESSMENT

Two categories of tests for assessing human AA status can be described: "static" tests, which measure the vitamin C body pool or levels in tissues or fluids, and functional measures, which quantitate an ascorbate-dependent function. Only static tests are currently practical for assessing AA status, because reliable functional measures have not been established. Functional measures are preferred because they relate directly to health or function, and the interpretation of results is not confused by variables unrelated to AA status, such as gender and cigarette smoking. Assessment of the total body AA pool provides a good marker of status, but practical methods for making this determination have not been devised. Lack of increase in serum AA or urinary AA excretion after an oral vitamin C load can provide a useful test of AA tissue deficit in individuals, but this type of test is not practical for use in nutrition surveys.[59]

### STATIC MEASURES

**Plasma and Leukocytes.** Measurement of plasma and leukocyte AA levels are currently the most practical and reliable tests for assessing human vitamin C status. Plasma AA levels have been shown to correlate with dietary AA intake and with leukocyte AA in both epidemiologic and experimental studies.[10,29,60,61] The direct response of plasma and leukocyte AA levels to changes in AA intake is shown in the top half of Figure 27–3 for 11 healthy adult men housed in a metabolic unit for 14 weeks.[60] Plasma AA levels are responsive to recent dietary intake, whereas leukocyte levels reflect tissue contents and the AA body pool more closely. Studies with monkeys and guinea pigs have confirmed that, of a variety of blood AA measures, leukocyte AA levels correlate best with liver AA and AA body pool.[7] Determination of leukocyte AA is technically complex, and leukocytes, e.g., the "buffy coat," constitute a heterogeneous mixture of cells for which interpretation of analytic results is far from being standardized (see *Interpretive Guidelines*). Plasma AA tests are preferred for large population studies because the test requires less blood and is easier to perform, and the results are interpreted rather easily.

The typical relationship between plasma AA and dietary AA intake is shown in Figure 27–4 for a healthy elderly population.[15] The curve is similar to those published from a variety of other studies, both experimental and population based, in which steady-state plasma AA levels plateau between 68 and 102 μmol/L (1.2 to 1.8 mg/dl) and vitamin C intakes include supplements,[15,60,62] or are from diet alone.[58]

**Whole Blood and Erythrocytes.** The pattern of changes in whole blood and erythrocyte AA levels after AA depletion in humans is qualitatively the same as for plasma levels, indicating a facile and relatively rapid exchange of the vitamin between plasma and red cells.[60] Whole blood or erythrocyte AA levels are considered a less sensitive indicator of AA deficiency, however, because they do not change as much or fall as low as plasma levels during AA deficiency. In subjects nearly depleted of the vitamin, in whom scurvy symptoms exist or are imminent (body pool is less than 300 mg of AA), whole blood AA levels will fall to 17 μmol/L (0.3 mg/dl) or

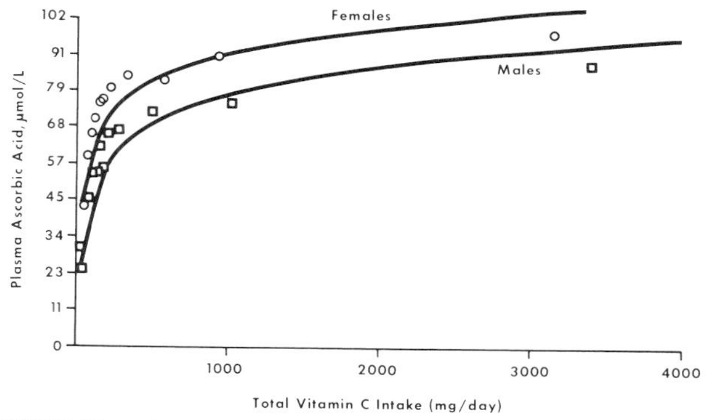
Females
Males
Plasma Ascorbic Acid, μmol/L
102
91
79
68
57
45
34
23
11
0
1000
2000
3000
4000
Total Vitamin C Intake (mg/day)

**FIGURE 27–4.** Plasma ascorbic acid versus total vitamin C intake (diet plus supplements) for elderly males (N = 235) and females (N = 442). Median plasma ascorbate values plotted at the median intakes for 12 percentiles of intake. (From Jacob, R.A., Otradovec, C.L., Russell, R.M., et al.: Am. J. Clin. Nutr., *48*:1436–1442, 1988.)

below, whereas plasma AA levels are less than 5.7 μmol/L (0.1 mg/dl).

**Urine.** The rate of excretion of AA in urine is not linear with AA intake because of efficient renal reabsorption at low AA intakes and renal clearance at high intakes. Healthy adults ingesting a normal Western diet containing 40 to 100 mg per day of AA would be expected to excrete some 5 to 50 mg per day of unmetabolized AA. At plasma AA levels exceeding the renal reabsorption threshold, about 80 μmol/L (1.4 mg/dl), excretion of AA increases abruptly with increased AA intake (see Fig. 27–3). At AA intakes below 40 mg per day, urine AA excretion falls dramatically, to less than 10 mg per day, and to nearly nondetectable levels in scurvy or in severe AA depletion. Hence, urinary AA content can be used to affirm a diagnosis of frank AA deficiency but is not useful for differentiating between subjects with normal or low (i.e., nonscorbutic) AA status. Measurement of urinary AA levels after an oral dose of 0.5 to 2 g of AA over 4 days can be useful for assessing a tissue ascorbate deficit.[59] Excretion of less than 60% of the dose indicates depletion of tissue AA.

**Other Static Measures.** The AA oral loading test just described represents an indirect measure of the AA body pool. The AA body pool has been determined directly by isotope dilution studies, using $^{14}C$- or $^{3}H$-labeled ascorbic acid as tracers.[30,32] After administration of oral doses of the tracer, total body AA can be calculated from measurements of the tracer and total AA in blood and urine, because the extent of dilution of the tracer is proportional to the existing AA body pool. Other parameters such as intestinal absorption, biologic turnover, and metabolic pathways can also be determined. General guidelines for interpreting levels of the AA body pool are listed in Table 27–4. Although valid for assessing vitamin C status, measures of the AA body pool are not practical for use in nutritional status assessment because a simple procedure has yet to be devised. Salivary AA content does not appear to be a good measure of vitamin C status, as low or nondetectable levels of salivary AA have been reported,[60] and salivary AA levels generally have not been found to correlate well with AA intake, plasma AA, or leukocyte AA levels.

**Interpretive Guidelines.** The reference ranges listed in Table 27–4 are general guidelines for interpreting biochemical AA measures. The guidelines for interpreting plasma AA levels are relatively well established. Little data on AA body pool measurements are available, however, and reported ranges of leukocyte AA vary greatly, in part because of the heterogeneous nature of blood cells, and in part because of technical difficulties in their analysis. Generally, the "deficiency" category represents frank vitamin C deficiency, in which clinical symptoms are either apparent or imminent. The "low" category represents a state of moderate risk for develop-

**TABLE 27–4.** GUIDELINES FOR INTERPRETING BIOCHEMICAL MEASURES OF ASCORBIC ACID STATUS*

| | PLASMA: μmol/L† (mg/dl) | BODY POOL: mg | MIXED LEUKOCYTES: nmol/10⁸ CELLS‡ (μg/10⁸ CELLS) | MONONUCLEAR LEUKOCYTES: nmol/10⁸ CELLS (μg/10⁸ CELLS) |
|---|---|---|---|---|
| Adequate | >23 (>0.4) | >600 | >114 (>20) | >142 (>25) |
| Low | 11.4–23 (0.2–0.4) | 300–600 | 57–114 (10–20) | 114–142 (20–25) |
| Deficient | <11.4 (<0.2) | <300 | <57 (<10) | <114 (<20) |
| Normal Range | 23–84 (0.4–1.5) | 500–1500 (10–22 mg/kg) | 114–301 (20–53) | 142–250 (25–44) |

*Upper end of ranges may be higher in subjects taking vitamin C supplements.
†μmol/L ÷ 56.8 = mg/dl.
‡nmol/$10^8$ cells ÷ 5.68 = μg/$10^8$ cells; mixed leukocytes are buffy coat or mixed cell fraction containing neutrophils and mononuclear cells; $10^8$ cells ~ 100 μl.

ing overt vitamin deficiency symptoms because of low AA intake and/or depleted body pool.

Unlike plasma, the interpretation of leukocyte AA levels is complicated by differing AA concentrations among the various cell types. Mononuclear (MN) cells contain some two to threefold higher AA levels than polymorphonuclear (PMN) cells. Other clinical and physiologic factors (e.g., infection, drugs, and glycemic state) affect leukocyte AA levels because of alteration either in cell populations or of their AA uptake.[63] Similarly, use of the heterogeneous "buffy coat" for assessing cellular vitamin C status has been criticized as being affected by diverse factors unrelated to AA nutriture.[63]

The oxidized form of the vitamin, DHAA, is present in negligible amounts in the plasma of healthy subjects.[38] In leukocytes, however, a dynamic relationship exists between AA and DHAA, especially in phagocytic cells, in which AA is active as an antioxidant and free radical scavenger attendant to the respiratory burst. Reported levels of DHAA in human leukocytes range from zero to nearly half of the total cellular content of vitamin C,[27,36,64] although the vitamin exists in isolated human neutrophils solely in the reduced form.[36] Increasing amounts of evidence suggest an effective intracellular reduction of DHAA by glutathione and/or NADPH-dependent reductases.[37] Thus, like in plasma, AA may be the predominant intracellular form of the vitamin in most cells. The extent to which reported leukocyte levels of DHAA truly exist in vivo, or result from methodologic (oxidative) artifacts, is not clear.

The leukocyte cell fraction that is most useful for assessing vitamin C status has not been determined. Although AA levels of the plasma and of the PMN cell fraction are more responsive to changes in AA intake, AA in the MN cell fraction represents a pool that is depleted more slowly than that from other blood compartments.[24,28,29]

**Effect of Gender, Smoking, and Age.** Typical effects of gender, age, and smoking on plasma AA levels are shown in Figure 27–5 for a population of healthy Boston area residents, ages 60 to 98 years.[15] Women had higher plasma AA levels than men for all subgroups of age, smoking, or AA supplement use, even though dietary AA intakes were approximately the same. Women show a higher plasma AA level throughout the entire range of AA intakes (see Fig. 27–4), and mean values for AA supplement users were higher in women (84 μmol/L (1.48 mg/dl)) than in men (76 μmol/L (1.34 mg/dl)).

In most studies, smokers show lower AA levels in plasma and leukocytes, and lower dietary AA intake of smokers only partially explains the lower levels.[14,15,58]

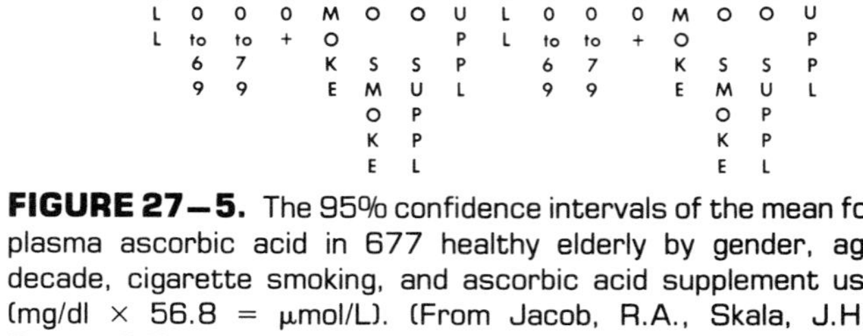

Plasma Ascorbic Acid, mg/dl
MALES
FEMALES
1.6
1.4
1.2
1.0
0.8
0.6
ALL
60 to 69
70 to 79
80+
SMOKE
NON SMOKE
NON SUPPL
SUPPL
ALL
60 to 69
70 to 79
80+
SMOKE
NON SMOKE
NON SUPPL
SUPPL

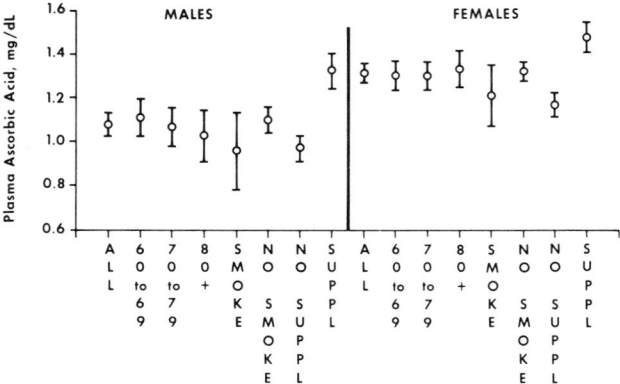


**FIGURE 27–5.** The 95% confidence intervals of the mean for plasma ascorbic acid in 677 healthy elderly by gender, age decade, cigarette smoking, and ascorbic acid supplement use (mg/dl × 56.8 = μmol/L). (From Jacob, R.A., Skala, J.H., Omaye, S.T., et al.: Biochemical methods for assessing vitamin C status of the individual. *In* Nutritional Status Assessment of the Individual. Edited by G.E. Livingston. Trumbull, CT, Food & Nutrition Press, 1989, pp. 323–338.)

The implications of these observations are discussed in the succeeding section.

No significant relationship between age and plasma AA levels exist in the data presented in Figure 27–5, although the trend of mean values is downward in aging men. The AA status of the elderly population has been discussed previously.

### FUNCTIONAL MEASURES

Despite its known or suspected role in a variety of biochemical reactions, no reliable functional markers of human AA status have been established. The role of AA in hydroxylating proline and lysine during collagen formation is well known, but the levels of these two amino acids (or their hydroxy forms) in serum or urine have not been shown to relate consistently to AA status. Decreases in gingival integrity during experimental AA depletion of adult men was accompanied by increases in urinary hydroxyproline excretion (see Fig. 27–3); however, such increases were not sufficiently distinct to provide a reliable measure of AA deficiency.[65] Despite the links between AA and carnitine biosynthesis (previously discussed), several studies have failed to show a relationship between AA deficiency and blood or urine carnitine levels. Evidence that AA plays an important role in antioxidant defense and immunocompetence continues to accumulate, although no AA-related measure of immune or antioxidant function has been shown to be sufficiently specific to serve as an index of AA status.[66,67]

## DIETARY REQUIREMENTS

The human dietary requirement for vitamin C continues to be controversial. The current recommended dietary allowances (RDA) of Western countries are designed to provide an AA intake that maintains a sufficient AA body pool to preclude classic scorbutic symptoms, even after several weeks of a deficient diet and/or stresses that might increase the requirement or turnover. It is assumed that no clear benefit exists in achieving AA tissue or body saturation, or in recommending higher intakes such that AA homeostasis is operating to limit intestinal absorption and to increase renal excretion of unmetabolized vitamin. On this basis, the recommended daily vitamin C intakes of Western countries range from 30 mg per day (United Kingdom and the World Health Organization (WHO)) to 75 mg per day (West Germany). The United States RDA has varied from 45 mg per day in 1974 to 60 mg per day in 1980 and 1989[14] (see Appendix Table A–2b). Given an AA turnover of about 3% of the body pool per day, and development of the first scorbutic symptoms and/or reduction of total AA body pool to 300 mg or less in 24 to 30 days for both men and women, the Committee considering the 1989 version (10th Edition) of the United States RDA set the RDA for adult men and women at 60 mg per day, the same as in the previous edition.[14] To cover 95% of the population, the 60 mg per day includes an increment of +2 SD above the mean intake estimated to provide adequate vitamin C reserves. The United Kingdom and WHO value of 30 mg per day represents an intake deemed adequate for the population in that it is about threefold what is needed to prevent scurvy. The 60 mg per day level of intake precludes the appearance of scorbutic symptoms for at least 4 weeks, even in the face of deficient AA intakes and/or increased use and needs. Such an intake would also provide plasma and leukocyte AA levels above the "at risk" or low levels listed in Table 27–4, i.e., >23 μmol/L (0.4 mg/dl) and >114 nmol/$10^8$ cells (>20 μg/$10^8$ cells) for most of the population. An AA intake of 60 mg per day is easily achieved in normal Western diets.

Because of frequently observed low blood AA levels, as well as possible increased needs from sickness and therapeutic drug use, it has been suggested to increase recommended AA intakes for elderly individuals. No increases in the vitamin C RDA for this population have been formally recommended, however, because the observed low blood AA levels may be explained in part by reduced AA intakes, and convincing evidence of an increased requirement or AA turnover related to aging alone has not been reported (see preceding discussion of elderly AA status). As discussed previously, additional dietary AA may significantly enhance nonheme iron absorption. This effect may be important in vegetarians or individuals with limited heme iron intakes, but the uncertain benefit of this effect to most omnivorous individuals does not justify increasing recommended AA intakes on a population basis.

Evidence that certain clinical conditions increase the body's requirement for AA is reviewed in the section on clinical aspects.

American nutritional scientists are not unanimous in their approval of the 1989 RDA values. In fact, the 1980 to 1985 RDA committee provided a report to the National Academy of Sciences in which the recommended RDA values for adult men and women were 40 and 30 mg AA, respectively. When that report was rejected by the National Academy of Sciences, a subcommittee of the Food and Nutrition Board was commissioned to revise the chapter on AA in light of the 1980 RDA value of 60 mg per day. The 1980 to 1985 RDA committee reasoned that intakes of 40 and 30 mg per day would provide a body pool of 900 mg per day, thus protecting against deficiency symptoms for at least 1 month; that no signs of AA deficiency have been shown at this pool size; and that higher body reserves have not been shown to provide increased health benefits.[68] Indeed, the worldwide conventional recommended allowances for vitamin C ranging from 30 to 70 mg per day are similar in that they are set basically to preclude classic vitamin C deficiency symptoms on a population basis. Currently, the data suggesting extrascorbutic health benefits for consumption of higher doses of vitamin C are not viewed as sufficiently rigorous or convincing to merit significantly increased RDA values.

### SMOKERS

As discussed previously, the lower plasma and leukocyte AA levels found in smokers compared to nonsmokers are explained only in part by lower AA intakes of smokers. Using radioisotope-labeled AA as a tracer in healthy men, Kallner et al. determined that the metabolic turnover of AA in smokers averaged about double that of nonsmokers (70.0 versus 35.7 mg per day).[31] The reason for this disparity has not been established (increased catabolism of AA because of oxidative stress of smoking has been suggested). The lower levels of AA and decreased AA half-life in smokers puts them at comparatively greater risk for development of AA deficiency. To allow for this propensity, an increased dietary intake of AA in smokers is deemed appropriate, and the United States RDA is 40 mg per day higher for smokers (to 100 mg per day) in the 1989 edition.[14]

### PREGNANCY AND LACTATION

Plasma AA levels of women decrease during pregnancy, primarily because of hemodilution. However, the plasma AA levels of the fetus and neonates are some 50% higher than those of the mother, indicating active transplacental transport and a relatively higher body pool of the vitamin. The increased maternal requirement for AA based solely on the weight of a near-term fetus would be about 3 to 4 mg per day, although AA turnover in the growing fetus is believed to be greater than that for adults. The RDA of 1989 therefore includes additional intake of 10 mg per day for pregnant women to compensate for AA losses during pregnancy and to maintain an adequate body pool.[14]

Human breast milk contains 170 to 568 μmol/L (3 to 10 mg/dl) of AA and average milk volumes are 750 ml (first 6 months) and 600 ml (7 to 12 months) per day. To allow for variation in AA level and milk production, the 1989 RDA committee recommends an additional intake of 35 mg per day during the first 6 months of lactation, and 30 mg per day thereafter.[14]

### INFANTS AND CHILDREN

On the basis of a complete lack of reports of scorbutic symptoms in breast-fed infants receiving 7 to 12 mg per day of AA and in formula-fed infants receiving about 7 mg per day, an intake of 30 mg per day is recommended to provide adequate vitamin C reserves plus a margin of safety in 95% of the population for infants during the first 6 months of life.[14] Beyond 6 months, the requirements gradually increase to the adult level.

## CLINICAL, PROPHYLACTIC, AND THERAPEUTIC ASPECTS

Whereas current recommended allowances for vitamin C are based on providing sufficient body reserves to preclude scorbutic symptoms plus a margin of safety, some authors reason that higher AA intakes should be recommended based on apparent extrascorbutic roles of AA, such as in antioxidant defense and immunocompetence.[34,56,69,70] Often the stated goal is to achieve tissue saturation of AA, i.e., to maximize the AA body pool, or to surpass the steady-state maximal levels by frequent ingestion of megadoses (more than 1 g) of AA. Such intakes are meant to satisfy proposed pharmacologic rather than physiologic roles for AA. Over the past two decades, suggestions for such roles have been varied and prolific. A brief review of proposed extrascorbutic and clinical roles follows. The reader is referred to other sources for expanded and detailed coverage.[33,34,56,71,72]

### IMMUNOCOMPETENCE

A variety of immune-related functions have been associated with AA status,[33,56] including decreased resistance to a variety of infectious agents during AA deficiency, and effects on neutrophil activity, lymphocyte blastogenesis, and immune modulators C1q and interleukin 1. Stimulation of neutrophil chemotaxis is suggested as the mechanism underlying improved antimicrobial activity after AA supplementation in conditions such as chronic granulomatous disease and Chediak-Higashi syndrome. Certain immune system modulators are affected by ingestion of AA, including levels of cyclic nucleotides in B and T cells and levels of histamine, prostaglandins, and prostacyclin.

Leukocyte AA levels in a patient with a cold fall to below normal levels, with only megadoses of AA being able to restore them during the illness. Use of megadoses of AA to prevent and treat the common cold has been recommended by Pauling,[73] although a review of the subject shows no clear and consistent benefit toward either cold prevention or duration.[74] The effect of AA in reducing blood histamine levels[55,56] may explain in part the belief among some individuals that AA supplements reduce the symptoms and duration of the common cold.

Results from studies of the effects of AA supplements on immune functions have not been consistent, perhaps in part because of unreliable techniques used to assess immunocompetence. The extrapolation of results from animal models and isolated cell studies to steady-state in vivo immune function in humans is not as straightforward as implied. Whereas the findings of many studies suggest that higher doses of AA have beneficial effects, those from other studies show no effects, or negative effects.[67,75–77] Indeed, because of active transport of AA into leukocytes, the effect of increasing dietary AA intakes on intracellular leukocyte AA levels is questionable. In a double-blind study of 24 healthy free-living women, ingestion of 1 or 4 g of AA daily produced increases in serum AA levels relative to the placebo group, but no differences were evident in the leukocyte AA levels or in leukocyte function.[78]

## ANTIOXIDANT DEFENSE

The important role of AA in the overall antioxidant defense system of the body has been reviewed.[79] The vitamin scavenges aqueous superoxide and hydroxyl radicals and acts as a chain-breaking antioxidant in lipid peroxidations. Ascorbic acid may also act indirectly in protecting lipid membranes by regenerating the active form of membrane-bound vitamin E; however, as discussed previously, not all data support this role. The vitamin appears to be important for antioxidant protection in plasma as well as in other extracellular fluids, for membranes, and intracellularly.

The high AA levels in neutrophils are believed to provide cellular and host tissue protection during the respiratory burst in which reactive oxidants and free radicals are produced.[36,80] Myeloperoxidase-derived hypochlorous acid is scavenged by AA, and lack of sufficient vitamin at sites of inflammation such as in the rheumatoid joint has been suggested to facilitate proteolytic damage.[81] Similarly, the high levels of AA in the humors of the eye may provide antioxidant protection to various ocular fluids and tissues, including the lens, cornea, vitreous humor, and retina.[82] Ascorbic acid was the only endogenous antioxidant that completely protected plasma lipids from detectable peroxidative damage induced by aqueous peroxyl radicals in vitro. Furthermore, lipid hydroperoxides were detected only after all plasma AA was used.[70] In healthy men fed low dietary AA levels (5, 10, or 20 mg per day), reducing substances (reduced glutathione and NADPH) are lowered in concentration and DNA bases of sperm are increasingly oxidized.[66,83] Thus, such intakes of AA, although sufficient to prevent overt scurvy, may permit increased oxidative damage. Ascorbic acid, in concert with iron, can enhance hydroperoxide-dependent lipid peroxidation in vitro, possibly by reduction of iron, which then catalyzes lipid peroxidation. This type of reaction is not believed to be important in vivo.[84]

## CANCER

Evidence suggesting a role for AA in cancer prevention has been reviewed.[72] Most evidence is from epidemiologic studies, which associate the occurrence of cancers in populations with AA status or dietary intakes, although evidence gleaned from animal model and laboratory studies has also been reported.

Possible anticarcinogenic effects of AA likely involve its ability to detoxify carcinogens or block carcinogenic processes (through antioxidant or free-radical scavenging actions) and to enhance immunocompetence. The established effectiveness of AA in preventing formation of carcinogenic nitrosamines in foods and in the gastrointestinal tract has been linked to prevention of gastric cancers. The vitamin has also been reported to detoxify other chemical carcinogens, including anthracene, benzpyrene, organochlorine pesticides, and heavy metals. As a free-radical scavenger, the vitamin is believed to be important in preventing oxidative damage to macromolecules such as proteins and DNA. Oxidative damage to human sperm DNA, as determined by levels of γ-hydroxy-2′-deoxyguanosine, was increased in men consuming low dietary intakes of AA and was inversely related to semen AA levels.[83] The possible roles of AA in immunocompetence were discussed previously. Lymphocytes can effectively destroy some types of cancer cells, and certain neutrophil functions are augmented by AA, suggesting that AA levels may play a role in immunosurveillance.

Evidence that AA provides an antitumorigenic effect in animals exposed to carcinogens is seen in many but not all animal studies (mice, rat, and hamster). Some protective effects of AA have also been seen in tumor cell transplant and cell culture experiments, but results have been inconsistent.

The bulk of data suggesting a link between AA intake and cancer prevention comes from epidemiologic studies, which provide indirect rather than cause-and-effect evidence. In most cases, consumption of foods is reported, not AA intake or status per se. Hence, which nutrient(s) might be responsible for an observed relation is not clear. On review, evidence for a protective effect of AA is strongest for cancers of the esophagus, oral cavity, and uterine cervix; suggestive but mixed for cancers of the stomach, rectum, larynx, bladder, and pancreas; and weak or nonexistent for cancers of the lung and prostate.[72] It is not likely, however, that associations of AA-containing foods and cancer occurrence can be attributed to the actions of AA alone, as numerous other nutritional factors may be involved, and interactions of AA with other putative anticarcinogenic micronutrients such as carotenoids, vitamin E, and folic acid have been noted.

Studies reporting a therapeutic use of AA for treatment of cancer have been neither abundant nor consistent. Prolongation of survival of colorectal cancer patients by AA megadosing has been claimed, but not replicated.[85] Current data suggests a possible role for the vitamin in cancer prevention, but no utility as a treatment agent.

## LIPID METABOLISM AND HEART DISEASE

Some experimental and epidemiologic evidence suggests possible roles for AA in the genesis or prevention of heart disease.[33,34,56,86] Evidence of AA effects on lipid metabolism, vascular tissue integrity, and thrombotic episodes has been reported. Effects of AA intake on cholesterol and triglyceride metabolism have been related to altered hepatic conversion of cholesterol to bile acids and tissue lipolytic activity, respectively. Some studies however, report no relation between AA status and blood lipid levels.[78] Inverse associations between AA intake or status and heart disease have been related to the effects of AA on the integrity of vascular tissue and changes in fibrinolytic activity.[33,56] Overall, the data are not sufficient to conclude that AA plays a significant role in the etiology or prevention of heart disease.

### OTHER CLINICAL ASPECTS

Evidence suggests a possible role for AA in a variety of other clinical conditions.[33,56] Like its suspected role in degenerative diseases and immunocompetence, the evidence is not sufficiently convincing to recommend vitamin-based therapies or widespread increases in intakes as a prophylactic measure.

Patients with asthma or hypersensitivity may benefit from AA supplements, as increased AA intakes have been shown to lower body histamine levels.[33,56,87] Vitamin C is important to wound healing, presumably because of its role in biosynthesis of mature cross-linked collagen, and in maintaining healthy gingival tissue, thus helping to prevent gingivitis (Fig. 27–3).[54] Ascorbic acid has been shown to ameliorate heavy metal toxicity effects, in some cases because of reductive action that reduces metal absorption or converts metals to less toxic forms. Large doses of AA have been reported to alleviate pain and provide clinical benefit in some bone diseases, including bone metastases, Paget's disease, and osteogenesis imperfecta.

Disturbed AA metabolism has been observed in animals made hyperglycemic and in patients with diabetes, ostensibly from antagonism of the structurally similar glucose molecule toward cellular AA transport.[88] Proposed benefits of AA in rheumatic diseases and cataract formation may be based on the vitamin's antioxidant function. Other conditions linked to AA status include anemia, mental depression, gastrointestinal ulcers and hemorrhage, menorrhagia, habitual abortion, premature birth, and premature rupture of fetal membranes.[56]

## PHARMACOLOGIC INTAKES

Possible harmful effects of pharmacologic intakes of AA in the range of 1 to 15 g per day have been suggested, although the relative paucity of harmful effects reported among a United States population wherein some 25% of individuals consume supplementary AA suggests that the vitamin is nontoxic even in large amounts. Homeostatic mechanisms—saturation of absorption at 2 to 3 g per day intake and renal clearance of excess unmetabolized vitamin—probably play the most important roles in preventing AA toxicity effects. Nausea and diarrhea that sometimes accompany megadose intakes are ascribed to osmotic effects of unabsorbed vitamin passing through the intestine.

The fact that oxalic acid is a metabolite of AA catabolism prompts concerns of hyperoxaluria and contributions to kidney stones, although excess AA is excreted into the urine unchanged and the amount metabolized to oxalate is limited regardless of intake. Most studies show that increased AA intakes do not significantly increase body oxalate levels,[13,42] and reports of stone formation linked directly to excess AA intake are rare. Nevertheless, patients with kidney stones, or renal disease, are advised to avoid excess intake of AA.

The effect of AA in facilitating intestinal iron absorption has been suggested as possibly contributing to iron overload in adult, especially elderly, men. A review of 24 studies in which iron absorption and status were assessed along with daily AA intakes of more than 60 mg suggests that iron absorption and body reserves were not affected and that the higher AA intakes are not a significant factor in iron overload.[89] Nevertheless, the results are not totally consistent, warranting further study and possible monitoring of iron reserves in certain individuals consuming AA supplements.

Suggestions that supplementary intakes of AA interfere with copper absorption and the metabolism of vitamins $B_6$ and $B_{12}$ have not been confirmed.[42,90]

The reductive action of large amounts of AA in urine and feces can interfere with certain laboratory diagnostic tests such as for glycosuria and fecal occult blood. A variety of blood tests based on redox chemistries, (e.g., cholesterol, glucose, and ceruloplasmin oxidases) are biased by high plasma AA levels that result from supplement consumption.[91] Large doses of AA may interfere with heparin or coumarin anticoagulant therapy.

As with many aspects of vitamin C actions, the question of a systemic conditioning effect of high AA intake and subsequent rebound deficiency after withdrawal of high intake is controversial. A recent review concludes that reports of rebound scurvy in humans, and infant scurvy induced in utero by high AA intakes of the mothers, do not establish credibly that a conditioning effect operates in humans.[92] However, recent studies with guinea pigs[93] and with adult men in a metabolic unit[94] indicate that a systemic conditioning effect does indeed operate, although the mechanism has not been determined. Until the question is resolved, persons are advised to withdraw gradually from high AA intakes over a period of 2 to 4 weeks.

## REFERENCES


1. Jukes, T.H.: J. Nutr., *118*:1290–1293, 1988.
2. Carpenter, K.J.: J. Nutr., *118*:1422–1423, 1988.
3. Carpenter, K.J.: The history of scurvy and vitamin C. New York, Cambridge University Press, 1986.
4. Jacob, R.A., Skala, J.H., Omaye, S.T., et al.: Biochemical methods for assessing vitamin C status of the individual. *In* Nutritional Status Assessment of the Individual. Edited by G.E. Livingston. Trumbull, CT, Food & Nutrition Press, 1989, pp. 323–338.
5. Pachla, L.A., Reynolds, D.L., Kissinger, P.T.: J. Assoc. Off. Anal. Chem., *68*:2–12, 1985.
6. Omaye, S.T., Turnbull, J.D., Sauberlich, H.E.: Selected methods for the determination of ascorbic acid in animal cells, tissues, and fluids. *In* Methods in Enzymology. Edited by D.B. McCormick and L.D. Wright. New York, Academic Press, 1979, pp. 3–11.
7. Omaye, S.T., Schaus, E.E., Kutnink, M.A., et al.: Ann. N. Y. Acad. Sci., *498*:389–401, 1987.
8. Sauberlich, H.E.: Ascorbic acid (vitamin C). *In* Clinics in Laboratory Medicine (Symposium on Laboratory Assessment of Nutritional Status). Edited by R.F. Labbe. Philadelphia, W.B. Saunders, 1981, pp. 673–684.
9. Sauberlich, H.E., Green, M.D., Omaye, S.T.: Determination of ascorbic acid and dehydroascorbic acid. *In* Advances in Chemistry Series, No. 200. Edited by P.A. Seib and B.M. Tolbert. Washington, D.C., American Chemical Society, 1982, pp. 199–221.
10. Sauberlich, H.E., Kretsch, M.J., Taylor, P.C., et al.: Am. J. Clin. Nutr., *50*:1039–1049, 1989.
11. Agricultural Research Service: Composition of Foods: Raw, Processed and Prepared. Revision of Agricultural Handbook No. 8–9 and 8–11. U.S. Department of Agriculture, Science and Education Administration. 1984, 1986.
12. Vanderslice, J.T., Higgs, D.J., Hayes, J.M., et al.: J. Food Comp. Anal., *3*:105–118, 1990.
13. Hornig, D.H., Moser, U., Glatthaar, B.E.: Ascorbic acid. *In* Modern Nutrition in Health and Disease. 7th Ed. Edited by M.E. Shils and V.R. Young. Philadelphia, Lea & Febiger, 1988, pp. 417–435.
14. Food and Nutrition Board, National Research Council: Water-soluble vitamins. *In* Recommended Dietary Allowances, 10th Ed. Washington, D.C., National Academy Press, 1989, pp. 115–123.
15. Jacob, R.A., Otradovec, C.L., Russell, R.M., et al.: Am. J. Clin. Nutr., *48*:1436–1442, 1988.
16. Kubler, W., Gehler, J.: Int. J. Vitam. Nutr. Res., *40*:442–453, 1970.
17. Kallner, A., Hartmann, D., Hornig, D.: Int. J. Vitam. Nutr. Res., *47*:383–388, 1977.
18. Kallner, A., Hornig, D., Pellikka, R.: Am. J. Clin. Nutr., *41*:609–613, 1985.
19. Sacharin, R., Taylor, T., Chasseaud, L.F.: Int. J. Vitam. Nutr. Res., *47*:68–74, 1977.
20. Pelletier, O., Keith, M.O.: J. Am. Diet. Assoc., *64*:271–275, 1974.
21. Yew, M.S.: Nutr. Rep. Int., *30*:597–601, 1984.
22. Vinson, J.A., Bose, P.: Am. J. Clin. Nutr., *48*:601–604, 1988.
23. Hornig, D.: Ann. N. Y. Acad. Sci., *258*:103–118, 1975.
24. Evans, R.M., Currie, L., Campbell, A.: Br. J. Nutr., *47*:473–482, 1982.
25. Lee, W., Hamernyik, P., Hutchinson, M., et al.: Clin. Chem., *10*:2165–2169, 1982.
26. Ikeda, T.: Tohoku. J. Exp. Med., *142*:117–120, 1984.
27. VanderJagt, D.J., Garry, P.J., Bhagavan, H.N.: Am. J. Clin. Nutr., *49*:511–516, 1989.
28. Blanchard, J., Conrad, K.A., Watson, R.R., et al.: Eur. J. Clin. Nutr., *43*:97–106, 1989.
29. Jacob, R.A.: J. Nutr., *120*:1480–1485, 1990.
30. Kallner, A., Hartmann, D., Hornig, D.: Am. J. Clin. Nutr., *32*:530–539, 1979.
31. Kallner, A.B., Hartmann, D., Hornig, D.H.: Am. J. Clin. Nutr., *34*:1347–1355, 1981.
32. Baker, E.M., Hodges, R.E., Hood, J., et al.: Am. J. Clin. Nutr., *24*:444–454, 1971.
33. Basu, T.J., Schorah, C.J.: Vitamin C in Health and Disease. Westport, CT, AVI Publishing, 1982.
34. Ginter, E.: Nutr. Health., *1*:66–77, 1982.
35. Moser, U.: Ann. N. Y. Acad. Sci., *498*:200–214, 1987.
36. Washko, P., Rotrosen, D., Levine, M.: J. Biol. Chem., *264*:18996–19002, 1989.
37. Anonymous: Nutr. Rev., *11*:360–361, 1989.
38. Dhariwal, K.R., Hartzell, W.O., Levine, M.: Am. J. Clin. Nutr., *54*:712–716, 1991.
39. Melethil, S., Mason, W.D., Chang, Y., et al.: Int. J. Pharmacol., *31*:83–89, 1986.
40. Spector, R.: N. Engl. J. Med., *296*:1393–1398, 1977.
41. Kinsey, V.E.: Am. J. Ophthalmol., *30*:1262–1266, 1947.
42. Jacob, R.A., Omaye, S.T., Skala, J.H., et al.: Ann. N. Y. Acad. Sci., *498*:333–346, 1987.
43. Englard, S., Seifter, S.: Annu. Rev. Nutr., *6*:365–406, 1986.
44. Barnes, M.J., Kodicek, E.: Vitam. Horm., *30*:1–43, 1972.
45. Feller, A.G., Rudman, D.: J. Nutr., *118*:541–547, 1988.
46. Hughes, R.E., Hurley, R.J., Jones, E.: Br. J. Nutr., *43*:385–387, 1980.
47. Nelson, P.J., Pruitt, R.E., Henderson, L., et al.: Biochim. Biophys. Acta, *672*:123–127, 1981.
48. Dunn, W.A., Rettura, G., Seifter, E., et al.: J. Biol. Chem., *259*:10764–10770, 1984.
49. Hughes, R.E.: Recommended daily amounts and biochemical roles-the vitamin C, carnitine, fatigue relationship. *In* Vitamin C (Ascorbic Acid). Edited by J.N. Counsell and D.H. Hornig. London, England, Applied Science Publishers, 1981, pp. 75–86.
50. Hallberg, L., Brune, M., Rossander-Hulthen, L.: Ann. N. Y. Acad. Sci., *498*:324–332, 1987.
51. Hunt, J.R., Mullen, L.A., Lykken, G.I., et al.: Am. J. Clin. Nutr., *51*:649–655, 1990.
52. Niki, E.: Ann. N. Y. Acad. Sci., *498*:186–199, 1987.
53. Burton, G.W., Wronska, U., Stone, L., et al.: Lipids, *25*:199–210, 1990.
54. Leggott, P.J., Robertson, P.B., Rothman, D.L., et al.: J. Periodontol., *57*:480–485, 1986.
55. Cheng, L., Cohen, N., and Bhagavan, H.N.: Vitamin C and the elderly. *In* Handbook of Nutrition in the Aged. Edited by R.R. Watson. Boca Raton, FL, CRC Press, 1985.
56. Clemetson, C.A.B.: Vitamin C. Vols. I–III. Boca Raton, FL, CRC Press, 1989.

57. Blanchard, J., Conrad, K.A., Mead, R.A., et al.: Am. J. Clin. Nutr., *51*:837–845, 1990.
58. Itoh, R., Yamada, K., Oka, J., et al.: Int. J. Vitam. Nutr. Res., *59*:365–372, 1989.
59. Sauberlich, H.E., Dowdy, R.P., Skala, J.H.: Laboratory tests for the assessment of nutritional status. Boca Raton, FL, CRC Press, 1974.
60. Jacob, R.A., Skala, J.H., Omaye, S.T.: Am. J. Clin. Nutr., *46*:818–826, 1987.
61. Bates, C.J., Rutishauser, I.H.E., Black, A.E., et al.: Br. J. Nutr., *42*:43–55, 1977.
62. Garry, P.J., Goodwin, J.S., Hunt, W.C., et al.: Am. J. Clin. Nutr., *36*:332–339, 1982.
63. Lee, W., Davis, K.A., Rettmer, R.L., et al.: Am. J. Clin. Nutr., *48*:286–290, 1988.
64. Schaus, E.E., Kutnink, M.A., O'Connor, D.K., et al.: Biochem. Med. Metab. Biol., *36*:369–376, 1986.
65. Hevia, P., Omaye, S.T., Jacob, R.A.: Am. J. Clin. Nutr., *51*:644–648, 1990.
66. Henning, S.M., Zhang, J.Z., McKee, R.W., et al.: J. Nutr., *121*:1969–1975, 1991.
67. Jacob, R.A., Kelley, D.S., Pianalto, F.S., et al.: Am. J. Clin. Nutr., *54*:1302S–1309S, 1991.
68. Olson, J.A., Hodges, R.E.: Am. J. Clin. Nutr., *45*:693–703, 1987.
69. Pauling, L.: Proc. Natl. Acad. Sci. U.S.A., *11*:4442–4446, 1974.
70. Frei, B., England, L., Ames, B.N.: Proc. Natl. Acad. Sci. U.S.A., *86*:6377–6381, 1989.
71. Burns, J.J., Rivers, J.M., Machlin, L.J. (Eds.): Third Conference on Vitamin C. Annals of the New York Academy of Sciences. Volume 498. New York, New York Academy of Sciences, 1987.
72. Block, G., Menkes, M.: Ascorbic acid in cancer prevention. *In* Nutrition and Cancer Prevention. Edited by T.E. Moon and M.S. Micozzi. New York, Marcel Dekker, 1989, pp. 341–388.
73. Pauling, L.: Vitamin C and the Common Cold. San Francisco, W.H. Freeman, 1970.
74. Linder, M.C.: Nutrition and metabolism of vitamins. *In* Nutritional Biochemistry and Metabolism with Clinical Applications. Edited by M.C. Linder. New York, Elsevier, 1985.
75. Shilotri, F.G., Bhat, K.S.: Am. J. Clin. Nutr., *30*:1077–1081, 1977.
76. Kennes, B., Dumont, I., Hubert, C., et al.: Gerontology, *29*:305–310, 1983.
77. Delafuente, J.C., Prendergast, J.M., Modigh, A.: Int. J. Immunopharmacol., *8*:205–211, 1986.
78. Hamilton Smith, C., Hansson, L.O., Stendahl, O.: Int. J. Vitam. Nutr. Res., *49*:160–165, 1979.
79. Bendich, A., Machlin, L.J., Scandurra, O., et al.: Adv. Free Rad. Biol. Med., *2*:419–444, 1986.
80. Anderson, R., Lukey, P.T.: Ann. N. Y. Acad. Sci., *498*:229–247, 1987.
81. Halliwell, B., Wasil, M., Grootveld, M.: FEBS Lett., *213*:15–18, 1987.
82. Varma, S.D.: Ann. N. Y. Acad. Sci., *498*:280–306, 1987.
83. Fraga, C.G., Motchnik, P.A., Shigenaga, M.K., et al.: Proc. Natl. Acad. Sci. U.S.A., *88*:11003–11006, 1991.
84. Laudicina, D.C., Marnett, L.J.: Arch. Biochem. Biophys., *278*:73–80, 1990.
85. Pauling, L.(Affirmative), Moertel, C.G.(Negative): Nutr. Rev., *44*:28–32, 1986.
86. Jacques, P.F., Hartz, S.C., McGandy, R.B., et al.: Ann. N. Y. Acad. Sci., *498*:100–109, 1987.
87. Oh, C., Nakano, K.: J. Nutr., *118*:639–644, 1988.
88. Pecoraro, R.E., Chen, M.S.: Ann. N. Y. Acad. Sci., *498*:248–258, 1987.
89. Bendich, A., Cohen, M.: Toxicol. Lett., *51*:189–201, 1990.
90. Jacob, R.A., Skala, J.H., Omaye, S.T., et al.: J. Nutr., *117*:2109–2115, 1987.
91. Young, D.S.: Lab. Med., *14*:278–282, 1983.
92. Gerster, H., Moser, U.: Nutr. Res., *8*:1327–1332, 1988.
93. Tsao, C.S., Leung, P.Y.: J. Nutr., *118*:895–900, 1988.
94. Omaye, S.T., Skala, J.H., Jacob, R.A.: Am. J. Clin. Nutr., *48*:379–381, 1988.

## SELECTED READINGS

Basu, T.J., Schorah, C.J.: Vitamin C in Health and Disease. Westport, CT, AVI Publishing, 1982.

Carpenter, K.J.: The History of Scurvy and Vitamin C. Cambridge, Cambridge University Press, 1986.

Englard, S., Seifter, S.: The biochemical functions of ascorbic acid. Annu. Rev. Nutr., *6*:365–406, 1986.

Jacob, R.A.: Assessment of human vitamin C status. J. Nutr., *120*:1480–1485, 1990.

Pachla, L.A., Reynolds, D.L., Kissinger, P.T.: Review of ascorbic acid methodology: analytical methods for determining ascorbic acid in biological samples, food products, and pharmaceuticals. J. Assoc. Off. Anal. Chem., *68*:2–12, 1985.

CHAPTER 28

# Choline

Steven H. Zeisel



Choline is a quaternary amine that is ubiquitously distributed in foods (Fig. 28–1). It is required to make the phospholipids phosphatidylcholine, lysophosphatidylcholine, choline plasmalogen, and sphingomyelin—essential components of all membranes. It is a precursor for the biosynthesis of the neurotransmitter acetylcholine and also is an important source of labile methyl groups.[1] Choline, first discovered by Strecker in 1862, was chemically synthesized in 1866.[2] It was known to be a component of phospholipids, but the pathway for its biosynthesis was first described in 1941 by du Vigneaud.[3] The route for its incorporation into phosphatidylcholine (lecithin) was not elucidated until 1956.[4] The importance of choline as a nutrient was first appreciated during the pioneering work on insulin.[5,6] Depancreatized dogs, maintained on insulin therapy, developed fatty infiltration of the liver and died. Administration of raw pancreas prevented hepatic damage; the active component was the choline moiety of pancreatic phosphatidylcholine. In 1935, the association between a low-choline diet and fatty infiltration of the liver in rats was recognized.[6] The term *lipotropic* was coined to describe choline and other substances that prevented deposition of fat in the liver. Subsequently, researchers suggested that the liver disease associated with alcoholism might respond to choline therapy. However, little data supported this hypothesis. The assays for choline available at the time were not particularly sensitive or specific, and the therapy did not prove to be effective.

In 1975, Wurtman and colleagues and Haubrich and associates reported that administration of choline accelerated the synthesis and release of the acetylcholine by neurons.[7–12] At the same time, technical breakthroughs in the assay of choline made it possible to accurately detect picomoles of the substance.[13] A revival of interest in choline ensued, resulting in a plethora of publications characterizing the metabolism, physiologic effects, and pharmacology of choline. Much attention has been given to the effects of supplemental choline on brain function. Still unresolved, however, is the question of whether choline is normally required as part of the human diet. Choline has been considered a dispensable nutrient for humans because of an endogenous pathway for the de novo biosynthesis of choline moiety via the sequential methylation of phosphatidylethanolamine,[14] and because a choline deficiency syndrome has been difficult to identify in healthy humans as most common foods contain choline.

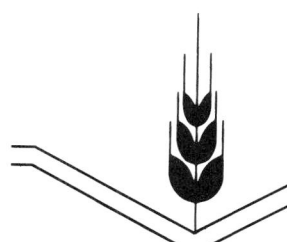

Several lines of evidence suggest that choline is indeed an essential nutrient for humans: (1) human cells grown in culture have an absolute requirement for choline;[15] (2) healthy humans fed diets deficient in choline have decreased plasma choline concentrations (discussed later in this review); (3) malnourished humans have diminished plasma or serum choline concentrations;[16,17] (4) humans fed intravenously with solutions containing little or no choline develop liver dysfunction that is similar to that seen in choline-deficient animals;[16] and (5) in other mammals, including the monkey, choline deficiency results in severe liver dysfunction.[1,18] These arguments clearly do not prove or disprove that humans require dietary choline. Diminished tissue levels of a nutrient associated with dietary deficiency are suggestive of a nutrient requirement, but deficiency should also be associated with deterioration of organ function if a nutrient is essential. The presence of a pathway for endogenous synthesis does not make a nutrient dispensable. This review includes a discussion of the expected biochemical and physiologic uses for choline, the ex-

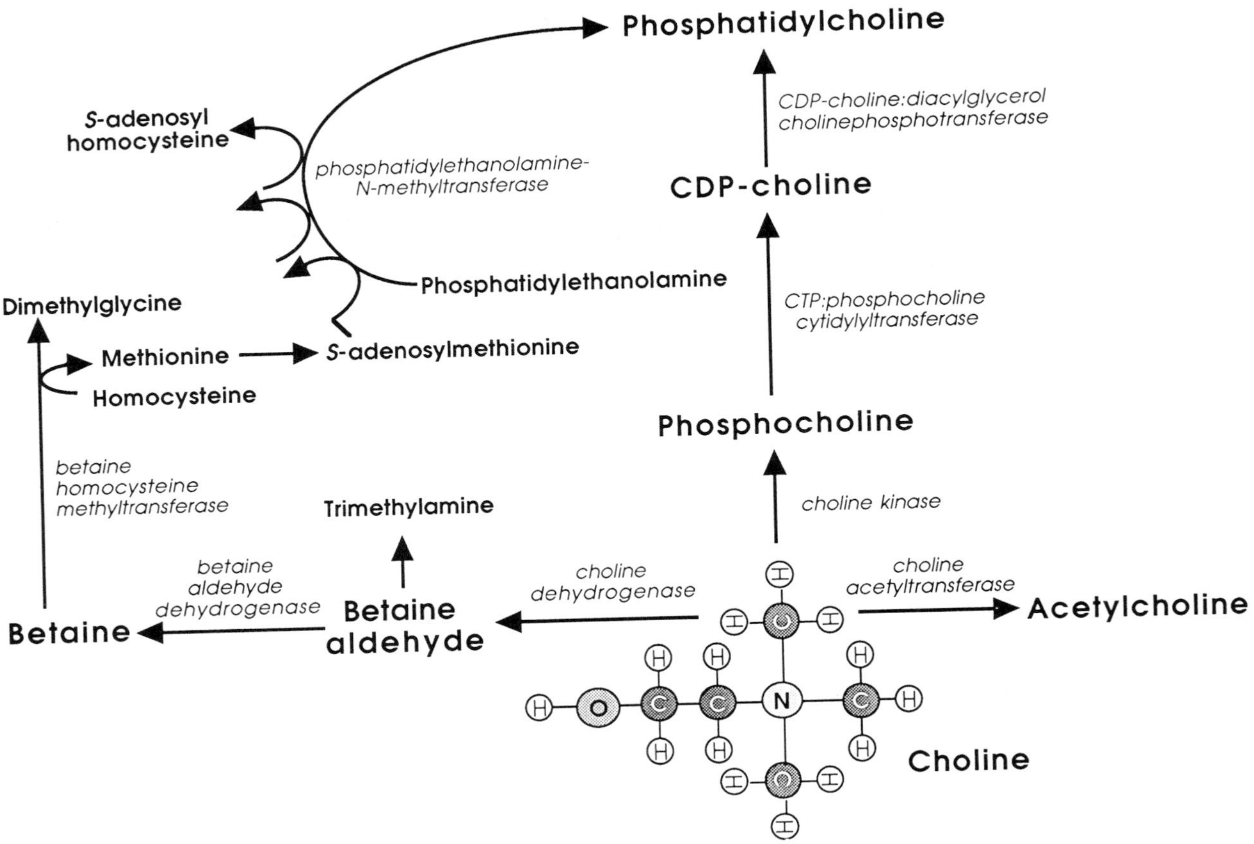
Phosphatidylcholine
CDP-choline:diacylglycerol cholinephosphotransferase
CDP-choline
CTP:phosphocholine cytidylyltransferase
Phosphocholine
choline kinase
S-adenosyl homocysteine
phosphatidylethanolamine-N-methyltransferase
Phosphatidylethanolamine
Dimethylglycine
Methionine
S-adenosylmethionine
Homocysteine
betaine homocysteine methyltransferase
Trimethylamine
betaine aldehyde dehydrogenase
Betaine aldehyde
choline dehydrogenase
choline acetyltransferase
Acetylcholine
Betaine
Choline

**FIGURE 28–1.** Metabolism of choline. The three major uses for choline are as a precursor for phosphatidylcholine biosynthesis, as a methyl donor, and as a precursor for acetylcholine biosynthesis. The molecular weight of choline is 104.17 g/mol.

pected effects of choline deficiency, and evidence of a requirement for choline in the human's diet.

## DIETARY SOURCES OF CHOLINE

In the adult human, serum choline concentrations fluctuate over an approximately two-fold range when common choline-containing foods are ingested.[19] Individuals in the United States probably ingest at least 6 g of phosphatidylcholine per day (100 mg/day of this amount deriving from addition to foods during processing). Total choline intake in the adult human (as free choline and the choline in phosphatidylcholine and other choline esters) probably is in excess of 6 to 10 mmol (600 to 1000 mg) per day. Consumption of choline is higher in humans ingesting phosphatidylcholine (also called lecithin), a dietary "health food" supplement. Calculations of dietary choline intake are based on estimates of the free choline and phosphatidylcholine content of foods.[20–24] Older assay procedures for choline were imprecise, making many of the available data unreliable. We measured the choline, phosphatidylcholine, and sphingomyelin contents of some foods using a gas chromatography/mass spectrometic assay (Table 28–1). Our own measurements of the lysophosphatidylcholine, glycerophosphocholine, and phosphocholine contents of rat tissues show that these choline-containing compounds are present in high concentrations in many tissues (e.g., muscle concentrations of these three esters were approximately 100 μmol/kg each).[25] Because the foods eaten by humans probably also contain significant amounts of these esters of choline, our estimates of choline intake may be low. Phosphatidylcholine is also often added to processed foods because it acts as an emulsifying agent or as an antioxidant.

Milk contains approximately 200 μmol/L each of free choline, phosphatidylcholine, and sphingomyelin (colostrum and transitional milk have three to four-fold higher free choline content than does mature milk; bovine milk and formula derived from it are similar in choline content to mature human milk; soy bean-derived formula can have three to four-fold higher choline concentration than does bovine milk). The mammary gland is capable of actively accumulating choline from maternal blood[26] and can synthesize choline molecules de novo.[27]

**TABLE 28–1.** CHOLINE CONTENT OF SOME COMMON FOODS

| FOOD | CHOLINE CONCENTRATION (μMOLES/KG)* Choline | Phosphatidylcholine | Sphingomyelin |
|---|---|---|---|
| Apple | 27 | 280 | 15 |
| Banana | 240 | 37 | 20 |
| Beef liver | 5,831 | 43,500 | 1,850 |
| Beef steak | 75 | 6,030 | 506 |
| Butter | 42 | 1,760 | 460 |
| Cauliflower | 1,306 | 2,770 | 183 |
| Corn oil | 3 | 12 | 5 |
| Coffee | 1,010 | 15 | 23 |
| Cucumber | 218 | 76 | 27 |
| Egg | 42 | 52,000 | 2,250 |
| Ginger ale | 2 | 4 | 3 |
| Grape juice | 475 | 15 | 5 |
| Iceberg lettuce | 2,930 | 132 | 50 |
| Margarine | 30 | 450 | 15 |
| Milk (bovine, whole) | 150 | 148 | 82 |
| Orange | 200 | 490 | 24 |
| Peanut butter | 3,895 | 3,937 | 9 |
| Peanuts | 4,546 | 4,960 | 78 |
| Potato | 511 | 300 | 26 |
| Tomato | 430 | 52 | 32 |
| Whole wheat bread | 968 | 340 | 11 |

*Choline, phosphatidylcholine, and sphingomyelin were measured using a gas chromatography/mass spectrometry assay[25] in foods prepared in the form that they would normally be consumed. 1 μmol choline = 104.17 μg.

For these reasons, choline concentrations in milk can be as high as 60 times those found in maternal plasma.[24] Neonatal animals and humans have exceptionally high blood choline concentrations.[28,29]

The extent to which dietary choline is bioavailable depends on the efficiency of its absorption from the intestine. Some ingested choline is metabolized before it can be absorbed from the gut. Gut bacteria degrade it to form betaine and to make methylamines.[30–33] The free choline surviving these fates is absorbed all along the small intestine.[31,34,35] At this time, no other component of the diet has been identified as competing with choline for transport by intestinal carriers.

Both pancreatic secretions and intestinal mucosal cells contain enzymes (phospholipases $A_1$, $A_2$, and B) capable of hydrolyzing phosphatidylcholine in the diet.[36–38] The free choline that is formed enters the portal circulation of the liver.[38]

## UPTAKE OF CHOLINE BY TISSUES

All tissues accumulate choline, but uptake by liver, kidney, mammary gland, placenta, and brain are of especial importance.[39,40,41] Most tissues take up choline by a combination of transport processes (diffusion and mediated transport) such as have been described in brain, liver, kidney, erythrocytes, placenta, and intestine.[34,40,42–46] Hepatectomy increases the half-life of choline and results in an increase in blood choline concentration. The rate at which liver takes up choline is sufficient to explain the rapid disappearance of choline injected systemically. The kidney also accumulates choline.[45–50] Some of this choline appears in the urine unchanged, but most is oxidized within kidney to form betaine,[51] which serves as an important osmoprotectant within kidney.[52] Mean free choline concentration in the plasma of azotemic humans is several times greater than that in normal control subjects, and hemodialysis rapidly removes choline from the plasma.[53] Renal transplantation in humans lowers plasma choline levels from 30 μmol/L in the azotemic patient to 15 μmol/L within 1 day.[54]

The placenta actively accumulates choline.[42,55–57] Specific transport systems for choline are on both sides of the syncytiotrophoblast.[58] A specific carrier mechanism transports free choline across the blood-brain barrier at a rate that is proportional to serum choline concentration.[59] In the neonate, this choline transporter has high capacity;[60] this capacity decreases as rats age.[61]

## CHOLINE METABOLISM

Only a small fraction of dietary choline is acetylated, catalyzed by the activity of choline acetyltransferase (EC 2.3.1.6).[41,62] This enzyme is highly concentrated in the terminals of cholinergic neurons,[63] but it is also present in such non-nervous tissues as the placenta.[64] The availability of choline and acetyl-coenzyme A (CoA) influence choline acetyltransferase activity.[7-10] In brain, it is unlikely that choline acetyltransferase is saturated with either of its substrates, so that choline (and possibly acetyl-CoA) availability determines the rate of acetylcholine synthesis.[65] Some investigators report that administration of choline or phosphatidylcholine results in the accumulation of acetylcholine within brain neurons,[7-10] whereas others observe that such acceleration of acetylcholine synthesis by choline administration can only be detected after pretreatments with agents that cause cholinergic neurons to fire rapidly.[66-70] Increased brain acetylcholine synthesis is associated with an augmented release into the synapse of this neurotransmitter. A temporal dissociation between choline administration and effects on brain acetylcholine synthesis and release has been observed,[67] suggesting that choline taken up by brain may first enter a storage pool (perhaps the phosphatidylcholine in membranes) before being converted to acetylcholine.

A major use for choline is through irreversible oxidation forming betaine, an important methyl donor. Once betaine is formed, it cannot be reduced to reform choline; however, it can donate a methyl group to homocysteine, thereby producing dimethylglycine and methionine. Dimethylglycine is converted to sarcosine and then to glycine, producing a one-carbon fragment. Thus, the oxidation pathway acts to diminish the availability of choline to tissues while, at the same time, scavenging some methyl groups. Much greater amounts of choline are oxidized to form betaine (9 μmol/hour/g) than are phosphorylated to form phosphocholine (1 μmol/hour/g) by rat liver.[71] Betaine is formed from choline via the intermediate betaine aldehyde. Choline dehydrogenase (EC 1.1.99.1) catalyzes the conversion of choline to betaine aldehyde and uses molecular oxygen as the electron acceptor.[72] Choline dehydrogenase in mammalian liver and kidney is mitochondrial, located on the matrix side of the inner membrane.[73-75] Another enzyme, betaine aldehyde dehydrogenase (EC 1.2.1.8), also catalyzes conversion of betaine aldehyde to betaine. This enzyme requires $NAD^+$, and is found in both mitochondria (this mitochondrial enzyme may be identical to choline dehydrogenase) and cytosol.[75]

The phosphorylation of choline is catalyzed by choline kinase (EC 2.7.1.32).[76-78] This enzyme is distributed widely in mammalian tissues including the liver, brain, kidney, and lung.[76-80] Phosphorylation of choline is the first step in the major pathway for phosphatidylcholine synthesis.[4,79] CTP phosphocholine cytidylyltransferase (EC 2.7.7.15) catalyzes the synthesis of CDP-choline form CTP and phosphocholine. The activity of this enzyme is rate limiting for the pathway.[79] In choline-deficient hepatocytes, cytidylyltransferase is activated.[81] We observed that, during choline deficiency, whatever choline was available was converted to phosphatidylcholine.[82] We suggest that when choline supplies are limited, phosphatidylcholine synthesis takes precedence over other uses for choline.

The only source of choline other than from diet is from the de novo biosynthesis of phosphatidylcholine catalyzed by phosphatidylethanolamine-*N*-methyltransferase (PeMT; EC 2.1.1.17). This enzyme synthesizes phosphatidylcholine through sequential methylation of phosphatidylethanolamine using S-adenosylmethionine as a methyl donor.[83-86] Most PeMT activity is found in the liver,[87] but significant activity is present in brain[84,88] and mammary tissue[27] and detectable activity is found in most other tissues.[89-98] No accurate estimates of the activity of phosphatidylethanolamine-*N*-methyltransferase in vivo are available. Best estimates, based on in vitro data, are that 15 to 40% of the phosphatidylcholine present in liver is synthesized by the PeMT pathway, with the remainder coming from the CDP pathway.[87,99] The PeMT pathway may be especially important in brain, where it provides choline for acetylcholine synthesis.[100] The regulation of PeMT activity has not been characterized completely. In adult liver, PeMT seems to be regulated by the availability of phosphatidylethanolamine, the S-adenosylmethionine/S-adenosylhomocysteine concentration ratio, and by the composition of the boundary lipids that surround this transmembrane protein.[101] The availability of S-adenosylmethionine relative to S-adenosylhomocysteine also determines PeMT activity.[102,103] S-adenosylmethionine, a product of the reactions, inhibits the methyltransferase.[102,103] The availability of S-adenosylmethionine in the liver of choline-deficient animals limits the activity of this pathway.[104,105]

## CHOLINE AND METHYL-GROUP METABOLISM

The demand for choline as a methyl donor is probably the major factor that determines how rapidly a diet deficient in choline induces pathologic change. The pathways of choline and one-carbon metabolism intersect at the formation of methionine from homocysteine (see Fig. 28–1).[106-108] Methionine is regenerated from homocysteine in a reaction catalyzed by betaine:homocysteine methyltransferase, in which betaine, a metabolite of choline, serves as the methyl donor.[107] The only alternative mechanism for regeneration of methionine is through a reaction catalyzed by 5-methyltetrahydrofolate:homocysteine methyltransferase (EC 2.1.1.13), which uses a methyl group generated de novo from the one-carbon pool.[107,109] Methionine is converted to S-adenosylmethionine in a reaction catalyzed by methionine adenosyl transferase. S-adenosylmethionine is the active methylating agent for many enzymatic methylations.

A disturbance in folate or methionine metabolism results in changes in choline metabolism and vice versa. During choline deficiency, hepatic choline concentration decreases rapidly.[110] At the same time, hepatic S-adenosylmethionine concentrations decrease.[110-113] It has been suggested that the availability of methionine limits S-adenosylmethionine synthesis during choline deficiency because the 5-methyltetrahydrofolate homocysteine methyltransferase reaction alone cannot fulfill the total requirement for methionine and the betaine-dependent remethylation of homocysteine is limited by the availability of betaine.[107] Methotrexate, which is used widely in the treatment of cancer, psoriasis, and rheumatoid arthritis, limits the availability of methyl groups by competitively inhibiting dihydrofolate reductase, a key enzyme in intracellular folate metabolism. When one-carbon metabolism is poisoned, the only alternative to choline as a source of methyl groups for regeneration of methionine is lost. Hepatic choline, phosphocholine, S-adenosylmethionine and betaine concentrations are diminished after treatment with methotrexate.[82,114-117] Choline supplementation reverses the fatty liver caused by methotrexate administration.[117-120]

## BIOCHEMICAL AND PHYSIOLOGIC CONSEQUENCES OF CHOLINE DEFICIENCY

Chronic ingestion of a diet deficient in choline has major consequences that include hepatic, renal, pancreatic, memory, and growth disorders. In the rat,[121] hamster,[122] guinea pig,[123] pig,[124,125] dog,[5,6,126] monkey,[18] trout,[127] quail,[128] and chicken,[129] choline deficiency results in liver dysfunction. Hepatocyte turnover is increased greatly during choline deficiency.[130,131] During choline deficiency, extremely large amounts of lipid (mainly triglycerides) can accumulate in the liver, eventually filling the entire hepatocyte.[121,132-135] Fatty infiltration of the liver starts in the central area of the lobule and spreads peripherally.[132] This process is different from that occurring in kwashiorkor or essential amino acid deficiency, in which fatty infiltration usually begins in the portal area of the lobule. The accumulation of triacylglycerol within hepatocytes begins within hours after rats begin a choline-deficient diet, peaks within the first 6 months (at greater than 2000 mg/liver compared to 28 mg/liver in controls), and then diminishes as the liver becomes fibrotic.[136] Triacylglycerol accumulation occurs because triglyceride must be packaged as very low density lipoprotein (VLDL) to be exported from liver. Phosphatidylcholine is an essential component of VLDL;[133,134] other phospholipids cannot act as a substitute.[133,134] Hepatocytes isolated from choline-deficient rats were unable to export VLDL until choline or methionine was made available.[133] Renal function is also compromised by choline deficiency, with abnormal concentrating ability, free water reabsorption, sodium excretion, glomerular filtration rate, renal plasma flow, and gross renal hemorrhage.[137-140] Infertility, growth impairment, bony abnormalities, decreased hematopoiesis, and hypertension have also been reported to be associated with diets low in choline content.[141-144]

The availability of choline during critical periods of brain development is crucial. Meck and colleagues observed two sensitive periods (embryonic days 12 to 17 and postnatal days 15 to 30) during development of the rat during which supplementation with choline results in significant long-lasting facilitation of spatial memory.[145] Maintaining adult rats on a choline-deficient diet lowered brain choline levels, but did not lower brain acetylcholine levels in some studies.[66,146] However, Nagler reported lower levels of choline and acetylcholine in brain, kidney, and intestine of choline-deficient rats.[147] Choline supplementation increases the number of dendritic spines in the cerebral cortex of old mice.[148,149] In these same animals, memory, as assessed by learning performance, was improved by choline supplementation.[150]

## CHOLINE DEFICIENCY AND CARNITINE

Carnitine is a cofactor for long-chain acetyl-CoA: carnitine acyltransferase; human deficiency syndromes have been identified.[151] Rats fed a choline-deficient diet had reduced levels of carnitine in liver, heart, and skeletal muscle,[152,153] which has been attributed to a methyl-group deficiency, i.e., carnitine is derived from trimethyllysine. However, a single injection of choline (but not of methionine, betaine, or sarcosine) was able to raise the concentration of hepatic carnitine in these animals to control values within 1.5 hours.[153] This result suggests that choline was capable of facilitating carnitine release from some storage pool, as de novo synthesis of carnitine would have taken more time. Paradoxically, plasma carnitine content was higher in choline-deficient rats,[153] probably because transport into tissues was inhibited. Perhaps a choline molecule must exit the cell in order to flip the carnitine carrier from the inside to the outside of the plasma membrane.

## CHOLINE DEFICIENCY AND HEPATOCARCINOGENESIS

Choline-deficient animals (fed diets just adequate in methionine and folate; i.e., lipotrope limited) are more likely to develop hepatocarcinomas.[130,131,136,154-162] Deficiency alone is sufficient to trigger carcinogenesis; no exposure to any known carcinogen is needed.[131,136,163] Several mechanisms have been suggested for the cancer-promoting effect of a choline devoid diet. In the choline-deficient liver, a progressive increase in cell proliferation occurs, related to regeneration after parenchymal cell death.[136,163,164] Cell proliferation, with associated increased rate of DNA synthesis, could be the cause of greater sensitivity to chemical carcinogens,[130] however, the overall rate of liver cell proliferation could be dissociated from the rate at which preneoplastic lesions formed during choline deficiency, suggesting that cell proliferation is not the sole condition acting as a promoter of liver cancer.[162] Methylation of DNA is important for the regulation of expression of genetic information. It has been suggested that the undermethylation of DNA (decreased 5-methylcytosine content in nuclear DNA) observed during choline deficiency (despite adequate dietary methionine) is responsible for carcinogenesis.[160] Hypomethylation of the c-*fos*, c-Ha-*ras* and c-*myc* genes occurs in methyl-group deficiency. Hypomethylation is associated with overexpression of these genes, which are thought to regulate cell growth.[185] Another proposed mechanism is based on the observation that, when rats are fed a choline deficient diet, increased lipid peroxidation occurs within liver (presence of diene conjugates in lipids isolated from purified hepatic nuclei[165]). Lipid peroxides in the nucleus could be a source of free radicals that could modify DNA and cause carcinogenesis.

1,2-*sn*-Diacylglycerol (1,2-DAG) accumulates in choline-deficient liver.[135] 1,2-DAG is an important intermediate for the biosynthesis of triacylglycerol and membrane phospholipids and is also a second messenger, formed when plasma membrane receptors for certain hormones, neurotransmitters, or growth factors are coupled to phospholipase C.[166] The 1,2-DAG molecule can activate a regulatory enzyme, protein kinase C (PKC).[167] Several lines of evidence indicate that cancers might develop secondary to abnormalities in PKC-mediated signal transduction. Some of the most potent mitogens and tumor promoters, the phorbol esters, are analogues of 1,2-DAG. Having a higher affinity than 1,2-DAG for the same site on PKC, phorbol esters might cause PKC translocation to membranes and long-lasting activation.[167] Gene expression abnormalities that are often associated with tumors can also be associated with alterations in 1,2-DAG- and PKC-mediated pathways. Fibroblasts normally respond to excess 1,2-DAG by activating diacylglycerol kinase activity (the enzyme translocates from cytosol to membranes); in erbB-transformed fibroblasts this activation does not occur.[168] 1,2-DAG levels are elevated in vivo in *ras*-transformed liver of neonatal transgenic mice bearing a hybrid gene construct consisting of mouse albumin enhancer/promoter fused to the coding sequence of an activated human Ha-*ras* oncogene.[169] NIH 3T3 cells transformed with the oncogenes Ha-*ras* or Ki-*ras*, v-*src*, and v-*fms* oncogenes have elevated 1,2-DAG levels as well as tonic activation and partial down-regulation of PKC.[170,171] Activated PKC, in turn, may participate in mechanisms leading to the induction of expression of the c-*myc* oncogene.[172,173] Fibroblasts, transfected with a gene for a mutant PKC that is constantly in the active conformation, become transformed and form tumors in mice.[174] This evidence is the strongest to date that activation of PKC is a key event in some forms of carcinogenesis. It is possible that the elevated hepatic concentrations of 1,2-DAG present during choline deficiency alter PKC activity and that this change results in carcinogenesis.

## PATHOPHYSIOLOGIC EVENTS THAT COULD RESULT IN CHOLINE DEFICIENCY

Choline and phosphatidylcholine are so ubiquitous in the food supply that a deficiency syndrome in humans has only recently been proven (see subsequent discussion). The rat requires cystine for hair formation. This requirement may increase the demand for methionine and the methyl groups of choline relative to the human. Certain clinical situations increase demands for choline, and therefore organ dysfunction might be more likely to result secondary to choline deficiency.

Hepatic complications associated with total parenteral nutrition (TPN), which include fatty infiltration of the liver and hepatocellular damage, have been reported by many clinical groups.[175] Frequently, TPN must be terminated because of the severity of the associated liver disease. It is possible that some of the liver disease associated with TPN is related to choline deficiency. When rats were fed intravenously with choline-free TPN solutions (4.25% FreAmine II in 25% glucose), they developed fatty infiltration of the liver and had elevated serum levels of conjugated bilirubin and transaminases.[176] Oral or intravenous supplements of choline in these animals were effective in reversing hepatic lipid accumulation. This finding suggests that these rats were choline deficient and that the methyl groups supplied by methionine within the TPN solution were not available in adequate amounts or were not used to spare choline requirements. Other investigators, however, have observed that intravenously administered choline did not prevent fatty liver in rats treated with TPN.[177]

Amino acid-glucose solutions used in TPN of humans contain no choline.[16,178] The lipid emulsions used to deliver extra calories and essential fatty acids during TPN contain choline in the form of phosphatidylcholine (20% emulsion contains 13.2 μmol/ml.)[16] Burt et al. reported that plasma choline concentrations were decreased in TPN patients at the same time that liver dysfunction was present.[179] Malnourished humans, at the time they were referred for TPN therapy, had significantly lower plasma choline concentrations than did well-fed control subjects.[16,178] Plasma choline concentrations in these patients declined further when they were treated with an amino acid-glucose solution lacking choline during the first week of therapy.[16] However, when patients were treated with lipid emulsion as well as an amino acid-glucose solution, their plasma choline concentrations rose slightly. Neither group received sufficient choline to restore plasma choline concentrations to normal values. We calculated that humans treated with TPN required 1000 to 1700 μmol of choline-containing phospholipid per day during the first week of TPN therapy to maintain plasma choline levels.[16] Enteral food supplements, which contained choline, contributed to the rising plasma choline value observed after the first week of TPN therapy. Malnourished humans with cirrhosis who were fed enterally also had diminished plasma choline content.[17]

Conditions that enhance hepatic triglyceride synthesis (such as carbohydrate loading) increase the requirement for the choline-containing lipoprotein envelope surrounding these compounds in plasma.[180] Thus, treatment of malnourished patients with high-calorie TPN solutions, at a time when choline stores are depleted, might cause hepatic dysfunction. The definitive experiment, in which supplemental choline (in the form of lecithin) was administered during TPN has recently been performed.[186] These investigators observed that 2 to 6 weeks of lecithin supplementation brought plasma choline levels back to normal and diminished the incidence of hepatic dysfunction as well as diminished hepatic steatosis. In subjects treated with placebo, liver dysfunction and hepatic steatosis did not improve. This finding strongly suggests that choline is an essential nutrient during long-term TPN.

Bypass surgery involving large segments of the bowel (i.e., to produce weight loss in obese humans) is associated with fatty liver. In obese rats that have had 90% of their small intestine bypassed, fatty liver develops. Choline supplementation prevents this development, and choline-deficient diets in such patients exacerbate the accumulation of fat in the liver.[181]

Pregnancy is associated with increased requirements for tissue (fetus) biosynthesis. As discussed previously, a placental transport system withdraws choline from mother into fetus. The choline concentration of the liver fell from a mean of 130 nmol/g in adult nonpregnant rats to 38 nmol/g in late pregnancy.[182] Pregnant women, especially those in their third trimester, are particularly susceptible to development of fatty liver, perhaps attributable to an increased choline requirement.[183]

## EXPERIMENTAL CHOLINE DEFICIENCY IN HUMANS

We characterized the effects of making normal humans choline deficient.[184] Male volunteers were hospitalized and fed for 1 week a semisynthetic diet that was devoid of choline but supplemented with 500 mg choline per day. Subjects were then divided randomly into two groups, one that continued to receive choline (control), and the other that received no choline (deficient) for three additional weeks. During the fifth week of the study, all subjects received choline. In the choline-deficient group, plasma choline and phosphatidylcholine concentrations decreased an average of 30% during the 3 weeks when a choline-deficient diet was ingested; no such changes occurred in the control group. In the choline-deficient group, serum alanine aminotransferase activity steadily increased from a mean of 0.42 μkat/L (25 U/L) to a mean of 0.62 μkat/L (37 U/L) during the 3 weeks when a choline-deficient diet was ingested; no such change occurred in the control group. Results of other tests of liver function and renal function were unchanged in both groups during the study. Serum cholesterol levels decreased an average of 15% in the deficient group and did not change in the control group. Healthy humans consuming a choline-deficient diet for 3 weeks had depleted stores of choline in tissues and developed signs of incipient liver dysfunction. Our observations support the conclusion that choline is an essential nutrient for humans.

## REFERENCES


1. Zeisel, S.H.: "Vitamin-like" molecules: Choline. *In* Modern Nutrition in Health and Disease. 7th ed. Edited by M.E. Shils and V.R. Young. Philadelphia, Lea & Febiger, 1988, pp. 440–452.
2. Strecker, A.: Ann. Chem. Pharmacie, *123*:353–360, 1862.
3. duVigneaud, V., Cohn, M., Chandler, J.P., et al.: J. Biol. Chem., *140*:625–641, 1941.
4. Kennedy, E.P., Weiss, S.B.: J. Biol. Chem., *222*:193–214, 1956.
5. Best, C.H., Huntsman, M.E.: J. Physiol., *75*:405–412, 1932.
6. Best, C.H., Huntsman, M.E.: J. Physiol., *83*:255–274, 1935.
7. Cohen, E.L., Wurtman, R.J.: Life Sci., *16*:1095–1102, 1975.
8. Cohen, E.L., Wurtman, R.J.: Science, *191*:561–562, 1976.
9. Haubrich, D.R., Wang, P.F., Clody, D.E., et al.: Life Sci., *17*:975–980, 1975.
10. Haubrich, D.R., Wedeking, P.W., Wang, P.F.: Life Sci., *14*:921–927, 1974.
11. Wecker, L.: Can. J. Physiol. Pharmacol., *64*:329–333, 1986.
12. Wood, J.L., Allison, R.G.: Fed. Proc., *41*:3015–3021, 1982.
13. Goldberg, A.M., McCaman, R.E.: J. Neurochem., *20*:1–8, 1973.
14. Bremer, J., Greenberg, D.: Biochim. Biophys. Acta, *46*:205–216, 1961.
15. Eagle, H.: J. Exp. Med., *102*:595–600, 1955.
16. Sheard, N.F., Tayek, J.A., Bistrian, B.R., et al.: Am. J. Clin. Nutr., *43*:219–224, 1986.
17. Chawla, R.K., Wolf, D.C., Kutner, M.H., Bonkovsky, H.L.: Gastroenterology, *97*:1514–1520, 1989.
18. Hoffbauer, F.W., Zaki, F.G.: Arch. Pathol. Lab. Med., *79*:364–369, 1965.
19. Zeisel, S.H., Growdon, J.H., Wurtman, R.J., et al.: Neurology, *30*:1226–1229, 1980.
20. Engel, R.W.: J. Nutr., *25*:441–446, 1943.
21. McIntire, M., Schweigert, B.S., Elvehjem, C.A.: J. Nutr., *28*:219–223, 1944.
22. Food and Nutrition Board: Comprehensive GRAS survey, usage levels reported for NAS appendix A substances (group 1) used in regular foods. Washington, D.C., National Academy Press, 1973.

23. Weihrauch, J.L., Son, Y.-S.: J. Am. Oil. Chem. Soc., *60:*1971–1978, 1983.
24. Zeisel, S.H., Char, D., Sheard, N.F.: J. Nutr., *116:*50–58, 1986.
25. Pomfret, E.A., daCosta, K.A., Schurman, L., et al.: Anal. Biochem., *180:*85–90, 1989.
26. Chao, C.K., Pomfret, E.A., Zeisel, S.H.: Biochem. J., *254:*33–38, 1988.
27. Yang, E.K., Blusztajn, J.K., Pomfret, E.A., et al.: Biochem. J., *256:*821–828, 1988.
28. Zeisel, S.H., Epstein, M.F., Wurtman, R.J.: Life Sci., *26:*1827–1831, 1980.
29. Zeisel, S.H., Wurtman, R.J.: Biochem. J., *198:*565–570, 1981.
30. De La Huerga, J., Popper, H.: J. Clin. Invest., *31:*598–603, 1952.
31. Flower, R.J., Pollitt, R.J., Sanford, P.A., et al.: J. Physiol., *226:*473–489, 1972.
32. Zeisel, S.H., Wishnok, J.S., Blusztajn, J.K.: J. Pharmacol. Exp. Ther., *225:*320–324, 1983.
33. Zeisel, S.H., daCosta, K.A., Youssef, M., et al.: J. Nutr., *119:*800–804, 1989.
34. Sheard, N.F., Zeisel, S.H.: Pediatr. Res., *20:*768–772, 1986.
35. Kuczler, F.J., Nahrwold, D.L., Rose, R.C.: Biochim. Biophys. Acta, *465:*131–137, 1977.
36. DeHaas, G.H., Postema, N.M., Nieuwenhuizen, W., et al.: Biochim. Biophys. Acta, *159:*103–117, 1968.
37. Subbaiah, P.V., Ganguly, J.: Indian J. Biochem. Biophys., *8:*197–203, 1971.
38. Lekim, D., Betzing, H.: Hoppe Seylers Z. Physiol. Chem., *357:*1321–1331, 1976.
39. Gardiner, J.E., Gwee, M.C.: J. Physiol., *239:*459–476, 1974.
40. Zeisel, S.H., Story, D.L., Wurtman, R.J., et al.: Proc. Natl. Acad. Sci. U.S.A., *77:*4417–4419, 1980.
41. Haubrich, D.R., Wang, P.F., Wedeking, P.W.: J. Pharmacol. Exp. Ther., *193:*246–255, 1975.
42. Welsch, F.: Biochem. Pharmacol., *25:*1021–1030, 1976.
43. Martin, K.: J. Gen. Physiol., *51:*497–516, 1968.
44. Simon, J.R., Kuhar, M.J.: J. Neurochem., *27:*93–99, 1976.
45. Acara, M., Rennick, B.: J. Pharmacol. Exp. Ther., *182:*1–13, 1972.
46. Lerner, J.: Comp. Biochem. Physiol. [C.] , *93:*1–9, 1989.
47. Acara, M.: Am. J. Physiol., *228:*645–649, 1975.
48. Acara, M., Rennick, B.: Am. J. Physiol., *225:*1123–1128, 1973.
49. Bean, G.H., Lowenstein, L.M.: J. Clin. Invest., *61:*1551–1554, 1978.
50. Besseghir, K., Pearce, L.B., Rennick, B.: Am. J. Physiol., *241:*F308–314, 1981.
51. Rennick, B., Acara, M., Glor, M.: Am. J. Physiol., *232:*F443–447, 1977.
52. Grossman, E.B., Hebert, S.C.: Am. J. Physiol., *256:*F107–F112, 1989.
53. Rennick, B., Acara, M., Hysert, P., et al.: Kidney Int., *10:*329–335, 1976.
54. Acara, M., Rennick, B., LaGraff, S. et al.: Nephron, *35:*241–243, 1983.
55. Jorswieck, I.: N.S. Arch. Pharmacol., *282(Suppl.):*R42, 1974.
56. Welsch, F.: Biochem. Pharmacol., *27:*1251–1257, 1978.
57. Sweiry, J.H., Yudilevich, D.L.: J. Physiol., *336:*251–266, 1985.
58. Sweiry, J.H., Page, K.R., Dacke, C.G., et al.: J. Dev. Physiol., *8:*435–445, 1986.
59. Cornford, E.M., Braun, L.D., Oldendorf, W.H.: J. Neurochem., *30:*299–308, 1978.
60. Cornford, E.M., Cornford, M.E.: Fed. Proc., *45:*2065–2072, 1986.
61. Mooradian, A.D.: Brain Res., *440:*328–332, 1988.
62. White, H.L., Cavallito, C.J.: Biochim. Biophys. Acta, *206:*343–358, 1970.
63. Malthe, S.D., Fonnum, F.: Biochem. J., *127:*229–236, 1972.
64. Rama Sastry, B.V., Henderson, G.I.: Biochem. Pharmacol., *21:*787–802, 1972.
65. White, H.L., Wu, J.C.: J. Neurochem., *20:*297–307, 1973.
66. Wecker, L., Dettbarn, W.D.: J. Neurochem., *32:*961–967, 1979.
67. Trommer, B.A., Schmidt, D.E., Wecker, L.: J. Neurochem., *39:*1704–1709, 1982.
68. Wecker, L.: J. Neurochem., *51:*497–504, 1988.
69. Miller, L.G., Greenblatt, D.J., Roy, R.B., et al.: J. Pharmacol. Exp. Ther., *248:*1–6, 1989.
70. Wecker, L., Cawley, G., Rothermel, S.: J. Neurochem., *52:*568–575, 1989.
71. Weinhold, P.A., Sanders, R.: Life Sci., *13:*621–629, 1973.
72. Tsuge, H., Nakano, Y., Onishi, H., et al.: Biochim. Biophys. Acta, *614:*274–284, 1980.
73. Kaiser, W., Bygrave, F.L.: Eur. J. Biochem., *4:*582–585, 1968.
74. Streumer-Svobodova, Z., Drahota, Z.: Physiol. Bohemoslov., *26:*525–534, 1977.
75. Wilken, D.R., McMacken, M.L., Rodriquez, A.: Biochim. Biophys. Acta, *216:*305–317, 1970.
76. Brophy, P.J., Choy, P., Toone, J., et al.: Eur. J. Biochem., *78:*491–496, 1977.
77. Weinhold, P.A., Rethy, V.B.: Biochemistry, *13:*5135–5141, 1974.
78. Haubrich, D.R.: J. Neurochem., *21:*315–328, 1973.
79. Pelech, S.L., Vance, D.E.: Biochim. Biophys. Acta, *779:*217–251, 1984.
80. Farrell, P.M., Lundgren, D.W., Adams, A.J.: Biochem. Biophys. Res. Commun., *57:*696–701, 1974.
81. Yao, Z., Jamil, H., Vance, D.E.: J. Biol. Chem., *265:*4326–4331, 1990.
82. Pomfret, E.A., daCosta, K.-A., Zeisel, S.H.: J. Nutr., Biochem., *1:*533–541, 1990.
83. Blusztajn, J.K., Zeisel, S.H., Wurtman, R.J.: Biochem. J., *232:*505–511, 1985.
84. Blusztajn, J.K., Zeisel, S.H., Wurtman, R.J.: Brain Res., *179:*319–327, 1979.
85. Zeisel, S.H.: Annu. Rev. Nutr., *1:*95–121, 1981.
86. Ridgway, N.D., Vance, D.E.: J. Biol. Chem., *262:*17,231–17,239, 1987.
87. Bjornstad, P., Bremer, J.: J. Lipid Res., *7:*38–45, 1966.
88. Crews, F.T., Calderini, G., Battistella, A., et al.: Brain Res., *229:*256–259, 1981.
89. Davis, P.B.: Pediatr. Res., *20:*1290–1296, 1986.
90. Fonlupt, P., Dubois, M., Gallet, H., et al.: C. R. Soc. Biol., *296:*1005–1007, 1983.
91. Harari, Y., Castro, G.A.: Mol. Biochem. Parasitol., *15:*317–326, 1985.
92. Laychock, S.G.: Mol. Pharmacol., *27:*66–73, 1985.
93. Nieto, A., Catt, K.J.: Endocrinology, *113:*758–762, 1983.
94. Niwa, Y., Sakane, T., Taniguchi, S.: Arch. Biochem. Biophys., *234:*7–14, 1984.
95. Panagia, V., Ganguly, P.K., Okumura, K., et al.: J. Mol. Cell. Cardiol., *17:*1151–1159, 1985.

96. Hirata, F., Tallman, J.F., Henneberry, R.C., et al.: Prog. Clin. Biol. Res., *63:*383–388, 1981.
97. Saceda, M., Garcia, M.P., Mato, J.M., et al.: Biochem. Int., *8:*445–452, 1984.
98. Robinson, B.S., Snoswell, A.M., Runciman, W.B., et al.: Biochem. J., *244:*367–373, 1987.
99. Sundler, R., Akesson, B.: J. Biol. Chem., *250:*3359–3367, 1975.
100. Blusztajn, J.K., Wurtman, R.J.: Nature, *290:*417–418, 1981.
101. Ridgway, N.D., Yao, Z., Vance, D.E.: J. Biol. Chem., *264:*1203–1207, 1989.
102. Hoffman, D.R., Haning, J.A., Cornatzer, W.E.: Lipids, *16:*561–567, 1981.
103. Ridgway, N.D., Vance, D.E.: J. Biol. Chem., *263:*16,864–16,871, 1988.
104. Haines, D.S.: Can. J. Biochem., *44:*45–57, 1966.
105. Pascale, R., Pirisi, L., Daino, L., et al.: FEBS Lett., *145:*293–297, 1982.
106. Mudd, S.H., Poole, J.R.: Metab. Clin. Exp., *24:*721–735, 1975.
107. Finkelstein, J.D., Martin, J.J., Harris, B.J., et al.: Arch. Biochem. Biophys., *218:*169–173, 1982.
108. Wong, E.R., Thompson, W.: Biochim. Biophys. Acta, *260:*259–271, 1972.
109. Finkelstein, J.D., Martin, J.J., Harris, B.J.: J. Biol. Chem., *263:*11,750–11,754, 1988.
110. Zeisel, S.H., Zola, T., daCosta, K., et al.: Biochem. J., *259:*725–729, 1989.
111. Shivapurkar, N., Poirier, L.A.: Carcinogenesis, *4:*1051–1057, 1983.
112. Poirier, L.A., Grantham, P.H., Rogers, A.E.: Cancer Res., *37:*744–748, 1977.
113. Barak, A.J., Beckenhauer, H.C., Tuma, D.J.: An. Biochem., *127:*372–375, 1982.
114. Barak, A.J., Kemmy, R.J.: Drug Nutr. Interact., *1:*275–278, 1982.
115. Barak, A.J., Tuma, D.J., Beckenhauer, H.C.: J. Am. Coll. Nutr., *3:*93–96, 1984.
116. Svardal, A.M., Ueland, P.M., Berge, R.K., et al.: Cancer Chemother. Pharmacol., *21:*313–318, 1988.
117. Freeman-Narrod, M., Narrod, S.A., Custer, R.P.: J. Natl. Cancer Inst., *59:*1013–1017, 1977.
118. Custer, R.P., Freeman-Narrod, M., Narrod, S.J.: J. Natl. Cancer Inst., *58:*1011–1015, 1977.
119. Aarsaether, N., Berge, R.K., Aarsland, A., et al.: Biochim. Biophys. Acta, *958:*70–80, 1988.
120. Freeman-Narrod, M.: J. Med. Pediatr. Oncol., *3:*9–14, 1977.
121. Lombardi, B.: Fed. Proc., *30:*139–142, 1971.
122. Handler, P., Bernheim, F.: Proc. Soc. Exp. Biol. Med., *72:*569, 1949.
123. Tani, H., Suzuki, S., Kobayashi, et al.: J. Nutr., *92:*317–324, 1967.
124. Fairbanks, B.W., Krider, J.L.: N. Am. Vet., *26:*18–23, 1945.
125. Blair, R., Newsome, F.: J. Anim. Sci., *60:*1508–1517, 1985.
126. Hershey, J.M., Soskin, S.: Am. J. Physiol., *93:*657–658, 1931.
127. Ketola, H.G.: J. Anim. Sci., *43:*474–477, 1976.
128. Ketola, H.G., Young, R.J.: Poult. Sci., *52:*2362–2363, 1973.
129. Ketola, H.G., Nesheim, M.C.: J. Nutr., *104:*1484–1486, 1974.
130. Ghoshal, A.K., Ahluwalia, M., Farber, E.: Am. J. Pathol., *113:*309–314, 1983.
131. Ghoshal, A.K., Farber, E.: Carcinogenesis, *5:*1367–1370, 1984.
132. Lombardi, B., Pani, P., Schlunk, F.F.: J. Lipid Res., *9:*437–446, 1968.
133. Yao, Z.M., Vance, D.E.: J. Biol. Chem., *263:*2998–3004, 1988.
134. Yao, Z.M., Vance, D.E.: J. Biol. Chem., *264:*11373–11380, 1989.
135. Blusztajn, J.K., Zeisel, S.H.: FEBS Lett., *243:*267–270, 1989.
136. Chandar, N., Lombardi, B.: Carcinogenesis, *9:*259–263, 1988.
137. Michael U.F., Cookson, S.L., Chavez, R., et al.: Proc. Soc. Exp. Biol. Med., *150:*672–676, 1975.
138. Baxter, J.H.: J. Nutr., *34:*333, 1947.
139. Best, C.H., Hartroft, W.S.: Fed. Proc., *8:*610, 1949.
140. Griffith, W.H., Wade, N.J.: J. Biol. Chem., *131:*567–573, 1939.
141. Chang, C.H., Jensen, L.S.: Poul. Sci., *54:*1718–1720, 1975.
142. Jukes, T.H.: J. Biol. Chem., *134:*789–792, 1940.
143. Kratzing, C.C., Perry, J.J.: J. Nutr., *101:*1657–1661, 1971.
144. Caniggia, A.: Haematologica, *34:*625–627, 1950.
145. Meck, W.H., Smith, R.A., Williams, C.L.: Dev. Psychobiol., *21:*339–353, 1988.
146. Haubrich, D.R., Wang, P.F., Chippendale, T., et al.: J. Neurochem., *27:*1305–1313, 1976.
147. Nagler, A.L., Dettbarn, E., Seifter, E., et al.: J. Nutr., *94:*13–19, 1968.
148. Mervis, R.F.: J. Neuropathol. Exp. Neurol., *41:*363–367, 1982.
149. Bertoni, F.C., Mervis, R.F., Giuli, C., et al.: Mech. Ageing Dev., *30:*1–9, 1985.
150. Bartus, R.T., Dean, R.L., Goas, J.A., et al.: Science, *209:*301–303, 1980.
151. Borum, P.R.: Annu. Rev. Nutr., *3:*233–259, 1983.
152. Corredor, C., Mansbach, C., Bressler, R.: Biochim. Biophys. Acta, *144:*366–374, 1967.
153. Carter, A.L., Frenkel, R.: J. Nutr., *108:*1748–1754, 1978.
154. Copeland, D.H., Salmon, W.D.: Am. J. Pathol., *22:*1059–1081, 1946.
155. Salmon, W.D., Copeland, D.H., Burns, M.J.: J. Natl. Cancer Inst., *15:*1549–1568, 1955.
156. Reddy, T.V., Ramanathan, R., Shinozuka, H., et al.: Cancer Lett., *18:*41–48, 1983.
157. Shivapurkar, N., Wilson, M.J., Hoover, K.L., et al.: J. Natl. Cancer Inst., *77:*213–217, 1986.
158. Rogers, A.E.: Cancer Res., *35:*2469–2474, 1975.
159. Giambarresi, L.I., Katyal, S.L., Lombardi, B.: Br. J. Cancer, *46:*825–829, 1982.
160. Locker, J., Reddy, T.V., Lombardi, B.: Carcinogenesis, *7:*1309–1312, 1986.
161. Mikol, Y.B., Hoover, K.L., Creasia, D., et al.: Carcinogenesis, *4:*1619–1629, 1983.
162. Shinozuka, H., Lombardi, B.: Cancer Res., *40:*3846–3849, 1980.
163. Newberne, P.M., Rogers, A.E.: Annu. Rev. Nutr., *6:*407–432, 1986.
164. Chandar, N., Amenta, J., Kandala, J.C., et al.: Carcinogenesis, *8:*669–673, 1987.
165. Rushmore, T., Lim, Y., Farber, E., et al.: Cancer Lett., *24:*251–255, 1984.
166. Blackshear, P., Nairn, A., Kuo, J.: FASEB J., *2:*2957–2969, 1988.
167. Nishizuka, Y.: Science, *233:*305–312, 1986.

**168.** Kato, M., Kawai, S., Takenawa, T.: FEBS Lett., *247*:247–250, 1989.
**169.** Wilkison, W.O., Sandgren, E.P., Palmiter, R.D., et al.: Oncogene, *4*:625–628, 1989.
**170.** Wolfman, A., Macara, I.G.: Nature, *325*:359–361, 1987.
**171.** Wolfman, A., Wingrove, T.G., Blackshear, P.J., et al.: J. Biol. Chem., *262*:16546–16552, 1987.
**172.** Rozengurt, E.: Science, *234*:161–166, 1986.
**173.** Kaibuchi, K., Tsuda, T., Kikuchi, A., et al.: J. Biol. Chem., *261*:1187–1192, 1986.
**174.** Megidish, T., Mazurek, N.: Nature, *342*:807–811, 1989.
**175.** Poley, J.R.: Liver and nutrition: Hepatic complications of total parenteral nutrition. *In* Textbook of Gastroenterology and Nutrition in Infancy. Edited by E. Lebenthal. New York, Raven Press, 1981, pp. 743–763.
**176.** Kaminski, D.L., Adams, A., Jellinek, M.: Surgery, *88*:93–100, 1980.
**177.** Hall, R.I., Ross, L.H., Bozovic, M.G., et al.: J. Parenter. Ent. Nutr., *9*:597–599, 1985.
**178.** Chawla, R.K., Berry, C.J., Kutner, M.H., et al.: Am. J. Clin. Nutr., *42*:577–584, 1985.
**179.** Burt, M.E., Hanin, I., Brennan, M.F.: Lancet, *2*:638–639, 1980.
**180.** Carroll, C., Williams, L.: Nutr. Rep. Int., *25*:773, 1982.
**181.** Kaminski, D.L., Mueller, E.J., Jellinek, M.: Am. J. Physiol., *239*:G358–362, 1980.
**182.** Gwee, M.C., Sim, M.K.: Clin. Exp. Pharmacol. Physiol., *5*:649–653, 1978.
**183.** Gwee, M.C.: Med. Hypotheses, *9*:157–162, 1982.
**184.** Zeisel, S.H., daCosta, K.-A., Franklin, P.D., et al.: FASEB J., *5*:2093–2098, 1991.
**185.** Dizik, M., Christman, J.K., Wainfan, E.: Carcinogenesis, *12*:1307–1312, 1991.
**186.** Buchman, A.L., Dubin, M., Jenden, D., et al.: Gastroenterology, *102*:1363–1370, 1992.

## SELECTED READINGS

Blusztajn, J.K., Holbrook, P.G., Lakher, M., et al.: "Autocannibalism" of membrane choline-phospholipids: Physiology and pathology. Psychopharmacol. Bull, *22*:781–786, 1986.
Blusztajn, J.K., Wurtman, R.J. Choline and cholinergic neurons. Science, 221:614–620, 1983.
Kennedy, E.P., Weiss S.B.: The function of cytidine coenzymes in the biosynthesis of phospholipids. J. Biol. Chem., *222*:193–214, 1956.
Newberne, P.M., Rogers, A.E.: Labile methyl groups and the promotion of cancer. Annu. Rev. Nutr., *6*:407–432, 1986.
Sheard, N.F., Tayek, J.A., Bistrian, B.R., et al.: Plasma choline concentration in humans fed parenterally. Am. J. Clin. Nutr., *43*:219–224, 1986.

Some of the work described was supported by grants from the National Institutes of Health (HD26553, AGO9525, and RR-00533), and the American Institute for Cancer Research.

CHAPTER 29

# Carnitine

Harry P. Broquist



Carnitine was discovered as a minor nitrogenous compound in muscle tissue in 1905, and its structure was subsequently shown to be L-β-hydroxy-γ-N-trimethylaminobutyric acid. It received little further attention until 1952, when Carter et al. established that vitamin $B_T$, a growth factor for the meal worm, Tennebrio molitor, was carnitine, thus implying a critical physiologic role for this growth factor.[1] Subsequent investigations of Fritz[2] and Bremer[3] led to the knowledge of a role for carnitine in the intramitochondrial transport of fatty acids, a process essential for subsequent fatty acid oxidation and energy release. It is now clear that carnitine plays several roles in mammalian metabolism involving conjugation of acyl residues to the β-hydroxyl group of carnitine with subsequent translocation from one cellular compartment to another. Such metabolism has considerable clinical interest, inasmuch as carnitine acyltransferase deficiencies, for example, are associated with particular metabolic disorders.

Animal foods are rich in carnitine, in contrast to plant-derived foods. Human requirements for carnitine are met from both endogenous biosynthesis and the diet. Much is known about the biosynthesis of carnitine from lysine and methionine and the cofactors required for such synthesis. Considerable nutritional and clinical interest is now focused on defining what is currently termed *conditional carnitine deficiency* in man. The carnitine economy in the body is well conserved and regulatory mechanisms and carnitine transport are under active study.

Numerous reviews concerning carnitine have appeared in the last decade; three of the most recent, which emphasize biochemical,[4] nutritional,[5] and clinical[6] aspects of the field, are cited, providing references to earlier reviews and original work.

## CARNITINE FUNCTION

L-Carnitine participates in transesterification reactions of the following type:*

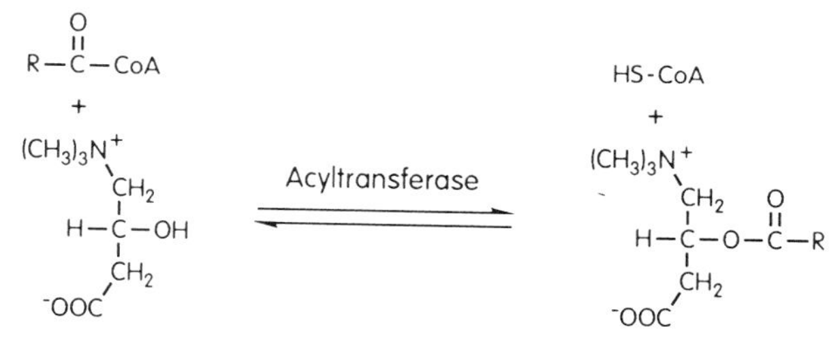
R—C—CoA
O
+
$(CH_3)_3N^+$
$CH_2$
H—C—OH
$CH_2$
$^-OOC$
Acyltransferase
HS-CoA
+
$(CH_3)_3N^+$
$CH_2$
H—C—O—C—R
O
$CH_2$
$^-OOC$

Coenzyme A (CoA) esters of varying chain length, branching, and substitution react with carnitine in a transesterification catalyzed by the appropriate fatty acyltransferase to give a carnitine ester and free coenzyme A. The reaction is fully reversible.

### CARNITINE PALMITOYLTRANSFERASE (CPT, LONG-CHAIN FATTY ACYLTRANSFERASE)

Fatty acyl-CoA esters cannot cross from the cytosol into the mitochondria; yet such esters are present in the mitochondria where they are subject to β-oxidation and

*(From Rebouche, C.J.: J. Appl. Nutr., *40*:99–111, 1988.)

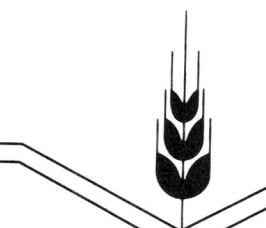

subsequent energy release. This problem of fatty acyl-CoA transport across the mitochondrial membrane is now understood (see reviews of Bieber[4] and Pande and Murthy[7]), as depicted by the events of Figure 29–1. CPT may in fact be two distinct enzymes. CPT I (also designated $CPT_o$ ) located on the outer membrane, and CPT II (or $CPT_i$) located on the inner membrane (Fig. 29–1), in concert with carnitine-acylcarnitine translocase in the intermembrane space, carry out the import of acyl groups into the mitochondria. $CPT_o$ catalyzes transesterification with acyl-CoA and carnitine giving acylcarnitine. The latter ester is transported across the inner mitochondrial membrane by way of carnitine-acylcarnitine translocase. A second transesterification with CoA by $CPT_i$ regenerates fatty acyl-CoA subject to β-oxidation. Free carnitine released is translocated by carnitine-acylcarnitine translocase back to the intermitochondrial space, where it can repeat catalysis of the fatty acylester transport process.

## CARNITINE PALMITOYLTRANSFERASE REGULATION

The CPT system, shown in Figure 29–1, is of great importance in relating lipid metabolism to energy metabolism, and it might likely be under tight physiologic regulation. In this regard, malonyl-CoA, the first committed intermediate in the conversion of carbohydrate to fat, is a competitive inhibitor of $CPT_o$, as depicted in Figure 29–1.[8] Under certain conditions, the estimated hepatic concentration of this metabolite relates inversely to the prevailing rates of fatty acid oxidation. Thus, after a high carbohydrate meal (low glucagon to insulin ratio), malonyl-CoA levels are elevated, fatty acid biosynthesis is brisk, and fatty acid oxidation is blocked. Conversely, when the glucagon to insulin ratio is high, or fatty acyl-CoA levels are elevated, malonyl-CoA concentrations decrease, lipogenesis concomitantly ceases, $CPT_o$ activity increases, and fatty acid oxidation occurs.

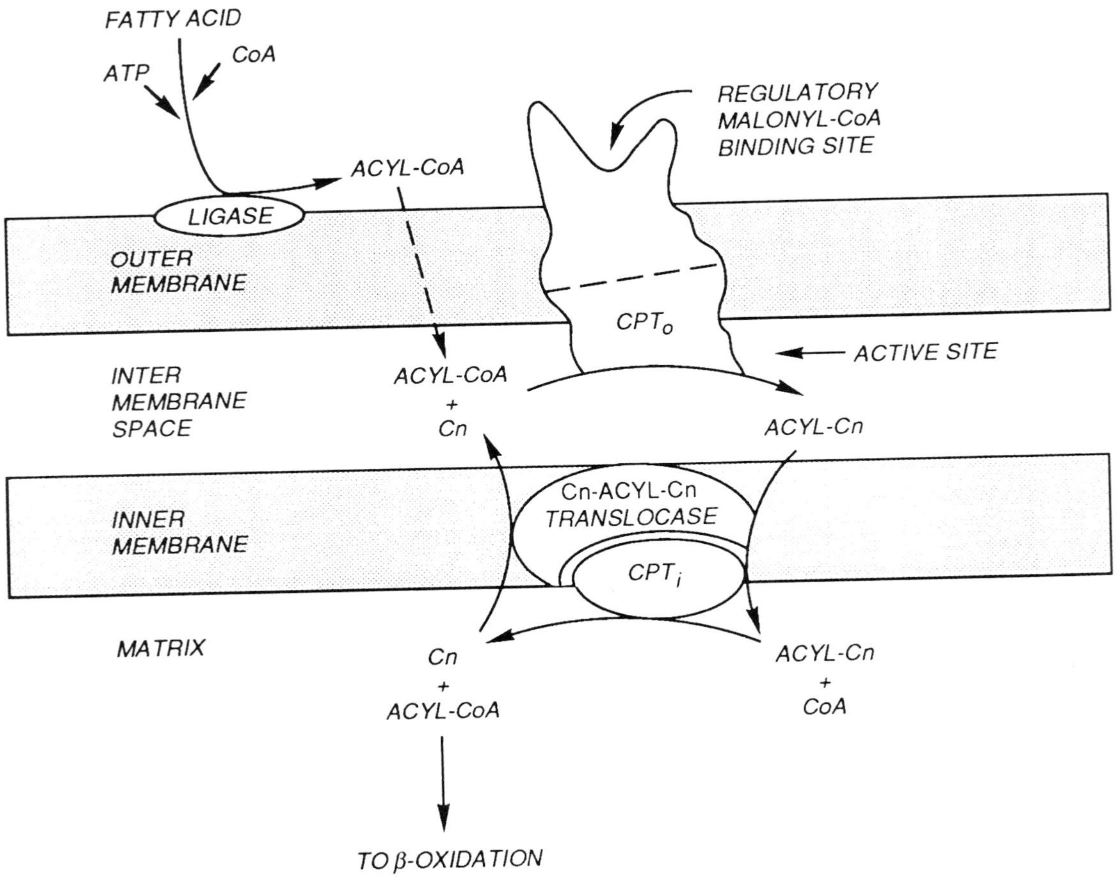
FATTY ACID
ATP
CoA
REGULATORY
MALONYL-CoA
BINDING SITE
ACYL-CoA
LIGASE
OUTER
MEMBRANE
CPTo
ACTIVE SITE
INTER
MEMBRANE
SPACE
ACYL-CoA
+
Cn
ACYL-Cn
INNER
MEMBRANE
Cn-ACYL-Cn
TRANSLOCASE
CPTi
MATRIX
Cn
+
ACYL-CoA
ACYL-Cn
+
CoA
TO β-OXIDATION

**FIGURE 29–1.** Schematic representation of the carnitine-dependent import of acyl groups into mitochondria. Being reversible, the same sequence allows also the export of acyl groups from the mitochondrial matrix. $CPT_o$, Outer CPT; $CPT_i$, inner CPT; Cn, carnitine. (From Pande, S.V., Murthy, M.S.R.: Biochem. Cell Biol., *67*:671–673, 1989.)

With the realization of the pivotal role of $CPT_o$ in fat metabolism, pharmacologic agents are being sought, such as analogues of carnitine that might inhibit the $CPT_o$ system and act as hypoglycemic agents, attenuating gluconeogenesis and stimulating peripheral glucose use. Aminocarnitine (3-amino-4-trimethylaminobutyrate) and several of its N-acyl derivatives have promise in this regard.[9,10] For example, in a rat liver mitochondrial system, in the presence of 1 mmol/L (1 mM) carnitine, 5 μmol/L (5 μM) aminocarnitine inhibited $CPT_o$ by 64%. In starved mice, liver and kidney triglyceride levels were elevated for up to 3 days after a single administration of acetyl-DL-carnitine.[9] This result is interesting in a clinical context because it has been suggested that excessive free fatty acid metabolism is a key factor in diabetes. Consequently, treatment of diabetes might be possible by correcting the abnormally high rate of free fatty acid oxidation (see discussion by Kanamaru et al.[10]).

## SHORT-CHAIN AND MEDIUM-CHAIN CARNITINE ACYLTRANSFERASES

Carnitine also facilitates removal from the mitochondrion of short- and medium-chain organic acids that accumulate as a result of normal or abnormal metabolism. The mechanism is thought to be by a reverse of the process shown in Figure 29–1, although whether the role of carnitine in this process is essential or just facilitory has been difficult to establish.

Carnitine octanoyltransferase has been found in three organelles of liver, namely peroxisomes, microsomes, and mitochondria, and has a broad specificity, e.g., the peroxisomal enzyme recognizes acyl groups varying in chain length from $C_6$ to $C_{20}$. Liver carnitine acetyltransferase is also present in these organelles and also possesses broad substrate specificity. The diverse activity of these acyltransferases has relevance to recent findings that some short-chain acids formed under certain pathologic conditions or after drug administration are excreted in the urine as carnitine esters (Table 29–1). The excretion of certain xenobiotics as carnitine esters suggests a detoxification role for carnitine, although if such urinary excretion is sustained for long periods, a secondary deficiency of carnitine may be induced.[6]

In addition to the role of short-chain and medium-chain carnitine acyltransferases in translocating acyl moieties across an acyl-CoA barrier, carnitine also modulates the availability of reduced CoASH in such processes. Extensive studies of mitochondrial carnitine acetyltransferase in heart muscle show that carnitine buffers the CoASH to acetyl-CoA ratio in the matrix of the mitochondria, thus allowing a shift of the "acetyl pressure" from the mitochondria to the cytoplasm.[3] For example, as the CoASH to acetyl-CoA ratio increases with mitochondrial acetyl-CoA oxidation, cytosolic acetyl groups enter the carnitine acetyltransferase system and the CoASH to acetyl-CoA ratio decreases.

## SOURCES OF CARNITINE: DIET AND SYNTHESIS

Table 29–2 outlines the carnitine content of selected foods and shows that carnitine levels are high in meat and dairy products. Vegetables, cereals, and fruits are negligible sources of carnitine. The average nonvegetarian diet has been estimated to provide 100 to 300 mg carnitine per day.

In mammals, carnitine is synthesized from the essential amino acids lysine and methionine (Fig. 29–2), in which carbon atoms 3, 4, 5, and 6 and the 6-amino group of lysine constitute the carbon-nitrogen backbone of

**TABLE 29–1.** EXCRETION OF SHORT- AND MEDIUM-CHAIN ORGANIC ACIDS AS CARNITINE ESTERS*

| ACID EXCRETED AS CARNITINE ESTER | CONDITIONS UNDER WHICH ORGANIC ACID ACCUMULATES |
|---|---|
| $CH_3CH_2COOH$ Propionic acid | Propionyl-CoA carboxylase and methylmalonyl-CoA mutase deficiencies |
| $(CH_3)_2CHCH_2COOH$ Isovaleric acid | Isovaleric acidemia |
| $HOOCCH_2CH(CH_3)CH_2COOH$ 3-Methylglutaric acid | 3-Hydroxy-3-methylglutaryl-CoA lyase deficiency |
| $CH_3(CH_2)_6COOH$ Octanoic acid | Medium-chain acyl-CoA dehydrogenase deficiency |
| $(CH_3)_3CCOOH$ Pivalic acid | Pivampicillin treatment |
| $(CH_3CH_2CH_2)_2CHCOOH$ Valproic acid | Valproic acid therapy |

*See references in article by Rebouche (reference 5) for details.

**TABLE 29–2.** CARNITINE CONTENT OF SELECTED FOODS*

| Food | Carnitine |
|---|---|
| **DAIRY PRODUCTS** | |
| Whole milk | 20.4 |
| Butter | 3.1 |
| American cheese | 23.2 |
| Cottage cheese | 7.0 |
| Ice cream | 23.0 |
| **VEGETABLES** | |
| Green beans (cooked) | 0.019 |
| Green peas (cooked) | 0.037 |
| Asparagus (cooked) | 1.21 |
| Beets (cooked) | 0.020 |
| Broccoli (fresh) | 0.023 |
| (cooked) | 0.011 |
| Carrots (fresh) | 0.041 |
| (cooked) | 0.039 |
| Potato (baked) | 0.080 |
| Lettuce | 0.007 |
| **FRUITS** | |
| Apples | 0.0002 |
| Bananas | 0.0056 |
| Strawberries | ND |
| Peaches | 0.0060 |
| Pineapple | 0.0063 |
| Pears | 0.0107 |
| **MEAT PRODUCTS†** | |
| Beef steak | 592 ± 260 (4) |
| Ground beef | 582 ± 32 (3) |
| Chicken breast | 24.3 ± 8.0 (3) |
| Cod fish | 34.6 ± 11.7 (3) |
| Pork | 172 ± 32 (3) |
| Bacon | 145 ± 24 (3) |
| **BREAD AND CEREAL** | |
| Whole-wheat bread | 2.26 |
| White bread | 0.912 |
| Rice (cooked) | 0.090 |
| Macaroni | 0.780 |
| Corn flakes | 0.078 |
| **NON-DAIRY BEVERAGES** | |
| Coffee | 0.009 |
| Orange juice | 0.012 |
| Tomato juice | 0.030 |
| Grape juice | 0.093 |
| Grapefruit juice | ND‡ |
| Cola | ND |
| **MISCELLANEOUS** | |
| Eggs | 0.075 |
| Peanut butter | 0.516 |

*Units are μmol/100 g (solid foods) or μmol/100 ml (liquids); 1 μmol = 0.161 mg. Values reported are for total carnitine (free plus esterified).

†Values for meat products are mean ± SD (number of determinations in parentheses) and are based on the precooked weight.

‡ND, not detectable.

(Adapted from Rebouche, C.J., Engle, A.G.: J. Clin. Invest., *73*:857–867, 1984, *in* Rebouche, C.J.: J. Appl. Nutr., *40*:99–111, 1988.)

carnitine. The N-methyl groups derive from methionine. The initial methylation reaction (reaction 1, Fig. 29–2) occurs as a post-translational modification of peptide-bound lysine in which S-adenosylmethionine (AdoMet) is the methyl donor. γ-N-Trimethyllysine covalently bound in proteins such as actin, myosin, and histones is subsequently released by way of lysosomal hydrolases and may then enter the carnitine pathway, which involves respective hydroxylation, aldolase cleavage, oxidation, and hydroxylation to yield carnitine. Details of the elucidation of the carnitine biosynthetic pathway and relevant enzymology are discussed elsewhere.[11] A unique circumstance is the presence of two distinct α-ketoglutarate, ascorbate, $Fe^{++}$-dependent dioxygenases, one mitochondrial and the other cytosolic (hydroxylases 2 and 5, respectively, see Fig. 29–2). Also, a requirement for pyridoxal phosphate in aldolase catalysis (reaction 3, Fig. 29–2) should be noted. In general, the liver of all mammals studied carries out reactions 2 to 5 (see Fig. 29–2). These reactions also occur in the kidney of certain higher animals, including the rhesus monkey and man. Knowledge of the substrates and cofactors of carnitine biosynthesis, together with relevant enzymology, have contributed importantly in investigations relating to "carnitine deficiency" in man.

## CARNITINE METABOLISM: ABSORPTION, RENAL CLEARANCE EXCRETION, REGULATION

Based largely on animal studies, dietary carnitine appears to be absorbed rapidly from the intestinal lumen across the mucosal membrane by both passive and active transport mechanisms. Carnitine is then taken up from the portal circulation by the liver and subsequently released into the systemic circulation. Most cells possess a stereospecific mechanism for transporting carnitine across the cell membrane, with a resulting 10- to 100-fold gradient between extracellular and intracellular concentration. Rebouche and Engel described the kinetics of carnitine metabolism in humans using a compartmental analysis technique (a three-compartment system—extracellular fluid, skeletal muscle, and other tissues).[12] L-[methyl-$^{14}C$] carnitine was administered (intravenously) and monitored in the compartments with time.

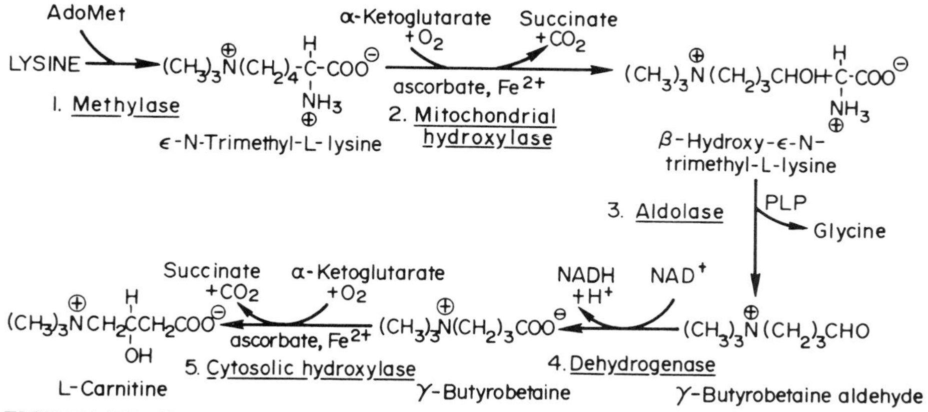
AdoMet
LYSINE
I. Methylase
ε-N-Trimethyl-L-lysine
α-Ketoglutarate +O2
Succinate +CO2
ascorbate, Fe2+
2. Mitochondrial hydroxylase
β-Hydroxy-ε-N-trimethyl-L-lysine
3. Aldolase
PLP
Glycine
NADH +H+
NAD+
4. Dehydrogenase
γ-Butyrobetaine aldehyde
γ-Butyrobetaine
Succinate +CO2
α-Ketoglutarate +O2
ascorbate, Fe2+
5. Cytosolic hydroxylase
L-Carnitine

**FIGURE 29–2.** The biogenesis of carnitine from lysine and methionine.

The tracer appeared more slowly in skeletal muscle (80% of the dose in 50 hours) than in the other tissues but remained high throughout the study (28 days). Calculations showed that skeletal muscle contains 95% of body carnitine stores and has a slow turnover rate (191 hours). Some evidence from tracer studies in rats[13] indicates that not all of dietary carnitine is absorbed intact. About 6.5% of the radioactivity of an orally administered dose of L-[methyl-$^{14}$C] carnitine was recovered as γ-butyrobetaine (feces) and trimethylamine oxide (urine), such metabolites having arisen from endogenous microflora of the gastrointestinal tract.

Renal clearance of carnitine is a highly conserved process; thus, in normal individuals, more than 90% of carnitine filtered by the glomerulus is reabsorbed. When plasma carnitine values are elevated, however, such reabsorption rapidly declines, suggesting that plasma carnitine levels may be regulated to a degree by renal clearance mechanisms.

Knowledge of the enzymes of carnitine biosynthesis together with the availability of certain of the intermediates, particularly trimethyllysine and γ-butyrobetaine, have permitted studies relating to possible rate-limiting steps in carnitine biosynthesis. Of interest is the observation that hepatic but not renal γ-butyrobetaine hydroxylase (see reaction 5, Fig. 29–1) in infant liver is only 25% of that in adult liver. However, both infants and adults were found to increase their rate of carnitine excretion by at least 30-fold after the addition of γ-butyrobetaine to the diet, indicating that γ-butyrobetaine is not rate limiting for either adults or infants.[14] Similar urinary excretion studies in humans after ingestion of dietary trimethyllysine indicated that exogenous trimethyllysine is not used effectively for carnitine synthesis, likely because it is poorly absorbed by the tissues and poorly reabsorbed by the kidneys. Although the availability of trimethyllysine deriving from protein-bound trimethyllysine appears to be rate limiting in rats, this concept has not been established conclusively in man.[5]

## NUTRITIONAL AND FUNCTIONAL DEFICIENCY

Because higher animals including man can synthesize carnitine, it has long been assumed that it is a nonessential nutrient. But much clinical nutrition research now indicates that carnitine should be viewed as a "conditionally essential nutrient." Rudman and Williams defined such a nutrient as, "a nutritionally dispensable compound for which, under a particular conditioning circumstance, dietary removal causes a demonstrable adverse effect."[15] In this context, Feller and Rudman listed seven causes for impairment of carnitine function within cells, some of which well illustrate this concept.[6] This list, abbreviated for space considerations, is given subsequently and is illustrated where relevant by examples from the nutrition literature.

1. *Reduced Capacity for Biosynthesis.* (1) Limiting amino acid precursors and/or cofactors for carnitine synthesis (see Fig. 29–2); (2) impairment by disease of organs concerned in carnitine biosynthesis (e.g., liver); (3) a congenital block in the biosynthetic pathway. In severely malnourished children and adults, in whom intake of carnitine and its precursors is very low, or in rats receiving diets simulating these conditions, carnitine levels in the plasma and the tissues are low, coupled with impaired fatty acid oxidation and lipid accumulation (see reference 16). In a study of carnitine nutriture in cirrhosis,[17] 20 of 60 patients had low serum and urinary levels of carnitine with severe fatty liver. The intakes of these cirrhotic patients of preformed carnitine, lysine, and methionine were only 30% of the intakes of normal individuals.
2. *Subnormal CPT I ($CPT_o$).* Important congenital disorders of carnitine metabolism are the lipid storage myopathies. The systemic type is characterized by low levels of carnitine in skeletal muscle, as well as in other tissues (heart, liver) and the plasma. In addition

to muscle weakness are abnormalities of the liver, central nervous system, and the heart. Both the skeletal muscle and liver are infiltrated with fat. The precise biochemical defect is not known, but it can be visualized from Figure 29–1, how limiting concentrations of carnitine in the CPT system would impair fatty acyl transport with concomitant lipid accumulation in the tissues.

3. *Alterations in Cellular Mechanisms for Carnitine Transport.* In the myopathic variant of the lipid storage myopathies, type I fibers are infiltrated extensively by fat, yet the enzymes of the carnitine acyltransferase and fatty acid oxidation systems are normal. However, the carnitine level in the muscle is low in contrast to normal levels in the plasma, suggesting a defect in carnitine transport. Many, but not all, individuals with either the myopathic or systemic disease have responded dramatically to carnitine supplementation.

4. *Excess Loss of Carnitine.* This cause is well illustrated by the loss of carnitine in body fluids and tissues that can occur, for example, after hemodialysis in patients with chronic renal failure, in enteral feedings with protein hydrolysate formulas, and in total parenteral nutrition (see reference 6). Such findings raise the question of the appropriateness of carnitine supplementation in these clinical situations. The possibility of loss of carnitine from the body in relation to the organic acidemias and xenobiotic administration also deserves mention (see Table 29–1).

5. *Raised Tissue Requirement for Carnitine.* At birth, the neonate shifts significantly from glucose to fatty acids for energy demands, and studies have shown that premature infants and neonates have low tissue levels of carnitine.[18] Furthermore, soy-based infant formulas are lacking in carnitine. For these reasons, infants may be considered at risk for carnitine deficiency, and a case can be made for carnitine supplementation of infant formulas.[19]

The foregoing examples by no means exhaust the diverse clinical and nutritional circumstances relating to conditional carnitine deficiency; a carnitine research symposium[20] focused on this subject in greater depth. One difficulty in this field from a clinical standpoint is that of interpreting the significance of "low" levels of carnitine in body fluids and tissues, i.e., to what degree do such figures indicate latent or existing pathologic change? In this regard, the carnitine status in vegetarians, who consume diets low in carnitine for prolonged periods (see Table 29–2), is of interest. In one study in adult vegetarians and lactovegetarians,[21] plasma and urinary carnitine levels were significantly lower than in adults with a mixed diet. Children showed more significant diet-related differences, but the study permitted no conclusions regarding the risk of overt carnitine deficiency. Clearly, carnitine biosynthesis and renal conservation operates efficiently in maintaining carnitine status in these instances in the face of low carnitine intakes.

## EVALUATION OF NUTRIENT STATUS

Recent developments in the methodology for carnitine assay, together with the identification and quantitation of the acylcarnitines, have been reviewed in detail.[22,23] Present methods for the determination of carnitine are based on the carnitine acetyltransferase (CAT) reaction:

$$\text{L-carnitine} + \text{acetyl-CoA} \xrightarrow{\text{CAT}} \text{acetyl-L-carnitine} + \text{CoASH}$$

In a spectrophotometric method, carnitine extracts are incubated with freshly prepared acetyl-CoA and CAT (a stable, commercially available enzyme preparation). The carnitine-dependent appearance of CoASH is determined spectrophotometrically with Ellman's reagent, dithiobisnitrobenzoic acid. In a radioisotope assay, which is at least 10 times as sensitive, [1-$^{14}$C] acetyl-CoA is used; radioactive acetylcarnitine formed is separated from residual [1-$^{14}$C] acetyl-CoA by cation exchange filtration, and radioactivity is counted. In these methods, mild alkaline hydrolysis is used such that the total amount of carnitine is measured. The difference between the values of total carnitine and free carnitine (before hydrolysis) yields the amount of O-acylcarnitine.

## REFERENCES


1. Carter, H.E., Bhattacharya, P.K., Weidman, K.R., et al.: Arch. Biochem. Biophys., *38:*405–416, 1952.
2. Fritz, I.B.: Adv. Lipid Res., *1:*285–334, 1963.
3. Bremer, J.: Physiol. Rev., *63:*1420–1468, 1983.
4. Bieber, L.L.: Annu. Rev. Biochem., *57:*261–283, 1988.
5. Rebouche, C.J.: J. Appl. Nutr., *40:*99–111, 1988.
6. Feller, A.G., Rudman, D.: J. Nutr., *118:*541–547, 1988.
7. Pande, S.V., Murthy, M.S.R.: Biochem. Cell Biol., *67:*671–673, 1989.
8. McGarry, J.D., Woeltje, K.F., Kuwajima, M., et al.: Diabetes Metab. Rev., *5:*271–284, 1989.
9. Jenkins, D.L., Griffith, O.W.: J. Biol. Chem., *260:*14,748–14,755, 1985.
10. Kanamaru, T., Shinagawa, S., Asai, M., et al.: Life Sci., *37:*217–223, 1985.
11. Broquist, H.P.: Fed. Proc., *41:*2840–2842, 1982.
12. Rebouche, C.J., Engel, A.G.: J. Clin. Invest., *73:*857–867, 1984.
13. Rebouche, C.J., Mack, D.L., Edmonson, P.F.: Biochemistry, *23:*6422–6426, 1984.
14. Olson, A.L., Rebouche, C.J.: J. Nutr., *117:*1024–1031, 1987.

15. Rudman, D., Williams, P.J.: Pathophysiologic principles of nutrition. *In* Pathophysiology, the Biological Principles of Disease. Edited by L.H. Smith and S.O. Thier. Philadelphia, W.B. Saunders, 1985.
16. Broquist, H.P., Borum, P.R.: Adv. Nutr. Res., *4:*181–204, 1982.
17. Rudman, D., Sewel, C.W., Ansley, J.D.: J. Clin. Invest., *60:*716–723, 1977.
18. Shenai, J.P., Borum, P.R.: Pediatr. Res., *18:*679–682, 1984.
19. Borum, P.R.: Nutr. Rev., *39:*385–390, 1981.
20. Borum, P.R. (ed.): Clinical Aspects of Human Carnitine Deficiency. New York, Pergamon, 1986.
21. Lombard, K.A., Olson, A.L., Nelson, S.E., et al.: Am. J. Clin. Nutr., *50:*301–306, 1989.
22. Bieber, L.L., Lewen, L.M.: Methods Enzymol., *72:*276–279, 1981.
23. Bieber, L.L., Kerner, J.: Methods Enzymol., *123:*264–284, 1986.

## SELECTED READINGS

Bieber, L.L.: Carnitine. Annu. Rev. Biochem., *57:*261–283, 1988.

Bremer, J.: Carnitine metabolism and function. Physiol. Rev., *63:*1420–1468, 1983.

Feller, A.G., Rudman, D.: Role of carnitine in human nutrition. J. Nutr., *118:*541–547, 1988.

Rebouche, C.J.: Carnitine metabolism and human nutrition. J. Appl. Nutr., *40:*99–111, 1988.

Rebouche, C.J., Paulson, D.J.: Carnitine metabolism and function in humans. Annu. Rev. Nutr., *6:*41–66, 1986.

# CHAPTER 30

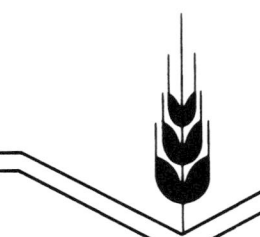

# Inositol and Pyrroloquinoline Quinone

## A. INOSITOL

Harold M. Aukema and Dr. Bruce J. Holub



Nutritional scientists have been interested in inositol (*myo*-inositol) as a nutrient since the early 1940s, when its essentiality in certain rodent models was first suggested. Inositol depletion resulted in alopecia in mice,[1] and in the accumulation of fat in the liver of rats fed certain diets.[2] Since then, however, it has become apparent that although inositol is a physiologically essential growth factor at the cellular level, it is only required as a dietary nutrient in certain species and under certain dietary conditions. Presently, interest in inositol nutrition is focused on its potential importance in clinical situations. It is now recognized that dietary inositol may have therapeutic potential in complementing the treatment of several disorders in which altered inositol metabolism occurs. Inositol and its derivatives are widely distributed in nature and occur in animals, higher plants, fungi, and bacteria where they perform essential metabolic functions. Inositol metabolism in mammalian cells has been the subject of many studies and has been reviewed in detail.[3,4] Present research interest in inositol biosynthesis and degradation is focused particularly on its role in inositol-containing phospholipids and their functions as cellular mediators of signal transduction, metabolic regulation, and growth. The pioneering contributions of Hokin and Hokin[5] and of Michell[6] are noteworthy in this regard. Interest in this rapidly expanding field is evidenced by the appearance of more than 50 new papers per month in the English scientific literature dealing with various facets of inositol phospholipid metabolism. Several in-depth reviews on this topic are available.[7–10]

## CHEMISTRY AND BIOLOGIC ACTIVITY

Of the nine possible isomers of hexahydroxycyclohexane, *myo*-inositol is by far the most common form in mammalian tissues and cells, and is the nutritionally significant isomer. Inositol occurs in mammalian tissues and cells in its free form, as a constituent of inositol phospholipid, and as part of glycosyl-phosphatidylinositol anchors of membrane proteins. The latter form, serving as a glycolipid anchor, is a recent discovery and represents a major form of post-translational modification of membrane proteins. The elucidation of the function(s) of this inositol form promises to be an exciting area of research (for review, see reference 11). Inositol exists in plants mainly as phytic acid (inositol hexaphosphate). Inositol phosphate isomers are also present at low levels in avian and fish erythrocytes and are postulated to play a role in allosteric regulation of oxygen affinity to the hemoglobins.[12]

Figure 30A–1 gives the structure of free *myo*-inositol and phosphatidylinositol (PI), the predominant form of

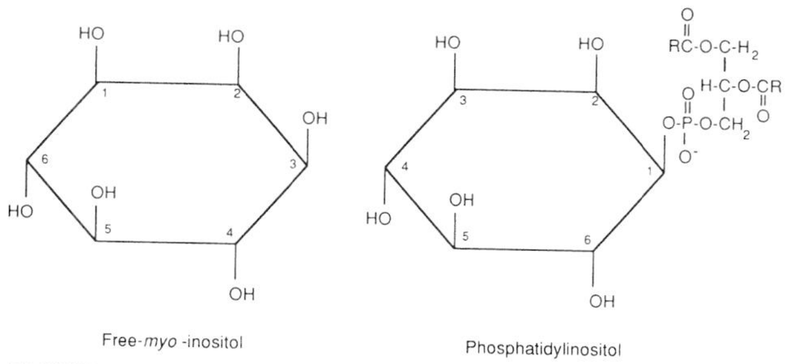
Free-myo-inositol
Phosphatidylinositol

**FIGURE 30A–1.** Structures of free *myo*-inositol and phosphatidylinositol. The molecular weight of inositol is 180.16 g/mol.

inositol phospholipid in mammalian tissues and cells. When inositol phospholipids and inositol phosphates are synthesized, phosphorylation on O-3 alters the numbering of the carbon atoms, reversing C-3 to C-1.[13] The existence of the polyphosphoinositides, PI-4-phosphate (PI-4-P) and PI-4, 5-bisphosphate (PI-4, 5-$P_2$), has been known for several years. Recently, however, there have been reports on the presence of several other isomers including PI-3-P,[14] PI-3,4-$P_2$,[15,16] and PI-3,4,5-trisphosphate (PI-3,4,5-$P_3$).[15,17,18] PI accounts for 2 to 12% of the total phospholipid of various mammalian tissues; the two major polyphosphoinositides, PI-4-P, and PI-4,5-$P_2$, exist at levels of 5 to 70% of PI; the other polyphosphoinositides are present at much lower concentrations. The diverse biologic activity of these compounds is presently the focus of much exciting research.

## METABOLISM

Inositol is present in the diet from both plant and animal sources, providing the adult human on a mixed North American diet with approximately 5.5 mmol (1 g) per day of total dietary inositol. In animal products such as fish, poultry, meats, and dairy products, inositol is present in both its free form and as inositol phospholipid. Inositol is present in high concentrations in breast milk,[19] and has also been added to some infant formulas. In plant foodstuffs, the predominant form of inositol exists as phytate, a compound known to form insoluble complexes with $Ca^{++}$, $Zn^{++}$, and $Fe^{++}$. High levels of dietary phytate therefore can significantly impair the gastrointestinal absorption of these nutrients. Conversely, high-$Ca^{++}$ diets also increase the amount of phytate excreted. Inositol in the form of inositol phospholipid is generally considered to be a readily available source of dietary inositol.

### DIGESTION AND ABSORPTION

Dietary phytate is dephosphorylated to produce free inositol, orthophosphate, and intermediary products (Fig. 30A–2) in the gut of monogastrics by phytase, an

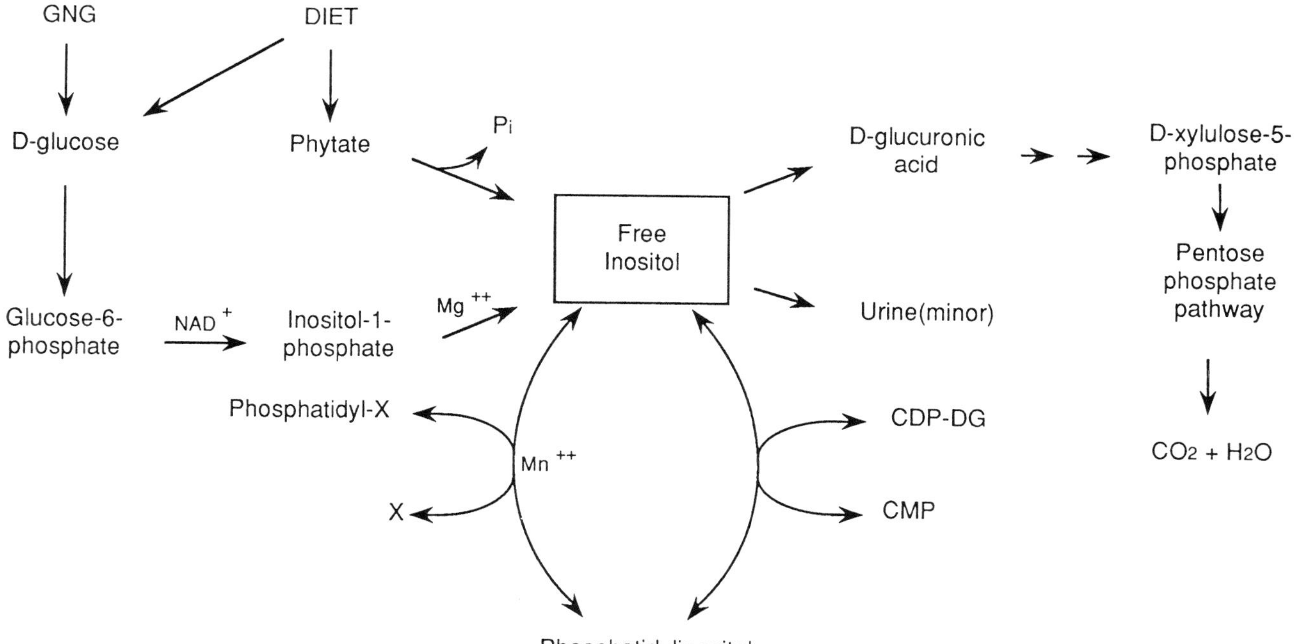
GNG
DIET
D-glucose
Phytate
Pi
Free Inositol
D-glucuronic acid
D-xylulose-5-phosphate
Pentose phosphate pathway
Glucose-6-phosphate
NAD +
Inositol-1-phosphate
Mg ++
Urine(minor)
Phosphatidyl-X
Mn ++
CDP-DG
X
CMP
CO2 + H2O
Phosphatidylinositol

**FIGURE 30A–2.** Pathways of free inositol metabolism. CDP-DG, Cytidine diphosphate-diacylglycerol; CMP, cytidine monophosphate; GNG, gluconeogenesis; Pi, orthophosphate; X, choline, ethanolamine, serine, or inositol (preferred substrate).

enzyme found in both plant material and in the intestinal mucosa of animals.[4,20] Inositol is actively transported across the intestinal wall, via a $Na^+$ and energy dependent mechanism that can be inhibited by glucose, but is different from the glucose transport system.[4,21] Although PI is a significant component of dietary inositol, its mode of digestion and absorption has not been studied. It is assumed that PI undergoes enzymatic digestion by intestinal phospholipase $A_2$ in a manner similar to phosphatidylcholine digestion. Following absorption, the resulting lyso-PI may then either be reacylated or further degraded upon entering the intestinal cell. Inositol is transported in human blood plasma in its free form at a concentration of approximately 29 μmol/L (0.5 mg/dl) in normal subjects.[22] The very small amount of PI present in plasma is associated with circulating lipoproteins.

### BIOSYNTHESIS, CATABOLISM, AND EXCRETION

In addition to dietary sources, free inositol is also synthesized in vivo in several tissues. In the rat, the testis, brain, liver, and kidney have exhibited the capacity to synthesize inositol from D-glucose. The internal cyclization of glucose-6-phosphate by inositol-1-phosphate synthase results in the production of inositol-1-phosphate, which is subsequently hydrolized by the $Mg^{++}$ requiring enzyme, inositol-1-phosphatase, to produce free inositol (Fig. 30A–2). Niacin is also required in the active form of $NAD^+$ (the oxidized form of nicotinamide-adenine dinucleotide) for this conversion of glucose to inositol. The relative contribution of the various tissues to the biosynthesis of inositol is not known. Approximately 50% of the free inositol in rabbit brain appears to be synthesized in vivo.[23] The liver and kidney are important contributors to the free inositol pool in the rat.[24] It is estimated that the two human kidneys synthesize approximately 22 mmol (4g) per day of inositol, which is considerably more than the average of 5.5 mmol (1 g) that is ingested daily. As in the rat, extrarenal tissues are also implicated as sources of endogenous inositol in the human.[22]

The kidney has been implicated as the principal regulator of inositol levels by its ability to catabolize excess inositol. Although normal rats are able to convert 16% of injected [$^{14}$C]inositol to respiratory [$^{14}$C]$CO_2$ in 5 hours, bilaterally nephrectomized rats are unable to degrade [$^{14}$C]inositol. Less than 1% of the administered radiolabeled inositol is released into the urine over the same period, indicating that catabolism of inositol by the kidney is much more significant than urinary excretion.[25] This is also the case in the human kidney, which has the capacity to catabolize approximately 40 mmol (7 to 8g) of inositol per day per kidney.[22] Inositol is catabolized to D-glucuronic acid, which is eventually converted to the pentose phosphate pathway intermediate D-xylulose-5-phosphate, and ultimately to $CO_2$ and $H_2O$ (Fig. 30A–2).

### CELLULAR UPTAKE AND INCORPORATION INTO PHOSPHOLIPID

Free inositol is taken up into most tissues against a concentration gradient in a $Na^+$ and energy dependent process that may be distinct from glucose transport. Inositol can then be incorporated within the microsomal fraction of the cell into PI via two biochemical mechanisms (Fig. 30A–2). Inositol reacts with cytidine diphosphate-diacylglycerol in the presence of PI synthetase in the de novo biosynthetic route. This pathway is the major route of PI synthesis. Inositol can also react with endogenous phospholipid and enter PI in a $Mn^{++}$-stimulated exchange, with PI being the preferred substrate for this reaction. The PI formed can subsequently be converted in an adenosine triphosphate (ATP)-dependent manner to PI-phosphate (PIP), PI-bisphosphate ($PIP_2$), and possibly PI-trisphosphate ($PIP_3$) by PI kinase, PIP kinase, and $PIP_2$ kinase, respectively. PI transfer proteins are believed to distribute the endogenously formed PI from the endoplasmic reticulum to the plasma membrane and other subcellular fractions.

## METABOLIC FUNCTIONS OF FREE INOSITOL AND INOSITOL PHOSPHOLIPIDS

Free inositol, its different phosphorylated forms, and various inositol phospholipids show different biologic activities within cells.

### FREE INOSITOL

The concentration of free inositol exceeds that of the inositol phospholipids in most tissues, indicating a possible biologic role for the free form. The organs of the male reproductive tract are particularly rich in free inositol, as is mammalian semen and seminal plasma. Inositol may play a role in the maturation of sperm cells as they pass through the epididymis, because pharmacologically induced reduction of inositol levels results in the disappearance of spermatids and spermatozoa.[26] Unbound inositol is also relatively enriched in neural tissue compared to plasma. The association of free inositol with microtubules in these tissues has led to speculation that microtubule function and stability may be modulated by inositol. It has been proposed that inositol acts as an osmoregulatory molecule in neural tissue, as well as in other cells.[27] In chronically hypernatremic mice, inositol accumulates in the brain, whereas in hyponatremic mice, brain inositol concentration decreases, allowing the brain to balance its intracellular osmolality with that of the plasma. This results in normal brain water content despite profound hyponatremia, and prevents edema.[28] With respect to microtubule stabilization, it has been suggested that inositol in the form of polyphosphoinositides may play a role in the regulation of microtubule polymerization.[29]

## INOSITOL PHOSPHOLIPIDS

Many of the physiologic and biochemical roles for inositol in mammalian tissues have been ascribed to the inositol phospholipids.[4] As an integral part of cellular and subcellular membranes, PI exerts its effect through membrane-mediated events. PI is able to modulate the activity of several enzymes, such as $Na^+K^+$ adenosine triphosphatase ($Na^+K^+$ ATPase), alkaline phosphatase, 5′nucleotidase, acetyl-CoA carboxylase, and tyrosine hydroxylase, an enzyme that catalyzes the rate-limiting step in the biosynthesis of catecholamines, dopamine, and norepinephrine.

Although PI is not present in large quantities in mammalian tissues and cells, its relative enrichment in arachidonic acid, plus its rapid degradation (by phospholipases $A_2$ and C—see Fig. 30A–3) upon agonist-stimulated activation, renders this inositol phospholipid a significant source of eicosanoids. The eicosanoids (including prostaglandins, thromboxanes, leukotrienes, and lipoxins) effect a wide range of physiologic responses in numerous cell systems.[30] Not only does the degradation of PI release the eicosanoid precursor, arachidonic acid, but the conversion of PI to polyphosphoinositides and their subsequent agonist-induced degradation also result in the release of a plethora of cellular second messengers, as reviewed recently.[7–10] Degradation of PI and the polyphosphoinositides (PIP, $PIP_2$, and possibly $PIP_3$) by phospholipase C results in the formation of diacylglycerol (DG) and a series of inositol phosphates, with the number of phosphates attached to the inositol ring dependent on the phosphate content of the parent compound (Fig. 30A–3). On the one side of this bifurcating pathway, the DG produced can modulate the activity of protein kinase C and associated protein phosphorylations.[31] DG itself may also be degraded to release arachidonic acid for subsequent conversion to biologically active eicosanoids, or it may be reconverted to PI via phosphatidic acid. On the other arm of the inositol phospholipid signaling system, a whole range of inositol phosphates are generated that play a role in $Ca^{++}$ mobilization. Protein kinase C activation, as well as a host of other cellular processes, can be regulated by $Ca^{++}$ concentrations, thus resulting in the possibility of intri-

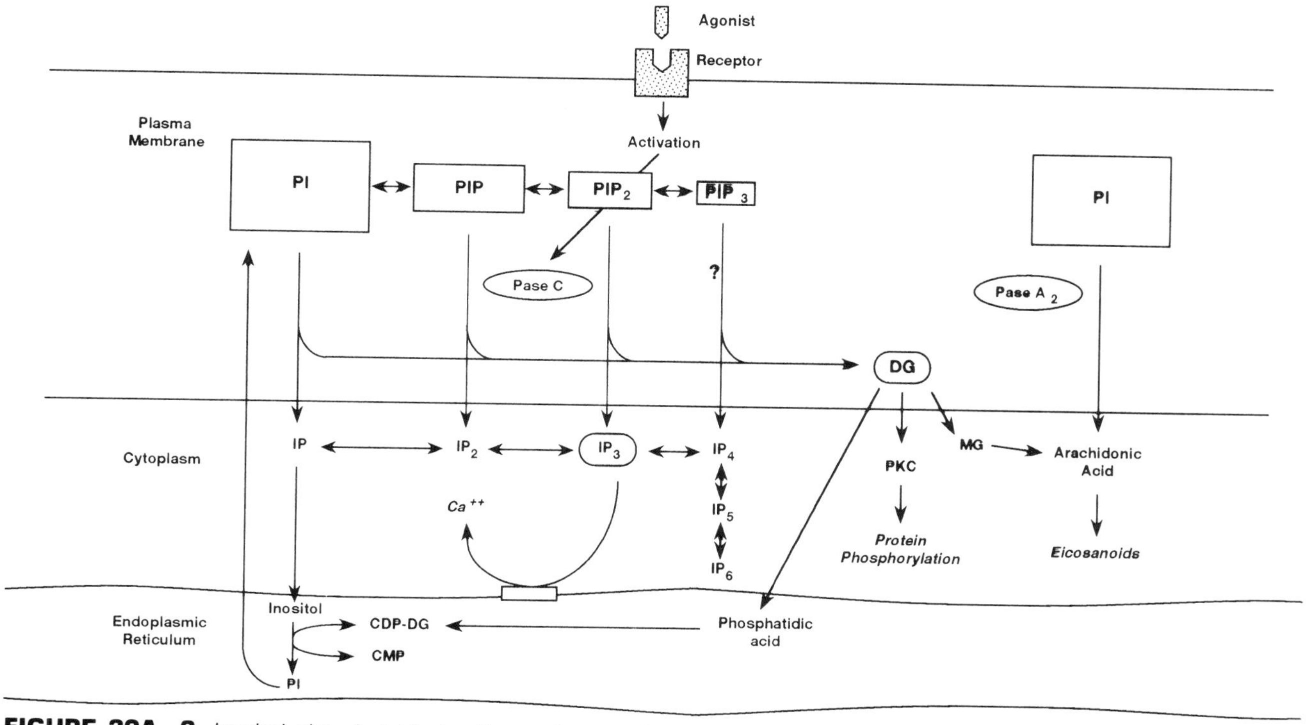

Agonist
Receptor
Plasma Membrane
Activation
PI
PIP
PIP2
PIP3
PI
Pase C
?
Pase A2
DG
Cytoplasm
IP
IP2
IP3
IP4
IP5
IP6
Ca++
MG
Arachidonic Acid
PKC
Protein Phosphorylation
Eicosanoids
Endoplasmic Reticulum
Inositol
CDP-DG
CMP
PI
Phosphatidic acid


**FIGURE 30A–3.** Inositol phospholipid signaling pathways. CDP-DG, Cytidine diphosphate-diacylglycerol; CMP, cytidine monophosphate; DG, diacylglycerol; IP, inositol phosphate; MG, monoacylglycerol; Pase, phospholipase; PI, phosphatidylinositol; PIP, PI-phosphate; $PIP_2$, PI-bisphosphate; $PIP_3$, PI-trisphosphate; PKC, Protein kinase C.

cate interactions between the two arms of the signaling system. Inositol-1, 4, 5-trisphosphate ($IP_3$) has the greatest $Ca^{++}$-mobilizing capacity; its rapid conversion to less potent inositol phosphates by kinases or phosphatases allows for fine-tuned control of the $Ca^{++}$ signal. It has been proposed that the interactions between $IP_3$ and inositol tetrakisphosphate ($IP_4$) modulate the oscillatory nature of $Ca^{++}$ influxes within cells.[32]

## EFFECTS OF DIETARY INOSITOL

Despite the capacity of certain animal tissues to synthesize and catabolize inositol in vivo, levels of this cyclitol can be readily altered with dietary inositol supplementation or deprivation.[3,4] In rats, the level of free inositol is significantly reduced in plasma, the testis, liver, heart, lens, lung, kidney, and small intestine, but not the cerebrum and cerebellum, when inositol-depleted diets are fed compared to controls. In the liver the inositol-containing phospholipid levels are also altered in inositol deficiency.[33] Inositol deprivation in the female gerbil results in lowering of both free and lipid-bound inositol in the liver and intestine, but only of free inositol in the kidney and pancreas. Oral doses of supplementary inositol can significantly elevate plasma inositol concentrations in human subjects.

The early work with dietary inositol suggested its nutritional efficacy as a lipotropic factor.[1,2] Depending on the composition of the overall diet and on other factors, accumulation of hepatic or intestinal triglyceride can occur in rats, gerbils, and other animals and fish deprived of adequate dietary inositol. Choline, another lipotrope, is unable to prevent this phenomenon when supplemented at levels considered to be nutritionally adequate. Hepatic accumulation of lipids may be due to the impaired ability of liver to secrete lipoproteins in inositol deficiency.[34] There is also evidence suggesting increased mobilization of fatty acid from adipose tissue to the liver in inositol-deficient rats,[35] as well as increased hepatic fatty acid synthesis.[36]

The experimental animal that has been demonstrated to be particularly sensitive to dietary inositol deficiency is the female gerbil.[37] When fed a semipurified diet containing coconut oil, this animal develops a severe intestinal lipodystrophy that can be prevented by the inclusion of inositol in the diet. In prolonged inositol deficiency, there is a progressive decline in body weight associated with alopecia, eventually leading to exudative dermatitis, inanition, and ultimately death. The small intestine from the inositol-deficient gerbil becomes greatly enlarged, and the serosal surface is unusually white, with the exposed mucosa appearing swollen and corrugated. A reduced biosynthesis of PI due to the lack of dietary inositol may be responsible for the impaired chylomicron assembly and secretion and the decreased intestinal lipid clearance in these animals. That castrated animals are also more susceptible to the symptoms of inositol deficiency suggests that the lower susceptibility of male gerbils to inositol deficiency may be due to the ability of the male reproductive tract to synthesize inositol.

## DIETARY REQUIREMENTS AND RECOMMENDED INTAKES

Inositol is not listed as an essential nutrient in the Recommended Dietary Allowances for humans, although possible therapeutic roles in diabetes mellitus, chronic renal failure, and galactosemia are indicated.[38] Although the nutritional requirements for the rat published by the National Research Council do not include inositol, numerous researchers routinely include inositol in their experimental diets.[3] Because inositol is regulated in vivo through endogenous synthesis and catabolism, only in specific circumstances does it appear to be essential as a nutrient. Intestinal flora also synthesize inositol and contribute to the metabolic pool of inositol in vivo. Serum inositol levels reflect dietary levels under normal conditions and can be measured accurately, most commonly by optical techniques or by gas chromatography.[39,40] High concentrations of inositol in human breast milk and higher levels in colostrum result in elevated serum inositol in neonates. Premature infants have even higher serum inositol levels than full-term infants. This suggests that research on the requirement for dietary inositol supplementation in neonatal and prenatal life is warranted. Excess dietary inositol appears not to be toxic, except in certain clinical situations where inositol metabolism is impaired.

## ALTERED INOSITOL METABOLISM IN CLINICAL SITUATIONS

Inositol metabolism is altered in several clinical conditions, including diabetes, renal disease, respiratory distress syndrome, and several other diseases.

### DIABETES

A reduction in neural inositol content in both spontaneously and experimentally induced diabetes has been associated with impaired polyol metabolism and metabolic and functional defects in nerve, including a reduced $Na^+K^+$ ATPase activity and decreased peripheral motor and sensory nerve conduction velocities.[41] Lower tissue inositol levels in diabetes may be due to several mechanisms. Hyperglycemia in diabetes inhibits inositol transport, resulting in cellular deficiency of free inositol.[42,43] Endogenous production of inositol may also be decreased, because the activity of inositol-1-phosphate synthase is reduced in streptozotocin-induced diabetic rats.[44] The enzyme that synthesizes PI from cytidine diphosphate-diacylglycerol and inositol, PI synthase, requires a high inositol concentration to achieve half-maximal activity[45] and thus may require high levels of free inositol to maintain cellular inositol phospholipid levels. A small drop in tissue free inositol could thus potentially contribute to alterations in inositol phospholipid levels and accompanying cellular functions. Abnormal turnover of $PIP_2$ has been documented in sciatic nerves from streptozotocin-induced diabetic rats.[46]

Treatment of diabetics with dietary inositol has been shown to normalize neural inositol levels, $Na^+K^+$ ATPase activity, and motor conduction velocity in many instances, [41,47,48] but not in all cases.[49] Amelioration of nerve conduction velocities occurs despite persistent hyperglycemia and elevated nerve sorbitol and fructose concentrations. Aldose reductase inhibitors reduce elevated polyol pathway metabolism, increase tissue inositol levels, and normalize neural abnormalities in diabetes, thus linking reduced tissue free inositol levels with altered polyol pathway metabolism and the associated neural defects in diabetes.[41,48] In addition to effects on neural tissue, dietary inositol supplementation may also have therapeutic potential in several other abnormalities associated with diabetes, such as elevated glomerular filtration rates, vascular alterations,[48] altered ascorbic acid metabolism,[50] and diabetes-related birth defects.[51] Although dietary inositol supplementation has therapeutic potential in diabetes, excess dietary inositol has been shown to be toxic in both normal and diabetic rats, reducing motor conduction velocities.[47]

## RENAL DISEASE

Hyperinositolemia is present in chronic renal failure, indicating that altered inositol metabolism occurs in human renal disease. Plasma inositol levels have been reported to be 7 to 15 times higher than in normal subjects.[4,22] Impairment of inositol catabolism may contribute significantly to the hyperinositolemia, because the kidney is the primary site of inositol breakdown. A decreased glomerular filtration rate and disturbed inositol reabsorption are also present in advanced forms of glomerulosclerosis. Thus, serum or urinary inositol levels may be useful indicators of renal function in renal disease patients. High levels of circulating inositol may show toxic effects on neural tissue; hyperinositolemia may also contribute to the pathogenesis of uremic polyneuropathy in subjects with chronic renal disease.

## RESPIRATORY DISTRESS SYNDROME

Inositol levels are high in neonates, and the concentration of inositol in human breast milk is approximately 1 mmol/L (18 mg/dl). Thus dietary inositol may well play an important role in prenatal and neonatal development and may be an essential nutrient in early infancy.[19] Maternal dietary inositol has been shown to modify lung development in immature fetal lung in response to exogenous hormones in rabbits.[52] In small preterm infants with respiratory distress syndrome, inositol supplementation appears to improve lung development.[53]

## OTHER DISEASES

Abnormal inositol metabolism may also occur in several other clinical situations, including galactosemia,[54] multiple sclerosis, and hypercholesterolemia.[3,4] In addition, altered inositol phospholipid metabolism has been implicated in cell proliferation and cancer. Dietary inositol has recently been shown to be antineoplastic in a rodent model of carcinogenesis.[55] As a consequence, much attention is currently focused on alterations of inositol phospholipid metabolism in various diseases. Because the concentrations, as well as the metabolic turnover, of free inositol and the inositol phospholipids are subject to nutritional modification, it will be of interest to determine whether normalization of inositol phospholipid metabolism by dietary modifications can be used clinically to alter the progression of associated disease states.

## REFERENCES


1. Woolley, D.W.: J. Biol. Chem., *139:*29–34, 1941.
2. Gavin, G., McHenry, E.W.: J. Biol. Chem., *139:*485, 1941.
3. Holub, B.J.: The nutritional significance, metabolism, and function of *myo*-inositol and phosphatidylinositol in health and disease. *In* Advances in Nutritional Research. Vol. 4. Edited by H.H. Draper. New York, Plenum Publishing, 1982.
4. Holub, B.J.: Annu. Rev. Nutr., *6:*563–597, 1986.
5. Hokin, L.E., Hokin, M.R.: Biochim. Biophys. Acta, *18:*102–110, 1955.
6. Michell, R.H.: Biochim. Biophys. Acta, *415:*81–147, 1975.
7. Berridge, M.J.: Annu. Rev. Biochem., *56:*159–193, 1987.
8. Downes, C.P., Macphee, C.H.: Eur. J. Biochem., *193:*1–18, 1990.
9. Rana, R.S., Hokin, L.E.: Physiol. Rev., *70:*115–164, 1990.
10. Auger, K.R., Cantley, L.C.: Cancer Cells, *3:*263–270, 1991.
11. Low, M.G.: Biochim. Biophys. Acta, *988:*427–454, 1989.
12. Izaacks, R.E., Harkness, D.R., Whitham, P.R.: Dev. Biol., *62:*344–353, 1978.
13. Nomenclature Committee of the International Union of Biochemistry: Eur. J. Biochem., *180:*485–486, 1989.
14. Whitman, M., Downes, C.P., Keeler, M., et al.: Nature, *332:*644–646, 1988.

15. Auger, K.R., Serunian, L.A., Soltoff, S.P., et al.: Cell, *57*:167–175, 1989.
16. Nolan, R.D., Lapetina, E.G.: J. Biol. Chem., *265*:2441–2445, 1990.
17. Traynor-Kaplan, A.E., Harris, A.I., Thompson, B.I., et al.: Nature, *334*:353–356, 1988.
18. Vadnal, R.E., Parthasarathy, R.: Biochem. Biophys. Res. Commun., *163*:995–1001, 1989.
19. Pereira, G.R., Baker, L., Egler, J., et al.: Am. J. Clin. Nutr., *51*:589–593, 1990.
20. Sandberg, A., Andersson, H.: J. Nutr., *118*:469–473, 1988.
21. Vilella, S., Reshkin, S.J., Storelli, C., et al.: Am. J. Physiol., *256*:G501–G508, 1989.
22. Clements, R.S., Jr., Diethelm, A.G.: J. Lab. Clin. Med., *93*:210–219, 1979.
23. Spector, R., Lorenzo, A.V.: J. Neurochem., *25*:353–354, 1975.
24. Hauser, G.: Biochim. Biophys. Acta, *70*:278–289, 1963.
25. Lewin, L.M., Yannai, Y., Sulimovici, S.: Biochem. J., *156*:375–380, 1976.
26. Morris, R.N., Collins, A.C.: J. Reprod. Fertil., *27*:201–210, 1971.
27. Garcia-Perez, A., Burg, M.B.: Physiol. Rev., *71*:1081–1115, 1991.
28. Hollowach Thurston, J.H., Sherman, W.R., Hauhart, R.E.: Pediatr. Res., *26*:482–485, 1989.
29. Forscher, P.: Trends Neurochem., *12*:468–474, 1989.
30. Needleman, P., Turk, J., Jakschik, A.: Annu. Rev. Biochem., *55*:69–102, 1986.
31. Nishizuka, Y.: Science, *233*:305–312, 1986.
32. Berridge, M.J., and Irvine, R.F.: Nature, *341*:197–205, 1989.
33. Burton, L.E., Ray, R.E., Bradford, J.R.: J. Nutr., *106*:1610–1616, 1976.
34. Hoover, G.A., Nicolosi, R.J., Corey, J.E.: J. Nutr., *108*:1588–1594, 1978.
35. Hayashi, E., Maeda, T., Tomita, T.: Biochim. Biophys. Acta, *360*:146–155, 1974.
36. Beach, D.C., Flick, P.K.: Biochim. Biophys. Acta, *711*:452–459, 1982.
37. Hegsted, D.M., Hayes, K.C., Galagher, A., et al.: J. Nutr., *103*:302–307, 1973.
38. National Research Council: Recommended Dietary Allowances. 10th Ed. Washington, D.C., National Academy Press, 1989.
39. Eades, D.M., Williamson, J.R., Sherman, W.R.: J. Chromatogr., *490*:1–8, 1989.
40. Palmer, S., Wakelam, J.O.: Biochim. Biophys. Acta, *1041*:239–246, 1989.
41. Greene, D.A., Lattimer, S.A., Carrol, P.B.: J. Clin. Invest., *85*:1657–1665, 1990.
42. Haneda, M., Kikkawa, R., Arimura, T.: Metabolism, *39*:40–45, 1990.
43. Olgemöller, B., Schwaabe, S., Schleicher, E.D.: Biochim. Biophys. Acta, *1052*:47–52, 1990.
44. Whiting, P.H., Palmano, K.P., Hawthorne, J.N.: Biochem. J., *179*:549–553, 1979.
45. Troyer, D.A., Schwertz, D.W., Kreisberg, J.I., et al.: Annu. Rev. Physiol., *48*:51–71, 1986.
46. Bell, M.E., Peterson, R.G., Eichberg, J.: J. Neurochem., *39*:192–200, 1982.
47. Greene, D.A., DeJesus, P.V., Winegrad, A.I.: J. Clin. Invest., *55*:1326–1336, 1975.
48. Pugliese, G., Tilton, R.G., Speedy, A., et al.: Diabetes, *39*:312–322, 1990.
49. Cameron, N.E., Cotter, M.A., Robertson, S.: Q. J. Exp. Physiol., *74*:917–926, 1989.
50. Yue, D.K., McLennan, S., Fisher, E.: Diabetes, *38*:257–261, 1989.
51. Wiegandsberg, M.J., Garcia-Palmer, F.J., Freinkel, N.: Diabetes, *39*:575–582, 1990.
52. Anceschi, M.M., Petrelli, A., Zaccardo, G.: Pediatr. Res., *24*:617–621, 1988.
53. Hallman, M., Arjomaa, P., Hoppu, K.: J. Pediatr., *110*:604–610, 1987.
54. Beyer-Mears, A., Bucci, F.A., Del Val, M., et al.: Pharmacology, *39*:59–68, 1989.
55. Shamsuddin, A., Ullah, A., Chakravarthy, A.K.: Carcinogenesis, *10*:1461–1463, 1989.


## SELECTED READINGS


Downes, C.P., Macphee, C.H.: *myo*-Inositol metabolites as cellular signals. Eur. J. Biochem., *193*:1–18, 1990.

Holub, B.J.: Metabolism and function of *myo*-inositol and inositol phospholipids. Annu. Rev. Nutr., *6*:563–597, 1986.

Holub, B.J.: The nutritional significance, metabolism, and function of *myo*-inositol and phosphatidylinositol in health and disease. *In* Advances in Nutritional Research. Vol. 4. Edited by H.H. Draper. New York, Plenum Publishing, 1982.

Rana, R.S., Hokin, L.E.: Role of phosphoinositides in transmembrane signaling. Physiol. Rev., *70*:115–164, 1990.

## B. PYRROLOQUINOLINE QUINONE

Francene M. Steinberg and Robert B. Rucker



### CHEMISTRY

Flavinoids and quinoline quinones have excited interest as bioactive quinones because of their potential as growth factors.[1] Recently pyrroloquinoline quinone (PQQ) has been identified as a potent growth factor and antioxidant. Although the status of PQQ as a vitamin requires considerable resolution, enough is known currently to suggest its tentative qualification as a "vitamin-like" molecule. For example, on a molar basis, PQQ is one of the most biologically potent quinones (according to bioassays) that involve growth and reproductive performance. Growth impairment is observed in neonatal mice and rat pups when PQQ is omitted from chemically defined diets. Normal growth is observed when PQQ is added to deficient diets in picomolar to nanomolar amounts, or when PQQ or PQQ-like compounds are detectable in fecal samples or urine.[1] PQQ also can serve as an antioxidant under conditions in which free-radical oxidative damage is easily measured without added PQQ or antioxidants.[2–4]

PQQ, also designated methoxatin, was identified in the 1970s as a cofactor for various dehydrogenases in methylotropic bacteria.[5,6] The identification of PQQ next led to an appreciation that certain bacteria also appeared to require a source of PQQ, which in turn led to the examination of eukaryotic systems for putative PQQ-containing enzymes. Among mammalian enzymes, the copper-containing amine oxidases were considered likely candidates.[7,8] Critical scrutiny of these enzymes, however, suggests that PQQ is not a covalently bound cofactor. Rather, post-translationally modified tyrosyl residues, such as peptidyl 6-hydroxydopa, or modified tryptophan residues appear to serve at catalytic sites.[7–9] Consequently, although PQQ appears to stimulate growth and improve reproductive performance, PQQ has not been directly linked to a specific cofactor function in mammalian tissues.

The structure and pathway for the synthesis of PQQ are given in Figure 30B–1. PQQ is a tricarboxylic acid *o*-quinone containing a dicarbonyl functional center at carbons 4 and 5. Carbon 5 is the more electrophilic of the two carbonyls, but both contribute to the ability of PQQ to act as a redox catalyst by accepting one or two electrons. PQQ also interacts easily with primary amines. Such properties are analogous to combining some of the best chemical features of riboflavin, ascorbic

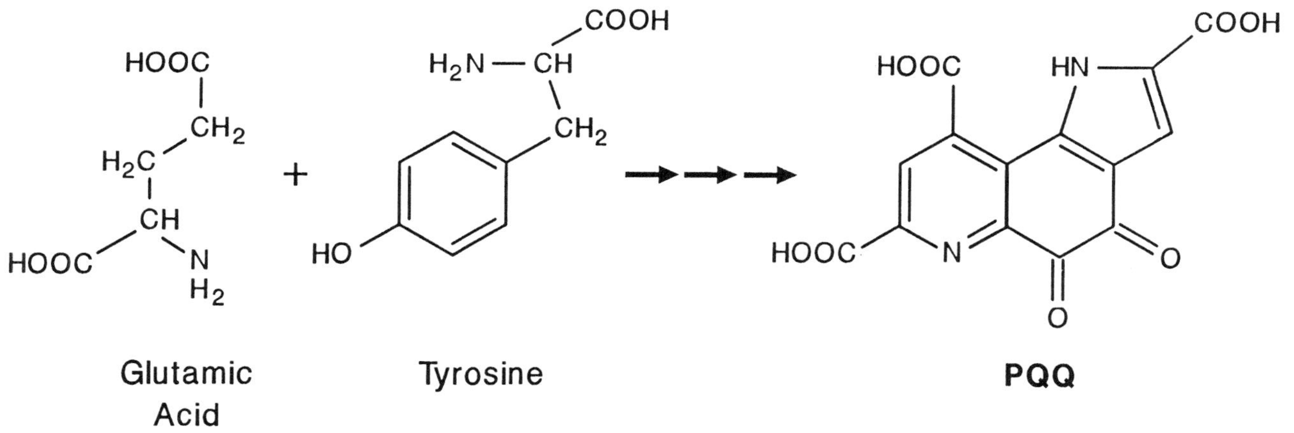

HOOC
CH2
H2C
CH
HOOC
N
H2
+
COOH
H2N — CH
CH2
HO
HOOC
HN
COOH
HOOC
N
O
O
Glutamic Acid
Tyrosine
PQQ


**FIGURE 30B–1.** Biosynthesis of pyrroloquinoline quinone (PQQ) from L-tyrosine or a dopa intermediate and L-glutamic acid or L-glutamine.

acid, and pyridoxal into one molecule. An important chemical feature is the ability of PQQ to carry out redox cycling. Picomolar amounts of PQQ are capable of generating micromolar amounts of product. PQQ can be reduced to $PQQH_2$ under aerobic and anaerobic conditions by the reduced form of nicotinamide adenine dinucleotide (NADH), the reduced form of NAD phosphate (NADPH), or ascorbic acid. Analogous to other quinones and enediols, PQQ can exist in a dehydro, semiquinone, as quinol form. PQQ also has unusual ultraviolet (UV) and fluorescent spectral characteristics. The molecular weight of PQQ is 330.22 g/mol.

## BIOSYNTHESIS AND METABOLISM

PQQ is synthesized in methlytropic bacteria utilizing steps that stem from the shikimic acid pathway.[10] For example, $^{14}$C-L-tyrosine is incorporated into PQQ. The process appears to involve the condensation of L-tyrosine with L-glutamate, followed by other metabolic steps (Fig. 30B–1). In mammalian cells, PQQ-like compounds also appear to be produced, although the evidence is indirect.

In mice, PQQ is readily absorbed, primarily from the large intestine, and accumulates to a limited extent in various tissues (skin and blood cells). It then appears to be excreted primarily via the kidney.[11] Because the normal intestinal microflora in the mouse does not synthesize a significant amount of PQQ,[12] the diet and possibly its endogenous synthesis are assumed to be major sources. PQQ is reported to be relatively ubiquitous and is found in rodent chow, commercial casein hydrolysates, and vegetable and yeast extracts.[12,13]

## PHYSIOLOGIC SIGNIFICANCE

When mice and rats are fed purified amino acid-based diets containing no added PQQ, a number of physiologic responses are observed that suggest that PQQ influences growth and development. Impaired growth is observed when a PQQ-free diet is fed throughout gestation and the postnatal period. In contrast, a normal growth response is observed when PQQ is added in amounts as little as 200 to 300 ng per gram of diet—about 1 nmol. A more striking observation is that reproductive failure and small litters result from PQQ deprivation.[1] Also, pups born of PQQ-derived dams are often cannibalized at birth. Taken together, the signs of poor growth, reproductive failure, and compromised survival are used as evidence that PQQ or a similar compound is required during perinatal development.[2]

Signs of PQQ deprivation also include friable skin, markedly impaired immune response, and signs of impaired connective tissue maturation.[1] Many of the signs are similar to those observed in lathrytic animals (i.e., animals fed lysyl oxidase inhibitors, such as β-aminoproprionitrile). Lysyl oxidase is a key enzyme involved in connective tissue maturation. A decrease in lysyl oxidase activity results in impaired cross-linking of collagen and elastin. In skin, decreased collagen cross-linking leads eventually to impaired collagen deposition and to an increase in collagen turnover. Of interest, the accumulation of lysyl oxidase in skin appears to be sensitive to PQQ status in neonates. Whether or not PQQ serves as a lysyl oxidase cofactor, however, is not known. It is obviously an important point to resolve, because lysyl oxidase is an example of a copper-containing amine oxidase, but is markedly dissimilar from the serum amine oxidases in chemical, physical, and biologic properties.

PQQ also influences oxidative defense systems in cells. Administration of PQQ to fertile chicken eggs protects developing embryos against the formation of lens cataracts and from oxidative damage induced in response to hydrocortisone treatment; PQQ also protects against carbon tetrachloride-induced and alcohol-induced liver damage.[2–4]

## PQQ DETECTION

The recognition that PQQ is a growth-stimulating factor and that it is utilized by bacteria has been important to the development of PQQ detection systems and assays.[13] Growth of Pseudomonas testeroni is stimulated by the addition of PQQ to culture medium. The use of apoenzymes such as apoglucose dehydrogenase, whose activity is restored upon reconstitution with PQQ, has been useful as an assay. The glucose dehydrogenase of certain strains of Escherichia coli exists mainly in the apoform and is membrane-bound. The functional activity of this dehydrogenase directly depends on PQQ concentration. Reconstitution to full enzymatic activity, however, may be influenced by the redox state of PQQ, oxamine or oxazole complex formation, and interactions with other strong redox catalysts.

Chromatographic separation of PQQ and chemical detection methods have also been described.[14] Reduction of PQQ with sodium borohydride followed by oxidation with sodium periodate yields fluorescent products; alternatively, reaction with phenylhydrazine has provided the basis for PQQ detection after chromatographic separation. PQQ may be estimated in the picomolar range by methods based on redox cycling[13] (Fig. 30B–2). Under alkaline conditions and in the presence of molar concentrations of glycine, PQQ catalyzes the reduction of dyes such as nitroblue tetrazolium ($T^+$). This assay functions independently of the initial redox state of PQQ. Thus, when PQQ is readily accessible to reagents, both bound and unbound forms of PQQ may be assayed. By adding sodium borate and metal chelating agents to assays, it is also possible to

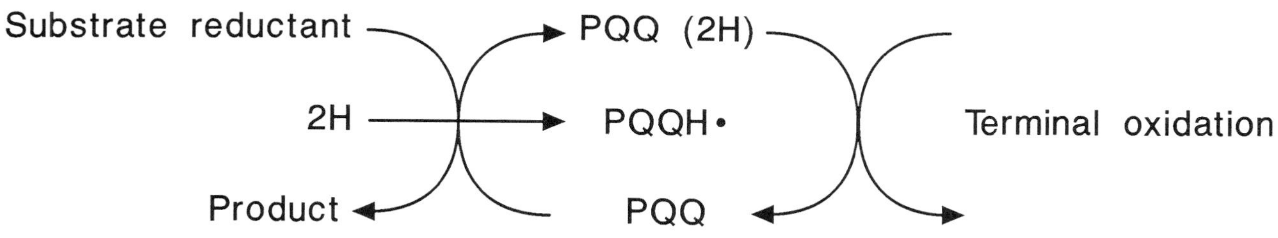
Substrate reductant
2H
Product
PQQ (2H)
PQQH•
PQQ
Terminal oxidation

**Reductant Sources Involving PQQ**

Amino acids and amines → NH=CH-R
Ascorbate → Dehydroascorbate
NADH (or NADPH) + $H^+$ → $NAD^+$ (or $NADP^+$)
Hydroquinone → Quinone
2 $Ferrocyanide^{4-}$ + $2H^+$ → 2 $Ferricyanide^{3-}$
Alcohol → Aldehyde

**Terminal Oxidations Involving PQQ (2H)**

$O_2 \rightarrow H_2O_2$
$T^+ \rightarrow TH + H^+$
$2\ O_2 \rightarrow 2\ O_2^-$ (superoxide) + $2H^+$
$2\ O_2 + T^+ \rightarrow 2\ O_2 + TH + H^+$
$R{-}H + O_2 \rightarrow R{-}OH + H_2O$

**FIGURE 30B–2.** Selected pyrroloquinoline quinone (PQQ) reactions that involve 2H reductant sources or terminal oxidations. As implied in this figure, the mechanisms for oxidation or reduction probably involve PQQ free radical intermediates (PQQH). Detection systems have been based on the estimation of $H_2O_2$, or the reduction of nitroblue tetrazolium ($T^+$) to formazan (TH).

reduce interfering side reactions, such as ascorbate-catalyzed reductions.

The high efficiency of redox cycling obtained with PQQ (up to $10^3$ to $10^4$ cycles) may be due to the multiple negative charges on the PQQ molecule, which may inhibit oxidative dimerization. In contrast to PQQ, in the presence of amines, most quinones and dicarbonyl compounds polymerize. As a consequence, other reductants and quinones are also required at substantially higher amounts to promote product formation at rates similar to those of PQQ.

## DIETARY CONSIDERATIONS AND TOXICITY

As noted, PQQ does not appear to be synthesized by the gut microflora but may be synthesized in some form by mammalian cells.[13] PQQ-like compounds have been isolated from human and bovine milk and blood cells.[13] As with substances such as carnitine or inositol, a requirement for PQQ-like compounds may well be conditional—that is, dependent on age, stress, or species of animals. In mice, the need for PQQ is most apparent during neonatal development. However, whether or not PQQ is substituting for quinoids derived from 6-hydroxydopa or analogous precursors is not clear.

Although the biologic effects of PQQ can be attributed in part to its chelation and anti-oxidant properties, the case for a functional role is strong, particularly in view of observations that picomolar to nanomolar amounts in diets seem to have positive effects on neonatal growth and development.

As a final point, toxicity in rats has been reported when PQQ is injected intraperitoneally at 10 mg/kg body weight, which is 100 to 1000 times the amount needed for optimal neonatal development. Degenerative changes of the proximal tubular epithelium and hematuria have also been observed.

## REFERENCES


1. Killgore, J., Smidt, C., Duich, L., et al.: Science, *245:*850–852, 1989.
2. Nighigori, H., Yasunaga, M., Mizumura M., et al.: Life Sci., *45:*593–598, 1989.
3. Watanabe, A., Hobara, N., Tsuji, T.: Curr. Ther. Res., *44:*896–901, 1988.
4. Hamagishi, Y., Murata, S., Kamei, H., et al.: J. Pharmacol. Exp. Ther., *255:*980–985, 1991.
5. Anthony, C., Zatman, L.J.: Biochem. J., *104:*960–969, 1967.
6. Salisburg, S.A., Forrest, H.S., Cruse, W.B.T., et al.: Nature, *280:*843–844, 1979.
7. McIntire, W.S., Wemmer, D.E., Christoserdov, A., et al.: Science, *252:*817–824, 1991.
8. Janes, S.M., Mu, D., Wemmer, D., et al.: Science, *248:*981–987, 1990.
9. Brown, D.E., McGuire, M.A., Dooley, D.M., et al.: J. Biol. Chem., *266:*4049–4051, 1991.
10. Houck, D.R., Hanners, J.L., Unkefer, C.J.: J. Am. Chem. Soc., *110:*6920–6921, 1988.
11. Smidt, C.R., Unkefer, C.J., Hovek, D.R., et al.: Proc. Soc. Expl. Biol. Med., *197:*27–31, 1991.
12. Smidt, C.R., Bean-Knudsen, D., Kirsch, D.G., et al.: Biofactors, *3:*53–59, 1991.
13. Paz, M.A., Book, A., Kagan, H.M., et al.: J. Biol. Chem., *266:*689–692, 1991.
14. van der Meer, R.A., Groen, B.W., van Kleef, M.A.G., et al.: Methods Enzymol., *188:*260–283, 1990.
15. Watanabe, A., Hobara, N., Ohsawa, T., et al.: Hiroshima J. Med. Sci., *38:*49–51, 1989.


## SELECTED READINGS


Jongejan, J.A., Duine, J.A. (eds.): PQQ and Quinoproteins. Dordrecht, Kluwer Academic Publishers, 1989.

Smidt, C.R., Myers-Steinberg, F., Rucker, R.B.: Physiologic importance of pyrroloquinoline quinone. Proc. Soc. Exp. Biol. Med., *197:*19–26, 1991.

CHAPTER **31**

# Taurine

**Kenneth C. Hayes and Elke A. Trautwein**



Although taurine has been recognized as a component of living organisms since 1827 when it was first isolated from ox bile (*Bos taurus*) and named accordingly,[1] it was long considered an inert end product of sulfur amino acid metabolism. Its potential importance in biologic functions other than bile acid conjugation has only recently been emphasized.[2–9] Interest in taurine metabolism and its nutritional requirement for humans has expanded in the past two decades since the discovery that retinal degeneration and blindness developed in taurine-deficient cats[3,4,10] and the observed depression in plasma and urine taurine concentration in infants fed taurine-free formulas[11] and in children and adults maintained on long-term parenteral nutrition.[12–16] The focus of current interest has centered on the addition of taurine to human infant formulas and its inclusion in solutions for parenteral nutrition to accommodate situations in which taurine has been considered a conditionally essential nutrient in humans.[17]

To date, evidence exists that taurine is involved in physiologic functions including development of the nervous system, neuromodulation, cell membrane stabilization, detoxification, and osmoregulation.[5,18]

## CHEMISTRY

Taurine, β-aminoethanesulfonic acid (Fig. 31–1), is unique among other natural amino acids because of its sulfonic acid group, which replaces the carboxylic group of what would normally be alanine. A colorless, crystalline compound with a molecular weight of 125, taurine is water-soluble up to 0.84 M solution. As a free amino acid without dissociable side groups, it exists as a true zwitterion at physiologic pH with a $pK_a$ of 1.5 (sulfonic acid group) and a $pK_b$ of 8.74 (amino group). Taurine takes part in few biochemical reactions and is not incorporated into proteins, nor is it a major source of organic sulfur or inorganic sulfate, but is found instead as a free amino acid in most animal tissues and biologic fluids, often as the most abundant free amino acid present—for example, in muscle, platelets, and the developing central nervous system (CNS).[3] Notable exceptions to its nonreactivity is its conjugation with bile acids through an amide linkage and its reactions with certain xenobiotics and with the powerful oxidant, hypochlorous acid, generated in leukocytes to form the relatively stable taurochloramine.[19] Taurine has also been described as a component of some low-molecular-weight peptides, isolated from the parathyroid gland and from brain synaptosomes. Glutaurine (γ-L-glutamyl-taurine), the most abundant of these peptides, appears to act as a neurotransmitter. Glutaurine also may function as an intracellular storage form of taurine involved in the stability of the intracellular taurine pool in the brain.[20,21]

$$H_2N\text{-}CH_2\text{-}CH_2\text{-}SO_3H$$

$$^{+}H_3N\text{-}\ CH_2\text{-}CH_2\text{-}SO_3^{-}$$

(Zwitterion at physiological pH)

**FIGURE 31–1.** Structure of taurine.

## BIOSYNTHESIS AND METABOLISM

### TAURINE SYNTHESIS

Taurine biosynthesis derives from the trans-sulfuration pathway in certain mammalian cells, but not usually in plant cells, which means that it is essentially absent from the plant kingdom. Taurine is the end product of sulfur amino acid metabolism in mammalian cells. Its sulfur moiety can be oxidized to sulfate by intestinal bacterial flora, but not by mammalian cells. The synthesis of taurine proceeds via several enzymatic reactions involving the enzymatic oxidation and conversion of cysteine either directly or following conversion of methionine to cysteine (Fig. 31–2). Although several possible pathways exist, the major pathway follows oxidation of cysteine to cysteinesulfinic acid (CSA), subsequent decarboxylation to hypotaurine, and oxidation to taurine (Fig. 31–2). Other pathways have been demonstrated, including the formation of taurine from cysteic acid by oxidation of CSA. A reaction between inorganic sulfate and serine can also form cysteic acid for further decarboxylation to taurine. Another possible synthesis of taurine includes the fixation of sulfate with serine to form cysteamine, which is further oxidized to hypotaurine and taurine.[2,3] Although all these pathways may exist in mammals, they are considered to be of minor metabolic significance, and it is generally agreed that the route involving enzymatic activity of cysteinesulfinic acid decarboxylase (CSAD) reflects the major pathway for taurine biosynthesis in different organs (tissues). Whereas the enzymatic involvement of CSAD is well characterized, other enzymes and biochemical conversions, such as the transformation of hypotaurine or cysteic acid to taurine, have not been carefully delineated. Enzymes in the transulfuration pathway to taurine biosynthesis heavily depend on vitamin $B_6$ as a cofactor (cystathionine synthase, cystathionase, and CSAD). A dietary deficiency of vitamin $B_6$ has a depressing effect on taurine synthesis and is accompanied by decreased urinary excretion of taurine.[3,6] The pathway utilizing CSAD is the dominant route of taurine synthesis in the liver and brain of many species and is age-dependent—that is, it may be poorly developed in the preterm and newborn infant, making the synthesis of taurine even more restricted in the neonate.[3]

On the basis of CSAD activity, various tissues from a number of species have been compared for their taurine synthetic capacity (Table 31–1). It is thought that humans (and primates in general) are species with poor synthetic ability, worse even than cats, in contrast to species such as the rat and the dog, in which hepatic

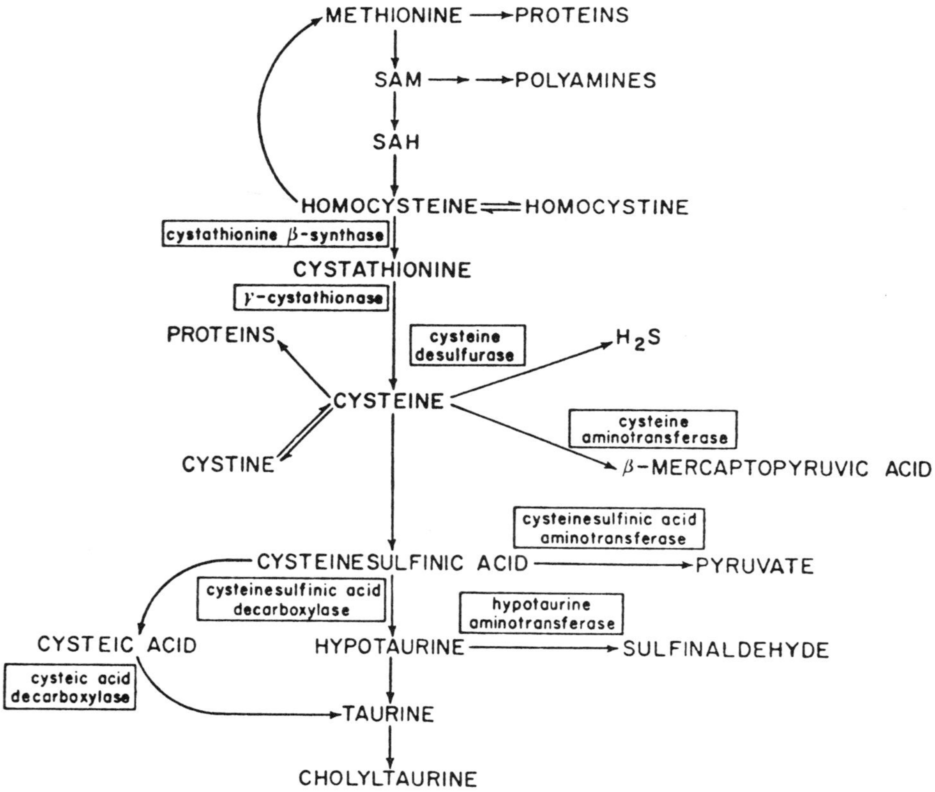
METHIONINE
PROTEINS
SAM
POLYAMINES
SAH
HOMOCYSTEINE
HOMOCYSTINE
cystathionine β-synthase
CYSTATHIONINE
γ-cystathionase
PROTEINS
cysteine desulfurase
$H_2S$
CYSTEINE
cysteine aminotransferase
CYSTINE
β-MERCAPTOPYRUVIC ACID
cysteinesulfinic acid aminotransferase
CYSTEINESULFINIC ACID
PYRUVATE
cysteinesulfinic acid decarboxylase
hypotaurine aminotransferase
CYSTEIC ACID
HYPOTAURINE
SULFINALDEHYDE
cysteic acid decarboxylase
TAURINE
CHOLYLTAURINE

**FIGURE 31–2.** Taurine biosynthesis derives from the transulfuration pathway involving methionine and cysteine. The three key enzymes depicted along this route require vitamin $B_6$ as cofactor.

**TABLE 31–1.** CYSTEINESULFINIC ACID DECARBOXYLASE ACTIVITY IN LIVER AND BRAIN OF VARIOUS SPECIES

| SPECIES | LIVER Adult | LIVER Fetus | BRAIN Adult | BRAIN Fetus |
|---|---|---|---|---|
| | nmol $CO_2$ produced/mg protein/hour | | | |
| Man | <1 | <1 | 5 | — |
| Monkey | | | | |
| Rhesus | 5 | 4 | 5 | trace |
| Cebus | 2 | — | 2 | — |
| Rat | 468 | 9 | 63 | 1 |
| Dog | 412 | — | 54 | — |
| Cat | 4 | 7 | 59 | 6 |
| Rabbit | 14 | 16 | 25 | 8 |
| Guinea pig | 3 | 2 | 6 | 4 |

(Data from Sturman, J.A., Hayes, K.C.: Adv. Nutr. Res., *3*:231–299, 1980; and Hayes, K.C., Sturman, J.A.: Annu. Rev. Nutr., *1*:401–425, 1980.)

synthesis is extremely high. However, by use of the stable isotope $^{18}O_2$, adult humans were shown in one study to synthesize an appreciable amount of taurine.[22] It is noteworthy that the CNS, including the retina, has moderate taurine synthetic capacity in most species, even though hepatic synthesis varies among species. In terms of available taurine it is not clear that the hepatic taurine pool is readily circulated as a donor pool for other tissues, because bile acids appear to constitute the primary demand for liver taurine.[6] For this reason and because most tissues appear to concentrate taurine against a concentration gradient, a low plasma concentration of taurine may not be a good indicator of individual tissue pools and likely reflects dietary intake most closely.[23]

Taurine is relatively inactive because of its sulfonyl group, the notable exception being the stable taurine conjugate of bile acids. Although only 1% of taurine in man is present in bile, conjugation of taurine with bile acids is an important physiologic function for lipid absorption and solubilization.[3–5] Although most species conjugate bile acids with glycine in addition to taurine, all seem to prefer taurine conjugation when supplemented with taurine. Noteworthy is the fact that cats conjugate bile acids almost exclusively with taurine and secrete free bile acids rather than reverting to glycine when hepatic taurine is exhausted. In primates depleted of taurine, chenodeoxycholic acid seems to have preferential access to the remaining taurine, whereas cholic acid conjugates readily with glycine. This preference depends on the species of primate,[4] suggesting that bile acid conjugation with taurine is more complex than the simple hepatic concentration of this amino acid.[6]

By use of $^{35}S$-taurine in man, a total body pool of 100 to 150 mmol (12 to 18 g) has been calculated, and a multicompartmental model for taurine metabolism has been suggested.[24] Turnover is best described by two exchangeable pools, a small (2 mmol), rapidly miscible pool (half-time, or $T\frac{1}{2}$, = 0.1 hours), and a larger (100 mmol) pool with a slow turnover rate ($T\frac{1}{2}$ = 70 hours).[24] Excretion occurs from the rapidly miscible plasma pool into the urine, resulting in loss of 0.5 to 2.0 mmol per day. Subcompartments of the actively exchangeable pool would include bile acids, the central nervous system, and "other" tissues, most of which actively take up taurine against a concentration gradient. Daily synthesis of taurine in adult humans has been estimated to be between 0.4 and 1 mmol, or about 50 to 125 mg.[22]

Under normal circumstances plasma taurine ranges from 30 to 70 μmol/L in humans with any excess being readily excreted via the kidney in the urine. Both urine and plasma concentrations are reduced when the combined dietary and synthetic contributions are inadequate.[2]

## KIDNEY-REGULATED TAURINE EXCRETION

Because taurine is excreted primarily in the urine, the kidney greatly impacts the total body taurine pool. High dietary taurine intake as well as conditions causing taurine release from cells, such as surgery, muscle disease, or radiation therapy, result in increased taurine excretion.[25] Urinary taurine values are usually high, 200 to 2000 μmol/L, or roughly 2 to 10 times the plasma taurine concentration. Taurine is a major urinary amino acid in humans because renal tubular reabsorption is ordinarily limited. This constant loss of circulating taurine reduces the efficacy of the plasma as an interorgan transport system, when dietary input or synthesis is reduced. Normal urinary values vary appreciably within and between individuals, with variation highly dependent on dietary intake. Conversely, reduced dietary intake of taurine, as in infants receiving taurine-free formula, patients maintained on total parenteral nutrition (TPN), and vegetarians lacking taurine in their diet, is normally compensated by enhanced renal conservation of taurine and reduced urinary excretion.[11,26–28]

Under normal conditions taurine is filtered through the glomerulus and partially reabsorbed by the tubular cell.[29] Reabsorption of taurine across the renal brush border membrane involves a high-affinity, low-capacity, $Na^+$-dependent, β-amino acid specific transport system.[29] In untreated essential hypertensives urinary taurine excretion was significantly lower (708 ± 57 versus 1594 ± 143 μmol per day, untreated hypertensives versus controls, respectively), and taurine clearance and the taurine/creatinine ratio were markedly decreased.[30]

Neonatal "physiologic aminoaciduria," which appears in all mammalian species including man, is a reflection of the immaturity of the renal tubular transport system. The high taurine excretions in taurine-depleted, very low-birth-weight infants is a result of the failure of the immature tubular cell to adjust to taurine depletion.[16] On the other hand, full-term infants and preterm infants weighing more than 1700 g are able to respond to taurine depletion by increasing taurine reabsorption and excreting less taurine.[11,31]

## PHYSIOLOGIC MODE OF ACTION

Although the mode of action for taurine is not adequately delineated, its ubiquitous presence (in most cells) and varied biologic activity (Table 31–2) suggest a prominent role for taurine in cell function. The high concentration in the developing nervous system, muscle, and platelets, along with its association with calcium, has fueled speculation that it functions as a modulator of cation flux, especially for calcium. In this capacity it may stabilize or sequester membrane calcium during depletion of electrolytes.[32] In platelets taurine has the effect of decreasing aggregation sensitivity, presumably by modulating calcium ion concentration—that is, the taurine affinity for calcium appears to be enhanced by increasing alkalinity. During taurine depletion, platelets become overly sensitive, whereas during taurine supplementation, their tendency to aggregate is depressed.[33]

**TABLE 31–2.** BIOLOGIC FUNCTIONS AFFECTED BY TAURINE

| |
|---|
| Retinal photoreceptor activity |
| Bile acid conjugation |
| White blood cell antioxidant activity |
| Pulmonary antioxidant activity (protects against oxidant injury) |
| CNS neuromodulation (depressant) |
| Platelet aggregation (reduces) |
| Cardiac contractility (enhances) |
| Sperm motility (enhances) |
| Growth (enhances) |
| Insulin activity (enhances) |
| Cell differentiation (lymphocytes) |

**TABLE 31–3.** INFLUENCE OF TAURINE ON THE HEART

| |
|---|
| Antiarrhythmic agent |
| Inotropic in regard to calcium ion |
| Enhancer of digitalis inotrophy |
| Enhancer of cardiac contractility |
| Osmotic agent |
| Hypotensive agent |

(Adapted from Huxtable, R.J., Sebring, L.A.: Prog. Clin. Biol. Res., *125*:5–11, 1983.)

In heart muscle, taurine increases the calcium available for contractions at low calcium concentrations, yet protects against intracellular calcium overload when calcium is abundant. This regulation is thought to be modulated by the sarcolemma, possibly by interacting with specific phospholipids, such as phospatidylinositol, or alternatively by taurine binding to specific high- and low-affinity protein receptors in the membrane.[32] The inotropic effect of taurine in cardiac muscle mediates contractility and work load to the extent that taurine has been considered effective therapy in congestive heart failure, where it can be lifesaving in cats.[34] Taurine is also thought to exert a hypotensive action on the cardiovascular system.[8] A summary of cardiac effects is presented in Table 31–3.

In the retina and CNS, taurine may serve a structural and functional role in stabilizing neural membranes, especially those situated in the lamellae of photoreceptor outersegments.[3,4,9] Van Gelder has postulated a centralized mechanism for taurine function involving the basic regulation of the excitation threshold.[35] In this model taurine would stabilize membranes by controlling mobilization of calcium ions during depolarization. Control is influenced by pH, bicarbonate ion availability, and a zinc-taurine membrane-associated complex that would interact with $CO_2$ and $NH_3$ to regulate glutamate generation, the latter then acting in its role as neurotransmitter. In this capacity taurine would function as a neuromodulator indirectly depressing neuroexcitation through its control over glutamate metabolism. Several aspects of the hypothesis remain to be tested.

Taurine may also act as a conjugator and detoxifier of certain xenobiotics and other exogenous toxins in addition to endogenous compounds such as secondary bile acids.[5] The amino group of taurine can react with partially degraded retinol to form retinotaurine in the liver, representing another potential detoxification function. Taurine also may act as an oxidant scavenger, including free radicals, to prevent severe cellular damage. For example, taurine has been shown to protect against $NO_2$-induced lung injury in hamsters[36] and may block membrane lipid peroxidation in rabbit spermatozoa.[5] In mollusks and other marine animals existing in environments with varying alkalinity, taurine seems to function as a cell-volume regulator by controlling osmolarity.[2,35] Taurine does not seem to play a similar role in freshwater species, but may act similarly in the mammalian CNS.

## DEFICIENCY

Taurine is not ordinarily a dietary essential nutrient for humans. Nonetheless, interest has been kindled by the fact that plasma and urinary taurine decreases in preterm and full-term infants fed synthetic formulas without taurine[11,31] and in infants and adults maintained by parenteral nutrition.[12,13] Interestingly, the taurine concentration is exceedingly high in colostrum in both human milk and cow's milk. Whereas human milk maintains an appreciable concentration (300 μmol/L or 40 mg/L) throughout lactation, cow's milk is not a rich source of taurine (30 μmol/L or 4 mg/L) because most such milk is obtained after prolonged lactation when taurine secretion has waned.

The strongest evidence for the biologic importance of taurine has been obtained in kittens,[4] a species in which taurine biosynthesis is limited and demand is relatively high because cat bile acids are conjugated almost exclusively with taurine. This requirement places an unusual demand on the body taurine pool, depleting most tissues to 10% or less of their normal concentration when kittens are fed a taurine-free diet. In kittens, bile acids, retina, and the olfactory bulb maintain their taurine concentration most avidly. However, when taurine in the retina has been depleted to approximately 50% of its normal concentration, electrical and morphologic changes are demonstrable in the photoreceptor cells. Continued depletion of taurine results in extensive, irreparable degeneration of the retina. Repletion with taurine in less advanced stages of degeneration allows restoration of photoreceptor outer segments and restored vision, although cone-timing delays and distorted cone morphology persist indefinitely. Similar, less clinically noticeable changes have been reported in monkeys raised on human infant formulas lacking taurine.[37]

Additional responses to taurine depletion include depressed body weight gain and a decrease in the taurine/glycine ratio of bile acid conjugates, both of which were observed in infant monkeys fed soy-based, human infant formula lacking taurine.[4] Weight depression was apparently not noted in a similar study with a larger species of infant monkey.[37] Following the original descriptions of retinal degeneration and clinical blindness in cats,[10] the taurine deficiency syndrome in this species has expanded to include reproductive failure and growth retardation, CNS dysfunction, dilated cardiomyopathy, platelet hyperaggregation, and impaired immune function.[6,38]

Whether these observations are relevant to humans is unclear because of difficulty in documenting physiologic evidence of human taurine deficiency, particularly in the premature infant, where the problem is most apt to occur. Preterm and full-term neonates develop reduced plasma and urinary concentrations of taurine when fed infant formulas without taurine compared to infants fed human breast milk or infant formula containing the same taurine concentration as breast milk.[11,31] However, the plasma taurine concentration in these depleted infants (35 μmol/L) was much higher than that in taurine-depleted cats (<10 μmol/L), and taurine supplementation had no effect on growth or nitrogen retention in preterm infants.[39–41] Unfortunately, the whole blood taurine concentration, which represents a better index of taurine status (see below), was not measured in these early studies.

Conflicting results have been obtained when the effect of taurine supplementation on cholesterol and bile acid metabolism and fat absorption was examined in low-birth-weight infants. Supplementation of the formula at 300 μmol/L of taurine (45 μmol/kg per day) for 3 weeks in premature infants weighing about 2300 g had no effect on either bile acid synthesis or primary or total bile acid pools, even though the taurine/glycine bile acid ratio was increased.[42] In what were described as "sicker" premature infants weighing between 1400 and 2100 g who were fed a taurine supplement of 250 μmol/L infant formula (also equivalent to 45 μmol/kg per day), their low plasma taurine values failed to increase, whereas urinary taurine concentrations showed a minor increase at the beginning of the study but revealed a decrease from the first to the fourth week of the study. The concentration of duodenal bile salts was higher and that of cholesterol lower in these "sicker" taurine-supplemented infants, suggesting a greater conversion of cholesterol into bile acids.[39] Thus, the smallest premature infants (unlike larger infants) may be subject to taurine manipulation of their bile metabolism.[42,43] In another study a 10-day intravenous supplementation of taurine failed to improve cholestasis induced by parenteral nutrition in premature infants weighing less than 1500 g.[44] No effect of taurine on fat absorption was detected in three studies,[39,45,46] whereas one study reported that supplemental taurine improved fat absorption, especially of saturated fatty acids.[41] Taurine supplementation also improved fat absorption in children with cystic fibrosis and led to increased growth in terms of both weight gain and bone growth.[47,48] A rationale for the taurine effect may be the tendency for taurine-conjugated bile acids to be absorbed lower in the small intestine, mostly in the ileum, thereby increasing the solubilization and absorption of fat, especially saturated fatty acids, which require a longer length of intestine to be absorbed.[6,49]

By contrast, adult human males fed 3.0 g per day of taurine revealed a modest but significant decrease (11%) in their bile acid pool size. The relative biliary lipid composition (i.e., biliary saturation index) and the distribution of primary bile acids were unaffected.[50] In another study taurine supplementation (3.2 g per day for 2 weeks) failed to affect serum lipids or biliary lipid composition, although taurine-conjugated bile acids were increased.[51]

With the exception of the effects on growth in children with cystic fibrosis and the improvement of fat absorption in preterm infants and in children with cystic fibrosis, taurine supplementation of infant formula generally failed to have an impact on infant growth, serum cholesterol, blood urea nitrogen (BUN), serum proteins, or blood acid-base balance,[40] which would suggest that the dietary taurine requirement is minimal in humans for most physiologic circumstances. More sophisticated measures of taurine function on the central nervous system must be used if an exogenous (dietary) requirement is to be identified. The likelihood of demonstrating such a requirement would seem to be greatest during parenteral nutrition of very low-birth-weight infants, who have limited ability to synthesize taurine, and in patients in whom the immature nephron fails to adapt to low taurine intake by increasing tubular reabsorption of taurine.[16]

Geggel et al. have expanded their original description of taurine depletion in humans receiving parenteral nutrition, emphasizing that children, as compared to adults, are at high risk of taurine depletion under these circumstances.[12,13] In children receiving long-term TPN, plasma taurine levels dropped to 26 ± 13 μmol/L (57 ± 16 μmol/L in controls), and abnormalities in the electroretinograms were found.[13] In adults undergoing long-term TPN with an estimated enteral caloric absorption less than 25% of their daily requirement, taurine concentrations were significantly reduced in plasma, platelets, lymphocytes, and erythrocytes.[52] Plasma, platelet, and urine taurine concentrations were significantly reduced and lymphocyte and erythrocyte taurine tended to be lower in children on long-term TPN compared to normal children.[26] It has been noted that infused parenteral solutions lack cysteine, the sulfur amino acid generating the substrate for the enzyme (cysteinesulfinic acid decarboxylase) leading to formation of taurine.[53] Furthermore, the flux through the transulfuration pathway is thought to be diminished in very young patients because of the limited activity of cystathionase, which is needed to convert methionine to cysteine.

## INDIVIDUALS AT RISK OF TAURINE DEPLETION

Based on the above information, and if we can extrapolate from kittens and monkeys, one might predict that taurine depletion depends on an inability to synthesize appreciable taurine (low CSAD activity) in the face of extreme demand or unusual loss (Fig. 31–3). A rationale for taurine depletion suggests that an organism is susceptible to depletion if taurine biosynthesis is inadequate when dietary supply is minimal and the demand (requirement) by tissues is high.[54] For instance, the carnivorous cat normally eats meat to ensure a dietary intake of taurine that compensates for poor hepatic synthesis. However, the bile acid pool in cats is extremely demanding (obligate taurine conjugator), such that most endogenous taurine becomes sequestered by bile to the detriment of other tissues when the dietary supply fails. The whole-body supply of taurine is further exacerbated by the extremely rapid growth rate in kittens, with its rapidly expanding muscle mass, in addition to the competition for cysteine in fur growth and in glutathione synthesis, all of which impact the taurine supply.[55] Thus, depletion occurs. Most species that grow rapidly, like the rat and dog, synthesize taurine avidly. Other species, that experience poor taurine synthesis, such as man and most monkeys, grow slowly or are able to conjugate bile acids with glycine and thereby relieve the demand for taurine. Thus, minimal synthesis is adequate. In human infants the supply/demand balance might be compromised when already limited synthesis is impaired by prematurity or hepatic dysfunction during periods when growth rate is maximal and an exogenous supply is nonexistent (tau-

| INPUT | = | DEMAND |
|---|---|---|
| biosynthesis | | bile acid conjugation |
| diet | | muscle growth |
| | | CNS development (brain, retina) |
| | | other cell functions (platelets, lymphocytes) |
| | | endocrine glands |
| | | glutathione synthesis |
| | | fur production |

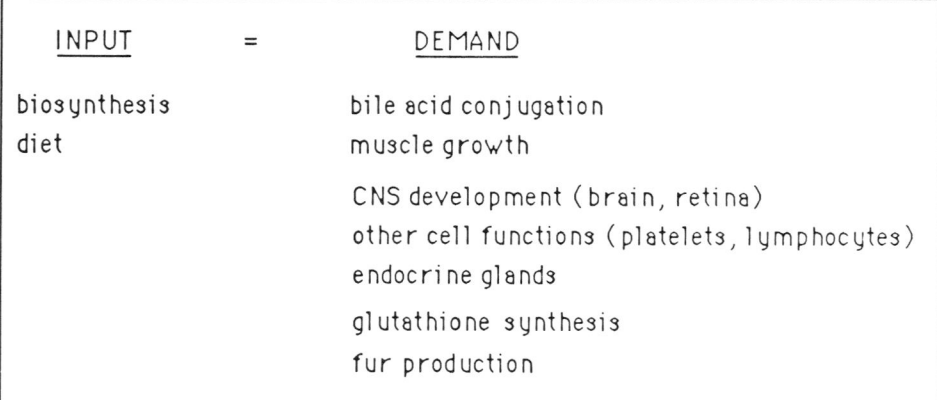

**FIGURE 31–3.** Requirements for whole-body taurine balance. (Adapted from Hayes, K.C., Sturman, J.A.: Adv. Exp. Med. Biol., *139*:79–87, 1982.)

rine-free infant formulas, parenteral nutrition). Once growth has been completed, it is difficult to imagine a situation in which taurine would become limiting in normal circumstances. Excessive taurine loss in association with bile acids (as in chronic malabsorption) or impaired synthesis (as in chronic hepatic disease in which synthesis is precluded) might be clinical situations wherein concern for taurine depletion would be real.

That dietary taurine might be most critical to the neonate is further suggested by numerous studies of placental and milk transfer of taurine in utero and during the suckling period, respectively, in rhesus monkeys and rats. The human fetus accumulates approximately 50 to 60 μmol per day (6 to 8 mg) of taurine during the last 4 weeks of pregnancy.[16] Therefore, the preterm infant, who is unable to benefit from this transfer into its taurine reserves, is at risk of taurine depletion. Thus, taurine seems to be of benefit during development, an observation that is underscored by the high concentration in fetal brain. These transfers are critical in the neonatal period because the synthetic pathway is limited in its capacity for taurine biosynthesis during development and during early life,[3] and because urinary loss may be excessive because of the inability of the immature kidney tubular cell to reabsorb taurine.[16] If the exogenous supply of taurine is limited (taurine-free formula, parenteral nutrition), depletion of the taurine body pool may occur during the first weeks of life, especially in preterm infants.

## DIETARY CONSIDERATIONS

The noteworthy relationship between taurine and diet is its absence from vegetable sources and its abundance in animal products, particularly in shellfish (Table 31–4). Thus, vegetarians would be at a disadvantage in terms of their taurine status if it were an essential nutrient for humans. Because vegetarians are not known to suffer unduly from lack of taurine and their plasma taurine concentrations are essentially normal,[27,28] adults apparently do not require a dietary supply of taurine under normal physiologic conditions. In such cases, the body pool of taurine derived from limited intake and biosynthesis seems to be conserved by enhanced renal taurine reabsorption.[27,28,56]

As mentioned earlier, a concern for the dietary taurine requirement in humans has arisen in infants fed substitute milk formulas or maintained by parenteral nutrition. In such infants plasma and urinary taurine are known to decline.[11–13,16,31] An actual dietary requirement for taurine may exist under these circumstances, especially in immature infants.

In contrast, cats fed commercial diets based on vegetable protein clearly suffer from retinal degeneration[4] and cardiomyopathy.[34] The dietary requirement for cats is thought to be 500 to 750 ppm (4 to 6 μmol/g) for the growing kitten and lactating queen. Based on the urinary excretion rate in the adult human, a dietary intake of 125 to 500 ppm (1 to 4 μmol/g) would suffice if diet were the exclusive source of taurine. For the cat the dietary

**TABLE 31–4.** DIETARY SOURCES OF TAURINE

| DIETARY SOURCE | WET WEIGHT in mg/100 g* | |
|---|---|---|
| | Mean | Range |
| Meat | | |
| Beef (lean round) | 36 | 15–47 |
| Beef (liver) | 19 | 14–27 |
| Pork (loin) | 50 | 39–69 |
| Pork (liver) | 17 | 11–23 |
| Lamb (leg) | 47 | 45–51 |
| Chicken (leg) | 34 | 30–38 |
| Seafood | | |
| Cod (frozen) | 31 | 23–40 |
| Clams (fresh) | 240 | 145–370 |
| Clams (minced, canned) | 152 | — |
| Oysters (fresh) | 70 | 39–124 |
| Tuna fish (canned) | 70 | — |
| | mg/L | |
| Cow's milk | | |
| Colostrum (1–3 days) | 70 | 39–98 |
| Early lactation (15–40 days) | 12 | 3–37 |
| Mid lactation (over 100 days) | 4 | 1–16 |
| Pasteurized milk | 6 | 3–11 |
| Human milk | 54 | 24–85 |

(Data from Roe, D.A., Weston, M.O.: Nature, *205*:287–288, 1965; and Erbersdobler, H.F., Braasch, S., Trautwein, E.A.: J. Anim. Physiol. Anim. Nutr., *63*:1–7, 1990.)

*1 mg taurine equals 8 μmol.

requirement is at least two or more orders of magnitude above most vitamins and an order of magnitude less than the typical essential amino acid requirement. The fact that taurine is synthesized to some extent by most tissues precludes its being a true vitamin and renders its dietary essentiality conditionally dependent on metabolic peculiarities of individual species, particularly reflecting age, growth status, and kidney maturity. The actual daily intake of taurine in humans is estimated to range between 40 and 400 mg or approximately 100 to 1000 ppm on a dietary basis.

To date no interrelationships have been described linking the requirement for taurine with that of other nutrients per se. However, because taurine synthesis depends on sulfur amino acid metabolism, limited intake of methionine or cysteine can increase the dietary requirement for taurine, at least in cats, and a high taurine intake may spare the requirement for cysteine or methionine. Because the transulfuration pathway also requires vitamin $B_6$, inadequate supply of this vitamin could theoretically increase the dependency on dietary taurine. In fact, evidence of vitamin $B_6$ deficiency has been found to precede any evidence of taurine depletion in cebus monkeys.[56]

## EVALUATION OF TAURINE STATUS

The most accurate and reliable estimate of taurine status is based on plasma and whole blood taurine concentrations. Although the taurine concentration in blood cells relative to plasma (100 times in lymphocytes, 300 times in granulocytes, and 400 times in platelets) is remarkable,[4,33,52] the measurement of the whole blood taurine pool, mainly representing intracellular taurine, has not been fully appreciated. However, the whole blood taurine pool is remarkably stable and varies only under extremes of depletion or sustained supplementation of taurine, whereas the fluctuating plasma taurine pool reflects acute changes in taurine availability.[23] The "physiologic normal" plasma taurine concentration is thought to range between 35 and 60 μmol/L.[23] Plasma taurine levels below 30 μmol/L may signal the onset of taurine depletion, although it is not known at what point a "low" plasma taurine concentration corresponds to sufficient depletion of whole blood or tissue stores to initiate deficiency in humans. Infants and children thought to be depleting their taurine pools still maintained plasma values in the 30 to 40 μmol/L range.[11,12] In very low-birth-weight infants (<28 weeks, birth weight ≦1000 g) plasma taurine concentrations ranging from 16 to 34 μmol/L were found between the third and seventh postnatal week.[16] Values of 1 to 10 μmol/L are common in taurine-depleted cats. Plasma taurine values exceeding 80 μmol/L in humans suggest "spillage" of intracellular taurine or sustained, excessive dietary taurine intake. Normal whole blood taurine in humans ranges between 160 and 320 μmol/L with a mean value of 225 ± 38 μmol/L.[23]

A recurring problem when assessing plasma taurine status is the spuriously high plasma concentration that derives from contamination by intracellular taurine, especially from platelets and white blood cells, a problem highly affected by sampling technique. The choice of anticoagulant in conjunction with sample handling also influences the taurine values obtained. Using ethylenediaminetetraacetic acid (EDTA) as anticoagulant and strict handling of blood samples at room temperature have routinely provided the most reliable and accurate measurement.[23,57]

Early techniques used for taurine analysis in biologic samples included thin-layer chromatography, paper chromatography, and colorimetric determination. More recently, techniques such as automated amino acid analysis based on ion-exchange chromatography and high-performance liquid chromatographic (HPLC) determination after precolumn fluorescence derivatization have been used successfully for taurine analysis in physiologic tissues and fluids.[57–59] The HPLC methods that include fluorescence detection are among the most sensitive and allow detection in the picomolar range while depending on minimal sample volume.

## TOXICITY

To our knowledge no evidence of taurine toxicity has been reported. Amounts as high as 0.8% taurine (16 times the recommended dietary allowance) have been fed to cats without untoward effect,[60] and 5% taurine was fed to mice without any difficulty.[61]

## REFERENCES

1. Tiedemann, F., Gmelin, L.: Ann. Physik. Chem., *9*:326–337, 1827.
2. Jacobsen, J.G., Smith, L.H.: Physiol. Rev., *48*:424–511, 1968.
3. Sturman, J.A., Hayes, K.C.: Adv. Nutr. Res., *3*:231–299, 1980.
4. Hayes, K.C., Sturman, J.A.: Annu. Rev. Nutr., *1*:401–425, 1980.
5. Wright, C.E., Tallan, H.H., Lin, Y.Y.: Annu. Rev. Biochem., *55*:427–453, 1986.
6. Hayes, K.C.: Nutr. Res. Rev., *1*:99–113, 1988.
7. Sturman, J.A.: J. Nutr., *118*:1169–1176, 1988.
8. Kendler, B.S.: Prev. Med., *18*:79–100, 1989.
9. Lombardini, J.B.: Brain Res. Rev., *16*:151–169, 1991.
10. Hayes, K.C., Carey, R.E., Schmidt, S.Y.: Science, *188*:949–951, 1975.

11. Gaull, G.E., Rassin, D.K., Raiha, N.C.R., Heinonen, K.: J. Pediatr., *90*:348–355, 1977.
12. Geggel, H.S., Heckenlively, J.R., Martin, D.A., et al.: Doc. Ophthalmol. Proc. Ser., *31*:199–207, 1982.
13. Geggel, H.S., Ament, M.E., Heckenlively, J.R., et al.: N. Engl. J. Med., *312*:142–146, 1985.
14. Ament, M.E., Geggel, H.S., Heckenlively, J.R., et al.: J. Am. Coll. Nutr., *5*:127–135, 1986.
15. Vinton, N.E., Laidlaw, S.A., Ament, M.E., et al.: Pediatr. Res., *21*:399–403, 1987.
16. Zelikovic, I., Chesney, R.W., Friedman, A.L., et al.: J. Pediatr., *116*:301–306, 1990.
17. Gaull, G.E.: J. Am. Coll. Nutr., *5*:121–125, 1986.
18. Sturman, J.A.: Ann. N.Y. Acad. Sci., *477*:196–213, 1986.
19. Weiss, S.J., Klein, R., Slivka, A., et al.: J. Clin. Invest., *70*:598–607, 1982.
20. Marnela, K.M., Morris, H.R., Panico, M., et al.: J. Neurochem., *44*:752–754, 1985.
21. Feuer, L.: Biological effects of gammal-I-glutamyl-taurine (glutaurine): A new parathyroid hormone. *In* The Effects of Taurine on Excitable Tissues. Edited by S.W. Schaffer, S.I. Baskin, and W. Kocsis. Jamaica, NY, Spectrum Publ., 1981, pp. 31–39.
22. Irving, C.S., Mark, L., Klein, P.D., et al.: Life Sci., *38*:491–495, 1986.
23. Trautwein, E.A., Hayes, K.C.: Am. J. Clin. Nutr., *52*:758–764, 1990.
24. Sturman, J.A., Hepner, G.W., Hofmann, A.F., et al.: J. Nutr., *105*:1206–1214, 1975.
25. Chesney, R.W.: Adv. Pediatr., *32*:1–42, 1985.
26. Vinton, N.E., Laidlaw, S.A., Ament, M.E., et al.: Pediatr. Res., *21*:399–403, 1987.
27. Rana, S.K., Sanders, T.A.B.: Br. J. Nutr., *56*:17–27, 1986.
28. Laidlaw, S.A., Shultz, T.D., Cecchino, J.T., et al.: Am. J. Clin. Nutr., *47*:660–663, 1987.
29. Chesney, R.W., Gusowski, N., Friedman, A.L.: Kidney Int., *24*:588–594, 1983.
30. Kohashi, N., Katori, R.: Jpn. Heart J., *24*:91–102, 1983.
31. Jarvenpaa, A.L., Rassin, D.K., Raiha, N.C.R., et al.: Pediatrics, *70*:221–230, 1982.
32. Huxtable, R.J., Sebring, L.A.: Prog. Clin. Biol. Res., *125*:5–11, 1983.
33. Hayes, K.C., Pronczuk, A., Addesa, A.A., Stephan, Z.F.: Am. J. Clin. Nutr., *49*:1211–1216, 1989.
34. Pion, P.D., Kittleson, M.D., Rogers, Q.R., et al.: Science, *237*:764–768, 1987.
35. Van Gelder, N.: J. Neurochem Res., *8*:687–699, 1983.
36. Gordon, R.E., Shaked, A.A., Solano, D.F.: Am. J. Pathol., *125*:585–600, 1986.
37. Sturman, J.A., Wen, G.Y., Wisniewski, H.M., et al.: Int. J. Dev. Neurosci., *2*:121–129, 1984.
38. Schuller-Levis, G., Mehta, P.D., Rudelli, P., et al.: J. Leukoc. Biol., *47*:321–331, 1990.
39. Okamoto, E., Rassin, D.K., Zucker, C.L., et al.: J. Pediatr., *104*:936–940, 1984.
40. Jarvenpaa, A.L., Raiha, N.C.R., Rassin, D.K., et al.: Pediatrics, *71*:171–178, 1983.
41. Galeano, N.F., Darling, P., Lepage, G., et al.: Pediatr. Res., *22*:67–71, 1987.
42. Watkins, J.B., Jarvenpaa, A.L., Szczepanik-Van Leeuwen, P., et al.: Gastroenterology, *85*:793–800, 1983.
43. Jarvenpaa, A.L., Rassin, D.K., Kuitunen, G.E., et al.: Pediatrics, *72*:677–683, 1983.
44. Cooke, R.J., Whitington, P.F., Kelts, D.: J. Pediatr. Gastroenterol. Nutr., *3*:234–238, 1984.
45. Jarvenpaa, A.L.: Pediatrics, *72*:684–689, 1983.
46. Bijleveld, C.M.A. Vonk, R.J., Okken A., et al.: Eur. J. Pediatr., *146*:128–130, 1987.
47. Darling, P.B., Lepage, G., Leroy, C., et al.: Pediatr. Res., *19*:578–582, 1985.
48. Belli, D.C., Levy, E., Darling, P.: Pediatrics, *80*:517–523, 1987.
49. Gaull, G.E.: Pediatrics, *83*:433–442, 1989.
50. Hardison, W.G.M., Grundy, S.M.: Gastroenterology, *84*:617–620, 1983.
51. Tanno, N., Oikawa, S., Koizumi, M., et al.: Tohoku J. Exp. Med., *159*:91–99, 1989.
52. Vinton, N.E., Laidlaw, S.A., Ament, M.E., et al.: Am. J. Clin. Nutr., *44*:398–404, 1986.
53. Vandewoude, M.F.J., De Leeuw, I.H.: N. Engl. J. Med., *313*:120–121, 1985.
54. Hayes, K.C., Sturman, J.A.: Adv. Exp. Med. Biol., *139*:79–87, 1982.
55. Hayes, K.C., Trautwein, E.A.: Vet. Clin. North Am. (Small Anim. Pract.), *19*:403–413, 1989.
56. Stephan, Z.F., Sturman, J.A., Hayes, K.C.: Nutr. Res., *4*:421–435, 1984.
57. Trautwein, E.A., Hayes, K.C.: J. Nutr. Biochem., *2*:571–576, 1991.
58. Larsen, B.R., Grosso, D.S., Chang, S.Y.: J. Chromatogr. Sci., *18*:233–236, 1980.
59. Porter, D.W., Banks, M.A., Castranova, V., et al.: J. Chromatogr., *454*:311–316, 1988.
60. Berson, E.L., Hayes, K.C., Rabin, A.R., et al.: Invest. Ophthalmol. Vis. Sci., *15*:52–58, 1976.
61. Nakamura-Yamanaka, Y., Tsuji, K., Ichikawa, T.: J. Nutr. Sci. Vitaminol., *33*:239–243, 1987.

## SELECTED READINGS

Chesney, R.W.: Taurine: Its biological role and clinical implications. Adv. Pediatr., *32*:1–42, 1985.

Hayes, K.C.: Taurine nutrition. Nutr. Res. Rev., *1*:99–113, 1988.

Huxtable, R.J.: Taurine in the central nervous system and the mammalian actions of taurine. Prog. Neurobiol., *32*:471–533, 1989.

Kendler, B.S.: Taurine: An overview of its role in preventive medicine. Prev. Med., *18*:79–100, 1989.

Lombardini, J.B.: Taurine: retinal function. Brain Res. Rev., *16*:151–169, 1991.

Sturman, J.A.: Taurine in development. J. Nutr., *118*:1169–1176, 1988.

# PART II

# Nutrition in Integrated Biologic Systems

CHAPTER 32

# Nutritional Regulation of Gene Expression

Alan G. Goodridge



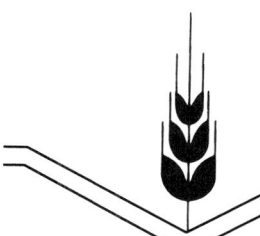

In vertebrate animals, the amount and composition of the diet regulate the activities of many enzymes. To understand the molecular bases of such phenomena requires knowledge of the plasma factor(s) that regulate the activity of a particular enzyme and the molecular nature of each event between binding of that plasma factor to its cellular receptor and altered activity of the relevant enzyme. Regulatory factors in plasma may be specific dietary components, such as heavy metals, or they may be fuels or hormones, the concentrations of which are regulated by the dietary intake of a component of the diet. Intracellular events may involve metabolism of a plasma fuel to an active metabolite or activation of a hormonally-regulated intracellular signaling pathway. Events in the intracellular signaling pathway start with hormone binding and include the regulated and all subsequent steps in the pathway of gene expression, a pathway that begins with transcription and ends with an active enzyme. In this chapter, a strategy will be outlined for analyzing the molecular basis of the regulation of gene expression by diet, and our current understanding of the molecular basis for nutritional regulation of the activity of two enzymes involved in lipogenesis will be described. The overall strategies illustrated in these studies of "lipogenic" enzymes are models for analyses of the nutritional regulation of expression of many genes.

The synthesis of long-chain fatty acids occurs primarily in the liver in many animals. The flux of carbon through this pathway is slow in starved animals and fast in fed ones, especially if the diet is high in carbohydrate and low in fat. The activities of several enzymes involved in lipogenesis, including L-type pyruvate kinase (L-PK) and malic enzyme (ME) have similar patterns. The regulation of these enzymes by starvation and refeeding and by altering the carbohydrate content of the diet will be described.

## RELEVANCE TO HUMAN HEALTH

Chronic hyperalimentation leads to obesity because the excess dietary energy is converted to fat. A significant fraction of human obesity appears to have a genetic basis. Even though the rate of fatty acid synthesis is low in humans, mainly because our diets are relatively high in fat, regulatory defects that result in higher-than-normal rates of fatty acid synthesis could lead to obesity. Such defects might involve correct responses of specific genes to inappropriate hormonal signals or incorrect responses of specific genes to appropriate regulatory signals. Interestingly, many of the components of the signaling pathways that regulate lipogenic genes also are involved in regulation of cell division. Thus, the molecular basis for the nutritional regulation of genes involved in fatty acid synthesis may be important in understanding the excessive growth of adipose tissue caused by obesity and the excessive growth of tumors caused by neoplastic transformation.

## HUMORAL FACTORS

Insulin, glucagon, glucocorticoids, and triiodothyronine ($T_3$) modulate the rate of fatty acid synthesis and the activities of the lipogenic enzymes. Evidence that these hormones are mediators of the effects of diet on hepatic enzyme activities is based on a variety of mainly correlative evidence.[1,2] The blood of animals fed high-carbohydrate diets has an elevated level of insulin and a decreased level of glucagon. The opposite is observed in starved animals—lowered insulin and elevated glucagon. In diabetic animals, insulin levels are low and glucagon levels high; the rate of lipogenesis and the activities of the lipogenic enzymes are low. In perfused liver, liver slices, and isolated hepatocytes, insulin stimulates and glucagon inhibits the rate of fatty acid synthesis. Increases in lipogenic flux and activities of the lipogenic enzymes caused by refeeding starved animals are blocked by the simultaneous administration of glucagon. Finally, in hepatocytes in culture, insulin stimulates and glucagon inhibits accumulation of the lipogenic enzymes.[1-3] These results suggest that insulin and glucagon play important roles in the metabolic transitions between the fed and starved states.

Although the level of thyroxine is not affected by starvation or feeding, the concentration of the active form of thyroid hormone, $T_3$, is regulated in a manner similar to that for insulin—decreased in starved animals and increased in fed ones.[4] Furthermore, in rats[5] and hepatocytes in culture,[6] $T_3$ is a potent inducer of ME. L-PK activity also is regulated by thyroid state in rats.[2,3] These results are consistent with a role for $T_3$ in the regulation of lipogenic enzyme activity during the transitions between the fed and starved states.

Glucocorticoids are another class of hormones involved in the regulation of lipogenic enzymes, but their role in nutritional regulation of these enzymes is not well understood. The involvement of glucocorticoids in the increased expression of both gluconeogenic enzymes in starved animals and lipogenic enzymes in fed animals makes it unlikely that they are signaling factors that communicate dietary status to the liver. The glucocorticoids may be permissive for the expression of a variety of hepatic enzymes involved in intermediary metabolism.

Changes in the levels of fuels derived directly or indirectly from dietary nutrients also regulate the activities of lipogenic enzymes. Thus, dietary fructose stimulates an increase in the activities of the lipogenic enzymes in starved rats, whether they are diabetic or not. Glucose is effective only in nondiabetic animals. Even in the nondiabetics, the stimulatory effect of fructose is unlikely to involve insulin because insulin secretion is increased only modestly by fructose and then only at high concentrations. In rat hepatocytes in culture, fructose and other sugars stimulate increased activities of the lipogenic enzymes.[7] The similarity of the effects of insulin-dependent glucose metabolism and insulin-independent fructose metabolism on hepatic lipogenesis has led some investigators to postulate that the lipogenic enzymes are regulated by an intracellular intermediate common to the metabolism of both sugars.[8,9]

Fat is a second major dietary component that influences the rate of lipogenesis. In rats, the activities of the lipogenic enzymes are decreased by diets enriched in polyunsaturated fats; regulation is probably at pretranslational steps.[10] The mechanisms by which dietary fat and fatty acids regulate abundance of the lipogenic mRNA are unknown and will not be discussed further in this review.

## PATHWAY FOR GENE EXPRESSION

Intracellular signaling pathways are often branching; binding of a hormone can lead to several different end-effects. The strategy that I and others have adopted is to trace each signaling pathway backwards from its distal end, altered enzyme activity, to its proximal end, binding of a hormone or metabolite to its receptor; thus the signaling pathways being analyzed were always those involved in regulating the relevant enzyme. The signaling pathways that regulate enzyme activity have part or all of two pathways. A distal limb involves information transfer, starting with transcription and ending with enzyme activity. The proximal limb involves transfer of regulatory information from the hormone receptor complex to the point in the information transfer pathway that is rate-limiting and controls enzyme activity. The first task, therefore, was to identify the step in the information transfer pathway regulated by nutritional state or hormone or metabolite.

In a metabolic pathway of an intact cell, unidirectional flux through an enzymatic step can be regulated by controlling either the amount of an enzyme or its catalytic efficiency. In our examples, activity is controlled by regulating enzyme concentration. Concentration, in turn, can be controlled by regulating synthesis or degradation of the enzyme (or both). Nutritional state and hormones control the concentrations of L-PK and ME by regulating the rate of enzyme synthesis. Enzyme synthesis is controlled by regulating either the amount of the relevant mRNA or the efficiency with which it is translated. In general, enzyme synthesis is determined by mRNA concentration because the translation factors required for the synthesis of proteins do not distinguish between different mRNAs. Sometimes the efficiency of translation of an mRNA is regulated, or the mRNA may be sequestered in a nontranslatable form. For most proteins, including L-PK and ME, rate of enzyme synthesis and abundance of enzyme mRNA are controlled coordinately, indicating pretranslational regulation.

Pretranslational control can be exerted at several different points between the initiation of transcription and the appearance of a mature cytoplasmic mRNA (Fig. 32–1). After a nascent RNA transcript is initiated, it is elongated, and then the completed primary transcript is terminated. Termination usually occurs downstream from the eventual 3′-end of the transcript. The nucleotide sequence, AAUAAA, is located upstream of the termina-

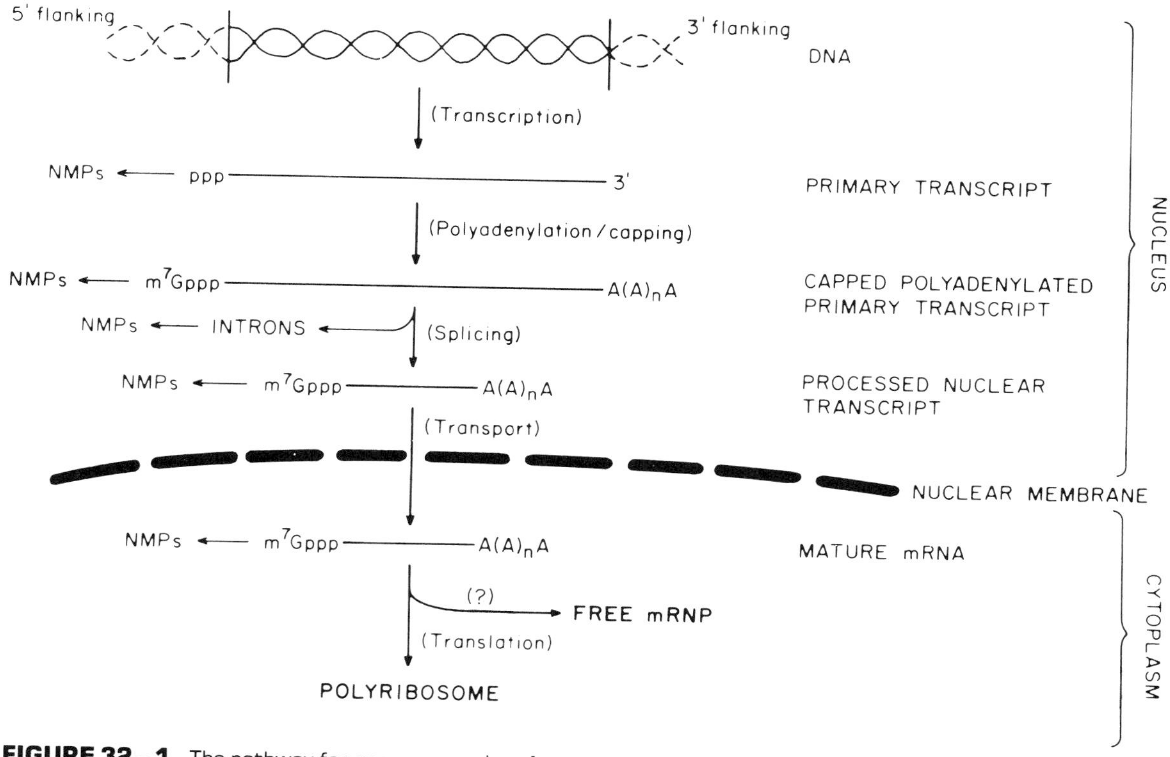
5' flanking
3' flanking
DNA
(Transcription)
NMPs
ppp
3'
PRIMARY TRANSCRIPT
(Polyadenylation/capping)
NMPs
m7Gppp
A(A)nA
CAPPED POLYADENYLATED PRIMARY TRANSCRIPT
NMPs
INTRONS
(Splicing)
NMPs
m7Gppp
A(A)nA
PROCESSED NUCLEAR TRANSCRIPT
(Transport)
NUCLEUS
NUCLEAR MEMBRANE
NMPs
m7Gppp
A(A)nA
MATURE mRNA
(?)
FREE mRNP
(Translation)
POLYRIBOSOME
CYTOPLASM

**FIGURE 32–1.** The pathway for gene expression. A generalized scheme for the transcription, processing, transport, and degradation of intermediate and final products in the synthesis of mRNA. NMP, Nucleoside monophosphate; $m^7$, 7-methyl guanosyl residue; mRNP, messenger ribonucleoprotein particle. (From Goodridge, A.G.: Annu. Rev. Nutr., 7:157–185, 1987.)

tion site and serves as a signal for cleavage and polyadenylation of the 3′-end of the RNA. Cleavage occurs about 29 bases downstream from the AAUAAA signal sequence. The 5′-end of the RNA is capped with 7-methyl guanylate in an unusual 5′-5′ triphosphate linkage. This completes formation of the primary transcript. Next, introns are removed in one or more splicing reactions, finally resulting in a mature nuclear mRNA that is then transported from the nuclear compartment to the cytoplasm. Each of the foregoing processes is a potential regulatory site at which the production of mRNA could be regulated. In addition, the steady-state level of the mature mRNA can be controlled by regulating degradation of that mRNA. Finally, degradation of the nuclear intermediates also can be regulated, thus controlling concentration of those intermediates and flux through the pathway.

The step most commonly observed to control the concentration of mature cytoplasmic mRNA is transcription initiation. Degradation of mature mRNA and its nuclear precursors also have been implicated in the regulation of mRNA concentration. Capping at the 5′-end and polyadenylation at the 3′-end may make the transcript resistant to degradation, but are unlikely to be involved in the modulation of production of specific mRNAs. The rare occurence of regulation at other steps is probably due to a combination of a low frequency of control at these sites and the difficulty of measuring the rates of those processes.

## IDENTIFYING REGULATED STEPS

Complementary DNAs (cDNAs) bind to their complementary mRNAs with very high affinities and specificities. This property makes them essential reagents for measuring the amount and rates of metabolism of specific mRNAs. The cDNAs corresponding to L-PK and ME mRNAs were isolated in several laboratories by standard molecular cloning techniques.[3] Under appropriate conditions, labeled cDNAs hybridize only to their corresponding mRNAs. In the commonest methods, an unknown mixture of mRNA is fixed to a solid support, either by adding a sample directly to a membrane ("dot" or "slot" blot) or by transfer from a gel after separating the RNAs by size by agarose electrophoresis ("Northern" blot). The intensity of the autoradiographic signal is proportional to the concentration of the mRNA.

Cloned complementary or genomic DNAs also are used to measure the rates of transcription initiation of specific genes in the "run-on" assay.[11] Nuclei are isolated from tissues of intact animals or from cells in culture. When the cells are broken and nuclei are isolated, RNA polymerases, with their nascent RNA chains attached, stop transcribing and remain bound to the DNA where they stopped. In vitro, the pre-existing nascent RNAs are elongated in the presence of $^{32}$P-UTP ($^{32}$P-uridine triphosphate) under conditions that do not permit significant initiation of new chains. The DNA probes are attached to a solid matrix and used to purify rapidly the corresponding specific RNA from other labeled RNAs. The RNA/DNA hybrids, still attached to the solid matrix, are treated with RNase to reduce background and remove single-stranded RNA not base-paired to probe DNA. Radioactivity incorporated into specific RNA is usually detected by autoradiography. The run-on assay thus provides a relative measure of the number of RNA polymerase molecules engaged in transcription at the time the tissue or cells were prepared; this, in turn, should be proportional to the rate of transcription initiation for the corresponding gene in the intact cell. This is the most commonly used assay to estimate transcription in animals or cells in culture.

## REGULATION OF PRODUCTION OF LIPOGENIC mRNAS

### L-TYPE PYRUVATE KINASE

L-PK (EC 2.7.1.40) catalyzes the conversion of phosphoenolpyruvate to pyruvate and plays an important role in directing pyruvate toward glucose synthesis in starved animals or toward oxidation and incorporation into long-chain fatty acids in fed animals. The level of L-PK decreases greatly in starved rats and is increased when starved rats are refed, particularly if the diet contains a high level of carbohydrate.[12] In diabetic animals, L-PK concentration is very low; treatment with insulin restores normal levels. Feeding a diet high in fructose, but not glucose, partly restores the normal level of L-PK in a diabetic rat.[13,14] These changes in concentration of L-PK are due to changes in the synthesis rate of the protein.[15] Thyroid hormone also stimulates accumulation of L-PK protein in thyroidectomized rats.[16]

When starved rats are fed a carbohydrate-rich diet, the abundance of L-PK mRNA in the liver is increased 40 to 100 times.[17,18] The three L-PK mRNAs expressed in liver (3.2, 2.2, and 2.0 kilobases) differ only by the lengths of their 3′-noncoding regions and are regulated by diet in the same manner.[19] Organ ablation studies indicate that thyroid hormone and glucocorticoids play permissive roles in the induction of L-PK mRNA in starved rats refed a high-carbohydrate diet,[20] although glucocorticoids were not required for the stimulation by fructose.[21] The level of L-PK mRNA is increased in rats treated with insulin and decreased in diabetic animals or animals treated with glucagon or cyclic adenosine monophosphate (cAMP).[17,20,22] Fructose and certain other simple sugars cause an increased accumulation of L-PK and its mRNA, even in diabetic animals.[13,23,24]

A common property of the active sugars is entry into the pathways of liver metabolism via enzymes other than hexokinase or glucokinase. A metabolite derived from the metabolism of simple sugars or a metabolic intermediate, the concentration of which is controlled by the rate of metabolism of sugars, may be the active compound. In hepatocytes in culture, both insulin and glucose are required to stimulate accumulation of L-PK and its mRNA.[25] Glucagon or dibutyryl cAMP block the effects of insulin plus glucose in rat hepatocytes in maintenance culture[25] and in an immortalized rat liver cell line in culture.[26] Regulation of the rate of synthesis of L-PK protein by hormones and metabolites is thus predominantly pretranslational.

Potential control steps involved in pretranslational regulation include gene transcription, processing of primary transcripts, or degradation of mRNA. Starvation, feeding a carbohydrate-rich diet, insulin, and cAMP (glucagon) exert their effects on the level of L-PK mRNA by regulating gene transcription.[21,27] Feeding fructose to diabetic animals stimulates accumulation of the mRNA but does not stimulate transcription of the gene.[21] Glucagon suppresses the increase in hepatic L-PK mRNA caused by a high-fructose diet. Because the increase in mRNA caused by fructose appears to be regulated post-transcriptionally, the inhibition by glucagon also may be post-transcriptional.[21] In vivo and in hepatocytes in culture, glucagon or dibutyryl cAMP also exerts post-transcriptional effects on the expression of this gene by stimulating degradation of L-PK mRNA[25,27,28] (Fig. 32–2). Thus, regulation of the level of L-PK mRNA is not exclusively transcriptional, and different hormones may regulate expression of this gene by regulating different reactions in the gene expression pathway.

### MALIC ENZYME

ME (EC 1.1.1.40) catalyzes the oxidative decarboxylation of malate to pyruvate and $CO_2$, simultaneously generating the reduced form of nicotinamide adenine dinucleotide phosphate (NADPH) from $NADP^+$. Much of the NADPH generated by this reaction is utilized in the de-novo synthesis of long-chain fatty acids. ME responds to dietary and hormonal manipulation in much the same way as L-PK does. The level of the hepatic enzyme is low in starved animals and high in fed animals, especially if the diet is high in carbohydrate.[29] The concentration of ME is controlled by regulating its synthesis rate,[30,31] which in turn correlates positively with abundance of ME mRNA,[32,33] indicating pretranslational regulation.

Steps involved in the nutritional regulation of abundance of the ME mRNA have been analyzed in young chicks, ducklings, and adult rats. A 50- to 100-fold increase in mRNA level is caused by refeeding starved chicks or ducklings; this is accompanied by about a

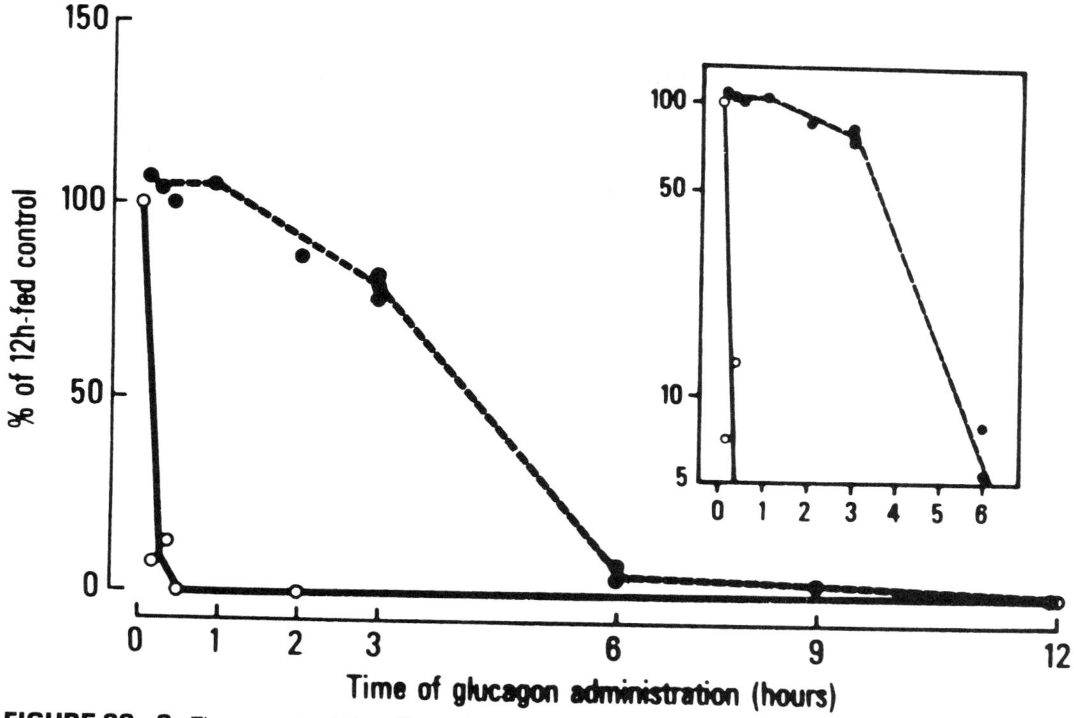
% of 12h-fed control
150
100
50
0
0 1 2 3 6 9 12
Time of glucagon administration (hours)
100
50
10
5
0 1 2 3 4 5 6

**FIGURE 32–2.** Time course of the effect of glucagon on transcription of the L-type pyruvate kinase (L-PK) gene and the level of L-PK mRNA in the liver of rats refed a carbohydrate-rich diet. Transcription of the L-PK gene (●-●) and mRNA abundance (o-o) were measured in nyctohemeral inverted rats given glucagon for varying periods of time ranging from 0 to 12 hours after refeeding for 12 hours. The animals ate adequately during the entire period of glucagon treatment. Data are expressed as a percentage of transcription of mRNA level at the time of glucagon administration. The *inset* shows the same results in a semilogarithmic representation. (From Vaulont, S., Munnich, A., Decaux, J.-F., et al.: J. Biol. Chem., *261*:7621–7625, 1986.)

50-fold increase in transcription of the ME gene[34] (Fig. 32–3). DNA probes specific for intronic regions of the primary transcript did not detect significant levels of nuclear precursors of ME mRNA in the livers of starved chicks but detected high levels in the livers of fed ones.[34] This finding is consistent with transcriptional regulation. Based on the kinetics with which ME mRNA approaches a new steady-state level,[35] the rate constant for degradation of the ME mRNA is 3 to 5 times higher in starved than in fed ducklings.[36] Thus, despite a small post-transcriptional component, transcription initiation appears to be the major regulated step for the nutritional control of chick or duckling ME. In rat liver, the increased abundance of ME mRNA caused by switching from chow to a high-carbohydrate, low-fat diet is accompanied by decreased degradation of the mature ME mRNA but no change in transcription.[37,38] The lack of effect of diet on transcription was analyzed using the transcription "run-on" assay and confirmed by measuring the levels of nuclear precursors with intron-specific probes. Abundant nuclear precursors were detected in the livers of both chow- and carbohydrate-fed rats.[38] The basis of the discrepancy between rats and chicks is not apparent.

Hormones also play an important role in regulating ME. The concentration of ME is low in diabetic and hypothyroid animals and restored to normal or higher levels by treatment with insulin or $T_3$, respectively.[29] In chick-embryo hepatocytes in culture in serum-free medium, $T_3$ stimulates about a 50-fold increase in the amount of ME.[39] Insulin has little effect by itself but amplifies the effect of $T_3$, such that the total increase is 100- to 150-fold.[39] IGF-1 (insulin-like growth factor I) has the same effects as insulin, no effect alone, and amplification of the $T_3$ effect. IGF-1 is effective at lower doses than insulin is; some of the effect of insulin might be via the IGF-1 receptor.[40] Insulin and $T_3$ also stimulate accumulation of ME in rat hepatocytes in culture, but to a smaller extent than observed in vivo[41,42] or in chick-embryo hepatocytes.

The small or nonexistent effect of insulin by itself and its relatively small (two- to three-fold) amplification of the stimulation caused by $T_3$ in hepatocytes from both chick embryos and rats are not in accordance with the large decrease in ME observed in the diabetic state and the postulated importance of insulin in the response of hepatic ME to refeeding a starved chick or to feeding a rat a high-carbohydrate diet. Thus, factors other than

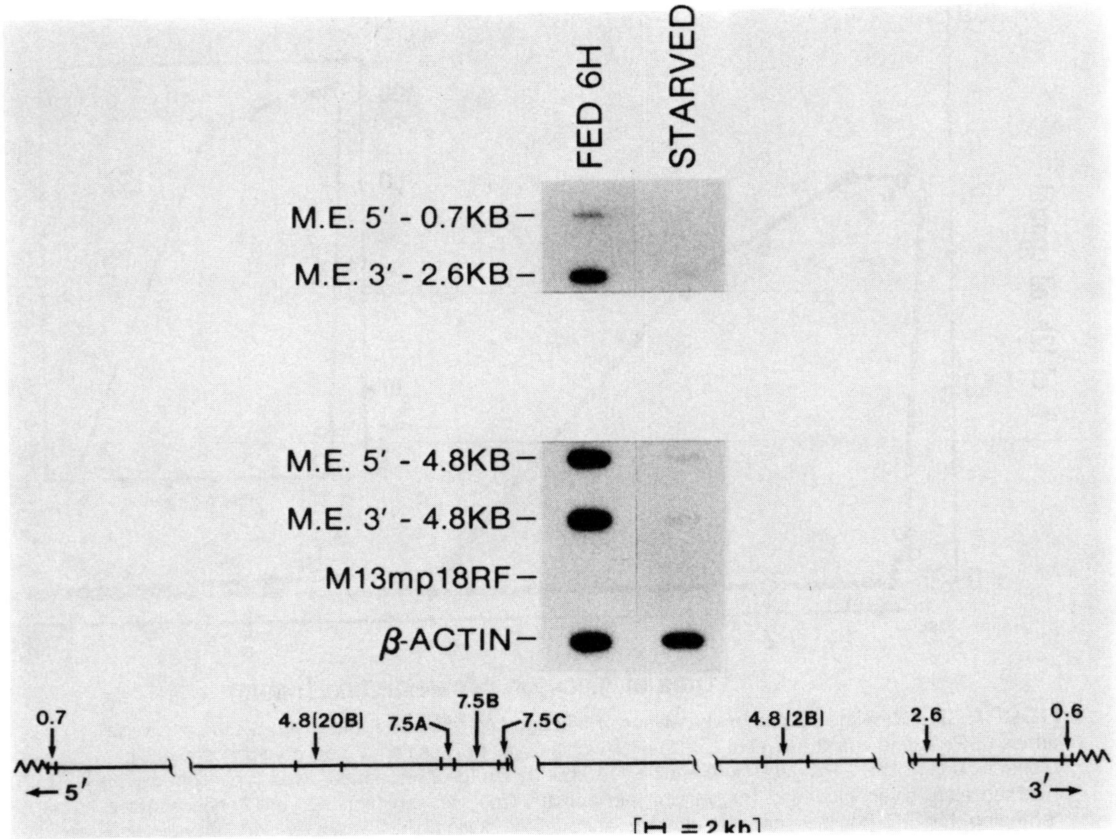
FED 6H
STARVED
M.E. 5' - 0.7KB–
M.E. 3' - 2.6KB–
M.E. 5' - 4.8KB–
M.E. 3' - 4.8KB–
M13mp18RF–
β-ACTIN–
0.7
4.8(20B)
7.5A
7.5B
7.5C
4.8(2B)
2.6
0.6
← 5'
3' →
[⊢ = 2 kb]

**FIGURE 32–3.** Stimulation of transcription of the malic enzyme (M.E.) gene by refeeding in chick liver. Nuclei were isolated from livers of 12- to 14-day chicks that were starved for 48 hours and then were either starved for an additional 6 hours or were refed for 6 hours. Nuclear run-on assays were performed as described.[34] Identical strips were hybridized with $2 \times 10^7$ cpm/ml each of $^{32}P$-labeled nascent RNA from liver nuclei from either starved or refed chicks. Vector DNA (M13mp18RF) was a control for nonspecific hybridization; the cDNA for β-actin was a control for selectivity; the level of hepatic β-actin is unaffected by starvation or refeeding. The map at the bottom of the figure indicates the location of the various DNA probes within the malic enzyme gene.

insulin may be involved in the decreased concentration of ME in diabetic animals. Levels of circulating glucagon are high in diabetic animals and are lowered by treatment of these animals with insulin.[43] Furthermore, glucagon, acting via cAMP, inhibits the induction of ME and its mRNA caused by insulin plus $T_3$ in hepatocytes in culture.[33,39,44] Thus, changes in circulating glucagon may be more important than changes in circulating insulin in mediating the effects of nutritional state on the activity of the lipogenic enzymes. Other hormones, growth factors, and plasma fuels also may play important roles in mediating the response of hepatic lipogenic enzymes to feeding and starvation.

One fuel that affects ME, apparently independently of insulin, is fructose. As with other lipogenic enzymes, dietary fructose increases the levels of ME and its mRNA even in diabetic animals.[45,46] In rat hepatocytes in culture, glucose, fructose, and other simple sugars stimulate increased accumulation of lipogenic enzymes.[7,42] Dichloroacetate, an activator of pyruvate dehydrogenase, also stimulates accumulation of ME in rat hepatocytes, suggesting that the active intermediate may be generated in mitochondria.[42] In chick-embryo hepatocytes, neither glucose nor fructose increases ME activity, with or without insulin in the medium, and $T_3$ is about 50% more effective in inducing ME in a medium containing glucose compared to a glucose-free medium.[47] The mechanisms whereby glucose or fructose or intermediates derived therefrom or intermediates affected by the metabolism thereof, control expression of ME, remain obscure.

Hormones control the synthesis of ME by regulating the abundance of its mRNA, indicating pretranslational control.[30,33,39,46,48] Based on Northern analyses, $T_3$ stimulates a 50- to 150-fold increase in the abundance of ME mRNA (Fig. 32–4). Glucagon, dibutyryl cAMP, or agents

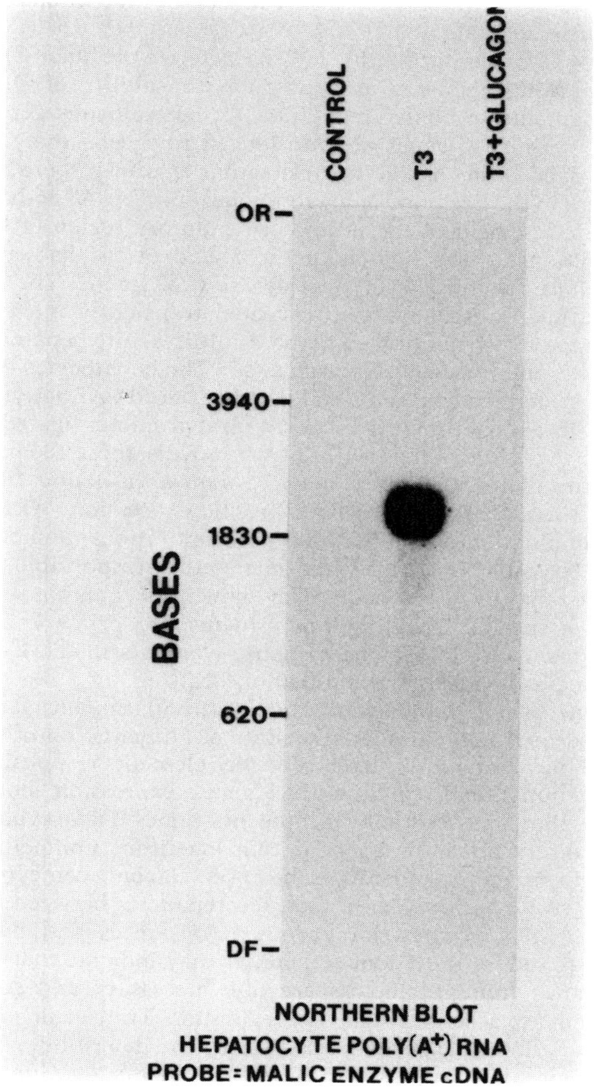
CONTROL
T3
T3+GLUCAGO
OR—
3940—
1830—
BASES
620—
DF—
NORTHERN BLOT
HEPATOCYTE POLY(A+) RNA
PROBE=MALIC ENZYME cDNA

**FIGURE 32–4.** The effects of $T_3$ and glucagon on the abundance of malic enzyme mRNA. RNA was extracted from hepatocytes that were isolated from the livers of 19-day-old chick embryos and then incubated for 3 days in serum-free Waymouth medium MD 705/1 containing insulin (300 ng/ml) (control), insulin plus $T_3$ (1 μg/ml) or insulin plus $T_3$ plus glucagon (1 μg/ml). Each lane contained 20 μg of RNA. DF, Dye front; Or, origin. (From Goodridge, A.G., Crish, J.F., Hillgartner, F.B., et al.: J. Nutr., *119*:299–308, 1989.)

that raise the intracellular concentration of cAMP virtually totally block the induction by $T_3$[33,34] (Fig. 32–4). Comparable changes in transcription were measured using genomic DNA probes and the transcription run-on assay.[49,50] Based on the rate of decrease in the abundance of mRNA in the presence of transcription inhibitors, glucagon stimulates degradation of the ME mRNA by about 7 times.[51] The magnitude of this effect is insufficient to account for the greater than 95% inhibition of mRNA level caused by glucagon. Thus, regulation of ME by both $T_3$ and glucagon is primarily transcriptional. Similarly, the amplifying effect of insulin or IGF-1 is also exerted at the transcriptional level.[49]

## CIS-ACTING SEQUENCE ELEMENTS IN LIPOGENIC GENES

Nutritional and hormonal treatments that regulate transcription of lipogenic genes control expression of specific, usually small, sets of genes and have little or no effect on other genes. The intracellular signaling machinery recognizes the regulated genes by virtue of short sequence elements, usually just upstream from the start site for transcription. Specific DNA-binding proteins interact with these regulatory elements. These DNA-binding proteins have two specificity domains, one for recognition of a component of the appropriate intracellular signaling pathway and the other to recognize the appropriate gene. They also have functional domains involved in regulation of transcription initiation. The nucleotide sequences recognized by specific DNA-binding proteins are called cis-acting regulatory elements because they are required in cis (same molecule) for regulation by a particular agent. Methods for identifying such DNA regulatory elements are based on sequence-specific binding of proteins or on the ability of the sequence element to bestow hormone responsiveness on a heterologous gene. Neither a binding assay nor a functional assay by itself is sufficient to characterize these elements. Together, however, these methods can provide convincing evidence for the importance of specific sequence elements in the regulatory process. Analyses of cis-acting sequence elements of lipogenic genes are just beginning.

Hormone regulatory elements usually involve very short stretches of DNA. Sometimes as few as 8 to 10 base pairs will make up a core sufficient to confer regulation on a heterologous gene. These core sequences show some variability from gene to gene. Thus, they cannot be recognized on the basis of sequence alone because modestly conserved sequences of 8 to 10 base pairs are apt to occur often in the genome. Such small regions also are difficult to localize in the hundreds of base pairs of potential regulatory DNA upstream and downstream from the start site for transcription. Furthermore, sequence flexibility implies that accessory factors, probably proteins recognizing nearby sequences and other proteins, play roles in determining specificity of the hormonal response. DNA structure also may be important.

Because the regulatory elements can be located almost anywhere within many kilobases of DNA, identifying smaller regions of DNA that have the potential to harbor cis-acting sequence elements can simplify the analysis. DNase I hypersensitive sites identify regions in DNA that are free of nucleosomes, regions that often are involved in the binding of regulatory proteins.[52] Therefore, a first step in the analysis of cis-acting elements is often the determination of DNase I hypersensitive sites in the region surrounding the start site for transcription.

## L-TYPE PYRUVATE KINASE

The rat L-PK gene uses two promoters. The L promoter is specific for liver, and the L'promoter is specific for erythroid tissue.[53] The rat liver L-PK gene contains two DNase I hypersensitive sites located upstream from the L promoter of the L-PK gene. The site at −24 to −40 base pairs is hypersensitive when transcription of the L-PK gene is stimulated and not hypersensitive when transcription is inhibited. The site at −3.2 to −3.0 kilobases is hypersensitive whether the gene is active or not. Factors may bind to the upstream site whether they are in their active conformations or not, whereas binding of factors at the downstream site may correlate with increased transcription.

DNase "footprinting" and the "band shift" assay are used to identify cis-acting sequence elements and to monitor purification of specific DNA-binding proteins. The DNase "footprinting" assay involves incubation of nuclear extracts or purified proteins with cloned DNA, followed by treatment of the DNA with sufficient DNase to introduce randomly about one cleavage per molecule. When the cleaved DNA is separated by size on a DNA sequencing gel, the random fragments appear as a "ladder" of bands of increasing molecular weight. Proteins binding to the DNA protect it from cleavage by DNase and result in a blank space in the ladder. The "band-shift" or "gel retardation" assay also involves incubation of cloned DNA with nuclear extracts or purified proteins. If the fragments of DNA are relatively small and binding is of high affinity, the protein will remain bound to the DNA during electrophoresis and retard its mobility relative to the DNA fragment without bound protein.[54]

The 183 base pairs upstream from the start site of transcription of the L promoter of the L-PK gene contain four sites protected specifically by nuclear extracts from rat liver.[55] Two of the four proteins that bind to this region are expressed mainly in the liver, and the other two are expressed in most tissues. Based on the nucleotide sequences at the binding sites, the liver-specific factors are hepatocyte nuclear factor 1 (HNF-1) and liver factor A1 (LF-A1), DNA-binding proteins that regulate transcription of genes expressed specifically in liver. The other two factors bind to sequences similar to those for ubiquitous nuclear factor 1 (NF-1) and another ubiquitous nuclear factor that binds to the major late promoter of adenovirus 2 and to some other genes. All of these DNA binding factors were present at similar levels in the nuclear extracts of livers from both carbohydrate-fed and starved rats, indicating that they do not regulate transcription of the L-PK gene via changes in their concentrations. It remains possible, however, that covalent modifications or allosteric effects could regulate activities of these factors as a function of nutritional or hormonal state.

Assays used to identify and characterize the function of cis-acting elements are based on the ability of DNA fragments to confer regulation on heterologous genes. The chimeric genes are introduced into cells that are derived from specific tissues or that exhibit responsiveness to the hormone or agent in question.[56,57] A 186-base pair fragment of the promoter/regulatory region of the L-PK gene was ligated to the 5′-end of the bacterial chloramphenicol acetyltransferase (CAT) gene. The resulting transgene was transfected transiently into rat hepatocytes maintained in mass cultures, into hepatoma cells, and into mouse fibroblasts.[58] The hepatocytes and liver-derived hepatoma cell lines produced CAT activity; the mouse fibroblasts did not. A viral promoter ligated to CAT was functional in all cell types. Thus, these 186 base pairs of the L-PK gene may contain a cis-acting DNA element that specifies liver-specific expression. With a combination of deletion and point mutations, it should be possible to identify the nucleotides responsible for liver-specific expression. The sequences that bind the liver-specific DNA binding proteins are prime candidates. As yet, hormone response elements in the L-PK gene have not been identified or localized.

According to the hypothesis that circulating hormones and fuels communicate the state of alimentation of the whole animal to the liver, sequence elements responsible for nutritional regulation of a gene's expression should be the same as those for the hormones that regulate transcription of that gene in cells in culture. Compelling evidence of their identities, however, can only come from in vivo experiments. In fact, discrepancies between the elements required for hormonal responses and those required for nutritional responses may indicate that the known humoral factors are not "necessary and sufficient" to account for in vivo regulation. Transgenic mice are suitable experimental systems for determining sequence requirements in vivo. Fragments of putative promoter/regulatory DNAs are ligated upstream of reporter genes and injected into fertilized mouse eggs. The foreign DNA can be integrated as a genetically stable component into the mouse's genomic DNA.

Tremp et al. have constructed a strain of transgenic mice containing a complete rat L-PK gene, including 3.2 kilobases of 5′-flanking DNA and 1.4 kilobases of 3′-flanking DNA.[53] In this instance, the rat L-PK mRNA is the reporter gene and can be distinguished experimentally from the corresponding mouse mRNA by hybridization analyses. Rat L-PK mRNA was expressed specifically in mouse liver, as would be expected if the sequences responsible for tissue specificity are in the first 186 base pairs of flanking DNA. In addition, abundance of the rat L-PK mRNA was regulated by nutritional state—low in starved mice and high in fed ones. Administration of glucagon concomitantly with refeeding blocked the increase in rat L-PK mRNA in these mice. Changes in the levels of the rat mRNA paralleled changes in abundance of the endogenous mouse mRNA. A second line of mice was constructed in which the transgene was considerably shortened, containing only exons 1, 10, and 11 plus the same 5′ and 3′ flanking DNA as in the first construction. Expression of the minigene form of rat L-PK was regulated in the same manner as that of the complete rat gene was. Thus, cis-acting sequences involved in regulation of mRNA by diet, glucagon, and tissue type are probably contained in the 3.2 kilobases of DNA upstream of the L-type promoter. Analysis of additional deletions and mutations will be necessary to eliminate completely the possibility of a role for 3′ sequences or for sequences in exons 1, 10, and 11 and to identify the specific nucleotides involved in these regulatory phenomena.

## MALIC ENZYME

The rat ME gene contains four DNase I hypersensitive sites in its 5′-flanking DNA at −50, −170, −310, and −4100 base pairs with respect to the start site for transcription.[59] The sites at −170 and −4100 base pairs were hypersensitive in liver nuclei from both hypothyroid and hyperthyroid rats. The sites at −50 and −310 base pairs were hypersensitive only in the hyperthyroid state. Thus, the three- to four-fold difference in transcription of the ME gene between hypothyroid and hyperthyroid rats was accompanied by a significant change in chromatin structure just upstream from the start site.

The ME gene in chick liver also contains DNase I hypersensitive regions in its 5′-flanking DNA (Fig. 32–5).[34] Four distinct sites centered about −100, −164, −270, and −350 base pairs were found in region I just upstream of the start site for transcription. Hypersensitivity in the region (I) closest to the start site was barely detectable after 48 hours of starvation but became intense upon refeeding. Three additional regions of hypersensitivity were located at about −1600, −3200, and −3900 base pairs. DNA at these sites was hypersensitive in nuclei from liver but not from heart or kidney, and hypersensitivity was not affected by nutritional status. DNase I hypersensitivity is often associated with the binding of regulatory proteins, so these regions may bind proteins involved in the tissue-specific expression of ME. Hypersensitive sites also were detected in nuclei from chick-embryo hepatocytes in culture. All four regions were hypersensitive to about the same extent (like nuclei from livers of fed chicks) in hepatocytes incubated with no hormones, insulin alone, insulin plus $T_3$, or insulin plus $T_3$ plus glucagon (or cAMP).[49]

The lack of responsiveness to $T_3$ of hypersensitive sites in the 5′-flanking DNA of the chick-embryo hepatocyte ME gene, despite a 30-fold or greater increase in transcription of the gene, contrasts with the $T_3$-stimulated change in hypersensitivity of sites in the rat gene correlated with only a three- to four-fold increase in transcription. The effects of thyroid status on DNase I hypersensitivity and transcription in intact animals may be due to agents other than $T_3$; circulating levels of these

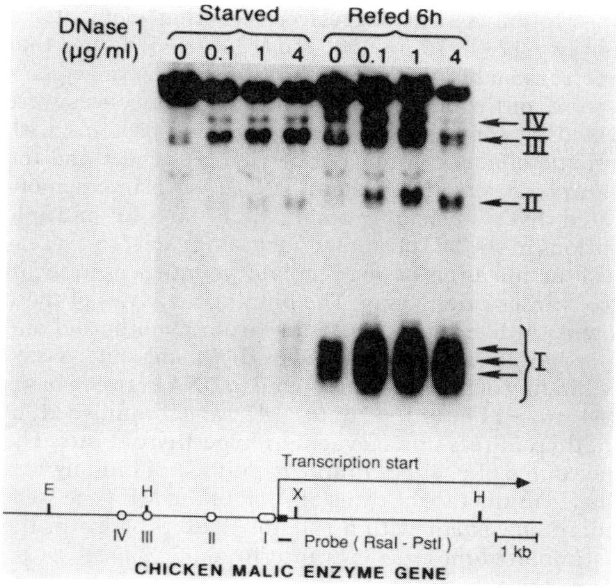
DNase 1
(µg/ml)
Starved
Refed 6h
0 0.1 1 4 0 0.1 1 4
IV
III
II
I
Transcription start
E
H
X
H
IV III
II
I
Probe ( Rsal - PstI )
1 kb
CHICKEN MALIC ENZYME GENE

**FIGURE 32–5.** DNase I hypersensitivity of the 5′ flanking region of the hepatic malic enzyme gene. The 5′ end and flanking region of the chick malic enzyme gene were tested for DNase I hypersensitivity by the indirect end-labeling strategy diagramed at the bottom of the figure. Restriction sites and the position of the probe (about 210 bp) are indicated. E, EcoRI; X, XhoI; H, HindIII. Nuclei were isolated from livers of 14-day chicks starved for 48 hours or starved for 48 hours and refed for 6 hours. Nuclei were digested with DNase I and the DNA was purified, was digested with EcoRI and XhoI to generate 5.9-kb fragments, and was Southern-blotted onto a nylon membrane. The probe was labeled with [$\alpha$-$^{32}$P]dCTP. Region I contains four discernible cleavage sites marked by arrows. Additional sub-bands were products of EcoRI star activity. (From Ma, X.-J., Salati, L.M., Ash, S.E., et al.: J. Biol. Chem., *265*18,435–18,441, 1990.)

other agents may be regulated by thyroid state. Similarly, the lack of effect of hormones on hypersensitivity in culture may mean that the large changes in hypersensitivity of the chick liver gene caused by refeeding starved chicks are not mediated primarily by $T_3$, insulin, or glucagon.

Cis-acting regulatory elements in the 5′-flanking DNA of the rat ME gene were localized by transfection of cells in culture[60] and then identified by virtue of their abilities to direct transcription in an in vitro system and to bind to nuclear proteins.[61] The transfection analysis defined three regions of the promoter. The region from the start site of transcription to −41 base pairs was essential for basal transcription. A substantial increase in expression was observed if sequences from −41 to −122 also were included in the construct. Finally, sequences between −122 and −145 or so resulted in another major increase in transcription. Sequences between −177 and −882 had no added effect. Unfortunately, malic enzyme in these cell lines is not responsive to hormones, so that the presence of hormone regulatory elements was not tested.[60] A deletion analysis combined with in vitro transcription assays suggested cis-acting elements at −144 to −123, −70 to −50, and −30 to +5, values that agree reasonably well with the transfection analysis.[61] Positions of the elements and their base sequences were verified by competition for DNA-binding proteins with synthetic oligonucleotides of defined sequences and the in vitro transcription system. DNase footprints demonstrated liver nuclear proteins that bind to multiple positions in the ME promoter, including each of the areas that function as cis-acting regulatory sequences in the in vitro transcription assay. The binding activities of these proteins in liver nuclear extracts from hypothyroid and hyperthyroid rats were assayed by the "band-shift" assay. The binding of proteins that bound to DNA between bases −144 to −114 and −76 to −47 was diminished in hypothyroid rats and elevated in hyperthyroid rats. The time course of changes in the magnitude of binding and changes in the rate of transcription of the ME gene were similar, consistent with a role for these proteins in the $T_3$-stimulated increase in transcription.

The lack of a cell line in which ME responds to $T_3$ or other hormones has hampered functional analysis of hormone regulatory elements in the mammalian system. In an effort to circumvent that difficulty, COS-7 cells were co-transfected with an expression vector containing the cDNA for the $T_3$ receptor ligated to the promoter/enhancer of Rous Sarcoma virus and test vectors containing fragments of the 5′-flanking DNA of the rat ME gene ligated to the CAT gene.[62] When the ME test construct contained 882 base pairs of 5′-flanking DNA, addition of $T_3$ to the culture medium caused a five-fold increase in CAT activity. A similar result was observed when the 5′ end was deleted to −315. When an additional 68 base pairs were deleted to position −248, $T_3$-responsiveness was completely abolished. Based on this functional assay, therefore, a triiodothyronine response element (TRE) lies between −315 and −248. Most of the effects of $T_3$ are thought to originate from the binding of $T_3$ to its receptor, a protein bound to its cis-acting DNA sequence whether hormone is present or not.[63] The mechanism whereby ligand alters the ability of the $T_3$ receptor to regulate transcription from a nearby gene is unknown.

Authentic $T_3$ receptor was synthesized in a reticulocyte lysate programmed with in vitro-synthesized mRNA for the $T_3$ receptor. Reticulocyte lysate programmed with either the rat α or human β form of the $T_3$ receptor was incubated with the −178 to −357 fragment. Specific retarded bands were observed in the "band-shift" assay. Unprogrammed lysates or lysates programmed with other mRNAs did not produce these specific retarded bands. The same pattern of band-shifts was obtained whether $T_3$ was present or not, which is consistent with the hypothesis that the $T_3$ receptor binds to its TRE in the liganded or unliganded form. When lysate programmed with receptor mRNA was used in a DNA footprint analysis (*o*-phenanthroline copper method),[64] protection was observed from −280 to −260. Short oligonucleotides containing this or related sequences competed for binding of the receptor in the "band-shift" assay. These results argue strongly that a TRE is located between base −280 and −260 in the 5′-flanking DNA of the rat ME. Thus, stimulation of the transcription of the ME gene may well involve a dual mechanism—direct stimulation by the ligand-activated $T_3$ receptor and indirect stimulation via a $T_3$-stimulated increase in binding of a stimulatory trans-acting protein(s).

Cis-acting hormone regulatory elements are much less well characterized in the chicken ME gene. In chick-embryo hepatocytes transfected with a 400-base pair fragment of the 5′-flanking region ligated to the CAT gene, CAT activity is not stimulated by $T_3$ but is inhibited by about 60% by cAMP.[65] If a 5800-base pair fragment of flanking DNA is used, addition of $T_3$ stimulates a 15- to 20-fold increase in CAT activity and cAMP inhibits the $T_3$-stimulated increase by about 60%. These data suggest that a TRE and a cAMP-regulatory element are located somewhere between −400 and −5800 base pairs and +31 and −5300 base pairs upstream from the start site for transcription, respectively.

In summary, tracing the gene expression pathway backwards to its intersection(s) with intracellular signaling pathways leads to the conclusion that both hormones and nutrition regulate lipogenic enzyme activity primarily by regulating transcription of the lipogenic genes. It is generally agreed that thyroid hormone exerts its transcriptional effects by binding to its TRE-bound receptor, which in turn regulates transcription initiation. Although many details remain to be worked out, this phase of the analysis is likely to be completed in the near future. Once the TRE are identified and characterized, much of the pathway will be complete for this hormone. The role of other proteins in determining the specificity of a response to $T_3$ remains to be explored. For lipogenic as well as for all other genes, the molecular detail of how the liganded receptor facilitates an increase in gene transcription is an area of intense current interest in molecular biology. For cAMP, insulin, IGF-1, and other as-yet unidentified agents, tracing the signaling pathway back to the interaction of hormone or agent with its receptor remains a substantial challenge. After the hormone regulatory elements (HRE) are identified, trans-acting proteins that interact with that sequence will be identified and purified using many of the techniques described in this chapter. The next problem will be to determine how the signaling pathway regulates either the binding of the factor to the HRE or the transcriptional regulatory activity of the factor. Does the hormone or agent alter the protein by covalent modification, by allosteric mechanisms, or by altering its concentration? A similar set of analyses will be carried out for each step in the signaling pathway, until we understand the molecular nature of each event between regulation of transcription and binding of hormone or agent to receptor. Nutritional regulation is likely to involve modulation via several different hormones or agents. Thus another challenge will be to determine how the various signaling pathways interact to bring about a particular rate of transcription.

## REFERENCES


1. Volpe, J.J., Vagelos, P.R.: Physiol. Rev., *56*:339–417, 1976.
2. Wakil, S.J., Stoops, J.K., Joshi, V.C.: Annu. Rev. Biochem., *52*:537–579, 1983.
3. Goodridge, A.G.: Annu. Rev. Nutr., *7*:157–185, 1987.
4. Danforth, E. Jr., Burger, A.G.: Annu. Rev. Nutr., *9*:201–227, 1989.
5. Tepperman, H.M., Tepperman, J.: Am. J. Physiol., *206*:357–361, 1964.
6. Goodridge, A.G.: Fed. Proc., *34*:117–123, 1975.
7. Mariash, C.N., Oppenheimer, J.H.: Metabolism, *33*:545–552, 1983.
8. Kaiser, F.E., Mariash, C.N., Schwartz, H.L., Oppenheimer, J.H.: Metabolism, *29*:767–772, 1980.
9. Volpe, J.J., Vagelos, P.R.: Proc. Natl. Acad. Sci. U.S.A., *71*:889–893, 1974.
10. Clarke, S.D.: Metabolic adaptations to dietary fats. *In* Dietary Fat and Cancer. Edited by C. Ip, D.F. Birt, A.E. Rogers, and C. Metlin. New York, Alan R. Liss, 1986.
11. McKnight, G.S., Palmiter, R.D.: J. Biol. Chem., *254*:9050–9058, 1979.
12. Tanaka, T., Harano, Y., Sue, F., Morimura, H.: J. Biochem., *62*:71–91, 1967.
13. Sillero, A., Sillero, M.A.G., Sols, A.: Eur. J. Biochem., *10*:351–354, 1969.
14. Weber, G., Stamm, N.B., Fisher, E.A.: Science, *149*:65–67, 1965.
15. Cladaras, C., Cottam, G.L.: Arch. Biochem. Biophys., *200*:426–433, 1980.
16. Böttger, I., Kriegel, H., Wieland, O.: Eur. J. Biochem., *13*:253–257, 1970.
17. Noguchi, T., Inoue, H., Chen, H.-L., et al.: J. Biol. Chem., *258*:15220–15223, 1983.
18. Weber, A., Marie, J., Cottreau, D., et al.: J. Biol. Chem., *259*:1798–1802, 1984.
19. Marie, J., Simon, M.-P., Lone, H.-C., et al.: Eur. J. Biochem., *158*:33–41, 1986.
20. Munnich, A., Marie, J., Reach, G., et al.: J. Biol. Chem., *259*:10228–10231, 1984.
21. Noguchi, T., Inoue, H., Tanaka, T.: J. Biol. Chem., *260*:14393–14397, 1985.
22. Vaulont, S., Munnich, A., Marie, J., et al.: Biochem. Biophys. Res. Commun., *125*:135–141, 1984.
23. Inoue, H., Noguchi, T., Tanaka, T.: J. Biochem., *96*:1457–1462, 1984.
24. Noguchi, T., Inoue, H., Tanaka, T.: Eur. J. Biochem., *128*:583–588, 1982.
25. Decaux, J.-F., Antoine, B., Kahn, A.: J. Biol. Chem., *264*:11584–11590, 1989.
26. Miller, B.C., Cottam, G.L.: Arch. Biochem. Biophys., *254*:66–78, 1987.
27. Vaulont, S., Munnich, A., Decaux, J.-F., et al.: J. Biol. Chem., *261*:7621–7625, 1986.
28. Meienhofer, M.C., de Medicis, E., Cognet, M., Kahn, A.: Eur. J. Biochem., *169*:237–243, 1987.
29. Frenkel, R.: Curr. Top. Cell. Regul., *9*:157–181, 1975.
30. Li, J.J., Ross, C.R., Tepperman, H.M., et al.: J. Biol. Chem., *250*:141–148, 1975.
31. Silpananta, P., Goodridge, A.G.: J. Biol. Chem., *246*:5754–5761, 1971.
32. Sul, H.S., Wise, L.S., Brown, M.L., et al.: J. Biol. Chem., *259*:555–559, 1984.
33. Winberry, L.K., Morris, S.M. Jr., Fisch, J.E., et al.: J. Biol. Chem., *258*:1337–1342, 1983.
34. Ma, X.-J., Salati, L.M., Ash, S.E., et al.: J. Biol. Chem., *265*:18,435–18,441, 1990.
35. Berlin, C.M., Schimke, R.T.: Mol. Pharmacol., *1*:149–156, 1965.
36. Goldman, M.J., Back, D.W., Goodridge, A.G.: J. Biol. Chem., *260*:4404–4408, 1985.
37. Dozin, B., Rall, J.E., Nikodem, V.M.: Proc. Natl. Acad. Sci. U.S.A., *83*:4705–4709, 1986.
38. Song, M.-K.H., Dozin, B., Grieco, D., et al.: J. Biol. Chem., *263*:17,970–17,974, 1988.
39. Goodridge, A.G., Adelman, T.G.: J. Biol. Chem., *251*:3027–3032, 1976.
40. Stapleton, S.R., Mitchell, D.A., Salati, L.M., et al.: J. Biol. Chem., *265* : 18,442–18,446, 1990.
41. Mariash, C.N., McSwigan, C.R., Towle, H.C., et al.: J. Clin. Invest., *68*:1485–1490, 1981.
42. Spence, J.T., Pitot, H.C.: Eur. J. Biochem., *128*:15–20, 1982.
43. Dobbs, R., Sakurai, H., Sasaki, H., et al.: Science, *187*:544–547, 1975.
44. Goodridge, A.G., Crish, J.F., Hillgartner, F.B., et al.: J. Nutr., *119*:299–308, 1989.
45. Fukuda, H., Iratani, N., Tanaka, T.: J. Nutr. Sci. Vitaminol., *29*:691–699, 1983.
46. Katsurada, A., Iritani, N., Fukuda, H., et al.: Biochem. Biophys. Res. Commun., *112*:176–182, 1983.
47. Goodridge, A.G.: Regulation of malic enzyme in hepatocytes in culture: a model system for analyzing the mechanism of action of thyroid hormone. *In* Molecular Basis of Thyroid Hormone Action. Edited by J.H. Oppenheimer and H.H. Samuels. New York, Academic Press, 1983, pp. 245–263.
48. Magnuson, M.A., Nikodem, V.M.: J. Biol. Chem., *258*:12712–12717, 1983.
49. Salati, L.M., Ma, X.-J., McCormick, C.C., Stapleton, S.R., et al.: J. Biol. Chem., *266*:4010–4016, 1991.
50. Goodridge, A.G.: The role of nutrients in gene expression. *In* World Review of Nutrition and Dietetics. Vol. 63. Genetic Variation and Nutrition. Edited by A.P. Simopoulos and B. Childs. Basel, Karger, 1990, pp. 183–193.
51. Back, D.W., Wilson, S.B., Morris, S.M. Jr., et al.: J. Biol. Chem., *261*:12555–12561, 1986.
52. Elgin, S.C.R.: J. Biol. Chem., *283*:19259–19262, 1988.
53. Tremp, G.L., Boquet, D., Ripoche, M.-A., et al.: J. Biol. Chem., *264*:19904–19910, 1989.
54. Revzin, A.: BioTechniques, *7*:346–355, 1989.
55. Vaulont, S., Puzenat, N., Levrat, F., et al.: J. Mol. Biol., *209*:205–219, 1989.
56. Wynshaw-Boris, A., Short, J.M., Hanson, R.W.: BioTechniques, *4*:104–109, 1986.
57. Felgner, P.L., Gadek, T.R., Holm, M., et al.: Proc. Natl. Acad. Sci. U.S.A., *84*:7413–7417, 1987.
58. Ginot, F., Decaux, J.-F., Cognet, M., et al.: Eur. J. Biochem., *180*:289–294, 1989.
59. Usala, S.J., Young, W.S. III, Morioka, H., et al.: Mol. Endocrinol., *2*:619–626, 1988.
60. Morioka, H., Tennyson, G.E., Nikodem, V.M.: Mol. Cell. Biol., *8*:3542–3545, 1988.
61. Petty, K.J., Morioka, H., Mitsuhashi, T., et al.: J. Biol. Chem., *264*:11483–11490, 1989.

62. Petty, K.J., Desvergne, B., Mitsuhashi, T., et al.: J. Biol. Chem., *265*:7395–7400, 1990.
63. Samuels, H.H., Forman, B.M., Horwitz, Z.D., et al.: Annu. Rev. Physiol., *51*:623–639, 1989.
64. Kuwabara, M.D., Sigman, D.S.: Biochemistry, *26*:7234–7238, 1987.
65. Klautky, S.A., Goodridge, A.G.: FASEB J., *4*:A2095, 1990.

## SELECTED READINGS

Goodridge, A.G.: Dietary regulation of gene expression: Enzymes involved in carbohydrate and lipid metabolism. Annu. Rev. Nutr., *7*:157–185, 1987.

Granner, D., Pilkis, S.: The genes of hepatic glucose metabolism. J. Biol. Chem., *265*:10173–10176, 1990.

Roesler, W.J., Vandenbark, G.R., Hanson, R.W.: Cyclic AMP and the induction of eukaryotic gene expression. J. Biol. Chem., *263*:9063–9066, 1988.

The work reported from my laboratory was supported in part by Grant DK21594 from the National Institutes of Health and by the Core Facilities of the Diabetes and Endocrinology Research Center (DK25295).

CHAPTER **33**

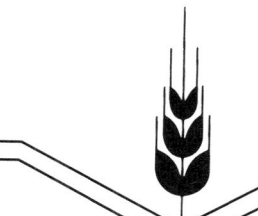

# Oxidative Stress, Oxidant Defense, and Dietary Constituents

**James A. Thomas**



Oxidative stress has been clearly implicated in human disease by a growing body of scientific evidence in recent years. Dietary constituents have likewise been implicated both as causative agents in oxidative stress and as protective agents in the antioxidant defense against stress. Foodstuffs contain both natural and added materials that participate in these processes, including vitamins and minerals, added antioxidants, pesticides, polyunsaturated lipids, and a variety of plant and microorganism-derived toxins. This chapter deals with our current understanding of the molecules that cause oxidative stress at the cellular level, with the antioxidant systems that function at the cellular and organismal level, and with the role of dietary materials in oxidative stress and human disease. Other chapters in this volume present more detailed information about individual vitamins and minerals and their potential participation in oxidative stress.

Oxidative stress has been defined as a disturbance in the equilibrium status of pro-oxidant/antioxidant systems in intact cells.[1] This definition of oxidative stress implies that cells have intact pro-oxidant/antioxidant systems that function continuously to generate and to detoxify oxidants during normal aerobic metabolism. When additional oxidative events occur, the proxidant systems may outbalance the antioxidant, resulting in oxidative damage to lipids, proteins, carbohydrates, and nucleic acids. Ultimately, cell death may occur from severe oxidative stress. Oxidative stress may also induce a rapid alteration in the antioxidant systems by inducing proteins that participate in these systems and by depleting cellular stores of antioxidant materials such as glutathione and vitamin E.

A disturbance in pro-oxidant/antioxidant systems results from a myriad of different oxidative challenges, including radiation, xenobiotic metabolism of environmental pollutants and other materials, and challenges to the immune system in human disease or in abnormal immune function. Clear evidence for the role of a variety of radical species in these processes has led to considerable interest in the reactions of partially reduced oxygen species and radical and nonradical species derived from them. A radical species is more specifically understood as any atom that contains one or more orbital electrons with unpaired spin states. The radical may be a very small molecule such as oxygen or it may be a part of a large biomolecule such as a protein, carbohydrate, lipid, or nucleic acid. Some radical species are very reactive with other biomolecules; others, like the normal triplet state of molecular oxygen, are relatively inert.

## RADICAL AND NONRADICALS IN OXIDATIVE STRESS

Radicals of oxygen (superoxide anion, and hydroxyl, alkyoxyl, and peroxyl radicals), reactive nonradical oxygen species (hydrogen peroxide and singlet oxygen), and radicals of carbon, nitrogen, and sulfur constitute the variety of reactive molecules that cause an oxidative stress to cells.[2,3] It has been estimated that a maximum of 5% of the total oxygen metabolism of liver cells results in the production of partially reduced oxygen species such as those shown in Figure 33–1. This is a significant stress by itself, but extracellular sources of these molecules may be even more significant. Therefore, much attention centers on the identification of excessive oxyradical-generating processes.

Atmospheric oxygen, although a radical, is not particularly reactive with biologic molecules because the two orbital electrons participating in oxidation reactions have the same spin state. Thus, electrons that might be added to these orbitals during reduction of oxygen must be added singly rather that as a pair of electrons with paired spins. This spin restriction prevents rapid reactions with compounds that could easily react without the spin restriction. A one-electron reduction of oxygen produces the more-reactive radical called superoxide anion. A second form of oxygen, singlet oxygen, is a much more reactive form with paired electrons. Reduction of this form of oxygen does not have the same spin-state restriction. Singlet oxygen is formed by oxidation of the other reactive oxygen intermediates in Figure 33–1 and itself may be an important reactant in oxidative stress. It has been identified in tissues under oxidative stress.

Superoxide anion is generated continuously by several cellular processes, the most important of which are the microsomal and mitochondrial electron transport systems. In addition, xanthine dehydrogenase/oxidase and other cellular oxidases may be important sources of this molecule. Myeloid cells have a special role in production of superoxide anion because they contain a plasma membrane-bound electron transfer complex that reduces oxygen with the reduced form of nicofinamide adenine dinucleotide phosphate (NADPH) to produce copious amounts of superoxide anion.[4] This process is a required component in the bactericidal action of these cells.

The presence of superoxide dismutase in both cytoplasm and mitochondria ensures that much of the superoxide is rapidly converted into hydrogen peroxide. Superoxide anion, which is not a particularly reactive molecule, can diffuse considerable distances from its site of production. It must be transported across membranes (by an anion transport mechanism), and in the vicinity of membranes it may be protonated to $HO_2$, becoming a much more reactive substance.

Hydrogen peroxide is generated by the same sources that produce superoxide anion because both enzymatic (superoxide dismutase) and nonenzymatic destruction of superoxide anion produces hydrogen peroxide. A number of other specific enzymes also produce hydrogen peroxide directly. These include peroxisomal enzymes associated with fatty acid metabolism and cytoplasmic enzymes responsible for the oxidation of a variety of cell metabolites. Hydrogen peroxide can diffuse over considerable distances and may pass through membranes readily. Thus, intracellular pools of hydrogen peroxide equilibrate rapidly across membrane boundaries.

Hydrogen peroxide and superoxide anion are found in extracellular space and in blood plasma as a result of the

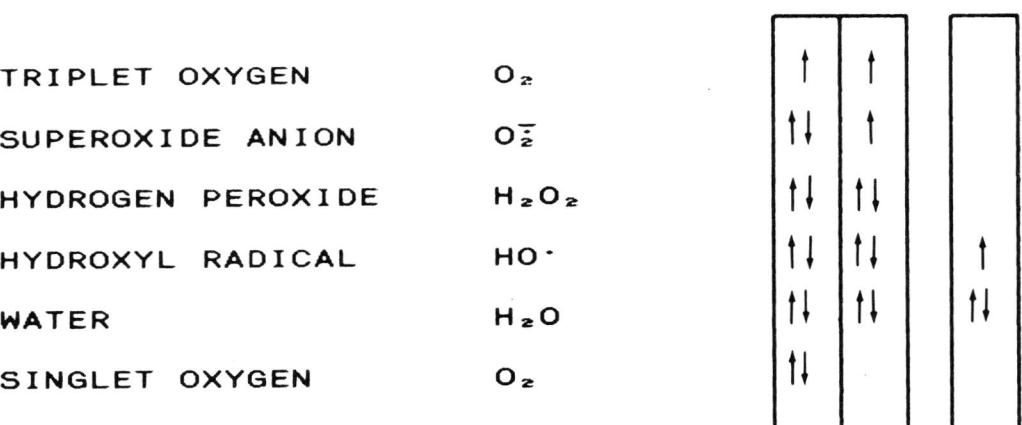

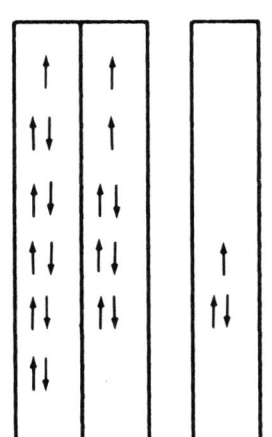

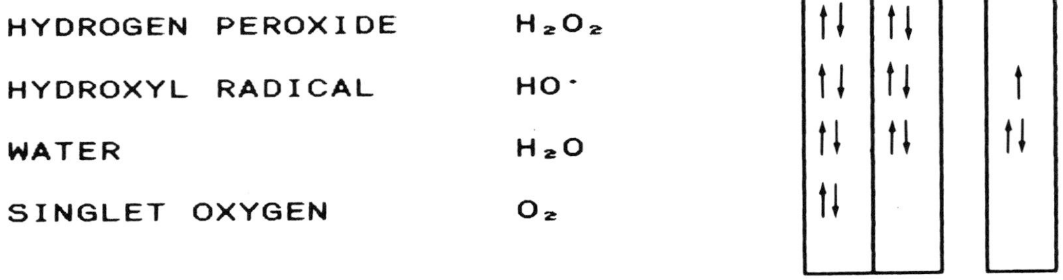
ELECTRON–ACCEPTING ORBITALS
π
σ
TRIPLET OXYGEN
O₂
SUPEROXIDE ANION
O₂⁻
HYDROGEN PEROXIDE
H₂O₂
HYDROXYL RADICAL
HO·
WATER
H₂O
SINGLET OXYGEN
O₂

**FIGURE 33–1.** Molecular species of oxygen in oxidative stress. Each relevant orbital electron is indicated by an arrow showing its spin state. Each molecular species (except for singlet oxygen) is obtained by a one electron reduction of the one above it in the table. In intact cells singlet oxygen is formed by oxidation of one of the partially reduced states of oxygen.

membrane-associated reaction of myeloid cells such as neutrophils and macrophages.[4] The membrane-associated NADPH-oxidase produces superoxide anion that rapidly dismutes to hydrogen peroxide as well.

In the presence of a transition cation such as iron or copper, superoxide anion can give rise to the highly reactive hydroxyl radical species by the Haber-Weiss reaction,[5,6] shown in the equation following. Some forms of bound iron are more efficient than free cationic iron in this process. Other complexes of iron prevent its participation in these reactions.

*Haber-Weiss Reaction*

$$O_2^{\overline{\cdot}} + H_2O_2 \rightarrow O_2 + HO^- + \underset{\text{Hydroxyl Radical}}{HO\cdot}$$

*Iron-Catalyzed Haber-Weiss Reaction*

$$Fe^{III} + O_2^{\overline{\cdot}} \rightarrow Fe^{II} + O_2$$
$$Fe^{II} + H_2O_2 \rightarrow Fe^{III} + HO^- + HO\cdot$$

Hydroxyl radical may be a principal actor in the toxicity of partially reduced oxygen species. It reacts with all kinds of biologic macromolecules and produces products that cannot be regenerated by cell metabolism (Fig. 33–2). The rate of reaction of hydroxyl radical is diffusion controlled, and it reacts close to its site of production. Therefore, damage by this radical is site-specific.

Peroxyl radicals occur during the oxidation of lipids in oxidative stress. They are associated with such processes as the iron-catalyzed destruction of lipid peroxides and the action of prostaglandin H synthase in prostaglandin synthesis.[7] These radicals may also be formed by a one-electron transfer from a carbon-centered radical to oxygen (reaction 1 below). The peroxyl radical species are not very reactive and may diffuse a considerable distance. They have been shown to react with sulfhydryl groups (thiols) to generate the thiyl radical (reaction 2 below).[8]

$$-\overset{|}{\underset{|}{C}}\cdot \longrightarrow -\overset{|}{\underset{|}{C}}OO\cdot \qquad (1)$$

$$\underset{\text{[thiolate anion]}}{R{-}S^-} + ROO\cdot \rightarrow \underset{\text{[thiyl radical]}}{R{-}S^{\overline{\cdot}}} + ROO^- \qquad (2)$$

Singlet oxygen is formed by oxidation of other partially reduced oxygen species, resulting in an oxygen with paired electrons in the reactive orbital.[2]

The variety of oxygen species described above indicates the complexity of the reactions that can result from an oxidative stress. Factors such as the site of production, the availability of transition metals, and the action of enzymes determine the fate of each radical species and its availability for reaction with cellular molecules. The $H_2O_2$ concentration under steady state conditions in liver has been estimated to be $10^{-7}$ to $10^{-9}$ mol/L, whereas superoxide anion may be approximately $10^{-11}$ mol/L.

## EFFECTS OF OXIDANTS ON MACROMOLECULES

### CARBOHYDRATES

Hydroxyl radicals react with carbohydrates by randomly abstracting a hydrogen atom from one of the carbon atoms, producing a carbon-centered radical.[9] This leads to chain breaks in important molecules such as hyaluronic acid in a process involving intermediates

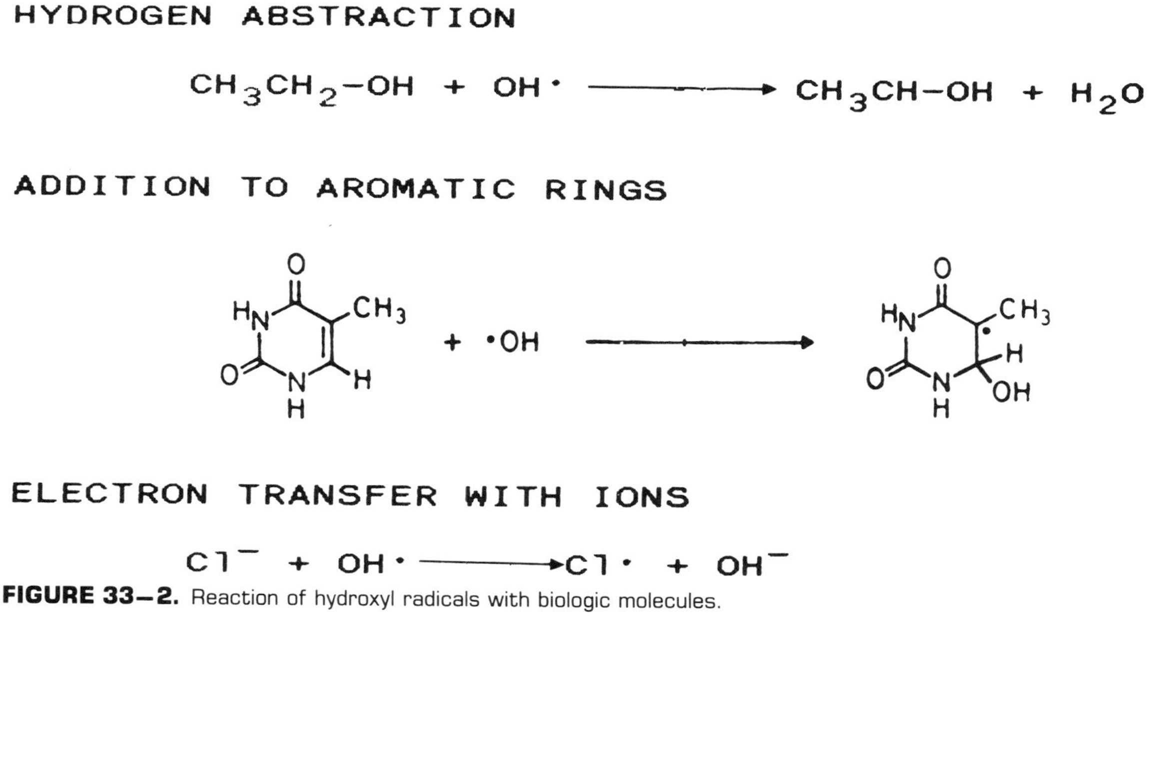
HYDROGEN ABSTRACTION
CH3CH2–OH + OH· → CH3CH–OH + H2O
ADDITION TO AROMATIC RINGS
+ ·OH
ELECTRON TRANSFER WITH IONS
Cl⁻ + OH· → Cl· + OH⁻

**FIGURE 33–2.** Reaction of hydroxyl radicals with biologic molecules.

such as peroxyl radicals (Fig. 33–3). In the synovial fluid surrounding joints, an accumulation and activation of neutrophils during inflammation produces significant amounts of oxyradicals. This phenomenon apparently accounts for a significant decrease in the synovial fluid of affected joints.

## NUCLEIC ACIDS

Nucleic acids are also carbohydrate polymers that can undergo reactions with hydroxyl radicals such as those depicted for hyaluronic acid[10] (Fig. 33–3). In addition, important examples of modifications to the base portion of the polymer have been demonstrated (Fig. 33–4). These base modifications may be responsible for genetic defects produced by oxidative stress. Recently, 8-hydroxy guanosine has generated considerable interest as a product of hydroxyl radical attack on DNA that can be used to estimate DNA damage in humans.[11,12] Oxidative damage to DNA has been estimated as $10^4$ hits per cell per day. Estimation of modified bases in urine is proving to be a useful means of assessing the amount of DNA damage in experimental animals. Products such as 8-hydroxy guanosine, thymine glycol, and uric acid are used in this manner. DNA damage has also been estimated by chain breaks and base modifications in cultured cells under oxidative stress. An important metabolic effect of DNA damage is the rapid induction of polyadenosine diphosphate ribose synthesis (ADP-ribosylation) in nuclei, resulting in extensive depletion of cellular NADH pools. ADP-ribosylation has been associated with repair of damaged DNA.

## PROTEINS

Proteins have many reactive sites that can be damaged during oxidative stress, but interest has centered on three measurable events. First, aggressive radicals such as hydroxyl radical can fragment proteins in plasma, and the fragmented products of specific proteins can be detected if these are known.[13] This fragmentation is associated with reactions at specific amino acids such as proline and histidine[14] (Fig. 33–5). Second, proteins may contain metal binding sites that are especially susceptible to oxidative events through interaction with the metals. These reactions usually produce irreversible modifications in amino acids that might be involved in metal ion binding, such as histidine. These modifications may produce signal sequences that are recognized by specific cellular proteases that degrade such proteins.[15,16] Finally, many intracellular proteins have "reactive" sulfhydryl groups on specific cysteine residues (see following sections on antioxidants) that can be modified (oxidized) to specific forms (disulfides), which can be reduced again by metabolic processes.[17] Similarly, some extracellular proteins have a "reactive" methionine that can undergo reversible modification.[18] These latter events may function as protection mecha-

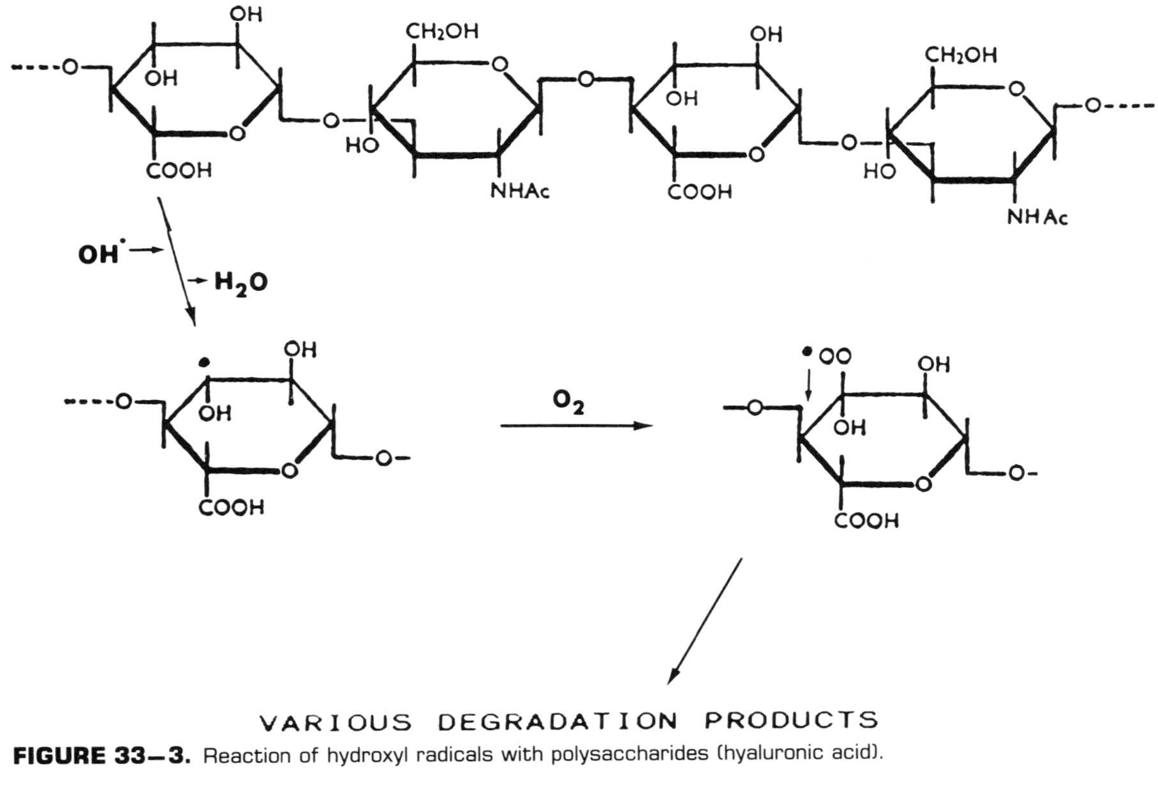
OH
CH₂OH
OH
CH₂OH
OH
OH
HO
HO
COOH
NHAc
COOH
NHAc
OH˙
H₂O
OH
OH
COOH
O₂
•OO
OH
OH
COOH
VARIOUS DEGRADATION PRODUCTS

**FIGURE 33–3.** Reaction of hydroxyl radicals with polysaccharides (hyaluronic acid).

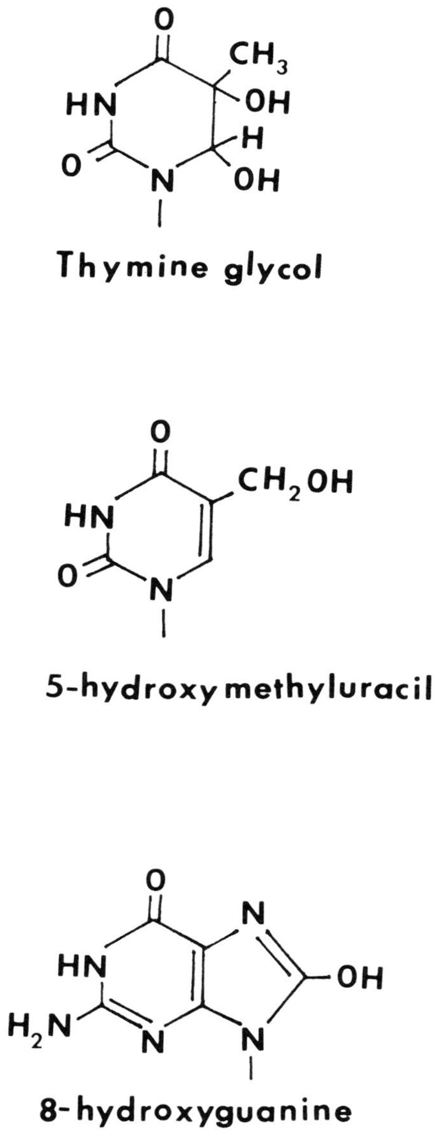
Thymine glycol
5-hydroxymethyluracil
8-hydroxyguanine

**FIGURE 33–4.** Some modified bases found in DNA after oxidative stress.

nisms for individual proteins, and may also act in an antioxidant capacity to protect other cell constituents that do not contain these sulfur constituents. The reversible nature of cysteine and methionine modification suggests that they may have a regulatory role in cellular metabolism during oxidative stress.

### LIPIDS

Lipid peroxidation is a facile process with polyunsaturated lipids, materials that are prevalent in dietary constituents and in cellular membranes.[19,20] Peroxidation of cellular lipid results in a variety of deleterious effects on important membrane functions. Most peroxidized lipid occurs as a result of oxidative stress in intact cells, but some peroxidized lipid in the diet may be directly incorporated into cell structures.[21] Lipid peroxidation is a radical-initiated chain reaction that is self-propagating in cellular membranes. As a result isolated oxidative events may have profound effects on membrane function. The reactions of this process are depicted in Figure 33–6.

The products of lipid peroxidation are easily detected in blood plasma and have been used as a measure of oxidative stress. The most commonly measured product is malondialdehyde (Fig. 33–6). In addition the unsaturated aldehydes produced from these reactions have been implicated in the modification of cellular proteins and other materials.[22] The peroxidized lipid can produce peroxy radicals and singlet oxygen by the reactions discussed above. Vitamin E is particularly effective as an antioxidant in lipid peroxidizing systems.

## CELLULAR ANTIOXIDANTS

The most effective antioxidant in oxidative stress depends on the specific molecules causing the stress (e.g., superoxide anion, lipid peroxides, iron-generated hydroxyl radical) and the cellular or extracellular location of the source of these molecules. As an example, damage to a cell membrane occurs from both internally and externally generated oxidative stress. This damage is most effectively prevented by vitamin E, which reacts with peroxyl and hydroxyl radicals; by carotenoids, which react with singlet oxygen; and possibly by membrane-bound proteins. The chain-breaking anti-oxidant function of vitamin E in membranes results from its close association with polyunsaturated components of the membrane.[23] Vitamin E radical can be reduced by cytoplasmic vitamin C and glutathione, or by membrane-bound quinols. Vitamin C is reduced by glutathione that is reduced by the glutathione cycle described below. Thus, a specific attack on membranes results in the participation of at least three different antioxidants. Similarly, when oxidative stress occurs in plasma, a variety of different antioxidants participate in the response. Many plasma proteins are affected by the process, causing either irreversible or reversible loss of functional protein activity. A good example is the oxidation of methionine residues in $\alpha_1$ protease inhibitor (an inhibitor of elastase). The modification can be reversed by a specific reductase enzyme that restores that activity of the inhibitor.[18]

### GLUTATHIONE AND PROTEIN SULFHYDRYLS

The low-molecular-weight thiol, glutathione, and "reactive" protein sulfhydryls (specific cysteines in many proteins), are primary participants in cellular antioxi-

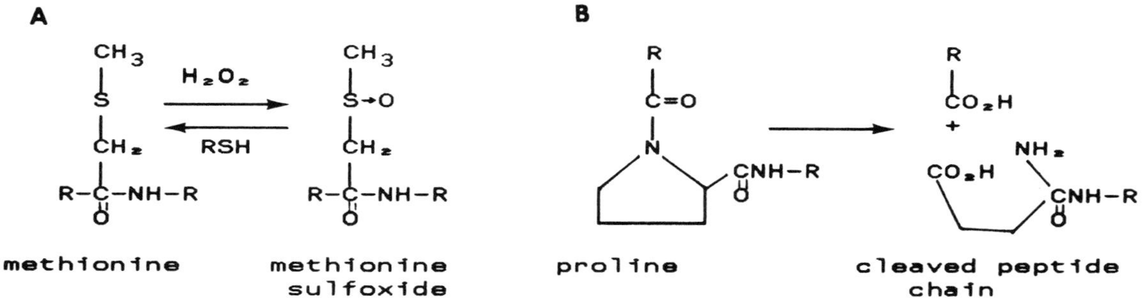
A
B
$H_2O_2$
RSH
methionine
methionine sulfoxide
proline
cleaved peptide chain

**FIGURE 33–5.** Methionine and proline oxidation. *A*, The reversible oxidation/reduction of methionine in some proteins. The reduction is an enzymatic process that requires a reduced thiol such as glutathione. *B*, The irreversible oxidation of proline. The result is a break in the polypeptide chain and the introduction of new carboxyl groups that can be measured to quantitate these events.

| | |
|---|---|
| INITIATION | LIPID + [R· / OH·] → LIPID· + [RH / $H_2O$] |
| PROPAGATION | LIPID· + $O_2$ → LIPID-OO· |
| | LIPID-OO· + LIPID → LIPID-OOH + LIPID· |
| TERMINATION | LIPID· + LIPID· → LIPID-LIPID |
| | LIPID-OO· + LIPID-OO· → LIPID-OO-LIPID + $O_2$ |
| | LIPID-OO· + LIPID· → LIPID-OO-LIPID |
| SCAVENGING | LIPID· + VIT E → LIPID + VIT E· |

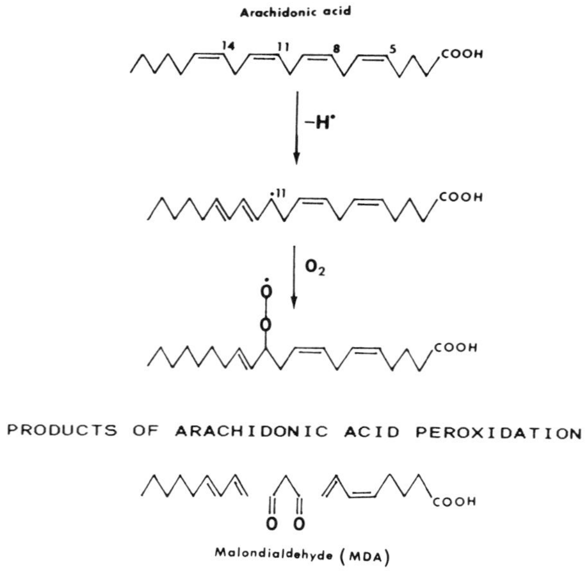
Arachidonic acid
14
11
8
5
COOH
-H·
·11
COOH
$O_2$
COOH
PRODUCTS OF ARACHIDONIC ACID PEROXIDATION
COOH
Malondialdehyde (MDA)

**FIGURE 33–6.** Reactions of lipid peroxidation.

dant systems. Glutathione is abundant (3 to 10 mmol/L) in cytoplasm, nuclei, and mitochondria (Fig. 33–7), and it is the major soluble antioxidant in these fractions.[24] The concentration of reactive protein sulfhydryls is equally high in both soluble proteins and in membrane-bound proteins.[25] "Reactive" protein sulfhydryls probably make up the largest pool of thiols in cells.

The sulfur atom in these sulfhydryls easily accommodates an extra electron (reaction 1 below), and the lifetime of radical species of sulfur (e.g., a thiyl radical) is

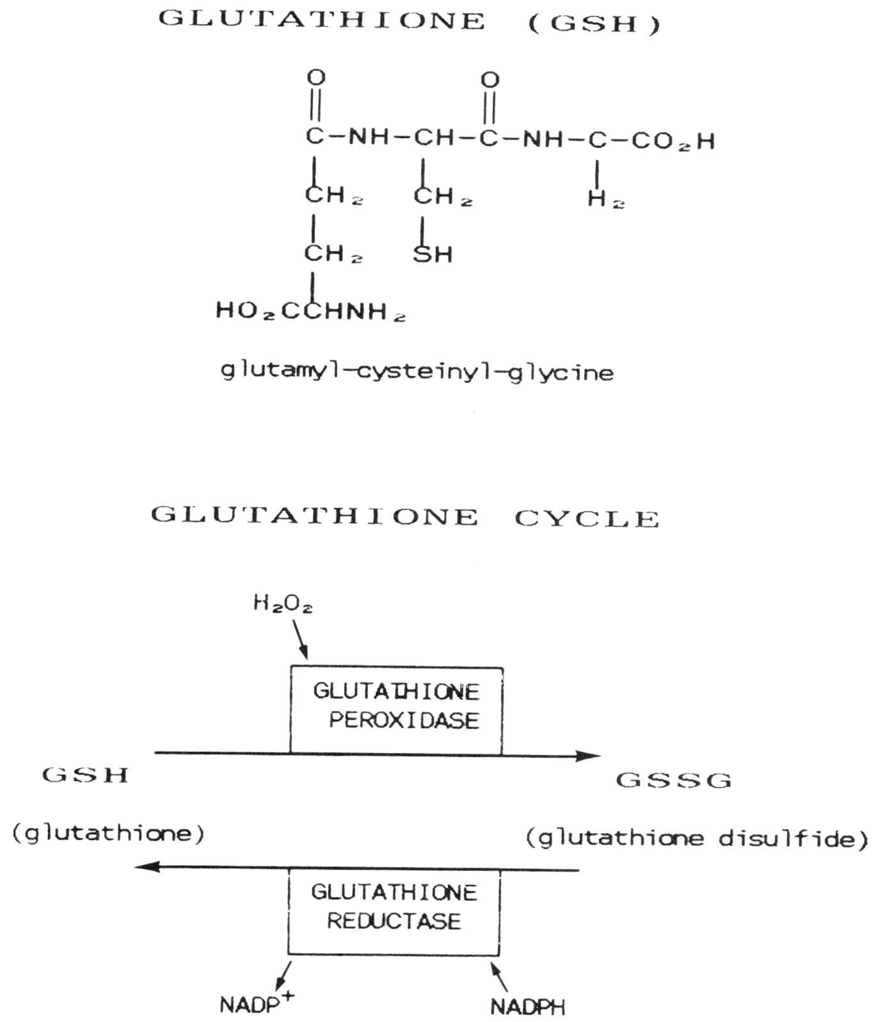
GLUTATHIONE (GSH)
glutamyl-cysteinyl-glycine
GLUTATHIONE CYCLE
$H_2O_2$
GLUTATHIONE PEROXIDASE
GSH
(glutathione)
GSSG
(glutathione disulfide)
GLUTATHIONE REDUCTASE
$NADP^+$
NADPH

**FIGURE 33–7.** Structure and metabolism of glutathione.

long compared to many other radicals that can be generated during stress. Many sulfhydryl groups are also partially ionized at cellular pHs, producing the very reactive, nucleophilic thiolate anion (reaction 2). The thiolate anion is responsible for the reactivity of thiols with a variety of foreign materials in conjugation reactions during xenobiotic metabolism. Thus, the reactions of sulfhydryls during oxidative stress include examples in which both sulfur radicals and thiolate anions are important.

$$\text{Glutathione–SH} \rightarrow \text{glutathione–S}\cdot \qquad (1)$$

$$\text{Protein–SH} \rightarrow \text{protein–S}\cdot$$

$$\text{R–SH} \rightarrow \text{R–S}^- + \text{H}^+ \qquad (2)$$

$$\text{Protein–SH} \rightarrow \text{protein–S}^-$$

The enzymes of the glutathione redox cycle are shown in Figure 33–7. In that cycle, glutathione is oxidized by hydrogen peroxide to glutathione disulfide by the selenium-containing enzyme, glutathione peroxidase, and by other enzymes that may use lipid peroxides rather than hydrogen peroxide as the oxidant. Thus, glutathione can detoxify both soluble and lipid peroxides. Glutathione disulfide is subsequently reduced by glutathione reductase, using NADPH as the reductant. Cellular NADPH, produced by the pentose phosphate pathway and by other cytoplasmic sources, provides the major source of reducing power for detoxifying many peroxides. As mentioned previously, glutathione can also act as a reductant for vitamin C, and it can directly reduce some protein-bound sulfhydryls. In combination with an enzyme called glutaredoxin (or thioltransferase), glutathione can reduce a larger number of protein sulfhydryls[26] (Fig. 33–8).

The concentration of cellular glutathione has a major effect on its antioxidant function. Nutrient limitation, exercise, and oxidative stress have major effects on

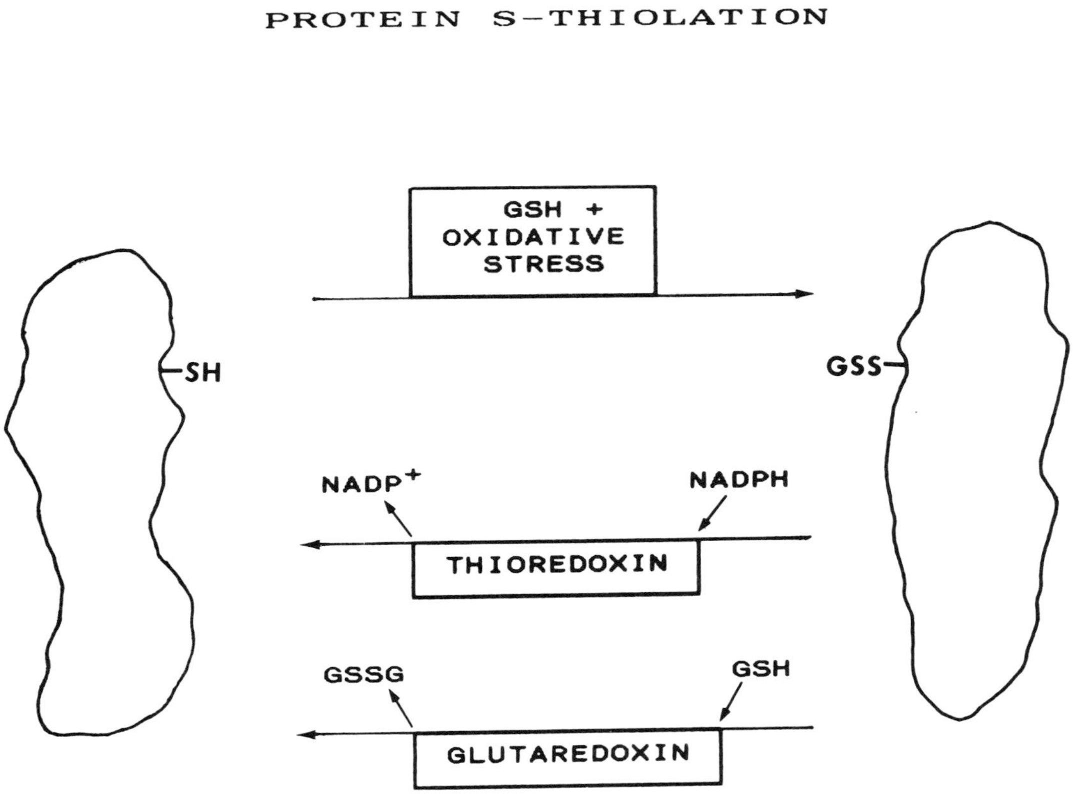
PROTEIN S–THIOLATION
GSH + OXIDATIVE STRESS
–SH
GSS–
NADP+
NADPH
THIOREDOXIN
GSSG
GSH
GLUTAREDOXIN

**FIGURE 33–8.** Protein sulfhydryl cycle in oxidative stress. The figure on the left shows a protein with a reduced "reactive" sulfhydryl (SH), and the figure on the right shows that protein in the S-thiolated state, i.e., with a molecule of glutathione (GSH) attached to the "reactive" sulfhydryl by a disulfide bond. The S-thiolated protein is formed during oxidative stress but can be reduced effectively by two different mechanisms that involve small dithiol proteins, i.e., thioredoxin and glutaredoxin.

glutathione concentration. Under oxidative conditions, glutathione can be considerably diminished through conjugation to xenobiotics, and by secretion of both the glutathione conjugates and glutathione disulfide from the affected cells. A considerable amount of glutathione may also become protein-bound during severe oxidative stress. Recently, compounds that can both increase and decrease the glutathione concentration when administered to animals have been developed.[27]

Protein sulfhydryls are also very reactive toward oxygen radicals and other oxidants formed during oxidative stress. During oxidative stress, a large number of proteins are modified by oxidation of the sulfhydryls, often producing protein mixed-disulfides with glutathione, a process called S-thiolation[17] (Fig. 33–8). Protein-protein disulfides and other oxidation states of the protein sulfhydryl (sulfenic and sulfonic acids) may also be produced during oxidative stress. S-thiolated proteins and protein disufides are easily reduced by cellular reductive processes, whereas sulfonic acids are not easily reduced. Figure 33–8 shows the reactions involved in the reversible modification of proteins by S-thiolation. Two low-molecular-weight proteins, such as glutaredoxin and thioredoxin,[26,28] can participate in the reduction of these proteins.

## VITAMIN E AND MEMBRANE PEROXIDATION

Vitamin E refers to a family of related compounds (tocopherols) that have hydroxylated aromatic rings (chromanol rings) and polyisoprenoid side chains. The molecule is highly lipophilic and resides almost exclusively in cell membranes. The chromanol ring may be at the surface of the membrane and the polyisoprenoid chain is inserted into the bilayer.[29] The chromanol ring is the active radical-quenching part of the vitamin. Because lipid peroxidation occurs on unsaturated fatty acid chains that reside within the lipid bilayer, the action of vitamin E as an antioxidant must involve considerable movement of the lipids and vitamin E to promote molecular interaction.[30] The reactions by which a chromanol ring can participate in these processes are shown in the Figure 33–9. Vitamin E is a chain reaction–breaking antioxidant because it quenches the intermediate in the chain reaction. The ascorbate radical formed in

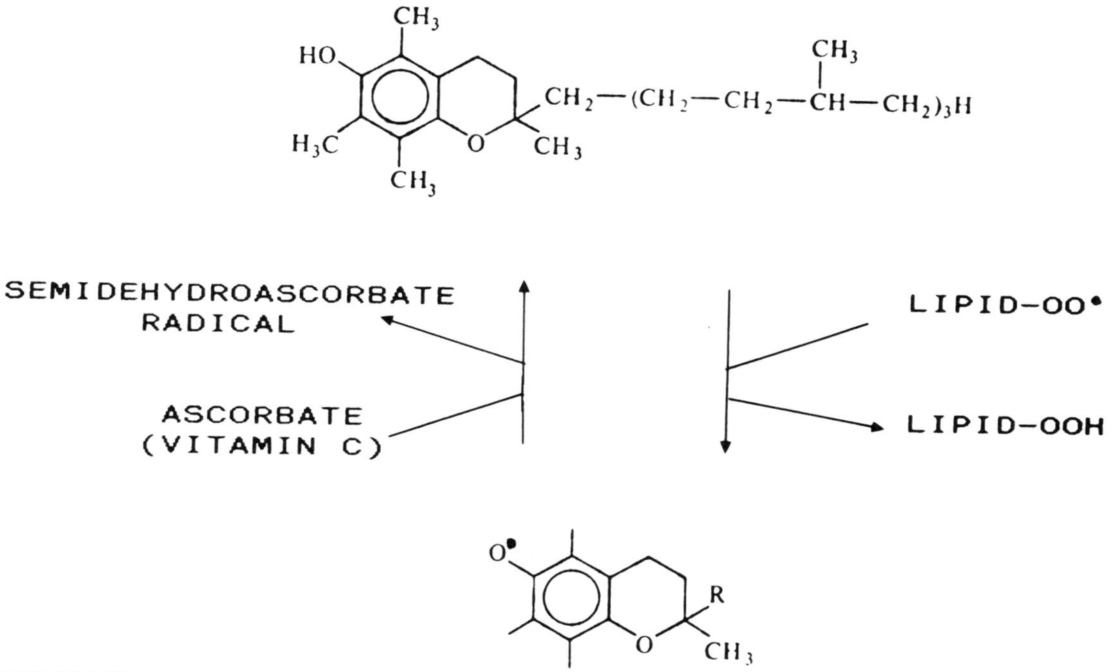
SEMIDEHYDROASCORBATE RADICAL
ASCORBATE (VITAMIN C)
LIPID-OO•
LIPID-OOH

**FIGURE 33–9.** Reaction of vitamin E with lipid radicals.

this process reacts rapidly with reduced glutathione, as discussed earlier.

## ENZYMES

Superoxide dismutase is one of the most important enzymes that function as cellular antioxidants.[31] It is present in cell cytoplasm (copper-zinc enzyme) and in mitochondria (manganese enzyme) in order to maintain a low concentration of superoxide anion.

$$2\ O_2^{\bar{}} + 2\ H^+ \rightarrow O_2 + H_2O_2 \text{ Superoxide dismutase}$$

The absence of this enzyme is lethal, but increasing its concentration in cells may not increase antioxidant protection. It has been suggested that an excess of this enzyme may produce hydrogen peroxide at a rate that makes it more toxic to cells in oxidative stress. Superoxide dismutase is increased by specific redox-sensitive genes in cells under continued stress.[32] An extracellular form of superoxide dismutase, different from the intracellular forms of the enzyme, occurs in plasma, lymph, and synovial fluid.[33] The extracellular enzyme may function at cell surfaces.

Catalase is a heme protein that catalyzes the reaction shown below. It is usually found in peroxisomes. In cells such as erythrocytes, which do not contain these organelles, it is a cytoplasmic enzyme.[34] Catalase provides a protective role that is similar to that of glutathione peroxidase in most cells. The relative contribution of catalase and glutathione peroxidase to hydrogen peroxide detoxification is variable.[35]

$$2\ H_2O_2 \rightarrow O_2 + 2\ H_2O \text{ Catalase}$$

Superoxide dismutase and catalase provide a rapid means of equilibrating and detoxifying superoxide anion and hydrogen peroxide in cells. In addition, both enzymes have considerable use as pharmacologic agents to decrease the effect of oxygen radicals in human disease. There has been interest in these enzymes for prevention of reperfusion injury (discussed later).[36]

## PLASMA ANTIOXIDANTS

Human plasma contains little catalase, superoxide dismutase, glutathione, or glutathione peroxidase; the antioxidant properties of this important fluid reside primarily in a number of small molecules and protein constituents. In studies using both artificially generated oxidants and natural oxidants such as cigarette smoke, ascorbate is among the first compounds that become oxidized in stress.[38,39] Other plasma components may become oxidized only when ascorbate is depleted. Oxidation affects thiol groups (mostly on proteins), bilirubin, urate, and finally vitamin E. Bilirubin (bound to albumin) and uric acid, both considered to be metabolic waste products in plasma, are potentially good scavengers of oxyradicals. Transport into and from erythocytes may provide additional antioxidant potential, because the reductive processes of these cells are vigorous.

The antioxidant proteins of plasma that are most important include ceruloplasmin, albumin, transferrin, haptoglobin, and hemopexin. The first three proteins may sequester iron and copper ions in forms that prevent their participation in reactions that generate the aggressive hydroxyl radical. Haptoglobin and hemopexin bind free heme, a source of iron that can participate in lipid oxidation reactions.

Oxidative stress also affects plasma lipid particles such as low-density lipoproteins (LDL).[39] The proteins and lipids in LDLs are good targets for oxidation, and the oxidized forms of LDL are now strongly implicated in formation of fatty lesions (atheromas) in artery walls. The apoprotein B component of these particles is fragmented by oxidation. A variety of lipid peroxidation products, including adducts of lipid and apoprotein B, are produced. LDL particles contain a significant amount of vitamin E and carotenoids that may serve as primary antioxidants.

## HUMAN DISEASE AND OXIDATIVE STRESS

### CANCER

Radicals of different kinds, including oxyradicals, are involved in both initiation and promotion in multistage cancer development.[40,41] In this process, DNA is damaged and the cellular antioxidant systems are modified as a result of the expression of different genetic components in precancerous and tumor cells. Because specific genes are apparently controlled by oxidation/reduction switching of important gene regulatory proteins, the effect of oxidative stress may be manifested directly by alterations in these specific proteins.[32,41] On the other hand, base modifications may also cause an altered response of certain genes during oxidative stress (see Fig. 33–4). Free radical scavengers function as inhibitors at both the initiation and promotion stage of carcinogenesis, thus protecting cells from the oxidative damage that occurs.[42] In tumors the enzymes involved in antioxidant systems are altered (i.e., tumors are low in manganese superoxide dismutase and possibly the copper-zinc enzyme, while glutathione peroxidase, reductase, and S-transferase are increased). In keeping with an increase in glutathione metabolism, one also finds increased glucose 6-phosphate dehydrogenase, a source of NADPH for the glutathione and protein S-thiolation cycles (see Figs. 33–7 and 33–8).

Some of the effective quinone-type anticancer drugs are also promoters of oxyradical production.[43] These drugs may be effective because of their ability to generate oxidative species that cause DNA, membrane, or enzyme damage in tumor cells.

### CATARACT AND EYE INJURY

The crystallins, the major proteins of the eye lens, are long-lived proteins that are unusually abundant in methionine and cysteine groups. These are easily oxidized protein components during oxidative stress and much work has implied a direct role of oxidative stress in the development of opacities in the lens.[44,45] The lens is a highly susceptible target, because it is continually exposed to the effects of light and a number of oxidizing metabolic products. The lens has a high concentration of both glutathione and glutathione reductase. There is good evidence that glutathione decreases substantially in lens lesions. The vitreous humor of the eye also contains hyaluronic acid that is depolymerized when exposed to oxyradicals. Dietary vitamin E has been shown to help prevent eye damage in infants exposed to high oxygen concentrations.

### REPERFUSION INJURY

There is growing evidence that oxyradicals can mediate tissue injury during ischemia and reperfusion.[46] This phenomenon has been implicated in the treatment of myocardial infarcts, and neutrophils have been implicated as a causative agent. The accumulation of neutrophils in the damaged tissue produces a significant oxidant stress to the surviving tissue cells, leading to irreversible injury to those cells as a result of the massive generation of superoxide anion and other neutrophil products.[47] This damage has been successfully prevented with inhibitors of oxyradical generation (e.g., allopurinol) and with materials that destroy the radicals after generation (e.g., superoxide dismutase or mannitol).[36]

### ARTHRITIS AND RHEUMATIC DISORDERS

These diseases are characterized by inflammatory responses in which extensive tissue damage can occur through oxidative stress. In rheumatoid arthritis, the effects of oxyradicals on the function of synovial fluid have been well documented (see Fig. 33–3). In addition, extensive cellular damage results in the release of clastogenic factors, and typical cellular damage products are detected in urine. Thus, materials such as peroxidized lipid or modified bases from cellular DNA have been found in urine of patients suffering from these diseases. It has been postulated that antigens may be created by oxyradical attack on biomolecules, thereby instigating development of autoimmune antibodies and a continuing inflammatory response to affected tissue.

## NUTRITIONAL EFFECTS ON OXIDATIVE STRESS

The idea that diet plays an important role in oxidative stress has been enhanced in recent years by studies on toxic dietary materials such as pesticides, alcohol, and carcinogens (both natural and synthetic), and on both natural and synthetic antioxidants.[48,49] Equally important, the biologic action of many essential nutrients has been related to oxidative stress and resultant disease. Minerals such as selenium, iron, copper, and zinc, vitamins such as A, C, and E, and other supplementary materials such as carotenoids, cholesterol, and unsaturated fats presumably play important roles in the balance between pro-oxidant and antioxidant systems in humans. It seems likely that some dietary supplements will have a relationship to the toxicity of other components of the diet.

Alcohol toxicity presents a good example of a dietary material that may directly increase cellular oxidative stress.[48] Ethanol produces lipid peroxidation in liver, and oxygen radicals have been directly demonstrated after ethanol ingestion by advanced spin-trapping techniques. Antioxidants can also prevent induction of ethanol-induced fatty liver. Several mechanisms have been suggested to account for the oxidative stress resulting from alcohol ingestion.

Lipid hydroperoxides and the decomposition products from lipid peroxidation are other examples of dietary components that have been studied as potential sources of oxidative stress.[21,50] With a diet high in unsaturated fats, lipid peroxides become an important dietary constituent; indeed, diets high in peroxidized lipid have toxic effects on growth and tissue function. However, dietary peroxides do not accumulate significantly in tissues, suggesting that the break-down products from these unstable materials may be more important than the peroxides themselves. Thus, addition of antioxidants to food decreases the amount of lipid peroxides and their break-down products. On the other hand, some antioxidants such as BHA (butylated hydroxyanisole) have carcinogenic effects in some animal models, suggesting that added antioxidants may have a complex action as dietary constituents.[42]

Dietary polyunsaturated fatty acids may also have a direct effect on the peroxidation of cellular lipids because these dietary lipids can alter the membrane composition of various cells, making them more or less susceptible to peroxidation damage during oxidative stress.[21]

It seems clear that the role of nutritional components in oxidative stress should be a continuing and important field of investigation in the near future. The importance of these experiments will be enhanced by continuing to study the cellular basis of oxidative stress and antioxidant protection. The mechanisms of cell injury by oxidative stress, and the protection of cells from this injury, potentially involve many dietary constituents that may diminish or enhance the role of oxidative stress in disease.

## REFERENCES

1. Sies, H.: Oxidative Stress: Introductory remarks. *In* Oxidative Stress. Edited by H. Sies. Orlando, FL, Academic Press, 1985, pp. 1–8.
2. Cardenas, E.: Annu. Rev. Biochem., *58:*79–110, 1989.
3. Slater, T.F.: Biochem. J., *222:*1–15, 1984.
4. Badwey, J.A., Karnovsky, M.L.: Curr. Topics Cell. Regul., *28:*183–208, 1986.
5. Halliwell, B., Gutteridge, J.M.C.: Biochem. J., *219:*1–14, 1984.
6. Sutton, H.C.: J. Free Radic. Biol. Med., *1:*195–202, 1985.
7. Marnett, L.J.: Carcinogenesis, *8:*1365–1373, 1989.
8. Willson, R.L.: Organic Peroxy Free Radicals as Ultimate Agents in Oxygen Toxicity. Edited by H. Sies. Orlando, FL, Academic Press, 1985, pp. 41–72.
9. von Sonntag, C.: Adv. Carbohydr. Chem. Biochem., *37:*7–77, 1980.
10. Shulte-Frohlinde, D., von Sonntag, C.: Radiolysis of DNA and Model Systems in the Presence of Oxygen. Edited by H. Sies. Orlando, FL, Academic Press, 1985, pp. 11–40.
11. Fraga, C.G., Shigenaga, J.P., Degan, P., Ames, B.N.: Proc. Natl. Acad. Sci. U.S.A., *87:*4533–4537, 1990.
12. Floyd, R.A.: FASEB J., *4:*2587–2597, 1990.
13. Wolff, S.P., Garner, A., Dean, R.T.: Trends Biochem. Sci., *11:*27–31, 1986.
14. Dean, R.T., Wolff, S.P., and McElligott, M.A.: Free Radic. Res. Commun., *7:*97–103, 1989.
15. Stadtman, E.R.: Free Radic. Biol. Med., *9:*315–325, 1990.
16. Davies, K.J.A.: J. Biol. Chem., *262:*9895–9901, 1987.
17. Miller, R.M., Sies, H., Park, E-M., Thomas, J.A.: Arch. Biochem. Biophys., *276:*355–363, 1990.
18. Brot, H., Weissbach, H.: Arch. Biochem. Biophys., *223:*271–281, 1983.
19. Gutteridge, J.M.C.: Lipid Peroxidation; Some Problems and Concepts. Edited by B. Halliwell. Bethesda, MD, FASEB for Upjohn Co., 1988.
20. Gardner, H.W.: Free Radic. Biol. Med., *7:*65–86, 1989.
21. Wills, E.D.: The Role of Dietary Components in Oxidative Stress in Tissues. Edited by H. Sies. Orlando, FL, Academic Press, 1985, pp. 197–220.
22. Witz, G.: Free Radic. Biol. Med., *7:*333–349, 1989.
23. Pascoe, G.A., Reed, D.J.: Free Radic. Biol. Med., *6:*209–224, 1989.
24. Meister, A.: J. Biol. Chem., *263:*17205–17208, 1988.
25. Ziegler, D.M.: Annu. Rev. Biochem., *54:*305–330, 1985.
26. Chai, Y-C., Jung, C-H., Lii, C-K., et al.: Arch. Biochem. Biophys., *284:*191–200, 1991.
27. Anderson, M.E., Meister, A.: Anal. Biochem., *183:*16–20, 1989.

28. Park, E.M., Thomas, J.A.: Arch. Biochem. Biophys., *272:*47–54, 1989.
29. Niki, E., Yamamoto, Y., Takahashi, M., et al.: Ann. N.Y. Acad. Sci., *570:*23–31, 1989.
30. Wayner, D.D.M., Burton, G.W., Ingold, K.U., et al.: Biochim. Biophys. Acta, *924:*408–419, 1987.
31. Fridovich, I.: J. Biol. Chem., *264:*7761–7764, 1989.
32. Storz, G., Tartaglia, L.A., Ames, B.N.: Science, *248:*189–194, 1990.
33. Marklund, S.L.: Proc. Natl. Acad. Sci. U.S.A., *79:*7634–7638, 1982.
34. Jones, D.P.: Archiv. Biochem. Biophys., *214:*806–814, 1982.
35. Thayer, W.S.: FEBS Lett., *202:*137–140, 1986.
36. Greenwald, R.A.: Free Radic. Biol. Med., *8:*201–209, 1990.
37. Halliwell, B., Gutteridge, J.M.C.: Arch. Biochem. Biophys., *280:*1–8, 1990.
38. Stocker, R., Glazer, A.N., Ames, B.N., Proc. Natl. Acad. Sci. U.S.A., *84:*5918–5922, 1987.
39. Steinbrecher, U.P., Zhang, H., Lougheed, M.: Free Radic. Biol. Med., *9:*155–168, 1990.
40. Sun, Y.: Free Radic. Biol. Med., *8:*583–599, 1990.
41. Abate, C., Patel, L., Raucher, F.J., Curran, T.: Science, *249:*1157–1161, 1990.
42. Ito, N., Hirose, M.: Adv. Cancer Res., *53:*247–303, 1989.
43. Powis, G.: Free Radic. Biol. Med., *6:*63–101, 1989.
44. Bloemendal, H.: CRC Crit. Rev. Biochem., *14:*1–38, 1982.
45. Mandel, K., Chakrabarti, B., Thomson, J., Siezen, R.J.: J. Biol. Chem., *262:*8096–8102, 1987.
46. Simpson, P.J., Fantone, J.C., Lucchesi, B.R.: Myocardial Ischemia and Reperfusion Injury: Oxygen Radicals and the Role of the Neutrophil. Edited by B. Halliwell. Bethesda, MD, FASEB for Upjohn, 1988.
47. Warren, J.S., Yabroff, K.R., Mandel, D.M., et al.: Free Radic. Biol. Med., *8:*163–172, 1990.
48. Cederbaum, A.I.: Free Radic. Biol. Med., *7:*537–539, 1989.
49. Ames, B.N., Magaw, R., Gold, L.S.: Science, *236:*271–280, 1987.
50. Kowalski, D.P., Feeley, R.M., Jones, D.P.: J. Nutr., *120:*1115–1121, 1990.

## SELECTED READINGS

Halliwell, B., Gutteridge, J.M.C.: Free Radicals in Biology and Medicine. Oxford, Clarendon Press, 1985.

Sies, H. (ed.): Oxidative Stress. London, Academic Press, 1985.

Sies, H. (ed.): Oxidative Stress: Oxidants and Antioxidants. London, Academic Press, 1991.

Simic, M.G., Taylor, K.A., Ward, J.F., von Sonntag, C. (eds.): Oxygen Radicals in Biology and Medicine. New York, Plenum Press, 1987.

CHAPTER 34

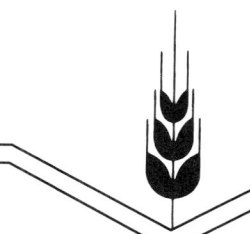

# Nutrition of Cells in Culture

Kathleen Shive Matthews



The culture of mammalian cells has developed over the past several decades to a point where this technique is an essential tool for the study of biochemical processes and developmental events. Growth in isolated systems provides the opportunity to examine metabolic pathways and nutritional requirements of cells in a controlled fashion. Bettger and McKeehan have reviewed the basic principles involved in cellular nutrition.[1] Essential nutrients, including an energy source, are required for cell survival, multiplication, and differentiation; these compounds correspond to those that cannot be produced by the cell in adequate quantities. In addition to essential nutrients, cells may require growth factors, generally protein in nature, hormones, or other compounds that play crucial roles in cellular processes. The ability to culture cells from a wide variety of sources in chemically defined media provides the potential to determine both the qualitative and quantitative requirements of each cell type and compare these singly and in aggregate to the intact organism.[2] Furthermore, growth of cells in culture allows exploration of problems not amenable to study in humans and reduces, but does not replace, the need for animal studies.

## HISTORICAL PERSPECTIVE

The first attempts to culture cells utilized supplements such as serum, plasma, and milk to provide unknown components required for cells to grow isolated from the in vivo milieu. The unknown composition and variability of commonly used supplements, notably serum, introduce complexities in interpretation of results, particularly with respect to definition of nutritional needs. Therefore, recent efforts in a number of laboratories have focused on the determination of specific growth requirements for cells in culture, with this area being investigated intensively.[1–4] Barnes has reviewed the different approaches used for developing defined, serum-free media,[3] typified by ground-breaking work in the laboratories of Ham and Sato who used complementary methods for elimination of serum. Ham and co-workers focussed on the improvement of basal media by optimizing the amounts of each component for growth of cells; this method yielded media that supported growth of cells with the elimination of serum supplementation.[5,6] A major contribution of this work was the demonstration that protein components in serum were necessary at least in part to compensate for imbalances in the basal nutritional components in the medium, and proper formulation of these components could eliminate the requirement for at least some of the hormonal signals derived from serum supplements. Sato and co-workers pursued a complementary course that involved identifying the specific components of serum that are required for the growth of cells in culture and providing these components in purified form.[4,7,8] The combination of these basic approaches provides a means to formulate an optimal basal medium with supplementation by the specific hormonal components that are required for a specific cell type in culture.

## APPLICATION AND UTILITY OF DEFINED MEDIA

Bettger and McKeehan have compared the development of defined media for cell culture with the formulation of semipurified and purified diets for studies of animal nutrition in the laboratory.[1] Cell culture in media of known composition allows definition of the experimental context, an essential prerequisite for rational design of experiments, and can be applied to a vast range of biologic problems in fields spanning most of the biomedical sciences. Cell culture isolates the biologic unit in a defined environment and allows exploration of the complex array of signals and intracellular processes that result in growth, differentiation, and association with other cells to form organs. In the context of nutrition, culture of cells in defined media can be utilized to determine individual nutritional requirements and to decipher individual metabolic characteristics. Thus, the tedious nature of determining the nutrient requirements of cells in culture is balanced by the significant advances that derive from this accomplishment. The remainder of this chapter will review in detail the defined media developed for growth of lymphocytes and summarize similar media that have been found to support growth of other cell types.

## CHEMICALLY DEFINED MEDIA FOR CULTURE OF LYMPHOCYTES

Both human peripheral blood lymphocytes and mouse splenocytes serve as excellent model systems for examining nutritional and biochemical/metabolic aspects of cell growth. Lymphocytes are resting cells that can be obtained readily and can be stimulated by a variety of mitogenic signals to progress through the cell cycle and proliferate. In addition to the mitogenic stimuli, lymphokines are required for cellular proliferation; these polypeptides are generally released by cells into the medium following mitogen exposure and do not need to be included in the growth medium. In particular, interleukin-1 produced by macrophages potentiates the response of T cells to mitogen and serves as a mediator of interleukin-2 production by subsets of T cells.[9] This complex intercommunication between macrophages and subsets of the lymphocyte population is a requirement for cell division following stimulation.[9] The metabolic activities of lymphocytes are generally in common with other cells, and a wide variety of receptors are found on their surface. These characteristics along with the ease of isolation render this cell class an ideal candidate for in vitro studies, particularly efforts to assess individual metabolic requirements.

### DEVELOPMENT OF SERUM-FREE MEDIA FOR LYMPHOCYTES

The medium used most commonly for studies of human lymphocytes in culture has been RPMI 1640 with fetal bovine serum supplementation in amounts dependent on the particular application.[10] The use of serum, however, precludes many types of informative experiments using this cell type.[7] These problems have led to the development of several different types of supplements for media that can be used to culture lymphocytes under serum-free conditions. A number of artificial serum substitutes have been produced commercially and will support proliferation of lymphocytes;[11] however, the levels of mitogen required for maximal response may differ from the corresponding levels in serum-containing media.[12] RPMI 1640 medium supplemented with glutamine, magnesium, and HEPES (N-[2-hydroxyethyl]piperazine-N′-[2-ethanesulfonic acid]) buffer will support growth of human lymphocytes, although higher cell concentrations are required than are needed in the presence of serum.[13] Lipoprotein and transferrin supplements to RPMI 1640 along with increased levels of glutamine have been shown to support mitogen-induced lymphocyte proliferation.[14]

The specific macromolecular components that were found to replace serum and provide a growth response comparable to or better than the serum-mediated level in several basal media included the following: transferrin, albumin, lipids, and in some cases growth factors.[15,16] Albumin and lipids could be eliminated from these media, provided insulin, ethanolamine, and selenium were provided.[17] The stimulatory properties of lipids on proliferation in albumin-free media suggest that sources of fatty acids may be requisite for the growth of cells; conversely, requirements for albumin, even at lower concentrations, may reflect the need for associated fatty acids.[15,17,18] The ability to replace albumin with casein is consistent with its postulated role as lipid source, because both proteins bind lipids.[19] Catalase has been shown to replace either albumin or casein in some cases, an observation that suggests that serum and supplemental proteins may play some role in protecting against oxidative damage to the cells.[19]

A defined basal medium for growth of murine T cells in vitro based on Iscove's modification of the formulation of Dulbecco's medium (IMDM) was reported by Gersten and Cohn.[20] Improved growth in this basal medium required only small amounts of supplementation with bovine serum albumin, transferrin, and insulin as well as mercaptoethanol and L-glutamine. Elimination of albumin and lipids from this medium did not significantly affect the growth response. Other workers have also modified IMDM, with inclusion of defined lipids, transferrin, bovine serum albumin, and α-thioglycerol (C-IMDM) to achieve increased response in serum-free medium.[21] One advantage observed in serum-free media with minimal protein supplements is a significant decrease in nonspecific T-cell proliferation.[20,22]

A distinction must be made between long-term and short-term culture of lymphocytes. A basal medium that combines Dulbecco's Modified Eagle's Medium, DMEM,[23] and Ham's F12 medium[5] in a 1:1 ratio supplemented with ethanolamine, transferrin, insulin, and selenium would not support long-term growth of IL-2 dependent human T cells or other permanent lymphocyte lines unless albumin and a source of lipid were provided.[17] This basal medium has been used with casein, insulin, testosterone, transferrin, and linoleic acid supplements for long-term culture of lymphocytes.[19] In the presence of conditioned medium from phytohemagglutinin-stimulated lymphocytes as a supplement, presumably to provide lymphokine signals, particularly interleukin-2, T lymphoblasts could be maintained for up to 5 weeks.[19] Ham's F12 medium supplemented with insulin, transferrin, albumin, and cholesterol will support a human lymphocyte cell line;[24] the presence of fatty acid and cholesterol in this medium may provide the crucial factors for maintenance of cells in long-term versus short-term culture.

The timing of exposure to serum can be crucial to the cellular response, as indicated by studies that demonstrate that the "requirement" for serum in T-cell proliferation occurs during the early phases of activation ($G_0$-$G_1$ transition) and serum is not required for later events.[25] Thus, defined media that obviate the need for serum early in the activation process may require more stringent nutritional definition than media that support lymphocyte growth later in the activation process.

Shive and co-workers have demonstrated growth of human lymphocytes in a chemically defined minimal medium (CFBI 1000) without serum or protein supplements;[22] this medium was formulated using as a starting point Ham's MCDB 104 medium and a closely related medium used to demonstrate a selenium requirement for human cells in culture.[26] Components that were not stimulatory for growth were eliminated from this defined medium, and concentrations of remaining components were adjusted to a level just sufficient to give optimal response. This use of the lowest concentration of a given component minimizes trace contaminants from the various ingredients and avoids imbalances between components that may result in growth inhibition. With this minimal medium, as well as others noted below for different cell types, growth responses can be influenced by the formulation of the mixture. Factors such as order of addition of components, method of pH adjustment, water quality (chlorine, organic compounds, ions), and chemical quality and source can influence the ability of the assembled medium to support growth of cells.[27] It should be noted that cells cultured in a minimal medium may be subject to inhibition by environmental effects, including airborne contaminants.

## COMPONENTS ESSENTIAL FOR GROWTH OF LYMPHOCYTES

The classes of compounds that are required for mitogen-induced lymphocyte proliferation (Table 34–1) include the following[22]: glucose (or related carbohydrate source), amino acids, vitamins, inorganic salts, and several basic components that are not synthesized by the cells in amounts adequate to support growth. The following sections discuss each of these components required for maximal growth of lymphocytes.

### *GLUCOSE*

Glucose or an alternate carbohydrate source is essential for growth of cells, including lymphocytes; almost all media formulations utilize concentrations of glucose comparable to those found in serum. In the CFBI 1000 medium, it has been found that mannose, galactose, and a few other sugars can replace glucose at least partially.[28] The ability of these sugars to substitute for glucose is presumably related to their utilization by the cell in glycolysis. Minimal information is available on the ability to metabolize more complex carbohydrates in these cells.

**TABLE 34–1.** ESSENTIAL MEDIA COMPONENTS FOR GROWTH OF LYMPHOCYTES

| | | |
|---|---|---|
| | Carbon/Energy Source | |
| Glucose | | |
| | Amino Acids | |
| Arginine | Isoleucine | Serine |
| Cysteine | Leucine | Threonine |
| Glutamine | Lysine | Tryptophan |
| Glycine | Methionine | Tyrosine |
| Histidine | Phenylalanine | Valine |
| | Vitamins | |
| Biotin | Nicotinamide | Riboflavin |
| Folinic Acid | Pantothenate | Thiamine |
| Hydroxocobalamin | Pyridoxine | |
| | Inorganic Ions | |
| Calcium | Magnesium | Sodium |
| Chloride | Phosphate | Sulfate |
| Iron (as EDTA complex) | Potassium | |
| | Other Components | |
| Adenine | Inositol | |
| Choline | Pyruvate | |
| Buffer | | |
| [Antibiotics] | | |
| | Mitogen | |
| Phytohemagglutinin | | |

*AMINO ACIDS*

Early studies demonstrated the requirement for glutamine and 12 additional amino acids in culture of cells in vitro.[29] The 13 required amino acids include arginine, cysteine, glutamine, histidine, isoleucine, leucine, lysine, methionine, phenylalanine, threonine, tryptophan, tyrosine, and valine. Lymphocytes from some human donors exhibit maximal growth in the presence of these amino acids; however, lymphocytes from other individuals require serine, glycine, or both for maximal growth. For this reason, these two amino acids were included in the formulation of CFBI 1000.[22] It is noteworthy that lymphocytes isolated from many individuals will exhibit maximal response, even in the absence of glycine and serine, provided the folinic acid concentration in the medium is increased and vitamin $B_6$ is present.[28] Thus, the availability of both folinic acid and vitamin $B_6$ is requisite for synthesis of serine and glycine.

The ratio of amino acids may be as crucial as concentration. In one study optimizing amino acid composition of RPMI 1640 for in vitro antibody response of mouse splenocytes resulted in concentration adjustments for a number of amino acids when tested singly.[30] Combining adjustments that individually provided improvement often resulted in diminished response.[30] Thus, the relative concentrations of amino acids must be considered along with the absolute levels. The effects of interacting components were observed a number of years ago in Eagle's Minimal Essential Medium (MEM).[31] In this serum-containing medium, either serine or glycine was required for growth response, and increased cell density enhanced growth in the absence of these amino acids. Studies of lymphocytes in RPMI 1640 supplemented with 10% dialyzed fetal calf serum have shown that insufficient serine synthesis occurs for optimal growth response to lectin stimulation.[32] Medium composition clearly affects the ability of lymphocytes to synthesize glycine and serine.

The glutamine requirement appears absolute for human B lymphocyte transformation and plasma cell formation; cells cultured in RPMI 1640 with dialyzed fetal bovine serum but deficient in glutamine fail to undergo DNA synthesis or morphologic transformation.[33] Similarly, concanavalin A in another study did not stimulate thymidine incorporation into rat T lymphocytes in the absence of glutamine.[34] Glutamine is metabolized at a rate four-fold greater than glucose in lymphocytes and produces glutamate, aspartate, lactate, and ammonia as products.[35] The role of glutamine utilization in lymphocytes is to generate nitrogen and carbon for macromolecular precursors (amino acids, purines, and pyrimidines) and energy for the cell; in addition, the high rate of glutamine utilization may also provide a mechanism to regulate the rate at which intermediates in this pathway are utilized for biosynthesis.[35] Asparagine and purines, end products of glutamine metabolism, diminish significantly the requirement for glutamine in the defined medium, CFBI 1000.[36]

The dependence of transformed human B lymphocytes and peripheral blood lymphocytes in culture on methionine in the medium has been observed.[37] The presence of homocysteine and methylfolate in the context of demonstrable levels of cobalamin-dependent methionine synthetase activity did not provide sufficient methionine to support growth. A further study showed that provision of cobalamin bound to transcobalamin II did elicit growth enhancement; however, the mechanism of this effect has not been elucidated.[38] It is noteworthy that lymphocytes from some human subjects can respond in CFBI 1000 medium to homocysteine in lieu of methionine provided adequate vitamin $B_{12}$ is available.[39]

*VITAMINS*

The eight B vitamins known to be required for animal growth are constituents of minimal medium developed for the growth of human lymphocytes.[22,27] Lipoic acid, although essential for other cell lines,[26] does not improve short-term lymphocyte growth.[22] The essential nature of the B vitamins can be demonstrated in a variety of ways. Omission of pantothenate results in a marked diminution in growth for lymphocytes in CFBI 1000 medium, whereas growth decrements in response to omission of other B vitamins are more variable and presumably reflect the nutritional status of the individual from whom the cells are obtained.[28]

Lymphocytes have been used as a marker of past nutritional state for folate and $B_{12}$ deficiencies.[40] In short-term cultures of lymphocytes stimulated with phytohemagglutinin, suppressed incorporation of radiolabeled thymidine into DNA was observed in the presence of deoxyuridine for cells from normal subjects. In contrast, this suppression did not occur for lymphocytes from patients with megaloblastic anemia consequent to folate or vitamin $B_{12}$ deficiency.[40] Although deoxyuridine suppression was restored by addition of the appropriate vitamin to these cells in vitro, diminished suppression values for lymphocytes grown in folate and vitamin $B_{12}$–limited medium persisted for up to 84 days following vitamin supplementation of the human subjects.[40] Based on these observations, the authors concluded that the lymphocyte deoxyuridine suppression test reflects vitamin status of the patient at the time of lymphocyte generation and therefore provides information on past nutritional status.[40] However, this method has been called into question because of the findings of experiments using lymphocytes from normal individuals.[41] Cells that are deficient in folate will exhibit diminished deoxyuridine suppression of radiolabeled thymidine incorporation compared to cells replete in folate; when intracellular folate levels fell below 1.1 pmol (~500 pg)/$10^6$ cells, lymphocytes from normal subjects grown in folate-free medium exhibited elevated deoxyuridine suppression values, similar to the pattern observed for subjects with megaloblastic anemia. Medium folate levels below 0.73 μmol/L (0.32 μg/ml) are inadequate to support proliferation following mitogen stimulation, and the dilution of folate as the cells grow results in acquired deficiency regardless of the initial status of the cells.[41] On the basis of this evidence for acquired folate deficiency in culture for lymphocytes from normal subjects, the utility of the deoxyuridine suppression assay for diagnosis of vitamin deficiencies has been questioned.[41] Although deoxyuridine suppression tests tend to be higher in megaloblastic anemia patients, the acquisition of folate deficiency during culture presents an obvious complication to unambiguous interpretation of results.[42] Despite these complexities, this method is used widely to evaluate vitamin $B_{12}$ and folate status.[43]

A different approach to determine folate/folinic acid, vitamin $B_{12}$, and vitamin $B_6$ responses was developed using CFBI 1000 minimal medium.[22,28] In glycine-free medium containing serine, the conversion of serine to glycine is the growth-limiting step, and this reaction requires folate/folinic acid and pyridoxal phosphate (vitamin $B_6$) as cofactors. By monitoring growth of cells in folate-free, glycine-free medium, the adequency of cellular reserves of folate for glycine synthesis from serine can be established.[22,28,44] Vitamin $B_6$ is also required for the synthesis of serine, a required amino acid for cell growth; by monitoring cellular proliferation in a medium free of both glycine and serine, provided sufficient folate is present, the adequacy of cellular reserves of vitamin $B_6$ for lymphocyte growth can be determined. Finally, the conversion of homocysteine to methionine is a vitamin $B_{12}$–dependent process. By monitoring the ability of cells to grow on homocysteine- rather than methionine-containing medium, vitamin $B_{12}$ status of the lymphocytes can be assessed; the requirement for vitamin $B_{12}$ to obtain effective replacement of methionine by homocysteine has been demonstrated previously in serum-containing media.[37]

A biotin requirement for cells in culture has been difficult to demonstrate in complex media, despite its essential role in reactions involving carboxylases.[45] In contrast, in the CFBI 1000 minimal medium, a direct dose-response effect of biotin has been observed on the growth of lymphocytes.[27] Other variations in the basal CFBI 1000 media can be used to determine vitamin status. For example, any diminished growth of lymphocytes in response to elimination of vitamin $B_1$ from the medium is magnified by utilization of a ribosyl derivative rather than glucose in the medium;[28] this effect presumably derives from cellular dependence on transketolase, which requires vitamin $B_1$ as a cofactor, for conversion of the alternate sugar to glucose. Metabolic antagonists also can be used to demonstrate the cellular requirement for vitamin cofactors.[39,44]

Although vitamin C is not requisite for the growth of lymphocytes in culture, it has been demonstrated recently that the intracellular levels of this compound are high in isolated lymphoid cells and are rapidly depleted by more than 96% during cell culture.[46] Provision of vitamin C in the medium resulted in reaccumulation of the intracellular level with large gradients of concentration across the plasma membrane. Most *in vitro* studies using lymphocytes use medium free of vitamin C and therefore examine cells depleted of this cofactor.[46] This observation may provide the basis for the development of an in vitro assay for vitamin C status and for understanding the requirements for ascorbic acid in immune cellular function.

Partly as a consequence of difficulty in solubilization and partly because of the lack of evidence for a requirement in cellular proliferation, the fat-soluble vitamins in general have not been included in media for the growth of human lymphocytes. In fact, several forms of vitamin D inhibit both B- and T-cell growth in vitro, at least in part due to suppression of interleukin-2 production.[47] These studies have been conducted largely in media containing serum, and the inhibitory effects of vitamin D compounds could be partially reversed by the addition of purified interleukin-2.[47] Addition of vitamin D at or later than 24 hours following mitogen exposure did not affect growth pattern significantly; thus, inhibition by vitamin D appears to be cell cycle-dependent.[47] The target population for the suppressive effects of vitamin D appears to be the T-helper cells.[48]

## *INORGANIC IONS*

In the minimal medium CFBI 1000, calcium, ferrous or ferric iron, potassium, magnesium, sulfate, and phosphate ions, in addition to sodium chloride, are required for activation and proliferation of lymphocytes.[22] Although not added to the medium, trace elements are presumably required as well for cellular metabolism. These elements might either be carried over in the cells themselves or be present in small quantities as contaminants in other media components.

CFBI 1000 is an iron-containing, protein-free medium; thus, it does not contain transferrin.[22,27] The level of iron in the medium (10 μmol/L) is high relative to the amount of transferrin that can be used to replace the iron salts (0.13 μmol/L, or ~10 μg/ml); this difference is presumably related to the efficiency with which iron can be delivered to the interior of the cell by transferrin receptors.[49] The role of transferrin appears to be exclusively to provide iron to cells that are rapidly dividing.[49,50] Lymphocyte subsets differ in their iron requirement and therefore in their dependence on transferrin/transferrin receptor interaction and turnover.[51] RPMI 1640 and other commonly used media do not contain iron salts, and thus transferrin is an essential component in these media for growth of lymphocytes in culture. Although elimination of transferrin increases definition of the medium by eliminating compounds that may bind to this protein, trace metal contaminants in the ferrous sulfate and ethylenediaminetetraacetic acid (EDTA) that are used in larger quantities may affect growth of cells in an unknown fashion, either inhibiting or providing small amounts of essential factors not present in the minimal medium.

Maximal lymphocyte DNA synthesis was observed in a serum-free medium at 270 μmol/L calcium ion and 100 μmol/L magnesium ion in one study,[52] whereas in a different system somewhat higher levels were requisite.[53,54] Although the responses of lymphocytes from different individuals vary, for most the level of 1 mmol/L used in CFBI 1000 is adequate for maximum proliferation.[22,28] In RPMI 1640 supplemented with glutamine and serum, reduced calcium levels resulted in suppressed proliferation, interleukin-2 production, and interleukin-2 receptor expression; below 10 μmol/L proliferation was eliminated, but interleukin-2 receptor expression was still measurable.[55]

Determination of growth requirements for trace metals have focussed primarily on copper and zinc; to execute such experiments, it is essential to remove these ions from the culture media and sera. Chelation utilizing metal binding compounds attached to solid matrices can be used to remove the ions and simultaneously to prevent exposure of the lymphocytes to the chelator.[54,56] Using this approach, it has been possible to demonstrate reduced T-lymphocyte proliferation in the absence of zinc, with restoration of response upon repletion of this ion to the culture medium. Depletion of copper, zinc, and magnesium from media resulted in suppression of T-lymphocyte but not B-lymphocyte growth in response to mitogen.[57] The phagocytic activity of macrophages also was suppressed in media deficient in zinc and magnesium. The sensitivity of cells to depletion of trace metals may depend in part on the cellular reserves and the size of the inoculum used for culture, as well as other factors.

Copper and zinc have been shown to have significant effects on lymphokine secretion, with the type of effect depending on the presence or absence of serum in the culture medium; it is concluded from these studies that these trace metals may be involved in regulating secretion of specific lymphokines.[58] Animal studies have been utilized to correlate zinc deficiency states in the animal with growth of cells in culture.[59] The decreased proliferation of T cells from animals following 6 weeks of dietary zinc deprivation was found to be due to an effect on macrophages; however, following 12 weeks of dietary zinc depletion, T-cell proliferative capacity itself was also diminished. These results suggest that T cells produced in the thymus prior to dietary depletion are unaffected in their ability to proliferate in response to appropriate signals, whereas those processed during dietary depletion are affected directly either in terms of maturational status or maintenance state.[59] The longevity of the T lymphocyte in a resting state provides a means to assess the nutritional history of an individual, and the higher metabolic state of the macrophage provides access to more-recent nutritional events in the life of the organism.

### *OTHER COMPONENTS*

Omission of pyruvate, choline, inositol, or adenine from CFBI 1000 medium results in diminished growth response for lymphocytes from most individuals.[22,28] Upon pyruvate elimination, the growth response observed for lymphocytes from some individuals is almost normal, whereas in others absence of this component results in nearly complete inhibition. This effect is presumably related to the varied effectiveness of the cells in executing glycolysis. Choline-deficient media result in a substantial decrease (70 to 90%) in growth response for lymphocytes, although certain precursors can alleviate this inhibition at least partially.[28] The synthesis of choline appears to be significantly restricted in lymphocytes. Inositol and purines are not produced by the lymphocytes in amounts sufficient to support maximal growth; thus, these components must be included in the basal medium.[22,28] Precursors of purines can enhance the response if adenine is removed from the medium. Stimulation with PHA results in rapid activation of purine salvage pathways in lymphocytes, significant increase in 5-phosphoribosyl-1-pyrophosphate levels, and increase in de novo purine biosynthesis.[60] This rapid increase in nucleotide production presumably correlates with the requisite increases in energy metabolism and nucleic acid synthesis upon activation.[60]

Intracellular glutathione availability has been shown to be directly related to lymphocyte proliferation in response to mitogenic stimuli.[61] Cysteine and mercaptoethanol in the medium, although providing some enhancement to intracellular glutathionine levels and promoting lymphocyte growth, do not substitute entirely in the presence of a glutathione inhibitor (buthionine sulfoximine).[61] The influence of glutathione on lymphocyte proliferation may be mediated in part by effects on interleukin-2 binding and metabolism.[62] The inclusion of cysteine in CFBI 1000 medium apparently provides the thiol requirement that has been observed in other studies, possibly by enhancing the level of intracellular glutathione, as observed in mouse spleen lymphocytes.[63] It is noteworthy that the replacement of the 2-mercaptoethanol requirement for mouse spleen lymphocyte proliferation by cysteine requires the presence of a selenium compound for maximum proliferation; the effects of cysteine and selenium compounds appear to be additive and independent, with sodium selenite and L-selenocysteine more effective than sodium selenate and L-selenomethionine.[64] The ability of cysteine to provide the thiol requirement for cellular proliferation in defined, minimal medium may be related to the presence of small contaminating levels of selenium in other medium components.

A requirement for lipoproteins or exogenous fatty acids has been demonstrated for lymphocytes grown in RPMI 1640 (supplemented with glutamine and transferrin).[14,65] The transferrin requirement is not surprising given the absence of iron salts in RPMI 1640. The stimulation by low-density lipoprotein and high-density lipoprotein appeared in one study to be both LDL receptor-mediated and LDL receptor-independent.[65] The absence of a requirement for fatty acids in CFBI 1000 may be related to the balance of other nutrients, because substitution of the amino acid mixture in RPMI 1640 for that in CFBI 1000 resulted in significant diminution of cellular proliferation (M. Glenn, W. Shive, and K.S. Matthews, unpublished data). These data illustrate the complexity of determining specific requirements for growth of cells, because the particular formulation and ratio of ingredients can have significant effects on cellular metabolism and consequently on the proliferation observed. Specific compounds may be required in the context of one medium that are nonessential in a different constellation of media components.

## CHEMICALLY DEFINED MEDIA FOR CULTURE OF OTHER TYPES OF MAMMALIAN CELLS

As indicated by the discussion of lymphocytes, successful formulation of a medium for serum-free culture of mammalian cells can be complex. A number of basal media have been developed that are used with modification for a variety of cell types. The basic requirements of cells are similar in general (see Table 34–1) and include the following: glucose, amino acids, B vitamins (including lipoate in some instances), inorganic ions (including trace metals in many cases), buffer, adenine, choline, inositol, pyruvate, and often fatty acid, putrescine (or similar compound), and acetate. What differs among cell types, as illustrated in the specific examples outlined below, is the amount of a particular component that yields optimal growth. In addition to the basic nutritional requirements of cells, on which we are focussing in this chapter, each cell type may depend on the presence of specific macromolecular growth factors that are essential to proliferation. Some of these factors are signals analogous to mitogens in the lymphocyte system, whereas others relate to attachment of the cells that may be crucial for growth; finally there are proteins such as insulin and transferrin, which are required for delivery of nutrients. Although a number of serum-free media are commercially available, the composition of these products is frequently unknown, as is that of many serum substitutes. Because formulation of medium from single components is an extraordinarily time-consuming and difficult task, most efforts begin with a previously formulated medium or combination of media, followed by attempts either to wean the cells from serum or to replace serum with specific components. In the process of screening media for a specific application, it is essential to define the parameters that are to be monitored (e.g., growth versus differentiation) and to establish criteria for assessing the effectiveness of a medium. As an example, thymocytes are unable to proliferate in the absence of exogenous mitogenic stimuli in RPMI 1640 containing serum, whereas use of a defined medium (KC2000, Hazleton, which contains salts, vitamins, and amino acids, and is supplemented with glutamine, mercaptoethanol, fetuin, transferrin, and albumin) with or without serum provided rapid proliferation in one study; from the results obtained, the authors concluded that thymocytes may have nutritional requirements unmet by commonly used media.[66] This situation may apply to other cell types as well.

In the following sections, a few specific examples of serum-free, chemically defined media applied to different systems are summarized.

### OLIGODENDROCYTES

In the presence of a basal medium composed of DMEM mixed in a 1:1 ratio with Ham's F12 medium and with sodium bicarbonate and HEPES as buffers, oligodendrocytes isolated in one study from primary neonatal rat cerebral cultures were grown with addition of insulin, transferrin, and fibroblast growth factor.[67] The elimination of insulin, transferrin, or fibroblast growth factor individually or provision of transferrin alone resulted in diminished survival after 5 days in culture. Insulin addition alone maintained cell viability but did not induce proliferation, whereas addition of fibroblast growth factor alone supported proliferation over a 5-day period comparable to that observed in the presence of 10% fetal calf serum.[67] It was noted that there was a requirement for pyruvate in the basal medium, presumed to be the result of low activities of pyruvate dehydrogenase and hexokinase.[67] The nature of the cells that proliferate was confirmed by ultrastructural, biochemical, and immunologic criteria. Growth of astrocytes (which requires prostaglandin $F_{2\alpha}$, putrescine, and hydrocortisone) was not supported by the medium developed for oligodendrocytes, emphasizing the distinction among cell types for specific constellations of nutrients and factors for growth.

### ADIPOCYTES

A medium containing a 1:1 mixture of DMEM and Ham's F12 basal medium was supplemented with bicarbonate, HEPES, biotin, pantothenate, insulin, and triiodothyronine to support differentiation of human stromal vascular cells into adipocytes in one study.[68] In this medium, more than 25% of the cells were able to undergo terminal differentiation within 18 days. The addition of glucocorticoids (notably cortisol) stimulated the differentiation process (up to 70% differentiation for samples from young adults) in a dose-dependent manner. The addition of serum to this basal medium yielded a much lower fraction of differentiated cells, although growth of the cells was maintained under these conditions, apparently induced by serum factors.[68] These studies noted that the fraction of differentiated cells depended on the age of the donor, a factor that may be important in studies of other cell types.[68] Another study showed that in a similar basal medium supplemented with insulin, transferrin, and triiodothyronine, up to 90% of young rat pre-epididymal and subcutaneous stromal-vascular cells underwent differentiation without glucocorticoids.[69] Up to 70% of cells from older animals also demonstrated the differentiation response, in contrast to behavior in serum-supplemented medium. The low mitogenic activity of serum-free, defined medium results in a high frequency of differentiated cells present as monolayers.

## KERATINOCYTES

This cell type was used in the initial studies by Ham and co-workers to define the low-molecular-weight medium components required for growth.[70,71] The inhibition of fibroblast growth in the medium developed for optimal proliferation of keratinocytes, MCDB 153, illustrates the differential requirements of differing cell types: adenine in the MCDB medium is about 20 times the amount optimal for fibroblasts, whereas calcium levels are too low.[70] In addition to the basal medium of inorganic ions, amino acids, vitamins (including lipoate), buffer, trace elements, linoleate and putrescine, acetate, adenine, choline, glucose, inositol, pyruvate, and thymidine, supplements of monoethanolamine, phosphoethanolamine, and hydrocortisone were made. Macromolecular components required for maximal growth included insulin and epidermal growth factor. Keratinocytes will undergo growth arrest at moderate densities, apparently at least partially because of depletion of amino acids in the medium.[70] The advantage of cells grown in this defined medium is the absence of complicating factors arising from serum, feeder layers, and similar items that are commonly used for epidermal cell growth. In addition, the effect of specific components on cell growth can be easily assessed and levels optimized for increased definition of experiments. For example, stratification and terminal differentiation of keratinocytes are observed with 1 mmol/L calcium in this medium.[71]

Using a different basal medium (M199) supplemented with bovine serum albumin, insulin, transferrin, hydrocortisone, triiodothyronine, and epidermal growth factor, the requirement for high levels of inositol and choline for optimal growth has been demonstrated.[72,73] Based on these data, it was suggested that inositol and choline may serve different functions, either quantitatively or qualitatively, in this cell type compared to others with a lower requirement.

## CARDIAC MYOCYTES

Cells from the intact myocardium include cardiac myocytes, smooth muscle cells, endothelial cells, and fibroblasts. Under most culture conditions in the presence of serum, the preferential growth of cells other than cardiac myocytes results in loss of cardiac myocytes in the culture.[74] Selection in favor of cardiac myocytes was improved by growth in a medium based on MCDB 107 supplemented with insulin and transferrin with culture on fibronectin-coated plates.[74] However, dexamethasone was necessary to observe maximum contractility in these cells. Other media formulations were not as effective as MCDB 107, developed originally for growth of fibroblasts,[75] in supporting growth of cardiac myocytes.[74] This result illustrates the importance of careful testing of media with different compositions for growth of specific cell types.

## HEPATOCYTES

From a survey of culture media, a 1:1 mixture of DMEM and Waymouth's medium MAB87/3 was found to support the growth of rat hepatocytes under serum-free conditions.[76] This medium permits the majority of hepatocytes to undergo DNA synthesis and mitosis in response to supplements of epidermal growth factor and insulin. Neither preplating with serum nor a collagen substratum is required for growth under these conditions.[76] It is noteworthy that insulin- and epidermal growth factor–stimulated hepatocyte cell division occurs in the 1:1 mixture of media indicated, but not in the parent media individually without serum. This observation underscores the importance of testing multiple media and their combinations or varying concentrations of individual components to determine optimum conditions for growth, proliferation, and differentiation in culture.

## MESENCHYME CELLS

Chicken limb mesenchyme cells at various stages in primary culture are used for studies of cell differentiation, and a serum-free, chemically defined medium has been developed to support growth and differentiation of stage-24 cells, particularly to chondrocytes.[77] The study illustrates an important aspect of media selection: the establishment of criteria for determining optimal media composition. The criteria selected for the mesenchyme cells were cell attachment, morphology, proliferation, synthesis of cartilage extracellular matrix, and differentiation. It was found that a mixture of 40% DMEM and 60% Ham's F12 medium yielded the optimal results for all cell densities; supplements of insulin, transferrin, and hydrocortisone 21-phosphate improved both growth and differentiation effects. Bovine serum albumin and hydrocortisone promoted cultures that gave cell morphology more similar to serum-containing "controls," and fibronectin coating of plates was necessary for attachment of the cells. The ability to generate differentiation with morphology characteristic of that observed in the presence of serum provides a culture system for discerning effects of a variety of stimuli on this complex process.

### OTHER SYSTEMS

Growth of human breast cancer cells in serum-free medium provides a mechanism for characterizing in vitro effects of hormone, growth factors, and other compounds on proliferation. A defined medium using a 1:1 mixture of Ham's F12 and DMEM supplemented with HEPES, transferrin, and bovine serum albumin was found in one study to support the growth of several types of human breast cancer cells.[78] Although proliferation was significantly slowed, multiple rounds of cell division were observed in response to known mitogens and tissue extracts for these cell types, and influence of specific components could be readily assessed. Insulin provided significant stimulation for two breast cancer cell types.[78] This medium underlies a method to examine the individual and potential synergistic and antagonistic effects of various growth factors on human breast cancer cells in culture. Using this medium, it was possible to demonstrate that seeding of cultures in serum for 24 hours followed by withdrawal of the serum can influence response to growth factors;[78] the long-term cellular consequences of serum exposure complicate interpretation of experiments that use serum in the initial preparation and plating of cells.

Mouse mammary cells transformed by bovine papillomavirus and the uninfected parent cell line were examined in MCDB 151 medium supplemented with epidermal growth factor, transferrin, hydrocortisone, ethanolamine, phosphoethanolamine, retinoic acid, trace metals, and insulin.[79] In this defined medium, the transformed cells divide more slowly than the parent cells, whereas in the presence of fetal bovine serum, the uninfected parent cell divides more slowly.[79] Papillomavirus-transformed cells exhibit more-stringent requirements for growth than the parental line, and the defined medium provides a system for deciphering the differences that arise because of viral infection and transformation.

## GENERALIZATIONS FROM MULTIPLE CELL TYPES

As reviewed recently,[80] several generalizations can be made regarding the nutritional requirements for cells in culture. First, a balanced set of common nutrients (Table 34–1) is required by most cell types. In addition, there may be nutrients that are required in unusual amounts by specific classes of cells or that are exclusive for a particular cell type. The challenge in defining a basal medium is identification of the specific levels and nutrients that yield optimal growth. The second group of broadly required media components includes insulin, transferrin, and serum albumin or other proteins as fatty-acid/lipid carriers. A third category of molecules required for growth of cells in culture are hormones, substrata, growth factors, and polypeptide signal molecules; this class of compounds is generally cell-specific, and the constellation of these components required for growth and differentiation must be identified. Finally, there may be specific, and sometimes exclusive, requirements for a particular cell type, and selection of media conditions may select for growth of one class of cells from a complex initial mixture. The success in culturing many different cell types provides a strong database to select a basal medium and to determine variations that optimize growth of cells for which a defined medium has not been formulated.

In conclusion, definition of the nutritional requirements of cells in culture provides a background against which experiments of many different types can be undertaken in a variety of fields.[80] The use of defined media in cell culture yields standardization and reproducibility, which in turn make transfer of technology among laboratories more straightforward, and place control of the experimental context in the hands of the investigator. Furthermore, media variations can be made systematically to address specific questions. As an example, the composition of CFBI 1000 minimal medium for lymphocytes can be varied in multiple ways to test the associated effects on growth of lymphocytes from a given individual; thus, this medium forms the basis for rational design of nutritional and metabolic tests for humans.[28,36] Because isolated lymphocytes reflect past nutritional history of the organism,[40,59] in vitro culture of these cells may be used to identify both previous deficits and present metabolic patterns. The development and application of defined media for growth of specific classes of cells provide essential experimental tools to address a wide array of questions over the complete range of biologic sciences.

## REFERENCES

1. Bettger, W.J., McKeehan, W.L.: Physiol. Rev., *66*:1–35, 1986.
2. Nutrition Reviews, *44*:245–247, 1986.
3. Barnes, D.: Wld. Rev. Nutr. Diet., *45*:167–197, 1985.
4. Barnes, D., Sato, G.: Anal. Biochem., *102*:255–270, 1980.
5. Ham, R.G.: Proc. Natl. Acad. Sci. U.S.A., *53*:288–293, 1965.
6. Ham, R.G., McKeehan, W.L.: Methods Enzymol., *58*:44–93, 1979.
7. Barnes, D., Sato, G.: Cell, *22*:649–655, 1980.

8. Bottenstein, J., Hayashi, I., Hutchings, S., et al.: Methods Enzymol., *58:*94–109, 1979.
9. Kouttab, N.M., Mehta, S., Morgan, J., et al.: Clin. Chem., *30:*1539–1545, 1984.
10. Moore, G.E., Gerner, R.E., Franklin, H.A.: JAMA, *199:*519–524, 1967.
11. Blaehr, H., Ladefoged, J.: J. Immunol. Methods, *111:*125–129, 1988.
12. Li, W., Kumar, R.K.: Immunol. Lett., *23:*235–236, 1990.
13. Needleman, B.W., Weiler, J.M.: J. Immunol. Methods, *44:*3–14, 1981.
14. Cuthbert, J.A., Lipsky, P.E.: J. Biol. Chem., *261:*3620–3627, 1986.
15. Iscove, N.N., Melchers, F.: J. Exp. Med., *147:*923–933, 1978.
16. Spieker-Polet, H., Polet, H.: J. Biol. Chem., *251:*987–992, 1976.
17. Mendelsohn, J., Caviles, A. Jr., Castagnola, J.: Culture of human lymphocytes in serum-free medium. *In* Methods for Serum-Free Culture of Neuronal and Lymphoid Cells. Edited by D.W. Barnes, D.A. Sirbasku, and G.H. Sato. New York, Alan R. Liss, 1984, pp. 207–214.
18. Spieker-Polet, H., Polet, H.: J. Immunol., *126:*949–954, 1981.
19. Darfler, F.J., Insel, P.A.: Growth of lymphoid cells in serum-free medium. *In* Methods for Serum-Free Culture of Neuronal and Lymphoid Cells. Edited by D.W. Barnes, D.A. Sirbasku, and G.H. Sato. New York, Alan R. Liss, 1984, pp. 187–196.
20. Gersten, M.J., Cohn, M.: Cell. Immunol., *91:*143–158, 1985.
21. Lipson, S.M.: Diagn. Microbiol. Infect. Dis., *4:*203–214, 1986.
22. Shive, W., Pinkerton, F., Humphreys, J., et al.: Proc. Natl. Acad. Sci. U.S.A., *83:*9–13, 1986.
23. Morton, H.J.: In Vitro, *6:*89–108, 1970.
24. Yen, A., Duigou, R.: Immunol. Lett., *6:*169–174, 1983.
25. Herzberg, V.L., Smith, K.A.: J. Immunol., *139:*998–1004, 1987.
26. McKeehan, W.L., Hamilton, W.G., Ham, R.G.: Proc. Natl. Acad. Sci. U.S.A., *73:*2023–2027, 1976.
27. Matthews, K.S., Pettit, F., Boghossian, J., et al.: Methods Enzymol., *150:*134–146, 1987.
28. Shive, W., Matthews, K.S.: Annu. Rev. Nutr., *8:*81–97, 1988.
29. Eagle, H.: J. Biol. Chem., *214:*839–852, 1955.
30. Zhu, D., Lefkovits, I.: In Vitro, *20:*615–622, 1984.
31. Dubrow, R., Pizer, L.I., Brody, J.I.: J. Natl. Cancer Inst., *51:*307–311, 1973.
32. Rowe, P.B., Sauer, D., Fahey, D., et al.: Arch. Biochem. Biophys., *236:*277–288, 1985.
33. Crawford, J., Cohen, H.J.: J. Cell. Physiol., *124:*275–282, 1985.
34. Ardawi, M.S.M., Newsholme, E.A.: Biochem. J., *212:*835–842, 1983.
35. Newsholme, E.A., Crabtree, B., Ardawi, M.S.M.: Br. J. Exp. Physiol., *70:*473–489, 1985.
36. Pettit, F.H., Boghossian, J.O., Shive, W.: Biochem. Biophys. Res. Commun., *164:*1348–1351, 1989.
37. Hall, C.A., Begley, J.A., Chu, R.C.: Proc. Soc. Exp. Biol. Med., *182:*215–220, 1986.
38. Hall, C.A., Chu, R.C., Begley, J.A.: Proc. Soc. Exp. Biol. Med., *189:*217–222, 1988.
39. Sterling, R.K.: Preliminary results on the development of assay for vitamin $B_1$ and $B_{12}$ status of human lymphocytes. M.A. Thesis, University of Texas, Austin, 1984.
40. Das, K.C., Herbert, V.: Br. J. Haematol., *38:*219–233, 1978.
41. Matthews, J.H., Wickramasinghe, S.N.: Br. J. Haematol., *63:*281–291, 1986.
42. Matthews, J.H., Wickramasinghe, S.N.: Eur. J. Haematol., *40:*174–180, 1988.
43. Town, G.I., Fitchett, A.C., Carter, J.M.: N.Z. Med. J., *99:*633–635, 1986.
44. Shive, W.: J. Int. Acad. Prev. Med., *8:*5–16, 1984.
45. Dakshinamurti, K., Chalifour, L., Bhullar, R.P.: Ann. N.Y. Acad. Sci., *447:*38–55, 1985.
46. Bergsten, P., Amitai, G., Kehrl, J., et al.: J. Biol. Chem., *265:*2584–2587, 1990.
47. Rigby, W.F.C., Stacy, T., Fanger, M.W.: J. Clin. Invest., *74:*1451–1455, 1984.
48. Lemire, J.M., Adams, J.S., Kermani-Arab, V., et al.: J. Immunol., *134:*3032–3035, 1985.
49. Brock, J.H., Mainou-Fowler, T., Webster, L.M.: Immunology, *57:*105–110, 1986.
50. Brock, J.H., Stevenson, J.: Immunol. Lett., *15:*23–25, 1987.
51. Kemp, J.D., Thorson, J.A., Gomez, F., et al.: Cell. Immunol., *122:*218–230, 1989.
52. Abboud, C.N., Scully, S.P., Lichtman, A.H. et al.: J. Cell. Physiol., *122:*64–72, 1985.
53. Carpentieri, U., Myers, J., Daeschner, C.W. III, et al.: Clin. Res., *35:*63A, 1987.
54. Carpentieri, U., Myers, J., Daeschner, C.W. III, et al.: J. Biochem. Biophys. Methods, *14:*93–100, 1987.
55. Modiano, J.F., Kelepouris, E., Kern, J.A., et al.: J. Cell. Physiol., *135:*451–458, 1988.
56. Messer, H.H., Murray, E.J., Goebel, N.K.: J. Nutr., *112:*652–657, 1982.
57. Flynn, A.: J. Nutr., *114:*2034–2042, 1984.
58. Scuderi, P.: Cell. Immunol., *126:*391–405, 1990.
59. James, S.J., Swendseid, M., Makinodan, T.: J. Nutr., *117:*1982–1988, 1987.
60. Barankiewicz, J., Cohen, A.: Arch. Biochem. Biophys., *258:*167–175, 1987.
61. Hamilos, D.L., Zelarney, P., Mascali, J.J.: Immunopharmacology, *18:*223–235, 1989.
62. Liang, C.-M., Lee, N., Cattell, D., et al.: J. Biol. Chem., *264:*13519–13523, 1989.
63. Ishii, T., Sugita, Y., Bannai, S.: J. Cell. Physiol., *133:*330–336, 1987.
64. Ishii, T., Sugita, Y., Bannai, S.: Cell Struct. Funct. *14:*287–297, 1989.
65. Cuthbert, J.A., Lipsky, P.E.: J. Biol. Chem., *264:*13468–13474, 1989.
66. Wood, G.W., Greenwood, J.H., Mauser, L.: Immunology, *69:*303–311, 1990.
67. Saneto, R.P., de Vellis, J.: Proc. Natl. Acad. Sci. U.S.A., *82:*3509–3513, 1985.
68. Hauner, H., Entenmann, G., Wabitsch, M., et al.: J. Clin. Invest., *84:*1663–1670, 1989.
69. Deslex, S., Negrel, R., Ailhaud, G.: Exp. Cell Res., *168:*15–30, 1987.
70. Shipley, G.D., Pittelkow, M.R.: Arch. Dermatol., *123:*1541a–1544a, 1987.
71. Boyce, S.T., Ham, R.G.: J. Invest. Dermatol., *81:*33s–40s, 1983.
72. Gordon, P.R., Gelman, L.K., Gilchrest, B.A.: J. Nutr., *118:*1487–1494, 1988.
73. Gordon, P.R., Mawhinney, T.P., Gilchrest, B.A.: J. Cell. Physiol., *135:*416–424, 1988.
74. Suzuki, T., Ohta, M., Hoshi, H.: In Vitro Cell. Dev. Biol., *25:*601–606, 1989.

75. McKeehan, W.L., McKeehan, K.A.: In Vitro, *16*:475–485, 1980.
76. Sand, T.-E., Christoffersen, T.: In Vitro Cell. Dev. Biol., *24*:981–984, 1988.
77. Kujawa, M.J., Lennon, D.P., Caplan, A.I.: Exp. Cell Res., *183*:45–61, 1989.
78. Ogasawara, M., Sirbasku, D.A.: In Vitro Cell. Dev. Biol., *24*:911–920, 1988.
79. Di Lorenzo, T.P., De Maro, J.A., Pumo, D.E.: In Vitro Cell. Dev. Biol., *25*:909–913, 1989.
80. McKeehan, W.L., Barnes, D., Reid, L., et al.: In Vitro Cell. Dev. Biol., *26*:9–23, 1990.

## SELECTED READINGS

Barnes, D.W., Sirbasku, D.A., Sato, G.H. (eds.): Cell Culture Methods for Molecular and Cell Biology. Vol. 1–4. New York, Alan R. Liss, 1984.

Fischer, G., Wieser, R.J. (eds.): Hormonally Defined Media. Berlin, Springer-Verlag, 1983.

Mather, J.P. (ed.): Mammalian Cell Culture: The Use of Serum-Free Hormone-Supplemented Media. New York, Plenum Press, 1984.

Sato, G.H., Pardee, A.B., Sirbasku, D.A. (eds.): Growth of Cells in Hormonally Defined Media, Cold Spring Harbor Conferences on Cell Proliferation. Vol. 9, Books A and B. Cold Spring Harbor, NY, Cold Spring Harbor Laboratory, 1982.

Waymouth, C., Ham, R.G., Chapple, P.J., (eds.): The Growth Requirements of Vertebrate Cells In Vitro. Cambridge, Cambridge University Press, 1981.

CHAPTER **35**

# Regulation of Food Intake

**G. Harvey Anderson**



The initiation and termination of feeding are complex processes that involve a large number of signals to the central nervous system (Fig. 35–1). In humans, cultural and social conventions can be major determinants of food intake, and are significant modifiers of the impact of metabolic and physiologic signals. However, the focus of this chapter is on the metabolic and physiologic cues that signal initiation or termination of feeding, at least in experimental animals. These cues may arise from the perception, ingestion, digestion, absorption, or metabolism of food and nutrients (Fig. 35–1). The brain serves as the organizer and integrator of these signals, balancing output and storage of nutrients with input (food intake). The purpose of this chapter is to illustrate that the metabolism of food for energy and nutrients is involved in food intake control mechanisms, and that, in the past 20 years, concepts have changed with respect to these signals and mechanisms.

Because the earlier theories of the regulation of total food intake and energy balance centered on the metabolism of glucose, fat, and amino acids, these theories and current views of their application will be examined first. Then the following sections will describe two relatively recent advances in our understanding of appetite regulation. First, it is now realized that food intake regulation involves not only the quantitative or energy content of food, but its composition as well. Therefore, evidence for the regulation of nutrient intake and of food selection, with specific reference to the control of fat, protein, and carbohydrate will be examined.

A second important advance has occurred with developments in the understanding of brain neurotransmitters and their function. This has resulted in identification of a large number of "appetite" signals and regulatory pathways within the brain. Therefore, in the final sections of this chapter current views of the involvement of brain centers and the role of brain neurotransmitters in control pathways determining energy balance and food selection is described.

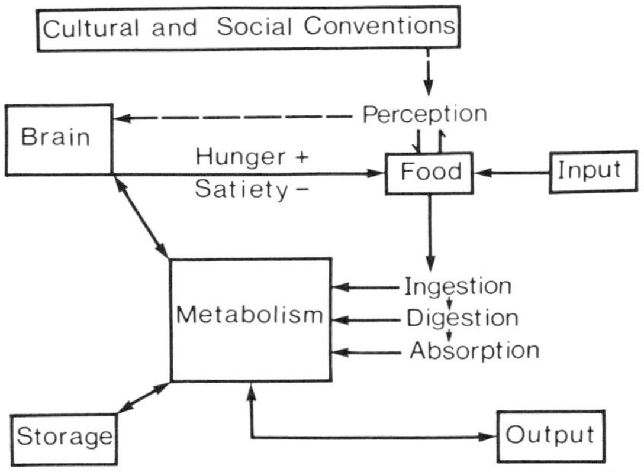
Cultural and Social Conventions
Perception
Brain
Hunger +
Satiety −
Food
Input
Metabolism
Ingestion
Digestion
Absorption
Storage
Output

**FIGURE 35–1.** An overview of sources of signals used by the brain in the regulation of body energy intake, output, and storage.

## REGULATION OF TOTAL FOOD INTAKE AND ENERGY BALANCE: MACRONUTRIENTS AS REGULATORS

Historically, the focus of research on the regulation of energy intake has been motivated by observations on the physiologic constancy of adult body weight[1] and concern with deviations from this, as occur in obesity and anorexia nervosa in the human. It is clear that when energy requirements are changed, food intake is rapidly and appropriately adjusted. For example, both cold exposure[2] and exercise[3] bring about a quantitative increase in food intake of rats. Also, after food deprivation, rats show compensatory overeating during the first few days of refeeding.[4] Thus, maintenance of energy balance appears to be a primary goal of the mechanism controlling feeding behavior.[5,6] It should not be surprising, therefore, that considerable scientific inquiry has been dedicated to elucidating the feeding control mechanisms regulating this easily defined motivation for feeding.

Because metabolic energy is ultimately derived from the three macronutrients, carbohydrate, fat, and protein, each has been investigated for a putative role in control mechanisms. Each of these nutrients, in addition to providing energy, has other properties that may also provide signals to the central nervous system.

### GLUCOSE

The enthusiasm for glucose as a primary metabolic substrate regulating food intake is related to its role as a ready source of cellular energy. Glucose is readily converted to energy (adenosine triphosphate, or ATP), $CO_2$, and $H_2O$ in all cells of the body. Not all cells require glucose as the energy substrate, but the brain and presumably the appetite regulatory centers depend on glucose under normal day-to-day conditions of feeding. Thus, fluctuations in blood glucose levels, seen as an indication of availability of glucose to nervous tissue and glucose utilization by brain cells, have been suggested as primary signals leading to regulation of food intake. This is known as the glucostatic theory of food intake.[6]

The role of blood glucose concentration in providing signals either indirectly or directly to the brain is uncertain, however. Although it has been reported that a 7% decrease in blood glucose concentration occurs prior to the initiation of meals in the rat,[7] and that with food consumption, blood glucose increases,[8] it is also clear that hypoglycemia does not consistently elicit eating. For example, infusion of fructose, a sugar that does not cross the blood-brain barrier,[9] to insulin-treated rats terminates feeding despite the presence of hypoglycemia.[10] This observation suggests that feeding after insulin treatments may not be purely a consequence of hypoglycemia but due to other effects of insulin. These effects may include a reduction in the concentration of plasma free fatty acids, ketone bodies, and amino acids, any one of which may influence, directly or indirectly, signals to the brain.[11] Conversely, hyperglycemia does not necessarily suppress feeding. Intravenous infusion of glucose sufficient to raise blood glucose by a constant 20 to 30 mg% did not in one study affect either frequency of eating or the amount consumed by rats.[12]

Uncertainty with respect to the role of blood glucose concentration in controlling feeding probably arises from the fact that blood concentration does not necessarily indicate the rate of glucose utilization by tissues. Therefore, it is encouraging for subscribers to the glucostatic hypothesis of feeding to find that brain cellular glucose utilization appears to be more closely related to feeding. A high rate of cellular glucose utilization after a meal corresponds with a state of satiation in animals,[13] whereas the converse is associated with eating.[14]

In the past 5 years, new evidence that transient declines in blood glucose serve as signals for initiation of feeding in nondeprived rats has been derived through continuous monitoring of blood glucose and feeding.[15] It is hypothesized that transient declines that follow a specified pattern, measured in magnitude and time, reliably predict the initiation of a meal. The mechanism underlying this relationship has not been defined and could be associated with either a decrease in brain utilization of glucose, or with brain stimulation by events of peripheral origin.

In addition to brain cellular energy utilization serving as an indicator of glucose availability, it has been proposed that glucose availability in the liver influences glucoreceptors, which provide signals to the brain via the vagus nerve.[16] This would explain the observation that when glucose utilization in the liver is blocked by infusion of 2-deoxy-D-glucose, an antimetabolite of glucose, into the portal vein of rabbits, eating is elicited. Systemic infusions are much less effective.[17] Further evidence that there is a relationship between the liver's metabolism of glucose and satiety has been provided from studies of the effects of hepatic-portal glucose infusions. A decrease in food intake after glucose infusion into the portal vein occurs in food-deprived but not fed rabbits,[17] suggesting that liver energy reserve (glycogen) modifies the sensitivity of the hepatic glucoreceptors.

A link between glucoreceptors in the liver and the brain's control of feeding probably involves messages transmitted via the vagus nerve. Subdiaphragmatic vagotomy blocks the food intake suppression caused by duodenal glucose infusion.[18] The dependence of long-term body energy balance or even meal size on hepatic glucoreceptors seems unlikely, however, because denervation of the liver in dogs and rats does not affect food consumption.[19] Thus, although glucose concentrations in plasma and tissues and glucose utilization appear to influence feeding under certain conditions, it is also clear that these factors do not offer as much of an explanation of the mechanisms of food intake regulation as originally expected.[6]

## LIPID

The lipostatic theory of food intake regulation is based on the observation that depot fat in animals serves as an energy reservoir, suggesting that variations in total energy storage (adiposity) should provide signals that cause animals to alter their energy intake.[20] Whether or not there is any direct link, neural or otherwise, between body fat stores and feeding control mechanisms in the brain has not been established. Similarly, the significance of fat mass per se and its regulation is uncertain because it is clear that food consumption, in excess, can occur in obese animals and humans.[21] It is probable, however, that circulating substrates derived from fat metabolism influence food consumption.

The mobilization of body fat, with the release of free fatty acids and glycerol, and the interaction with glucose metabolism provide a possible explanation of circadian fluctuation of food intake in the rat, as well as some evidence of a link between brain function and lipid metabolism. On a day-to-day basis, lipid metabolism is synchronized with the circadian fluctuation in food intake[22] and appears to be under the influence of the ventromedial hypothalamus (VMH), a brain region involved in feeding control and historically called the "satiety" center. Stimulation of the VMH enhances lipolysis in white adipose tissues,[23,24] which in turn is associated with decreased feeding. Furthermore, electrical activity in the VMH, but not in the lateral hypothalamus (the "feeding" center) of rats, is enhanced during the light period when they do not eat and when lipolysis is occurring, but is suppressed during the dark hours when they do eat.[25] Consistent with the link between lipid metabolism and feeding is the observation that a day-time feeding pattern can be induced during the dark hours by stimulating lipid breakdown with adrenaline infusion.[26] Conversely, if lipid synthesis is stimulated during the light period by insulin infusions, rats develop a meal pattern consisting of hyperphagia and increased meal frequency similar to that normally observed at night.[27]

Mobilization of body fat during the light hours has been suggested as the reason that rats ingest only two to three meals, accounting for less than 25% of their daily intake, throughout the light period of a 24-hour light-dark cycle.[28] Those who emphasize a role for glucose in the initiation and termination of feeding suggest that the expected initiation of a meal by a fall in blood glucose is delayed during the light portion of the day because there is an endogenous supply of energy from lipolysis.[29] In contrast, during the dark hours, the rat's insulin response to a glucose load is enhanced, as is lipogenesis and glucose utilization. This results in a rapid fall in blood glucose after each eating episode, reduced levels of substrates from fat breakdown, and more meals initiated at night. In this way it is proposed that metabolism of glucose and lipid interact in signaling the brain's regulation of feeding.[22,29] Clearly, however, body lipid stores, or plasma lipid content, do not independently control feeding behavior.

There is no readily apparent product of lipid metabolism that can be used to explain feeding behavior.[23,30,31] Plasma levels of the products of lipid metabolism, including free fatty acids, glycerol, triglycerides, and ketone bodies (β-hydroxy-butyrate, acetoacetate) fluctuate with feeding and fasting. During and immediately after a meal triglycerides predominate, and are the primary vehicle of transport of fat from the gut and liver to adipose tissue. Because of concurrent insulin release, free fatty acids, glycerol, and ketone bodies are very low. Gradually, however, as availability of the products of digestion is depleted, adipose tissue switches from taking up fat to releasing it. This release results in an increase in plasma free fatty acids, glycerol, and ketone bodies. As pointed out earlier, it is thought that, in the rat, the presence of these energy substrates reduces frequency of eating during the day.[22] Similarly, it has been proposed that the loss of acute hunger associated with fasting or very restricted food intake of greater than 2 or 3 days in man is specifically due to the presence of ketone bodies in plasma. This view does not appear to withstand examination, however, because no correlation was found between plasma and urinary ketone levels and subjective hunger in obese men on an energy-restricted diet in one study.[30] Advocates of the lipostatic theory have also suggested that an increase in plasma free fatty acids, such as that which occurs when adipose tissue is mobilized, signals that food consumption should begin.[31] This hypothesis obviously contradicts the view that the presence of free fatty acids explains the rat's lack of eating during the light hours.

Possibly the mechanism of fat storage and mobilization is in itself a signal to the brain, although, as pointed out earlier, a direct link has not been made between adipose tissue and the brain. The activity of adipose tissue lipoprotein lipase (LPL), the enzyme that breaks down triglycerides for ultimate storage in adipose tissue, appears to correlate with food intake. For example, ovariectomy, which decreases LPL activity, decreases fat storage and food intake.[32] Because an increase in LPL activity preceeds the increased food intake in genetically obese rats, the possibility exists that capacity for fuel storage has some effect on food consumption.[33] Overall, however, one can only conclude that the roles of fat metabolites, fat stores, and fat synthesis as components of food intake control mechanisms merit considerable further investigation.

## AMINO ACIDS

Amino acids, like fat and glucose, provide energy to body cells. Their primary role, however, is in the formation of body proteins and in the provision of substrates for the synthesis of several important regulators of metabolism, including creatine, carnitine, polyamines, purine, pyrimidine, and neurotransmitters. Studies of the role of amino acids in regulating feeding behavior illustrate clearly that the production of energy is not the only aspect of macronutrient metabolism significant to appetite control.

The concept that plasma amino acids influence feeding behavior was introduced in the early 1950s by Mellinkoff et al.[34] They observed an inverse relationship between serum amino acid concentration and appetite in man, and proposed that the brain is sensitive to amino acids, through mechanisms independent of their energy-producing property. This postulate is known as the aminostatic theory of feeding control. In the following years, considerable work has been undertaken to identify the shifts in plasma and brain amino acids that may influence the brain's regulation of feeding.[35]

The inhibition of food intake by high-protein or imbalanced diets has been associated with shifts in the plasma[35] and brain[36] amino acid patterns in rats. For example, rats fed high-protein diets display a marked and sustained increase in plasma branched-chain amino acids,[37,38] which may be of significance to appetite control. Branched-chain amino acids could influence feeding behavior either directly because of their elevation in brain free amino acid pools, or indirectly by blocking brain uptake of other large neutral amino acids that share a common system for uptake across the blood-brain barrier.[39] As will be shown later, some of the amino acids occurring in decreased concentrations in the brain serve as precursors for the synthesis of neurotransmitters involved in control mechanisms of feeding.[39,40] Thus, amino acid deficits may signal the brain through their effect on neurotransmitter synthesis, but this is not necessarily the only mechanism by which appetite regulating centers are signaled by amino acids, as is illustrated by the effect of feeding imbalanced diets.

The decreased feeding induced by imbalanced diets may be due to decreased availability of a growth-limiting amino acid to the brain rather than to excesses of amino acids.[41] Imbalanced diets are created by adding to a low-protein diet, usually 6% casein, an equal quantity of an amino acid mixture that does not contain one of the essential amino acids.[35] Feeding activity can be restored if the supply of the growth-limiting amino acid is increased by its injection into the carotid artery. In contrast, the same quantity of amino acid injected into the jugular vein, and hence distributed to other tissues as well as to the brain, has no effect on food intake.[41]

Depression of food intake has been reported to occur in response to individual amino acids, based on studies conducted with individual amino acids added in excess (1 to 10% of the diet) to a low-protein diet fed to rats.[35] However, large amounts of tryptophan, tyrosine, or phenylalanine given individually by gavage have little effect. Other amino acids have not been tested for their acute effects on food intake.[42] However, there is now an indication that relatively small amounts of amino acids affect feeding behavior in humans. For example, a mixture of four amino acids (phenylalanine, 3 g; valine, 2 g; methionine, 2 g; tryptophan, 1 g) taken by overweight subjects 1 half-hour before a midday meal reduced their food intake by 22.5%.[43] Tryptophan alone, in amounts of 2 or 3 g, also reduced lunch-time intake of normal-weight young men and women.[44]

Brain regions sensitive to alterations in plasma amino acid patterns or levels appear to lie outside the hypothalamus, the center traditionally recognized in the regulation of food intake. Lesions of the VMH have little effect on the food intake depression observed following consumption of imbalanced diets.[45] Rather, it appears that the amygdala and prepyriform cortex may be involved in mediating the response to amino acid imbalanced and deficient diets. Rats with prepyriform cortex lesions failed to depress food intake of amino acid imbalanced and deficient diets, whereas rats with amygdala lesions failed to respond to imbalanced diets.[41] Bilateral injection of the dietary limiting amino acid into the prepyriform cortex restores feeding.[46] These are not the only brain regions sensitive to plasma amino acids, however, because both lesioned groups showed depressed food intake after consumption of high-protein diets.

## INTEGRATION OF FUELS

As has been shown previously, a variety of mechanisms based on individual glucostatic, lipostatic, or aminostatic signals have been proposed as the metabolic basis of energy intake regulation. However, an integrative view of the role of carbohydrate, fat, and protein in feeding control has been proposed, based on their property of energy production. This hypothesis states that the initiation of feeding occurs when the brain receives a message of a generalized decreased rate of utilization at the cellular level of all of the energy-producing substrates.[47] Support for the integrated control of food intake based on the oxidation of metabolic fuels arises from evidence that simultaneous inhibition of glucose and fatty acid metabolism in the liver produces a synergistic increase in food intake.[48] It is unclear, however, how the brain receives information arising from fuel oxidation and the extent to which the liver or other sites are the source of the information.

Although the mechanism is not understood, animals regulate energy balance on diets of widely differing macronutrient content and density if the conditions are such that protein and other nutrient requirements can be met. For example, animals fed high-protein diets will initially show a food intake depression, but will quickly increase their metabolic capacity to catabolize amino acids, and as a result food intake returns to normal.[35,39] Hence, it would seem that the ingestion of sufficient food to achieve energy balance is a priority within appetite regulatory systems, and that the system must be able to detect total energy flow and storage. It is reasonable therefore to ask why metabolites derived from each of the macronutrients appear to be involved in control mechanisms regulating food intake, but yet can be so easily ignored in the achievement of energy balance. An answer to this question may be found in the fact that animals have the ability to regulate quality in addition to quantity of food intake.

## REGULATION OF NUTRIENT INTAKE AND FOOD SELECTION

Animals survive and reproduce in a variety of nutritional environments. This suggests that they are able to choose from this environment foods that maximize their chance of survival by being adequate in essential nutrients and free of poisonous or harmful substances. It is clear that animals have adapted to their environments by a variety of anatomic and physiologic developments, so that, for example, some animals are principally herbivores and others carnivores. In addition, food selection is appropriate, suggesting that mechanisms have been developed to link internal metabolic processes to needs and to consequences of eating.

Despite the situation existing in nature, most scientists have chosen to feed their test animals single diets of fixed composition. Thus, the majority of literature on appetite regulation is made up of reports describing whether or not the animal eats the one diet chosen by the investigators. Because only one diet is fed, it is easy to translate the feeding response into one indicating that the role of control mechanisms relates solely to the goal of achieving energy balance.

Yet, the early literature has also provided a clear indication of nutrient specific appetites in animals. In 1918, Osborne and Mendel observed that rats ate little of a protein-free diet when also provided an 18% casein diet.[49] They wrote: "It is therefore interesting to have this evidence that the desire of a young animal for food is something more than the mere satisfaction of its calorific needs."

The concept of nutrient-specific appetites was more extensively investigated in the 1940s. Curt Richter demonstrated that rats offered a wide choice of foods survived and grew as well as rats fed a standard laboratory chow.[50] He suggested that rats were able to maintain relatively constant daily intakes of most nutrients by adjusting their food choices according to nutrient requirements and nutrient availability.

### SPECIFIC APPETITES FOR VITAMINS AND MINERALS

For some vitamins and minerals, specific appetites have been illustrated in a food choice situation and under circumstances in which nutrient deficiencies or abnormal metabolisms occur. One of the best-known examples of this is presented by the adrenalectomized rat. These animals experience high sodium loss, but compensate for deficits in body sodium by choosing to drink a salt solution rather than water.[50] Similarly, rats that are parathyroidectomized and unable to maintain plasma calcium levels by mobilization of stores show a preference for a dietary source of calcium.[51]

Vitamin deficiencies can also be detected and appropriate diets can be chosen, as illustrated in the case of thiamine. Thiamine-deficient rats quickly learned to detect a thiamine-containing diet and ignore the deficient one. If the rats are maintained on a thiamine-adequate diet, however, they do not illustrate a strong preference.[52] Although these examples illustrate that specific appetites for vitamins and minerals can be demonstrated under certain conditions of metabolic deficiencies, they do not show that there is a quantitative regulation of micronutrient intake. That is, the fact that animals fed deficient diets make appropriate choices, perhaps on the basis of gross metabolic disturbances, and learn to choose a food that alleviates the disturbances, does not necessarily indicate that in normal rats metabolism guides their choice.

An excellent demonstration of a quantitative regulation of a micronutrient intake by well nourished, healthy rats is that shown for phosphorus.[53,54] When given a choice of high- or low-phosphorus diets, growing or adult rats selected a remarkably constant 0.23 to 0.24% or 0.64 to 0.69%, respectively, of their diet as phosphorus.[54] Why phosphorus should be so precisely regulated on a day-to-day basis, whereas calcium is not, is presently unexplained. Whether or not intake of other micronutrients can be regulated in accordance with physiologic needs remains to be determined.

In contrast to current information on micronutrient intake regulation, the better-defined regulation of macronutrient consumption has offered some direction toward a definition of metabolically based control mechanisms regulating food intake. In particular, the fact that the animal is able to regulate intakes of protein, carbohydrate, or fat if offered dietary choices shows the benefit of metabolic signals arising from each of these food constituents.

### REGULATION OF MACRONUTRIENT INTAKE

Despite earlier investigation, the presence of macronutrient-specific appetites was not clearly established until the past decade. The early efforts by Richter[50] and others[55] were likely confounded because of the then-existing lack of knowledge of the nutrient needs of the rat. As a result, although the rats were given food choices, the dietary circumstances were often such that it was impossible for the rat to obtain a nutritionally complete diet. It would be predicted then that metabolic signals arising in the brain from the micronutrient deficiencies would not allow the rat to provide the investigator with evidence for macronutrient-specific appetites. In the past 10 years, macronutrient-specific appetites have been reinvestigated and their presence has been firmly established.

## *PROTEIN INTAKE*

As pointed out earlier, the concept of protein intake regulation is not new; the first investigation of the rat's ability to regulate this component of the diet can be dated back to 1918.[49] Since then, studies designed to examine this aspect of food intake regulation have used the approach of allowing the rats an opportunity to select for protein as well as for energy.[39] As a result, evidence has emerged that protein intake is regulated not only on a day-to-day basis[56] but also within the day[28] and even within a meal.[57]

A systematic investigation of the rat's ability to regulate protein intake on a day-to-day basis was reported in 1974 by Musten et al.[56] In their studies, young rats were simultaneously presented with two diets differing only in protein and carbohydrate content. One diet of the choice was low in protein and high in carbohydrate, whereas the other was high in protein and low in carbohydrate. By substituting carbohydrate for protein (or vice versa) the diets formed were kept isocaloric. As well, both diets were complete with respect to vitamins and minerals and contained identical nutrient-to-energy ratios.

From a number of dietary choices (e.g., 0 and 50%, 15 and 55%, 25 and 65% protein), rats regulated their protein intake at a constant proportion of their food consumed, averaging 33 to 35% of the dietary energy. Furthermore, this regulation was almost as precise as the regulation of total energy intake.[56] Other studies have shown that a constant energy density of the diets is not essential because the rat seeks a constant protein intake under a variety of circumstances. When diets containing the protein sources were diluted with noncaloric materials such as water or agar, methyl cellulose and water, or non-nutritive fiber, both adult and weanling rats compensated by adjusting their intake of the protein-containing diet so that protein consumption remained relatively constant.[58,59]

Although it is now generally agreed that experimental animals regulate their intake of protein if they are fed dietary choices, the precision of this regulation has little agreement. This problem arises from the low external validity of procedures used within any one laboratory. Depending on many factors, including diet composition, sex, and age of the rats, protein intake may be as high as 40% or as low as 15% of the total calories. Furthermore, variability among rats in a group can be high, even though the individual rat maintains a relatively constant selection pattern.[59]

Because the amount of protein selected is usually at or above the required level of 13 to 15% of dietary energy,[60] the existence of a protein intake regulatory mechanism in the rat might serve to ensure an intake of protein adequate to provide for its needs. In general, the quantity of protein consumed is a characteristic of the particular protein fed and the animal's usual intake.[58,59] By adding certain amino acids to the protein, the quantity consumed can be manipulated while energy intake remains unaffected. For example, adding lysine to gluten, tryptophan to casein and to zein, or methionine to casein causes the rat to select a lower proportion of food energy as protein, but calorie intake is usually unaffected.[60,61] Whether this decrease in protein intake caused by amino acid additions is due to an improvement of protein quality or is the specific effect of the amino acids added awaits future investigation.

A dissociation between the control mechanisms that regulate protein and energy intake also occurs. When adjustment in energy intake is necessary the rat's protein intake is usually unaffected. For example, animals selectively increase their energy intake while maintaining a constant intake of protein when their energy requirement is increased by either cold exposure[56] or increased activity.[3] Similarly, hyperphagia in rats given ventromedial hypothalamus lesions and in the genetically obese Zucker rats is characterized by overconsumption of total food energy as carbohydrate and fat, whereas protein intake is similar to that of appropriate control animals.[62] Although these findings indicate a functional separation of the controls of protein and energy intake, it is reasonable to assume that both mechanisms must interact to determine food intake.

An ability to quantitatively regulate protein intake has been demonstrated for species other than the rat, including mice,[63] dogs,[64] and chickens.[65] A protein intake regulatory mechanism might exist in humans, but the evidence is weak. Whenever a diverse and adequate food supply is available, man consumes 14 to 16% of the dietary calories as protein, even though food varies in protein concentration from 0 to 96%, and the proportions of fat and carbohydrate calories consumed vary markedly.[66] More-direct evidence comes from one study of the dietary patterns of monozygotic versus dizygotic twins. Dietary records obtained from each of twin pairs raised in separate home environments showed that dietary protein concentration selected by monozygotic identical twin pairs was similar. In contrast, the diets of dizygotic twins raised in different home environments were dissimilar, suggesting that a primitive, genetically determined control mechanism may underlie protein intake in man.[67] The only current evidence for physiologic determinants of protein intake arises from the demonstration of enhanced taste preference for protein solutions by protein-malnourished elderly persons.[68] Perhaps the depleted protein state was a signal for the brain to increase sensory identification of protein sources.

Protein intake by the rat is regulated not only on a day-to-day, but a meal-to-meal basis. Evidence for meal-to-meal regulation emerged from studies in which selection of protein and of total food energy was monitored throughout the day. Rats given simultaneous access to a high-protein and a protein-free diet showed different circadian patterns of protein and energy intake.[28] Energy intake, mainly from the protein-free, primarily carbohydrate diet, showed large circadian fluctuations, with the largest intake occurring in meals consumed during the dark period. In contrast, average protein intake at a meal is relatively constant throughout the day. However, small variations in protein consumed within a meal occur and appear to be of significance in determining both size and time of onset of the subsequent meal.[28] That is, a positive correlation is present between the quantity of protein in a meal and the postprandial interval. Moreover, the calories derived from the nonprotein components of a meal are directly related to the length of the interval immediately preceding that meal. Taken together, this information shows that after a low-protein meal the rat will take a shorter-than-average time to start another meal and, consequently, this meal will be selected so that it contains relatively more protein and fewer carbohydrate calories than average.

The effect of recently ingested food composition on subsequent food choice and macronutrient preference has been more-precisely defined by providing rats a choice of diets after they were fed either carbohydrate or protein meals. In one study, high-protein meals suppressed total food intake in the absence of food choice,[35] and another study showed that, in the presence of a food choice, high-protein meals led to decreased preference for protein (or a relatively increased preference for carbohydrate) in a subsequent meal.[57]

## CARBOHYDRATE INTAKE

The notion of a regulated carbohydrate appetite has also been with us for some time. By using a variation of the self-selection method of feeding, Soulairac attempted to quantitate the rat's ability to regulate carbohydrate intake.[69] He allowed rats access to carbohydrate-containing fluids, as well as to food. His observations had the benefit of showing that modification of carbohydrate metabolism can affect appetite for carbohydrate. Unfortunately he did not report data on either total energy or carbohydrate intake, but only on amount of carbohydrate solution consumed.

Evidence for carbohydrate as a regulated variable driving diet selection is indirect and much less convincing than for protein. However, diet selection studies have been used to provide evidence for carbohydrate intake regulation.[70] Under a given set of conditions carbohydrate intake can be shown to be relatively constant, but depending on the conditions, rats select from 10 to 80% of their diets as carbohydrate. The level chosen is influenced by taste, texture, and composition of the diet choices, and whether or not the rat has a choice of all three macronutrients or of some combination of two diets.[71] In contrast to their willingness to work to maintain protein intake, rats will do little work for carbohydrate.[72] Carbohydrate intake by humans is also highly variable, ranging from 40 to 80% of the habitual diets, depending on the composition of the food supply.[66] Possibly the distinguishing feature between protein and carbohydrate as regulated variables relates to the fact that protein is an essential nutrient, whereas there is no evidence of a requirement for carbohydrate, except perhaps in very small quantities (e.g., 50 g to prevent ketosis in humans).

The absence of a dietary requirement for carbohydrate does not exclude the possibility that food selection is guided by its carbohydrate composition. As is the situation for protein consumption, carbohydrate consumption has immediate effects on food selection. Food choice has been examined in fasting animals allowed to consume a small (25-kJ) premeal supplement containing either carbohydrate or carbohydrate and protein. Ninety minutes later the rats were allowed access to a pair of isoenergetic, isoprotein 25% and 75% carbohydrate diets. Those eating the carbohydrate premeal supplement chose to eat less of the high-carbohydrate diet, even though they ate the same number of calories as those eating the mixed premeal supplement.[70]

## FAT INTAKE

There is little information on regulation of fat intake. Again, however, in a given set of circumstances, relative constancy of fat selection has been described.[71,73] For example, when the protein concentration of a high-fat and a high-carbohydrate diet choice was kept at 32% protein energy, rats selected approximately 60% of the daily intake as fat. However, if the protein provided only 10% of the protein energy in both diets, the rats switched to the high-carbohydrate diet, and consumed only 20% of the diet as fat energy.[73] This switch to carbohydrate from fat energy when protein is limiting may offer further proof that protein intake is regulated closely to requirements. Carbohydrate, compared to fat, is known to be protein sparing, and hence its consumption when protein is limiting would be an obvious advantage to the rat.

An examination of the literature will lead the reviewer to conclude that the absolute intake of protein, carbohydrate, and fat selected by rats varies considerably among reports. This variation cannot be readily explained and is in contrast to energy intake, which is found to be relatively constant, when expressed relative to body size, for animals fed different diets in different locations. Overall, however, it is clear that within a constant set of experimental conditions the selection of macronutrients by the rat is remarkably consistent. As a result, control mechanisms regulating each of these appetites are being examined. Studies to date have established the principle that control mechanisms previously thought to be involved only in regulating energy intake are also possible regulators of nutrient-specific appetites.

## BRAIN MECHANISMS AND THE REGULATION OF FOOD INTAKE

For metabolic events to affect feeding behavior, they must first be detected by the nervous system. Thus, the role of various brain regions in the control of feeding behavior has been extensively studied. From this work, the central role of the hypothalamus in the control of feeding has been identified. Originally, on the basis of lesion studies, the VMH was identified as the satiety center because its destruction resulted in overeating and increased body weight. The lateral hypothalamus (LH) was identified as the feeding center because its destruction caused starvation. Although oversimplified, this concept of the hypothalamus having two control centers has served as a useful working model in the study of feeding mechanisms. At this time, however, it is more appropriate to recognize the hypothalamus as an integrative unit functioning in the brain's reception and organization of the many signals arising from food ingestion.

The brain serves as the organizer and integrator of the many signals arising from food (Fig. 35–1). Signals begin at the cognitive level, arising from the sight, smell, or thought of food. These signals initiate the cephalic phase of appetite, during which time there is a stimulation of hunger and increased sympathetic outflow from the brain, resulting in metabolic activity designed to prepare the system for the ingestion of food.[74,75] For example, salivation, gastric secretions, and hormone activity increase. Satiation is brought about by a sequence of events arising from the sensory, postingestive, and postabsorptive consequence of food.[74] These factors combine to terminate the meal, and to determine the time of onset, composition, and size of the next meal. Ultimately the brain must relate these short-term, meal-to-meal events to the goal of balancing input on the longer term with output and storage of nutrients and energy.

### SENSORY SIGNALS

The sensory qualities (taste, smell, texture, and appearance) of food are strong determinants of eating behavior.[76] Humans begin life with innate taste preferences, with a preference for sweet taste, rejection of bitter and sour substances, and an indifferent response to salty taste. Taste preferences are modified by experience resulting in either increased or decreased acceptability of foods. For example, food preferences of children are strongly influenced by their parents and by their social environments. Thus it is unlikely that biologic factors alone can account for the observation of large individual variation in food preference.

The sensory properties of food play a role, however, in not only determining its consumption but also in determining the satiety value of the food and total food intake and food selection during a meal. In general, the pleasantness of a food is greater during hunger than when sated. Furthermore, the observation that the hedonic value of a food or of foods similar in sensory properties decline as they are consumed suggests that satiety is not a general phenomenon, but during a meal is specific to the particular foods consumed.[76] As a result, this may be a mechanism that encourages the consumption of a variety of foods for the purpose of increasing the opportunity for the ingestion of all essential nutrients. That is, if the pleasantness of a food declines as it is consumed, this will encourage a choice of other uneaten foods, which will appear relatively more palatable.

The largest changes in hedonic property of foods occur rapidly and thus before much of the meal is absorbed. Thus, it is not surprising that the hedonic value of foods can modify the size of the meal consumed. Increasing the variations in flavor, appearance, and mouth feel of a specific food enhances food intake by 15%, whereas giving meals containing several different foods can enhance intake by 60% over when only a single food item is provided.[76]

How these short-term meal responses to the sensory properties of foods in a meal relate to the longer-term regulation of energy and nutrient balances is unclear. Whether or not the sensory properties of food reflected in the variety of foods available today account for the increased prevalence of obesity in the population, suggesting an override of food intake control mechanisms, is a matter of debate. Rats fed cafeteria-type diets, composed of a variety of foods appealing to humans, become obese. On the other hand, there is no evidence that obese humans consume excess calories because of preference for any one food property (e.g., sweetness) or because of the availability of sensorily appealing foods.[76]

### PREABSORPTIVE SIGNALS

With the ingestion and digestion of food causing gastric distension and the release of fat, amino acids, and glucose, preabsorptive information is provided to the brain via the vagus nerve. Evidence has been obtained for the presence of gastrointestinal mechanoreceptors, osmoreceptors, and chemoreceptors.[58,74] Glucose, amino acids, and fat also signal the release of gastrointestinal hormones, 10 of which have been shown to inhibit feeding (cholecystokinin, bombesin, gastrin, secretin, glucagon, insulin, somatostatin, neurotensin, substance P, and pancreatic polypeptide).[77]

Of the gut hormones, cholecystokinin (CCK) is the most studied modulator of food intake. The satiety effect of intravenous CCK has been demonstrated in mice, rats, rabbits, rhesus monkeys, and humans. CCK is released from the small intestine by fatty acids and intact protein.[78] It has a rapid onset of action and shortens the duration of eating without affecting the rate of eating. The peripheral action of the hormone in some species appears to depend on the vagus nerve, specifically the afferant branch arising from the stomach. If this branch of the nerve is cut in rodents, CCK injections do not bring about reductions in food intake. Whether or not CCK or any of the other gut peptides are physiologic satiety agents remains uncertain.[79]

### POSTABSORPTIVE SIGNALS

Postabsorptively—that is, after entry into the portal vein and passage to the liver—nutrients may also provide, via the vagus nerve, information to the brain. For example, as reviewed earlier, glucose entry to the liver and its storage are known to influence feeding behavior.[16]

Plasma fluctuations in nutrients are clearly useful to the brain in monitoring the "milieu interior." These fluctuations create changes in brain concentrations because of the activity of many blood-brain barrier transport systems.[80,81] Neurons sense change in availability of a nutrient by a variety of mechanisms including direct interaction with receptors (e.g., glucose[82] and amino acids[83]), recognition of a change in rate of nutrient utilization for energy production (e.g., glucose[6]), and recognition of altered neurotransmitter activity because of precursor (e.g., tyrosine or tryptophan), or cofactor (e.g., B, iron) roles of nutrients in neurotransmitter synthesis.[84] With altered neuronal activity, a large number of neuronal systems become involved, and may utilize many monoamine and neuropeptide neurotransmitters. Eventually, the information provided becomes integrated, and feeding behavior is regulated to maintain the nutritional homeostasis of the organism.[74]

To fully understand the brain's regulation of feeding behavior, a determination of what brain signals initiate a meal, as well as those which terminate a meal, is of fundamental importance. Classic theories of feeding behavior have suggested that the LH is always providing a tonic signal for the rat to eat, and appetite regulation is primarily an inhibition of this signal. However, both endogenous and exogenous opioid peptides have been shown to stimulate food intake, and it has been proposed that stress-induced eating in both human beings and experimental animals may be stimulated by opiate release.[86] The attractive hypothesis has been stated that obesity may result from an autoaddiction to endogenous opioid peptides, but this remains to be proved. Nevertheless, this information raises the possibility that eating is initiated by specific signals, rather than by a decreased presence of appetite-suppressive signals.

The large number of signals already identified that influence feeding suggests that there is redundancy in feeding-control mechanisms. Alternatively, it has been proposed that all of these factors may in some way be involved, in a cascade of events.[74] If so, many of the appetite signals identified to date may not be of independent significance, but may be interdependent components of a complex system.

## BRAIN MECHANISMS AND THE REGULATION OF MACRONUTRIENT INTAKE

Confusion with respect to the importance of each of the putative signals influencing feeding may also arise from the experimental design of the majority of feeding studies. As indicated previously, most studies of control mechanisms have utilized energy balance and total food intake, without regard to meal composition, as measures of feeding behavior. However, the determination of nutrient-specific appetites has indicated that some control mechanisms that were previously proposed as being involved in the determination of energy balance may also be nutrient-specific. For example, the hypothalamus and many neuronal systems are involved in the regulation of macronutrient intake.

The hypothalamus plays a role in the regulation of macronutrient selection, in addition to its established role in the regulation of energy balance. Ventromedial hypothalamic lesions and parasagittal knife cuts through the medial hypothalamus cause hyperphagia. However, in a situation in which the rat is allowed access to separate sources of protein, carbohydrate, and fat, the hyperphagia is expressed by a preferred consumption of carbohydrate.[86] This increase in carbohydrate appetite could be due to hyperinsulinemia, which also occurs with these lesions. However, rats with paraventricular hypothalamic (PVH) lesions are not hyperinsulinemic,[87] but also have increased carbohydrate appetites, suggesting that the hypothalamic neuronal circuitry is directly involved in the regulation of carbohydrate intake.

Of the neurotransmitters now known to influence food choice, which include serotonin (5-hydroxytryptamine, 5-HT), norepinephrine, and the opiates, the role of serotonin has received the closest examination. Based on studies in which rats were allowed access to single diets while serotonergic systems were pharmacologically manipulated, its action has been described as inhibitory.[74] More recent research, however, suggests that a role of 5-HT may be to regulate the composition of food consumed in such a way as to achieve an adequate intake and balance of protein and carbohydrate. This role of 5-HT may be predicted for two reasons. First, brain 5-HT synthesis is under control by the availability of its tryptophan precursor. The rate-limiting enzyme in the pathway of conversion of tryptophan to serotonin is tryptophan hydroxylase. Because this enzyme, which converts tryptophan to 5-hydroxytryptophan, the first product in the pathway to serotonin, is not fully saturated by normal brain tryptophan concentrations, fluctuations in tryptophan availability influence serotonin synthesis.[39,40,74] Thus, events that influence plasma tryptophan concentration and brain uptake can be expected to modify brain serotonin synthesis. A second reason for predicting that 5-HT may be involved in the regulation of food selection arises from the fact that brain tryptophan availability is modulated in opposite directions by carbohydrate and protein consumption.[88]

Tryptophan (TRP), a dietary essential amino acid, appears in the blood as a result of protein ingestion and body protein breakdown. It is transported across the blood-brain barrier via a carrier mechanism specific for the large neutral amino acids (NAAs), which include tryptophan, tyrosine, phenylalanine, valine, isoleucine, and methionine.[81] Because of the competitive nature of amino acid uptake, the effect of food ingestion on brain tryptophan is not simply related to its tryptophan content. Because tryptophan is present in protein in relatively small amounts, a meal of protein causes a greater increase in plasma large neutral amino acids relative to tryptophan, decreasing the ratio of plasma TRP/NAA and therefore brain tryptophan uptake.[88] Conversely, a carbohydrate meal increases the plasma TRP/NAA ratio.[39,84] This is due to carbohydrate-induced insulin release, which increases the uptake of all amino acids into tissues; insulin, however, has a lesser effect on tryptophan, which is carried in plasma both in free form and bound to albumin.[89] Insulin reduces the free fatty acid content of plasma, and consequently the amount available to bind with albumin is decreased. Because tryptophan and fatty acids have the same binding site on albumin, tryptophan binding increases after a carbohydrate meal, and tends to be retained in plasma. Tryptophan is released, however, as albumin transverses the brain capillaries, and because of tryptophan's competitive advantage in the blood and hence at the blood-brain barrier, more tryptophan enters the brain relative to other competing amino acids. Thus, protein ingestion decreases brain serotonin level by limiting brain tryptophan uptake, whereas tryptophan administration and carbohydrate ingestion increase the concentration of brain tryptophan and serotonin.

On the basis of the observations that rats are capable of regulating macronutrient intake, and that brain serotonin synthesis can be affected in opposite directions by carbohydrate and protein ingestion, a serotonin hypothesis of food selection was advanced.[59,90] In this hypothesis, diet-induced changes in brain serotonin metabolism are described as components of a feedback regulatory loop that controls protein and carbohydrate selection (Fig. 35–2). This hypothesis has been the subject of considerable debate,[91] and the physiologic significance of the susceptibility of serotonergic neurons to respond to diet composition remains unresolved.[92]

Some support for physiologic relevance is derived from observation that rats fed a meal rich in carbohydrate emphasize protein in the next meal[70] and vice versa.[57] Increases in rat brain 5-HT concentrations and turnover occur after the carbohydrate meal and are further increased if the meal contains a small amount (15 mg) of TRP.[93] The addition of TRP also causes a greater preference for protein than if carbohydrate is given alone. Consistent with the hypothesis that 5-HT is involved in the change on food preference is the observation that para-chlorophenylalanine, an inhibitor of tryptophan hydroxylase and therefore of 5-HT synthesis, blocks the diet-induced changes in food preference.[93] On the other hand, others have vigorously argued that 5-HT is not involved in food selection, based on the failure to describe the expected associations among diet composition, the plasma amino TRP/NAA ratio, and brain 5-HT.[94] This opposing view has support from data showing that the administration of the precursor TRP alone, by either the peritoneal cavity[42,95] or the gastric route,[42] has little to no effect on food selection.

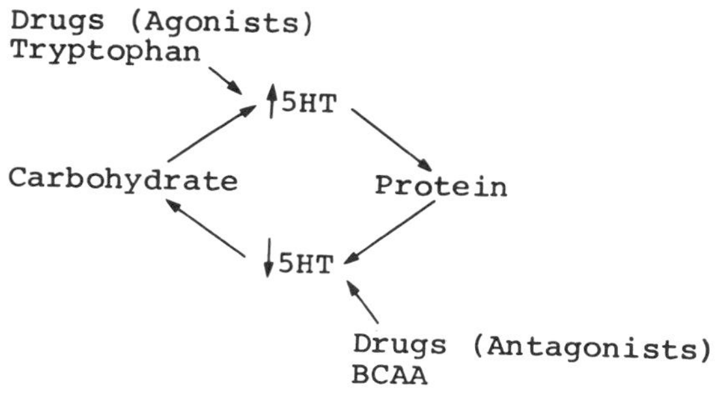
Drugs (Agonists)
Tryptophan
↑5HT
Carbohydrate
Protein
↓5HT
Drugs (Antagonists)
BCAA

**FIGURE 35–2.** Brain serotonin (5-HT) as a regulator of macronutrient preference. The hypothesis is that foods or drugs that increase brain 5-HT cause the animal to prefer protein relative to carbohydrate. Conversely, when brain 5-HT is decreased, a preference for carbohydrate relative to protein occurs.

Better evidence for an association between brain serotonergic activity and food selection based on its macronutrient composition is shown by the use of pharmacologic and surgical techniques that manipulate serotonergic neurons. In early studies, relatively crude techniques were used to lower brain serotonin concentrations. Surgical or chemical ablation of serotonergic neurons[96] or vagotomy[97] have been associated with the rat's increased intake of carbohydrate and decreased intake of protein. More-recent studies have involved drugs that activate or inhibit serotonergic neurons. When rats are given small quantities of the serotonin agonists dexfenfluramine or fluoxetine they selectively decrease carbohydrate relative to protein intake in the next meal.[98] Conversely, buspirone and 8-hydroxy-2-(di-n-propylamino)-tetralin, which inhibit the serotonin system, cause nondeprived self-selecting rats to increase intake exclusively from carbohydrate.[99] Because quantities of these drugs can be identified that affect food selection without modifying total food intake, the possibility exists that small changes in brain serotonin arising after food ingestion are physiologically relevant.

The role of other neurotransmitters, which are known to be involved in feeding control mechanisms, might also be elucidated by experiments in which the food choice paradigm is utilized. For example, the catecholamines and opioid peptides, primarily through a neuronal system coordinated by the hypothalamus, also influence food choice and meal composition. Rats selectively increased carbohydrate intake after microinjection of norepinephrine into the PVH.[100] Carbohydrate, however, is not the only nutrient whose selection is modified by activity of catecholaminergic neurons. When catecholaminergic tone was suppressed by clonidine, a presynaptic α-receptor agonist, rats increased their intakes of both protein and total food.[101] Conversely amphetamine, a central catecholaminergic agonist, decreased total food intake, with a greater effect on protein intake.[102] Although the synthesis of the catecholamines has been reported to be influenced by tyrosine availability under certain circumstances,[84,103] variations in brain tyrosine caused by tyrosine administration do not appear to influence food choice.[42] One might speculate, however, that the elevated norepinephrine synthesis that occurs after protein consumption[103] might reflect activation in neurons involved in feeding and thus direct the animal to prefer carbohydrate in the next meal.

In addition to norepinephrine and serotonin, the opiates also influence food choice. A selective preference for fat can also be induced by morphine[104] and decreased by naloxone, an opiate antagonist.[105] The site of action of the opiates appears to be in the hypothalamus with the feeding response involving norepinephrine-containing neurons.

Many if not all of the gut hormones are present in the brain.[75] At the present time the view is that their presence in the brain is due to endogenous synthesis rather than to active transport from the bloodstream and that they function in some way as neuromodulators. Despite the strong effect on food intake of systemic injections of some of these peptides, preliminary reports suggest that at least CCK does not influence macronutrient choice.[97]

Clearly, the role of neurotransmitters and the many physiologic events that occur in response to both the quantity and composition of food ingested awaits elucidation. Nevertheless, the hypothesis that animals select diets based in part on the composition of food has stimulated research aimed at elucidating the relationships among food composition, energy balance, and eating behavior of humans. There is now evidence that biologic factors are relevant in determining both quantity and composition of the food selected by humans exhibiting normal feeding behavior.[92] Furthermore, abnormalites in these biologic systems may be causative factors in obesity or in the abnormal feeding behaviors presented by patients with anorexia nervosa and bulimia nervosa.

The serotonergic hypothesis of food selection has been favored as the mechanism regulating food-selective appetites, especially those associated with the carbohydrate composition of food (for review, see reference 92). Food selection, with enhanced food intake from snacks and desserts, has been observed (1) during the luteal phase, compared with the follicular phase, of the menstrual cycle in normal women, (2) in those suffering from premenstrual syndrome, (3) during the full depressive phase of the seasonal affective disorder, (4) in obese subjects classified as "carbohydrate cravers," and (5) during food binges of bulimia nervosa patients. For each of these a link between feeding behavior and altered serotonin has been proposed.[106] Currently, serotonin agonists are the most favored drugs for management of feeding behavior in these circumstances. For a complete review on pharmacologic approaches to appetite suppression see Blundell.[74]

In summary, an integrative view of the concepts presented in this review is provided in Figure 35–3. Feeding results in the ingestion of food containing energy and nutrients. The presence of macronutrient breakdown products in the gastrointestinal tract, particularly amino acids and fat, may directly, or indirectly by hormone release, stimulate vagal receptors and hence provide impulses directly to the brain. The products of digestion and hormones released from the gut and entering the liver also affect the brain, through stimulation of the vagus nerve. Nutrients and hormones passing the liver result in changes in plasma concentrations, which in turn may signal the brain in some indirect manner without uptake across the blood-brain barrier, or more directly as a result of brain uptake and changes in brain nutrient concentration and availability. Both energy utilization and storage in tissues also provide signals to the brain, although their mechanism is unknown. Through a complex system of neurotransmitters the brain organizes the information arising from the metabolism of food and directs feeding so that the animal's intake of both energy and macronutrients is quantitatively regulated.

Many metabolic factors are involved in the central regulation of appetite. The evolutionary process would appear to have generated a complex control system. As a result, it seems unlikely that appetite control will be understood within the near future. Indeed we seem further away from a unifying answer than three decades ago when hunger and satiety centers of the hypothalamus and the glucostatic theory were being explored. Given the complexity of the mechanism of regulation of food intake and its responsiveness to so many signals, however, one can only be amazed that in most animals and man it works as effectively as it does.

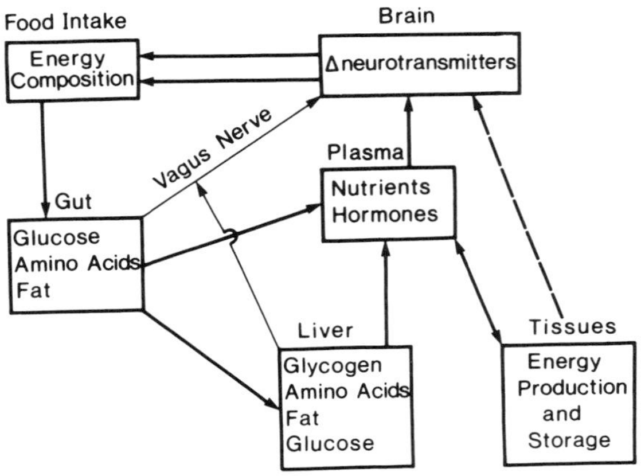
Food Intake
Energy
Composition
Brain
Δneurotransmitters
Vagus Nerve
Plasma
Nutrients
Hormones
Gut
Glucose
Amino Acids
Fat
Liver
Glycogen
Amino Acids
Fat
Glucose
Tissues
Energy
Production
and
Storage

**FIGURE 35–3.** An integrative view of the regulation of intake of food quantity (energy) and of composition. Signals arrive in the brain via many sources and are integrated in a manner that leads to food selection as well as to quantitative intake.

## REFERENCES


1. Durnin, J.G.V.A.: J. Physiol., *156*:294–299, 1961.
2. Sellers, E.A., You, R.W., Moffat, N.W.: Am. J. Physiol., *177*:367–371, 1954.
3. Collier, G., Leshner, A.I., Squibbs, R.L.: Physiol. Behav., *4*:79–82, 1969.
4. Adolph, E.F.: Am. J. Physiol., *151*:1110–1125, 1947.
5. Hamilton, C.L.: J. Am. Diet. Assoc., *62*:35–40, 1973.
6. Mayer, J.: Physiology of hunger and satiety. *In* Modern Nutrition and Disease. 6th Ed. Edited by R.S. Goodhart and M.E. Shils. Philadelphia, Lea & Febiger, 1980.
7. Louis-Sylvestre, J., Le Magnen J.: Neurosci. Biobehav. Rev., *4(Suppl.)*:13–15, 1980.
8. Strubbe, J.H., Steffens, A.B.: Physiol. Behav., *19*:303–308, 1977.
9. Rapoport, S.I.: Blood-brain barrier. *In* Physiology and Medicine. New York, Raven Press, 1976.
10. Stricker, E.M., Rowland, N., Saller, C.F.: Science, *196*:78–81, 1977.
11. Friedman, M.I., Ramirez, E., Wade, G.N., et al.: Physiol. Behav., *29*:515–518, 1982.
12. Rezek, M., Havlicek, V., Novin, D.: Am. J. Physiol., *299*:545–548, 1975.
13. Glick, Z., Mayer, J.: Nature, *219*:1374, 1968.
14. Muller, E.E., Paneri, A., Cocchi, D., et al.: Experientia, *29*:874–875, 1973.
15. Campfield, L.A., Smith, J.F.: Int. J. Obes., *14(Suppl. 3)*:15–33, 1990.
16. Russek, M.: Neurosci. Res., *4*:213–282, 1971.
17. Novin, D.: Visciral mechanisms in the control of food intake. *In* Hunger: Basic Mechanism and Clinical Implications. Edited by D. Novin, W. Wyrwicka, and G. Bray. New York, Raven Press, 1976.
18. Novin, D., Sanderson, J.D., Vanderweele, D.A.: Physiol. Behav., *13*:3–8, 1974.
19. Mayer, J.: N. Engl. J. Med., *249*:13–16, 1953.
20. Faust, I.M.: Signals from adipose tissue. *In* The Body Weight Regulatory System: Normal and Disturbed Mechanisms. Edited by L. Cioffi, W.P.T. James, and T.B. Van Italie. New York, Raven Press, 1981, pp 39–43.
21. Mrosovsky, N., Powley, T.L.: Behav. Biol., *20*:205–223, 1977.
22. Le Magnen, J., Devos, M.: Physiol. Behav., *5*:805–814, 1970.
23. Shimazu, T.: Diabetologia, *20(Suppl)*:343–356, 1981.
24. Takahashi, A., Shimazu, T.: J. Auton. Nerv. Syst., *4*:195–205, 1981.
25. Schmitt, M.: Am. J. Physiol., *225*:1096–1101, 1973.
26. Danquir, J., Nicolaidis, S.: Am. J. Physiol., *228*:E223–E228, 1980.
27. Larue-Achagiotis, C., Le Magnen, J.: Physiol. Behav., *22*:435–440, 1979.
28. Johnson, D.J., Li, E.T.S., Coscina, D.V., et al.: Physiol. Behav., *22*:777–782, 1979.
29. Le Magnen, J.: Physiol. Rev., *63*:314–386, 1983.
30. Cahill, G.F. Jr.: N. Engl. J. Med., *1282*:668–675, 1970.
31. Harris, R.B.S., Martin, R.J.: Nutrit. Behav., *1*:253–275, 1984.
32. Wade, G.N., Gray, J.M.: Physiol. Behav., *22*:583–593, 1979.
33. Greenwood, M.R.C., Cleary, M., Steingrimsdotter, L., et al.: Adipose tissue metabolism and genetic obesity: the LPL hypothesis. *In* Recent Advances in Obesity Research III. Edited by P. Bjorntorp, M. Cairella, and A.N. Howard. London, John Libbey, 1981, pp 75–79.
34. Mellinkoff, S.M., Franklin, M., Boyle, D. et al.: J. Appl. Physiol., *8*:535–538, 1956.
35. Harper, A.E., Benevenga, N.J., Wohlhueter, R.M.: Physiol. Rev., *50*:428–558, 1970.
36. Peng, Y., Tews, J.K., Harper, A.E.: Am. J. Physiol., *222*:314–321, 1972.
37. Anderson, H.L., Benevenga, N.J., Harper, A.E.: Am. J. Physiol., *214*:1008–1013, 1968.
38. Johnson, D.J., Anderson, G.H.: Am. J. Physiol., *243*:R99–R103, 1982.
39. Anderson, G.H., Li, E.T.S., Glanville, N.T.: Brain Res. Bull., *12*:167–173, 1984.
40. Anderson, G.H. Bialik, R.J., Li, E.T.S.: Amino acids in the regulation of food intake and selection. *In* Amino Acid Availability and Brain Function in Health and Disease. Edited by G. Huethr. Berlin, Springer-Verlag, 1988, p 245–257.
41. Rogers, Q.R., Leung, P.M.B.: Fed. Proc. Fed. Am. Soc. Exp. Biol., *32*:1709–1719, 1973.
42. Ng, L.T., Anderson, G.H.: J. Nutr., *122*:283–293, 1992.
43. Butler, R.M., Davis, M., Gehling, N.J., et al.: Am. J. Clin. Nutr., *34*:2045–2047, 1981.
44. Hrboticky, N., Leiter, L., Anderson, G.H.: Nutr. Res., *5*:595–607, 1985.
45. Scharrer, E., Baile, C.A., Mayer, J.: Am. J. Physiol., *218*:400–404, 1970.
46. Beverly, J.L., Gietzen, D.W., Rogers, Q.R.: Am. J. Physiol., *259 (Regulatory Integrative Comp. Physiol. 28)*:R709–R715, 1990.
47. Nicolaidis, S., Even, P.C.: Int. J. Obesity, *14(Suppl. 3)*:3552, 1990.
48. Friedman, M.I.: Int. J. Obes., *14(Suppl. 3)*:53–67, 1990.
49. Osborne, T.B., Mendel, L.B.: J. Biol. Chem., *35*:19–27, 1918.
50. Richter, C.P.: Harvey Lect., *38*:63–103, 1943.
51. Richter, C.P., Eckert, J.: Am. J. Med. Sci., *198*:9–16, 1939.
52. Harris, L.J., Clay, J., Hargreaves, F.J., et al.: Proc. R. Soc. Lond.[ Biol.], *113*:161–190, 1933.
53. Siu, G.M., Hadley, M., Draper, H.H.: J. Nutr., *111*:1681–1685, 1981.
54. Siu, G.M., Hadley, M., Agwu, D.E., et al.: J. Nutr., *114*:1059–1105, 1984.
55. Lat, J.: Handbook of Physiology. Section 6. Vol. 1. Washington, D.C., American Physiology Society, 1967.
56. Musten, B., Peace, D., Anderson, G.H.: J. Nutr., *104*:563–572, 1974.
57. Li, E.T.S., Anderson, G.H.: Physiol. Behav., *29*:779–783, 1982.
58. Li, E.T.S., Anderson, G.H.: Nutr. Abstr. Rev. Clin. Nutr. Series A, *53*:169–181, 1983.
59. Anderson, G.H., Ashley, D.V.M.: Plasma amino acids, brain mechanisms and the control of protein intake. *In* Nutrition in Transition; Proceedings of the Western Hemisphere Nutrition Congress V. Edited by P.L. White and N. Selvey. Munroe, WI, Am. Med. Assoc., 1978.
60. Ashley, D.V.M., Anderson, G.H.: J. Nutr., *105*:1405–1411, 1975.

61. Ashley, D.V.M., Anderson, G.H.: Life Sci., *21*:1235–1244, 1977.
62. Anderson, G.H., Leprohon, C.E., Chambers, J.H., et al.: Physiol. Behav., *22*:777–780, 1979.
63. Chee, K.M., Romsos, D.R., Bergen, W.G.: J. Nutr., *111*:668–677, 1981.
64. Romsos, D.R., Ferguson, D.J.: Am. Vet. Med. Assoc., *182*:41–43, 1983.
65. Summers, J.D., Leeson, S.: Br. Poult. Sci., *19*:425–430, 1978.
66. FAO/WHO: Joint Expert Committee on Energy and Protein Requirement. World Health Organization Technical Report Series, No. 522, Geneva, 1973.
67. Wade, J., Milner, J., Krondl, M.: Am. J. Clin. Nutr., *34*:143–147, 1981.
68. Murphy, C., Withee, J.: J. Gerontol., *42*:73–78, 1987.
69. Soulairac, A.: Bull. Biol. Fr. Belg., *81*:273–432, 1947.
70. Wurtman, J.J., Moses, P.L., Wurtman, R.J.: J. Nutr., *133*:70–78, 1983.
71. Kanarek, R.B.: Am. J. Clin. Nutr., *42*:940–950, 1985.
72. Ashley, D.V.M.: Brain Res. Bull., *15*:411–415, 1985.
73. Ashley, D.V.M., Leathwood, P.D.: Nestle Research News 1982/83. La Toux-De-Peilz, Switzerland, Nestle Products Technical Assistance Co., 1983.
74. Blundell, J.L.: Trends Pharm. Sci., *12*:147–157, 1991.
75. Friedman, M., Richardson, C.T.: The cephalic phase of gastric secretion. *In* Interaction of the Chemical Senses with Nutrition. Edited by M.R. Kare, and J.D. Brand. New York, Academic Press, 1986, pp. 181–192.
76. Rolls, B.E. Changing hedonic responses to foods during and after a meal. *In* Interaction of the Chemical Senses with Nutrition. Edited by M.R. Kare, and J.D. Brand. New York, Academic Press, 1986.
77. Smith, G.P., Gibbs, J.: Brain-gut peptides and the control of food intake. *In* Neurosecretion and Brain Peptides. Edited by J.B. Martin, S. Rechlin, and K.L. Bick. New York, Raven Press, 1981.
78. Lewis, L.D., Williams, J.A.: Am. J. Physiol., *258*:G512–518, 1990.
79. Silver, A.T., Morley, J.E.: Prog. Neurobiol., *36*:23–34, 1991.
80. Pardridge, W.M.: Adv. Exp. Med. Biol., *291*:43–53, 1991.
81. Smith, Q.R.: Adv. Exp. Med. Biol., *291*:55–71, 1991.
82. Oomura, Y.: Significance of glucose, insulin and free fatty acids in the hypothalamic feeding and satiety neurons. *In* Hunger: Basic Mechanism and Clinical Implications. Edited by D. Novin, W. Wyrwicka, and G. Bray. New York, Raven Press, 1976.
83. Wayner, M.J., Ono, T., Young De, A., et al.: Pharmac. Biochem. Behav., *3(Suppl. 1)*:85–90, 1975.
84. Anderson, G.H., Johnston, J.L.: Can. J. Physiol. Pharmacol., *61*:271–281, 1983.
85. Kanarek, R.B., Feldman, P.G., Hanes, C.: Physiol. Behav., *27*:337–343, 1981.
86. Sclafani, A., Aravich, P.F.: Am. J. Physiol., *244*:R686–R694, 1983.
87. Wurtman, R.J., Fernstrom, J.D.: Biochem. Pharmacol., *25*:1692–1696, 1976.
88. Teff, K.L., Young, S.N.: Can. J. Physiol. Pharmacol., *66*:683–688, 1988.
89. McMenamy, R.H., Oncley, J.L.: J. Biol. Chem., *233*:1436–1447, 1978.
90. Anderson, G.H.: Can J. Physiol. Pharmacol., *57*:1043–1057, 1979.
91. Fernstrom, J.D.: Appetite, *8*:163–184, 1987.
92. Anderson, G.H., Black, R.M., Li, E.T.S.: Physiological determinants of food selection: Association with protein and carbohydrate. *In* Feast and Famine: Relevance to Eating Disorders. Edited by G.H. Anderson and S.H. Kennedy. New York, Academic Press, 1992.
93. Li, E.T.S., Anderson, G.H.: Life Sci., *34*:2453–2460, 1984.
94. Harper, A.E., Peters, J.C.: J. Nutr., *119*:677–689, 1989.
95. Morris, P., Li, E.T.S., MacMillam, M., Anderson, G.H.: Physiol. Behav., *40*:155–163, 1987.
96. Ashley, D.V.M., Coscina, D.V., Anderson, G.H.: Life Sci., *24*:973–984, 1979.
97. Li, E.T.S., Anderson, G.H.: Am. J. Physiol., *247*:E815–E821, 1984.
98. Luo, S., Ransom, T., Li, E.T.S.: Life Sci., *46*:1643–1648, 1990.
99. Luo, S., Li, E.T.S.: Brain Res. Bull., *24*:729–733, 1990.
100. Leibowitz, S.F.: Neurochemical systems of the hypothalamus in control of feeding and drinking behavior and water-electrolyte excretion. *In* Handbook of the Hypothalamus. Vol. 3A. Edited by P.J. Morgane and J. Panksepp. New York, Dekker, 1980.
101. Mauron, C., Wurtman, J.J., Wurtman, R.J.: Life Sci., *27*:781–791, 1980.
102. Blundell, J.E., McArthur, R.A.: Br. J. Pharmacol., *67*:436–438, 1979.
103. Gibson, C.J., Wurtman, R.J.: Life Sci., *22*:1399–1406, 1978.
104. Marks-Kaufman, R.M., Kanarek, R.B.: Pharmacol. Biochem. Behav., *12*:427–430, 1980.
105. Marks-Kaufman, R.M., Kanarek, R.B.: Psychopharmacology (Berlin), *74*:321–324, 1981.
106. Leibowitz, S.F.: Drugs, *39(Suppl.)*:33–48, 1990.

CHAPTER 36

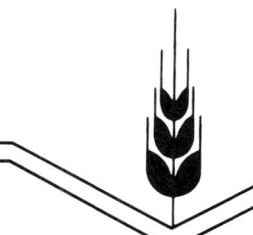

# Nutrition and the Chemical Senses

Richard D. Mattes and Morley R. Kare*



Undoubtedly, the chemical senses evolved, in part, to facilitate the location and identification of foods and to promote their ingestion. The first treatise formally considering the mechanisms of taste dates back to the Greek physician Alcmaeon in the middle of the sixth century B.C.[1] Aristotle also studied taste, linking the sensations to physiologic conditions. A student of Aristotle, Theophrastus, authored the first treatise on olfaction and recognized the utility of the sense, which can operate over distances, in food acquisition.[2] Work from that time to the 1940s was largely preoccupied with questions about the anatomy and physiology of the systems. Basic and applied research on the sensory properties of foods dates back to the mid-1940s, being prompted largely by military and commercial interests. Despite almost 50 years of study, understanding of the nutritional implications of the chemical senses remains wanting.

*Morley R. Kare died on July 30, 1990. He was an internationally noted pioneer in chemosensory research who founded the Monell Chemical Senses Center and served as its director for 23 years. His investigations made a major contribution towards understanding the relationship of taste and smell to nutrition. Dr. Mattes dedicates this chapter to his co-author in recognition of the important influence Dr. Kare had on his professional pursuits.

## OVERVIEW OF THE ANATOMY AND PHYSIOLOGY OF THE CHEMICAL SENSES

The flavors of foods are an amalgam of input from the chemical senses: gustation (taste), olfaction (smell), and chemesthesis (chemical sensitivity of the somatosensory system). These sensory systems are distinct anatomically, have different functional characteristics, and contribute unique information.

### GUSTATION

The gustatory system is composed of specialized epithelial cells located on the tongue, hard and soft palate, and esophagus, as well as the neurons that synapse with these peripheral cells and relay information about taste stimuli to the central nervous system. On the tongue, taste cells coalesced in onion-shaped taste buds occur in fungiform, foliate, and circumvallate papillae. The fungiform papillae are mushroom-shaped structures (appearing as red bumps) on the anterior two thirds of the tongue and contain an average of 1.8 taste buds. Taste cells in these structures receive innervation from the chorda tympani nerve (lingual branch of the facial, or seventh cranial, nerve). Foliate papillae appear as three to eight folds on the posterior lateral margins of the tongue and contain an average of 120 taste buds per papillae. These structures are innervated anteriorly by the chorda tympani nerve and by the glossopharyngeal (lingual branch of the ninth cranial nerve) posteriorly. Eight to twelve circumvallate papillae are arranged in a "V" configuration on the posterior dorsal tongue. Each papilla is surrounded by a trench where 200 to 250 taste buds arranged in tiers on the lower two thirds of the papillae face the opposing wall of the trench. Innervation of these taste cells is provided by the glossopharyngeal nerve. Taste buds on the epiglottis are innervated by the superior laryngeal branch of the vagus nerve (tenth cranial nerve). The greater superficial petrosal nerve subserves taste buds on the soft palate.[3,4] All gustatory neurons synapse in the nucleus of the solitary tract, but projections to other sites where coding may occur remain poorly characterized in humans.[5]

The responsivity of taste cells to sapid stimuli varies in different regions of the oral cavity. However, subjective reports and electrophysiologic recordings following stimulation of single taste cells with varying taste qualities demonstrate that individual cells and regions respond to multiple taste qualities.[6] Consequently, damage to a specific region of the tongue or to a specific gustatory nerve does not result in the loss of responsivity to a specific taste quality.

The issue of whether taste is a synthetic or analytic sense has yet to be resolved. The former view holds that there are taste primaries, commonly identified as sweet, salty, sour, and bitter (although the Japanese include "umami" or "meat flavor"), which in combination can account for the full range of taste sensations. Vision is an example of a synthetic sense. The analytic view is that there are multiple tastes which, even in combination, are distinguishable. Audition is an example of an analytic sense. This issue is fundamental because the prevailing acceptance of the synthetic view has focused research on taste transduction mechanisms that may account for the four to five primaries. Present knowledge indicates that salt taste is largely mediated through active epithelial channels in the taste cell membrane; sour stimuli are perceived by proton inhibition of outward-going potassium channels; transduction of sweet taste involves receptor-mediated production of cyclic adenosine monophosphate (cyclic AMP); and bitterness is mediated by modulation of potassium channels, alterations in intracellular second messengers, or both.[7] Work on transduction mechanisms is extremely complex, owing to the wide diversity of chemical structures that elicit similar sensations. For example, sucrose (a carbohydrate), aspartame (a dipeptide), monellin (a 10,000-kd protein), saccharin (an aromatic compound), and cyclamate (a heterocyclic compound) are all sweet.

### OLFACTION

A 2 to 4 cm$^2$ patch of olfactory epithelium is located at the apex of the nasal cavities. It contains approximately $10^7$ receptor cells. These receptor cells are first-order neurons that merge into the olfactory nerve (first cranial nerve), pass through the cribriform plate, and synapse directly with the olfactory bulb.

Olfactory stimuli consist of volatile molecules, but the characteristics responsible for quality discrimination remain elusive. There are currently two predominant hypotheses. One holds that quality is determined by specificity of receptors for the physiochemical properties of the myriad ambient olfactory stimuli. The other argues that physiochemical properties of olfactory stimuli determine their temporal and spatial distribution across the olfactory epithelium and that activation of neurons in different areas provides quality information.

### CHEMESTHESIS

Sensitivity to chemical irritants (e.g., capsaicin, the burning compound in chili peppers) in the oral and nasal cavities is mediated by elements of the somatosensory system. This subpopulation of fibers is often referred to as the "common chemical sense." The primary somatosensory pathway in the nose and mouth is the trigeminal nerve (fifth cranial nerve), although in the oral cavity both the chorda tympani and glossopharyngeal nerves also contain fibers that respond to temperature and touch. The chemosensitive afferent sensory neurons of this sensory system are believed to compose subsets of fibers associated with the senses of pain and temperature.[8] Input from chemical stimuli is primarily transduced by polymodal nociceptors. However, cold fibers also respond to some chemical irritants such as menthol. Presently, there is only suggestive evidence that warm-sensitive fibers respond to chemical stimuli. Although there may be specific protein receptors for some compounds, stimulation probably also occurs nonspecifically when irritants disturb neural membranes or act directly on ion channels.

## MEASURES OF SENSORY FUNCTION

The senses of taste and smell convey intensity and quality information about appropriate stimuli. The most traditional measure of function is threshold sensitivity, which may be determined as the "detection" or the "recognition" threshold. The former represents the lowest concentration of a stimulus that can be detected in a given medium, and the latter is the lowest concentration that can be recognized with respect to its quality (e.g., NaCl is salty). Intensity ratings are also frequently obtained and reflect the strength of sensation elicited by suprathreshold stimulus concentrations. It is argued that intensity ratings are more nutritionally relevant than thresholds because stimuli are presented at levels more commonly encountered under normal eating conditions. However, attempts to demonstrate associations between intensity ratings and either food preferences or intake have generally been unsuccessful. Suprathreshold concentrations of stimuli are also used in identification tasks in which subjects are asked to indicate the quality of unlabeled simple compounds or foods. Each of these measures provides unique functional information. Correlations between the measures are not generally strong.

One additional clinical measure focuses on hedonic attributes of stimuli. Judgments about acceptability rely on higher-order processing of input from the periphery. Commonly evaluated hedonic dimensions include, but are not limited to, preferred frequency of stimulus intake, preferred concentration of the stimulus in a medium, and preference for stimuli with a characteristic quality. Individually, these hedonic attributes are more strongly related to intake than threshold and intensity ratings, but only in combination can predictions about intake be made with some confidence.[9]

Chemesthesis in the oral and nasal cavities is not routinely evaluated in clinical research centers. This stems from the limited array of stimuli that selectively stimulate this sensory system (e.g., carbon dioxide for nasal and capsaicin for oral stimulation), logistical difficulties with stimulus administration, the persistence of their effects, rarity of complaints about this component of the chemical senses, and uncertainty about the contribution of this set of sensory attributes to food selection and quality of life. The nutritional importance of other information conveyed by the somatosensory system, such as thermal sensation, is recognized, but this input is not chemically induced. The ability of chemesthesis to convey stimulus quality information remains controversial. The importance of interactions between chemesthesis, gustation, and olfaction in food preferences and intake have not been explored.

## RELATIONSHIPS BETWEEN NUTRIENT INTAKE AND THE CHEMICAL SENSES

There is a reciprocal relationship between nutrient intake and chemosensory function. Gustatory and olfactory tissues are composed of specialized epithelial and neural cells with relatively high turnover rates (i.e., 10 to 12 days for taste and 30 to 45 days for olfaction) and metabolic requirements. Provision of adequate nutrients is vital for proper function. At the same time, the functional status of these sensory systems can strongly influence food and nutrient intake. Despite longstanding recognition of this association, little is known about the nutrient requirements of these tissues.[10] Present knowledge stems largely from clinical observations of sensory abnormalities associated with various pathologic processes and treatment regimens. Insights have also been acquired from various animal models, but because of interspecies differences in the characteristics and uses of the chemical senses, the interpretation of much of this work is unclear.

### EFFECTS OF NUTRITIONAL STATUS ON CHEMOSENSORY FUNCTION

#### *VITAMIN A*

Vitamin A deficiency leads to increased keratinization of the oral and nasal epithelia. In addition, mucopolysaccharide synthesis is diminished, leading to reduced cleansing of the perireceptor area and drying of the epithelia. Blockage of stimulus access to chemosensory receptors ensues (Fig. 36–1). Vitamin A depletion results in a gradual loss of taste in rats[11] that is reversible with vitamin repletion. Chemosensory deficits are not a common feature of vitamin A deficiency in areas where this problem is endemic, although hypogeusia and hyposmia have been reported in normal adults made vitamin A–deficient and in patients with cirrhosis, acute viral hepatitis, and malabsorption disorders who were depleted of the vitamin.[12] Supplementation with vitamin A reverses these chemosensory losses. It is important to recognize the role of zinc in maintaining normal plasma vitamin A levels, especially among patients with liver disorders. Zinc administration has also been reported effective at reducing taste deficits in alcoholic cirrhosis patients.[13] Given the potential toxicity of vitamin A, it is vital that its probable etiologic role in a sensory disorder be established before therapeutic supplementation is initiated.

#### *B VITAMINS*

Studies in dogs reveal that diet-induced deficiencies of niacin, riboflavin, pyridoxine, pantothenic acid, and folic acid result in noninflammatory lesions of the oral mucosa, especially on the dorsal tongue surface.[14] Papillary atrophy and degeneration is also observed, particularly on the anterior tongue, though in niacin deficiency the entire tongue surface may be involved (Fig. 36–2). Fungiform papillae are the most severely affected; no abnormalities have been noted in circumvallate papillae. Pathologic changes are progressively worse with successive deficiency trials. Replacement therapy results in prompt restoration of the epithelium. Improvement is apparent in 2 to 3 days and is complete within a week. Recovery of connective tissue is slower. Distinct lesions are apparent in animals with specific vitamin deficiencies, and these identifiable lesions are superimposed in animals with multiple deficiencies.

Findings similar to those reported in dogs have been observed in humans.[15] In addition, deficiencies of pyridoxine, riboflavin, and cobalamin lead to peripheral neuropathies. However, it should be emphasized that

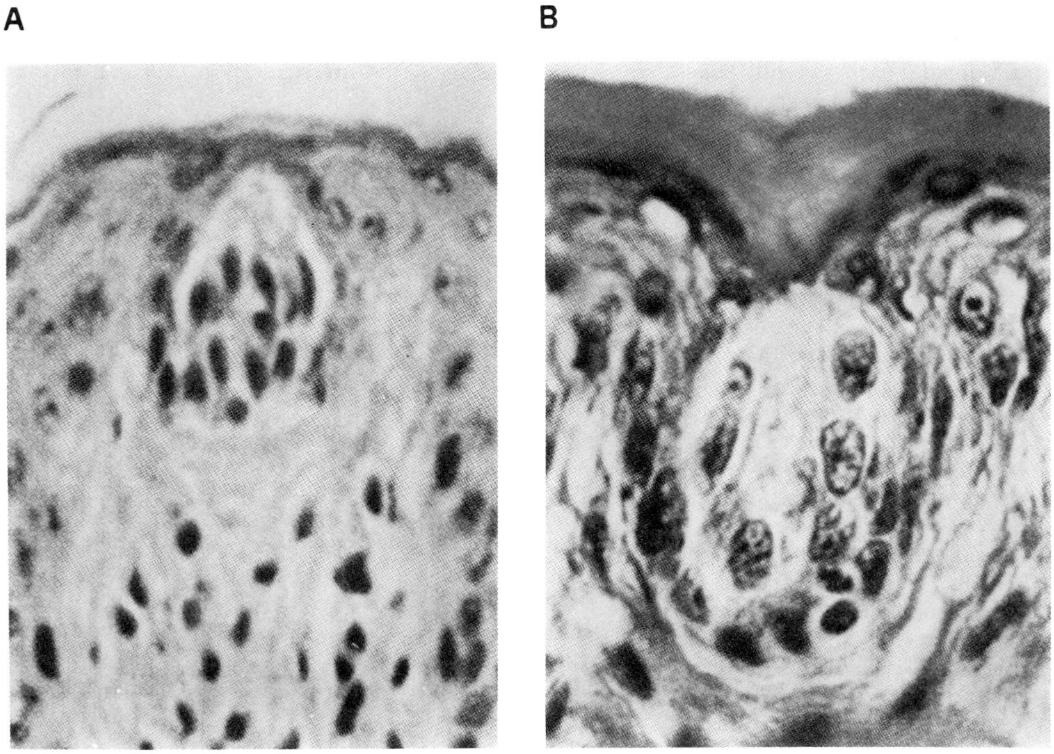
A
B

**FIGURE 36–1.** *A*, Longitudinal section of single taste bud in a fungiform papilla from a vitamin A–replete rat. *B*, Comparable section from a vitamin A–deficient rat. The taste bud pore is infiltrated with keratin. (From Bernard, R.A., Halpern, B.P.: J. Gen. Physiol., *52*:459, 1968. Reproduction from the *Journal of General Physiology* by copyright permission of the Rockefeller University Press).

such changes are only associated with marked depletions. There are only case studies of chemosensory changes in patients with B vitamin deficiencies.[16] Importantly, although repletion of pyridoxine has reportedly corrected chemosensory disturbances in patients with subclinical pellagra,[16] high levels of pyridoxine have also been associated with peripheral neuropathy.[17] In such patients, nonspecific axonal degeneration has been observed with a loss of sensory-nerve action potentials in response to an electromyogram. Thus, indiscriminate use of high levels of B vitamins to treat chemosensory disorders is inappropriate.

### *COPPER*

Rats treated with penicillamine exhibit a heightened preference for NaCl, which may reflect a decrement in salt taste.[18] Withdrawal of the drug or treatment with copper corrects the shift in salt preference. A more general hypogeusia has been reported in humans treated with the same drug that also was reversible.[19] The taste decrements were associated with low ceruloplasmin levels. Administration of penicillamine to patients with Wilson's disease does not lead to chemosensory complaints, indicating that the drug-related alteration of taste was likely due to low copper levels rather than to some other drug action. Because indices of other trace elements potentially involved in taste have not been monitored in patients treated with penicillamine, the specificity of the purported copper effect is unknown. Penicillamine also binds zinc, nickel, and other cations that share an affinity for many binding sites, possibly including ones on taste cells. Indeed, both copper and zinc have been reported to improve taste sensitivity in patients treated with this drug.

### *IODINE*

Diminutions of taste and olfactory sensitivity or dysgeusias have been documented in hypothyroid patients.[20] The reported incidence of sensory complaints in such patients ranges from a few percent to over 80%. This may be attributable to the generally slow onset of symptoms and consequent lack of subjective awareness. Replacement hormone therapy generally results in correction of the chemosensory disorder. Treatment of hyperthyroid patients with antithyroid agents (e.g., me

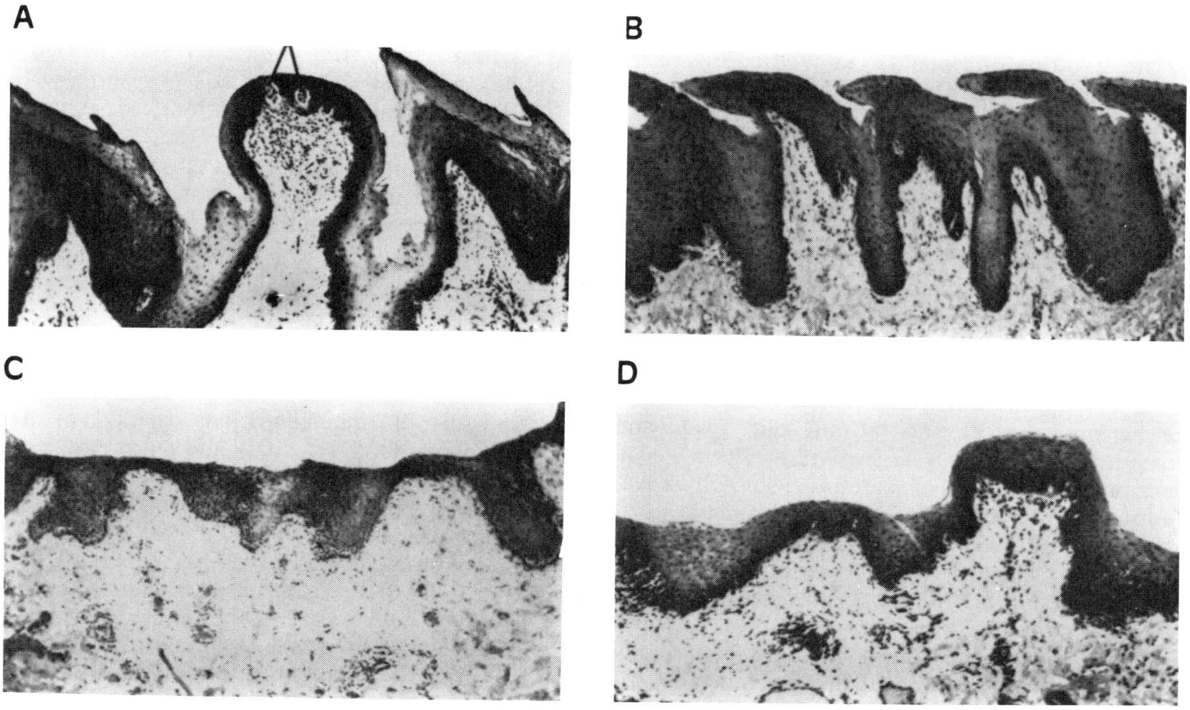
A
B
C
D

**FIGURE 36–2.** *A*, Longitudinal section of a normal fungiform papilla containing two taste buds in a dog. On either side of the fungiform papilla are filiform papillae. *B*, Papillae atrophy in a niacin-deficient dog. *C*, Late stage papillae atrophy in a dog deficient in pyridoxine. *D*, The absence of filiform papillae and atrophied fungiform papilla of dog made riboflavin deficient for the first time. (From Afonsky, D.: Ann. N. Y. Acad. Sci., *85*:364 and 365, 1960.)

thimazole, methylthiouracil) has also led to partial or complete loss of taste and smell that resolves upon cessation of drug use. It is presumed that thyroid-related chemosensory problems are related to impaired iodine trapping in the thyroid gland or to diminished iodination of tyrosine, rather than to altered activity of thyroxin in target organs or changes in sensory neurons. However, in a rat model of hypothyroidism with concomitant anosmia, differentiation of presumptive olfactory neurons is disrupted.[21] Altered levels or chelation of other nutrients (e.g., zinc) involved in chemosensation could also be involved.

A higher prevalence of goiter has been reported in a subgroup of patients relatively insensitive to the taste of selected goitrogenic compounds (e.g., thiocarbamide, propylthiourea), prompting speculation that this genetically determined dimorphism may play an etiologic role in the development of goiters. That is, insensitive tasters will consume higher levels of unpleasant bitter dietary goitrogens. However, the overwhelming majority of diet-related goiters stem from low iodine intake in regions where the limited diversity of available foods precludes a significant impact of discretionary intake. Even where a wide array of foods is available, discrepancies in consumption of biologically active goitrogens by tasters and nontasters has not been observed.[22]

### *IRON*

Iron deficiency in rats has been associated with a heightened preference for NaCl and KCl without any shift in response to sodium saccharin, hydrochloric acid, or quinine sulfate.[23] This relationship has not been studied in humans. Cravings and pica have been reported in iron-depleted individuals, but there is presently no evidence that this is related to shifts in chemosensory function.

### *ZINC*

Zinc depletion or abnormalities of zinc metabolism have been documented in a number of clinical disorders (e.g., acute infectious hepatitis, chronic cirrhosis of the liver, Crohn's disease, chronic renal disease). Taste abnormalities have also been reported among patients with these disorders. In addition, low levels of plasma zinc have been noted in some hypogeusic patients. Normal taste function returned in some of these patients following zinc repletion. These observations have lead to a hypothesis that zinc plays an integral role in taste transduction.[24] Additional support for this view stems from work, primarily from one laboratory, indicating that zinc is present in taste buds as a component of the enzyme alkaline phosphatase as well as in the protein "gustin," a constituent of saliva that bathes the taste cells. Gustin reportedly posses trophic properties for taste cells.

While the foregoing findings represent an important testable hypothesis in an area where few treatment approaches have been identified, the preponderance of data fails to support a role for zinc in all but severly zinc-depleted individuals. Much of the evidence cited previously was drawn from small numbers of patients. For example, clinical support for the role of gustin in taste stems from assessment of only three hypogeusic patients. Secondly, the studies focused on zinc levels in the various clinical populations, but levels and the bioavailability of other critical nutrients also vary in these patient groups. For example, as noted above, zinc is required for vitamin A transport from the liver, and taste changes have been documented in vitamin A–deficient rats.[11] Zinc deficiency attributable to administration of penicillamine has been associated with parakeratosis and keratitis, symptoms of vitamin A deficiency. Shifts in zinc levels are also known to induce changes in concentrations and activities of other cations because of common affinities for binding sites. Indeed, copper and nickel appear to be as effective as zinc in the treatment of hypogeusia. Finally, changes in trace element–dependent enzymes in saliva, blood, neural tissue, and other body compartments that may influence taste and smell also undoubtedly occur in these clinical groups.

Despite its clinical popularity, there is little evidence that zinc supplements will benefit the majority of patients with chemosensory disorders. In a randomized, double-blind crossover study of 106 patients with taste and smell abnormalities of multiple causes, treatments with $ZnSO_4$ proved no more effective than placebo.[25] Similar findings have been reported from a study evaluating responses of the elderly to zinc supplementation for 95 days,[26] and from a 12-month double-blind, pair-matched study of 60 5- to 7-year-old boys.[27] Zinc may be effective among individuals in whom zinc nutriture is compromised, and this is the etiologic factor underlying the chemosensory problem. However, because there is evidence that levels of zinc recommended for use with chemosensory patients (i.e., 1530 μmol (100 mg) per day) may lead to anemia, neutropenia, and impaired immune function,[28] this therapeutic approach must only be used with caution.

### *HEAVY METALS*

Studies with mice demonstrate that application of heavy metal salts (i.e., $CuCl_2$, $ZnCl_2$, $FeSO_4$, $MnCl_2$, $CoCl_2$, $CdCl_2$, $NiCl_2$) to the dorsal tongue surface can diminish chorda tympani nerve responses to prototypical sweet, sour, salty, and/or bitter stimuli.[29] The specific nature of the inhibition varies across the series of metals, with each eliciting a different pattern of depression for different taste qualities. It has been hypothesized that the mechanism involves competitive inhibition. Case studies in humans indicate that accidental exposure to mercury or lead as well as parenteral administration of gold can produce taste abnormalities. The mechanisms in these cases remain unexplored.

## EFFECTS OF CHEMOSENSORY FUNCTION ON FOOD INTAKE

Under normal conditions, the chemical senses may influence food selection and ingestion by a variety of mechanisms ranging from transduction of selected innately preferred and aversive types of stimulation to conveyance of relevant dietary information derived from previous ingestive experiences. The relative importance of this source of input under normal conditions is reviewed in Chapter 35. Much less is known about the nutritional implications of taste and smell disorders. Chemosensory abnormalities reportedly afflict about two million Americans,[30] though the reliability of this figure is uncertain. It has been an enigma that no marked or consistent changes in dietary behavior or nutritional status have been noted in this population. However, recent work indicates that subgroups of patients do experience dietary or nutritional disorders, but that they tend to be offsetting, thereby obscuring important effects. For example, over 75% of patients with chemosensory disorders complain of decreased enjoyment of foods, and a majority indicate they have made compensatory modifications of their customary diet. Some individuals increase intake to mask undesirable tastes or odors and others do so to achieve a level and type of missed stimulation. In contrast, others decrease intake because of the loss of appeal of foods or because foods may provoke their problem. One report noted that among those patients who indicated that they decreased intake, about 45% had lost more than 10% of their initial body weight and 24% were underweight (based on a body mass index of less than 20.0).[31] On the other hand, approximately 45% of patients who compensated by increasing intake had gained more than 10% of their initial body weight, and this group had an incidence of being overweight of 76% (based on a body mass index greater than 25.0). In addition, individual patients in each of these groups had adopted highly inappropriate eating strategies. Another important distinction lies in the nature of the chemosensory complaint. Distortions (phantom, persistent, obnoxious, or inappropriate tastes and smells) appear more problematic nutritionally than do diminutions or losses of sensation.[31–33] Weight loss is more common in patients with distortion than in patients with losses of sensation.

## CHEMICAL SENSES AND NUTRIENT UTILIZATION

A potential role of sensory stimulation on the digestion, absorption, and utilization of nutrients has been recognized since the work of Pavlov, but remains poorly characterized. Sensory, especially chemosensory stimulation, elicits digestive responses that anticipate the arrival of food in the gut that are termed preabsorptive or cephalic phase responses. These responses are vagally mediated. Cephalic phase salivary, gastric, pancreatic exocrine, and endocrine responses have been documented in various animals and in humans.[34] There are other preabsorptive responses to sensory stimulation with nutritional implications as well. These include changes in thermogenesis and cardiovascular function.

### CEPHALIC PHASE SALIVARY RESPONSE (CPSR)

The efficacy of purely chemosensory stimulation on salivary release in humans is uncertain because of a contribution of cognitive and visual input. Voluntary manipulation of salivary flow in response to verbal suggestion has been observed.[35] In addition, following visual presentation of a variety of foods, salivary flow is greatest with items that provoke the largest release during ingestion,[36] indicating that the response may be a consequence of prior associative learning. However, the magnitude of the CPSR is greatest following chemosensory, especially gustatory, stimulation. Under normal eating conditions, chemosensory stimulation results in a reliable rise in whole-mouth salivary flow from typical basal levels of about 0.3 ml per minute to over 1.0 ml per minute. Generally, paradigms involving delivery of calorically discrepant preloads, varying periods of energy restriction, or adherence to diets of different energy value indicate that the magnitude of the CPSR is directly related to an individual's state of hunger.[37] Restrained dieters purportedly exhibit heightened responsiveness. Presentation of unpalatable stimuli has elicited little differential response in some,[38] but not all[36] studies, which suggests a possible contribution of stimulus palatability as well.

### CEPHALIC PHASE GASTRIC RESPONSE (CPGR)

Studies of human sham feeding and modified sham feeding (i.e., chewing and expectorating food) demonstrate an effect of taste and smell on release of gastrin and gastric acid.[39] Approximately a third of total acid secretion under normal dietary conditions may be contributed by cephalic stimulation. Following antrum bulb resection, the gastrin release is abolished and acid levels are reduced in response to cephalic stimulation.[40] This indicates the presence of a direct or primary cephalic response on acid release as well as an indirect or secondary response through an influence on gastrin release. Cognitive influences on gastric acid release have also been documented[41] and may contribute to the reported chemosensory-related effects. Thus, quantitation of chemosensory stimulation is problematic. Nevertheless, it appears that gustatory stimulation is more potent than olfactory stimulation. A role for food palatability has been exemplified in a study showing that modified sham feeding of gruel, a self-selected hospital meal, or a freely selected meal resulted in progressively increasing levels of acid output.[42] Given the generally excess capacity of the gastric phase of digestion to carry out its functions, the nutritional importance of the cephalic component is unclear.

### CEPHALIC PHASE PANCREATIC EXOCRINE RESPONSE (CPExR)

Combined olfactory, trigeminal, and visual stimulation elicits an exocrine pancreatic response, although not as large as that following gustatory stimulation.[43] According to one study, relative to baseline in a sham-feeding paradigm, lipase and trypsin were elevated by 10 to 75% and 13 to 40%, respectively. Chymotrypsin and amylase levels were more variable, rising 10 to 89% for the former and from −16% (in one subject) to +75% for the latter. Bicarbonate and water showed little change.[44] Consequently, cephalic stimulation yields an especially enzyme-rich secretion. This response probably has a primary and secondary component. It is well-recognized that passage of gastric contents into the duodenum promotes pancreatic exocrine secretion; the CPGR may account for a portion of the CPExR. A primary response has also been demonstrated in humans using a balloon between the stomach and duodenum to block the flow of gastric acid and by studying patients with achlorhydria.

An influence of stimulus palatability or subject expectations has also been demonstrated. In dogs sham-fed a basal diet that was modified with an acceptable or unpleasant taste compound, a larger pancreatic flow and protein output were observed with the more palatable food.[45] Repeated elicitation of this effect requires the inclusion of swallowing.[46] An enhanced CPExR has also been noted in humans when foods customarily ingested at a given time of day were presented at that time, as compared to a different time.[43]

The nutritional implications of the CPExR have not been evaluated. The secretion of enzymes may facilitate digestion, although in dogs, protein release during sham feeding represents only a small fraction (i.e., 10 to 15%) of the level observed during meal ingestion.[47] There is evidence, though controversial, that cholecystokinin possesses satiety properties in humans,[48] and sham-feeding studies in rats suggest that oral stimulation enhances the satiety properties of cholecystokinin.[49] However, the extent to which gut hormones are released and influence an individual's level of hunger and satiety is unclear.

### CEPHALIC PHASE PANCREATIC ENDOCRINE RESPONSE (CPEnR)

A cephalic phase release of insulin (CPIR) and pancreatic polypeptide has been documented in humans. A release of glucagon has been reported in rats and dogs,[50,51] but not in humans. Partitioning the relative effects of different sensory stimuli is problematic, again because of a cognitive influence. Elevations of plasma insulin may occur in response to the thought of preferred foods.[52] Visual, olfactory, and gustatory stimulation are also sufficient stimuli for an insulin response.[52,53] Modified sham-feeding and sham-feeding protocols have been used to document the pancreatic polypeptide response, so the relative contributions of olfactory, gustatory, and tactile stimulation are uncertain.[54] Importantly, a greater response was noted in sham-feeding subjects, indicating the importance of swallowing in cephalic phase hormone release.

The endocrine response has been characterized as highly variable, prompting speculation that there may be responders and nonresponders. However, recent work that entailed repeated testing every other day for 5 days using a visual, olfactory, gustatory, and trigeminal stimulus (strawberry-flavored mousse containing dairy fat) revealed a 90% response rate (defined as a rise in plasma insulin exceeding one standard deviation of each subject's own baseline level within 6 minutes).[55] Thus, failure to acclimate subjects to the testing paradigm may account for the apparent response fragility. Subject and stimulus characteristics may also influence responses. For example, a heightened response has been noted in the obese compared to the lean,[52,56] although this may be related to their elevated basal insulin levels. Palatable stimuli elicit a larger response than less palatable items,[57] and previous experience with a stimulus can alter its efficacy. That is, pairing an effective stimulus with a noxious compound may abolish the stimulatory efficacy of the former.[53]

The functional significance of the CPEnR is unclear. Especially in the case of insulin, the response is only a fraction of that noted postabsorptively, and rarely is a decrease in plasma glucose observed. However, declines in plasma fatty acids are observed more commonly in humans.[58] Animal studies suggest that the insulin response may be important in regulating the glycemic response to meals. Relative to orally fed rats, animals receiving comparable meals intragastrically display marked hyperglycemia and hyperinsulinemia.[59] Prolonged elevation of plasma glucose is also observed.[60] Whether these observations apply to humans is not known, as the issue has not been tested directly. However, in one study, glucose tolerance was improved by 63% in men allowed to sham-feed while receiving a glucose infusion.[61] Moreover, simultaneous delivery of insulin and meals has been associated with a two-fold decrease in incremental blood glucose among insulin-dependent diabetics[62] and with a 33% lower glycemic response among noninsulin-dependent diabetics, relative to the condition where insulin delivery was delayed.[63]

### OTHER CEPHALIC PHASE RESPONSES

Cephalic phase thermogenic and cardiovascular responses have also been identified. Dogs that were sham-fed or merely exposed to the sight and smell of food exhibit a rise in heat production within the first 15 minutes of exposure, which is comparable to that noted when food is ingested.[64] Intragastric feeding fails to elicit a rise. This phenomenon has been attributed, in part, to sympathetic stimulation because it is associated with elevations of catecholamine levels. Parasympathetic stimulation is also involved because sectioning the vagus nerve or treatment with atropine diminishes the response.[65] The parasympathetic contribution is probably a secondary effect mediated by insulin.[66] A similar response has been reported in humans.[67] The work with human subjects has also demonstrated a role for food palatability because no substantial increase in thermogenesis was noted when an unpalatable meal was provided.[68] Interestingly, the gastrointestinal phase (occurring 30 minutes or longer after stimulus exposure) is diminished if the cephalic component is reduced by somatostatin infusion.[69] The extent to which the thermic effect of foods influences energy balance remains controversial.

There is a transient rise in aortic blood pressure, heart rate, and cardiac output in response to meal presentation and initiation of its ingestion. In addition, an increased resistance has been noted in the mesenteric vasculature by some but not all researchers.[70] Within 5 to 30 minutes, the cardiovascular effects begin to diminish and mesenteric blood flow rises. Sympathetic stimulation has again been implicated because administration of a sympathetic blocking agent can diminish the response.[71] These effects may hold nutritional implications in light of evidence that intestinal absorption of substances is directly related to blood flow.[72]

## CHEMICAL SENSES AND DIET IN AGING AND SELECTED CHRONIC DISEASES:

### AGING

Statistically significant declines in taste and especially smell sensitivity have been reported in many but not all studies of the elderly.[73] However, the functional significance of these changes is unclear because the absolute magnitude of decline is small. For example, data in Figure 36–3, representing an age- and sex-stratified sample of healthy adults, reveal a statistically significant decline in sucrose taste and phenyl ethyl alcohol odor thresholds with age, but the more striking feature of these data are the number of elderly persons with normal function.[74] The elderly also perform more poorly on

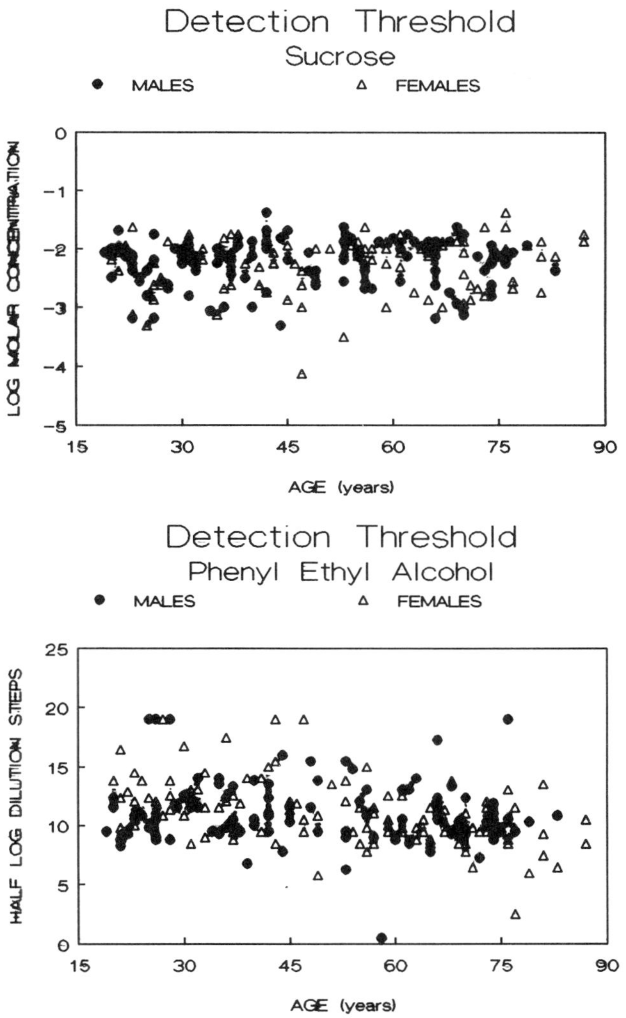
Detection Threshold
Sucrose
MALES
FEMALES
LOG MOLAR CONCENTRATION
0
−1
−2
−3
−4
−5
15
30
45
60
75
90
AGE (years)
Detection Threshold
Phenyl Ethyl Alcohol
MALES
FEMALES
HALF LOG DILUTION STEPS
25
20
15
10
5
0
15
30
45
60
75
90
AGE (years)

**FIGURE 36–3.** *A*, Scatterplot of sucrose taste detection thresholds for healthy adults 19 to 87 years of age. *B*, Scatterplot of olfactory detection thresholds of healthy adults 19 to 87 years of age for phenyl ethyl alcohol.

food-recognition tests, although recent studies using familiar odors and short delays in response time diminish differences. This suggests that deficits attributed to aging may largely be attributable to losses of memory, cognition, and testing skills. Increased use of medications and a higher prevalence of health disorders that may influence sensory function may also contribute to the belief that aging is associated with marked declines in chemosensory function.

## HYPERTENSION

The view that sodium intake is related to hypertension has prompted studies of salt taste in various high-risk populations including different classes of hypertensives (e.g., low versus high renin), normotensive offspring of hypertensives, and salt-sensitive individuals. Individual studies have revealed small differences between some of these groups and control subjects on isolated measures of salt taste (i.e., recognition thresholds but not detection thresholds). However, the preponderance of work has failed to reveal any meaningful associations.[75,76] More generally, a link between salt taste preferences (not thresholds or intensity scaling) and intake has been elucidated.[77] In this regard it has been demonstrated that preferred levels of salt in foods are a function of salt exposure. After 6 to 8 weeks of adherence to a reduced-sodium diet, preferred salt levels in food decline.[78] Similarly, experimentally imposed increases for 6 to 8 weeks have led to higher preferred levels.[79] Importantly, this occurred only among individuals who tasted the extra dietary salt and was not observed among individuals consuming equivalent amounts via enteric-coated tablets. Thus, the shift in preferred salt levels of foods appears to be attributable to sensory exposure rather than to absolute level of intake.

## DIABETES

Disturbances of taste and smell in diabetics have long been recognized.[80] Estimates on the prevalence of these complications vary, but experimental studies suggest that over 60% of patients experience a diminution of chemosensory function. Speculative mechanisms include nerve degeneration, alterations in salivary glucose levels, and various biochemical changes. Evidence that the severity of hypogeusia increases with progressing neuropathy[81] supports the former interpretation. However, the most consistent sensory changes involve alterations in glucose taste thresholds among noninsulin-dependent diabetics and their nondiabetic first-degree relatives. This suggests that the sensory changes may reflect a general abnormality of glucose receptors. However, these two mechanisms are not mutually exclusive—the latter may prevail until complications of hyperglycemia result in more generalized sensory impairment due to peripheral neuropathy. The extent to which these chemosensory changes may influence food selection and adherence to prescribed diets has not been established.

## CANCER

Changes of chemosensory function (sensitivity and preferences) are frequently reported by untreated patients with cancer. Systematic study of these complaints has failed to identify any consistent pattern of change with respect to the nature of the sensory complaint (e.g., quality-specific versus general loss, loss versus distortion) and the site, severity, or duration of disease. Similarly, no clear association between sensory function and anorexia has been established in this patient population.[82,83] More problematic for the sensory systems than the disease are various treatment modalities. Radiotherapy involving gustatory and olfactory tissues results in a profound loss of function from damage to the sensory end organs and supporting tissues (e.g., salivary glands).[84,85] Among patients with head and neck cancer receiving radiotherapy, there is a strong association between loss of sensory function, anorexia, and weight loss. Altered chemosensory function may also result from chemotherapy regimens, but the impact of these changes on diet are less clear.[86]

It is commonly argued that learned food aversions (LFAs) contribute to anorexia and weight loss in cancer patients. LFAs are aversions that patients form towards previously acceptable foods following their association with malaise. The incidence of such aversions ranges from about 40 to 65% in the general population.[87,88] In untreated cancer patients the incidence is about 50%, but following the onset of either chemotherapy or radiotherapy, approximately 50 to 55% of patients form new LFAs. High-protein items, sweets, caffeinated beverages, and high-fat items are particularly problematic, but any item, including water, may be targeted.[89] Typically, treatment-related aversions are specific (a mean of three to four items per individual) and transient (often less than 1 month in duration); consequently, they hold little dietary significance. Their principal impact may be on quality of life. Several approaches aimed at preventing the formation of LFAs have been explored. First, patients may be counseled to refrain from eating prior to treatments, but evidence that LFAs may form towards items consumed the day before or following treatment indicates that such advice is often not practical. Antiemetics administered to reduce the adverse side effects of treatments (the purported conditioning stimulus) have also proven ineffective. One approach that appears promising involves exposing patients to a nutritionally inconsequential food just prior to their first treatment. This may interfere with the formation of LFAs towards wholesome foods in the patient's customary diet.[88,91] Such an approach has reduced the incidence of treatment-related LFAs from 55 to 11%.[91]

## OBESITY

Although small differences in sensory responses to aqueous solutions of taste stimuli or experimentally prepared foods have been noted between the obese and the lean,[92,93] the preponderance of studies fail to support an association between body weight and chemosensory responses.[94–96] Whether the generally negative evidence accurately reflects a lack of difference or may be attributable to methodologic issues is uncertain. The failure to control for effects of recent dieting and dietary restraint may confound such studies. If more careful studies reveal a significant association between sensory measures and body weight regulation, sensory responses may provide useful diagnostic or prognostic insights. Given the lack of compelling evidence that the eating behaviors of lean and obese individuals differ,[94] and the paucity of data indicating that sensory responses among the obese actually influence their eating behavior, assumptions that sensory factors play an etiologic role in the onset or maintenance of obesity are not currently appropriate.

## REFERENCES


1. Bartoshunk, L.M.: History of taste research. *In* Handbook of Perception. Edited by E.C. Carterette and M.P. Friedman. New York, Academic Press, 1978.
2. Cain, W.S.: History of research on smell. *In* Handbook of Perception. Edited by E.C. Carterette and M.P. Friedman. New York, Academic Press, 1978.
3. Sandick, B., Cardello, A.V.: Chem. Sen., *6:*197–214, 1981.
4. Mistretta, C.M.: Gerodontology, *3:*131–136, 1984.
5. Norgren, R.: Chem. Sen., *10:*143–161, 1985.
6. Nilsson, B.: Acta Odontol. Scand., *35:*51–62, 1977.
7. Teeter, J.H., Brand, J.G.: Peripheral mechanisms of gustation: Physiology and biochemistry. *In* Neurobiology of Taste and Smell. Edited by T.E. Finger. Philadelphia, John Wiley & Sons, 1987.
8. Green, B.G.: Effects of thermal, mechanical, and chemical stimulation on the perception of oral irritation. *In* Chemical Senses. Vol. 2: Irritation. Edited by B.G. Green, J.L. Mason, and M.R. Kare. New York, Marcel Dekker, 1990.
9. Mattes, R.D., Mela, D.J.: Chem. Sen., *11:*523–539, 1986.
10. Gershoff, S.N.: The role of vitamins and minerals in taste. *In* The Chemical Senses and Nutrition. Edited by O. Maller and M.R. Kare. New York, Academic Press, 1977.
11. Bernard, R.A., Halpern, B.P.: J. Gen. Physiol., *52:*444–464, 1968.
12. Garrett-Laster, M., Russell, R.M., Jacques, P.F.: Hum. Nutr. Clin. Nutr., *38C:*203–214, 1984.
13. Weismann, K., Christensen, E., Dreyer, V.: Acta Med. Scand., *205:*361–366, 1979.
14. Afonsky, D.: Ann. N. Y. Acad. Sci., *85:*362–367, 1960.
15. Afonsky, D., Changsha, H.: Oral Surg. Oral Med. Oral Pathol., *3:*1299–1327, 1950.
16. Green, R.F.: JAMA, *218:*1303, 1971.
17. Schaumburg, H., Kaplan, J., Windebank, A., et al.: N. Engl. J. Med., *309:*445–448, 1983.
18. Kare, M.R., Henkin R.I.: Proc. Soc. Exp. Biol. Med., *131:*559–565, 1969.
19. Henkin, R.I., Keiser, H.R., Jaffe, I.R., et al.: Lancet, *2:*1268–1271, 1967.
20. Mattes, R.D., Heller, A.D., Rivlin, R.S.: Abnormalities in suprathreshold taste function in early hypothyroidism in humans. *In* Clinical Measurement of Taste and Smell. Edited by H.L. Meiselman and R.S. Rivlin. New York, Macmillan, 1986.

21. Mackay-Sim, A., Beard, M.D.: Dev. Brain Res., *36:*190–198, 1987.
22. Mattes, R.D., Labov, J.: J. Am. Diet. Assoc., *89:*692–694, 1989.
23. Chan, M., Brand, J.G., Ingle, D.E., et al.: Nutr. Res., *3:*511–518, 1983.
24. Henkin, R.I.: Biol. Trace Element Res., *6:*263–280, 1984.
25. Henkin, R.I., Schecter, P.J., Friedewald, W.T., et al.: Am. J. Med. Sci., *272:*285–299, 1976.
26. Greger, J.L., Geissler, A.H.: Am. J. Clin. Nutr., *31:*633–637, 1978.
27. Gibson, R.S., Vanderkooy, P.D.S., MacDonald, A.C., et al.: Am. J. Clin. Nutr., *49:*1266–1273, 1989.
28. Fosmire, G.J.: Am. J. Clin. Nutr., *51:*225–227, 1990.
29. Iwasaki, K., Sato, M.: Jnp. J. Physiol., *34:*907–918, 1984.
30. U.S. Department of Health, Education, and Welfare, National Institute of Neurological and Communicative Disorders and Stroke: Report of the Panel on Communicative Disorders to the National Advisory Neurological and Communicative Disorders and Stroke Council. NIH publication 79–1914. Washington, D.C., U.S. Government Printing Office, 1979.
31. Mattes, R.D., Cowart, B.J., Schiavo, M.A., et al.: Am. J. Clin. Nutr., *51:*233–240, 1990.
32. Ferris, A.M., Schlitzer, J.L., Schierberl, M.J.: Nutrition and taste and smell deficits: A risk factor or an adjustment? *In* Clinical Measurement of Taste and Smell. Edited by H.L. Meiselman and R.S. Rivlin. New York, Macmillan, 1986.
33. Mattes-Kulig, D.A., Henkin, R.I.: J. Am. Diet. Assoc., *85:*822–826, 1985.
34. Brand, J.G., Cagan, R.H., Naim, M.: Annu. Rev. Nutr., *2:*249–276, 1982.
35. Winer, R.A., Barber, T.X., Chauncey, H.H.: Proc. Soc. Exp. Biol. Med., *119:*1–4, 1965.
36. Christensen, C.M., Navazesh, M.: Appetite, *5:*307–315, 1984.
37. Wooley, O.W., Wooley, S.C.: Appetite, *2:*331–350, 1981.
38. Wooley, S.C., Wooley, O.W.: Psychosom. Med., *35:*136–142, 1973.
39. Feldman, M., Richardson, C.T.: Gastroenterology, *90:*428–433, 1986.
40. Knutson, U., Bergegardh, S., Olbe, L.: Scand. J. Gastroenterol., *9:*357–365, 1974.
41. Moore, J.G., Schenkenberg T.: Gastroenterology, *66:*954–959, 1974.
42. Janowitz, H.D., Hollander, F., Orringer, D., et al.: Gastroenterology, *16:*104–116, 1950.
43. Sarles, H., Dani, R., Prezelin, G., et al.: Gut, *9:*214–222, 1968.
44. Novis, B.H., Banks, S. Marks, I.N.: Scand. J. Gastroenterol., *6:*417–422, 1971.
45. Behrman, H.R., Kare, M.R.: Proc. Soc. Exp. Biol. Med., *129:*343–346, 1968.
46. Naim, M., Kare, M.R., Merritt, A.M.: Physiol. Behav., *20:*563–570, 1978.
47. Crittenden, P.J., Ivy, A.C.: Am. J. Physiol., *119:*724–733, 1937.
48. Kissileff, H.R., Pi-Sunyer, X., Thornton, J., et al.: Am. J. Clin. Nutr., *34:*154–160, 1981.
49. Forsyth, P.A., Weingarten, H.P., Collins, S.M.: Physiol. Behav., *35:*539–543, 1985.
50. Nilsson, G., Uvnas-Wallensten, K.: Acta Physiol. Scand., *100:*248–302, 1977.
51. DeJung, A., Strubbe, J.J., Steffens, A.B.: Am. J. Physiol., *233:*E380–E388, 1977.
52. Johnson, W.G., Wildman, H.E.: Behav. Neurosci., *97:*1025–1028, 1983.
53. Louis-Sylvestre, J., LeMagnen, J.: Neurosci. Biobehav. Rev., *4(Suppl. 1):*43–46, 1980.
54. Schwartz, T.W., Stenquist, B., Olbe, L.: Scand. J. Gastroenterol., *14:*313–320, 1979.
55. Teff, K.L., Mattes, R.D., Engelman, K.: Am. J. Physiol., *261:*E430–E436, 1991.
56. Sjostrom, L., Garellick, G., Krotkiewski, M., et al.: Metabolism, *29:*901–909, 1980.
57. Lucas, F., Bellisle, F., DiMaio, A.: Physiol. Behav., *40:*631–636, 1987.
58. Parra-Covarrubias, A., Rivera-Rodriguez, I., Almaraz-Ugalde, A.: Diabetes, *20:*800–802, 1971.
59. Steffens, A.B.: Am. J. Physiol., *230:*1411–1415, 1976.
60. Proietto, J., Rohner-Jeanrenaud, F., Ionescu, E., et al.: Diabetes, *36:*791–795, 1987.
61. Lorentzen, M., Madsbad, S., Kehlet, H., et al.: Acta Endocrinol., *115:*84–86, 1987.
62. Kraegen, E.W., Chisholm, D.J., McNamara, M.E.: Horm. Metab. Res., *13:*365–367, 1981.
63. Bruce, D.G., Chisholm, D.J., Storlien, L.H., et al.: Diabetes, *37:*736–744, 1988.
64. Diamond, P., Brondel, L., LeBlac, J.: Am. J. Physiol., *248:*E75–E79, 1985.
65. Nacht, C.A., Christin, L., Temler, E., et al.: Am. J. Physiol., *253:*E481–E488, 1987.
66. Deriaz, O., Nacht, C.A., Chiolero, R., et al.: Metabolism, *38:*1082–1088, 1989.
67. LeBlanc, J., Cabanac, M.: Physiol. Behav., *46:*479–482, 1989.
68. LeBlanc, J., Brondel, L.: Am. J. Physiol., *248:*E333–E336, 1985.
69. Calles-Escandon, J., Robbins, D.C.: Diabetes, *36:*1167–1172, 1987.
70. Vatner, S.F., Patrick, T.A., Higgins, C.B., et al.: J. Appl. Physiol., *36:*524–529, 1974.
71. Fronek, K., Stahlgren, L.H.: Circ. Res., *23:*687–692, 1968.
72. Winne, G.I.: J. Pharmacol. Exp. Ther., *6:*333–393, 1979.
73. Murphy, C., Cain, W.S., Hegsted, D.M. (Eds.): Ann. N. Y. Acad. Sci., *561*, 1989.
74. Cowart, B.J.: Ann. N. Y. Acad. Sci., *561:*39–55, 1989.
75. Mattes, R.D.: J. Chron. Dis., *37:*195–208, 1984.
76. Mattes, R.D., Falkner, B.: Chem. Sen., *14:*673–679, 1989.
77. Mattes, R.D.: Assessing salt taste preference and its relationship with dietary sodium intake in humans. *In* Food Acceptance and Nutrition. Edited by J. Solms, D.A. Booth, R.M. Pangborn, and O. Raunhardt. New York, Academic Press, 1987.
78. Bertino, M., Beauchamp, G.K., Riskey, D.R., et al.: Appetite, *2:*67–73, 1981.
79. Bertino, M., Beauchamp, G.K., Engelman, K.: Physiol. Behav., *38:*203–213, 1986.
80. Settle, R.G.: Diabetes mellitus and the chemical senses. *In* Clinical Measurement of Taste and Smell. Edited by H.L. Meiselman and R.S. Rivlin. New York, Macmillan, 1986.
81. Abbasi, A.A.: Geriatrics, *36:*73–78, 1981.
82. Trant, A.S., Serin, J., Douglass, H.O.: Am. J. Clin. Nutr., *36:*45–58, 1982.
83. Carson, J.A.S., Gormican, A.: Research, *70:*361–365, 1977.
84. Mossman, K., Shatzman, A., Chencharick, J.: Int. J. Radiat. Oncol. Biol. Phys., *8:*991–997, 1982.
85. Mossman, K.L.: Br. J. Cancer, *53(Suppl.* 7):9–11, 1986.
86. Bruera, E., Carraro, S., Roca, E., et al.: Cancer Treat. Rep., *68:*873–876, 1984.

**87.** Garb, J.L., Stunkard, A.J.: Psychiatry, *131*:1204–1207, 1974.
**88.** Midkiff, E.E., Bernstein, I.L.: Physiol. Behav., *34*:839–841, 1985.
**89.** Mattes, R.D., Arnold, C., Boraas, M.: Cancer, *60*:2576–2580, 1987.
**90.** Broberg, D.J., Bernstein, I.L.: Cancer, *60*:2344–2347, 1987.
**91.** Mattes, R.D., Arnold, C., Boraas, M.: Cancer Treat. Rep., *71*:1071–1078, 1987.
**92.** Rodin, J., Moskowitz, H.R., Bray, G.A.: Physiol. Behav., *17*:591–597, 1976.
**93.** Drewnowski, A., Brunzell, J.D., Sande, K., et al.: Physiol. Behav., *35*:617–622, 1985.
**94.** Spitzer, L., Rodin, J.: Appetite, *2*:293–329, 1981.
**95.** Frijters, J.E.R., Rasmussen-Conrad, E.L.: J. Gen. Psychol., *107*:233–247, 1982.
**96.** Pangborn, R.M., Bos, K.E.O., Stern, J.S.: Appetite, *6*:25–40, 1985.

## SELECTED READINGS

Friedman M.I., Tordoff M.G., Kare M.R. (Eds.): Chemical Senses: Appetite and Nutrition. New York, Marcel Dekker, 1991.

Getchell T.V., Doty R.L., Bartoshuk L.M., et al. (Eds.): Smell and Taste in Health and Disease. New York, Raven Press, 1991.

Meiselman H.L., Rivlin R.S. (Eds.): Clinical Measurement of Taste and Smell. New York, MacMillan, 1986.

Solms J., Booth D.A., Pangborn R.M., et al. (Eds.): Food Acceptance and Nutrition. New York, Academic Press, 1987.

CHAPTER **37**

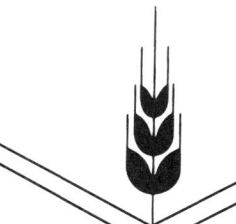

# The Gastrointestinal Tract: Regulator of Nutrient Absorption

**Harry L. Greene and J. Roberto Moran**



The gastrointestinal tract is a complex organ system whose primary functions are to carry out digestion and absorption of ingested nutrients and simultaneously to protect the body from ingested microorganisms and noxious substances. After ingestion, food is mechanically divided, mixed with digestive enzymes, and cleaved into readily absorbable particles. Nutrients are then absorbed through specialized mucosa and nonabsorbed substances are expelled. More than 95% of ingested carbohydrate, fat, and protein is usually absorbed during passage through a normally functioning gastrointestinal tract, although absorption of certain vitamins, minerals, and trace elements may be less efficient.[1]

Protection against harmful, non-nutritive substances is provided first by the practice of food selection and preparation before ingestion, and to some extent by sensory discrimination at the time of ingestion. The chemical action of saliva and production of mucus, gastric acid, and digestive enzymes further alter potentially harmful substances.[2] A complex immune system that involves the production of luminal antibodies to neutralize many ingested parasites, bacteria, and viruses adds further protection. Additional protective mechanisms include vomiting, which is coordinated by the brain stem vomiting center sensitive both to the influence of central chemoreceptors and to afferent impulses from the gastrointestinal tract,[3] and diarrhea. Prostaglandins also appear to aid this protective action by modulating the motor and secretory activity of the intestine.[4] Inhibition of prostaglandin synthesis by agents, such as nonsteroidal anti-inflammatory drugs, appears to disrupt the functional integrity of the gastric and duodenal mucosa creating the potential for ulcer formation.

## INTEGRATION OF THE GASTROINTESTINAL TRACT WITH OTHER ORGANS

The gastrointestinal tract is an extremely active metabolic organ. Although it contains most of the enzymes that are present in the liver, the metabolic pathways are generally less active than those of the liver. Its metabolic functions are therefore directed primarily toward supporting digestion and delivery of ingested nutrients to the liver for further processing. This function demands substantial quantities of energy in the postabsorptive state. In order to meet these energy demands, the gastrointestinal tract consumes 30% of the cardiac output from two major arteries.[2] Together they carry more blood than any other branch of the aorta; the blood flow may increase even further with eating. In fact, postprandial increases in blood flow may produce cardiac and mesenteric angina in susceptible subjects.

**Liver.** The liver is the organ most responsible for metabolic homeostasis of absorbed nutrients. The liver participates in the absorption of lipids through secretion of bile and in the modulation of blood nutrient levels through the clearance of absorbed nutrients from the portal vein and subsequent release into the hepatic vein. Other hepatic functions include detoxification of drugs and noxious chemicals, modulation of certain circulating hormones, and elimination of pathogenic organisms.

Venous blood from the gastrointestinal tract is carried to the liver via the portal vein. With the exception of intestinal chylomicrons that enter the lymphatics, all absorbed products pass initially through the liver and, in most instances, are extracted or modified before passage into the systemic circulation. Many nutrients and some drugs are subject to an enterohepatic circulation through their excretion in bile and subsequent reabsorption by the small intestine. Interruption of this cycle by biliary diversion or failure of reabsorption accounts for a more rapid onset of specific deficiencies than might otherwise be anticipated. Examples of substances with enterohepatic circulation include bile salts, vitamin D, vitamin $B_{12}$, folate, cholesterol, and drugs such as methotrexate. The enterohepatic circulation of methotrexate increases the liver and intestinal exposure to the drug and contributes to its tendency toward hepatic and intestinal toxicity.[5]

**Pancreas.** The endocrine and exocrine activity of the pancreas is integrally related to gastrointestinal and hepatic handling of nutrients. Insulin is released from beta cells in response to a rise in plasma amino acids or glucose, vagal stimulation, or a rise in circulating gastrin, cholecystokinin (CCK), or secretin. All such postprandial signals appear to originate in the intestine. The anabolic actions of insulin facilitate intracellular transfer of glucose, amino acids, and fatty acids and increase glucose oxidation, glycogenesis, lipogenesis, and protein synthesis. Glucagon, which is secreted by alpha islet cells in response to rises in circulating alanine, ketones, and CCK, or a fall in blood glucose levels of values, balances the actions of insulin. Pancreatic exocrine function, which is stimulated by hormones released from the small bowel mucosa in response to luminal nutrients, aids in the digestion and absorption of food. The exocrine pancreas also produces somatostatin and possibly other hormones that may further modulate metabolic and functional activities of the intestine by as yet unidentified mechanisms. Table 37–1 is a list of several clinical syndromes associated with pancreatic tumors.

**TABLE 37–1.** SYNDROMES ASSOCIATED WITH PANCREATIC TUMORS

| TUMOR PRODUCT | CLINICAL MANIFESTATION |
|---|---|
| Gastrin | Peptic ulcer, diarrhea |
| VIP | Secretory diarrhea |
| Insulin | Fasting hypoglycemia |
| Pancreatic polypeptide | Skin disease, hyperglycemia |
| Somatostatin | None |
| ACTH | Cushing's syndrome |
| GH | Acromegaly |

VIP, Vasoactive intestinal peptide; ACTH, adrenocorticotropic hormone; GH, growth hormone.

**Brain.** The relationship between the brain and the gastrointestinal tract is more complex than initially supposed. More than 15 peptides with dual distribution in brain and intestine have been described.[6] Apart from hormonal and neurotransmitter functions in the intestine, several of these peptides show paracrine activity between adjacent cells. Many of these same peptides also appear to act as neurotransmitters at central nerve ganglia. A new term has therefore evolved to describe this system of common transmission in brain and in gastrointestinal tract—the "peptidergic nervous system."[7] Peptide transmitters include vasoactive intestinal peptide (VIP), motilin, CCK, and somatostatin. In addition, many opiate peptides or endorphins are also found in both the brain and the intestinal mucosa. In the brain, these transmitters may modulate pain; in the gut, they appear to inhibit gastrointestinal motility and secretion. Although the integrated function of these peptides in the control of intestinal function is unclear at present, some of the peptides have been studied individually.

Appetite plays a major role in food-seeking behavior, and although it is incompletely understood, it is apparently regulated by the central nervous system, particularly the hypothalmus.[6,8] Studies based on the postulated relationship between appetite regulation and these peptide transmitters should represent a fruitful area of investigation.

**Immune System.** The gut is an important interface between the internal and external environment. In protecting the body from potentially harmful foreign substances, the immune system may favorably influence nutrient absorption, but conversely, malnutrition or certain dietary toxins adversely affect immune function. The intestinal immune system acts to reduce the amount of antigen absorbed by the intestine and, by humoral communication, may prevent undesirable immune reactions from otherwise harmless antigenic substances that have managed to cross the intestinal mucosa. Impairment of the intestinal immune system is implicated in the genesis of several diseases that affect gut function and nutritional status.[9] These diseases include gluten-sensitive enteropathy, food allergies, immunodeficiency syndromes, and possibly inflammatory bowel disease. The role of the immune system is discussed in detail in Chapter 41.

## STRUCTURE AND DEVELOPMENT OF THE GASTROINTESTINAL TRACT

### EMBRYOLOGY

The primitive gut forms during the fourth week of gestation from the foregut, midgut, and hindgut. The foregut gives rise to the pharynx, esophagus, stomach, duodenum (proximal to the ampulla of Vater), liver and biliary apparatus, and the pancreas. The blood supply for these organs derives from the celiac artery. Because the trachea and esophagus have a common origin, incomplete partitioning may lead to stenoses, atresias, and fistulas. Duodenal atresia occurs when vacuolization between the foregut and the midgut fails to occur.

The derivatives of the midgut are the small intestine (below the opening of the common bile duct), the cecum, the appendix, the ascending colon, and the proximal part of the transverse colon. Blood is supplied to these structures by the superior mesenteric artery. Omphaloceles, malrotations, and abnormalities of fixation occur when the midgut fails to return from the umbilical cord or fails to rotate appropriately.

The hindgut begins at the distal part of the transverse colon and extends through the descending and sigmoid colon, the rectum, and the superior portion of the anal canal. Hindgut derivatives are supplied by the inferior mesenteric artery.

### ANATOMY AND GROWTH

The gastrointestinal tract is a musculomembranous tube that stretches from the mouth to the anus. Accessory organs include the salivary glands, liver, gallbladder, and pancreas (Fig. 37–1).

The wall of the gastrointestinal tract contains a series of cellular layers. These layers are the epithelium (including glands), lamina propria, muscularis mucosae, submucosa (containing blood vessels, nerves, lymphatics), muscularis externa, and serosa. The two nerve plexuses of the enteric nervous system lie within the submucosa and between the two muscle layers of the bowel, the circular and longitudinal layers of the muscularis externa.

The stomach is a food reservoir where digestion begins. Although its capacity is normally 1000 to 1500 ml, under unusual circumstances as much as 6000 ml may be present. The area just below the lower esophageal sphincter is designated the cardia; the fundus is

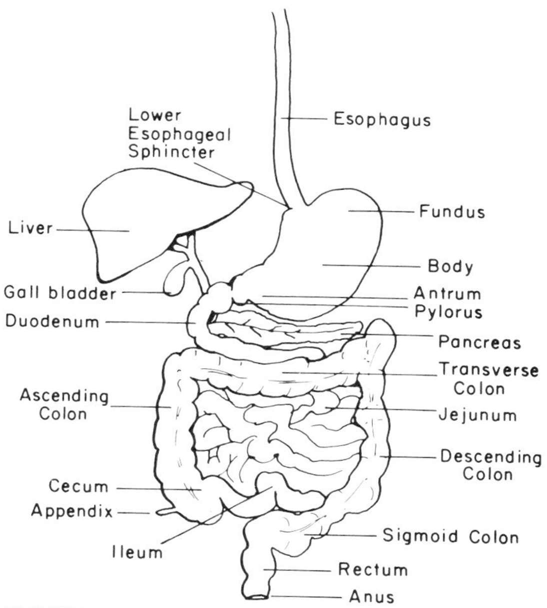

Lower Esophageal Sphincter
Esophagus
Fundus
Liver
Body
Gall bladder
Antrum
Pylorus
Duodenum
Pancreas
Transverse Colon
Ascending Colon
Jejunum
Descending Colon
Cecum
Appendix
Sigmoid Colon
Ileum
Rectum
Anus


**FIGURE 37–1.** Diagram of the major parts of the gastrointestinal tract.

that portion of the stomach that continues lateral to and above the cardia, and the body extends from the cardia to the antrum, which stretches from the angulus to the pylorus. The antrum, which differs dramatically from the remainder of the stomach in function, may be distinguished grossly by the absence of rugae as well as by its histologic appearance. The pylorus, a muscular sphincter between the stomach and the duodenum, controls gastric emptying and limits reflux of bile.

Gastric epithelium contains numerous glands lined by mucous cells, parietal (acid-producing) cells, and chief (pepsinogen-producing) cells. In the cardia and antrum, these glands contain predominantly mucous cells. Gastrin cells are located in the antral epithelium and have surface microvilli that monitor the intragastric pH. These cells secrete gastrin into the blood in response to rises in intragastric pH. Adjacent to gastrin-producing cells are D cells, which produce somatostatin and may modulate gastrin production.[10]

The pancreas is a triangular compound racemose gland lying deeply between the duodenum, bile duct, stomach, colon, and spleen. Pancreatic acini produce exocrine secretions that drain into a branching duct system and eventually into the duodenum to aid in primary digestion of food. Scattered throughout the pancreas are islets of Langerhans, which produce insulin, glucagon, somatostatin, and possibly other peptide hormones.

The liver is a large bilobular organ in the right upper abdomen. It receives 30% of its blood supply from the hepatic artery and the remainder from the portal vein

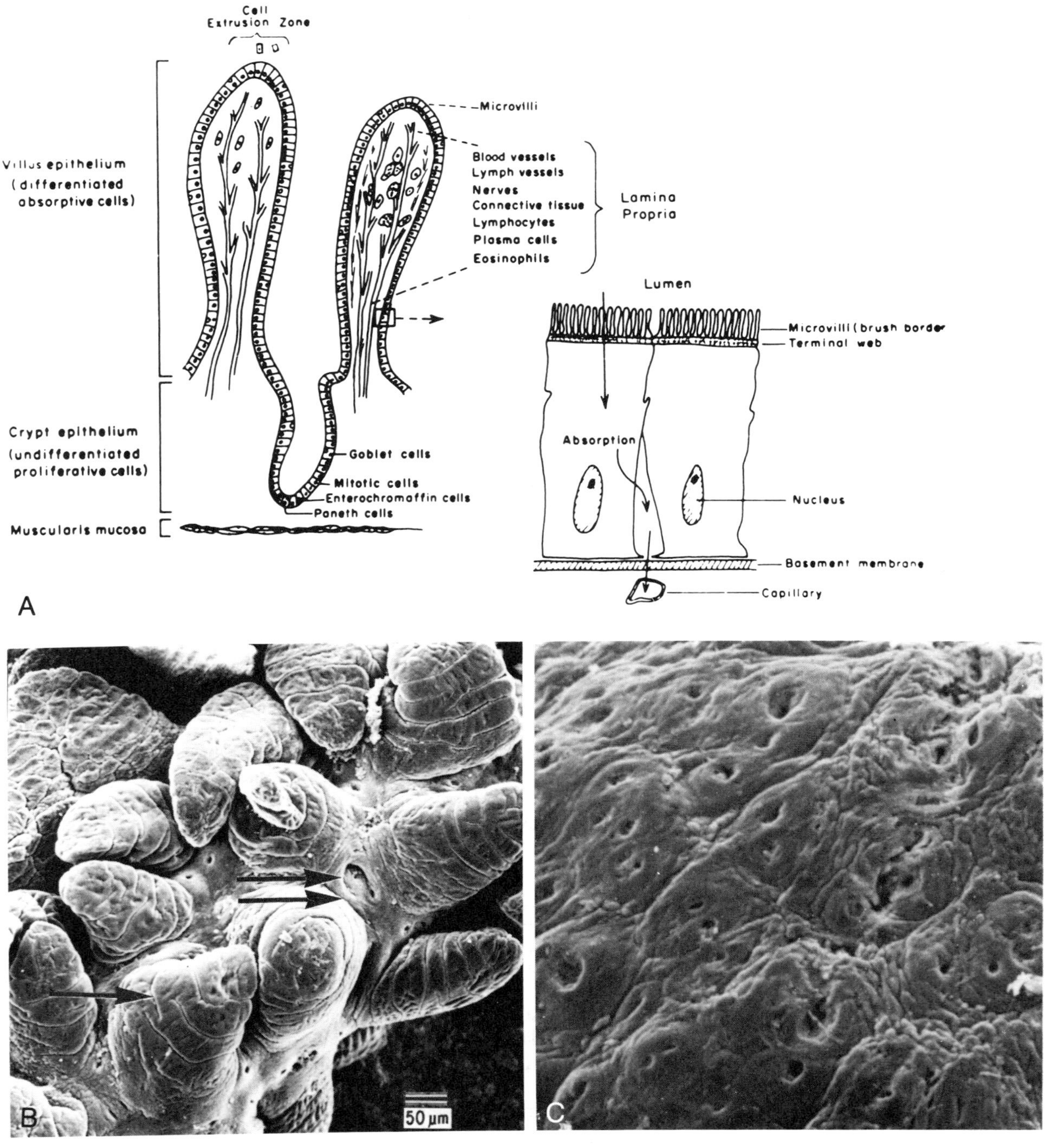

Cell Extrusion Zone
Microvilli
Villus epithelium (differentiated absorptive cells)
Blood vessels
Lymph vessels
Nerves
Connective tissue
Lymphocytes
Plasma cells
Eosinophils
Lamina Propria
Lumen
Microvilli (brush border
Terminal web
Absorption
Nucleus
Basement membrane
Capillary
Crypt epithelium (undifferentiated proliferative cells)
Goblet cells
Mitotic cells
Enterochromaffin cells
Paneth cells
Muscularis mucosa
A
B
50 µm
C


**FIGURE 37–2.** *A*, Diagram of the functional units of the intestine (magnified about 1000 ×) and two epithelial cells showing the brush border and primary direction of nutrient transport through the cell into the capillary. *B*, Scanning electron micrograph of jejunal villi with crypts (magnified about 500 ×) apparent between and at the base of the villi. *C*, Scanning electron micrograph showing the epithelium of a patient with severe, untreated gluten-sensitive enteropathy with complete absence of villi and only crypts remaining (magnified about 800 ×).

that carries blood from the stomach, intestines, pancreas, and spleen. The liver is composed of microscopic lobules. In each lobule, the blood flows from the hepatic artery and portal vein through sinusoids lined with cords of liver cells (hepatocytes) to central veins and eventually to hepatic veins that drain into the vena cava. The difference in oxygen and nutrient content in blood at the periportal areas versus that at the central vein areas accounts for certain differences in metabolic activity between the periportal and central lobular cells. Bile flows from the hepatocyte through microscopic bile canaliculi to bile ductules and then along the biliary system to the duodenum.

The adult small intestine measures about 22 feet long at post mortem, although it may appear less than half that length at surgery. The jejunum is arbitrarily defined as the upper 40% and the ileum as the remainder. The epithelial lining of the small bowel has a far greater surface area than the muscle coat to which it is attached, the result of many invaginations (crypts) and projections (villi), as shown in Figure 37–2. Each villus cell has its own microscopic projections (microvilli), which in turn are covered by a fuzzy coat or glycocalyx containing many digestive enzymes. Several cell types have been identified within the intestinal mucosa, but their functions are incompletely established. The villus epithelial cells have digestive as well as absorptive function. Rapidly dividing cells at the base of the crypts are responsible for secretion, but as they migrate to the villus, they mature into absorptive cells and eventually are extruded from the villus tip. Small intestinal cell turnover time (48 to 72 hours) is one of the most rapid of any tissue. Consequently, malnutrition and compounds (such as methotrexate[7]) that interfere with protein synthesis or cell replication may adversely affect intestinal function. Figure 37–2 illustrates normal-appearing villi, as compared to those seen in severe villus atrophy present in a child with gluten-sensitive enteropathy.

The colon is a large-diameter muscular organ that frames the small intestine. The vermiform appendix, which is attached to the cecum, contains specialized lymphatic structures. The epithelial surface of the normal colon is composed of absorptive cells that predominantly absorb water and electrolytes. Goblet (mucus-producing) cells line the glandular crypts. Endocrine cells are also present, but hormonal function as related to the colon is not well understood. The turnover time of colonic mucosa is 3 to 8 days, substantially longer than that of the small intestine.

The gastrointestinal tract grows in length and caliber until somatic growth ceases after puberty. This visceral growth appears to depend on the same general factors as somatic growth (nutritional adequacy, insulin, growth hormone, thyroid hormone, cortisol, androgens, and estrogens) as well as specified factors such as the direct effect of ingested nutrients, gastrointestinal hormones, and secretions.[11] The principal factors affecting the growth of the gastrointestinal mucosa are shown in Figure 37–3. Several of the hormones affecting growth, secretion, and contractility are shown in Table 37–2.

## INTESTINAL IMMUNE SYSTEM

Elements of the intestinal immune system include (1) lymphocytes scattered between the cells of the gastrointestinal epithelium, (2) lymphocytes and macrophages scattered diffusely in the lamina propria of the stomach and intestine, and (3) differentiated lymphoid structures located along the course of the gastrointestinal tract. The latter, which include the tonsils, the Peyer's patches, and the lymphoid structures of the appendix, are the initial site of interaction between many antigens and the immune system. The overlying epithelial surface contains T lymphocytes, which appear to facilitate the binding and entry of antigens. Memory cells produced in response to antigens migrate to other parts of the body and the intestine via the general circulation. Re-exposure to antigens leads to differentiation of these memory cells into plasma cells that produce type-specific IgA or IgE.[12]

Plasma cells in the lamina propria of the gut synthesize and secrete immunoglobulins including antibodies directed against antigens present in the gut lumen. Plasma cells produce IgA in contrast to other lymphoid tissues in which IgG is the predominant immunoglobulin produced. IgA enters the intestinal lumen with two additional peptide chains: one of these, the secretory component, protects the IgA from luminal digestion; the second facilitates polymerization. Secretory IgA may prevent bacterial adherence to the mucosal surfaces, but it does not appear to fix complement. Details of the immune system are discussed in Chapter 41.

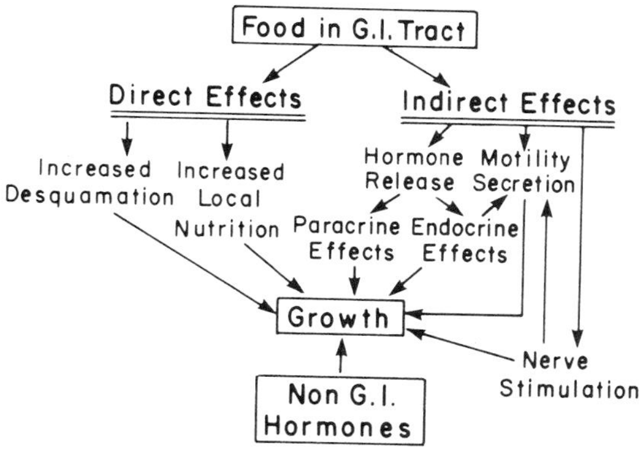
Food in G.I. Tract
Direct Effects
Indirect Effects
Increased Desquamation
Increased Local Nutrition
Hormone Release
Motility Secretion
Paracrine Effects
Endocrine Effects
Growth
Nerve Stimulation
Non G.I. Hormones

**FIGURE 37–3.** Factors influencing growth of the gastrointestinal mucosa. (Redrawn from Johnson, L.R.: Regulation of gastrointestinal growth. *In* Physiology of the Gastrointestinal Tract. Edited by L.R. Johnson. New York, Raven Press, 1981.)

## FUNCTIONS OF THE GASTROINTESTINAL TRACT

After ingestion, food is chewed and swallowed. Integrated motility and secretion subsequently enhance digestion and mucosal contact for ultimate absorption. Secretion and motility are subject to exogenous influences but organized primarily by autonomous intrinsic neurologic and hormonal systems.

### NEURAL AND HORMONAL CONTROL OF INTESTINAL ACTIVITY

The functions of eating and evacuation are controlled by the central nervous system through its somatic division and modulated by numerous hormonal interactions.

Autonomic innervation of the gastrointestinal tract (efferent sympathetic fibers arising from the ganglia of the sympathetic trunk and parasympathetic fibers in the vagus, pelvic, and splanchnic nerves) modifies motility and secretions but is not essential for coordinated function. The usual autonomic neurotransmitters appear to have only a limited role in the intrinsic nervous system of the gut, which is maintained primarily by a different set of transmitters described subsequently.

The enteric nervous system (ENS) contains more than $10^8$ neurons in humans (roughly equivalent to all the neurons in the spinal cord).[13,14] The physiologic independence of the ENS was described with considerable precision by Bayliss and Starling in 1899.[15] The ENS contains sensory receptors, primary afferent neurons, interneurons to carry reflexes, and motor neurons to relax or excite smooth muscle. Loss of certain intrinsic components of the ENS, as is seen in Hirschsprung's or Chagas' diseases, is associated with functional obstruction and proximal dilatation. Propulsive movement of the bowel thus depends on local reflex activity mediated by ganglia of the ENS.

The ENS is composed of two interconnected ganglionated plexuses (neuroglial sheaths) lying in the submucosa and between the longitudinal and circular muscle layers. Nerve endings and muscle fibers are widely separate with consequent nondiscrete control—the gut does not twitch but shows broad regional responses. Putative neurotransmitters (in addition to catecholamines and acetylcholine) include serotonin,[16] purines,[17] VIP,[18] substance P,[19] somatostatin,[20] encephalins,[21] bombesin,[22] pancreatic polypeptide, and neurotensin.[23] Acetylcholine appears to act as an excitatory transmitter between vagal fibers and enteric neurons, between enteric interneurons, and between enteric neurons and intestinal smooth muscle. Intestinal motility is thus vulnerable to interruption by ganglion-blocking agents such as hexamethonium and by muscarinic antagonists such as atropine. Noradrenergic innervation is concentrated at the periphery of the myenteric and submucosal plexuses,

**TABLE 37–2.** HUMAN GASTROINTESTINAL REGULATORY PEPTIDES: MAIN ANATOMIC SOURCE, MODE OF ACTION, AND POSSIBLE MAIN PHYSIOLOGIC ACTION

| REGULATORY PEPTIDE | MAIN SOURCE(S) | MODE OF ACTION | MAIN ACTION |
|---|---|---|---|
| Gastrin | Antrum | Hormone | Stimulates gastric acid secretion |
| Cholecystokinin | Upper small intestine and CNS | Hormone/ neurotransmitter | Gallbladder contraction and pancreatic enzyme secretion |
| Secretin | Upper small intestine | Hormone | Pancreatic bicarbonate secretion |
| Pancreatic glucagon | Pancreas | Hormone | Stimulates hepatic glucose output |
| Gastric inhibitory polypeptide | Upper small intestine | Hormone | Enhancement of insulin secretion |
| Motilin | Upper small intestine | Hormone | Stimulates gastrointestinal motility |
| Vasoactive intestinal polypeptide | All tissues | Neurotransmitter | Neurotransmitter (secretomotor, vasodilator, and smooth muscle relaxation) |
| Bombesin | Gut, CNS, and lung | Neurotransmitter/ paracrine | Stimulates gut hormone release |
| Somatostatin | Gut and CNS | Paracrine/ neurotransmitter | Inhibits hormone release and hormone target tissues |
| Neurotensin | Ileum and CNS | Hormone/ neurotransmitter | Inhibits gastric emptying and acid secretion |
| Substance P | Gut, CNS, and skin | Neurotransmitter | Sensory neurotransmitter (especially pain) |
| Leu-enkephalin and ?met-enkephalin | Gut and CNS | Neurotransmitter | Opiate-like (endorphin system) |
| Peptide HI | Gut and CNS | Unknown | Unknown |
| Peptide YY | Gut and CNS | Hormone | Inhibits gastric acid secretion and gut motility |

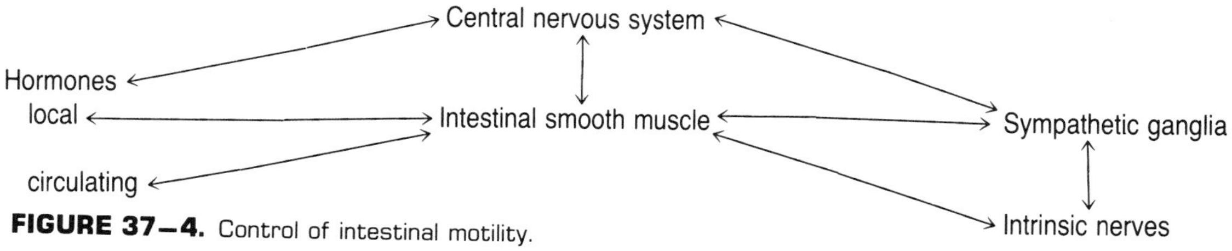
Central nervous system
Hormones
local
circulating
Intestinal smooth muscle
Sympathetic ganglia
Intrinsic nerves

**FIGURE 37–4.** Control of intestinal motility.

although sympathetic axons may directly activate neuroendocrine cells and affect absorption. Norepinephrine inhibits gastrointestinal motility by direct beta and indirect alpha actions. More powerful than sympathetic inhibition of gastrointestinal motility is the inhibition mediated by the ENS. This inhibition is unrelated to norepinephrine, but a specific ENS neurotransmitter has not yet been identified. Candidates include adenosine triphosphate (ATP) and VIP, both of which cause gut relaxation.

Many different types of endocrine cells are found in the epithelial lining of the gastrointestinal tract.[24] These cells characteristically have villi on the luminal surface, and contain secretory granules that can be released and cross the basolateral membrane. Their contents may then act locally or be transported to targets by the systemic circulation (see Table 37–2).

## INTEGRATION OF CONTROL OF MOTILITY

As described previously, many potential agents are involved in the control of intestinal motility. These mechanisms appear to act in concert to produce the various patterns of contractility seen in intact humans. Figure 37–4 illustrates the integration of the controlling influences on intestinal motility.

The primary unit of contractile activity is the smooth muscle cell. This unit can contract on its own and in a regular fashion. At least two other factors can modulate these intrinsic contractions, namely, circulating and locally released chemicals or "hormones," and neurotransmitters from either intrinsic or extrinsic neural fibers. Each system is capable of either excitatory or inhibitory influences to produce various patterns of contractions. Thus, the classification of motility into only two distinct types, segmental and propulsive, does not cover the wide spectrum of motility patterns of which the intestine is capable. On the other hand, the complexities of this system and its overall control are so poorly understood that the simplistic classification continues to serve as a practical approach to evaluation of clinical problems relating to gastrointestinal motility.

Esophageal motor contractions begin at the upper end of the esophagus with each conscious swallow and travel toward the lower esophageal sphincter. A second wave of spontaneous peristalsis usually follows if the primary wave fails to empty the esophagus. The lower esophageal sphincter (LES) relaxes to allow the bolus of food to pass.

Although the resting pressure in the body of the esophagus is lower than that of the stomach, reflux of gastric contents, even in the head-down position, is prevented by the higher resting pressure of the LES, which only relaxes to allow a food bolus to pass. The LES appears to be subject to the influence of the vagus nerve, neurohormonal agents (gastrin, secretin, and other gastrointestinal hormones), and prostaglandins, although their exact physiologic roles are uncertain.

Gastric motility is coordinated by the ENS but is sensitive to vagal and hormonal factors. Gastric emptying depends on antral motility, proximal gastric tone, pyloric resistance, and the consistency of the gastric contents. These factors are further modified by duodenal feedback (to protect against volume, tonicity, irritant, or pH overload) and gastric distention. The stomach normally empties exponentially at around 3% per minute. Gastric emptying of fluid can be influenced by several conditions, some of which are listed in Table 37–3. In the fasting state, infrequent migrating motor complexes (peristaltic waves) originate in the gastric antrum or upper small intestine and travel down the small intestine, clearing secretions and sloughed cells. This activity aborts in the fed state (but not with total parenteral nutrition) and is replaced by irregular bursts of contractions (segmentation and peristalsis) interspersed with transient quiescence.

In the small intestine, rhythmic segmentation is weaker than peristalsis, but it occurs more frequently. Segments become ballooned between contraction rings, facilitating mixing and increasing lymph flow. These segmentations occur 10 to 12 times per minute in the duodenum with a progressive decrease in rate to 6 to 8 per minute in the terminal ileum. These segmental contractions are mediated by the myenteric plexus. Peristaltic contraction waves (which may be preceded by a relaxation wave) travel aborally for only a few centimeters. Their speed is faster in the proximal than in the terminal intestine. Peristalsis depends on the myenteric plexus and is abolished by atropine, removal of the mucosa, or plexus degeneration.

Motor activity (both peristalsis and segmentation) increases with entry of chyme into the duodenum, gastric distention, mucosal irritation, and intestinal distention. The latter produces powerful peristaltic rushes.

Colonic contractions are either mixing or propulsive. Mixing movements are segmental contractions of 10 to 60 seconds duration found in the cecum, colon, and rectum. Propulsive contractions are most frequent in the midtransverse colon, and their net effect is to move

**TABLE 37–3.** FACTORS DETERMINING THE RATE OF GASTRIC EMPTYING

| DECREASE EMPTYING | INCREASE EMPTYING |
|---|---|
| Foods | Foods |
| Fats > protein > carbohydrate | In Stomach |
| Thicker consistency (solids >liquids) | Liquids |
| High osmolality > 800 mosm/L | Change in temperature |
| | In Duodenum |
| | High osmolality |
| | High volume |
| | Low pH |
| | Irritant |
| Drugs | Drugs |
| Anticholinergics | Cholinergics |
| Ganglion blockers | Metoclopramide |
| Gastrointestinal (GI)Hormones | GI Hormones |
| Secretin | Gastrin |
| Cholecystokinin | Motilin |
| Glucagon | |
| Diseases or Surgery | Diseases or Surgery |
| Vagotomy | "Irritable colon" |
| Pseudo-obstruction | Pyloroplasty |
| Diabetic neuropathy | Partial gastrectomy |
| Autonomic neuropathy | |
| Scleroderma | |
| Mechanical | Mechanical |
| Peptic ulcer | Gravity |
| Extrinsic pressure | Gastric distention |

colonic contents toward the rectum. Propulsion, which occurs several times daily, especially postprandially, is preceded by loss of segmental contractions. Eating produces an increase in the amplitude and frequency of colonic propulsive movement. Colonic movements are coordinated by intrinsic enteric nerves, but are subject to autonomic modulation, which can be blocked by anticholinergic drugs and increased by opiates.

Anal continence is maintained by cortical suppression of the urge to defecate that comes with rectal stimulation. When colonic contents pass into the rectum, cortical perception of rectal distention produces contraction of the external anal sphincter to counteract reflex relaxation of the internal sphincter. If defecation is convenient, the external anal sphincter relaxes, the glottis closes, the diaphragm and abdominal muscles contract, and the increased intra-abdominal pressure leads to evacuation of feces.

## MEMBRANE TRANSPORT

Substances are transported across the epithelial membranes by either passive (through electrochemical gradients) or active transport (energy-dependent mechanisms). The diffusional transport depends on both size and fat solubility of the substrate. Carrier mediation increases the transport capabilities of some substrates.[25]

**Passive Transport.** The permeability of the gastrointestinal mucosa primarily governs passive transport. The principal force driving this passive transport of solutes, as well as water, is the electrochemical or concentration gradient across the gastrointestinal mucosa.[26] Because the membranes are composed of a lipid layer sandwiched between two protein layers, lipid solubility also plays a facilitative role in passive solute transport.

Movement of electrically charged particles through membranes presents special problems. These charged particles are generally fat-insoluble and can permeate the membrane only through aqueous channels. The passive distribution of charged particles across the membrane depends on the prevailing chemical and electrical difference.[27] The rate of passive solute transport depends on the size as well as the charge of the aqueous channels. The size of the channels ranges from about 15 nm in the jejunum to only 4 nm in the less permeable colon. The net charge in the channels depends on the ratio of carboxyl to amino groups. For example, the anionic carboxyl groups outnumber the cationic amino groups in the gallbladder, giving the channels a net negative charge. This makes the gallbladder more permeable to cations because opposite charges attract one another. In the stomach, the reverse is true.

Another characteristic of the gastrointestinal tract is the variability of the microenvironment immediately adjacent to the luminal membrane. This fluid layer is not identical to the fluid in the middle of the lumen. Because no amount of peristaltic movement can affect this layer, it has been termed the "unstirred layer." Its presence has two important consequences: (1) Because it is aqueous, it comprises the principal diffusion barrier for lipid absorption. (2) Owing to the acidic groups in the glycocalyx, the lower pH of the layer influences absorption of weak electrolytes, including many drugs.[28]

Finally, in considering passive transport in the gastrointestinal tract, permeability paths between the epithelial cells must be discussed. These intercellular or paracellular "shunt" pathways are mainly of importance to small electrolytes and water. The protein cement of cellular junctions serves as an alternate channel for passive diffusion. In the ileum, about four times as much water and electrolytes traverse the paracellular pathways as cross the cellular membranes, and the gallbladder is even a looser epithelium, having a paracellular shunt 20 times that of the transcellular pathway.

In summary, many factors influence the permeability and therefore passive transport of water and substrate across the gastrointestinal epithelium. These factors are illustrated in Figure 37–5.

**Active Transport.** Active transport is distinguished by the interaction of the permeating substance with one of the protein components of the membrane. This interaction has all the characteristics of the interaction between an enzyme and substrate: i.e., the reaction is saturable, shows competition between structurally similar substrates, has specificity to stereoisomers of substrates, and is inhibited by metabolic poisons. Thus, the "carrier" protein that shuttles substrate from one side of the membrane to another may be considered a specialized membrane enzyme. This class of transport is termed "carrier-mediated" transport.

Carrier-mediated transport serves the needs of the gastrointestinal cell by allowing larger, water-soluble substances to cross the membrane. It can allow essential substrates to move against the prevailing diffusional forces of chemical and electrical differences.[27]

If mediated transport uses energy and operates the uphill shuttle across the membrane, it is termed "active" transport. The metabolic energy for this active movement of substances across the membrane is adenosine triphosphate (ATP). The release of energy is provided by an ATPase that hydrolyzes the terminal phosphate from ATP to form adenosine diphosphate (ADP). Thus, each active transport process is driven by the activity of membrane ATPase.[28] The ATPases are not necessarily specific for that substance being transported. For example, the active transport of sugars and amino acids lacks specific ATPases, and their active transfer comes about by specific coupling to the active transport of $Na^+$. Thus, the carrier protein for sugars and amino acids has specific sites for glucose (or amino acids) and also for $Na^+$. The binding of both $Na^+$ and sugars or $Na^+$ and amino acids occurs on the luminal side of the membrane where they then diffuse to the intracellular side for release.[29,30]

The requirements for metabolic energy mentioned previously occur at the opposite side of the cell at the basolateral membrane. Here, $Na^+$ is actively extruded from the cell by the $Na^+/K^+$ pump, which thus conserves the $Na^+$ gradient across the mucosal membrane. The outward movement of sugar and amino acids across the basolateral membrane is energetically downhill and could, in principle, occur by simple diffusion (Fig. 37–6).

Virtually all substances enter or leave the cells of the gastrointestinal tract partly or wholly by simple passive transport. Most classes of substances are transported in the absence of sodium coupling, and several are transported in more than one way. The various types of transport used in transfer across the intestinal membranes are listed in Table 37–4.

The table demonstrates that whole proteins may be transported by pinocytosis. This process may be important in the absorption of small amounts of immunoglobulins from breast milk. This process requires energy and is classified as active.

## SECRETION

Secretions entering the gastrointestinal tract contain electrolytes, bile salts, digestive enzymes, antibodies, and other organic molecules. Table 37–5 lists mean concentrations of major electrolytes in these secretions. Normal adults ingest about 1 to 2 L of fluid and secrete an additional 6 to 10 L of fluid into the gastrointestinal tract daily. Because only about 1 L leaves the small

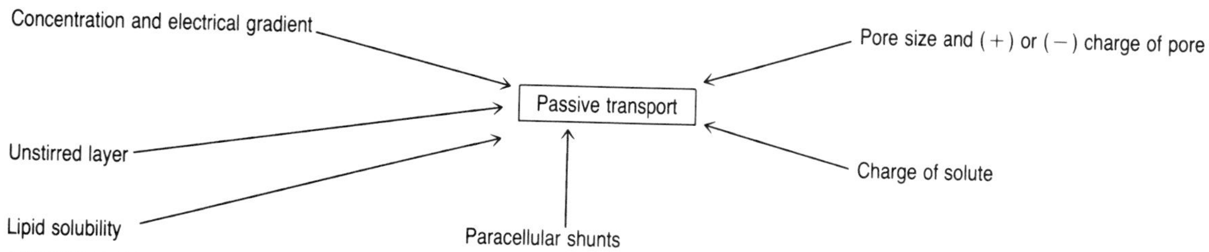
Concentration and electrical gradient
Pore size and (+) or (−) charge of pore
Passive transport
Unstirred layer
Charge of solute
Lipid solubility
Paracellular shunts

**FIGURE 37–5.** Factors that influence the permeability and passive transport of water and substrate across the gastrointestinal epithelium.

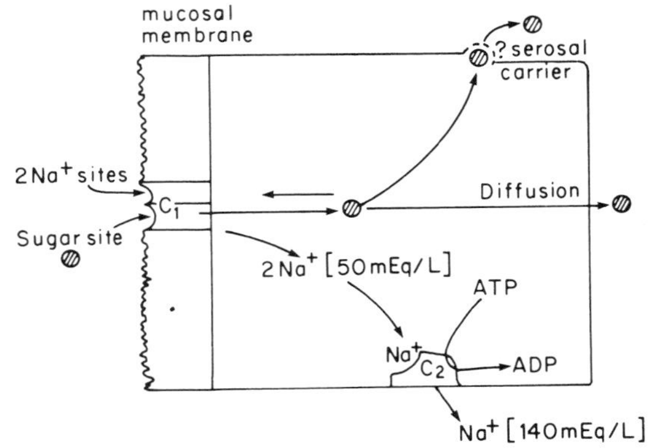
mucosal membrane
? serosal carrier
2Na+ sites
C1
Sugar site
Diffusion
2 Na+ [50 mEq/L]
ATP
Na+
C2
ADP
Na+ [140 mEq/L]

**FIGURE 37–6.** Diagram of the proposed mechanism of sodium-coupled, active transport mechanism. C1, Carrier 1 for coupled transport into the cell; C2, carrier 2 for transport of sodium out of the cell.

intestine for the colon, the small intestine absorbs 200 to 400 ml of water per hour with a maximum rate of about 700 ml per hour. With a normal meal of 645 ml of food, the volume increases to about 1500 ml by mid-duodenum, decreases to 750 ml by midjejunum, and is only 250 ml in the lower small bowel. The colon absorbs additional fluid so that only about 75 ml, or 10% of the original intake, is excreted.

Saliva functions to moisten the mouth, maintaining oral hygiene. It contains thiocyanate and lysozyme, both of which are strongly bactericidal. Saliva is an effective buffer that contains calcium to minimize calcium loss from teeth. It also contains an amylase and hormones such as epidermal growth factor, nerve growth factor, and somatostatin. Secretion of saliva is controlled by conditioned cortical reflexes (made famous by Pavlov) and nonconditioned oral and gastrointestinal reflexes.

Gastric secretions contain acid, pepsins (proteolytic enzymes), mucus, and intrinsic factor. The parietal cell is responsible for secretion of hydrogen ion at concentrations of about 4 million times that of plasma (the highest ion gradient known in physiology). Three substances in the body are capable of acting directly on the parietal cell to increase acid secretion. These substances are acetylcholine (from the vagus nerve), histamine, and gastrin.[31] Histamine is abundant in mast-like cells of the lamina propria of the oxyntic gastric mucosa and, after release, diffuses into adjacent parietal cells. Its role in physiologic control of acid secretion is uncertain, although the introduction of all H2 antagonist, such as cimetidine, suggests it may play an important physiologic role in acid secretion. Cimetidine also inhibits the response to gastrin,[32] as do the cholinomimetics.[33] Table 37–6 summarizes several modulating effects of agents affecting gastric acid secretion. Secretin, CKK, and motilin may also play a modulating role in acid secretion.

**TABLE 37–4.** TYPES OF TRANSPORT USED IN TRANSFER ACROSS INTESTINAL MEMBRANES

| Passive Transport | Active Transport |
|---|---|
| Simple | Active |
| Water | Electrolytes |
| Fats | Sugars |
| Drugs | Amino acids |
| Electrolytes | Dipeptides |
| Sugars | Vitamins |
| Amino acids | Bile acids |
| Vitamins | Coupled Active |
| Sterols | Electrolytes |
| Facilitated | Sugars |
| Sugars | Amino acids |
| Amino acids | Vitamins |
| Electrolytes | Pinocytosis |
| | Proteins |

Pepsinogen is secreted by gastric chief cells. Gastric acid converts the pepsinogen to the active enzyme, pepsin. Pepsin is principally secreted by cells in the acid-secreting part of the stomach. Somatostatin and glucose-dependent insulin-releasing peptide (GIP) reduce pepsin secretion. Mucoproteins produced by the neck cells of the gastric glands provide a lubricant and mucosal buffer. Mucus secretion is increased by food, acid, and ethanol in the stomach and by vagal and sympathetic stimulation.

Intragastric food, especially protein breakdown products, promotes secretion of gastric juice. This effect is mediated in part by the local intrinsic plexus but predominantly through the dorsal motor nucleus of the vagus. Gastrin is the major factor stimulating gastric acid release; its release in response to food is not blocked by atropine or vagotomy. In response to intragastric food, acid secretion occurs at a rate of approximately 200 ml per hour for 2 to 3 hours.

Within the small intestine, the crypts of Lieberkühn produce small intestinal juice that contains electrolytes, bicarbonate, mucus, traces of brush border enzymes, and other contents of shed cells. Secretion of water and electrolytes is mediated by cyclic AMP. Cholera enterotoxin, by stimulating production of cyclic AMP, increases sodium and water excretion through its action on the NaCl pump at the cell-lumen interface. Other hormones that increase intestinal secretions are prostaglandins, calcitonin, and antidiuretic hormone (ADH), as well as the intestinal hormones listed in Table 37–2.

Bile is an isotonic fluid that is concentrated in the gallbladder and is released after stimulation by CCK. It contains bile salts, lecithin, cholesterol, and electrolytes.

Pancreatic secretions contain enzymes, bicarbonate, and electrolytes. The enzymes are responsible for digestion of protein, carbohydrate, lipids, and nucleic acids. They are secreted in an inactive form and activated in the duodenum, mostly by trypsin. Enterokinase from intestinal brush border activates trypsinogen to its

**TABLE 37–5.** ELECTROLYTE CHARACTERISTICS OF ENTERIC SECRETIONS

| ORGAN OR FLUID | VOLUME* (ML/24 HR) | $H^+$ (MEQ/HR) | $NA^+$ (MEQ/L) | $K^+$ (MEQ/L) | $CA^+$ (MEQ/L) | $CL^-$ (MEQ/L) | $HCO3^-$ (MEQ/L) |
|---|---|---|---|---|---|---|---|
| Saliva | 1,200 | — | 10 | 26 | 2 | 10 | 8 |
| Stomach† | 1,500 | 2 (basal)<br>17 (peak) | 150 | 15 | 2 | 130 | — |
| Pancreas‡ | 1,500 | — | 157 | 7.0 | 4 | 50 | 110 |
| Bile§ | 1,000 | — | 146 | 5.0 | 4 | 110 | 46 |
| Duodenum and small bowel‖ | 4,000 | — | 140# | 6.3 | 3 | 100 | 17 |
| Stool | 125 | — | 25 | 60 | 1 | 20 | 3 |

*Unstimulated volume.
†Stimulated by histamine. Data from Hunt, J.N.: Physiol. Rev., 491, 1959 and Trudeau, W.L., McGuigan, J.E.: N. Engl. J. Med., *284*:408, 1971.
‡Data from Swanson, C.H. Soloman, A.K.: J. Gen. Physiol., *62*:407,1973.
§Data from Erlinger, S.: *In* The Liver Biopsy and Pathobiology. New York, Raven Press, 1982, p. 407.
‖Data from Krejs, G.J., Fortran, J.S.: *In* Gastrointestinal Disease. Philadelphia, W. B. Saunders., 1978, p. 297.
#This value for $Na^+$ is higher than that generally given by others (see Chap. 6).

**TABLE 37–6.** FACTORS MODULATING THE PRIMARY AGENTS INCREASING GASTRIC SECRETION

| MODULATOR | ACETYLCHOLINE (VAGAL STIMULUS) | HISTAMINE | GASTRIN |
|---|---|---|---|
| Atropine | Decrease | 0 | 0 |
| Calcium | Increase | 0 | 0 |
| Lanthanum | Decrease | 0 | 0 |
| Cimetidine | Mild decrease[33] | Decrease | Mild decrease[32] |
| $PGE_2$ | 0 | Decrease | 0 |

active enzyme, trypsin. Trypsin inhibitors present in acinar cells and ducts adsorb and inactivate free trypsin.

A cephalic phase of pancreatic secretion (before the ingestion of food) results in direct vagal stimulation of pancreatic enzyme secretion without increased flow. This process fills the duct system with a viscous enzyme-rich fluid. As gastric juice enters the duodenum, acidity stimulates the release of secretin from the intestinal mucosa. This process promotes an increase in volume and bicarbonate output. Intraduodenal protein (or protein components), fat, carbohydrate, and luminal distention all stimulate release of CCK, which stimulates further secretion of enzymes. Pancreatic secretions are suppressed by intravenous administration of amino acid and dextrose. Less stimulation occurs with intraduodenal free amino acids than with peptides or intact protein. Thus, parenteral nutrition or the administration of a formula containing low fat, high carbohydrate, and amino acid may provide less stimulus to pancreatic secretion than food or a defined formula with intact or hydrolyzed protein and fat. This finding may be important in management of patients with pancreatitis. Intragastric feeding provokes acid secretion and, through secretin, increases the volume and bicarbonate output. Small bowel distention also activates the pancreas by vagovagal reflex.

## DIGESTION OF CARBOHYDRATE, PROTEIN, AND LIPID

Secretions from the mouth, stomach, small intestine, liver, and pancreas are mixed with food. Complex molecules are consequently hydrolyzed to simple components that can then be absorbed.

**Carbohydrate.** The chief dietary forms of carbohydrate are polysaccharides (starches and components of dietary fiber), disaccharides (sucrose and lactose), and monosaccharides (glucose and fructose). Digestion and absorption of carbohydrate occur in the mouth, stomach, and small intestine[34–38] as illustrated in Figure 37–7*A*. In addition, carbohydrates not absorbed in the small bowel may provide substantial calories to some animal species,

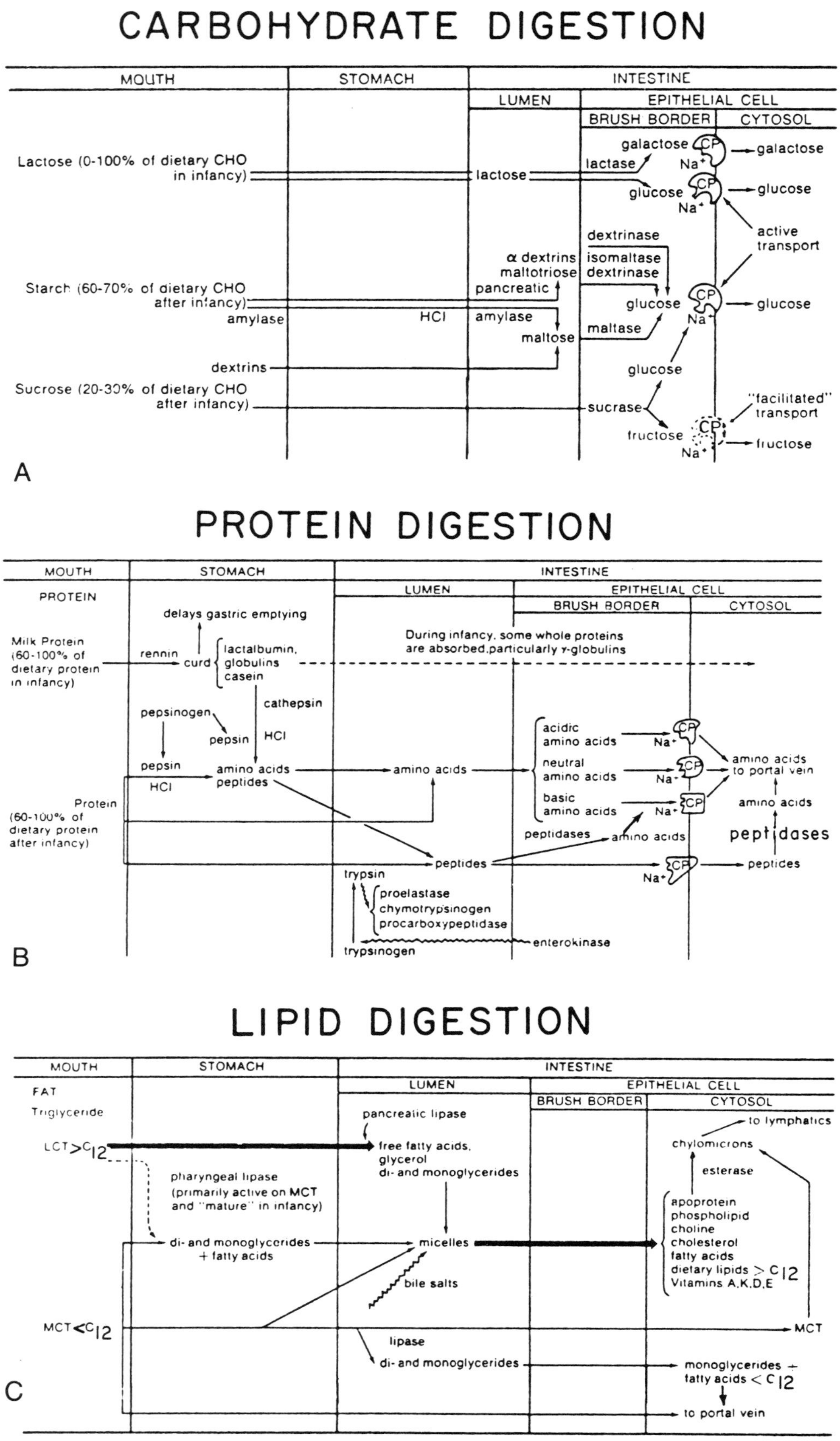
CARBOHYDRATE DIGESTION
MOUTH
STOMACH
INTESTINE
LUMEN
EPITHELIAL CELL
BRUSH BORDER
CYTOSOL
Lactose (0-100% of dietary CHO in infancy)
lactose
lactase
galactose
glucose
CP
Na+
galactose
glucose
active transport
dextrinase
α dextrins
maltotriose
isomaltase
dextrinase
Starch (60-70% of dietary CHO after infancy)
amylase
HCl
pancreatic amylase
maltose
maltase
glucose
dextrins
glucose
Sucrose (20-30% of dietary CHO after infancy)
sucrase
fructose
"facilitated" transport
fructose
A
PROTEIN DIGESTION
MOUTH
STOMACH
INTESTINE
LUMEN
EPITHELIAL CELL
BRUSH BORDER
CYTOSOL
PROTEIN
delays gastric emptying
Milk Protein (60-100% of dietary protein in infancy)
rennin
curd
lactalbumin, globulins casein
During infancy, some whole proteins are absorbed, particularly γ-globulins
cathepsin
pepsinogen
pepsin
HCl
pepsin
HCl
amino acids
peptides
amino acids
acidic amino acids
neutral amino acids
basic amino acids
amino acids to portal vein
amino acids
peptidases
Protein (60-100% of dietary protein after infancy)
peptidases
amino acids
peptides
peptides
trypsin
proelastase
chymotrypsinogen
procarboxypeptidase
trypsinogen
enterokinase
B
LIPID DIGESTION
MOUTH
STOMACH
INTESTINE
LUMEN
EPITHELIAL CELL
BRUSH BORDER
CYTOSOL
FAT
Triglyceride
LCT>C12
pancreatic lipase
free fatty acids, glycerol di- and monoglycerides
to lymphatics
chylomicrons
esterase
pharyngeal lipase (primarily active on MCT and "mature" in infancy)
apoprotein
phospholipid
choline
cholesterol
fatty acids
dietary lipids > C12
Vitamins A,K,D,E
di- and monoglycerides + fatty acids
micelles
bile salts
MCT<C12
MCT
lipase
di- and monoglycerides
monoglycerides + fatty acids < C12
to portal vein
C

**FIGURE 37–7.** Schema of carbohydrate, protein, and lipid digestion. CP, Carrier protein. (Reprinted with permission of Ross Laboratories, Columbus, OH, from Developmental Nutrition.)

bacterial fermentation appears to provide an insignificant energy source for humans.

Simple sugars (glucose, fructose, and galactose) are absorbed by carrier-mediated saturable processes.[36,37] Deficiency of the brush-border enzymes may result in carbohydrate malabsorption. The resulting diarrhea is often accompanied by flatulence related to bacterial fermentation of unabsorbed disaccharides in the cecum, producing gas and osmotically active particles.[39] Dietary fiber, which is composed predominantly of carbohydrate, is resistant to human digestive enzymes but is broken down by bacteria, resulting in increased stool volume and stool water. If fiber is consumed in excess, diarrhea with flatulence results.

**Protein.** Digestion of protein occurs in the stomach and small intestine, and the final products are amino acids and di- and tripeptides (Fig. 37–7*B*). In the stomach, activated pepsins hydrolyze protein to polypeptides of diverse size. Within the small intestine, pancreatic endopeptidases (trypsin, chymotrypsin, and elastase) split peptide bonds within the protein to produce smaller peptides. Exopeptidases (carboxypeptidase A and B) cleave the terminal bonds of large peptides to produce single amino acids and peptide fragments. These enzymes have an optimum pH of 8.0, and hypersecretion of gastric acid (as with the Zollinger-Ellison syndrome) may impair their function. Brush-border and cytosolic peptidases hydrolyze small peptides to produce amino acids.

**Lipid.** The chief forms of dietary lipid are triglycerides, phospholipids, cholesterol, and cholesterol esters (Fig. 37–7*C*). Pharyngeal lipase hydrolyzes some triglyceride intragastrically to fatty acids and diglycerides. Within the small intestine, pancreatic lipase continues this hydrolysis to produce free fatty acids and glycerol. Colipase is a pancreatic polypeptide that acts as cofactor for pancreatic lipase, improving its activity in the presence of bile salts. An intestinal lipase has also been identified, but its precise function is uncertain. Bile salts, which have both hydrophilic and hydrophobic ends, form micelles, which have an external hydrophilic layer and are water-soluble. This process facilitates the absorption of their fat-soluble contents (fatty acids, cholesterol, fat-soluble vitamins). Triglycerides containing fatty acids of less than 12 carbons can be absorbed directly without undergoing hydrolysis, although this may not be quantitatively important because infants with lipase-colipase deficiency respond less well to medium-chain triglyceride formulas than to pancreatic enzyme extracts.

## ABSORPTIVE FUNCTION OF THE GASTROINTESTINAL TRACT

Glucose, ethanol, aspirin, and water can be absorbed from the oral and gastric mucosa. However, absorption of nutrients and most drugs occurs primarily in the small intestine. The colon absorbs principally water and electrolytes. A descending gradient of absorption exists for most nutrients, with most absorption occurring in the first 4 feet of intestine in normal adult humans. Substances actively transported are absorbed mainly in the jejunum.

**Carbohydrate.** As discussed previously, sodium entering from the luminal side of the cell provides the driving force for carbohydrate transfer.[34–38] Glucose is thus cotransported into the cell against a concentration gradient (see Fig. 37–6). Glucose freed from the carrier complex accumulates in the cell and establishes a concentration gradient for facilitated diffusion across the basolateral membrane into the intracellular spaces and ultimately the blood. Other water-soluble organic substrates that are transported by similar $Na^+$-dependent gradient coupling include amino acids, di- and tripeptides, ascorbic acid, sulfate and phosphate, bile salts, bilirubin, and riboflavin.[40–43] This transport mechanism appears to be ubiquitous throughout the animal and plant kingdoms. Amino acids and glucose reciprocally inhibit absorption of one another by competing for a limited supply of energy from this electrochemical gradient. An increase in the luminal concentration of $Na^+$ results in improved absorption of glucose and amino acids and vice versa. Knowledge of this phenomenon has led to the use of sodium-glucose solutions to aid in the management of patients with cholera or acute diarrheal syndromes.

**Peptides and Amino Acids.** As described with absorption of glucose, amino acid absorption is a sodium-dependent, carrier-mediated, and saturable process. Di- and, to some extent, tripeptides may be absorbed intact. Cytoplasmic peptidases hydrolyze the di- and tripeptides and limit the amount of dietary protein reaching the liver as anything but amino acids. Single amino acids are transported across the basolateral membrane by both simple passive diffusion and carrier-mediated diffusion (see Fig. 37–6).

**Fat.** Fat absorption is generally a passive process,[43–46] although fatty acids or triglycerides with less than 12 carbon atoms (short- and medium-chain triglycerides) can pass directly into the portal blood. Long-chain fat (more than 12 carbon atoms) requires digestion to fatty acids and monoglycerides for micellar solubilization and efficient absorption. Bile and pancreatic enzymes greatly facilitate fat absorption, but brush-border lipase and simple diffusion in a healthy intestine allow absorption of a considerable proportion of ingested fat. This absorptive fraction is relatively unaffected by the total amount ingested; under usual circumstances, the more fat ingested, the more will be absorbed. Unsaturated fats are more readily absorbed than saturated fats. Within the enterocyte, fatty acids and other lipid particles from within the micelle are packaged and released into lymphatics as chylomicrons.[47,48]

**Water and Ions.** The $Na^+$-$K^+$ ATPase-dependent pump located on the basolateral membrane extrudes $Na^+$ and thus maintains intracellular electronegativity.[49] Sodium is absorbed passively by diffusion from luminal chyme into enterocytes along an electrochemical gradient, and chloride follows passively. A small amount of $Cl^-$ is actively reabsorbed in exchange for excreted $HCO3^-$.[50] This process occurs mainly in the lower ileum and large intestine. Intracellular sodium is actively transported into the extracellular space. Water moves passively according to the prevailing osmotic gradient and follows sodium into the extracellular space. Chyme remains isotonic during its passage through the small and large intestine. Sudden delivery of large volumes of hypertonic fluids into the small intestine results in a rapid water flux *into* the lumen, which may produce circulating hypovolemia and the dumping syndrome. As the water and sodium move into the extracellular space, the hydrostatic pressure increases and flow occurs into the lymphatics and capillaries of the villi.[51]

Calcium is absorbed most actively in the duodenum. The low relative efficiency of this process (30%) is increased by 1,25-dihydroxycholecalciferol (calcitriol). Passive absorption also occurs in the jejunum and ileum. Absorption is impaired by multiple luminal factors and by high levels of circulating cortisol, thyroxine, and estrogen. Absorption is facilitated by parathormone, hypocalcemia, and increased duodenal acidity. See Chapters 7 and 17 for details of calcium metabolism.

**Water-Soluble Vitamins.** Water-soluble vitamins are predominantly absorbed passively and are carrier-mediated at physiologic intakes. Results of some studies suggest that ascorbate,[52,53] riboflavin,[54] and thiamine[55] are absorbed by sodium-dependent mechanisms. Folate polyglutamate is hydrolyzed by zinc-dependent intestinal brush-border conjugase from dietary polyglutamates to monoglutamate and is then absorbed predominantly in the duodenum by a pH-dependent, carrier-mediated transport system. Absorption is reduced during intestinal damage, folate deficiency, or vitamin $B_{12}$ deficiency by ethanol, sulfasalazine, and phenytoin.[56]

Vitamin $B_{12}$ is absorbed with approximately 10% efficiency. It initially binds to R protein (present in saliva and gastric juice) from which it is separated by pancreatic enzymes in the duodenum.[57] Free $B_{12}$ then binds to intrinsic factor (IF) released from gastric mucosa,[57] which facilitates active $B_{12}$ absorption at specific sites on the brush border of cells in the distal ileum. Approximately 99% of $B_{12}$-IF absorption occurs in the distal ileum, and passive absorption in the jejunum and proximal ileum accounts for only 1% of absorption. Impaired absorption and clinical deficiency may occur after gastric resection or atrophy (resulting in loss of IF), small intestinal bacterial or parasitic overgrowth (resulting in consumption of the ingested $B_{12}$), pancreatic exocrine failure, or terminal ileal disease (regional enteritis, ileal resection, or congenital absence of ileal $B_{12}$ and IF receptors). Large oral doses of vitamin $B_{12}$ may allow adequate absorption in the absence of IF or in the presence of terminal ileal disease, although parenteral therapy usually is preferred. Selective familial vitamin $B_{12}$ malabsorption has been described, but the specific defect has not been clearly defined.[58]

**Fat-Soluble Vitamins.** The absorption of fat-soluble vitamins parallels the absorption of fat, although only about 50% of the ingested dose is generally retained.[59] These lipid-soluble molecules are absorbed in micelles and leave the intestine in chylomicrons. Vitamin E absorption is facilitated by a bile salt-dependent luminal esterase of pancreatic origin.[60,61] Absorption of fat-soluble vitamins is impaired in any disease-producing fat malabsorption such as pancreatic insufficiency, cholestasis, or nonspecific malabsorption, as seen with bacterial overgrowth or gluten-sensitive enteropathy.

**Trace Elements.** Absorption of iron occurs predominantly in the duodenum. Absorption is passive and relatively inefficient with only 5 to 15% of ingested iron absorbed. Absorption is subject to modification by luminal agents and to mucosal influences, including reduced iron stores, active erythropoiesis, and idiopathic hemochromatosis. Iron is best absorbed as heme (organic) iron, although the inorganic ferrous ion is also well absorbed.

Zinc is absorbed by facilitated diffusion throughout the small intestine with an efficiency of 20 to 40%. Absorption improves in zinc deficiency. Organic zinc is better absorbed than inorganic zinc, and the latter is more sensitive to interference by luminal factors such as phytates, dietary fiber, phosphate, other cations, and products of the Maillard reactions.[62] The absorption of zinc is facilitated by zinc-binding ligands found in human milk and in pancreatic secretions.[63] Although 1 to 2 mg of zinc may be secreted via the pancreas each day, it is reabsorbed by the small bowel. Patients with malabsorptive diseases are prone to zinc deficiency. If the malabsorption results from exocrine pancreatic failure, however, clinical signs of zinc deficiency are uncommon. This phenomenon is possibly related to simultaneous decrease in zinc output by the pancreas. During zinc absorption, the intestinal cell retains a large amount of the absorbed zinc, which is bound to an intracellular protein, metallothioneine. This bound zinc is eventually sloughed with the cell and lost in the feces. Metallothionein may, therefore, contribute to the regulation of absorption or retention of zinc, as well as other cations such as copper.[64]

Little is known about absorption of other trace elements such as iodine, chromium, manganese, selenium, and molybdenum. Each appears to be passively absorbed with varying degrees of efficiency. Except in geographic areas where the soil is severely deficient in iodine or selenium, deficiency of these minerals is extremely uncommon and is generally associated with

**TABLE 37–7.** GASTRIC FLUID ANALYSIS

| AGE | HCl PRODUCTION* (mEq/L:mEq/hr/kg of wt—mean) | VOLUME GASTRIC JUICE* (ml/hr—mean) | PEPSIN* (ng/hr/kg of wt—mean) | IF† (mean) | SERUM GASTRIN‡ (pg/ml—mean ± SEM) |
|---|---|---|---|---|---|
| Birth | 8.1:0.01 | 3.3 | 0.40 | 8 | 64 ± 125 |
| 3–8 days | 14.4:0.02 | 3.7 | 0.06 | 17.8 | 151 ± 15.8 |
| 10–17 days | 34.4:0.12 | 4.0 | 0.15 | 29.2 | — |
| 25–32 days | 26.4:0.02 | 6.4 | 0.24 | 27.9 | 193 ± 28 |
| 60–90 days | 34.8:0.01 | 13.4 | 0.28 | 34.4 | — |
| 4–9 years | 114.2:–0.1 | 42.5 | — | 79.5 | 215 ± 37 |
| Adult | 91.2:0.19 | 143.2 | 0.60 | 78.7 | <90 |

*Tritratable acid obtained during 1 hour of intermittent suction after 1.0 mg/kg body weight of histalog. Data from Agunod, M., et al.: Am. J. Dig. Dis., *14*:400, 1969.
†IF, intrinsic factor.
‡Data from Rogers, I.M., et al.: Arch Dis. Child., *49*:796, 1974 and Rogers, I.M., et al.: Arch Dis. Child., *50*:467, 1975.

severe bowel disease and/or the use of prolonged total parenteral nutrition.

**The Colon.** The colon has a large absorptive capacity, particularly for water. It absorbs about 850 ml of the average 1000 ml that daily crosses the ileocecal valve. Indiscriminate use of enemas over a few hours may lead to water intoxication. Colonic absorption of glucose, amino acids, and vitamins is minor, but short-chain fatty acids (the products of colonic bacterial metabolism of unabsorbed carbohydrate) are readily absorbed. The rectal mucosa also provides a route for administration of certain drugs including antiemetics, sedatives, antipyretics, and steroids.

## FACTORS AFFECTING GASTROINTESTINAL FUNCTION

### MATURATION

The newborn gastrointestinal tract undergoes many maturational changes during the first months of life. Several of these changes are illustrated in Tables 37–7 and 37–8. During the first 3 to 4 months, sucking reflexes are present, while extrusion reflexes protect against introduction of potentially indigestible solids. Esophageal motility is present at birth, but coordination of propulsive waves does not develop until after four months of postnatal life. The LES pressure remains low, and the intragastric pressure often exceeds the esophageal and LES pressure. This results in a high incidence of "spitting" of gastric contents for the first 3 to 6 months of life. Gastric motility is poorly coordinated for 3 to 4 months, which leads to poor antral mixing and therefore less digestion of solid foods than after 4 months of age. Usually at 12 weeks, intestinal peristalsis of a type seen in older children and adults develops, but it is approximately one third slower. The slower transit may serve to increase exposure time to the intestinal mucosa and thereby improve nutrient digestion and absorption. The motor function in the large intestine appears to be fully mature at birth.

Intestinal mucosal permeability is greatest during the neonatal period, and many large molecules, including proteins such as immunoglobulins, tend to be absorbed intact. This process provides a mechanism for passive transfer of antibodies from mother's milk but also permits the passage of whole proteins with a potential to provoke allergic responses. The relationship between ingestion of whole cow's milk and anemia from chronic intestinal blood loss during the first few months of life appears to result from this mechanism. Other nonhuman protein foods may also cause similar changes in the first 6 months of life.

Secretory and absorptive functions of the intestine mature during the first 2 years of life (see Tables 37–7 and 37–8). In general, animal fat is less well digested and absorbed than vegetable oils by infants. The intestinal mucosal α-glucosidases (sucrase, maltase, isomaltase) are well developed by 32 weeks of gestation and are present at near adult levels at the time of the term delivery. By contrast, the β-galactosidase lactase develops late in fetal life and does not reach maximal activity until feeding begins. In spite of the relatively low lactase activity, formulas containing lactose are well tolerated by term infants and many infants over 34 weeks gestation. For extremely premature infants (27 to 32 weeks gestation), formulas with less than 60% of total carbohydrate calories as lactose are generally best tolerated.

### SENESCENCE

Age-related changes in intestinal function occur simultaneously with loss of lean body mass.[65] Impaired glucose homeostasis, decreased clearance of drugs, variability in temperature control, and deterioration in

**TABLE 37–8.** DUODENAL FLUID ANALYSIS IN 36 PREMATURE INFANTS AND IN CHILDREN

| AGE | VOLUME* (ml) | αAMYLASE*‡ (U) | TRYPSIN*‡ (mg) | Lipase* (IU) |
|---|---|---|---|---|
| Premature (wt 2.0–2.4 kg) | | | | |
| birth, before feeding | 44(4.3–152) | 0.88(0–3.6) | 60(0–482) | 77(3–343) |
| 24 hr after first feeding | 55(16–98) | 0.62(0.2–1.4) | 43(1.6–148) | 66(2–209) |
| 1 wk | 82(17–168) | 2.07(0.2–8.2) | 233(5–660) | 329(7–1,249) |
| 4 wk | 90(34–187) | 1.67(0–4.6) | 196(0.9–660) | 284(11–730) |
| Children (9 mos–13 yrs)† | 390(180–810) | 665(160–2,150) | 765(215–2,000) | 1,465(350–5,000) |

*Data from Zoppi, G., et al.: Pediatr. Res., *6*:880, 1972. Values expressed on basis of body weights (kg) and represent mean and (range), during 50 min after injections of pancreozymin (2 units/kg) and secretin (2 units/kg).
†Data from Zoppi, G., et al.: Acta Paediatr. Scand., *59*:692, 1970.
‡Term infants had slightly lower enzyme activities 1 week after birth.

immunologic function also occur with the alteration in gastrointestinal function.[66] Other changes include loss of dentition, reduced taste and smell acuity, esophageal dysmotility and delayed gastric emptying, hypochlorhydria, a tendency to ischemia, and intestinal amyloidosis. These factors and the frequent use of medication in elderly individuals may all contribute to impaired gastrointestinal tract function and an increased tendency toward malnutrition. Many of the physiologic changes observed with aging (immune senescence, reduction in visceral protein levels, and decreased lean body mass) are similar to those observed in malnutrition in younger subjects,[20] although normal aging alone does not appear to impair protein-energy absorption substantially. Gastric emptying and intestinal transit are slowed, and the efficiency of absorption, particularly of vitamin A, may be improved as a result. On the other hand, absorption of vitamin $B_{12}$,[67] calcium,[68] and zinc seems to be impaired in the elderly population.

## ADAPTATION

The gastrointestinal tract is capable of extensive adaptation, particularly in children. Where intestinal function is marginal (as may occur after extensive resection), the residual intestine is capable of considerable dilation, increase in rugosity, and hypertrophy of villi and microvilli. Increased surface area and absorptive capacity result. Cell turnover and enzyme activities increase. These adaptive changes can be maximized by mucosal exposure to nutrients, pancreatic and biliary secretions, and by certain hormonal factors that remain unidentified. The search for trophic hormones has important therapeutic implications, but no candidates have shown conclusive growth-stimulating activity in the small intestine. Gastrin's trophic action affects primarily the esophagus, stomach, colon, and pancreas and may play some role in adaptation of the small intestine. Cholecystokinin (CCK) and secretion are mildly trophic to the small intestine, but this reaction may result from their stimulation of bile and pancreatic secretions.[69] Factors that limit intestinal adaptation include inadequate blood supply, poor nutritional status, and the presence of residual disease. The ileum is better able to adapt than the jejunum, which cannot assume certain specialized functions of the ileum such as active absorption of vitamin $B_{12}$ and bile salts. Slower transit in the ileum may improve absorptive capacity, but conversely provides a better milieu for bacterial overgrowth.

## NUTRITION

Food appears to play a pivotal role in maintenance of intestinal function. As indicated in Figure 37–3, gastrointestinal function is affected by multiple agents which respond to diet. Several models to evaluate food and some of its components have been evaluated.

**Starvation and Malnutrition.** With infantile malnutrition and protracted diarrhea, steatorrhea and poor tolerance to carbohydrate is characteristic.[70] Bowel changes after a moderate reduction in dietary intake not associated with malnutrition has not been fully evaluated. It is recognized, however, that dietary restriction for the purpose of weight loss is associated with transient, mild to moderate gastrointestinal symptoms with refeeding. These symptoms probably result from the aggregate reduction in gastric, biliary, pancreatic, and intestinal secretions and mucosal enzyme content. However, the symptoms are transient and minimal, if any, malabsorption is present. Severe protein deficiency predisposes to immune dysfunction, leading to diarrhea from ingestion or overgrowth of bacteria in the small intestine. The latter may result in a further decline in intestinal function because of impaired motility and depressed mucosal enzyme activity. Vitamin $B_{12}$

deficiency may further complicate function. Bacterial translocation to lymph nodes may also represent a significant risk.

**Lack of Enteral Intake.** Exclusion of dietary foods, despite the maintenance of adequate nutrition by parenteral feeding, is associated with atrophic changes in the muscular as well as mucosal layers of the bowel.[71] Similar changes have also been described in segments of bowel that have been bypassed.[72] Thus, exposure to food, as well as the presence of upper gastrointestinal secretions, are necessary to maintain optimal gastrointestinal morphology and function.

**Glutamine as an Intestinal Fuel.** The nonessential amino acid glutamine has been the focus of extensive interest in maintenance of mucosal epithelium. It appears to be the preferred fuel for rapidly proliferating cells such as enterocytes and lymphocytes.[73] Some experimental evidence suggests that during critical illness, endogenous synthesis of glutamine may not meet the needs of the organism and supplements may enhance medical management. Additionally, the administration of glutamine-containing parenteral feedings has resulted in attenuation of the usual degree of bowel atrophy associated with parenteral feedings.[74,75] Although glutamine is relatively unstable as a free amino acid, future studies may find it to be advantageous given in the form of a peptide additive in parenteral nutrition. A symposium on the nutritional aspects of glutamine has been published.[76]

**Fiber in Maintenance of Bowel Function.** Some types of dietary fiber are known to affect bowel motility in the human.[77] For example, gastric emptying rate is retarded by pectins, whereas colonic transit is shortened by wheat bran. The addition of dietary fiber to enteral diets has also been shown to improve intestinal mucosal growth and anastomotic healing after colonic resection as well as absorptive adaptation after massive bowel resection.[78,79] Results of recent studies suggest that the loss of bowel mass associated with the use of a defined formula diet can be prevented by the addition of either glutamine or fiber to the regimen. However, neither agent appears to reduce cecal bacterial overgrowth or bacterial translocation to mesenteric lymphatics.[80]

The multiplicity of fiber types coupled with the various conditions associated with bowel growth, atrophy, and hypertrophy (see Fig. 37–3) make it difficult to identify any single dietary variable as most important in the maintenance of bowel function in disease. It does seem clear that food in its usual complex composition is the most important ingredient in maintenance of bowel mass and efforts to feed real foods to patients should not be abandoned in favor of technologic formulations until the newer formulations have been fully evaluated.

## ABSORPTION OF WATER AND IONS

The intestinal epithelium controls the exchange of water, electrolytes, and other water-soluble solutes between the bowel lumen and the circulation. The small bowel mucosa is freely permeable to water, which follows the movement of electrolytes, and water-soluble solutes are dragged in turn by the movement of water. This free movement of fluid and solute allows the osmotic pressure of the jejunal contents to equilibrate with that of the plasma; it further illustrates that the active uptake of electrolytes from the intestine into the plasma plays a pivotal role in the maintenance of fluid balance as well as nutrient (solute) absorption. These transport processes were summarized previously.

In contrast with the small intestine, the colon is less permeable and is more active in conservation of water and ions. The Na and Cl ions are actively absorbed and K ion is secreted into the lumen. Because colonic epithelium has a lower passive permeability to ions and water than does the small intestine, the differences in concentration created by the active transport processes are not easily dissipated by simple diffusion back across the mucosa. Thus, stool concentrations of electrolytes are normally different from plasma concentrations. Despite the relatively high concentrations of electrolytes in feces, the amounts lost each day are trivial because of the small volume of stool. These trivial losses, coupled with the ability of the kidney to conserve electrolytes, help to explain the capacity of humans to survive on an extremely low intake of salt. Predictably, a patient who has a colectomy is less able to conserve enteric losses of electrolytes.

Regulation of ion transport influences the movement of water between the environment and the body. The balance between secretion and absorption is a dynamic process represented by the enterosystemic water cycle.[80,81] During fasting, water that enters the lumen is reabsorbed after Na absorption. Therefore, little water is lost in stools. During a meal, as much as 7 L of water may enter the intestinal lumen as a consequence of digestive secretions. Water is reabsorbed during electrolyte and solute absorption, mainly through the solute-Na cotransport system.

### ORAL REHYDRATION SALT SOLUTIONS (ORS)

It is generally accepted that the intestine maintains an active process of absorption as well as an active process of secretion, and that these systems are present in two separate epithelial cell types; absorption is predominant in villus cells and secretion in the crypt cells (see Fig. 37–2). This spacial distribution in cell types is further complicated in the functioning intestine because crypt cells differentiate into villus cells. The balance of absorption and secretion therefore depends not only on the relative mass of villus to crypt cells, but also on the rate of cell turnover and differentiation. Thus, it would follow that disease entities affecting predominantly crypt cells will primarily affect the secretory rate and diseases predominantly affecting the more mature villus cells will alter primarily the absorptive capacity. In either case, the remaining villus cells could be used to promote maximum absorption of water and solute presented to it. Knowledge of the normal mechanisms of fluid, electrolyte and solute absorption and secretions, coupled with the general principles of how various diseases affect these processes has led to the development of oral solutions designed to take maximum advantage of any remaining absorptive epithelial function.

In a practical sense, the benefits of oral rehydration salt solutions (ORS) for treatment of infants, children, and adult patients with dehydration has been extensively documented. The physiologic basis of ORS is the coupled transport of sodium and glucose or other actively transported small organic molecules, as discussed in the previous section. To avoid hypertonicity, which would by itself induce additional fluid loss, these solutions are composed of approximately equimolar concentrations of glucose and sodium. Oral replacement solutions supplemented with glucose or amino acids in general do not diminish diarrhea and new formulations, particularly rice-based ORS are being investigated, which might have this advantage over the formulation used currently.

## GUIDELINES FOR THE USE OF ORS

The general principles for optimum use of ORS are: (1) correct existing water and electrolyte deficits, (2) replace ongoing abnormal diarrheal losses, (3) provide daily fluid requirements, and (4) allow early feeding during fluid therapy. Rehydration therapy is usually achieved except in cases of severe dehydration, uncontrollable vomiting, or a serious complication (such as sepsis or thrombosis). Solutions are usually given orally, but in unusual situations, a continuous nasogastric infusion may be necessary.

The World Health Organization (WHO) has made recommendations for the general use of ORS. Although its use is still evolving and future recommendations may differ with the accumulation of more experience, the following is a description of the current recommendations. ORS is used in two phases: initial replacement of deficit, and subsequent replacement of ongoing losses. The safety and efficacy of the single WHO formula for both phases of treatment has been documented, although a solution containing less sodium (50 to 70 mmol/L; 70 mEq/L) may be used in patients minimally dehydrated. Calculation of the initial fluid dosage is based on the estimated degree of dehydration (i.e., a 9-kg infant with estimated 10% dehydration requires 1000 ml of ORS). This dose is administered over 4 to 6 hours. Ongoing stool losses are measured and added to the amount given. At the end of the 4 to 6 hours of rehydration, the patient is re-examined and the child is placed in either a maintenance phase of treatment or an additional period of rehydration. In the maintenance phase, a general rule of thumb is that for the first 10 kg of body weight, a child requires 4 ml/kg per hour, 2 ml/kg per hour for the second 10 kg, and 1 ml/kg per hour for each 10 kg over 20 (i.e., a 30-kg child requires 40 + 20 + 10 = 70 ml/kg per hour for maintenance). Institution of appropriate oral feedings early in the course of the treatment is recommended. Infants being breast-fed should resume breast-feeding during the maintenance phase and those being formula-fed should resume feeding with formula as tolerated. Table 37–9 lists fluids used in rehydration.

**TABLE 37–9** SOLUTIONS COMMONLY USED FOR FLUID AND ELECTROLYTE REPLACEMENT

| FLUID | CHO (g/L) | NA$^+$ | K$^+$ | CL$^-$ (mEq/L)† | BASE* |
|---|---|---|---|---|---|
| Rehydration | | | | | |
| WHO ORS | 20 | 90 | 20 | 80 | 30 |
| Rehydralyte‡ | 25 | 75 | 20 | 65 | 30 |
| Maintenance | | | | | |
| Pedialyte‡ | 25 | 45 | 20 | 35 | 30 |
| Ricelyte§ | 30§ | 50 | 25 | 45 | 34 |
| Apple juice | 119 | 0.43 | 25 | — | — |
| Gatorade | 40 | 23.5 | 2.5 | 17 | — |

Various fluids in common use for rehydration and maintenance in infants and children with dehydrating diarrhea. Oral solutions listed under *Rehydration* may also be used for replacement of losses during maintenance, provided that adequate additional fluid as breast-milk formula is also taken. Juice and Gatorade are shown for comparison; neither is recommended for use because of high osmolarity. ORS, Oral rehydration salt solutions.

*mEq potential bicarbonate, e.g., may be, citrate, acetate.

†For Na$^+$, K$^+$, and Cl$^-$, SI units, expressed as mmol/L, are equivalent to mEq values, whereas for base, SI units, expressed as mmol/L, are equivalent to one third of mEq values (e.g., 30 mEq = mmol/L).

‡Ross Laboratories.

§Mead Johnson Nutritionals: carbohydrate source: rice syrup solids.

Future studies for advanced ORS formulations are aimed at providing solutions that would reduce the volume and/or duration of stool output. For example, increasing the concentration of glucose might increase the rate of salt and water cotransport; however, the increased osmotic load promotes a higher stool water output. The idea of achieving a higher glucose content without increasing the osmotic load may be circumvented by using glucose polymers. A growing body of information indicates that cereal-based polymers (particularly rice-based) promote a reduction in both volume and duration of diarrhea as well as an earlier return to appetite.[82,83]

Another theoretic approach is to use other systems that cotransport with sodium, such as amino acids, peptides, or small proteins from grain sources. Such studies are in the early stages of evaluation.

## REFERENCES


1. Robert, A., Nezamis, J.E., Lancaster, C., et al.: Gastroenterology, *77:*433–443, 1979.
2. Donaldson, R.M.: The relation of enteric bacterial populations to gastrointestinal junction and disease. *In* Gastrointestinal Disease. 3rd Ed. Edited by M.H. Sleisenger and J.S. Fordtran. Philadelphia, W.B. Saunders Co., 1983, p. 79.
3. Bukhave, K., Rask-Madsen, J.: Gastroenterology, *78:*32–42, 1980.
4. Tarnawski, A., Stachura, J., Ivey, K.T., et al.: Prostaglandins (Suppl.), *21:*147–159, 1980.
5. Trier, J.S.: Gastroenterology, *42:*295–305, 1962.
6. Smith, G.P.: Lancet, *2:*88–89, 1983.
7. Wood, J.D.: Physiology of the enteric nervous system. *In* Physiology of the Gastrointestinal Tract. Edited by L.R. Johnson. New York, Raven Press, 1981.
8. Morley, J.E., Levine, A.S.: Lancet, *1:*398–401, 1983.
9. Kagnoff, M.F.: Immunology and allergic responses of the bowel. *In* The Role of the Gastrointestinal Tract in Nutrient Delivery. (Edited by M. Green and H.L. Greene.) New York, Academic Press, 1984.
10. Pearse, A.G.E., Polak, J.M., Bloom, S.R.: Gastroenterology, *72:*746–761, 1977.
11. Johnson, L.R.: Regulation of intestinal growth. *In* Physiology of the Gastrointestinal Tract. Edited by L.R. Johnson. New York, Raven Press, 1981.
12. Doe, W.F., Hapel, A.J.: Clin. Gastroenterol., *12:*415–436, 1983.
13. Gershon, M.D., Erde, S.M.: Gastroenterology, *80:*1571–1594, 1981.
14. Furness, J.B., Costa, M.: Neurosciences, *5:*1–20, 1980.
15. Wood, J.D.: Physiology of the enteric nervous system. *In* Physiology of the Gastrointestinal Tract. Edited by L.R. Johnson. New York, Raven Press, 1987.
16. Gershon, M.D., Robinson, R.G., Ross, L.L.: J. Pharmacol. Exp. Ther., *198:*548–561, 1976.
17. Burnstock, G., Campbell, G., Satchell, D., et al.: Br. J. Pharmacol., *40:*668–688, 1970.
18. Said, S.I., Mutt, V.: Science, *169:*1217–1218, 1970.
19. von Euler U.S., Gaddum, J.H.: J. Physiol., *72:*74–87, 1931.
20. Costa, M., Patel, Y., Furness, J.B., et al.: Neurosci. Lett., *6:*215–222, 1977.
21. Hughes, J., Kosterlitz, H.W., Smith, T.W.: Br. J. Pharmacol., *61:*639–647, 1977.
22. Bloom, S.R., Ghatei, M., Warton, J.W., et al.: Gastroenterology, *76:*1103–1107, 1979.
23. Polak, J.M., Sullivan, S.N., Bloom, S.R., et al.: Nature, *270:*183–186, 1977.
24. Tatemoto, K.: Chemical assay for natural peptides: Application to the isolation of candidate hormones. *In* Gastrointestinal Hormones. Edited by G.B.J. Glass. New York, Raven Press, 1980.
25. Aynsley-Green, A.: Endocrine function of the gut in early life. *In* Pediatric Gastrointestinal Disease. Edited by W.A. Walker, P.R. Durie, J.R. Hamilton, et al. Philadelphia, B.C. Decker, 1991.
26. Schultz, S.G., Zalusky, R.: J. Gen. Physiol., *47:*1567–1584, 1964.
27. Schultz, S.G., Zalusky, R.: J. Gen. Physiol., *47:*1043–1059, 1964.
28. Wilson, F.A., Dietchy, J.M.: Biochim. Biophys. Acta, *363:*112–117, 1974.
29. Kimmich, G.A., Cater-Su, C.: Am. J. Physiol., *235:*C78, 1978.
30. Kimmich, G.A., Randles, J.: Biochim. Biophys. Acta, *596:*439–444, 1980.
31. Gardner, J.D., Jackson, M.J., Batzvi, S., et al.: Gastroenterology, *74:*348–354, 1978.
32. Grossman, M.I., Konturek, S.G.: Gastroenterology, *66:*517–521, 1974.
33. Grossman, M.I.: Vagal stimulation and inhibition of acid secretion and gastrin released: Which aspects are cholinergic? *In* Gastrins and the Vagus. Edited by J.F. Rehfeld, and Andrup. New York, Academic Press, 1979.
34. Cezard, J-P., Conklin, K.A., Das, B.C., et al.: J. Biol. Chem., *254:*8969–8975, 1979.
35. Conklin, K.A., Yamashiro, K.M., Gray, G.M.: J. Biol. Chem., *250:*5735–5741, 1975.
36. Crane, R.K.: Fed. Proc., *24:*1000–1006, 1965.
37. Crane, R.K., Malathi, P., Preiser, H.: Biochem. Biophys. Res. Commun., *71:*1010, 1976.
38. Fogel, M.R., Gray, G.M.: J. Appl. Physiol., *35:*262–267, 1973.
39. Gray, G.M.: Intestinal disaccharidase deficiencies and glucose-galactose malabsorption. *In* Metabolic Basis of Inherited Disease. 4th Ed. Edited by J.B. Stanbury, J.B. Wyngaarden, and D.S. Fredrickson. New York, McGraw-Hill Book, 1982.
40. Adibi, S.A.: J. Clin. Invest., *50:*2266–2275, 1971.
41. Rivier, D.: Experientia, *29:*1443–1446, 1973.
42. Reichen, J., Baumgartner, G.: Am. J. Physiol., *231:*734–742, 1976.
43. Wilson, F.A., Dietschy, J.M.: J. Clin. Invest., *51:*3015–3025, 1972.
44. Wilson, F.A., Treanor, L.L.: J. Membr. Biol., *33:*213–230, 1977.
45. Sallee, V.L., Dietschy, J.M.: J. Lipid Res., *14:*475–484, 1973.

46. Chow, S.L., Hollander, D.: Lipids, *13*:239–245, 1978.
47. Vodovar, H., Flanzy, J., Francois, A.C.: Ann. Biol. Anim., *9*:219–232, 1968.
48. Norum, K.R., Lilljeqvist, A.C., Helgerud, P., et al.: J. Clin. Invest., *9*:55–62, 1979.
49. Stirling, C.E.: J. Cell Biol., *53*:704–714, 1972.
50. Liedke, C.M., Hopfer, U.: Biochem. Biophys. Res. Commun., *76*:579–585, 1977.
51. Diamond, J.M., Bossert, W.H.: J. Gen. Physiol., *50*:2061–2083, 1967.
52. Rose, R., Nahrwold, D.: Int. J. Vitam. Nutr. Res., *48*:382–386, 1978.
53. Siliprandi, L., Vanni, P., Kessler, M., et al.: Biochim. Biophys. Acta, *552*:129–142, 1979.
54. Rivier, D.: Experientia, *29*:1443–1446, 1973.
55. Rindi, G., Ferrari, G.: Experientia, *33*:211–213, 1977.
56. Rosenberg, I.H.: Intestinal absorption of folate. *In* Physiology of the Gastrointestinal Tract. Edited by L.R. Johnson. New York, Raven Press, 1981, pp. 1221–1230.
57. Allen, R.H., Seetharam, B., Podell, E., et al.: J. Clin. Invest., *61*:47–54, 1978.
58. Mackenzie, I.L., Donaldson, R.M., Trier, J.S., et al.: N. Engl. J. Med., *286*:1021–1025, 1972.
59. Thompson, G.R.: J. Clin. Pathol., *24*: Suppl. R. Coll. Pathol., *5*:85–89, 1971.
60. Gallo-Torres, H.E.: Lipids, *5*:379–384, 1970.
61. Thompson, G.R., Scott, M.L.: J. Nutr., *100*:797–809, 1970.
62. Reinhold, J.G., Faradji, B., Abadi, P., et al.: Effects of cellulose comsumption on zinc, calcium and phosphorus in man. *In* Trace Elements in Human Health and Disease. Edited by A.S. Prasad. New York, Academic Press, 1976.
63. Duncan, J.R., Hurley, L.S.: Am. J. Physiol., *235*:556–559, 1978.
64. Hunt, D.M.: Nature, *249*:852–854, 1974.
65. Bowman, B.B., Rosenberg, I.H.: Am. J. Clin. Nutr., *37C*:75–78, 1983.
66. Shock, N.: Sci. Am., *206*:110–116, 1962.
67. King, C.E., Liebach, J., Toskes, P.P.: Dig. Dis. Sci., *24*:397–402, 1979.
68. Gallagher, J.C., Riggs, B.L., Eisman, J., et al.: J. Clin. Invest., *64*:729–732, 1979.
69. Johnson, L.R.: Regulation of gastrointestinal growth. *In* Physiology of the Gastrointestinal Tract. Edited by L.R. Johnson. New York, Raven Press, 1981.
70. Greene, H.L., McCabe, D.R., Merenstein, G.B.: J. Pediatr., *87*:695–704, 1975.
71. Johnson, L.R., Copeland, E.M., Dudrick, S.J.: Gastroenterology, *68*:1177–1183, 1975.
72. Gronqvist, B., Engstrom, B., Grimelius, L.: Acta Chir. Scand., *141*:208–217, 1975.
73. Souba, W.W., Smith, R.J., Wilmore, D.W.: JPEN J. Parenter. Enteral Nutr., *9*:608–617, 1985.
74. Hwang, T.L., O'Dwyer, S.T., Smith, R.J., et al.: Surg. Forum, *37*:56–59, 1986.
75. Grant, J.P., Snyder, P.J.: J. Surg. Res., *44*:506–513, 1988.
76. Proceedings of an International Glutamine Symposium: Glutamine Metabolism in Health and Disease: Basic Science and Clinical Aspects. JPEN J. Parenter. Enteral Nutr., *14(Suppl.)*:395–1375, 1990.
77. Kirwan, W.O., Smith, A.N.: Scand. J. Gastroenterol., *12*:331–335, 1977.
78. Koruda, M.J., Rolandelli, R.H., Settle, R.G., et al.: JPEN J. Parenter. Enteral Nutr., *10*:343–350, 1986.
79. Barber, A.E., Jones, W.G., Minei, J.P., et al.: JPEN J. Parenter. Enteral Nutr., *14*:335–343, 1990.
80. Desjeux, J.F.: Transport of water and ions. *In* Pediatric Gastrointestinal Disease. Edited by W.A. Walker, P.R. Durie, J.R., Hamilton, et al.: Philadelphia, B.C. Decker, 1991.
81. Desjeux, J.F., Tannenbaum, C., Tai, Y.H., et al.: Am. J. Dis. Child., *131*:331–340, 1977.
82. Carpenter, C.J.C., Greenough, W.B., Pierce N.F.: N. Engl. J. Med., *319*:1346–1348, 1988.
83. Pizarro, D., Posada, G., Sandi, L. et al.: N. Engl. J. Med., *324*:517–521, 1991.


## SELECTED READINGS


Bloom, S.R., Polak, J.M.: Gut Hormones. Edinburgh, Churchill Livingstone, 1981.

Johnson, L.R.: Physiology of the Gastrointestinal Tract, 2nd Ed. New York, Raven Press, 1988.

Grand, R.J., Sutphen, J.L., Dietz, W.H.: Pediatric Nutrition: Theory and Practice. Boston, Butterworth, 1987.

McCaughan, G., Basten, A.: Immune system of the gastrointestinal tract. *In* Gastrointestinal Physiology IV. International Review of Physiology 28. Edited by J.A. Young. Baltimore, University Park Press, 1983.

Mutt, V.: Scand. J. Gastroenterol., *17(Suppl.77)*:133–152, 1982.

Sleisenger, M.H., Fordtran, J.S.: Gastrointestinal Disease. 4th Ed. Philadelphia, W.B. Saunders, 1989.

Spiro, H.M.: Clinical Gastroenterology. 3rd Ed. New York, Macmillan, 1983.

Thomas, H.C., Jewell, D.P.: Clinical Gastrointestinal Immunology. Oxford, Blackwell Scientific, 1979.

CHAPTER 38

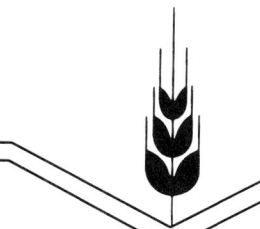

# Nutritional and Metabolic Roles of Intestinal Flora

Barry R. Goldin, Alice H. Lichtenstein, and Sherwood L. Gorbach



The intestinal microflora of humans represents a rich ecosystem composed of metabolically active microorganisms in close proximity to an absorptive mucosal surface. Substrates for bacterial transformation can reach the colonic flora through direct oral ingestion, by biliary secretion into the upper segments of bowel, or by secretion across the mucosa. This chapter is a review of the current knowledge of the relationship between the intestinal microflora and the physiology and biochemistry of the host in health and disease.

## COMPOSITION AND DISTRIBUTION OF MICROFLORA

The bacterial inhabitants of the human gastrointestinal tract constitute a complex ecosystem. More than 400 bacterial species have been identified in feces of a single subject.[1,2] Anaerobic bacteria are the predominant microorganisms in the gastrointestinal tract, outnumbering aerobes by a factor of $10^2$ to $10^4$. The most prevalent anaerobic bacteria are bacteroides, bifidobacterium, fusobacterium, clostridium, eubacterium, peptococcus, and peptostreptococcus. Numerous other species are present in varying but lesser degrees.

In healthy humans, the upper gastrointestinal tract is sparsely populated with microorganisms. Bacteria from the oral cavity are washed along with saliva into the stomach where most microorganisms are destroyed by gastric juice.[3] The most commonly isolated bacteria in the stomach are gram-positive facultative forms such as streptococcus, staphylococcus, and lactobacillus (Table 38–1).

The small intestine constitutes a zone of transition between the sparsely populated stomach and the luxuriant bacterial flora of the distal ileum and colon. The microflora of the proximal small bowel is similar to that of the stomach. Here, the concentration of bacteria increases to between $10^3$ and $10^4$ colony-forming units (CFU) per milliliter of intestinal contents. The most common organisms are gram-positive aerobes, although coliform and anaerobic bacteria can be isolated in low concentrations. In the distal ileum, the concentration of bacteria increases to between $10^6$ and $10^7$ CFU per milliliter, and gram-negative bacteria outnumber gram-positive organisms. Coliforms are consistently present, and anaerobic bacteria, such as bacteroides, bifidobacterium, fusobacterium, and clostridium, are found in substantial concentrations.[4]

**TABLE 38–1.** DISTRIBUTION AND COMPOSITION OF THE INTESTINAL FLORA

| SITE | COMPOSITION* | TOTAL NUMBER OF ORGANISMS PER MILLILITER OF CONTENTS |
|---|---|---|
| Stomach | Streptococcus<br>Lactobacillus | $10^1–10^2$ |
| Duodenum and jejunum | Similar to stomach | $10^2–10^4$ |
| Ilium-cecum | Bacteroides<br>Clostridium<br>Streptococci<br>Lactobacilli | $10^4–10^8$ |
| Colon | Bacteroides<br>Clostridium ($10^{10}$)<br>Eubacterium ($10^{10}$)<br>Peptococcus ($10^{10}$)<br>Bifidobacterium ($10^9–10^{10}$)<br>Streptococcus ($10^{10}$)<br>Fusobacterium ($10^9–10^{10}$) | $10^{11.5}–10^{12}$ |

*Organisms listed represent only the major species from the different sites.

Distal to the ileocecal sphincter, bacterial concentrations increase sharply. Within the colon, the bacterial concentration is between $10^{11}$ and $10^{12}$ CFU per milliliter of fecal material. One third of the fecal dry weight consists of viable bacteria. A summary of the distribution and composition of the gastrointestinal flora is presented in Table 38–1.

## EFFECT OF DIET ON COMPOSITION OF MICROFLORA

Numerous animal and human studies have been designed to investigate the effect of diet on the composition of the intestinal microflora. In this section, results of some of the human studies are summarized; subsequent sections also include relevant examples.

The data are conflicting regarding the ability of diet to alter specific microbial components of the human adult flora. Moore et al. reported no change in the predominant organisms in the fecal flora of individuals shifted from an omnivorous to a vegetarian diet.[5] In another study, Maier et al. investigated four subjects fed a meatless diet for 4 weeks, and then a high-meat diet for 4 weeks.[6] Increased fecal counts of bacteroides and lower counts of coliforms were noted when subjects were eating the high-meat diet. However, a statistical analysis was not performed and the changes were not big. Reddy et al. reported a similar study in which eight volunteers, initially consuming a high-meat diet, were shifted for 4 weeks to a nonmeat diet.[7] The shift resulted in a lower number of total anaerobic bacteria, including decreased counts of bacteroides, bifidobacterium, and peptococcus, when the nonmeat diet was consumed.

Intercountry studies performed in the early 1970s showed that people living in Britain or the United States eating a Western diet had more bacteroides and fewer enterococci and other aerobic organisms than people eating a largely vegetarian diet in Uganda, India, and Japan.[8] In such large cross-cultural studies, however, it is difficult to eliminate factors other than diet that may influence the microflora.

The most detailed studies of the human microflora have been performed by Finegold and co-workers. Subjects eating a Western diet were compared with subjects eating a Japanese diet, and with vegetarian and nonvegetarian Seventh-Day Adventists.[9] The subjects eating a Japanese diet had significantly higher fecal counts of Streptococcus faecalis, Eubacterium lentum, and E. contortum; they also had a lower count of bacteroides, although the values were not significantly different. The data were also evaluated in terms of populations at low and high risk for colon cancer.[9] The low-risk group included subjects eating a Japanese diet and the vegetarian and nonvegetarian Seventh-Day Adventists; the high-risk group included people eating a Western diet and patients with colonic polyps. The low-risk group had higher counts in their feces of Klebsiella pneumoniae and various lactobacillus species, whereas the high-risk group had greater numbers of bififobacterium, peptococcus, and clostridium.

Draser et al. studied the effect of fiber on the fecal flora of four volunteers.[10] Crude wheat fiber was increased from 3.6 to 11.7 g per day by adding wheat bran to the diet. These investigators reported no change in the microbial composition of the fecal flora as a result of this dietary modification.

In summary, studies of dietary influence on specific bacteria in intestinal flora indicate that people eating low-meat, high complex-carbohydrate diets have higher fecal counts of aerobic bacteria and lower numbers of certain anaerobic bacteria. The overall shifts in the composition of the flora are hardly dramatic, and in some studies, no alterations are seen.

These studies of fecal microflora are based on classic principles of bacterial taxonomy, by which bacteria are named for their morphologic characteristics and their ability to perform certain biochemical reactions, usually having no relation to the physiology of the host. Because the flora is so complex (consisting of over 400 species), based on standard taxonomy, with a concentration of $10^{11}$ bacteria/g, it is difficult to show changes in any specific bacterium. Another approach, outlined in subsequent sections, deals with the metabolic activity of the microflora as a whole in relation to specific substrates. By this criterion, diet can, indeed, alter the metabolic activity of the flora. These changes may be more relevant to the host than the Latin or Greek name of the microorganisms.

## EFFECT OF DIET ON BACTERIAL REACTIONS

Variations in bacterial metabolic activity can result from a variety of environmental factors.[11] Hill reported that feces from United States and English subjects contained higher levels of steroid nuclear dehydrogenating Clostridium than feces from African and Asian subjects.[12] The incriminated enzyme is involved in the production of unsaturated steroids from saturated steroids such as androgens and bile acids.

The microbial metabolism of bile acids and neutral steroids, as well as microbial β-glucuronidase, has been measured in the feces of various groups of people in the United States consuming diets of different compositions in order to assess the degree of microbial activity.[13] These measurements were performed among Americans consuming a mixed Western diet as well as among American vegetarians and Seventh-Day Adventists (lacto-ovo vegetarians). When compared to the vegetarians, the Americans consuming a mixed Western diet had fecal microflora with a greater ability to hydrolyze glucuronide conjugates, to metabolize bile acids to lithocholic and deoxycholic acids, and to reduce cholesterol.

In Seventh-Day Adventists and subjects consuming a mixed Western diet MacDonald et al. studied the fecal nicotinamide adenine dinucleotide (NAD) and NAD phosphate (NADP)-dependent 7-α-hydroxysteroid dehydroxylase that converts hydroxy steroids to ketosteroids.[14] The activity of fecal 7-α-hydroxysteroid dehydroxylase was lower in the Seventh-Day Adventists.

Goldin and Gorbach reported that rats fed a high-fat (meat) diet for 1 month had higher levels of fecal bacterial enzymes, β-glucuronidase, nitroreductase, and azoreductase, than rats on a low-fat (no meat) diet.[15] These results were confirmed and extended in a subsequent study in which investigators found that a high-fat diet, independent of the meat content, elevated the activity of these fecal bacterial enzymes.[16] Goldin et al. also studied these fecal bacterial enzymes, as well as 7-α-steroid dehydroxylase, in humans eating a Western diet and in lacto-ovo vegetarians and vegans.[17] Levels of all four bacterial enzymes were lower in the nonmeat-eating vegetarian subjects. These results confirm that the metabolic activity of the intestinal microflora can be altered by the nature of the diet. More detailed studies are required to determine the relationship of specific dietary components to the activity of different bacterial reactions.

Lindop et al. compared intestinal bacterial β-glucuronidase activities in rats given a fiber-free diet or a diet containing pectin or cellulose.[18] They found pectin and cellulose significantly reduced β-glucuronidase activity of cecal contents. Cellulose also lowered the β-glucuronidase activity of the jejunal and ileal contents while pectin reduced the activity in the ileum. Dietary fiber components had no effect on jejunal or ileal mucosal β-glucuronidase activity.

Wyatt et al. described a study in which 10 g of gum arabic were fed daily to a female volunteer.[19] Gum arabic is a water-soluble complex polysaccharide that is classified as a dietary fiber because of the inability to digest the gum. They reported that 6.5% of the fecal flora from the volunteer was initially capable of hydrolyzing gum arabic, after 18 days of feeding the percentage had increased to 53.6%; however, no increase in the number of anaerobic organisms in the feces was noted. Analysis of the feces indicated that bacteroides and bifobacterium were the principal gum-arabic fermenters. Findings of this study indicate that specific substrates introduced into the diet can cause elevation of fecal bacterial enzymes that can catalyze these substrates without altering the composition of the flora.

## METABOLIC ACTIVITIES OF MICROFLORA

The metabolic capacity of the gut bacteria is extremely diverse. Any compound taken orally or any substance entering the intestine through the biliary tract or the blood or by secretion directly into the lumen is a potential substrate for bacterial transformation. Table 38–2 contains a partial list of reactions that can be performed by the intestinal bacteria as well as examples of substrates for these reactions.

### GLYCOSIDES

Hydrolysis of glycosidic bonds is one of the best-known examples of bacterial metabolism. Glycosides are compounds consisting of a nonsugar moiety (aglycone)

**TABLE 38–2.** BIOCHEMICAL REACTIONS BY INTESTINAL BACTERIA

| REACTION | REPRESENTATIVE SUBSTRATE |
|---|---|
| Hydrolysis | |
| Glucuronides | Estradiol-3-glucuronide |
| Glycosides | Cycasin |
| Sulfamates | Cyclamate, amygdalin |
| Amides | Methotrexate |
| Esters | Acetyldigoxin |
| Nitrates | Pentaerythritol trinitrate |
| Dehydroxylation | |
| C-hydroxy groups | Bile acids |
| N-hydroxyl groups | N-Hydroxyfluorenylacetamide |
| Decarboxylation | Amino acids |
| D-demethylation | Biochanin A |
| Deamination | Amino acids |
| Dehydrogenase | Cholesterol, bile acids |
| Dehalogenation | DDT |
| Reduction | |
| Nitro groups | P-nitrobenzoic acid |
| Double bonds | Unsaturated fatty acids |
| Azo groups | Food dyes |
| Aldehydes | Benzaldehydes |
| Alcohols | Benzyl alcohols |
| N-oxides | 4-Nitroquinoline-1-oxide |
| Nitrosamine formation | Dimethylinitrosamine |
| Aromatization | Quinic acid |
| Acetylation | Histamine |
| Esterification | Galic acid |

bound to a sugar by either an α- or β-glycosidic linkage. Glycosides enter the gut from two major sources: diet or the liver (through the bile). The diet contains a large number of plant glycosides, predominantly flavonoids. Glycosides coming from the liver include compounds that are detoxified by glucuronide formation and subsequently secreted into the bowel by way of the bile. The intestinal flora can then hydrolyze the β-glucuronide bond leading to the release of the biologically active aglycones, some of which are potentially toxic or carcinogenic.

The principal glycosidase produced by the intestinal flora is β-glucuronidase.[3] On the basis of studying 50 strains each of four bacterial species commonly found in the bowel, Hawksworth et al. concluded that, on a per-cell basis, Escherichia coli and clostridium had the highest β-glucuronidase activity and lactobacillus and bifidobacterium had the lowest activity.[20] The relative activities were different for β-glucosidase; Escherichia coli had the lowest activity, and bacteroides and Streptococcus faecalis had the highest activity.

There are a number of interesting examples of the role of bacteria in the metabolism of glycosides. Cycasin methylazoxymethanol-β-D-glucoside is a naturally occurring compound that is a constituent of cycad plants, also known as tropical ferns. Much of the interest in cycasin stems from the finding that the aglycone, methylazoxymethanol, caused tumors in conventional but not in germfree rats. These results suggested that the hydrolysis was a result of the intestinal microorganisms. This hypothesis was confirmed by monocontaminating germfree rats with bacteria having different levels of β-glucosidase activity. Toxicity after feeding cycasin was positively correlated with the β-glucosidase levels of the particular bacterial strain implanted.[21] A more detailed discussion of the interaction of the bacterial flora with cycasin is presented in a subsequent section.

Rutin is a plant glycoside that is not mutagenic in tests, such as the Salmonella test. On hydrolysis of the glycosidic linkages, however, the hydrolysate becomes mutagenic. Several authors have reported that mixed fecal cultures[22] or fecal isolates, such as Streptococcus faecalis,[23] can convert rutin (quercetin-3-0-B-D-glucose-y-L-rhamnose) to quercetin, a compound that is mutagenic in the Salmonella liver homogenate test. Beverages such as red wine and tea contain glycosides of quercetin. In addition, cell-free extracts from fecal cultures grown in the presence of bile acids have increased ability to form quercetin from rutin.[24]

The cathartic agent cascara sagrada is a mixture of glycosides. The glycosides themselves have no pharmacologic action; however, on bacterial hydrolysis, the active aglycone is released. Hawksworth et al. found that the β-glucosidase of S. facealis can hydrolyze cascara sagrada.[20]

The metabolism of the cardiac glycoside digoxin has been studied by Lindenbaum et al.[25] To produce pharmacologic effects, the bacterial flora must remove a trisaccharide from the parent compound, releasing diagoxigenin. The intestinal flora of approximately 36% of Americans in New York City given digoxin further reduce the double bond in the lactone ring, resulting in the formation of dihydrodigoxigenin.[26] This compound is pharmacologically inactive. A total of 14% of New Yorkers tested excreted large amounts of digoxin metabolites. Therefore, at least 14% and likely a greater percentage receiving digoxin will not achieve predicted serum levels as a result of bacterial inactivation. In contrast, only 13.7% of Indians living in urban southern India metabolized digoxin, with only 1% excreting large amounts of metabolites.[26] Similarly 13.8% of Bangladeshi living in Dhaka metabolized digoxin.[27] These results indicate a large interethnic variation exists in the metabolic capacity of the intestinal flora. The microorganism Eubacterium lentum is exclusively responsible for this reduction.[28]

The bacterial hydrolysis of disaccharides is another example of a hydrolytic glycosidic reaction. The dietary disaccharides, sucrose, lactose, and maltose, are normally hydrolyzed by mammalian enzymes in the intestinal mucosal brush border in the upper segment of the small bowel. This arrangement minimizes contact of the disaccharides with the high bacterial populations in the colon. Those individuals who, either by genetic design or by an acquired disorder, lack mucosal disaccharidase have resultant insufficient absorption of related sugars in the upper part of the small intestine. The sugars are transported to the ileum and large bowel where the bacterial enzymes lactase (β-galactosidase), maltase (α-glucosidase), and sucrase (α-glycosidase) hydrolyze the disaccharides. The monosaccharides produced from this hydrolysis are further metabolized by bacteria to short-chain acids in a classic fermentation reaction. The production of these acids leads to an osmotic imbalance, and water flows into the bowel lumen causing diarrhea. The acid production also lowers the pH of the fecal stream, causing irritation of the colonic wall. The most common disaccharidase disorder is lactase deficiency leading to the well-known disorder of lactose intolerance. Deficiencies in sucrase or isomaltase, which produce similar symptoms, also occur, but are rarer.

## AMINES

Bacteria can deaminate or remove amino groups from amines by four direct pathways. Also, an indirect route of removal of amino groups is by way of the Strickland reaction. These deamination reactions are discussed in greater detail with respect to amino acid metabolism in a later section.

The contribution of ammonia from bacterial deamination of amino acids is small, relative to the total intestinal pool. The major source of ammonia production in the intestine is deamination of the primary amine urea. Bacterial urease catalyzes the production of carbon dioxide and ammonia from urea. Urease is present in a wide range of organisms found in the intestinal tract, including both aerobes and anaerobes.[29] Intestinal bacteria hydrolyze approximately 40% of the urea synthesized by the liver.[3]

Intestinal bacteria can esterify primary amino groups to a variety of compounds. This reaction is an important mechanism by which bacteria can inactivate sulfonamides and certain aminoglycoside antibiotics. The bacterial esterification of histamine is the major source for N-acetyl linkage of secondary amines. An example of this reaction is the de-esterification of the antibiotic chloramphenicol, with release of the dichloracetyl group.

The intestinal flora can also remove alkyl groups from secondary amines. The demethylation of methylamphetamine to produce amphetamine is an example of this reaction.

The bacterial flora can also add a nitroso group to secondary amines, producing nitrosamines, an addition known as N-nitrosation. Bacteria can use nitrate as the nitrosating agent. Aerobes such as Streptococcus faecalis and the common anaerobes, clostridium, bacteroides, and bifidobacterium, can catalyze the N-nitrosation of diphenylamine. (The implication of this reaction to human health is discussed subsequently.)

## AZOCOMPOUNDS

Most artificial coloring additives used in foods and in the textile industry are dyes containing a single azo bond (mono azo dyes). American consumption of azo dyes has been increasing steadily during the past 20 years. During that time, more than a dozen dyes have been taken off the market after laboratory testing indicated they may be toxic and carcinogenic. The water-soluble dyes are not well absorbed from the intestine and are subject to bacterial action in the large bowel, which contributes to their detrimental effects. Results of several studies showed that the bacterial flora can reductively hydrolyze the azo bond, resulting in the formation of substituted aromatic amines.[30] This class of bacterially generated compounds contains a number of well-established carcinogens.[31] For example, orange II can be reductively cleaved, leading to the formation of the bladder carcinogen 1-amino-2-naphthol.[32] Ponceau 3R,[33] methyl yellow, and methyl orange, formerly used as food colorants, can be transformed by intestinal anaerobes into mutagens.[34]

## SULFATES

Bacterial sulfatase activity in the intestine has been reported.[35] The intestinal flora can hydrolyze C-sulfonates, O-sulfates, and N-sulfonates.[36] An example of the significance of these reactions is the bacterial hydrolysis of cyclamate. Cyclamate (cyclohexylamine N-sulfonate) was used as an artificial sweetening agent until it was banned in 1969. Initially, researchers believed that cyclamate could not be metabolized in the body. It was shown subsequently that cyclamate could be converted to the bladder carcinogen cyclohexylamine through an N-sulfate ester hydrolysis by the bacterial flora.[37,38] Cyclohexylamine was absorbed and excreted in the urine. Prolonged feeding of cyclamate to rats increased the amount of metabolite; removal of cyclamate from the diet led to a loss of hydrolytic activity of the flora within 5 days.[39]

## STEROIDS

The bacterial deconjugation and dehydroxylation of bile acids are examples of the importance of the intestinal flora in the metabolism of endogenous compounds. Bile acids are synthesized in the liver and excreted in the bile into the small intestine. Before entering the small intestine, they are conjugated to the amino acids taurine or glycine. The intestinal bacteria hydrolyze the conjugates, releasing the free bile acids. Most bile acids have a hydroxyl group at the 7 position of the steroid nucleus. The bacterial enzyme 7-α-steroid dehydrogenase can remove this hydroxyl group. About 80% of the cholic and chenodeoxycholic primary bile acids undergo 7-α-dehydroxylation to yield deoxycholic and lithocholic acid, respectively. The implications of this reaction in relation to the etiology of large bowel cancer are discussed later.

The nuclear dehydrogenation of steroids by intestinal microorganisms represents another class of bacterial intestinal reaction. In this case, double bonds are introduced into the steroid structure. When androgens are substrates for this reaction, the double bonds are introduced in the 1 and 4 position, giving rise to 1,4 androgens.

### AROMATIZATION

Quinic acid is present in many food products, including coffee, tea, vegetables, and fruits. The compound has an aliphatic cyclic structure. Quinic acid is aromatized when taken orally and excreted in urine as hippuric acid. The aromatization does not occur when quinic acid is given parenterally, and the reaction is inhibited by the action of the antibiotic neomycin in the rat and man.[40] These data suggest that aromatization is a bacterially catalyzed event in the bowel.

### C-RING AND CARBON-CARBON BOND CLEAVAGE

The human intestinal flora can cleave the carbon-carbon bond between two of the rings of the plant product sennidin, which is found in senna and rhubarb.[41] The final product of this reaction is rhein anthrone. The physiologic importance of this reaction derives from the observation that the plant sennosides have a laxative action; however, the parent compounds are inactive, and thus the metabolic action of the intestinal microflora is necessary for the observed laxative effect. A more complete discussion of intestinal bacterial metabolism is provided in review articles by Scheline.[35,42]

## ENTEROHEPATIC CIRCULATION

A substance is said to undergo an enterohepatic circulation when it is metabolized in the liver, excreted into the bile, passed into the lumen of the intestine, reabsorbed through the intestinal wall, and then returned to the liver in the portal circulation. Many endogenous compounds have an enterohepatic circulation, including estrogens, folic acid, vitamin $B_{12}$, bile acids, cholesterol, protoporphyrin, and the metabolites of vitamin D.[43,44] Enterohepatic circulation has also been demonstrated for drugs and chemicals, including ouabain, promazine, morphine, colchicine, diethystilbestrol, digoxin, rifampin, and iopanoic acid.[43]

Several factors determine whether a compound is secreted from the liver into the bile. The compound generally is conjugated to a polar group such as glucuronic acid, sulfate, taurine, glycine, or glutathione before secretion into bile. In addition, a compound that undergoes an enterohepatic circulation tends to have a molecular mass in excess of 200. Once secreted into the small intestine, the microflora plays an important role in the next phase of the enterohepatic circulation. The conjugated compounds themselves are not well absorbed; they cannot undergo an enterohepatic circulation unless hydrolyzed by the enzymes of the bacterial flora. These bacterial enzymes include β-glucuronidase, sulfatase, and various glycosidases. These enzymes can hydrolyze a variety of conjugates resulting in the release of the nonconjugated compounds in the intestine with subsequent reabsorption.

An example of the physiologic implications of diet-mediated alteration of the enterohepatic circulation has been reported by Goldin et al.[45] These investigators found that American vegetarian women excreted between two and three times more estrogen in their feces and had between 20 and 40% lower plasma levels of estrogen than American omnivores eating a Western diet. An inverse correlation existed between fecal excretion of estrogen and plasma estrogen levels.

In summary, the enterohepatic circulation contributes to an increased half-life and elevated plasma levels for these substances, which is advantageous for certain compounds but not for others. The composition of the diet can alter the enterohepatic circulation by affecting bacterial deconjugating enzymes.

## VITAMINS

The conversion of vitamin K, a member of the naphthoquinone family, is a classic example of the involvement by the bacterial flora in the metabolism of a vitamin. The prothrombin complex, a blood-clotting factor, is synthesized by the liver. The peptides that become the glycoproteins of the prothrombin complex cannot be synthesized on the appropriate RNA unless the liver contains menaquinone, a substituted naphthoquinone. Because animals cannot synthesize the substituted naphthoquinone ring, they depend on vegetables in the diet for their supply.

Bacteria found in the intestinal tract also synthesize homologues of vitamin $K_2$ (menaquinone-7). These homologues range from menaquinone-6 (6 isoprene units in the side chain) to menaquinone-13.[46,47] The bacterial metabolism apparently occurs, at least in part, in the ileum, where the menaquinone can be absorbed.

The importance of bacterial synthesis of vitamin K has been demonstrated in studies in which healthy adult subjects were given low vitamin K diets for several weeks without causing a deficiency. Treatment of subjects on low vitamin K diets with bowel-sterilizing antibiotics, such as neomycin, caused a significant decrease in plasma prothrombin levels.[48,49]

In contrast, vitamin $B_{12}$ (cyanocobalamin) is synthesized solely by microorganisms. Vitamin $B_{12}$ is synthesized by the microflora of ruminants, and is absorbed in the small intestine of these animals. The meat and milk from these animals are a major dietary source of vitamin $B_{12}$ for humans. The human microflora also synthesizes significant amounts of vitamin $B_{12}$, and approximately 5 μg are excreted in the feces daily. However, the primary site for the synthesis of vitamin $B_{12}$ in humans is the large bowel. Absorption from this site is poor or nonexistent because of a lack of receptors in the mucosa. The ileum is the major location of vitamin $B_{12}$ absorption in humans. Albert et al. reported the synthesis of vitamin $B_{12}$ in the jejunum and ileum of healthy Southern Indian subjects.[50] At least two organisms, Pseudomonas and Klebsiella, were shown to synthesize significant amounts of vitamin $B_{12}$ in the small intestine.

Biotin is synthesized to a major extent by the intestinal flora of animals and humans.[51] Large doses of antibiotics can cause biotin deficiency in laboratory animals. The administration of antibiotics also lowers urinary biotin levels in humans. Germfree rats require biotin in their diet, whereas conventional rats appear to have sufficient bacterial synthesis to satisfy systemic requirements for biotin.

Several other B complex vitamins, such as folic acid and thiamine, are synthesized by bacteria in the gastrointestinal tract,[52] although this pathway does not provide adequate absorbable amounts to eliminate the requirement for a dietary source for these vitamins.

## AMINO ACIDS AND PROTEINS

In monogastric animals, the microflora of the lower intestine hydrolyzes digested food proteins incompletely. Similarly, proteins from the epithelial cells and digestive secretions such as enzymes and glycoproteins (mucins), secreted too far down in the gastrointestinal tract to be acted on by intestinal protease, are metabolized by intestinal bacteria. The ability of the flora to destroy ABO blood antigens in the gut could be a measure of mucin degradation.[53] In addition, intestinal bacteria can ferment most amino acids. The initial reactions involve either deamination or decarboxylation. Many amines derived from amino acid metabolism by the gut flora are found in the urine, indicating subsequent resorption of the metabolites. Piperidine and pyrrolidine are examples of cyclic secondary amines that are formed from lysine and arginine by way of cadaverine and putrescine.

Five mechanisms of bacterial deamination have been described. Nonoxidative deamination by aspartate ammonia-lyase catalyzes the conversion of aspartate to fumarate; histidine ammonia-lyase produces urocanic acid from histidine; and cystathione-γ-lyase forms pyruvate from cysteine. Oxidative deamination is a minor pathway in bacteria. Only a few organisms use this pathway on a restricted range of amino acids such as glycine, alanine, and glutamic acid. Reductive deamination, producing a saturated fatty acid from an amino acid, is a major bacterial pathway. By this mechanism, aspartic acid is deaminated to succinic acid, and tryptophan is deaminated to indopropionic acid. Bacterial hydrolysis of amino acids is exemplified by the deamination of aspartic acid to yield malic acid. This route of metabolism generates α-hydroxy acids from amino acids. Another mechanism of deamination is the indirect removal of ammonia by the mixed amino acid, or Strickland reaction. Clostridia primarily catalyze this reaction in which two amino acids react to yield a keto acid and a saturated fatty acid.

The bacterial degradation of proteins and metabolism of the resulting amino acids cause the formation of a wide range of different amines and short-chain organic acids. The short-chain fatty acids can be absorbed across the colonic mucosa, and to some extent, this helps the body reclaim energy that would otherwise be lost in the stool. The overproduction of short-chain fatty acids or poorly absorbed hydroxy short-chain fatty acids can cause an osmotic diarrhea similar to that observed for nonabsorbable carbohydrates (i.e., lactose).

## LIPIDS

In humans and monogastric animals, most of the fatty acids from dietary lipids are absorbed in the small intestine. Some unsaturated fatty acids do reach the lower segments of the small intestine and colon. The cecum of the rabbit has the capacity to hydrogenate these unsaturated fatty acids.[51] Evidence in humans shows that anaerobic bacteria, in addition to hydrogenating, can also hydrate unsaturated fatty acids.[54] Small amounts of 10-hydroxystearic acid have been identified in human feces. In general, lipid metabolism by intestinal bacteria is important in ruminants, but has only minor significance in humans.

## CARBOHYDRATES

The anaerobic intestinal flora is capable of fermenting carbohydrate to short-chain fatty acids. Acetate, propionate, and butyrate are the major end products in the feces of humans. Carbon dioxide, hydrogen, methane, and water are also end products of the fermentation process. Acetate usually is formed by the oxidative decarboxylation of pyruvate and butyrate, and by reduction of acetoacetate from acetate. The production of propionate is by two pathways, involving fixation of carbon dioxide to form succinate, which is subsequently decarboxylated, or formation of lactate and acrylate (the "acrylate pathway"). Lactate may also be formed from pyruvate by anaerobic bacteria, but lactate is not a key intermediate in fermentation, and significant amounts are rarely found in the human colon.

The major source of fermentable carbohydrates in the human colon is plant cell-wall polysaccharides, such as cellulose pectins, and hemicellulose, the major components of dietary fiber. Starch, intestinal mucus, and mono- and disaccharides can also be fermented in significant quantities. It is estimated that between 20 and 70 g of carbohydrate are fermented per day, depending on the fiber content of the diet. The higher values occur in populations consuming a diet consisting predominantly of plant sources. The plant cell-wall polysaccharides are composed of glucose, galactose, xylose, arabinose, and uranic acid monomers, which are fermented by bacteria along various anaerobic pathways. Hexose breakdown is mainly via the Embden-Meyerhof-Parnas glycolytic pathway to pyruvate. Alternatively, hexose is converted to 6-phosphogluconate and then metabolized by the pentose monophosphate shunt.

The short-chain fatty acids produced as a result of bacterial fermentation of carbohydrate can be absorbed by the colonic mucosa.[54] In the rabbit, these organic acids contribute 30 to 40% of the basal energy requirement.[55] In humans eating a low-fiber diet (10 g per day), the short chain fatty acids provide 25 kcal (105 kJ) of energy per day; however, in populations eating a high-fiber diet, this source of energy could provide 150 to 200 kcal (635 to 845 kJ) per day.[55] The rate of absorption is between 6 and 12 mol/cm$^2$ per hour and is more rapid than sodium transport.[55] Substantial amounts of these absorbed fatty acids are metabolized within the colonic epithelial cells. In isolated epithelial cells from human colon, butyrate is an important energy source for colonic mucosa, accounting for the major part of energy needs even in the presence of glucose.[54] The short-chain fatty acids can be further metabolized to acetyl-coenzyme A (CoA). Propionate is converted into propionyl-CoA, which by oxidative decarboxylation is converted into acetyl-CoA. Butyrate can be converted into acetyl-CoA by a fatty acid thiokinase.

## BILE ACIDS

The bile acids synthesized in the liver and secreted in bile are substituted C-24 cholanic acids conjugated to glycine or taurine. In Table 38–3, the principal bile acids and the various side-chain substitutions are presented. The free bile acids are absorbed either by active transport from the terminal ileum or, to a lesser extent, by passive diffusion from the small or large intestine. The absorbed bile acids return to the liver through the portal circulation and are reconjugated and re-secreted in the bile. Approximately 5% of the bile acids are lost in the feces in each cycle.[43] The bile acids found in the feces are deconjugated. Primary bile acids are synthesized by the liver, and they are converted to secondary bile acids by intestinal bacteria. Studies with germfree animals show an absence of secondary bile acids in the feces.

The principal bacterial reactions involved in the conversion of bile acids include three separate classes: the hydrolysis of the amide bond to release the free bile acid from its glycine or taurine conjugates; an oxido-reduction reaction of the hydroxyl groups at C-3, C-7, and C-12 to give either oxo-bile acids (hydroxyl to keto group) or β-hydroxyl groups after the reduction of the keto group (inversion products); and dehydroxylation at C-7, and to a smaller extent at the C-3 and C-12 positions. The hydroxyl groups of the primary bile acids are in the α-configuration. The formation of a keto group and subsequent reduction of this group can lead to the formation of a β-hydroxyl group. The source and properties of these bacterial enzymes are discussed in detail by Draser and Hill.[3]

## CHOLESTEROL

The range of the amount of fecal cholesterol excreted is between 75 and 200 mg/day. The three primary sources of this cholesterol are as follows: unabsorbed from the diet, which contributes about 20%; bile, which contributes the bulk of the cholesterol or 67%; and the intestinal epithelium or lining of the small intestine, which contributes 13%.[56]

Cholesterol, the precursor of bile acids, is a substituted neutral (e.g., no charged groups) C-27 cholestene. Two principal fecal metabolites of cholesterol are coprostanone and coprostanol, and one minor product is cholestenone. The production of coprostanol involves a steroid nuclear hydrogenation of the 5,6 double bond. The conversion of cholesterol to coprostanone results from the reduction of the 4,5 bond and a C-3 oxidoreduc-

**TABLE 38–3.** MAJOR FECAL BILE ACIDS IN HUMANS

| NATURE OF SUBSTITUENT AT POSITION | | | |
|---|---|---|---|
| 3 | 7 | 12 | TRIVIAL NAME* |
| OH | OH | OH | Cholic acid |
| OH | OH | — | Chenodeoxycholic acid |
| OH | — | OH | Deoxycholic acid |
| OH | — | — | Lithocholic acid |
| β-OH | — | — | Isolithocholic acid |

*All are substituted 5 β-cholanic acids.

tase converting the hydroxyl group to a keto group. The sequence of these reactions has not been elucidated fully. Coprostanone may be synthesized by cholestenone (4-cholesten-3-one). In general, coprostanol accounts for 50% of the total amount of fecal neutral sterols, coprostanone 10 to 15%, and unmetabolized cholesterol most of the remainder. In germfree rats, cholesterol is the only neutral sterol in the feces, indicating that the intestinal flora is solely responsible for the metabolism of cholesterol in the intestine. The percentage conversion of intestinal cholesterol to its metabolites varies from 70 to 85% in Americans and Western Europeans to 55 to 65% in Africans and Asians.[13]

## BILE PIGMENTS

Bile pigments, the end products of the breakdown of hemoglobin and heme-containing enzymes, are normal constituents of bile. Between 200 and 300 mg of bilirubin, the product derived from heme, are excreted daily in the bile. Approximately 90% of the bilirubin is conjugated as a glucuronide into the bile. The glucuronide conjugate of bilirubin is hydrolyzed by the gut flora, releasing the free compound, which can be reabsorbed in the intestine. Alternately, bilirubin can be reduced by intestinal bacteria to urobilinogen. Approximately 20% of the urobilinogen is reabsorbed from the intestine of humans. Further nonenzymatic oxidation of urobilinogens results in the formation of pigmented urobilins that can also be reabsorbed from the small intestine. Urobilins and bilirubin are the principal pigments of urine, bile, and feces.

The four major components of bile (cholesterol, bile acids, bile pigments, and lecithin) as well as androgens and estrogens, which also are excreted by this route, are subject to bacterial action in the intestine. The physiologic importance of these reactions constitutes an area of ongoing research.

## BACTERIAL OVERGROWTH ("BLIND LOOP") SYNDROME

Anatomic and physiologic derangements of the gastrointestinal tract can lead to proliferation of bacteria in the upper segment of the small intestine. This condition, known as "bacterial overgrowth," may cause a variety of metabolic disorders, including steatorrhea, vitamin deficiencies, and carbohydrate malabsorption.[57]

One cause of bacterial overgrowth in the upper small bowel relates to gastric acid production. Gastric acid normally limits bacterial growth in the stomach and upper small intestine. However, a number of situations, such as atrophic gastritis, pernicious anemia, surgical resections, and therapy with drugs (e.g., cimetidine), can cause hypochlorhydria. These conditions usually are accompanied by overgrowth of bacterial populations in the stomach and upper small intestine.

Small-bowel bacterial overgrowth also can result from inadequate clearance of microorganisms because of disordered peristalsis. This situation can result from anatomic disorders such as small-bowel diverticula, surgically created blind loops, or strictures with partial small-bowel obstruction. Scleroderma and diabetic autonomic neuropathy are associated with ineffective peristalsis and bacterial overgrowth.

A complex flora is present in the upper small bowel of patients with bacterial overgrowth. More than 20 different species of bacteria have been identified, at concentrations ranging from $10^7$ to $10^9$ CFU/ml. Counts as high as $10^{11}$/ml have been reported,[58] which are considerably greater than the $10^2$ to $10^4$ CFU/ml in the normal state.

The most common clinical manifestation of small-bowel overgrowth is malabsorption of fat, along with the related malabsorption of fat-soluble vitamins. The major cause of fat malabsorption involves deconjugation of bile salts. Normally, the conjugated bile salts, which contain a hydrophobic and hydrophilic region (conferring detergent-like properties), solubilize fatty acids and monoglycerides by forming mixed micelles. In the setting of bacterial overgrowth, particularly with anaerobic bacteria, the concentrations of conjugated bile acids in the upper small bowel are reduced by bacterial hydrolysis. This process results in impaired micelle formation, fat malabsorption, and steatorrhea.

In addition to the low concentration of conjugated bile salts associated with small-bowel overgrowth is a corresponding increase in the number of free bile acids. Free bile acids can cause intestinal tissue damage and dysplasia.[59,60] Free bile acids, particularly deoxycholic acid, can also inhibit the esterification of fatty acids by the intestinal tissue during absorption. The combination of impaired micelle formation, altered intestinal cell structure and kinetics, and decreased intestinal esterification contributes to a malabsorption syndrome.

Small-bowel bacterial overgrowth is also associated with megaloblastic anemia that occurs with vitamin $B_{12}$ deficiency. Reduced vitamin $B_{12}$ absorption is related to binding of the vitamin to the bacteria present in the proximal small bowel, thereby preventing vitamin $B_{12}$ absorption in the distal ileum.[61] Vitamin $B_{12}$ malabsorption in rats with surgically created blind loops was corrected by the administration of metronidazole,[62] an antibiotic that acts against anaerobic bacteria. In vitro studies have demonstrated that bacteroides bind the intrinsic factor-cobalamin complex. Patients with bacterial overgrowth syndrome have high levels of vitamin $B_{12}$ in the lumen of the small intestine, not only from nonabsorbed dietary sources but also from local bacterial synthesis. Yet they still suffer from vitamin $B_{12}$ deficiency because no vitamin is available for intestinal absorption.

Amino acid and carbohydrate absorption is impaired in patients with small-bowel bacterial overgrowth. Fecal nitrogen content is increased, serum proteins are low, and, on occasion, a clinical picture of protein-calorie malnutrition is present.[63] These patients also have abnormally low D-xylose absorption resulting from bacterial metabolism of this pentose sugar and from impaired mucosal transport. Elevated levels of volatile fatty acids, degradation products of bacterial carbohydrate metabolism, have been demonstrated in the jejunal aspirates from patients with small-bowel bacterial overgrowth, suggesting bacterial use of ingested carbohydrates.[64]

## COLON CANCER: ROLE OF MICROFLORA

More than 150,000 cases of large-bowel cancer are diagnosed annually in the United States. It has become the cancer of internal organs diagnosed most frequently in the United States, surpassing even lung and breast cancers. Epidemiologic studies have shown that the incidence of colon cancer is higher among North Americans and Western Europeans than among Africans, Asians, and South Americans. The critical factor that may account for these differences is the characteristic "Western" diet, which is high in beef, fat, and protein, and low in dietary fiber. Armstrong and Doll,[65] Howell,[66] and Draser and Irving[67] demonstrated, by using intercountry comparisons, positive correlation between the consumption of beef, total fat, animal fat, and animal protein and the incidence of colon cancer.

Studies of migrant populations indicate that their cancer incidence approximates the prevailing rates in the place of residence, rather than the place of birth. Dunn compared the incidence of cancer in Japan with that among Japanese in California.[68] The incidence of stomach cancer, which is high in Japan, has undergone a stepwise reduction, with intermediate rates in immigrant Japanese, to lower rates in American-born Japanese. In contrast, cancer of the colon has shown the opposite trend: among American-born Japanese, the incidence of colon tumors is approaching that observed in native white Americans.

In the past 10 years, several investigators have proposed that the effect of diet on cancer development is indirect, primarily by affecting the ability of the host to metabolize procarcinogens to proximate carcinogens. In the case of colon cancer, however, activation of carcinogens may be mediated by the bacterial flora in the large bowel. Several bacterial enzymes have been implicated in generating mutagens, carcinogens, and various tumor promoters: β-glucuronidase, β-glucosidase, β-galactosidase, nitroreductase, azoreductase, 7-α-steroid dehydrogenase, and 7-α-hydroxy-steroid dehydroxylase.[15,16,21,69]

The carcinogenic potential of bacterial enzymes in the intestinal microflora has been illustrated in a series of studies involving experimental colon cancer induced by cycasin. This substance is a naturally occurring β-glucoside of the methylazoxymethanol, extractable from the seed and roots of cycad plants. Laqueur et al. discovered that feeding cycasin to infant rats caused hepatomas, renal sarcomas, squamous cell carcinomas of the ear duct, and, in greatest frequency, intestinal adenocarcinomas that were almost exclusively located in the large bowel.[21] The genetic strain of rat had little influence on the carcinogenic effect of cycasin; similar tumors were induced in Osborne-Mendel, Sprague-Dawley, Fischer, and Wistar rats.[21] The intestinal flora was required for the carcinogenic activity of cycasin because the compound was completely inactive when given orally to germfree rats.

The age of the animal was a critical factor. Cycasin was inactive when given parenterally to adult conventional animals. Newborn conventional and newborn germfree rats, however, developed tumors after subcutaneous or intraperitoneal injection of cycasin. A tissue (host) or bacterial (microflora) β-glucosidase is required to hydrolyze the glycolytic bond in cycasin in order to release the active aglycone methylazoxymethanol. The observation that subcutaneous or intraperitoneal injections of cycasin caused tumors in infant rats, but not in older rats, supported the view that young animals have a tissue β-glucosidase that is required for hydrolysis.

The discovery of the carcinogenicity of cycasin led Druckery et al. to test the precursors azoxymethane, azomethane, and dimethylhydrazine.[70] These compounds were carcinogenic in conventional and germfree animals.[71] The route of administration was not critical because tumors developed after oral or subcutaneous administration.[21]

### BACTERIAL ENZYMES

Bacterial β-glucuronidase seems to play an important role in colon carcinogenesis. This substance has a wide substrate specificity and, consequently, can hydrolyze many different glucuronides. These reactions are potentially important in the generation of carcinogenic and toxic substances, inasmuch as many compounds are detoxified by glucuronide formation in the liver and subsequently enter the bowel by way of bile. Deconjugation in the intestine then regenerates the carcinogenic or toxic compound. Several studies have shown that intestinal β-glucuronidase can alter or amplify the biologic activity of exogenous and endogenous compounds. For example, toxic aglycones can be regenerated in situ in the bowel by bacterial β-glucuronidase. Fisher et al. investigated the metabolic fate of diethylstilbestrol-β-D-glucuronide.[72] When given orally to germfree rats, the compound was recovered rapidly in the feces as a result of poor absorption of the glucuronide in the intestine. In contrast, when this compound was fed to conventional animals, both the rate and the amount of compound recovered in the feces decreased. These changes were accounted for by intestinal absorption of free diethylstilbestrol. In animals with conventional microflora, diethylstilbestrol makes approximately 1.5 passes through the enterohepatic circulation. This increased exposure can amplify the biologic activity of this compound, which is believed to be a carcinogen for vaginal and mammary tissue.

Weisburger et al. studied the metabolism of the carcinogen N-hydroxyfluorenylacetamide, administered parenterally to conventional and germfree rats.[73] Germfree rats excreted appreciably larger amounts of the glucuronide of N-hydroxyfluorenylacetamide in their feces than did conventional animals. The cecal and fecal metabolites in conventional rats were mostly free, unconjugated compounds, whereas the major fraction in germfree animals was conjugated with glucuronic or sulfuric acid.

Morotomi et al. reported that cell-free extracts of some strains of intestinal bacteria, including Bacteroides fragilis, B. vulgatus, B. thetaiotaomicron, Eubacterium lentum, Peptostreptococcus, and Escherichia coli, enhanced the mutagenicity of bile from rats given 1-nitropyrene by using stomach tube.[74] These bacterial cell-free extracts hydrolyzed the synthetic β-D-glucuronides of phenolphthalein and/or p-nitrophenol. Cell-free extracts of bacteria not capable of increasing mutagenicity did not hydrolyze the glucuronides of 1-nitropyrene. Metabolites secreted into the bile can be hydrolyzed in the intestine by bacterial β-glucuronidases to potent mutagenic aglycones.

Nitroreductase and azoreductase are responsible for reducing nitro and azo compounds, respectively, to aromatic amines. The highly reactive intermediates and end products are known mutagens and carcinogens in animals. These enzymes are mostly confined to bacteria residing in the bowel. Azo dyes are used widely in the textile, printing, and food dye industries and in laboratories. Water-soluble azo dyes are degraded by intestinal microorganisms in the gastrointestinal tract.[74] Large-bowel cancer occurs more commonly in highly industrialized countries, and the extent of the use of azo dyes is related to the degree of industrialization of the country. A possible connection may exist between the number of cancer cases and the use of azo dyes.[75]

A 90% correlation exists between carcinogenicity and mutagenicity for aromatic amines and azo dyes tested with the Salmonella/microsomal mutagenicity test.[76] The transformation of azo dyes by intestinal bacteria may be a necessary prerequisite of carcinogenicity.

The reduction of azocompounds by azoreductase is believed to be mediated through a free radical mechanism that produces intermediates that react with proteins and nucleic acids. Azoreductase also can reduce food dyes, releasing phenyl- and naphthyl-substituted amines. These compounds have been implicated as chemical carcinogens.[77] The amines generated in the bowel through the azoreductase reaction are probably further oxidized by microbial enzymes in the intestinal mucosa to carcinogens.

The role of bacteria in the generation of mutagens from a number of azo dyes is noteworthy. Trypan blue is used widely as a biologic stain and is not mutagenic, but reduction by a cell-free extract of Fusobacterium produces a mutagen, O-toluidine,[78] which is mutagenic in the Ames assay and also is carcinogenic.[79] Ponceau 3R, another biologic stain, is reduced in vitro by Fusobacterium to a 2,4,5-trimethylaniline, which has been determined to be mutagenic.[80] Incubation of methyl orange or methyl yellow with intestinal anaerobes and testing with a Salmonella TA 1538 in the presence of a microsomal activating system have proved positive for mutagenicity. Both dyes are reductively cleaved to the mutagen N,N-dimethyl-p-phenylene diazine.[81] Other azo dyes that have been shown to undergo bacterial reduction to mutagenic or carcinogenic products are direct black 38, direct red 2, and direct blue 15. These dyes are converted to benzidine, 3-3-dimethylbenzidine, and 3,3-dimethoxybenzidine, respectively. Congo red is also reduced by rat cecal bacteria to benzidine.[82] In the absence of a bacterial reductase system, however, preincubation of Congo red with cecal bacteria has resulted in a positive mutagenic response.

Nitroreductase causes the formation of reactive nitroso and N-hydroxy intermediates in the course of converting aromatic nitro compounds to aromatic amines. The precursor aromatic nitro compounds are found commonly in factory effluents as industrial chemical pollutants. Wheeler et al. studied a similar reaction, the reduction of p-nitrobenzoic acid, in conventional and germfree rats.[83] Conventional animals rapidly converted p-nitrogenzoic acid, whereas germfree rats reduced little of the nitrocompound.

The nitrated polynuclear aromatic hydrocarbon called 1-nitropyrene is readily formed by reaction of nitrogen oxides with the combustion product pyrene. Its presence in diesel engine exhaust represents a potential health hazard because of its high mutagenicity in bacterial test systems and its carcinogenicity in rats. When 1-nitropyrene was administered orally to conventional rats, 5 to 6% of the dose was detected in the feces as 1-aminopyrine.[84] When a similar experiment was performed on germfree rats, no 1-aminopyrine appeared in the feces. Because reduction of 1-nitropyrene to 1-aminopyrine is an activation process, the results indicate that intestinal microflora are important in the metabolic activation of 1-nitropyrene.

A mixed culture of bacteria obtained from a human fecal specimen has been shown to metabolize the carcinogen 6-nitrochrysene in a semicontinuous culture system.[85] One of the products was 6-aminochrysene, which is carcinogenic in mice. In addition, the intermediate nitrosopolyclic aromatic hydrocarbons formed in this reaction are similar to other biologically active compounds. The results indicate that the ability of the intestinal flora to generate genotoxic compounds from 6-nitrochrysene may be important in the carcinogenicity of this compound. Miller and Miller[86] and Weisburger,[87] after reviewing the evidence, suggested that the products of these reactions are extremely important in chemical carcinogenesis.

The effect of diet on fecal bacterial nitroreductase and azoreductase activity has been studied in rats.[15] Rats initially maintained on a grain diet, then shifted after several weeks to a meat diet, showed a twofold rise in fecal nitroreductase activity on the meat diet. This increase started within 6 days, although the total effect required 12 to 17 days. Fecal azoreductase activity also increased approximately twofold when rats were shifted to the meat diet. An increase in specific activity of this enzyme was noted between 4 and 10 days after the dietary change.

Studies involving human populations have revealed that American vegetarians have lower levels of fecal nitroreductase than Americans eating a Western diet.[17] Fiber supplements to the Western diet do not affect the levels of fecal azoreductase or nitroreductase.

### BILE ACIDS, BEEF, AND BACTERIA

Bile acids have been studied extensively as candidate carcinogens because of their structural similarity to the carcinogenic polycyclic aromatic hydrocarbons. The concentration of fecal bile acids is increased in people eating a beef (high-fat) diet. This concentration induces colonic bacteria to produce larger amounts of 7-α-dehydroxylase, the enzyme involved in conversion of primary to secondary bile acids.[88] Salvioli and co-workers found increased fecal concentrations of choleic and chenodeoxycholic acid and decreased fecal concentrations of secondary bile acids after daily administration of lyophilized Streptococcus faecalis to normal volunteers.[89]

Demographic studies have demonstrated a correlation between high fecal concentrations of secondary bile acids and the Western high-beef diet.[19] Hill et al. noted that the fecal microflora of North Americans and Western Europeans contained more bacterial strains capable of 7-α-dehydroxylation than did those from Ugandans or Indians.[14] In studies by Mower et al. involving Japanese living in Akita, Japan, and Japanese living in Hawaii who adopted a Western-style diet, the latter group had higher levels of fecal deoxycholic acid; however, little difference was noted in levels of the other fecal bile acids.[90] In contrast to these studies, fecal concentrations of coprostanol and coprostanone, degradation products of cholesterol, are higher in people eating a Western-style diet. Mastromarino and co-workers studied patients with colon cancer and found elevated levels of both 7-α-dehydroxylase and cholesterol dehydrogenase compared with normal controls.[88] Elevations of both enzymes also were noted in patients with nonhereditary colonic polyps.[91]

MacDonald et al. studied in vegetarian Seventh-Day Adventists and subjects consuming a mixed Western diet the fecal NAD- and NADP-dependent 7-α-hydroxysteroid dehydrogenase, which converts hydroxy-bile acids to keto-bile acids.[14] The activity was lower in the vegetarian group, suggesting that increased fecal NAD- and NADP-dependent 7-α-hydroxysteroid dehydrogenase is associated with risk of large-bowel cancer.

### BACTERIAL REACTIONS AS PROTECTION AGAINST TUMORS

Most reports dealing with the relationship between the intestinal flora and cancer have emphasized the generation of carcinogens. Evidence exists, however, that the opposite, an inactivation of carcinogenic compounds, also occurs. For example, Rowland and Grasso have shown that E. coli, lactobacillus, bifidobacterium, and bacteroides can degrade the carcinogens dimethylnitrosamine and diphenylnitrosamine to nitrite and the corresponding amine.[92] The reaction could counteract the generation of N-nitroso compounds formed nonenzymatically in the stomach or by bacterial action in the lower intestine.

Williams et al. indicated that bacteria in the cecum of the rat have the ability to dehydroxylate N-hydroxylacetamide.[93] The dehydroxylation of N-hydroxyamines may reverse the activation of amines to proximal carcinogens.

Other studies by Wheeler et al. demonstrated that the intestinal flora can dehydroxylate. N-hydroxyl-4-acetylaminobiphenyl to acetylaminobiphenyl.[94] The reversal of the metabolic activation of the parent carcinogen can be demonstrated in cultures of some bacteria that are indigenous to the intestinal tract. The flora of the cecum is particularly active in this reduction. These experiments may explain the observation that rats fed this compound develop tumors in the forestomach, but not in the cecum.

## REFERENCES


1. Finegold, S.M., Attebery, H.R., Sutter, V.L.: Am. J. Clin. Nutr., *27:*1456–1469, 1974.
2. Moore, W.E.C., Holderman, L.V.: Appl. Environ. Microbiol., *27:*961–979, 1974.
3. Draser, B.S., Hill, M.J.: Human Intestinal Flora. New York, Academic Press, 1974.
4. Draser, B.S., Skinner, M., McLeod, G.M.: Gastroenterology, *56:*71–79, 1969.
5. Moore, W.E.C., Holderman, L.V.: Cancer Res., *35:*3418–3420, 1975.
6. Maier, B.R., et al.: Am. J. Clin. Nutr., *27:*1470–1474, 1974.
7. Reddy, B.S., Weisburger, J.H., Wynder, E.L.: Science, *183:*416–417, 1974.
8. Hill, M.J., et al.: Lancet, *1:*95–100, 1971.
9. Finegold, S.M., et al.: Am. J. Clin. Nutr., *30:*1781–1792, 1977.
10. Draser, B.S., Jenkins, D.J.A., Cummings, J.H.: J. Med. Microbiol., *9:*423–431, 1975.
11. Goldin, B.R., Gorbach, S.L.: Microbial factors and nutrition in carcinogenesis. *In* Advances in Nutritional Research. Edited by H.H. Draper. New York, Plenum Press, 1979.
12. Hill, M.J.: Cancer Res., *35:*3398–3402, 1975.

13. Reddy, B.S., Wynder, E.L.: J. Natl. Cancer Inst., *52*:1437–1442, 1973.
14. MacDonald, L.A., Webb, G.R., Mahoney, D.C.: Am. J. Clin. Nutr., *31*:5233–5238, 1978.
15. Goldin, B.R., Gorbach, S.L.: J. Natl. Cancer Inst., *57*:371–375, 1976.
16. Goldin, B.R., Sullivan, C.E., Gorbach, S.L.: Etiologic factors in the development of colonic cancer: Bacteria, beef and animal fat. *In* Nutrition in Gastrointestinal Diseases. Edited by R.C. Kurtz. New York, Churchill Livingstone, 1981.
17. Goldin, B.R., Swenson, L., Dwyer, J., et al.: J. Natl. Cancer Inst., *64*:255–261, 1980.
18. Lindop, R., Tasman-Jones, C., Thomsen, L.L., et al.: Br. J. Nutr., *54*:21–26, 1985.
19. Wyatt, G.M., Bayliss, C.E., Holcroft, J.D.: Br. J. Nutr., *55*:261–266, 1986.
20. Hawksworth, G., Draser, B.S., Hill, M.J.: J. Med. Microbiol., *4*:451–459, 1971.
21. Laqueur, G.L., Spatz, M.: Cancer Res., *28*:2262–2264, 1968.
22. Tamura, G., Fold, C., Ferro-Luzze, A., et al.: Proc. Natl. Acad. Sci. USA, *77*:4961–4965, 1980.
23. MacDonald, L.A., Bussard, R.G., Hutchinson, D.M., et al.: Appl. Environ. Microbiol., *47*:350–355, 1984.
24. Mader, J.A., MacDonald, L.A.: Mutat. Res., *155*:99–104, 1985.
25. Lindenbaum, J., Rund, D.L., Butler, V.P., et al.: N. Engl. J. Med., *305*:789–794, 1981.
26. Mathan, V.I., Wiederman, J., Dobkin, J.F., et al.: Gut, *30*:971–977, 1989.
27. Alam, A.N., Saha, J.R., Dobkin, J.F., et al.: Gastroenterology, *95*:117–123, 1988.
28. Lindenbaum, J.: Bacterial inactivation of digoxin. 8th International Symposium on Intestinal Microecology, Boston, 1983.
29. Suzuksi, K., Benno, Y., Mitsuoka, T., et al.: Appl. Environ. Microbiol., *37*:379–382, 1979.
30. Parkinson, T.M., Brown, J.P.: Annu. Rev. Nutr., *1*:175–205, 1981.
31. Combes, R.D., Haveland-Smith, R.B.: Mutat. Res., *98*:101–248, 1982.
32. Bonser, G.M., Bradshaw, L., Clayson, D.B., et al.: Br. J. Cancer, *10*:539–546, 1956.
33. Hartman, C.P., Andrews, A.W., Chung, K.T.: Infect. Immun., *23*:686–689, 1979.
34. Chung, K.T., Fulk, G.E., Andrews, A.W., et al.: Mutat. Res., *58*:375–379, 1978.
35. Scheline, R.R.: Pharmacol. Rev., *25*:451–523, 1973.
36. Kojima, S., Ichibagose, H.: Chem. Pharm. Bull. (Tokyo), *14*:971–974, 1966.
37. Renwick, A.G., Williams, R.T.: Biochem. J., *129*:869–879, 1972.
38. Wallace, W.C., Lethco, E.T., Brouwer, E.A.: J. Pharmacol. Exp. Ther., *175*:325–330, 1970.
39. Van Edlere, J., Robben, J., De Pauw, G., et al.: Appl. Environ. Microbiol., *54*:2112–2117, 1988.
40. Asatoor, A.M.: Biochim. Biophys. Acta, *199*:200–202, 1965.
41. Hattori, M., Namba, T., Akoo, T., et al.: Pharmacology, 36(Suppl 1):172–179, 1988.
42. Scheline, R.R.: Monogr. Pharmacol. Physiol., *5*:551–580, 1980.
43. Plaa, G.L.: The enterohepatic circulation. *In* Handbook of Experimental Pharmacology. Edited by J.R. Gillette. New York, Springer, 1975.
44. Kumar, R., Nagubandi, S., Mattox, V.R., et al.: J. Clin. Invest., *65*:277–284, 1980.
45. Goldin, B.R., Adlercreutz, H., Gorbach, S.L., et al.: N. Engl. J. Med., *307*:1542–1547, 1982.
46. Matschiner, J.T., Taggart, W.V., Amelotti, J.M.: Biochemistry, *6*:1243–1248, 1967.
47. Pennock, J.F.: Vitam. Horm., *24*:307–329, 1966.
48. Udall, J.A.: JAMA, *194*:127–129, 1965.
49. Frick, P.G., Riedler, G., Brogli, H.J.: J. Appl. Physiol., *23*:387–389, 1967.
50. Albert, M.J., Mathan, V.I., Baker, S.J.: Nature, *283*:781–783, 1980.
51. Coates, M.E., Fuller, R.: The gnotobiotic animal in the study of gut microbiology. *In* Microbial Ecology of the Gut Flora. Edited by R.T.J. Clarke, T. Bauchop. New York, Academic Press, 1977, pp. 311–342.
52. Wostman, B.S.: Annu. Rev. Nutr., *1*:257–279, 1981.
53. Hoskins, L.C., Boulding, E.T.: J. Clin. Invest., *57*:63–73, 1976.
54. Cummings, J.H.: Gut, *22*:763–779, 1981.
55. McNeil, N.I., Cummings, J.H., James, W.P.T.: Gut, *19*:819–822, 1978.
56. Ferezou, J., Coste, T., Chevallier, F.: Digestion, *21*:232–243, 1981.
57. Simon, G.L., Gorbach, S.L.: Dig. Dis. Sci., *31*:147S–162S, 1986.
58. Tabaqchali, S., Booth, C.C.: Lancet, *2*:12–16, 1966.
59. Fry, R.J.M.: Nature, *203*:1396–1398, 1964.
60. Raicht, R.F.F., Deschner, E., Salem, G.: Gastroenterology, *68*:979, 1975.
61. King, C.E., Toskes, P.P.: Gastroenterology, *76*:1035–1055, 1979.
62. Welkos, S., Toskes, P.P., Baker, H.: Gastroenterology, *80*:313–320, 1981.
63. Gracey, M.: Am. J. Clin. Nutr., *32*:234–243, 1979.
64. Prizont, R., Whitehead, J.S., Kim, Y.S.: Gastroenterology, *69*:1254–1264, 1975.
65. Armstrong, B., Doll, R.: Int. J. Cancer, *15*:617–631, 1975.
66. Howell, M.A.: J. Chron. Dis., *28*:67–80, 1975.
67. Draser, B.S., Irving, D.: Br. J. Cancer, *27*:167–172, 1973.
68. Dunn, J.E.: Cancer Res., *35*:3240–3245, 1975.
69. Mastromarino, A., Reddy, B.S., Wynder, E.L.: Am. J. Clin. Nutr., *29*:1455–1460, 1976.
70. Druckery, H., Preussman, R., Matzbies, F., et al.: Naturwissenschaften, *54*:285–286, 1967.
71. Laqueur, G.L., McDaniel, E.G., Matsumoto, H.: J. Natl. Cancer Inst., *39*:355–371, 1967.
72. Fisher, L.K., Millburn, P., Smith, R.L.: Biochem. J., *100*:69, 1966.
73. Weisburger, J.H., Grantham, P.H., Horton, R.E.: Biochem. Pharmacol., *19*:151–162, 1970.
74. Morotomi, M., Nanno, M., Watanrobe, T., et al.: Mutat. Res., *149*:171–178, 1985.
75. Chung, K.T.: Mutat. Res., *114*:269–281, 1983.
76. Wolff, A.W., Oehme, F.W.J.: Am. Vet. Med. Assoc., *164*:623–629, 1974.
77. Weisburger, J.J., Weisburger, E.K.: Pharmacol. Rev., *25*:1–66, 1973.
78. Hartman, C.P., Falk, C.E., Andrews, A.W.: Mutat. Res., *58*:125–132, 1978.
79. Weisburger, J.J., Weisburger E.K.: Chem. Eng. News, *44*:124–142, 1966.
80. Hartman, C.P., Andres, A.W., Chung, K.T.: Infect. Immun., *23*:686–689, 1979.
81. Chung, K.T., Fulk, C.E., Andrews, A.W.: Mutat. Res., *58*:375–379, 1978.
82. Reid, T.M., Morton, K.C., Wang, C.Y., et al.: Mutat. Res., *117*:105–112, 1983.

**83.** Wheeler, L.A., Soderberg, F.B., Goldman, P.: J. Pharmacol. Exp. Ther., *194:*135–144, 1975.
**84.** El-Bayoumy, K., Fharma, C., Louis, Y.M., et al.: Cancer Lett., *19:*311–316, 1983.
**85.** Manning, B.W., Campbell, W.L., Franklin, W., et al.: Appl. Environ. Microbiol., *54:*197–203, 1988.
**86.** Miller, J.A., Miller, E.C.: Prog. Exp. Tumor Res., *11:*273–301, 1969.
**87.** Weisburger, J.H.: Cancer, *28:*60–70, 1971.
**88.** White, B.A., Lipsky, R.L., Prieke, R.J., et al.: Steroids, *35:*103–109, 1980.
**89.** Salvioli, G., et al.: Digestion, *23:*80–88, 1981.
**90.** Mower, H.F., et al.: Cancer Res., *39:*328–331, 1979.
**91.** Mastromarino, A.J., Reddy, B.S., Wynder, F.L.: Cancer Res., *38:*4458–4462, 1978.
**92.** Rowland, L.R., Grasso, P.: Appl. Environ. Microbiol., *29:*7–12, 1973.
**93.** Williams, J.R., Grantham, P.H., Marsh, H.H., et al.: Biochem. Pharmacol., *19:*173–188, 1970.
**94.** Wheeler, L.A., Soderberg, F.B., Goldman, P.: Cancer Res., *35:*2962–2968, 1975.

CHAPTER **39**

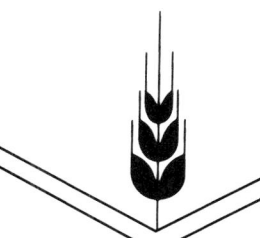

# Diet Factors Affecting Nutrient Absorption and Metabolism

**David J.A. Jenkins, Thomas M.S. Wolever, and Alexandra L. Jenkins**



In the treatment of gastrointestinal disease, emphasis has been placed on improving absorption of nutrients in conditions such as Crohn's disease, celiac disease, short bowel and stagnant loop syndromes, radiation enteropathy, postgastrectomy disorders, and Whipple's disease. In other situations, however, therapies have attempted to reduce the rate or amount of nutrients absorbed. These include the treatment of diabetes, hyperlipidemia, or obesity using, for example, high-fiber diets, enzyme inhibitors, nonabsorbable food substitutes, or gastric stapling.

Manipulations that increase or decrease the rate of absorption are likely to have certain physiologic consequences, as illustrated in Figures 39–1 and 39–2. Where the absorption rate is reduced, a larger length of small intestine is likely to be exposed to the nutrient, with an increased proportion absorbed more distally (see Fig. 39–1*A*). On the other hand, rapidly absorbed foods are likely to be taken up more proximally in the small intestine and over a shorter segment (see Fig. 39–1*B*). After oral intake, the consequences of the slower flux of nutrient into the system will result in lower circulating nutrient levels and consequently lower endocrine responses (see Fig. 39–2*A*), as opposed to the sharper rises and falls seen with the more rapid fluxes (see Fig. 39–2*B*). In addition, differences can be expected in nutrient absorption characteristics (e.g., chylomicra synthesis), depending on the region of the bowel in which this takes place. Regional specialization also occurs in terms of gut endocrine responses to nutrients absorbed in different parts of the bowel. For example, more gastric inhibitory polypeptide (GIP) will be secreted when carbohydrates are absorbed proximally and more enteroglucagon will be secreted when they are absorbed distally.

The food factors that influence the absorption of nutrients relate not only to the nature of the nutrients themselves, but also to their interaction with each other and with the nonabsorbable components of the food, the dietary fiber, and associated antinutrients. All these factors combined produce the form or physical state of the food, which itself exerts a major influence on the handling of a food by the gastrointestinal tract. Some of these effects are short term, but food constituents also have long-term effects. They may influence the absorptive capacity of the gut either by enzyme induction or by effects that may be stimulatory, inhibitory, or toxic to mucosal cell growth, turnover, and villus structure.

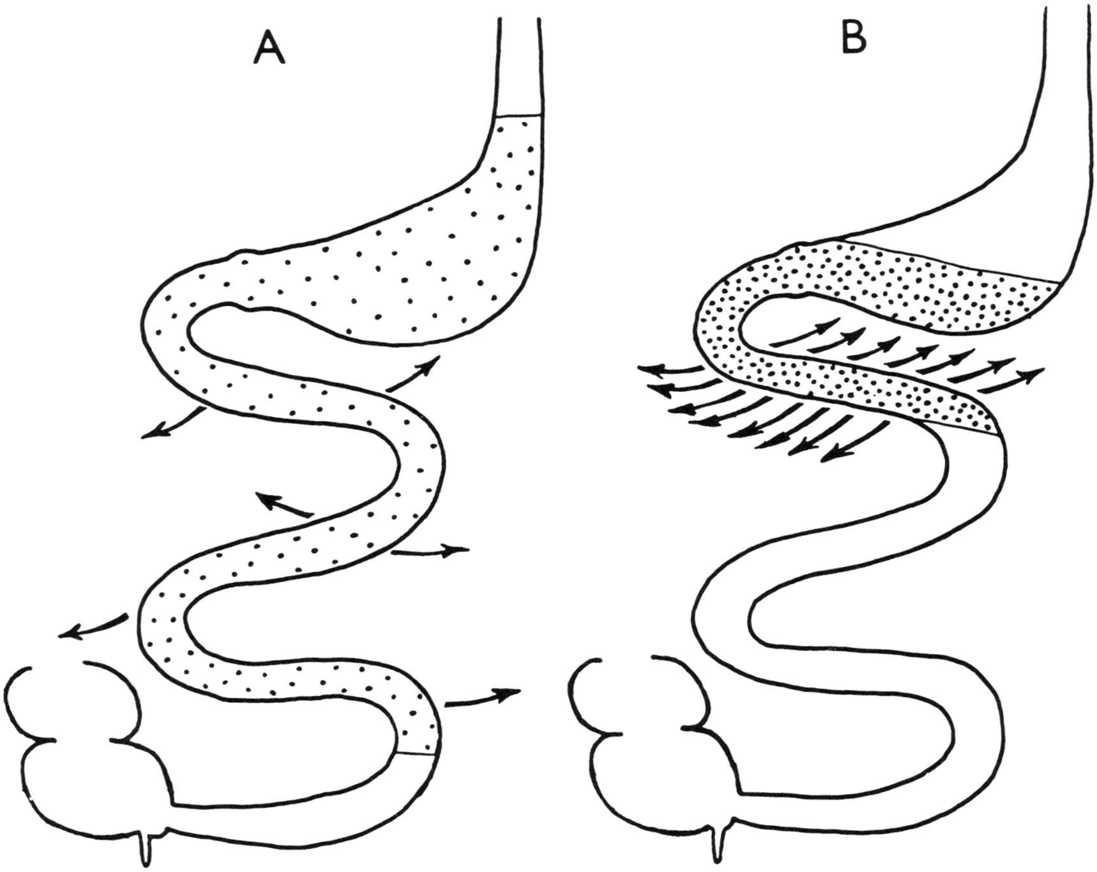
A
B

**FIGURE 39–1.** Schematic representation of stomach and small intestine showing *(A)* slow digestion and absorption of energy-dilute food in a "fiber-rich" diet and *(B)* rapid digestion and absorption of energy-dense food from a low-fiber diet.

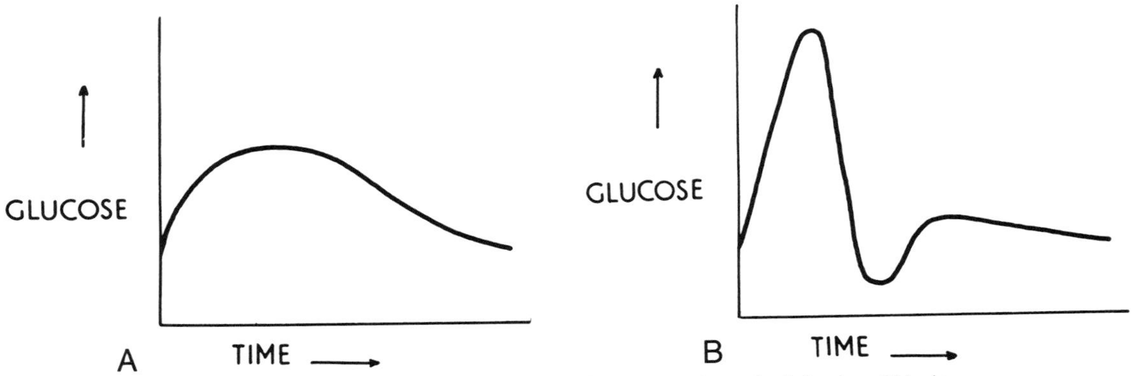
GLUCOSE
A
TIME
GLUCOSE
B
TIME

**FIGURE 39–2.** Schematic representation of the postprandial glycemia following *(A)* slow absorption of starchy fiber-rich meals and *(B)* rapid absorption with undershoot due to excessive insulin release following refined, fiber-depleted carbohydrate foods.

## EFFECT OF MACRONUTRIENTS AND FIBER

Before discussing the effects of food form and the so-called antinutrients on the absorbability of natural diets, it is useful to consider both the similarities and the differences that exist within the three macronutrient groupings and their relationships to each other and to fiber.

### CARBOHYDRATE

Traditionally, it was held that "complex" carbohydrates (starches) are absorbed more slowly than "simple" carbohydrates.[1] Meals therefore that contain a higher proportion of their carbohydrates as sugars were considered to result in more rapid absorption and higher blood glucose rises.[2] This view has been challenged by several studies. Using solutions of starch (a glucose polymer), caloreen (predominantly 5 glucose units), and glucose itself, Wahlquist and colleagues demonstrated similar glucose and insulin rises following consumption of 50-g carbohydrate loads of each of these glucose sources by healthy volunteers.[3]

#### *STARCH*

Such results should have been predictable because earlier work of Dahlquist and Borgstrom and Fogel and Gray had indicated that luminal hydrolysis of starch is not rate-limiting for starch digestion.[4,5] Fogel and Gray had stated that even patients with chronic pancreatitis and significant exocrine pancreatic insufficiency (10% amylase secretion rate compared with normal) nevertheless hydrolyzed starch in vivo at a rate similar to that of normal subjects.[5] Their studies involved feeding 50-g starch loads and aspirating the residual hydrolytic contents at the ligament of Treitz (duodenojejunal junction). Nevertheless, this finding does not indicate that luminal events are unimportant in the digestion of foods of complex composition. Rather, it indicates that differences in absorption are unlikely to be seen among meals containing sugars or highly processed, low amylose, or soluble starches (25 to 30% amylose and 70 to 75% amylopectin).[6] Such a statement does not cover the important effects of differences in food form or indigestible food components that may have a profound effect on the rate of luminal digestion.

If, however, the proportion of amylose (1-4 linked straight chain starch) to amylopectin (1-6 linked branched starch) varies in a food, then alterations in digestibility may be seen. Traditionally, such branching was considered nutritionally significant because α-amylase has poor specificity for 1-6 branch points and produces α-limit dextrins.[7] Digestion was considered to proceed more slowly for this reason. It now appears, however, the brush border α-glucosidases are so efficient that it makes no difference in terms of rates of uptake whether the substrate for absorption is glucose, maltose, or α-limit dextrins.[8] Some evidence even indicates that absorption is more rapid as chain length increases up to 10 glucose units.[8] Part of the explanation may be related to the reduced osmotic effect.

Nevertheless, differences do exist between amylose and amylopectin, but opposite to what was originally expected. This phenomenon may relate to the more compact structure and hydrogen bonding of the glucose chains in amylose, which render it physically less accessible to amylolytic attack than the more open and branched amylopectin.[9] In this respect, raw legume starch (higher in amylose) has been shown in rats to be less digestible than cornstarch (higher in amylopectin), and the rate of hydrolysis of legume starch in vitro is less than that of cornstarch.[10,11] Possible differences in the nature of starches from different foods have been emphasized by Crapo and co-workers.[12–15] In vivo studies of whole legumes (30 to 40% amylose) have indicated that they produce lower glycemic responses than cereals (25 to 30% amylose).[16,17] They are also digested less rapidly in vitro than other starchy foods.[18,19] As expected from their higher amylose content, they produce more glucose and less maltotriose on digestion. Studies with high-amylose long-grain rice have demonstrated that the amylose content relates to the glycemic effect of the rice. The greater the amylose content, the flatter the response.[20] High-amylose diets have been shown to reduce insulin secretion and serum lipids in healthy volunteers.[21]

Furthermore, the degree of hydration of the starch is a major determinant of digestibility,[22] and this is a function of both cooking and other forms of processing. Cooked starch produced higher blood glucose responses than raw starch (Fig. 39–3).[23] This effect may be due to the degree of gelatinization of starch. The uptake of water by the starch molecule may render it more accessible to enzymatic digestion. In addition, processing (milling) prior to cooking legumes was more effective in increasing digestibility than grinding after cooking,[24] and damp heat had more effect than dry heat in making both the carbohydrate[24–26] and protein[27,28] more easily absorbed.

Comparisons of legumes and cereal foods illustrate many facets of foods that influence absorbability. Studies have clearly demonstrated the slower digestibility of legumes by comparison with cereal products and the relationship of digestibility with the glycemic response in both normal and diabetic volunteers.[19,29] Nevertheless, such studies also highlight the other factors of possible importance including food form, fiber, and non-nutritive food factors (including the so-called antinutrients) in determining absorbability of carbohydrate from foods.

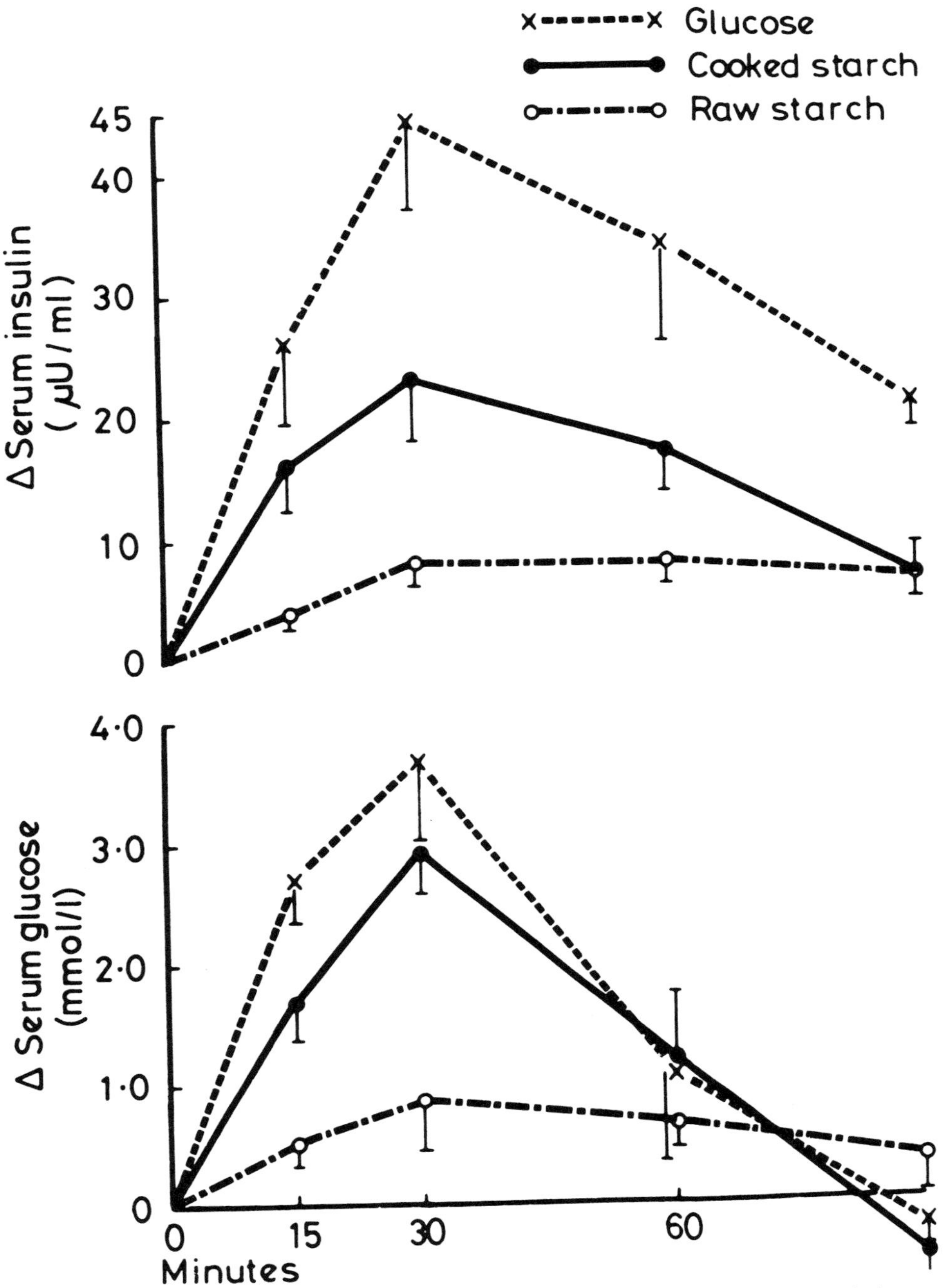

Glucose
Cooked starch
Raw starch
Δ Serum insulin (μU / ml)
45
40
30
20
10
0
Δ Serum glucose (mmol/l)
4·0
3·0
2·0
1·0
0
0
15
30
60
Minutes


**FIGURE 39–3.** Mean serum insulin and glucose concentrations after ingestion of glucose monohydrate (1.1 g/kg body weight) and cooked and raw cornstarch (0.91 g/kg body weight) in healthy volunteers. Conversion (SI to traditional units): glucose: 1mmol/L ≈ 18 mg/dl. (From Collings, P., Williams, C., MacDonald, I., Br. Med. J., *282*:1032, 1981.)

*SUGARS*

Efficient transport systems exist for maltose, maltotriose, α-limit dextrins, sucrose, lactose, glucose, and galactose. Fructose absorption is less efficient and the transport maxima may be exceeded with large amounts of this sugar. The pentose, D-xylose, is only approximately 50% absorbed, and considerable malabsorption is found with the sugar alcohols or polyols, sorbitol and xylitol.[30] Therefore, great differences exist among sugars in the rate and proportions likely to be absorbed.

Investigators have shown much interest in the comparative effects of sugars and starches on metabolic responses. Contrary to many previous assumptions, numerous studies have shown that the response to sucrose in both normal and diabetic volunteers is less than that after an equivalent amount of starch.[16,31] Nevertheless, large differences are apparent in the degree to which different sugars raise the blood glucose concentration: fructose causes a comparatively small rise, lactose and sucrose are intermediate, and glucose and maltose cause the highest rises.[16,32–35] This effect appears to relate to the proportion of the sugar molecule that is glucose, with nonglucose components raising the blood glucose minimally. On the other hand, it is becoming apparent that fructose may raise serum lipids by comparison with starch and so may offset the advantage of slower absorption and flatter glycemic response.[36]

## FATS

Although much work has been done on the absorption of fatty acids, most fat in the human diet is in the form of triglycerides. Studies by Calloway, Kurtz et al. indicated comparable digestibility of many edible fats including butter, lard, and soybean, coconut, corn, and cottonseed oils.[37] Early work had already demonstrated that butter, lard, shortening, and cod liver and corn oils were all absorbed to the same extent, with maximum absorption occurring within 6 to 8 hours at a time when the chylomicra rise would also have peaked.[16,31–35,37–41] It was estimated that 24 to 41% of the fat was absorbed by 2 hours, 53 to 71% by 4 hours, 68 to 86% by 6 hours, and 97 to 99% after 12 hours.[38] In comparisons of lymphatic absorption of long-chain fatty acids, including palmitic, oleic, linoleic, and stearic acids in man, there was a slight discrimination against triglyceride synthesis from stearic acid and in favor of cholesterol ester synthesis from oleic acid.[42] In addition, other studies suggest that triglycerides composed of the saturated dietary fatty acids (palmitic and stearic) are less well absorbed in the presence of high calcium, whereas triglycerides containing the unsaturated fats of lower melting point (oleic and linoleic) are unaffected.[43,44] Investigators have suggested that, in general, either palmitic or stearic acid in the 1,3 positions of the triglyceride molecule reduces the absorption of that fat.[45,46]

Through the use of medium-chain triglycerides (MCT) in drinks, baked foods, and enteral feedings, however, attempts have been made to increase the absorption of dietary fat. Their advantage lies in their direct absorption without micelle formation with uptake as the fatty acid into the portal vein and clearance by the liver. They can therefore be absorbed even in the absence of bile salts or when lipoprotein synthesis necessary for chylomicra production is impaired or absent. Animal studies suggest that the efficiency of absorption of MCT is four times that of long-chain triglycerides.[47]

The use of MCT has been advocated in various situations, including small intestinal disease or damage, short bowel syndrome, pancreatic and biliary insufficiency (biliary atresia), and α-β-lipoproteinemia (Tangier disease). Their disadvantages are several. They do not stimulate chylomicra formation, and fat-soluble vitamins are therefore not transported out of the enterocyte.[48] In addition, in experiments on rats, dietary substitution of MCT for corn oil resulted in 20% less weight gain, largely through lack of deposition of carcass fat. In man, weight gain has been variable,[42] and the early clinical use of MCT was in the control of obesity.[49,50] The increased absorptive efficiency of the gut for MCT was questioned on the grounds that the widely used solvent system for stool lipid extraction in the Van de Kamer method[51] only extracts up to 68% of the medium- to short-chain fatty acids;[52] however, it was noted that in the titrimetric determination, where the assumed mean fatty acids molecular weight is 284, the conversion factor is twice that which should be applied to the MCT (mean molecular weight, 144) to derive the grams of fat malabsorbed. The two errors should therefore balance out.[53] Cramping abdominal pain and increased diarrhea together with increased steatorrhea have been reported in the short bowel syndrome following MCT use, however.[54] In addition, MCT should not be used in decompensated cirrhosis because poor clearance of short- and medium-chain fatty acids may exacerbate encephalopathy.[55,56] Further cautioning against possible associations with liver disease is a report of two instances in which cirrhosis evolved in young patients with α-β-lipoproteinemia who were fed diets high in MCT on a long-term basis.[57]

Thus, in terms of dietary fats, foods and dishes containing oleic or linoleic acid appear to be well absorbed. MCT may have an advantage in specific states, but it should be monitored with caution. As the dietary fat load is increased, proportionate increases in fecal fat losses occur.[58]

## PROTEIN

Comparatively little is known of the intrinsic digestibility of proteins from different food sources independent of other factors in the food such as enzyme inhibitors. Some recent data suggest that differences exist among such common protein foods as, for example, eggs, meats, poultry, fish, and cheeses that might favor their specific incorporation into the therapeutic diets of patients with limited absorptive capacity. In general, evidence indicates that animal proteins are more rapidly absorbed and metabolized than vegetable proteins.[59] Surprisingly, in patients with cirrhosis, nitrogen balance studies have indicated no advantage of conventional animal protein foods over protein from cereal and legumes.[60–62]

Although foods may be processed in ways that may influence the digestibility of their constituent proteins, studies have focused on the total amount absorbed or retained, rather than on how the rate of absorption may be modified.

When protein foods are heated, cross-linking may occur among amino acids or between amino acid side chains and sugars. In this last reaction, the free $NH_2$ groups on the lysine chains combine with the reducing groups of sugars, especially in the presence of heat, such as in baking of breads or cereal products and the manufacture of breakfast cereals. This synthesis (Maillard reaction) reduces the effectiveness of tryptic digestion and in experimental animals reduces the biologic value of the protein. The effect on blood amino acid responses in man remains to be assessed.

In addition, much work is being done on modifying proteins such as those of soy,[63] fish,[64] casein, and whey[65] to improve such functional properties as solubility, emulsifying capacity, and heat stability, so they may be used in human foods. Their nutritional and digestibility properties will be reduced, however, because common methods involve succinylation or acetylation of the ϵ-amino group of lysine, the hydroxyl group of serine and threonine, the sulfhydryl group of cysteine, the phenol group of tyrosine, or the imidazole group of histidine.[66] In vitro, succinylated proteins have low digestibility, owing to resistance of the succinyl-lysyl bonds to pancreatic digestion.[66,67]

In terms of processing, the predominant effect is therefore to reduce the digestibility of the proteins. Nevertheless, these same processes (e.g., heat) may be essential to remove the antinutrients from other food sources (e.g., legumes, cereals, and tubers) and to enhance digestibility. Thus, use of heat in the achievement of this latter objective is likely to have a net positive rather than negative nutritional impact.

## DIETARY FIBER

Many of the differences in the digestibility of foods that cannot be explained by intrinsic differences in their macronutrient components are attributable to differences in their dietary fiber or antinutrient constituents. Large differences exist in the physical form and the physiologic effect of various classes of dietary fiber. In general, purified viscous fibers such as the gums, gels, and mucilages reduce the rate of nutrient absorption, whereas the particulate fibers (e.g., cereal brans) have little effect on nutrient absorption in the small intestine but have a major impact on colonic function (see later in this section).

Dietary fibers of the viscous type, such as the gums and pectic substances, delay gastric emptying[68–71] and slow small intestinal uptake of sugars, amino acids,[72,73] and drugs such as acetaminophen and digoxin.[68,74] Fiber is also associated with increased fecal losses of bile acids.[75,76] The effect of fiber on the small intestine is thought to be due to its ability to increase the thickness of the unstirred water layer, which acts as a barrier to diffusion of nutrients to the enterocyte brush border. Studies using pectin have supported this concept.[77] It has also been suggested, however, that the effect of viscous fibers in slowing absorption is due simply to impedance of diffusion in the bulk phase. The mechanism may also differ along the length of the small intestine as water is absorbed. Use of a triple-tube lumen and balloon tamponade to isolate a segment of human small intestine in vivo has shown that addition of guar to the perfusate reduces the rate of small intestinal absorption of glucose.[78] Nevertheless, although slow absorption has been observed, malabsorption has not resulted, as judged by urinary recoveries of xylose,[73] acetaminophen,[68] and the lack of breath $H_2$ evolution.[79] In addition, only minimally raised fat and protein losses have been reported, as judged by the marginally increased outputs of protein and fat from the terminal ileum[80] after bran supplementation. Viscous fiber preparations, possibly because of their lipid emulsion stabilizing property, are associated with enhanced chylomicronemia and higher postprandial fat-soluble vitamin levels.[81,82] Similar enhanced vitamin A absorption has been seen with cholestyramine at a low level,[83] but not at high levels where fat absorption is depressed.[84]

Viscous fiber preparations have been used in the management of diabetes,[85–88] as well as to reduce serum cholesterol levels in hyperlipidemia.[89–91] These preparations also improve symptoms in the dumping syndrome following gastric surgery.[70,92,93] Detailed studies have demonstrated that the addition of viscous fiber to test meals resulted in blunting of the glucose, insulin, and GIP responses when taken with a glucose load,[93] less of an undershoot in blood glucose,[92] and less hemoconcentration assessed by hematocrit.[94]

The results are less clear in terms of the effect of fiber in foods on reducing the rate of absorption and altering associated metabolic events. No significant differences were found between white bread, pasta, and rice and their wholemeal or bran equivalents in terms of glycemic response[94,95] (Fig. 39–4) or digestibility.[19] In addition, when over 50 foods of equivalent carbohydrate content were compared, the flattening in postprandial glycemia was significantly negatively related to their fat and protein contents, but not to fiber (Fig. 39–5).[16] This may have been due to the large number of high-cereal fiber foods examined. Because cereal fiber appears to have little effect on small intestinal absorption, the effect of

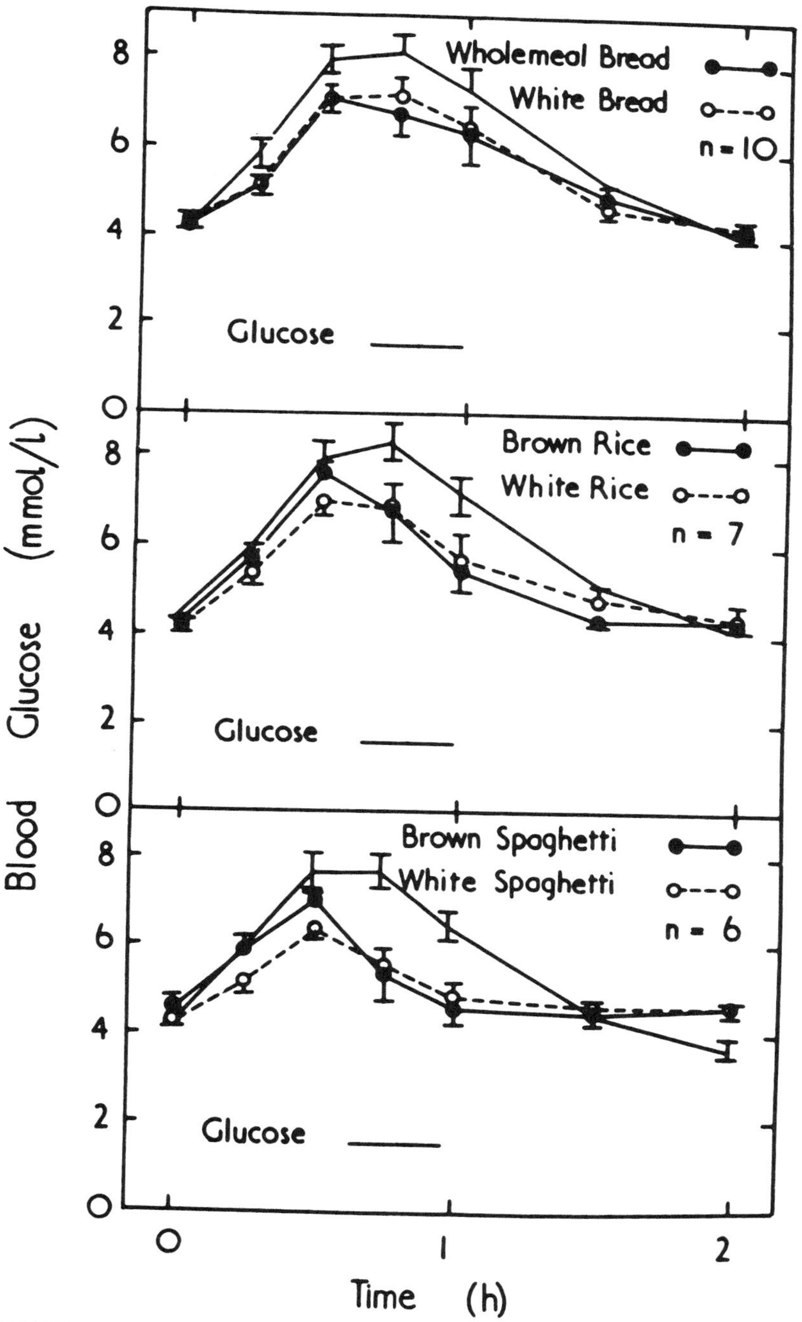
Wholemeal Bread
White Bread
n = 10
Glucose
Brown Rice
White Rice
n = 7
Glucose
Brown Spaghetti
White Spaghetti
n = 6
Glucose
Blood Glucose (mmol/L)
8
6
4
2
0
0
1
2
Time (h)

**FIGURE 39–4.** Effect of fiber depletion on the mean blood glucose curves after eating 50-g carbohydrate portions of bread, rice, and spaghetti compared with 50-g glucose tolerance tests. (From Jenkins, D.J.A., Wolever, T.M.S., Taylor, R.H., et al.: Diabetes Care, *4*:509–513, 1981.)

other types of fiber may have been obscured. The selection of fiber sources may be all important because this debate continues, with some,[96] but not all,[97] workers finding a fiber-glycemic index relationship.

Studies with purified fibers therefore indicate that certain types of fiber may affect the absorbability of foods. Fiber in unprocessed foods is also likely to influence the absorption of the macronutrient components in a Western diet through its effect on food form however, (discussed later).

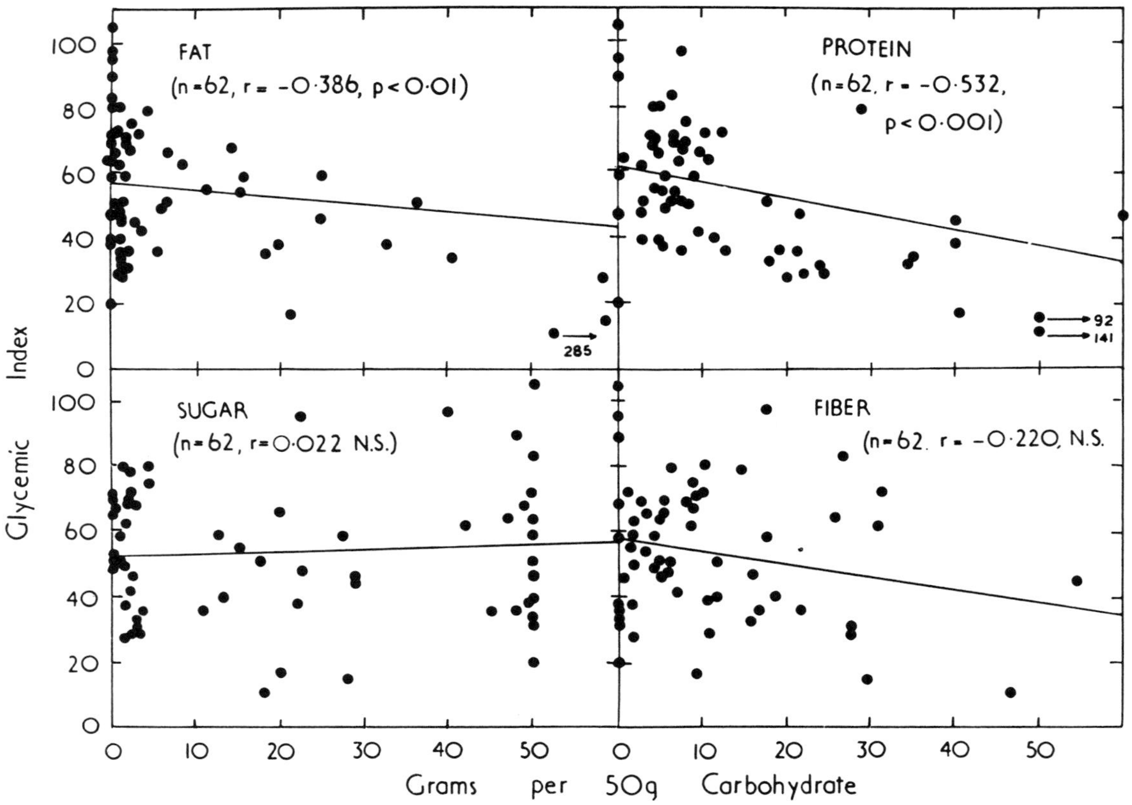
FAT
(n=62, r= -0·386, p<0·01)
PROTEIN
(n=62, r= -0·532, p<0·001)
SUGAR
(n=62, r=0·022 N.S.)
FIBER
(n=62, r= -0·220, N.S.
285
92
141
Glycemic Index
Grams per 50g Carbohydrate

**FIGURE 39–5.** Relationship of fat, protein, and fiber content of 62 foods and sugars with the glycemic index of 50-g carbohydrate portions. (From Jenkins, D.J.A., Wolever, T.M.S., Taylor, R.H.: Am. J. Clin. Nutr., *34*:362–366, 1981.)

## NUTRIENT-NUTRIENT INTERACTIONS IN FOODS

The nutrient-nutrient interactions have a significant effect on the digestibility of foods. Studies using breath hydrogen measurement to assess carbohydrate malabsorption have indicated significant (10 to 20%) malabsorption from white bread and other farinaceous products.[98] When gluten-free flour was used, no malabsorption was seen, nor was malabsorption produced by adding back purified gluten to the same level as found originally in the white bread (Fig. 39–6). The investigators concluded that the natural physical interaction of the starch and protein in wheat limited its rate of digestion, resulting in malabsorption of a proportion.[98] The implication of this study is that patients without definite evidence of celiac disease who are placed on a gluten-free diet and appear to improve may do so because of the enhanced availability of dietary starch, rather than the elimination of the gliadin component of wheat protein. Such a measure may therefore have general therapeutic applicability where malabsorption of carbohydrate (starch) is a problem. Of additional interest in this respect is the finding that the in vitro digestion rate of gluten-free or gluten-reconstituted bread was more rapid than that of regular bread and the in vivo glycemic response to feeding breads made of these flours (gluten reduced) was also higher.[99]

Conversely, the presence of protein in the small intestine aids in the stabilization of fat emulsions and enhances micelle formation and fatty acid uptake.[39,100] This finding has been demonstrated with casein given with olive oil to dogs,[39,100] in mixtures of proteins (bovine albumin and bovine hemaglobin/ovalbumin mixture), and in various digests of these administered to rats.[100] In addition, the effect of fiber in reducing the glycemic response to carbohydrate has been reported to diminish as the level of dietary protein increases.[101]

Fat, on the other hand, has long been recognized for its ability to delay gastric emptying,[102] and thus it slows the digestion and absorption of other nutrients. The degree to which this is achieved, however, may depend on the stability of the fat-food mixture because separation of fat into an upper lipid phase may cause the fat to have little effect on the gastric emptying of the carbohydrate and protein lying below.

A starch-lipid interaction has been described in which the hydrocarbon chain of a monoglyceride becomes

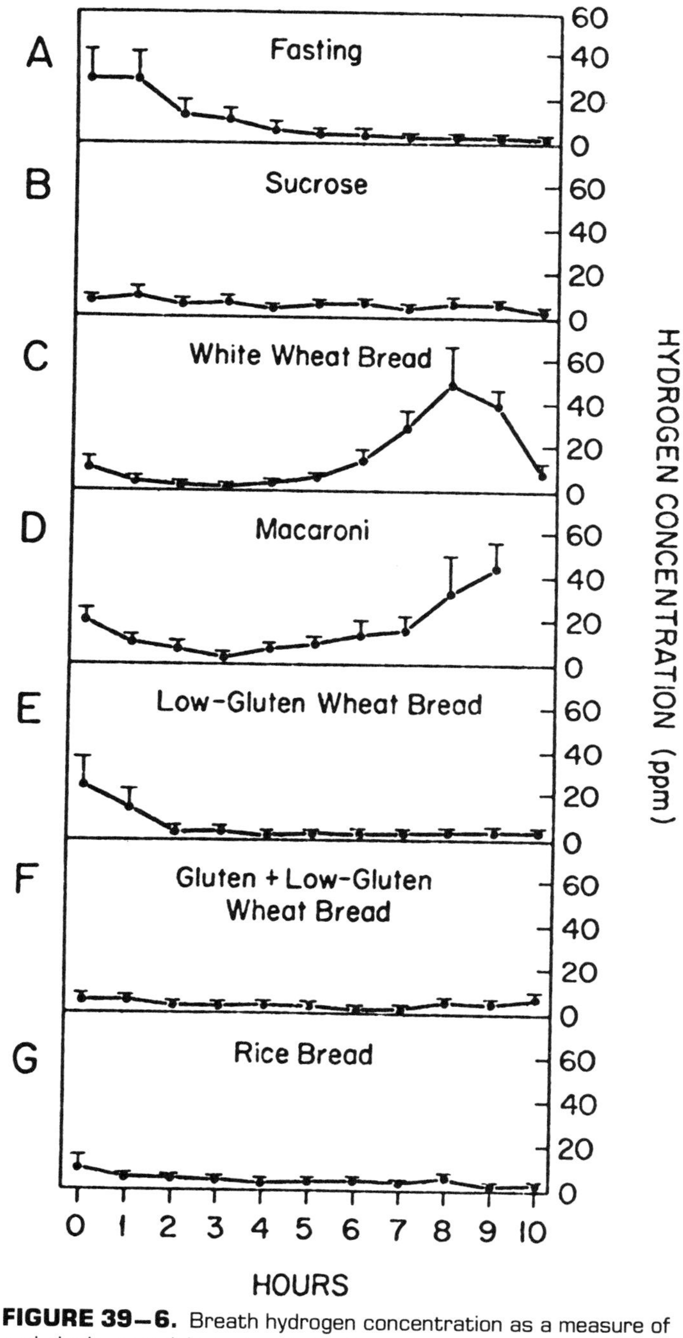
A
Fasting
B
Sucrose
C
White Wheat Bread
D
Macaroni
E
Low-Gluten Wheat Bread
F
Gluten + Low-Gluten Wheat Bread
G
Rice Bread
0 1 2 3 4 5 6 7 8 9 10
HOURS
0 20 40 60
HYDROGEN CONCENTRATION (ppm)

**FIGURE 39–6.** Breath hydrogen concentration as a measure of carbohydrate malabsorption in healthy volunteers during a 10-hour fast (A) and after ingestion of 100 g carbohydrate (B through G). (Ref. 90 with permission N. Engl. J. Med.) (From Anderson, I.H., Levine, A.S., Levitt, M.D.: N. Engl. J. Med., *304*:891–892, 1981, by permission of the New England Journal of Medicine.)

embedded within the relatively hydrophobic internal portion of the amylose α-helical structure.[103] Investigators have suggested that starch-lipid interactions may form in the upper part of the small intestine during fat ingestion and may slow the rate of starch digestion and reduce the glycemic response.

Lipid-lipid interactions are also important. For example, lecithin may enhance triglyceride absorption by facilitating micelle formation.[39,104] Similarly, owing to their effect in stimulating chylomicra formation, long-chain fatty acids increase cholesterol absorption[105] and, most important, the absorption of fat-soluble vitamins.[106]

### MICRONUTRIENT INTERACTIONS

The discussion has so far focused on the factors affecting the absorption of the so-called macronutrients from foods, rather than the minerals, trace elements, and vitamins. At this level is another series of interrelationships. Evidence indicates that fiber binds minerals in vitro.[107] Various types of fiber have been shown to reduce the absorbability of calcium ($Ca^{++}$), iron ($Fe^{++}$), and magnesium ($Mg^{++}$).[108–111] Phytate, a fiber-associated antinutrient, may also be an important factor, although the relation of this substance to deficiency states is not clear. Results are affected by the kind of fiber and by the presence of other agents that occur in foods. Responses to test meals given human subjects indicate that fiber may decrease absorption of iron and zinc.[112] Responses were affected by amounts of fiber and minerals and by the presence of protein and phytate in test meals. Although fiber intakes by vegetarians have been reported to be higher than those for omnivores, studies do not reveal differences in blood mineral levels between the two groups.[112]

Results of human balance studies involving fiber and mineral bioavailability are controversial. Many factors influence the outcome of such studies and they are therefore difficult to evaluate. Phytate and oxalate in food can also bind minerals and may contribute to decreased mineral balances.[113] The relative levels of fiber, minerals, protein, and other substances in the diet are important and contribute to the confusion in attempts to compare different studies. The type of fiber is also a variable, and indications are that insoluble fibers are more likely than soluble fibers to have an adverse effect on mineral bioavailability.

The length of the study period is another important factor in evaluating the results of human balance studies.[114] Adaptation to a different level of mineral intake or to a different level of availability may take considerable time, depending on the magnitude of the change. Thus, study subjects fed a lower level of intake of a mineral than in their usual diets may develop negative mineral balance at the beginning of the study, but they may become adapted to the new level of intake if sufficient time is allowed.

From reports of balance studies in the literature, it appears that an intake of 25 g per day of insoluble fiber does not have an adverse effect on mineral nutrition when adequate levels of mineral intake are maintained.

Consumption of long-chain fatty acids facilitates fat-soluble vitamin uptake. High levels of fat in the diet may increase $Ca^{++}$ losses in the feces.[115] Raising the dietary protein intake may diminish the absorption of zinc ($Zn^{++}$), copper ($Cu^{++}$), and $Ca^{++}$ all in the presence of modest amounts of fiber.[101] In the colon, the reduction of pH by carbohydrate fermentation favors the absorption of $Mg^{++}$[116] and vitamin K.[117] Many other such interrelationships are discussed in their respective sections of this book.

## INFLUENCE OF FOOD FORM AND NON-NUTRIENT FOOD COMPONENTS

Many of the studies showing differences in the absorbability of natural diets have been carried out in relation to those factors concerned with the absorption of carbohydrate from foods. Much of the present discussion therefore concentrates on carbohydrate digestibility as an illustration of the general principles. Factors include food form, fiber content, and the presence of lectins, tannins, saponins, and phytates. The possible role of fiber has already been mentioned.

### FOOD FORM

The form in which a food is eaten is a major determinant of its rate of digestion and absorption. Apples eaten whole, as opposed to blended, produced flatter blood glucose and insulin responses as an indication of the slower rate of absorption.[118] Crapo and co-workers demonstrated differences in glucose and insulin responses to a range of starchy foods including baked potato, boiled rice, bread, and corn that in part might be attributed to food form.[12,13] Maize and rice produced the least responses, representing whole seeds, whereas baked potato, a less "compact" food, approximated the blood glucose rise seen when the equivalent amount of carbohydrate was given as glucose.[12–14] The importance of this finding was further brought out by studies demonstrating that rice that was ground and then cooked gave rises in blood glucose and insulin approximating those for glucose,[119] together with a more rapid rate of in vitro digestion compared with whole rice.

Particle size, an important aspect of food, is not detected by assessment of chemical composition of the diet. Many traditional foods with low glycemic indices have large particle sizes. Such foods include whole-grain barley, as used in traditional soups, cracked wheat or tabouli, a staple food in North Africa and throughout the Middle East, and pumpernickel bread with 80% whole rye grains, as commonly used in Northern Europe.

The proportion of whole grain (wheat or barley) in a bread mix determines the glycemic effect and the in vitro rate of digestion; more whole grain in the bread produces a slower absorption rate and a flatter glycemic response.[120] The concept has been applied by Heaton and colleagues to explain possible health benefits of traditionally milled flours independent of their fiber content.

Their studies have shown that traditional coarse-milled flours with large particle sizes produce flatter postprandial glucose and insulin responses.[121]

A further factor that appears to influence the digestibility of cereal grains is "parboiling," i.e., the precooking of a grain in its husk before dehusking. Possibly because of prevention of swelling and hence a reorganization of the starch molecule, subsequent cooking fails to hydrate the dehulled grain, which, although perfectly acceptable for consumption, produces a lower glycemic response.[122] This is a traditional way of processing rice.

Although food form is a determinant of digestibility, application of this principle may not be universal. Studies with lentils indicated that blending to a smooth paste after cooking made no difference to the in vitro rate of digestion or the glycemic response,[123] nor did boiling for an additional 40 minutes. Heat treatment for 12 hours was required to increase the digestibility of the lentils.[123]

## ENZYME INHIBITORS

Enzyme inhibitors in foods, although common in storage organs such as seeds, cereal grains, and beans, are usually effectively destroyed by the heat treatment of conventional cooking practices.[124] Their relevance to human nutrition is therefore likely to be limited. In terms of animal nutrition, however, the antitryptic activity of uncooked bean meal has attracted attention because it limits the protein quality of animal feeds. In rats it was associated with impaired growth and pancreatic hypertrophy.[102]

On the positive side, purified enzyme inhibitors are beginning to find a use in modifying small intestinal absorption. Inhibitors of carbohydrate absorption have been developed specifically to control the rate of carbohydrate absorption. An anti $\alpha$-amylase isolated from wheat was shown to reduce the rate of starch digestion and the glycemic response to a starch meal in rats, dogs, and man.[125] Subsequently, commercial development of an $\alpha$-glycoside hydrolase inhibitor with antisucrase, antimaltase, and antiamylase activity was shown to have application in the treatment of diabetes,[126] as well as in the dumping syndrome.[127] In the dumping syndrome, relief was obtained despite enhanced carbohydrate losses.[127] Presumably, the reduction in glycemic excursions caused by dampening the carbohydrate flux offered a large measure of relief to patients and outweighed the discomfort of carbohydrate malabsorption to which they were already accustomed. Thus, although enzyme inhibitors may be of little relevance in the context of commonly eaten foods and dietetic manipulations, the pharmacologic development of these agents may in future provide a further means of modifying small intestinal absorption in the same way that enzymes are currently added to enhance absorption of foods in pancreatic insufficiency.

## SAPONINS

These steroidal or triterpenoid amphiphilic glycosides with surface active and emulsion stabilizing properties are relatively heat resistant, and thus, their levels are maintained in fat-containing plant foods and oils. Under normal circumstances, they are not absorbed. They have attracted attention by possibly precipitating cholesterol and interfering with micelle formation in the small intestine by enhancing the binding of bile acids to fiber.[128] There is no suggestion that they would induce major changes in fat absorption, but in view of their effects on cholesterol absorption, they may possibly interfere with fat-soluble vitamin uptake. The exact effect of these surface active agents on the enterocyte or digestive enzymes remains to be documented.

## TANNINS

These large condensed polyphenols are powerful reducing agents widely distributed in plant food. Because they are heat stable, however, they survive cooking procedures and have been shown to complex with dietary proteins and to reduce protein digestibility.[129] They are also known to reduce the activity of the digestive enzymes trypsin and amylase.[130,131] Tannins may therefore reduce the rate or total absorption of both dietary starch and protein from foods. Although tannins occur in high concentrations in certain natural diets, their effects have not been studied directly in man. Their concentration in foods has been shown to relate negatively with the digestibility and glycemic response of a wide range of foods tested, however.[132]

## PHYTATES

The most important of these substances is *myo*-inositol 1,2,3,4,5,6 hexakis dihydrogen phosphate. It is found in relatively high concentrations in many high-fiber foods (cereals, legumes, and vegetables). Its levels are reduced by the action of yeast in the leavening of bread. Nevertheless, phytates have the ability to bind metal ions and to bind to protein,[133,134] and possibly to starch, thereby reducing macro- and micronutrient digestibility. As a consequence, phytates have been implicated in calcium and zinc deficiency in man.[135] Their exact role, however, seems to be of lesser importance in relation to macronutrient absorption than that of fiber.[136] Nevertheless, phytates have been shown to reduce carbohydrate digestibility when they are added to white bread in the same concentration as found in legumes (Fig. 39–7).[137] This effect is likely to be due to the binding of $Ca^{++}$, which catalyzes the action of amylase[138] because the addition of excess $Ca^{++}$ minimizes the effect.[137] Although phytate may also bind to proteins and so reduce protein digestibility,[133,134] the significance of this effect

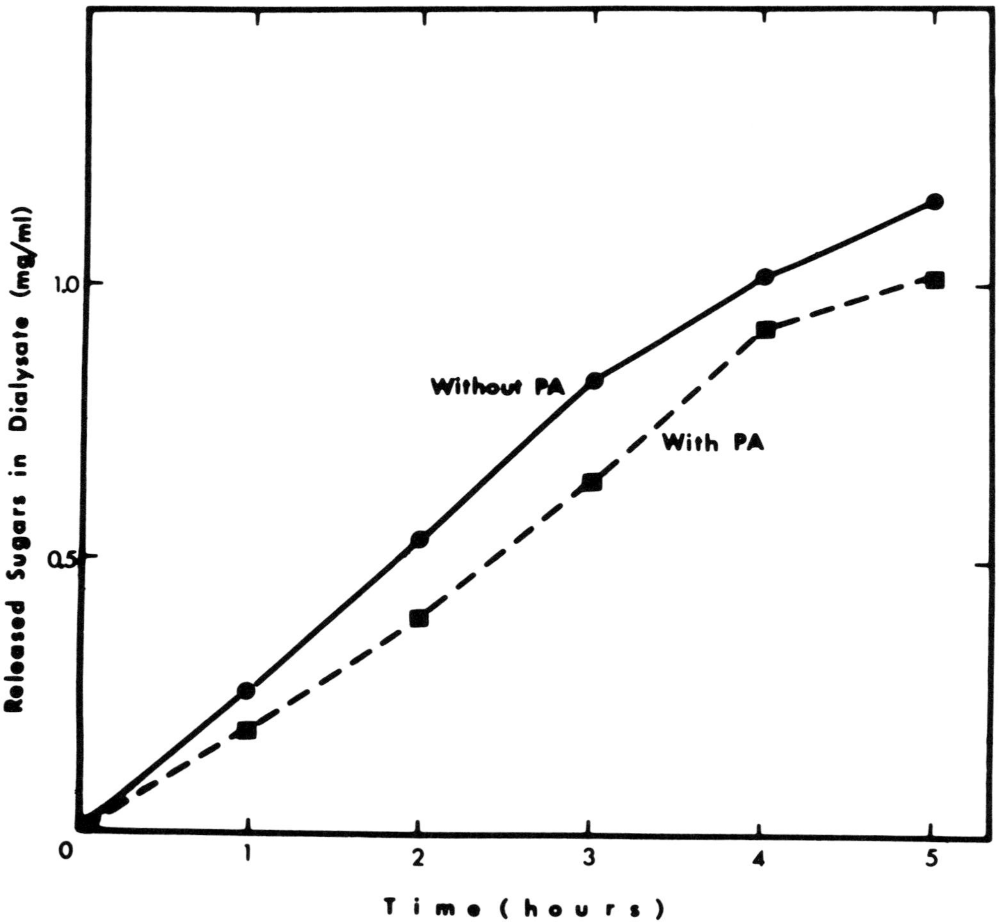

Released Sugars in Dialysate (mg/ml)
1.0
0.5
0
1
2
3
4
5
Time (hours)
Without PA
With PA


**FIGURE 39–7.** Rate of digestion of starch in unleavened breads with and without addition of sodium phytate (PA). (From Yoon, J.H., Thompson, L.U., Jenkins, D.J.A.: Am. J. Clin. Nutr., *38*:835–842, 1983.)

in commonly eaten foods is not clear. Phytates may possibly play a major role in determining starch digestibility in foods because they have been shown to have a highly significant negative relationship with digestibility and glycemic response to many foods tested in man.[137] Their levels are especially high in legumes, which show some of the slowest rates of in vitro digestion.[19]

## LECTINS

These substances are a diverse family of proteins and glycoproteins found ubiquitously in plant foods.[139] Lectins bind to carbohydrate receptors on cell surfaces and, in extremely high concentrations, have caused small intestinal mucosal damage in rats.[140] Apart from retrospective studies by Noah, Bender et al. concerning raw kidney bean consumption,[141] no toxic effects have been reported in man at levels commonly found in the diet; however, preliminary studies indicate that, as with many antinutrients, the lectin content of a food and its digestibility both in vitro and in vivo are related.[142] The exact significance of this finding awaits further elaboration.

## RATE OF FOOD INGESTION AND MEAL FREQUENCY

Finally, the rate of nutrient delivery to the organism can be slowed simply by reducing the rate and prolonging the time over which food is ingested (Fig. 39–8). In many ways, this also provides the least complicated model for examining the physiologic effects of reducing the rate of absorption. In short-term studies of glucose or mixed meals, possibly the most notable effect has been the reduction in postprandial insulin levels.[143–145] This economy in insulin secretion has been seen in longer-term studies (Fig. 39–8*A*), and it has been associated with reduced serum lipid and lipoprotein levels, notably

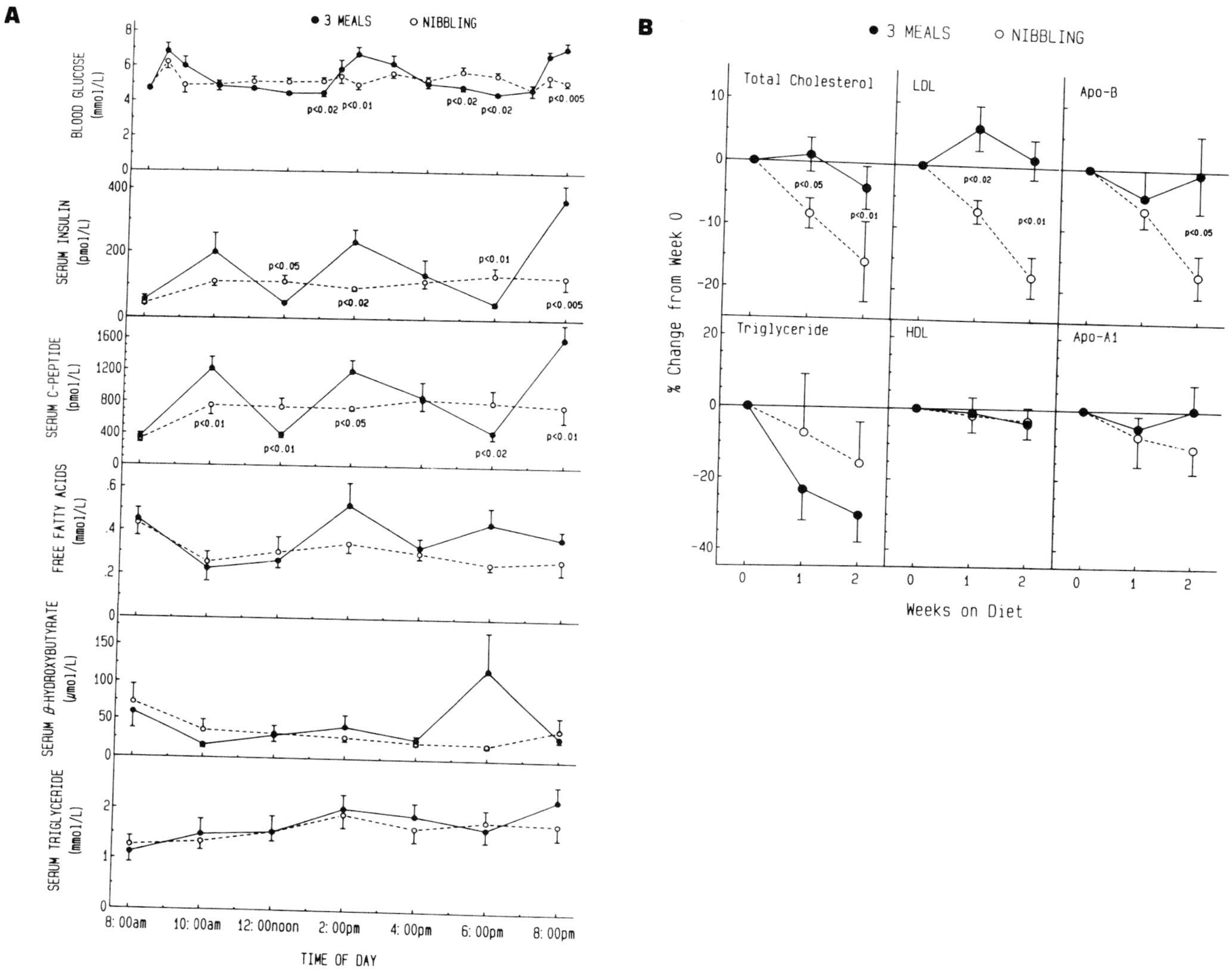
A
• 3 MEALS
○ NIBBLING
BLOOD GLUCOSE (mmol/L)
SERUM INSULIN (pmol/L)
SERUM C-PEPTIDE (pmol/L)
FREE FATTY ACIDS (mmol/L)
SERUM β-HYDROXYBUTYRATE (μmol/L)
SERUM TRIGLYCERIDE (mmol/L)
p<0.02
p<0.01
p<0.005
p<0.05
8:00am
10:00am
12:00noon
2:00pm
4:00pm
6:00pm
8:00pm
TIME OF DAY
B
• 3 MEALS
○ NIBBLING
Total Cholesterol
LDL
Apo-B
Triglyceride
HDL
Apo-A1
% Change from Week 0
Weeks on Diet

**FIGURE 39–8.** *A*, Mean (±SE) blood glucose levels and serum cncentrations of insulin, C-peptide, free fatty acids, 3-hydroxybutyrate, and triglyceride in seven men on day 13. During the nibbling diet, meals were eaten hourly from 8 A.M. onward, and during the three-meal diet, 8 A.M., 1 P.M., and 7 P.M. *B*, Mean (±SE) percentage of change from time 0 in serum lipid and apolipoprotein (apo) concentrations in seven men during the nibbling diet and the three-meal diet. (From Jenkins, D.J.A., Wolever, T.M.S., Vuksan, V., et al.: N. Engl. J. Med., *321*:929–934, 1989, by permission of the New England Journal of Medicine.)

LDL cholesterol and apolipoprotein B (Fig. 39–8*B*). Indeed, for over a quarter of a century, evidence has accumulated on the beneficial effect of meal frequency on serum lipids.[146–148] In addition to reduced insulin levels, and hence a lesser stimulus to hydroxymethylglutaryl coenzyme A (HMGCoA) reductase,[149,150] the rate-limiting step in cholesterol synthesis, it is also possible that alteration or expansion of the bile salt pool, secondary to more frequent enterohepatic cyclying, is also a factor in the lower lipid levels. These beneficial effects of increased meal frequency on serum lipids and coronary heart disease[151] have not been seen in relation to cancer where increased cancer incidence has been noted.[152,153] In the cancer studies, the determining factor may be the nature of the snack foods used (high fat, high salt, etc.) in uncontrolled diets. These findings emphasize the need for more research into the physiologic and pathologic consequences of alterations in food frequency and by inference factors that prolong absorption time in general.

## DIFFERENCES IN DIGESTIBILITY OF FOODS AND PHYSIOLOGIC IMPLICATIONS

Owing to the many factors that may alter the digestion and absorption of foods, the present state of knowledge is not sufficiently comprehensive to predict the rate at which a food will be digested simply by knowing its constituents. Nevertheless, as illustrated by starch-containing foods, large differences are seen among different foods (Table 39–1).[28] Predictably, the legumes that are relatively high in soluble fiber and antinutrients are digested more slowly than the cereal foods and potato.[28] In addition, they release a greater proportion of glucose and maltose and a smaller proportion of maltotriose. As mentioned earlier, this effect, in turn, may reflect their higher content of the less readily digested amylose form of starch. On the other hand, the content of cereal fiber in white and wholemeal bread demonstrates clearly the lack of effect of this form of fiber in reducing the rate of digestion of bread. Again, by contrast, foods of similar composition (e.g., white bread and white spaghetti) differ markedly, presumably because of differences in food form. Because the rate of digestion relates well to the glycemic response to foods,[19] the physiologic implications of these differences are great. Flatter glycemic responses are seen (expressed as a glycemic index) in response to feeding foods that are digested less rapidly (Fig. 39–9).[19] As data accumulate, it should be possible to select diets on the basis of rates of digestion to achieve the desired physiologic and metabolic effects.

### GLYCEMIC INDEX

Because many factors in foods may influence their rates of digestion and glycemic responses, and because most of these factors are not listed in food tables and many have nothing to do with food composition, it is not possible to predict the physiologic effect of a food on the basis of its chemical composition. Therefore, the glycemic index was developed as an index of the physiologic effect of foods to supplement information on chemical composition.[16] It was reasoned that such information may allow a better understanding of the effects of carbohydrate foods and aid in the selection of appropriate foods for therapeutic diets. The glycemic index is defined as the blood glucose response to a 50-g available carbohydrate portion of a food expressed as a percentage of the response to the same amount of carbohydrate from a standard food, which has been either glucose or white bread. Bread is the preferred standard and gives glycemic index values 1.38 times greater than if glucose is the standard (because glucose produces a glycemic response 138% that of white bread). The glycemic index value obtained also depends on the method of calculating the area under the glycemic response curve and, to a lesser extent, on other methodologic variables, discussed fully elsewhere.[154]

Over 75 different foods have been tested in various centers (see Appendix Table A–24a).[155] For most foods tested more than once in different centers there is reasonable agreement, with an average coefficient of variation of the mean glycemic index values of 16%.[154] The variability of certain foods in many cases has been found

**TABLE 39–1.** DIFFERENCES IN DIGESTION RATES AND SUGARS RELEASED FROM COMMON FOODS*

| FOOD | SUGAR CONCENTRATION (MG/L) AT 3 HOURS TOTAL | % OF TOTAL AS | | |
|---|---|---|---|---|
| | | GLUCOSE | MALTOSE | MALTOTRIOSE |
| White bread standard | 866 | 6.9 | 76.6 | 16.5 |
| Whole wheat bread | 811 | 6.2 | 17.2 | 17.2 |
| Rice | 652 | 3.9 | 71.7 | 24.4 |
| Cornflakes | 954 | 4.9 | 73.5 | 21.7 |
| Porridge oats | 424 | 6.3 | 76.5 | 17.3 |
| Spaghetti | 583 | 5.6 | 73.4 | 21.0 |
| Potato | 638 | 8.8 | 74.2 | 17.1 |
| MEAN | 707 | 6.0 | 74.6 | 19.4 |
| Kidney beans | 263 | 6.9 | 79.8 | 13.3 |
| Chick peas | 263 | 8.7 | 79.1 | 12.3 |
| Lentils | 258 | 10.6 | 84.0 | 5.4 |
| MEAN | 261 | 8.7 | 81.0 | 10.3 |
| Significance of difference between beans and other foods | 0.005 | 0.05 | 0.005 | 0.005 |

*Mean concentration and percentage of sugars released into 800 ml dialysate after 3 hours of salivary digestion of 2-g carbohydrate portions of 10 foods.

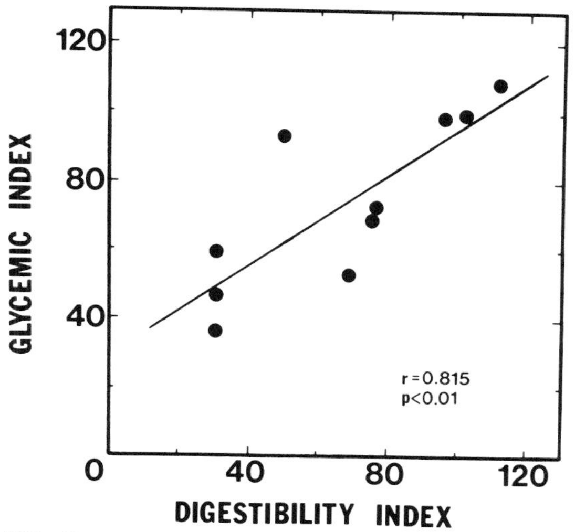
GLYCEMIC INDEX
120
80
40
0
40
80
120
DIGESTIBILITY INDEX
r=0.815
p<0.01

**FIGURE 39–9.** Relationship between the mean glycemic index and mean digestibility index for each of the 10 foods studied. The glycemic and digestibility indices were calculated by ascribing to white bread a value of 100 both for the glycemic response areas observed over 3 hours after consumption of the test foods and for the total sugars liberated at 3 hours during in vitro digestion (descending order of digestibility: cornflakes, white and wholemeal breads, rice, potato, spaghetti, porridge, kidney beans, chick peas, and lentils). (From Jenkins, D.J.A., Ghafari, H., Wolever, T.M.S.: *22*:450–455, 1982.)

subsequently to be due to subtle differences among foods, such as the method of rice processing (parboiled versus polished),[122] different varieties of potato,[154] and the ripeness of banana.[156] Different individuals may have vastly different absolute glycemic responses to a food, depending upon their glucose tolerance status. The glycemic index normalizes each subject's response to that of a standard food, however, so differences among individuals are removed.[157] Thus, the glycemic index values of foods are the same in normal and diabetic subjects.

In individual subjects, blood glucose responses vary from day to day. For this reason, the glycemic index cannot be applied quantitatively in individual subjects who test foods only once. One can predict the ranking of glycemic responses, however, with the chance of a correct prediction determined by the variation of glycemic responses within the subject tested, the expected glycemic index difference, and the number of times the subject repeats the tests.[158] The glycemic index can be applied to mixed meals if appropriate methods are used.[154,159] Briefly, the meal glycemic index is the weighted average of the glycemic index value of all the individual carbohydrate foods in the meal, with the weighting based on the proportion of the total meal carbohydrate contributed by each food. The percentage differences among meal glycemic index values accurately predicts the percentage differences among the mean incremental glycemic response areas of mixed meals taken by groups of subjects, provided accurate glycemic index values are known for the individual foods.

The clinical relevance of the glycemic index has been demonstrated in studies where the types of starchy carbohydrate foods in the diet have been altered without changing the overall composition of the diet in terms of fat, protein, carbohydrate, and dietary fiber (see Chap. 70). A low glycemic index diet has been shown to reduce blood lipids in hypertriglyceridemic subjects,[160,161] to reduce insulin secretion,[162] to improve overall blood glucose control in insulin-dependent and noninsulin-dependent diabetic subjects,[163–166] to reduce abnormal blood glucose, insulin, and amino acid levels in patients with cirrhosis,[167] and to reduce urinary urea excretion, presumably by increasing nitrogen trapping by colonic bacteria.[162] In addition, some evidence indicates that low glycemic index foods enhance satiety[168] and increase athletic endurance.[169]

## COLONIC ABSORPTION

Food residues not completely absorbed in the small intestine may be absorbed in the colon. In terms of overall protein metabolism, ammonia and the bacterial metabolites of amino acids may have little impact apart from their deleterious effects in the genesis of encephalopathy in liver disease. In the case of malabsorbed carbohydrate, however, the situation is different. A small proportion of the starch in many commonly consumed foods escapes absorption in the small intestine and enters the colon. This is especially true for foods that are slowly absorbed. Breath $H_2$[105,123] and ileostomy studies[170,171] indicate that 7 to 20% of the starch in bread enters the colon. With other foods, such as legumes, the percentage lost may be higher. Although these losses relate to the in vitro rate of digestion, the differences in the percentage of carbohydrate malabsorbed among foods are of a much smaller magnitude than the percentage differences in their glycemic responses.[16,17,172] Carbohydrate losses therefore do not appear to account for the flatter glycemic responses of starchy foods of low glycemic index.

In terms of energy losses from carbohydrate foods (starch, sugars, and fiber), much may be salvaged by colonic absorption of the resulting volatile fatty acids.[173,174] These have been estimated to contribute 10% or more of dietary calories.[174] Therefore, factors that alter the rate of carbohydrate digestion may not be reflected in malabsorption, so much as an altered balance of nutrient absorption from different parts of the gut including the colon.

## SHORT-CHAIN FATTY ACIDS (SCFA): LOCAL AND SYSTEMIC METABOLISM

The major products of carbohydrate fermentation in the colon are the short-chain fatty acids (SCFA), acetate, propionate, and butyrate. These anions are taken up rapidly from the colonic lumen and may exert local and systemic effects on metabolism. Studies indicate that SCFA may enhance the uptake of divalent metal ions,[175] and investigators have suggested that the colon may be a major organ for salvaging minerals and trace elements trapped by fiber that is fermented in the colon.[176] In man, colonic $Ca^{++}$ absorption is enhanced by incorporating acetate and propionate into the perfusate. SCFA are also considered valuable energy sources for the host. Butyrate is a preferred substrate for the colonocyte and has been suggested to have antineoplastic properties.[177] Butyrate has been used in enemas to treat exclusion (diversion) colitis.[178] Propionate is largely extracted by the liver. It is gluconeogenic and may have an inhibitory effect on cholesterol synthesis.[179] Acetate is taken up by both liver and peripheral tissues. Of the three SCFA mentioned, acetate is the only one to appear in significant quantities in the peripheral circulation.

Colonic SCFA may influence systemic carbohydrate and lipid metabolism, but the exact effects are not fully known, and this is an area of current research.

Acetate has no effect on intravenous or oral glucose tolerance or glucose turnover rates.[180,181] It may influence glucose utilization indirectly by its effect in reducing serum free fatty acid levels, however. The effect of acetate on serum free fatty acids was first described in studies suggesting that acetate accounted for the free fatty acid-lowering effect of alcohol.[182] Recently, investigators have demonstrated that colonic acetate also has the same effect in reducing serum free fatty acids.[183] Propionate has been shown to have direct effects on carbohydrate metabolism. Evidence indicates that, as in ruminants, propionate is gluconeogenic in humans.[183] Feeding propionate has been shown to improve carbohydrate tolerance, an effect that may be related, in part, to an inhibitory effect of propionate on starch digestion.[184]

The potential effects of colonic SCFA on lipid metabolism have been of major interest, especially as a mechanism for the lipid-lowering effect of soluble fiber. In vitro, propionate inhibits cholesterol synthesis in slices of hepatic tissue;[185] however, the concentration of propionate required may be greater than that ever reached in the portal vein.[186] In human feeding studies, propionate has been found to have no effect on serum cholesterol.[184,187] Nevertheless, propionate does have the ability to inhibit the incorporation by isolated hepatocytes of acetate into cholesterol and triglyceride.[188] This may be significant in humans because rectal infusion of acetate results in an increase in serum cholesterol within 1 hour, an effect partly blocked by the addition of a physiologic amount of propionate.[183] The serum cholesterol-raising effect of acetate was further suggested by the finding that feeding lactulose for 2 weeks to healthy subjects increased serum total and LDL cholesterol, apolipoprotein B, and triglyceride concentrations (Fig. 39–10).[189] Therefore, the influence of propionate on lipid metabolism cannot be determined until the importance of colonic acetate as a substrate for cholesterol synthesis is known.

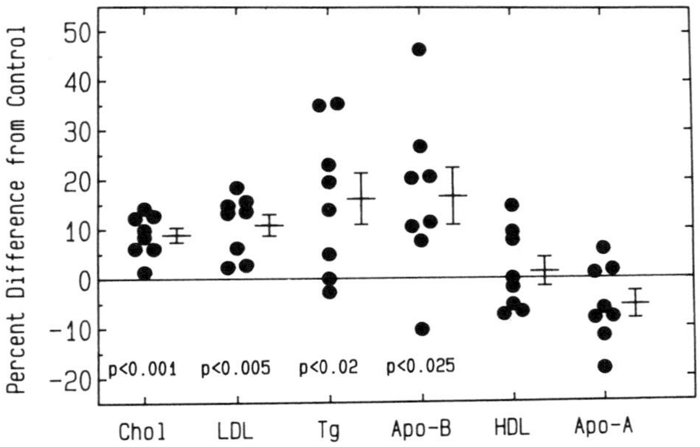
Percent Difference from Control
50
40
30
20
10
0
-10
-20
p<0.001
p<0.005
p<0.02
p<0.025
Chol
LDL
Tg
Apo-B
HDL
Apo-A

**FIGURE 39–10.** Mean 2-week lactulose values for blood lipids and apolipoproteins expressed as the percentage difference from the corresponding control values. Bars represent the Mean ± SE of the lipid and lipoprotein categories for subjects. (From Jenkins, D.J.A., Wolever, T.M.S., Jenkins, A.L., et al.: Am. J. Clin. Nutr, *54*:141–147, 1991.)

## LONG-TERM EFFECTS

Not only is it possible to identify specific short-term effects in terms of gastrointestinal function and absorption by using specific foods or food processes, but also important long-term effects may be associated with specific diets and dietary components. For example, feeding diets high in carbohydrate induces sucrase-isomaltase and enhances the absorption of sucrose, whereas removal of carbohydrate from the diet rapidly reverses this trend.[190] Diets high in specific dietary fibers have reduced sucrase levels in rats.[191] Pectin reduced sucrase and lactase, tannin and galactomannan reduced lactase, and cellulose was without effect.[191] Other studies have demonstrated that increasing the protein or the carbohydrate in the diets of diabetic rats either decreased or increased the absorption of cholesterol respectively.[192] Changes in small intestinal morphology may also be produced by diet. In view of the broad leaf-like jejunal villi seen in inhabitants of areas where high-fiber are common but are not associated with tropical sprue, researchers wondered what effect unprocessed vegetable material had on villous structure. Studies in rats demonstrated that standard chow and pectin feeding resulted in a flattening of villous structure that was not seen when cellulose or cholestyramine were the only unabsorbable component of the diet.[193] An unexplored but possibly analogous situation might be seen in subjects habitually consuming diets high in the glycoproteins (lectins). Certainly, this is evident in extreme form in susceptible individuals (celiacs) following exposure to the glycoprotein, gliadin, of wheat.

Dietary components apparently may be used to induce changes not only in morphology, enzyme levels, and absorptive function of the upper gastrointestinal tract, but also in motor activity. Studies have indicated that after 4 weeks of pectin supplementation, gastric emptying of a pectin-free meal in healthy volunteers was decreased by twofold by comparison with the original control. This, too, may have important nutritional and metabolic consequences. Cellulose supplementation was without effect.[194]

In summary, the nature of dietary carbohydrates, fats, and proteins is acutely important in influencing the absorption of natural diets. Perhaps less well recognized is the role of food form and food preparation procedures, especially those that alter either the absolute amount of fiber and antinutrients within a food or their relationship with the macronutrients. Increasingly, factors that alter carbohydrate absorption can be viewed not simply as causing or reducing malabsorption, but as altering the rate of absorption. Thus, factors that reduce the rate of absorption result in absorption at sites increasingly further along the small intestine. Finally, carbohydrate that is not absorbed in the small intestine may still be salvaged as SCFA in the colon. The endocrine and metabolic effects of these changes can be considerable, as are the effects on the absorption of other nutrients. In addition, the long-term adaptation of small intestinal and, indeed, colonic function to the maneuvers described is only now beginning to be explored. Active modification of small intestinal absorption probably has the potential for becoming an important therapeutic technique in future.[195]

## REFERENCES


1. Allen, F.M.: J. Exp. Med. Balt., *31:*381–402, 1920.
2. Christakis, G., Miridjanian, A.: *In* Diabetes Mellitus. Theory and Practice. Edited by M. Ellenberg and H. Ritkin. New York, McGraw-Hill, 1970, pp. 594–623.
3. Wahlquist, M.L., Wilmshurst, E.G., Richardson, E.N.: Am. J. Clin. Nutr., *31:*1988–2001, 1978.
4. Dahlquist, A., Borgstrom, B.: Biochem. J., *81:*411–418, 1961.
5. Fogel, M.R., Gray, G.M.: J. Appl. Physiol., *35:*263–267, 1973.
6. Wolfrom, M.L., Khoden, H.E.: *In* Chemistry and Technology. New York, Academic Press, 1965, p. 254.
7. Gray, G.M., Fogel, M.R.: *In* Modern Nutrition in Health and Disease. 6th Ed. Edited by R.S. Goodhart and M.E. Shils. Philadelphia, Lea & Febiger, 1980, pp. 99–112.
8. Silk, D.B.A., Sawson, A.M.: International Reviews of Physiology: Gastrointestinal Physiology III. Vol. 19. Edited by R.H. Crane. Baltimore, University Park Press, 1979, pp. 151–204.
9. Leach, H.W.: *In* Starch Chemistry and Technology. New York, Academic Press, 1965, p. 292.
10. Geervani, P., Theophilus, F.: J. Food Sci., *46:*817–828, 1981.
11. Shurpalekar, K.S., Sunderavalu, D.E., Rao, M.N.: Nutr. Rep. Rev., *19:*111–117, 1979.
12. Crapo, P.A., Reaven, G., Olefsky, J.: Diabetes, *25:*741–747, 1976.
13. Crapo, P.A., Reaven, G., Olefsky, J.: Diabetes, *26:*1178–1182, 1977.
14. Crapo, P.A., Kolterman, O.G. Waldeck, N., et al.: Am. J. Clin. Nutr., *33:*1723–1728, 1980.
15. Crapo, P.A., Insel, J., Sperling, M., et al.: Am. J. Clin. Nutr., *34:*184–190, 1981.
16. Jenkins, D.J.A., Wolever, T.M.S., Taylor, R.H., et al.: Am. J. Clin. Nutr., *34:*362–366, 1981.
17. Jenkins, D.J.A., Wolever, T.M.S., Jenkins, A.L., et al.: Diabetologia, *24:*257–264, 1983.
18. Jenkins, D.J.A., Wolever, T.M.S., Taylor, R.H., et al.: Br. Med. J., *281:*14–17, 1980.
19. Jenkins, D.J.A., Ghafari, H., Wolever, T.M.S., et al.: Diabetologia, *22:*450–455, 1982.
20. Juliano, B.O., Goddard, M.S.: Plant Foods Hum. Nutr., *36:*35–41, 1986.
21. Behall, K.M., Scholfield, D.J., Canary, J.: Am. J. Clin. Nutr., *47:*426–432, 1988.
22. Bocher, C.E., Behan, I., McNeans, E.: J. Nutr., *45:*75, 1951.
23. Collings, P., Williams, C., MacDonald, I.: Br. Med. J., *282:*1032, 1981.
24. Kon, S., Wagner, J.R., Booth, A.N., et al.: J. Food Sci., *36:*635–639, 1971.
25. Geervani, P., Theophilius, F.: J. Sci. Food Agric., *32:*71–78, 1981.
26. Devados, R.P., Leela, R., Chanchasilearan, K.N.: J. Nutr. Diet., *1:*84–86, 1964.
27. Alli, I., Baker, R.E.: J. Sci. Food Agric., *31:*1316–1322, 1980.
28. Pak, C.W., Belea, C.S., Bartter, F.C.: N. Engl. J. Med., *290:*175–178, 1974.
29. Jenkins, D.J.A., Wolever, T.M.S., Thorne, M.J., et al.: Am. J. Clin. Nutr., *40:*1125–1191, 1984.
30. Felber, J.-P.: Beta Release, *7:*6–9, 1983.
31. Bantle, J.P., Laine, D.C., Castle, G.W.: N. Engl. J. Med., *309:*7–12, 1983.
32. Schauberger, G., Brinck, U.C., Guldner, G., et al.: Diabetes, *26:*415, 1977.
33. Crapo, P.A., Scarlett, J.A., Kolterman, O.G., et al.: Diabetes Care, *5:*512–517, 1982.
34. Swan, D.C., Davidson, P., Albrink, M.J.: Lancet, *1:*60–63, 1966.
35. Bohannon, N.V., Karana, J.H., Forsham, P.H.: Diabetes, *27(Suppl. 2):*438, 1978.
36. Swanson, J.E., Laine, D.C., Thomas, W., et al.: Am. J. Clin. Nutr., *55:*851–856, 1992.
37. Calloway, D.H., Kurtz, G.W., McMullen, J.J., et al.: Food Res., *21:*621, 1956.
38. Steenbock, H., Irwin, M.H., Weber, J.: J. Nutr., *12:*103–111, 1936.
39. Turner, D.A.: Am. J. Dig. Dis., *3:*594–708, 1958.
40. Jenkins, D.J.A., Gassull, M.A., Leeds, A.R., et al.: Int. J. Vitam. Nutr. Res., *46:*226–230, 1976.
41. Gassull, M.A., Blendis, L.M., Jenkins, D.J.A., et al.: Int. J. Vitam. Nutr. Res., *46:*211–214, 1976.

42. Bloomstrand, R., Gurtler, J., Werner, B.: J. Clin. Invest., *44:*1766–1777, 1965.
43. Werner, M., Lutwak, L.: Fed. Proc., *22:*553–563, 1963.
44. Cheng, A.L.S., Morehouse, M.G., Davel, H.J.: J. Nutr., *37:*237–250, 1949.
45. Tomarelli, R.M., Meyer, B.J., Waeber, J.R., et al.: J. Nutr., *95:*583–590, 1968.
46. Filer, L.J., Mattson, F.H., Formon, S.J.: J. Nutr., *99:*293–298, 1969.
47. Bennett, S.: Q. J. Exp. Physiol., *49:*210–218, 1964.
48. Geliebter, A., Torbay, N., Braeco, E.F., et al.: Am. J. Clin. Nutr., *37:*1–4, 1983.
49. Winawer, S.J., Broitman, S.A., Wolochow, D.A.: N. Engl. J. Med., *274:*72–78, 1966.
50. Kaunitz, H., Slanetz, C.A., Johnson, R.E., et al.: J. Nutr., *64:*513, 1958.
51. Van de Kamer, J.H., ten Bokkel Huinink, H., Weyers, H.A.: J. Biol. Chem., *177:*347–355, 1949.
52. Saunders, D.R.: Gastroenterology, *52:*135–136, 1967.
53. Senior, B.: *In* Medium Chain Triglycerides. Edited by B. Senior, T.B. Van italie, and N. Greenberger. Philadelphia, University of Pennsylvania Press, 1968, p. 38.
54. Greenberger, N.J., Ruppert, R.D., Tzagousis, M.: Ann. Intern. Med., *66:*727–734, 1967.
55. Muto, Y., Takahaski, Y.: Postgrad. Med., *37:*A158, 1965.
56. Zieve, L.: Arch. Intern. Med., *118:*211–223, 1966.
57. Partin, J.S., Partin, J.C., Schubert, W.K., et al.: Gastroenterology, *67:*107–118, 1974.
58. Cummings, J.H., Wiggins, H.S., Jenkins, D.J.A., et al.: J. Clin. Invest., *61:*953–962, 1978.
59. Gannon, M.C., Nattall, F.G., Neil, B.J., et al.: Metabolism, *37:*1081–1088, 1988.
60. Uribe, M., Marquez, M.A., Ramos, G.G., et al.: Dig. Dis. Sci., *27:*1109–1116, 1982.
61. de Bruijn, K.M., Blendis, L.M., Zilm, D.H., et al.: Gut, *24:*53–60, 1983.
62. Shaw, S., Wroner, T.M., Lieber, C.S.: Am. J. Clin. Nutr., *38:*59–62, 1983.
63. Franzen, K., Kinsella, J.E.: J. Agric. Food Chem., *24:*788–795, 1976.
64. Mehychyn, P., Stapley, R.B.: United States Patent 3764711, 1973.
65. Creamer, L.K., Roeper, J., Lahrey, E.N.: N.Z. J. Dairy Sci. Technol., *6:*107, 1971.
66. Siu, M., Thompson, L.U.: J. Agric. Food Chem., *30:*743–747, 1982.
67. Matoba, T., Doi, E.: J. Food Sci., *44:*537, 1979.
68. Holt, S., Heading, R.C., Carter, D.C., et al.: Lancet, *1:*636–639, 1979.
69. Leeds, A.R., Ralphs, D.N.L., Bonlos, D., et al.: Proc. Nutr. Soc., *37:*33, 1978.
70. Leeds, A.R., Ralphs, D.N.L., Ebied, F., Metz, G., Dilawari, J.B.: Lancet, *1:*1075–1078, 1981.
71. Taylor, R.H.: Lancet, *1:*872, 1979.
72. Elsenhans, B., Sufke, V., Blume, R., et al.: Clin. Sci., *59:*373–380, 1980.
73. Jenkins, D.J.A., Wolever, T.M.S., Leeds, A.R., et al.: Br. Med. J., *1:*1392–1394, 1978.
74. Kasper, H., Zilly, W., Fassl, H., et al.: Am. J. Clin. Nutr., *32:*2436, 1979.
75. Eastwood, M.A., Hamilton, D.: Biochim. Biophys. Acta, *152:*165–173, 1968.
76. Kay, R.M., Truswell, A.S.: Am. J. Clin. Nutr., *30:*171–175, 1977.
77. Florie, B., Vidon, N., Florent, C.H., et al.: Gut, *25:*936–941, 1984.
78. Blackburn, N.A., Redfern, J.S., Jarjis, H., et al.: Clin. Sci., *66:*329–336, 1984.
79. Sandberg, A.S., Andersson, H., Hallgren, B., et al.: Br. J. Nutr., *45:*283–294, 1981.
80. Jenkins, D.J.A.: *In* International Conference on Atherosclerosis. Edited by L.A. Carlson, R. Paoletti, C.R. Sirtori, et al. New York, Raven Press, 1978, pp. 173–182.
81. Kasper, H., Rabast, U., Fassl, H., et al.: Am. J. Clin. Nutr., *38:*1847–1849, 1979.
82. Weintraub, M.S., Eisenberg, S., Breslow, J.L.: J. Clin. Invest., *79:*1110–1119, 1987.
83. Jenkins, D.J.A., Leeds, A.R., Gassull, M.A., et al.: Ann. Intern. Med., *86:*20–23, 1972.
84. Barnard, D.L., Heaton, K.W.: Gut, *14:*316–318, 1973.
85. Jenkins, D.J.A., Wolever, T.M.S., Hockaday, T.D.R., et al.: Lancet, *2:*779–780, 1977.
86. Jenkins D.J.A., Wolever, T.M.S., Nineham, R., et al.: Br. Med. J., *2:*1744–1746, 1978.
87. Aro, A., Uusitupa, M., Voutilainen, E., et al.: Diabetologia, *21:*29–33, 1981.
88. Doi, K., Matsuura, M., Kuwara, A., et al.: Lancet, *1:*987–988, 1979.
89. Fahrenbach, M.J., Riccardi, B.A., Saunders, J.L., et al.: Circulation, *31/32 (Suppl. 2):*1141, 1965.
90. Miettinen, T.A., Tarpila, S.: Clin. Chim. Acta, *79:*471–477, 1977.
91. Jenkins, D.J.A., Reynolds, D., Slavin, B.: Am. J. Clin. Nutr., *33:*575–581, 1980.
92. Jenkins, D.J.A., Gassull, M.A., Leeds, A.R., et al.: Gastroenterology, *73:*215–217, 1977.
93. Jenkins, D.J.A., Bloom, S.R., Albuquerque, R.H., et al.: Gut, *21:*574–579, 1980.
94. Jenkins, D.J.A., Wolever, T.M.S., Taylor, R.H., et al.: Diabetes Care, *4:*509–513, 1981.
95. Jenkins, D.J.A., Wolever, T.M.S., Jenkins, A.L., et al.: Diabetes Care, *6:*155–159, 1981.
96. Nishimune, T., Yakushiji, T., Sumimoto, T., et al.: Am. J. Clin. Nutr., *54:* 414–419, 1991.
97. Wolever, T.M.S.: Am. J. Clin. Nutr., *51:*72–75, 1990.
98. Anderson, I.H., Levine, A.S., Levitt, M.D.: N. Engl. J. Med., *304:*891–892, 1981.
99. Jenkins, D.J.A., Thorne, M.J., Wolever, T.M.S., et al.: Am. J. Clin. Nutr., *45:*946–951, 1987.
100. Meyer, J.H., Stevenson, E.A., Watts, H.D.: Gastroenterology, *70:*232–239, 1976.
101. Monoz, J.M.: *In* Dietary Fiber in Health and Disease. Edited by G.V. Vahouny and D. Kritchevsky. New York, Plenum, 1982, pp. 85–89.
102. Thomas, E.J.: Physiol. Rev., *37:*453–474, 1957.
103. Holm, J., Bjorck, I., Ostrowska, S., et al.: Starch/Starke, *35:*294–297, 1983.
104. Augur, V., Rollman, H.S., Deuel, H.J.: J. Nutr., *33:*177–186, 1947.
105. Sylven, C., Borgstrom, B.: J. Lipid Res., *10:*351–355, 1969.
106. Roels, D.A., Trout, H., Dujacquier, R.: J. Nutr., *65:*115–127, 1958.
107. Kelsay, J.L.: Update on Fiber and Mineral Availability. Edited by G.V. Vahouny and D. Kritchevsky. New York, Plenum, 1985, pp. 361–372.
108. Reinhold, J.G., Faradji, B., Abadi, P., et al.: J. Nutr., *106:*493–503, 1976.

109. Cummings, J.H., Hill, M.J., Jivraj, T., et al.: Am. J. Clin. Nutr., *32*:2086–2093, 1979.
110. Jenkins D.J.A., Hill, M.J., Cummings, J.H.: Am. J. Clin. Nutr., *28*:1408–1411, 1975.
111. Kelsay, J.: *In* Dietary Fiber in Health and Disease. Edited by G.V. Vahouny and D. Kritchevsky. New York, Plenum, 1982, pp. 91–103.
112. Life Sciences Research Office, Federation of American Societies for Experimental Biology (FASEB): Physiological Effects and Health Consequences of Dietary Fiber. Edited by S.M. Pilch. FASEB, 1987, pp. 136–146.
113. Kelsay, J.L.: Am. J. Gastroentero., *82*:983–986, 1987.
114. Kelsay, J.L., Prather, E.S., Clark, W.M., et al.: J. Nutr., *118*:1197–1204, 1988.
115. Nicolaysen, R., Eeg-Larsen, N., Malm, O.J.: Physiol. Rev., *33*:424–444, 1953.
116. Rayssiguier, Y., Remesy, C.: Ann. Rech. Vet., *8*:105–110, 1977.
117. Hollander, D., Rim, E., Ruble, P.E.: Gastroenterology, *72*:A48/1071, 1977.
118. Haber, E.B., Heaton, K.W., Murphy, D., et al.: Lancet, *2*:679–682, 1977.
119. O'Dea, K., Nestel, P.J., Antionoff, L.: Am. J. Clin. Nutr., *33*:760–765, 1980.
120. Jenkins, D.J.A., Wesson, V., Wolever, T.M.S., et al.: Br. Med. J., *297*:958–960, 1988.
121. Heaton, K.W., Marcus, S.N., Emmett, P.M., et al.: Am. J. Clin. Nutr., *47*:675–682, 1988.
122. Wolever, T.M.S., Jenkins, D.J.A., Kalmunsky, J., et al.: Nutr. Res., *6*:349–357, 1986.
123. Jenkins, D.J.A., Thorne, M.J., Camelon, K., et al.: Am. J. Clin. Nutr., *36*:1093–1101, 1982.
124. Leiner, I.E.: Proc. Nutr. Soc., *38*:109–113, 1979.
125. Puls, W., Keup, V.: Diabetologia, *9*:97–101, 1973.
126. Walton, R.J., Sherif, I.T., Noy, G.A., et al.: Br. Med. J., *1*:220–221, 1979.
127. Jenkins, D.J.A., Barker, H.M., Taylor, R.H., et al.: Lancet, *1*:109, 1982.
128. Oakenfull, D.G., Fenwick, D.E.: Br. J. Nutr., *40*:299–309, 1978.
129. Bressani, R., Elias, L.G.: *In* Polyphenols in Cereals and Legumes. Edited by J.H. Hulse. Ottawa, International Development Research Centre, 1980.
130. Singh, D., Jambunathan, R.: J. Food Sci., *46*:1364–1367, 1981.
131. Griffiths, D.W., Moseley, G.: J. Sci. Food Agric., *31*:255–259, 1980.
132. Thompson, L.U., Yoon, J.H., Jenkins, D.J.A., et al.: Am. J. Clin. Nutr., *39*:745–751, 1984.
133. Erdman, J.W.: J. Am. Oil Chem. Soc., *56*:736–740, 1979.
134. Cheryan, M.: CRC Crit. Rev. Food Sci. Nutr., *13*:297–335, 1980.
135. Reinhold, J.G., Lahimgarzodeh, A., Nasr, K., et al.: Lancet, *1*:28–33, 1973.
136. James, W.P.T.: *In* Medical Aspects of Dietary Fiber. Edited by G.A. Spiller and R.M. Kay. New York, Plenum Publishing, 1980, pp. 239–259.
137. Yoon, J.H., Thompson, L.U., Jenkins, D.J.A.: Am. J. Clin. Nutr., *38*:835–842, 1983.
138. Alfonsky, D.: *In* Saliva and its Relation to Oral Health. Birmingham, University of Alabama Press. 1966.
139. Nachbar, M.S., Oppenheim, J.D.: Am. J. Clin. Nutr., *33*:2338–2345, 1980.
140. Puzstai, A., Clarke, E.M.W., King, T.P.: Proc. Nutr. Soc., *38*:115–120. 1979.
141. Noah, N.D., Bender, A.L., Reaidi, G.B., et al.: Br. Med. J., *281*:236–237, 1980.
142. Rea, R., Thompson, L.U., Jenkins, D.J.A.: Nutr. Res., *5*:919–929, 1985.
143. Jenkins, D.J.A., Wolever, T.M.S., Vuksan, V., et al.: N. Engl. J. Med., *321*:929–934, 1989.
144. Jenkins, D.J.A., Wolever, T.M.S., Ocana, A.M., et al.: Diabetes, *39*:775–781, 1990.
145. Jenkins, D.J.A., Ocana, A.M., Jenkins, A.L., et al.: Am. J. Clin. Nutr., *55*:461–467, 1992.
146. Gwinup, G., Byron, R.C., Roush, W., et al.: Am. J. Clin. Nutr., *13*:209–213, 1963.
147. Irwin, M.I., Feeley, R.M.: Am. J. Clin. Nutr., *20*:816–824, 1967.
148. Young, C.M., Frankel, D.L., Scanlan, S.S., et al.: J. Am. Diet. Assoc., *59*:473–480, 1971.
149. Lakshmanan, M.R., Nepokroeff, C.M., Ness, G.C., et al.: Biochem. Biophys. Res. Commun. *50*:704–710, 1973.
150. Jaganathan, S.N., Connon, W.F., Beveridge, J.M.R.: Am. J. Clin. Nutr., *15*:90–93, 1964.
151. Fabry, P., Tepperman, J.: Am. J. Clin. Nutr., *23*:1059–1068, 1970.
152. Potter, J.D., McMichael, A.J.: JNCI, *76*:557–569, 1986.
153. Young, T.B., Wolf, D.A.: Int. J. Cancer, *42*:167–175, 1988.
154. Wolever, T.M.S., Jenkins, D.J.A., Jenkins, A.L., et al.: Am. J. Clin. Nutr., *54*:846–854, 1991.
155. Wolever, T.M.S.: World Rev. Nutr. Diet., *62*:120–185, 1990.
156. Wolever, T.M.S., Jenkins, D.J.A., Jenkins, A.L., et al.: J. Clin. Nutr. Gastroenterol., *3*:85–88, 1988.
157. Wolever, T.M.S., Jenkins, D.J.A., Vuksan, V., et al.: Diabetes Care, *13*:126–132, 1990.
158. Wolever, T.M.S., Csima, A., Jenkins, D.J.A., et al.: J. Am. Coll. Nutr., *8*:235–247, 1989.
159. Wolever, T.M.S., Jenkins, D.J.A.: Am. J. Clin. Nutr., *43*:167–172, 1986.
160. Jenkins, D.J.A., Wolever, T.M.S., Kalmusky, J., et al.: Am. J. Clin. Nutr., *42*:604–617, 1985.
161. Jenkins, D.J.A., Wolever, T.M.S., Kalmusky, J., et al.: Am. J. Clin. Nutr., *46*:66–71, 1987.
162. Jenkins, D.J.A., Wolever, T.M.S., Collier, G.R., et al.: Am. J. Clin. Nutr., *46*:968–975, 1987.
163. Collier, G.R., Giudici, S., Kalmusky, J., et al.: Diabetes Nutr. Metab., *1*:11–19, 1988.
164. Fontvieille, A.M., Acosta, M., Rizkalla, S.W., et al.: Diabetes Nutr. Metab., *1*:139–143, 1988.
165. Brand, J.C., Colagiuri, S., Crossman, S., et al.: Diabetes Care, *14*:95–101, 1991.
166. Wolever, T.M.S., Jenkins, D.J.A., Vuksan, V., et al.: Diabetes Care, *15*:562–564, 1992.
167. Jenkins, D.J.A., Thorne, M.J., Taylor, R.H., et al.: Am. J. Gastroenterol., *82*:223–230, 1987.
168. Brand, J.C., Holt, S., Saveny, C., et al.: Proc. Nutr. Soc. Aust., *15*:209, 1990.
169. Thomas, D.E., Brotherhood, J.R., Brand, J.C.: Med. Sci. Sports Med. Exercise, *22(Suppl.)*:S121, 1990.
170. Wolever, T.M.S., Thorne, M.J., Thompson, L.U., et al.: Proc. Nutr. Soc., *5*:919–929, 1985.
171. Stephen, A.M., Haddad, A.C., Phillips, S.F.: Gastroenterology, *85*:589–595, 1983.
172. Steinhart, A.H., Jenkins, D.J.A., Mitchell, S., et al.: Am. J. Gastroenterol., *87*:48–54, 1992.

173. Bond, J.A., Currier, B.E., Buchwald, H., et al.: Gastroenterology, *78:*444–447, 1980.
174. Cummings, J.H.: Gut, *22:*763 –779, 1981.
175. James, W.P.T.: Dietary Fiber and Mineral Asborption: Medical Aspects of Dietary Fiber. Edited by G.A. Spiller and R. McPherson-Kay. New York, Plenum, 1980, pp. 237–259.
176. Thompson, L.U., Trinidad, T., Wolever, T.M.S.: Calcium Absorption in the Colon of Man. Seventh International Symposium on Trace Elements in Man and Animals, Dubrovnik, May 20–25, 1990. Edited by B. Momčilovič. Zagreb, Institute for Medical Research and Occupational Health, 1990.
177. Kruk, J.: Mol. Cell. Biochem., *42:*65–82, 1982.
178. Haing, J.M., Soergel, K.H., Komorowski, R.A., et al.: N. Engl. J. Med., *320:*23–28, 1987.
179. Thacker, P.A., Solomon, M.O., Aheme, F.X., et al.: Can. J. Anim. Sci., *61:*969–975, 1981.
180. Scheppach, W., Cummings, J.H., Branch, W.J., et al.: Clin. Sci., *75:*355–361, 1988.
181. Scheppach, W., Wiggins, H.S., Halliday, D., et al.: Clin. Sci., *75:*363–370, 1988.
182. Crouse, J.R., Gerson, C.D., DeCarli, L.M., et al.: J. Lipid Res., *9:*509–512, 1968.
183. Wolever, T.M.S., Spadafora, P., Eshuis, H.: Am. J. Clin. Nutr., *53:*681–687, 1991.
184. Todesco, T., Rao, A.V., Bozello, O., et al.: Am. J. Clin. Nutr., *54:*860–865, 1991.
185. Chen, W.-J.L., Anderson, J.W., Jennings, D.: Proc. Soc. Exp. Biol. Med., *175:*215–218, 1984.
186. Illman, R.J., Topping, D.L., McIntosh, G.H., et al.: Ann. Nutr. Metab., *32:*97–107, 1988.
187. Venter, C.S., Vorster, H.H., Cummings, J.H.: Am. J. Gastroenterol., *85:*549–553, 1990.
188. Nishina, P.M., Freedland, R.A.: J. Nutr., *120:*668–673, 1990.
189. Jenkins, D.J.A., Wolever, T.M.S., Jenkins, A.L., et al.: Am. J. Clin. Nutr., *54:*141–147, 1991.
190. Rosensweig, N.S., Herman, R.: J. Clin. Invest., *47:*2253, 1968.
191. Thomsen, L.L., Tasman-Jones, C.: Digestion, *23:*253, 1982.
192. Thomson, A.B.R., Rajotte, R.: Am. J. Clin. Nutr., *37:*244–252, 1983.
193. Tasman-Jones, C., Owne, R.L., Jones, A.L.: Dig. Dis. Sci., *27:*519, 1982.
194. Schwartz, S.E., Levine, R.A., Singh, A., et al.: Gastroenterology, *83:*812–817, 1982.
195. Creutzfeldt, W.: *In* Delaying Absorption as a Therapeutic Principle in Metabolic Diseases. Edited by W. Creutzfeldt and U.R. Folsch. New York, Thieme-Stratton, 1983, p. 1.

CHAPTER 40

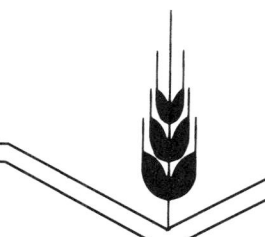

# Hormone and Nutrient Interactions

Irwin G. Brodsky and John T. Devlin



This chapter examines the effects of various hormones on the metabolism of macronutrients. In addition to providing updated information on the effects of pancreatic islet, thyroid, adrenal, pituitary, and gonadal hormones, the scope of the chapter in previous editions is extended by examining the function of immune cells as hormone-elaborating cells that mediate changes in metabolism during severe illness. Figure 40–1 and Table 40–1 distinguish the effects of hormones primarily affecting nutrient storage (Fig. 40–1) and hormones mediating nutrient mobilization (Fig. 40–2). Table 40–2 summarizes the influence of various hormones on circulating concentrations of glucose, free fatty acids, and amino acids.

## PANCREATIC HORMONES: INSULIN, GLUCAGON, AND SOMATOSTATIN

### CARBOHYDRATE METABOLISM

Carbohydrate metabolism is finely regulated by interactions between insulin, the hormone promoting fuel storage, and the counter-regulatory hormones, such as glucagon, epinephrine, cortisol, and growth hormone. Glucose homeostasis is maintained in the presence of widely varying quantities and compositions of food intake. Because the brain requires a constant supply of glucose even in the absence of available carbohydrate, the importance of these homeostatic mechanisms is apparent.

The central role of insulin in regulating glucose metabolism has long been recognized. Insulin, like other peptide hormones, initiates its metabolic effects by binding to a cell-surface receptor. These effects depend on the activation of a tyrosine-specific protein kinase, which is contained in the β-subunit of the receptor.[1,2] After binding to its cell-surface receptor, insulin accelerates the membrane transport of sugars. Increases in maximal glucose transport rates in response to insulin vary from 3.2-fold in skeletal muscle to 30-fold in adipocytes.[3–5] This effect is produced by insulin-mediated translocation of glucose transporter proteins from intracellular membrane pools to plasma membrane in insulin-sensitive tissues.[6,7] Transporters located in the insulin-sensitive tissues (e.g., adipose tissue, skeletal

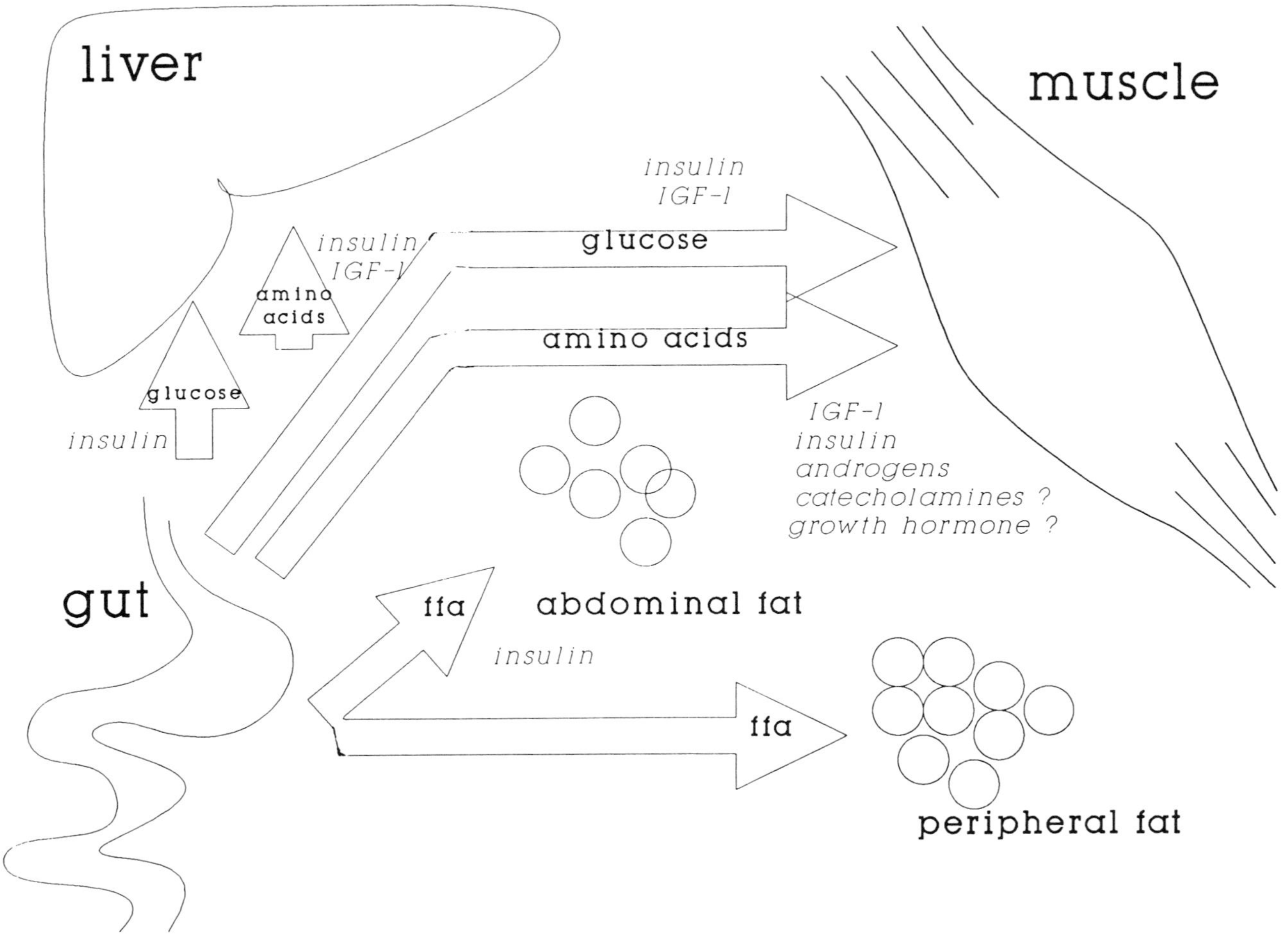
liver
muscle
insulin
IGF-1
insulin
IGF-1
glucose
amino acids
amino acids
glucose
insulin
IGF-1
insulin
androgens
catecholamines ?
growth hormone ?
gut
ffa
abdominal fat
insulin
ffa
peripheral fat

**FIGURE 40–1.** Hormones promoting nutrient storage. Arrows represent the release of ingested nutrients from the gut to storage sites in liver, skeletal muscle, and adipose tissue. The hormones promoting storage of particular nutrients are presented in italics juxtaposed to the appropriate arrows. IGF-1, Insulin-like growth factor; ffa, free fatty acids.

muscle, and heart muscle) are sodium independent, facilitative transporters named GLUT1 and GLUT4.[8] GLUT4 is the primary protein involved in insulin-stimulated translocation.[9] Patients who are insulin resistant have been shown to have decreased expression of the GLUT4 transporter in skeletal muscle.[10] Insulin rapidly increases membrane glucose transport, within 1 to 2 minutes, with a maximal effect in 15 to 20 minutes.

Many tissues, including brain and liver, maintain glucose uptake independent of insulin concentrations.[11] This ability corresponds to the predominance in those tissues of glucose transporters such as GLUT1 (a ubiquitous transporter) and GLUT3 (brain) or GLUT2 (liver), respectively, which have plasma membrane activities known to be independent of insulin concentrations.[12] The hypothalamus may represent a brain region with some dependence on insulin for glucose use, particularly in the glucose-sensitive areas of the ventromedial and lateral nuclei.[13,14] Conversely, skeletal muscle (generally an "insulin-sensitive" tissue) may take up glucose without insulin stimulation under circumstances of contractile stimulation.[15]

In addition to increasing glucose transport, insulin also has major effects on intracellular glucose metabolism (Fig. 40–3). In experimentally induced diabetes, activities of enzymes involved in glycolysis and glucose oxidation, such as glucokinase, phosphofructokinase, and pyruvate kinase, are decreased, and activities of gluconeogenic enzymes, such as glucose-6-phosphatase, fructose 1,6-bisphosphatase, phosphoenolpyruvate carboxykinase, and pyruvate carboxylase, are increased. These abnormalities are corrected by insulin replacement. Insulin also promotes glycogen synthesis, by promoting the conversion of glycogen synthase to its active, glucose-6-phosphate independent ("I") form, and by decreasing the activity of phosphorylase. Insulin causes rapid decreases in phosphorylase activity and

**TABLE 40–1.** EFFECT OF HORMONES ON NUTRIENT STORES

| HORMONES | CARBOHYDRATE | LIPID | PROTEIN |
|---|---|---|---|
| Pancreatic Hormones | | | |
| Insulin | ↑ | ↑ | ↑ |
| Glucagon | ↓ | ↓ | ↓ |
| Somatostatin | * | * | * |
| Thyroid Hormones | | | |
| Thyroxine(T4)/ Triiodothyronine (T3) | * | ↓ | * |
| Glucocorticoid/ACTH | | | |
| ACTH | * | ↓ | * |
| Cortisol | * | * | ↓ |
| Growth Hormone/IGF-1 | | | |
| Growth hormone | * | * | ↑ |
| Insulin-like Growth factor-1 (IGF-1) | ↑ | ↑ | ↑ |
| Catecholamines | | | |
| Epinephrine/ Norepinephrine | ↓ (α + β) | ↓ (β1) | * |
| Gonadal Hormones/Prolactin | | | |
| Estrogen | * | * | * |
| Progesterone | * | * | * |
| Testosterone | ↓ | * | ↑ |
| Prolactin | * | ↓ | * |
| Cytokines/Eicosanoids | | | |
| Thromboxane A2 (TXA2)/prostaglandin E2, and F2α (PGE2, PGF2α) | ↓ | * | * |
| Tumor necrosis factor-α (TNF-α) | * | ↓ | ↓ |
| Interleukin 6 | * | * | ↑ |

*, no effect, variable effects, or unknown; see text.

more gradual increases in synthase I activity, although the hormonal effect is brief in vivo.[16]

Insulin generates an enzymatic profile that decreases glucose carbon recycling, seen during insulin deficiency, and promotes glucose use for energy storage.[17] Some data suggest that elevations in plasma glucose levels may play a more important role than insulin concentrations in activation of glycogen synthase and glycogen deposition in the liver, whereas insulin has a key role in the regulation of skeletal muscle glycogen metabolism.[18] However, results of studies with cultured hepatocytes indicate that glucose-stimulated glycogen deposition plateaus within 2 hours of exposure to high-glucose medium, and insulin is required to continue glycogen accumulation beyond that time.[19] Insulin stimulates glycolysis and lipogenesis in adipose tissue and both glycolysis and glycogen synthesis in skeletal muscle tissue, and inhibits gluconeogenesis in the renal cortex and liver.[20]

The ingestion of carbohydrate produces a prompt increase in plasma insulin and a decrease in glucagon concentrations.[21] The rise in insulin occurs before the rise in arterial glucose concentrations, comprising the so-called "enteroinsular axis" and cephalic phase insulin release, which are mediated through hormonal[22,23] and parasympathetic[24,25] mechanisms. This early insulin release creates a "priming effect" in which the action of insulin begins concurrently with the absorption of glucose to minimize the extent of hyperglycemia after a meal. As glucose is absorbed, the hepatic production of glucose is decreased through the hormonal changes just mentioned, and glucose uptake by the liver, muscle, and adipose tissues increases. Approximately 75% of glucose taken orally bypasses hepatic metabolism and is taken up peripherally.[26] Skeletal muscle is the predominant tissue for disposal of an oral glucose load.

During periods of starvation, the maintenance of euglycemia is critically important to the organism. In the nonketotic state, the energy needs of the brain can only be met by glucose, and its absence results in the death of central nervous system tissues. Because the glucose pool can provide only 15 to 20 g in the adult, and glycogen that can be mobilized to provide circulating glucose (i.e., hepatic glycogen) averages 70 g, performed glucose can only provide for less than an 8-hour supply of glucose on average. Thus, gluconeogenesis is important for the maintenance of postabsorptive plasma glucose concentrations and becomes the sole source of glucose

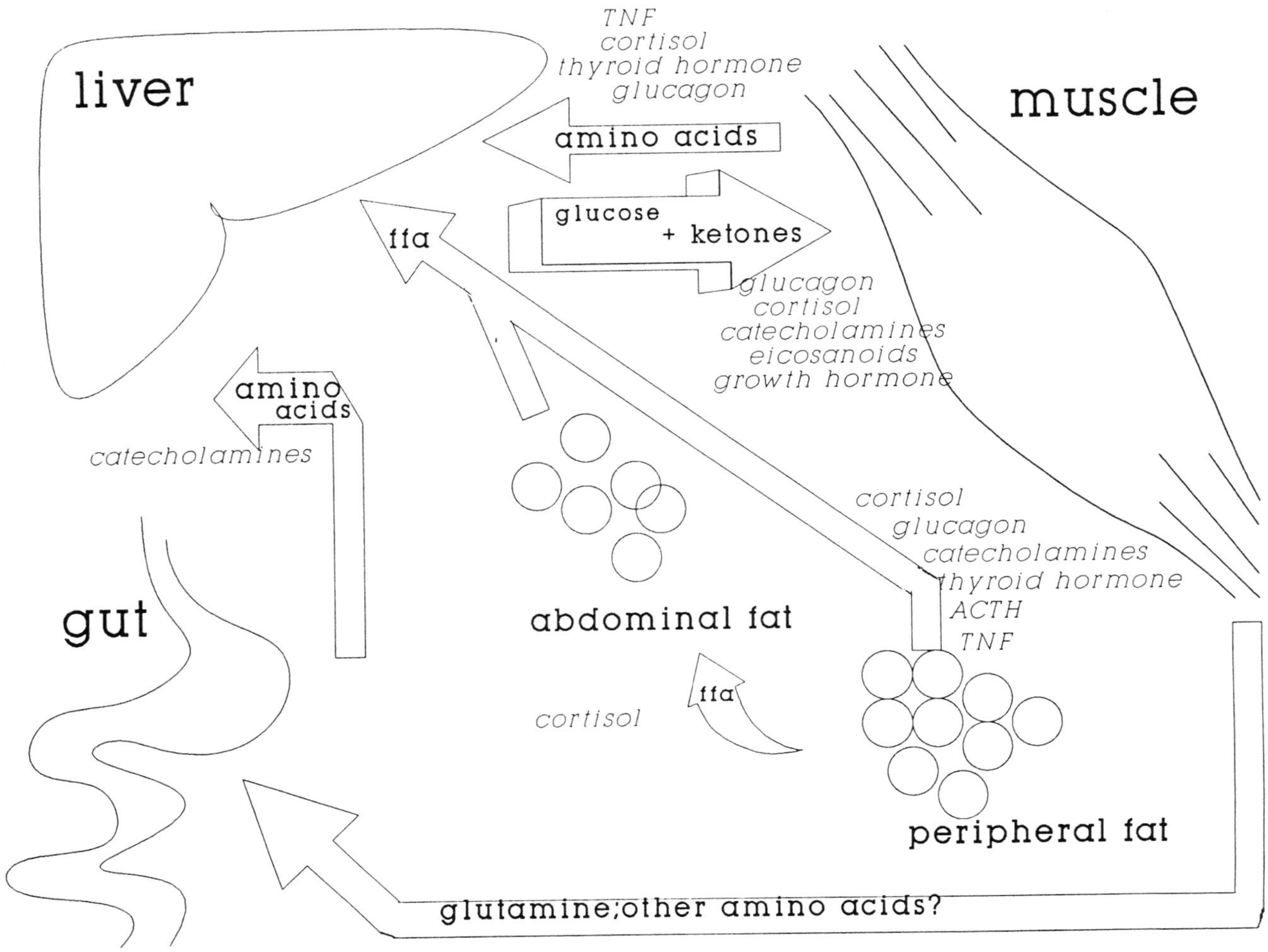
liver
muscle
TNF
cortisol
thyroid hormone
glucagon
amino acids
glucose
+ ketones
ffa
glucagon
cortisol
catecholamines
eicosanoids
growth hormone
amino acids
catecholamines
cortisol
glucagon
catecholamines
thyroid hormone
ACTH
TNF
gut
abdominal fat
ffa
cortisol
peripheral fat
glutamine;other amino acids?

**FIGURE 40–2.** Hormones promoting nutrient mobilization from tissue stores. Arrows represent the release of nutrients from storage sites in skeletal muscle, adipose tissue, gut, and liver. The hormones stimulating the release of particular nutrients are indicated in italics next to the appropriate arrows. TNF, Tumor necrosis factor; ACTH, adrenocorticotropic hormone; ffa, free fatty acids.

production beyond a 24- to 48-hour fast. Only the liver and kidneys contain glucose-6-phosphatase, the enzyme necessary for the release of glucose into the circulation. The liver and kidneys also contain the enzymes necessary for gluconeogenesis (pyruvate carboxylase, PEP carboxykinase, and fructose 1,6-bisphosphatase). Except after prolonged starvation when renal gluconeogenesis becomes important, the liver is the sole source of endogenous glucose production (EGP). Starvation is associated with a decline in insulin and a rise in glucagon concentrations,[27] which result in increased rates of gluconeogenesis. Decreased plasma insulin concentrations allow decreased glucose use by peripheral tissues and enhanced lipolysis; free fatty acids are thus more available for use as an oxidative fuel during starvation. These changes in serum insulin and glucagon concentrations also result in increased conversion of free fatty acids to the ketone bodies, acetoacetate and β-hydroxybutyrate, which can substitute for glucose as an energy supply for the brain.[28] The change from a glucose- to a lipid-based (free fatty acids and ketone bodies) energy supply in prolonged starvation helps to minimize skeletal muscle protein catabolism by reducing the need for amino acid-derived gluconeogenesis.[29] β-Hydroxybutyrate also directly increases skeletal muscle protein synthesis in humans while simultaneously decreasing leucine oxidation.[30] Similarly, studies in dogs have demonstrated that increased free fatty acid availability decreases whole-body leucine oxidation rate and leucine carbon flux (an estimate of protein degradation rate).[31]

The effects of insulin deficiency are exemplified by type I, insulin-dependent diabetes mellitus (IDDM). As stated previously, this disorder is associated with increased activities of enzymes involved in gluconeogenesis, and decreased activities of glycolytic and oxidative enzymes. In addition, IDDM often is associated with relative or

**TABLE 40–2.** EFFECTS OF HORMONES ON CIRCULATING CONCENTRATIONS OF METABOLITES

| HORMONES | GLUCOSE | FREE FATTY ACIDS | AMINO ACIDS |
|---|---|---|---|
| Pancreatic Hormones | | | |
| Insulin | ↓ | ↓ | ↓ |
| Glucagon | ↑ | ↑ | ↓ |
| Somatostatin | ↑ | ↑ | * |
| Thyroid Hormones | | | |
| Thyroxine (T4)/ Triiodothyronine (T3) | ↑ | ↑ | * |
| Glucocorticoid/ACTH | | | |
| ACTH | * | ↑ | * |
| Cortisol | ↑ | ↑ | ↑ |
| Growth Hormone/IGF-1 | | | |
| Growth Hormone | * | * | * |
| Insulin-like growth factor (IGF-1) | ↓ | ↓ | ↓ |
| Catecholamines | | | |
| Epinephrine/ norepinephrine | ↑ | ↑ | ↓ |
| Estrogen | * | * | * |
| Progesterone | * | * | * |
| Testosterone | ↑ | * | * |
| Prolactin | ↑ | ↑ | * |
| Cytokines/Eicosanoids | | | |
| Thromboxane A2 (TXA2), prostaglandin E2 PGE2, and PGF2α | ↑ | * | * |
| Tumor necrosis factor (TNF-α) | * | ↑ | ↑ |
| Interleukin 6 (Il-6) | * | * | * |

*, no effect, variable effects, or unknown; see text.

absolute hyperglucagonemia,[32,33] resulting from loss of the restraining influence of insulin[34] on the secretion of glucagon by the pancreatic alpha cell.[35] An increase in glucose concentration also fails to inhibit glucagon secretion[36,37] as it normally does, and may paradoxically increase glucagon release.[38] Glucagon responses to protein are also excessive in association with IDDM[20] and are not blunted by hyperglycemia.[39] Control of the plasma glucose concentration to near normal levels with insulin therapy corrects the basal hyperglucagonemia[40] and the exaggerated response to protein ingestion.[38]

Inappropriate hyperinsulinemia, as seen in insulin-producing islet cell adenomas or hyperplasia, results in postabsorptive hypoglycemia. In this condition, insulin secretion probably does not decrease as the plasma glucose declines in the postabsorptive state. The result is a low rate of EGP with rates of glucose uptake that are not high in the absolute sense but are inappropriately high relative to the plasma glucose concentration. The hypoglycemic effect of insulin is potent, and when present in sufficient quantity, it can cause hypoglycemia despite the actions of all known counter-regulatory factors. Postabsorptive hypoglycemia may also occur when both glucagon and epinephrine are deficient and insulin is present.[41] This situation occurs in some patients with IDDM,[42,43] but has not been demonstrated convincingly in other conditions.

Glucagon is secreted from the alpha cells of the pancreatic islets into the hepatic portal circulation, and is thought to act exclusively on the liver under physiologic conditions. Glucagon exerts its effects through activation of adenyl cyclase.[44] Cyclic adenosine monophosphate (AMP) concentrations in liver rise within seconds after the administration of glucagon. Glucagon is a potent activator of glycogenolysis and gluconeogenesis and is able to increase EGP within minutes, although the effect is transient. Glucagon decreases levels of fructose-2, 6-diphosphate, a key regulator of gluconeogenesis and glycolysis. Despite ongoing hyperglucagonemia, EGP decreases toward basal levels within 90 minutes. Glucagon-induced hyperglycemia is transient because the increase in glycogenolysis does not persist. This transient response is not the result of glycogen depletion, but more likely glucagon-induced insulin secretion coupled with an autoregulatory effect of hyperglycemia to inhibit EGP.

During fasting in humans, about 75% of EGP is mediated by glucagon.[45] In circumstances of combined

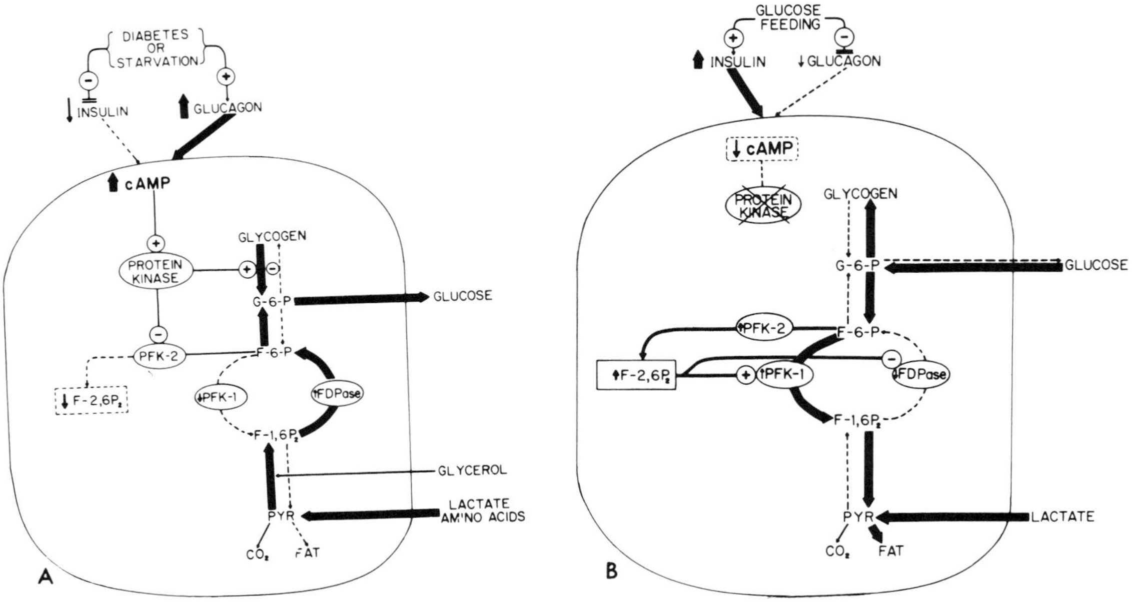
DIABETES OR STARVATION
INSULIN
GLUCAGON
cAMP
PROTEIN KINASE
GLYCOGEN
G-6-P
GLUCOSE
PFK-2
F-6-P
F-2,6P2
PFK-1
FDPase
F-1,6P2
GLYCEROL
PYR
LACTATE AMINO ACIDS
CO2
FAT
A
GLUCOSE FEEDING
INSULIN
GLUCAGON
cAMP
PROTEIN KINASE
GLYCOGEN
G-6-P
GLUCOSE
PFK-2
F-6-P
F-2,6P2
PFK-1
FDPase
F-1,6P2
PYR
LACTATE
CO2
FAT
B

**FIGURE 40–3.** *A*, Enhancement of gluconeogenesis and glycogenolysis by glucagon in diabetes and starvation. Both processes are activated by increases in cyclic adenosine monophosphate (cAMP) in the hepatocyte. Phosphofructokinase-1 (PFK-1) catalyzes formation of fructose 1,6-biphosphate (F-2, 6-$P_2$) in the glycolytic pathway, whereas PFK-2 synthesizes F-2, 6-$P_2$, a regulator of PFK-1 activity; cAMP-induced phosphorylation of the enzyme decreases PFK-1 and increases PFK-2. Decreased F-2, 6-$P_2$ decreases glycolysis and increases gluconeogenesis. *B*, Inhibition of gluconeogenesis and activation of glycogen synthesis and lipogenesis by insulin. Insulin decreases cAMP, deactivates protein kinase, and reverses changes in F-2, 6-$P_2$ and substrate flux over the glycolytic-gluconeogenic pathway produced by glucagon. Glycogen synthesis and lipogenesis are also increased. (From Unger, R.H., Foster, D.W.: *In* Williams Textbook of Endocrinology. 7th Ed. Edited by J. Wilson and D.W. Foster. Philadelphia, W.B. Saunders, 1985.)

glucagon and insulin deficiency, the decreased glucose production may not be balanced by decreased insulin-mediated glucose use because only about 40% of glucose use occurs in insulin-sensitive tissues. Therefore, plasma glucose concentrations would remain constant or even fall. The major effect of insulin on the liver is to oppose the effect of glucagon.[46] Insulin deficiency has a minimal influence on hepatic glucose and ketone metabolism in the absence of glucagon, and significant overproduction of glucose and ketones by the liver does not occur without glucagon.[47]

Glucagon deficiency, produced experimentally by infusion of somatostatin with partial insulin replacement, reduces nadir glucose concentrations after glucose ingestion by approximately 30%. Patients who have glucagon deficiency from pancreatectomy have been shown to manifest decreased rates of glucose "recyling" (measured as the difference between 6-$^3$H-glucose and 1-$^{14}$C-glucose turnover rates, an index of gluconeogenesis) and increased serum concentrations of gluconeogenic precursors such as alanine and lactate.[48] However, prolonged hypoglycemia does not occur because it is prevented by epinephrine secretion. As noted previously, combined glucagon and epinephrine deficiency, as seen in some longstanding IDDM subjects, totally disrupts the counter-regulatory process and results in hypoglycemia late after glucose ingestion. Recent evidence suggests that diminished glucagon response to insulin-induced hypoglycemia is in part related to concomitant insulin-induced hypoaminoacidemia.[49]

Exercise requires increased glucose production to counterbalance the increased glucose use that occurs with muscular work. Approximately 60 to 70% of the increased glucose production is mediated by increased glucagon secretion coupled with inhibited insulin release; another 30 to 40% is the result of epinephrine secretion.[50,51] The changes in glucagon and insulin are associated with decreased fructose-2,6-diphosphate concentration in liver with resultant increased gluconeogenesis; simultaneous increases in epinephrine concentration produce increased concentrations of fructose-2,6-diphosphate in nonexercising muscle with resultant stimulation of glycolysis and lactate production for use in gluconeogenesis.[52] Combined glucagon deficiency and adrenergic blockade during exercise at 60% of maximal oxygen consumption produces profound hypoglycemia between 30 and 60 minutes of the exercise bout.[50]

Glucagon excess, as seen in islet-cell glucagonoma, is

associated with glucose intolerance, hypoaminoacidemia, and a characteristic skin rash, "necrolytic migratory erythema," thought to be the result of either the hyperglucagonemia or the decreased plasma amino acid levels.[53,54] The glycogenolytic and gluconeogenic actions of glucagon result in mild hyperglycemia that can usually be controlled by dietary therapy. The syndrome is also characterized by increased resting energy expenditure that is blunted by insulin infusion.[55] The cause of the hypermetabolism is unknown.

In the somatostatinoma syndrome,[56] seen in somatostatin-producing islet cell adenomas, suppression of both insulin and glucagon causes mild diabetes mellitus. Neither the hyperglycemia nor the hyperketonemia is severe, most likely because of glucagon and growth hormone suppression. The somatostatin analogue, octreotide, can similarly blunt postprandial glycemic excursions in IDDM patients and decrease prandial insulin requirements.[57]

## LIPID METABOLISM

Insulin and glucagon also play important roles in lipid metabolism; increased insulin concentrations stimulate lipogenesis and lipid storage, and the decreased insulin and increased glucagon levels seen in fasting promote lipolysis and lipid oxidation.[58] The major function of stored triglyceride in adipose tissue is to act as an efficient energy reserve. Triglyceride stores can serve as a fuel to support many weeks of fasting, whereas stored carbohydrate is able to support a fast lasting only several hours. Stored triglyceride yields over two times as many calories per gram as either carbohydrate or protein, and requires less than one half the intracellular water for storage.

In the fed state, insulin and glucose are required for lipogenesis. Glucose use is needed for fatty acid synthesis and esterification, and supplies the following: (1) acetyl coenzyme A (CoA) as a precursor of long-chain fatty acids, (2) α-glycerophosphate for esterification to fatty acids to form triglycerides, and (3) nicotinamide adenine dinucleotide phosphate (NADPH). Insulin stimulates carrier-mediated glucose transport, and (1) activates pyruvate dehydrogenase for conversion of glucose to acetyl CoA,[59] and (2) inhibits lipolysis, thereby reducing palmitoyl CoA, an inhibitor of lipogenesis.[60] In humans, however, less than 1% of ingested carbohydrate is converted to lipid.[61] The mixed fat and carbohydrate intake of humans allows dietary fat to supply lipid for storage in a more thermically efficient process than would be achieved if significant lipogenesis from carbohydrate occurred (i.e., 2% versus 23% of ingested calories, representing the cost of storing these nutrients as lipid, respectively).[62]

Fatty acids stored in adipose tissue as triglyceride are derived from either dietary (chylomicrons) or endogenous (hepatic very low-density lipoproteins [VLDL]) sources. Preformed triglycerides are transported from the gastrointestinal tract and liver to adipose tissue, where they are hydrolyzed by the enzyme lipoprotein lipase (LPL) on the cell surface of the capillary endothelium. Insulin has an important role in maintaining and stimulating the activity of LPL.[63] In addition, insulin has a direct stimulatory effect on free fatty acid uptake by adipose tissue. During insulin deficiency, LPL activity is reduced and uptake of free fatty acids by adipose tissue is diminished.[64]

In humans, liver as well as adipose tissue is a major site of lipid synthesis, occurring when dietary fat is replaced by carbohydrate. The liver removes a large proportion of circulating free fatty acids delivered from adipose tissue in a concentration-dependent manner. Fatty acids synthesized in the liver are converted mainly to VLDL, which are secreted into plasma and then cleared from the circulation within minutes to hours by mechanisms similar to those involved in the removal of chylomicron triglycerides (see Chap. 3). During insulin deficiency, hexose monophosphate shunt activity is impaired, and NADPH is not provided for fatty acid synthesis.[65] In addition, decreased glucose use reduces the availability of acetyl CoA and citrate, which retards lipogenesis.

Lipolysis, with a net release of free fatty acids and glycerol from adipose tissue, occurs during periods of fasting, exercise, stress, and uncontrolled diabetes mellitus. Low levels of insulin and increased glucagon concentrations enhance this mobilization of lipid from adipose tissue.[58] Several hormones, including glucagon, catecholamines, thyroid stimulating hormone (TSH), and adrenocorticotrophic hormone (ACTH), play important roles in lipolysis (Fig. 40–2) through cyclic-AMP mediated stimulation of "hormone-sensitive lipase." Insulin reduces catecholamine-stimulated cAMP concentrations in adipose tissue,[66] by either decreasing adenylate cyclase and/or increasing phosphodiesterase activity.[67] With lipolysis, glycerol diffuses out of the adipocyte, because adipose tissue lacks the enzyme glycerolkinase and cannot reuse glycerol. Free fatty acids can either be released into the circulation or re-esterified with glycerol phosphates into triglycerides in adipose tissue. Part of the antilipolytic action of insulin is to stimulate re-esterification of fatty acids.

After release from adipose tissue, the glycerol and free fatty acids circulate briefly in the plasma. Glycerol is metabolized primarily in the liver and kidney, where it is phosphorylated and either re-esterified to triglyceride or used for gluconeogenesis. Free fatty acids are taken up by tissues in proportion to local blood flow and plasma concentrations. The potential fate of those taken up by the liver includes re-esterification to triglyceride, oxidation, or conversion to ketone bodies, depending on the hormonal milieu. In the absence of either glucose or insulin, and in the presence of glucagon, only a small proportion of the free fatty acids taken up by the liver is re-esterified to triglyceride and released as VLDL. The insulin-glucagon ratio[68] appears to be critical in regulating the hepatic metabolism of free fatty acids.

Activated fatty acids must be transported into the mitochondria for oxidation or conversion to ketone bodies, and neither free fatty acids nor their CoA derivatives can penetrate the inner mitochondrial membrane. Carnitine palmitoyl transferase I is an enzyme present on the inner mitochondrial membrane, which reversibly transfers fatty acyl groups from CoA to carnitine and allows entry into the mitochondria. A second enzyme, carnitine palmitoyl transferase II, irreversibly transfers the fatty acyl groups to mitochondrial CoA, allowing them to undergo either β-oxidation or conversion to the ketone bodies acetoacetate and β-hydroxybutyrate. The activity of the key enzyme, carnitine palmitoyl transferase I, is regulated through the effects of insulin and glucagon on malonyl CoA concentrations.[69] In addition to their effects on carnitine palmitoyl transferase I activity, low insulin and high glucagon concentrations also contribute to increased lipid oxidation and ketogenesis by increasing adipose tissue lipolysis and free fatty acid delivery. Ketone bodies circulate in plasma and are metabolized in skeletal muscle and heart and brain tissues.

Alterations in lipid metabolism are frequently present in subjects with diabetes mellitus, with hypertriglyceridemia occurring in approximately one third of patients. This finding is related to the key role insulin plays in both hepatic triglyceride production and in removal of triglyceride-rich lipoproteins.[70] Insulin is essential for the normal function of lipoprotein lipase (LPL); with severe insulin deficiency, hypertriglyceridemia is secondary to acquired LPL deficiency. "Diabetic lipemia," with milky plasma and eruptive xanthoma, may be the result of coexistent poorly controlled IDDM and a familial form of hypertriglyceridemia.[71] This defect is promptly reversed with appropriate insulin replacement. Withdrawal of insulin from subjects with IDDM can produce decreased LPL activity and hypertriglyceridemia within 48 hours.

Obese subjects, both with and without diabetes, have higher than normal rates of VLDL triglyceride production.[72,73] This increased rate is probably related to an increased flow of glucose and free fatty acids to the liver as part of an insulin resistance syndrome.[74] This form of hypertriglyceridemia responds dramatically to weight reduction.[75]

The predominant insulin deficiency of IDDM and the predominant insulin resistance of NIDDM have other widespread effects on lipoprotein metabolism.[76] In IDDM, this may include increased low-density lipoprotein (LDL) from decreased insulin-stimulated LDL receptor activity. In NIDDM, these include (1) low levels of high-density lipoprotein (HDL) from decreased transfer of surface components of triglyceride-rich lipoproteins to HDL, (2) triglyceride enrichment of LDL and VLDL particles, and (3) accumulation of VLDL remnant particles, related perhaps in part to an increased ratio of apoprotein CIII to CII. Nonenzymatic glycosylation of lipoproteins in both forms of diabetes may further alter their clearance characteristics such that LDL catabolism is decreased and HDL catabolism is increased.[77]

The effect of dietary composition on lipoprotein metabolism in diabetes remains controversial. Current recommendations for a low-fat, high-carbohydrate diet are based on the decreased total and LDL cholesterol values seen with this approach.[78] Some investigators suggest that a moderate carbohydrate intake with expanded use of monounsaturated fats provides the most effective control of the VLDL elevation and low HDL of NIDDM.[75,79]

## PROTEIN METABOLISM

Insulin and other hormones play an important role in *protein metabolism*. In as small a period as several hours of starvation, protein catabolism is increased to provide amino acids for gluconeogenesis. With more prolonged starvation, metabolic adjustments occur that spare muscle protein, such as increased reliance by the central nervous system on ketone bodies as an oxidative fuel (see Chap. 56). Nonetheless, muscle continues to yield a net release of amino acids as plasma insulin levels fall during prolonged starvation; the phenomenon can be reversed completely when insulin delivery is increased.[80] When fuel supplies become plentiful, protein synthesis is restored.

Insulin lowers blood concentrations of several amino acids in normal as well as in diabetic subjects in a time pattern that is similar to that for glucose concentration. The serum insulin concentrations required to produce half-maximal suppression of plasma amino acid concentrations are similar to those required for half-maximal stimulation of peripheral glucose disposal.[81] The lowering of plasma levels of the essential amino acids occurs in a pattern that corresponds to their relative concentrations in muscle protein. Isolated muscle preparations incubated in vitro liberate amino acids; the rate of release is depressed by the addition of insulin. The presence of glucose may be necessary for insulin-mediated inhibition of heart muscle proteolysis.[82] Insulin also inhibits intracellular protein degradation in isolated hepatocytes, an effect that depends on internalization of insulin by the cells.[82] In addition to inhibiting release, insulin also stimulates accumulation of amino acids in skeletal muscle. Of the six identified amino acid transport systems in human fibroblasts, insulin strongly stimulates two, the A and the $X_c$ systems (transporters for neutral amino acids and long-chain anionic amino acids, respectively).[83] System A is similarly regulated by insulin in hepatocytes.[84] The primary effect of insulin is to increase the $V_{max}$ of transport, felt to represent an increase in plasma membrane transporter number. Insulin regulates amino acid transport in many other tissues, including muscle, bone, and lymphocytes, but the transport systems involved are not well characterized.

Prior exercise may potentiate the ability of insulin to increase amino acid uptake by muscle tissues.[85] Exercise additionally inhibits amino acid release from skeletal muscle protein, but the effect appears limited to nonmyofibrillar proteins.[86] When added to isolated muscle preparations, insulin promotes incorporation of labeled amino acids into tissue protein.[87] At the subcellular level, protein synthesis appears to be stimulated in both cytoplasm and mitochondria.[88]

Insulin stimulates the incorporation of labeled precursors into nucleic acid.[89] Although insulin increases RNA synthesis in muscle, the increase does not appear to be a requisite for hormone-mediated stimulation of protein synthesis; actinomycin, an inhibitor of RNA synthesis, does not impair the ability of insulin to increase protein synthesis.[90]

The importance of insulin in the regulation of protein balance has been demonstrated most clearly in subjects with IDDM who rapidly develop negative nitrogen balance with the cessation of insulin therapy. In heart and most skeletal muscles studied, the absolute protein content, i.e., the quantity of protein per tissue or organ, was significantly less in diabetic than in control animals. In contrast, the protein content of liver was unaffected in those with diabetes.[91] The most significant loss of protein in vivo, as the result of insulin deficiency, occurs in muscle. Studies with stable isotopes of amino acids used to examine rates of whole-body protein turnover and oxidation have demonstrated increased rates of protein degradation and leucine oxidation in insulin-deprived IDDM subjects, which could be decreased by insulin infusions.[92] In vitro[93] and animal[94] studies have demonstrated decreased rates of protein synthesis in diabetes. In contrast, increased rates of protein synthesis were found in insulin-deprived IDDM human subjects, although protein breakdown was more accelerated.[95] The postulated mechanism for this increase in protein synthesis in vivo, not found in vitro, is that accelerated protein degradation provides increased intracellular free amino acid concentrations as precursors for protein synthesis. Conversely, insulin administration to insulin-dependent diabetic patients decreases intracellular free amino acid concentrations through inhibition of protein degradation in skeletal muscle, resulting in an inability of insulin to increase muscle protein synthesis in vivo.[96,97] Some authors have reported resistance to insulin-mediated suppression of branched-chain amino acid (BCAA) plasma concentrations,[98] and rates of BCAA turnover and oxidation[99] in IDDM. Other investigators show normalization of whole-body amino acid metabolism in IDDM with prolonged tight glycemic control.[100]

The effects of glucagon on amino acid metabolism are threefold: (1) to increase membrane transport of amino acids, (2) to decrease protein synthesis and increase catabolism (when accompanied by insulin deficiency, both protein degradation and amino acid oxidation rates increase); and (3) to increase amino acid conversion into glucose (gluconeogenesis).[101,102]

Glucagon increases gluconeogenesis in perfused liver, an effect that can be reproduced by perfusion with cyclic AMP. Glucagon increases hepatic use of glycine, alanine, glutamate, and phenylalanine for gluconeogenesis. In addition, glucagon also increases the rate of ureagenesis.

During early starvation, plasma glucagon and insulin concentrations increase and decrease, respectively, resulting in increased rates of gluconeogenesis and ureagenesis. Splanchnic extraction of alanine is increased from 43% in the postabsorptive state to 71% after 3 days of fasting, but this value decreases to 53% after 6 weeks of fasting.[103] These effects of fasting are mimicked by glucagon infusion.[104] With prolonged starvation, the brain adapts by developing the capacity to use ketone bodies as an energy source, thereby decreasing the need for increased rates of gluconeogenesis.

Glucagon is able to increase liver protein catabolism in the intact animal. Liver protein content is decreased and branched-chain amino acid release from the liver is increased by glucagon. This increased protein catabolism can be suppressed by the administration of insulin or a mixture of amino acids.

When protein is ingested without accompanying carbohydrate, insulin concentrations increase slightly, allowing skeletal muscle protein retention, with a parallel rise in glucagon[21] that prevents hypoglycemia.[105]

As mentioned previously, a common feature of patients with glucagonoma syndrome is hypoaminoacidemia. When similar degrees of hyperglucagonemia are produced by infusions of glucagon in normal volunteers, reductions in blood amino acid concentrations are similar.[106] High-protein diets can normalize the plasma amino acid profile and result in a positive nitrogen balance in patients with glucagonoma syndrome.[107] When glucagon deficiency is produced by infusions of somatostatin with insulin replacement, amino acid concentrations are increased.[108] Urinary urea nitrogen and total nitrogen excretion rates are lower during glucagon deficiency than during glucagon excess, suggesting that alterations in the rate of gluconeogenesis constitute one mechanism by which glucagon influences blood amino acid levels.

## THYROID HORMONES

### CARBOHYDRATE METABOLISM

Thyroid hormones exert multiple effects on *carbohydrate metabolism.* Patients with hyperthyroidism frequently (30 to 50%) display mild to moderate degrees of glucose intolerance.[109–111] Part of this abnormality is attributable to more rapid gastric emptying and intestinal absorption of glucose in hyperthyroidism,[112] whereas glucose absorption is delayed in hypothyroidism. Additionally, insulin secretion is reduced in hyperthyroidism in response to oral but not intravenous administration of glucose,[113] and may be accompanied by impaired processing of proinsulin to insulin.[114]

Rates of hepatic glucose production are increased by 20% in the basal state, and the liver is less sensitive to insulin infusions in hyperthyroid human subjects.[115] Hepatic glycogen stores are reduced in states of thyroid hormone excess. Thyroid hormones appear to modulate the magnitude of the glycogenolytic and hyperglycemic actions of epinephrine and norepinephrine, possibly by enhancing the responsiveness of the adenylate cyclase-cyclic AMP system. In rats, thyroid hormone exerts a biphasic effect on liver glycogen. Small doses of thyroid hormone increase glycogen synthesis in the presence of insulin, whereas large doses augment hepatic glycogenolysis. Small doses of thyroid hormone enhance, and large doses depress, the glycogenolytic response to epinephrine.[116] The glycogen content of liver and muscle tissues is decreased in hypothyroidism, possibly reflecting a new balance between simultaneously decreased rates of glycogen synthesis and degradation.[117]

Rates of gluconeogenesis are also increased in hyperthyroidism, in part because of an increase in substrate supply from protein breakdown and lipolysis. The splanchnic uptake of gluconeogenic precursors is also increased by 20 to 120% in hyperthyroidism.[115] Glyconeogenesis is suppressed in hypothyroidism. In vitro, the addition of $T_3$ to hypothyroid hepatocytes stimulates hepatic gluconeogenesis by approximately 80 to 90% within 30 to 40 minutes.[117]

Rates of total glucose disposal during euglycemic, hyperinsulinemic clamp studies were normal, suggesting that skeletal muscle is not insulin-resistant in hyperthyroidism.[118] However, in vitro skeletal muscle preparations from hyperthyroid rats display rates of insulin-stimulated glucose oxidation that are significantly (twofold) increased, whereas rates of glycogen synthesis are reduced.[119] Oxidative glucose use appears to be synergistically stimulated by exercise and thyroid hormones.

Total body glucose turnover rates are increased in thyrotoxicosis. A major fraction of the increased glucose turnover is accounted for by increases in glucose recycling. Recycling through both the Cori (glucose-lactate) and the glucose-alanine cycles is increased in hyperthyroidism and decreased in hypothyroidism.[116] In addition, patients with hyperthyroidism form hexose intermediates of both glycolysis and gluconeogenesis simultaneously at increased rates (i.e., glucose $\leftrightarrow$ glucose-6-P and fructose-6-P $\leftrightarrow$ fructose-1,6-di-P).[120] In part, thyroid hormone facilitates these cycling phenomena by stimulating glucose transporter gene expression and enhancing glucose transport across the plasma membrane in muscle and liver cells.[121,122]

## LIPID METABOLISM

Thyroid hormones also have an impact on multiple aspects of *lipid metabolism*, including lipid synthesis, mobilization, and degradation. Degradation is affected more than synthesis, so the net effect of excess thyroid hormone is a decrease in total body lipid stores and plasma concentrations. Thyroid hormones increase lipolysis in adipose tissue by both directly stimulating cyclic AMP production and increasing the sensitivity to other lipolytic agents (catecholamines, TSH, ACTH, growth hormone, glucocorticoids, and glucagon). Conversely, lipolysis is impaired in hypothyroidism.

The delivery of free fatty acids to peripheral tissues and the liver is increased in hyperthyroidism. Free fatty acid turnover rates are increased approximately twofold in thyrotoxicosis.[123] Lipid oxidation rates are also increased in thyrotoxicosis, which may contribute to the calorigenic action of thyroid hormones.

Hepatic triglyceride synthesis is increased in hyperthyroidism, in large part because of the increased delivery of free fatty acids and glycerol to the liver. The synthesis and clearance of cholesterol and triglyceride are accelerated in hyperthyroidism, with the latter effect predominating. Serum cholesterol and triglyceride levels are usually modestly reduced.[124] Conversely, serum lipid levels may be increased in hypothyroidism because of impaired clearance. HDL cholesterol levels decrease in hypothyroidism even at a subclinical stage and revert to normal with thyroxine therapy.[125] Both hepatic and adipose tissue lipoprotein lipase activity have been reported to be low in hypothyroidism.[126,127]

At a cellular level, lipid transfer into and out of membranes is altered by thyroid hormone. Cholesterol is transfered out of erythrocyte plasma membranes into plasma in hyperthyroidism, resulting in a higher relative phospholipid content of the erythrocyte membrane.[128] The change in lipid content of mitochondrial membrane induced by hyperthyroidism allows increased phosphate transport[129]—teleologically, a favorable compensation for partially uncoupled electron transport in this condition.

## PROTEIN METABOLISM

With regard to *protein metabolism*, short-term administration of thyroid hormones produces increased liver protein and RNA content, with a concomitant decrease in muscle protein. With more prolonged administration, both liver and peripheral tissues decrease in size.[130] Thyroid hormone increases amino acid uptake by the liver, and increases incorporation of amino acids into protein by isolated liver microsomes and mitochondria.[131] The latter does not occur in the presence of actinomycin, suggesting that these effects of thyroid hormone are mediated by DNA transcription and RNA translation.[132]

Clinically, a great excess of thyroid hormone appears to have the opposite effect, with suppressed rates of protein synthesis,[133] increased catabolism of collagen,[134] and increased forearm amino acid release[135] in human subjects. Nitrogen excretion is increased in thyrotoxicosis, and nitrogen balance may be normal or negative depending on whether intake is sufficient to meet the increased demand.

In hypothyroidism, rates of protein synthesis and degradation are both decreased. Patients are usually in positive nitrogen balance. Treatment of myxedema is accompanied by mobilization of extracellular protein and a significant temporary negative nitrogen balance.

Total serum protein concentrations are usually normal in hypothyroidism.

## GLUCOCORTICOIDS

### CARBOHYDRATE METABOLISM

Corticosteroids in excess are known to produce increases in plasma insulin and glucose concentrations, i.e., a state of insulin resistance. This resistance is out of proportion to the degree of obesity seen in patients with Cushing's syndrome.[136–138] Glucose intolerance in association with Cushing's syndrome has been reported in 80 to 90% of patients, although overt diabetes occurs in only 15 to 20% of subjects.[139,140]

Glucocorticoids counteract the effects of insulin at numerous steps in glucose homeostasis. First, rates of gluconeogenesis may be augmented by several mechanisms: (1) increased release of gluconeogenic precursors, i.e., amino acids[141] and lactate,[142] from peripheral tissues; (2) increased activity of key gluconeogenic enzymes,[143] including pyruvate carboxylase and phosphoenolpyruvate (PEP) carboxykinase, the unidirectional, rate-limiting enzyme in the initiation of the gluconeogenic cascade from pyruvate; and (3) stimulation of glucagon secretion by pancreatic alpha cells.[141,144] The latter effect may be the result of increased proteolysis and hyperaminoacidemia. Corticosteroids act in conjunction with glucagon to increase rates of gluconeogenesis in perfused rat liver.[145] Recent in vivo human studies have shown increased activity of glucose-6-phosphatase rather than gluconeogenesis as the cause of increased hepatic glucose output in response to dexamethasone.[146] Thus, the subject remains controversial.

The second way in which glucocorticoids may affect glucose tolerance is by decreasing production of glucose transporters and promoting their sequestration in intracellular pools rather than at the plasma membrane, an effect reported in rat adipocytes[147] and fibroblasts.[148] Third, glucocorticoids decrease insulin binding to its receptor through decreases in receptor affinity[149,150] and number.[147] Finally, postreceptor defects in insulin action induced by glucocorticoids may exist and are not yet characterized.[137,151] The hyperglycemic action of glucocorticoids is amplified if increases in glucagon, catecholamines, or growth hormone are also present.[152,153] However, in regard to epinephrine, this synergism may only occur when epinephrine levels are elevated briefly in the presence of increased cortisol and not during prolonged (72-hour) elevation of levels of both hormones.[154]

Glucocorticoids stimulate hepatic glycogen deposition, and in this regard resemble the action of insulin. The carbon source for this new liver glycogen is derived from breakdown of muscle protein with release of amino acids. The activity of glycogen synthase, the rate-limiting enzyme for glycogen synthesis, is decreased in adrenalectomized rats, and restored to normal by corticosteroid treatment.

### LIPID METABOLISM

Glucocorticoids appear to exert a permissive effect on lipolysis through activation of cyclic AMP-dependent hormone-sensitive lipase in the adipocyte. Epinephrine-induced lipolysis is promoted by cortisol,[155] which appears necessary for the full stimulation of lipolysis by catecholamines.[156] Glucocorticoids are similarly required for the maximal lipolytic action of growth hormone. The lipolytic action of cortisol is prevented by inhibitors of protein synthesis.[157]

Prolonged treatment with glucocorticoids may result in increased plasma triglyceride concentrations.[158] This effect is seen most often in the presence of diabetes mellitus and primarily reflects impaired triglyceride removal. However, hepatocytes in culture increase triglyceride production and VLDL apoprotein synthesis when incubated with glucocorticoids.[159] LDL uptake and degradation by cultured fibroblasts and smooth muscle cells are also impaired by high doses of glucocorticoids.[160] Chronic glucocorticoid treatment may result in a "fatty liver," because of increased lipolysis and free fatty acid delivery associated with enhanced hepatic uptake of free fatty acids.

A chronic excess of corticosteroids also produces increases in total body fat in humans and in laboratory animals. Pair-feeding experiments suggest that increased food intake is the major factor contributing to obesity in steroid-treated rats.[161] Changes in body fat distribution are also characteristic of Cushing's syndrome, with accumulations of fat in the supraclavicular, truncal, and facial areas.[162] The altered fat distribution in humans with Cushing's syndrome is associated with enhanced adipocyte LPL activity and diminished lipolytic response to catecholamines in abdominal fat as compared with femoral region fat.[163] In addition, glucocorticoid receptor number and its mRNA are increased in abdominal region subcutaneous as opposed to femoral region subcutaneous fat; they are increased to an even greater extent in omental adipose tissue.[164]

The administration of ACTH stimulates lipolysis through cyclic AMP-mediated activation of adipose tissue hormone-sensitive lipase. This result is a direct action of ACTH, because it is demonstrable in adrenalectomized animals.[165]

### PROTEIN METABOLISM

One of the major metabolic effects of glucocorticoids is to stimulate skeletal muscle protein breakdown. Many of the clinical features of Cushing's syndrome, such as the loss of bone density, increased capillary fragility and dermal atrophy, muscle wasting, and growth retardation in children, are attributable, in part, to this augmented proteolysis. In addition to increasing protein breakdown, corticosteroids also appear to inhibit incorporation of amino acids into muscle protein.[166,167] Elevations of cortisol levels within the physiologic range have been shown to increase muscle proteolysis, with increased activation of muscle branched-chain ketoacid dehydrogenase and BCAA oxidation,[168,169] de novo alanine synthesis,[170] and muscle glutamine release.[171] Corticosteroid inhibition of muscle protein synthesis is sustained during prolonged elevation of glucocorticoid levels in the rat, whereas muscle proteolysis shows adaptation toward normal levels within a few days.[172] Thus, diminished protein synthesis rather than proteolysis may account for long-term effects of glucocorticoids to produce muscle wasting. The mechanism of adaptation of muscle myofibrillar protein breakdown is unknown; nonmyofibrillar muscle proteins may be spared by adaptive increases in insulin.[173]

In contrast to these effects on muscle tissues, corticosteroids can increase liver protein content. The administration of glucocorticoids results in increased protein and RNA contents of liver and other viscera.[174] Amino acids delivered as a result of enhanced muscle proteolysis and decreased peripheral use for protein synthesis are transported to the liver where they can be used for protein synthesis. The administration of cortisol to rats results in enhanced hepatic uptake of α-aminoisobutyric acid[167] and increased free amino nitrogen concentrations in the liver.[175] These effects of glucocorticoids depend on the diet, with increased protein synthesis occurring when the caloric and protein contents of the diet are adequate. Under circumstances of systemic inflammatory processes, glucocorticoids increase hepatocyte receptors for interleukin 6, a potent stimulator of synthesis of acute phase proteins such as C-reactive protein and fibrinogen.[176]

## GROWTH HORMONE AND INSULIN-LIKE GROWTH FACTOR-1 (IGF-1; SOMATOMEDIN-C)

When discussing the metabolic effects of growth hormone, it is important to distinguish the direct effects of growth hormone from those of IGF-1. The latter is synthesized by liver and other tissues in response to stimulation by growth hormone, although nutritional intake appears to have a direct effect on IGF-1 production. In normal human volunteers, IGF-1 levels decline 60 to 70% during a 5-day fast.[177] Studies in the rat have shown that both adequate dietary protein and total energy contents are necessary to produce IGF-1-stimulated cartilage growth.[178] The "somatomedin hypothesis" states that many of the anabolic, growth-promoting effects of growth hormone are mediated by IGF-1 (somatomedin-C), whereas growth hormone has direct catabolic effects on glucose and lipid metabolism.

### CARBOHYDRATE METABOLISM

The acute administration of growth hormone elicits a biphasic response. During the initial 2 hours after administration, growth hormone exhibits an insulin-like effect, lowering plasma glucose levels by directly stimulating beta-cell insulin secretion[179] and also by stimulating glucose use in peripheral tissues. Nonetheless, growth hormone does not produce hypoglycemia in normal subjects. It does have such an effect, however, in hypophysectomized animals that also have an impaired pituitary-adrenal axis.[180] From 2 to 12 hours after acute administration, growth hormone exhibits anti-insulin effects. This state of insulin resistance results from a postreceptor defect in peripheral glucose use, coupled with hepatic insulin resistance.[181,182]

With chronic administration in animals and humans, growth hormone results in an insulin-resistant state. Glucose intolerance in association with acromegaly has been reported in 60 to 70% of patients, although elevations in fasting plasma glucose concentrations are reported to occur in only 6 to 25% of acromegalic patients.[183–186] Even more striking than glucose intolerance is the hyperinsulinemia and resistance to insulin that occur in acromegaly[184] and in patients receiving growth hormone by injection.[187] In most patients, increased insulin secretion is able to compensate for the insulin-resistant state. A chronic excess of growth hormone results in increased rates of hepatic glucose production and decreased glucose use by peripheral tissues,[188,189] largely the result of decreased glucose oxidation.[190] Controversy exists as to whether the insulin resistance of acromegaly derives from defects at the level of the insulin receptor or entirely postreceptor. Decreased peripheral glucose use in acromegaly is associated with a decreased number of insulin receptors on peripheral blood monocytes.[191] However, the defect is not reproduced by incubation of monocytes with acromegalic plasma or growth hormone. Furthermore, porcine adipocytes show no defects in insulin binding or insulin receptor tyrosine kinase activity with chronic growth hormone treatment.[192] Elevations in the concentration of plasma free fatty acids and ketone bodies inhibit glucose use by muscle tissue, and may in part explain the postreceptor defect seen in acromegaly.[193] Successful treatment of acromegaly results in improved glucose tolerance and reductions in serum insulin concentrations in most patients.[184,194,195] In contrast to acromegaly, chronic growth hormone deficiency produces increased insulin sensitivity.

Whereas chronic elevations in growth hormone concentrations produce anti-insulin effects, many of the actions of IGF-1 mimic those of insulin. This fact is not surprising given the structural similarities in tertiary configuration between IGF-1 and proinsulin.[196] IGF-1 acts through a specific cell-surface receptor with substantial homology to the insulin receptor but is capable of stimulating the insulin receptor itself.[197] IGF-1 has been shown to increase glucose transport[198] and rates of glycolysis and glycogen synthesis[199] in heart and skeletal muscle tissues.

### LIPID METABOLISM

The acute effects of growth hormone administration on *lipid metabolism* are similar in their insulin-like nature to those described for glucose. Within the first few hours after growth hormone is given, reductions in plasma free fatty acid concentrations are seen. In addition, reduced rates of epinephrine-stimulated lipolysis have been described in hypophysectomized rats during this early period after growth hormone administration.[200]

Free fatty acid levels and ketone body levels are increased as the result of longer term growth hormone administration. Increased glycerol concentrations after in vivo administration of biosynthetic growth hormone in humans suggests stimulation of lipolysis.[185] Growth hormone-mediated lipolysis is similar to that induced by glucocorticoids, in that a lag time of at least 1 hour is required before the effect can be observed, and the lipolytic actions can be blocked by inhibitors of protein synthesis.[201] Some investigators have shown significant growth hormone-mediated lipolysis to occur only in the presence of insulin deficiency.[202–205] No lipolytic response to growth hormone is seen in vivo or in vitro in the growth hormone-deficient mouse.[206] Rather, fatty acid synthesis is inhibited by growth hormone, suggesting a primary role for blunted lipogenesis in the deranged fat metabolism in this model. Ketogenesis occurs in response to increased free fatty acid delivery to the liver and as the result of a direct hepatic effect of growth hormone on ketone production.[207]

In humans, regional differences exist in the response of adipocyte lipolysis and lipogenesis to growth hormone such that abdominal cells are more affected than peripheral (e.g., gluteal) cells. This variation results in fat redistribution from "android" (truncal) to "gynoid" (hip/thigh) deposition in patients treated with growth hormone.[208]

In contrast to the effects of growth hormone on lipid metabolism, IGF-1 has been shown to increase lipogenesis and to inhibit epinephrine-stimulated lipolysis in adipose tissue.[209] IGF-1 infusion in humans decreases serum triglyceride levels and the ratio of total to HDL cholesterol.[210]

### PROTEIN METABOLISM

One of the major effects of growth hormone is the promotion of linear growth and skeletal maturation. IGF-1 has been shown to be responsible for these effects, producing increased synthesis of DNA, RNA, and protein in fibroblasts and chondrocytes.[211] Extraskeletal effects include increased rates of protein synthesis and cell proliferation. IGF-1 secretion is found in multiple tissues and may serve as an anabolic factor in tissue hypertrophy and repair by autocrine and paracrine actions.[212,213] Animals made growth hormone-deficient by hypophysectomy develop a negative nitrogen balance, and protein and RNA contents decrease in various tissues. Growth hormone administration stimulates amino acid uptake and incorporation into protein in both liver and skeletal muscle tissues.[214] In humans, local administration of growth hormone to forearm skeletal muscle stimulates amino acid uptake.[215] This response may occur without increases in systemic IGF-1 levels. Nonetheless, the extent to which growth hormone can stimulate protein anabolism directly and independently of IGF-1 paracrine or autocrine actions remains controversial.

## CATECHOLAMINES

The catecholamines are epinephrine, norepinephrine, and dopamine. Norepinephrine is secreted from the sympathetic neurons throughout the body, and to a limited extent from the adrenal medulla. The principal secretory product of the adrenal medulla is epinephrine. Both epinephrine and norepinephrine have α- and β-agonist activities, although norepinephrine predominantly produces α-adrenergic effects. The major stimuli to sympathetic nervous system stimulation and adrenomedullary secretion are physical exercise, circulatory dysfunction, trauma, cold exposure, pain, emotional stress, and hypoglycemia. Although combined increases in epinephrine and norepinephrine secretion occur with most stresses, hypoglycemia predominantly augments epinephrine secretion.[216] However, epinephrine appears to be critical for recovery from hypoglycemia only in the absence of glucagon.[217]

### CARBOHYDRATE METABOLISM

Catecholamines have multiple effects on *carbohydrate metabolism.* α-Adrenergic stimulation inhibits insulin secretion, whereas β-adrenergic stimulation augments insulin release. The α-adrenergic inhibitory effects on pancreatic beta-cell function generally prevail under conditions of stress or sympathetic nerve stimulation. Both α- and β-adrenergic stimulation appear to augment pancreatic glucagon secretion.[218,219]

Catecholamines increase glycogen breakdown in liver and muscle tissues. β-Adrenergic stimulation activates phosphorylase, and inhibits glycogen synthase, through a cAMP-dependent mechanism. In addition, the α-adrenergic system is able to activate phosphorylase and inhibit glycogen synthase through a cAMP-independent mechanism involving membrane calcium transport.[220–223] Liver glycogenolysis appears to be mediated predominantly through α-adrenergic, cAMP-independent mechanisms. This conclusion is derived from in vitro data showing inhibition of catecholamine-mediated hepatic glycogenolysis (and gluconeogenesis) by α-adrenergic, but not β-adrenergic, blocking drugs.[222–224] A study in conscious dogs, however, yielded contradictory findings.[225] In contrast, skeletal muscle glycogenolysis is mediated by β-adrenergic stimulation of adenylate cyclase[226] and does not appear to be affected by α-adrenergic mechanisms.[220,227] The effects of catecholamines on muscle glycogen metabolism are antagonized by insulin and depend on glucocorticoids.[228–230]

As mentioned, catecholamines also stimulate hepatic gluconeogenesis through α-adrenergic mechanisms. Catecholamines increase the delivery of gluconeogenic precursors to the liver through their lipolytic (glycerol) and muscle glycogenolytic (lactate and pyruvate) actions. In addition, α-adrenergic agonists increase hepatic uptake of amino acids and possibly lactate.[231,232] The decreases in circulating insulin and increases in glucagon concentrations after sympathetic stimulation also promote glycogenolysis and gluconeogenesis. However, dose-related increases in such activity occur as the result of direct hepatic effects of epinephrine when plasma insulin and glucagon are maintained at fixed concentrations.[233]

Infusions of epinephrine resulting in physiologic elevations of plasma concentrations inhibit insulin-stimulated glucose uptake by peripheral tissues, even when plasma glucose and insulin concentrations are controlled by using the insulin clamp technique.[234,235] This effect is primarily associated with diminished insulin-stimulated glycogen deposition as glucose oxidation is slightly increased.[236] Additionally, skeletal muscle oxygen consumption during insulin infusion is increased, at least in part because of expansion of tricarboxylic acid cycle intermediates and NADH.[237] In contrast to these acute responses, chronic administration of terbutaline, a $\beta_2$-adrenergic agonist, resulted in significant increases in peripheral insulin sensitivity through increased nonoxidative glucose use (glycogen deposition) during insulin clamp studies.[238] Chronic infusion of norepinephrine, an α- and $\beta_1$-agonist, produces similar increases in peripheral insulin sensitivity in the rat.[239]

### LIPID METABOLISM

The major effect of catecholamines on *lipid metabolism* is augmentation of lipolysis. Both epinephrine and norepinephrine activate hormone-sensitive lipase in adipose tissue, liver, heart, and skeletal muscle. Stimulation of lipolysis is cAMP-dependent and is mediated through $\beta_1$-adrenergic stimulation of adenlyate cyclase.[240,241] $\alpha_2$-Adrenergic stimulation has an antilipolytic effect,[240] although this fact may not be of physiologic importance. Many other hormonal factors affect catecholamine-induced lipolysis, with insulin producing a major opposing role. Thus, catecholamine inhibition of insulin secretion plays an important role in promoting lipolysis.

Catecholamines also increase lipogenesis and ketogenesis. Hepatic triglyceride synthesis is increased by adrenergic stimulation, although this effect is predominantly related to increased free fatty acid delivery resulting from enhanced lipolysis.[226] Augmented ketogenesis is also partly the result of increased free fatty acid delivery to the liver, although other mechanism(s) coexist. Norepinephrine produces dose-dependent increases in ketogenesis in isolated rat hepatocytes, without increasing free fatty acid uptake.[242]

Catecholamines also produce increases in plasma lipid levels. Cholesterol synthesis and plasma levels increase after epinephrine administration, through activation of the rate-limiting enzyme controlling cholesterol synthesis, 3-hydroxy-3-methylglutaryl CoA reductase.[243–245] Triglyceride levels increase acutely during catecholamine infusions,[246] but are not elevated after chronic administration.

### PROTEIN METABOLISM

Catecholamines have insulin-like effects on plasma amino acid levels. Infusions of epinephrine resulting in plasma concentrations similar to those seen during acute stress result in a decrease in total amino acid levels, although alanine concentrations are unchanged.[247] This effect occurs in the absence of insulin secretion (in type I diabetics), and can be prevented by β-adrenergic blockade with propranolol. In contrast to insulin, epinephrine increases splanchnic uptake of gluconeogenic amino acids as well as increases peripheral de novo alanine synthesis and hepatic alanine delivery.[248,249] During recovery from insulin-induced hypoglycemia in dogs, amino acids are released from the gut into the portal circulation, providing gluconeogenic precursors;[250] the amino acid release is suppressed by α-adrenergic blockade.[251] Stimulation of lactate uptake by liver during hypoglycemia occurs after α-adrenergic blockade and is inhibited by β-adrenergic blockade.[252] Paradoxically, epinephrine has not been shown to increase nitrogen excretion despite the enhancement of gluconeogenesis.

## SEX STEROIDS AND PROLACTIN

### CARBOHYDRATE METABOLISM

Estrogen therapy as used in oral contraceptive preparations has been reported to exacerbate mild diabetes mellitus. However, recent reports suggest that it is the progestogen component, specifically the 19-nortestosterone derivatives, of oral contraceptives that alters glucose tolerance. The effect is seen with some, but not all, of these compounds and is less prominent in low-dose formulations.[253,254] The administration of testosterone to female rats produces decreases in insulin-stimulated glucose transport, increases in plasma insulin levels, decreased muscle glycogen synthesis, and decreased capillarization and number of type 1 muscle fibers (associated with insulin resistance).[255]

### LIPID METABOLISM

Pharmacologic doses of estrogens influence the production and removal rates of plasma lipoproteins. Plasma concentrations of VLDL-cholesterol are increased because of enhanced hepatic production rates.[256] In contrast, the clearance of LDL is enhanced by estrogens, in part because of increased hepatic excretion of cholesterol in the bile.[257] This effect has led to the therapeutic use of estrogens in some types of familial hypercholesterolemia, with the most striking results seen in women with familial dysbetalipoproteinemia (type III), and in some postmenopausal women with heterozygous familial hypercholesterolemia (type II).[258] Whereas estrogens produce significant increases in plasma HDL-cholesterol levels, the progestogens of the 19-nortestosterone series, often combined with estrogen in oral contraceptives, may lower HDL concentrations.[259] A large-scale clinical study of the use of combined estrogen/progestin oral contraceptives indicated that levonogestrel produced a dose-dependent increase in LDL-cholesterol and a decrease in HDL-cholesterol (particularly the HDL2 subfraction).[260] In contrast, norethindrone had opposite effects, indicating that lipoprotein changes related to progestogens may vary with their molecular side chain configurations.

Despite the pharmacologic effects of sex hormones on plasma lipids, epidemiologic evidence does not support a major role for sex hormones as the cause of abnormalities of lipoprotein levels in otherwise healthy people.[261,262] However, relationships between sex hormones and lipids may be obscured by the fact that hyperinsulinemia and upper-body obesity, commonly associated with syndromes of hyperlipidemia, tend to decrease levels of sex hormone binding globulin (SHBG), thereby decreasing the ratio of total to free hormone.[263–265] An interesting corollary to this observation is that Western-style refined carbohydrate, low-fiber, high-fat diets, also associated with hyperlipidemia, appear to increase the availability of sex hormones, raising total concentrations while decreasing SHBG.[266]

### PROTEIN METABOLISM

Testosterone administration to hypogonadal or castrated men decreases urinary nitrogen excretion and results in weight gain.[267] A major component of this weight gain is augmentation of skeletal muscle mass, most prominently in the pectoral and shoulder girdle areas. In normal men, pharmacologic doses of androgens produce only about half the nitrogen retention seen in hypogonadal men, and the effect is short-lived. Attempts to improve the rate of nitrogen repletion with androgens in patients suffering from catabolic illness have resulted in minimal or no therapeutic benefit.[268] Effects of androgens to increase weight in such individuals are probably related to stimulation of appetite and increased food intake.

Estrogens in pharmacologic doses inhibit somatic growth. This effect may be mediated through suppression of IGF-1 generation, which has been demonstrated in growth hormone-treated hypopituitary subjects.[269]

Prolactin has a weak stimulatory effect on IGF-1 generation in patients with prolactin-secreting pituitary tumors.[270] Prolactin administration to growth hormone-deficient human subjects mimics many of the actions of growth hormone, producing nitrogen retention, lipid mobilization, glucose intolerance, and modest skeletal growth.

## CYTOKINES AND EICOSANOIDS

The severely injured or infected patient shows dramatic metabolic responses characterized by mobilization of stored carbohydrate, fat, and protein substrates. As mentioned previously, these phenomena occur, in part, because of elaboration of classic "stress hormones" such as cortisol and catecholamines from endocrine organs such as the adrenal. It is now recognized that cells of immune origin such as macrophages, monocytes, and lymphocytes, well known to mediate tissue repair and elimination of infecting organisms, also mediate some of the metabolic responses to injury and infection. (See Chapters 3, 41, and 69 for more information on cytokines and growth factors.)

### CARBOHYDRATE METABOLISM

Thromboxane A2 (TXA2), prostaglandin F2α (PGF2α), and PGE2, derivatives of arachidonic acid, increase glycogenolysis when secreted by Kupffer cells in the liver.[176] These prostanoids are released in response to stimulation by phagocytosis and bacterial lipopolysaccharide, explaining in part the glucose intolerance and insulin resistance associated with infection and inflammation.

### LIPID METABOLISM

The peptide cytokine tumor necrosis factor-α (TNF-α), also known as cachectin, produces many of the metabolic and nutritional perturbations associated with the critically ill patient.[271] Specifically with regard to lipid metabolism, it induces anorexia and lipolysis while inhibiting lipogenesis. These effects are mediated by the ability of TNF-α to stimulate adipocyte hormone-sensitive lipase while suppressing expression of LPL, fatty acid binding protein, and glycerol-3-phosphate dehydrogenase.[272]

## PROTEIN METABOLISM

TNF-α promotes catabolism of skeletal muscle protein, in large part by its promotion of anorexia with resultant starvation. TNF-α stimulates skeletal muscle proteolysis in vivo independent of starvation.[273] However, the effect may be mediated by another, undefined factor, because it does not occur when skeletal muscle is incubated with TNF-α in vitro. In contrast to skeletal muscle, visceral protein content and cell proliferation is enhanced by TNF-α such that liver, heart, and lung weight are all increased.[274] Production of circulating proteins such as albumin and transferrin is depressed by TNF-α. Albumin gene transcription and steady state albumin mRNA levels are decreased by TNF-α.[275] However, acute-phase circulating proteins may be increased by TNF-α, probably resulting in large part from stimulation of interleukin 6 formation. Interleukin 6 is the most potent stimulator of hepatic acute-phase protein synthesis currently known.[276] Thus, elaboration of cytokines from immune cells helps to explain further the peripheral wasting and visceral preservation noted after prolonged critical illness. The effects are opposite to those seen during adequate nutrition and health in which insulin and IGF-1 promote peripheral storage of nutrients. Interestingly, some investigators have found that the administration of insulin to TNF-α-treated rats may reverse the catabolic effects of that cytokine.[277]

## REFERENCES


1. Kahn, C.R.: Clin. Res., *31*:326–335, 1983.
2. Kasuga, M., Zick, Y., Blithe, D.L., et al.: Nature, *298*:667–669, 1982.
3. Sternlicht, E., Barnard, R.J., Grimditch, G.K.: Am. J. Physiol., *254*:E633–638, 1988.
4. Cushman, S.W., Wardzala, L.J.: J. Biol. Chem., *255*:4758–4762, 1980.
5. Suzuki, K., Kono, T.: Proc. Natl. Acad. Sci. U.S.A., *77*:2542–2545, 1980.
6. Wardzala, L.J., Cushman, S.W., Salans, L.B.: J. Biol. Chem., *253*:8002–8005, 1978.
7. Wardzala, L.J., Jeanrenaud, B.: J. Biol. Chem., *256*:7090–7093, 1981.
8. Charron, M.J., Brosius, F.C. III, Alper, SL., et al.: Proc. Natl. Acad. Sci. U.S.A., *86*:2535–2539, 1989.
9. Klip, A., Paquet, M.R.: Diabetes Care, *13*:228–243, 1990.
10. Dohme, G.L., Elton, C.W., Friedman, J.E., et al.: Am. J. Physiol., *260*:E459–E463, 1991.
11. Hertz, M.M., Paulson, O.B., Barry, D.I., et al.: J. Clin. Invest., *67*:597–604, 1981.
12. Bell, G.I., Kayano, T., Buse, J.B., et al.: Diabetes Care, *13*:198–208, 1990.
13. Debons, A.F., Krimsky, I., From, A., et al.: Am. J. Physiol., *217*:1114–1118, 1969.
14. Oomura, Y., Kita, H.: Diabetologia, *20*:290–298, 1981.
15. Goodyear, L.J., King, P.A., Hirschman, M.F., et al.: Am. J. Physiol., *258*:E667–672, 1990.
16. Curnow, R.T., Rayfield, E.J., George, D.T., et al.: Am. J. Physiol., *228*:80–87, 1975.
17. Benn, J.J., Rai, R., Sonksen, P.H.: Diabetologia, *33*:158–162, 1990.
18. Parkes, J.L., Grieninger, G.: J. Biol. Chem., *260*:8090–8097, 1985.
19. Agius, L., Peak, M., Alberti, K.G.: Biochem. J., *266*:91–102, 1990.
20. Taunton, O.D., Stifel, F.B., Greene, H.L., et al.: J. Biol. Chem., *249*:7228–7239, 1974.
21. Muller, W.A., Faloona, G.R., Aguilar-Parada, E., et al.: N. Engl. J. Med., *283*:109–115, 1970.
22. Unger, R.H., Ketterer, H., Dupre, J., et al.: J. Clin. Invest., *46*:630–645, 1967.
23. Andersen, D.K., Elahi, D., Brown, J.C., et al.: J. Clin. Invest., *62*:152–161, 1978.
24. Bloom, S.R., Vaughan, N.J.A., Russell, R.C.G.: Lancet, *2*:546–549, 1974.
25. Berthoud, H., Bereiter, D.A., Trimble, E.R., et al.: Diabetologia, *20*:393–401, 1981.
26. Katz, L.D., Glickman, M.G., Rapoport, S., et al.: Diabetes, *32*:675–679, 1983.
27. Aguilar-Parada, E., Eisentraut, A.M., Unger, R.H.: Diabetes, *18*:717–723, 1969.
28. Owen, O.E., Morgan, A.P., Kemp, H.G., et al.: J. Clin. Invest., *46*:1589–1595, 1967.
29. Cahill, G.F., Herrera, M.G., Morgan, A.P., et al.: J. Clin. Invest., *45*:1751–1769, 1966.
30. Nair, K.S., Welle, S.L., Halliday, D., et al.: J. Clin. Invest., *82*:198–205, 1988.
31. Tessari, P., Nissen, S.L., Miles, J.M., et al.: J. Clin. Invest., *77*:575–581, 1986.
32. Aguilar-Parada, E., Eisentraut, A.M., Unger, R.H.: Am. J. Med. Sci., *257*:415–419, 1969.
33. Unger, R.H., Aguilar-Parada, E., Muller, W.A., et al.: J. Clin. Invest., *49*:837–848, 1970.
34. Samois, E., Tyler, J.M., Marks, V.: Glucagon-insulin interrelationships. *In* Glucagon: Molecular Physiology, Clinical and Therapeutic Implications. Edited by P.J. Lefebvre and R.H. Unger. New York, Pergamon Press, 1972, pp. 151–173.
35. Samols, E., Weir, G.C., Bonner-Weir, S.: Intraislet insulin-glucagon-somatostatin relationships. *In* Glucagon. Vol. 2. Edited by P.J. Lefebvre. Berlin, Springer, 1983, pp. 133–173.
36. Unger, R.H.: Diabetologia, *20*:1–11, 1981.
37. Unger, R.H., Madison, L.L., Muller, W.A.: Diabetes, *21*:301–307, 1972.
38. Buchanan, K.D., McCarroll, A.M.: Lancet, *2*:1394–1395, 1972.
39. Raskin, P., Aydin, I., Yamamoto, T., et al.: Am. J. Med., *64*:988–997, 1978.
40. Raskin, P., Pietri, A., Unger, R.H.: Diabetes, *28*:1033–1035, 1979.
41. Rosen, S.G., Clutter, W.E., Berk, M.A.: J. Clin. Invest., *73*:405–411, 1984.
42. White, N.H., Skor, D., Cryer, P.E., et al.: N. Engl. J. Med., *308*:485–491, 1983.

43. Santiago, J.V., White, N.H., Skor, D.A., et al.: Am. J. Physiol., *247*:E215–E220, 1984.
44. Rodbell, M.: The actions of glucagon at its receptor: Regulation of adenylate cyclase. *In* Glucagon. Vol. 1. Edited by P.J. Lefebvre, Berlin, Springer, 1983, pp. 263–290.
45. Liljenquist, J.E., Mueller, G.L., Cherrington, A.D., et al.: J. Clin. Invest., *59*:369–374, 1977.
46. Boyd, M.E., Albright, E.B., Foster, D.W., et al.: J. Clin. Invest., *68*:142–152, 1981.
47. Dobbs, S., Sakurai, H., Sasaki, H., et al.: Science, 187:544–547, 1975.
48. de Kreutzenberg, V.S., Maifreni, L., Lisato, G., et al.: J. Clin. Endocrinol. Metab., *70*:1023–1029, 1990.
49. Nair, K.S., Welle, S.L., Tito, J.: Diabetes, *39*:376–382, 1990.
50. Marker, J.C., Hirsch, I.B., Smith, L.J., et al.: Am. J. Physiol., *260*:E705–E712, 1991.
51. Hirsch, I.B., Marker, J.C., Smith, L.J., et al.: Am. J. Physiol., *260*:E695–E704, 1991.
52. Winder, W.W., Fisher, S.R., Gygi, S.P., et al.: Am. J. Physiol., *260*:E756–E761, 1991.
53. Mallinson, C.M., Bloom, S.R., Warin, A.P., et al.: Lancet, *2*:1–5, 1974.
54. Wood, S.M., Polak, J.M., Bloom, S.R.: Glucagonoma syndrome. *In* Glucagon. Vol. 2. Edited by P.J. Lefebvre. Berlin, Springer, 1983, pp. 411–430.
55. Devlin, J., Calles-Escandon, J., Poehlman, E., et al.: Diabetes, *38 (Suppl. 2)*:224A, 1989.
56. Krejs, G.J., Orci, L., Conlon, J.M., et al.: N. Engl. J. Med., *301*:285–292, 1979.
57. Nosari, I., Lepore, G., Querci, F., et al.: J. Endocrinol. Invest., *12*:413–417, 1989.
58. Felig, P.: N. Engl. J. Med., *283*:149–150, 1970.
59. Taylor, S.I., Mukherjee, C., Jungas, R.L.: J. Biol. Chem., *248*:73–81, 1973.
60. Weber, G., Lea, M.A., Stamm, N.B.: Lipids, *4*:388–396, 1969.
61. Bjorntorp, P., Sjostrom, L.: Metabolism, *27*:1853–1865, 1978.
62. Acheson, K.J., Schutz, Y., Bessard, T., et al.: Am. J. Physiol., *246*:E62–E70, 1984.
63. Bagdade, J.D., Porte, D., Bierman, E.L.: N. Engl. J. Med., *276*:427–433, 1967.
64. Kessler, J.I.: J. Clin. Invest., *42*:362–367, 1963.
65. Siperstein, M.D., Fagan, V.M.: J. Clin. Invest., *37*:1185–1195, 1958.
66. Butcher, R.W., Baird, C.E., Sutherland, E.W.: J. Biol. Chem., *243*:1705–1712, 1968.
67. Keirns, J.J., Freeman, J., Bitensky, M.W.: Am. J. Med. Sci., *268*:62–91, 1964.
68. Unger, R.H.: Diabetes, *20*:834–838, 1971.
69. McGarry, J.D., Wright, P.H., Foster, D.W.: J. Clin. Invest., *55*:1202–1209, 1975.
70. Bierman, E.L.: Isr. J. Med. Sci., *8*:303–308, 1972.
71. Chait, A., Brunzell, J.D.: Metabolism, *32*:209–214, 1983.
72. Grundy, S.M., Mok, H.Y.I., Zech, L., et al.: J. Clin. Invest., *63*:1274–1283, 1979.
73. Kissebah, A.H., Alfarsi, S., Evans, D.J., et al.: Diabetes, *31*:217–225, 1982.
74. Dunn, F.L.: Med. Clin. North Am., *72*:1379–1398, 1988.
75. Hollenbeck, C.B., Coulston, A.M.: Diabetes Metab. Rev., *3*:669–689, 1987.
76. Betteridge, B.J.: Br. Med. Bull., *45*:285–311, 1989.
77. Steinbrecher, U.P., Witztum, J.L.: Diabetes, *33*:130–134, 1984.
78. American Diabetes Association- position statement: Diabetes Care., *14 (Suppl. 2)*:20–27, 1991.
79. Garg, A., Bonanome, A., Grundy, S.M., et al.: N. Engl. J. Med., *319*:829–834, 1988.
80. Fryburg, D.A., Barrett, E.J., Louard, R.J., et al.: Am. J. Physiol., *259*:E477–E482, 1990.
81. Fukagawa, N.K., Minaker, K.L., Young, V.R., et al.: Am. J. Physiol., *250*:E13–E17, 1986.
82. Sugden, P.H., Smith, D.M.: Biochem J., *206*:467–472, 1982.
83. Longo, N., Franchi-Gazzola, R., Bussolati, O., et al.: Biochim. Biophys. Acta, *844*:216–223, 1985.
84. Shotwell, M.A., Kilberg, M.S., Oxender, D.: Biochim. Biophys. Acta, *737*:267–284, 1983.
85. Zorzano, A., Balon, T.W., Garetto, L.P., et al.: Am. J. Physiol., *248*:E546–E552, 1985.
86. Rodnick, K.J., Reaven, G.M., Azhar, S., et al.: Am. J. Physiol., *259*:E706–E714, 1990.
87. Jefferson, L.S., Robertson, J.W.: Diabetes, *21 (Suppl. 1)*:341, 1972.
88. McKee, E.E., Grier, B.L.: Am. J. Physiol., *259*:E413–E421, 1990.
89. Wool, I.G.: Am. J. Physiol., *199*:719–721, 1960.
90. Davidson, M.B., Goodner, C.J.: Diabetes, *15*:835–838, 1966.
91. Manchester, K.L.: Sites of hormonal regulation of protein metabolism. *In* Mammalian Protein Metabolism. Vol. 4. Edited by H.N. Munro. New York, Academic Press, 1970, pp. 229–298.
92. Umpleby, A.M., Boroujerdi, M.A., Brown, P.M., et al.: Diabetologia, *29*:131–141, 1986.
93. Jefferson, L.J., Rannels, D.E., Munger, B.L., et al.: Fed. Proc., *33*:1098–1104, 1974.
94. Sloan, G.M., Norton, J.A., Brennan, M.F.: J. Surg. Res., *28*:442–448, 1980.
95. Nair, K.S., Garrow, J.S., Ford, C., et al.: Diabetologia, *25*:400–403, 1983.
96. Pacy, P.J., Nair, K.S., Ford, C., et al.: Diabetes, *38*:618–624, 1989.
97. Bennett, W.M., Connacher, A.A., Smith, K., et al.: Diabetologia, *33*:43–51, 1990.
98. Trevisan, R., Nosadini, R., Avogaro, A., et al.: J. Clin. Endocrinol. Metab., *62*:1155–1162, 1986.
99. Tessari, P., Nosadini, R., Trevisan, R., et al.: J. Clin. Invest., *77*:1797–1804, 1986.
100. Luzi, L., Castellino, P., Simonson, D., et al.: Diabetes, *39*:38–48, 1990.
101. Marliss, E.B., Aoki, T.T., Cahill, G.F.: *In* Glucagon: Molecular Physiology, Clinical and Therapeutic Implications. Edited by P.J. Lefebvre and R.H. Unger. New York, Pergamon Press, 1972.
102. Nair, K.S., Halliday, D., Matthews, D.E., et al.: Am. J. Physiol., *253*:E208–E213, 1987.
103. Felig, P., Owen, O.E., Wahren, J., et al.: J. Clin. Invest., *48*:584–594, 1969.
104. Boden, G., Tappy, L., Jadali, F., et al.: Am. J. Physiol., *259*:E225–E232, 1990.
105. Unger, R.H., Ohneda, A., Aguilar-Parada, E., et al.: J. Clin. Invest., *48*:810–822, 1969.
106. Liljenquist, J.E., Lewis, S.B., Cherrinton A.D., et al.: Metabolism, *30*:1195–1199, 1981.
107. Abraira, C., DeBartolo, M., Katzen, R., et al.: Am. J. Clin. Nutr., *39*:351–355, 1984.

108. Boden, G., Rezvani, I., Owen, O.E.: J. Clin. Invest., *73*:785–793, 1984.
109. Kreines, K., Jett, M., Knowles, H.C.: Diabetes, *14*:740–744, 1965.
110. Doar, J.W.H., Stamp, T.C.B., Wynn, V., et al.: Diabetes, *18*:633–639, 1984.
111. Maxon, H.R., Kreines, K.W., Goldsmith, R.E., et al.: Arch. Intern. Med., *139*:1477–1480, 1975.
112. Holdsworth, C.D., Besser, G.M.: Lancet, *2*:700–702, 1980.
113. Ikeda, T., Fujiyama, K., Hoshino, T., et al.: Metabolism, *39*:633–637, 1990.
114. Beer, S.F., Parr, J.H., Temple, R.C., et al.: Clin. Endocrinol. (Oxf.), *30*:379–383, 1989.
115. Wennlund, A., Felig, P., Hagenfeldt, L., et al.: J. Clin. Endocrinol. Metab., *62*:174–180, 1986.
116. Ingbar, S.H.: The thyroid gland. *In* Textbook of Endocrinology. Edited by J.D. Wilson and D.W. Foster. Philadelphia, W.B. Saunders, 1985, pp. 682–815.
117. Muller, M.J., Seitz, H.J.: Klin. Wochenschr., *62*:11–18, 1984.
118. Randin, J.-P., Tappy, L., Scazziga, B., et al.: Diabetes, *35*:178–181, 1986.
119. Dubaniewicz, A., Kaciuba-Usciko, H., Budohoski, L.: Biochem. J., *263*:243–247, 1989.
120. Shulman, G.I., Ladenson, P.W., Wolfe, M., et al.: J. Clin. Invest., *76*:757–764, 1985.
121. Brodie, C.: J. Neurochem., *55*:186–191, 1990.
122. Weinstein, S.P., Watts, J., Graves, P.N., et al.: Endocrinology, *126*:1421–1429, 1990.
123. Saunders, J., Hall, S.E.H., Sonksen, P.H., et al.: Clin. Endocrinol. (Oxf.), *13*:33–44, 1980.
124. Agdeppa, D., Macaron, C., Mallik, T., et al.: J. Clin. Endocrinol. Metab., *49*:726–729, 1979.
125. Caron, P., Calazel, C., Parra, H.J., et al.: Clin. Endocrinol. (Oxf.), *33*:519–523, 1990.
126. Krauss, R.M., Levy, R.I., Fredrickson, D.S.: J. Clin. Invest., *54*:1107–1124, 1974.
127. Pykalisto, O., Goldbert, A.P., Brunzell, J.D.: J. Clin. Endocrinol. Metab., *43*:591–600, 1976.
128. Ruggiero, F.M., Cafagna, F., Quagliariello, E.: Lipids, *25*:529–533, 1990.
129. Paradies, G., Ruggiero, F.M.: Biochim. Biophys. Acta, *1019*:133–136, 1990.
130. Munro, H.N.: General aspects of the regulation of protein metabolism by diet and hormones. *In* Mammalian Protein Metabolism. Vol. 1. Edited by H.N. Munro. New York, Academic Press, 1964, pp. 381–481.
131. Roche, J., Dumazert, C., Emond, Y., et al.: C. R. Soc. Biol., *136*:326, 1942.
132. Sokoloff, L., Kaufman, S., Gelboin, H.V.: Biochim. Biophys. Acta, *52*:410–412, 1961.
133. Crispell, K.R., Parson, W., Hollifield, G.: J. Clin. Invest., *35*:164–169, 1956.
134. Kivirikko, K.I., Laitinen, O., Aer, J., et al.: Endocrinology, *80*:1051–1061, 1967.
135. Foley, T.H., London, D.R., Prenton, M.A.: J. Clin. Endocrinol. Metab., *26*:781–785, 1966.
136. Wajchenberg, B.L., Leme, C.E., Lerario, A.C., et al.: Diabetes, *33*:455–459, 1984.
137. Nosadini, R., Del Prato, S., Tiengo, A., et al.: J. Clin. Endocrinol. Metab., *57*:529–536, 1983.
138. De Pirro, R., Green, A., Kao, M.Y.-C., et al.: Diabetologia, *21*:149–153, 1981.
139. Plotz, C.M., Knowlton, A.J., Ragan, C.: Am. J. Med., *13*:597–614, 1952.
140. Pupo, A.A., Wajchenberg, B.L., Schnaider, J.: Diabetes, *15*:24–29, 1966.
141. Wise, J.K., Hendler, R., Felig, P.: J. Clin. Invest., *52*:2774–2782, 1973.
142. Issekutz, B., Allen, M.: Metabolism, *21*:48–59, 1972.
143. Wicks, W.D., Barnett, C.A., McKibbin, J.B.: Fed. Proc., *33*:1105–1111, 1974.
144. Marco, J., Calle, C., Roman, D., et al.: N. Engl. J. Med., *288*:128–132, 1973.
145. Eisenstein, A.B., Strack, I.: Endocrinology, *83*:1337–1348, 1968.
146. Wajngot, A., Khan, A., Giacca, A., et al.: Am. J. Physiol., *259*:E626–E632, 1990.
147. Kahn, B.B., Flier, J.S.: Diabetes Care, *13*:548–564, 1990.
148. Horner, H.C., Munck, A., Lienhard, G.E.: J. Biol. Chem., *262*:17,696–17,702, 1987.
149. Olefsky, J.M., Johnson, J., Liu, F., et al.: Metabolism, *24*:517–527, 1975.
150. Kahn, C.R., Goldfine, I.D., Neville, D.M., et al.: Endocrinology, *103*:1054–1066, 1978.
151. Olefsky, J.M.: J. Clin. Invest., *56*:1499–1508, 1975.
152. Shamoon, H., Hendler, R., Sherwin, R.S.: J. Clin. Endocrinol. Metab., *52*:1235–1241, 1983.
153. Eigler, N., Sacca, L., Sherwin, R.S.: J. Clin. Invest., *63*:114–123, 1979.
154. Martin, I.K., Christopher, M.J., Alford, F.P., et al.: Am. J. Physiol., *260*:E148–E153, 1991.
155. Nayak, R.V., Feldman, E.B., Carter, A.C.: Proc. Soc. Exp. Biol. Med., *111*:682–686, 1962.
156. Shafrir, E., Steinberg, D.: J. Clin. Invest., *39*:310–319, 1960.
157. Fain, J.N.: Science, *157*:1062–1064, 1967.
158. Bagdade, J.D., Porte, D., Bierman, E.L.: Arch. Intern. Med., *125*:129–134, 1970.
159. Martin-Sanz, P., Vance, J.E., Brindley, D.N.: Biochem. J., *271*:575–583, 1990.
160. Henze, K., Chait, A., Albers, J.J., et al.: Eur. J. Clin. Invest., *13*:171–177, 1983.
161. Kroteiwski, M., Bjorntorp, P.: Acta Endocrinol. (Copenh.), *80*:667–675, 1975.
162. Lamberts, S.W.J., Birkenhager, J.C.: J. Clin. Endocrinol. Metab., *42*:864–868, 1976.
163. Rebuffe-Scrive, M., Krotiewski, M., Elfverson, J., et al.: J. Clin. Endocrinol. Metab., *67*:1122–1128, 1988.
164. Rebuffe-Scrive, M., Bronnegard, M., Nilsson, A., et al.: J. Clin. Endocrinol. Metab., *71*:1215–1219, 1990.
165. Engel, F.L.: Vitam. Horm., *19*:189–227, 1961.
166. Kostyo, J.L.: Endocrinology, *76*:604–613, 1965.
167. Noall, M.W., Riggs, T.R., Walker, L.M., et al.: Science, *126*:1002–1005, 1957.
168. Block, K.P., Richmond, W.R., Mehard, W.B., et al.: Am. J. Physiol., *252*:E396–E407, 1987.
169. Block, K.P., Buse, M.G.: Med. Sci. Sports Exerc., *22*:316–324, 1990.
170. Simmons, P.S., Miles, J.M., Gerich, J.E., et al.: J. Clin. Invest., *73*:412–420, 1984.
171. Muhlbacher, F., Kapadia, C.R., Colpoys, M.F., et al.: Am. J. Physiol., *247*:E75–E83, 1984.
172. Kayali, A.G., Young, V.R., Goodman, M.N.: Am. J. Physiol., *252*:E621–626, 1987.
173. Kayali, A.G., Goodman, M.N., Lin, J., et al.: Am. J. Physiol., *259*:E699–E705, 1990.
174. Clark, I.: J. Biol. Chem., *200*:69–76, 1953.
175. Weber, G., Srivasta, S.K., Singhal, R.L.: J. Biol. Chem., *240*:750–756, 1965.

176. Decker, K.: Eur. J. Biochem., *192*:245–261, 1990.
177. Isley, W.L., Underwood, W.E., Clemmons, D.R.: J. Clin. Invest., *71*:175–182, 1983.
178. Phillips, L.S., Orawski, A.T., Belosky, D.C.: Endocrinology, *103*:121–127, 1978.
179. Frohman, L.A., MacGillivray, M.H., Aceto, T.: J. Clin. Endocrinol. Metab., *27*:561–567, 1967.
180. Kostyo, J.L., Reagan, C.R.: Pharmacol. Ther. (B), *2*:591–604, 1976.
181. Bratusch-Marrain, P.R., Smith, D., DeFronzo, R.A.: J. Clin. Endocrinol. Metab., *55*:973–982, 1982.
182. Ng, S.F., Storlien, L.H., Kraegen, E.W., et al.: Metabolism, *39*:264–268, 1990.
183. Beck, P., Schalch, D.S., Parker, M.L., et al.: J. Lab. Clin. Med., *66*:366–379, 1965.
184. Sonksen, P.H., Greenwood, F.C., Ellis, J.P., et al.: J. Clin. Endocrinol. Metab., *27*:1418–1430, 1967.
185. Boden, G., Soeldner, J.S., Steinke, J., et al.: Metabolism, *17*:1–9, 1968.
186. Emmer, M., Gorden, P., Roth, J.: Med. Clin. North Am., *55*:1057–1064, 1971.
187. Seng, G., Galgoti, C., Louisy, P., et al.: Am. J. Clin. Nutr., *50*:1348–1354, 1989.
188. Weil, R.: Acta Endocrinol., *98 (Suppl.)*:7–92, 1965.
189. Kipnis, D.M.: *In* The Nature and Treatment of Diabetes. Edited by B.S. Leibel and G.A. Wrenshall. New York, Exerpta Medica, 1965, p. 258.
190. Moller, N., Jorgensen, J.O., Alberti, K.G., et al.: J. Clin. Endocrinol. Metab., *70*:1179–1186, 1990.
191. Muggeo, M., Bar, R.S., Roth, J., et al.: J. Clin. Endocrinol. Metab., *48*:17–25, 1979.
192. Magri, K.A., Adamo, M., Leroith, D.: Biochem. J., *266*:107–113, 1990.
193. Randle, P.J., Garland, P.B., Hales, C.N., et al.: Lancet, *1*:785–789, 1963.
194. Luft, R., Cerasi, E., Hamberger, C.A.: Acta Endocrinol., *56*:593–607, 1967.
195. Eastman, R.C., Gordon, P., Roth, J.: J. Clin. Endocrinol. Metab., *48*:931–40, 1979.
196. Blundell, T.L., Bedarkar, S., Rinderknecht, E., et al.: Proc. Natl. Acad. Sci. U.S.A., *75*:180–184, 1978.
197. Nissley, S.P., Rechler, M.M.: Clin. Endocrinol. *13*:43–68, 1984.
198. Meuli, C., Froesch, E.R.: Eur. J. Clin. Invest., *5*:93–99, 1975.
199. Froesch, E.R., Muller, W.A., Burgi, H., et al.: Biochim. Biophys. Acta, *121*:360–374, 1966.
200. Goodman, H.M.: Metabolism, *19*:849–855, 1970.
201. Fain, J.N., Dodd, A., Novak, L.: Metabolism, *20*:109–118, 1971.
202. Gerich, J.R., Lorenzi, M., Bier, D.M.: J. Clin. Invest., *57*:875–884, 1976.
203. Metcalfe, P., Johnston, D.G., Nosadini, R., et al.: Diabetologia, *20*:123–128, 1981.
204. Schade, D.S., Eaton, R.P., Peake, G.T.: Diabetes, *27*:916–924, 1978.
205. Luft, R., Ikkos, D., Gemzell, C.A., et al.: Lancet, *1*:721, 1958.
206. Ng, F.M., Adamafio, N.A., Graystone, J.E.: J. Mol. Endocrinol., *4*:43–49, 1990.
207. Villar-Pilasi, C., Larner, J.: Annu. Rev. Biochem., *39*:639–672, 1970.
208. Rosenbaum, M., Gertner, J.M., Leibel, R.L.: J. Clin. Endocrinol. Metab., *69*:1274–1281, 1989.
209. Zapf, J., Schoenle, E., Waldvogel, M., et al.: Eur. J. Biochem., *113*:605–609, 1981.
210. Guler, H.P. Schmid, C., Zapf, J., et al.: Acta Paediatr. Scand., *367 (Suppl.)*:52–54, 1990.
211. Zapf, J., Schoenle, E., Froesch, E.R.: Eur. J. Biochem., *87*:285–296, 1978.
212. Daughaday, W.H., Rotwein, P.: Endocr. Rev., *10*:68–91, 1989.
213. Skottner, A., Arrhenius-Nyberg, V., Kanje, M., et al.: Acta Paediatr. Scand., *367 (Suppl.)*:63–66, 1990.
214. Nutting, D.F.: Endocrinology, *98*:1273–1283, 1976.
215. Fryburg, D.A., Gelfand, R.A., Barrett, E.J.: Am. J. Physiol., *260*:E499–E504, 1991.
216. Garber, A.J., Cryer, P.E., Santiago, J.V., et al.: J. Clin. Invest., *58*:7–15, 1976.
217. Clarke, W.L., Santiago, J.V., Thomas, L., et al.: Am. J. Physiol., *236*:E147–E152, 1979.
218. Smith, P.H., Madson, K.L.: Diabetologia, *20*:314–322, 1981.
219. Smith, P.H., Porte, D.: Annu. Rev. Pharmacol. Toxicol., *16*:269–285, 1976.
220. Exton, J.H.: Am. J. Physiol., *238*:E3–E12, 1980.
221. Kneer, N.M., Bosch, A.L., Clark, M.G., et al.: Proc. Natl. Acad. Sci. U.S.A., *71*:4523–4527, 1974.
222. Hutson, N.J., Brumley, F.T., Assimacopoulos, F.D., et al.: J. Biol. Chem., *251*:5200–5208, 1976.
223. Cherrington, A.D., Assimacopoulos, F.D., Harper, S.C., et al.: J. Biol. Chem., *251*:5209–5218, 1976.
224. Tolbert, M.E.M., Butcher, F.R., Fain, J.N.: J. Biol. Chem., *248*:5686–5692, 1973.
225. Steiner, K.E., Stevenson, R.W., Green, D.R., et al.: Metabolism, *34*:1020–1023, 1985.
226. Himms-Hagen, J.: Effects of catecholamines on metabolism. *In* Catecholamines: Handbook of Experimental Pharmacology. Vol. 33. Edited by H. Blaschko and E. Muscholl. Berlin, Springer, 1972, pp. 363–462.
227. Dietz, M.R., Chiasson, J.-L., Soderling, T.R., et al.: J. Biol. Chem., *255*:2301–2307, 1980.
228. Shikama, H., Chiasson, J.-L., Exton, J.H.: J. Biol. Chem., *256*:4450–4454, 1981.
229. Foulkes, J.G., Cohen, P., Strada, S.J.: J. Biol. Chem., *257*:12,493–12,496, 1982.
230. Green, G.A., Chenoweth, M., Dunn, A.: Proc. Natl. Acad. Sci. U.S.A., *77*:5711–5715, 1980.
231. Exton, J.H., Park, C.R.: J. Biol. Chem., *243*:4189–4196, 1968.
232. Le Cam, A., Freychet, P.: Endocrinology, *102*:379–385, 1978.
233. Stevenson, R.W., Steiner, K.E., Connoly, C.C., et al.: Am. J. Physiol., *260*:E363–E370, 1991.
234. Abramson, E.A., Arky, R.A.: Diabetes, *17*:141–146, 1968.
235. Chiasson, J.-L., Shikama, H., Chu, D.T.W., et al.: J. Clin. Invest., *68*:706–713, 1981.
236. Raz, I., Katz, A., Spencer, M.K.: Am. J. Physiol., *260*:E430–E435, 1991.
237. Spencer, M.K., Katz, A., Raz, I.: Am. J. Physiol., *260*:E436–E439, 1991.
238. Scheidegger, K., Robbins, D.C., Danforth, E.: Diabetes, *33*:1144–1149, 1984.
239. Lupien, J.R., Hirshman, M.F., Horton, E.S.: Am. J. Physiol., *259*:E210–E215, 1990.
240. Fain, J.N., Garcia-Sainz, J.A.: J. Lipid Res., *24*:945–966, 1983.
241. Belfrage, P., Fredrickson, G., Olsson, H., et al.: Control of adipose tissue lipolysis by phosphorylation/dephosphorylation of hormone-sensitive lipase. *In* The Adipocyte and Obesity: Cellular and Molecular Mechanisms. Edited by A.

Angel, C.H. Holberg., and D.A.K. Ronicari. New York, Raven Press, 1983, pp. 217–224.
242. Oberhaensli, R.D., Schwendimann, R., Keller, U.: Diabetes, *34*:774–779, 1985.
243. Edwards, P.A.: Arch. Biochem. Biophys., *170*:188–203, 1975.
244. Edwards, P., Lemongello, D., Fogelman, A.M.: J. Lipid Res., *20*:2–7, 1979.
245. George, R., Ramasarma, T.: Biochem. J., *162*:493–499, 1977.
246. Miller, H.I.: Metabolism, *16*:1096–1105, 1967.
247. Shamoon, H., Jacob, R., Sherwin, R.S.: Diabetes, *29*:875–881, 1980.
248. Miles, J.M., Nissen, S.L., Gerich, J.E., et al.: Am. J. Physiol., *247*:E166–E172, 1984.
249. Del Prato, S., DeFronzo, R.A., Castellino, P., et al.: Am. J. Physiol., *258*:E878–E887, 1990.
250. Hourani, H., Williams, P., Morris, J.A., et al.: Am. J. Physiol., *259*:E342–E350, 1990.
251. Abumrad, N.N., personal communication, 1991.
252. Hourani, H., Lacy, D.B., Nammour, T.M., et al.: J. Trauma, *30*:1116–1123, 1990.
253. Spellacy, W.N., Ellingson, A.B., Tsibris, J.C.: Adv. Contracept., *6*:185–191, 1990.
254. Brooks, P.G.: J. Reprod. Med., *29 (Suppl.)*:539–546, 1984.
255. Holmang, A., Svedberg, J., Jennische, E., et al.: Am. J. Physiol., *259*:E555–E560, 1990.
256. Glueck, C.J., Fallat, R.W., Scheel, D.: Metabolism, *24*:537–545, 1975.
257. Everson, G.T., McKinley, C., Kern, F.: J. Clin. Invest., *87*:237–46, 1991.
258. Tikkanen, M.J., Nikkila, E.A., Vartiainen, E.: Lancet, *2*:490–491, 1978.
259. Wahl, P., Walden, C., Knopp, R., et al.: N. Engl. J. Med., *308*:862–867, 1983.
260. Godsland, I.F., Crook, D., Simpson, R., et al.: N. Engl. J. Med., *323*:1375–1381, 1990.
261. Duell, P.B., Bierman, E.L.: Arch. Intern. Med., *150*:2317–2320, 1990.
262. Cauley, J.A., Gutai, J.P., Kuller, L.H., et al.: Am. J. Epidemiol., *132*:884–894, 1990.
263. Pasquali, R., Casimirri, F., Cantobelli, S., et al.: Metabolism, *40*:101–104, 1991.
264. Nestler, J.E., Powers, L.P., Matt, D.W., et al.: J. Clin. Endocrinol. Metab., *72*:83–89, 1991.
265. Weaver, J.U., Holly, J.M., Kopelman, P.G., et al.: Clin. Endocrinol. (Oxf.), *33*:415–422, 1990.
266. Adlercruetz, H.: Scand. J. Clin. Lab. Invest., *201 (Suppl.)*:3–23, 1990.
267. Wilson, J.D., Griffin, J.E.: Metabolism, *29*:1278–1295, 1980.
268. Tweedle, D., Walton, C., Johnston, I.D.A.: Br. J. Clin. Pract., *27*:130–132, 1972.
269. Wiedemann, E., Schwartz, E.: J. Clin. Endocrinol. Metab., *34*:51–58, 1972.
270. Clemmons, D.R., Underwood, L.E., Ridgway, E.C., et al.: J. Clin. Endocrinol. Metab., *52*:731–735, 1981.
271. Van Der Poll, T., Romijn, J.A., Endert, E., et al.: Am. I. Physiol., *261*:E457–E465, 1991.
272. Beutler, B., Cerami, A.: Endocr. Rev., *9*:57–66, 1988.
273. Goodman, M.N.: Am. J. Physiol., *260*:E727–E730, 1991.
274. Hoshino, E., Pichard, C., Greenwood, C.E., et al.: Am. J. Physiol., *260*:E27–E36, 1991.
275. Brenner, D.A., Buck, M., Feitelberg, S.P., et al.: J. Clin. Invest., *85*:248–255, 1990.
276. Andus, T., Geiger, T., Hirano, T., et al.: Eur. J. Biochem., *173*:287–293, 1988.
277. Fraker, D.L., Merino, M.J., Norton, J.A.: Am. J. Physiol., *256*:E725–E731, 1989.

CHAPTER 41

# Immunology and Nutrition

**Quentin N. Myrvik**



Immunology, as a biologic subject, can be defined as a study of the immunity of living organisms to harmful agents. Early on it was recognized that mammals produced specifically reacting glycoproteins against foreign substances. These protective glycoproteins were called antibodies, because they reacted and neutralized the "foreign bodies," which induced the production of the specific antibodies. The foreign molecules capable of inducing the formation of antibodies were called antigens because they generated antibody in the host.

Because serum antibodies are special glycoproteins, or globulins, and are concerned with immunity, they are called immunoglobulins. Five classes of immunoglobulins are recognized, namely, IgG, IgM, IgA, IgE, and IgD. The production of antibodies by a host is commonly referred to as the humoral immune response. (See *Selected Readings* for further information.)

Early developments in immunology took place within the discipline of microbiology, because of the numerous observations that individuals who recovered from infectious diseases were specifically resistant to subsequent infections by the same microorganism.

Before the turn of the century, it was observed that the serum of animals that had recovered from experimental diphtheritic infection contained specific glycoprotein molecules that neutralized the potent toxin produced by Corynebacterium diphtheriae, the etiologic agent of diphtheria. These glycoprotein molecules were referred to as antitoxins.

B lymphocytes are the cells responsible for antibody formation. In addition, another class of lymphocytes, designated T lymphocytes, can mediate cell-mediated immunity (CMI) directly as cytotoxic immune cells (tissue graft and tumor immunity) or through macrophages that are mobilized and activated by T-lymphocyte products (lymphokines). Lymphokines are cytokines or mediator products that act on many cell types (see subsequent discussion). This latter system is primarily involved in antimicrobial immunity.

The scope of immunology has extended to essentially every aspect of biology and medicine. Subdisciplines now include immunochemistry, immunogenetics, immunopathology, immunopharmacology, immunohematology, and immunotoxicology.

Because the immune system is a complex interplay of many cell types, which results in cell proliferation and synthesis of a wide variety of chemical moieties, it is not surprising that nutritional status can influence the immune response. Studies on the effects of nutrition on the immune response have spawned a new subdiscipline.

## FUNDAMENTALS OF IMMUNOLOGY

### EVOLUTION OF THE IMMUNE SYSTEM

The biologic world comprises a multitude of plant and animal species. Although some species benefit from association with other species, each competes with and may be harmed by other species as well. Every individual is endowed with attributes for self-preservation and preservation of the species to which it belongs. It is almost axiomatic that every multicellular animal possesses mechanisms to distinguish between components of self and foreign substances and to oppose invasion of its body by potentially harmful foreign agents. In mammals, the ability to distinguish between foreign antigens and antigens of self is vested in the lymphocyte and is one of many of the important expressions whereby cells can recognize foreign substances.

Cell recognition rests primarily on specific molecular cell surface configurations that represent discrete and intrinsic components imbedded within the fluid matrix of the cell membrane; these components can move independently within the membrane. Some of these moieties function as receptors, which endow cells with the ability to respond to various stimuli and mediate such diverse events as hormone stimulation, phagocytosis, organogenesis, and the immunologic activities of cells.

Early in evolution, the multicellular animals developed a primitive circulation called the hemolymph system, which included phagocytic cells capable of recognizing, engulfing, and often destroying foreign agents. Cells that carry out the specialized function of phagocytosis are commonly referred to as professional phagocytes, to distinguish them from certain other cells that under special circumstances can engage in limited phagocytosis. Ultimately, in the course of evolution, the lower animals developed the ability to synthesize nonspecific humoral factors of defense, especially antimicrobial factors.

Concomitant with the development of higher animals, complex lymphoreticular organs and specialized cells called lymphocytes emerged that were capable of mounting specific immune responses to foreign agents. This ability also included the unique capacity to respond specifically with accelerated and enhanced responsiveness on re-exposure to the same agent (anamnesis or memory). Anamnesis is mediated by special lymphocytes that are generated during the immune response and are referred to as memory cells.

The manner by which higher animals exercise such an astounding ability to mount a specific immune response to a nearly infinite number of different antigens is not totally understood. It is known, however, that large numbers of clones of lymphocytes exist and that the cells of each clone can possess surface receptors of unique configuration that bind specifically to a complementary structure on the antigen molecule called the antigen determinant or epitope. Accordingly, specific binding of antigen molecules to specifically immunocompetent lymphocytes that possess complementary surface receptors can trigger the lymphocyte to replicate, expand the number of cells in the specific clone, and induce differentiation to an antibody-secreting plasma cell. T cells multiply and expand the clones in the same way; however, the receptor responsible for specific responsiveness is intrinsic to the membrane of the T cell and is not an immunoglobulin.

The total immune response consists of three phases. The first is the afferent phase during which the antigen is bound to the immunocompetent cell; during the central phase, the stimulated cell differentiates and proliferates; and during the efferent or effector phase, immune T cells and/or antibodies are generated by B cells and react with residual antigen or reintroduced antigen.

Total immunity represents the sum of innate immunity, which is mediated by constitutive nonspecific humoral and cellular mechanisms and specific acquired or adaptive immunity. Acquired immunity depends principally on the specific activities of antibodies and immune T cells.

The terms antimicrobial immunity and antitissue immunity are often used. The former designates immunity against microorganisms; the latter designates immunity against cells of foreign grafts or autochthonous (of self) tumors. In some instances, individuals can mount a specific immune response against their own tissues and unfortunately destroy them (autoimmunity).

### CELLS OF THE IMMUNE SYSTEM

Conceptually, the mammalian immune system is divided into the central lymphoid system and the peripheral lymphoid system. The terms lymphoid and lymphatic are used synonymously. The central lymphoid system comprises the bone marrow, thymus, and the theoretic bursa equivalent, whereas the peripheral lymphoid system comprises the spleen, lymph nodes, tonsils, mucous membrane-associated lymphoid tissue (MALT), and other diffuse lymphoid tissues of the body. The differentiation and proliferation of lymphocytes within the central lymphoid system do not involve antigen-sensitive stem cells and are not antigen driven; however, these events are antigen driven in the peripheral lymphoid system.

Immune responses are mediated by numerous cell types and complex cell interactions. These cells include lymphocytes, macrophages, granulocytes, mast cells, and dendritic cells (accessory cells for antigen presentation). As noted subsequently, these cell interactions usually take place within the specialized microenvironment of the various organ systems involved in the immune response. The following cells have various important functions with respect to the affector and effector mechanisms of total immunity.

### *GRANULOCYTES*

Blood granulocytes, which comprise neutrophils, eosinophils, and basophils, are found in the blood as fully differentiated and short-lived cells 12 to 15 μm in diameter. They originate from a common progenitor in the bone marrow. Neutrophils are usually multilobed and are referred to as polymorphonuclear leukocytes, whereas eosinophils and basophils tend to possess bilobed nuclei.

Neutrophils comprise about 75% of the circulating blood leukocytes. They are short-lived cells that persist in circulation for only a few days at most and constantly leave vessels in small numbers to migrate into the tissues. They have a number of functions including the liberation of the fever-producing agent referred to as endogenous pyrogen, and are active in the digestion of foreign material and dead tissue. Neutrophils provide the first line of phagocytic defense against many microorganisms, as will be noted. Neutrophils, as well as eosinophils, are attracted by antigen-antibody (immune) complexes, particularly when the complement factor C5a (see subsequent discussion) is generated. Neutrophils and eosinophils engulf immune complexes mainly because they possess receptors for the Fc segment of the IgG molecule and a receptor for the C3b component of complement.

The human adult produces about 126 billion neutrophils every day. Possibly 25 billion neutrophils circulate in the blood and equal numbers are attached to the endothelium of the blood vessels in the process of moving out to the extravascular tissues. For every circulating neutrophil, 100 more are in reserve in the bone marrow. Within 1 hour, 20 times the number of neutrophils in the blood can be mobilized from the bone marrow reserve.

Eosinophils comprise about 2 to 6% of the circulating leukocytes. They are characterized by coarse membrane-invested cytoplasmic granules that stain with the acid dye eosin. The granules are rich in hydrolytic enzymes, peroxidase, and a major basic protein as well as eosinophilic cationic protein. Although their ability to inhibit or kill ingested microorganisms is limited, they can be an important effector cell in immunity against several animal parasitic infections.

The basophil normally comprises about 0.05 to 1% of the circulating leukocytes. It possesses receptors that bind to the Fc segment of the IgE antibody molecule. The cytoplasm of the basophil is characterized by coarse basophilic cytoplasmic granules containing stores of various biologically active molecules. The mast cell, which is the functional counterpart of the basophil in tissues, is abundant in perivascular and peribronchiolar connective tissue adjacent to smooth muscle. Basophils and mast cells become activated and release mediators when IgE molecules are bound to the Fc receptors and are cross-linked by reacting with specific antigen. Mast cell rupture resulting from tissue trauma can also result in the release of mediators that can cause significant inflammation.

### *MACROPHAGES*

Macrophages are large, long-lived mononuclear phagocytic cells that range in diameter from about 12 to 25 μm. They arise from radiosensitive promonocytes in the bone marrow. Macrophage precursors (promonocytes) pass continually from the bone marrow to the blood as small (12 to 15 μm) nonactivated cells. They comprise about 5% of the blood leukocytes. Many of the monocytes in the blood become fixed to vessel walls within organs such as the liver and the spleen, where they engage in phagocytic and pinocytic activity, which in turn induces their activation and maturation. Some monocytes migrate through the tight junctions of vessel walls to reach extravascular sites and tissues such as body cavities, lung alveoli, lymphoid organs, and even the brain. Macrophages possess various surface receptors including Fc receptors that bind antibodies of the human subclasses IgG1 and IgG3, as well as the C3b receptor, which binds the opsonic C3b complement component. Antibodies can bind to macrophages, which enables the macrophage to adhere and attack the membranes of foreign mammalian cells containing the corresponding antigens. Macrophages play a major role in acquired antimicrobial CMI. Antigen-triggered immune T cells secrete lymphokines that can mobilize and activate macrophages to the site of infection; such activated macrophages have an enhanced capability to kill microorganisms. In addition, they also have elevated levels of hydrolytic enzymes packaged in lysosomes. These enzymes include plasminogen activator, collagenase, elastase, proteases, and lysozyme. Macrophages can also function in processing and presenting antigens to lymphocytes for induction of the immune response.

### *LYMPHOCYTES*

Lymphocytes play the central role in the specific immune response. A normal human adult possesses approximately $10^{12}$ lymphocytes, most of which reside in the lymphoid organ systems. The stem cell progenitor of all lymphocytes resides in the bone marrow.

The three major groups of lymphocytes are B cells, T cells, and null cells. The latter group lacks most of the surface characteristics of either B or T cells. Null cells appear to play an important role as killer cells in antitissue immunity. The overall specific immune response is divided into two major types of responses: the humoral and the cell-mediated immune response. The immune cell responsible for the humoral antibody response is the B cell, whereas the T cell is responsible for mediating cell-mediated immune responses.

B cells are responsible for the production of all the immunoglobulins. However, certain antigens, referred to as thymus-dependent (TD) antigens, can induce antibody formation by B cells only if T helper cells (CD4) are present. Accordingly, T helper cells can react with the antigen determinants of the antigen that is also stimulating the B cells. In contrast, when thymus-independent (TI) antigens are introduced to the host, B cells can be activated without the need of T helper cells. Null cells have been demonstrated to contain two subsets, one referred to as killer (K) cells, which can destroy mammalian cells when specific antibodies are bound to the surface antigens of the target cell. The second subset is classified as natural killer (NK) cells, which are capable of killing tumor cells directly in the absence of any immunoglobulin.

Plasma cells are the end cells of antigen-stimulated B cells. These are highly specialized, fully differentiated cells derived from B cells that produce and secrete immunoglobulin. Plasma cells are found only in extravascular sites and do not circulate in the vascular compartment. The plasma cells are characteristic because of enormous amounts of dilated endoplasmic reticulum in the cytoplasm.

## TISSUES AND ORGANS OF THE IMMUNE SYSTEM

### *RETICULAR TISSUE AND ASSOCIATED CELLS*

Reticular cells possess dendrite-like cytoplasmic processes and are commonly found in lymphoreticular organs. These cells are particularly important in the presentation of antigens to immunocompetent lymphoid cells. There are three cell types: dendritic cells, interdigitating reticular cells, and Langerhans' cells. Dendritic cells appear to be associated with the B cell-dependent areas of lymphoid tissue, whereas interdigitating reticular cells usually are associated with T cell-dependent areas. Langerhans' cells are located abundantly in the thymus, eye, and epidermis. They have also been observed in the T cell-dependent areas of lymph nodes. These cells as a group are important in antigen presentation and the induction of humoral or cell-mediated immunity.

### *THYMUS AND T CELL DIFFERENTIATION*

The thymus originates as an epithelial outgrowth of an embryonic structure, the bronchial pouch, and is the principal lymphoid organ of the early embryo. The major function of the thymus is to provide the environment in which precursor lymphoid cells undergo differentiation and become T cells. Several hormones are produced by the thymus, including thymopoietin, thymosin, and thymulin. The thymic hormones presumably promote differentiation of precursor cells into T cells. The thymus is well developed at birth and begins to diminish in size or involute after puberty. During early embryonic life, and thereafter, the thymus seeds the peripheral lymphoid system with differentiated T cells that express a high degree of clone diversity with respect to antigen recognition. In adulthood, the organ seems to play a lesser role because adult thymectomy depresses T cell function only after a delay of weeks to months. This delay is probably related to the extensive seeding of T cells in peripheral lymphoid organs and the long life of certain T cell subsets.

### *POTENTIAL SITES OF B CELL MATURATION*

The bursa of Fabricius, the central lymphoid organ in birds, is involved in the early nonantigen-driven differentiation of B cells. Accordingly, the term bursa cell is the origin of the term B cell or B lymphocyte. In the case of the mammal, a bursa equivalent has not been defined precisely. Mammalian B cell maturation most likely occurs at multifocal sites in the peripheral lymphoid system.

### *LYMPH NODES*

The lymph node is an encapsulated lymphoreticular ovoid organ traversed by supporting trabeculae, connective tissue, and a radial arrangement of lymph sinuses that lead from the subcapsular marginal sinus to the medulla. The cells in the node are principally lymphocytes with lesser numbers of macrophages, plasma cells, and a few granulocytes. The paracortical area is populated largely by aggregates of T cells that emigrate from the thymus. Interdigitating reticular cells and a few Langerhans' cells are also present in the paracortex. The other portions of the node represent B cell-dependent areas (Fig. 41–1). Lymph nodes contribute to systemic as well as local defense by serving as important sites for production of antibodies and immune T cells. The slow percolation of lymph through the intricate network of lymphatic sinuses provides ample opportunity for soluble antigens, antigen-antibody complexes, and foreign particulates to come in contact with the surfaces of macrophages, dendritic cells, and lymphocytes. More than 99% of a soluble antigen can be trapped in the draining lymph nodes of an unprimed animal. Lymph nodes have both efferent and afferent lymph vessels. The lymph circulation is complex and allows for an orderly return of extravascular fluid, proteins, and lymphoid cells to the blood compartment through the thoracic duct.

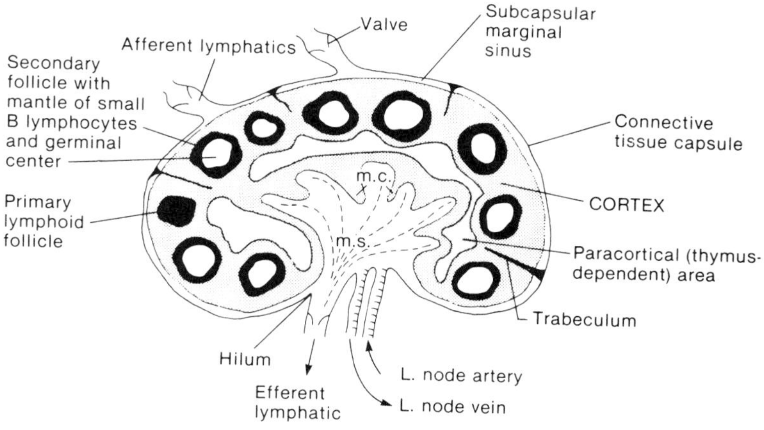
Afferent lymphatics
Valve
Subcapsular
marginal
sinus
Secondary
follicle with
mantle of small
B lymphocytes
and germinal
center
Connective
tissue capsule
m.c.
CORTEX
Primary
lymphoid
follicle
m.s.
Paracortical (thymus-
dependent) area
Trabeculum
Hilum
L. node artery
Efferent
lymphatic
L. node vein

m.c. Medullary cords
m.s. Medullary sinuses

**FIGURE 41–1.** Diagrammatic representation of a typical lymph node. Note B cell-dependent and T cell-dependent areas. (From Myrvik, Q.N., Weiser, R.S.: Fundamentals of Immunology. 2nd Ed. Philadelphia, Lea & Febiger, 1984.)

### *LYMPHOID FOLLICLES*

Lymphoid follicles occur in lymphoreticular structures, including lymph nodes, and comprise collections of B cell clones. Primary lymphoid follicles that characterize the newborn consist of uniform clusters of small lymphocytes. Secondary follicles develop as a consequence of exposure to foreign antigens. Germinal centers arising from progenitor B cells derived from the bone marrow are commonly associated with the evolution of secondary follicles. Events that occur in germinal centers include trapping and presentation of antigen to lymphocytes, expansion of specifically reactive clones of antibody-forming cells, and production of memory B cells; however, most of the plasma cells that are generated in the humoral response develop outside the germinal centers.

### *SPLEEN*

The spleen is a large lymphoreticular organ located within the circulation of the vascular compartment, where it serves as a filter for blood (Fig. 41–2). The spleen is pervaded by a reticular network the organization of which varies in different segments of the organ. The capsule and trabeculae are rich in flexible tissue that lends elasticity to the organ. The small central arteries are surrounded by a cylindric collar of lymphatic tissue called the white pulp. The structural function of the white pulp resembles that of the lymph node. The white pulp contains lymphoid follicles rich in B cells, whereas the nonfollicular area is a T cell-dependent area. The red pulp is a large matrix rich in red cells and thin-walled vena sinuses. Lymphocytes leave the spleen through efferent lymphatics as well as the vena sinuses. The spleen is a storehouse for blood and is a major site for the destruction of effete red blood cells. It can compensate for blood loss by contracting and expelling enormous numbers of red blood cells into the circulation.

### *THE MUCOUS MEMBRANE-ASSOCIATED LYMPHOID TISSUE (MALT)*

This highly specialized lymphoid system comprises lymphoid tissue directly associated with the mucosal surfaces of the body. The MALT possesses efferent but not afferent lymph vessels. It comprises both diffuse and organized lymphoid tissues containing essentially all the types of cells and fine structure that characterize major lymphoid organs. The effectors of specific immunity in the MALT include immune T cells, secretory IgA antibody, and lesser amounts of antibody of the other classes. Secretory IgA, which is uniquely resistant to digestive enzymes, is formed chiefly by plasma cells in the lamina propria of the mucosa of the gastrointestinal and bronchial tracts as well as the mammary gland. Undoubtedly, the secretory IgA found at all mucosal surfaces plays an important part in protecting the mucosal surfaces against microbial agents.

### *CIRCULATION OF LYMPHOCYTES*

Certain populations of lymphocytes, especially virgin cells and memory cells, continually recirculate from the blood to lymph and back again to the blood. The

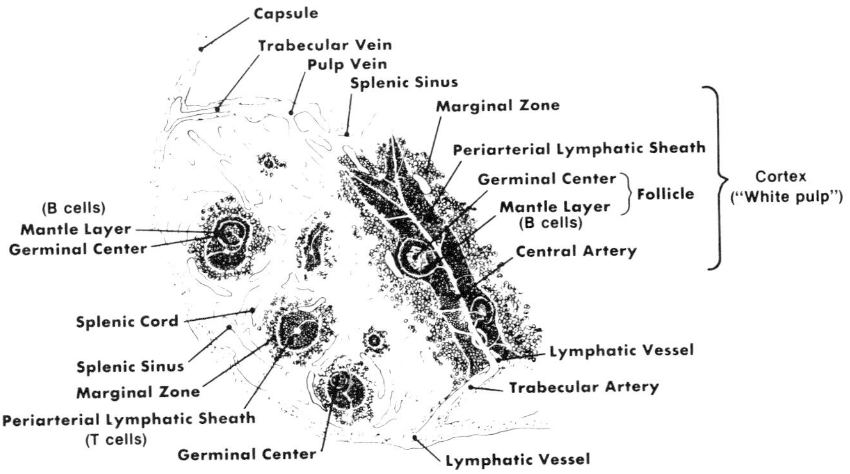
Capsule
Trabecular Vein
Pulp Vein
Splenic Sinus
Marginal Zone
Periarterial Lymphatic Sheath
Germinal Center
Mantle Layer
(B cells)
Follicle
Cortex
("White pulp")
Central Artery
(B cells)
Mantle Layer
Germinal Center
Splenic Cord
Splenic Sinus
Marginal Zone
Periarterial Lymphatic Sheath
(T cells)
Germinal Center
Lymphatic Vessel
Trabecular Artery
Lymphatic Vessel

**FIGURE 41–2.** Diagrammatic representation of the spleen. Note T cell and B cell areas. (From Myrvik, Q.N., Weiser, R.S.: Fundamentals of Immunology. 2nd Ed. Philadelphia, Lea & Febiger, 1984.)

recirculating interval of T cells is about 30 hours; for B cells, it is probably somewhat less. Most lymphocytes in the thoracic duct lymph and in the blood of normal adults are long-lived recirculating T cells.

Lymphocyte recirculation is of obvious importance: (1) it permits the rapid mobilization of specifically competent lymphocytes to the site of antigen deposition; (2) it ensures that committed cells can leave the organ and distribute the efferent specific immune response systemically to distant lymphoid tissues; and (3) it maintains a large number of mobile memory cells in the immune cell population that can be deployed readily to mount either an afferent or an efferent response at any site where antigen may reappear.

### *IMMUNOLOGIC ASPECTS OF PHAGOCYTOSIS*

Steps that lead to phagocytosis include directional movement of the phagocyte toward the particle (chemotaxis), recognition of the particle, adherence of the particle to the phagocyte, and, finally, engulfment. Some microorganisms resist phagocytosis, and specific antibody is necessary for the phagocytic event to take place. As a rule, phagocytosis of pathogenic bacteria is Fc and C3b receptor dependent.

## STRUCTURAL AND FUNCTIONAL CHARACTERISTICS OF HUMAN IMMUNOGLOBULINS

The gammaglobulins were first recognized and designated as a distinct group of serum proteins by Tiselius in 1937. He termed these proteins gammaglobulins because they migrated more slowly in an electric field than globulins of two other groups called alpha and beta. Five classes of immunoglobulins are recognized: IgG, IgM, IgA, IgD, and IgE (Fig. 41–3). The IgG molecule has been studied intensively and is a model of the basic structural unit of all immunoglobulins. It is a Y-shaped monomeric four-chain polypeptide complex containing two identical light chains and two identical heavy chains (either κ or λ) held together by noncovalent and covalent disulfide bonds. Extensive studies have been made of the amino acid sequence of various immunoglobulins. Each chain has a constant region and a variable region. The variable (V) regions represent the site of the antibody molecule that reacts with the antigen determinants. Domains also have been identified on the respective chains. For example, in the IgG molecule, each heavy chain has one V region domain referred to as the $V_H$ domain and three-heavy chain domains called $C_H1$, $C_H2$, and $C_H3$ (Fig. 41–4). The $C_H2$ and $C_H3$ domains have a number of biologic activities, including complement activation, transplacental transfer of IgG, and binding of the molecule to phagocytic cells and certain lymphoid cells possessing Fc receptors. Whereas the $C_H2$ domain is the site where complement components first interact to initiate the complement activation cascade, the $C_H3$ domain possesses sites that bind the molecule to Fc receptors on macrophages, granulocytes, and certain lymphocytes. The properties of human immunoglobulins can also be found in Tables 41–1 and 41–2. The various classes of immunoglobulins are described as follows.

### *IMMUNOGLOBULIN G*

Human IgG can be subdivided into four subclasses, IgG1, IgG2, IgG3, and IgG4. They comprise 66%, 23%, 7%, and 4%, respectively, of the IgG in the blood. Whereas IgG3, IgG1, and IgG2 can fix complement in

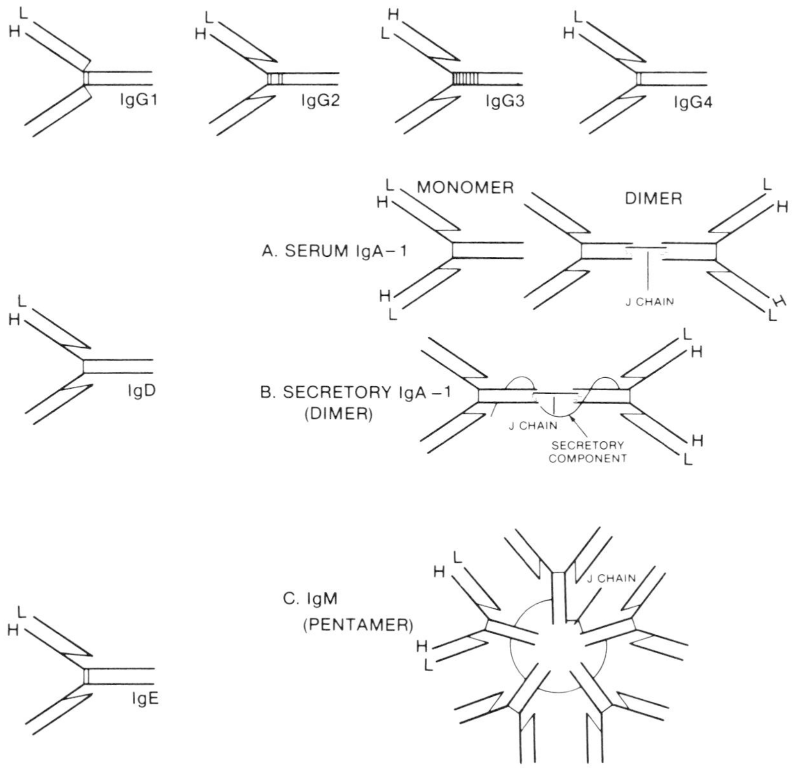
IgG1
IgG2
IgG3
IgG4
MONOMER
DIMER
A. SERUM IgA-1
J CHAIN
IgD
B. SECRETORY IgA-1
(DIMER)
J CHAIN
SECRETORY
COMPONENT
C. IgM
(PENTAMER)
J CHAIN
IgE

**FIGURE 41–3.** Diagram illustrating human immunogiobulins. Human immunoglobulins belong to five classes: IgG, IgA, IgM, IgD, and IgE. Basic monomers of all immunoglobulin molecules are composed of two L and two H chains. All immunoglobulins have either identical kappa (κ) or lambda (λ) chains. Heavy chains of each immunoglobulin class are designated by Greek letters corresponding to the capital letter identifying the class. (From Fudenberg, H.H., Stites, D.P., Caldwell, J.L., et al. (Eds.): Basic and Clinical Immunology. 3rd Ed. Los Altos, CA, Lange Medical Publications, 1980.)

that order, the IgG4 subclass cannot activate the classic complement pathway.

*IMMUNOGLOBULIN A*

Immunoglobulin A comprises two subclasses, IgA1 and IgA2, which occur in the serum in the ratio of 40 to 1. IgA has two basic molecular forms, serum IgA and secretory IgA. Serum IgA is, for the most part, a monomeric four-chain polypeptide unit, whereas secretory IgA consists of a J chain-coupled dimer to which secretory component, a product of epithelial cells, is added.

*IMMUNOGLOBULIN M*

The IgM molecule is a 19S, star-shaped polymer composed of five basic monomers held together by disulfide bonds and a J chain. Each H chain carries four domains on the constant segment. Although the molecule has 10 potential antigen-binding sites, only 5 can readily be demonstrated to bind high-molecular weight antigens. Because of its multivalence, IgM possesses high avidity for antigens carrying repeating (identical) antigen determinants such as polysaccharides. It is an efficient agglutinin as well as efficient complement activating antibody.

*IMMUNOGLOBULIN D*

This immunoglobulin class comprises only about 0.2% of the total immunoglobulins in serum. Although its role in acquired immunity is unknown, IgD is found commonly on the surface of precursor immature lymphocytes in conjunction with monomeric IgM.

*IMMUNOGLOBULIN E*

This immunoglobulin is found in low concentrations in human serum. It is a potent antibody in terms of mediating anaphylactic hypersensitivity reactions such as hay fever, allergic asthma, and food allergies, based

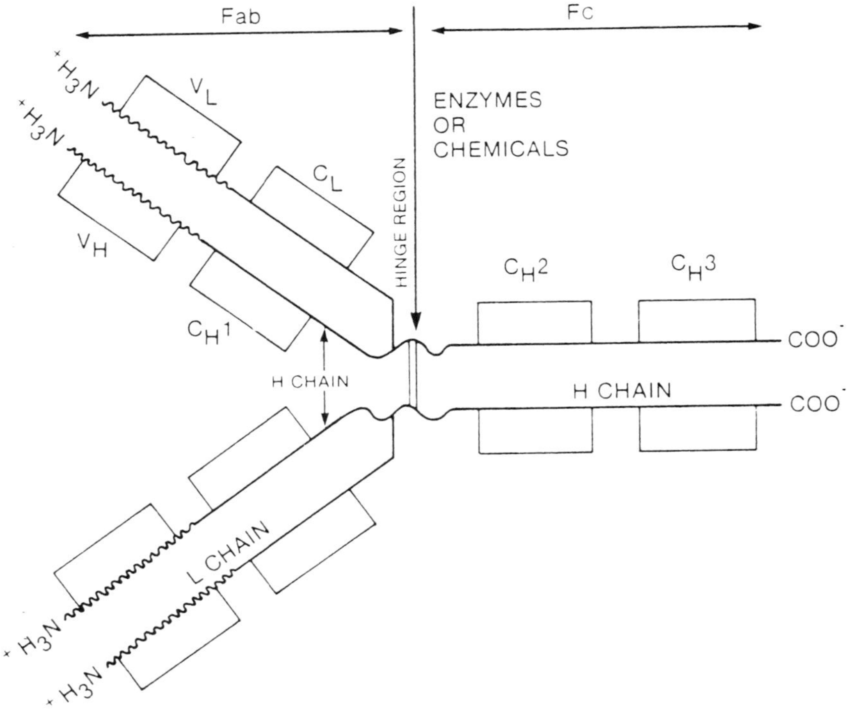
Fab
Fc
ENZYMES
OR
CHEMICALS
HINGE REGION
$^{+}H_3N$
$^{+}H_3N$
$V_L$
$C_L$
$V_H$
$C_H1$
$C_H2$
$C_H3$
COO⁻
COO⁻
H CHAIN
H CHAIN
L CHAIN
$^{+}H_3N$
$^{+}H_3N$

**FIGURE 41–4.** A simplified model for an IgG1 human Ab molecule showing the 4-chain basic structure and domains. V, Variable region; C, constant region; vertical arrow, hinge region. Thick lines represent H and L chains; thin lines represent disulfide bonds. (Modified from Fudenberg, H.H., Stites, D.P., Caldwell, J.L., et al. (Eds.): Basic and Clinical Immunology. 3rd Ed. Los Altos, CA, Lange Medical Publications, 1980.)

**TABLE 41–1.** PROPERTIES OF HUMAN IMMUNOGLOBULINS

| CLASS | HALF-LIFE (days) | SERUM CONCENTRATION (mg/dl) | DISTRIBUTION (% of Total in Intravascular Space) | SYNTHETIC RATE (mg/kg/day) | TOTAL IMMUNO-GLOBULIN (%) |
|---|---|---|---|---|---|
| IgG | 23 | 1000 | 45 | 33 | 80 |
| IgA (serum) | 6 | 200 | 42 | 24 | 16 |
| IgM | 5 | 120 | 76 | 6–7 | 4 |
| IgD | 3 | 3 | 75 | 0.4 | 0.001 |
| IgE | 3 | 0.05 | 51 | 0.02 | 0.00003 |

(From Myrvik, Q.N., Weiser, R.S.: Fundamentals of Immunology. 2nd Ed. Philadelphia, Lea & Febiger, 1984.)

largely on its affinity for mast cells and basophils through its Fc segment. When specific antigen reacts with IgE bound to mast cells, they undergo degranulation, releasing potent mediators such as histamine, serotonin, bradykinin, and the leukotrienes.

## THEORIES TO EXPLAIN ANTIBODY DIVERSITY

The specificity of an antibody molecule is attributable to the amino acid sequences of the variable regions of the L and H chains. Accordingly, the germ line theory has emerged as a major possible mechanism responsible for antibody diversity in terms of specificity for antigenic determinants. Because somatic mutation of these genes is frequent, this mechanism probably contributes importantly to the fine tuning of antibody specificity through a clonal selection process.

The heavy-chain V (variable) genes in man comprise at least four subgroups, and the gene products of any one of these genes can combine with the products of the constant-region gene. In addition, some four to six respective V-region gene subgroups have been tentatively identified for human light chains. Individually,

**TABLE 41–2.** PROPERTIES OF HUMAN IMMUNOGLOBULINS

| CLASS | IMMUNOLOGIC ACTIVITIES | OPSONIC ACTIVITY | PLACENTAL PASSAGE | ORDER OF APPEARANCE OF SYNTHETIC ABILITY IN INFANTS | FUNCTIONAL VALENCE |
|---|---|---|---|---|---|
| IgG | Late response to Ag; antibacterial; antitoxic; antiviral; blood group Abs | + | Yes (all subclasses) | Late | 2 |
| IgA (serum) | Block bacterial adherence; viral defense | – | No | Intermediate | 2 (monomer) |
| IgA (secretory) | Activity in mucous secretions; block bacterial adherence; viral defense | – | No | Intermediate | 2–4 (dimer) |
| IgM | Early response to Ag; antibacterial; antiviral; blood group Abs | + | No | Early | 5 (10)* |
| IgD | Present on lymphocyte surface | + | No | | 2 |
| IgE | Allergic (anaphylactic) reactions; possible respiratory tract defense; mast cell fixation; raised in parasitic infections; cytophilic, for basophils and mast cells | + | No | | 2 |

*A valence of 10 is the theoretic maximum and could only be achieved with low-molecular-weight hapten. (From Myrvik, Q.N., Weiser, R.S.: Fundamentals of Immunology. 2nd Ed. Philadelphia, Lea & Febiger, 1984.)

these gene products also can combine with the constant-region genes through recombination events.

With respect to the L chain, this recombination takes place between a germ-line V-region gene and a distinct segment of DNA on the same chromosome, referred to as a joining (J) gene, which encodes a 13 amino acid sequence. The J gene is responsible for at least two important signals, one for DNA recombination and one for ribonucleic acid (RNA) splicing. The RNA splicing is required even after DNA transcription because the L and H chain genes remain at different discrete coding segments separated by intervening sequences of DNA (introns).

Whereas L chains are encoded by three genes (V, J, and C genes), the encoding of H chains involves the additional D gene for diversity. Thus, the functional H chain gene complex represents a combination of V, D, J, and C genes in that order. Multiple different D genes exist, but the exact numbers are unknown. The combinatorial possibilities of the genes for L and H chains can account theoretically for the large number of specificities expressed in the immune responses to the large number of antigen determinants that are foreign to the host.

## THE COMPLEMENT SYSTEM

The complement system consists of 17 different plasma proteins. Nine major components comprise the classic pathway of complement activation and cell lysis initiated by certain antigen-antibody interactions on the cell surfaces. The nine major components of the classic pathway are designated C1 through C9 in the order of their discovery, which is not the order of their reaction sequence. C1 consists of three subunits: C1q, C1r, and C1s. A second pathway of complement activation, called the alternative pathway, is initiated nonspecifically by extrinsic agents other than antigen-antibody complexes such as bacterial endotoxin and high-molecular weight polysaccharides. Serum factors unique to the alternative pathway are designated by the capital letters B, D, and P (properdin). Two other components of the complement system are C3bINA, which inactivates C3b, and BIH, which enhances the activity of C3bINA. A summary of the classic and alternative pathway reactions is presented in Figure 41–5. The classic pathway as well as the alternative pathway can generate the chemotactic factor C5a and the opsonic factor C3b. In addition, if the complement factors C5b through 9 are activated by either pathway, the lysis of cells can result. The alternative pathway is initiated with the C3 moiety of complement. Accordingly, C1, C2, and C4 are not involved in the alternative pathway.

The C3b component of complement bound to bacterial membranes as well as the Fc moiety of IgG antibodies bound to their corresponding antigenic epitope on bacteria can react with the C3b and Fc receptors on phagocytes and produce a synergistic action in terms of mediating opsonin-mediated phagocytosis of bacteria. Complement can also aid in the clearance of circulating

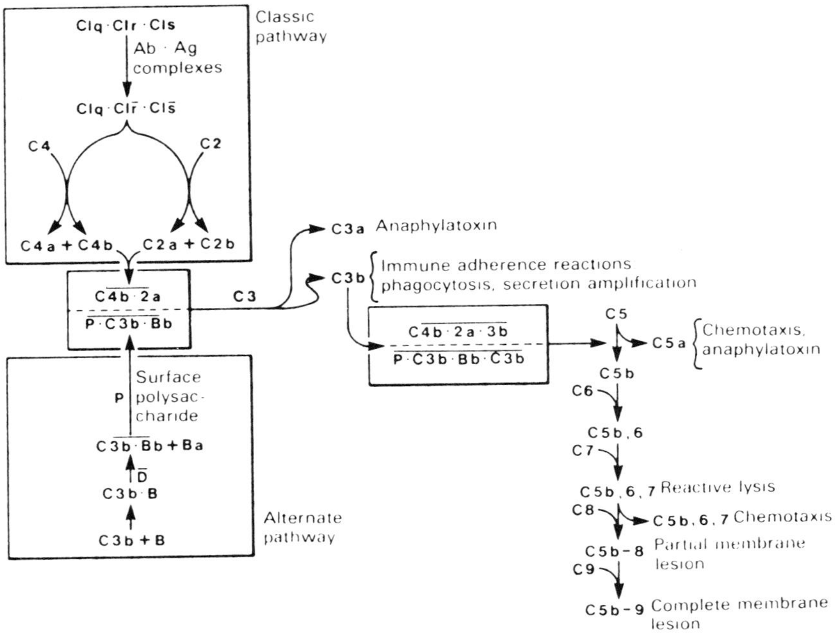

Classic pathway
Ab · Ag complexes
C4
C2
C4a + C4b
C2a + C2b
C3
C3a Anaphylatoxin
C3b
Immune adherence reactions phagocytosis, secretion amplification
C5
C5a
Chemotaxis, anaphylatoxin
C5b
C6
C5b,6
C7
C5b,6,7 Reactive lysis
C8
C5b,6,7 Chemotaxis
C5b-8 Partial membrane lesion
C9
C5b-9 Complete membrane lesion
Surface polysaccharide
C3b + B
Alternate pathway


**FIGURE 41–5.** Reaction sequence of the classic and alternative complement system. Note that C4b2a and PC3bBb are the C3 convertases for the classic and alternative C pathways, respectively. (From Eisen, H.N.: Immunology. 2nd Ed. Hagerstown, MD, Harper & Row, 1980.)

immune complexes by way of the C3b and Fc receptors on phagocytes.

Individuals genetically deficient in C2 exhibit increased susceptibility to infection. Because C2 is not involved in the alternative pathway, this finding suggests that the alternative pathway alone is not sufficient for normal function of antimicrobial mechanisms of defense. In particular, patients with C3 deficiencies are highly susceptible to infections, particularly pulmonary infections, indicating the importance of C3b in complement-mediated opsonic action.

## INTERACTIONS OF ANTIGENS AND ANTIBODIES IN VITRO

Antibodies of all the major immunoglobulin classes and subclasses can participate in various types of antigen-antibody interactions in vitro. Numerous studies have involved the use of haptens as monovalent determinants (epitopes) on proteins to study antigen-antibody interactions in vitro. An antigen determinant will react with the antibody-reacting site in a highly specific way. The typical antibody-reacting site on an antibody molecule is a three-dimensional cavity comprising approximately 500 to 700 $A^2$ in area. Antigen-antibody bonds generally are weak and range from 7 to 20 kcal/mol; however, the reactions can be highly specific.

If antigens and antibodies react in soluble state, a precipitate usually forms. The antibody in this case is referred to as a precipitin. If the antigen is particulate or if it is on the surface of a cell, the specific antibody can produce agglutination or aggregation. Such antibodies are commonly referred to as agglutinins. A large array of gel precipitation tests use the reactions of soluble antigens and antibodies. In addition, immunoelectrophoresis is used commonly as a technique to separate antigen preparations in mixtures followed by developing precipitin arcs with appropriate antibodies. Discrete antigen-antibody systems can be visualized with this technique. Other immunologic techniques involve radioimmunoassays, immunofluorescence, immobilization tests, complement fixation tests, and virus neutralization tests. Enzyme immunoassays, as well as crossed immunoelectrophoresis, are other techniques developed and used in in vitro interactions of antigens and antibodies. Descriptions of these techniques are readily available in standard immunologic textbooks.

## CELLULAR BASIS OF AFFERENT IMMUNE RESPONSES

### *ONTOGENY OF B LYMPHOCYTES*

The early development and differentiation of B cells are not antigen-driven events. Differentiation proceeds from a pluripotential bone marrow stem cell that is unable to form immunoglobulin to a family of line progenitor cells called pre-B cells. These cells synthesize but do not secrete IgM, the first immunoglobulin to be synthesized by differentiating B cells. Two types of pre-B cells exist, a rapidly dividing large cell type and a slowly dividing small cell type. In the adult bone marrow, the large pre-B cell differentiates into a small pre-B cell. Both cell types contain a small amount of cytoplasmic IgM (monomeric) but little or no surface IgM. The small pre-B cell continues to differentiate to become an immature B cell possessing intrinsic surface monomeric IgM but no cytoplasmic IgM. Immature B cells leave the bone marrow and move to peripheral lymphoid tissues where they differentiate rapidly to become mature immunocompetent cells carrying both surface IgM and surface IgD but no cytoplasmic immunoglobulin. Before their experience with antigens, the mature B cells are commonly called virgin B cells. Most B cells carry surface immunoglobulin. On encountering antigen, a virgin B cell can differentiate to become a memory cell, an antibody-secreting end cell (plasma cell), or a tolerized cell. A summary depicting the ontogeny of B cells is presented in Figure 41–6.

### *ONTOGENY OF T LYMPHOCYTES*

Progenitor T cells migrate from the bone marrow to the thymus to differentiate and proliferate in the thymus cortex and pass to the medulla. Human T-lymphocyte antigens that characterize human T cells first appear at the pre-T cell stage together with the receptor for peanut agglutinin. Changes in the enzyme patterns of human thymocytes occur during maturation. For example, terminal deoxynucleotide transferase is present only in progenitor hematopoietic cells and immature thymocytes, whereas α-naphthol acetate esterase is present in mature T cells. One human T cell subset, the Tμ cell, which possesses receptors for the Fc segment of IgM, is a precursor of the T helper cell. Another T cell subset that possesses receptors for the Fc segment of IgG (Tγ cells) is the precursor of the T suppressor cell. Additional subsets of T cells possess Fc receptors for IgA (Tα cells) and IgE (Tϵ cells). A summary of the ontogeny of T cells is presented in Figure 41–7. A third group of lymphoid cells is referred to as null cells because they lack the characteristic B and T lymphocyte markers. One subset of this group possesses Fc receptors for both IgG and IgG-containing immune complexes and is referred to as killer (K) cells. A second set is referred to as natural killer (NK) cells. The K cells can act as killer cells against tumor cells in cooperation with specific antibody, whereas the NK cells can act as killer cells without immunoglobulin using some undefined primitive recognition system.

The immune responses in the fetus and neonate are relatively weak and tolerance is induced easily. During fetal life, an excess of suppressor T cells apparently exist in the fetus, which down-regulate the maternal immune response. It has been suggested that this process prevents the mother from rejecting the fetus as a foreign graft.

### *B CELL ACTIVATION AND THE HUMORAL RESPONSE*

The nonantigen-driven events in B cell maturation result in randomization of a large number of clones that fortuitously can react with antigens encountered by the host. The genetic repertoire of specificities resides within

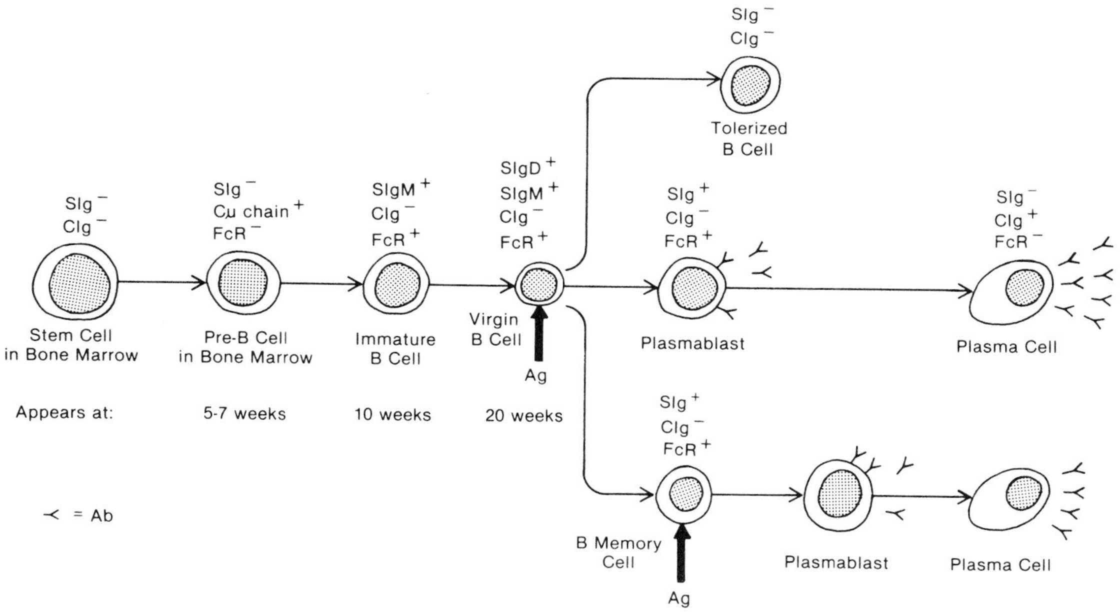
SIg⁻
CIg⁻
Tolerized
B Cell
SIg⁻
CIg⁻
SIg⁻
Cu chain⁺
FcR⁻
SIgM⁺
CIg⁻
FcR⁺
SIgD⁺
SIgM⁺
CIg⁻
FcR⁺
SIg⁺
CIg⁻
FcR⁺
SIg⁻
CIg⁺
FcR⁻
Stem Cell
in Bone Marrow
Pre-B Cell
in Bone Marrow
Immature
B Cell
Virgin
B Cell
Ag
Plasmablast
Plasma Cell
Appears at:
5-7 weeks
10 weeks
20 weeks
SIg⁺
CIg⁻
FcR⁺
= Ab
B Memory
Cell
Plasmablast
Plasma Cell
Ag

**FIGURE 41–6.** Ontogeny of B cells. Note that surface IgM (SIgM) first appears on the immature B cell with loss of cytoplasmic Ig (CIg). The virgin B cell possesses SIgD and SIgM. Fc receptors (FcR) appear at the immature B cell stage. (From Myrvik, Q.N., Weiser, R.S.: Fundamentals of Immunology. 2nd Ed. Philadelphia, Lea & Febiger, 1984.)

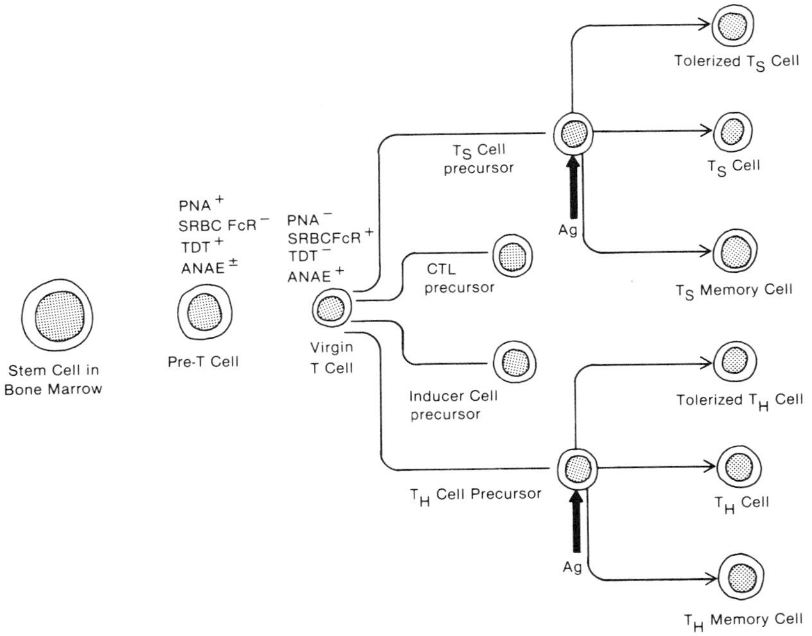
Tolerized $T_S$ Cell
$T_S$ Cell precursor
$T_S$ Cell
Ag
PNA +
SRBC FcR −
TDT +
ANAE ±
PNA −
SRBCFcR +
TDT −
ANAE +
CTL precursor
$T_S$ Memory Cell
Stem Cell in Bone Marrow
Pre-T Cell
Virgin T Cell
Inducer Cell precursor
Tolerized $T_H$ Cell
$T_H$ Cell Precursor
$T_H$ Cell
Ag
$T_H$ Memory Cell

**FIGURE 41–7.** Ontogeny of T cells. Note that pre-T cells are peanut agglutinin (PNA) positive and positive for terminal deoxynucleotidyltransferase (TDT). Virgin T cells, however, are negative for PNA and TDT but carry Fc receptors (FcRs) for sheep red blood cells and are positive for α-naphthol acetate esterase (ANAE). (From Myrvik, Q.N., Weiser, R.S.: Fundamentals of Immunology. 2nd Ed. Philadelphia, Lea & Febiger, 1984.)

the genome of the responding cell. When cross-linked, antigen determinants react with a specifically reacting surface IgM molecule on a mature immunocompetent B cell, the B cell replicates, and a clone is generated that subsequently synthesizes IgM antibodies with that single specificity. A second type of B cell activation involves T helper cells, in which case cross-linked antigen determinants are not required. Subsets of specifically reacting T helper cells likely are responsible for the switch to other immunoglobulin classes. Switching may occur as follows: IgM to IgG, IgM to IgA, and IgM to IgE. As a rule, switching only occurs with TD antigens. As previously stated, TI antigens only stimulate production of IgM and do not require T helper cells.

As summarized subsequently, several growth factor-like molecules are involved in B cell activation. Interleukin 4 (IL-4) stimulates activation of B cells in conjunction with cross-linked antigen determinants, whereas IL-5 functions as a B cell growth factor for activated B cells. IL-2 and IL-6 cause B cells to differentiate into antibody-secreting cells.

## *ROLE OF T CELLS IN THE CELL-MEDIATED IMMUNE RESPONSE*

The cell-mediated immune (CMI) response can only be induced by TD antigens. Intracellular parasites like Mycobacterium tuberculosis and Histoplasma capsulatum develop good CMI responses because their antigens persist and are slowly released from the parasitized macrophages. Water-insoluble antigen complexes are apparently more effective in producing a CMI response than are water-soluble proteins. Effector CMI responses in humans are mediated by at least two subsets of T cells: (1) human T lymphocytes expressing the CD4 surface antigen and mediating an antimicrobial CMI response through mediated macrophage deployment and activation, and (2) precursor T lymphocytes expressing CD8 surface antigen and mediating antitissue CMI. The CD8-lymphocyte subset is referred to as a cytotoxic T lymphocyte (CTL).

## *ACTIVATION OF SUPPRESSOR T CELLS*

As indicated previously, the two prominent T lymphocyte subsets comprise T helper/inducer cells (CD4) and T suppressor/cytotoxic cells (CD8). The intravenous injection of antigen tends to favor the development of T suppressor cells that become abundant in the spleen. Suppressor cells can be involved in suppressing the B cell response as well as the T cell response. Clearly, suppressor T cells play an important role in the regulation of the immune response.

## *CONTRIBUTIONS OF ACCESSORY CELLS TO LYMPHOCYTE ACTIVATION*

Macrophages play an important role as accessory cells and are effective in processing and presenting antigens to immunocompetent lymphocytes. Macrophages are also important in the production of interleukin-1 (IL-1) which activates T cells and induces them to replicate. Interleukins are mediators that function as the communication system of immune cells.

Macrophages contribute to the humoral response to TD antigens by processing antigen and presenting it to specifically competent T helper cells and virgin B cells. In accord with these events, IL-1, which is produced by macrophages, stimulates the activation and replication of T cells. In turn, activated T cells secrete IL-2, which plays an important role in the activation and replication of additional T cells during an immune response. As mentioned previously, other cells also can function as accessory cells. In particular, the Langerhans' cells and the interdigitating reticular cells play an important role in the induction of the CMI response, whereas dendritic cells appear to play an important role in the activation of the humoral immune response. These accessory cells, as well as macrophages, always contain HLA-DR antigens on their surface when functioning as antigen-presenting cells. The human HLA-DR system is equivalent in the mouse Ia system, which is involved in antigen presentation, to immunocompetent lymphocytes.

### *CYTOKINES AND THE CELL COMMUNICATION SYSTEMS*

During the last 20 years, a substantial body of information has accumulated that delineates the integrated systems of communication between cells that participate in the immune response. The chemical moieties involved in the major events include the interleukins (IL), interferons (IFN), tumor necrosis factor (TNF) and granulocyte-macrophage colony-stimulating factor (GM-CSF).

**Interleukin 1(IL-1).** Activated macrophages appear to be the main source of secreted IL-1, although fibroblasts, endothelial cells, and keratinocytes can produce this cytokine.[1] The two forms of IL-1 are termed α and β. IL-1 can regulate T and B lymphocyte activation as well as maturation of T cell and B cell precursors. IL-1 appears to induce lymphokine receptor synthesis as well as lymphocyte proliferation. IL-1 also plays important roles in inflammation by the stimulation of arachidonic acid metabolism and the secretion of plasminogen activator as well as neutral proteases.[2] IL-1 also functions as a pyrogen, causing elevation of temperature. IL-1 also can stimulate cAMP production in fibroblast cultures.

**Interleukin 2 (IL-2).** IL-2 was originally referred to as T cell mitogenic or growth factor. However, IL-2 also stimulates growth of B cells, NK cells, and lymphokine-activated K cells.[3,4] Normally, resting T cells do not express the IL-2 receptor except in the presence of an antigen-presenting cell and antigen. It has been suggested that IL-2 stimulates T cell mitogenesis through activation of protein kinase C(PKC).

**Interleukin 3 (IL-3).** IL-3 promotes the development of a large number of hemopoietic cell types such as granulocytes, macrophages, mast cells, erythroid cells, megakaryocytes, and B and T lymphocytes.[5,6] It seems likely that the IL-3 produced during immune responses recruits additional cells to amplify the immune response. However, no evidence shows that IL-3 is required for baseline hemopoiesis. IL-3 reacting with its receptor also appears to activate PKC.

**Interleukin 4 (IL-4).** This lymphokine can act as a co-stimulant of B cell proliferation and enhance expression of class II major histocompatibility antigens on resting B cells. It can enhance the responses of B cells to other B cell stimulants.[7] In addition, IL-4 enhances IgG1 and IgE production by B cells. IL-4 also stimulates T cells, granulocytes, macrophages, erythroid precursors, megakaryocytes, and mast cells. In particular, IL-4 can stimulate macrophage antitumor activity and act synergistically with granulocyte colony-stimulating factor (G-CSF) to enhance growth of granulocyte or erythroid cell precursors emerging from bone marrow cultures.[8] With respect to immediate hypersensitivity, IL-4 apparently can induce isotype switching to IgE production. It also induces a low affinity receptor for IgE (FcεII) on resting B cells.

**Interleukin 5 (IL-5).** IL-5 can enhance the in vitro synthesis of IgM, IgG1, and IgA by previously stimulated B cells. In addition, IL-5 can induce maturation of eosinophils and induce receptors for IL-2 on T and B cells.[9] It can also induce the formation of cytotoxic T cells in the presence of IL-2.

**Interleukin 6 (IL-6).** IL-6 is a glycoprotein with a broad spectrum of activity.[10,11] For example, it can function as a growth factor for plasmacytomas, hepatocytes, and mouse hybridomas. It has been suggested that IL-6 functions as an autocrine growth factor for human multiple myelomas. It can also induce immunoglobulin production and IL-2 receptors in T cells. IL-1 and IL-6 can cause a synergistic induction of T cell proliferation as well as acute-phase protein production by hepatocytes. IL-6 also functions as a pyrogen.

**Interleukin 7 (IL-7).** IL-7 is primarily a growth-promoting factor that appears to function in stimulating growth of immature pre-B cells from the bone marrow.[12] IL-7 appears to be one of the most potent stimulators of proliferation of immature B cells as well as immature T cells. It is of special interest that daily treatment with IL-7 of mice given radiation resulted in a substantial increase in the number of B cells in the blood and lymphoid organs.

**Interleukin 8 (IL-8).** The culture of human endothelial cells with IL-1, TNF, or bacterial endotoxin induces the production of endothelial-leukocyte adhesion molecules. Adhesion of leukocytes to endothelial cells promotes emigration of inflammatory cells to the perivascular space, which can result in endothelial injury. However, activated endothelial cells also secrete a soluble leukocyte adhesion inhibitor that can reduce or attenuate adhesive reactions. This molecule has been named IL-8, and may be important in attenuating inflammation at the endothelial cell-blood interface.[13]

**Interferon-α, $\beta_1$ (IFN-α, $\beta_1$).** Leukocytes are probably the dominant source of IFN-α, whereas fibroblasts appear to be the major source of IFN $\beta_1$. IFN-α, $\beta_1$ inhibit cell proliferation, tumor cell growth, viral replication, and fibroblast differentiation. They also stimulate macrophage accessory activity, cytokine production, as well as expression of FcR and class I and II major histocompatibility complex (MHC) antigens. In vivo effects include induction of autoimmune and inflammatory reactions. In addition, antiviral, antibacterial, antifungal, and antitumor effects also can be demonstrated in vivo.[14]

**Interferon-γ (IFN-γ).** IFN-γ was first recognized by its capacity to block viral replication in fibroblasts, a property common to all interferons.[15] In addition, IFN-γ could prime or activate macrophages to a highly effective antibacterial potential. It is of special interest that IFN-γ is a potent inducer of NK activity, which has suggested also that it has a role in tumor resistance.[16]

**Tumor Necrosis Factor (TNF).** Certain tumor cells are killed by activated macrophages and, in some instances, it appears that a macrophage-produced cytokine, TNF, is responsible.[17] NK cells may also effect killing of tumor cells with TNF and possibly other cytokines. TNF functions as a major mediator of inflammation. In this regard, TNF appears to mediate endotoxin shock. In addition, TNF probably mediates antiparasitic host defense. Other properties of TNF include cachectic activity and wasting partially attributable to suppression of lipoprotein lipase activity in adipocytes; pyrogenic activity similar to IL-1; stimulating activity of activated T cells by increasing IL-2 receptor expression and inducing IFN-γ production; antiviral effects most likely resulting from induction of IFN production; and inhibition of bone synthesis and induction of bone resorption.

**Granulocyte-Macrophage Colony-Stimulating Factor (GM-CSF).** This T cell-derived cytokine plays an important role in controlling hematopoiesis.[18] Similar to IFN-γ, GM-CSF also can activate or prime macrophages to express tumoricidal activity as well as increased superoxide production.[19] GM-CSF can stimulate in vitro maturation and development of granulocyte-macrophage colonies.

**Migration Inhibition Factors (MIF) and Macrophage Activation Factors (MAF).** Culture fluids of antigen-stimulated T cells inhibit the migration of normal macrophages using an in vitro capillary tube migration assay. Initially, this test was used extensively as an in vitro correlate of delayed hypersensitivity. Subsequently, it was noted that MIF also activated macrophages and it was postulated to be IFN-γ or the main macrophage activation factor (MAF).[20] The availability of recombinant lymphokines has now clarified this complex problem to some degree.

It is now apparent that IFN-γ, IL-4, and GM-CSF can activate macrophages and induce identical changes in macrophage function. When macrophages are activated, they exhibit migration inhibition. The redundancy in macrophage activation factors carries out a common and familiar pattern in biology, particularly in critical areas such as CMI.[21]

**Transforming Growth Factor (β (TGF-β).** This cytokine is produced by several cell types, including platelets, T and B cells, kidney cells, and activated macrophages. It appears to play an important role in negative feedback based on the observation that it inhibited the growth of fibroblasts under conditions of anchorage-independent noncontact growth. This antiproliferative effect occurs with a wide variety of neoplastic and normal cells. However, it can function as a chemoattractant for fibroblasts and macrophages. TGF-β counteracts the proliferative effects of IL-2 on T and B cells and of IL-1 on thymocytes.[22] Although TGF-β can activate macrophages to produce IL-1, it inhibits the production of oxygen intermediates.

**Connective Tissue Growth Factors.** Other growth factors have been described, such as platelet-derived growth factor (PDGF), epidermal growth factor (EGF), and fibroblast growth factor (FGF), which can participate in inflammatory and immune responses.[23] PDGF is produced by endothelial cells and macrophages. All three factors can enhance immunologic responses by augmenting the production of IFN-γ. These factors appear to stimulate wound healing and enhance immunologically mediated inflammatory responses.

**Low Molecular Weight Inflammatory Cytokines.** A new family of low molecular weight cytokines (8 to 10 kd) have been purified. These include monocyte-derived neutrophil chemotactic factor (MDNCF), β-thromboglobulin (β-TG), PF4, a platelet factor chemotactic for fibroblasts, IP10, 9E3, and GR0. The function of the latter three cytokines is unknown. β-TG induces fibroblast proliferation and collagen production.

It is becoming increasingly apparent that the families of cytokines play a critical and important role in linking inducer and effector cells that participate in immune and inflammatory responses. Macrophages functioning as antigen-presenting cells interacting with T cells that express a receptor for the processed form of the antigen results in IL-1 and IL-6 production by macrophages, which in turn induces synthesis of other interleukins by $CD4^+$ T cells. T helper cells can be divided into two subsets, TH1 and TH2. Although both subsets respond to antigen-presenting cells, they have different patterns of interleukin synthesis. In this regard, TH1 cells can be induced to express high affinity IL-2 receptors as well as production of IL-2, IL-3, and IFN-γ. Accordingly, IL-2 functions as an autocrine molecule that stimulates proliferation of T cells as well as NK cells. IL-3 stimulates hemopoiesis, which increases the numbers of effector cells. The production of IFN-γ by TH1 cells induces activation of macrophages as well as the activity of CD8 (suppressor/cytotoxic) cells and NK cells.

In contrast, activated TH2 cells secrete IL-3, IL-4, IL-5, and IL-6. IL-1 plus IL-4 induce proliferation of TH2 cells. IL-4 together with IL-5 and IL-6 induce proliferation and terminal differentiation of B cells into antibody-secreting plasma cells. Furthermore, the combined actions of IL-1, IL-3, IL-4, IL-7, and IFN-γ can promote recruitment of additional B cells.

### *GENETIC BASIS FOR AFFERENT IMMUNE RESPONSES*

Specific immune responses are controlled by two genetic systems in mammals. Genes of the first system, which encode for immunoglobulin structure, are present in three distinct unlinked loci on three respective chromosomes. Genes of the second system, which regulate the immune response to TD antigens, are associated with the major histocompatibility complex (MHC), so named because it contains genes encoding antigens concerned with allograft rejection. In the mouse, the genes that determine the immune responses to TD antigens are located in the I region situated between the K and D regions of chromosome 17 and are called immune response (Ir) genes. No genes controlling the specific immune responses to TI antigens have been found in the MHC.

After the identification of Ir genes, researchers observed that serologically distinct Ir gene products are present in various types of cells, particularly, the cells of the immune system. They are low-molecular weight polymorphic glycoproteins that can be identified with alloantisera. Because these gene products are antigenic, they were called I region-associated antigens (Ia antigens). The I region has been divided into five subregions, including I-A, I-B, I-C, and I-E based on the mapping of Ir genes, most of which are present in the I-A subregion. The fifth subregion, I-J, is based on the serologic identification of a distinct gene product on T suppressor cells called Ia 4. Both macrophages and certain B cells carry Ia antigens encoded by I-A and I-C subregion genes. I-A genes also code for Ia antigens in certain T cell subsets and are present in the helper factor complexes shed by T helper cells.

An animal that is a nonresponder to a given TD antigen may (1) lack T cells that bear that specific antigen receptor, (2) have defects in handling and presentation of antigens by accessory cells, (3) lack certain Ia antigens on T cells, or (4) have B cells that lack a receptor for the specific helper factor produced by T helper cells. In addition, excess suppressor cell function can dampen the immune response to the point where it may appear to be partially defective. This situation is particularly noticeable during the fetal and neonatal period. On the other hand, old animals tend to lack normal suppressor cell function, which in turn appears to lead to the development of autoimmune diseases in which the immune system begins reacting to antigens of self.

### *ANAMNESTIC (MEMORY) RESPONSE*

One of the most important responses with respect to the function of the immune system is the secondary antibody response or anamnestic response to TD antigens. The secondary response is distinguished readily from the primary response by a shortened induction phase, an earlier appearance of antibodies in serum, a more rapid rate of antibody synthesis, particularly IgG antibody, a higher peak of total serum antibody, and a delay in the phase of decline in the serum levels of IgG. These characteristics are attributable to increased numbers of B cells and T helper memory cells that play a major role in the secondary response. Virgin B cells likely play only a minor role in the secondary antibody response because of feedback suppression by IgG antibody (Fig. 41–8).

Any antibody still present in serum when the second dose of antigen is given declines or disappears rapidly (negative phase) owing to its almost immediate reaction with antigen to form immune complexes that are removed by the reticuloendothelial system. If the dose of antigen is adequate but low enough to allow its full incorporation into antigen-antibody complexes, antigen is cleared rapidly from the blood and the titer of antibody formed later rises to levels of 10 to 100 times the serum level attained in the normal primary response. If the secondary dose of antigen is in subpicogram quantities, an antibody response may not occur, presumably because antigen-antibody complexes formed would be meager and would be rapidly reduced by phagocytic destruction to substimulatory levels. Serum antibodies generated during the secondary antibody response are for the most part high-affinity IgG antibodies because most of the antibody-forming cells participating in the response are the progeny of memory cells that have been selected to have high-affinity antigen receptors. Low doses of antigen preferentially activate those lymphocytes that have receptors with the highest affinity. The ability of an animal to mount a rapid secondary response yielding high-affinity antibodies is of great practical importance, because it can result in the elimination of a viral or bacterial infection before clinical manifestations develop.

### *ABNORMALITIES OF THE IMMUNE SYSTEM*

Immunodeficiencies can be characterized by decreased or abnormal function in one or more components of the immune system, which usually results in increased susceptibility to infection. As a rule, the primary immune deficiencies are hereditary or congenital and are considered to result from defects in the development of

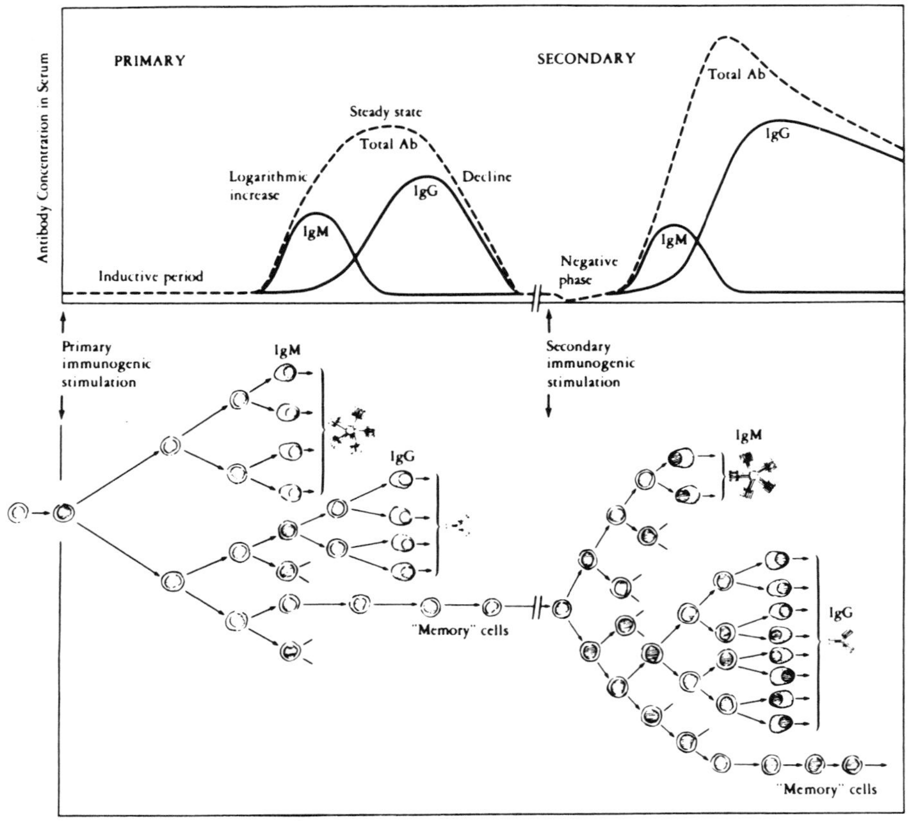

Antibody Concentration in Serum
PRIMARY
SECONDARY
Steady state
Total Ab
Logarithmic increase
Decline
IgG
IgM
Inductive period
Negative phase
Total Ab
IgG
IgM
Primary immunogenic stimulation
Secondary immunogenic stimulation
IgM
IgG
"Memory" cells
IgM
IgG
"Memory" cells


**FIGURE 41–8.** Primary and secondary antibody responses. Note the kinetics of IgM and IgG responses. (From Bellanti, J.A.: Immunology III. Philadelphia, W.B. Saunders, 1985.)

the immune system. In contrast, secondary immune deficiencies are the consequence of some other systemic disorder that indirectly causes a defect in the response of the immune system. A third category of immunodeficiency diseases can be referred to as "physiologic," which can affect any individual, although to different degrees. Such deficiencies could be age dependent because of increased susceptibility to infection in the first few months of life as well as certain defects in the immune system that occur with old age. A physiologic immunodeficiency could also be the result of malnutrition at any age. This topic is discussed further in this chapter.

### *IMMUNODEFICIENCIES OF THE T CELL SYSTEM*

These abnormalities are characterized by the classic DiGeorge syndrome, which is the prototype of a selective T cell deficiency. This immunodeficiency is manifested by increased susceptibility to infections of microorganisms of low virulence, such as Pneumocystis carinii and Candida albicans. Although the levels of immunoglobulins and the number of B cells can approach normal levels, secondary responses generally are depressed because of the lack of adequate numbers of T helper cells. A nucleoside phosphorylase deficiency has also been associated with this T cell deficiency and, in this case, the enzyme nucleoside phosphorylase is missing. As a consequence, patients accumulate inosine, guanosine, and the respective deoxy compound. These metabolites can exert inhibitory effects on normal T cell function in vitro.

### *IMMUNODEFICIENCIES OF THE B CELL SYSTEM*

These abnormalities can include panhypogammaglobulinemia (Bruton's agammaglobulinemia) and several dysgammaglobulinemias. With the latter, patients can have selective IgA deficiency, selective IgM deficiency, deficiencies of IgG and IgA with increased IgM, and selective deficiencies of any of the IgG subclasses. In panhypogammaglobulinemia, the almost total lack of B cells suggests a developmental defect in B cell precursors. Inherited hypogammaglobulinemia is characterized by recurring sinus and pulmonary infections with Haemophilus influenzae and Streptococcus pneumoniae. The B cell-dependent areas of lymphoid tissue usually are depleted of lymphocytes with germinal centers and lymphoid follicles lacking in the lymph nodes. The lamina propria of the intestinal mucosa is also devoid of plasma cells.

*COMBINED IMMUNODEFICIENCIES*

Combined immunodeficiencies are associated with syndromes such as reticular dysgenesis, ataxia-telangiectasia, Wiskott-Aldrich syndrome, and short-limbed dwarfism. Combined immunodeficiency disease has also been associated with adenosine deaminase deficiency, in which case patients suffer from an inborn error in purine metabolism. This disorder is inherited in an autosomal recessive manner. Lack of adenosine deaminase, which metabolizes adenosine and deoxyadenosine, results in accumulation of metabolites, such as cAMP and deoxy-ATP, which can depress lymphocyte function in vitro.

*COMBINED IMMUNODEFICIENCIES WITHOUT ASSOCIATED ADENOSINE DEAMINASE DEFICIENCY OR SPECIFIC CLINICAL SYNDROMES*

Patients with Nezelof's syndrome reveal severe T-lymphocyte depletion, although immunoglobulin levels may be close to normal. The antibody response to immunization usually is poor, and the serum antibodies frequently have restricted heterogeneity. This immunodeficiency may result from developmental arrest at the level of the stem cell or at early stages of lymphocyte differentiation.

*IMMUNODEFICIENCIES OF THE COMPLEMENT (C) SYSTEM*

Primary deficiencies of C1q, C1r, C1s, C2, and C4 are frequently associated with autoimmune diseases. In addition, C2 and C4 deficiencies are also associated with increased frequency of certain histocompatibility antigens. Deficiencies of C3 and C5 are associated with increased susceptibility to infection that usually can be corrected by replacement therapy. Deficiency of C5, which commonly involves the presence of nonfunctional C molecules, has also been reported to be associated with autoimmune diseases. The generation of C3b and C5a is apparently an important component in opsonization and chemotactic functions. A host deficient in the production of these components will show increased susceptibility to infections.

*ACQUIRED IMMUNE DEFICIENCY SYNDROME (AIDS)*

This disease surfaced in the United States about 1980 in male homosexuals and drug abusers. AIDS is a sexually transmitted disease that can be transmitted by body fluids, including contaminated blood and contaminated needles. It is caused by a retrovirus designated as human immunodeficiency virus (HIV), which infects T cells and monocytes/macrophages resulting in severe depression of immune functions with devastating consequences for the affected individuals.

A major target cell in AIDS is the $CD4^+$ cell, which contains $CD4^+$ (the surface marker that serologically defines the $CD4^+$ cell population), the cellular receptor for HIV. This disease leads to a progressive depletion of $CD4^+$ cells and onset of immunodeficiency.[24] In addition, patients appear to have a general loss of T cell function. Also, HIV can replicate in certain B cells as well as monocyte/macrophages.[25] Recent evidence suggests that monocyte/macrophages may be the most important target cell, and indicates that HIV can infect bone marrow stem cells.

In a recent communication, Moseson et al. summarizes some current observations of malnutrition that pertain to AIDS patients.[26] For example, the administration of supplemental vitamin E decreased the number of $CD8^+$ (suppressor/cytotoxic) cells and increased the $CD4^+/CD8^+$ ratio. In addition, β-carotene increased the number of $CD4^+$ (helper/inducer) cells. Because malnutrition, low serum zinc levels, and intestinal malabsorption occur in AIDS patients, more research is needed to determine whether malnutrition contributes significantly to the rapid breakdown of the immune system in some patients.

## PRINCIPLES OF INNATE AND ACQUIRED IMMUNITY TO PARASITES

Immunity to a given agent may be complete or partial depending on two variables, the virulence of the parasite and the resistance of the host. It is useful to outline host immunity as set forth in Table 41–3.

**TABLE 41–3.** HOST IMMUNITY

| TYPE OF IMMUNITY | | | EXAMPLE OF IMMUNITY EXHIBITED |
|---|---|---|---|
| | Innate or Constitutive | | During early stages of primary infection |
| Acquired | Acquired naturally | Active | Following a case of whooping cough |
| | | Passive | Result of placental transfer of immunity from mother to fetus, e.g., immunity to diphtheria |
| | Acquired artificially | Active | Result of tetanus toxoid vaccination |
| | | Passive | Result of injection of tetanus antitoxin |

### *INNATE IMMUNITY*

Defined as immunity that is constitutive for the species, innate immunity is expressed in the early stages of primary infection before acquired immunity develops. The major factors responsible for innate immunity include anatomic barriers, phagocytes, special antimicrobial substances, and the basic phagocytic response associated with inflammation.

### *ACQUIRED IMMUNITY*

This immunity may be nonspecific as well as specific. For example, immunity naturally acquired by infection by one parasite may be nonspecifically operative concomitantly against another antigenically unrelated parasite.

### *ARTIFICIAL ACTIVE IMMUNITY*

This form results from purposeful vaccination with immunogenic antigens derived from or associated with a specific or related microorganism.

### *ARTIFICIAL PASSIVE IMMUNITY*

Artificial passive immunity usually is accomplished by injection of an immune serum that contains antibodies capable of conveying specific immunity against the microbe to the recipient.

### *NATURAL PASSIVE IMMUNITY*

For the most part, this immunity is mediated by specific antibodies of the class IgG in humans because immunity is transferred almost exclusively to the human fetus by way of the placenta. Artificial passive immunity may be mediated by IgM and IgA, as well as IgG antibodies, all of which are present in injectable commercial human immunoglobulin preparations. However, IgG is the dominant and most important immunoglobulin.

### *INTERNAL CELLULAR ORGAN SYSTEMS OF DEFENSE*

Inflammation is important in antimicrobial defense because it creates a fibrin network to trap microorganisms and promotes the movement of fluid and leukocytes into the area of inflammation.

Phagocytosis, a major mechanism of internal defense against invading microbes, can function in both innate and specific acquired immunity. The neutrophil or polymorphonuclear neutrophil leukocyte (PMN) represents the first line of defense against many microbes. Certain microorganisms, particularly encapsulated strains, can resist phagocytosis unless opsonized with specific antibody. Polymorphonuclear cells possess high levels of acid hydrolases as they emerge from the bone marrow to populate the blood. Hydrolases are packaged in membrane-bound structures called lysosomes. Polymorphonuclear cells express two classes of antimicrobial systems, oxygen-dependent and oxygen-independent. The toxic oxygen-derived radicals (superoxide, hydrogen peroxide, and hydroxyl radical) generated by a burst in the hexose monophosphate shunt at the time of phagocytosis are particularly important bactericidal agents in the course of phagocytosis.

The mononuclear phagocyte system involves large circulating mononuclear cells of the blood (monocytes) and tissue phagocytes (macrophages), such as alveolar macrophages of the lung, pleural macrophages, peritoneal macrophages, Kupffer cells of the liver, and microglial cells in the brain. The macrophage is a highly adaptive cell that differentiates according to need. Because the macrophage can undergo limited mitosis in the local lesion, it is not wholly dependent on blood-borne cells. In CMI, macrophages are mobilized and activated by T-lymphocyte products referred to as lymphokines. Once macrophages are immunologically active, they possess an increased capacity to inhibit and kill bacteria in a nonspecific manner. Oxygen-derived metabolites such as superoxide ion and hydrogen peroxide probably play major roles in microbial killing within macrophages.

### *NONANTIBODY BIOCHEMICAL AGENTS IN SYSTEMS OF DEFENSE*

The host can exert many nonspecific systems in the defense against microorganisms. The following substances illustrate this point.

Lysozyme hydrolyzes the muramic acid from the mucopeptide in the cell walls of gram-positive bacteria. It can also act synergistically with antibody and complement in the lysis of gram-negative bacteria because a thin inner mucopeptide layer is present. Lysozyme normally is present in most of the body fluids as well as neutrophils and macrophages.

Beta-lysin (serum bactericidin) system is activated by the clotting mechanism and is potent against several gram-positive organisms. Basic polypeptides, which have been isolated from PMN lysosomes, can inhibit or kill several microorganisms. Spermine is a polyamine found in renal tissue and semen. It is particularly inhibitory and lethal for tubercle bacilli and staphylococci. Lactoferrin and transferrin are iron-binding compounds that can deprive bacteria of adequate supplies of iron and consequently exert bacteriostasis. Organic acids can be bacteriostatic and are particularly toxic at low pH when they are in the nonionized state. Hematin and mesohematin are iron porphyrins that have antibacterial properties owing largely to their ability to compete with other porphyrins in bacterial metabolism.

Peroxidase, thiocyanate, and hydrogen peroxide ($H_2O_2$) form an antimicrobial system that inhibits the growth of a number of species of microorganisms. Lactoperoxidase, which is present in bovine milk, and myeloperoxidase, which is present in PMN, can participate in this system. Thiocyanate is a constituent of extracellular fluids including serum, saliva, and milk. Microorganisms that accumulate $H_2O_2$ (and lack catalase) are inhibited by the addition of thiocyanate and peroxidase, whereas microorganisms that possess catalase are inhibited only if a $H_2O_2$ -generating system is present. Accordingly, when leukocytes generate $H_2O_2$ during phagocytosis, the peroxidase-thiocyanate system can be activated.

### *ACQUIRED IMMUNITY TO BACTERIA*

Classes of bacterial pathogens comprise (1) extracellular parasites such as Staphylococcus aureus, Streptococcus pyogenes, and Klebsiella pneumoniae; (2) facultative intracellular parasites such as Mycobacterium tuberculosis, Francisella tularensis, and Brucella abortus; and (3) obligate intracellular parasites such as Rickettsia rickettsii, Rickettsia typhi, and Coxiella burnetii. As a rule, pathogenic extracellular bacteria are resistant to humoral antimicrobial factors but are fully susceptible to killing by phagocytes. Accordingly, they usually express virulence factors that subvert and block phagocytosis. However, specific antibodies of acquired immunity can reverse the virulent effects by neutralizing toxins (IgG, IgA, and IgM) and functioning as opsonins (IgG, IgM). The term opsonin refers to antibodies that promote the uptake and phagocytosis of microbial agents.

On the other hand, facultative intracellular parasites characteristically are resistant to intracellular killing by both PMN and macrophages. As a consequence, the CMI system evolved to provide special phagocytes with superior killing powers. This system involves T helper cells that synthesize lymphokines that attract and activate macrophages to a level of antibacterial activity far above that expressed by normal macrophages. Obligate intracellular bacterial pathogens are also handled by activated macrophages and, in some instances, by an interplay with the humoral mechanisms.

### *HUMORAL MECHANISMS OF ANTIBACTERIAL DEFENSE*

Antibodies of various classes play important and fundamental roles in acquired immunity against many bacterial pathogens.

**Chemotaxis.** The major factors of chemotaxis are derived from complement in which C5a and the complex C5b67 are formed. Oxidation products from arachidonic acid can also serve as important chemotaxins as well as certain chemotactic polypeptides that are liberated during inflammation.

**Opsonic Action.** Antibodies of the classes IgM and IgG play the major role in promoting phagocytosis of bacteria; human PMN and macrophages have Fc receptors for IgG1 and IgG3. Accordingly, IgG can function even in the absence of complement in the system. However, complement augments opsonization by way of C3b generated on the surfaces of bacteria and the C3b receptor on phagocytes.

**Antibacterial Action of Antibody plus Complement.** Specific antibody, particularly IgM plus complement, can be highly bactericidal against some gram-negative organisms, especially Escherichia coli, a member of the gut flora. However, gram-positive bacteria are totally resistant to this mechanism. It is of special interest that lysozyme can act synergistically with the antibody-complement system when the antibody is specific for gram-negative organisms.

**Neutralization of Toxin.** One of the major roles of specific antibody in acquired immunity is to neutralize bacterial toxins. Specific IgG, IgA, or IgM can effect toxin neutralization in toxigenic diseases such as diphtheria and tetanus.

**Blocking of Bacterial Colonization.** Certain bacteria must adhere to host cells to produce disease; e.g., Vibrio cholerae organisms that colonize the surfaces of intestinal epithelial cells. If specific IgA antibodies are present in the gut and can react with surface antigens of the V. cholerae, colonization of this organism is blocked and the disease is prevented.

### *ACQUIRED ANTIBACTERIAL CELL-MEDIATED IMMUNITY*

In the development of CMI, the host produces an enormous expansion of clones of specifically reactive T memory cells. These circulating immune memory cells can be activated by specific antigen(s) in the course of a subsequent infection with the corresponding intracellular parasite. This activation results in clonal expansion, lymphokine production and secretion, followed by mobilization and activation of macrophages. As mentioned previously, the macrophages that are immunologically activated are far superior to the normal macrophage in terms of killing intracellular parasites. Immunologically activated macrophages can exhibit a 10- to 20-fold burst in the production of hydrogen peroxide in the course of phagocytosing intracellular parasites. T memory cells can migrate to interstitial tissues and probably remain there for extended periods without recirculating. Accordingly, if microorganisms invade and infect tissue, interstitial T memory cells (immune) can activate the whole process of CMI.

### *EXAMPLES OF INTERPLAY OF SPECIFIC AND NONSPECIFIC MECHANISMS*

Total immunity depends on the interplay between the factors of specific acquired immunity and those of innate immunity, as exemplified by the following:

1. Antibody, complement, and lysozyme can act synergistically against gram-negative bacteria. The opsonic action of antibody interplays with the bactericidal action of phagocytes. Opsonic action can also interplay with the bactericidal activity of complement and lysozyme.
2. Synergism also can exist between humoral immune and cell-mediated immune mechanisms. For example, opsonization can interact and interplay with immunologically activated macrophages that are destined to engulf facultative intracellular parasites.

### *ACQUIRED IMMUNITY TO FUNGI*

The process of CMI appears to be the major mechanism of acquired immunity against fungi, a finding that reflects the chronic nature of most fungal infections. In addition, odd-numbered fatty acids in skin, as well as the integuments, can be natural barriers to infection. The mononuclear phagocyte system and immune T cells play major roles in intracellular infections caused by fungi such as Histoplasma capsulatum, Candida albicans, and Coccidioides immitis.

One of the potential problems of chronic fungal infections is the generation of T suppressor cells ($CD8^+$) that can negate acquired CMI.

### *ACQUIRED IMMUNITY TO VIRUSES*

The major elements that participate in nonspecific internal defense against viral infections include the interferons, NK cells, and macrophages. During virus replication, the virus induces the production of interferon, which can passively cause neighboring cells to become resistant. Macrophages can destroy virus if the virus does not replicate in the macrophage (nonpermissive). Natural killer cells can destroy virus-infected cells.

Antibody-mediated immunity involves specific antibodies (IgG, IgA, and IgM) that neutralize extracellular virus and block infection; complement can enhance viral neutralization in the case of IgG and IgM. Specific IgG and IgM plus complement can also destroy virus-infected cells, because, with some viruses, viral antigen is inserted in the membrane of the infected cell before virus maturation is completed. Hence, the infection can be aborted.

Cell-mediated immunity against virus-infected cells is mediated by specific cytotoxic T cells (CD8) that can also react with the viral antigen in the cell membrane and abort the infection before mature virus is made. Other CMI mechanisms can involve NK cells, K cells, and macrophages. The NK cell can effect antibody-independent killing, whereas the latter two cell types can participate in an antibody-dependent cell cytotoxic reaction.

## LABORATORY TESTS TO QUANTIFY IMMUNOLOGIC RESPONSES

### *PLAQUE-FORMING ASSAY*

This assay is useful experimentally to quantify the number of B lymphocytes in the spleen of laboratory animals, such as mice, that produce IgM or IgG antibody after administration of sheep red blood cells (SRBC). For example, IgM-producing B cells are dispersed in agar containing a lawn of SRBC to which complement is added. IgM specific for SRBC lyse the surrounding SRBC in the presence of complement, forming a "clear plaque" around the lymphocyte (Fig. 41–9). The plaque-forming cells can be counted, and the kinetics of the number of specific IgM-producing cells can be plotted.

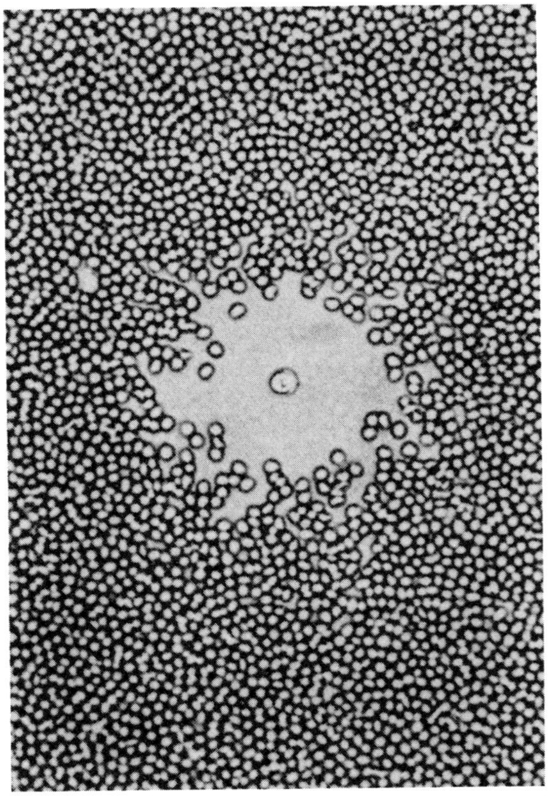

**FIGURE 41–9.** Plaque-forming cell embedded in a layer of sheep red blood cells. Antibody secreted by the cell combines with the surrounding red cells. Addition of complement reacting with the antibody-red cell complex caused lysis of the red cells. (From Garvey, J.S., Cremer, N.E., Sussdorf, D.H.: Methods in Immunology. 3rd Ed. Reading, MA, W.A. Benjamin, 1977.)

The quantitation of the IgG-producing B cells requires an overlay of IgM specific for the IgG (anti-SRBC) molecules made by the individual B cells. This step is required because the IgG-complement lysis of SRBC is less efficient than that of IgM. Accordingly, the addition of IgM specific for IgG plus complement provides an amplification of SRBC lysis. The resulting plaques can be scored as the number of B cells producing IgG after subtracting the number of plaques that are formed only by IgM antibodies specific for SRBC.

### *BLASTOGENIC RESPONSES OF LYMPHOCYTES TO MITOGENS*

Both B and T lymphocytes can proliferate when incubated with certain mitogens. For example, phytohemagglutinin (PHA) and concanavalin A (Con A) cause T cells to proliferate, whereas lipopolysaccharide (LPS) and pokeweed mitogen cause B cells to proliferate. The proliferative responses are polyclonal responses with respect to antigenic specificity.

Proliferation usually is quantified by measuring the incorporation of tritiated thymidine, which reflects DNA synthesis. These tests measure important functional characteristics of lymphocytes, including the relative number of immunocompetent cells. The same principle is applied during attempts to measure the specific proliferative response to antigens, except that the uptake of tritiated thymidine is less with antigens than with polyclonal mitogens because the responses in this case are specific and clonal.

### *CELL-MEDIATED HYPERSENSITIVITY (DELAYED HYPERSENSITIVITY)*

This immune effector response is commonly monitored by a skin test. Skin test antigens can include candidin, tuberculin, SK-SD, and so forth. A positive skin test response is characterized by an infiltration of lymphocytes and macrophages that peaks at 24 to 30 hours. Another approach involves the production of migration inhibition factor (MIF) when immune T cells (peripheral blood) are incubated with their specific antigen. The lymphocyte product(s) or lymphokine(s) cause activation and migration inhibition of macrophages. As one might expect, incubation of T cells with the polyclonal mitogens Con A or PHA also induces production of MIF. These tests are useful in obtaining relative data on changes in immunocompetence with respect to CMI mechanisms.

### *T CYTOTOXIC (KILLER) CELL ACTIVITY*

Specific cytotoxic T cells are induced as a consequence of allogeneic tissue transplants, transplantable tumors, and certain viral infections. This arm of the CMI response can be evaluated readily in vitro using a chromium-51 release test. The target cells are first incubated with chromium-51 to allow endocytosis of the isotope, and then they are incubated with immune cytotoxic T cells. Release of chromium-51 indicates lysis of target cells.

### *CYTOTOXIC ANTIBODIES*

These antibodies can lyse or destroy allogeneic target cells, virus-infected cells, or certain tumor cells when complement is present. The antibodies are specific and usually of the class IgM or IgG.

### *BLOCKING ANTIBODIES*

These antibodies do not activate complement and have no demonstrable effect on target cells. They can block the activity of cytotoxic antibodies or cytotoxic T cells because of steric effects.

### *ENUMERATION OF T HELPER AND T SUPPRESSOR LYMPHOCYTES*

It is common practice to quantify the numbers of T helper and T suppressor cells. This task is readily accomplished by using specific fluoresceinated monoclonal antibodies that are specific for CD4 (helper) or CD8 (suppressor) T cells or mouse Ly1 (helper) or Ly2,3 (suppressor) (T cells). Fluoresceinated cells can be counted by fluorescence microscopy or by a cytofluorograph (laser cell sorter).

### *QUANTITATION OF SERUM IMMUNOGLOBULINS*

The levels of serum immunoglobulin can be quantified by the use of radial immunodiffusion plates. These plates contain specific antibodies against IgG, IgM, or IgA. Sera are added to the wells and a precipitin ring is formed that relates to the amount of the respective immunoglobulin present in the serum (Fig. 41–10). Because IgE is in low levels, a radioimmunoassay is required that is based on allowing an immobilized anti-IgE (IgG) to react with the total IgE present in the serum. After washing, a radiolabeled anti-IgG is added that specifically reacts with the complex. The bound radioactive counts relate to the amount of IgE present in the serum.

## EFFECT OF MALNUTRITION ON IMMUNE RESPONSES

Results of numerous studies reveal that severe protein deficiencies suppress antibody formation.[27] In addition, deficiencies of pyridoxine, pantothenic acid, and pteroylglutamic acid also result in suppressed antibody responses. Deficiencies of components of the vitamin B complex also can cause some depression in antibody formation.

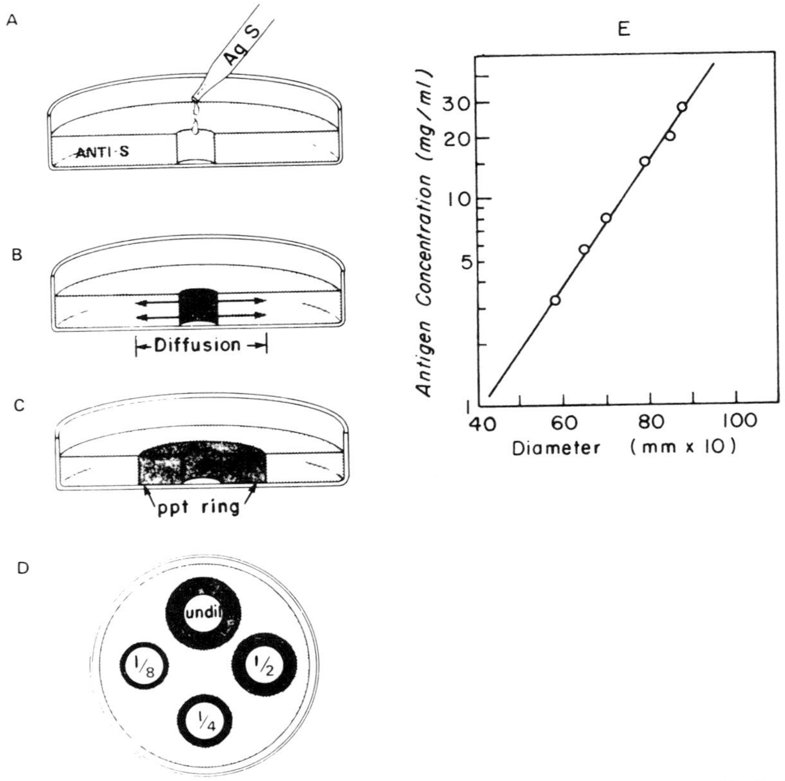
A
Ag S
ANTI-S
B
Diffusion
C
ppt ring
D
undil
1/8
1/2
1/4
E
Antigen Concentration (mg/ml)
30
20
10
5
1
40
60
80
100
Diameter (mm x 10)

**FIGURE 41–10.** Radial immunodiffusion in agar. *A,* Petri dish is filled with semisolid agar solution containing antibody (Ab) to antigen (Ag) S. The center well is filled with a precisely measured concentration of Ag S. *B,* Antigen S is allowed to diffuse radially from the center well. *C,* After reaction proceeds to completion, a sharp ring is formed. *D,* By serial dilution of a known standard quantity of Ag S in a defined measure of time (24 hours), rings of progressively decreasing size are formed. The amount of Ag S in unknown specimens can be calculated and compared with a standard Ag (24 hours) (1/1, 1/4, 1/8). *E,* Relation of the log of Ag concentration to the diameter of immune precipitate. (From Fudenberg, H.H., Stites, D.P., Caldwell, J.L., et al. (Eds.): Basic and Clinical Immunology. Los Altos, CA, Lange Medical Publications, 1976.)

The number of papers published concerning the effect of malnutrition on the immune responses has increased greatly during the last decade. However, many questions remain unanswered or only partially answered.

## COMPLEXITIES IN INTERPRETING DATA

Naturally occurring states of malnutrition are difficult to interpret, largely because deficiencies usually involve multiple dietary factors. This problem is compounded further by infection, anorexia, debilitation, and severe negative nitrogen balances that occur in various combinations. For example, a reduction in food intake is commonly associated with vitamin and mineral deficiencies, thus contributing to the effects of protein-energy undernutrition.

Single nutrients can only be analyzed in defined and controlled animal experiments. Even in this context, a word of caution is in order because synergism may occur between two or more required nutrients. Another issue concerns the degree of suppression of immunologic functions that reflect true significant immunodeficiencies. Accordingly, caution must be exercised in the analysis of data from all nutritional experiments. Emphasis must be placed on proper controls, appropriate evaluation of immunologic assays, and careful scrutiny of perturbing influences such as infection and proper housing.

## EFFECT OF PROTEIN AND PROTEIN-ENERGY MALNUTRITION

The studies by Cooper et al. revealed that the number of plaque-forming lymphocytes that became activated and the corresponding amount of antibody synthesized were directly correlated with protein or protein-energy intake when three levels of dietary protein were given (6%, 12%, or 27%).[28] In contrast, under moderate conditions of chronic protein or protein-calorie deprivation, some T cell-mediated immunologic functions were increased.[28,29] These functions included proliferative responses to Con A and PHA, development of delayed hypersensitivity, and formation of MIF.[30]

Studies of tumor immunity further illustrate the depression of the B cell system and sparing of the T cell system when moderate protein-calorie restriction occurred. For example, T killer cell activity was normal or heightened in nutritionally deprived mice and rats using experimental tumor systems, whereas the formation of cytotoxic and blocking antibodies was reduced. However, with only a 3% protein intake, tumor cell killing was reduced in mice. Similar results were noted with guinea pigs.[30]

Wunder et al. carried out a malnutrition study in guinea pigs using two different protocols.[31] In the first, test animals started on a normal diet that was reduced weekly by 25% for 4 weeks. In the second, groups of animals were given 5%, 30%, and 60% casein; other dietary components were constant. In the first experiment and in the group that received 5% casein, comparable declines in phagocytic function occurred by the third week. A depression of opsonization was also evident. Serum C3 was significantly lower, and mitogenic responses to PHA were 85% lower in these malnourished animals.

Sakamoto et al. reported that complement components C1, C4, C2, and C3 were lower in the 0.5% protein rat group compared to the 18% protein group.[32] In addition, the $CH_{50}$ complement titers were also lower in the 0.5% protein group. Sakamoto et al. also found that rats maintained on 0.5% protein diet for 4 weeks exhibited reduced tuberculin skin reactivity.[33] Tuberculin reactivity disappeared completely in all rats after they were on a 0.5% protein diet for 8 weeks.

Severe protein-energy malnutrition in humans affects many systems and usually is complicated by multiple simultaneous nutrient deficiencies that also can be aggravated by infection. Nevertheless, a significant body of knowledge is available that can be helpful in the dissection of this complex problem. In this regard, the weight of evidence now indicates that severe protein or calorie malnutrition in humans results in impairment of both humoral and cell-mediated immune functions.[34–38] Severe thymic atrophy and associated T cell deficiencies are particularly common in undernourished children.[39] A depression of T helper cells and possibly an increase in T suppressor cells also can occur in protein-energy malnutrition. Salimonu et al.[40] and Schlesinger et al.[41] reported decreased K cell activity decreased production of IFN in children with protein-energy malnutrition and patients with marasmus, respectively. Several investigators have observed reduced levels of secretory IgA in pharyngeal secretions, tears, and saliva that could be responsible for the compromised resistance to organisms that cause respiratory infections.[42–45] Impairment of secretory IgA is thought to represent depression of IgA synthesis in the submucosa, impaired synthesis of secretory component, or both.[38] These observations are compatible with the findings in protein-energy malnutrition of the loss of intestinal epithelium, mucosal thinning, and atrophy of gut-associated lymphoid tissue.[46] A summary of the reported changes in the immune system resulting from protein-calorie malnutrition is presented in Table 41–4.[47]

Clinical studies of protein-energy malnourished hospital patients have revealed an impaired release of IL-1 from stimulated peripheral blood monocytes.[48–51] Comparable results were noted in the impaired release of IL-1 from stimulated peritoneal macrophages procured from rats with protein deficiency.[52] It is of interest that decreased IL-1 release after protein deficiency can be corrected by inhibitors of prostaglandin secretion.[53] Protein-depleted guinea pigs do not produce fever, granulocytosis, or acute-phase protein responses after administration of IL-1. Accordingly, the ability of stimulated macrophages to release IL-1 as well as the hepatic and hypothalamic responses to IL-1 are impaired by protein deficiency. In view of the central role IL-1 plays in the immune response, one of the primary defects may reside at this step in the immune system.

It appears that MIF and IL-2 production is minimally affected by protein-energy malnutrition, whereas IFN, prostaglandin $E_2$, and IL-1 production appear to be significantly impaired.

Serum factors occur in protein-energy malnutrition that have varying effects on immune cell function. Salimonu et al. described an E rosette-inhibitory substance in the sera of 9 of 22 children with kwashiorkor but only 3 of 15 children with marasmus.[54] The nature of this factor is unknown.

## SINGLE-NUTRIENT DEFICIENCIES

Most clinical studies of nutrition-related immunodeficiencies in humans have been complicated by multiple-deficiency states as well as by infection. Although data from animal studies are probably more reliable, selected clinical data have been helpful in arriving at a consensus of how single nutrients affect the immune system.

### *AMINO ACIDS*

Although the data concerning the effects of amino acid deficiencies are somewhat limited, the clear indication is that deficiencies of essential amino acids can result in impairment of the humoral response. On the other hand, as might be expected, it appears that deficiencies of single nonessential amino acids may have little effect on the immune system. However, there may be some exceptions, as in the case of giving supplemental argin-

**TABLE 41–4.** SUMMARY OF EFFECTS OF PROTEIN-CALORIE MALNUTRITION ON IMMUNE FUNCTIONS

| | HUMAN | ANIMAL |
|---|---|---|
| Lymphoid anatomy | | |
| Thymus | ↓ | ↓ |
| Spleen | ↓ | ↓ |
| Lymph nodes | ↓ | ↓ |
| Other lymphoid tissue | ↓ | ↓ |
| Total circulating lymphocytes | ↓ | ↓ |
| Humoral immunity | | |
| Circulating B lymphocytes | ↓ or N | |
| Serum Ig levels | ↑ or N | ↓ |
| Serum Ab, response to Ag | ↓ | ↓ |
| Secretory IgA | ↓ | |
| Splenic plaque-forming cell responses | | ↓ |
| Cellular immunity | | |
| Circulating T-lymphocytes | ↓ | |
| Delayed cutaneous hypersensitivity | ↓ | ↓ |
| Allograft rejection | | N or ↑ or ↓ |
| Tumor cytotoxicity | | ↑ |
| Immunity to intracellular organisms | ↓ | |
| Lymphocyte proliferation | | |
| (a) Concanavilin A | ↓ or N | |
| (b) PHA | ↓ or N | N or ↑ or ↓ |
| (c) PWM | ↑ or N | |
| Lymphokine production | ↓ | |
| Phagocytic function | | |
| Monocyte chemotaxis | ↓ | ↓ |
| PMN chemotaxis | N | ↑ |
| PMN phagocytosis | N | |
| RES function | | ↑ or ↓ |
| Intracellular killing | ↓ or N | N |
| Complement | ↓ | ↓ |

PMN, Polymorphonuclear leukocyte; RES, reticuloendothelial system; N, normal; ↓, depressed: ↑, increased.
(From Dowd, P.S., Heatley, R.V.: Clin. Sci., *66*:241, 1984, by permission of the Biochemical Society, London.)

ine.[55] Chronic deficiencies of branched chain or sulfur-containing amino acids result in a depletion of cells from lymphoid tissues.[56]

Rats with tryptophan-deficient diets exhibit depressed IgG and IgM hemolysin titers after immunization with SRBC.[57] This impairment could be reversed by resupplying tryptophan to the diet.

Collectively, several studies indicate that tryptophan is vital in the maintenance of normal antibody production.[58,59] A phenylalanine deficiency also impaired the ability of rats to express a normal antibody response.[60] A combined deficiency of phenylalanine and tyrosine depressed antibody responses to tumor cells in rats, whereas cytotoxic cell-mediated immune responses were unaffected.[59]

Jose and Good fed rats diets deficient in single amino acids.[59,61] Diets were given at 50% of the dietary level of amino acids; leucine deficiency resulted in a reduction of the tumor cytotoxic response, whereas serum blocking and hemagglutinating antibody levels were intact. Tryptophan deficiency resulted in depressed cytotoxic function, with further reduction with leucine deficiency at the 25% dietary level. Significant depression of serum blocking and hemagglutinating antibody levels was noted with single deficiencies of methionine-cystine, valine, tryptophan, threonine, and phenylalanine-tyrosine reduced to the 25% dietary level.

Most amino acid deficiencies apparently result in more severe suppression of humoral antibody synthesis than of CMI.[61,62] When dietary protein was reduced to 4% in the diet or phenylalanine was reduced to 0.2% of the diet, the reticuloendothelial system of mice exhibited impaired clearance of labeled polyvinyl+pyrrolidone.[63,64] Tryptophan deficiency produced similar results.

A dietary overload (7%) of leucine in rats fed a 4% casein diet reduced antibody responses as well as splenic plaque-forming cells and the numbers of T cells that form rosettes. This dietary regimen also produced suppression of body weight, lymphopoiesis, and serum IgG levels.[65] The effects of this imbalance (7% leucine) were prevented by adding only 0.2% of both valine and isoleucine.

It has been reported that L-arginine, an amino acid considered essential only during active growth, has immunostimulatory effects in adult animals. For example, supplementary L-arginine reduced the growth and spread of several experimentally induced tumors in animals.[66,67] Also, arginine has been observed to enhance lymphocyte transformation responses to polyclonal mitogens.[68] Park et al. reported that L-arginine enhanced human NK and lymphokine-activated killer (LAK) cell activity employing an in vitro system.[69] These authors suggest that large doses of L-arginine could be useful in certain immunosuppressed states such as in malignant diseases and AIDS.

It is not surprising that deficiencies of essential amino acids can impair antibody synthesis. It is of special interest, however, that amino acid imbalances also can impair the immune response. More studies are indicated to determine if some special pattern or combination can produce similar effects with immunostimulatory and other combinations of amino acids. Additional studies on the effects of L-arginine also are needed.

## *ZINC*

Zinc deficiency causes atrophy of lymphoid tissue and produces abnormalities in both cellular and humoral immunity (Table 41–5).[70–72]

Zinc deficiency may be one of the most prevalent nutritional problems worldwide. The average adult must obtain about 15 mg of zinc per day from the diet. Because the body stores of this element are limited, a constant steady-state intake of zinc is required. Zinc deficiencies can result from inadequate dietary intake, disease, or known and unknown factors that interfere with intestinal absorption (see Chapter 10). Zinc deficiency is caused by diets that contain large amounts of grains, cereals, and unleavened bread, and in countries where little animal products are eaten. Because these foods contain high amounts of the zinc chelator phytic acid, zinc is less available for absorption.

In view of the large number of zinc-dependent enzymes, it is understandable how zinc deficiency affects the immune response. Zinc is a cofactor for at least 90 metalloenzymes, including enzymes required for transcription and translation. Because cells of the immune system are under continuous proliferation and differentiation and require numerous enzymes that use zinc as a cofactor, this deficiency not surprisingly can affect both the affector and effector responses. T cell maturation and replication are absolute requirements for normal function. A summary of the potential roles of zinc as a cofactor in immune-related enzymes is presented in Chapter 10.

**TABLE 41–5.** EFFECT OF ZINC DEFICIENCY ON THE IMMUNE RESPONSE

| |
|---|
| Lymphopenia, thymic atrophy |
| Reduced capacity to exhibit delayed hypersensitivity |
| Reduction in IgM and IgG plague-forming cells |
| Impaired secondary antibody responses |
| Reduced responses of lymphocytes to mitogens |
| Depressed levels of facteur thymique serique |
| Impaired cell-mediated immunity |
| Impaired T cell maturation |

Clinically, zinc-deficient children present with lymphopenia, retarded wound healing, thymic atrophy, reduced capacity to exhibit delayed hypersensitivity, and increased susceptibility to disease. A similar pattern of immune defects has been observed in children with acrodermatitis enteropathica, which is an inherited defect in intestinal absorption of zinc. This clinical entity, which was described in 1942,[73] can be cured by giving a zinc supplement.[74] Children with this disease tend to be plagued with severe skin disturbances, central nervous system disorders, gastrointestinal malfunction, and recurrent infections, particularly with fungi. A similar disease has been found in the A-46 mutant of black pied Danish cattle, a variant of the Holstein-Friesian line.[75] Calves born with this trait have alopecia, hyperkeratosis, and a severely involuted thymus, and they usually die of infections. The administration of zinc cures this syndrome.

Fraker et al. observed that young adult mice maintained on a zinc-deficient diet (1 μg zinc/g/day) for 30 days exhibited only 10 to 30% as many IgM and IgG plaque-forming cells per spleen in response to SRBC when compared to mice receiving 25 μg zinc/g/day.[76,77] Zinc-deficient mice also experienced severe thymic atrophy. In addition, they responded poorly to TI antigens. Secondary responses also were reduced, even if the primary immunization was given prior to zinc deprivation.[76] Taste acuity and appetite were gradually lost because of the zinc deficiency, which resulted in anorexia. Anorexia is a serious problem in such experiments because it always raises the potential for superimposed protein-energy malnutrition. To control this potential problem, the investigators included a group of mice given a diet that contained adequate amounts of zinc, but was given a restricted total diet, limited to the average amount consumed by the mice receiving the zinc-deficient diet. The diet-restricted mice experienced no suppression of their immune capacity compared to controls for 30 days. However, inanition became evident, and the immune response deteriorated when the animals were monitored for an additional 10 days.[78]

In this regard, in vitro studies reveal that splenocytes from zinc-deficient mice gave depressed responses to Con A but exhibited enhanced responses to LPS. These observations suggest a reduced response of T cells with an enhanced response by B cells. Furthermore, the responses of lymphocytes of zinc-deficient mice to allogeneic cells (mixed lymphocyte reaction) were enhanced 100% compared to control or diet-restricted mice. These results indicate that greater numbers of immature T cells occur in the spleens of zinc-deficient mice, suggestive of an arrest of T cell maturation.[79]

Hildebrandt et al. reported that the avidities of antibodies in plaques produced by zinc-deficient, 17-day-old neonates in response to trinitrophenol conjugated to LPS were lower than those of the normal control subjects.[80] These data suggest an interference with differentiation and expansion of nonantigen-driven B cell clones. Accordingly, zinc deficiency may suppress and delay ontogeny of lymphoid cells.

DePasquale-Jardieu and Fraker noted that splenocytes from zinc-deficient mice gave suboptimal secondary responses.[81] Their data suggest that zinc deficiency appears to destroy or block the development of memory cells. Other studies by the same authors revealed that plasma levels of corticosterone were elevated in zinc-deficient mice [3,208 nmol/L (115 μg/dl) compared to 827 nmol/L (30 μg/dl)] for controls.[81–85] Furthermore, they noted that in adrenalectomized, zinc-deficient mice, the thymus did not involute and appeared to contain normal numbers of thymocytes. However, these mice had only marginally better responses to SRBC than intact zinc-deficient mice. Again, the idea emerges that zinc deficiency results in an arrest of T cell maturation. Thymus involution appears to be stress induced under conditions of zinc malnutrition.

The thymic hormone facteur thymique serique (FTS) exists in two forms. The first form has no zinc and is biologically inactive. The second form contains zinc and is biologically active; this form is termed thymulin.[86] Investigators from at least two laboratories have reported that FTS levels drop sharply after the onset of zinc deficiency.[87,88]

Results of studies to date indicate that restoration of zinc to a zinc-deficient diet results in a return of normal immune function within 2 weeks.[89] However, it is puzzling that the kinetics of repair demonstrate a period of augmentation. For example, Zwickl and Fraker observed that previously zinc-deficient mice immunized 4 days after beginning a normal diet produced 2.5 times more plaque-forming cells per spleen after immunization with SRBC than did controls.[90]

Zinc deficiency also can lead to a breakdown in CMI, particularly killer T cell function[91] and helper T cell function.[92] In addition, plaque-forming cell responses also drop dramatically. Because terminal deoxyribonucleotidyltransferase is a zinc-containing DNA polymerase required by immature T cells for replication and function, the unique sensitivity of the T cell system to zinc deficiency can be explained in part.[93] Cook-Mills et al. proposed that zinc plays an important role in the oxidative burst of mononuclear phagocytes, and that zinc deficiency results in impairment of mononuclear phagocytes to kill Trypanosoma cruzi.[94]

### *IRON*

Human subjects with iron deficiency exhibit impaired delayed hypersensitivity reactions as well as defective neutrophil and macrophage killing functions.[95] Severely malnourished patients with coexisting deficiencies of protein and iron exhibit low concentrations of iron-binding proteins in plasma. Such patients may experience a clinical activation of intracellular infections (malaria, tuberculosis, or brucellosis) during iron repletion therapy because iron is freely available to the infectious organisms, stimulating their growth in the face of impaired CMI (see also Chap. 69).[96]

Antia et al. reported that the mean level of the iron-binding protein of serum transferrin in patients with kwashiorkor was only 34% of control levels,[97] whereas patients with marasmus had mean transferrin levels that were 71% of those of controls. McFarlane et al. noted that transferrin levels correlated with subsequent survival of children with kwashiorkor.[98] Survivors had transferrin levels about fourfold higher than the levels for those who did not survive. Because low levels of transferrin might make iron more available to bacteria, a low transferrin level might impede the natural antibacterial properties of transferrin even if normal levels of free iron were available. Researchers have suggested that, because transferrin levels are depressed in patients with severe protein-energy malnutrition, this nutritional deficit must be corrected before iron is administered.[99] Accordingly, hyperferremia or hypotransferrinemia are conditions that can result in increased susceptibility to infection, because iron is readily available to stimulate the growth of the infectious organism.[100]

Iron deficiency results in atrophy of lymphoid tissues and depletion of lymphocytes with a subsequent decrease in antibody production.[101,102] Evidence shows that infants receiving adequate iron and vitamins experienced only one half the incidence of respiratory infections compared to control subjects who were iron deficient but received vitamins only.[103]

The defects of the immune system that occur during iron deficiency are not well delineated.[104–107] Some authors have suggested that any effect of iron must occur by way of an indirect mechanism that involves perturbation of folate metabolism.[108,109] However, because lymphocytes require iron for normal cytochrome and enzyme function (ribonucleoside reductase) for DNA synthesis, it is likely that the effects of iron deficiency are expressed in this critical step, and so could account for the depressed T and B cell functions observed. The role of iron in increased susceptibility to infection as well as its role in lymphocyte and phagocyte function is still unresolved in part, principally because of problems relating to coexisting nutrient deficiencies.

Oppenheimer et al. observed that iron-deficient infants from New Guinea had fewer malarial infections than infants given iron-dextran injections.[110] An increase in the incidence of gram-negative meningitis and septicemia occurred in human neonates within 1 week of an injection of iron dextran.[111,112] Also, protein-deficient patients given supplemental iron, which fully saturated serum transferrin and provided free iron, exhibited increased susceptibility to infection.[113]

Iron also plays a critical role in neutrophils, which use iron-dependent enzymes and proteins like myeloperoxidase and cytochrome *b* of NADPH-oxidase in its killing action of phagocytosed bacteria.[114] Good evidence reveals that iron deficiency results in an impaired oxidative burst and subsequent production of superoxide, hydrogen peroxide, and hydroxyl radicals that play a critical role in the killing of bacteria.

With respect to iron deficiency on cytokine activities, Kuvibidila et al. reported a decrease in IL-1 production by peritoneal cells of iron-deficient rats.[115] Joynson et al.[116] and Swarup-Mitra and Sinha[117] reported that blood lymphocytes from humans with iron-deficient anemia produced less MIF in response to challenge with purified protein derivative or Candida than did control lymphoid cells. On the other hand, excess iron results in enhanced responses of lymphocytes to pokeweed mitogen but suppression of responses to PHA and Con A; suppression of cytotoxic T cell generation, and suppressed chemotactic, phagocytic, and bactericidal activity.[55,118,119]

Collectively, the data on iron deficiencies indicate the following: (1) reduced blastogenic responses of lymphocytes; (2) reduced numbers of circulating T cells; (3) reduced antibody titers; (4) long-term impairment of humoral immunity in pre- and postnatal iron-deficient rats if not corrected by proper iron administration; (5) impaired CMI, and (6) impaired microbial killing by neutrophils.[120–122]

Iron overload also appears to impair antigen-specific immune responses and reduces the number of helper precursor cells. For example, serum iron overload concentrations in patients results in impaired generation of cytotoxic T cells, enhanced suppressor T cell activity, and reduced proliferative capacity of helper T cells. A common tumor seen in patients with iron overload is hepatocellular carcinoma. Although the role of cirrhosis in the etiology of primary liver cancer is not clear, it may be of importance that primary liver cancer is seen more frequently in patients with hemochromatosis than in those with other types of cirrhosis.[123]

### *MANGANESE*

Little information is available on the effects of manganese on the immune response. Manganese apparently can stimulate macrophage spreading on antigen-antibody coated surfaces.[124] An excess of manganese can cause elevated antibody titers and other nonspecific resistance factors. On the other hand, animals fed a marginally deficient level of manganese exhibited decreased levels of IgG agglutinins and the 19S fraction of immunoglobulin.[125]

### *COPPER*

Deficiencies of copper appear to prevent the reticuloendothelial system from reacting normally to infection. For example, control spleens increased from 0.21 to 0.92% of body weight during the course of infection, whereas in copper-deficient animals, the increase was only from 0.17 to 0.22%.[126,127]

Lipsky and Ziff[128] reported an inhibition of T cell mitogen responses, especially T helper activity, in association with copper deficiency. Copper deficiency has also caused an increase in infections controlled by T cell-mediated immunity.[129]

Copper deficiency appears to impair maturation and formation of erythrocytes and neutrophils. It is also thought that copper is required for lymphocyte development.[130]

### *MAGNESIUM*

Limited studies reveal that rats depleted of magnesium for 6 to 12 weeks exhibited thymic hyperplasia.[131] In addition, serum IgG levels were 40 to 50% of control levels.[132] Subsequent studies suggested that peak serum hemagglutinin and hemolysin responses were depressed in magnesium-deficient rats (45% of control titers).

Rats fed a magnesium-deficient diet developed persistent leukocytosis with increased numbers of neutrophils, mononuclear cells, and eosinophils. Eosinophil numbers increased as much as 10-fold. Mast cells have also been reported to have an abnormal distribution and reduced numbers of granules concomitant with increased histamine levels in urine.[133–136]

### *SELENIUM*

The role of selenium in the immune response is not clear. A moderate increased intake of selenium appears to enhance the immune response in animals.[137] On the other hand, a selenium deficiency that results in a suppressed antibody response can be reversed by giving vitamin E.[138] Other findings reveal that a selenium deficiency also affects the secondary antibody response to T cell-dependent antigens.[139]

Selenium is an important component of the selenoprotein enzyme glutathione peroxidase, which probably is the major site for its function. This enzyme catalyzes the reduction of organic and inorganic hydroperoxides using glutathione as the electron donor, which in turn functions as a potent antioxidant.[140] Because neutrophils and macrophages generate large amounts of reactive oxygen species during an oxidative burst, it is important for the cell to neutralize an excess of these oxidants. It is possible that a selenium deficiency could result in a dysfunction of this peroxidase, reducing the ability of cells to protect themselves against the damage by oxidants generated during the burst. Therefore, selenium appears to function as an important antioxidant in the metabolism of phagocytes, which allows them to control autotoxic damage.[141]

Spallholz et al. reported that a deficiency of dietary selenium in mice caused a reduction in the HA antibody titers against SRBC.[142–144] Diets containing 1.25 to 2.25 PPM selenium were found to increase the primary immune response to SRBC in terms of plaque-forming splenic cell numbers as well as serum antibody titers. However, the mechanisms concerning the function of selenium in the immune response are not known.

## OTHER MINERALS

Minerals like cadmium, lead, chromium, mercury, nickel, vanadium, and gold are not required but are of potential importance because of their toxicity for cells and their potential deleterious effects on the immune system. Any significant intake of these minerals, either real or suspected, must be taken into account in evaluating the status of the immune system.

## SPECIAL MINERAL INTERACTIONS

An excess of either copper or zinc causes a reciprocal decrease of serum and hepatic levels of the other element. For example, patients with sickle cell disease who receive large doses of zinc in treatment subsequently develop a copper deficiency.[144] Also, it has been shown experimentally that high levels of manganese causes reduced iron stores as well as reduced hemoglobin synthesis. Supplemental administration of iron can reverse this effect.

## EFFECTS OF THE B COMPLEX VITAMINS ON THE IMMUNE RESPONSE

Because the B complex vitamins are involved in a broad spectrum of cell metabolic reactions, it is not surprising that vitamin deficiencies of this group can have an effect on resistance and the immune response.[145] As early as 1921, Cramer et al. observed that deficiencies of the water-soluble group B vitamins in rats or mice resulted in lymphopenia and atrophy of peripheral lymphoid tissue.[146] Deficiencies of pyridoxine, pantothenic acid, riboflavin, folate, and vitamin $B_{12}$ have the greatest effect, whereas biotin, thiamin, and pteroylglutamic acid have lesser effects (Table 41–6).

**TABLE 41–6.** EFFECTS OF VITAMIN DEFICIENCIES ON THE IMMUNE RESPONSE

| VITAMIN | EFFECTS |
|---|---|
| Pyridoxine ($B_6$) | Decreased lymphocyte responses to mitogens |
| | Impaired antibody responses |
| | Impaired cell-mediated responses |
| | Reduction of serum thymic hormones |
| | Atrophy of lymphoid tissue |
| Pantothenic acid | Impaired antibody response |
| Riboflavin ($B_2$) | Impaired antibody responses |
| | Decrease in thymic weights |
| Folic acid | Impaired neutrophil function |
| | Impaired responses of lymphocytes to PHA |
| | Impaired cytotoxic T cell function |
| | Impaired antibody responses |
| Vitamin $B_{12}$ | Impaired lymphocyte responses to PHA |
| | Impaired neutrophil function |
| Biotin | Impaired antibody responses |
| | Impaired cell-mediated responses |
| | Thymic atrophy |
| Thiamin ($B_1$) | Modest impairment of antibody response |
| Vitamin C | Impaired inflammatory responses |
| | Impaired cytotoxic T cell activity |
| | Impaired phagocytic function of neutrophils and macrophages |
| Vitamin A | Impaired antibody responses |
| | Impaired responses of lymphocyte responses to PHA, Con A, and LPS |
| | Increased susceptibility to some tumors |
| Vitamin E | Impaired antibody responses |
| | Impaired responses of lymphocytes to mitogens |
| | Impaired phagocytic function |

## *PYRIDOXINE ($B_6$)*

Pyridoxine functions as a coenzyme for many metabolic synthetic steps in the transformation of amino acids (including decarboxylation and deamination) and conversion of methionine to cysteine.

In the late 1940s, Stoerk et al. convincingly demonstrated that pyridoxine-deficient animals produced less antibody than controls.[147] In this regard, Pruzansky and Axelrod noted that pyridoxine deficiency had the greatest impairment on the anamnestic response.[148] In a clinical study, Hodges et al. observed that experimental pyridoxine deficiency resulted in only slight impairment of antibody formation against tetanus toxoid and typhoid vaccine.[149] However, when human volunteers were deficient in both pyridoxine and pantothenic acid, the impairment of the antibody response was substantial, resulting in hypogammaglobulinemia.[150]

Pyridoxine deficiency also affects CMI. For example, pyridoxine deficiency increased allogeneic graft survival.[151–153] Pyridoxine-deficient guinea pigs also expressed a profound depression of delayed hypersensitivity to purified protein derivative.[154,155] The afferent limb of the immune response apparently remains intact during the period of a pyridoxine deficiency because restoration of pyridoxine to deficient animals results in a normal response.[154]

Ha et al. reported that pyridoxine deficiency in mice depressed the immune response to P815 tumor cells.[156] On the other hand, phagocytosis of SRBC by macrophages and NK cell activity against YAC tumor cells were not affected. These authors also reported that a pyridoxine deficiency did not affect complement-dependent antibody-mediated cytotoxicity against P815 cells. They concluded that high doses (7×) of pyridoxine did not increase the immune response in animals. T and B lymphocyte responses appear to be affected to a greater degree than NK cell and macrophage functions, probably a reflection of their requirement of pyridoxine for nucleic acid and protein synthesis as in cell multiplication.

In summary, $B_6$ deficiency causes atrophy of lymphoid tissue, depressed primary and secondary antibody responses, reduced mixed lymphocyte responses, prolonged allograft survival, and decreased dermal hypersensitivity.[157]

## *PANTOTHENIC ACID*

Pantothenic acid deficiencies impair primary antibody responses to SRBC.[158] This effect has been observed by quantifying plaque-forming cells after immunization. Stoerk and Zucker observed a decrease in thymic weights of rats given a pantothenic acid-deficient diet.[159] No impairment of reticuloendothelial system function has been noted in pantothenic acid-deficient rats.[160] Specific symptoms resulting from pantothenic acid deficiency in humans have not been described. Human studies are limited and, for the most part, controversial.

## *RIBOFLAVIN*

Deficiencies of riboflavin in dogs resulted in increases in PMN but a decrease in peripheral lymphocytes.[161] In other reports, riboflavin-deficient rats and swine had impaired agglutinin responses to human red blood cells. In addition, riboflavin-deficient mice were more susceptible than control animals to Salmonella typhimurium.[162,163]

Rats given a riboflavin-deficient diet exhibited a decrease in thymic weight[159] as well as antibody responses to diphtheria toxoid.[164] On the other hand, high levels (7×) of riboflavin did not enhance immunologic responses in an elderly population.[165]

## *FOLIC ACID*

In folic acid deficiency, synthesis of thymidylate is inhibited, which results in megaloblastic changes of replicating cells. Because body stores of folic acid are depleted fairly rapidly in the face of insufficient intake, megaloblastic changes are evident in a few weeks.[166] Little doubt remains that a folic acid deficiency can lead to decreased responses of T cells to PHA as well as to decreased cytotoxic T cell function.[167,168]

Other studies indicate that rats on a folic acid-deficient diet had reduced skin responses to PHA as well as a decrease in the T cell populations in the spleen and peripheral blood.[169] Delayed hypersensitivity responses to dinitrochlorobenzene as well as impaired responses to PHA were noted in patients with megaloblastic anemia associated with a folic acid deficiency.[170]

Boles et al. reported significant impairment of phagocytosis by neutrophils obtained from patients with low serum folic acid levels.[171] The addition of folic acid to neutrophil cultures restored their phagocytic capacity.[171,172]

Impairment of antibody responses to diphtheria toxoid and human red blood cells has been reported to occur in rats with folate deficiency.[164,173]

## *VITAMIN $B_{12}$*

Vitamin $B_{12}$ is essential for nucleic acid synthesis, which is needed for cell growth and division. Low levels of $B_{12}$ also can result in decreased transport and use of folic acid. Deficiency of vitamin $B_{12}$ results in megaloblastic changes, particularly in the bone marrow. Das and Hoffbrand noted that the lymphocytes from subjects deficient in $B_{12}$ were more "megaloblastic" than normal cells.[174] They found that the lesion involves methylation of deoxyuridylate to thymidylate. MacCuish et al. found significant depression of lymphocyte transformation to PHA in patients with pernicious anemia.[175] However, T and B cell levels were normal in peripheral blood.

Because $B_{12}$ deficiency cannot be induced in animals, most studies depend on using patients with untreated primary pernicious anemia. Kaplan and Basford observed that neutrophils from pernicious anemia patients had an impaired ability to phagocytose and kill Staphylococcus aureus.[176]

In a study by Katka, the administration of $B_{12}$ caused negative tuberculin skin tests to revert to positive in five of seven patients.[177] Collectively, these studies indicate that vitamin $B_{12}$ is needed for DNA synthesis, which could explain the improved responsiveness of lymphocytes from patients receiving vitamin $B_{12}$ therapy.

### *BIOTIN*

Biotin deficiency has been clearly associated with impaired humoral and cell-mediated responses.[169] Biotin is a coenzyme for several enzyme-mediated carboxylation reactions required for fat and carbohydrate metabolism.

Lewis rats on a biotin-deficient diet exhibited a significant reduction in the size of the thymus. In addition, these rats had a depressed immune response to SRBC.[178]

### *THIAMIN (VITAMIN $B_1$)*

Thiamin functions as a coenzyme in decarboxylation reactions resulting in energy derived from glucose. As a consequence of a thiamin deficiency, increased levels of pyruvic acid and impairment of erythrocyte transketolase activity occurs.

Gross and Newberne reported that a thiamin deficiency resulted in increased susceptibility to Salmonella typhimurium in mice.[169] In addition, decreased antibody responses to human red blood cells in rats were observed. No significant increases in the normal immune parameters (neutrophil count, T lymphocyte response to PHA, delayed hypersensitivity to skin tests) were noted in elderly human subjects receiving high levels (up to 17,000× the RDA) of thiamin.[165]

Other reports suggest that thiamin reverses inhibition of neutrophil migration caused by the peroxidase-$H_2O_2$-halide system.[179,180,181] These observations suggest that thiamin has an antioxidant effect.

## OTHER VITAMINS (TABLE 41–6)

### *VITAMIN C*

Vitamin C deficiency clearly suppresses dermal delayed hypersensitivity responses.[182] In this regard, scorbutic guinea pigs also fail to develop allergic encephalitis after immunization with brain tissue and complete Freund's adjuvant.[183] Scorbutic guinea pigs cannot manifest a normal inflammatory response even though their T cells can transfer delayed hypersensitivity to normal animals.[184] Furthermore, these animals can produce normal levels of antibody but are incapable of expressing an Arthus-type skin reaction.[185] Anthony et al. also reported that lymphoid cells from scorbutic guinea pigs expressed impaired cytotoxic activities even though the number of T cells capable of forming rosettes was normal.[186]

A substantial body of information indicates that vitamin C plays an important role in phagocytic function of neutrophils and macrophages. Vitamin C appears to have an important role in cell motility. It has been observed that vitamin C functions by effecting the synthesis and assembly of microtubules of phagocytes.[187,188] This basic function could explain some of the defects of the cells that participate in inflammation and/or the effector mechanisms of immunity. The large concentrations of vitamin C normally present in phagocytic cells suggest a direct role.

The use of megadoses of vitamin C to prevent the common upper respiratory diseases remains an unproven claim.[189] Fourteen studies have been reviewed of which eight were considered acceptable.[190,191] Only minor and insignificant effects were noted in terms of the prophylactic benefit of administering megadoses of vitamin C. In some cases, it appears that vitamin C may have slightly reduced the severity of the symptoms. In another study, an excess of 80 mg of vitamin C per day achieved the same results as megadoses (1 to 2 g/day).[192] Based on the data available, there appears to be little justification for administering megadoses of vitamin C as a prophylactic regimen against the common cold.

### *VITAMIN A*

Vitamin A plays a major role in maintaining the functional integrity of epithelial and mucosal surfaces and promotes the production of mucous secretions as well as salivary and sweat gland lysozyme.[193] Rats with vitamin A deficiency have reduced resistance to Angiostrongylus cantonensis.[194] Vitamin A-deficient chickens have been observed to be more susceptible than controls to Newcastle disease virus administered intranasally.[195,196]

Impaired antibody responses occurred in vitamin A-deficient rats.[197,198] In addition, vitamin A deficiency causes a reduction in lymphocyte responses to PHA, Con A, or LPS.[199] However, little or no information is available on the effect of vitamin A on phagocytic cell function.

It has also been reported that an increased incidence of liver and colon cancer occurred in vitamin A-deficient rats treated with dimethylhydrazine or aflatoxin B.[200]

Some information suggests that supplemental or increased doses of vitamin A given to cancer patients increases the mitogenic responses of their lymphocytes.[201] Enhancement of skin graft rejection in mice as well as stimulation of cytotoxic T cells in mice given large quantities of vitamins has also been reported.[202–204] On the other hand, extremely high doses appear to suppress certain immune responses.[205,206]

Increased levels of retinoids can mediate resistance to some carcinogenic agents. Whether retinoids inhibit initial malignant cell growth or stimulate antitumor immune mechanisms is not known.

In one report, the authors found that large doses of trans-retinoic acid induced complete remission of acute promyelocytic leukemia; the patients experienced only small or modest side effects.[207]

In this regard, macrophage function has been reported to be enhanced by high levels of vitamin A to produce increased amounts of IL-1.[208]

### *VITAMIN E*

Vitamin E has important antioxidant properties and can be a potent immunoenhancing vitamin. Because the immune response depends on extensive cell activity requiring energy, it can be readily demonstrated that antioxidants like vitamin E, vitamin C, and β-carotene (provitamin A) are important in protecting cells from harmful free radicals. Vitamin E is an essential component of all cell membranes including nuclear and mitochondrial membranes.[209]

T and B lymphocytes procured from laboratory animals on a vitamin E-deficient diet have been reported to have severely depressed responses in terms of mitogen responses, mixed lymphocyte reaction, and plaque-forming cells.[209–212] In addition, Chavance et al. reported an association between high plasma vitamin E levels more than [31.3 μmol/L (1.35 mg/dl)] and a lower number of infections in a healthy human population exceeding 60 years of age.[212]

Other findings indicate that neutrophil and macrophage chemotaxis is impaired when the cells are procured from vitamin E-deficient rats; phagocytosis of complement-coated beads also is reduced.[213] Of particular interest is the observation that neutrophil-induced oxidative damage to lung tissue resulting from burn injuries was reduced in rats given vitamin E prior to the injury.[214] Splenic NK cell capacity to lyse tumor cells was not altered by vitamin E deficiency.[215] However, tumor cells grew faster in vitamin E-deficient mice than in control mice.[216]

A growing body of data indicates that vitamin E also interacts and neutralizes the metabolites of lipid peroxidation, the oxidation of arachidonic acid and prostaglandin formation, and interacts with vitamin C to regenerate the reduced form of vitamin E by oxidation of vitamin C. Vitamin E also plays some type of interactive role with selenium, a constituent of the metalloenzyme glutathione peroxidase, which can scavenge free radicals found in the cytoplasm.[217]

Support is good for concluding that supplemental vitamin E enhances both humoral and cellular immunity and augments phagocyte efficiency.[218]

## FATTY ACIDS AND THE IMMUNE RESPONSE

Essential fatty acids (EFA) clearly play a role in the modulation of the immune response. For example, EFA deficiencies can result in both enhanced cell-mediated and humoral immune responses. The effect can also be achieved by the administration of cyclooxygenase inhibitors, particularly when excess linoleic acid is given.

Thomas and Erickson (219) noted that delayed type hypersensitivity reactions to B16-BL6 melanoma cells were depressed in BALB/c mice fed a 20% coconut oil (saturated fat) or 20% polyunsaturated fatty acid (PUFA)-containing diet compared to control animals fed a minimal EFA diet.

The observations to date on the modulatory effects of dietary lipids on the immune system suggest that dietary fats may influence the immune responses through the modulation of eicosanoid synthesis, alterations in the quantity of cell receptors, and selective stimulation of some cell subsets. Unfortunately, many studies are not definitive and few conclusions can be made. The most attractive possibility may be the effects on eicosanoid synthesis. For example, increased prostaglandin levels can suppress lymphocyte blastogenic responses and also enhance tumor migration, resulting in a promotion of metastasis and suppression of antitumor defenses. Most evidence indicates that diets high in PUFA and EFA of the n-6 family (linoleic acid) enhance tumor growth.[220,221] It is of special interest that the tumor-promoting effects of high levels of fatty acid diets were abrogated by including indomethacin in the drinking water. A consensus exists that the incidence of tumors is increased by high levels of dietary PUFA of the n-6 types such as safflower and corn oils.

Murphy et al. reported that fish oils cause production of the pentaene form (LTB5) of leukotriene, which is less active than the tetraene (LTB4) form of leukotriene.[222] For example, LTB4 is 10- to 30-fold more active than LTB5 as a chemotaxin for human neutrophils.[223] The studies of Lee et al. suggest that diets containing fish oil fatty acids may have anti-inflammatory effects by inhibiting the 5-lipoxygenase pathway in neutrophils and monocytes and by inhibiting LTB4-mediated functions in neutrophils.[224]

Regulation of eicosanoid synthesis depends on free, unesterified fatty acids. In this regard, most long chain PUFA are esterified in the sn-2 position of glycerophospholipids in tissues; accordingly, the precursor fatty acids must be released by phospholipases before eicosanoids can be synthesized. Arachidonic acid (AA) is the major 20-carbon PUFA in tissues that is the precursor of eicosanoids. By increasing the dietary n-3 fatty acids, a reduction of AA occurs in the tissue lipids because of inhibition of the synthesis of AA from 18:2(n-6). This effect can be explained by a competition of linoleic acid [18:2(n-6)], linolenic acid [18:3(n-3)], and oleic acid [18:1(n-9)] for desaturases that mediate the synthesis of PUFA.[225] In addition, n-3 PUFA can competitively inhibit the oxygenation of AA by cyclooxygenase.[226] Accordingly, the ingestion of a long-chain n-3 PUFA, which is in high concentration in certain fish oils, can cause a reduction in tissue AA and a parallel decrease in the synthesis of eicosanoids.[227]

It is of special interest that rats fed an EFA-deficient diet had a resulting depletion of class II Ia-positive macrophages that present antigen to initiate an immune response.[228] Also, mice fed EFA-deficient diets exhibited accelerated allograft (skin) rejection, whereas the skin grafts showed prolonged survival after oral supplementation of linoleic acid.[229]

The prostaglandin E group apparently can exert negative feedback on the immune response. In addition, macrophages represent a major source of eicosanoids. Therefore, dietary EFA can have an influence on eicosanoid synthesis and the status of the immune response. Much research is still needed to determine the effects of other cyclooxygenase products on the immune response, the effects of lipoxygenase products on the immune response, and the true magnitude of whether EFA dietary manipulation can be used to manage some chronic diseases.

## EFFECT OF DIETARY OXIDIZED OILS ON IMMUNOCOMPETENT CELLS

Unsaturated lipids in foods can readily undergo spontaneous autoxidation, which leads to peroxides that polymerize and degrade to give several oxidation products.[230] In a study to determine the effect of oxidized oils on the responses of immunocompetent cells, Oarada et al. fed autoxidized methyl linoleate to mice.[231] They observed that the DNA synthesis of thymocytes was inhibited, whereas the mitogenic responses of splenocytes to Con A were increased. In addition, low molecular weight compounds generated by autoxidation damaged lymphocytes more than the peroxides.[232] The main components in the low molecular weight compounds were short-chain aldehydes like 4-hydroxynonenal.[233] Additional studies are needed to determine the identity and minimal amounts of rancid oil components needed to toxify the immune system.

## PRENATAL AND POSTNATAL MALNUTRITION

The developing thymolymphatic system of the fetus is highly sensitive to malnutrition involving deficiencies of protein, calories, lipotropic factors, vitamins, and iron. In utero, malnutrition can result in profound defects of immunologic function in the face of only a slightly reduced birth weight.

Experimental maternal protein deficiency resulted in decreased thymus weights, as well as cellularity, DNA, RNA, and protein in the thymuses of rat offspring, even when the postnatal diet was normal.[234] Thymus weights remained suppressed for 4 months even though the postnatal diet was adequate.[235]

Although the data are somewhat uncertain, it is potentially important that humans can suffer apparent long-term immunologic defects as a consequence of in utero or early postnatal malnutrition.[236] For example, maternal malnutrition during the third trimester had significant effects on fetal body weight and organ development. In particular, low-birth-weight infants from nutritionally deficient mothers had impressive reductions in spleen and thymus weights.[237] Immunologic defects that result from intrauterine malnutrition may be as severe as those associated with postnatal protein-calorie malnutrition.[238–241] Because of the low cord-blood levels of IgG in newborn infants having experienced intrauterine malnutrition, placental transfer of maternal IgG may be impaired.[240]

Long-term studies on the effects of intrauterine malnutrition have revealed decreased T cell levels as well as impaired delayed hypersensitivity.[241] Collectively, the results indicate that immunologic defects resulting from intrauterine malnutrition may be more refractory to reversal than the defects that accrue after any postnatal undernutrition.

Infants with only slight fetal growth retardation attributable to malnutrition have exhibited minimal immunologic impairment, whereas those infants who suffered from severely retarded intrauterine growth have exhibited substantial impairment of delayed hypersensitivity. Deficiency of protein or calories usually results in chronic suppression of both humoral and cell-mediated immunity.

## IMMUNOLOGIC SEQUELAE IN MALNOURISHED CHILDREN

One of the early changes noted in severely malnourished children is thymic atrophy.[242] Decreased cellularity was evident in certain areas of the spleen and lymph nodes usually populated by T lymphocytes. Postmortem studies on African children with marasmus and kwashiorkor revealed greatly reduced weights of thymuses, spleens, Peyer's patches, and appendices. In particular, paracortical areas were depleted and germinal centers were absent. The histopathologic picture correlated well with the reduced level of responsiveness to dinitrochlorobenzene (DNCB) and lowered blastogenic activity of their lymphocytes to PHA.[243]

Neumann et al. examined the immune status of Ghanaian children with moderate or severe malnutrition.[244] Dramatic depression of CMI responses was noted in all severely malnourished children with either marasmus or kwashiorkor. The authors found close correlations between delayed hypersensitivity to streptokinase-streptodornase and candidin and levels of serum albumin, carotene, vitamin C, and total serum protein. Whereas relatively rapid recovery of normal CMI responses has been observed with nutritional rehabilitation, impairment of CMI responses in some instances has persisted for several years.[245] For example, Dutz et al. reported that orphans who had been severely malnourished with infection during early infancy exhibited depression of CMI responses for at least 5 years, even though they were free of intercurrent disease and were well nourished.[246] McMurray et al. demonstrated that severely protein-malnourished children did not exhibit normal CMI responses even after nutritional rehabilitation.[247] Moderately malnourished children have responded with significantly less delayed hypersensitivity to purified protein derivative after bacille Calmette-Guérin vaccination.[248] Most CMI parameters are impaired in malnourished children, whereas some of the same parameters are normal or enhanced in moderately malnourished laboratory animals.

It has been demonstrated conclusively that serum complement levels are reduced in children with protein-calorie malnutrition followed by an increase during nutritional rehabilitation.[247,249,250] Children with moderate and severe protein malnutrition experience significant suppression (50%) of lysozyme secretion into tears.[251] In addition, the synthesis and secretion of secretory IgA also are reduced. Severely protein-malnourished Thai,[252] Indian,[253] and Colombian[254] children had 35 to 50% reduction of secretory IgA in secretions. However, levels of IgG or albumin were not reduced. A summary of secretory IgA levels in malnourished children is found in Table 41–7.

Numerous pressing questions remain unanswered as to the duration of immunologic impairment of a neonate who experiences intrauterine malnutrition, as well as the degree and reversibility in terms of timing and qualitative nature of the deficiency.

## OVERNUTRITION

Definitive studies that elucidate the effects of obesity or overnutrition on the immune system are lacking. It appears that excess intake of saturated and unsaturated fatty acids interferes with normal reticuloendothelial system functions. Excess intake of polyunsaturated fatty acids causes suppression of CMI functions. In contrast, low intake causes some potentiation of the immune response.

A moderate excess of vitamin A and vitamin E seems to exert an adjuvant-like effect on humoral and cell-mediated immunity. Excess sugar intake or hyperglycemia, as in diabetes, has been reported to impair phagocyte function. In general, the incidence of lower respiratory tract infections is higher in obese infants than in infants of normal weight.[255,256]

## INTERACTION OF NUTRITION AND INFECTION

The effect of infection on an existing state of malnutrition is poorly understood. Infection causes negative balances of nitrogen, zinc, iron, potassium, phosphates, magnesium, and sulfates as well as plasma amino acids.[257] For example, bacterial diarrhea is associated with malabsorption and possible nutrient deficiencies.[258] Infection also can cause anorexia, which can result in undernutrition or, in some instances, an unexplainable temporary resistance to infection.[259,260] Gopalan theorized that marasmus is an extreme degree of adaptation to malnutrition in which organs and body functions are protected at the expense of muscle tissue, whereas kwashiorkor develops when this adaptation breaks down.[261] Beisel suggested that infection may be a common factor that triggers the breakdown.[262]

Malnourished populations have impaired resistance to certain infections. Accordingly, it is understandable how anorexia and a negative nitrogen balance brought on by

**TABLE 41–7.** SECRETORY IMMUNOGLOBULIN A (SIgA) AND ANTIBODY TITERS IN MALNOURISHED HUMANS

| | WELL NOURISHED | MALNOURISHED |
|---|---|---|
| Indian children | | |
| SIgA in nasopharyngeal secretions | 2.8 mg/dl (20)* | 1.56 mg/dl (20)† |
| Neut. measles antibody titer | 1:64 titer (20) | 1.4 titer (20)† |
| Neut. poliovirus antibody titer | 1:64 titer (20) | 1:4 titer (20)† |
| Thai children | | |
| SIgA in nasal washings | 28.5 ± 3.4 mg/dl (23) | 11.5 ± 7.8 mg/dl (24)† |
| Indian children | | |
| SIgA in duodenal fluid | 42 ± 4 mg/dl (12) | 7 ± 2 mg/dl (16)† |
| | 120 ± 17 mg/g protein | 25 ± 9 mg/g protein† |
| SIgA in saliva | 24 ± 7 mg/dl (12) | 4 ± 2 mg/dl (16)† |
| | 60 ± 14 mg/g protein | 13 ± 8 mg/g protein† |
| SIgA in tears | 31 ± 14 mg/dl (12) | 10 ± 2 mg/dl (16)† |
| | 91 ± 15 mg/g protein | 32 ± 8 mg/g protein† |
| Indonesian children | | |
| SIgA in duodenal fluids | 15.1 ± 2.5 mg/dl (6) | 42.7 ± 6 (29) |

*Number studied.
†Significantly reduced.
(Adapted from Stiehm, E.R.: Fed. Proc., *39*:3093, 1980, by permission.)

infection could aggravate even a moderate state of malnutrition.[262–264] Subclinical infections produced with living vaccines can induce measurable deficits in the nutritional status of apparently healthy children, a finding that is also reflected in subnormal weight gain (see also Chapters 44, 46, and 69).[265]

## MODULATING INFLAMMATION AND IMMUNE FUNCTIONS WITH ARGININE, RNA, AND n-3 PUFA

The concept has emerged that certain "specialty nutrients" can be used to modulate inflammatory and immune responses favorably to counteract a state of inflammation-induced hypermetabolism in patients responding to diverse injuries such as trauma, burns, major surgery, sepsis, shock, and noninfectious pancreatitis.[266] It has been noted that states of persistent inflammation are commonly associated with immunosuppression.

**Arginine.** This amino acid is not classified as an essential amino acid (referred to as semiessential) except during growth and conditions that result in persistent inflammation.[267] Arginine can stimulate the release of prolactin, insulin, growth hormone, and glucagon and is an essential component of polyamine and nucleic acid synthesis. It is a major source of nitric and nitrous oxide in vivo as well as in vitro, which are mediators of protein synthesis, vascular dilatation, and electron transport.[268]

In humans, arginine administration has produced increased numbers of peripheral blood lymphocytes as well as increased responses to mitogens in vitro. Arginine supplementation has also been associated with reduced hospital stays after major operations.[267–269]

**RNA.** Purines and pyrimidines are not considered essential dietary nutrients because of synthesis from amino acids as well as through salvage pathways from bases and nucleosides.[270] However, restriction of dietary nucleotides can result in prolongation of allografts as well as suppression of CMI responses. T lymphocytes from nucleotide-deprived animals have an impaired ability to respond to antigenic stimuli.[271] The administration of uracil has been reported to restore these functions. These observations suggest that endogenous purines and pyrimidine stores may be limited and are required nutrients during states of metabolic stress or hypermetabolism.

**n-3 PUFA.** The major PUFA constituent in cell membranes in human populations that derive their PUFA from vegetable oils is n-6 PUFA. The n-3 PUFA, a major constituent in fish oils, can exchange with n-6 PUFA.[272] When macrophages have incorporated significant amounts of n-3 PUFA and reduced the n-6 to n-3 PUFA ratio, less dienoic eicosanoids are produced. In contrast, as the n-6 to n-3 ratio is increased, more TNF, IL-1, and dienoic eicosanoids are released. For example, linoleic acid increases the n-6 to n-3 ratio and as a consequence, more prostaglandin $E_2$ is produced, which in turn suppresses IL-2 synthesis and the proliferative responses of T cells to lectins and antigens.

## EFFECTS OF COMBINED THERAPY

Human trials involving the use of the three immune modulators just mentioned are of special interest. It has been reported that these nutrients restored T cell proliferative responses of patients to levels higher than those of normal nonstressed subjects.[266,272,273] Such favorable results apparently occurred independent of restored visceral protein synthesis and a proper nitrogen balance.

Arginine apparently stimulates lymphocyte numbers as well as responses. In addition, nucleotides, particularly uracil, seemed to restore CMI responses and possibly increased the capacity of lymphocytes to respond to antigens. The third nutrient, n-3 PUFA, appears to produce anti-inflammatory activity through suppression of some key inflammatory mediators and cytokines. These exciting possibilities require extensive study. Whether commercial preparations like Impact (Sandoz) can serve as the food regimen to correct the exaggerations and imbalances of the inflammatory and immune responses of patients remains to be established. This approach to modulating the harmful effects of exaggerated host responses to injury warrants more research because of the encouraging results obtained to date.

## PROBLEM OF FADDISH NUTRITION AND CORPORATE ZEAL

The theory behind numerous reports and convictions is that many essential nutrients, if given in gross excess, will achieve miraculous results compared to amounts considered adequate based on our knowledge of daily requirements. This thought has promoted an aggressive marketing posture by companies hoping to capitalize on new unconfirmed and poorly controlled laboratory discoveries. Unfortunately, a few researchers have exploited modest cause and effect changes in immune function to foster new regimens in nutrition. Unfounded zeal must be tempered with judicious caution. There is no basis for believing that taking megadoses of a micronutrient is significantly better than following the RDA or at most a modest supplementary dosage. In fact, megadoses of micronutrients are potentially dangerous and should be rejected totally as a scientifically valid approach to nutritional problems.[274]

Future knowledge can come only from carefully controlled animal experiments and well-planned double-blind clinical studies. A new area of study indicates that supplemental doses of nonessential nutrients like arginine, nucleic acids, and omega fatty acids can favorably modulate the immune response in patients experiencing extensive and sustained injury. These preliminary findings raise a new principle that suggests that endogenous biosynthetic pathways need help during conditions of extensive injury and physiologic stress. Undoubtedly, other nutrients also may be in limiting concentrations in such situations. Current studies with Impact (Sandoz), a new enteral diet formulation, should indicate whether this approach is scientifically sound and beneficial in restoring the immune response to an optimal level.[266,272] Much work is needed to clarify and elucidate the limiting factors involved in these special hypermetabolic states.

In summary, protein-calorie malnutrition has a greater effect on CMI than on humoral immunity, although this point is somewhat controversial. Some of this controversy may be the result of simultaneous, uneven multicomponent nutritional deficiencies. For example, a concurrent zinc deficiency could cause an exaggerated impairment of the CMI response. Single amino acid deficiencies such as tryptophan also could exaggerate a marginal protein-calorie deficiency.

Aside from impairment of the B and T lymphocyte network and resultant defective afferent responses, it is likely that impaired phagocyte function also becomes a sequela of malnutrition. This fact alone could explain increased incidence of infection in malnourished children. Phagocyte defects associated with protein-calorie malnutrition can include impaired chemotaxis, phagocytosis, bactericidal action, and metabolic responses, including the hexose monophosphate shunt and generation of oxygen-derived radicals.

Little doubt remains that single vitamin deficiencies can impair the immune response. This issue takes on great importance when one considers that 88% of a United States hospital population had at least one deficiency based on the results of a survey.

Of the so-called trace elements, zinc plays an essential role in the mononuclear phagocyte and lymphocyte systems. It is plausible that this deficiency is more common than realized, particularly in the aging population. The need for iron is well recognized.

An important area for future research involves the quantitative and qualitative nature of the effects of intrauterine malnutrition. The suggestion that impaired immune function in this case may be irreversible, at least in part, calls for extensive research of this problem.

Immunologists and nutritionists should be cautioned in drawing conclusions concerning nutrient effects based on small shifts in immunoglobulin levels, T and B cell counts, and phagocytic functional assays. It is always tempting to generalize from minor significant deviations of normal values. More research is needed to determine what shifts of immunologic parameters are valid predictors of a risk of infection or disease. Furthermore, infections can aggravate an already nutrition-compromised host and exacerbate immunologic functional impairment. In this regard, "hospital malnutrition" is an established phenomenon that is undoubtedly the result of synergism between marginal nutrition and an already existing disease complicated by medical interventions such as surgery, radiation, and immunosuppressive drugs.

Researchers need to examine carefully why the incidence of infection is not more extensive in patients with severe undernutrition considering the gross alterations of immunologic parameters that have been observed. Questions that remain unanswered include the following: (1) Are infectious organisms less aggressive or virulent in a host that provides a poor nutritional environment, and (2) is there compensatory nonspecific activation of the mononuclear phagocyte system when specific acquired immune mechanisms are compromised by undernutrition?

Essential nutrients and their respective daily requirements have been reasonably well established in normal healthy humans. However, an emerging concept holds that supplementation of certain nutrients that are not considered essential may modulate the inflammatory and immune responses in patients sustaining chronic or extensive injury. This theory implies that biosynthetic rates are inadequate to synthesize certain dietary components in chronically ill patients even though those components are adequately supplied through endogenous pathways in normal healthy subjects. This concept is exemplified by the beneficial effects achieved by supplemental arginine and uracil, particularly in ill patients. Modulation of the inflammatory response by n-3 PUFA indicates how a single class of nutrients can also modulate the inflammatory and immune responses through the attenuation of prostanoid synthesis. These findings are exciting and potentially important. Research in nutrition and immunology should have a highly productive future.

## REFERENCES

1. Durum, S.K., Schmidt, J.A., Oppenheim, J.J.: Annu. Rev. Immunol., *3:*263–287, 1986.
2. Durum, S.K., Oppenheim, J.J., Neta, R.: Immunophysiological role of interleukin 1. *In* Textbook of Immunophysiology. Edited by J.J. Oppenheim and E.M. Shevach. New York, Oxford University Press, 1988.
3. Smith, K.A.: Science, *240:*1169–1176, 1988.
4. Kuribayashi, K., Gillis, S., Kern, D.E., et al.: J. Immunol., *126:*2321–2327, 1981.
5. Schrader, J.W.: Annu. Rev. Immunol., *4:*205–230, 1986.
6. Ihle, J.N., Weinstein, Y.: Adv. Immunol., *39:*1–50, 1986.
7. Paul, W.E., Ohara, J.: Annu. Rev. Immunol., *5:*429–459, 1987.

8. Mitchell, L.C., Davis, L.S., Lipsky, P.E.: J. Immunol., *142:*1548–1557, 1989.
9. Sanderson, C.J., Campbell, H.D., Young, I.G.: Immunol. Rev., *102:*29–58, 1988.
10. Billiau, A., Van Damme, J., Ceuppens, J., et al.: Interleukin 6, a ubiquitous cytokine with paracrine as well as endocrine functions. *In* Lymphokine Receptor Interactions. Edited by D. Fradelizi and J. Bertoglio. London, John Libby Eurotext, 1989.
11. Kishimoto, T., Hirano, T.: Annu. Rev. Immunol., *6:*485–512, 1988.
12. Goodwin, R.G., Lupton, S., Schmierer, A., et al.: Proc. Natl. Acad. Sci. U.S.A., *86:*302–306, 1989.
13. Gimbrone, M.A., Jr., Obin, M.S., Brock, A.F., et al.: Science, *246:*1601–1603, 1989.
14. Friedman, R.M., Merigan T., Sreevalsan, A. (eds.): Interferons as Cell Growth Inhibitors and Antitumor Factors. New York, Alan R. Liss, 1986.
15. Gray, P.W., Goeddel, D.V.: Nature, *298:*859–863, 1982.
16. Herberman, R.R., Ortaldo, J.R., Bonnard, G.D.: Nature, *277:*221–223, 1979.
17. Decker, T., Lohmann-Matthes, M.-L., Gifford, G.E.: J. Immunol., *138:*957–962, 1987.
18. Rifkin, R.M., Hersh, E.M., Salmon, S.E.: Behring Inst. Mitt., *83:*125–133, 1988.
19. Klausmann, M., Pfluger, K.H., Krumwiek, D., et al.: Blut, *54:*307–312, 1987.
20. Roberts, W.K., Vasil, A.: J. Interferon Res., *2:*519–532, 1982.
21. Adams, D.O., Hamilton, T.A.: Annu. Rev. Immunol., *2:*283–318, 1984.
22. Kehrl, J.H., Roberts, A.B., Wakefield, L.M., et al.: J. Immunol., *137:*3855–3860, 1986.
23. Johnson, H.M., Torres, B.A.: Prog. Allergy *43:*37–67, 1988.
24. Dalgleish, A.G., Beverly, P.C.L., Clapham, P.R., et al.: Nature, *312:*763–767, 1984.
25. Ho, D.D., Rota, T.R., Hirsch, M.S.: J. Clin. Invest., *77:*1712–1715, 1986.
26. Moseson, M., Zeleninck-Jacqotte, A., Belsito, D.V., et al.: J. Acquired Immune Defic. Syndr., *2:*235–247, 1989.
27. Axelrod, A.E., Pruzansky, J.: Vitam. Hormo., *13:*1–27, 1955.
28. Cooper, W.C., Good, R.A., Mariani, T.: Am. J. Clin. Nutr., *27:*647–664, 1974.
29. Jose, D.G., Good, R.A.: Nature, *231:*323–325, 1971.
30. Kramer, T.R., Good, R.A.: Clin. Immunol. Immunopathol., *11:*212–228, 1978.
31. Wunder, J.A., Stinnett, J.D., Alexander, J.W.: Surgery, *84:*542–550, 1978.
32. Sakamoto, M., Ishii, S., Nishioka, K., et al.: Infect. Immun., *32:*553–556, 1981.
33. Sakamoto, M., Nishioka, K., Shimada, K.: Immunology, *38:*413–420, 1979.
34. Watson, R.R., Petro, T.M.: CRC Crit. Rev. Microbiol., *10:*297–315, 1984.
35. Neumann, C.G., Lawlor, G.J., Jr., Stiehm, E.R., et al.: Am. J. Clin. Nutr., *28:*89–104, 1975.
36. McMurray, D.N., Loomis, S.A., Casazza, L.J., et al.: Am. J. Clin. Nutr., *34:*68–77, 1981.
37. Bistrian, B.R., Blackburn, G.L., Scrimshaw, N.S., et al.: Am. J. Clin. Nutr., *28:*1148–1155, 1975.
38. Chandra, R.K., Newberne, P.M.: Nutrition, Immunity and Infection: Mechanism of Interactions. New York, Plenum Publishing, 1977.
39. Chandra, R.K.: Adv. Exp. Med. Biol., *262:*13–18, 1990.
40. Salimonu, L.S., Ojo-Amaize, E., Williams, A.I.O., et al.: Clin. Immunol. Immunopathol., *24:*1–7, 1982.
41. Schlesinger, L., Ohlbaum, A., Grez. L., et al.: Am. J. Clin. Nutr., *29:*758–761, 1976.
42. Stiehm, E.R.: Fed. Proc., *39:*3093–3097, 1980.
43. Salimonu, L.S., Johnson, A.O.K., Williams, A.I.O., et al.: Br. J. Nutr., *48:*7–14, 1982.
44. Schlesinger, L., Stekel, A.: Am. J. Clin. Nutr., *27:*615–620, 1974.
45. Rafii, M., Hashemi, S., Nahani, J., et al.: Clin. Immunol. Immunopathol., *8:*1–6, 1977.
46. Beatty, D.W., Dowdle, E.B.: Clin. Exp. Immunol., *35:*433–442, 1979.
47. Dowd, P.S., Heatley, R.V.: Clin. Sci., *66:*241–248, 1984.
48. Kaufman, C.A., Jones, P.G., Kluger, M.I.: Am. J. Clin. Nutr., *44:*449–452, 1986.
49. Keenan, R.A., Moldawer, L.L., Yang, R.D., et al.: J. Lab. Clin. Med., *100:*844–857, 1982.
50. Bhaskaram, P., Sivakumar, B.: Arch. Dis. Child, *61:*182–185, 1986.
51. Hoffman-Goetz, L.: Lymphokines and monokines in protein malnutrition. *In* Nutrition and Immunology. Edited by R.K. Chandra. New York, Alan R. Liss, 1988.
52. Bradley, S.F., Kauffman, C.A.: J. Leukocyte Biol., *43:*36–40, 1988.
53. Hoffman-Goetz, L., Keir, R.: Nutr. Res., *8:*89–93, 1988.
54. Salimonu, L.S., Johnson, A.O.K., Williams, A.I.O., et al.: Clin. Exp. Immunol., *47:*626–634, 1982.
55. Barbul, A.: Nutrition, *6:*59–62, 1990.
56. Gross, R.L., Newberne, P.M.: Physiol. Rev., *60:*188–302, 1980.
57. Kenney, M.A., Magee, J.L., Piedad-Pasqual, F.: J. Nutr., *199:*1063–1072, 1970.
58. Gershoff, S.N., Gill, T.J., Simonian, S.J.: J. Nutr., *95:*184–189, 1968.
59. Jose, D.G., Good, R.A.: J. Exp. Med., *137:*1–9, 1973.
60. Suskind, R.M., Shrisinha, S., Edelman, R., et al.: Immunoglobulins and antibody response in Thai children with protein-calorie malnutrition. *In* Malnutrition and the Immune Response. Edited by R.M. Suskind. New York, Raven Press, 1977.
61. Jose, D.G., Good, R.A.: Cancer Res. *33:*807–812, 1973.
62. Jose, D.G., Good, R.A.: Nature, *231:*323–325, 1971.
63. Coovadia, H.M., Soothill, J.F.: Clin. Exp. Immunol., *23:*373–377, 1976.
64. Coovadia, H.M., Soothill, J.F.: Clin. Exp. Immunol., *23:*562–567, 1976.
65. Ashkenasy, A.: J. Nutr., *109:*1214–1222, 1979.
66. Barbul, A.: J. Parenter. Enteral Nutr., *10:*227–238, 1986.
67. Reynolds, J.V., Daly, J.M., Shou, J., et al.: Ann. Surg., *211:*202–210, 1990.
68. Barbul, A., Sisto, D.A., Wasserkrug, H.L., et al.: Surgery, *90:*244–251, 1981.
69. Park, K.G.M., Hayes, P.D., Garlick, P.J., et al.: Lancet, *337:*645–646, 1991.
70. Dreizen, S.: Int. J. Vitam. Nutr. Res., *49:*220–228, 1978.
71. Beisel, W.R.: Malnutrition and the immune response. *In* Biochemistry of Nutrition I. Edited by A. Neuberger and T.H. Jukes. Baltimore, University Park Press, 1979.
72. Edelman, R.: Cell-mediated immune response in protein-calorie malnutrition—a review. *In* Malnutrition and the Immune Response. Edited by R.M. Suskind. New York, Raven Press, 1977.
73. Danbolt, N., Closs, K.: Acta Derm. Venereol. (Stockh.), *23:*127, 1942.

74. Moynahan, E.J., Barnes, P.M.: Lancet, *1*:676–677, 1973.
75. Khalil, M., Kabiel, A., El-Khateeb, S., et al.: Am. J. Clin. Nutr., *27*:260–267, 1974.
76. Fraker, P.J., Haas, S.M., Luecke, R.W.: J. Nutr., *107*:1889–1895, 1977.
77. Fraker, P.J., DePasquale-Jardieu, P., Zwickl, C.M., et al.: Proc. Natl. Acad. Sci. U.S.A., *75*:5660–5669, 1978.
78. Luecke, R.W., Simonel, C.E., Fraker, P.J.: J. Nutr., *108*:881–887, 1978.
79. Nash, L., Iwata, T., Fernandes, G., et al.: Cell. Immunol., *48*:238–243, 1979.
80. Hildebrandt, K.J., Luecke, R.W., Fraker, P.J.: J. Nutr., *112*:1921–1928, 1982.
81. DePasquale-Jardieu, P., Fraker, P.: J. Nutr., *114*:1762–1769, 1984.
82. Jardieu, P., Fraker, P.J.: Fed. Proc., *41*:218a, 1982.
83. DePasquale-Jardieu, P., Fraker, P.J.: J. Nutr., *109*:1847–1855, 1979.
84. DePasquale-Jardieu, P., Fraker, P.J.: J. Immunol., *124*:2650–2655, 1980.
85. Fraker, P.J.: Surv. Clin. Immunol., *2*:155–163, 1983.
86. Dardenne, M., Pleau, J., Lefrancier, P., et al.: C.R. Seances Acad. Sci. III, *292*:793–796, 1981.
87. Iwata, T., Incefy, G.S., Tanaka, T., et al.: Cell. Immunol., *47*:100–105, 1979.
88. Chandra, R.K., Heresi, G., Au, B.: Clin. Exp. Immunol., *42*:332–335, 1980.
89. Fraker, P.J., Zwickl, C.M., Luecke, R.W.: J. Nutr., *112*:309–313, 1982.
90. Zwickl, C.M., Fraker, P.J.: Immunol. Commun., *9*:611–626, 1980.
91. Fernandes, G., Nair, M., Onoe, K., et al.: Proc. Natl. Acad. Sci. U.S.A., *76*:457–461, 1979.
92. Luecke, R.W., Fraker, P.J.: J. Nutr. *109*:1373–1376, 1979.
93. McCaffrey, R., Smoler, D.F.: Proc. Natl. Acad. Sci. U.S.A., *70*:521–525, 1973.
94. Cook-Mills, J.M., Wirth, J.J., Fraker, P.J.: Adv. Exp. Med. Biol., *262*:111–121, 1990.
95. Chandra, R.K., Au, B., Woodford, G., et al.: Iron status, immune response and susceptibility to infection. *In* Iron Metabolism. Edited by H. Kies. Ciba Foundation Symposium 51. Amsterdam, Elsevier/Excerpta Medica/North Holland, 1977.
96. Murray, M.J., Murray, A.B., Murray, M.B., et al.: Br. Med. J., *2*:1113–1115, 1978.
97. Antia, A.U., McFarlane, H., Soothill, J.F.: Arch. Dis. Child., *43*:459–462, 1968.
98. McFarlane, H., Reddy, S., Adcock, K.J., et al.: Br. Med. J., *4*:268–270, 1970.
99. Weinberg, E.D.: Am. J. Clin. Nutr., *30*:1485–1490, 1977.
100. Powanda, M.C.: Am. J. Clin. Nutr., *30*:1254–1268, 1977.
101. Chandra, R.K.: Nutr. Rev., *34*:129–132, 1976.
102. Nalder, B.N., Mahoney, A.W., Makrishnan, R., et al.: J. Nutr., *102*:535–542, 1972.
103. Andelman, M.G., Sered, B.R.: Am. J. Dis. Child, *111*:45–55, 1966.
104. Gross, R.L., Reid, J.V.O., Newberne, P.M., et al.: Am. J. Clin. Nutr., *28*:225–232, 1975.
105. Kulapongs, P., Suskind, R.M., Vithayasai, V., et al.: Lancet, *2*:689–691, 1974.
106. Suskind, R.M., Kulapongs, P., Vithayasai, V., et al.: Iron deficiency anemia and the immune response. *In* Malnutrition and the Immune Response. Edited by R.M. Suskind. New York, Raven Press, 1977.
107. Dhur, A., Galan, P., Herzberg, S.: Comp. Biochem. Physiol., *94A*:11–19, 1989.
108. Hershko, C., Karasi, A., Eylon, L., et al.: Blood, *36*:321–329, 1970.
109. Toskes, P.P., Smith, G.W., Bensinger, T.A., et al.: Am. J. Clin. Nutr., *27*:355–361, 1974.
110. Oppenheimer, S.J., Gibson, F.D., Macfarlane, S.B., et al.: Trans. R. Soc. Trop. Med. Hyg., *80*:603–612, 1986.
111. Barry, D.M., Reeve, A.W.: Pediatrics, *60*:908–912, 1977.
112. Becroft, D.M., Dix, M.R., Farmer, K.: Arch. Dis. Child., *52*:778–781, 1977.
113. McFarlane, H., Reddy, S., Adcock, K.J., et al.: Br. Med. J., *4*:268–270, 1970.
114. Moore, L.L., Humbert, J.R.: Pediatr. Res., *18*:789–794, 1984.
115. Kuvibidila, S.R., Baliga, B.S., Suskind, R.M.: Am. J. Clin. Nutr., *34*:2635–2640, 1981.
116. Joynson, D.H., Walker, D.M., Jacobs, A., et al.: Lancet, *2*:1058–1059, 1972.
117. Swarup-Mitra, S., Sinha, A.K.: Indian J. Med. Res., *79*:354–362, 1984.
118. Van Asbeck, B.S., Verbrugh, H.A., Van Oost, B.A., et al.: Br. Med. J., *284*:542–544, 1982.
119. Weinberg, E.D.: Microbiol. Rev., *42*:45–66, 1978.
120. Fletcher, J., Mather, J., Lewis, M.J., et al.: J. Infect. Dis., *131*:44–50, 1975.
121. MacDougall, L.O., Anderson, R., McNab, G.M., et al.: J. Pediatr., *86*:833–843, 1975.
122. Kochanowski, B.A., Sherman, A.R.: Am. J. Clin. Nutr., *41*:278–284, 1985.
123. Good, M.F., Powell, L.F., Halliday, J.W.: Blood Rev., *2*:43–49, 1988.
124. Rabinovitch, M., Destefano, M.J.: Exp. Cell Res., *79*:423–430, 1973.
125. McCoy, J.H., Kenney, M.A.: J. Nutr., *105*:791–797, 1975.
126. Newberne, P.M., Gebhardt, B.M.: Nutr. Rep. Int., *7*:407–420, 1973.
127. Newberne, P.M., Hunt, C.E., Young, V.R.: Br. J. Exp. Pathol., *49*:448–457, 1968.
128. Lipsky, P.E., Ziff, M.: J. Clin. Invest., *65*:1069–1076, 1980.
129. Bazhora, I.I., Shtefan, E.E., Timoshevski, I.V.: Mikrobiol. Zh., *36*:771, 1974.
130. Pedroni, F., Bianclin, F., Vgazio, A.L., et al.: Lancet, *1*:1303–1304, 1975.
131. Alcock, N.W., Shils, M.E., Lieberman, P.H., et al.: Cancer Res., *33*:2196–2204, 1973.
132. Alcock, N.W., Shils, M.E.: Proc. Soc. Exp. Biol. Med., *145*:855–858, 1974.
133. Kashiwa, H.K., Hungerford, G.F.: Proc. Soc. Exp. Biol. Med., *99*:441–443, 1958.
134. Hungerford, G.F., Karson, E.F.: Blood, *16*:1642–1650, 1960.
135. McCreary, P.A., Battifora, H.A., Laing, G.H., et al.: Proc. Soc. Exp. Biol. Med., *121*:1130–1133, 1966.
136. McCreary, P.A., Battifora, H.A., Hahneman, B.M., et al.: Blood, *29*:683–690, 1967.
137. Levander, O.A.: Ann. N.Y. Acad. Sci., *393*:70–82, 1982.
138. Chandra, R.K.: Can. J. Physiol. Pharmacol., *61*:290–294, 1983.
139. Mulhern, S.A., Vessey, A.R., Taylor, G.L., et al.: Proc. Soc. Exp. Biol. Med., *180*:453–461, 1985.
140. Forstrom, J.W., Zakowski, J.J., Tappel, A.L.: Biochemistry, *17*:2639–2644, 1978.
141. Serfass, R.E., Ganther, H.E.: Life Sci., *19*:1139–1144, 1976.

142. Spallholz, J.E., Martin, J.L., Gerlack, M.L.: Proc. Soc. Exp. Biol. Med., *143:*685–689, 1973.
143. Spallholz, J.E., Martin, J.L., Gerlack, M.L.: Infect. Immun., *8:*841–842, 1973.
144. Spallholz, J.E., Martin, J.L., Gerlack, M.L.: Proc. Soc. Exp. Biol. Med., *148:*37–40, 1975.
145. Bendich, A., Cohen, M.: B vitamins: Effects on specific and nonspecific immune responses. *In* Nutrition and Immunology. Edited by R.K. Chandra. New York, Alan R. Liss, 1988.
146. Cramer, W., Drew, A.H., Mottram, J.C.: Lancet, *1:*1202–1208, 1921.
147. Stoerk, H.C., Eisen, H.N., John, H.M.: J. Exp. Med., *85:*365–371, 1947.
148. Axelrod, A.E., Traketellis, A.C.: Vitam. Horm., *22:*591–607, 1964.
149. Hodges, R.E., Bean, W.B., Ohlson, M.A. et al.: Am. J. Clin. Nutr., *11:*180–186, 1962.
150. Hodges, R.E., Bean, W.B., Ohlson, M.A. et al.: Am. J. Clin. Nutr., *11:*187–199, 1962.
151. Parkes, A.S.: Nature, *184:*699–701, 1959.
152. Axelrod, A.E., Fisher, E.B., Fisher, E., et al.: Science, *127:*1388–1389, 1958.
153. Herr, N.G., Coursin, D.B.: J. Nutr., *88:*273–279, 1966.
154. Axelrod, A.E., Trakatellis, A.C., Block, H., et al.: J. Nutr., *79:*161–167, 1963.
155. Stinebring, W.R., Trakatellis, A.C., Axelrod, A.E., et al.: J. Immunol., *91:*39–45, 1963.
156. Ha, C., Miller, L.T., Kerkvliet, N.I.: Cell. Immunol., *85:*318–329, 1984.
157. Chandra, R.K., Sudhakaran, L.: Ann. N.Y. Acad. Sci., *585:*404–423, 1990.
158. Ludovici, P.P., Axelrod, A.E.: Proc. Soc. Exp. Biol. Med., *77:*526–530, 1951.
159. Stoerk, H.C., Zucker, T.F.: Proc. Soc. Exp. Biol. Med., *56:*151–153, 1944.
160. Lederer, W.H., Kumar, M., Axelrod, A.E.: J. Nutr., *105:*17–25, 1975.
161. Morgan, A.F., Groody, M., Axelrod, A.E.: Am. J. Physiol., *146:*723–733, 1946.
162. Axelrod, A.E., Carter, B., McCoy, R.H.: Proc. Soc. Exp. Biol. Med., *66:*137–140, 1948.
163. Harmon, B.G., Miller, E.R., Hoefer, J.A., et al.: J. Nutr., *79:*269–275, 1963.
164. Pruzansky, J., Axelrod, A.E.: Proc. Soc. Exp. Biol. Med., *89:*323–325, 1955.
165. Goodwin, J.S., Garry, P.J.: Clin. Exp. Immunol., *51:*647–653, 1983.
166. Chanarin, I.: The Megaloblastic Anaemias. Oxford, Blackwell, 1969.
167. Gross, R.L., Newberne, P.M.: Malnutrition, the thymolymphatic system and immunocompetence. *In* The Reticuloendothelial System in Health and Disease. Vol. B. Edited by H. Friedman, M.R. Escobar, and S.M. Reichard. New York, Plenum Press, 1976.
168. Hollingsworth, J.W., Carr, J.: Cell. Immunol., *8:*270–279, 1973.
169. Gross, R.L., Newberne, P.M.: Physiol. Rev., *60:*188–302, 1980.
170. Gross, R.L., Reid, J.V.O., Newberne, P.M., et al.: Am. J. Clin. Nutr., *28:*225–232, 1975.
171. Boles, J.M., Youinou, P., Garre, M., et al.: Rev. Med. Interne, *3:*51–56, 1982.
172. Youinou, P.Y., Garre, M.A., Menez, J.F., et al.: Am. J. Med., *73:*652–657, 1982.
173. Beisel, W.R.: Am. J. Clin. Nutr., *36(Suppl.):*417–468, 1982.
174. Das, K.C., Hoffbrand, A.V.: Br. J. Haematol., *19:*459–468, 1970.
175. MacCuish, A.C., Urbaniak, S.J., Goldstone, A.H., et al.: Blood, *44:*849–855, 1974.
176. Kaplan, S.S., Basford, R.E.: Blood, *47:*801–805, 1976.
177. Katka, K.: Scand. J. Haematol., *32:*76–82, 1984.
178. Rabin, B.S.: J. Nutr., *113:*2316–2322, 1983.
179. Bendich, A., Cohen, M.: B Vitamins: effects on specific and nonspecific immune responses. *In* Nutrition and Immunology. Edited by R.K. Chandra. New York, Alan R. Liss, 1988.
180. Theron, A., Anderson, R., Grabow, G., et al.: Clin. Exp. Immunol., *44:*295–303, 1981.
181. Jones, P.T., Anderson, R.: Int. J. Immunopharmacol., *5:*377–389, 1983.
182. Perla, D., Marmorston, J.: Natural Resistance and Clinical Medicine. Boston, Little, Brown, 1941.
183. Mueller, P.S., Kies, M.W., Alvord, E.C., Jr., et al.: J. Exp. Med., *115:*329–338, 1962.
184. Zweiman, B., Besdine, R.W., Hildreth, E.A.: J. Immunol., *96:*672–675, 1966.
185. Kumar, M., Axelrod, A.E.: J. Nutr., *98:*41–44, 1969.
186. Anthony, L.E., Kurahara, C.G., Taylor, K.B.: Am. J. Clin. Nutr., *32:*1691–1699, 1979.
187. Boxer, L.A., Watanabe, A.M., Rister, M., et al.: N. Engl. J. Med., *295:*1041–1045, 1976.
188. Hayward, A.R., Harvey, B.A.M., Leonard, J., et al.: Lancet, *1:*1099–1101, 1979.
189. Pauling, L.: Vitamin C and the Common Cold. San Francisco, W.H. Freeman and Company, 1970.
190. Chalmers, T.C.: Am. J. Med., *58:*532–536, 1975.
191. Thomas, W.R., Holt, P.G.: Clin. Exp. Immunol., *32:*370–379, 1978.
192. Baird, I.M., Hughes, R.E., Wilson, H.K., et al.: Am. J. Clin. Nutr., *32:*1686–1690, 1979.
193. Axelrod, A.E.: Am. J. Clin. Nutr., *24:*265–271, 1971.
194. Darip, M.D., Sirisinha, S., Lamb, A.J.: Proc. Soc. Exp. Biol. Med., *161:*600–604, 1979.
195. Bang, B.G., Bang, F.B., Foard, M.A.: Am. J. Pathol., *68:*147–162, 1972.
196. Bang, F.B., Bang, B.G., Foard, M.A.: Am. J. Pathol., *78:*417–426, 1975.
197. Nauss, K.M., Mark, D.A., Suskind, R.M.: J. Nutr., *109:*1815–1823, 1979.
198. Newberne, P.M., Suphakarn, V.: Cancer, *40:*2553–2556, 1977.
199. Micksche, M., Cerni, C., Kokron, O., et al.: Oncology, *34:*234–238, 1977.
200. Floersheim, G.L., Bollog, W.: Transplantation, *14:*564–567, 1974.
201. Dennert, G., Lotan, R.: Eur. J. Immunol., *8:*23–29, 1978.
202. Malkovsky, M., Edwards, A.J., Hunt, R., et al.: Nature, *302:*338–340, 1983.
203. Glaser, M., Lotan, R.: Cell. Immunol., *45:*175–181, 1979.
204. Eremin, O., Ashby, J., Rhodes, J.: Int. Arch. Allergy Appl. Immunol., *75:*2–7, 1984.
205. Watson, R.R., Rister, M., Baehner, R.L.: J. Nutr., *106:*1801–1808, 1976.
206. Machlin, L.J.: Vitamin E. *In* Handbook of Vitamins. Edited by L.J. Machlin. New York, Marcel Dekker, 1984.
207. Warrell, R.P., Frankel, S.R., Miller, W.H., Jr., et al.: N. Engl. J. Med., *324:*1385–1393, 1991.
208. Trechsel, U., Evequoz, V., Fleisch, H.: Biochem. J., *203:*339–344, 1985.

209. Corwin, L.M., Gordon, R.K.: Ann. N.Y. Acad. Sci., *393*:437–451, 1982.
210. Corwin, L.M., Gordon, R.K., Shloss, J.: Scand. J. Immunol., *14*:565–571, 1981.
211. Gebremichael, A., Levy, E.M., Corwin, L.M.: J. Nutr., *114*:1297–1305, 1984.
212. Chavance, M., Brubacher, G., Herbeth, B., et al.: Immunological and nutritional status among elderly. *In* Lymphoid Cell Functions in Aging. Edited by A.L. deWeck. Rijswijk, Eurage, 1984.
213. Harris, R.E., Boxer, L.A. Baehner, R.L.: Blood, *55*:338–343, 1980.
214. Till, G.O., Hatherill, J.R., Tourtelotte, W.W., et al.: Am. J. Pathol., *119*:376–384, 1985.
215. Bendich, A., D'Apolito, P., Gabriel, E., et al.: J. Nutr., *114*:1588–1593, 1984.
216. Kurek, M.P., Corwin, L.M.: Nutr. Cancer, *4*:128–139, 1982.
217. Shamberger, R.J.: Biochemistry of Selenium. New York, Plenum Press, 1983.
218. Tengerdy, R.P.: Ann. N.Y. Acad. Sci., *587*:24–33, 1990.
219. Thomas, I.K., Erickson, K.L.: J. Nutr., *115*:1528–1534, 1985.
220. Clinton, S.K., Imrey, P.B., Alster, J.M., et al.: J. Nutr., *114*:1213–1223, 1984.
221. Erickson, K.L., Thomas, I.K.: J. Natl. Cancer Inst., *75*:333–340, 1985.
222. Murphy, R.C., Pickett, W.C., Culp, B.R., et al.: Prostaglandins, *22*:613–622, 1981.
223. Goldman, D.W., Pickett, W.C., Goetzl, E.J.: Biochem. Biophys. Res. Commun., *117*:282–288, 1983.
224. Lee, T.H., Hoover, R.L., Williams, J.D., et al.: N. Engl. J. Med., *312*:1217–1224, 1985.
225. Mohrhauer, H., Holman, R.T.: J. Nutr., *91*:528–534, 1967.
226. Hwang, D.: FASEB J., *3*:2052–2061, 1989.
227. Von Schacky, C., Fischer, S., Weber, P.C.: J. Clin. Invest., *76*:1626–1631, 1985.
228. Lefkowith, J.B., Schreiner, G.: J. Clin. Invest., *80*:947–956, 1987.
229. Mertin, J., Hunt, R.: Proc. Natl. Acad. Sci. U.S.A., *73*:928–931, 1976.
230. Esterbauer, H., Benedetti, A., Lang, J., et al.: Biochim. Biophys. Acta, *876*:154–166, 1986.
231. Oarada, M., Miyazawa, T., Fugimoto, K., et al.: Agric. Biol. Chem., *52*:2101–2102, 1988.
232. Oarada, M., Miyazawa, T., Kaneda, T.: Lipids, *21*:150–154, 1986.
233. Oarada, M., Majima, T., Miyazawa, T., et al.: Biochim. Biophys. Acta, *1012*:156, 1989.
234. Zeman, F.J., Stanbrough, E.C., Shrader, R.E.: Fed. Proc., *28*:488, 1969.
235. Olusi, S.O., McFarlane, H.: Pediatr. Res., *10*:707–712, 1976.
236. Naeye, R.L., Blanc, W.B., Paul, C.: Pediatrics, *52*:494–503, 1973.
237. Jelliffe, D.B.: J. Trop. Pediatr., *20*:232–238, 1974.
238. Chandra, R.K.: Lancet, *2*:1393–1394, 1974.
239. Chandra, R.K.: Am. J. Dis. Child, *1299*:450–454, 1975.
240. Chandra, R.K.: Cell-mediated immunity in fetally and postnatally malnourished children from India and Newfoundland. *In* Malnutrition and the Immune Response. Edited by R.M. Suskind. New York, Raven Press, 1977.
241. Chandra, R.K., Ali, S.K., Kutty, K.M., et al.: Biol. Neonate, *31*:15–18, 1977.
242. Watts, T.: J. Trop. Pediatr., *15*:155–158, 1969.
243. Smythe, P.M., Schonland, M., Brereton-Stiles, G.G., et al.: Lancet, *2*:939–943, 1971.
244. Neumann, C.G., Lawlor, G.J., Stiehm, E.R., et al.: Am. J. Clin. Nutr., *28*:89–104, 1975.
245. Watson, R.R., McMurray, D.N.: CRC Crit. Rev. Food Sci. Nutr., *12*:113–159, 1979.
246. Dutz, W., Rossipal, E., Ghavami, H., et al.: Eur. J. Pediatr., *122*:117–130, 1976.
247. McMurray, D.N., Watson, R.R., Reyes, M.A.: Am. J. Clin. Nutr., *34*:2117–2126, 1981.
248. Ziegler, H.D., Ziegler, P.B.: Johns Hopkins Med. J., *137*:59–64, 1975.
249. Sirsinha, S., Suskind, R.M.: The complement system in protein-calorie malnutrition—a review. *In* Malnutrition and the Immune Response. Edited by R.M. Suskind. New York, Raven Press, 1977.
250. McMurray, D.N., Reyes, M.A., Watson, R.R.: Fed. Proc., *36*:1171, 1977.
251. McMurray, D.N., Rey, H., Casazza, L.J., et al.: Am. J. Clin. Nutr., *30*:1944–1948, 1977.
252. Sirsinha, E., Edelman, R., Asvapaka, C., et al.: Pediatrics, *55*:166–170, 1975.
253. Chandra, R.K., Br. Med. J., *2*:583–585, 1975.
254. McMurray, D.N., Rey, H., Casazza, L.J., et al.: Fed. Proc., *35*:588, 1976.
255. Hutchinson-Smith, B.: Med. Off., *123*:257–262, 1970.
256. Leonard, P.J., MacWilliam, K.M.: J. Endocrinol., *29*:273–279, 1964.
257. Beisel, W.R.: Adv. Nutr. Res., *1*:125, 1977.
258. Ghadimi, H., Kumar, S., Abaci, R.: Pediatr. Res., *7*:161–168, 1973.
259. Wing, E.J., Young, J.B.: Infect. Immun., *28*:771–776, 1980.
260. Murray, J., Murray, A.: Prospect. Biol. Med., *20*:471–483, 1977.
261. Gopalan, C.: Am. J. Clin. Nutr., *23*:35–51, 1970.
262. Beisel, W.R.: Am. J. Clin. Nutr., *30*:1236–1247, 1977.
263. Scrimshaw, N.S.: Bibl. Nutr. Dieta., *18*:153–164, 1973.
264. Arbeter, A., Echeverri, L., Franco, D., et al.: Fed. Proc., *30*:1421–1428, 1971.
265. Kielmann, A.A.: Am. J. Clin. Nutr., *30*:592–598, 1977.
266. Cerra, F.B.: Am. J. Surg., *161*:230–234, 1991.
267. Stuehr, D.J., Gross, S.S., Sakuma, I., et al.: J. Exp. Med., *169*:1011–1020, 1989.
268. Reynolds, J.V., Shou, J.A., Sigal, R., et al.: Cell. Immunol., *128*:569–577, 1990.
269. Sonoda, T., Tatibana, M.: Biochim. Biophys. Acta, *521*:55–66, 1978.
270. Kulkarni, A.D., Fanslow, W.C., Rudolph, F.B., et al.: J. Parenter. Enteral Nutr., *10*:169–171, 1986.
271. Kinsella, J., Lokesh, B., et al.: Crit. Care Med., *18*:S94–113, 1990.
272. Cerra, F.B., Lehman, S., Lonstantinides, N., et al.: Nutrition, *6*:84–87, 1990.
273. Lieberman, M., Shou, J., Torres, B.S., et al.: Nutrition, *6*:88–91, 1990.
274. Chandra, R.K.: Ann. N.Y. Acad. Sci., *587*:9–16, 1990.

## SELECTED READINGS

Alexander, J.W., Peck, M.D.: Future prospects for adjunctive therapy: pharmacologic and nutritional approaches to immune system modulation. Crit. Care Med., *18(Suppl)*:159–164, 1990.

Bendich, A., Phillips, M., Tengerdy, R.P. (eds.): Antioxidant nutrients and immune functions. Adv. Exp. Med. Biol., *262*:1–165, 1988.

Bower, R.H.: Nutrition and immune function. Nutr. Clin. Pract., *5*:189–195, 1990.

Chernoff, R. (ed.): Nutrition and immune function. Clin. Appl. Nutr., *1*, 1991.

Chandra, R.K. (ed.): Nutrition and immunology. Contemp. Issues Nutr., *11*, 1988.

Myrvik, Q.N., Weiser, R.S.: Fundamentals of Immunology. 2nd Ed. Philadelphia, Lea & Febiger, 1984.

Panush, R.S., Delafuente, J.C.: Vitamins and immunocompetence. World Rev. Nutr. Diet., *45*:97–132, 1985.

Paul, W.E. (ed.): Fundamental Immunology. 2nd Ed. New York, Raven Press, 1989.

Spiller, G.A., Scala, J.: New Protective Roles for Selected Nutrients. New York, Alan R. Liss, 1989.

Wan, J.M., Haw, M.P., Blackburn, G.L.: Nutrition, immune function and inflammation: an overview. Proc. Nutr. Soc., *48*:315–335, 1989.

CHAPTER 42

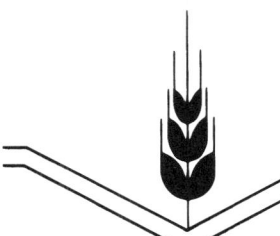

# Work and Exercise

Eric Hultman, Roger C. Harris, and Lawrence L. Spriet



Interest in the relationship between diet and activity, whether athletic, combative, or occupational, is not new, although the current explosion of literature in the field would suggest the opposite. An adequate intake of foodstuffs is fundamental to the maintenance of health and to the survival of the individual. Reportedly both the Greeks and Romans were interested in the best foodstuffs for maximal performance, but it would be surprising if even earlier, man did not have a similar interest in such matters. Understanding the significance of different foodstuffs and rationalization of this information to the energy requirements of different levels of activity, however, only really began in the last century with the work of the German physiologist von Liebig.[1] He considered that muscle proteins were the main provider of energy in working skeletal muscle, although by the end of the nineteenth century, it was clear that this conclusion was incorrect and the main sources were in fact carbohydrate and possibly also fat.[2,3]

The first positive evidence of the importance of fat as a substrate for energy production during contraction of muscle was presented by Himwich and Rose.[4] They performed respiratory quotient (RQ) measurements of muscle in dogs, which in the well-fed state was 0.92 at rest and 0.94 during exercise. After 5 to 15 days of starvation, these values decreased to 0.80 both at rest and during exercise. If one remembers that oxidation of carbohydrates results in an RQ of 1.00 and that of fat is 0.70, the results clearly indicated increased use of fat by the muscle after starvation. A decade later, Christensen and Hansen in their now classic study of the influence of diet on work performance in man similarly observed a lower RQ both at rest and during exercise after a high fat diet, and a 30% reduction in endurance time compared to that when a mixed diet was given.[5] In contrast, a high carbohydrate diet resulted in an increase in exercise RQ, and although this value decreased during the course of exercise (showing an increase in fat use), it never went below the resting value measured after the mixed diet. Endurance time after the carbohydrate diet was about twice that after the mixed diet.

Today, it is accepted that some of the energy expenditure during exercise can also be derived from protein use, especially when the work time is prolonged. The amount of energy covered, however, is only a few percent of the total, and in the isocaloric state, carbohydrate and fatty acids constitute the major energy sources. Final proof was eventually provided by direct measurement of the different substrates in the working muscles using the needle biopsy technique introduced by Bergström and Hultman in the middle of the 1960s. Initially, for the purpose of studying water and electrolytes in kidney patients,[6] the biopsy technique was subsequently used in the study of muscle glycogen in diabetic patients[7] and in studies of the local energy stores in normal muscle at rest and during exercise.[8–21] The introduction of the needle biopsy technique had a major, almost catalytic effect on the growth of exercise biochemistry and physiology as scientific disciplines. In 1970, the closely similar liver biopsy technique was used to measure the second major carbohydrate store in the body.[22–26] In combination with muscle, blood, and respiratory measurements, it became possible to obtain an almost complete picture of substrate use in exercising man.

An understanding of substrate use by the body during exercise and work is, of course, basic to a rational assessment of the nutritive needs of an individual. Today, with the rapid growth of recreational exercise, awareness of the effects of adequate nutrition on work performance is perhaps greater than ever before. However, even among the most fastidious—the elite athletes and their trainers—exists a plethora of nutritive practices that would seem to owe more to the early work of von Liebig than to subsequent studies.

## ENERGY SUBSTRATES AVAILABLE FOR WORK

When a muscle such as the quadriceps femoris is stimulated from rest to near maximal activity, the increase in the rate of energy expenditure is approximately 300-fold. The energy used by the body to perform work is chemical, and the immediate energy source for the muscle contraction is adenosine triphosphate (ATP). ATP, however, is stored only in small amounts in the muscle cells (circa 5.5 $mmol{\cdot}kg^{-1}$) and must be continually resynthesized from adenosine diphosphate (ADP). The energy for rephosphorylation can be derived from several reactions that can be divided into those requiring oxygen, i.e., aerobic metabolism, and those that can proceed in the absence of oxygen, i.e., anaerobic metabolism.

Aerobic resynthesis of ATP occurs only within the mitochondria of the cells, the rate of synthesis being governed largely by the size and number of mitochondria per muscle cell and the rate of oxygen uptake. Basic fuels that can supply substrates for oxidation are glucose transported from the liver by the blood, locally stored glycogen, and free fatty acids (FFA) taken up from the blood or to a limited extent derived from triglyceride depots within the muscle. Each of these fuels may be metabolized within the cytoplasm to smaller subunits, which then enter the tricarboxylic cycle within the mitochondria.

When the oxidative energy production is insufficient to cover the expenditure, as in the early stages of exercise before full readjustment of the blood supply or during high intensity exercise, resynthesis of ATP is essentially anaerobic, and involves two metabolic pathways. The first is from phosphocreatine (PCr), which in the presence of creatine kinase can directly rephosphorylate ADP to ATP. The second route is from glycogen or glucose with formation of lactate. This process is energetically far less efficient than when either substrate is metabolized completely to $CO_2$ and $H_2O$; anaerobic metabolism generates only 3 ATP compared to 38 to 39 ATP per glucose unit when oxidized.

The contribution of the different fuel supplies to the total energy output by the muscle varies with both the intensity and duration of the exercise and is influenced further by the fitness of the individual, the nutritional status both before and during exercise, the level of anxiety, and even the environment (altitude, temperature, and humidity). Morphologic differences between individuals in their muscle fiber make-up may also affect their use of the different fuels available during a standard exercise.

The maximum theoretic rate of use of a particular fuel for muscle contraction is determined by the activity of those enzymes involved in its metabolism. Estimates of the maximum power available from phosphagen, carbohydrate, and fat use by muscle are presented here both as the maximum rate of high energy phosphate ($\sim$P) that may be generated per kilogram of fresh muscle per second, and as the maximum rate calculated for the whole muscle mass. This value is assumed to be 28 kg in a 70-kg man. Values in this latter case are given as moles $\sim$P per minute.

$$\text{ATP, PCr} \rightarrow \text{ADP, Cr} \qquad (1)$$

a. Max. rate of degradation: 2.6 mmol $\sim$P (kg muscle)$^{-1}{\cdot}s^{-1}$ corresponding totally to 4.4 mol $\sim P{\cdot}min^{-1}$.
b. Amount available (quadriceps muscle): 24 mmol $\sim$P (kg muscle)$^{-1}$ or totally 0.67 mol in 28 kg of muscle.

The estimate of 2.6 mmol $\sim$P (kg muscle)$^{-1}{\cdot}s^{-1}$ has been calculated from direct measurements in needle biopsy samples obtained from human quadriceps muscle during near maximum voluntary isometric contraction[27,28] or during tetanic electrical stimulation.[29] Other workers have suggested a figure nearer to 6 mmol $\sim$P (kg muscle)$^{-1}{\cdot}s^{-1}$ based on less direct measurements.[30–32] This is close to the maximum velocity of creatine kinase measured in human muscle.[33]

$$\text{Glycogen} \rightarrow \text{lactate} \quad (2a)$$

a. Max. rate of $^{\sim}$P generation: 1.4 mmol $^{\sim}$P (kg muscle)$^{-1}$·s$^{-1}$ corresponding totally to 2.35 mol $^{\sim}$P·min$^{-1}$.
b. Amount available (quadriceps muscle): 240 mmol $^{\sim}$P·kg$^{-1}$ or totally 6.7 mol in 28 kg of muscle.

The estimate of 1.4 mmol $^{\sim}$P (kg muscle)$^{-1}$·s$^{-1}$ was calculated from direct measurements of the metabolite changes during near maximum isometric contraction of the quadriceps muscle.[27,28] The total amount of $^{\sim}$P available from glycogen was calculated, assuming that 90% of the normal store (i.e., 80 mmol glucose units·kg$^{-1}$) is used[13] and that 3 mmol·$^{\sim}$P is formed per mole of glucose in glycolysis. Total use of the muscle glycogen stores, however, never occurs, because of increased acidosis within the muscle. According to Margaria et al., the accumulation of 1 mol of lactate is the maximum the body is able to tolerate.[34] This amount would limit the total amount of $^{\sim}$P from anaerobic use of glycogen to 1.5 mol during heavy continuous work.

$$\text{Glycogen} \rightarrow CO_2 + H_20 \quad (2b)$$

a. Max. rate of $^{\sim}$P generation: 0.51 to 0.68 mmol $^{\sim}$P (kg muscle)$^{-1}$·s$^{-1}$ corresponding totally to 0.85 to 1.14 mol $^{\sim}$P·min$^{-1}$.
b. Amount available (quadriceps femoris): 3.000 mmol $^{\sim}$P·kg$^{-1}$ or totally 84 mol in 28 kg of muscle.

The limiting factor for the rate of glycogen oxidation is most probably mitochondrial electron transport determined by the activity of the oxygen transfer mechanisms. The rates of 0.51 to 0.68 were calculated assuming maximum rates of oxygen use available for glycogen oxidation of 3 L·$O_2$·min$^{-1}$ in an untrained individual and 4 L·min$^{-1}$ in a marathon runner. Aerobic glycogen degradation gives 38 mol $^{\sim}$P per mole glucose.

$$\text{Glucose} \rightarrow CO_2 + H_2O \quad (2c)$$

a. Max. rate of $^{\sim}$P generation: 0.22 mmol $^{\sim}$P (kg muscle)$^{-1}$·s$^{-1}$ corresponding totally to 0.16 mol $^{\sim}$P·min$^{-1}$.
b. Total amount available: 18 mol $^{\sim}$P.

The maximum rate of use is approximate and assumes maximum output from the liver of 5 mmol glucose per minute of which 4 mmol·min$^{-1}$ are available to the working muscles (calculated in this study as 11 kg).[20,35] During a short period of exercise, most of this glucose is derived from the use of liver glycogen, which corresponds to 500 mmol glucose totally in the resting state after a mixed diet.[36] This quantity will amount to 18 mol $^{\sim}$P.

$$\text{Fatty acids} \rightarrow CO_2 + H_2O \quad (3)$$

a. Max. rate of $^{\sim}$P generation: 0.24 mmol $^{\sim}$P (kg muscle)$^{-1}$·s$^{-1}$ corresponding totally to 0.4 mol $^{\sim}$P·min$^{-1}$.
b. Amount available: in adipose tissues, about 4.000 mol $^{\sim}$P.

The maximum rate of $^{\sim}$P generation, which was calculated by McGilvery,[37] is based on experimental results published by Pernow and Saltin.[38] As noted by McGilvery, the low rate of $^{\sim}$P generation from FFA oxidation must be the result of a limiting step located before formation of acetyl coenzyme A (CoA), because the later steps are also used when carbohydrates are oxidized.

## SUBSTRATE USE IN RELATION TO WORK LOAD

The mechanisms by which the muscle cells regulate the use of the different fuels are complex. In essence, FFA constitute the main energy substrate at rest and are used in preference to carbohydrate, principally muscle glycogen, while at supramaximal work loads, phosphagens are the major fuels. At no one work load, however, does muscle use just one fuel.

Some examples of energy demands during different types of exercise are given in Table 42–1. The rate of energy expenditure and the amount of energy needed for the activity determine the choice of substrate. Estimates of the energy requirement used in different activities are derived from Fox.[39] Estimates of maximum rates available from the different fuel sources together with the total amount available are drawn from our own work based on direct measurements from biopsy studies, with

**TABLE 42–1.** ENERGY REQUIREMENT FOR DIFFERENT ACTIVITIES AND THE MAX RATE OF ENERGY PROVISION AND AMOUNTS AVAILABLE FROM DIFFERENT SUBSTRATES (~P MOL·MIN$^{-1}$ AND $^{\sim}$P MOL, RESPECTIVELY)

| | ENERGY REQUIREMENT | | AVAILABLE FROM SUBSTRATES | | |
|---|---|---|---|---|---|
| ACTIVITY | rate | amount | max. rate | amount | |
| 100-m sprint | 2.6 | 0.43 | 4.4 | 0.50 | ATP+PCr |
| 400-m sprint | 2.3 | 1.72 | — | — | |
| 800-m run | 2.0 | 3.43 | 2.35 | 1.50 | Glucolysis* (anaerobic) |
| 1500-m run | 1.7 | 6.00 | 0.85–1.14 | 85 | Glucose oxidation |
| Marathon | 1.0 | 150.00 | 0.4–0.6 | 4000 | All of the above plus fat oxidation |
| Rest | 0.07 | 0.36 | — | — | |

*Available amount from glucolysis is calculated from the amount of lactate tolerated by the body, i.e., 1 mol totally.

the exception of the estimates for fat oxidation. Values for fat oxidation are recalculated by McGilvery from studies by Pernow and Saltin. The maximum rate during 100-m sprint has been estimated to be 2.6 mol ~P·min$^{-1}$. This value is below the maximum rate obtainable from PCr breakdown but above that from anaerobic glucolysis. On energetic grounds, therefore, ATP and PCr are obligatory fuels for this level of activity, although supply is augmented by anaerobic glucolysis. It was held previously that, during intense exercise, an alactic acid period of up to 10 seconds occurred, but we have shown that lactic acid accumulation may in fact begin within as little as 1.3 sec.[29] Other athletic activities that depend mainly on PCr breakdown are shot-put, high-jump, javelin, tossing the caber, and the hammer throw.

During a 400-m sprint, PCr breakdown again is used to meet the rate of ~P expenditure (2.3 mol·min$^{-1}$) but is in itself insufficient to cover the total energy requirement of 1.72 mol ~P. To meet this demand, further energy is required from anaerobic glucolysis with, in practice, an increasing contribution from aerobic glucolysis as the race continues. The same is true both for 800- and 1500-m runs, but in these races, total expenditure exceeds even the combined total possible from PCr breakdown and tolerance from the accumulation of lactate. At these distances, energy demand by necessity also requires oxidative use of muscle glycogen. At ultra long distances, such as the marathon, the ATP turnover rate in an elite athlete lies just below the rate sustainable by aerobic use of carbohydrate; however, the total demand would require considerable use of fat as well. When all available carbohydrate has been used, running speed is dictated by the maximum rate of fat use. This point is probably reached in marathon runners at around 15 to 20 miles, depending on how the race is run, and is synonymous with "hitting the wall." From then on, the race is run on fat oxidation as the only fuel available, with little or no possibility for acceleration of pace.

The preceding calculations are of course drawn from athletic performances, but undoubtedly, the same spectrum of fuel use also exists in occupational work ranging from light office work to hard intermittent manual labor.

Because of delays in the mobilization of the different fuel sources and adjustments of the circulation, some use of PCr occurs whenever the rate of energy demand is suddenly increased. When the rate of energy demand, however, is less than the maximum rate from anaerobic glucolysis, resynthesis of PCr, even during continuation of the work, is possible. The increase in lactate and resultant decrease in pH also affects the PCr level, because the increase in hydrogen ions displaces the equilibrium of the creatine kinase reaction toward creatine. Net use of PCr therefore always occurs when lactate is accumulating.

Accumulation of lactate is, however, self-limiting, because the decrease in muscle pH in turn inhibits further glycolysis and/or muscle contraction at the end of work with maximum power output. Under these conditions, total use of the glycogen store never occurs. At work rates close to the subject's maximum oxygen uptake ($VO_2$max), total glycogen use in the working muscles can occur (Fig. 42–1), and the amount of glycogen initially present is a determinant of work capacity. If work continues beyond this point, the work rate will decline as the muscles become progressively more dependent on FFA and blood-borne glucose for their supply of energy. As previously discussed, the maximum rate of ~P production from these two sources is appreciably lower than that from local muscle glycogen degradation.

During any form of prolonged exercise in excess of 1 hour, the use of fat progressively increases with time because of the increased availability of FFA. For instance, in a study by Ahlborg et al., a 4-hour exercise at a work load corresponding to 30% of $VO_2$max resulted in an energy contribution by FFA of 37% during the first 40 minutes, and this amount increased to 62% during the final hour (Fig. 42–2).[40]

The estimates of maximal fuel use given previously were calculated for a normal individual. In endurance-trained subjects, maximum fuel use from FFA can be higher because of an increased capacity to oxidize FFA.[41–44] Thus, the maximum power output that can be sustained by FFA use is higher, increasing from 55 to 65% of the subject's $VO_2$max. Above this level, however, work performance is still limited by availability of muscle glycogen. The relationship between glycogen degrada-

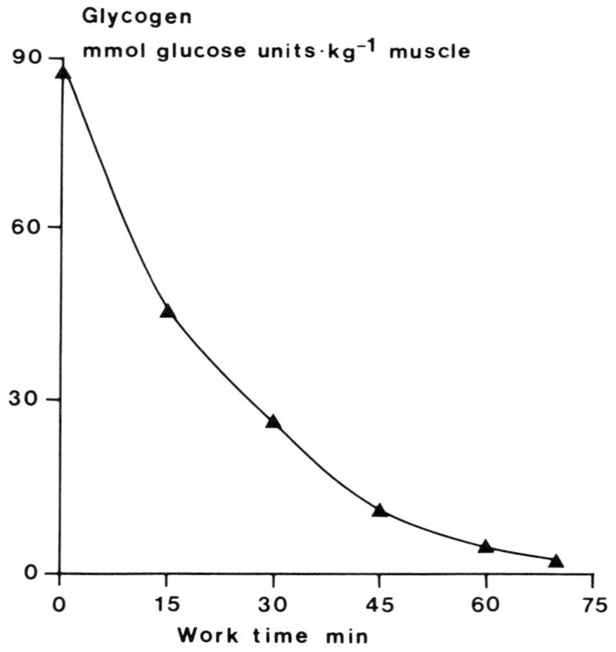
Glycogen
mmol glucose units·kg⁻¹ muscle
90
60
30
0
0
15
30
45
60
75
Work time min

**FIGURE 42–1.** The glycogen content in the quadriceps femoris muscle during continuous bicycle exercise maintained at a load corresponding to 80% $VO_2$max.[14] Each point is the mean value determined on 10 subjects. In each case the exercise was continued until exhaustion, at which time depletion of the muscle glycogen stores was virtually complete. (From Bergström, J., Hultman, E.: Scand. J. Clin. Lab. Invest., *19*:218–228, 1967.)

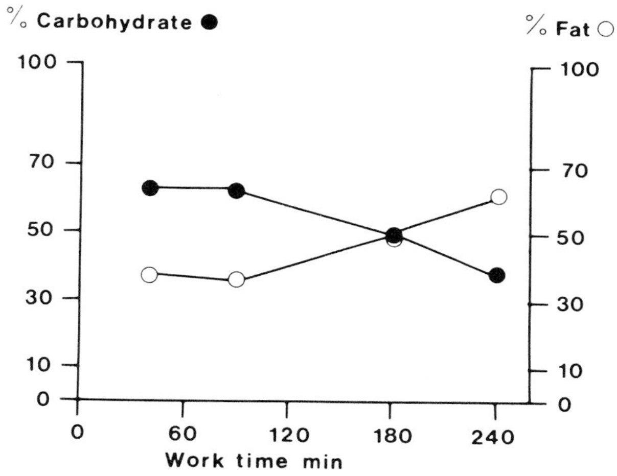
% Carbohydrate ●
% Fat ○
100
70
50
30
10
0
0
60
120
180
240
Work time min

**FIGURE 42–2.** The utilization of carbohydrate (predominantly muscle glycogen) and fat during prolonged exercise, i.e. bicycle exercise at a work load of 40% $VO_2$max. (From Ahlborg, G., Felig, G., Hagenfeldt, L., et al.: J. Clin. Invest., *53:*1080–1090, 1974.)

tion rate and work intensity is shown in Figure 42–3. The almost exponential rise in rate of glycogen degradation with increase in work load is consistent with: (1) high use of other energy sources (predominantly fat) at low work loads; (2) principally oxidative use of glycogen at middle loads; and (3) rapid but energetically inefficient anaerobic use of glycogen at the highest work loads.

## USE OF PROTEIN

The quantitative role of protein as an energy substrate in the isocaloric state is small, contributing at most about 5 to 10% of the total energy turnover.[46,47] Nonetheless, during periods of prolonged exercise or training, the degradation of protein can be of importance with respect to whole body homeostasis, and as such merits further discussion.

Results of studies have shown that the extracellular level of urea nitrogen increases during prolonged exercise,[46,48–50] and urinary output of urea increases during the rest period immediately after exercise.[49–52] In addition, measurements of the uptake and release of amino acids over the working muscles and over the splanchnic area, and of the metabolism of isotopically labeled amino acids also indicate a significant contribution by protein to total energy turnover during exercise. Transport of amino acids from the working muscles in the form of alanine and glutamine was first shown by Felig and co-workers.[53–55] The carbon skeletons of alanine and glutamine apparently were derived from pyruvate and glutamate and the amino groups from the deamination of amino acids in the muscle. The alanine and glutamine are converted to glucose in the liver.[53] It was also shown that branched amino acids were released from the liver and taken up by working muscle.[40]

Findings of studies have also suggested that branched-chain amino acids are oxidized during prolonged exercise to exhaustion at 75% $VO_2$max, and that a significant amount of the ammonia released from muscle is derived from amino acid degradation.[56,57] When a low carbohydrate diet was ingested before exercise at 75% $VO_2$max, resting plasma branched amino acid concentrations were elevated and the exercise-induced decrease in these amino acids was greater, suggesting that amino acid oxidation was higher.[58] Plasma ammonia levels were also elevated during exercise, suggesting that a significant amount of the released ammonia was derived from amino acid metabolism.

It also has been shown that the carbon skeleton of the branched chain amino acid leucine is used for production of $CO_2$ during exercise,[59–61] and that the rate at which this occurs is related to the work output.[62,63] Use of leucine, however, is modified by the amount of glycogen available in the muscles; a high glycogen content depresses the rate of leucine use.[46] Glucose infusion during exercise also decreases the use of leucine,[62] whereas increased availability of FFA can have

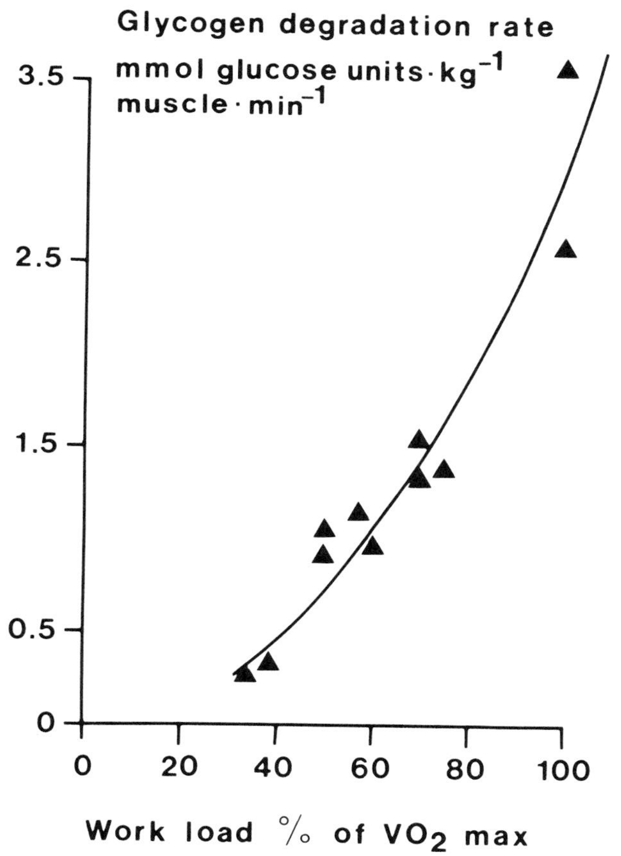
Glycogen degradation rate
mmol glucose units·kg⁻¹ muscle·min⁻¹
3.5
2.5
1.5
0.5
0
0
20
40
60
80
100
Work load % of VO2 max

**FIGURE 42–3.** The rate of muscle glycogen degradation during bicycle exercise sustained at different work loads. (From Hultman, E.: Muscle glycogen store and prolonged exercise. *In* Frontiers of Fitness. Edited by E.J. Shephard. Springfield, IL, Charles C Thomas, 1971.)

the opposite effect.[64] Increased oxidation of fat as a result of increased availability of FFA or decreased use of carbohydrate during prolonged exercise apparently increases the oxidation of the carbon skeleton of branched chain amino acids, possibly by direct stimulation of the oxidative decarboxylation of the ketoacids formed.[64]

Possible sources of amino acids for energy production are the free amino acid pool in muscle or plasma or those released from protein catabolism. A decrease of the amino acids in plasma has been observed during prolonged exercise.[51,65,66] Similarly, Rennie et al. found a decrease in the content of free amino acids in muscle at the end of prolonged exercise, and calculated that the decrease in the amino acid pool in plasma and muscle corresponded to 20% of the total nitrogen loss.[50] Thus, 80% of the nitrogen in this study must have been derived from the degradation of body protein. The origin of this protein, however, is not known. Studies of 3-methylhistidine excretion as a marker of muscle protein turnover have given conflicting results,[51,62,67] but generally they indicate that the contractile proteins are not broken down in exercise bouts if no apparent damage occurs to the muscle cells. Millward et al. indicated that the liver may be an important source of protein for use by the working muscles.[62] Most probably, the use of protein as a fuel represents a general effect in which the normal protein synthesis rate (about 300 g protein/day$^{-1}$)[68] is decreased and part of the amino acids released through normal protein degradation is directed to the supply of energy in working muscle cells. During recovery after prolonged exercise, an increase in the rate of protein synthesis has been observed.[50]

## ENERGY STORES AND EXERCISE CAPACITY

### PHOSPHAGEN

At supramaximum loads with endurance times of just a few seconds, energy supply is mainly derived from the use of phosphagen supplemented by anaerobic glucolysis. The phosphagen stores, however, are seemingly impervious to dietary manipulation and are unaffected by training.[69,70] Consequently, no easy way is known to increase maximum power output by this means.

### CARBOHYDRATE

At work intensities close to or above the subject's $VO_2max$, lactate accumulation, with attendant decrease in muscle pH, inhibits work output and energy production before depletion of the local glycogen stores. However, at work intensities corresponding to 65 to 85% $VO_2max$, the whole muscle store of glycogen may be used if the exercise is sufficiently prolonged; the power output from the muscle then declines. Onset of hypoglycemia can limit prolonged performance if the liver glycogen store at the start of exercise is low and no carbohydrate is taken during the work. In this range, any increase in the muscle glycogen store helps to improve performance. Increased glycogen storage can, as will be discussed, be achieved by one or more regimens of exercise and diet.

### FAT

Because of the almost limitless stores of FFA in the well-fed individual, no grounds exist for supposing that increase in the lipid stores will increase endurance even during excessively prolonged exercise periods. The limitation to work at low work loads appears to be related to factors other than the lack of substrate.

### PROTEIN

In contrast to fat and carbohydrates, no evidence exists of any specific body protein store available for exercise that can be increased by diet. A dietary effect related to protein, however, is the protein-sparing effect of carbohydrates as shown by a lower use of protein when blood glucose levels and muscle glycogen content are high.[46,62] Lemon and Mullin have shown that the protein share of the energy substrates used during a 60-minute exercise was 4% if the glycogen store in the muscle was increased, but 10% if it was depleted before the start of exercise.[46] Therefore, it is important that athletes engaged in frequent training sessions increase their total energy intake to meet the needs of the training. The majority of the increased energy intake should be in the form of carbohydrate.

## NUTRITION FOR INCREASED WORK PERFORMANCE

### MUSCLE GLYCOGEN STORE AND DIET

Initial studies on the influence of diet on the muscle glycogen stores showed that the feeding of a carbohydrate-rich diet or a carbohydrate-poor diet or even total starvation over a period of days had little effect on the stores at rest (Fig. 42–4).[16] However, a remarkable difference was noted between diets in the rate of glycogen synthesis when feeding was preceded by depletion of the stores by exercise. Total starvation or a carbohydrate-free diet resulted in low rates of resynthesis, and normal values were not achieved for several days, whereas a carbohydrate-rich diet resulted in a rapid resynthesis to values above the normal range (Fig. 42–5). Results of studies in which one leg only was exercised showed that rapid resynthesis of glycogen to supernormal values was a local phenomenon restricted to the exercised muscles (Figs. 42–6 and 42–7).[9]

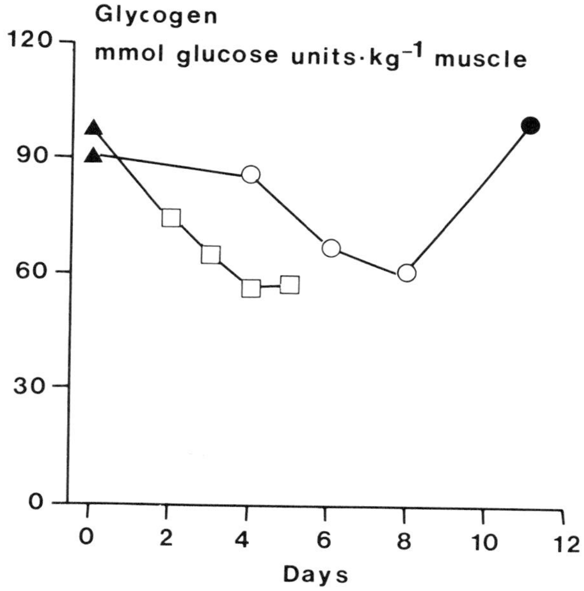
Glycogen
mmol glucose units·kg-1 muscle
120
90
60
30
0
0
2
4
6
8
10
12
Days

**FIGURE 42–4.** Glycogen content in the quadriceps femoris muscle after mixed diet (solid triangles), during 5 days of total starvation (open squares), and during 8 days of carbohydrate-free diet (open circles) followed by a carbohydrate-rich diet (solid circle). (From Hultman, E., Bergström, J.: Acta Med. Scand., *182*:109–117, 1967.)

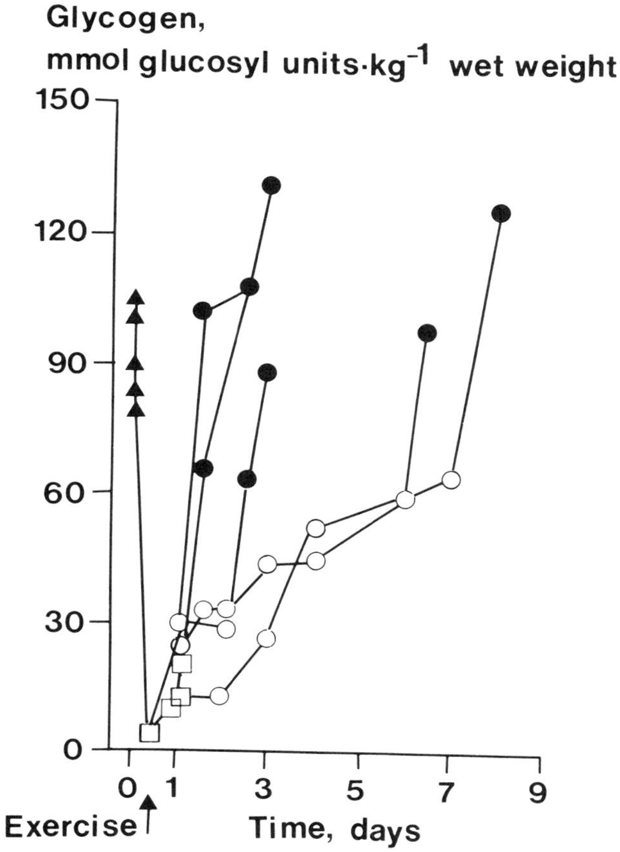
Glycogen,
mmol glucosyl units·kg-1 wet weight
150
120
90
60
30
0
0
1
3
5
7
9
Exercise
Time, days

**FIGURE 42–5.** Muscle glycogen content before and after exercise. Before exercise the diet was normal mixed (solid triangles), and on the following days either total starvation (open squares) or a carbohydrate-free diet (open circles) was followed by 1 or 2 days of carbohydrate-rich diet (solid circles).[16] Note the slow rate of glycogen resynthesis when the diet is carbohydrate free compared to the rate when the diet is rich in carbohydrate (see also Fig. 42–7).

The mechanism by which "supercompensation" in glycogen is brought about is not known. Enzyme studies have revealed that the enzyme, glycogen synthetase, responsible for glycogen formation is transformed from inactive D form to active I form when the glycogen store is depleted. After 1 day of carbohydrate refeeding, the I form is decreased to normal.[71] Other forms of the enzyme, intermediate between active and inactive, however, have been described,[72] and these forms could account for the continuation of glycogen synthesis to supernormal values.

The dramatic effect of increased muscle glycogen content on work capacity is illustrated in Figure 42–8. In this study, exhaustive exercise was repeated three times with an interval of 3 days between bouts. The diet given before the first exercise was a normal mixed diet, which was followed by a carbohydrate-free diet and finally (before the last exercise) by a carbohydrate-rich diet.[18] The effect of the different diets was an increase in work time from 1 hour after the carbohydrate-free diet to 3 hours or more after the carbohydrate-rich diet. The study was done originally to demonstrate the relationship between work capacity and the size of the muscle glycogen stores, but the method used to increase the muscle glycogen content has since been adopted as a procedure by athletes to increase these stores. A drawback to this regimen is that it leaves athletes with extremely low muscle glycogen stores for a period of 2 to 3 days, and this state could interfere with training. Sherman et al. proposed a modified regimen of diet and exercise that avoids any period of carbohydrate-free diet, yet still results in equally high glycogen levels.[73] For subjects in regular training, it is probably sufficient if they perform a depleting exercise twice during a period of mixed diet and thereafter change to a carbohydrate-rich diet during the final 3 days before competition. During the first two of these days, light exercise is possible, leaving only the last day for total rest.

Glycogen is stored in muscle together with water and potassium ions, 1 g (6 mmol) being associated with 2.7 g of water and 0.45 mmol of potassium.[21,74,75] As a result, supercompensation in glycogen results in considerable increases in muscle water content, which increases body weight and may induce feelings of heaviness and stiffness in the muscle. Supercompensation cannot therefore be recommended for athletes needing only limited supplies of glycogen, e.g., sprinters.

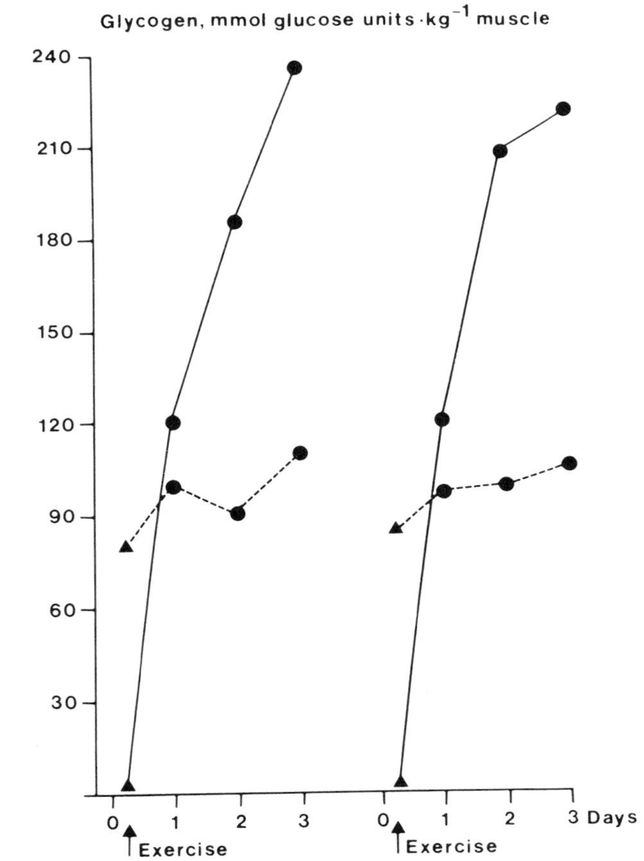
Glycogen, mmol glucose units·kg⁻¹ muscle
240
210
180
150
120
90
60
30
0 1 2 3 0 1 2 3 Days
Exercise
Exercise

**FIGURE 42–6.** One-leg exercise study showing the glycogen content of the exercised (solid lines) and the rested (broken lines) leg in two subjects. Biopsies were obtained immediately after the exercise and during 3 days when subjects were fed a carbohydrate-rich diet.

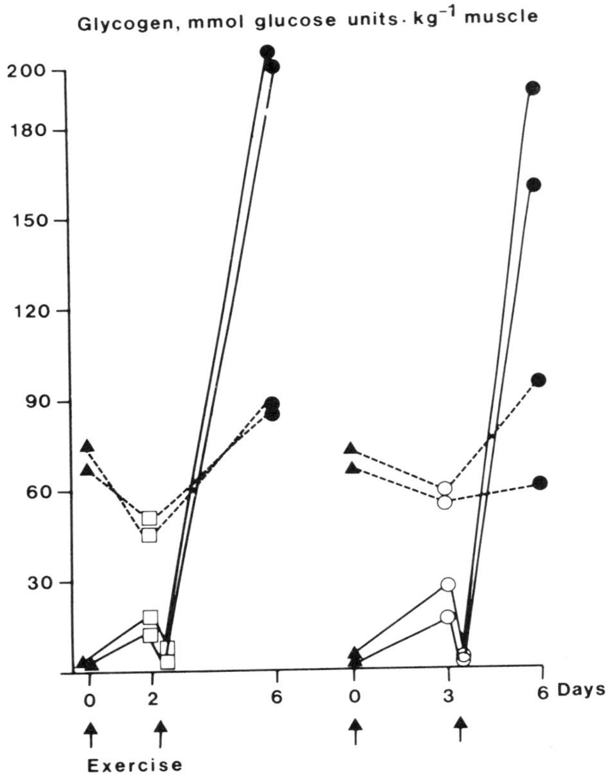
Glycogen, mmol glucose units·kg⁻¹ muscle
200
180
150
120
90
60
30
0 2 6 0 3 6 Days
Exercise

**FIGURE 42–7.** The some "one-leg exercise" procedure as in Figure 42–6 showing the glycogen content in the exercised (solid lines) and the rested leg (broken lines). The diet was either total starvation (open squares) or carbohydrate free (open circles) during 2 and 3 days, respectively. This was followed by a second one-leg exercise, and thereafter a carbohydrate-rich diet (solid circles) was given. The solid triangles represent a normal diet.

## LIVER GLYCOGEN STORE—EFFECT OF DIET

In contrast to muscle, the liver glycogen store is extremely labile, even in the resting state. The glycogen content after an overnight fast varies from 90 to 500 mmol glucose units·kg$^{-1}$ liver tissue (about 14 to 80 g glycogen).[36] This value corresponds to a total glycogen store of 160 to 900 mmol glucose units in a 1.8-kg liver, which is the normal weight. Measurements of glycogen in repeated liver biopsy samples taken in the postprandial state showed a continuous decrease, amounting to 0.3 mmol glucose units·min·kg$^{-1}$ liver, from which it can be calculated that just 1 day of starvation would empty the liver glycogen stores.[23] This situation was found in two subjects from whom biopsies were taken after 1 day without food intake. The liver glycogen stores decreased from 155 to 24 and 345 to 48 mmol glucose units·kg$^{-1}$. In one of the two subjects, the period of starvation was continued for a further 2 days with biopsies performed each morning. Liver glycogen contents in these biopsy samples were 15 and 21 mmol glucose units·kg$^{-1}$ (Fig. 42–9).[23]

It is known, however, that during even short periods of starvation, an increase occurs in both fat and protein degradation, which results in an increase in gluconeogenic substrate brought to the liver. Evidently, this increase is not sufficient for de novo synthesis of glycogen to occur in the liver. To increase the supply of gluconeogenic substrates, we gave a diet consisting of protein and fat with a caloric content of 8.400 kilojoules (kJ) per day. Still no increase in liver glycogen content occurred during a 10-day period (Fig. 42–9).[23] When the diet was changed to one rich in carbohydrates with the same caloric content, an immediate increase occurred in the liver glycogen content (up to 500 to 600 mmol glucose units·kg$^{-1}$). Carbohydrate intake through the diet is obviously necessary for preservation of the liver glycogen store. In these studies, the fat and protein diet consisted of bacon, eggs, meat, vegetable oils, butter, and small amounts of tomatoes and lettuce, whereas the carbohydrate-rich diet contained 90% carbohydrate in the form

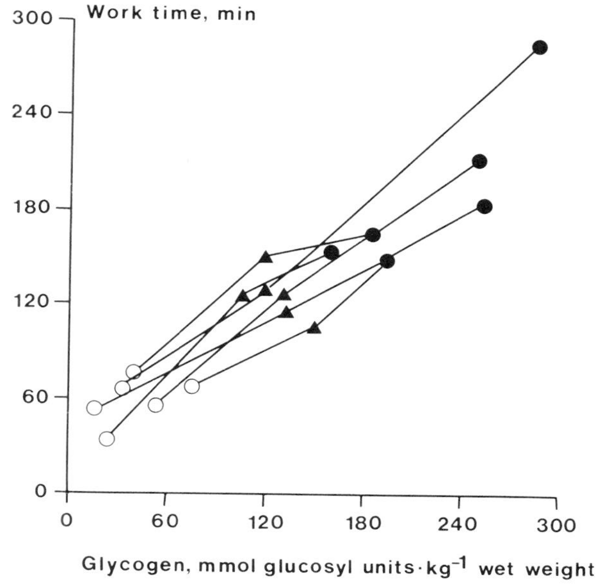

Work time, min
300
240
180
120
60
0
0
60
120
180
240
300
Glycogen, mmol glucosyl units·kg$^{-1}$ wet weight


**FIGURE 42–8.** The relationship between the initial glycogen content in the quadriceps femoris muscle and work time. Bicycle work was performed to exhaustion at a work load corresponding to 75% of $VO_2$max. Each subject worked three times and the experiments were preceded by 3 days of a dietary regimen: initially a mixed normal diet (solid triangles), followed by a carbohydrate-free diet (open circles) and thereafter a carbohydrate-rich diet (solid circles). The energy content of the diets was the same. (From Bergström, J., Hermansen, L., Hultman, E., et al.: Acta Physiol. Scand., *71*:140–150, 1967.)

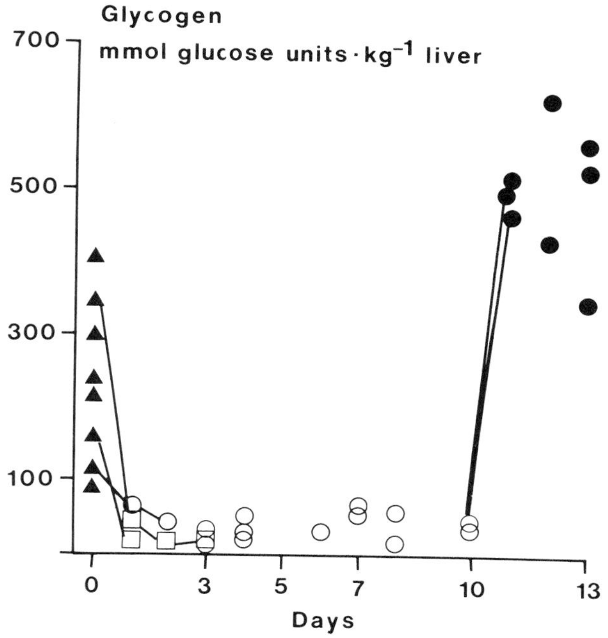

Glycogen
mmol glucose units·kg$^{-1}$ liver
700
500
300
100
0
3
5
7
10
13
Days


**FIGURE 42–9.** The glycogen content in the liver determined in needle biopsy specimens from normal subjects after different diets. A normal mixed diet (solid triangles) was followed by 1 or 3 days of starvation (open squares) or 1 to 10 days of a carbohydrate-free diet (open circles). The period was ended by 1 or 3 days of a carbohydrate-rich diet (closed circles).

of bread, spaghetti, potatoes, sugar, fruit, and juice. Spices and meat extract were added for taste.

The blood glucose concentration during fasting or during the period of carbohydrate-free diet decreased only marginally, from 5.2 to 4.3 mmol·L$^{-1}$ after 10 days with the lowest value being recorded on day 5 (3.8 mmol·L$^{-1}$). Only light office work was done during the experimental period. The glucose output by the liver decreased, however, by 60%, which corresponds to the share normally derived from glycogen degradation.[24] The fact that the blood glucose concentration shows only a small change is the result of various adaptations in body metabolism, including an increased output of ketone bodies from the liver[24] and a shift from glucose use to ketone body oxidation by the brain.[76,77] Seemingly, the adaptation by the brain is a rapid process.

## LIVER GLYCOGEN STORE—GLUCOSE RELEASE AND EFFECT OF EXERCISE

During exercise, glucose output from the liver increases. In one study of heavy bicycle exercise, a continuous increase in output was seen from 1 mmol·min$^{-1}$ before exercise up to 5 mmol·min$^{-1}$ during the last minute of the work.[20] The average output over the whole of the exercise period was 2.4 mmol·min$^{-1}$. In a further study in which liver biopsies were taken, 1 hour of hard bicycle exercise resulted in a mean glycogen degradation rate of 2.1 mmol glucose units·min$^{-1}$·kg$^{-1}$ liver.[25] This result means that up to one half of the normal liver glycogen store is lost during 1 hour of heavy exercise, and that most of the glucose output is derived from liver glycogen and only a small fraction from the uptake and use of lactate, amino acids, and glycerol.

If exercise is performed after a carbohydrate-free diet, glucose output from liver glycogen is decreased and is compensated only in part by increased gluconeogenesis. The effect, therefore, is a decrease in the blood glucose concentration during exercise. This process is illustrated in the study of Bergström et al. mentioned previously in which a pronounced decrease in blood glucose concentration was seen shortly after the start of the exercise performed after the period of carbohydrate-free diet.[18] In this study, the mean glucose content decreased during the first hour of exercise from 5.0 to 2.8 mmol·L$^{-1}$ blood, and several of the subjects suffered from headache and dizziness during the later part of the exercise. For one subject, the work had to be stopped because of hypoglycemic effects on the central nervous system. The blood glucose concentration was 1.7 mmol·L$^{-1}$, and the subject could not continue the exercise because of severe dizziness and headache. The corresponding blood glucose level after the carbohydrate-rich diet was 4.4 mmol·L$^{-1}$

after 1 hour of exercise and 3.5 mmol·L$^{-1}$ at the end of the work (after 3 hours).

Glucose production through gluconeogenesis normally is not increased during short-term exercise, but it can increase during prolonged work to values nearly twice the resting level.[40] An increased rate of gluconeogenesis, however, does occur during short intervals of hard exercise preceded by a period of carbohydrate-free diet,[35,78] although total glucose output, as previously mentioned, is still lower than after a normal mixed diet. After a carbohydrate-free diet, approximately 50% of the glucose release from the liver can be accounted for by use of gluconeogenic substrates, whereas after a carbohydrate-rich diet, the corresponding share is only 5 to 10%. After the carbohydrate-free diet, an increase in oxygen uptake by the liver was observed,[78] which is consistent with the increased rate of gluconeogenesis, this being an energy-consuming process.

In summary, dietary increase of the liver glycogen stores would be beneficial in most types of continuous or prolonged intermittent exercise/work. During work of several hours duration, a high liver glycogen level acts as a buffer against the development of hypoglycemia, which may lead to deleterious effects on central nervous function and exhaustion. One day of carbohydrate-rich diet before a competition is sufficient to produce high levels of glycogen in the liver.

## ENERGY REQUIREMENTS

### DURING OCCUPATIONAL WORK

The caloric need at rest has been calculated by Passmore and Durnin to be 105 kJ·kg$^{-1}$ body weight (BW)·day$^{-1}$ for men and 100 kJ·kg$^{-1}$ BW·day$^{-1}$ for women.[79] The FAO/WHO recommendations on the energy needs for men and women in occupational work are indicated in Table 42–2.[80] These estimates are for subjects with body weights of 65 and 55 kg, respectively, and aged 20 to 39 years. Energy requirement decreases with increasing age; subjects aged 40 to 49 years require 95% of the preceding estimates; 50 to 59 years, 90%; 60 to 69 years, 80%; and above 70 years old, 70%. Energy needs increase with activity (see Fig. 42–2). The figures in Table 42–2 are similar to those presented by other authors such as Norgan and Ferro-Luzzi for Italian shipyard workers engaged in occupational work requiring light activity.[81] The same authors also studied horticulturists in Papua-New Guinea and found a similar requirement in dietary energy of 160 to 190 kJ·kg$^{-1}$ BW·day$^{-1}$. Total energy requirements are obtained by multiplying the preceding estimates by body weight. Thus, for occupational work with light activity, total daily requirements for a 65-kg man and 55-kg woman would be 10.9 mega joules (MJ)* and 8.4 MJ, respectively.[80] More recent FAO/WHO data are available expressing energy costs per minute for various activities and are summarized in Appendix Table A–8d; energy costs as multiples of BMR are given in Appendix Table A–8e (see also Chap. 5).

### DURING EXERCISE

The energy requirement during athletic performance or training is of course determined by the type of activity and its duration. Several studies of the relative caloric costs of different sports have been published.[79,82] No details are given here, however, except to note that requirements vary from 12.5 to 25 MJ, the higher values associated with high-intensity endurance sports such as cross-country running or skiing and marathon running. High-energy intakes of the same order are also required in the course of sports requiring intense repetitive effort such as team sports (football, ice hockey, basketball), tennis, and fencing. In sports requiring sustained intense effort but over shorter periods, such as swimming events over 100 yd, wrestling, downhill skiing, and running for 1 to 2 miles, the average daily expenditure is on the order of 12.5 to 21 MJ. The lowest energy requirement, up to 16.7 MJ per day, is observed in low intensity sports of long duration such as baseball or golf, and when strenuous or maximal efforts are produced only during short periods, i.e., hurdles, long-jump, 50- to 100-yd swimming events, discus, hammer throw, high-jump, and javelin.

The total caloric need is influenced also by the body weight, the frequency of repetition of the event, and the length of practice during training. Training itself increases the daily caloric need by 5 to 40% depending on the nature of the exercise and the length of practice (for further details, see references[82]). The preceding estimates of energy expenditure have been adapted from Buskirk and are calculated to cover the caloric needs of

*1 MJ = 1000 kJ.

**TABLE 42–2.** ENERGY NEEDS FOR OCCUPATIONAL WORK

| ACTIVITY | MEN | WOMEN |
|---|---|---|
| Light | 167 kJ·kg$^{-1}$·day$^{-1}$ | 157 kJ·kg$^{-1}$·day$^{-1}$ |
| Moderate | 192 kJ·kg$^{-1}$·day$^{-1}$ | 167 kJ·kg$^{-1}$·day$^{-1}$ |
| High | 225 kJ·kg$^{-1}$·day$^{-1}$ | 194 kJ·kg$^{-1}$·day$^{-1}$ |
| Exceptionally high | 257 kJ·kg$^{-1}$·day$^{-1}$ | 225 kJ·kg$^{-1}$·day$^{-1}$ |

(From FAO/WHO Expert Committee Report: WHO Tech. Rep. Ser. *52*:1–118, 1973.)

75% of all male subjects.[82] Women athletes require 10% fewer calories to cover the energy need for each type of sport, or during training.

## RECOMMENDED USE OF MACRONUTRIENTS DURING WORK

Estimates of energy expenditure during normal occupational work were given in the previous section. This energy can be derived from a variety of combinations of fat and carbohydrate. Protein is used as a significant energy source only when the carbohydrate stores have been exhausted and then only during prolonged work periods. Use of available free amino acids, may occur although as indicated previously, their contribution to the total amount of energy used is probably small.

As seen in Table 42–3, the amount of energy stored as fat in the body is far in excess of that stored as carbohydrate. Theoretically, fat is capable of sustaining light work for long periods without supplementation. In contrast, the body's glycogen store would be exhausted within half a day if used exclusively. In practice, light occupational work relies mainly on fat use delaying considerably the exhaustion of the carbohydrate stores. At exceptionally high work loads, the capacity to oxidize fats is insufficient to meet the energy needs. At these work rates, carbohydrate therefore plays the central role in energy provision. Only carbohydrate use is adequate in matching the high rates of energy expenditure necessary to fulfil the work task. In practice, intense labor is interspersed with periods of lighter activity with lower energy demand sustainable through fat oxidation. The limited availability of the carbohydrate store in the body (Table 42–3), however, ultimately determines the duration of the work. This fact emphasizes the importance of a regular intake of carbohydrate in amounts sufficient to keep the body's stores high.

### CARBOHYDRATE

Dietary carbohydrate is essential both for the maintenance of the liver glycogen store and for the rapid resynthesis of muscle glycogen. A loss of liver glycogen results in decrease in the blood glucose content, and a lack of muscle glycogen decreases the work capacity. Omitting carbohydrate from the diet for more than 1 day will result in increased ketone-body production, degradation of body protein, and loss of cations and water. These effects are counteracted by a minimum intake of about 100 g of carbohydrate (600 mmol glucose units) per day.

Generally, however, it is recommended that 55 to 60% of the energy content of the diet should consist of carbohydrate. In a 70-kg man given a normal mixed diet, 70 to 150 g carbohydrate are stored as glycogen in the liver and 300 to 500 g in the muscles. The energy equivalents of these stores are 1.25 to 2.5 MJ and 5.0 to 8.3 MJ, respectively. As discussed previously, these stores may be greatly increased by using a combination of diet and exercise. If the carbohydrate intake is higher than the capacity for storage and its immediate requirements as an energy source, transformation to fat and subsequent storage as such will occur.

To obtain optimal usage of carbohydrates, the following foods should be included in the diet as complex saccharides, such as starch in bread, pasta, potatoes, rice, and cereals, and not as simple sugars, such as glucose and sucrose. Starch and other complex carbohydrates are digested more slowly in the intestine and are absorbed over a longer time, with the result that a larger fraction is deposited in the glycogen stores and less as fat.

### FAT

Fat in the form of FFA can be used directly as an energy substrate by most of the tissues in the body. Exceptions are the cells in the central nervous system and the red blood cells. Central nervous system cells are able to use both carbohydrate and ketone bodies if available, but the red blood cells and some other small cell compartments rely totally on carbohydrate. FFA constitutes the largest energy reserve in the body and is stored in the form of triglycerides in adipose tissue. The store in an average 70-kg man amounts to about 9 kg, which corresponds to approximately 338 MJ. It is generally recommended that the diet should contain 8 to 10% of the total energy in the form of polyunsaturated fatty acids, and the total fat intake should not exceed 30% of the dietary energy.

**TABLE 42–3.** FUEL STORES IN THE AVERAGE MAN

| | FUEL RESERVES | | DAYS RESERVES LAST IF USED AS EXCLUSIVE SOURCE | |
|---|---|---|---|---|
| FUEL | g | kJ | Light Exercise | Exceptionally High Activity |
| Adipose tissue | 9000 | 337,570 | 29 | 18.8 |
| Liver glycogen | 100 | 1,660 | 0.14 | 0.09 |
| Muscle glycogen | 350 | 5,800 | 0.5 | 0.3 |
| Blood glucose | 3 | 48 | — | — |

## PROTEIN

Dietary proteins provide amino acids for the de novo synthesis of proteins and other tissue constituents in the body. Replacement of protein is an ongoing process in the body. The result is a daily loss of nitrogen in the form of urea and amino acids, which must be covered by the intake of nitrogen-containing nutrients.

Amino acids taken up in the diet are used primarily for protein synthesis, but in excess, they are degraded rapidly because the body has no protein or amino acid store. An intake in excess of the need for synthesis of proteins results in increased formation of urea, which is excreted in urine and sweat. The carbon skeleton of the amino acids, however, is retained and used as an energy substrate. The carbon skeleton in some cases can also be converted to glucose in the liver. If protein and energy intake are greater than required, the extra amino acids may be converted to fat and carbohydrate and stored.

Energy production by the body is fundamental to life, and amino acids are used preferentially as an energy source if the total intake of energy is lower than the amount needed. Calculation of the minimum requirement of protein in the diet thus requires that the caloric need is adequately met by other sources in the food. The mean daily use of body protein in a normal individual fed a protein-free diet is of the order of 0.45 $g \cdot kg^{-1}$ BW.[83] When a high-quality protein is given, such as egg protein, the efficiency of use is about 70%, which increases the estimate of protein required to 0.59 $g \cdot kg^{-1}$ BW. For the North American diet, the average efficiency of use for the mixture of protein ingested is still lower, with the result that the recommended protein intake is increased to 0.8 $g \cdot kg^{-1}$ BW.[83] A 70-kg man would thus require 56 g protein a day, and a 55-kg woman would require 44 g.

## DIETARY PROTEIN INTAKE IN DIFFERENT DIETS

The actual protein intake in the average Swedish diet with an energy content of 11.7 MJ is 84 g of protein, corresponding to 1.2 $g \cdot kg^{-1}$ BW for a 70-kg man. This amount is 50% higher than the recommendations by the Committee on Dietary Allowances, Food and Nutrition Board (RDA).[83] The energy value of the protein intake corresponds to 12% of the total content in the Swedish diet. The corresponding value for protein intake for Italian shipyard workers is 12.5 to 12.8%,[84] the mean Japanese diet is reported to contain 14.4% of the energy in the form of protein,[85] the West German diet contains 11.1%,[86] and the American diet about 12%.[83]

## PROTEIN REQUIREMENT FOR ATHLETES DURING TRAINING

As discussed previously, the increase in the use of protein during exercise is only marginal. According to RDA, no increase in protein intake is needed when energy output is increased during training and competition, or even during heavy exercise.[83] The increased loss of protein during prolonged heavy exercise/work was estimated by Lemon and Mullin to amount to only 4% of the total energy expenditure when performed with adequate levels of glycogen in both muscle and liver, but about 10% when these were depleted.[46] Similar figures were presented by Rennie et al., who calculated the contribution of amino acid oxidation as 4 to 8% of the total energy expenditure during prolonged exercise (3 ¾ hours).[50] In recent studies examining the protein requirements of untrained subjects initiating a training program at 40 to 50% $VO_2max$, investigators found an initial decline in nitrogen balance that reached equilibrium within 2 weeks while ingesting 0.57 mg egg white $protein \cdot kg^{-1}$ $BW \cdot day^{-1}$.[87,88] The protein requirement for trained endurance runners maintained on an adequate energy intake and either 1.1 or 2.4 g mixed food $protein \cdot kg^{-1} \cdot day^{-1}$ during alternate 10-day periods was measured and compared to a sedentary control group.[89] The predicted nitrogen intake required for equilibrium was 1.37 and 0.73 $g \cdot kg^{-1} \cdot day^{-1}$ in the athlete and sedentary group, respectively.

These results suggest that athletes engaged in endurance training require more protein than sedentary individuals. However, the requirement is still well within the amount that the average North American consumes, so extra protein supplements are not required. Also, the protein requirements derived from high protein intakes may result in inflated values; however, the relative relationship of protein requirements between sedentary and trained individuals appears valid.[90] Thus, if protein is to be increased during heavy endurance training, it seems reasonable to limit the increase to 10% of the extra requirement of energy intake. Because the protein content of a normal diet constitutes 11 to 14% of the total energy, it will be sufficient to simply increase the amounts consumed to comply with the increase in energy requirement. No adjustment to the actual makeup of the diet is required. This recommendation is probably still true even when the daily energy requirement is far above that of normal athletes, as in ultraendurance events. An example is a study that simulated the 22-day Tour de France and demonstrated that these cyclists require in excess of 1.5 g of $protein \cdot kg^{-1} \cdot day^{-1}$.[91] This amount could be achieved by increasing the energy intake without altering the proportion of protein consumed.

In calculating the increase in protein required, however, it was assumed no preferential loss of any one essential amino acid (possible exception, leucine) occurred. If such a loss did occur, it would result in a negative nitrogen balance during longer periods of training, because the normal protein synthesis rate would decrease because of a lack of essential amino acids. Although findings of a few studies support this hypothesis,[48,52] most results indicate that nitrogen balance is maintained during training,[92–96] and may even be positive during heavy weight training,[97] when subjects are given a moderate protein intake of 0.8 to 1.4

$g \cdot kg^{-1} \cdot day^{-1}$. In the study of Marable and colleagues, an increase in lean body mass of 2 kg was observed after 28 days of heavy weight training with a protein intake of 0.8 $g\ kg^{-1} \cdot day^{-1}$.[97] A protein intake of 2.4 $g \cdot kg^{-1}$ resulted in a large increase in urinary nitrogen loss but the same rate of body protein synthesis. Similarly, Torún et al. found that total body potassium, an indicator of muscle mass, was unchanged or increased after 4 to 6 weeks of isometric exercise training when the subjects were given an egg protein intake of 1 $g \cdot kg^{-1} \cdot day^{-1}$.[92]

Much higher intakes of protein, however, are often seen in athletes. A dietary survey of Italian athletes showed an intake of protein corresponding to 17 to 18% of the energy content of the food or 2.2 to 2.8 $g \cdot kg^{-1}$ BW.[84] Laritcheva et al. reported a protein intake of 2.12 to 2.76 $g \cdot kg^{-1}$ in weight lifters during training, although this amount decreased to 1.36 to 1.80 $g \cdot kg^{-1}$ between training sessions.[98] Russian athletes studied by Rogozkin had a recommended intake of 13% of the dietary nutrients as protein for a total intake of 18.8 to 21 MJ, 12% for 23 to 27 MJ, and 11% at about 33 MJ.[99]

The excess of protein in the food of an athlete is often on the order of 100 g a day. If the protein was used for muscle protein synthesis, muscle mass would increase by 500 g a day. This of course is not the case. The extra protein consumed only increases the production and release of urea and thus increases the metabolic and excretory work by the liver and kidney. The calculation shows that extra intake of protein concentrates and protein pills, which is usual today among athletes and muscle builders, is of no meaning when the normal diet already contains protein in excess of that needed for both energy production and muscle protein synthesis.

### DIET COMPOSITION

Depending on work rate, the recommended daily energy intake for men is 160 to 250 kJ per kilogram BW, and 130 to 220 kJ per kilogram BW for women. Between 55 and 60% of the energy intake should be in the form of complex carbohydrates, 30% as fat (about half of which should be supplied as vegetable fat), and the remaining 12 to 15% in the form of high-quality protein. Athletes in training can use essentially the same diet but with an increase in energy intake to meet the increase in energy expenditure. Exceptions to this statement are long-distance runners, cyclists, and cross-country skiers, who during prolonged bouts of training need especially to increase their carbohydrate intake. For such individuals, 70 to 75% of the extra energy should be in the form of carbohydrate and a maximum of 10% as protein.

## DIET IN PREPARATION FOR COMPETITION

When the athlete is preparing for a competition involving prolonged heavy exercise of more than 60 minutes' duration, the muscle glycogen stores may be increased to maximum if the following program of diet and exercise is adopted. On the first day, i.e., 6 days before the competition, an exhausting exercise is performed, followed by 2 days of a low-carbohydrate diet with further bouts of exhausting exercise. Thereafter, a carbohydrate-rich diet (75 to 80% carbohydrate) is given for 3 days, during which no hard exercise is performed. To avoid excessive depletion of the muscle glycogen stores, Sherman et al. recommends a normal mixed diet for the first 3 days (50% carbohydrate) after which the carbohydrate-rich diet is given. At the same time, shorter periods of exercise are performed also on days 4 and 5, and rest is taken only on the day preceding the competition. This procedure is probably sufficient for athletes in regular training.

For competitions lasting less than 1 hour, a normal mixed diet is adequate during the final day of preparation. The protein intake recommended in the normal diet is sufficient for resistance sports, even during intensive training periods, provided the total caloric intake is adequate to meet the energy needs.

On the day of competition, a carbohydrate-rich meal should be given, preferably at least 2 hours before the start of the event. Intake of rapidly absorbed sugars, notably glucose, before and during competition may result in increased release of insulin leading to a decrease in blood glucose levels, inhibition of FFA release,[100] and, in the long run, greater use of the muscle glycogen stores. In longer events of 2 hours or more, in which replacement of water and electrolytes also is necessary, it has been shown that repeated intake of glucose polymer solution can delay the onset of fatigue.[101,102] These findings demonstrate that glucose ingestion is important for the maintenance of the blood glucose concentration, a fall in which may inhibit sustained prolonged exercise because of the effect of hypoglycemia on the central nervous system and/or decreased carbohydrate availability in the working muscle. Hypoglycemia is a result of the increased glucose use by exercising muscle when the local glycogen store is depleted and the emptying of the liver glycogen store during prolonged exercise.

The carbohydrate solution, taken in small amounts at frequent intervals, counteracts hypoglycemia and depletion of the liver glycogen store.

## WATER AND ELECTROLYTE BALANCE IN PHYSICAL ACTIVITY

Water is of great importance to those performing physical activity. Indeed, it is the only nutrient the lack of which presents an immediate and serious health risk, or even the possibility of death to the participants.[103,104] Without question, dehydration can bring about a decrease in performance.[105–107] Water balance, therefore, should be of concern to all involved with physical activity.

## ROLE OF WATER

The central role of water in the performance of exercise is a direct consequence of its involvement in the cardiovascular, metabolic, and thermoregulatory systems of the human body. During exercise, oxygen and fuel substrates must be delivered to the working cell, and metabolites must be removed. Consequently, a redistribution of cardiac output to the working muscles must occur. A consequence of the elevated rate of work is additional heat production. Heat production in contracting muscles during intense physical exercise can be 15 to 20 times that of basal metabolism. This rate of heat production is sufficient to raise core body temperature in an average person by 1° C every 5 to 8 minutes if no temperature-regulating mechanisms are activated.[104,108] The metabolic heat must be dissipated to prevent hyperthermia from occurring in 15 to 25 minutes. Fortunately, the body does not let this happen as it activates heat loss mechanisms. One of these mechanisms is to dilate the skin blood vessels and therefore redistribute the cardiac output to the periphery.[109] Skin temperature increases because of the increased skin blood flow that permits heat to be lost from the skin to the environment by radiation and convection. A second heat loss mechanism is the activation of sweating. Sweat glands secrete sweat on to the surface of the skin where it can evaporate. Because sweat rates can be as high as 2 to 2.8 L/hour, nearly all of the heat produced during exercise can be dissipated through this mechanism under ideal conditions.

When the weather is cool, most of the required heat loss during exercise occurs through radiation and convection from the exposed skin. Extensive sweating is not needed and does not occur, making the risk of dehydration relatively low. As the environmental temperature increases and approaches the skin temperature, heat transfer by radiation and convection cannot occur to any great extent. This condition leaves evaporation of sweat as the only effective means of dissipating heat. Consequently, the sweat rate is high during exercise in hot environments and the loss of body fluids must be replenished to maintain exercise performance and to prevent fatigue and hyperthermia.[110–112] The extent to which body fluid loss affects performance is governed by many factors, including the type and the mode of exercise, the intensity and duration of the work, the environmental conditions under which the work is performed, and the physical characteristics of the athlete (age, sex, weight, height, state of nutrition, hydration, and training).

Water metabolism during activity cannot be separated from the body's mineral balance. Water shifts between intracellular and extracellular spaces are also accompanied by shifts in sodium, potassium, magnesium, and chloride ions ($Na^+$, $K^+$, $Mg^{2+}$, $Cl^-$, respectively). Sweat losses also provide a means for electrolyte loss.[106,113,114] Disturbance of water and electrolyte balance occurs not only during single exercise bouts, but also over prolonged periods of training.

## TYPES OF STRESS

Two different situations stress water balance. In "make weight" sports such as wrestling, the competitor deliberately restricts intake of food and fluid and strives to lose water by exercise, heat exposure, laxatives, and diuretics, ostensibly to meet a smaller and weaker opponent.[115,116] This practice has been rejected for health reasons by professional associations.[105] Even so, the abuse continues and is prevalent in intense activities of brief duration that emphasize strength and coordination.

In contrast to such activities are endurance events such as road racing. These events may last for several hours, and the exertional and environmental heat load imposed on the body may produce rectal temperatures in excess of 40.6° C.[104] Under such conditions, athletes may lose fluid at rates of 2.0 to 2.8 $L \cdot hour^{-1}$, resulting in a water deficit of 6 to 8% of body weight.[117,118]

## EFFECTS OF DEHYDRATION

Numerous studies have been performed to assess the effects of dehydration on performance; the data reported include physiologic and biochemical variables and measures of muscular strength and endurance, anaerobic capacity, and aerobic power. Dehydration states have been produced thermally or in combination with exercise. The results depend on the extent of the dehydration, which is expressed as the % body weight loss (%BWL).

As little as 2% BWL imposes an increased strain on the cardiovascular[119] and thermoregulatory systems.[114] A 2.5% decrease in plasma volume and a 1% decline in muscle water typically occurs for each 1% BWL. Plasma water accounts for 10 to 11% of the total water deficit.[106] Rectal temperature increases 0.4 to 0.5° C for each 1% BWL.[120] A 4% BWL has been shown to result in an approximate 30% decline in isometric and isotonic strength, although peak isokinetic torque declined only 13% when an 8% BWL was induced by food and fluid restriction.[116] However, 5% BWL was without effect in an anaerobic cycling test and no impairment was noted at 8% BWL in an anaerobic running test.[116] A 4 to 5% BWL produced no change in $VO_2max$, although a decrease in the maximal work time was seen.[119] Similarly, during activities of long duration, dehydration has invariably been reported to result in a decreased ability to work.[105,111,119,121,122] In other studies, a decreased capacity is strongly suggested.[113,120] No positive benefits of weight reduction by hypohydration have been shown.

Electrolyte losses occur together with water loss, but because sweat is hypotonic, the loss in water exceeds the loss of $Na^+$, $K^+$, $Mg^{2+}$, or $Cl^-$. The net result is that the plasma becomes hypertonic. The principal ions lost in sweat are $Na^+$ and $Cl^-$.[106] A sweat loss causing a 5.8% BWL was found to produce a deficit of 5.7% in body $Na^+$ and $Cl^-$, but a 1% loss of $K^+$ and $Mg^{2+}$.[111] This small reduction in body stores is unlikely to lead to any impairment in neuromuscular function.

## REPLACEMENT STRATEGIES

Rehydration strategies to prevent, compensate for, or replace water loss are important in avoiding hypohydration. The aim of rehydration is either to quickly replace and re-establish water and electrolyte balance, as in the case of dehydrated performer about to enter an event, or to prevent or retard water loss that occurs during an endurance event. Studies reveal that several factors are involved in fluid replacement, such as fluid composition, drinking frequency, volume intake, and fluid temperature.[123] The rate of gastric emptying provides a measure of rehydration efficiency, because almost all absorption of sugar, electrolytes, and water proceeds from the intestine.[124]

**Effect of Fluid Composition.** It is often necessary during endurance exercise to not only supplement fluid stores but also to supplement carbohydrate stores through oral ingestion of glucose, fructose, sucrose, or carbohydrate polymers. These carbohydrate solutions can provide a slow release of energy substrate to the body over a prolonged period.[111] However, results of initial studies revealed that carbohydrate concentrations above 140 mM (25 g/L) significantly retard gastric emptying, which is detrimental for rapid rehydration.[123] Findings of more recent studies demonstrated that both carbohydrate and water delivery to the duodenum were at near maximal rates when the carbohydrate concentration of the drink was 440 to 560 mM (80 to 100 g/L).[124–126] During these studies, subjects exercised for 2 hours and drank 120 ml every 15 minutes. Therefore, if water replacement is the major concern during exercise, solutions with lower carbohydrate contents should be ingested, and if water replacement is not a priority, more concentrated carbohydrate solutions can be ingested. Most sports beverages routinely contain carbohydrate concentrations of 280 to 560 mM (50 to 100 g/L).

Many fluid replacement drinks also contain small amounts of salt. The addition of 10 to 30 mM NaCl may help replace body stores of $Na^+$ and $Cl^-$, the major ions lost in sweat.[106] Low levels of $Na^+$ are also reported to improve gastric emptying and to assist in maintaining the osmotic drive for drinking.[127] Drinking water only rapidly dilutes the blood, removes the drive for drinking, and stimulates urine output. However, large amounts of NaCl increase the osmolality of the drink and may actually cause fluid shifts into the gastrointestinal tract, thereby hindering gastric emptying.[121] Potassium supplements are not needed in replacement drinks because little $K^+$ is lost in sweat and these supplements are considered dangerous.[128]

**Fluid Volume.** Although large volumes of ingested fluid (up to 600 ml) increase the emptying rate, gastric discomfort may result. Drinking 100 to 200 ml every 10 to 15 minutes seems appropriate.[123,125,126]

**Fluid Temperature.** Chilled fluids (6 to 12° C) empty from the stomach more quickly than warm ones and can reduce body temperatures.[120,123]

**Drinking Schedule.** It is recommended to take 400 to 500 ml of fluid 10 to 15 minutes before competition, although this step does not replace the need for drinking during the event.[120] Hyperhydration 40 to 80 minutes before an event can precipitate diuresis, and rapid rehydration after exercise-induced dehydration can produce the same result.[129]

The consensus of reviews on this topic is to drink 100 to 200 ml of solution containing 280 to 560 mM (50 to 100 g/L) carbohydrate and 10 to 30 mM NaCl every 15 to 20 minutes when engaging in prolonged exercise lasting longer than 1 hour.[106,124,130,131] It is also beneficial if the solution is chilled to 6 to 12° C. Tremendous individual variation exists in the ability to tolerate carbohydrate-electrolyte drinks during prolonged strenuous exercise. This variation necessitates that each individual experiment with these drinks before competition to develop his or her own optimal strategy.

## EFFICACY OF REHYDRATION

Rehydration before or during an event has been shown to be of significant benefit. Consuming 150 ml of fluid every 10 minutes during a 2-hour cycling task in the heat dramatically limits the reduction in plasma volume, elevation of heart rate, and increase in body temperature.[111] Rectal temperature was about 0.7° C lower at the end of 2 hours of exercise when 200 ml of fluid was consumed every 20 minutes.[120]

The problems of dehydration may be alleviated in part during activity by the availability of water produced by metabolism and liberated during the breakdown of glycogen. Similarly, $K^+$ is released as glycogen is used.[11,21,74] These effects should help in maintaining fluid and electrolyte balance during exercise. Glycogen degradation and oxidation provide more water than does fat metabolism because of the release of stored water as well as metabolic water. As the fuel source shifts in favor of muscle glycogen at higher work loads, plasma volume and thermoregulatory control are maintained. In practice, however, production of metabolic water has been shown to play only a minor role.[132]

Unfortunately, rehydration often is only partially complete during exercise; during moderate to heavy work, a water deficit occurs that cannot be matched by increased fluid intake.[118,123,133] Inevitably, a delay in drinking sufficient fluid occurs because of increased exercise/thermal stress; this is termed involuntary dehydration.[134] Rules of a given event may also impede drinking.[101] Between 800 to 1500 ml·hour$^{-1}$ of fluid can be replaced,[121,123] but fluid deficits of 400 to 800 ml during even light exercise (with free drinking) have been reported.[134] Forced drinking before the onset of thirst may be undertaken to minimize dehydration.[111]

After thermal dehydration, even a 4-hour rehydration period is insufficient to restore fluid and electrolyte balances.[129] During repeated, heavy exercise, normal fluid balance was regained within 12 hours, but sodium conservation by the kidneys continued for 24 hours.

### TRAINING ADAPTATION AND ITS IMPLICATIONS

In response to endurance training, heat-exposed athletes adapt and improve their work-heat tolerance.[135] Hypervolemia develops over several days of prolonged training or with three or more bouts of intense, intermittent work. This expansion of plasma volume may contribute to the cardiovascular and thermoregulatory adaptations resulting from training.[136–138] These adaptations reduce the extent of body fluid shifts during exercise in the trained person.[110] Sweat rates increase as an adaptive response,[134,135,138] but water and electrolyte balances appear to be maintained. Together with an increase in voluntary fluid ingestion, the effect is a reduction in fluid deficit during work.[134] Hormonal control mechanisms operate to cause renal conservation and minimize the disturbance of water and electrolyte balance.[133,137] Given free access to food and fluid, trained runners are able to maintain body weight and normal fluid balance during 20 days of severe prolonged exercise in warm temperatures.[133]

## IRON BALANCE IN PHYSICAL ACTIVITY

Iron balance and metabolism in humans at rest and during exercise has been the topic of several reviews.[139–142] The subject is complex and presently is still not fully understood. Its importance to persons engaged in physical activity derives from the central role of iron in cell metabolism. Iron is essential in the transport and delivery of $O_2$ to the mitochondria of the working cell through the proteins hemoglobin and myoglobin. It is also a component of many other protein systems, including the cytochromes and α-glycerophosphate oxidase.[143] Iron deficiency, with or without anemia, is widespread in the population and is generally associated with decreased work performance[144] and other discomforting symptoms.[139]

### INCIDENCE OF IRON DEFICIENCY IN ATHLETES

Surveys of athletic groups have shown that both males and females, particularly those involved in intense endurance sports, have hemoglobin concentrations in the low and mid range of the population norms.[144–150] This state is often referred to as "sports anemia," but this term is imprecise and a misnomer.[151] In most athletes, the lower hemoglobin concentration is caused by a training-induced increase in plasma volume that dilutes the red blood cells.[136,137] The increase in blood plasma is a beneficial adaptation to aerobic exercise and should be called dilutional pseudoanemia. Some athletes, however, develop true anemia (iron deficiency anemia), which is a deficiency in the total amount of circulating hemoglobin or red blood cells. The number of athletes with true anemia is low, although significant. In one study, 11% of the females in a small group were anemic,[148] and in a second study, 10% of the males and none of the women had anemia.[146]

Serum ferritin, transferrin saturation, and bone marrow iron levels are sensitive indicators of prelatent and latent iron deficiency and are used in assessing the state of the tissue iron stores.[139] From these measurements it has been determined that many male and female endurance runners, although not anemic, are at risk for depletion of the iron stores. In studies including a range of sample sizes, investigators report 8 to 58% of male athletes and 40 to 80% of female athletes are iron deficient.[146,148,152–155] The extent of iron deficiency in athletes appears to be far higher than in the general population.[148] Without question, elite runners have lower plasma ferritin levels (protein-bound iron) than the general population. This difference may be related to hemodilution, transfer of stored iron into larger muscles and red blood cells, or altered iron metabolism, but regardless of the cause, this is the norm for these people. In a comprehensive examination of iron metabolism and dilutional pseudoanemia in male endurance athletes, the authors concluded that no sports anemia or iron deficiency existed when all markers of iron status were considered.[152,156,157]

### FACTORS INFLUENCING IRON STATUS

Several mechanisms have been proposed to account for iron deficiency anemia in athletes. This situation is most commonly caused by iron deficiency secondary to inadequate ingestion of iron to meet the body needs,[141,142] and typically occurs in rapidly growing adolescents involved in athletics, females involved in athletics, and those athletes engaged in activities that encourage low energy intakes and low body weights.[146,148] A second and far less important cause is footstrike hemolysis.[158,159] Several other factors also may contribute to iron status and ultimately iron deficiency anemia, but most are considered minor. Exercise has been shown to increase the elimination of iron and to interfere with the normal increase in iron absorption when iron stores are depleted.[150] Iron loss from gastrointestinal bleeding has been noted in some athletes associated with racing, but this condition is not a major cause of iron loss in most athletes.[142] The focus of some studies has been on iron loss in sweat,[150,153] but findings of one detailed study suggest these losses are trivial.[160]

### EFFECTS ON PERFORMANCE

Investigators have studied the ability to work aerobically over a wide range of hemoglobin concentrations, ranging from severe anemia to blood doping or induced erythrocythemia.[161–163] It is clear the $VO_2$max and the capacity for intense endurance exercise are correlated with hemoglobin concentration when the hemoglobin levels are below the mean of the population, including when anemia is present. Blood doping studies have also shown that increasing the hemoglobin concentration by about 10%, without altering blood volume, increases $VO_2$max and aerobic performance.[163–166] Reinfusion of red blood cells into trained athletes was shown first by Buick et al. to increase $VO_2$max by 5% and work performance by 35%.[165] Also, some evidence shows that iron deficiency anemia has detrimental effects on the endurance and productivity of workers.[161,167]

Controversy exists regarding whether iron depletion without anemia adversely affects athletic performance. Results of some studies suggest that performance is adversely affected only when anemia is present. Iron deficiency was induced without anemia in healthy males and had no effect on $VO_2$max or endurance performance.[168] In addition, iron therapy in female marathoners with low ferritin levels did not improve performance.[169]

### TREATMENT OF IRON DEFICIENCY

When iron deficiency anemia has been diagnosed in athletes, oral iron therapy has corrected the condition, and athletic performance has improved.[147,148] Oral iron treatment for iron deficiency without anemia has shown more inconsistent results. Hematologic variables of elite long-distance runners failed to show uniform improvement with iron therapy over 2 years during which a rich dietary source and supplemental iron were given. Iron stores remained depleted, although iron balance was maintained,[150] suggesting again that iron metabolism in endurance athletes is unlike that of the normal population. Iron supplementation restored measures of mild iron deficiency to normal and lowered blood lactate levels during maximal exercise, but it had no effect on performance.[170] When iron deficiency has not been diagnosed, iron supplementation has had little or no effect on hematologic measures or performance.[144,149]

Endurance athletes of both sexes, particularly runners who undergo prolonged, intense training, are susceptible to iron deficiency, with or without anemia. Impairment of performance may result. Iron status should be monitored regularly by serum ferritin and hemoglobin analysis. If latent or manifest iron deficiency is seen, supplemental oral iron treatments appear justified. When several measures of iron status reveal no true iron deficiency, routine iron supplementation is not indicated.[157] Iron deficiency can be prevented in most athletes by manipulating the diet to increase iron intake, such as eating more lean red meat and dark meat of chicken; drinking a source of vitamin C instead of coffee or tea when eating bread and cereal to improve iron absorption; cooking in cast iron pans; and eating dried beans or peas with poultry or seafood to increase iron absorption from the vegetables.

## VITAMINS, TRACE MINERALS, AND EXERCISE

The use of vitamins and minerals remains controversial. The conservative recommendations of most recognized scientific authorities contrast sharply with the practice of athletes and coaches who experiment with a wide range of diets and supplements in the hope of maximizing performance. Clearly, physical work capacity is reduced by deficient nutrition and an adequate diet is an important base for optimal work performance.

Results of studies suggest that exercise increases the need for some vitamins and minerals and that certain groups of athletes have specific vitamin and mineral deficiencies.[171,172] However, findings also show that the increased need can be met and the deficiencies can be corrected by a well-balanced diet. The most common method of assessing vitamin and mineral status in athletes is to monitor dietary intake. Unfortunately, this method relies on the accuracy of the recollection of the subject and records from only a few days may not be representative for some minerals and vitamins. Clinical signs are also used in evaluating a vitamin and mineral status. However, the most accurate methods are direct biochemical assessment of blood and, in many individuals, tissue vitamin and mineral levels.

Although controversy exists, few authors have documented any beneficial effect of vitamin and mineral supplementation in subjects who are not deficient. In addition, large doses of certain vitamins and minerals can be toxic. Reviews on this topic consistently agree with the preceding conclusions and note that most studies in this area have weak experimental designs and are poorly controlled.[171–174] Some of the problems are lack of control and placebo groups, lack of double blind and cross-over designs, inappropriate measurements of performance for the vitamin or mineral studied, and lack of an initial assessment of subject fitness.[171] It is appreciated that properly designed, well-controlled studies are difficult to perform in this area.

This chapter does not include an examination of all the vitamins and trace minerals that may relate to exercise for several reasons: the numerous reviews that exist in this area,[171–174] the large number of poorly designed and controlled studies, and the lack of investigations examining the relationship between exercise and some vitamins and minerals.

### FAT-SOLUBLE VITAMINS

This group includes vitamins A, D, and E. Vitamins A and E may be related to exercise in an antioxidant manner and vitamin D is instrumental in bone mineral metabolism. No evidence exists that these compounds enhance performance in nutritionally adequate individuals. Overdoses of vitamin A may lead to anorexia, hypercalcemia, and liver and kidney damage and overdoses of vitamin D can produce hypercalcemia and hypercalciuria.[171,175]

### WATER-SOLUBLE VITAMINS

Evidence suggests that exercise may affect the need for vitamin C, riboflavin, and thiamin.[172,176,177] Vitamin C supplementation did improve the ability to train in subjects who were vitamin C depleted.[178] However, in nutritionally balanced sedentary individuals and athletes, supplementation with thiamin, riboflavin, vitamin $B_6$ (pyridoxine), pantothenic acid, vitamin $B_{12}$ (cobalamin), so-called "vitamin $B_{15}$" ("pangamic" acid) and vitamin C had no effect on performance.[171,179–184] No study has been made of the effects of folate and biotin supplementation on exercise performance. The intake of a niacin supplement is known to inhibit the release of FFA from adipose tissue.[185] The result is an increase in muscle glycogen degradation during prolonged exercise, which leads to an earlier onset of fatigue.[186] Therefore, niacin supplements should be avoided.

### TRACE MINERALS

Many trace elements are involved directly in energy metabolism or in other functions related to exercise or recovery from exercise. Zinc is involved in carbohydrate (e.g., lactate dehydrogenase), fat, and protein metabolism, and in tissue repair. Copper is involved in oxidative phosphorylation (e.g., cytochrome *aa₃*), erythropoiesis, and catecholamine regulation. Chromium potentiates the effect of insulin and is involved in carbohydrate and fat metabolism. Selenium is an antioxidant and iron has a well-known role in oxygen delivery to tissues.

Iron status is examined in an earlier section of this chapter, and no studies have assessed the effects of chromium and selenium supplementation on athletic performance. Small amounts of zinc are known to be lost in sweat, and reports have indicated that some athletes ingest inadequate amounts of zinc.[187,188] Some endurance athletes have low resting blood levels of zinc,[187,189] whereas others have adequate levels.[190,191] One investigation measured plasma and red blood cell concentrations of zinc and copper and reported no relationship with $VO_2$max in athletes.[192] Surprisingly, few studies have examined the effect of zinc supplementation on exercise performance. However, this may be due to the negative effects of excessive zinc consumption; impaired copper absorption from the diet and hypocupremia, reduced circulating high-density lipoproteins and impaired immune responses.[171,193]

Several studies have also attempted to assess the potential benefits of supplementation with multivitamin/mineral combinations because several vitamins and minerals act synergistically. Two studies demonstrate no effects of 1 to 3 months of multivitamin/mineral ingestion on $VO_2$max and metabolic profiles during submaximal endurance tests to exhaustion in well-trained athletes.[194,195]

All athletes should eat a varied and well-balanced, nutrient-dense diet to ensure adequate vitamin and mineral intake. No evidence supports the ideas that consuming large doses of vitamin and mineral supplements improves athletic performance and that some vitamins/minerals decrease performance or produce negative side effects. The most recent United States[83] and Canadian dietary recommendations[196] review data concerning needs for thiamin, riboflavin, and niacin in relation to energy expenditure (see also Appendix Tables A–2b and A–3a). If the demands of training increase the need for energy, the intake of vitamins and minerals also increases. Therefore, the most logical way to ensure that both of these conditions are met is simply to increase the daily energy intake. However, many groups of athletes limit their energy intake, including those concerned with the cosmetic and performance aspects of extra weight (gymnasts, dancers, figure skaters, and divers) and those who must "make weight" to compete (wrestlers, boxers, jockeys, and light-weight class sports participants). For these people and any athletes, who for a number of reasons do not consume an adequate diet, a basic daily multivitamin/mineral tablet is appropriate, but megadose supplements are not.

## CONCLUSION

The recent interest concerning nutrition and diet in work and exercise stems not so much from our interest in occupational work but from those of high caliber training and competition in sports. It seems we have come full circle from the times of the Greeks and Romans. Elite athletes now experiment with a wide range of so-called ergogenic acids, including nutrients and foodstuffs, in what is often an irrational attempt to succeed.[197] It is at this level of exercise, which in the modern world places the greatest degree of physical stress on the human body, that the connection between nutrition and performance is best seen.

Scientific investigations have provided a sound understanding of the physiologic and biochemical events that occur in a variety of exercise situations; these studies form the basis for the recommendations on energy and fluid intake for optimization of performance and avoidance of exertional injury. Research has shown that dietary supplementation with vitamins and minerals above physiologic needs is both ineffective and an unnecessary ergogenic aid and, with abuse, may actually impair performance and health.

Results of studies have shown, however, that physical activity can make an individual susceptible to micronutrient deficiency states that ultimately may impair performance. Accompanying any increase in energy requirement is an increased need for thiamin, riboflavin, and niacin. Thus, the diet of an athlete must maintain a proper nutrient density as well as energy content. Exercise, by affecting absorption and/or elimination of nutrients, can upset the nutritional balance. Examples include riboflavin and minerals such as iron. At present, the risk of iron deficiency is best documented in young athletes. Continued research in this area is needed to better define the proper analytic measures as they relate to exercise performance, the effect of exercise on nutrient balance, and the means of preventing the occurrence of a suboptimal nutritional state.

A factor complicating general recommendations on nutrition and diet for athletes is the variety of activities constituting what is known as sport. This variety is highlighted in a detailed 4-year study of the dietary intake of university athletes.[198] At one extreme are strength sports (American football) in which one 118-kg player consumed 61.2 MJ in 1 day. At the other end of the continuum are light-weight wrestlers, gymnasts, and dancers with small bodies and dietary patterns that fluctuate widely in energy content but average 8.5 MJ daily. This extensive analysis of athletic diets across the range of sports revealed two points: that proper diet can provide the nutrition required for performance across the sports spectrum and that many of the athletes were at risk because of poor intake of one or more nutrients. Trends in these athletic diets reflect certain modern concerns, such as a high intake of saturated fat, cholesterol, and sodium and appreciable vitamin and mineral supplementation.[199] Studies reveal the need for more education programs about nutrition for athletes, trainers, and coaches and show that these groups are eager for factual information.[198,200]

Nutritional advice must be tailored to the demands of the specific work and exercise.[198] The statement by the American Dietetic Association provides a good model.[201] Recommendations for the general public and for athletes involved in training or competition are separated, yet span the categories of athletic, combative, or occupational activity. The recommendations and overall viewpoint within the present review are in basic agreement with the succinct recommendations contained in the statement. The significance of diet, nutrition, work, and exercise are best summarized as follows:

1. An adequate, balanced diet is necessary for an effective performance but does not guarantee it, because nutrition is but one aspect of performance.
2. A poor diet, on the other hand, guarantees substandard performance.
3. Being a fit, trained athlete does not alter the dietary requirements for most nutrients. Energy (carbohydrates), water, iron, and certain B vitamins are possible exceptions. These increased needs may, however, still be met through a balanced diet.
4. Ingestion of one or more nutrients in amounts much greater than body needs will not enhance performance and may actually impair it.

## REFERENCES


1. von Liebig, J.: Animal Chemistry or Organic Chemistry in Its Application to Physiology and Pathology. London, Taylor and Walton, 1842.
2. Zuntz, N.: Pflugers Arch., *68:*191, 1897.
3. Zuntz, N.: Arch. Gesamte Physiol. Menschen Tiere, *83:*557–571, 1901.
4. Himvich, H.E., Rose, M.I.: Am. J. Physiol., *81:*485–486, 1927.
5. Christensen, E.H., Hansen, O.: Scand. Arch. Physiol., *81:*160–175, 1939.
6. Bergström, J.: Scand. J. Clin. Lab. Invest., *14(Suppl. 68):*1–110, 1962.
7. Bergström, J., Hultman, E., Roch-Norlund, A.E.: Nature, *198:*97–98, 1963.
8. Bergström, J., Hultman, E.: Scand. J. Clin. Lab. Invest., *18:*16–20, 1966.
9. Bergström, J., Hultman, E.: Nature, *210:*309–310, 1966.
10. Hultman, E., Bergström, J., McLennan-Anderson, N.: Scand. J. Clin. Lab. Invest., *19:*56–66, 1967.
11. Ahlborg, B., Bergström, J., Ekelund, L.-G., et al.: Acta Physiol. Scand., *70:*129–142, 1967.
12. Hultman, E.: Circ. Res., *20 & 21(Suppl. 1):*1–99, 1967.
13. Hultman, E.: Scand. J. Clin. Lab. Invest., *19:*209–217, 1967.
14. Bergström, J., Hultman, E.: Scand. J. Clin. Lab. Invest., *19:*218–228, 1967.
15. Bergström, J., Hultman, E.: Acta Med. Scand., *182:*93–107, 1967.
16. Hultman, E., Bergström, J.: Acta Med. Scand., *182:*109–117, 1967.
17. Hermansen, L., Hultman, E., Saltin, B.: Acta Physiol. Scand., *71:*129–139, 1967.
18. Bergström, J., Hermansen, L., Hultman, E., et al.: Acta Physiol. Scand., *71:*140–150, 1967.
19. Ahlborg, B., Bergström, J., Brohult, J., et al.: Försvarsmedicin, *3:*85–100, 1967.
20. Hultman, E.: Scand. J. Clin. Lab. Invest., *19(Suppl. 94):*1–63, 1967.
21. Bergström, J., Beroniade, V., Hultman, E., et al.: Symposium Über Transport und Funktion Intracellulärer Elektrolyte. 3–4 Juni, Schüren/Saar, 1967, pp. 108–117.
22. Nilsson, L.H.: Studies on Liver Glycogen Metabolism in Man with Special Reference to Diet and Sugar Infusion. Thesis, Karolinska Institutet, Stockholm 1974.

23. Nilsson, L.H., Hultman, E.: Scand. J. Clin. Lab. Invest., *32*:325–330, 1973.
24. Nilsson, L.H., Fürst, P., Hultman, E.: Scand. J. Clin. Lab. Invest., *32*:331–337, 1973.
25. Hultman, E., Nilsson, L.H.: Adv. Exp. Med. Biol., *11*:143–151, 1971.
26. Nilsson, L.H., Hultman, E.: Scand. J. Clin. Lab. Invest., *33*:5–10, 1974.
27. Bergström, J., Harris, R.C., Hultman, E., et al.: Adv. Exp. Med. Biol., *11*:341–355, 1971.
28. Harris, R.C.: Muscle Energy Metabolism in Man in Response to Isometric Contraction. A Biopsy Study. Thesis, University of Wales, 1981.
29. Hultman, E., Sjöholm, H.: Substrate availability. *In* International Series on Sports Sciences. Vol. 13. Edited by H.G. Knuttgen, J.A. Vogel, J. Poortmans. Champaign, Il, Human Kinetic, 1983.
30. Fletcher, J.G.L., Lewis, H.K.: Ergonomics, *2*:114–115, 1959.
31. Wilkie, D.R.: Ergonomics, *3*:1–8, 1960.
32. Davies, C.T.M.: Ergonomics, *14*:245–256, 1971.
33. Kleine, T.O.: Z. Klin. Chem., *5*:244–247, 1967.
34. Margaria, R., Cerretelli, P., Mangili, F.: J. Appl. Physiol., *19*:623–628, 1964.
35. Hultman, E.: Regulation of carbohydrate metabolism in the liver during rest and exercise with special reference to diet. Third International Symposium on Biochemistry of Exercise. Vol. 3. Edited by F. Landry, W.A.R. Orban. Miami Symposia Specialists, 1979.
36. Nilsson, L.H.: Scand. J. Clin. Lab. Invest., *32*:317–323, 1973.
37. McGilvery, R.W.: The use of fuels for muscular work. *In* Metabolic Adaptation to Prolonged Physical Exercise. Edited by H. Howald, J.R. Poortmans. Basel, Birkhäuser Verlag, 1973.
38. Pernow, B., Saltin, B.: J. Appl. Physiol., *31*:416–422, 1971.
39. Fox, E.L.: Sports Physiology. 2nd Ed. Philadelphia, W.B. Saunders Company, 1984.
40. Ahlborg, G., Felig, G., Hagenfeldt, L., et al.: J. Clin. Invest., *53*:1080–1090, 1974.
41. Holloszy, J.O.: Biochemical adaptations to exercise: Aerobic metabolism. *In* Exercise and Sport Science Review. Edited by J.H. Wilmore. New York, Academic Press, 1973.
42. Holloszy, J.O., Booth, F.W.: Annu. Rev. Physiol., *38*:273–291, 1976.
43. Holloszy, J.O., Winder, W.W., Fitts, R.H., et al.: Energy production during exercise. *In* Regulatory Mechanisms in Metabolism During Exercise. Edited by F. Landry, W.A.R. Orban. Miami, Symposia Specialists, 1978.
44. Holloszy, J.O.: Arch. Phys. Med. Rehabil., *63*:231–234, 1982.
45. Hultman, E.: Muscle glycogen store and prolonged exercise. *In* Frontiers of Fitness. Edited by E.J. Shephard. Springfield, IL, Charles C Thomas, 1971.
46. Lemon, P.W.R., Mullin, J.P.: J. Appl. Physiol., *48*:624–629, 1980.
47. Brooks, G.A.: Med. Sci. Sports Exerc., *19*:S150–S156, 1987.
48. Yoshimura, H., Inoue, T., Yamada, T., et al.: World Rev. Nutr. Diet, *35*:1–86, 1980.
49. Refsum, H.E., Strömme, S.B.: Scand. J. Clin. Lab. Invest., *33*:247–254, 1974.
50. Rennie, M.J., Edwards, R.H.T., Krywawych, S., et al.: Clin. Sci., *61*:627–639, 1981.
51. Décombaz, J., Reinhardt, P., Anantharaman, K., et al.: Eur. J. Appl. Physiol., *41*:61–72, 1979.
52. Gontzea, I., Sutsesco, R., Dimitrache, S.: Nutr. Rep. Int., *11*:231–236, 1975.
53. Felig, P.E., Wahren, J.: J. Clin. Invest., *50*:2703–2714, 1971.
54. Felig, P.: Metabolism, *22*:179–207, 1973.
55. Felig, P.: Annu. Rev. Biochem., *44*:933–955, 1975.
56. Graham, T.E., Pedersen, P.K., Saltin, B.: J. Appl. Physiol., *63*:1457–1462, 1987.
57. MacLean, D.A., Spriet, L.L., Hultman, E., et al.: J. Appl. Physiol., *70*:2095–2103, 1991.
58. MacLean, D.A., Spriet, L.L., Graham, T.E.: Can. J. Physiol. Pharmacol., *70*:420–427, 1992.
59. Young, V.R., Bier, D.M.: Stable isotopes ($^{31}C$ and $^{15}N$) in the study of human protein and amino acid metabolism and requirements. *In* Nutritional Factors: Modulating Effects on Metabolic Processes. Edited by R.F. Beers, E.G. Bassett. New York, Raven Press, 1981.
60. Hägg, S.A., Morse, E.L., Adibi, S.A.: Am. J. Physiol., *242*:407–410, 1982.
61. Wolfe, R.R., Goodenough, R.D., Wolfe, M.H., et al.: J. Appl. Physiol., *52*:458–466, 1982.
62. Millward, D.J., Davies, C.T.M., Halliday, D., et al.: Fed. Proc., *41*:2686–2691, 1982.
63. White, T.P., Brooks, G.A.: Am. J. Physiol., *240*:155–165, 1981.
64. Buse, M.G., Biggers, J.F., Friedrici, K.H., et al.: J. Biol. Chem., *247*:8085–8096, 1972.
65. Haralambie, G., Berg, A.: Eur. J. Appl. Physiol., *36*:231–236, 1976.
66. Refsum, H.E., Gjessing, L.R., Strömme, S.B.: Scand. J. Clin. Lab. Invest., *39*:407–413, 1979.
67. Dohm, G.L., Williams, R.T., Kasparek, G.J., et al.: J. Appl. Physiol., *52*:26–33, 1982.
68. Munro, H.N.: Control of plasma amino acid concentrations. Ciba Found. Symp., *221*:5–18, 1974.
69. Boobis, L.H., Williams, C., Wootton, S.A.: J. Physiol., *342*:36P–37P, 1983.
70. Nevill, M.E., Boobis, L.H., Brooks, S., et al.: J. Appl. Physiol., *67*:2376–2382, 1989.
71. Hultman, E., Bergström, J., Roch-Norlund, A.E.: Adv. Exp. Med. Biol., *11*:273–288, 1971.
72. Brown, J.H., Thompson, B., Mayer, S.E.: Biochemistry, *16*:5501–5508, 1977.
73. Sherman, W.M., Costill, D.L., Fink, W.J., et al.: Int. J. Sports Med., *2*:114–118, 1981.
74. Bergström, J., Guarnieri, G., Hultman, E.: J. Appl. Physiol., *30*:122–125, 1971.
75. Bergström, J., Guarnieri, G., Hultman, E.: Changes in muscle water and electrolytes during exercise. *In* Limiting Factors of Physical Performance. Edited by J. Keul. Stuttgart, Georg Thieme, 1973.
76. Owen, O.E., Morgan, A.P., Kemp, H.G., et al.: J. Clin. Invest., *46*:1589–1595, 1967.
77. Owen, O.E., Felig, P., Morgan, A.P., et al.: J. Clin. Invest., *48*:574–583, 1969.
78. Hultman, E., Nilsson, L.: Liver glycogen as a glucose-supplying source during exercise. *In* Limiting Factors of Physical Performance. Edited by J. Keul. Stuttgart, Georg Thieme, 1973.
79. Passmore, J.V.G.A., Durnin, J.V.: Energy, Work and Leisure. London, Heineman, 1967.
80. FAO/WHO Expert Committee Report: Energy and Protein Requirements. WHO Tech. Rep. Ser., *52*:1–118, 1973.

81. Norgan, N.G., Ferro-Luzzi, A.: Int. Ser. Sport Sci., *7:*167–193, 1978.
82. Buskirk, E.R.: Nutrition for the athlete. *In* Sports Medicine. Edited by A.J. Ryan, F.L. Allman Jr. New York, Academic Press, 1974, pp. 141–159.
83. National Research Council, Food and Nutrition Board: Recommended Dietary Allowances. 10th Ed. Washington, D.C., National Academy of Sciences, 1989.
84. Ferro-Luzzi, A., Venerando, A.: Int. Ser. Sport Sci., *7:*145–154, 1978.
85. Suzuki, S., Oshima, S., Tsuji, E., et al.: Int. Ser. Sport Sci., *7:*194–214, 1978.
86. Wirths, W.: Int. Ser. Sport Sci., *7:*227–235, 1978.
87. Butterfield, G.E., Calloway, D.H.: Br. J. Nutr., *51:*171–184, 1984.
88. Todd, K.S., Butterfield, G.E., Calloway, D.H.: J. Nutr., *114:*2107–2118, 1984.
89. Tarnapolsky, M.A., MacDougall, J.D., Atkinson, S.A.: J. Appl. Physiol., *64:*187–193, 1988.
90. Butterfield, G.E.: Amino acids and high protein diets. *In* Perspectives in Exercise Science and Sports Medicine. Vol 4. Edited by D.R. Lamb, R. Williams. Carmel, IN, Benchmark Press, 1991.
91. Brouns, F., Saris, W.H.M., Stroecken, J., et al.: Int. J. Sports Med., *10:*S32–S40, 1989.
92. Torún, B., Scrimshaw, N.S., Young, V.R.: Am. J. Clin. Nutr., *30:*1983–1993, 1977.
93. Consolazio, C.R., Johnson, H.L., Nelson, R.A., et al.: Am. J. Clin. Nutr., *28:*29–35, 1975.
94. Darling, R.C., Johnson, R.E., Pitts, G.C., et al.: J. Nutr., *28:*273–281, 1944.
95. Pitts, G.C., Johnson, R.E., Consolazio, F.C., et al.: Am. J. Physiol., *142:*253–259, 1944.
96. Rasch, P.J., Pierson, W.R.: Am. J. Clin. Nutr., *11:*530–532, 1962.
97. Marable, N.L., Hickson Jr, J.F., Korslund, M.K., et al.: Nutr. Rep. Int., *19:*795–805, 1979.
98. Laritcheva, K.A., Yalovaya, N.I., Shubin, V.I., et al.: Int. Ser. Sports Sci., *7:*155–163, 1978.
99. Rogozkin, V.A.: Int. Ser. Sports Sci., *7:*119–123, 1978.
100. Koivisto, V.A., Karonen, S.-L., Nikkilä, E.A.: J. Appl. Physiol., *51:*783–787, 1981.
101. Coyle, E.F., Hagberg, J.M., Hurley, B.F., et al.: J. Appl. Physiol., *55:*230–235, 1983.
102. Coyle, E.F., et al.: J. Appl. Physiol., *61:*165–172, 1986.
103. Canadian Association of Sports Sciences: Can. J. Appl. Sport Sci., *6:*99–100, 1981.
104. American College of Sports Medicine: Med. Sci. Sports Exerc., *19:*529–533, 1987.
105. American College of Sports Medicine: Med. Sci. Sports Exerc., *15:*ix–xiii, 1983.
106. Saltin, B., Costill, D.L.: Fluid and electrolyte balance during prolonged exercise. *In* Exercise, Nutrition, and Energy Metabolism. Edited by E.S. Horton, R.L. Terjung. New York, Macmillan, 1988.
107. Sawka, M.N., Pandolf, K.B.: Effects of body water loss on physiological function and exercise performance. *In* Perspectives in Exercise Science and Sports Medicine. Vol. 3. Edited by C.V. Gisolfi, D.R. Lamb. Carmel, IN, Benchmark Press, 1990.
108. Nadel, E.R., Wenger, C.B., Peters, M.F., et al.: Ann. N. Y. Acad. Sci., *301:*98–109, 1977.
109. Rowell, L.B., Marx, H.J., Bruce, R.A., et al.: J. Clin. Invest., *45:*1801–1816, 1966.
110. Senay, L.C., Jr.: Med. Sci. Sports Exerc., *11:*42–48, 1979.
111. Costill, D.L., Miller, J.M.: Int. J. Sports Med., *1:*2–14, 1980.
112. Sawka, M.N., Young, A.J., Fransesconi, R.P., et al.: J. Appl. Physiol., *59:*1394–1401, 1985.
113. Sjogaard, G.: Am. J. Physiol., *245:*R25–R31, 1983.
114. Senay Jr, L.C.: J. Appl. Physiol., *47:*1–7, 1979.
115. Brownell, K.D., Nelson Steen, S., Wilmore, J.H.: Med. Sci. Sports Exerc., *19:*546–556, 1987.
116. Houston, M.E., Martin, D.A., Green, H.J., et al.: Phys. Sportsmed., *9:*73–78, 1981.
117. Costill, D.L.: Ann. N. Y. Acad. Sci., *301:*175–189, 1977.
118. Myhre, L.G., Hartung, G.H., Nunneley, S.A., et al.: J. Appl. Physiol., *59:*559–563, 1985.
119. Saltin, B.: J. Appl. Physiol., *19:*1125–1132, 1964.
120. Gisolfi, C.V., Copping, J.R.: Med. Sci. Sports Exerc., *6:*108–113, 1974.
121. Bergström, J., Hultman, E.: JAMA, *221:*999–1006, 1972.
122. Armstrong, L.E., Costill, D.L., Fink, W.J.: Med. Sci. Sports Exerc., *17:*456–461, 1985.
123. Costill, D.L., Saltin, B.: J. Appl. Physiol., *37:*679–683, 1974.
124. Costill, D.L.: Gastric emptying of fluids during exercise. *In* Perspectives in Exercise Science and Sports Medicine. Vol. 3. Edited by C.V. Gislofi, D.R. Lamb. Carmel, IN, Benchmark Press, 1990.
125. Mitchell, J.B., Costill, D.L., Houmard, J.A., et al.: Med. Sci. Sports Exerc., *20:*110–115, 1988.
126. Mitchell, J.B., Costill, D.L., Houmard, J.A., et al.: Med. Sci. Sports Exerc., *21:*269–274, 1989.
127. Nose, H., Mack, W.G., Schi, X., et al.: J. Appl. Physiol., *65:*325–331, 1988.
128. Knochel, J.P.: Ann. N. Y. Acad. Sci., *301:*175–189, 1977.
129. Costill, D.L., Sparks, K.E.: J. Appl. Physiol., *34:*299–308, 1973.
130. Hultman, E., Spriet, L.L.: Dietary intake prior to and during exercise. *In* Exercise, Nutrition and Energy Metabolism. Edited by E.S. Horton, R.L. Terjung. New York, Macmillan, 1988.
131. Maughan, R.: Carbohydrate-electrolyte solutions during prolonged exercise. *In* Perspectives in Exercise Science and Sports Medicine. Vol. 4. Edited by D.R. Lamb, M. Williams. Carmel, IN, Benchmark Press, 1991.
132. Pivarnik, J.M., Leeds, E.M., Wilkerson, J.E.: J. Appl. Physiol., *56:*613–618, 1984.
133. Wade, C.E., Dressendorfer, R.H., O'Brien, J.C., et al.: J. Appl. Physiol., *50:*709–712, 1981.
134. Greenleaf, J.E., Brock, P.J., Kiel, L.C., et al.: J. Appl. Physiol., *54:*414–419, 1983.
135. Gisolfi, C.V., Wilson, N.C., Claxton, B.: Ann. N. Y. Acad. Sci., *301:*129–150, 1977.
136. Green, H.J., Thomson, J.A., Ball, M.E., et al.: J. Appl. Physiol., *56:*145–149, 1984.
137. Convertino, V.A., Brock, P.T., Kiel, L.C., et al.: J. Appl. Physiol., *48:*665–669, 1980.
138. Convertino, V.A.: Med. Sci. Sports Exerc., *15:*77–82, 1983.
139. Conrad, M.E., Barton, J.C.: Am. J. Hematol., *10:*199–225, 1981.
140. Finch, C.A., Huebers, H.: N. Engl. J. Med., *306:*1520–1528, 1982.
141. Haymes, E.M.: Med. Sci. Sports Exerc., *19:*S197–S200, 1987.
142. Eichner, E.R.: Other medical considerations in prolonged exercise. *In* Perspectives in Exercise Science and Sports Medicine. Vol. 1. Edited by D.R. Lamb, R. Murray. Indianapolis, Benchmark Press, 1988.

143. Finch, C.A., Gollnick, P.D., Hlastala, M.P., et al.: J. Clin. Invest., *64:*129–137, 1979.
144. Pate, R.R.: Phys. Sportsmed., *11:*115–131, 1983.
145. Clement, D.B., Asmundson, R.C., Medhurst, C.W.: Can. Med. Assoc. J., *17:*614–616, 1977.
146. Clement, D.B., Asmundson, R.C.: Phys. Sportsmed., *10:*37–43, 1982.
147. Hunding, A., Jordal, R., Paulev, P.E.: Acta Med. Scand., *209:*315–318, 1981.
148. Nickerson, H.J., Tripp, A.D.: Phys. Sportsmed., *11:*60–66, 1983.
149. Brotherhood, J., Brozovic, B., Pugh, L.G.C.: Clin. Sci., *48:*139–145, 1975.
150. Ehn, L., Carlmark, B., Högland, S.: Med. Sci. Sports Exerc., *12:*61–64, 1980.
151. Eichner, E.R.: Phys. Sportsmed., *14:*122–130, 1986.
152. Magnusson, B., Hallberg, L., Rossander, L., et al.: Acta Med. Scand., *216:*149–155, 1984.
153. Paulev, P.E., Jordal, R., Pedersen, N.S.: Clin. Chim. Acta, *127:*19–27, 1983.
154. Par, R.B., Bachman, L.A., Moss, R.A.: Phys. Sportsmed., *12:*81–86, 1984.
155. Wishnitzer, R., Vorst, E., Berrebi, A.: Int. J. Sports Med., *4:*27–30, 1984.
156. Hallberg, L., Magnusson, B.: Acta Med. Scand., *216:*145–148, 1984.
157. Magnusson, B., Hallberg, L., Rossander, L., et al.: Acta Med. Scand., *216:*157–164, 1984.
158. Yoshimura, H.: Nutr. Rev., *10:*251–253, 1970.
159. Eichner, E.R.: Am. J. Med., *78:*321–325, 1985.
160. Brune, M., Magnusson, B., Persson, H., et al.: Am. J. Clin. Nutr., *43:*438–443, 1986.
161. Gardner, G.W., Edgerton, V.R., Senewiratne, B., et al.: Am. J. Clin. Nutr., *30:*910–917, 1977.
162. Perkkiö, M.V., Jansson, L.T., Brooks, G.A., et al.: J. Appl. Physiol., *58:*1477–1480, 1985.
163. Gledhill, N.: Med. Sci. Sports Exerc., *14:*183–189, 1982.
164. Gledhill, N.: The influence of altered blood volume and oxygen transport capacity on aerobic performance. *In* Exercise and Sport Science Reviews. Edited by R.L. Terjung. New York, Macmillan, 1985.
165. Buick, F.J., Gledhill, N., Froese, A.B., et al.: J. Appl. Physiol., *48:*636–642, 1980.
166. Spriet, L.L., Gledhill, N., Froese, A.B., et al.: J. Appl. Physiol., *61:*1942–1948, 1986.
167. Edgerton, V.R., Gardner, G.W., Ohira, Y., et al.: Br. Med. J., *2:*1546–1549, 1979.
168. Celsing, F., Blomstrand, E., Werner, B., et al.: Med. Sci. Sports Exerc., *18:*156–161, 1986.
169. Matter, M., Stittfall, T., Graves, J., et al.: Clin. Sci., *72:*415–422, 1987.
170. Schoene, R.B., Escourrou, P., Robertson, H.T., et al.: J. Lab. Clin. Med., *102:*306–312, 1983.
171. Clarkson, P.M.: Vitamins and trace minerals. *In* Perspectives in Exercise Science and Sports Medicine. Vol. 4. Edited by D.R. Lamb, R. Williams. Carmel, IN, Benchmark Press, 1991.
172. Belko, A.Z.: Med. Sci. Sports Exerc., *19:*S191–S196, 1987.
173. Williams, M.H.: Vitamins, iron and calcium supplementation: Effect on human physical performance. *In* Nutrition and Athletic Performance. Edited by W. Haskell, J. Scala, J. Whittan. Palo Alto, Bull, 1982.
174. Wilmore, J.H., Freund, B.J.: Nutr. Abst. Rev., Rev. Clin. Nutr., *54:*1–16, 1984.
175. DiPalma, J.R., Ritchie, D.M.: Annu. Rev. Pharmacol. Toxicol., *17:*133–148, 1977.
176. Belko, A.Z., Obarzanek, K., Kalkwarf, H.J., et al.: Am. J. Clin. Nutr., *37:*509–517, 1983.
177. Leklem, J.E., Schultz, T.D.: Am. J. Clin. Nutr., *38:*541–548, 1983.
178. Buzina, K., Buzina, R., Brubacker, G., et al.: Int. J. Vitam. Nutr. Res., *54:*55–60, 1984.
179. Montoye, H., Spata, P.J., Pinckney, V., et al.: J. Appl. Physiol., *7:*589–592, 1955.
180. Tin-May-Than, Ma-Win-May, Khin-Sann-Aung, et al.: Br. J. Nutr., *40:*269–273, 1978.
181. Keren, G., Epstein, Y.: J. Sports Med. Phys. Fitness, *20:*145–148, 1980.
182. Keith, R.E., Driskell, J.A.: Am. J. Clin. Nutr., *36:*840–845, 1982.
183. Gray, M.E., Titlow, L.W.: Med. Sci. Sports Exerc., *14:*424–427, 1982.
184. Tremblay, A., Boilard, B., Breton, M.F., et al.: Nutr. Res., *4:*201–208, 1984.
185. Herbert, V., Jacob, E.: JAMA, *230:*241–242, 1974.
186. Bergström, J., Hultman, E., Jorfeldt, L., et al.: J. Appl. Physiol., *26:*170–176, 1969.
187. Deuster, P.A., Kyle, S.B., Moser, P.B., et al.: Am. J. Clin. Nutr., *44:*954–962, 1986.
188. Peters, A.J., Dressendorfer, R.H., Rimar, J., et al.: Phys. Sportsmed., *14:*63–70, 1986.
189. Dressendorfer, R.H., Sockolov, R.: Phys. Sportsmed., *8:*97–100, 1980.
190. Weight, L.M., Noakes, T.D., Labadarios, D., et al.: Am. J. Clin. Nutr., *47:*186–191, 1988.
191. Bazzarre, T.L., Marquart, L.F., Izurietz, M., et al.: Med. Sci. Sports Exerc., *18:*S90, 1986.
192. Lukasi, H.C., Bolonchuk, W.W, Klevay, L.M., et al.: Am. J. Clin. Nutr., *37:*407–415, 1983.
193. McDonald, R., Keen, C.L.: Sports Med., *5:*171–184, 1988.
194. Weight, L.M., Myburgh, K.H., Noakes, T.D.: Am. J. Clin. Nutr., *47:*192–195, 1988.
195. Barnett, D.W., Conlee, R.K.: Am. J. Clin. Nutr., *40:*586–590, 1984.
196. Health and Welfare Canada: Nutrition Recommendations. Report of the Scientific Review Committee. Ottawa, Suppy and Services, 1990.
197. Percy, E.C.: Med. Sci. Sports Exerc., *10:*298–303, 1978.
198. Short, S.H., Short, W.R.: J. Am. Diet. Assoc., *82:*632–645, 1983.
199. Ellsworth, N.M., Hewitt, B.F., Haskell, W.L.: Phys. Sportsmed., *13:*78–92, 1985.
200. Bedgood, B.L., Tuck, M.B.: J. Am. Diet. Assoc., *83:*672–677, 1983.
201. American Dietetic Association: J. Am. Diet. Assoc., *76:*437–443, 1980.

## SELECTED READINGS

Horton, E.S., Terjung, R.L. (eds.): Exercise, Nutrition, and Energy Metabolism. New York, MacMillan, 1988.

Parizkova, J., Rogozkin, V.A. (eds.): Nutrition, Physical Fitness and Health. Baltimore, University Park Press, 1978.

Perspectives in Exercise Science and Sports Medicine. Carmel, IN, Indiana Benchmark Press. Vol. 1: Edited by D.R. Lamb and R. Murray, 1988; Vol. 3: Edited by C.V. Gisolfi and D.R. Lamb, 1990; Vol. 4: Edited by D.R. Lamb and M. Williams, 1991.

Symposium: Maximizing performance with nutrition. Med. Sci. Sports Exerc., *19:*S179–S200, 1987.

CHAPTER 43

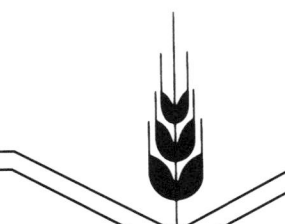

# Nutrition in Space

Paul A. Lachance



Since 1957, over 3000 successful space launches have occurred. The first manned spaceflight began on April 12, 1961 (Yuri Gagarin, Vostok 1). The first American flight in earth orbit was that of John Glenn, Jr. on February 20, 1962 in Friendship 7. Manned space launches now exceed 125. The longest American experience in microgravity is 84 days (Skylab 4, 1974). The longest Soviet experience (December, 1988) is 1 year (the duration of a mission to Mars and return is 2 years). The largest crew has been eight on an American Space Shuttle (STS-61-A, 1985). Table 43–1 gives program names and ranges of dates of the manned spaceflights mentioned in this chapter. Tentative National Aeronautics and Space Administration (NASA) plans are, by the year 2000, to assemble and occupy a space laboratory in earth orbit with a multinational crew of up to a dozen men and women (Space Station Freedom).

Every American mission has medical supervision, but on only a few selected missions were biomedical research data collected during flight as well as pre- and postflight (Gemini 7, Skylab 2, 3, and 4). Selected additional missions included significant pre- and postflight tests (Gemini 4, 5, and Apollo 14, 15, and 16) and a few shuttle missions. The reader must understand that the topic of this chapter is based primarily on American data collected on a limited number (24 to 30) of astronauts on flights lasting 4 to 84 days.

Before the first manned spaceflight, discussions focused on food and water requirements and the appropriate guidelines to be adopted.[1–6] Although actual and potential stresses and hazards of spaceflight could be enumerated,[7,8] no adequate and reliable spaceflight experience was available on which to base concrete estimates. The three possibilities considered were: (1) with prolonged weightlessness, energy demands and associated nutritional requirements would be decreased and approach the basal metabolic state; (2) a considerable increase in requirements, particularly energy, would occur, attributable to the increased toll of motion and work tasks in a low friction environment;[9] and (3) food and water needs would be essentially those of moderately active, Earth-bound men.[10] The latter view was adopted.

The reality of experience has shown that the energy cost of extravehicular activity (EVA); functioning in larger habitable volumes, (e.g., Salyut, Skylab, and Shuttle), and the increased duration of required in-flight exercise regimens has led to an upward revision in energy allowances for both cosmonauts (2800 kcal per day to 3150 kcal per day) and astronauts (2500 kcal per day to 3000 kcal per day) even in longer missions.

Little debate surrounded the critical need for water and it was agreed that water supplies should not be compromised. The Soviets allow 2.2 to 2.5 L of water from food and water in nominal operations but double the allowance for periods of EVA. Usage of palatable water on Skylab 2 (28 days) was 2.6 L per day, and it rose to 3.15 L per day on the Skylab 3 (59 days) and Skylab 4 (84 days) missions.

**TABLE 43–1.** MANNED SPACE FLIGHT EXPERIENCE

| LAUNCH ERA | COUNTRY | NAME | CREW SIZE | NUMBER OF MISSIONS | MAXIMUM DURATION |
|---|---|---|---|---|---|
| 1961–1963 | USSR | Vostok | 1 | 6 | 119 hours |
| 1961–1962 | USA | Mercury | 1 | 6 | 34 hours |
| 1964–1965 | USSR | Voskhod | 2–3 | 2 | 26 hours |
| 1965–1966 | USA | Gemini | 2 | 10 | 13.75 days |
| 1967–1979 | USSR | Soyuz | 1–3 | 15 | 18 days |
| 1968–1972 | USA | Apollo | 3 | 10 | 12.6 days |
| 1971–1979 | USSR | Soyuz/Salyut* | 2–3 | 22 | 185 days |
| 1973 | USA | Skylab | 3 | 2 | 59 days |
| 1974 | USA | Skylab | 3 | 1 | 84 days |
| 1980–1985 | USSR | Soyuz/Salyut* | 2–3 | 13 | 211 days |
| 1981–1983 | USA | Shuttle (STS Series) | 2–6 | 9 | 10 days |
| 1984–1988 | USA | Shuttle | 5–8 | 4 series 41<br>8 series 51†<br>3 series 61 | 8 days |
| 1986–1990 | USSR | Soyuz/MIR* | 2–3 | 6 | 326 days‡ |
| 1989–1990 | USA | Shuttle | 5–7 | 11 | 11 days |

*Space Station (MIR in orbit since February, 1986).
†Challenger exploded January 28, 1986.
‡Two astronauts.

## PROVISION OF FOOD AND WATER

### HISTORY AND EVALUATION

The Mercury foods were revised versions of items developed by the United States Army for United States Air Force space-oriented programs,[3] which predated NASA as well as the Air Force Manned Orbital Laboratory that was terminated. These foods included freeze-dried meat entrees, low-moisture cereal products, and compressed bite-size foods.[11] NASA accelerated the development of a feeding system specifically directed toward the Gemini and Apollo missions of up to 14 days, providing for specific environmental constraints and increasing the variety of foods.[12,13] New developments featured rehydratables of higher caloric density such as freeze-dried salads,[14] puddings,[15] and bite-size freeze-dried sandwiches.[15,16]

The feeding system for the Gemini and initial Apollo missions was designed to serve two or more men for up to 14 days and longer, if necessary. About one half of the available menu items were freeze-dried; the remaining were other types of dried low-moisture foods, some formed by compression. A typical menu consisted of approximately 50% rehydratables (foods requiring added water before ingestion), and the other 50% were bite-size items to be rehydrated in the mouth.[17] Ready-to-eat foods of normal moisture content were introduced as experimental foods early in the Apollo program,[18] including irradiated bread and meats sterilized by short-time, high-temperature (thermostabilized) methods. Adjustment of viscosity of food products allowed later Apollo crews to eat many foods with spoons in the normal way,[18] an idea first advanced by Calloway and colleagues[19] and developed by the Army Natick Laboratories in Natick, MA. Formulation and processing for all the space foods were described in Space Food Production Guides[20] used by industry in the production of flight food. More than 100 American food companies provided food ingredients/foods and/or packaging in compliance with these stringent requirements.

The number of available food items permitted a menu of at least a 4-day cycle of 3 to 4 meals per day or any combination of meals and snacks. The aim in the Gemini program was to assemble a menu providing at least 2500 kcal per day. In the Apollo Lunar Landing Program, provision of 2800 to 3200 kcal per day was possible. In a typical menu, 17% of calories were derived from protein, 33% from fat, and 50% from carbohydrate. Fiber (high residue)-containing or foods such as dairy items were minimized to decrease intestinal gas production, stool volumes, and frequency. The final menu for a given flight is affected by the need for nutritional balance, storage configuration in allocated areas, and astronaut preferences. A separate paragraph in this chapter is a discussion of waste collection and management.

The nutrient intake of Gemini 4, 5, and 7 crew members was calculated from the food consumption data and corresponding analytic data (Table 43–2).[21] The analytic data used were derived from analyses of representative lots of identical food items. The "amount provided" (the total quantity of food loaded on the spacecraft) can be misleading because crew members cannot possibly remove every fraction of food from the

**TABLE 43–2.** INTAKE OF KEY NUTRIENTS ON GEMINI 4, 5, AND 7

| FLIGHT | AMOUNT (per 24 hr) | ENERGY (kcal) | PROTEIN (g) | CALCIUM (mg) | CHLORIDES (g) |
|---|---|---|---|---|---|
| Gemini 4 | | | | | |
| June 3–7, 1965 | Provided: | 2549 | 108.9 | 847 | 10.35 |
| Days: hr: | Consumed by: | | | | |
| min: 4:0:56 | White | 2230 | 89.2 | 739 | 7.96 |
| | McDivitt | 2066 | 90.7 | 676 | 8.17 |
| Gemini 5 | | | | | |
| Aug. 21–29, 1965 | Provided: | 2755 | 96.4 | 849 | 10.29 |
| Days: hr: | Consumed by: | | | | |
| min: 7:22:55 | Cooper | 1075 | 41.9 | 373 | 4.70 |
| | Conrad | 915 | 35.8 | 333 | 4.06 |
| Gemini 7 | | | | | |
| Dec. 4–18, 1965 | Provided: | 2333 | 90.2 | 1194 | 8.70 |
| Days: hr: | Consumed by: | | | | |
| min: 13:18:35 | Borman | 1774 | 67.6 | 945 | 6.66 |
| | Lovell | 1804 | 68.3 | 922 | 6.88 |

(From Lachance, P.A., Nanz, R.A., Klicka, M.V.: Food Consumption and Gemini IV, V, and VII. Technical Memo X-58010. Houston, National Aeronautics and Space Administration, Manned Spacecraft Center, 1967.)

rehydrated food containers. Food residue can be as much as 20% (wet weight) of the amount provided. With bite-size food, the individual bites are either ingested completely or not eaten.

Fruit-flavored drinks were fortified with calcium lactate for the calcium balance experiment, which resulted in the desired calcium intake approaching 950 mg per day by the Gemini 7 crew. Compared with Gemini 4 results, proportionally fewer calories and other nutrients were consumed by the Gemini 7 crew. Without such fortification, the calcium intake of the Gemini 7 crew would have been considerably less than desired for the experiments conducted on this flight concerning bone demineralization[22] and calcium balance.[23]

The Apollo missions afforded increased volume and weight allowances for food as well as hot and cold water for rehydration, which permitted an increase in the variety of foods from 49 to 70 and a "pantry" concept. The use of spoon-bowl packaging (rehydrate and eat with spoon rather than squeeze from the container) was introduced. Packaged bread previously baked with irradiated flour made in-flight sandwich preparation possible when bread was combined with thermostabilized or natural spreads.[24] Commercially available thermostabilized foods in aluminum, pull-tab lid cans were tested on Apollo 10. Foods such as thermostabilized chicken salad and beef and gravy were incorporated into the menus of Apollo 14 and subsequent Apollo missions.[25]

The Lunar Module had similar foods but a defined menu. Mechanisms for access to the liquid and semiliquid foods for emergency nourishment over several days were devised for eating through a port in the pressurized suit (but never needed). A fluid drink and a food bar were incorporated into the interior of the helmet ring of the spacesuit for consumption, by sucking or biting, respectively, during periods exceeding 4 hours on the surface of the moon.[26]

Skylab, with durations of 28, 59, and 84 days in earth orbit, had significant space and power to permit the meal-like warmer tray and a 6-day menu cycle of food. Foods in the tray could be heated to 65 ± 3° C within 2 hours (in absence of convection). The prevailing atmospheric pressure was 250 mm Hg and thus the boiling point was 72.2° C. Although the food system was intended to ensure about 100% of RDA nutrients (Table 43–3), the 59- and 84-day missions incorporated the use of a daily vitamin supplement (Table 43–4).[27]

With the exception of beverages (rehydrated in a bellows-type container), foods were assembled on a tray and included thermostabilized easy-open containers and spoon-bowl dehydrated food. Astronauts were no longer required to hold each individual food container and thus could select from several foods, all open at the same eating occasion, and use knives and forks. Skylab had both refrigeration and freezing space. Frozen, dehydrated, thermostabilized, and intermediate-moisture preserved foods were part of the prescribed menu. In addition, condiments included liquid garlic, Tabasco sauce, and dehydrated horseradish and dry salt.[28]

The Space Shuttle is both a spacecraft and an aircraft (lands as a glider aircraft). The size of the crew has varied from two to eight and has a potential mission duration of 30 days. No refrigerator or freezer is on board. The food system is designed around commercially available food that is individually packaged for handling and use in microgravity. A fresh-food locker contains fresh foods (e.g., apples, oranges, carrots, and bread) that must be used within 2 to 3 days. As in Apollo and Skylab, rehydratable, natural, thermostabilized and intermedi-

**TABLE 43–3.** AVERAGE DAILY NUTRIENT INTAKES OF SKYLAB CREW MEMBERS (± SD)

| | UNITS | PREFLIGHT | IN-FLIGHT | POSTFLIGHT |
|---|---|---|---|---|
| Energy | kcal | 3128 ± 441 | 3130 ± 488 | 3265 ± 499 |
| Nitrogen | g | 18.6 ± 3.1 | 18.3 ± 3.8 | 18.6 ± 3.4 |
| Fat | g | 109.4 ± 22.0 | 86.8 ± 32.0 | 110.6 ± 25.0 |
| Carbohydrate | g | 363.0 ± 69.4 | 413.2 ± 89.3 | 397.4 ± 93.9 |
| Crude fiber | g | 6.1 ± 1.9 | 6.2 ± 2.1 | 6.4 ± 2.2 |
| Water | ml | 2991 ± 771 | 2819 ± 685 | 3093 ± 948 |
| Calcium | mg | 853 ± 170 | 913 ± 196 | 886 ± 194 |
| Phosphorus | mg | 1717 ± 290 | 1780 ± 332 | 1756 ± 321 |
| Sodium | mEq | 222 ± 46 | 236 ± 53 | 224 ± 45 |
| Potassium | mEq | 99.2 ± 18.4 | 98.1 ± 18.6 | 99.8 ± 19.3 |
| Magnesium | mEq | 25.0 ± 4.8 | 25.6 ± 6.5 | 26.4 ± 5.4 |
| Chloride | mEq | 189 ± 41 | 195 ± 44 | 189 ± 36 |
| Iron | mg | 17.0 ± 3.2 | 17.2 ± 3.9 | 17.4 ± 3.5 |
| Zinc | mg | 13.7 ± 3.4 | 13.1 ± 3.7 | 14.1 ± 3.4 |
| Copper | mg | 1.59 ± 0.48 | 1.64 ± 0.57 | 1.60 ± 0.50 |

(From Smith, M.C., Rambaut, P.C., Stadler, C.R.: Skylab nutritional studies. *In* Proceedings of the Skylab Life Sciences Symposium. Edited by R.S. Johnson, L.F. Dietlein. NASA TM X-58154. Washington, D.C., National Aeronautics and Space Administration, 1974, pp. 193–197.)

**TABLE 43–4.** COMPOSITION OF VITAMIN SUPPLEMENT CONSUMED DAILY BY CREW MEMBERS OF 59- AND 84-DAY MISSIONS

| | |
|---|---|
| Vitamin A | 5000 IU |
| Vitamin D | 500 IU |
| Vitamin E | 15 IU |
| Thiamine mononitrate | 10 mg |
| Riboflavin | 10 mg |
| Ascorbic acid | 313 mg |
| Niacinamide | 100 mg |
| Pyridoxine hydrochloride | 2 mg |
| Calcium pantothenate | 20 mg |
| Cobalamine | 4 μg |
| Folic acid | 33 μg |

(From Smith, M.C., Rambaut, P.C., Stadler, C.R.: Skylab nutritional studies. *In* Proceedings of the Skylab Life Sciences Symposium. Edited by R.S. Johnson, L.F. Dietlein. NASA TM X-58154. Washington, D.C., National Aeronautics and Space Administration, 1974, pp. 193–197.)

ate-moisture foods are used, and variety has increased to over 100 foods.[29,30] Four-day cycle menus are preselected and color coded (Table 43–5). About one half of the foods are rehydratable to conserve weight. Water for rehydration is obtained as a by-product of the fuel cells. A supplementary food pantry of 3 days of food is also provided. Meats were irradiated to ensure sterility and thus stability at ambient temperature. During EVA, in-suit fruit bars (170 kcal/50 g) are available for consumption within the pressure suit (grasp with teeth and bite off section) as well as a beverage with a one-way "straw."[29] These supplies are modeled on the lunar in-suit food/drink system.[26]

## FOOD SAFETY

Biologic, operational, and engineering constraints affect the selection, processing criteria, preparation, and use of food.[12,31] These constraints peak in applications where space, weight, and power are limited. The astronaut(s) are subjected to risks, some of which can be avoided, such as food-related infections or intoxications. The microbiologic criteria applied to space foods[12] were unique in that pathogens and not indicator organisms were specified, and standards invariably exceeded those for commercial foods. These criteria coupled with the Critical Control Point engineering management mandates of the Apollo program has led to the establishment of the Hazard Analysis Critical Control Point (HACCP) food safety rationale now being adopted by the food industry and government regulators.[32] During the early lunar landing flights, fear of the possible back contamination of a mutant infectious disease organism from the moon to the earth was controlled and studied by the isolation of the crew from recovery to several days in a specially constructed lunar material- and personnel-receiving facility in Houston. No risks were identified and instead man has littered the moon.

Because recovery from earth orbit is accomplished more readily and space, weight, and power constraints are lower, the introduction of fresh foods with minimal biohazard potential has been introduced in the Space Shuttle program. Initially, bread and a few other foods (meats) were irradiated to ensure sterility and enhance shelf life. This practice has since been limited to bread and rolls.[29]

The Soviet space foods from the outset have been based substantially on natural foods—fresh, canned, dehydrated, and fermented. Pureed foods in aluminum

**TABLE 43–5.** SHUTTLE STANDARD MENU

| MEAL | DAYS 1,* 5 | | DAYS 2, 6 | | DAYS 3, 7 | | DAYS 4, 8 | |
|---|---|---|---|---|---|---|---|---|
| A | Peaches | (T)† | Applesauce | (T) | Dried peaches | (IM) | Dried apricots | (IM) |
| | Beef pattie | (R) | Dried beef | (NF) | Sausage | (R) | Breadfast roll | (I)(NF) |
| | Scrambled eggs | (R) | Granola | (R) | Scrambled eggs | (R) | Granola w/blueberries | (R) |
| | Bran flakes | (R) | Breakfast roll | (I)(NF) | Cornflakes | (R) | Vanilla inst. brkfast | (B) |
| | Cocoa | (B) | Choc. inst. brkfst | (B) | Cocoa | (B) | Grapefruit drink | (B) |
| | Orange drink | (B) | Orange-grapefruit drk | (B) | Orange-pineapple drink | (B) | | |
| B | Frankfurters | (T) | Corned beef | (T)(I) | Ham | (T) | Ground beef w/ pickle sauce | (T) |
| | Turkey tetrazzini | (R) | Asparagus | (R) | Cheese spread | (T) | Noodles & chicken | (R) |
| | Bread (2×) | (I)(NF) | Bread (2×) | (I)(NF) | Bread (2×) | (I)(NF) | Stewed tomatoes | (T) |
| | Bananas | (FD) | Pears | (T) | Gr. beans & broccoli | (R) | Pears | (FD) |
| | Almond crunch bar | (NF) | Peanuts | (NF) | Crushed pineapple | (T) | Almonds | (NF) |
| | Apple drink (2×) | (B) | Lemonade (2×) | (B) | Shortbread cookies | (NF) | Strawberry drink | (B) |
| | | | | | Cashews | (NF) | | |
| | | | | | Tea w/lemon & sugar (2×) | (B) | | |
| C | Shrimp cocktail | (R) | Beef w/BBQ sauce | (T) | Cr. mushroom soup | (R) | Tuna | (T) |
| | Beef steak | (T)(I) | Cauliflower w/cheese | (R) | Smoked turkey | (T)(I) | Macaroni & cheese | (R) |
| | Rice pilaf | (R) | Gr. beans w/mushrooms | (R) | Mixed Italian vegetables | (R) | Peas w/butter sauce | (R) |
| | Broccoli au gratin | (R) | Lemon pudding | (T) | Vanilla pudding | (T) | Peach ambrosia | (R) |
| | Fruit cocktail | (T) | Pecan cookies | (NF) | Strawberries | (R) | Chocolate pudding | (T) |
| | Butterscotch pudding | (T) | Cocoa | (B) | Tropical punch | (B) | Lemonade | (B) |
| | Grape drink | (B) | | | | | | |

*Day 1 (launch day) consists of Meals B and C only.

†Abbreviations; T, thermostabilized: IM, Intermediate moisture; R, rehydratable; I, irradiated; FD, freeze-dried; NF, natural form; B, beverage (rehydratable).

(From Bourland, C.T., Fohey, M.F., Rapp, R.M., et al.: J. Food Protect., *44*:313–319, 1981.)

tubes that can be heated and several types of meat, poultry, and cheese are preserved in 100-g cans. Fermented milks (yogurts) and semidehydratd fruits are used.[33,34] Packaging is not as sophisticated and emphasis is placed on four meals per day. In long-term missions, the resupply "Provider" cargo craft carries apples, onions, garlic, oranges, lemons, and cranberries. Hot and cold recycled water is used. Tables 43–6 and 43–7 provide interesting contrasts between the American and Soviet food systems reflecting attitudes toward nutrient supplements and "psychologic" foods.[34] In contrast to the American emphasis on short-term missions, the Union of Soviet Socialist Republics has up to 1 year of experience in orbit (one half the duration of a flight to Mars).

## FEEDING SYSTEMS FOR EXTENDED DURATIONS

The psychology of food has greater importance as a mission's duration increases. When periodic resupply is not possible, however, such as during a 2-year or longer mission to Mars, the constraints of space, weight, and power necessitate alternate approaches to the complete provisioning of needed food and water supplies.

A highly motivated crew would accept fuel-cell water and a limited menu of highly defined foods. The freezing of thermostabilized and/or irradiated foods would provide a shelf life exceeding 2 years. Supplementation with the capability to bake bread and other novel, psychologically enhancing techniques would provide sufficient alternate presentations of common foods to give variety. Micronutrients would be supplied by supplements.

Closed ecologic life-support systems[35] can be implemented with increasing degrees of closure. The initial closure with a major saving requires the recycling of water (urine and atmosphere). The recycling of water from feces is psychologically difficult to accept; it also increases health risks and requires engineering sophistications that are practical only at a stationary base (lunar base).

A further degree of closure would provide selected high-density hydroponically grown higher plant materials (wheat, soy, and sugar beets), which can be processed readily into food. This capability of farming in space provides psychologic diversion in addition to fresh food. This capability may or may not be coupled with a waste

**TABLE 43–6.** DIFFERENCES IN RECOMMENDED NUTRIENT INTAKE OF COSMONAUTS AND ASTRONAUTS

| NUTRIENTS | COSMONAUTS | ASTRONAUTS |
|---|---|---|
| Kilocalories | 3200 kcal | 2300–3100 kcal |
| Protein | 1.5 g/kg b.w. (140 g)* | 0.8 g/kg b.w. (56 g) |
| Fat | 1.4 g/kg b.w. (100 g) | 1.3 g/kg b.w. (93 g) |
| Carbohydrates | 4.5 g/kg b.w. (395 g) | 4.8 g/kg b.w. (350 g) |
| Calcium | 1.7 g | 0.8 g |
| Sodium | 4.5 g | 3.5 g |
| Iron | 50 mg | 18 mg |

*b.w., body weight.
(From Lachance, P.A.: Activities Rep., *19:* 133–136, 1967.)

**TABLE 43–7.** OTHER DIFFERENCES IN FOOD INTAKE OF COSMONAUTS AND ASTRONAUTS

| FOOD | COSMONAUTS | ASTRONAUTS |
|---|---|---|
| Plant extract (Eleutherococcus); 500 mg/day or 1.0 g every other day | Used to increase stamina and to resist stress | None |
| Garlic | As food seasoning | None |
| Vodka | Small amount | None |
| Brandy | Small amount | None |
| Fresh fruits and vegetables | Supplied by "Progess" cargo ship | Stored 16 hours before launch on shuttle |
| Onion, dill, parsley | Cultivated in on-board vegetable garden | None |
| Multivitamin | Supplement, twice daily | Optional (shuttle) |
| Essential amino acids (methionine) | Supplements, increased amount | None |
| Glutamic acid | Supplement | None |

(From Lachance, P.A.: Activities Rep., *19:* 133—136, 1967.)

processing system and biomass production. Complete closure would provide oxygen and uptake carbon dioxide. Systems that are completely closed are feasible for stationary or orbited space stations. Extensive research is required to attain fully operational closed ecologic life-support systems.

## WASTE MANAGEMENT AND RESEARCH

Waste management and the biologic sampling of waste are "one of the greatest challenges to crew life support."[36] Initially, all urine and feces were collected in "intimate contact devices," such as in-suit bladders and in-suit diaper-type underwear. The bladder could be vented to space if full. In the Gemini and Apollo programs, a shared udder-shaped cone collected urine, which could be vented overboard, and a colostomy-type bag was used for feces.

In the Gemini biomedical experiments, an interrupter bag was placed in-line with an isotope dispenser (to monitor volume by dilution) and a representative 75-ml sample of each voiding was collected for storage. The remainder of the urine was vented overboard. Fecal containers were treated with an enclosed squeeze-to-open disinfectant and stored. The Skylab and Shuttle used a module resembling a seat that incorporates cabin air for pneumatic collections (artificial gravity and thus causing separation from the body and transport to storage). For in-flight experiments, the volume of urine and the mass measurement of feces were recorded and fecal samples were freeze-dried for return. Excess urine is vented to the vacuum of space. Feces on the Shuttle are collected into a single container, vacuum-dried, and returned to earth. Positive separation of feces from the anal area is a continuing flight problem.

A major source of error in all of the in-flight balance studies has been the quantification of urine volume and the collection of truly representative samples. Creatinine values proved to be a significant reference indicator of adequate sampling. Ingested markers for feces for the separation of collection periods have been adequate when the stool is formed.

## BODY COMPOSITION CHANGES

### WEIGHT LOSS

Weight loss has characterized practically all Soviet and American space missions (Fig. 43–1). Weight loss by the command pilot during Gemini 4 (4 days) was 2.0 kg, whereas that of the pilot was 3.9 kg. During Gemini 7 (14 days), the command pilot lost 4.5 kg and the pilot lost 2.9 kg. On the Gemini 5 flight (8 days), the command pilot lost 3.3 kg. and the pilot lost 3.9 kg.

The caloric deficit per mission, calculated from food consumption data and carbon dioxide absorbed by lithium hydroxide canisters,[12] is given in Table 43–8. Of the three Gemini missions discussed here, calculated oxygen consumption was lowest on Gemini 5 and probably reflects the low level of crew activity. Little food was consumed on Gemini 5, which the crew attributed to anorexia. The daily prospect of impending re-entry may have prompted the crew to postpone eating and to unstow as little food as possible to minimize housekeeping and permit re-entry on short notice. During the last few days of the mission, both crew members experienced a significant depression of appetite. Food consumption on Gemini 4 and 7 was good but obviously was not sufficient. Although weight loss may occur before flight because of the tension and work load,[37] in-flight weight loss usually occurs the first day and then stabilizes over 10 to 15 days.

The most comprehensive metabolic experiments were conducted during three Skylab missions lasting 28, 59, and 84 days. However, no direct measurements of body composition changes have been conducted. Through the analysis of a continuous time profile of daily total body changes in water, protein, and fat from metabolic balance data, indirect estimates of in-flight tissue and fluid losses were computed by Leonard.[38] The highlights of these findings follow.

The major components of body composition (water, protein, and fat) undergo significant changes. About 60% of the weight loss observed during all three Skylab missions could be attributed to loss of lean body mass, with the remainder derived from fat stores.

### BODY WATER

An obligatory loss of at least 1 L of body water occurs within the first few days of space flight. The initial water deficit is primarily a result of reduced fluid intake because urine and evaporative water losses, on the average, were equal to or below control preflight lev-

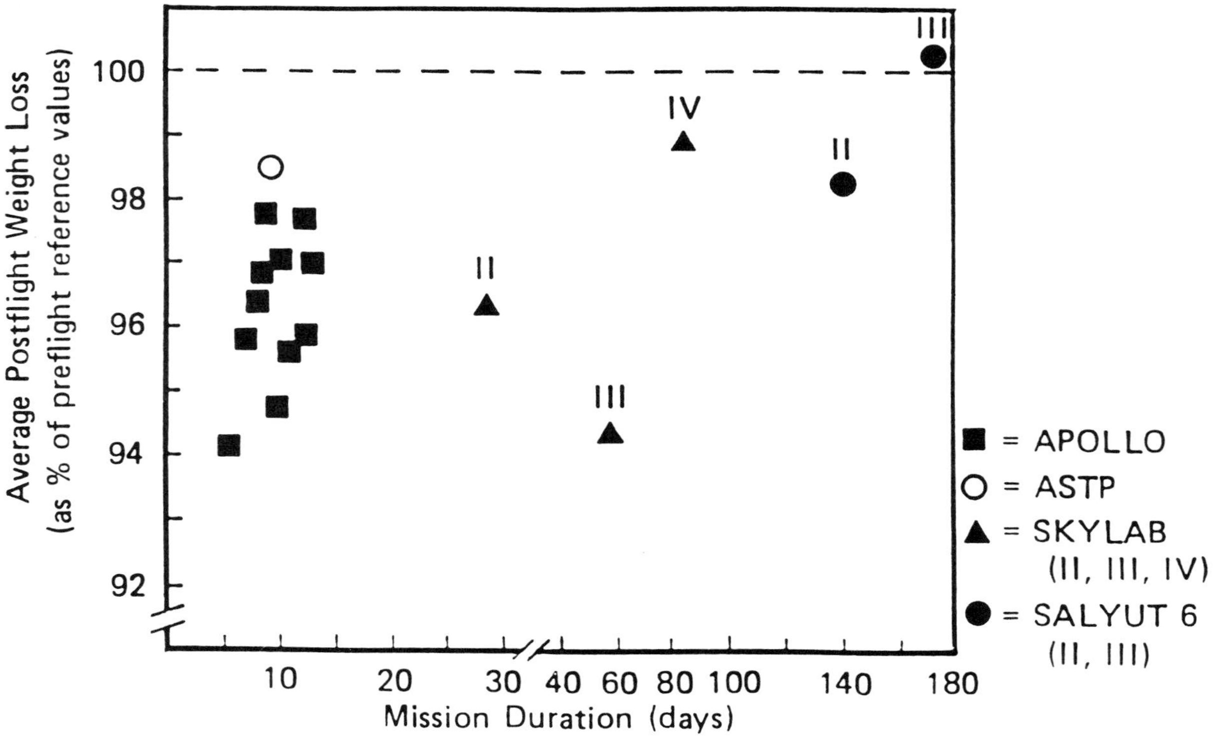
Average Postflight Weight Loss
(as % of preflight reference values)
100
98
96
94
92
10
20
30
40
60
80
100
140
180
Mission Duration (days)
IV
II
III
II
III
■ = APOLLO
O = ASTP
▲ = SKYLAB
(II, III, IV)
● = SALYUT 6
(II, III)

**FIGURE 43–1.** Weight losses found after flight in space missions. (From Nicogossian, A.E., Huntoon, C.L., Pool, S.L. (Eds.): Space Physiology and Medicine. 2nd Ed. Philadelphia, Lea & Febiger, 1989.)

**TABLE 43–8.** CALCULATED CALORIE DEFICIT ON GEMINI 4, 5, AND 7

| | GEMINI-TITAN | | |
|---|---|---|---|
| CALORIES PER DAY* | 4 | 5 | 7 |
| Stowed on board | 2550 | 2755 | 2333 |
| Expended (calculated from recovered $CO_2$)[44] | 2410 | 2010 | 2219 |
| Consumed | 2148 | 995 | 1789 |
| Deficit | −262 | −1015 | −430 |
| Accumulated deficit per mission | −1048 (4 days) | −8120 (8 days) | −6020 (14 days) |

*Average for two astronauts.
(From Lachance, P.A.: Environ. Biol. Med., *1*:205–228, 1971.)

els.[39,40] The crew members exhibiting severe space motion sickness symptoms reduced their fluid intake by the greatest amount and lost the greatest amount of body water. As motion sickness waned and normal intake was resumed, some body water repletion became evident in these susceptible crew members. The reduction in body water was maintained throughout the flight in spite of ad libitum drinking. Shifts of up to 2 L of fluid from the legs, observed on Skylab,[41,42] can easily account for the body water losses, assuming a large fraction of this fluid (when translocated to the upper body) is excessive in microgravity and is eliminated from the body. Measurements of the body fluid compartments before and after each mission, using isotope tracers, revealed mean net losses of plasma volume (−0.41 L) and intracellular fluid volume (−0.49 L).[43] Almost one half of the intracellular fluid loss can be traced to loss of red cell mass (−0.23 L).[44,45] Thus, most of the loss in total body water (−.82 L) measured during the first day of recovery (after some fluid replenishment had taken place) can be attributed to these compartments.

## BODY FAT

The Skylab results support the premise that body fat is the material preferentially used to compensate for energy deficits resulting from inadequate energy intake.[46] On average, about three times more weight as body fat was lost as was body protein; because the caloric value of fat is slightly more than twice that of protein, the body derived nearly six times as much energy from the metabolized fat as from protein. These proportions were twice as great for the crews of the two shorter missions during which energy intake was "controlled." Caloric intake probably was inadequate for the crews on the 28- and 59-day Skylab missions; the extent of their fat losses averaged about 50% of their total mass loss, a value similar to that estimated for the Apollo crews returning from 2-week space missions.[47] On the other hand, the crew with the highest caloric intake (84-day mission) exhibited a mean gain in body fat, implying a sufficient diet. The 84-day crew also exercised the most of all Skylab astronauts, and exercise by itself is capable of decreasing fat depots. Only part of the exercise performed could be quantitated, but on that basis, it appeared that the excess calories in the diet (compared to the two preceding Skylab crews) were greater than the extra work performed by this crew which could account for the small gain in fat (Table 43–9). Leonard used caloric values as obtained in bomb calorimetry.

Caloric intake was less than adequate for at least two reasons: (1) in the case of the crews on 28- and 59-day missions, a strictly controlled diet was used, based on the assumption that in-flight requirements should be less than those for a 1-G environment;[47] and (2) during the first week of each flight, a significant degree of anorexia occurred coinciding with motion sickness symptoms. As a result of the anorexia, fat losses were particularly rapid during the week after launch. In general, the changes in body fat appear to be explained by the balance between caloric intake and energy expenditure and do not appear to have been influenced by weightlessness per se.

## BODY PROTEIN

Atrophy of skeletal muscle occurs in response to disuse, inadequate functional load, insufficient food intake, and lack of exercise.[48,49] Spaceflight may be associated, at various times, with one or more of these conditions. The most important findings of the analysis by Leonard[38] with respect to body protein changes are that protein loss begins almost immediately after entering weightlessness and, during the first month, the rate of loss decreases exponentially. Protein loss stabilizes after the first month of flight. The initial losses occur in spite of a high protein diet and in the presence of exercise training. These observations are consistent with the hypothesis that the postural muscles virtually are unused in weightlessness with resultant atrophy.[48] Furthermore, the exercise performed on Skylab was not sufficient to maintain the entire mass of antigravity muscles.[50] A reduced caloric intake appears to be capa-

**TABLE 43–9.** IN-FLIGHT ENERGY BALANCE (KCAL/DAY) ON SKYLAB 1, 2, AND 3

| ENERGY BALANCE COMPONENT | SKYLAB MISSIONS | | | | | | | | |
|---|---|---|---|---|---|---|---|---|---|
| | 28 Days | | | 59 Days | | | 84 Days | | |
| Astronaut | 1 | 2 | 3 | 4 | 5 | 6 | 7 | 8 | 9 |
| Total diet | 2888 | 3031 | 2873 | 2888 | 2860 | 3927 | 3271 | 3149 | 3361 |
| Excreta | | | | | | | | | |
| Urine | 132 | 150 | 135 | 111 | 138 | 186 | 152 | 146 | 160 |
| Feces | 106 | 107 | 104 | 111 | 131 | 181 | 161 | 102 | 146 |
| Total excreta | 238 | 257 | 239 | 222 | 269 | 367 | 313 | 247 | 306 |
| Body tissue loss | | | | | | | | | |
| Protein | 34 | 79 | 60 | 35 | 28 | 28 | 44 | 24 | 2 |
| Fat | 178 | 720 | 274 | 348 | 551 | 90 | −160 | 48 | −26 |
| Total Tissue | 212 | 798 | 334 | 383 | 579 | 118 | −116 | 72 | −24 |
| Net energy utilization | 2861 | 3572 | 2968 | 3049 | 3170 | 3678 | 2842 | 2974 | 3031 |

Notes

Diet (kcal/day) = 4.182 diet carbohydrates (g/day) + 9.461 × diet fat (g/day) + 5.65 × protein (g/day).

Urine energy = 8.32 × urine nitrogen (g/day)

Energy from protein tissue loss = 5.65 kcal/g

Energy from fat tissue lost = 9.461 kcal/g

**Minus sign denotes gain in body tissue**

Net energy utilization = diet − excreta + energy from body tissue lost

(From Leonard, J.I.: Energy Balance and the Composition of Weight Loss during Prolonged Space Flight. NASA Contract NA59–16328. Houston, National Aeronautics and Space Administration, 1982.)

ble of increasing the loss of muscle mass, but increased caloric intake may not necessarily prevent this loss. These conclusions are stated guardedly because the assessment of nitrogen balance, on which the in-flight behavior of muscle metabolism is based, is prone to experimental error,[51] and the difficulties of in-flight sample collections are considerable. Also, differences in nitrogen balance between Skylab crew members who exercised at different levels were small and not statistically significant.

The rapid loss of muscle, which levels off within a month, is supported by other in-flight evidence, including the behavior of potassium balance (Fig. 43–2) and leg volume loss.[52,53] The exercise devices used in Skylab (bicycle ergometer, "bungee" cords and treadmill) were designed primarily to condition the leg muscles. The total muscle mass, comprising about 40% of body mass, is located in the hips, back, and neck. The most compelling conclusions of Thornton were based on analysis of lower limbs only,[53] whereas Leonard used whole-body data.[38] Therefore, it is possible that lean body mass in the legs was maintained during intensive local exercise conditioning in 0-G while upper body lean mass degenerated. This contention is supported by the Soviet success in slowing muscle loss and bone loss.[54]

In summary, the findings of Leonard[38] for the Skylab crews suggest that the major components of body composition (water, protein, and fat) undergo significant changes in spaceflight:

1. Water losses are obligatory as a result of normal physiologic responses to acute headward shifts of fluid in weightlessness and are independent of flight duration.
2. Protein losses are primarily a result of disuse atrophy of postural muscles and may be obligatory in weightlessness. Although overall body protein losses were independent of exercise levels on Skylab, data indicate that locally applied exercise may help to maintain protein mass in specific areas, particularly the legs.
3. Fat losses are more variable and probably depend on the usual 1-G influences of energy balance, i.e., fat stores increase with caloric intake and decrease with exercise. Also, changes in body fat depend on the cumulative effects of a positive or negative energy balance and are therefore highly time dependent.
4. Anorexia of varying degrees appears to be associated with the initial period of weightlessness and is related only in part to symptoms of frank motion sickness. If present, the anorexia of spaceflight augments tissue losses by virtue of a caloric deficiency and enhances water loss as a result of reduced fluid intake.
5. Energy requirements in a working spaceflight environment do not appear to be less than required for similar activities on the ground, contrary to former expectations. Leonard estimated that a caloric intake of 46 to 50 kcal/kg/day body weight would have prevented significant tissue loss (primarily fat) for the Skylab astronauts.[38]

Thornton, a scientist/physician/astronaut, has suggested the following guidelines for understanding the combined effects of exercise and diet on tissue storage based on experiences found in a 1-G environment.[53] His guidelines are compared to those of Leonard in paren-

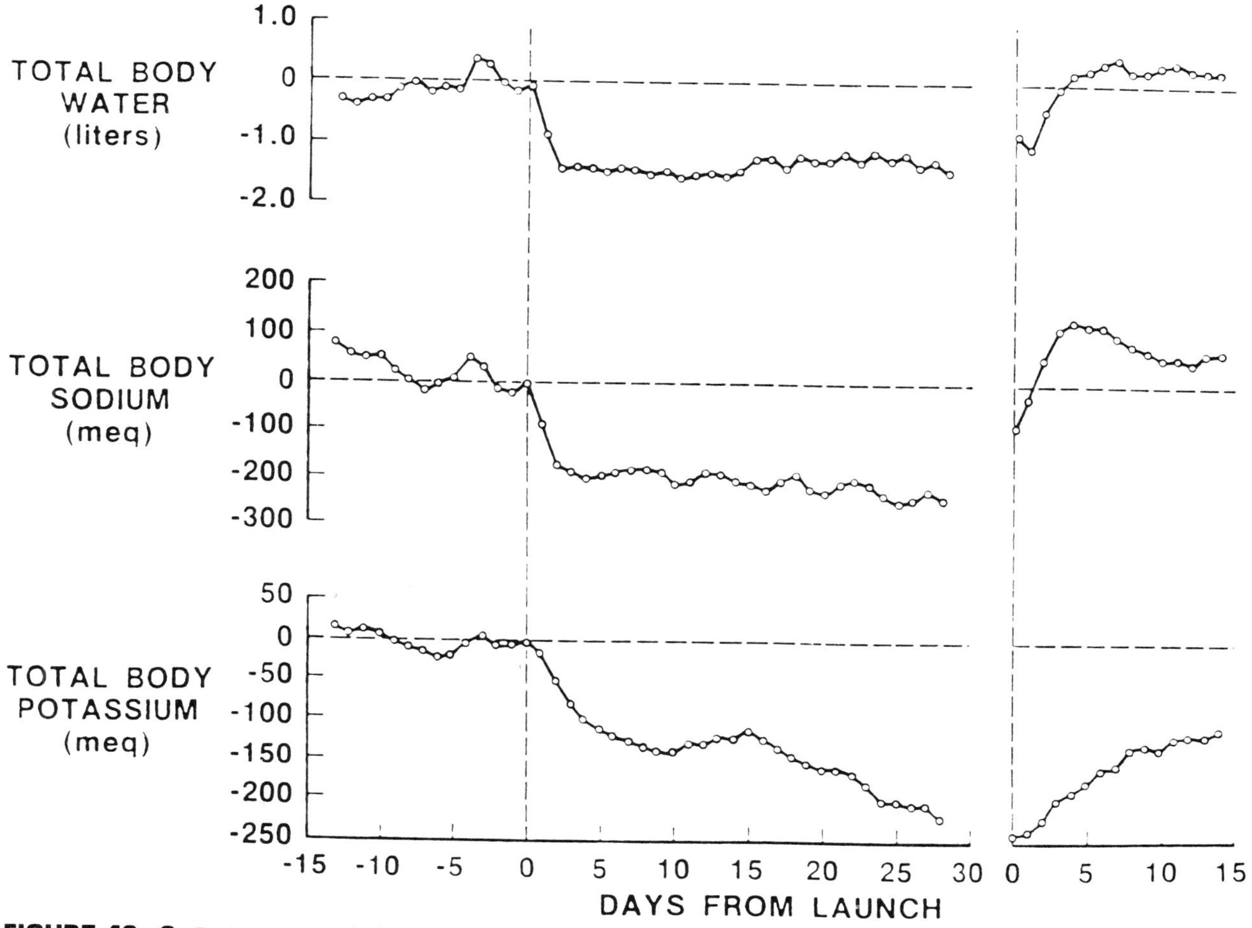
TOTAL BODY
WATER
(liters)
1.0
0
-1.0
-2.0
TOTAL BODY
SODIUM
(meq)
200
100
0
-100
-200
-300
TOTAL BODY
POTASSIUM
(meq)
50
0
-50
-100
-150
-200
-250
-15 -10 -5 0 5 10 15 20 25 30 0 5 10 15
DAYS FROM LAUNCH

**FIGURE 43–2.** Body water and electrolyte changes during prolonged spaceflight in Skylab (mean n=9). (From Leonard, J.I.: Energy Balance and the Composition of Weight Loss during Prolonged Space Flight. NASA Contract NA59–16328. Houston, National Aeronautics and Space Administration, 1982.)

theses, which were the in-flight changes estimated from the Skylab mission series results.

1. A calorically inadequate diet results in fat and muscle losses, with the ratio depending on individual body fat percentages. (Significant losses of fat and muscle were observed, but no strong correlations were found between preflight body fat and 0-G losses).
2. An inadequate diet coupled with insufficient exercise results in even more rapid muscle loss. (Protein loss was most severe when in-flight dietary protein intake decreased from preflight levels. However, within the limits of experimental accuracy, whole body protein losses, as reflected by several indices, did not appear to be related to the amount of exercise performed.)
3. With diet adequate to maintain body mass but insufficient exercise, the muscles atrophy and fat is deposited. From a caloric point of view, this condition represents the conversion of muscle into fat. (This phenomenon may have been observed in the crew of the 84-day mission). In two Soviet missions lasting 6 months, three of four cosmonauts had increases in body mass of 2 to 5%, plateauing around day 140 to 160. The gains were in adipose tissue, which more then offset losses in lean body mass.[54]

## MUSCLE ATROPHY

Increased protein catabolism, including breakdown of skeletal muscle, has been a consistent finding in spaceflight. A reduction of the volume of the lower extremities and a persistent rise in urinary nitrogen, phosphorus, amino acids, and 3-methylhistidine levels are some typical associated findings.[55,56] Whether these changes were caused by 0-G or other factors in the spaceflight environment has not been fully established, but weightlessness is thought to be the main etiologic factor.[57] Despite attempts at intervention such as diet and exercise, skeletal muscle atrophy continues to some extent throughout orbital flight, manifesting progressive muscle loss and negative nitrogen balance.[55,56,58–60]

In the Skylab missions (28, 59, and 84 days), nitrogen and phosphorous balances were negative during the first 2 to 3 weeks, then negative or slightly positive for the remainder of each mission.

Changes in strength of the arm and leg extensors and flexors of each of the three Skylab crews were estimated by pre- and postflight dynamometry.[50] Muscle strength of the crew of Skylab 2, whose sole in-flight exercise device was the bicycle ergometer, was measured 5 days after flight. Leg extensor strength was about 25% below preflight levels. Decrements in arm extensor strength were considerably less than in the legs. No loss in arm extensor strength was noted in the commander, who had pedaled the bicycle by hand as well as by leg.[50] In the Skylab 3 mission (59 days), average loss of strength was about 18% in the leg flexors and about 21% in the leg extensors. Again, losses of strength in the arm extensors and flexors were generally less than in the lower extremities, which probably reflects the relatively greater workload for the arms during flight.

Kozlovskaya et al.[61] reported the following muscular effects in crew members of the 75-, 140-, 175-, and 185-day Salyut missions: (1) "atony" of the calf muscles rear group and atrophy of the long muscles of the back; (2) slight "subatrophy" of the latissumus dorsi muscles; (3) slight decrease in strength of the gastrocnemius muscles at velocities of 0 and 60° per second; (4) a noticeable decrease in strength of the tibialis anticus muscle at all velocities tested, except at 180° per second; and (5) a significant decrease in strength/velocity relationship of the neck muscles.

Muscular deconditioning may have contributed to the tachycardia noted during EVA in the Gemini, Apollo, and Skylab astronauts, and to the cardiac arrhythmias and fatigue experienced during lunar surface activities and return to Earth in the Apollo 15 mission. Full recovery of muscular strength after spaceflight requires from several days to several weeks. Data are not available to show conclusively whether full recovery of muscle bulk takes place.[48]

United States astronauts and Soviet cosmonauts typically have developed negative potassium balance during flight (Fig. 43–2). After flight, they had decreased values of serum and urinary potassium, total body content of potassium 40, and exchangeable potassium.[43,57,58] This negative balance has been ascribed to a reduction of the intracellular potassium depot as a result of a decrease in cell mass, particularly in skeletal muscle. The negative potassium balance has persisted for as long as 6 days after flight.[57]

NASA flight crew schedules include less than 1 hour of daily exercise. On the other hand, the typical Soviet crew schedule in long-term missions specifies between 1.3 and 2.5 hours per day for exercise.[62,63] In addition, the cosmonauts wear an elasticized garment, the "penguin suit," which opposes body movement and, to an extent, compensates for the lack of gravity on the antigravitational parts of the musculoskeletal system in the trunk and lower extremities.[55,64] Load (penguin) suits have not been used operationally by American astronauts.

## BONE LOSS

**Earth-Bound Subjects.** Bone loss during spaceflight invariably occurs, but the mechanisms are poorly understood because they are complex. Various attempts have been made to identify suitable ground-based and inflight countermeasures. Exercise regimens have been associated with slower bone loss in patients with osteoporosis.[65] Stimulated by the 1949 finding of a reduction in calcium excretion of about 50% when bed rest subjects were placed on an oscillating bed through an arc of 25° once every 2 minutes for 8 hours,[66] 3- to 6-week bed-rest experiments with young men were sponsored from 1962 to 1966 by the United States Air Force.[67–69] Physical work capacity was preserved but head-up tilt intolerance and hypercalciuria persisted in spite of vigorous exercise while supine (upsidedown bicycle ergometer at 600 kpm of work for 30 minutes twice a day). Hypercalciuria persisted even when the supine exercise was increased to 2 to 4 hours per day. In contrast, quiet standing 3 hours per day for 3 weeks in four of five subjects resulted in a slow decline in calcium output to the basal range from the hypercalciuria induced by 3 to 4.6 weeks of bed rest. Neither lying nor sitting exercise for 1 hour daily (as just described), nor quiet sitting in a chair for 8 hours daily (as in nursing and rest homes), in the presence of 16 hours of bed rest prevents hypercalciuria in healthy young men. Quiet sitting did reduce orthostatic hypotension but did not preserve physical work capacity.[69]

Preliminary research with a "penguin suit" (an elastic harness compressing the spine and lower legs when legs are extended) for 3 hours in 30-minute intervals of skeletal pressure equal to body weight to simulate standing while in the supine position (bed rest) decreased the hypercalciuria previously induced by 22 days of bed rest in one of two subjects.[69] Three hours of daily standing equivalence appears to be the minimum duration effective for reversing bed rest-induced tilt intolerance and hypercalciuria. Schneider et al. studied the effects of 4 hours of ambulation during 6 weeks of bed rest and found that calcaneal density and calcium balance return to normal, whereas 3 hours resulted in less negative but incomplete amelioration of the negative calcium balance.[70] Twenty or 40 minutes of upright exercise on a bicycle ergometer did not improve the hypercalciuria in the studies of Birkhead et al.[69] nor the negative calcium balance observed by Schneider et al.[70] Compression loadings of 25 to 40 lb to each heel and compression by a "penguin suit" of 80% of body weight to the axial skeleton for 6 to 8 hours per day during otherwise supine bed rest (20 hours per day) did not ameliorate calcium loss but did maintain calcaneal density.[71,72] An important observation was that 3 hours of random daily ambulation (not just standing) resulted in less negative calcium balance. Four hours of controlled ambulation on a measured course during 6 weeks of bed rest (20 hours per day) was necessary to completely alleviate negative calcium balance.[72] These results appear to indicate that both exercise and weight bearing are necessary to counteract the bone mineral loss of prolonged bed rest.

Increasing protein intake to 156 g per day in five ambulatory subjects in the studies of Schneider et al.[71] increased calcium losses, and decreasing protein intake to 69 g per day lowered urinary calcium excretions, resulting in a slightly more positive calcium balance. Supplemental phosphorus (1.3 g per day as the potassium salt) prevented the hypercalciuria of bed rest but failed to prevent negative calcium balance or loss of os calcis density.[73] Calcium and phosphate supplementation (1.8 g calcium as calcium lactate and 3.0 g phosphorus) led to less negative calcium balance in 12 weeks of bed rest, and mean negative balance fell to 100 mg per day.[74] Fluoride supplements (10 mg per day) did not prevent calcium losses during bed rest.[75]

**In-flight and Postflight Observations.** Studies of animals and astronauts in spaceflight have documented altered bone metabolism.[76] Bone loss was first observed by x-ray densitometry during three Gemini missions[22] and was reported in Apollo experiments.[77] In-flight metabolic balance studies[23,56] with negative calcium balance (up to 0.5 g per day) indicate the possibility of a loss of 0.4% of bone calcium per month. Such a relentless loss over 2 years could lead to nephropathy and demineralization of clinical consequence. The three Skylab missions (28, 54, and 84 days) provide evidence of a relationship between the duration of weightlessness and bone demineralization (Fig. 43–3). No significant losses in bone density were found in the Skylab 2 (28 days) crew, but did occur in one of three astronauts in Skylab 2 (59 days) and in two of three astronauts in Skylab 4 (84 days) flights. Urinary excretion of calcium and phosphorous as a result of spaceflight follows the same pattern of increase and is of the same magnitude as that of healthy male bed-rest subjects.[67,71,78,79] In the 59-day Skylab mission, calcium balances returned to postflight values in 17 days for two of three astronauts, but they had not returned for the 84-day Skylab crew at the 18-day postflight evaluation (Fig. 43–4).[80]

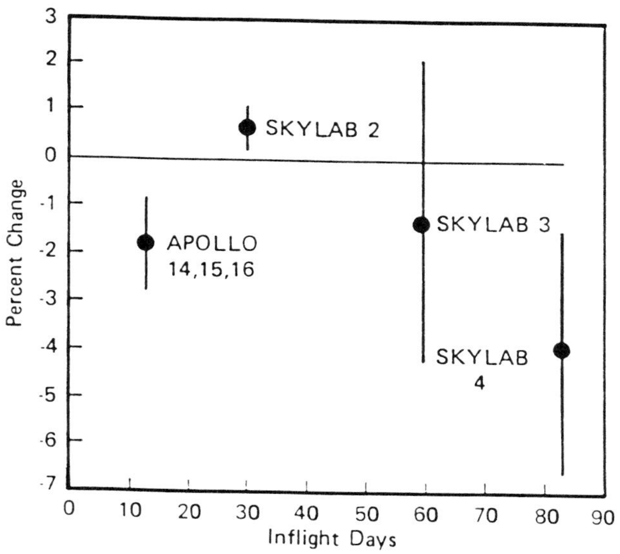
3
2
1
0
-1
-2
-3
-4
-5
-6
-7
Percent Change
SKYLAB 2
APOLLO
14,15,16
SKYLAB 3
SKYLAB
4
0 10 20 30 40 50 60 70 80 90
Inflight Days

**FIGURE 43–3.** Postflight bone mineral changes in spaceflight crews. (From Nicogossian, A.E., Huntoon, C.L., Pool, S.L. (Eds.): Space Physiology and Medicine. 2nd Ed. Philadelphia, Lea & Febiger, 1989.)

The os calcis mineral of two of the three Skylab 4 (84 days) astronauts had not returned to preflight values 95 days after flight. Tilton et al. re-evaluated the os calcis mineral content of the nine Skylab astronauts and seven controls 5 years after flight.[81] Compared to the original preflight data, a statistically significant loss in bone mineral was found in all but one of the crew members who had flown, but not in the control subjects. No information on diet and exercise during this 5-year postflight period is available.

Five to 8% loss in os calcis density has been reported by the Soviets in the 175-day Salyut mission, but did not extend to the lumbar vertebrae in four exercising cosmonauts. Ironically, the amount of daily exercise increased in each successive Skylab mission and slowed losses in lower body muscle mass but did not prevent the occurrence of a negative calcium balance. However, the lower body exercise, which places a load on the foot (ergometer/treadmill), may have had a sparing effect on the rate of os calcis bone loss.

After more than 1 day of weightlessness, urinary calcium content increased (see Fig. 43–3). Within 10 days, negative calcium balance ensued.[82] Within 30 days, the quantity of urinary calcium had approximately doubled that of control preflight levels and continued at this level. After flight, urinary calcium content decreased to levels below those before flight. At the end of 84 days in flight, the Skylab 4 crew had lost an average 25 g of calcium or 2.5% of the body pool. The loss initially was slow (50 mg per day) and rose to almost 300 mg per day on day 84. Fecal calcium excretion invariably increased.[23,56] The data suggest the development of progressive malabsorption, but the possibility of increased calcium secretion into the gut cannot be discounted. Mean urinary hydroxyproline excretion was increased 30% during the Skylab missions (with significant individual differences observed).[56,83]

Plasma levels of parathyroid hormone, 25 hydroxy cholecalciferol, and calcitonin measured in Apollo and Skylab flight crews did not change and, thus, did not account for the mobilization of bone calcium. Plasma levels of cortisol, insulin, and human growth hormone increased during flight. During spaceflight, plasma calcium and phosphate levels were within ranges considered normal.[76]

The fundamental mechanism in bone loss is presumed to be increased bone resorption rather than decreased bone formation. Yet data on weightless rats suggest complete cessation of bone growth occurs with zero gravity exposure.[84] However, animal food intake was lower and weight gain was retarded in these experiments and restricted energy alone is known to cause decreased animal skeletal growth.[85]

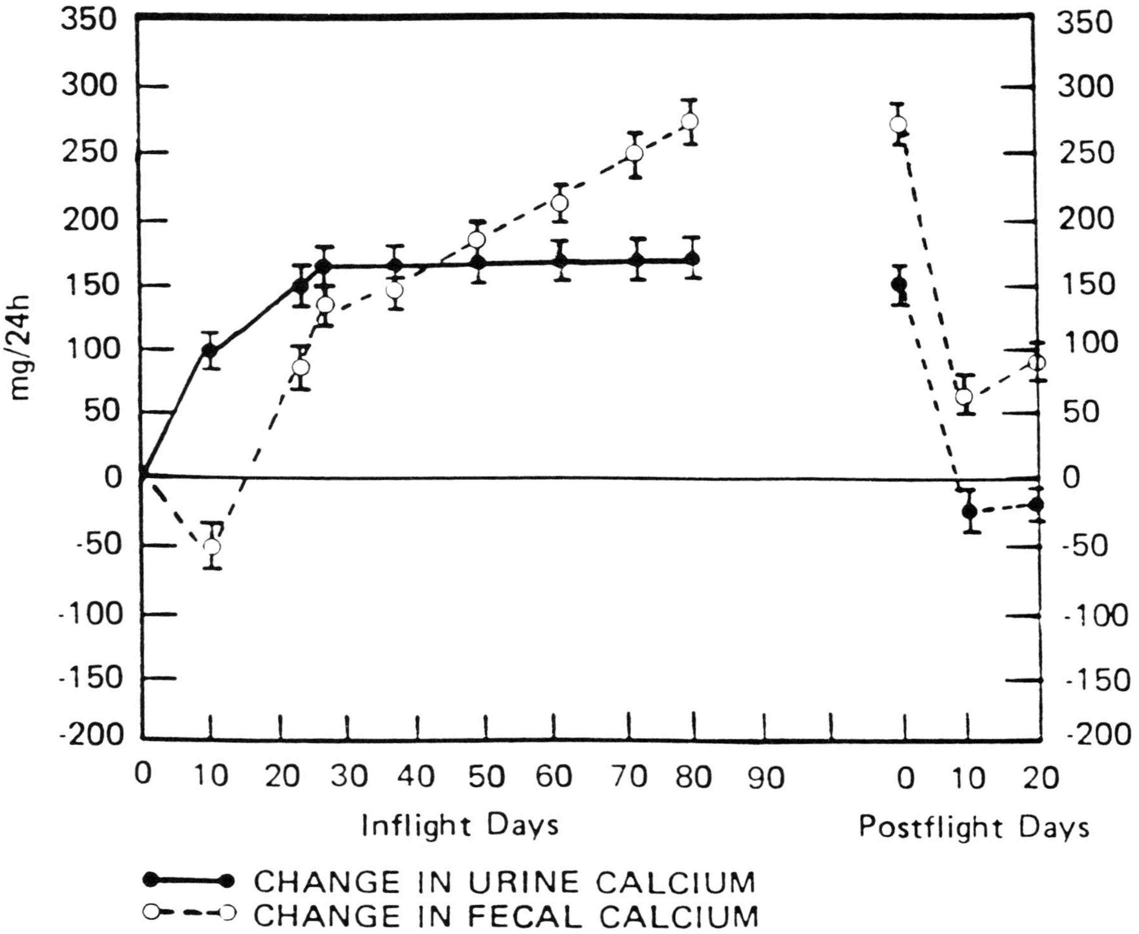
350
300
250
200
150
100
50
0
-50
-100
-150
-200
mg/24h
0 10 20 30 40 50 60 70 80 90
Inflight Days
0 10 20
Postflight Days
CHANGE IN URINE CALCIUM
CHANGE IN FECAL CALCIUM

**FIGURE 43–4.** Change in urine and fecal calcium concentration as a function of Skylab flight duration (mean ± SE). (From Nicogossian, A.E., Huntoon, C.L., Pool, S.L. (Eds.): Space Physiology and Medicine. 2nd Ed. Philadelphia, Lea & Febiger, 1989.)

In 1974, Whedon et al. stated, "it is reasonable to predict musculoskeletal safety for at least 6 months and probably for 9 months . . . unless protective measures can be developed . . . Completely lost trabecular bone cannot be restored."[82] Soviet scientists have accepted the need to slow the process, probably because of their pursuit of long-duration (1 year) manned spaceflight.

The Soviets have demonstrated that with a combination of pre, in-flight, and postflight countermeasures (diet, "penguin suit," vigorous treadmill, and other exercise), man can function in weightlessness 1 year or more without serious clinical consequences, such as spontaneous fractures.

The Soviets have conducted 120- and 182-day head-down (6°) bed-rest studies (20 subjects) demonstrating a continued negative calcium balance averaging 5.6 g per month. Levels of parathyroid hormone increased and those of calcitonin initially increased and thereafter decreased. Calcium lactate loading during bed rest increased renal calcium excretion as compared to baseline. On bed-rest day 116, iliac crest spongy bone showed a 15% calcium decrease. The calcium-phosphorus ratio of the bone decreased significantly.[86] Subsequently, a study designed to compare results of individuals after 120 days (15 males) and 370 days (10 males) of bed rest with 36 control subjects and 15 osteoporosis patients has been undertaken in the Soviet Union. The effect of various countermeasures (exercise, medication, and a combination) are being studied for changes including the ability of mononuclear blood cells to produce humoral mediators activating resorption in bone tissue.[87]

As the results of this research become available, the question of whether a maximum life-time dose of weightlessness needs to be established may be answered. The significance of this aerospace-driven biomedical research to everyday physical rehabilitation medicine and the clinical management of osteoporosis has yet to be appreciated fully. The Soviets have taken a "can do" attitude and appear convinced that a combination of protective diet, exercise, and other regimens will permit the manned exploration of Mars and other planets in the near future.

**TABLE 43–10.** IN-FLIGHT CHANGES IN VARIOUS HORMONES

| HORMONE | SKYLAB | SHUTTLE |
|---|---|---|
| Plasma | | |
| HGH* | Increase (first few days) | Not measured |
| Insulin | Decrease (after 2 weeks) | Not measured |
| PTH* | No change | Not measured |
| Catecholamines | Decrease | Not measured |
| Urine | | |
| Catecholamines | No change | No change† |

*HGH, human growth hormone; PTH, parathyroid hormone.
†One subject.
(From Nicogossian, A.E., Huntoon, C.L., Pool, S.L. (Eds.): Space Physiology and Medicine. 2nd Ed. Philadelphia, Lea & Febiger, 1982.)

**TABLE 43–11.** POSTFLIGHT (LANDING DAY) CHANGES IN VARIOUS HORMONES

| HORMONE | ASTP* | SKYLAB | SHUTTLE | SALYUT/SOYUZ |
|---|---|---|---|---|
| Plasma | | | | |
| HGH* | Increase | Increase | No change | No change |
| Insulin | Increase | No change | Increase | Increase |
| PTH* | Not measured | No change | Not measured | Not measured |
| $T_3$ | Not measured | Decrease | No change | No change |
| $T_4$ | Not measured | Increase | Increase | Increase |
| TSH* | No change | Increase | increase | No change |
| Urine | | | | |
| Catecholamines | Decrease in norepinephrine | Increase | Increase | Increase |

*ASTP, Apollo-Soyuz Test Project; HGH, human growth hormone; PTH, parathyroid hormone; TSH, thyroid-stimulating hormone.
(From Nicogossian, A.E., Huntoon, C.L., Pool, S.L. (Eds.): Space Physiology and Medicine. 2nd Ed. Philadelphia, Lea & Febiger, 1982.)

### HORMONAL CHANGES

Biomedical investigators and flight physicians have had a necessary interest in measuring hormonal changes in astronauts in order to understand both the effects of spaceflight on metabolism and the response of astronauts to the expense and stress of performing in this novel environment. The nature of hormone assays demands considerable emphasis on when, where, and how samples are taken for assay. In the Mercury, Gemini, Apollo, and most Shuttle missions, sampling of blood and urine was limited to pre- and postflight opportunities.[43,88] Furthermore, the number of crew members and the number of assays for interpretations are limited. The individual response is not necessarily comparable to those obtained from others on the same missions. Some blood samples were collected in flight during Skylab, but immediate assay was not possible.[80] The net result has been that changes in cortisol, insulin, growth hormone, thyroxine, and other hormones have not provided a consistent coherent pattern of change (Tables 43–10 and 43–11).[88] Changes in the number and distribution of hormonal receptors needs to be studied with corrections for changes in blood compartment and protein metabolism. Specific emphasis is needed on the hormonal assay protocols and assay techniques. Ideally, an astronaut specialist who is a clinical chemist would be a part of the crew. Coupled with in-flight assay hardware, a real-time chronobiology of hormonal changes would provide valuable and needed insights.

## OTHER EFFECTS AND RISKS

### MOTION SICKNESS

Motion sickness and vestibular dysfunction are reported to occur in a substantial percentage of astronauts, with some individuals more susceptible than others.[37,89,90] Microgravity limits the sensory input to movements of the head and body. The symptoms of nausea, vertigo, and disorientation occur shortly after lift-off and last 3 to several days. The symptoms can be ameliorated by drugs (L-scopolamine, D-amphetamine,

**TABLE 43–12.** PHYSIOLOGIC CHANGES RELATED TO SPACE FLIGHT

| PHYSIOLOGIC PARAMETER | SHORT-TERM FLIGHTS* (1–14 Days) | LONG-TERM FLIGHTS† (>2 Weeks) |
|---|---|---|
| Nitrogen and phosphorous balances | | Negative early IF, less negative or slightly positive later IF; rapid return to positive PF.‡ |
| Calcium balance | Increasing negative IF. | Positive preF, becoming increasingly negative IF; negative PF becoming less negative by day 10 but still slightly negative by day 20; several weeks to return to preF baseline. |
| Bone density | Os calcis density decreased PF; variable changes in radius and ulna. | Os calcis density decreased PF; amount of loss correlated with mission duration; little or no loss from nonweightbearing bones; recovery time about same as mission duration. |
| Muscle strength | Decreased IF and PF; RPB in 1-2 weeks. | PF decreases, particularly in leg extensors; increased exercise IF appears to reduce PF strength losses regardless of mission duration; arm strength normal or slightly decreased PF. |
| Electromyogram (EMG) analysis | PF EMG from gastroenemius suggest increased susceptibility to fatigue and reduced muscular efficiency. EMG from arm muscles show no change. | PF EMG suggest deterioration of muscle tissue and increased susceptibility to fatigue; RPB in about 4 days. |
| Achilles tendon reflex | Duration decreased PF. | Duration decreased 30% or more PF; reflex magnitude increased; compensatory increase in duration about 2 weeks PF; RPB in about one month. |
| Limb volume | IF leg volume decreases exponentially during first day and plateaus within 3 to 5 days; rapid increase immediately PF, followed by slower RPB. | Early IF period same as short missions; leg volume may continue to decrease slightly throughout mission; arm volume decreases slightly; rapid increase in leg volume immediately PF, followed by slower RPB. |
| Total body volume | Decreased PF. | Decreased PF; center of mass has shifted toward head. |
| Body composition | | Large losses of $H_2O$, protein, and fat during first month IF; fat probably regained; muscle mass partially preserved depending on food intake and amount of exercise. |
| Mass | PF weight losses average about 3.4% with about two thirds from $H_2O$ loss, remainder from loss of lean body mass and fat. | IF weight losses average 3 to 4% during first 5 days; thereafter, weight gradually declines for remainder of mission; early IF losses probably from loss of fluids and later losses are metabolic; rapid weight gain first 5 days PF mainly from replenishment of fluids; PF weight loss inversely related to IF caloric intake. |
| Total body water | Decreased PF. | Decreased PF. |
| Plasma volume | Decreased PF, except in Gemini 7 and 8. | Significantly decreased PF; RPB in 2 weeks. |

and ephedrine). Adaptation occurs as the visual system replaces vestibular function. Milder symptoms may occur for 24 hours after return to earth. During these periods of dysfunction, appetite is suppressed, which contributes to weight loss.

## BODY FLUID SHIFT

The lack of gravity leads to fluid shifts and anthropometric changes.[41,42] Within 3 to 6 hours in microgravity, up to 2 L of fluid shifts headward. Calf and thigh volume decreases 10% or more. The thoracolumbar spine straightens, with expansion of intervertebral disks. Astronauts experience an increase in height and a reduction in girth of abdomen and chest. The center of mass shifts upward by 3 or 4 cm. In-flight spacesuits and flightsuits, therefore, must be larger.

## HEMOCONCENTRATION

Hemoconcentration and a fall in plasma volume occur within a few days in microgravity.[91] The body responds by a loss of water, sodium, and potassium (see Fig.

**TABLE 43–12.** PHYSIOLOGIC CHANGES RELATED TO SPACE FLIGHT *continued*

| PHYSIOLOGIC PARAMETER | SHORT-TERM FLIGHTS* (1–14 Days) | LONG-TERM FLIGHTS† (>2 Weeks) |
|---|---|---|
| Plasma proteins | Occasional PF elevations in globulin, from increases of haptoglobin, ceruloplasmin, and $\beta_2$-macroglobin; elevated IgA and C3 factor. | No significant changes PF. |
| Serum/plasma electrolytes | Decreased K and Mg PF. | IF decreased Na, Cl, and osmolality, but slight increase in K and $PO_4$; PF decreases in Na, K, Cl, Mg, but increase in $PO_4$ and osmolality. |
| Serum/plasma hormones | PF increase in HGH, thyroxine, insulin, angiotensin I, sometimes aldosterone. | IF increase in cortisol, and decrease in ACTH, insulin; PF increase in angiotensin, aldosterone, thryoxine, TSH, GH, and decrease in ACTH. |
| Serum/plasma metabolites and enzymes | PF increase in BUN, creatinine, glucose; decrease in lactic acid dehydrogenase, creatine phosphokinase, albumin, triglycerides, cholesterol, uric acid. | PF decrease in cholesterol, uric acid. |
| Urine volume | Decreased PF. | Decreased early IF; normal or slightly increased PF. |
| Urine electrolytes | PF increase in Ca, creatinine, $PO_4$, osmolality; decrease in Na, K, Cl, Mg. | IF increase in osmolality, Na, K, Cl, Mg, Ca, $PO_4$, and decrease in uric acid; PF increase in Ca, and initial decrease in Na, K, Cl, Mg, $PO_4$, uric acid; Na and Cl increase week 2 and 3 PF. |
| Urinary hormones | IF decrease in OH-corticosteriods and increase in aldosterone; PF increase in cortisol, aldosterone, ADH, pregnanediol, and decrease in epinephrine, 17-OH-corticosteriods, androsterone, etiocholanolone. | IF increase in cortisol, aldosterone, total 17-ketosteroids, and decrease in ADH; PF increase cortisol, aldosterone, norepinephrine and decrease in total 17-OH-corticosteriods, ADH. |
| Behavior and performance | Initial IF slowness in accomplishing tasks (or a reduced work efficiency) and diminished motor coordination and precision of movement during adaptation to weightlessness; adjustment is rapid, but PF motor dysfunction can be debilitating for days or weeks. | Same as for short-term flights. |

*Data compiled from several reports on Mercury, Gemini, Apollo, ASTP, Vostock, Voskhod, and Soyuz missions.

†Data compiled from several reports on Skylab, and Salyut missions.

‡Abbreviations: preF, preflight; IF, inflight; PF, postflight; RPB, return to preflight baseline; HGH, human growth hormone; ACTH, adrenocorticotropic hormone; TSH, thyroid-stimulating hormone; GH, growth hormone; ADH, antidiuretic hormone.

(From Office of Space Science and Application, NASA: Research Opportunities in Nutrition and Metabolism in Space. Washington, D.C., National Aeronautics and Space Administration, 1986.)

43–2). The shift is reversible, beginning within 1 hour after landing. The electrolyte response is complicated by the fluid shift headward, the tendency of crew members to reduce fluid intake before launch,[92] and a decrease in thirst possibly resulting from cellular overhydration with headward fluid translocation.[91] A preliminary conclusion was that water diuresis occurred; however, the limited results of in-flight metabolic experiments to date indicate that the excretion of urine was normal and fluid intake was reduced.

Although clinically and functionally innocuous, red blood cell mass (RCM) loss averaging 10 to 15% has been observed consistently after spaceflight. Postflight recovery of RCM requires 4 to 6 weeks.[44] Oxygen toxicity is an unlikely cause because that phenomenon persisted when the cabin atmosphere of 100% oxygen at 258 mm Hg in Mercury, Gemini, and early Apollo missions was changed to 70% oxygen and 30% nitrogen at 258 mm Hg in late Apollo, Skylab, and the Shuttle programs. Reductions in lean body mass correlated with the decreased

RCM.[45] Erythrocyte life span was unaltered in the 211-day Salyut (Soviet) flight.

### ORTHOSTATIC INTOLERANCE

Another consistent occurrence that developed within 4 days of weightlessness was orthostatic intolerance, i.e., hypotension with return to gravity (or tilt after bed rest). Return to normal required several weeks after flight.[93] Preflight endurance training may not provide an advantage.[94] Vigorous in-flight exercise did not prevent orthostatic intolerance.[95] The most effective re-entry countermeasure is application of the antigravity suit.[96] Its use is critical in the Space Shuttle, because the crew is seated as in an aircraft during re-entry (+1.2 to 1.5 $G_{z(\text{footward})}$ for 20 minutes).

### IONIZING RADIATION

The hazardous effects of ionizing radiation are well known and depend on total dose and dose rate.[97,98] They can range from acute radiation illness and death, to cataracts and irreversible genetic damage, with an increased risk of early cancers. The van Allen belts include an inner zone of high intensity electrons. From the solar system, high-energy particles (mostly protons) approach velocities of the speed of light. Most of the radiation in a low earth orbit comes from protons at about 4 to 10 millirem per day. The inner radiation belt drops to within 300 km of the surfaces of the poles, and thus an orbital space mission tilted more toward the poles could increase the amount of radiation exposure about ten times. Orbits in the polar regions where the electromagnetic shield is absent would also expose the spacecraft to solar and galactic particles.

The exposure limit for a more highly exposed radiation worker on the ground is 5 rem per year, or 250 rem per lifetime. Radiation standards have permitted no more than 400 rem to the bone marrow during an astronauts career and no more than 25 rem during any single year. The highest dose received by an American astronaut has been 7 rem. United States astronauts on moon missions received 1 to 2 rem. No American or Soviet crew member has been exposed during a solar flare (which occurs every 5 to 10 years). The United States space station will be in a low orbit and occupants would be subject to 36 rem per year. A mission to Mars could entail 100 rem.

Increasing spacecraft/module wall thickness from 0.125 inches to about 0.25 inches aluminum equivalence would reduce the dose by a factor of 1.2,[36] but this countermeasure is expensive; 1000 lb of thrust are needed to insert 1 lb of payload into orbit. The shielding afforded by the present Space Shuttle spacesuit assembly (average 0.5/cm$^2$ aluminum equivalence) would be inadequate when EVA duration, such as in the assembly of a Space Station, would be lengthy. A more advanced spacesuit (under development) is designed to provide shielding of over 1.5 g/cm$^2$ aluminum equivalence over the entire body. A value of 2.0 g/cm$^2$ has been calculated to provide sufficient protection against all but the largest solar flares.[36] The aluminum and stainless steel walls of the Apollo Command Module actually had a protective value of no less than 2.75 g/cm$^2$, but the Lunar Module had walls with a density of only 1.5 g/cm$^2$. The technology exists for active physical protection provided by inducing a magnetic field around a spacecraft.[37] Both increased shielding and the use of special antiradiation supplementation (ascorbic acid, vitamin E, and β-carotene) to enhance cellular repair to injury would be practical. Of all the hazards, none appears more challenging to long-term habitation in space than protection against radiation. It has been the area least studied.

In summary, the data available make it impossible to write a concise and succinct summary of the physiologic and metabolic changes related to spaceflight Table 43–12 provides the most comprehensive summary available. The reader is urged to read the pertinent sections of this chapter for more extensive documentation. A decreased emphasis on the role of humans in space exploration is likely. Changes in the political and economic structure of the Soviet Union will probably severely curtail its space exploration program. Social needs in the United States and reallocations of the "peace dividend" have forced NASA to reassess its manned space operations[99] and to re-emphasize unmanned space explorations. Hopefully, funds will not be diverted from the much needed continuation of ground-based experimentations including bed-rest studies. The in-flight emphasis of Space Station Freedom on space biology and medicine in microgravity has been urged.[99] The results have considerable relevance not only to further explorations but also to rehabilitative medicine and the pathogenesis of various disease processes.

## REFERENCES

1. Martin Co.: General Human Factors Considerations. Vol. III, ASD-R-61-211. Dayton, OH, Wright-Patterson Air Force Base, 1961, p. 33.
2. Clamann, H.C.: Fed. Proc., *18*:1249–1255, 1959.
3. Taylor, A.A., Finkelstein, B., Hayes R.I.: Food for Space Travel: An Examination of Current Capabilities and Future Needs. ARDC Tech. Rep. 60–8. Washington, D.C., Andrews Air Force Base, 1960.

4. Space Science Board: A Revue of Space Research. Report of the Summer Study Conducted by the Space Science Board. Iowa City, State University of Iowa, 1962; Washington, D.C., National Academy of Sciences, National Research Council, 1962 (Publ. No. 1079, out of print).
5. Symposium: Fed. Proc. *22:*1424–1459, 1963.
6. Lachance, P.A.: Nutrition and the stresses of short-term space flight. *In* Conference on Nutrition in Space and Related Waste Problems. NASA SP-70. Washington, D.C., National Aeronautics and Space Administration, 1965, pp. 71–78.
7. Calloway, D.H., Bosley, J.H., Reynolds, O.R.: Am. Sci., *50:*362A–370A. 1962.
8. Springer, W.E., Stephens, T.L., Streimer, I.: Aerospace Med., *34:*486–488, 1963.
9. Webb, P., Ed.: NASA Life Sciences Data Book 1962. Reprinted as Bioastronautics Data Book, NASA SP-3006 (N65-15594). Washington, D.C., National Aeronautics and Space Administration, 1964.
10. Anonymous: Nutr. Rev., *25:*301–304, 1967.
11. Finkelstein, B.: J. Am. Diet. Assoc., *40:*529–531, 1962.
12. Lachance, P.A.: Environ. Biol. Med., *1:*205–228, 1971.
13. Nanz, R.A., Michel, E.L., Lachance, P.A.: Food Technol., *21:*1596–1602, 1967.
14. Tuomy, J.M.: Food Technol., *19:*46–50, 1965.
15. Klicka, M.V.: J. Am. Diet. Assoc., *44:*358–361, 1964.
16. Lachance, P.A., Klicka, M.V., Hollender, H.A.: Cereal Sci. Today, *13:*49–54, 1968.
17. Lachance, P.A., Berry, C.A.: Nutr. Today, *1:*2–11, 1967.
18. Smith, M., Berry, C.A.: Nutr. Today, *4:*37–42, 1969.
19. Calloway, D., Mathews, R., Hon, T., et al.: Development of a Feeding System for Project Apollo. Final Rep. Contr. NAS 9–150 Menlo Park, Stanford Research Institute, 1965.
20. Lachance, P.A.: Gemini Flight Food Specifications CSD-G-079. Houston, National Aeronautics and Space Administration Manned Spacecraft Center, 1964.
21. Lachance, P.A., Nanz, R.A., Klicka, M.V.: Food Consumption and Gemini IV, V and VII. Technical Memo X-58010. Houston, National Aeronautics and Space Administration Manned Spacecraft Center, 1967.
22. Mack, P.B., Lachance, P.A., Vose, G.P., et al.: AJR, *3:*503–505. 1967.
23. Lutwak, L., Whedon, G.D., Lachance, P.A., et al.: J. Clin. Endocrinol. Metab., *29:*1140–1156, 1969.
24. Hartung, T.E., Bullerman, L.R., Arnold, R.G., et al.: J. Food Sci., *38:*129–132, 1973.
25. Smith, M.C. Jr., Huber, C.S., Heidelbaugh, N.D.: Aerospace Med., *42:*1185–1192, 1971.
26. Huber, C.S., Heidelbaugh, N.D., Rapp, R.M., et al.: Aerospace Med., *44:*905–909, 1973.
27. Smith, M.C., Rambaut, P.C., Stadler, C.R.: Skylab nutritional studies. *In* Proceedings of the Skylab Life Sciences Symposium. Edited by R.S. Johnston, L.F. Dietlein. NASA TM X-58154. Washington, D.C., National Aeronautics and Space Administration, 1974, pp. 193–197.
28. Stadler, C.R., Sanford, D.D., Reid, J.M., et al.: J. Am. Diet. Assoc., *62:*390–393, 1973.
29. Stadler, C.R., Rapp, R.M., Bowland, C.T. et al.: Space Shuttle Food System Summary, 1981–1986. NASA Tech. Memo 100469. Houston, National Aeronautics and Space Administration, 1988.
30. Bourland, C.T., Fohey, M.F., Rapp, R.M., et al.: J. Food Protect., *44:*313–319, 1981.
31. Heidelbaugh, N.D., Romley, D.B., Powers, E.M., et al.: Appl. Environ. Microbiol., *25:*55–61, 1973.
32. Bauman, H.E.: Food Technol., *28:*30, 1974.
33. Lachance, P.A.: Activities Rep., *19:*133–136, 1967.
34. Ahmed, S.: Comparison of Soviet and U.S. Space Food and Nutrition Programs. Contract NGT-44-001-800 (N89-20059). Houston, Johnson Space Center, 1988, pp. 1–16.
35. Lachance, P.A., Vanderveen, J.F.: Food Technol., *17:*59–64, 1963.
36. Nicogossian, A.E., Huntoon, C.L., Pool, S.L. (Eds.): Space Physiology and Medicine. 2nd Ed. Philadelphia, Lea & Febiger, 1989. (Compare NASA-SP-477, Washington, D.C., 1982.)
37. Harding, R.: Survival in Space: Medical Problems of Manned Spaceflight. London, Routledge, 1989.
38. Leonard, J.I.: Energy Balance and the Composition of Weight Loss during Prolonged Space Flight. NASA Contract NA59–16328. Houston, National Aeronautics and Space Administration, 1982.
39. Leonard, J.I.: Skylab Water Balance Analysis. NASA Contract Report CR-167461, Washington, D.C., National Aeronautics and Space Administration, 1977.
40. Leach, C.S., Leonard, J.I., Rambaut, P.C., et al.: J. Appl. Physiol., *45:*430–436, 1978.
41. Thornton, W.E., Hofler, G.W., Rummel, J.A.: Anthropometric changes and fluid shifts. *In* Biomedical Results from Skylab. Edited by R.S. Johnston, L.F. Dietlein. NASA SP-377. Washington, D.C., National Aeronautics and Space Administration, 1977, pp. 330–338.
42. Thornton, W.E., Moore, T.P., Pool, S.L.: Aviat. Space Environ. Med., *58(Suppl. 9):*A86–A90, 1987.
43. Leach, C.S., Rambaut, P.C.: Biochemical response of the Skylab crewmen: An overview. *In* Biomedical Results from Skylab. Edited by R.S. Johnston, L.F. Dietlein. NASA SP-377. Washington, D.C., National Aeronautics and Space Administration, 1977, pp. 204–217.
44. Talbot, J.M., Fisher, K.D.: Fed. Proc., *45:*2285–2290, 1986.
45. Dunn, C.D.R., Johnson, P.C., Leonard, J.I.: Physiologist, *24(Suppl.):*55–56, 1981.
46. Grande, F.: Ann. Intern. Med., *68:*467–480, 1968.
47. Rambaut, P.C., Heidelbaugh, N.D., Reid, J.M., et al.: Aerospace Med., *44:*1264–1269, 1973.
48. Life Science Research Office: Research Opportunities in Muscle Atrophy. Edited by G.J. Herbison, J.M. Talbot. NASA-CR-175422 (N84-20135). Washington, D.C., National Aeronautics and Space Administration, January 1984.
49. Greenleaf, J.E.: J. Appl. Physiol., *57:*619–633, 1984.
50. Thornton, W.E., Rummel, J.A.: Muscular deconditioning and its prevention in space flight. *In* Biomedical Results from Skylab. Edited by R.S. Johnston, L.F. Dietlein. NASA SP-377. Washington, D.C., National Aeronautics and Space Administration, 1977, pp. 191–197.
51. Hegsted, D.M.: J. Nutr., *106:*307–331, 1976.
52. Leonard, J.I.: Analysis of Metabolic Energy Utilization of the Skylab Astronauts. NASA-CR-160402. Washington, D.C., National Aerospace and Space Administration, 1977.
53. Thornton, W.E.: Anthropometric changes in weightlessness. *In* Anthropometry for Designers. Vol. I. Edited by the Staff of Webb Associates, (Yellow Springs, Ohio). NASA RP-1024, Washington, D.C., National Aeronautics and Space Administration, 1978, pp. 1–613.
54. Gazenko, O.G., Genin, A.M., Egorov, A.D.: Acta Astronautica, *8:*907–917, 1981.
55. Nicogossian, A.E., Parker, J.F. (Eds): Space Physiology and Medicine. NASA SP-447. Washington, D.C., National Aeronautics and Space Administration, 1982.

56. Whedon, G.D., Lutwak, L., Rambaut, P.C., et al.: Mineral and nitrogen metabolic studies-Experiment M071. *In* Biomedical Results from Skylab. Edited by R.S. Johnston, L.F. Dietlein. NASA SP-377. Washington, D.C., National Aeronautics and Space Administration, 1977, pp. 423–430.
57. Gazenko, O.G., Grigoryev, A.I., Natochin, U.V.: Space Bioi. Aerospace Med., *14:*1–11, 1980.
58. Leach, C.S., Alexander, W.C., Johnson, P.C.: Endocrine electrolyte and fluid volume changes associated with Apollo missions. *In* Biomedical Results of Apollo. Edited by R.S. Johnston, L.F. Dietlein, C.A. Berry. NASA Sp-368. Washington, D.C., National Aeronautics and Space Administration, 1975, pp. 163–184.
59. Rambaut, P.C., Leach, C.S., Wheeler, H.O.: Nutritional studies. *In* Biomedical Results of Apollo. Edited by R.S. Johnston, L.F. Dietlein, C.A. Berry. NASA SP-368. Washington, D.C., National Aeronautics and Space Administration, 1975, pp. 277–302.
60. Whedon, G.D.: Physiologist, *25(Suppl.):*S41–S44, 1982.
61. Kozlovskaya, I.B., Kreidich, Y.V., Rakmanov, A.S.: Physiologist, *24*(Suppl.):S59–S64, 1981.
62. Kakurin, L.I.: US/USSR Joint Working Group on Space Biology and Medicine. Washington, D.C., National Aeronautics and Space Administration, 1981.
63. Yegorov, A.D.: Results of Medical Research During the 175-Day Flight of the Third Crew of the Salyut-6-Soyuz Orbital Complex. Edited by O.C. Gazenko, A.M. Genin. Moscow, 1980. (Compare NASA TM 76450, Washington, D.C., 1981.)
64. Gurowskiy, N.N., Yeremin, A.V., Gazenko, O.G., et al.: Space Biol. Aerospace Med., *92:*79–87, 1975.
65. Aloia, J.F., Cohn, S.H., Ostuni J.A., et al.: Ann. Intern. Med., *89:*356–358, 1978.
66. Whedon, G.D., Deitrick, J.E., Shorr, E.: Am. J. Med., *5:*684–711, 1949.
67. Issekutz, B. Jr., Blizzard, J.J., Birkhead, N.C., et al.: J. Appl. Physiol., *21:*1013–1020, 1966.
68. Birkhead, N.C., Blizzard, J.J., Daly, J.W., et al.: Cardiodynamic and Metabolic Effects of Prolonged Bedrest with Daily Recumbent or Sitting Exercise and with Sitting Inactivity. AMRL-TR-64-61. Wright-Patterson Air Force Base, Ohio, August, 1964.
69. Birkhead, N.C., Blizzard, J.J., Issekutz, B. Jr., et al.: Effect of Exercise, Standing, Negative Trunk and Posture Skeletal Pressure on Bed-Rest Induced Orthostasis and Hypercalciuria. AMRL-TR-66-6. Wright-Patterson Air Force Base, Ohio, January, 1966, pp. 1–36.
70. Schneider, V.S., Quan, L., McDonald, J.: Prevention of Disuse Osteoporosis of Bed Rest: Effect of Four-Hour Daily Normal Ambulation. Final Report NASA Contract T-66D. Houston, National Aeronautics and Space Administration, 1981, pp. 160–192.
71. Schneider, V.S., Burrill, K., Vogel, J.M., et al.: Modification of Negative Calcium Balance and Bone Mineral Loss During Prolonged Bed Rest: (1) Impact Loading; (2) Dietary Protein Manipulations. Final Report NASA Contract T-66D. Houston, National Aeronautics and Space Administration, 1981, pp. 5–72.
72. Schneider, V.S., Quan, L., McDonald, J.: Modification of Calcium Balance and Bone Mineral Loss During Prolonged Bed Rest: Impact Loading 25 or 40 Pounds Thrust or 6 or 8 Hours/Day, Respectively. Final Report NASA Contract T-66D. Houston, National Aeronautics and Space Administration, 1981, pp. 73–133.
73. Hulley, S.B., Vogel, J.M., Donaldson, C.L., et al.: J. Clin. Invest., *50:*2506–2518, 1971.
74. Hantman, D.A., Vogel, J.M., Donaldson, C.L., et al.: J. Clin. Endocrinol. Metab., *36:*845–858, 1973.
75. Maheshwari, U.R., Schneider, V.S., McDonald, J.T., et al.: Am. J. Clin. Nutr., *36:*211–218, 1982.
76. Life Sciences Research Office, FASEB: Research Opportunities in Bone Demineralization. Edited by S.A. Anderson, S.H. Cohn. NASA CR 3795. Washington, D.C., National Aeronautics and Space Administration, 1984, pp. 1–21.
77. Vogel, J.M.: Bone Mineral Measurement Apollo 15-Experiment M078. NASA Contract T-93591. Houston, National Aeronautics and Space Administration, 1974.
78. Deitrick, J.E., Whedon, G.D., Schorr, E.: Am. J. Med., *4:*3–36, 1948.
79. Donaldson, C.L., Hulley, S.B., Vogel, J.M., et al.: Metabolism, *19:*1071–1084, 1970.
80. Whedon, G.D., Leach, C.S., Rambaut, P.C.: Metabolic and endocrine balance studies in manned space flights. *In* Molecular Proceedings of Endocrinology. Edited by I. MacIntyre, M. Szelke. Amsterdam, Elsevier, 1979, pp. 229–250.
81. Tilton, F.E., Degioanni, J.J.C., Schneider, V.S.: Aviat. Space Environ. Med., *51:*1209–1213, 1980.
82. Whedon, G.D., Lutwak, L., Reid, J., et al.: Trans. Assoc. Am. Physicians, *137:*95–110, 1974.
83. Whedon, G.D.: Physiologist, *25(Suppl.):*S41–S44, 1982.
84. Morey, E.R., Baylink, D.J.: Science, *201:*1138–1141, 1978.
85. Handlerr, P., Baylin, G.J., Pollis, R.H.: J. Nutr., *34:*677–682, 1947.
86. Morukov, B.V., Orlov, O.I., Grigoriev, A.I.: Physiologist, *32:*S37–S40, 1989.
87. Lesniak, A.T., Konstantinova, J.V., Bodjikov, N.V., et al.: Physiologist, *32:*S53–S56. 1989.
88. Leach, C.S.: Acta Astronautica, *8:*977–988, 1981.
89. Graybiel, A.: Aviat. Space Environ. Med., *51:*814–822, 1980.
90. Young, L.R., Oman, C.M., Watt, D.G.D., et al.: Science, *225:*205–208, 1984.
91. Greenleaf, J.E.: J. Appl. Physiol., *60:*60–62, 1986.
92. Leach, C.S., Johnson, P.C., Cintron, N.M.: The regulation of fluid and electrolyte metabolism in weightlessness. *In* Space Physiology. Edited by J.J. Hunt. Toulouse, European Space Agency, SP-237, 1986, pp. 31–36.
93. Bonting, S.L.: Trends Biochem. Sci., *8:*265–269, 1983.
94. Greenleaf, S.E., Dunn, E.R., Nesvikck, C., et al.: Aviat. Space Environ. Med., *59:*152–159, 1988.
95. Garshnek, V.: Am. Soc. Grav. Space. Biol. Bull., *1:*67–80, 1988.
96. Levy, M.N., Talbot, J.M.: Physiologist, *26:*297–303, 1983.
97. Warren, S., Grohn, D.: Ionizing radiation. *In* Bioastronautics Data Book. 2nd Ed. Edited by J.F. Parker, V.R. West. NASA SP-3006. Washington, D.C., National Aeronautics and Space Administration, 1973, pp. 417–422.
98. Goode, A.W., Rambaut, P.C.: The metabolic consequences of space travel. *In* The Metabolic and Molecular Basis of Acquired Diseases. Vol. 1. Edited by R.D. Cohen, B. Lewis, K.G.M.M. Albert, A.M. Demman. London, Bailliere Tindall, 1990, pp. 417–422.
99. Albeson, P.H.: Science, *251:*357, 1991.

CHAPTER 44

# Nutrition in Pregnancy and Lactation

William J. McGanity, Earl B. Dawson, and Ann Fogelman



Significant changes in the female life cycle have occurred over the past 150 years (Table 44–1). The decline in average age of the onset of menarche has apparently stabilized at about 12.5 years. The average age of menopause is now more than 50 years of age. Consequently, the span of female reproductive potential has expanded to nearly 40 years.

During the last two decades, a slight decrease in the number of live births to women younger than 20 years of age has occurred, as well as a significant increase in the number of women delaying the first pregnancy until they are over 30 years of age. In the United States, of the more than 5.0 million pregnancies annually, only 75% result in live births. The remainder end in induced abortions or spontaneous miscarriages before the twentieth week of pregnancy.

The ever-improving level of obstetric and neonatal care has produced a downward trend in perinatal and infant mortality in the United States; however, rates persist among the black population that are twice those of the white population. Little change has occurred in the incidence of low birth weight (less than 2500 g), which remains at 7%, but is twice as high among the black population. Unfortunately, between 25 and 30% of all pregnant patients do not enter into prenatal care before the second trimester of pregnancy.[1] Few public-sector patients achieve the recommended standard of 14 prenatal visits, and they average fewer than 8 visits, most of which occur in the third trimester of pregnancy.

Nationally, approximately 40% of all pregnant women receive their prenatal care and delivery services in the public sector. Health-care coverage available through

**TABLE 44–1.** HISTORICAL TRENDS IN THE FEMALE LIFE CYCLE IN THE UNITED STATES FROM 1843 TO 1987

| YEAR | 1843–1858 | 1900 | 1930–1935 | 1960 | 1985–1987 |
|---|---|---|---|---|---|
| Life span (years)* | 42.0 | 47.3 | 59.7 | 69.7 | 74.9 |
| Menarche (age)† | 16.5 | 14.2 | 13.9 | 12.8 | 12.5 |
| Menopause (age) | | | <45.0 | 45.0 | 50.0 |
| Maternal mortality* | | | 0.3% | | 0.01% |
| Infant mortality* | 15% | | 5.6% | | 1.1% |

*Data from Hiatt, N., Hiatt, J.R.: Pharos, *Spring*: 2–6, 1992.
†Tanner, J.M.: Nutr. Rev., *39*:43–55, 1981.

the expanded Medicaid program covers most pregnant women with incomes lower than 185% of the poverty level. During the past 10 years, the number of family physicians who will accept any patient for prenatal care and/or delivery has seriously declined particularly in rural areas of the country. This problem has had a more severe impact on the public-sector Medicaid patient. This loss of available medical manpower is being replaced by physician extenders—certified nurse midwives, clinical nurse practitioners, and physician assistants.

What are mothers' expectations in the 1990s? The number of pregnancies per reproductive career has decreased by 25% in the past 30 years (from 3.2 to 2.3 children per reproductive career). The present-day American mother expects a perfect outcome to each pregnancy. If any question arises about the condition of her fetus, she is likely to exercise her option to interrupt the pregnancy. When the outcome is not perfect, she is predisposed to blame her health-care team for the failures that result and frequently seeks legal recourse.

Several reviews of the current states of prenatal nutrition emphasize that the goals for the mother and her offspring remain constant:[2,3] (1) for the mother, freedom from complications and intercurrent diseases throughout pregnancy and post partum, and a return to her normal, healthy nonpregnant state free of sequelae; and (2) for the infant, a mature baby of normal gestational age and birth weight, free of any anomalies or disabilities and able to thrive in the external environment.

## OPTIMAL NEEDS FOR REPRODUCTIVE PERFORMANCE

If the common goals of the mother and her health-care team are to be achieved, one must identify and eliminate as many maternal risk factors as possible by careful evaluation and appropriate treatment and prevent or ameliorate as many of the actual risks as possible *before the pregnancy begins*. Usual prenatal care in the United States consists of an initial visit for pregnancy confirmation and health examination after the individual's second missed menstrual period, followed by 12 periodic examinations at 4-, 2-, and 1-week intervals during the remaining course of the pregnancy, plus a minimum of one postpartum visit 4 to 6 weeks after delivery. A well-planned pregnancy should include the initial health examination 8 to 12 weeks before conception. Those initial 60 to 90 days of care are essential to controlling all maternal risk factors. For example, if a prospective mother desires to have her baby in January of 1994, her pregnancy preparation should have started in January 1993, and care should extend through at least 6 weeks after delivery. This regimen covers 54 weeks or more from the time that she should have discontinued her nonbarrier forms of contraception. It is desirable to have two or more normal, spontaneous menstrual cycles before finally removing barrier contraception for the purpose of conceiving. Similarly, after delivery she will require time for reproductive involution and maternal nutritional repletion to occur.

### PREREQUISITES FOR OPTIMAL PERFORMANCE

At least nine such prerequisites for optimal maternal reproductive performance are recognized (Table 44–2).

**Pregnancy is Optimal When the Mother is Biologically Mature.** A biologically mature female is a young woman who is at least 5 years postmenarchal, and this has greater impact on pregnancy than her chronologic age. Thus, if a 14-year-old girl began menstruating when she was 9 years old, she is 5 years postmenarchal and as

**TABLE 44–2.** NEEDS FOR OPTIMAL REPRODUCTIVE PERFORMANCES

| |
|---|
| Biologic maturity of the prospective mother |
| Preparation begun at conception minus 60 days |
| Protection from all preventable diseases |
| Tight control of all chronic and metabolic disorders |
| Eradication of all habits harmful to the fetus |
| Early and frequent prenatal care |
| Body weight within an acceptable range |
| Adequate nutrient intake and transport system |
| Working placental transfer and lactation delivery system |

biologically mature as she will ever become. Certainly, she may not be emotionally, economically, educationally, or psychosocially mature, but she is as biologically mature as a 20-year-old counterpart. If another 14-year-old girl were to become pregnant in the first year after menarche, however, she would be biologically immature. The growth demands of the pregnancy and fetus superimposed on the growth demands of an adolescent 1 year after menarche may result in an undesirable outcome.

**Prevent Everything That You Possibly Can.** The risk of German measles in the first trimester of pregnancy has been all but eliminated by an effective immunization program whereby all young girls are vaccinated against German measles before menarche. Recently, as discussed later, it has been shown that an intake of 400 μg* folic acid per day, from diet and/or as a supplement before conception and throughout the first trimester of pregnancy, significantly reduces the primary and secondary risk of neural tube defects in the fetus.

**Control Maternal Chronic and Metabolic Disorders.** Pregnancy in the diabetic mother requires a level of dietary and insulin control, so blood levels of glucose only fluctuate within the normal range of the nondiabetic patient. The expected perinatal mortality associated with diabetic mothers is now 4%, a fourfold reduction in the last 20 years. Unfortunately, the risk of fetal congenital malformation in the diabetic remains fourfold higher.

The patient with a phenylalanine metabolism disorder (PKU) who was on special diet until she was 8 or 9 years of age is now able to manage on a regular diet; however, she must be returned to strict dietary control before and throughout her pregnancy. Otherwise, the probability that the offspring will develop either a form of congenital malformation or another developmental abnormality is higher than 80%. All female patients must be specifically asked whether they have ever been on a special diet.

*All pregnancies should be started with a maternal height/weight relationship between 90 and 120% of standard, equivalent to a body mass index (BMI) of 20 to 26 because maternal and fetal consequences occur at both extremes* (BMI is discussed in Chapter 59; a nomograph is given in Appendix Table A–11i). One calculates a patient's percentage of standard weight (PSW) by first measuring her nude height and weight. One then adapts the American Diabetes Association's method to calculate PSW. Based on 1983 height/weight standards (see Appendix Table A–5b), 105 lb are allotted for the first 5 ft of height, and one adds 5 lb for every additional inch. That weight will give the 100% value of what the patient's standard weight should be. The patient's actual weight is then divided by this calculated ideal weight to give her PSW. When a woman is underweight when her child is conceived, her infant will have some degree of reduced birth weight, particularly if weight gain is also inadequate during pregnancy. On the other hand, prepregnant weight that is more than 135% of standard weight (BMI greater than 29) predisposes patients to maternal hypertension, pregnancy-induced toxemia, cesarean section, diabetes, and other maternal and fetal complications. Thereafter, maternal weight gain targets for the patient during her pregnancy should be based on the prepregnancy PSW or BMI category, as discussed later in this chapter.

**Eliminate and/or Reduce All Substance Abuse, Be It Tobacco, Alcohol, or Drugs.** All these substances have an impact on the maternal and/or fetal outcome of pregnancy. This impact may operate directly or indirectly through the pocketbook, through physiologic alterations, or by metabolic competition with nutrient intake.

## PROVISION OF ADEQUATE NUTRITION

A pregnant woman can provide the nutrients for herself and her fetus to meet the demands during her pregnancy in three ways. The most common and most desirable is the oral ingestion of adequate food through the mother's mouth when there is normal digestion, absorption, and transport into maternal circulation, normal metabolism, and transfer of simple nutrient building blocks from mother to fetus across the placenta. Individual nutrients cross with assistance of maternal transport carriers and are released within placental cell(s) to be picked up by their fetal counterparts.[4] For this system to work, one must have a functioning cardiovascular system and adequate uterine blood flow with an ample concentration of nutrients on the maternal side, to transfer the building blocks to the fetal side. Without these essential components, there will be some degree of intrauterine fetal growth retardation. The same thing results with respect to the normal lactational system in the nursing mother. Second, where necessary, the provision of nutrients may be replaced or augmented by the use of enteral[5] and/or parenteral[6] feeding, even for prolonged periods of time. A third and undesirable pathway is the mobilization of the mother's body reserves of the required calories, proteins, minerals, and vitamins for growth and development needs of both mother and fetus.

To ensure the expectant mother an adequate diet there must be an available food supply and functioning distribution system, as well as the necessary economic capacity to produce and/or procure the food. Without a dependable and abundant supply of all food needs, the woman has no way to provide the nutrients for her pregnancy. Among the public-sector patients are two important supplemental food programs—the Food Stamp Program, which serves over 24.0 million patients per month, and the Supplemental Feeding Program for Women, Infants, and Children (WIC), which monthly

*Conversion units to SI units of various nutrients are given in Appendix Table A–1a.

serves over 5.0 million persons per month, of whom 25% are pregnant or lactating women.

### ADDITIONAL RISK FACTORS

**Low Hemoglobin.** For a woman living *at sea level,* the hemoglobin should be above 110 g/L (11 g/dl) or her hematocrit should be above 331 (33%). This hemoglobin level should be above 110 g/L (11 g/dl), whether she be pregnant, not pregnant, or lactating, for adequacy of the patient's oxygen transport system. The odds of detecting any type of nutrient-deficiency anemia with a hemoglobin above 11 g/dl are less than 1%. This standard needs to be increased 1 g/dl for every 5000 feet of elevation above sea level, to provide for the needed expansion of oxygen-carrying capacity of the red cells during pregnancy. This hemoglobin standard is 20 g/L (2 g/dl) higher than those used in many developing countries, where mothers may have some unique capacity to compensate for the lower levels of hemoglobin; however, their maternal risks are enhanced and their margin of safety is compromised. That the hematologic condition of the fetus may be protected during pregnancy and lactation is one of the few nutritional illustrations of fetal parasitism.

**Pregnancy is the Occasion for the Mother to Gain Weight.** Maternal weight gain should be based on the prepregnant weight status and should occur in an orderly manner during the second and third trimesters of pregnancy. Of all the biologic factors that influence the birth weight of the fetus, maternal weight gain has the strongest influence.

Weight gains larger than 1 kg per week are cause for concern. A weight gain above 1 kg per week solely from the ingestion of food would require an intake of 7000 kcal (1000 kcal per day) in excess of need. This amount is unlikely because it represents almost 50% more than the usual total daily caloric intake during pregnancy. Hence this level of weight gain suggests an abnormal accumulation of tissue fluid.

Weight losses or weight gains of less than 1 kg per month are also cause for concern. The impact of weight loss on the mother or the fetus is discussed later in this chapter.

**Weight Gain and Lactation.** The decision and plans for breast-feeding should be made when the mother first feels her baby move, or at approximately 20 weeks of gestation, rather than at or after the delivery. Making the decision to nurse at this time provides sufficient opportunity for weight gain to be targeted to accumulate body stores for utilization during lactation. If the expectant mother is not going to nurse, then her maternal weight gain goals need to be decreased a modest degree. This will facilitate her return to her prepregnant weight status. Under ideal circumstances, breast-feeding is the method of choice in our developed society as well as in the developing societies of the world. Such is currently not the case in the United States. Most recent data indicate a downward trend in breast-feeding among all segments of our American society, but more pronounced in the black population.[1] At the time of hospital discharge, only 50% of mothers are breast-feeding their babies, and only one third of those continue breast-feeding for 6 months.

## ASSESSMENT OF THE PREGNANT WOMAN: HISTORY AND PHYSICAL EXAMINATION

General obstetric care requires, at the initial visit, a thorough evaluation of the pregnant woman, including a careful and complete history of her obstetric and medical characteristics, followed by a comprehensive physical examination. Before this, the patient has been weighed, has had her pulse taken, her respiration and blood pressure recorded, and a urine sample obtained to be checked by dip stick for 15 items of diagnostic value. A blood sample is drawn to provide a Health Survey File (HSP) to permit detection of any abnormalities that may exist in her hematologic, serologic, immunologic, and metabolic status. A few simple items relating to nutritional assessment can readily be added that are not time consuming and can performed by the dietician/nutritionist members of the health-care team. Both height and weight measurements are an essential part of the initial clinical anthropometry. Together, these measurements permit the calculation of PSW and proper targeting of weight gain throughout pregnancy.

A detailed nutritional assessment requires:

1. A physical examination of the appropriate exposed portions of the body including the arms, legs, and face and neck for evidence of clinical nutritional deficiencies.
2. A dietary food intake assessment based on either a food frequency utilization or a dietary history of a 3-, 5-, or 7-day food intake.
3. Basic anthropometric measurements of height, weight, and, on occasion, skin fold thickness.
4. A biochemical assessment of the nutrients as measured in blood and urine.

All of these measurements on an individual obstetric patient are usually not needed. A rapid nutritional assessment is needed for every patient, however, to identify any significant nutritional problems that may exist. If evidence of depletion is found, further assessments by the dietician and/or nutritionist colleagues will be needed for recommendations for nutritional therapies.

The physician in solo practice must be able to identify available personnel in the community who can provide a detailed nutritional assessment. Such individuals may be within the hospital setting as a part of its dietary department, they may be associated with the local health clinic and/or WIC program, or they may be in private practice.

Most pregnant women are normal, healthy females without disorders that interfere with the ingestion, digestion, absorption, metabolism, or utilization of a normal, well-balanced diet. If the hematology data and HSP are normal, it is unlikely that they will have evidence of either biochemical or clinical manifestations of any nutritional disorder; hence a more detailed assessment by trained nutrition personnel is not necessary.

National dietary goals are that 15% of total calorie intake come from protein, 30% from fat, and the remainder from carbohydrates, primarily starches. The United States Department of Agriculture has recently issued a food guide pyramid format to guide choices of various food groups, to achieve the proper mix to provide adequate calories and healthier sources of proteins, fats, and carbohydrates with the necessary amounts of minerals, vitamins, and fiber.[7] The prescription is fairly simple—an average daily intake of 6 to 11 servings of breads, cereals, rice, and pasta, 2 to 4 servings of various fruits; 3 to 5 servings of various vegetables; 2 or 3 servings of dairy products, and a similar number of servings of meats, fish, poultry, legumes, eggs, or nuts; fats, oils, and sweets are to be used sparingly.

It has been convenient to presume that the average prepregnant and pregnant woman in America has a more than adequate nutrient intake of calories, proteins, minerals, and vitamins. The results of 1980 and 1986 market basket surveys by the United States Department of Agriculture provide cause to question that conclusion.[8] This survey showed that 50 to 60% of the female population failed to ingest 70% of the recommended nutrient intake (Table 44–3). When the patient's dietary intake is poor in green leafy vegetables, fruits, and dairy products and is consistently less than 50% of the recommended dietary allowance (RDA), we should anticipate finding early clinical manifestations of nutritional disorders. These will not be the full-blown picture of classic nutritional deficiency, but rather the early manifestation of abnormalities such as evidence of protein and/or energy malnutrition (including muscle wasting, abnormal skin and hair texture, cheilosis, angular stomatitis), lesions of the gums associated with low vitamin C, and hyperkeratosis of the skin over the arms associated with vitamin A deficits. Such a patient is probably consuming less than half of her RDA for vitamins A and C, calcium, and riboflavin, respectively. She needs more than a supplemental mineral/vitamin pill; she needs nutritional counseling. The responsibility of physicians and other members of the health-care team should be to prove that their patients have an adequate nutrient intake. The nutrition/biochemical assessment is designed to help in that determination. Needed help can be given in group education classes, or, in specific circumstances, it may require individual therapeutic dietary instruction.

## PHYSIOLOGIC AND METABOLIC CHANGES IN PREGNANCY

Pregnancy is a normal physiologic process associated with major alterations affecting every maternal organ system and metabolic pathway. Every single blood and urine measurement—nutrients included—is significantly altered from nonpregnant values as a result of these changes. Values may change as the pregnancy advances from first to third trimester and to delivery and then return toward normal during the postpartum period. The two major physiologic forces driving these changes are (1) the 50% expansion of plasma volume with the 20% increase in hemoglobin mass; the former peaks in the middle of the third trimester, whereas the latter continues onto term (Fig. 44–1); and (2) the ever-increasing levels of estrogen and progesterone as well as other placenta-related hormones; these have a particular impact on the maternal lipids (cholesterol), carotene, and vitamin E, as well as on blood-clotting factors. These two physiologic modifications result in two dominant patterns of change: the first reduces

**TABLE 44–3.** PERCENTAGE OF WOMEN WITH DIETARY INTAKES FOR SELECTED MINERALS AND VITAMINS THAT ARE <50, <70, <100, OR ≥100% OF THE RECOMMENDED DIETARY ALLOWANCES (RDA)

| | 1979 RDA | <50% | <70% | <100% | ≥100% |
|---|---|---|---|---|---|
| Calcium | 800 mg | 27 | 50 | 78 | 22 |
| Iron | 18 mg | 44 | 79 | 95 | 5 |
| Zinc | 15 mg | 41 | 77 | 96 | 4 |
| Vitamin A | 800 μg | 21 | 39 | 55 | 45 |
| Vitamin E | 8 mg | 23 | 47 | 76 | 24 |
| Vitamin C | 60 mg | 16 | 28 | 44 | 56 |
| Vitamin $B_6$ | 2.0 mg | 44 | 74 | 94 | 6 |
| Folate | 400 μg | 63 | 87 | 96 | 4 |

(From United States Department of Agriculture: Nationwide Food Consumption Survey. Report No. 85–1. Hyattsville, MD, Nutrition Monitoring Division, Human Nutrition Information Service, U.S. Department of Agriculture, 1985.)

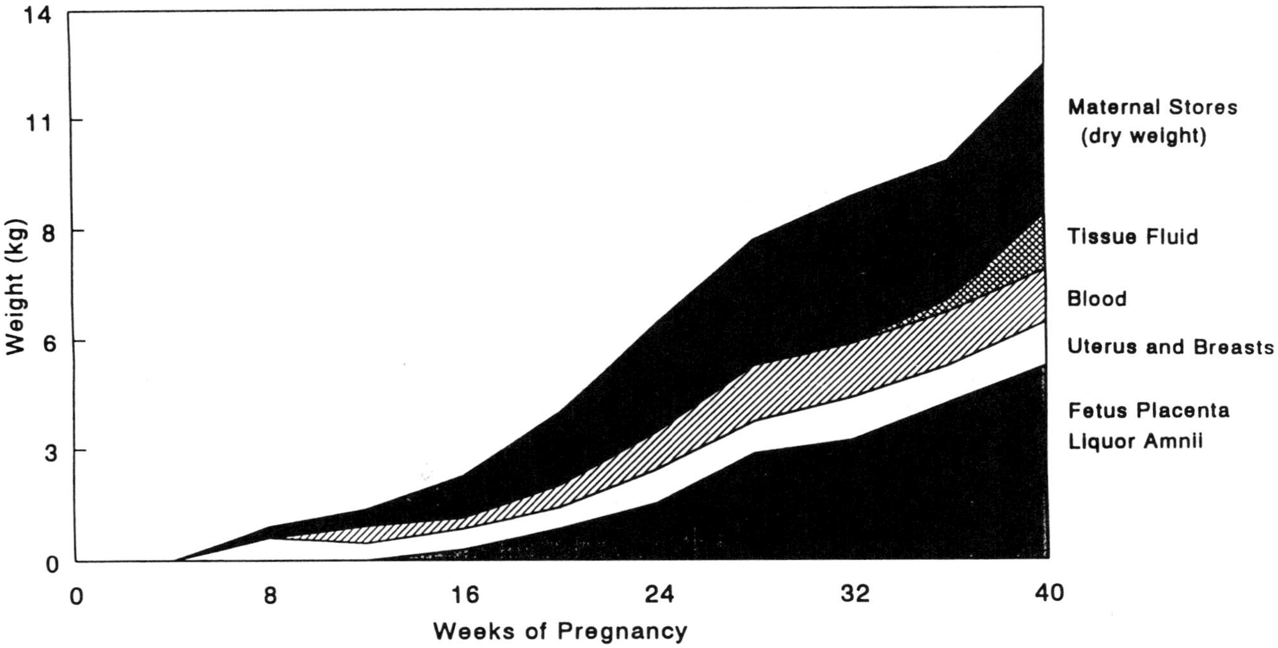

14
11
8
6
3
0
Weight (kg)
0
8
16
24
32
40
Weeks of Pregnancy
Maternal Stores
(dry weight)
Tissue Fluid
Blood
Uterus and Breasts
Fetus Placenta
Liquor Amnii


**FIGURE 44–1.** Components of weight gain in normal pregnancy. (From Hytten, F.E., Leitch, I.: Physiology of Human Pregnancy. Oxford, Blackwell Scientific, 1964.)

biochemical levels of substances such as albumin and hemoglobin during pregnancy, with a return to normal 8 to 10 weeks post partum; second, the estrogen-progesterone, placental hormone changes cause lipids to rise during pregnancy and return to baseline levels post partum.

## BIOCHEMICAL CHANGES AND LABORATORY MEASUREMENTS

The 30 to 40% expansion of overall blood volume during the last trimesters (with the plasma component expanding 50%) reaches a peak between weeks 32 and 34 of gestation. The red cell mass also increases about 20% and peaks at the time of delivery. The physiologic dilution accompanying the expansion of blood volume results in a 12 to 15% decrease in hemoglobin and hematocrit per deciliter of blood. Despite these changes, the mean corpuscular volume (MCV) and mean corpuscular hemoglobin concentration (MCHC) remain relatively unchanged in the nonanemic patient.

Other adaptations include progressive increases in cardiac output that peak at 28 weeks, accumulation of body water, and changes in renal, respiratory gastrointestinal and genitourinary functions (Table 44–4). These physiologic adaptations during pregnancy alter the blood levels of many nutritional components.

Generally, those nutrients that are water soluble follow the decline of serum albumin level, for example, the serum levels of vitamin C, folic acid, vitamin $B_6$, and vitamin $B_{12}$ (Tables 44–5 and 44–6). In addition, the urinary excretion of end products of folate, niacin, and pyridoxine metabolism are increased, as is the intact riboflavin. In contrast, the fat-soluble nutrients such as serum carotene and vitamin E are increased as much as 50% during pregnancy; however, vitamin A levels are relatively unchanged.

To provide proper management of the patient with these physiologic changes, it is necessary to conduct suitable biochemical studies at suitable intervals.

The initial assessment of hematologic status is a complete automated profile that provides more information than a hemoglobin or hematocrit level. Such data allow detection of iron-deficiency anemia or of macrocytic anemia. One of the first clues to macrocytic anemia, when associated with a low hemoglobin, is a decrease in the total number of RBC. An erythrocyte

**TABLE 44–4.** MAJOR PRENATAL PHYSIOLOGIC ALTERATIONS

| | |
|---|---|
| ↑↑ | Plasma volume |
| ↑ | Red blood cell volume |
| ↑ | Cardiac output |
| ↑ | Body water |
| ↑↑ | Renal glomerular filtration rate |
| ↑ | Respiratory tidal volume |
| ↓ | Gastrointestinal and Genitourinary motility |

**TABLE 44–5.** CALCULATED PERCENTAGE RATIO OF NUTRIENTS IN MATERNAL AND FETAL SERUM BY GESTATIONAL AGE

| Serum | MATERNAL NP/NL* | 3rd Trimester | Delivery | Lactating | FETAL Birth | Infant |
|---|---|---|---|---|---|---|
| Glucose | 100 | 90 | 85 | 100 | 105 | 118 |
| Protein | 100 | 90 | 90 | 88 | 77 | 77 |
| Albumin | 100 | 85 | 81 | 104 | 71 | 71 |
| Globulin | 100 | 95 | 122 | 108 | 67 | 92 |
| Lipids | 100 | 140 | 150 | 139 | 94 | 134 |
| Metals | | | | | | |
| Calcium | 100 | 90 | 90 | 80 | 110 | 90 |
| Iron | 100 | 70 | 70 | 100 | 100 | 100 |
| Zinc | 100 | 70 | 100 | 100 | 100 | 80 |
| Vitamins | | | | | | |
| A | 100 | 90 | 70 | 130 | 40 | 40 |
| β-carotene | 100 | 160 | 200 | 105 | 40 | 80 |
| D | 100 | 220 | 80 | 50 | 60 | 62 |
| E | 100 | 130 | 160 | n/a | 40 | 130 |
| C | 100 | 73 | 50 | 40 | 110 | 160 |
| Thiamin | 100 | 60 | 60 | 80 | 110 | 110 |
| Riboflavin | 100 | 40 | 90 | 100 | 190 | 170 |
| Niacin | 100 | 150 | 160 | 83 | 120 | 122 |
| $B_6$ | 100 | 40 | 70 | 80 | 220 | 130 |
| Folate | 100 | 70 | 40 | 120 | 150 | 80 |
| $B_{12}$ | 100 | 90 | 30 | 60 | 100 | 80 |
| Hemoglobin | 100 | 90 | 96 | 100 | 139 | 83 |
| Mean corpuscular volume | 100 | 100 | 100 | 100 | 116 | 89 |
| Mean corpuscular hemoglobin concentration | 100 | 100 | 100 | 100 | 92 | 97 |

(Data compiled from 18 literature references.) * Nonpregnant, not lactating.

**TABLE 44–6.** MAJOR PRENATAL NUTRITION ALTERATIONS

- ↓ Hematologic status
- ↑ White blood cells
- ↓↓ Serum albumin
- ↓ Serum vitamin C, folic acid, $B_{12}$
- ↑ Serum carotene
- → Vitamin A
- ↑ Serum tocopherol
- ↑ Urinary N′-methylnicotinamide
- ↑ Urinary riboflavin
- ↑ Urinary xanthuric-acid excretion

count at or near the 3 million/ml level is due to one of three possible problems: (1) macrocytic anemia; (2) hemolysis that is destroying the red cells; or (3) recent significant acute blood loss. These abnormalities result in an MCV in excess of 100.

As noted earlier, a screening profile is necessary to provide several different biochemical measurements by which to monitor organ and hormonal functions. Among them are measurements of direct nutritional significance, namely, electrolytes, glucose, magnesium, calcium, cholesterol, lipids, liver enzymes, albumin, urea nitrogen, and ferritin.

Table 44–7 identifies the key metabolic alterations, which include increases in the plasma levels of $T_3$ and $T_4$, so a physiologic state of mild hyperthyroidism exists. The changes in plasma insulin result in variations in metabolism of glucose and the occurrence of gestational diabetes. No other "stress test" can match this pronounced challenge of pregnancy for the identification of subsequent onset of adult diabetes. Calcium, iron, and zinc are probably required in proportionally greater quantity because of the requirements of the placental transport enzymes early in pregnancy and the size of the fetal skeletal and blood-forming tissue. As noted later,

**TABLE 44–7.** MAJOR PRENATAL METABOLIC ALTERATIONS

- ↑ Plasma $T_3$ and $T_4$
- ↑ Plasma insulin
- ↑ Abnormal glucose tolerance test
- ↑ Calcium and iron absorption
- ↑ Nitrogen retention (anabolic)
- ↑ Triglyceride, cholesterol, fibrinogen

folate catabolism increases, with resultant increased requirements.

The pregnant woman becomes anabolic for protein, with significant nitrogen retention particularly during the first 24 weeks of gestation. As noted previously, enhanced alterations in the lipid metabolic pathways occur, with doubling of the serum levels of triglycerides and cholesterol, as well as almost all of blood-clotting factors. The intestinal absorption of all nutrients is enhanced to a degree dependent on the amount presented, in maternal body stores, and the progressively increasing fetal requirements. By converting blood values to levels per unit of hematocrit, one can partially adjust for expansion of maternal blood volume for a measure of absolute nutrient change in gestation.[9]

## PLACENTAL TRANSFER OF NUTRIENTS

All nourishment is provided by the mother across the placental barrier during intrauterine life and, if the infant is breast-fed, by the mother and her mammary transfer system during extrauterine life. Both supply systems depend on an adequate maternal nutrient intake. These nutrient delivery systems are impeded if the mother is unable to ingest, absorb, metabolize, utilize, and transport these nutrients to the placenta or breast. Maternal complications such as (1) chronic cardiovascular and renal disease, (2) diabetes, and (3) pregnancy-induced toxemia compromise the maternal capacity to deliver nutrients, as well as oxygen across the placenta to her fetus. Normal fetal growth reaches 30 g per day during the last 16 weeks of gestation, 50% more than at any time during the infant's neonatal period.

Placental transfer of nutrients depends on their concentration in the maternal plasma and the adequacy of the uterine blood flow perfusing the placenta. The transfer of nutrients increases up to sixfold as pregnancy advances. As shown in Table 44–8, most of the electrolytes, gases, and fat-soluble vitamins cross by simple diffusion; carbohydrates cross by facilitated diffusion; and active transport is required for amino acids, water-soluble vitamins, and minerals such as calcium and iron.

As a result of three pathways, we find gradients in concentration of nutrients on the maternal and fetal side of the placenta creating a maternal/fetal nutrient ratio. Certain items are lower in the fetus and higher in the mother (see Table 44–5); other items have equal concentration on both sides of the placenta barrier; and some items are lower in the mother and higher in the fetus. Levels of the water-soluble vitamins and some of the essential metals tend to be lower in the mother than in the fetus in the unsupplemented pregnant woman. Levels of the fat-soluble vitamins, in contrast, are higher in the mother than in the fetus, maintaining the diffusion gradient. Maternal supplementation of some of the water-soluble vitamins such as folic acid, pyridoxine, and vitamin $B_{12}$ may significantly alter but not not eliminate these maternal/fetal ratios.[10]

## NUTRITION PROBLEMS AMONG PREGNANT TEENAGERS

As noted previously, the onset of menses ranges between 9 and 16 years of age in the United States, with a mean of slightly less then 13 years. Improved nutritional status, particularly calories, has been a contributing factor to the decrease of about 2.5 years that has occurred over many years. A difference of intake of 200 kcal per day between 2 groups of young girls resulted in a 1.5-year earlier onset of menarche in the group with the higher intake.[11] Frisch's study of 38 young female runners and swimmers who were in training for the 1980 Olympics also emphasizes the importance of adequate intake at this period.[12] Those who began their strenuous athletic training program before the onset of their menses had a 2.5-year delay in menarche, as compared with the age of onset of menses of those who began the same intensity of physical training after menarche (Table 44–9). The intake of the "before" group was significantly lower in total calories, protein, and calcium than that of their "after" counterparts.

The United States has the highest frequency of teenage pregnancy of all industrialized countries in the world, and Texas ranks second among the states. About 16% of all live births occur to young women who are younger than 20 years of age, with a little over one third (6%) of

**TABLE 44–8.** METHODS OF PLACENTAL TRANSFER OF NUTRIENTS

| DIFFUSION | | |
|---|---|---|
| SIMPLE | FACILITATED | ACTIVE TRANSPORT |
| Gases | Carbohydrates | Amino acids |
| Free fatty acids | | Water-soluble vitamins |
| Electrolytes | | Sodium/calcium/iron |
| Fat-soluble vitamins | | |
| Plus: Pinocytosis, solute drag, breaks in villi | | |

**TABLE 44–9.** MENARCHAL AGE AMONG FEMALE ATHLETES

| N | | 18 | 20 |
|---|---|---|---|
| ONSET OF TRAINING | | BEFORE | AFTER |
| Mean age years | Chronologic | 18.7 | 19.4 |
| | Menarche | 15.1 | 12.8 |
| | Biologic | 3.6 | 6.6 |
| Mean height (cm) | | 168.1 | 165.0 |
| Mean weight (kg) | | 57.1 | 57.7 |
| Mean % standard weight | | 92.0 | 98.0 |
| Mean calorie intake (kcal) | | 1773 | 2288 |
| Calculated kcal/kg | | 31 | 40 |
| Mean protein intake (g) | | 71 | 92 |
| Calculated g protein/kg | | 1.3 | 1.6 |
| Percentage amenorrheic | | 22 | 0 |
| Percentage with irregular menses | | 61 | 40 |

Adapted from Frisch, R.E.: Biol. Rev., *59*:161–188, 1984.)

those births occurring in young women younger than 18 years of age, many of whom are less then 5 years postmenarchal. The results of the Texas section of the *Ten State Nutrition Survey Report* (1968 to 1970) provided convincing evidence that significant numbers of adolescent females failed to ingest 50% of the RDA of all nutrients (Table 44–10);[13] in addition, 10 to 30% of the adolescent females surveyed showed inadequate biochemical levels of seven key nutrients. One third of all these 10- to 16-year-old girls had two or more "low" or "deficient" nutritional biochemical levels per individual. Our evidence indicates no real improvement in the intervening years. In general, teenagers currently appear to be in poorer overall health and nutritional condition than their parents.[14] They continue to have significant excesses and deficits in calories, fat, calcium, and iron; calcium intake remains below half the RDA, with 40% of the females not regularly ingesting dairy products. Their diets are high in fat, both as total fat and as saturated components. In 1968, 10% of the Texas teenage population were obese (over 120% of standard weight). In comparison, 1990 data indicate an obesity problem in the range of 15 to 25%.[15]

All obstetric and fetal performance studies of teenage pregnancies, particularly among those younger than 18 years of age (less than 5 years postmenarchal), have reported three common trends: (1) a decrease in mean infant birth weight that results in an increased percentage of low birth weight newborns; (2) an increase in the perinatal mortality rate; and (3) an increase in pregnancy-induced toxemia. These pregnant teenagers are part of a population group that receives its health care primarily in the public sector.

## OLDER PRIMIGRAVIDAS

Over the past 25 years, we have seen a significant twofold increase in the number of 30-year-old women who are delivering their first child. The older primigravida patient usually receives her care in the private sector.

**TABLE 44–10.** PERCENTAGE OF WOMEN WITH DIETARY INTAKES FOR SELECTED MINERALS AND VITAMINS THAT ARE <50, <70, OR ≥100% OF THE 1980 RECOMMENDED DIETARY ALLOWANCES (RDA)

| | <50% RDA | | <70% RDA | | ≥100% RDA | |
|---|---|---|---|---|---|---|
| | TNS* | USDA† | USDA† | | USDA† | |
| | 1968 | 1985 | 1980 | 1985 | 1980 | 1985 |
| Calcium | 26 | 27 | 42 | 50 | 32 | 22 |
| Iron | 26 | 44 | 32 | 79 | 43 | 5 |
| Vitamin A | 17 | 21 | 31 | 39 | 50 | 45 |
| Vitamin C | 20 | 16 | 26 | 28 | 59 | 44 |

*Data from McGanity, W.J., Dawson, E.B.: Unpublished data, Ten State Nutrition Survey, 1968–1970.
†United States Department of Agriculture: Nationwide Food Consumption Survey. Report No. 85–1. Hyattsville, MD, Nutrition Monitoring Division, Human Nutrition Information Service, U.S. Department of Agriculture, 1985.

How nutritionally well prepared is the older patient for pregnancy? Upwards of 40% of women in this age group are on, or have been on, some type weight-reduction diet for the previous 5 to 6 months.[16] Of the 10 most popular types of diets evaluated in 1987, 90% had fewer than 1500 calories, 70% had more than 20% of their calories coming from protein, and 60% had more than 30% coming from fat.[17] Seven out of 10 of these diets had inadequate content of the 5 essential minerals and the 8 vitamins. For many, their nutritional status before their first pregnancy is not better than that of many teenagers. Pregnant women over 35 years of age have an increase in chronic hypertension, a threefold increase in diabetes, twice the incidence of third-trimester bleeding—placenta previa and abruptio placentae, and an increased rate of cesarean sections that are not necessarily associated with obstructive labor problems.[18]

## RECOMMENDED DIETARY ALLOWANCES FOR PREGNANCY AND LACTATION

During the half-century that successive editions of the RDA have been published, changes have occurred in recommendations for nutrients, minerals, and vitamins based on the then current status of nutritional knowledge. For example, energy recommendations for nonpregnant adult women have varied from a low of 2000 kcal per day in 1948 and 1968 to a high of 2300 kcal in 1953 and 1958. Data based on the 1983 revision of the Metropolitan Life height, age, and weight tables and on data derived from the National Health and Nutrition Examination Survey (NHANES) II indicate that women of reproductive age are about 2 cm taller and 2 kg heavier than the RDA reference woman of the 1960s.[19] Since 1974, the recommendations for increased energy need during pregnancy and lactation have remained constant at 300 and 500 kcal per day, respectively.

The 1989 revision of the RDA has several significant changes in the recommendation for the nonpregnant, pregnant, and lactating woman (Table 44–11; see also Appendix Table A–2b).[20] Compared to 1980,[21] the 1989 allowances for *nonpregnant* women recommend a small increase in protein and decreased need for iron, zinc, folate, and $B_6$ in the face of a 5% increase of 100 kcal per day from 2100 to 2200 kcal. The 1989 recommendations for the *pregnant* woman include a 15 to 25% increase above the recommendations for the nonpregnant woman for calories, protein, magnesium, iodine, zinc, selenium, vitamin E, vitamin C, thiamin, and niacin, and more than 50% increase for iron and folic acid, as well as the same amount of calcium as for a teenager (1200 mg).

**TABLE 44–11.** 1989 RECOMMENDED DIETARY ALLOWANCES FOR PREGNANT AND LACTATING WOMEN 15 TO 25+ YEARS OLD

| PERCENTAGE OF CHANGE* | PREGNANT | NONPREGNANT | NUTRIENT | LACTATING, 1–6 MONTHS | PERCENTAGE OF CHANGE* |
|---|---|---|---|---|---|
| 114 | 2,500 | 2,200 | Energy (kcal) | 2,700 | 123 |
| 120 | 60 | 44–50 | Protein (g) | 65 | 130 |
| 150 | 1,200 | 800 | Calcium (mg) | 1,200 | 150 |
| 150 | 1,200 | 800 | Phosphorus (mg) | 1,200 | 150 |
| 200 | 30 | 15 | Iron (mg) | 15 | 100 |
| 114 | 320 | 280 | Magnesium (mg) | 355 | 127 |
| 117 | 175 | 150 | Iodine (μg) | 200 | 133 |
| 125 | 15 | 12 | Zinc (mg) | 19 | 158 |
| 118 | 65 | 55 | Selenium (μg) | 75 | 136 |
| 100 | 800 | 800 | Vitamin A (μg RE) | 1,300 | 162 |
| 100 | 10 | 10 | Vitamin D (μg) | 10 | 100 |
| 125 | 10 | 8 | Vitamin E (mg & TE)‡ | 12 | 150 |
| 100 | 55 | 55 | Vitamin K (μg) | 65 | 118 |
| 117 | 70 | 60 | Vitamin C (mg) | 95 | 158 |
| 136 | 1.5 | 1.1 | Thiamin (mg) | 1.6 | 145 |
| 123 | 1.6 | 1.3 | Riboflavin (mg) | 1.8 | 138 |
| 113 | 17 | 15 | Niacin (mg NE) | 20 | 133 |
| 222 | 400 | 180 | Folate (μg) | 280 | 108 |
| 138 | 2.2 | 1.6 | Vitamin $B_6$ (mg) | 2.1 | 131 |
| 110 | 2.2 | 2.0 | Vitamin $B_{12}$ (μg) | 2.6 | 130 |

*Allowances for pregnancy and lactation ÷ nonpregnant women 15 to 25+ years old.
†300 kcal above the nonpregnant woman in the second and third trimesters only.
‡As miligrams of α-tocopherol.
RE, Retinol equivalents; NE, niacin equivalents.
(From Food and Nutrition Board, National Research Council: Recommended Dietary Allowances. 10th Ed. Washington, D.C., National Academy Press, 1989.)

During the first 6 months of lactation, there is a further increase for protein, zinc, vitamins A, E, and C, and niacin when compared to the pregnant status and a decreased requirement for iron and folic acid.

Concern has been expressed that excessive caloric intake during and after pregnancy and lactation may be a major contributor to obesity. Pregnant and lactating women do need additional energy, but whether the 300 and 500 kcal recommended are needed in addition to the nonpregnant need of 1800 or 2200 kcal remains unresolved.

In developing countries, pregnant and lactating women with caloric intakes of 60 to 80% and 50 to 72%, respectively, of the 1989 RDA are supporting pregnancies and lactation.[19,22] Depressed BMR during the first 18 weeks of gestation was noted in chronically and marginally undernourished Gambian women.[65] In western and northern European and in Australian studies, actual caloric intakes for pregnant women averaged 78 to 100% (mean 2140 kcal) per day of the RDA and 85 to 109% (mean 2480 kcal) of the RDA for women during lactation, with superior maternal and fetal performance.[22] However, this summary included also data from a study in the United States of lactating women,[23] which had the lowest average of any of the studies listed. Appendix Table A–3a shows that the 1990 Canadian recommendations for pregnant and lactating women averaged 200 and 250 kcal per day lower than those of the United States RDA. United Kingdom standards are also appreciably lower than the RDA (see Appendix Table A–4a).

Since the 1970s, the usual reference standard for the pregnant woman has been based on Hytten's calculation that pregnancy requires an additional 80,000 kcal,[24] believed to accumulate in the course of pregnancy, as illustrated in Figure 44–2.[25] This figure of 80,000 is based on a pregnancy in which the mother gained 12.5 kg and gave birth to an infant weighing 3.3 kg. This estimate was used by the World Health Organization (WHO) in 1973 for the energy allowances for pregnancy with a rise from an extra 150 kcal per day for the first trimester to 350 kcal per day for the second and third trimesters; in the 1985 revision, an additional 250 kcal per day were recommended throughout pregnancy, with a reduction to 200 kcal per day throughout pregnancy when the expectant mother is able to reduce physical activity proportionately.[26] One of the major components of the energy cost is the accumulation of approximately 3.5 kg of fat, most of which is laid down by the thirtieth week (Fig. 44–2); this occurs during the time that the fetus and maternal reproductive organs are increasing weight slowly and was considered a protection against the high energy costs of the last trimester and lactation. The other major cost component concerns the increased energy requirements for maintenance metabolism that occur in the latter half of pregnancy.

Alternative assumptions have been made, based on further analyses of composition of the new tissues and more detailed observations of both energy intakes and expenditures of pregnant woman and their resting metabolism. Such calculations have led to estimates of the cost of pregnancy in healthy, well-nourished women as

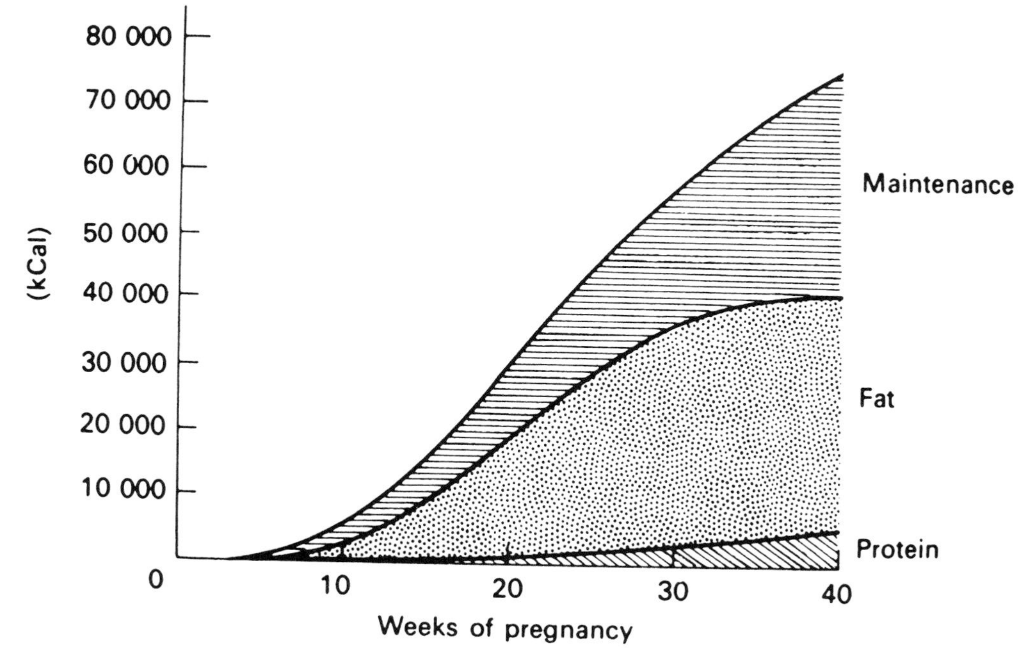
80 000
70 000
60 000
50 000
40 000
30 000
20 000
10 000
0
(kCal)
Maintenance
Fat
Protein
10
20
30
40
Weeks of pregnancy

**FIGURE 44–2.** The cumulative energy cost of pregnancy and its components. (From Hytten, F., Chamberlain, G.: Clinical Physiology in Obstetrics. Oxford, Blackwell Scientific Publications, 1980.)

low as 45,000 kcal[27] or 68,000 kcal,[28] and as high as 110,000 kcal.[29] The lower figures are based on the decreased activity of the pregnant woman during the third trimester of pregnancy.

For the healthy woman, achievement of an adequate intake (with some supplementation of iron, folate, and perhaps zinc) is accomplished by choosing among a variety of foods in the proportions recommended by the United States Department of Agriculture pyramid, with weight gain management in accordance with appropriate weight targets, as described in a later section of this chapter. Individuals who prefer an ethnic dietary pattern (e.g., Far Eastern, Near Eastern, Hispanic, vegetarian, and others) can meet their nutrient needs with proper food selection. Food exchange lists for a variety of food patterns are given in Appendix Table A–23. A strict vegan has nutrient deficits in hematologic components, particularly vitamin $B_{12}$; during pregnancy, she must be willing to ingest regularly a mineral/vitamin supplement that contains at least iron, zinc, folate, and $B_{12}$.

Not all the members of our society have the economic capacity to support their family's needs for food, clothing, and shelter. Ten percent of our population receive food stamps and their children participate in the school lunch program, and another 1 million women and 4 million of their children are enrolled in the WIC program. The WIC Food Package V for pregnant and breast-feeding women provides more than 840 kcal per day, which is more than 30% of the total recommended caloric intake, 65% of protein needs, and 100% of almost all the mineral and vitamin requirements except for iron and zinc during pregnancy and lactation. Apparently, not all this supplemental food is ingested by the mother, but is assimilated into the total food availability of the family unit. Evidence indicates an increase in mean infant birth weight of only 30 to 100 g for those infants whose mothers receive the WIC supplement during pregnancy.[2]

## MATERNAL WEIGHT GAIN

Maternal weight gain during pregnancy is an essential component of the normal growth and development of the mother and her fetus. Over the past 100 years, the medical profession has adopted acceptable/optimal weight gain guidelines. In the late 1890s, under the fear of maternal mortality associated with overly large infants and the risks of a cesarean section delivery, our German predecessors initiated the pattern of trying to restrict maternal weight gain deliberately in an attempt to reduce infant size and weight, therefore expediting the vaginal birth process. This pattern existed in one form or another through the 1960s. In 1970 the National Research Council's *Report on Maternal Nutrition and the Course of Pregnancy* increased these weight gain targets to a modest upward adjustment of 5 to 8 pounds per pregnancy.[30]

Today, the pendulum has swung towards "ad lib feeding" and further maternal weight gain to the extent that it may be a major contributor to the ever-increasing incidence of obesity among the female population of the United States. Over 25% of young women below 20 years of age are obese, and one third of all females have weights greater than 120% of standard weight.[16] On any given day, 40% of the adult women of the United States are on a diet and have been for 6 months.

The birth weight of the offspring depends on two maternal weight-related factors: (1) How much weight did she put on during her pregnancy? and (2) What was her initial height/weight relationship (PSW or BMI) when she began her pregnancy?

In its 1990 report on maternal weight gain, the National Research Council recommended that all pregnant women have a BMI calculation at the time of entry into prenatal care.[2] If a woman has a BMI of less than 20, her weight gain target should be 1.1 lbs of weight gain per week during the second and third trimester, in comparison to the woman whose BMI is greater than 26, with a weight gain target of only 0.7 lb per week. As noted previously, another method of weight/height expression if PSW of the American Diabetes Association, where a PSW of less than 90% of standard weight equals a BMI of less than 20, and a PSW of 135 equals a BMI of over 29.

### COMPONENTS OF WEIGHT GAIN

During normal pregnancy, these components consist of the fetus, placenta, amniotic fluid, enlarged uterine and breast tissue, and expanded maternal blood volume (see Fig. 44–1).[31] Together, they comprise the "obligatory" weight gain associated with pregnancy. In addition are highly variable accumulations of tissue fluid and adipose tissue and protein stores (Fig. 44–2). In studies from industrialized countries, obligatory weight gain amounts to about 7.5 kg (16.5 lb). Among developing countries, obligatory maternal weight gain is about 20% less (6 kg or 13.2 lb), with lesser accumulation of tissue fluid and adipose tissue and protein stores.[32]

If a woman begins her pregnancy at 65 in. (1.67 m) and 128 lb, (58.2 kg) over the 40 weeks of pregnancy her PSW will increase 13% (16.5 lb = 7.5 kg) from the obligatory weight gain alone. If, however, she puts on 32 pounds, her PSW will increase almost 26%, of which 1 to 2 kg will be tissue fluid and 7 kg in the form of fat. If she desires to return to her prepregnant weight after delivery or nursing, this will require at least 12 weeks of reduced calories and increased exercise to achieve that goal. For a primiparous mother who gains over 40 pounds (18.2 kg) it may well take a year to return to her initial weight status.

### INDIVIDUAL WEIGHT GAIN TARGETS

No single maternal weight gain target meets the needs of all types of pregnant women. Individualized pattern(s) of weight gain should be adjusted for (1) height/weight relationship or PSW, (2) biologic age, (3) plans to breast-feed, and (4) whether more than one fetus is being carried.

Does a biologically immature female need more weight gain during pregnancy to produce an equivalent-weight offspring? Garn, examining the data from the National Perinatal Study, found that for white and black women 14 years of age, the mother required almost 4 g of maternal weight to yield 1 g of baby; this was in contrast to her fully mature counterpart, who produced 200-g heavier infants on only 3 g of maternal weight for every 1 g of baby (Table 44–12).[33] These findings translate into an additional need for 150 kcal per day (3 kg in overall weight gain) for the biologically immature pregnant woman.

## GENERAL TARGETS OF APPROPRIATE WEIGHT GAIN

Five maternal weight gain targets have been developed (Fig. 44–3). These are as follows:

1. For the woman who enters her pregnancy at more than 120% of standard weight: the target an obligatory weight gain of 7 to 8 kg at a weekly rate of no more than 300 g per week (target I).
2. For the woman of normal PSW who is not going to nurse: the target is 10 kg overall at a rate of 350 g per week (target II).
3. For the woman who enters her pregnancy between 90 and 110% of standard weight and is planning to nurse her baby: the target is 12 kg overall with about 400 g per week during the second and third trimester (target III).
4. For the adolescent and the woman less than 90% of standard weight: the target is 14 to 15 kg (32 lb) at a rate of 500 g per week (target IV).
5. For the woman who is going to have twins: the target is 18 kg of weight gain with a weekly rate of 650 g during the last 20 weeks of her pregnancy (target V).

## RISKS OF EXCESSIVE WEIGHT GAIN

As noted previously, the 1990 maternal nutrition report of the National Research Council recommended an additional 5- to 10-lb increase above the 1980 targets for maternal weight gain to produce heavier but not necessarily more mature newborns.[30] This recommendation implies that the benefits of a heavier baby outweigh the costs associated with increased problems with delivery, as well as the maternal health costs associated with ever-increasing residual obesity. The wisdom of this recommendation merits discussion.

No convincing evidence indicates that an infant who is biologically mature at birth and who weighs over 3200 g would be better or healthier if he or she were to weigh 3500 g. This situation is different with respect to neonatal morbidity and mortality when an infant weighs 1000, 1250, 1500, or 2000 g, when weight gain is far more important than when the weight differential is between the 3000- and 4000-g range.

Furthermore, excessive maternal weight gain has been associated with increased rates of labor problems, cesarean section, fetal macrosomia, late delivery dates, and meconium staining of the fetus.

## OBESITY, AGE, AND PARITY

Cross-sectional data from the Texas Nutritional Survey of 1968 showed a progressive increase in the incidence of female obesity associated with advancing maternal age from 10% in the 15 to 19 year olds to as much as 60% in the age group from 40 to 44 years.[13]

**TABLE 44–12.** RELATIONSHIP OF WEIGHT STATUS IN ADOLESCENT MOTHERS AND THEIR INFANTS BY RACE

| WHITE | | | | | | BLACK | | | | |
|---|---|---|---|---|---|---|---|---|---|---|
| Weight Gain (kg) | Birth (g) | M/B‡ Ratio | Percentage of Standard Weight | BA* | CA† | Weight Gain (kg) | Birth (g) | M/B Ratio | Percentage of Standard Weight | BA* |
| 13.8 | 3,098 | 4.4 | 94 | 2.4 | 14 | 10.6 | 2,939 | 3.6 | 97 | 1.8 |
| 12.0 | 3,188 | 3.8 | 95 | 2.7 | 15 | 10.1 | 2,970 | 3.4 | 98 | 2.5 |
| 11.2 | 3,206 | 3.5 | 96 | 3.6 | 16 | 10.1 | 2,962 | 3.4 | 97 | 3.3 |
| 11.2 | 3,216 | 3.4 | 96 | 4.3 | 17 | 9.7 | 2,973 | 3.3 | 98 | 4.1 |
| 10.6 | 3,227 | 3.3 | 97 | 5.2 | 18 | 9.8 | 2,981 | 3.3 | 99 | 5.1 |
| 10.4 | 3,259 | 3.2 | 99 | 6.0 | 19 | 9.7 | 3,003 | 3.2 | 100 | 6.0 |
| 9.5 | 3,290 | 2.9 | 101 | n/a | 20–29 | 9.5 | 3,079 | 3.1 | 107 | n/a |

*Corrected biologic age (BA) = menarche + 0.5 years.
†Chronologic age (CA) at entry to prenatal care
‡Maternal weight gain (g) to baby weight (g)
(Adapted from Garn, S.M., Ridella, S.A., Petzold, A.S., et al.: Semin. Perinatol., *5*:155–162, 1981.)

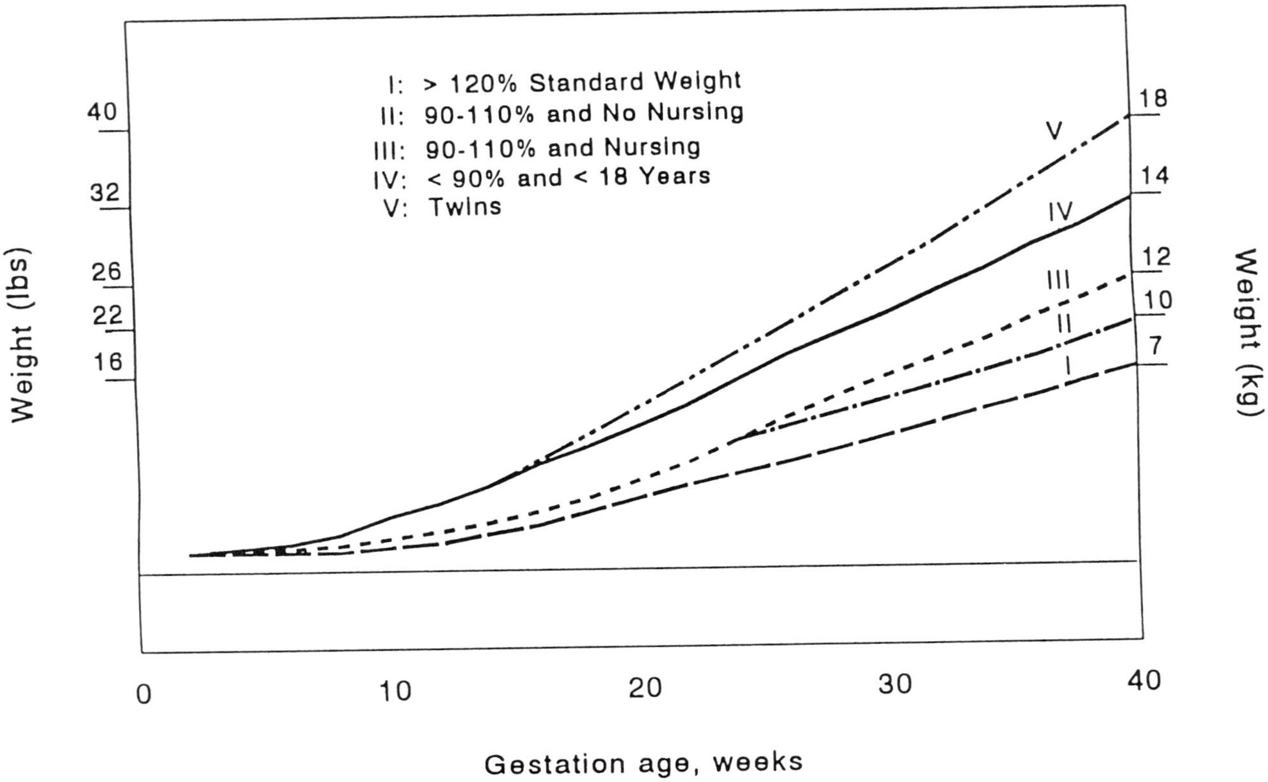
I: > 120% Standard Weight
II: 90-110% and No Nursing
III: 90-110% and Nursing
IV: < 90% and < 18 Years
V: Twins
V
IV
III
II
I
40
32
26
22
16
Weight (lbs)
18
14
12
10
7
Weight (kg)
0
10
20
30
40
Gestation age, weeks

**FIGURE 44–3.** Maternal weight gain targets.

Although obesity is directly related to advancing age, a much higher correlation exists between obesity and the number of times the same woman has been pregnant (gravidity). There was a 16% obesity rate among those who were never pregnant; this rate rose to a prevalence of 50 to 68% among grand multiparous women (Table 44–13).[13] An average of 2.5 kg (5.5 lb) is permanently added to the woman's body for each pregnancy.

Longitudinal data from two separate national collaborative studies of over 1200 and 600 women also found residual weight gain correlated with the number of prior pregnancies. Weiss et al. reported a 3-lb increase among black mothers and 3.8-lb increase in white mothers from one pregnancy to the next.[34] Garn et al. found an increase greater than 5 kg from the first to the third pregnancy, with lesser gains among smoking women.[33]

Our team has encouraged pregnant women to increase their dietary intake by 300 kcal or more per day for almost 200 days of pregnancy and by 500 kcal during the first 6 months of lactation; however, unless the patient has sustained guidance from her health-care team with instructions to *specifically reduce her caloric intake and increase her activity,* particularly if she is not going to nurse her baby, we anticipate her continuing to eat according to an appetite geared to a 2500-kcal level but with an energy need down to about 1800 kcal per day.

Lactation itself does not help the mother to return to her prepregnant weight status. Recent evidence suggests that the nonlactating female loses more weight and at a faster rate than the lactating mother.[35] These data also suggest that greater prenatal weight gain is associated with greater weight loss.

**TABLE 44–13.** PERCENTAGE UNDER- AND OVERWEIGHT BY GRAVIDITY

| PERCENTAGE OF STANDARD WEIGHT | | <80 | ≥120 |
|---|---|---|---|
| No. Pregnancy | N | | |
| 0 | 286 | 7.5 | 15.7 |
| 1 | 57 | 5.4 | 33.3 |
| 2 | 65 | 7.7 | 36.9 |
| 3 | 72 | 4.2 | 47.2 |
| 4 | 73 | 1.4 | 47.9 |
| 5 | 67 | 3.0 | 55.2 |
| 6 | 57 | — | 45.6 |
| 7 | 38 | — | 50.0 |
| 8 | 33 | 3.1 | 66.6 |
| 9 | 22 | — | 68.2 |
| 10 | 70 | — | 52.9 |

(From McGanity, W.J., Dawson, E.B.: Unpublished data, Ten State Nutrition Survey, 1968–1970.)

## ANEMIA PREVENTION

"Low" hemoglobin is the most common nutritional biochemical problem encountered in everyday prenatal care. If not accounted for by the normal hemodilution effect, nine times out of ten a true nutrient deficit problem will be related to iron, and one time out of ten it will be related to folic acid.

Except in those few individuals who are absolute "vegans" and a minimal number of other patients who have had a vitamin $B_{12}$ problem diagnosed and treated before their pregnancy, pregnancy anemia due to inadequate vitamin $B_{12}$ is uncommon. The commonest cause of a hemoglobin less than 110 g/L (11 g/dl) is due to hemodilution caused by the expansion of blood volume. When *nutritional anemia* develops, consider the following: (1) an inadequate intake of one or more hemopoietic nutrients; (2) an excess loss of blood secondary to external or internal bleeding; (3) inadequate iron stores to maintain hemoglobin production; (4) inadequate folate stores to maintain red cell maturation.

### IRON

The process of change from full iron stores with an adequate dietary intake to a classic chronic iron-deficiency anemia (with its small cells, poorly filled with hemoglobin) has many steps. A red cell distribution width, as provided by the automated Coulter Counter CBC, above 15 is one of the earliest indicators of iron-deficiency anemia. Another key is the serum ferritin level, which reflects the adequacy of the body's iron stores; levels lower than 12 μg/L (ng/ml) have generally been considered deficient, and levels lower than 35 μg provide little margin of safety in meeting the iron demands of mother and fetus during pregnancy.

In the typical American diet containing between 6 and 7 mg iron per 1000 kcal, an average of only 10% of the ingested $Fe^{++}$ is transported into the portal circulation. Table 44–14 indicates the milligrams of iron required to be transported into the maternal circulation during the various stages of the reproductive cycle from nonpregnant, through the trimesters of pregnancy, and during lactation. As a result of the cessation of menses, the amount of iron required in the first trimester decreases. In response to maternal and fetal demands, however, requirement increases throughout both the second and third trimesters. As long as lactation is total, the mother will remain amenorrheic, and her postpartum requirement for iron will remain low. In the third trimester of pregnancy, an average of 4 mg iron per day needs to cross into the maternal circulation. Because of fetal demands, however, the requirements may be as high as 7 mg for a short period of time during the middle of the third trimester.

How much iron is required in the diet in order to transport 4 to 7 mg iron across the intestinal barrier? Based on the current RDA, that might require 50% absorption if iron was available only from dietary sources. Various investigators have found that the pregnant woman has an enhanced ability to absorb iron across the intestinal mucosa.[36] The usual rate of 10% of iron transfer can increase up to three times (30%) that amount in response to a variety of levels of iron given during pregnancy. If the woman has 15 mg iron from dietary sources plus another 30 mg available in an iron supplement, she should have no difficulty meeting the iron requirements for pregnancy and her developing fetus. If the maternal hemoglobin level is more than 110 g/L (11 g/dl) at sea level, there is no need for more than the 30-mg supplement. If both a typical prenatal mineral/vitamin supplement containing 30 mg and an additional three tablets of 60 mg ferrous sulfate are prescribed, the patient will be ingesting over 200 mg elemental iron to get 7 mg across the gut. This is iron excess and can lead to gastric irritation. If the mother's hemoglobin is less than 100 g/L (10 g/dl) with low MCV and MCHC—classic iron-deficiency anemia—she will need 120 to 150 mg elemental iron per day to meet those demands until her hemoglobin returns to over 120 g/L (12 g/dl) and the serum ferritin levels are higher than 35 μg/L (ng/mL).

From NHANES II and other studies, it is known that hemoglobin and serum transferrin levels of black women are about 10% lower than those of either white or Hispanic women (Table 44–15). Similarly, hemoglobin levels are 12% higher in the first trimester of pregnancy than in the third; they are also higher in obese pregnant women than in those who are underweight.[37] In a

**TABLE 44–14.** PROVISIONAL REQUIREMENTS OF DIETARY IRON IN WOMEN

| AGE | | DAILY REQUIREMENTS (MG) | MG IRON AVAILABLE IN DAILY DIET | | |
|---|---|---|---|---|---|
| | | | 10% | 20% | 30% |
| 11–50 years, nonpregnant, nonlactating | | 1.8 | 18.0 | 9.0 | 6.0 |
| Pregnant | 1st trimester | 1.0 | 10.0 | 5.0 | 3.0 |
| | 2nd trimester | 3.0 | 30.0 | 15.0 | 10.0 |
| | 3rd trimester | 4.0 | 40.0 | 20.0 | 13.0 |
| Lactating | | 1.5 | 15.0 | 7.5 | 5.0 |

**TABLE 44–15.** HEMATOLOGIC LEVELS IN FEMALES (12–17 YEARS)

| HEMOGLOBIN (g/L) | TOTAL | WHITE | BLACK |
|---|---|---|---|
| Mean | 13.2 | 13.3 | 12.4 |
| Percentile | | | |
| 5 | 11.5 | 11.9 | 11.0 |
| 50 | 13.2 | 13.4 | 12.5 |
| 95 | 14.8 | 14.9 | 13.8 |
| TRANSFERRIN SAT (%) | | | |
| Mean | 25.7 | 26.1 | 24.1 |
| Percentile | | | |
| 10 | 13.7 | 14.1 | 12.1 |
| 50 | 24.6 | 24.7 | 23.4 |

(Data from National Health and Nutrition Examination Survey II, U.S. Department of Health, Education and Welfare, 1976–1980.)

**TABLE 44–16.** HEMATOLOGIC OUTCOME VERSUS SERUM FERRITIN AT 20 WEEKS' GESTATIONAL AGE

| IRON SUPPLEMENTATION GROUP | N | GESTATIONAL (n=61) Ferritin > 35 | GESTATIONAL (n=61) Ferritin <35 | THERAPEUTIC FAILURE (n=14) Ferritin >35 | THERAPEUTIC FAILURE (n=14) Ferritin <35 |
|---|---|---|---|---|---|
| A (0 mg)* | 21 | 4 | 17 | 0 | 9 |
| B (18 mg)* | 19 | 11 | 8 | 1 | 4 |
| C (65 mg)† | 21 | 10 | 11 | 0 | 0 |
| Total | 61 | 25 | 36 | 1 | 13 |

1 mg iron = 18 μmol
*+400 μg (0.91 μmol) folate
†+800 μg (1.82 μmol) folate
(Adapted from Sauberlich, H.E.: Evaluation of folate nutrition in population groups. *In* Folic Acid Metabolism in Health and Disease. Edited by M.F. Picciano, E.L.R. Stokstad, and J.F. Gregory, III. New York, Wiley-Liss, 1990, pp. 211–235.)

longitudinal study among three groups of adolescent pregnant females, all with over 11.0 g/dl hemoglobin, Dawson and McGanity et al conducted a 39-week therapeutic trial using a mineral/vitamin supplement containing three dosage levels of iron and two levels of folate[38] (Table 44–16). The young women were studied from the sixteenth week of their pregnancy through the remainder of the pregnancy, delivery, and first 12 weeks postpartum. Figure 44–4 illustrates that the mean serum ferritin in each group dropped significantly from their initial values at entry into the study to delivery, and all showed recovery in the postpartum period. Only group C, who were receiving the 65-mg iron supplement, returned to their initial entry levels by the twelfth week post partum, however. None of these three levels of maternal iron supplementation were able to overcome the dilutional effect of blood volume expansion and/or the demands for iron by the mother and fetus during the second and third trimester, in contrast to the response when the supplement was given before the pregnancy commences and during the weeks after the delivery.

Table 44–16 compares the study groups by level of iron supplementation, the initial serum ferritin level, and the number who failed to maintain their hemoglobin above 110 g/L (11 g/dl) throughout the pregnancy. Forty percent of group A, who were not receiving additional iron in their daily supplement, dropped below the 11-g/dl lower limit; 20% of group B, receiving 18 mg, were in this category, but none of group C, receiving 65 mg per day, fell below 11 g/dl. Only one of 15 (7%) individuals receiving either 0 or 18 mg iron fell below 11-g/dl if her serum ferritin level at 20 weeks of gestation was higher than 35 μg/L (ng/mL), whereas 13 of 25 (52%) did so if their initial serum was less than 35 μg/L (ng/mL).

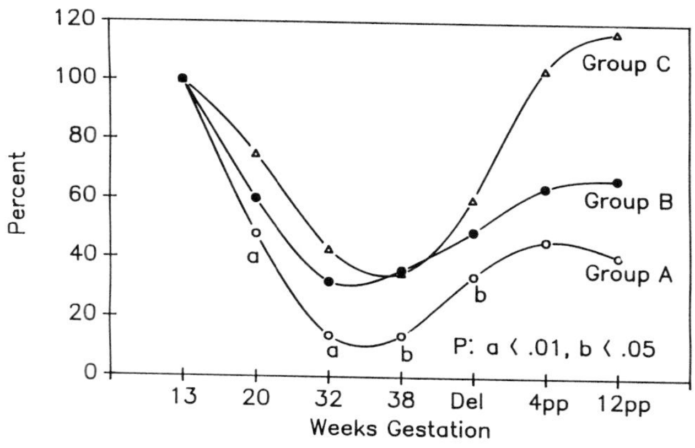

120
100
80
60
40
20
0
Percent
Group C
Group B
Group A
a
b
a
b
P: a < .01, b < .05
13
20
32
38
Del
4pp
12pp
Weeks Gestation


**FIGURE 44–4.** Mean relative percentage of change from prestudy baseline of serum ferritin (adjusted for serum volume) for groups A, B, and C who were given the supplement listed in Table 44–16.
pp, Post partum.

Deficient serum ferritin levels lower than 12 μg/L (ng/mL) have been associated with a two- to threefold increase in the incidence of low birth weight and preterm deliveries. These data suggest that pregnant women with serum ferritin levels lower than 35 μg/L (35 ng/mL) during the first trimester are also at risk without an adequate level of iron supplementation during the last half of their pregnancy. Routine assessment of the serum ferritin status before 20 weeks of gestation should indicate the need for an appropriate level of elemental iron supplement throughout the remainder of the pregnancy and for 100 days post partum.

### FOLIC ACID

Deficiency of folic acid (folate) is associated with an increased incidence of low birth weight babies and megaloblastic anemia in mothers.[39] Because the calculated total fetal and placental folate content is about 800 μg at term,[40] it is unlikely that the increased demand for this vitamin is due merely to fetal transfer; the latter represents a drain of less than 5 μg per day. Investigators have demonstrated, in normal pregnant women, that the urinary concentration of a breakdown product of folate (*p*-acetamidobenzoylglutamate) rose significantly in the second trimester and returned to baseline post partum.[41] It was estimated that the increase rate of folate metabolism produces an extra demand for dietary folate of about 200 to 300 μg per day in pregnant women.[41]

The role of folic acid in prevention of neural tube defects is reviewed later.

Folate supplementation given to the same three groups noted in Table 44–16 increased levels of tissue storage, measured as the folate in maternal red cell in all groups during gestation. The higher 800-μg per day folate supplement reached higher levels throughout the pregnancy and beyond.

### HOMEOSTASIS OF IRON STATUS IN THE FETUS AND NEWBORN INFANT

Over the last 60 years, various investigators have demonstrated the ability of the maternal hematopoietic system to protect the fetus in the face of a range of severe hematologic deficits.[42–44] Hemoglobin, serum iron, and serum ferritin all can be low during pregnancy and lactation, and the newborn infant's iron status and breast milk content remain unaffected.

As noted in Chapter 9 (Table 9–2), the total iron cost of an uncomplicated pregnancy, plus that lost in milk during lactation for 6 months, is in the broad range of 420 to 1030 mg or 1.2 to 2.5 mg per day over this 15-month period, with the major need in the third trimester, as noted previously. Adequate maternal iron stores need to be created before pregnancy, not by trying to do catch-up during gestation. An adequate dietary intake and/or iron supplementation should begin in the months before conception. The typical well-balanced American diet does not provide an adequate supply of iron to meet the maternal and fetal needs during the last half of pregnancy, nor does it replenish the 600 to 1000 ml blood lost at delivery. The nonlactating, postpartum woman needs to be continued on supplemental iron for 100 days (12 weeks) after delivery to replenish her own body stores.

## INFANT AND PERINATAL MORTALITY

Infant mortality rates have been lowered from 15% to less than 1% as sanitation, immunizations, antibiotics, and blood replacements became generally available.

### INFANT MORTALITY

Before the mid-1980s, the leading cause of infant mortality in the United States had been associated with low birth weight and prematurity. Both the infant and perinatal mortality rates in the United States and the percentage of low birth weight infants have decreased over 20% since 1980.[1] As compared with other countries, the United States remains in the mid twentieth rankings. This decrease has occurred more in the white population; African-Americans still have twice the mortality rate of each indicator of our maternal and infant health-care programs.

### PERINATAL MORTALITY

Perinatal mortality, on the other hand, is primarily associated with the fetus's birth weight and gestational age at the time of delivery. As noted in Chapter 46, approximately 7% of all infants born in the United States weigh less than 2500 g at birth. For example, with a newborn infant who weighs less than 700 g and has a biologic age less than 24 weeks of gestation, one can expect a perinatal mortality of 80%, whereas an infant of 2000 g and over 34 weeks' gestation has a perinatal mortality risk of <1.5%. How much of this improvement may be due to maternal nutrition status before and during pregnancy? Certainly, the amount of maternal weight gain is inversely correlated with the rate of perinatal mortality. Poor maternal weight gain during pregnancy increases the risks of the fetus in utero. Increased perinatal mortality rates have also been associated with consistently low levels of serum vitamin C.[45]

## CONGENITAL MALFORMATIONS

Since 1986, almost one fourth of all infant mortality in the United States has been associated with birth defects.[46] As a percentage of infant deaths, congenital malformations have increased from an 8% problem in 1916 to a 24% one in the late 1980s.

We have known since the late 1940s that single maternal nutrient deficits in the experimental laboratory animal can result in an increased frequency of congenital malformations in their offspring. To date, deficiencies of seven essential minerals, five of eight water-soluble vitamins, and three of four fat-soluble vitamins are reported to cause neural, cardiac, or renal birth defects.[47] In the human, it has taken over 40 years to confirm the role of a single nutrient, folic acid, in the primary and secondary prevention of neural tube defects.

Congenital malformations have their origin about 20% of the time in mendelian errors, 10% are chromosomal problems, and 5% are accountable by environmental factors. The remaining 65% have multifactorial or "unknown" contributing factors. In normal intrauterine growth and development of the embryo from the time of conception through implantation and early fetal development, almost all the cleavages and fusions necessary in the formation of the normal fetal architecture and their basic functions have been established by the tenth week of gestation. In fact, the most critical period for neural tube closures occurs in the first 4 weeks of the fetus's gestational life. During this period, the pregnant woman is usually not being followed medically because entry into prenatal care occurs usually about the time of her second missed menstrual period, which is 50 to 60 days from the time of conception. *If we are to do anything about the prevention of congenital malformation, we must actively address the problem in the 8 to 10 weeks before conception.*

The following are three examples of areas in which nutrition intervention before conception can play a major preventive role.

**Diabetes Mellitus.** The level of hemoglobin A1c in the diabetic patient is maintained at acceptable normal values by tight dietary control and insulin regulation as needed. Such proper management can lead to significant improvement in overall reproductive well-being, a decrease in the rate of spontaneous abortions, and a reduction in the three to four times greater frequency of congenital malformations in the offspring of the diabetic mother.

**Phenylketonuria.** Over 3000 young American women are now of reproductive age with an abnormality in their phenylalanine metabolism. If such a patient is returned to the required dietary control before she conceives a child, and if her serum phenylalanine level is kept below 605 μ mol/L (10 mg/dl), one can significantly reduce the risk of congenital and developmental problems in her newborn offspring.[48] The expectant mother with uncontrolled PKU faces an 80 to 90% possibility that the baby will have some type of congenital defect or cranial maldevelopment.

**Spina Bifida and Other Neural Tube Defects.** Each year in the United States about 2500 infants are born with the neural tube defects spina bifida and anencephaly; in addition, an unknown number of fetuses affected by these birth defects are aborted. All infants with anencephaly die shortly after birth, whereas the majority of babies born with spina bifida grow to adulthood with, in severe cases, paralysis and varying degrees of bowel and bladder incontinence.

Evidence has been accumulating for several years that consumption of folic acid before conception (the preconceptual period) and during early pregnancy can reduce the number of neural tube defects. In the randomized controlled trials sponsored by the British Medical Research Council, relatively high-dose folic acid supplements (4.0 mg per day) were taken by women who had a prior pregnancy affected by a neural tube defect, and this vitamin supplement reduced the risk of subsequent pregnancy affected by the disorder by 70%.[49] Increasing numbers of observations have also indicated a lower risk of such defects for women without a prior pregnancy affected by neural tube defect who consumed multivitamin/mineral supplements that included 0.4 to 0.8 mg (400 to 800 μg) folic acid.[50,51] The United States Centers for Disease Control have reviewed this literature.[52] On the basis of such evidence, The United States Public Health Service has recommended

> that all women of childbearing age in the United States who are capable of becoming pregnant should consume 0.4 mg of folic acid per day for the purpose of reducing their risk of having a pregnancy affected with spina bifida or other NTD's. Because the effects of high intakes are not well known but include complicating the diagnosis of vitamin $B_{12}$ deficiency, care should be taken to keep total folate consumption at <1 mg per day, except under the supervision of a physician. Women who have had a prior NTD-affected pregnancy are at high risk of having a subsequent affected pregnancy. When these women are planning to become pregnant, they should consult their physicians for advice.[52]

Women who have had an pregnancy affected by a neural tube defect are advised to consume 0.4 mg folic acid per day *unless* they are planning a pregnancy; in that instance they are advised to consult their physicians about the desirability of using 4.0 mg folic acid per day.[52]

## LOW BIRTH WEIGHT PREGNANCIES: PREVENTIVE ASPECTS

Low birth weight (less than 2500 g) in the newborn infant continues to be a problem that has resisted solution. The percentage of low birth weight infants delivered in the United States between 1980 and 1992 has not changed, remaining around 7% of live births; twice as many such infants are born to black mothers as to white or Hispanic mothers.

The rate of intrauterine fetal growth follows an straight line progression between weeks 24 and 38 of pregnancy, with the infant gaining an average of about 30 g of weight per day, or 0.21 kg (almost half a pound) per week.[53] In the obstetric management of a patient in the third trimester with premature labor and intact membranes, every effort will be made to quiet the contractions, to stabilize the uterus, and to allow the intrauterine fetal growth to continue as long as the placental transfer system is well functioning. The 30-g of weight gain per day while inside the uterus is 50% more than the best that can be accomplished after delivery with the infant in an intensive neonatal care nursery.

Perinatal survival improves 50% between weeks 24 and 27 of gestation (700 to 1000 g in birth weight). By 34 weeks (2000 g), the perinatal survival rate is over 98%. It is critical that we use the best incubator and nutrient delivery system yet designed, called "the uterus and placenta," until complete fetal maturation has been achieved.

As obstetricians, can we intervene and prevent the occurrence of prematurity and low birth weight infants? Remember that the target is the delivery of an undamaged infant who is more than 2500 g in weight, whose biologic age is more than 37 weeks of gestation, and who will be able to survive in its external environment once the umbilical cord has been severed. Weiss and Jackson have identified over 30 obstetrically related factors that influenced the birth weight of both black and white infants.[34] The items most positively associated with the birth weight of both black and white infants were the following: (1) How much weight did the mother gain during her pregnancy? (2) What was her original height/weight status (percentage of standard weight [PSW] or body mass index [BMI]) at the time she became pregnant? (3) Had she ever given birth to a low birth weight infant before (the hereditary or genetic background); and (4) Does she or does she not smoke a package or more of cigarettes a day? (5) Early entry into prenatal care and frequent periodic visits (10 to 14 per pregnancy). These are also associated with an improved mean birth weight and fewer infants who weigh less than 2500 g. This is true regardless of the mother's age, marital status, or ethnic background.

The highest incidence of low birth weight infants occurs in the youngest mothers, be they younger than 16 or 18 years of age, as a consequence of their biologic immaturity as well as inadequate nutrient status and dietary intake and late entry into prenatal care. When the mother was underweight at conception (less than 90% of standard weight or 20 BMI), Edwards et al. found an almost 230-g difference in the birth weight of the offspring when compared to matched controls.[54] This increase was associated with a 50% reduction in the low birth weight rate and a 60% decrease in the prematurity rate (Table 44–17).

### SMOKING

Smoking of one or more packages of cigarettes per day costs the infant's potential weight about 220 to 250 g.[55] In addition are increases in the number of abortions, preterm deliveries, and perinatal mortality rate. This impact of cigarette smoking is dose related. How does cigarette smoking interfere with an infant's birth weight at delivery? First, smokers have up to a 10% reduction in their oxygen-carrying capacity because of the amount of carboxyhemoglobin found as a byproduct of smoking. Second, smoking causes vascular constriction, which decreases blood flow to placenta and interferes with the fetal nutrient delivery system. Third, smokers require almost twice as much vitamin C intake per day to

**TABLE 44–17.** COMPARISON OF NEONATAL COMPLICATIONS UNDERWEIGHT (<90%) VERSUS CONTROL

| MATERNAL PREGNANT STATUS | UNDERWEIGHT | CONTROLS |
|---|---|---|
| N | 354 | 354 |
| Birth weight: sample mean | 2,977 g | 3,208 g |
| <2,500 g | 15.3% | 7.6% |
| ≥4,000 g | 3.1% | 4.5% |
| Gestational prematurity: | | |
| <37 Weeks | 23.0% | 14.0% |

(Data from Edwards, L.G., et al.: Am. J. Obstet. Gynecol., *135*:297–302, 1979.)

maintain the same serum concentration of vitamin C as do nonsmokers[56] (see Chap. 27). Serum levels of carotene, vitamin $B_{12}$, and zinc tend to be lower. Finally, consistently low vitamin C intakes and serum levels have been associated with a higher frequency of low birth weight infants.[45]

One third of single pregnant women and one fifth of married expectant mothers smoke at least a pack a day during pregnancy; more of them are white and are spread evenly throughout the age range. To stop smoking completely is no easier for a woman who is pregnant than otherwise. If usage can be reduced to fewer than five cigarettes per day, the nutritional and fetal consequences will disappear from a statistical point of view. Unpublished, fragmentary reports suggest that the use of nicotine patches by the mother have not had adverse maternal or fetal outcomes. Some of the maternal and fetal nutritional consequences of smoking are mentioned earlier in this chapter.

### AVOIDANCE OF WEIGHT REDUCTION DURING PREGNANCY

A weight-reduction regimen should not be instituted at any time during pregnancy or lactation. A dramatic demonstration of the severe risk to pregnant women and their offspring occurred with the semistarvation imposed by the siege of Rotterdam in 1944 and 1945. A reduction of almost 50% in the intake of calories and protein, especially during the second and third trimesters, interfered with normal intrauterine growth and development of the fetus.[57] The result was a 10% (330-g) reduction in the mean birth weights of the newborn (Table 44–18). When the city was freed and maternal refeeding resumed during the second and/or third trimester, partial fetal weight catch-up was attained.

The American equivalent of wartime intrauterine starvation of the 1990s is chronic cocaine abuse by some pregnant women. It causes a most severe impact on an infant's birth weight potential, as much as a 500-g deficit. In addition, these newborns are severely developmentally immature. Whether these are the consequences of drug use alone or whether they are a byproduct of the financial cost that prevents an adequate nutrient intake has not yet been full determined.

In Table 44–19, we developed estimates of the cost to the potential birth weight of the fetus for each of nine nutrition-related maternal insults. Combinations of two or more have an additive, not concurrent, effect, which in total could produce as much as a 2-lb reduction in the potential weight of the developing infant. If identified in the months before conception, each of these maternal factors is correctable and the fetal consequence preventable.

## NUTRIENT SUPPLEMENTS, CAFFEINE, ALCOHOL, DRUGS, AND EXERCISE

### MINERAL AND VITAMIN SUPPLEMENTS

Both calcium and zinc supplements have been reported to improve maternal reproductive outcome. An additional calcium intake of 2000 mg per day decreased systolic and diastolic blood pressure and the development of pregnancy-induced toxemia;[58] 22 mg of added zinc[59] per day has been associated with less abruptio placentae, fewer preterm deliveries, and a lower rate of perinatal mortality.

No evidence indicates that the daily ingestion of a prenatal mineral/vitamin supplement containing less than twice the RDA is hazardous to either the mother or her fetus/infant during pregnancy and/or lactation. There is added protection in the ingestion of a daily prenatal mineral/vitamin supplement that contains no more than one times the RDA for only the essential minerals and vitamins. Such formulas are available "over the counter" at less than three cents per day.

### CAFFEINE

Most pregnant women (74%) consume caffeine from multiple sources each day—coffee, tea, soft drinks, and chocolate. Their average total daily intake ranges from

**TABLE 44–18.** CHANGES IN MEAN BIRTH WEIGHT IN DUTCH WOMEN BEFORE AND AFTER FAMINE CONDITIONS

| | POSTPARTUM MATERNAL WEIGHT (kg) | BIRTH WEIGHT (g) |
|---|---|---|
| Before famine | 59.0 | 3,338 |
| Famine during third trimester | 57.6 | 3,220 |
| Famine during second and third trimester | 56.5 | 3,011 |
| Famine during first and third trimester | 61.0 | 3,370 |
| Famine during first trimester | 61.6 | 3,312 |
| After famine | 62.0 | 3,308 |

(Adapted from Stein, Z., Suzzer, M.: Pediatr. Res., *9*:70–83, 1975.)

**TABLE 44–19.** ESTIMATED IMPACT OF MATERNAL RISKS ON BIRTH WEIGHT OF FETUS

| MATERNAL FACTORS | FETAL EFFECTS |
|---|---|
| <5 years postmenarchal | ↓ 100–130 g |
| <90% standard weight | ↓ 230 g |
| Excessive work and/or exercise | ↓ 200 g |
| 50% ↓ in kcal in 2nd and 3rd trimesters | ↓ 330 g |
| 50% ↓ in kcal in 3rd trimester | ↓ 120 g |
| >20 cigarettes per day | ↓ 250 g |
| Chronic cocaine addiction | ↓ 500 g |
| "Social alcohol use" | ↓ 100–140 g |
| ↑ Altitude from 0 to 10,000 ft | ↓ 2.0 g/L hemoglobin |
| 8- to 10-km run body temperature | ↑ 2° C |

100 to 150 mg caffeine per day. Caffeine, which acts as a central nervous system stimulant, has a greatly lengthened half-life during pregnancy and among oral contraceptive users; however, caffeine ingestion does not appear to effect a woman's fertility or her ability to conceive. It is not metabolized by the fetus or during the early months of infant life. Early reports raised concerns about its safe use citing increased risks of birth defects and intrauterine growth retardation. More recent studies, however, found that moderate caffeine use (less than 300 mg per day) does not increase risks of spontaneous abortion, fetal growth retardation, or birth defects.[60] A cup of coffee or its equivalent two to three times a day is not detrimental to the well-being of the mother or the fetus.

## ALCOHOL

Half of all women have an occasional drink during their pregnancy and even more during lactation, less than 5% have a drink every day, and another 3% have a drink three times a week. It is estimated that 2 to 3% of all pregnant women are chronic heavy drinkers. Alcoholism is more common in white than either Hispanic or black women, and the incidence is higher in older and more educated women. (The caloric content of various alcoholic beverages is given in Appendix Table A–17.)

Fetal alcohol syndrome is the end result of chronic alcohol abuse during pregnancy, but not all fetal outcomes are at that degree of severity.[61] The consequences range across the spectrum from no apparent fetal sequelae to intrauterine growth retardation to severely damaged infants. Alcohol provides calories that are more difficult for the mother to metabolize and are devoid of protein, minerals, and vitamins. When the mother is ingesting 1500 kcal per day from alcohol, it is impossible to meet her other nutrient requirements from the other third of her food intake. Impaired absorption, metabolism, and utilization of nutrients decrease maternal protein synthesis and the placental transfer of amino acids, as well as the availability of zinc, vitamin A, folic acid, and thiamin (see Chap. 64). Although an occasional glass of wine with food has not yielded maternal and/or fetal consequences, one should be on the lookout for the binge drinker.

## DRUGS

Drugs come in all forms and enter the body by various routes—from over-the-counter items, to prescription medications, to street drugs. Whether they enter the body by mouth or by injection, they all reach equilibrium between mother, fetus, and infant within 30 minutes of entry. Most are readily transferred across the placenta and carried in breast milk to the nursing infant. The typical pregnant woman may well have four or more medications prescribed during her pregnancy. Several of these may have drug/nutrient interactions that interfere with both the effectiveness of the drug and the availability of the nutrient(s) (see Chap. 78).

From 10 to 27% of pregnant woman acknowledge their use of marijuana during pregnancy.[62] Its metabolites cross the placenta; they are fat soluble and extremely slowly excreted. Like tobacco, marijuana tends to reduce the oxygen-carrying capacity of hemoglobin. It increases the heart rate and blood pressure, resulting in decreased uterine blood flow and placental perfusion. Infant birth weights are lower and preterm deliveries are increased. Fertility in the male is reduced secondary to oligospermia. Direct drug/nutrient interference has not been confirmed.

No street drug has had as severe an impact on the maternal and fetal outcome of pregnancy as cocaine and crack cocaine. Reports indicate that around 10% (3 to 17%) of all pregnant women have used these drugs during pregnancy and 6% within the past month.[63] Use of these drugs is higher among Hispanic and black pregnant women and those who live in the inner city. Cocaine readily crosses the placenta, and once on the fetal side, it may be detected in the meconium for up to 8 weeks. Chronic users have decreased appetite, food intake, and uptake of tryptophan. The resultant fetus and newborn are likely to be growth retarded, and the mothers are more susceptible to abruptio placentae and premature labor.

All these types of street drugs are not used in isolation, but complicated further by other abuses and risk behaviors of which HIV infection is currently the most serious.

## EXERCISE

The maternal and fetal effects of exercise during pregnancy have been comprehensively reviewed.[64] Walking, cycling, climbing stairs, and swimming are excellent types of activity for the normal, healthy pregnant woman when done in moderation by time and cardiovascular response. With severe exercise comes a temperature response and circulatory redistribution that takes away from the uterus and placenta and directs to the lower extremities. The pregnant woman needs to build up her conditioning program gradually and specifically to avoid trauma-prone exercises, high altitudes, dehydration, and serious competition. Among women with complicated pregnancies, rest, not exercise, may be the prescription of choice. Postdelivery or postweaning exercise is an essential component along with caloric restriction in the woman regaining her prepregnant weight status.

## YEAR 2000 GOALS FOR MATERNAL AND CHILD HEALTH

These identify 10 targets in need of improvement, 6 with direct or indirect nutritional implications, as we have discussed in this chapter, are given here, whereas others are given in Appendix Table A–16d on nutrition priority areas: (1) to reduce the LBW rate; (2) to reduce fetal alcohol syndrome; (3) to improve adequate maternal weight gain; (4) to double the number of nursing mothers at 6 months; (5) to decrease tobacco, alcohol, and drug use; and (6) to decrease late entry into prenatal care.

## REFERENCES


1. U.S. Department of Health and Human Services: Child Health USA 1991. Publication No. HRS-M-CH91-1. Washington, D.C., U.S. Department of Health and Human Services, 1991.
2. Institute of Medicine: Nutrition During Pregnancy. Washington, D.C., National Academy of Sciences, 1990.
3. Worthington-Roberts, B., Williams, S.R.: Nutrition in Pregnancy and Lactation. 4th Ed. Boston, Times Mirror/Mosby, 1989.
4. Harris, E.D.: Nutr. Rev., *50:*329–331, 1992.
5. Barclay, B.A.: Nutr. Clin. Pract., *5:*153–155, 1990.
6. Wolk, R.A., Rayburn, W.F.: Nutr. Clin. Pract 5: 139–152, 1990.
7. U.S. Department of Agriculture, Human Nutrition Information Service: The Food Guide Pyramid. Home and Garden Bulletin No. 252, Hyattsville, MD, U.S. Department of Agriculture, 1992.
8. United States Department of Agriculture: Nationwide Food Consumption Survey. Report No. 85–1. Hyattsville, MD, Nutrition Monitoring Division, Human Nutrition Information Service, U.S. Department of Agriculture, 1985.
9. Dawson, E.B., Clark, R.R., McGanity, W.J.: Am. J. Obstet. Gynecol., *104:*953–958, 1969.
10. King, J.C.: Nutrition in Pregnancy. London, Royal College of Obstetricians/Gynaecologists, 1982.
11. Mitchell, H.S., Reed, R.B., Valeadian, I., et al.: Proceedings of the 7th International Congress of Nutrition. Vol. 4. Oxford, Pergamon Press, 1966, pp. 132–139.
12. Frisch, R.E.: Biol. Rev., *59:*161–188, 1984.
13. McGanity, W.J., Dawson, E.B.: Unpublished data, Ten State Nutrition Survey, 1968–1970.
14. Meredith, C.N., Dwyer, J.T.: Annu. Rev. Public Health, *12:*309–333, 1991.
15. Story, M., Alton, I.: Top. Clin. Nutr., *6:*51–58, 1991.
16. Atkinson, R.L.: Nutr. Rev., *50:*338–345, 1992.
17. Lachance, P.A., Fisher, M.C.: J. Am. Diet. Assoc., *85:*451–454, 1985.
18. Chervenak, J.L., Kardon, N.B.: Female Patient, *16:*17–24, 1991.
19. National Health and Nutrition Examination Survey II: Unpublished data. Hyattsville, MD, National Center for Health Statistics, Public Health Service, U.S. Department of Health, Education and Welfare, 1976–1980.
20. Food and Nutrition Board, National Research Council: Recommended Dietary Allowances. 10th Ed. Washington, D.C., National Academy Press, 1989.
21. Recommended Dietary Allowances. 9th Ed. Washington, D.C., National Academy of Sciences, 1980.
22. Whitehead, R.G.: Pregnancy and lactation. *In* Modern Nutrition in Health and Disease. 7th Ed. Edited by M.E. Shils and V.R. Young. Philadelphia, Lea & Febiger, 1988, pp. 931–943.
23. Sims, L.S.: J. Am. Diet. Assoc., *73:*139–146, 1978.
24. Hytten, F.E., Leitch, I.: The Physiology of Human Pregnancy. 2nd Ed. Oxford, Blackwell Scientific, 1971.
25. Hytten, F., Chamberlain, G.: Clinical Physiology in Obstetrics. Oxford, Blackwell Scientific, 1980.
26. Food and Agriculture Organization/World Health Organization (WHO)/United Nations University: Energy and Protein Requirements WHO, Tech. Rep. Ser. No. 724. Geneva, WHO, 1985.
27. Durnin, J.V.G.A.: Energy requirements of pregnancy: an integration of the longitudinal data from the 5-country study. *In* Nestle Foundation Annual Report. Lausanne, Switzerland, Nestle Foundation, 1986, pp. 147–154; see also Lancet, *2:*897–903, 1987.

28. van Raaij, J.M.A., Schonk, C.M., Vermaat-Miedema, S.H., et al.: Am. J. Clin. Nutr., *49:*765–772, 1989.
29. Forsum, E., Sadurkis, A., Wagner, J.: Am. J. Clin. Nutr., *47:*942–947, 1988.
30. Committee of Maternal Nutrition: Maternal Nutrition and the Course of Pregnancy. Washington, D.C., National Academy of Sciences, 1990.
31. Hytten, F.E., Leitch, I.: Physiology of Human Pregnancy. Oxford, Blackwell Scientific, 1964.
32. Hurley, L.S.: Developmental Nutrition. Englewood Cliffs, NJ, Prentice Hall, 1980.
33. Garn, S.M., LaVelle, M., Pesick, S.D., et al.: Am. J. Dis. Child., *138:*32–34, 1984.
34. Weiss, W., Jackson, E.C.: Perinatal Factors Affecting Human Development. Washington, D.C., Pan American Health Organization, 1969, pp. 54–69.
35. Potter, S., Hannum, S., McFarlin, B., et al.: J. Am. Diet. Assoc., *91:*441–446, 1991.
36. Hahn, P.F., Carothers, E.L., Darby, M.D., et al.: Am. J. Obstet. Gynecol., *61:*477–486, 1951.
37. Garn, S.M., Ridella, S.A., Petzold, A.S., et al.: Semin. Perinatol., *5:*155–162, 1981.
38. Dawson, E.B., McGanity, W.J.: J. Reprod. Med., *32:*475–496, 1987; unpublished data, 1990.
39. Sauberlich, H.E.: Evaluation of folate nutrition in population groups. *In* Folic Acid Metabolism in Health and Disease. Edited by M.F. Picciano, E.L.R. Stokstad, and J.F. Gregory, III. New York, Wiley-Liss, 1990, pp. 211–235.
40. Iyengar, L., Apte, S.V.: Br. J. Nutr., *27:*313–317, 1972.
41. McPartlin, J., Halligan, A., Scott, J.M., et al.: Lancet, *341:*148–149, 1993.
42. Strauss, M.B.: J. Clin. Invest., *12:*345–353, 1933.
43. Woodruff, C.W., Bridgeforth, E.B.: Pediatrics, *12:*681–685, 1953.
44. Murray, M.J., Murray, A.B., Murray, N.J., et al.: Br. J. Nutr., *39:*627–630, 1978.
45. Martin, M.P., Bridgeforth, E., McGanity, W.J., et al.: J. Nutr., *62:*201–225, 1957.
46. Centers for Disease Control: MMWR, *38:*633–685, 1989.
47. Basu, T.K.: Int. J. Environ. Stud., *17:*31–35, 1981.
48. Platt, L.D., Koch, R., Azen, C., et al.: Am. J. Obstet. Gynecol., *166:*1150–1162, 1992.
49. Medical Research Council Vitamin Study Research Group: Lancet, *338:*131–137, 1991.
50. Czeizel, A.E., Dudas, I.: N. Engl. J. Med., *327:*1832–1835, 1992.
51. Rosenberg, I.H.: N. Engl. J. Med., *327:*1875, 1992. (editorial).
52. Centers for Disease Control. MMWR, *41:*81–85, 1992.; *41*(NORR-14):1–7, 1992.
53. Widdowson, E.M.: Biology of Gestation. New York, Academic Press, 1968, pp. 1–49.
54. Edwards, L.E., et al.: Am. J. Obstet. Gynecol., *135:*297–302, 1979.
55. Butler, N.R., Goldstein, H., Ross, E.M.: Br. J. Med., *2:*127–130, 1972.
56. Smith, J.L., Hodges, R.E.: Ann. N.Y. Acad. Sci., *498:*144–152, 1987.
57. Stein, Z., Susser, M.: Pediatr. Res., *9:*70–83, 1975.
58. Anon: Nutr. Rev., *50:*233–236, 1992.
59. Kuhnert, B.R., Kuhnert, P.M., Groh-Wargo, S.L., et al.: Am. J. Clin. Nutr., *55:*981–984, 1992.
60. Mills, J.L., Holmes, L.B., Aarons, J.H., et al.: JAMA, *269:*593–597, 1993.
61. Russell, M.: Bull. N.Y. Acad. Med., *67:*207–222, 1991.
62. Zuckerman, B., Frank, D.A., Hingson, R., et al.: N. Engl. J. Med., *320:*762–768, 1989.
63. Lutiger, B., Graham, K., Einarson, T.R., et al.: Teratology, *44:*405–414, 1991.
64. Revelli, A., Durando, A., Massobrio, M.: Obstet. Gynecol. Surv., *47:*355–367, 1992.
65. Pappit, S.D., Prentice, A.M., Jéquier, E., et al.: Am. J. Clin. Nutr., *57:*353–364, 1993.

CHAPTER **45**

# Nutrition and Cell and Organ Growth


**Elsie M. Widdowson**




All mammals start life as a single cell, the fertilized ovum. During the early part of gestation, this cell divides and redivides many times, and different kinds of cell develop during the process of differentiation and arrange themselves to form part of the various organs of the body. No two types of cell and no two organs are the same and, moreover, within any one organ often are several kinds of cell. Some cells have a single nucleus, those of the kidney for example; others, like muscle fibers, have many nuclei, and others again such as the red blood cells have no nuclei at all. Some cells, such as the neuronal and glial cells of the brain, are relatively stable, but others, like the cells of the intestinal mucosa, are continually being removed and new cells take their place. Thus, cell growth and organ growth are complex processes, and broad generalizations may be misleading. However, certain principles apply to all cells, whatever their situation and function. Cells are the metabolically active part of the body, and they are surrounded by extracellular fluid. All transport of nutrients and waste products to and from the cell must take place through the extracellular fluid, for no direct exchange occurs between one cell and another. Mechanisms are necessary to replenish the nutrients by absorption from the digestive tract and to remove the waste products through the kidneys if the extracellular fluid is to remain constant in volume and composition. Because all exchanges between cell and extracellular fluid have to take place through the surface of the cell, there must be a limit to the volume a cell can attain if its more slowly expanding surface is to fulfill the demands made on it by the metabolism of the inclusions within it.

The fluid inside and outside the cells is in osmotic equilibrium, but the composition of the two fluids is different: potassium is the cation of the cells and sodium of the fluid surrounding them (Table 45–1). Within the past 10 to 15 years, it has gradually been realized, however, that the relatively minute amounts of calcium within the cells and their mitochondria are of vital importance to function. Phosphorus is the main cellular anion, and chloride is the extracellular one. A large part of the protein in the body is inside the cells.

The composition of the intra- and extracellular fluid remains remarkably constant in many respects, not only from age to age, but also from species to species. However, the relative amounts of the two fluids within the body vary greatly from one age and one organ to another and may alter in malnutrition and disease. The immature organism is characterized by having a large volume of extracellular fluid in all its organs and tissues

**TABLE 45–1.** COMPOSITION OF PLASMA AND INTRACELLULAR FLUID

| | PLASMA (mEq/L water) | INTRACELLULAR FLUID (mEq/L water) |
|---|---|---|
| Na | 169 | 8 |
| K | 6 | 151 |
| Ca | 6 | 2 |
| Mg | 6 | 28 |
| Cl | 123 | — |
| $HCO_3$ | 32 | 10 |
| $PO_4$ | 2 | 100 |
| $SO_4$ | 1 | 10 |

(From Black, D.A.K.: Essentials of Fluid Balance. 2nd Ed. Oxford, Blackwell Scientific Publications, 1960.)

in relation to the cell mass. As development proceeds and the cells increase in number and size, the proportion of the tissue taken up by the cells increases, and the percentage of extracellular material decreases. This is true of all the separate parts of the body and of the body as a whole. However, some organs develop earlier in this respect than others, the fetal heart and kidney, for example, being nearer their adult composition than skeletal muscle at the time of birth.

## CELL AND ORGAN GROWTH

Growth in the early stages of gestation is brought about entirely by cell division. Because the first divisions of the ovum are not preceded by any increase in size, the individual cells become successively smaller. By the time the blastocyst is implanted in the wall of the uterus, the cells begin to enlarge before they divide. A change also occurs in the timing of the divisions. The first few occur almost simultaneously, but after a few days, cell division becomes staggered, so that only a small proportion of the cells is dividing at the same time. Cell division goes on more rapidly in the first weeks after conception in some species than in others. It has been estimated that the rat increases from a single cell to 3000 million during its first 3 weeks of development,[2] whereas the human fetus increases only to 1.3 thousand million after 8 weeks of gestation.[3] These figures are rough, but they are confirmed by body weight. The rat emerges from the uterus at 3 weeks weighing 5 g, whereas the human fetus takes 8 weeks to reach a weight of 1 g. The rate of cell division just after conception sets the pace for growth later and is genetically determined; nutrition plays little part at this stage of development. The time comes, however, when cells begin to increase in size and Winick and Noble described three phases of cellular growth: first, increase in number without any increase in average size; then, increase in size and number; finally, increase only in size of cells.[4] This concept has been criticized by Sands, Dobbing, and Gratrix,[5] and is discussed in more detail later. Obviously, the description of the last stage could not be strictly true, because some organs, like the liver, pancreas, and adrenal cortex, are capable of almost unlimited cellular division when occasion demands, for example, after surgical removal of part of the organ. Further, as already explained, cells cannot go on increasing in size in an unlimited way, so once the maximum size has been attained, further growth of the organ can only be by increase in number of cells.

### MEASUREMENT OF NUMBER AND SIZE OF CELLS

Up to the 1940s, the only method of measuring the number and size of cells in a tissue was to count them in a section of tissue in a field of known dimensions under a microscope. This technique had been in use for many years for red blood cells, and it remained the only method until the introduction of the Coulter counter. For nucleated cells, however, another method became available with the description by Schneider[6] and Burton[7] of chemical methods for the determination of DNA. These involved smashing up the cells so that all the cell walls were broken down and the chemical reagents could get at the contents of the nuclei, including the DNA, and react with it so that it could be measured. It was proposed by Boivin, Vendrely, and Vendrely that all the diploid nuclei of a given animal species contain the same amount of DNA,[8] 6 pg for man and 6.2 pg for the rat. Davidson and Leslie suggested that if the total amount of DNA was measured in an organ or tissue, which has mononuclear cells with only diploid nuclei within them, the number of nuclei and hence of cells in an organ could be calculated.[9] The constancy of DNA may not be strictly true,[10] but in view of all the other inaccuracies of this kind of work, minor variations in the amount of DNA within the nucleus are probably not important.

Because most of the protein within soft tissues, except skin, is in the cells, a measurement of protein gives an index of the amount of cytoplasm, so the ratio of protein to DNA, or of protein per nucleus, gives an index of the average size of the cell. Intracellular protein is sometimes measured, and this figure is in theory more accurate, but in practice does not make much difference, especially when comparisons are being made. Some investigators have measured RNA, which is responsible for protein synthesis within the cell, and this method gives a more dynamic approach to cellular growth than the measurement of the protein that is already there. However, although the total RNA in an organ increases during growth, it increases in parallel with the DNA, that is, with the number of nuclei, and so gives no indication of the amount of cytoplasm associated with each nucleus.

The speed with which determinations of DNA, RNA, and protein can be made has enabled us to learn a great deal about the quantitative side of cellular growth and multiplication, which we should never have been able to get with a microscope. But the method has its limitations. Perhaps the most important of these is related to the fact that the cells within an organ or tissue are rarely homogenous. The cells of the liver, kidney, and pancreas, for example, and above all of the brain, are functionally highly differentiated, but a measurement of DNA gives no clue about this or to the way the different structures within the organ develop and begin to function. Further, the cells may or may not represent the functional units within an organ. In the kidney, the number of cells goes on increasing long after the number of nephrons is complete. Even among the same type of cell within an organ is often a wide range in the size of the cells. Other difficulties arise because some tissues have many nuclei within a cell, the most obvious being the skeletal muscle fiber. In this case, DNA gives a measure of the number of nuclei, but not the number of muscle fibers, which must still be determined by histologic methods.

Adipose tissue presents other problems. Adipocytes are nucleated and are specialized connective tissue cells localized mostly in the subcutaneous tissue and around the internal organs. Adipose tissue contains other nucleated cells, fibroblasts, some but not all of which are designated preadipocytes, which become adipocytes when they start to fill with fat. A measurement of DNA, therefore, gives a falsely high number of adipose cells. In fact, this is no different from the problem encountered in other tissues, for example, the brain, where a measurement of DNA gives no indication of the number of nuclei present in the different types of cell. However, investigators concerned with the cellular development of adipose tissue have generally been interested in one type of cell, that containing lipid, and other methods that detect only lipid-containing cells were therefore devised. These techniques depend on the measurement of the size of the actual cells. The size of the adipocytes depends in turn on the amount of lipid within them. In one method, the fat in a known weight of adipose tissue is fixed with osmium tetroxide. The little balls of fixed lipid are then freed from connective tissue, suspended in glycerin and saline, and counted in a Coulter counter. In the other method, frozen sections are cut, and the mean volume of cells in the adipose tissue is determined from their diameter measured under the microscope. Volume of lipid is converted to weight, and the number of cells in a known weight of tissue is determined chemically so that the number of adipocytes containing that lipid can be calculated. Then, if it is desired to know the total number of fat cells in the whole body, the amount of fat in the body is determined, either by calculation from the body density determined by weighing in air and under water, or from skinfold measurements, using a formula such as that suggested by Durnin and Womersley for relating skinfold measurements at four sites to total body fat.[11] Alternatively, lean body mass is calculated from a measurement of the amount of water or of potassium in the body and the amount of fat is obtained by difference. By extrapolation from the number of cells in, say, 20 mg of adipose tissue obtained by biopsy from one site, the number of adipocytes in the adipose tissue of the whole body is calculated. The adipose tissue in an obese person may weigh 100 kg.

The assumptions and inaccuracies in calculating the number of fat cells in an individual from the measurements just described are now accepted as so great that the whole concept of relating obesity to number and size of fat cells in childhood or in later life has largely been abandoned. However, it was pursued with great enthusiasm in the early 1970s and, even if only for historical reasons, the more important of the difficulties are briefly described. Quite apart from all the inaccuracies involved in measuring total body fat, we now know that the mean fat cell size is not the same all over the body, so a biopsy from one site will not be representative of all the adipose tissue in the body. In the full-term infant, for example, cells in the gluteal region averaged 68 μm in diameter, and those in the anterior abdominal wall 50 μm.[12] Because of the relation between the diameter of a sphere and its volume, the amount of fat in a cell differs more than its diameter. The average cell in these two sites contained 0.17 and 0.06 μg of fat, respectively. Thus, the number of fat cells calculated to be present in the body might vary by a factor of 3, depending on which site was chosen for a biopsy.

The other serious problem arises because, if the Coulter counter is used to measure the number of fat cells in a sample of adipose tissue, then the cell must contain a minimum of 0.01 μg of lipid to register on the machine. The average lipid content of the adipocyte in the human adult is 0.5 to 0.8 μg, with a maximum of about 1.2 μg. However, a lean individual may well have millions of potential fat cells that contain less than 0.01 μg lipid, and these would never appear in an adipose cell count, but are ready to be filled if the intake of energy becomes greater than the expenditure and the capacity of storage of energy in cells already containing fat is exhausted.

## GROWTH OF THE BODY AND ITS TISSUES

Figures 45–1 to 45–3 show the weights of skeletal muscle, heart, liver, brain, and kidney throughout the growth period[13,14] and also of the body as a whole. Because the dimensions of the body and its tissues are so different, the weight at full-term birth has been taken as unity and all other values are expressed in relation to this amount. Weights at birth that have been taken as unity and all other values are expressed in relation to this amount. Weights at birth that have been taken as unity are shown in Table 45–2.

The largest soft tissue in the body is skeletal muscle. It

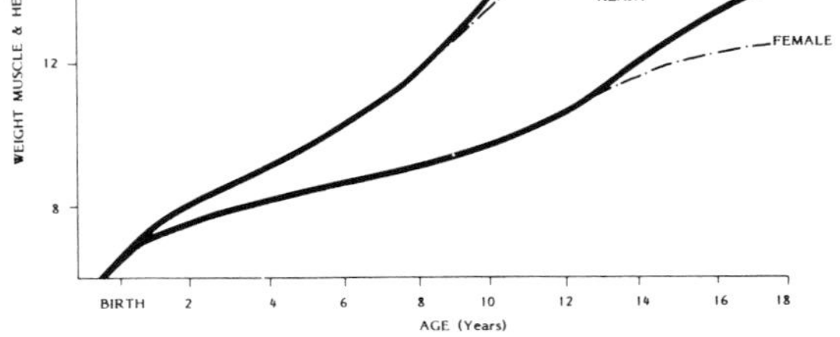
SKELETAL MUSCLE
MALE
FEMALE
HEART
MALE
FEMALE
36
28
20
12
8
WEIGHT MUSCLE & HEART (WEIGHT AT BIRTH = 1)
BIRTH
2
4
6
8
10
12
14
16
18
AGE (Years)

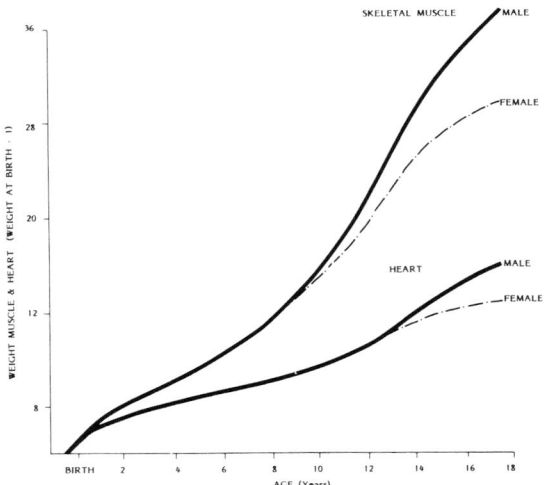

**FIGURE 45–1.** Weight of skeletal muscle and heart. Weight at birth = 1. (From Documenta Geigy Scientific Tables. 7th Ed. Edited by K. Diem and C. Lentner. Basel, J.R. Geigy, 1970.)

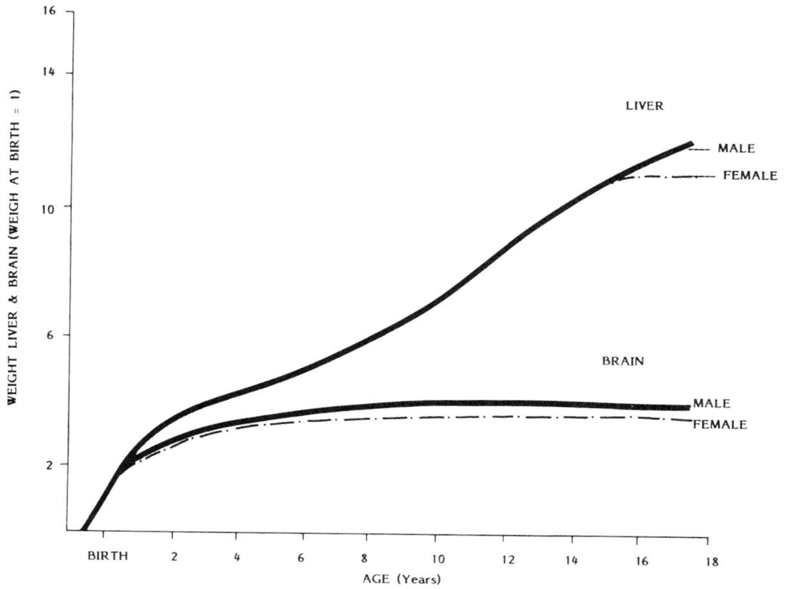
WEIGHT LIVER & BRAIN (WEIGH AT BIRTH = 1)
16
14
10
6
2
LIVER
MALE
FEMALE
BRAIN
MALE
FEMALE
BIRTH
2
4
6
8
10
12
14
16
18
AGE (Years)

**FIGURE 45–2.** Weight of liver and brain. Weight at birth = 1. (From Documenta Geigy Scientific Tables. 7th Ed. Edited by K. Diem and C. Lentner. Basel, J.R. Geigy, 1970.)

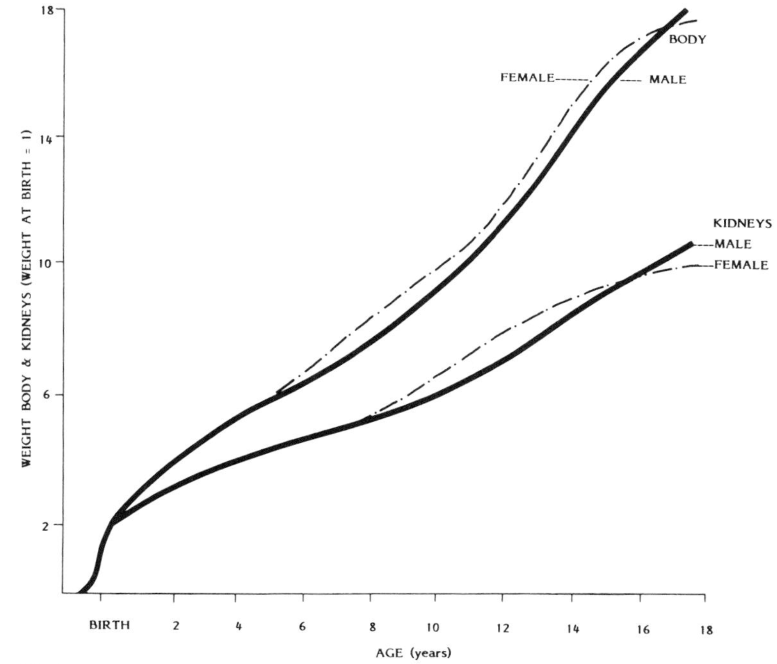
WEIGHT BODY & KIDNEYS (WEIGHT AT BIRTH = 1)
18
14
10
6
2
BODY
FEMALE
MALE
KIDNEYS
MALE
FEMALE
BIRTH
2
4
6
8
10
12
14
16
18
AGE (years)

**FIGURE 45–3.** Weight of whole body and kidneys. Weight at birth = 1. (From Documenta Geigy Scientific Tables. 7th Ed. Edited by K. Diem, and C. Lentner. Basel, J.R. Geigy, 1970.)

makes up 24% of the weight of the fetus at 20 to 24 weeks gestation, 24% of the infant at term, and 40 to 50% of the adult.[15] Men have more muscle than women; muscle is approximately 50% of the weight of the "average" man and 40% of the weight of the "average" woman. The figures show that skeletal muscle increases more in weight after birth than the body as a whole or any of the other tissues considered here, and from the age of 10 years, the increase in weight of the muscle is greater in boys than in girls.

**TABLE 45–2.** WEIGHT OF BODY AND ORGANS AT BIRTH

| | BOYS | GIRLS |
|---|---|---|
| Skeletal muscle (kg) | 0.82 | 0.77 |
| Heart (g) | 20 | 20 |
| Liver (g) | 124 | 124 |
| Brain (g) | 353 | 347 |
| Kidneys (g) | 24 | 24 |
| Whole body (kg) | 3.4 | 3.2 |

Compiled from references 13, 14, and 15. Weights are taken as unity in Figures 45–1 to 45–3.

The rate in growth of heart muscle (Fig. 45–1) is less than that of skeletal muscle. The hearts of boys increase more in weight than those of girls, but the difference is not apparent until age 14 years.

The increase in weight of the liver and brain is shown in Figure 45–2. The liver increases in weight by 10 or 11 times between birth and age 18 years, and gender-related differences are small.

The growth of the brain is different. The rapid period of brain growth, or "growth spurt," occurs from midgestation to 18 months after birth, by which time the brain has reached a weight of about 1 kg, or more than 70% of its adult weight. At birth the brains of boys are slightly heavier than those of girls, and this difference persists throughout life. The increase in weight after birth is marginally greater in boys and in girls.

The kidneys increase in weight in a similar fashion to the liver (Fig. 45–3). Both liver and kidneys increase in weight after birth less than the body so that they come to form a smaller percentage of the body weight.

## CELLULAR DEVELOPMENT OF SPECIFIC ORGANS AND TISSUES

**Skeletal Muscle.** Skeletal muscle changes considerably in chemical, anatomic, and cellular structure during development. Muscle fibers are believed to be formed from elongated precursor cells, called myoblasts, with single nuclei. During fetal development, these fuse to form myotubes, which are long narrow cells with many nuclei. The nuclei are situated centrally in the myotubes and are large in proportion to the diameter of the cell. The spaces between the myotubes are filled with the ground substance of the extracellular phase. The myotubes are converted to muscle fibers, the nuclei move to the periphery and lie immediately under the sarcolemma, and the muscle fibers become arranged in bundles. As in other tissues, the number of cells or fibers increases up to the time of a full-term birth and probably into the first year. MacCallum[16] and Montgomery[17] considered that the adult number of fibers is reached early in postnatal development, but others believe that the number of fibers goes on increasing.[18] Stickland's study of fetal muscle suggests that the rate of increase in number of myofibers in the sartorius muscle starts to slow down at about 21 weeks gestation and by term has become very slow indeed (Fig. 45–4).[19] The mean cross-sectional area of a myofiber, on the other hand, increases rapidly throughout gestation, reaching 90 $\mu m^2$ at term, and continues to increase all through the period of growth. At adolescence, the mean area is about 2000 $\mu m^2$[20]

Evidence exists that the number of muscle fibers in an individual is genetically determined within species as well as between them.[21,22] Muscle fibers are much the same width in adult mammals of such different sizes as mice and cattle, 50 μm, which corresponds to an area of about 2000 $\mu m^2$, the same as is found in man. The interspecies difference in size of muscles relates to a difference of several orders of magnitude in the number of fibers.[23] Growth of muscle after birth in man is caused primarily by an increase in the size of the fibers that already exist at birth, and this is influenced by nutrition and activity. As the muscle fibers grow in diameter and length, the extracellular material between them becomes less and less. Table 45–3 shows the chloride or extracellular space of human skeletal muscle at various ages and the intracellular fluid and protein per 100 g of muscle.[24] The number of nuclei within the muscle fibers increases as the muscle grows; this increase is brought about by both mitosis and incorporation of satellite cells into the fiber. Figure 45–5 shows the total amount of DNA in two gastrocnemius muscles of the human fetus before and up to term. The amount of DNA and hence the number of nuclei in the gastrocnemius muscles increased by 10 between weeks 13 and 22 of gestation.[25] Between 22 and 40 weeks of gestation, a further four-fold increase occurred, but the rate of increase was already slowing down. No values are available for individual muscles after birth, but Cheek has calculated the amount of DNA and hence the number of nuclei in the total muscle mass of infants soon after birth and of older infants and children up to the age of 17 years.[13] The amount of DNA in a weighed biopsy sample of gluteal muscle was determined, and it was assumed that this amount was representative of all the muscle of the body, which may or may not be true.[26] The weight of muscle in the individual was estimated from the excretion of creatinine, taking each gram of urinary creatinine in 24 hours as being equivalent to 20 kg of muscle. Cheek's results suggest that the amount of DNA and the number of nuclei in muscle increase six-fold between birth and 11 years of age in both sexes. A further 50% increase occurs in girls between 11 and 17 years, but a 2½-fold increase is noted in boys, which parallels the greater amount of skeletal muscle they lay down during adolescence.

The ratio of protein to DNA (mg/mg) in gastrocnemius muscle increased from 20 at 13 weeks gestation to 120 at term (Fig. 45–5).[25] The ratio at adolescence was about 300.[13] Thus, the amount of cytoplasm, as indicated by protein, that is associated with one nucleus, as indicated by DNA, increased six-fold in the last 26 weeks of

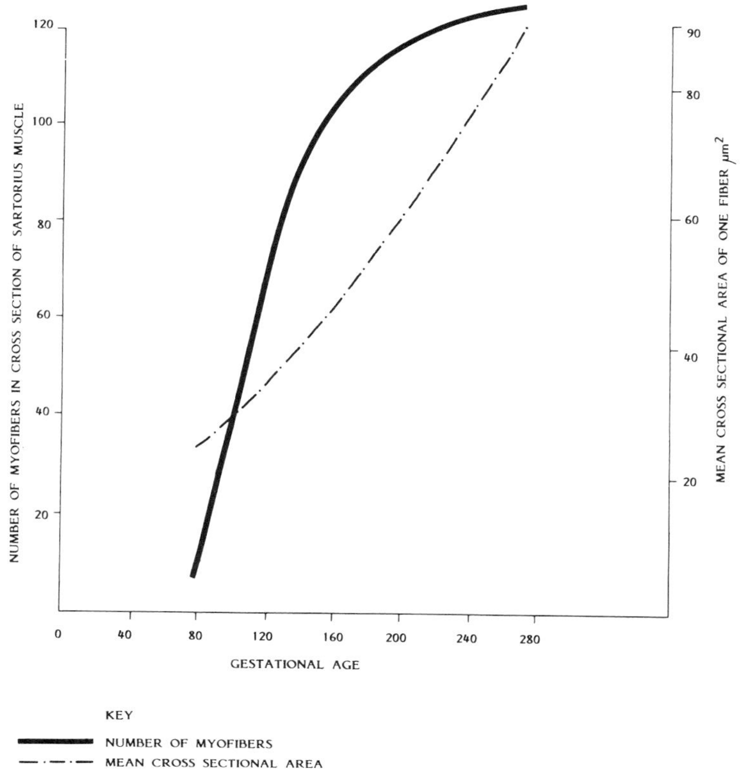
NUMBER OF MYOFIBERS IN CROSS SECTION OF SARTORIUS MUSCLE
120
100
80
60
40
20
MEAN CROSS SECTIONAL AREA OF ONE FIBER $\mu m^2$
90
80
60
40
20
0
40
80
120
160
200
240
280
GESTATIONAL AGE
KEY
NUMBER OF MYOFIBERS
MEAN CROSS SECTIONAL AREA

**FIGURE 45–4.** Number and mean cross-sectional area of myofibers in sartorius muscle of the human fetus (age in days). (From Stickland, N.C.: J. Anat., *132*:557–579, 1981.)

**TABLE 45–3.** EXTRACELLULAR AND INTRACELLULAR COMPARTMENTS OF SKELETAL MUSCLE

| | FETUS | | INFANT | | ADULT |
|---|---|---|---|---|---|
| | 13–14 weeks | 20–22 weeks | Newborn at term | 4–7 months | |
| Chloride or extracellular fluid space g/100g muscle | 67.2 | 57.7 | 35.0 | 29.3 | 18.3 |
| Intracellular fluid space g/100g muscle | 23.5 | 31.0 | 45.4 | 49.2 | 60.9 |
| Intracellular protein g/100g muscle | 6.6 | 7.5 | 9.1 | 13.6 | 16.9 |

(From Widdowson, E.M., Dickerson, J.W.T.: Chemical composition of the body. *In* Mineral Metabolism. Vol. 2A. Edited by C.L. Comar and F. Bronner. New York, Academic press, 1964, pp. 1–247.)

gestation, but barely trebled between birth and maturity.

**Heart.** The heart is fully formed at 11 weeks of gestation, and heart sounds usually can be heard by 18 to 20 weeks. It develops early, too, in its chemical composition; the proportions of water and protein at birth are not much different from those of adult heart.

Figure 45–6 shows the amount of DNA found in the whole heart of human fetuses between 13 weeks of gestation and term.[25] A rapid increase occurs between 13 and 30 weeks, the amount of DNA approximately doubling each 3 weeks. Then, the rate of cell division fell off, and at the same time, the ratio of protein to DNA rose from 10 to 13 weeks gestation to 30 at 30 weeks and 70 at term. There was a further increase of about five-fold in DNA to 250 mg in adult heart, and more than a doubling of the protein/DNA ratio to 190 mg in the adult organ.

**Kidney.** The kidneys, like the heart, develop and begin to function early in fetal life, and by 9 weeks of gestation, they are already beginning to secrete urine. Kidney tissue always includes the fluid that was in the tubule at the time of death, and in the adult, who produces a

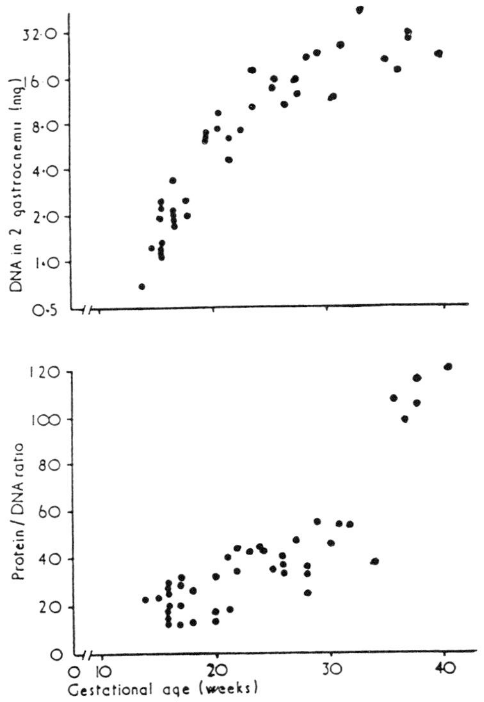

32·0
16·0
8·0
4·0
2·0
1·0
0·5
DNA in 2 gastrocnemii (mg)
120
100
80
60
40
20
0
Protein / DNA ratio
0 10
20
30
40
Gestational age (weeks)


**FIGURE 45–5.** DNA and protein/DNA ratio in gastrocnemius muscle of the human fetus. (From Widdowson, E.M., Crabb, D.E., Milner, R.D.G.: Arch. Dis. Child., *47*:652–655, 1972.)

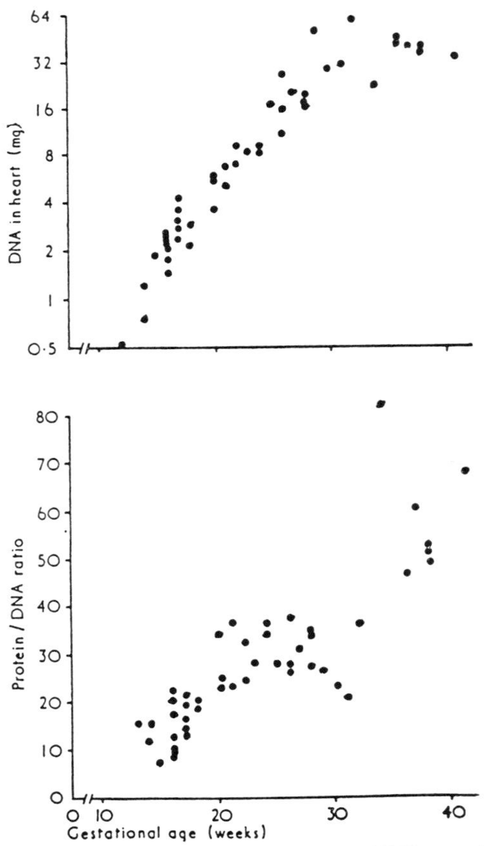

64
32
16
8
4
2
1
0·5
DNA in heart (mg)
80
70
60
50
40
30
20
10
0
Protein / DNA ratio
0 10
20
30
40
Gestational age (weeks)


**FIGURE 45–6.** DNA and protein/DNA ratio in heart of human fetus. (From Widdowson, E.M., Crabb, D.E., Milner, R.D.G.: Arch. Dis. Child., *47*:652–655, 1972.)

hypertonic urine, the concentration of chloride is likely to be higher than the true value in the kidney tissue itself. In fetal life, the urine is hypotonic with respect to sodium and chloride, which may make fetal kidney tissue appear to contain less chloride and extracellular fluid than it really does. The concentration of protein increased from 9 g/100 g at 20 to 22 weeks of gestation to 12 g/100 g at term and further to 15 g/100 g in the adult.[27]

Figure 45–7 shows the total amount of DNA in the two kidneys before birth.[28] By 13 weeks gestation, the two kidneys already had about 1 mg of DNA in them, or the amount in the nuclei of 200 million cells. Five further divisions and redivisions were required to bring the amount of DNA to 40 mg at 26 weeks of gestation and perhaps one more division to arrive at the amount of 80 to 100 mg at term. Among the kidneys, there was often one with twice as much DNA and therefore presumably twice as many cells as another of the same gestational age. Just the same was true of the heart, and indeed also of the gastrocnemius muscle. Those with the most DNA at any given age were in fact one cell division ahead of those with the least. In the adult, too, wide variation was noted in the amount of DNA in the organs from one individual to another. The mean value for DNA in adult kidneys was 736 mg, but the range was from 505 to 803 mg. In the adult, however, the bigger the body the bigger the organ, and on the whole, the bigger the organ the more cells in it, but this was not necessarily true in the active period of cell division before birth.

The ratio of protein to DNA in the kidneys rose fairly steadily from about 8 to 13 weeks gestation to 35 at term and 45 in the adult. Thus, in the kidneys, as in the heart and muscle, there was a far greater increase in number of nuclei or cells between birth and adult life than there was in the size of the cells, which in the kidneys only increased by about 30%.

Results of morphologic studies of the development of the human kidney show that the number of functional units or nephrons is complete at the time of full-term birth.[28] The glomeruli are about one half the adult size, and the tubules are short and not completely differentiated. They are all there, however, about 82,000 in each kidney, by the time the fetus reaches term; yet, the cells have reached less than 20% of the adult number.

**Liver.** Difficulties arise when using the total DNA and the protein/DNA ratio to measure the number and size of liver cells. The liver cells are not all diploid, and polyploidy occurs in hepatocytes at all ages. Further, some cells are binucleate, and both mononucleate and binucleate cells exhibit polyploidy. Evidence exists, however, that the amount of cytoplasm in hepatocytes is proportioned to the ploidy of the cell,[29] so that the

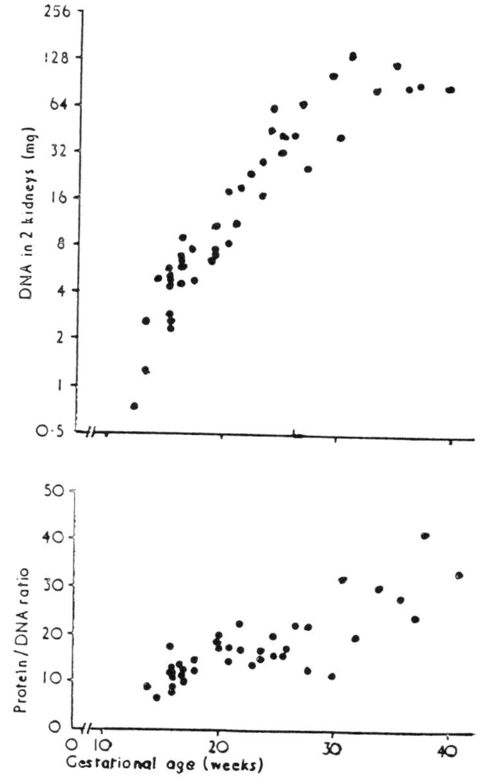
DNA in 2 kidneys (mg)
256
128
64
32
16
8
4
2
1
0·5
Protein / DNA ratio
50
40
30
20
10
0
0 10
20
30
40
Gestational age (weeks)

**FIGURE 45–7.** DNA and protein/DNA ratio in kidneys of human fetus. (From Widdowson, E.M., Crabb, D.E., Milner, R.D.G.: Arch. Dis. Child., *47*:652–655, 1972.)

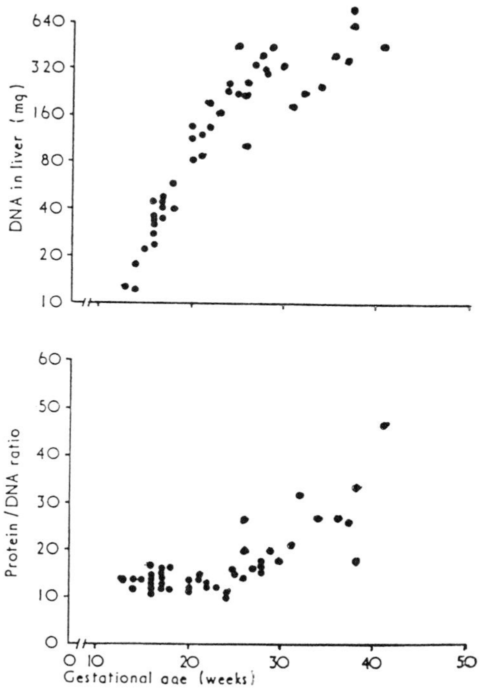
DNA in liver (mg)
640
320
160
80
40
20
10
Protein / DNA ratio
60
50
40
30
20
10
0
0 10
20
30
40
50
Gestational age (weeks)

**FIGURE 45–8.** DNA and protein/DNA ratio in liver of human fetus. (From Widdowson, E.M., Crabb, D.E., Milner, R.D.G.: Arch. Dis. Child., *47*:652–655, 1972.)

protein/DNA ratio may still be a valid index of changes in mean cell size. The fetal liver, however, is heterogeneous, containing both hepatic and hemopoietic tissue. Clearly, a chemical approach to measurement of cellular growth of the liver is limited in value, for this method can take no account of the differential growth of the different kinds of cells within the organ.

The liver increases in weight about 13-fold between birth and maturity; its protein content increases rather more because the percentage of the organ that is occupied by cells increases. The amount of DNA in the livers of human fetuses increased from about 12 mg at 13 weeks gestation to 320 mg at 30 weeks[25] (Fig. 45–8), and then the rate of increase slowed, while the ratio of protein to DNA began to rise. Little change in the protein/DNA ratio in the liver occurred up to 30 weeks gestation, but then it rose from about 15 to 30 at term. Thus, bearing in mind the complication arising from polyploidy and mononucleate and binucleate cells, it is perhaps unwise to make statements about the number of cells in the liver, but the amount of DNA in the liver, like that in the kidneys and heart, appeared to increase rapidly up to 25 or 30 weeks gestation, and the rate of increase slowed at about the same time as the ratio of protein to DNA began to increase. A 6-fold increase in DNA and a 2½-fold increase in protein/DNA ratio were evident between the time of birth and adulthood, which suggests that more of the growth of the liver after birth is caused by an increase in the number of cells and less by an increase in their size.

We do not know when cell division normally ceases in the human liver, but we do know that, unlike skeletal muscle, the liver is capable of considerable cell division after birth, and in fact, the cells retain the capacity to divide and arrange themselves into new functional units after growth has ceased. During pregnancy,[30] and to a much greater extent during lactation,[31] the liver of the rat enlarges in response to the increased food intake, and this change is brought about by an increase in number and a small increase in size of cells. If part of the liver of a rat is surgically removed, the remainder grows by cell division to the original size and functional efficiency, and this operation has been repeated 12 times in the same animal in 1 year, each time followed by cellular division and liver growth.[32]

**Brain.** Much of our information about the cellular development of the human brain comes from the work of Dobbing and Sands.[33] They analyzed the brains of fetuses from 10 weeks gestation to term, and from children of various ages up to maturity. They studied 148 brains in all, and most of those of children after birth were from infants up to 1 year of age. The brains were from fetuses and children who were apparently growing normally when they died.

Much of Dobbing and Sands' interest was in cellular development in the three main regions of the brain, the forebrain or cerebrum, the cerebellum, and the brain stem. In the cerebrum, the total number of cells, as measured by DNA, rises rapidly during fetal life, and this rise continues after birth until the second year (Fig. 45–9). Then, cell multiplication slows, but it continues throughout the remainder of childhood, so that the total number of cells is approximately doubled between 2 years and maturity. The cells in the cerebellum begin their rapid multiplication later in fetal life than those in the forebrain, but the process is faster during the first year after birth, and the adult number of cells in the cerebellum is reached between 1 and 2 years (Fig. 45–10). The increase in number of cells in the brain stem follows a similar course to that of the cerebrum.

The two main types of cells in the brain are those of the neurons and those of the glia. Dobbing and Sands were able to identify two phases of rapid cell multiplication in the forebrain (Fig. 45–11). The first lasted from 10 to 18 weeks of gestation and corresponds to the multiplication of the neuroblasts; this process ceases at about 18 weeks of gestation when the neuroblasts are differentiated into neurons. About this time, glial multiplication begins, and further increase in number of cells results from an increase in number of glia. As already stated, cell multiplication in all parts of the brain has slowed by 2 years. Myelination follows glial multiplication, because the constituent lipids are synthesized by the glia. This process continues at a fairly rapid rate until about 4 years of age and then more gradually throughout childhood into adolescence.[34]

One striking point that arises from the results of Dobbing and Sands is the wide variation in number of cells in the forebrain from one individual to another of the same age. One child of 2 years had twice as much DNA in its forebrain as another. It was the larger brains that had the most DNA, but no evidence exists of any relationship between mental ability and the size of the brain or the number of cells in it.

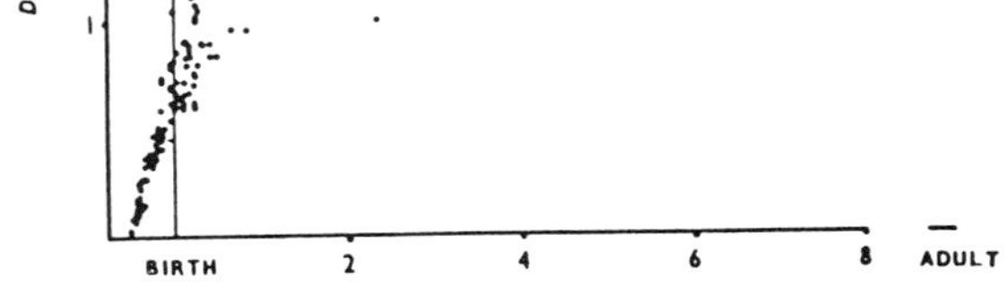
HUMAN FOREBRAIN
DNA-P (mmol)
3
2
1
BIRTH
2
4
6
8
ADULT

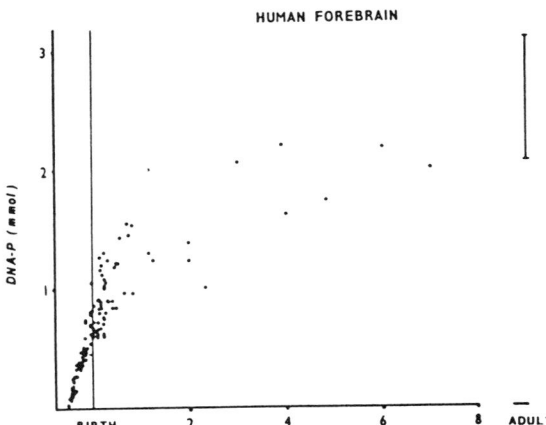

**FIGURE 45–9.** DNA-P in human forebrain during growth. (From Dobbing, J., and Sands, J.: Arch. Dis. Child., *48*:757–767, 1973.)

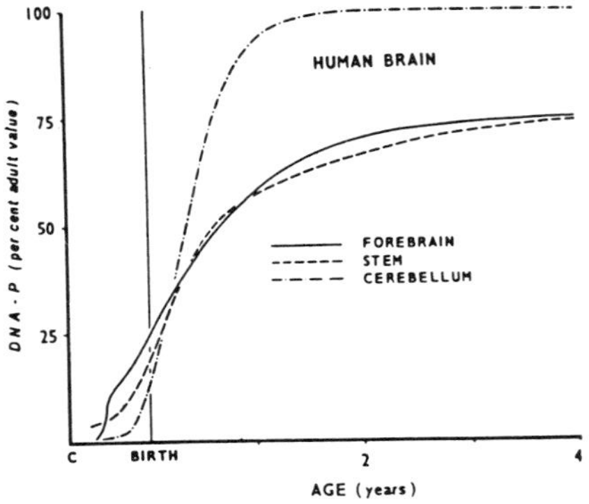
100
75
50
25
DNA - P (per cent adult value)
HUMAN BRAIN
FOREBRAIN
STEM
CEREBELLUM
C
BIRTH
2
4
AGE (years)

**FIGURE 45–10.** DNA-P in human forebrain, cerebellum, and brain stem as a percentage of adult value. (From Dobbing, J., and Sands, J.: Arch. Dis. Child., *48*:757–767, 1973.)

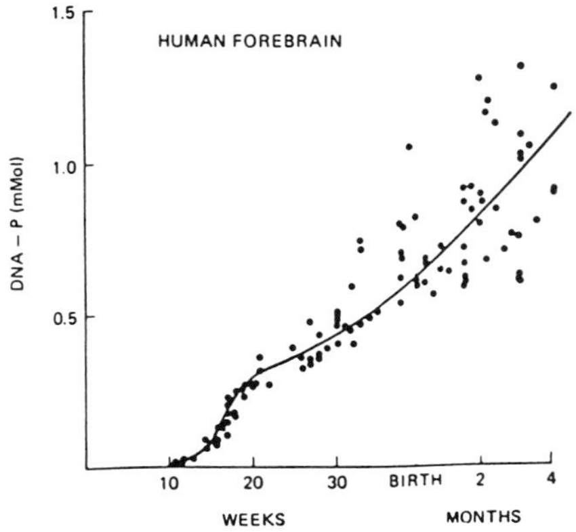
HUMAN FOREBRAIN
1.5
1.0
0.5
DNA – P (mMol)
10
20
30
BIRTH
2
4
WEEKS
MONTHS

**FIGURE 45–11.** DNA-P in human forebrain before and after birth. (From Dobbing, J., Sands, J.: Arch. Dis. Child., *48*:757–767, 1973.)

**Adipose Tissue.** White fat, in the form of triglycerides, is contained in a specific type of connective tissue cells, which have a particular distribution in the body, in the subcutaneous tissue and around the internal organs. At about 6 months of gestation, the rate of deposition of triglycerides begins to increase. Most of the fat cells are unilocular by this time and contain a single fat droplet. They are smaller than the cells at term, with a mean cell diameter of about 40 μm and a fat content of 0.03 μg.[12] As already stated, in the term infant, the cells in the gluteal region averaged 68 μm in diameter and contained 0.17 μg lipid. In the anterior abdominal wall, the corresponding figures were 50 μm and 0.06 μg. After birth, the cells of adipose tissue from both regions continued to increase in size to about 120 μm in diameter and 0.9 μg lipid between 6 and 12 months. Thus, in the gluteal region, a five-fold increase was noted in the amount of lipid in the average cell, and in the adipose tissue from the abdominal wall, a 14-fold increase occurred. The total fat content in the body increases about four-fold during the first year after birth, which suggests that no increase in number of cells is required to accommodate it.

Between 1 year and maturity, the amount of fat in the bodies of males increases by about five times and in females seven to eight times, whereas the mean fat content per cell rises by about 50%. Therefore, a considerable increase in number of adipocytes during childhood and adolescence must occur to accommodate all this fat. Brook reported a five-fold increase in the number of cells containing fat in normal children between 1 and 15 years of age.[35]

## CESSATION OF GROWTH

At a predetermined age for each species, growth slows and ultimately stops. The skeleton is the tissue above all that determines the dimensions of the body, and in man, the growth of the skeleton ceases when the epiphyses fuse at the end of the puberty growth spurt around 18 years. In some species, however, such as the rat, which reach puberty long before they reach their adult stature, the epiphyses never fuse, yet growth of the skeleton ultimately slows and virtually ceases. In other species, such as the pig, which reaches puberty while still growing rapidly, the epiphyses do eventually fuse and growth of the skeleton ceases, but this occurs at 2 to 3 years, whereas puberty is reached at around 7 months when the pig is only one half its adult weight.

The length of a muscle depends on the distance between its two points of attachment, most obvious in the limbs. Muscles attached to the long bones can grow only as long as the bones to which they are attached, and the size of the skeleton determines the length of the individual muscles. They too, therefore, cease growing in length when the skeleton reaches its final size. Excessive activity of particular parts of the body in all species leads to an increase in the width of the muscles, but not in their length.

Generally speaking, the internal organs of man and animals are appropriate to the size of the body. Thus, a genetically small man, a Yorkshire terrier, or a pony has smaller organs than a tall man, a Labrador dog, or a Shire horse. Some organs, the liver, the pancreas, adrenals, ovaries and testes, for example, can go on growing and multiplying the number of their cells long after growth of the skeleton has ceased. Yet they too stop growing when they have reached the appropriate size and functional capacity for the body they have to serve. How this is brought about still remains to be discovered.

## EFFECTS OF UNDER- AND OVERNUTRITION ON ORGAN AND CELL GROWTH

### UNDERNUTRITION

Undernutrition retards growth in all the different parts of the body. Some parts are affected more than others, adipose tissue losing its fat, and muscle and liver some of their protein. If the undernutrition is severe, the adipocytes become unrecognizable as cells and the spaces between the empty cells fill with an extracellular "gel." The muscle fibers shrink, and again the spaces between them are occupied with extracellular material. There is less change in the composition of the kidneys and heart, and the brain is the least affected of all.

If undernutrition is imposed early in life, when growth is at its most rapid, then complete recovery in size may never be possible, even though the undernutrition is temporary and plentiful food is supplied thereafter. Winick and Noble explained this concept at a cellular level.[36] They postulated that if the animal is undernourished at the stage of development when the cells are dividing rapidly, cell division is hindered, and the cell divisions lost during the period of undernutrition will never be regained. Thus, organs will have a smaller number of cells than they would have had the animal been well nourished throughout, and they therefore cannot grow as large as those of their well-nourished counterparts, even after rehabilitation. Winick and Noble demonstrated that the smaller organs of rats undernourished during the first 3 weeks after birth by being suckled in large numbers on one mother and then given plentiful food did indeed contain less DNA and hence fewer cells than those of larger animals originally suckled in groups of 3.[36] Rats undernourished for 3 weeks at a later stage of development do recover completely when rehabilitated. Winick and Noble's suggestion, which was based on their own observations[4] and those of Enesco and Le Blond[2] that cellular growth takes place in three stages, hyperplasia, hyperplasia and hypertrophy, and then hypertrophy alone, seemed to be a breakthrough in our understanding of the observed effects of undernutrition and rehabilitation at different ages. But with time, it has been realized that matters are not quite as simple as they seemed. From what has been said earlier, it is clear that there is a physiologic limit to the size an individual cell can grow, and the major contributor to growth of organs after birth, in man at any rate, is in the number of cells in them. Sands, Dobbing, and Gratrix[5] repeated Winick and Noble's[4] original study on rats, and their results were somewhat different. In their animals, the ratio of weight to DNA, which they took as a measure of cell size, had reached its mature value by 8 weeks after birth in the kidney, heart, and liver, but the total DNA was still increasing when the experiment terminated at 16 weeks. They concluded that cell multiplication continues until growth of the body comes to an end. Thus, they did not confirm Winick and Noble's[4] third stage of cellular growth consisting only of enlargement of already existing cells. However, an early phase of rapid cell multiplication undoubtedly does occur, and this may well be the stage of development when the organism is particularly vulnerable to undernutrition.

Another problem that arises over the attempt to explain the failure of rats to recover completely after a period of undernutrition just after birth is that it is not the internal organs or even skeletal muscle that determines the dimensions of the body, but the skeleton. It is the failure of the skeleton to show "catch-up" growth after early undernutrition that results in the small body, and the small body has organs that are appropriate to its size. There is no reason to suppose that the livers of rats that are small because they were undernourished early in life could not regenerate themselves by hyperplasia after partial hepatectomy just as well as those of rats that were well nourished throughout their lives. The small kidneys of the small animals are perfectly capable of maintaining the constancy of the volume and composition of the body fluids even though, taken out of the body and analyzed, they might be condemned as having too few cells. We have to be careful when drawing conclusions about the efficiency of an organ from its size or the number of cells in it without considering its size, structure, and performance relative to the body from which it came. Organs of animals undernourished early in life and then rehabilitated may be small, but this is the consequence and not the cause of the failure of the body as a whole to show "catch-up" growth.

### OVERNUTRITION

Just as it was believed in the early 1970s that a small number of cells in the internal organs somehow conferred a disadvantage on the individual, so it was thought that a large number of adipose cells did the same thing. Papers were published suggesting that obese children and adults have more fats cells than leaner ones.[37–39] The suggestion was made that fat cells are formed early in life and never lost later, so that fat infants tend to become fat adults, and adults whose obesity dated from infancy had an excess of fat cells that were inevitably with them for the rest of their lives. Brook et al. found that children who became obese during their first year had more cells with fat than those who had been of average weight, but this was not true of those who became obese later, although the amount of fat was similar in the two obese groups.[38] Those that became fat later had more fat in each cell. Salans et al. came to a similar conclusion,[40] and they and Brook et al.[38] agreed that once an excessively large number of adipose cells had been achieved, this excess was not reduced when weight was lost by dieting. Häger did not confirm these observations, and he could not find any relationship between the age of onset of obesity and the number of cells containing fat.[41] Knittle showed that it was not until 2 years that obese children had a significantly greater number of detectable adipose cells than those that were of normal size.[42] Moreover, fat is not necessarily lost from all cells equally when an individual becomes slim, and Ashwell and Garrow demonstrated in one obese patient who lost weight that the mean cell size actually increased because small cells lost what little fat they had and so disappeared from the reckoning.[43]

The errors involved in estimating the total number of fat cells in the body have already been discussed, and it is now generally held that weight and fatness and number of adipocytes during the first year after birth may not be an important determinant of shape, size, and obesity during later childhood.[44–46]

## HARMONY OF GROWTH

"The growth of a living organism is a highly complex affair, involving as it does a multitude of different processes working in harmony, each cutting in and cutting out at the appropriate time. . . . The general principles about growth apply to all species, but species vary very much among themselves, most obviously perhaps in the rate at which the body grows and the ultimate size that it becomes. . . . The rate of cell division is genetically determined, but its fulfilment depends upon the supply of food and to the ability of the animal to make use of it. . . . Within each species, the growth and development of each part of the body is in perfect harmony with that of the rest, and it is exactly attuned at each age to the function it has to perform."[47]

## REFERENCES


1. Black, D.A.K.: Essentials of Fluid Balance. 2nd Ed. Oxford, Blackwell Scientific Publications, 1960.
2. Enesco, M., LeBlond, C.P.: J. Embryol. Exp. Morphol., *10:*530–564, 1962.
3. Osgood, E.E.: Pediatrics, *15:*733–751, 1965.
4. Winick, M., Noble, A.: Dev. Biol., *12:*451–466, 1965.
5. Sands, J., Dobbing, J., Gratrix, C.A.: Lancet, *2:*503–505, 1979.
6. Schneider, W.D.: J. Biol. Chem., *161:*293–303, 1945.
7. Burton, K.: Biochem. J., *62:*315–323, 1956.
8. Boivin, A., Vendrely, R., Vendrely, C.: C.R. Acad. Sci. (III), *226:*1061–1063, 1948.
9. Davidson, J.N., Leslie, I.: Nature, *165:*49–53, 1950.
10. Brachet, J.: Biochemical Cytology. New York, Academic Press, 1957.
11. Durnin, J.V.G.A., Womersley, J.: Br. J. Nutr., *32:*77–79, 1974.
12. Dauncey, M.J., Gairdner, D.: Arch. Dis. Child., *50:*286–290, 1975.
13. Cheek, D.B.: Muscle cell growth in normal children. *In* Human Growth. Edited by D.B. Cheek. Philadelphia, Lea & Febiger, 1968.
14. Documenta Geigy Scientific Tables. 7th Ed. Edited by K. Diem, C. Lentner. Basel, J.R. Geigy S.A., 1970.

15. Wilmer, H.A.: Proc. Soc. Exp. Biol. Med., *43*:545–547, 1940.
16. MacCallum, J.B.: Bull. Johns Hopkins Hosp., *9*:208–215, 1898.
17. Montgomery, R.D.: Nature, *195*:194–195, 1962.
18. Adams, R.D., DeRueck, J.: Basic Research in Myology. Proceedings of the II International Congress on Muscle Diseases. Part I. ICN Series No. 294. Amsterdam, Excerpta Medica, 1973.
19. Stickland, N.C.: J. Anat., *132*:557–579, 1981.
20. Hartman, W.H.: Histologic study of muscle cell size. *In* Human Growth. Edited by D.B. Cheek. Philadelphia, Lea & Febiger, 1968, pp. 372–381.
21. Luff, A.R., Goldspink, G.: Life Sci., *6*:1821–1826, 1967.
22. Stickland, N.C., Widdowson, E.M., Goldspink, G.: Br. J. Nutr., *34*:421–428, 1975.
23. Burleigh, I.G.: Biol. Rev., *49*:267–320, 1974.
24. Widdowson, E.M., Dickerson, J.W.T.: Chemical composition of the body. *In* Mineral Metabolism Vol. 2A. Edited by C.L. Comar, F. Bronner. New York, Academic Press, 1964, pp. 1–247.
25. Widdowson, E.M., Crabb, D.E., Milner, R.D.G.: Arch. Dis. Child., *47*:652–655, 1972.
26. Enesco, M., Puddy, D., Am. J. Anat., *114*:235–244, 1964.
27. Widdowson, E.M., Dickerson, J.W.T.: Biochem. J., *77*:30–43, 1960.
28. Potter, E.L., Thierstein, S.T.: J. Pediatr., *22*:695–706, 1943.
29. Epstein, C.J.: Proc. Natl. Acad. Sci. USA, *57*:327–334, 1967.
30. Campbell, R.M., Fell, B.F., Mackie, W.S.: J. Physiol. (Lond.), *241*:699–713, 1972.
31. Kennedy, G.C., Pearce, W.M., Parrott, D.M.: J. Endocrinol, *17*:158–160, 1958.
32. Ingle, D.J., Baker, B.L.: Proc. Soc. Exp. Biol. Med., *95*:813–815, 1957.
33. Dobbing, J., Sands, J.: Arch. Dis. Child., *48*:757–767, 1973.
34. Hoar, R.M., Monie, I.W.: Comparative development of specific organ systems. *In* Developmental Toxicology. Edited by C.A. Kimmel, J. Buelke-Sam. New York, Raven Press, 1981, pp. 13–33.
35. Brook, C.D.G.: Lancet, *2*:624–627, 1972.
36. Winick, M., Noble, A.: J. Nutr., *89*:300–406, 1966.
37. Hirsch, J., Knittle, J.L.: Fed. Proc., *29*:1516–1521, 1970.
38. Brook, C.G.D.: Lloyd, J.K., Wolff, O.H.: Br. Med. J., *2*:25–27, 1972.
39. Brook, C.G.D.: Arch. Dis. Child., *46*:182–184, 1971.
40. Salans, L.B., Cushman, S.W., Weismann, R.E.: J. Clin. Invest., *52*:929–941, 1973.
41. Häger, A.: Postgrad. Med. J., *53*:101–107, 1977.
42. Knittle, J.L.: Adipose tissue development in man. *In* Human Growth. Vol. 2. Edited by F. Falkner, J.M. Tanner. London, Baillière Tindall, 1977, pp. 295–315.
43. Ashwell, M., Garrow, J.S.: Lancet, *2*:1036–1037, 1973.
44. Melbin, T., Viulle, J.C.: Br. J. Prev. Soc. Med., *27*:225–235, 1973.
45. Fisch, R.O., Bilek, M.K., Ulstrom, R.: Pediatrics, *56*:521–528, 1975.
46. Poskitt, E.M.E., Cole, T.J.: Br. Med. J., *1*:7–9, 1977.
47. Widdowson, E.M.: Lancet, *1*:901–905, 1970.

CHAPTER 46

# Nutritional Requirements During Infancy and Childhood

William C. Heird



The nutritional requirements of infants and children reflect the unique needs of this population to support growth and developmental changes in organ function and body composition as well as their maintenance needs. Moreover, because the metabolic rate of infants and children is greater and the turnover of nutrients more rapid than in the adult, the unique nutritional needs for growth and development are superimposed on higher maintenance requirements than those of the adult. In addition, the impact of intake during early life on later development and health must be considered. Finally, provision of these greater needs, particularly to the smaller members of this population, is hindered by their lack of teeth as well as their limited digestive and metabolic processes.

In this chapter, the nutritional needs of normal infants as well as those of low-birth weight (LBW) infants are discussed. Because the nutritional management of LBW infants presents some of the most pressing problems encountered by those involved in the feeding of infants and children, the nutritional needs of this subpopulation are discussed more fully. The nutritional needs of infants and children with acute or chronic disease as well as those with some specific disease states are detailed in another chapter, which also includes a general discussion of approaches to providing the nutritional needs of compromised infants and a detailed discussion of parenteral nutrition in pediatric patients.

## THE NORMAL INFANT

The nutritional requirements of the normal infant have been addressed by investigators over many years, and recommended dietary allowances (RDA) for most nutrients have been established. The most recent recommendations are summarized in Table 46–1.[1] The requirements and recommended intakes of some nutrients are discussed briefly here.

### ENERGY

Per unit of body weight, the daily energy requirements of the normal newborn infant are three to four times greater than those of the adult, i.e., 90 to 120 kcal/kg versus 30 to 40 kcal/kg. These greater needs reflect both the infant's relatively high resting metabolic rate and the special needs for growth and development. However, even in the normal infant, relatively inefficient intestinal absorption contributes to these requirements. Individual variations in energy requirements, of course, can be considerable.

With respect to the source of energy, there is no evidence that either carbohydrate or fat is superior, provided total energy intake is adequate. Sufficient

**TABLE 46–1.** RECOMMENDED DAILY ALLOWANCES OF NUTRIENTS FOR NORMAL INFANTS

| NUTRIENT | RECOMMENDED INTAKE PER DAY 0–6 Months (Weight = 6 kg) | 6–12 Months (Weight = 9 kg) |
|---|---|---|
| Energy (kcal) | 650 | 850 |
| Fat (g) | | |
| Carbohydrate | | |
| Protein (g) | 13 | 14 |
| Electrolytes and minerals: | | |
| Calcium (mg) | 400 | 600 |
| Phosphorus (mg) | 300 | 500 |
| Magnesium (mg) | 40 | 60 |
| Sodium (mg)* | 120 | 200 |
| Chloride (mg)* | 180 | 300 |
| Potassium (mg)* | 500 | 700 |
| Iron (mg) | 6 | 10 |
| Zinc (mg) | 5 | 5 |
| Copper (mg)† | 0.4–0.6 | 0.6–0.7 |
| Iodine (μg) | 40 | 50 |
| Selenium (μg) | 10 | 15 |
| Manganese (μg)† | 0.3–0.6 | 0.6–1.0 |
| Fluoride (mg)† | 0.1–1 | 0.2–1 |
| Chromium (μg)† | 10–40 | 20–60 |
| Molybdenum (μg) | 15–30 | 20–40 |
| Vitamins: | | |
| Vitamin A (μg RE) | 375 | 375 |
| Vitamin D (μg) | 7.5 | 10 |
| Vitamin E (mg α-TE) | 3 | 4 |
| Vitamin K (μg) | 5 | 10 |
| Vitamin C (mg) | 0.3 | 0.4 |
| Thiamine (mg) | 0.3 | 0.4 |
| Riboflavin (mg) | 0.4 | 0.5 |
| Niacin (mg NE) | 5 | 6 |
| Vitamin $B_6$ (mg) | 0.3 | 0.6 |
| Folate (μg) | 25 | 35 |
| Vitamin $B_{12}$ (μg) | 0.3 | 0.5 |
| Biotin (μg)† | 10 | 15 |
| Pantothenic acid (mg)† | 2 | 3 |

*Minimum requirements (mg/day) rather than recommended.
†Estimated safe and adequate daily intake.
(Data from Food and Nutrition Board, National Research Council: Recommended Dietary Allowances. 10th Ed. Washington, D.C., National Academy Press, 1989.)

carbohydrate intake to avoid development of ketosis and/or hypoglycemia is required (less than 5.0 g/kg per day), as is enough fat to avoid development of essential fatty acid deficiency (0.5 to 1.0 g/kg per day of linoleic acid plus a smaller amount of linolenic acid).

In concert with the recommendation of reducing the dietary fat intake of the general population, particularly that of cholesterol and saturated fat, some agencies have suggested that this guideline be applied to infants. However, because fat is a major source of energy as well as a source of essential fatty acids, groups responsible for making recommendations for infants have not endorsed this recommendation. After 1 to 2 years of age, however, attention to this general guideline is warranted.

## PROTEIN

The protein requirement of the normal infant per unit of body weight also is greater than that of the adult, but not as great as the requirement of the LBW infant. The infant also requires a higher proportion of essential amino acids than the adult (Table 46–2).[2] The minimal intakes of essential amino acids consistent with normal growth were determined under conditions of maximal nitrogen sparing. Thus, if the required intakes of the essential amino acids are met, the total intake of nitrogen probably is more important than the particular mixture of amino acids provided. Indeed, the overall protein requirement is some two to three times the

**TABLE 46–2.** ESSENTIAL AMINO ACID REQUIREMENTS OF THE TERM INFANT

| AMINO ACID | MINIMUM REQUIREMENT (mg/kg per day) |
|---|---|
| Leucine | 76–229 |
| Isoleucine | 102–119 |
| Lysine | 88–103 |
| Methionine (with cyst(e)ine) | 33–45 |
| Phenylalanine (with tyrosine) | 47–90 |
| Threonine | 45–87 |
| Tryptophan | 15–22 |
| Valine | 85–105 |
| Histidine | 16–34 |

(From Holt, L.E., Jr., Snyderman, S.E.: JAMA, *175:*100–103, 1961.)

aggregate requirement for essential amino acids. Obviously, the required intake of a specific protein is a function of its quality or how closely its amino acid pattern resembles that of human milk. It also follows that the overall quality of a specific protein can be improved by supplementing it with the essential amino acid(s) that is lacking. An example is soy protein; in the native state, it has insufficient methionine, but when fortified with methionine, soy protein approaches or equals the overall quality of bovine milk protein.[3]

Whereas the amino acid composition of human milk is ideal, its overall protein content, approximately 1.0 g/dl, is such that ingestion of 180 to 200 ml/kg per day is required to ensure a protein intake equal to the recommended daily intake of 2.0 to 2.2 g/kg. This fact has led some to question the adequacy of the protein content of human milk and others to question the validity of the recommended intake. On balance, the high quality and easy digestibility of human milk protein appear to compensate for any quantitative deficiency. On the other hand, bovine milk protein, the protein source of most infant formulas, also is a high quality protein and, if properly processed, is utilized nearly as well as human milk protein. Thus, the actual requirement for protein when bovine milk is the source may be only slightly higher, if at all, than when human milk is the source.[4]

## ELECTROLYTES, MINERALS, AND VITAMINS

The electrolyte, mineral, and vitamin requirements of the normal infant are not as well defined as those for energy and protein. Nonetheless, recommended intakes for most have been established (see Table 46–1), and infants who receive these intakes experience few problems. In recent years, the concept that limitation of sodium intake may decrease the incidence of hypertension later in life has received some attention; however, few hard data are available on which to base a definitive conclusion.[5]

Iron deficiency is the most common nutrient deficiency syndrome in infancy. This fact is somewhat surprising because the normal infant at birth has sufficient stores of iron to meet requirements for 4 to 6 months. However, these stores as well as the absorption of iron are quite variable. Although human milk contains less iron than most formulas, iron deficiency is less common in breast-fed infants. To prevent development of iron deficiency, routine iron supplementation of most formula-fed infants over 2 months of age is recommended.[6] Some individuals also recommend supplementation of infants less than 2 months of age. As discussed more fully in the section addressing the iron requirement of LBW infants, the amount required may be related to the vitamin E and polyunsaturated fat contents of the diet.

If protein intake is adequate, vitamin deficiencies are rare; if not, deficiencies of nicotinic acid and choline, which are synthesized, respectively, from tryptophan and methionine, may develop. In contrast, if bovine milk and bovine milk formulas were not supplemented with vitamin D, hypovitaminosis D would be endemic among formula-fed infants, particularly those with limited exposure to sunlight. The breast-fed infant may be relatively better protected from development of vitamin D deficiency,[7] but vitamin D supplementation of breast-fed infants also is recommended. Routine perinatal administration of vitamin K is recommended as prophylaxis against hemorrhagic disease of the newborn.

## WATER

The normal infant's absolute requirement for water probably is 75 to 100 ml/kg per day. However, because of higher obligate renal, pulmonary, and dermal water losses as well as a higher overall metabolic rate, the infant is more susceptible to development of dehydration, particularly with vomiting and/or diarrhea. Thus, provision of 150 ml/kg per day is recommended. The typical breast-fed infant as well as the typical formula-fed infant usually consumes at least this volume for the first several weeks of life.

## HUMAN MILK VERSUS ARTIFICIAL FORMULA

Because of its ready availability, its relative safety, and the possibility that it may enhance intestinal development, resistance to infection, and bonding between the mother and infant, human milk is considered the perfect food for the normal infant.[8] This statement undoubtedly is true for the majority of infants, but certain theoretical and practical hazards of breast-feeding must be considered.

The major nutritional concern is that human milk may contain too little calcium and phosphorus for optimal skeletal development of the growing infant. Indeed, breast-fed infants have a less well-mineralized skeleton throughout the early months of life than infants fed formulas of higher calcium content.[9] On the other hand, unlike the situation in LBW infants, these lower calcium and phosphorus intakes and the less mineralized skeleton secondary to these intakes apparently are not detrimental to the normal infant.

Another potential hazard of human milk is its association in some infants with hyperbilirubinemia. This phenomenon usually is transient and is limited to the first few days to weeks of life; thus, unless hyperbilirubinemia persists or plasma bilirubin concentration exceeds 12 to 15 mg/dl, most clinicians think proscription of breast-feeding is not necessary.

The possibility that certain noxious or infectious agents may be present in breast milk (e.g., chemicals, drugs, foreign proteins, and viruses) also must be borne in mind. However, the risk of infection secondary to mode of feeding is far greater in formula-fed than breast-fed infants, particularly if the artificial formula is prepared under less than optimal hygienic conditions.

The most important potential disadvantage of breast-feeding concerns the lack of constancy and adequacy of maternal milk supply. With proper counseling, an adequate supply usually is not a problem. Nonetheless, breast-fed infants must be followed closely over the first few days to weeks of life to ensure that growth and development is proceeding normally. This requirement is crucial for first-born infants.

In large part, the historical problems associated with feeding the infant who cannot be breast-fed have been solved. In fact, considering the safety and easy digestibility of modern infant formulas, it is difficult to understand the emphasis placed by governmental and nongovernmental agencies on the promotion of breast-feeding. Although the economic advantages and microbiologic safety of breast-feeding for less developed and less affluent societies are obvious, these factors are of lesser importance in affluent, developed countries in which the majority of the current generation were fed artificial formulas during infancy. Thus, a reasonable and conservative approach is to allow the mother to make an informed choice of how she wishes to feed her infant and support her in that decision. Some evidence suggests that breast-fed infants in affluent societies have fewer common and serious infections during early life than formula-fed infants[10]; if this difference is proven to be attributable to breast-feeding rather than to a myriad of other possible factors (e.g., socioeconomic status), the current emphasis on promoting breast-feeding, clearly, is warranted.

Many formulas are available for feeding the normal infant. The composition of those used most commonly is shown in Table 46–3. Most are available in both a "ready to use" and a concentrated liquid form. Powdered products also are available; although used rarely in the United States, these products are the only ones available in many parts of the world.

The most commonly used formulas contain either unmodified or modified bovine milk protein in a concentration of 1.5 g/dl. Thus, the infant who receives 180 ml/kg daily receives a daily protein intake of 2.7 g/kg, 35 to 50% more than the breast-fed infant and also somewhat more than the most recent recommended intake. Unmodified bovine milk protein has a whey to casein ratio of 18:82, whereas modified bovine milk protein has a whey to casein ratio of 60:40, which is similar to that of human milk. The latter products are prepared from either a mixture of bovine milk protein and bovine milk whey proteins or a mixture of bovine milk whey proteins and caseins. For the normal term infant, there is no convincing evidence that either the modified or unmodified bovine milk protein is more efficacious than the other. Formulas containing soy protein as well as formulas containing partially hydrolyzed bovine milk proteins are available for feeding infants who are intolerant of bovine milk protein (Table 46–4).

The major carbohydrate of the most common bovine milk formulas is lactose. The soy protein formulas, however, contain either sucrose or a glucose polymer; thus, they are useful for the infant with either transient or congenital lactase deficiency. The fat content of both bovine milk and soy protein formulas usually comprises about 50% of the nonprotein energy. In general, the blend of vegetable oils present in most formulas is easily absorbed; results of most studies suggest that intestinal absorption is at least 90%.

The electrolyte, mineral, and vitamin contents of most formulas are similar. When fed in adequate amounts (150 to 180 ml/kg per day), all provide the recommended daily allowances of these nutrients. Both iron-supplemented (about 12 mg/L) and nonsupplemented (about 1 mg/L) formulas are available. As mentioned previously, clinicians usually recommend that infants receive iron-supplemented formulas, particularly after 2 to 3 months of age. Vitamin supplementation, although frequently recommended, is not required if intake of these formulas is adequate.

The goal of both breast-feeding and formula-feeding is to deliver enough milk to support adequate growth. As a rule of thumb, the weight of the normal term infant should double over the first 3 to 5 months of life and triple over the first 12 months. For the breast-fed infant, adequacy of intake can be assessed by periodic weighing immediately before and after feeding (1 g of weight gain = 1 ml of milk ingested); for the formula-fed infant, intake can be assessed by recording the quantity of formula ingested.

Demand feeding may be preferable during the early weeks of life, but most infants adjust easily to an every 4-hour schedule; after 2 months of age, night feedings usually can be omitted. Introduction of solid foods and administration of multivitamin supplements are unnecessary before about 4 months of age; thereafter, the addition of a multivitamin supplement as well as strained or blenderized foods is recommended. The latter should be added stepwise, beginning with cereals, vegetables, and fruits. By approximately 1 year of age, most infants should have graduated successfully to table food and be eating 3 to 4 meals daily. Once teeth have erupted

**TABLE 46–3.** COMPOSITION (AMOUNT/100 KCAL) OF STANDARD FORMULAS FOR NORMAL INFANTS

| COMPONENT | SIMILAC* | ENFAMIL† | SMA‡ | GERBER§ | GOOD START‖ |
|---|---|---|---|---|---|
| Protein (g) | 2.14 (bovine milk) | 2.2 (bovine milk; whey) | 2.2 (bovine milk; whey) | 2.2 (bovine milk) | 2.4 (whey) |
| Fat (g) | 5.4 (soy and coconut oils) | 5.6 (coconut and soy oils) | 5.3 (oleo; coconut, oleic and soy oils) | 5.4 (palmoleic, coconut, soy, and high-oleic safflower oils) | 5.1 (palm-oleic, coconut, soy, and high-oleic safflower oils) |
| Carbohydrate (g) | 10.7 (lactose) | 10.3 (lactose) | 10.6 (lactose) | 10.7 (lactose) | 11.0 (lactose; maltodextrin) |
| Electrolytes and minerals | | | | | |
| Calcium (mg) | 73 | 69 | 63 | 75 | 64 |
| Phosphorus (mg) | 56 | 47 | 42 | 58 | 36 |
| Magnesium (mg) | 6 | 7.8 | 7 | 6 | 6.7 |
| Iron (mg) | 0.22(1.8)# | 0.16(1.88)# | 0.2(1.8)# | 0.48(1.8)# | 1.5 |
| Zinc (mg) | 0.75 | 0.78 | 0.8 | 0.75 | 0.75 |
| Manganese (μg) | 5 | 15.6 | 15 | 5 | 7 |
| Copper (μg) | 90 | 94 | 70 | 90 | 80 |
| Iodine (μg) | 14 | 10.2 | 9 | 8 | 8 |
| Selenium (μg) | 2.2 | 1.77 | 1.8 | – | – |
| Sodium (mg) | 27 | 27 | 22 | 33 | 24 |
| Potassium (mg) | 120 | 108 | 83 | 108 | 98 |
| Chloride | 64 | 63 | 55.5 | 70 | 59 |
| Vitamins | | | | | |
| Vitamin A (IU) | 300 | 310 | 300 | 300 | 300 |
| Vitamin D (IU) | 60 | 63 | 60 | 60 | 60 |
| Vitamin E (IU) | 3.0 | 3.1 | 1.4 | 3 | 2 |
| Vitamin K (μg) | 8 | 8.6 | 8 | 8 | 8.2 |
| Thiamine (μg) | 100 | 78 | 100 | 100 | 60 |
| Riboflavin (μg) | 150 | 156 | 150 | 150 | 135 |
| Vitamin $B_6$ (μg) | 60 | 63 | 62.5 | 60 | 75 |
| Vitamin $B_{12}$ (μg) | 0.25 | 0.23 | 0.2 | 0.25 | 0.22 |
| Niacin (μg) | 1050 | 1250 | 750 | 1050 | 750 |
| Folic acid (μg) | 15 | 15.6 | 7.5 | 15 | 9 |
| Pantothenic acid (μg) | 450 | 470 | 315 | 450 | 450 |
| Vitamin C (mg) | 9 | 8.1 | 8.5 | 9 | 8 |
| Biotin (μg) | 4.4 | 2.3 | 2.2 | 4.4 | 2.2 |
| Choline (mg) | 16.0 | 15.6 | 15.0 | 16 | 12 |
| Inositol (mg) | 4.7 | 4.7 | 4.7 | 4.7 | 18 |

*Ross Laboratories, Columbus, OH.
†Mead-Johnson Nutritionals, Evansville, IN.
‡Wyeth-Ayerst Laboratories, Philadelphia, PA.
§Gerber Products Company, Fremont, MI.
‖Carnation Nutritional Products, Glendale, CA.
#Content of iron fortified formula in parentheses.

and solid food is tolerated without difficulty, weaning should have been completed.

## THE 6- TO 12-MONTH-OLD CHILD

Considerably less attention has been paid to the nutritional needs of the 6- to 12-month-old child than to those of the younger infant. In fact, the RDA for the various nutrients for this age group (see Table 46–1) rely heavily on extrapolations from data obtained in younger infants, taking into account the developmental differences between the younger and the older infants as well as the greater level of activity and somewhat slower rate of growth of children 6 to 12 months of age. Despite the lack of specific data, few participants in a recent symposium on the nutritional needs of the 6- to 12-month-old child thought that the most recent RDA for this age group required extensive revision.[11]

One exception concerns energy, the RDA for which is somewhat higher than the current energy intake of apparently normal infants.[12] Although infants receiving the lower intakes exhibit lower rates of weight gain as well as lower rates of increase in skinfold thicknesses

**TABLE 46–4.** COMPOSITION OF SOY AND HYDROLYZED PROTEIN FORMULAS

| COMPONENT | ISOMIL* | PROSOBEE† | NURSOY‡ | NUTRAMIGEN† | PREGESTIMIL† | ALIMENTUM* |
|---|---|---|---|---|---|---|
| Protein (g) | 2.66 (soy protein isolate) | 3 (soy protein isolate and L-methionine) | 3.1 (soy protein isolate) | 2.8 (casein hydrolysate, cystine, tyrosine and tryptophan) | 2.8 (casein hydrolysate, cystine, tyrosine, and tryptophan) | 2.75 (casein hydrolysate, cystine, tyrosine, and tryptophan) |
| Fat (g) | 5.46 (soy and coconut oils) | 5.3 (coconut and soy oils) | 5.3 (oleo, coconut, oleic, and soy oils) | 3.9 (corn oil) | 5.6 (medium-chain triglycerides; corn and high oleic safflower oils) | 5.54 (medium-chain triglycerides; safflower and soy oils) |
| Carbohydrate (g) | 10.1 (corn syrup; sucrose)§ | 10 (corn syrup solids) | 10.2 (sucrose) | 13.4 (corn syrup solids) | 10.3 (corn syrup solids; dextrose) | 10.2 (sucrose) |
| Electrolytes and minerals | | | | | | |
| Calcium (mg) | 105 | 94 | 90 | 94 | 94 | 105 |
| Phosphorus (mg) | 75 | 74 | 63 | 63 | 63 | 75 |
| Magnesium (mg) | 7.5 | 10.9 | 10 | 10.9 | 10.9 | 7.5 |
| Iron (mg) | 1.8 | 1.88 | 1.7 | 1.88 | 1.88 | 1.8 |
| Zinc (mg) | 0.75 | 0.78 | 0.8 | 0.78 | 0.94 | 0.75 |
| Manganese (μg) | 30 | 25 | 30 | 31 | 31 | 30 |
| Copper (μg) | 75 | 94 | 70 | 94 | 94 | 75 |
| Iodine (μg) | 15 | 10.2 | 9 | 7 | 8 | 15 |
| Selenium (μg) | 2.1 | 2.3 | 1.0 | 2.3 | 2.3 | 2.8 |
| Sodium (mg) | 44 | 36 | 30 | 47 | 39 | 44 |
| Potassium (mg) | 108 | 122 | 105 | 109 | 109 | 118 |
| Chloride | 62 | 83 | 56.5 | 86 | 86 | 80 |
| Vitamins | | | | | | |
| Vitamin A (IU) | 300 | 310 | 300 | 310 | 380 | 300 |
| Vitamin D (IU) | 60 | 63 | 60 | 63 | 75 | 45 |
| Vitamin E (IU) | 3.0 | 3.1 | 1.4 | 3.1 | 3.8 | 3.0 |
| Vitamin K (IU) | 15 | 15.6 | 15. | 15.6 | 18.8 | 15 |
| Thiamin (μg) | 60 | 78 | 100 | 78 | 78 | 60 |
| Riboflavin (μg) | 90 | 94 | 150 | 94 | 94 | 90 |
| Vitamin $B_6$ (μg) | 60 | 63 | 62.5 | 63 | 63 | 60 |
| Vitamin $B_{12}$ (μg) | 0.45 | 0.31 | 0.3 | 0.31 | 0.31 | 0.45 |
| Niacin (μg) | 1350 | 1250 | 750 | 1250 | 1250 | 1350 |
| Folic acid (μg) | 15 | 15.6 | 7.5 | 15.6 | 15.6 | 15 |
| Pantothenic acid (μg) | 750 | 470 | 450 | 470 | 470 | 750 |
| Biotin (μg) | 4.5 | 7.8 | 5.5 | 7.8 | 7.8 | 4.5 |
| Vitamin C (mg) | 9 | 8.1 | 8.5 | 8.1 | 11.7 | 9.0 |
| Choline (mg) | 8 | 7.8 | 13.0 | 13.3 | 13.3 | 8 |
| Inositol (mg) | 5 | 4.8 | 4.1 | 4.7 | 4.7 | 8 |

*Ross Laboratories, Columbus, OH.
†Mead Johnson Nutritionals, Evansville, IN.
‡Wyeth-Ayerst Laboratories, Philadelphia, PA.
§Isomil-SF (sucrose free) has similar composition with exception that glucose polymers are substituted for corn syrup and sucrose.

than the National Center for Health Statistics (NCHS) standard rates, increase in length and head circumference are not compromised. Thus, proponents of a lower RDA for energy i.e., 85 versus 95 kcal/kg per day, argue that the growth response of infants ingesting the lower energy intake reflect the current concepts of parents regarding appropriate body size and proportions and, also, that these responses are appropriate for current feeding practices (e.g., delayed introduction of solid foods). More data are needed concerning this issue, but there is no evidence that the lower energy intake apparently characteristic of many modern infants is harmful.

By 6 months of age, the infant's previously compromised capacity to digest and absorb a variety of dietary components as well as to metabolize, utilize and excrete the absorbed products of digestion is near the capacity of the adult.[13] Moreover, teeth are beginning to erupt and the infant is more active and is beginning to explore his or her surroundings. Hence, during this interval, diet plays a variety of roles other than delivery of required nutrients. A number of concerns also emerge during this period. For example, with the eruption of teeth, the role of diet in development of dental caries must be considered.[14] Consideration of the long-term effects of inadequate or excessive intakes during infancy also assumes greater importance, as does consideration of the psychosocial role of foods during development.

These concerns, rather than concerns about delivery of adequate amounts of nutrients, are the basis for most recommendations for feeding during the second 6 months of life. While all nutrient needs during this period can be met with reasonable amounts of currently available infant formulas, although perhaps not with exclusive breast-feeding, the addition of weaning foods to the diet of infants 4 to 6 months of age usually is recommended.

Although weaning, or "follow-up", formulas with a somewhat higher protein content than regular infant formulas are popular in Europe, these formulas have not been popular in the United States. This situation may change with the recent introduction of such a formula (Carnation Follow-Up Formula, Carnation Nutritional Products, Glendale, CA). This formula contains 3 g of bovine milk protein per 100 kcal. Fat content is 3.9 g/100 kcal (a mixture of corn, palm, and high-oleic safflower oils). Carbohydrate content is 13.2 g/100 kcal (a mixture of lactose and corn syrup solids).

Aside from the association of bottle feeding with dental caries,[14] little is known about the various issues related to the non-nutritional role of diet during the second half of the first year of life. Thus, a wide variety of feeding practices are observed during this period. Nonetheless, most recent surveys indicate that infants fed according to current practices receive the RDA for most nutrients.[15]

One current feeding practice, i.e., the use of bovine milk, particularly low-fat bovine milk, deserves comment. Although current recommendations are to limit the intake of bovine milk and to avoid low-fat or skimmed milk before 1 year of age,[16] recent surveys suggest that a sizable percentage of 6- to 12-month-old infants, albeit still fewer than 20 years ago, are fed bovine milk rather than infant formula.[17,18] More important, almost half of these infants are fed low-fat or skimmed milk, often, interestingly, on the advice of their physician.

The consequences of this practice are not known with certainty. However, infants fed bovine milk ingest, on average, roughly three times the recommended daily allowance for protein and 1.5 times the upper limit of the "safe range" of sodium intake but only two thirds of the recommended daily intake of iron and only one half of the recommended intake of linoleic acid. The protein and sodium intakes of infants fed skimmed rather than whole bovine milk are even higher, the iron intake is equally low, and, most important the intake of linoleic acid is less than one half of the amount recommended. Interestingly, whereas the most common reasons for substituting low-fat or skimmed milk for whole milk or formula are to reduce fat and energy intakes, the energy intake of infants fed skimmed milk is not lower than that of infants fed whole milk or formula.[18] Rather, they appear to compensate for the lower energy density of low-fat or skimmed milk by increasing intake of other foods.

Current knowledge is insufficient to support definitive statements concerning the consequences of the high protein and sodium intakes associated with feeding either whole or skimmed milk. The low iron intake clearly is not desirable but probably can be overcome by the use of medicinal iron supplementation. The low intake of linoleic acid is more problematic. Although signs and/or symptoms of essential fatty acid deficiency appear to be uncommon in infants fed either whole or skimmed milk, an exhaustive search for such symptoms has not been made. Moreover, because essential fatty acid deficiency develops in both younger and older infants fed special formulas providing roughly the same linoleic acid intake, it is likely that such a search would uncover a reasonably high incidence of essential fatty acid deficiency. On the other hand, older infants fed formulas of high linoleic acid content prior to 6 months of age may have sufficient body stores to limit the consequences of a low intake between 6 and 12 months of age. However, simply assuming that this is true could have undesired consequences; although biochemical essential fatty acid deficiency may not result in clinically detectable symptoms, it may result in long-term deleterious effects on development.[19]

Addressing the concerns raised by the practice of feeding bovine milk is important for practical as well as health reasons. For example, the cost of bovine milk is roughly one third that of infant formula, a difference of sufficient magnitude to have important economic consequences for most families, particularly those with limited income. In addition, if the Women, Infants, and Children (WIC) program were to provide bovine milk rather than formula to infants over 6 months of age, current funds would permit expansion of benefits to many more of the country's most needy infants. While clearly desirable, this change obviously cannot occur until data substantiating the safety of feeding bovine milk during the second 6 months of life are available.

The questions raised by the increasingly common practice of substituting skimmed or low-fat milk for whole milk or formula are even more complex. The suggestion that infants fed skimmed milk increase their intake of other foods raises the important question of whether food intake during infancy may, in some way, imprint intake patterns throughout life. If so, this apparent attempt to improve longevity or at least cardiovascular health, paradoxically, may be more detrimental to both than a less prudent diet during infancy.

## THE 1- TO 10-YEAR-OLD CHILD

The 1-year-old child has several teeth and the various digestive and metabolic systems are functioning at adult or near-adult capacity. Thus, the earlier restrictions with respect to source of nutrients are no longer applicable. Indeed, by 1 year of age, most children tolerate table foods either as presented to other family members or with minimal alterations. Although coordination remains poor until 3 to 4 years of age, most children begin attempting to feed themselves during the early part of the second year of life. Until coordination improves, however, these attempts usually result in as much food on the table or floor as in the child's stomach.

Most children are walking or beginning to walk by 1 year of age. Hence, with improved coordination over the next few years, activity increases dramatically. This greater activity, in turn, increases energy needs. Concurrently, however, the rate of growth decreases, e.g., whereas the birth weight triples over the first year of life, it does not quadruple until about 3 years of age (Table 46–5). Thus, although the energy requirements incident to activity increases dramatically after the first year of life, the requirements for nutrients that are stored in the process of growth decrease. These changing nutrient needs are reflected in the RDA for the various nutrients for children from 1 to 3, 4 to 6, and 7 to 10 years of age (Table 46–6).

As demonstrated by Davis[20] more than 50 years ago and more recently by Birch et al.,[21] most young children, if provided access to a varied diet including items from each of the major food groups, will consume adequate amounts of all nutrients. However, most children, particularly those less than 5 to 6 years of age, are finicky eaters. Moreover, many tend to use eating (or not eating) to exert control over parents or caretakers. Thus, the intake of most children at a single meal, or even over an entire day, is not necessarily well balanced. Rather, a balanced intake is achieved over a period of several days.

The erratic eating pattern of most young children usually is of considerable concern to parents, particularly those who have not witnessed this behavior previously. Unfortunately, their efforts to control the child's intake usually make matters worse. They should be reassured and instructed to present the child with well-balanced meals and snacks throughout the day, to remove the food after a reasonable period of time, and to avoid coaxing and cajoling, particularly offering preferred foods or treats as rewards.

The importance of providing items from most or all of the major food groups cannot be overemphasized. If the child does not have access to items from all food groups on a regular basis, self-selection of a balanced diet either within 1 day or over several days is impossible. It also is important to limit intake between regular meals and snacks; the child will not likely be hungry when the regularly scheduled meal or snack is offered. Alternatively, if the appetite is not dampened, the intake between regular meals and snacks will increase total energy intake disproportionally and contribute to development of obesity. A major distinction between meals and snacks also should be avoided, thereby assuring that the child has access to an adequate amount and variety of food when he or she is hungry or willing to eat rather than only at conventional meal times.

As the child matures and begins to socialize more, it becomes increasingly difficult to control the content of snacks or meals. Many children, in fact, eat as much or more away from home as at home, a practice that most likely contributes to the development of obesity. Perhaps the best that can be done, short of changing modern lifestyles, is to counsel parents concerning the potential problem and advise them to devise ways of assessing their children's intake when away from home. Regular monitoring of weight and height should alert the clinician to the existence of a potential problem.

Perhaps the major controversy concerning the nutrient needs of the 1- to 10-year-old child concerns the extent to which the currently advocated dietary guidelines are appropriate for this population. Although the American Heart Association,[22] the American Health Foundation,[23] and the National Institutes of Health Consensus Devel-

**TABLE 46–5.** WEIGHT AND LENGTH OF MALE CHILDREN FROM 1 TO 10 YEARS OF AGE

| | WEIGHT (kg) | | | LENGTH (cm) | | |
|---|---|---|---|---|---|---|
| AGE (YR) | 5% | 50% | 95% | 5% | 50% | 95% |
| 1 | 8.43 | 10.15 | 11.99 | 71.7 | 76.1 | 81.2 |
| 2 | 10.49 | 12.34 | 15.50 | 82.5 | 86.8 | 94.4 |
| 3 | 12.05 | 14.62 | 17.77 | 89.0 | 94.9 | 102.0 |
| 4 | 13.64 | 16.69 | 20.27 | 95.8 | 102.9 | 109.9 |
| 5 | 15.27 | 18.67 | 23.09 | 102.0 | 109.9 | 117.0 |
| 6 | 16.93 | 20.69 | 26.34 | 107.7 | 116.1 | 123.5 |
| 7 | 18.64 | 22.85 | 30.12 | 113.0 | 121.7 | 129.7 |
| 8 | 20.40 | 25.30 | 34.51 | 118.1 | 127.0 | 135.7 |
| 9 | 22.25 | 28.13 | 39.58 | 122.9 | 132.2 | 141.8 |
| 10 | 24.33 | 31.44 | 45.29 | 127.7 | 137.5 | 148.1 |

**TABLE 46–6.** RECOMMENDED DAILY ALLOWANCES (RDA) OF NUTRIENTS FOR NORMAL CHILDREN

| NUTRIENT | RECOMMENDED INTAKE PER DAY 1–3 Years (Weight = 13 kg) | 4–6 Years (Weight = 20 kg) | 7–10 Years (Weight = 28 kg) |
|---|---|---|---|
| Energy (kcal) | 1300 | 1800 | 2000 |
| Fat (g) | | | |
| Carbohydrate | | | |
| Protein (g) | 16 | 24 | 38 |
| Electrolytes and minerals | | | |
| Calcium (mg) | 800 | 800 | 800 |
| Phosphorus (mg) | 800 | 800 | 800 |
| Magnesium (mg) | 80 | 120 | 170 |
| Sodium (mEq)* | 13 | 20 | 28 |
| Chloride (mEq)* | 13 | 20 | 28 |
| Potassium (mEq)* | 26 | 36 | 40 |
| Iron (mg) | 10 | 10 | 10 |
| Zinc (mg) | 10 | 10 | 10 |
| Copper (mg)† | 0.7–1.0 | 1.0–1.5 | 1–2 |
| Iodine (μg) | 70 | 90 | 120 |
| Selenium (μg) | 20 | 20 | 30 |
| Manganese (μg)† | 1–1.5 | 1.5–2 | 2–3 |
| Fluoride (mg)† | 0.5–1.5 | 1–2.5 | 1–2.5 |
| Chromium (μg)† | 20–80 | 30–120 | 50–200 |
| Molybdenum (μg) | 25–50 | 30–75 | 50–150 |
| Vitamins | | | |
| Vitamin A (μg RE) | 400 | 500 | 700 |
| Vitamin D (μg) | 0.10 | 10 | 10 |
| Vitamin E (mg α-TE) | 6 | 8 | 7 |
| Vitamin K (μg) | 15 | 20 | 30 |
| Vitamin C (mg) | 40 | 45 | 45 |
| Thiamin (mg) | 0.7 | 0.9 | 1.0 |
| Riboflavin (mg) | 0.8 | 1.1 | 1.2 |
| Niacin (mg NE) | 9 | 12 | 13 |
| Vitamin $B_6$ (mg) | 1 | 1.1 | 1.4 |
| Folate (μg) | 50 | 75 | 100 |
| Vitamin $B_{12}$ | 0.7 | 1.0 | 1.4 |
| Biotin (μg)† | 20 | 25 | 30 |
| Pantothenic acid (mg)† | 3 | 3–4 | 4–5 |

*Minimal requirements rather than recommended.
†Estimated safe and adequate daily intake.
(Data from Food and Nutrition Board, National Research Council: Recommended Dietary Allowances. 10th Ed. Washington, D.C., National Academy Press, 1989.)

opment Panel[24] recommend that the current guidelines be applied to children over the age of 1 to 2 years, the Committee on Nutrition of the American Academy of Pediatrics[25] expresses some concerns, chief among which is the safety of a diet emphasizing lower intakes of fat, cholesterol, and salt along with higher intakes of bulky cereal grains and plant products. Such a diet, the Committee points out, could result in lower than desired intakes of energy as well as many other essential nutrients (e.g., essential fatty acids, amino acids, calcium, vitamins, iron, and other trace minerals).

The efficacy of such a diet during childhood in lowering serum cholesterol and, hence, the risk of atherosclerosis later in life also is questioned. Although fatty streaks are present in the aorta of most 10-year-old children, the distribution of fibrous plaques, the characteristic lesion of atherosclerosis, is less ubiquitous.[26] Moreover, it is not certain that fatty streaks progress to fibrous plaques.[27] The Committee also emphasizes that the frequency of atherosclerotic lesions in casualties of the Vietnam war was about 40% lower than the frequency of such lesions in casualties of the Korean war (45% versus 77.3%), and that this change occurred without a major change in childhood dietary habits.[28,29] The decreasing incidence of atherosclerotic disease over the past several decades[30] is cited as yet another example of the lack of compelling evidence for the necessity of the proposed dietary changes during childhood.

Nonetheless, the Committee concludes that the current dietary trends toward decreased consumption of saturated fats, cholesterol, and salt and increased consumption of polyunsaturated fats, if followed with moderation, are sensible for children over 2 years of age. A total fat intake of 30 to 40% of calories is considered reasonable for adequate growth and development. The Committee also advocates counseling children and their parents on maintenance of ideal weight and adoption of other aspects of lifestyle likely to reduce the risks of atherosclerosis (e.g., exercise, avoidance of tobacco, and the like). Screening of children over 2 years of age with a family history of atherosclerosis is recommended. If serum cholesterol concentration is elevated and is not attributable to high-density lipoprotein cholesterol, appropriate dietary therapy and/or medication to lower serum cholesterol is endorsed.

## THE LOW-BIRTH WEIGHT INFANT

Approximately 7% of all infants born in the United States each year weigh less than 2500 g at birth and, over the past few decades, their survival has improved steadily. Today, for example, up to 75% of even the smallest such infants (i.e., those weighing less than 1000 g at birth) survive, and survival of larger low-birth weight (LBW) infants approaches 100%. This increasing number of surviving LBW infants must be fed, thus heightening awareness of the problems encountered in meeting their nutritional needs.

The importance of adequate early nutritional management of the LBW infant is best illustrated by considering the energy metabolism of the fasted infant. As in the adult, energy to meet ongoing needs during fasting is derived from endogenous stores of various nutrients. Although hepatic glycogen stores are used initially, these stores are limited and hence are soon depleted. Thus, fat stores become the major source of endogenous energy, although protein stores also are used to provide amino acids from which glucose can be synthesized (i.e., gluconeogenesis) for use by those tissues with an absolute requirement for glucose. Therefore, if hydration is adequate, the available endogenous stores of fat and protein are the ultimate determinants of the length of time a fasting infant can survive.

As illustrated in Table 46–7, the body content of both protein and fat, particularly fat, increases throughout gestation.[31] Thus, an infant weighing 3500 g at birth has more extensive endogenous nutrient reserves than one weighing 2000 g and an infant weighing 1000 g has very limited reserves, that is, the smaller the infant, the greater its inability to withstand starvation. Under conditions of total starvation, the 1000-g infant has sufficient endogenous reserves to survive for only 4 to 5 days, the 2000-g infant has sufficient reserves to survive for approximately 12 days, and the term infant has sufficient reserves to survive for approximately 1 month.[32] Daily provision of glucose intravenously (e.g., 7.5 g/kg per day, the amount provided by 150 ml/kg per day of a 5% glucose solution or 75 ml/kg per day, of a 10% glucose solution), theoretically, will prolong survival of the 1000-g, 2000-g, and 3500-g infant, respectively, by 7, 18 and 50 days.[32]

These theoretical calculations depict in a semiquantitative manner the general clinical observations concerning the susceptibility of the LBW infant to starvation and, hence, the necessity for careful attention to early nutritional management. In addition to this practical role of early adequate nutrition, there is concern that inadequate nutrition at any time during the period of cellular proliferation of various organ systems, particularly the central nervous system, may result in nonrecoupable cellular deficits. This concern is based on evidence obtained primarily in rodents,[33] but is thought to be applicable to all species.[34] If so, the prematurely born infant, whose brain would have grown considerably during the last trimester of intrauterine life, may be

**TABLE 46–7.** INTRAUTERINE ACCRETION RATES OF VARIOUS NUTRIENTS DURING THE LAST TRIMESTER OF PREGNANCY

| | ACCUMULATION DURING VARIOUS STAGES OF GESTATION* | | |
|---|---|---|---|
| COMPONENT | 26–30 wk | 30–34 wk | 34–38 wk |
| Weight (g) | 600 | 750 | 930 |
| Protein (g) | 68 | 97 | 126 |
| Fat (g) | 60 | 95 | 145 |
| Water (g) | 459 | 539 | 627 |
| Calcium (g) | 3.4 | 5.12 | 8.7 |
| Phosphorus (g) | 2.2 | 3.3 | 5.4 |
| Magnesium (mg) | 93 | 131 | 193 |
| Sodium (mEq) | 46 | 53 | 64 |
| Potassium (mEq) | 25 | 31 | 39 |
| Chloride (mEq) | 35 | 37 | 37 |

*Body weight increases from 880 g at 26 weeks to 1480 g at 30 weeks, 2230 g at 34 weeks and 3160 g at 38 weeks.

(Adapted from Ziegler, E.E., O'Donnell, A.M., Nelson, S.E., et al.: Growth, *40:*329–340, 1976.)

particularly vulnerable to inadequate nutrition. Although the period of cellular proliferation of the entire human brain encompasses at least the first 18 months of life,[35] and although transient cellular deficits apparently can be reversed if adequate nutrition is provided before the end of this period,[36] little is known concerning the duration of cellular proliferation within specific regions of the brain. This uncertainty, coupled with the persistently high incidence of neurodevelopmental deficits in surviving LBW infants,[37] suggests that better nutritional management not only might decrease mortality but also might improve neurodevelopmental outcome.

The factors just discussed are recognized by neonatologists, and the importance of early adequate nutritional management of the LBW infant is generally accepted. As a result, the general subject of the nutritional requirements of LBW infants is an area of active investigation. The discussion that follows is an attempt to summarize the present state of knowledge.

## GOALS OF NUTRITIONAL MANAGEMENT

The most generally accepted goal is to provide sufficient amounts of all nutrients to support, at a minimum, continuation of the intrauterine growth rate.[38] Thus, the minimal requirements for various nutrients are assumed to be the amounts necessary to allow their accumulation at intrauterine rates (see Table 46–7). This concept figures prominently in the recommended nutrient intakes for LBW infants proposed by the Committee on Nutrition of the American Academy of Pediatrics (Table 46–8) as well as the composition of formulas designed for feeding the hospitalized LBW infant (Table 46–9).

Opposing views concerning the goals for nutritional management of LBW infants include, on the one hand, the fear that failure to provide human milk will deprive the infant of factors needed for optimal development of the gastrointestinal tract and immune system and, on the other, the desire to produce the most rapid growth

**TABLE 46–8.** RECOMMENDED NUTRIENT INTAKES FOR LOW-BIRTH WEIGHT INFANTS*

| NUTRIENT | RECOMMENDED INTAKE (amount/100 kCal) |
|---|---|
| Protein (g) | 2.7–3.1 |
| Fat (g) | 4.3–5.4 (300 mg essential fatty acids) |
| Carbohydrate | — |
| Electrolytes and minerals | |
| Sodium (mEq) | 2.3–2.7 |
| Potassium (mEq) | 1.8–1.9 |
| Calcium (mg) | 140–160 |
| Magnesium (mg) | 6.5–7.5 |
| Phosphorus (mg) | 95–108 |
| Chloride (mEq) | 2–2.4 |
| Iron† | |
| Zinc (mg) | 0.5 |
| Copper (μg) | 90 |
| Manganese (μg) | 5 |
| Iodine (μg) | 5 |
| VITAMINS | AMOUNT/DAY |
| Vitamin A (IU) | 1400 |
| Vitamin D (IU) | 500 |
| Vitamin E (IU) | 5–25 (1.0 IU/g linoleic acid) |
| Vitamin C (mg) | 35 |
| Thiamin (μg) | 300 |
| Riboflavin (μg) | 400 |
| Niacin (mg) | 6 |
| Vitamin $B_6$ | 300 (15 μg/g protein) |
| Folic acid (μg) | 50 |
| Vitamin $B_{12}$ (μg) | 0.3 |
| Pantothenic acid (mg) | 2 |
| Biotin (μg) | 35 |

*Lower values are the recommended intakes for larger infants; higher values are the recommended intakes for smaller infants (birth weight less than 1/250 g).

†See text.

(From Committee on Nutrition, American Academy of Pediatrics: Pediatrics, *65*:657–658, 1980.)

**TABLE 46–9.** COMPOSITION (AMOUNT/100 KCAL) OF STANDARD FORMULAS FOR LOW-BIRTH WEIGHT INFANTS

| COMPONENT | SIMILAC SPECIAL CARE* | ENFAMIL PREMATURE† | SMA PREMIE‡ |
|---|---|---|---|
| Protein (g) | 2.71 (bovine milk; whey) | 3 (bovine milk; whey) | 2.4 (bovine milk; whey) |
| Fat (g) | 5.43 (medium-chain triglycerides; soy and coconut oils) | 5.1 (medium-chain triglycerides; soy and coconut oils) | 5.4 (coconut, oleic and soy oils; oleo, medium-chain triglycerides |
| Carbohydrate (g) | 10.6 (lactose; glucose polymers) | 11.1 (lactose; corn syrup solids) | 10.5 (lactose; glycose polymers) |
| Electrolytes and minerals | | | |
| Calcium (mg) | 180 | 165 | 90 |
| Phosphorus (mg) | 90 | 83 | 50 |
| Magnesium (mg) | 12 | 7.6 | 8.6 |
| Iron (mg) | 0.37 | 1.88 | 0.38 |
| Zinc (mg) | 1.5 | 1.56 | 1.0 |
| Manganese (mg) | 12 | 13 | 25 |
| Copper (μg) | 250 | 130 | 86 |
| Iodine (μg) | 20 | 7.9 | 10 |
| Selenium (μg) | 1.9 | 1.66 | 1.7 |
| Sodium (mg) | 43 | 39 | 40 |
| Potassium (mg) | 129 | 100 | 90 |
| Chloride (mg) | 81 | 85 | 66 |
| Vitamins | | | |
| Vitamin A (IU) | 680 | 1200 | 300 |
| Vitamin D (IU) | 150 | 270 | 60 |
| Vitamin E (IU) | 4.0 | 4.6 | 1.9 |
| Vitamin K (μg) | 12 | 13 | 8.6 |
| Thiamin (μg) | 250 | 250 | 100 |
| Riboflavin (μg) | 620 | 250 | 160 |
| Vitamin $B_6$ (μg) | 250 | 250 | 60 |
| Vitamin $B_{12}$ (μg) | 0.55 | 0.3 | 0.3 |
| Niacin (μg) | 5000 | 4000 | 750 |
| Folic acid (μg) | 37 | 35 | 12.5 |
| Pantothenic acid (μg) | 1900 | 1200 | 450 |
| Vitamin C (mg) | 37 | 35 | 8.6 |
| Biotin (μg) | | 2 | |
| Choline (mg) | | 7.6 | |
| Inositol (mg) | | 4.7 | |

*Ross Laboratories, Columbus, OH.
†Mead Johnson Nutritionals, Evansville, IN.
‡Wyeth-Ayerst Laboratories, Philadelphia, PA.

rate possible, thereby permitting more rapid recoupment of the roughly 10 to 15% of body weight usually lost over the first several days of life and possibly reducing the duration of, and hence the cost of, hospitalization. Proponents of the former view advocate feeding human milk because of its alleged non-nutritional benefits, e.g., enhanced maternal infant bonding and protection against infection. They also point out that the lower protein content of human milk is less likely to overwhelm the LBW infant's limited capacity to catabolize excess protein. Proponents of the latter view stress the potential advantages of catch-up growth and point out that protein intakes well in excess of those from human milk do not appear to tax the ability of the LBW infant to catabolize protein.

Results from a multicenter study conducted for the last decade in England are beginning to appear[39] and are likely to provide considerable insight into this longstanding controversy. In this study, infants whose mothers elected to provide milk for feeding her infant were assigned randomly to receive supplements of either banked human milk or formula and infants whose mothers elected not to provide milk were assigned randomly, at some centers, to receive either formula or banked human milk and, at other centers, to receive a preterm or term formula. Thus, to some extent, the usual confounding factor of the mother's intent to breast-feed or not breast-feed her infant was controlled and infants also received a variety of protein intakes. Results published to date indicate that infants fed human milk, either as the sole diet or with formula, have a lower incidence of necrotizing enterocolitis during the neonatal period[40] and also appear to be more resistant to infection.[41] In addition, whereas developmental indices at 18 months of age are higher in infants who received greater protein intakes during the neonatal period,[42] those fed human milk were less adversely affected.[41] On the other hand, length at 9 and 18 months of age was lower in those who had the highest serum alkaline phosphatase activity during the neonatal period (usually those fed human milk[32]).

## ENERGY

It is usually assumed that LBW infants require approximately 120 kcal/kg per day,[44] 75 kcal/kg per day for resting expenditure and the remainder for specific dynamic action (10 kcal/kg), replacement of inevitable stool losses (10 kcal/kg), and growth (25 kcal/kg).

The usual allotment for resting needs (75 kcal/kg per day) includes the basal requirement (about 50 kcal/kg) as well as additional requirements imposed by activity and response to cold stress. However, LBW infants are relatively inactive and, with careful control of environmental temperature, energy expenditure in response to cold stress is minimal. In fact, recent data from relatively inactive infants maintained in a strictly thermoneutral environment suggest that the resting energy requirement is closer to 60 kcal/kg per day.[45–49]

The energy required for specific dynamic action, or the thermic effect of food (i.e., the difference between resting energy expenditure of the fed infant and that of the fasted infant), may be a function of the composition of the diet. At one time, protein intake was considered the primary determinant of this component, but more recent studies suggest that the energy intake may be equally important.[47–49]

Fecal losses of nutrients, especially fat, appear to be inevitable in the fed LBW infant. The extent of these losses is a function of the infant's stage of development and the nature of the fat intake (see subsequent discussion). In infants fed either human milk or modern formulas, stool fat losses rarely exceed 15% of the fat intake, or less than 7.5% of the total energy intake.

The precise energy requirement for growth is unknown. This requirement includes two components, i.e., the energy cost of synthesizing new tissue, which probably is measured as a part of resting expenditure, and the energy value of stored nutrients. Values of 3 to 6 kcal/g weight gain have been reported for the latter component. Because this amount depends on the composition of the newly synthesized tissue (e.g., deposition of calorically dense fat tissue requires more calories than deposition of lean body mass), such a range is to be expected. The calculated energy value of tissue deposited by the fetus between weeks 30 to 38 of gestation is 2.0 to 2.5 kcal/g (see Table 46–5), whereas the calculated energy value of tissue deposited by the normally growing term infant between birth and 4 months of age is approximately 4.5 kcal/g.[50]

Thus, the energy requirement of the LBW infant may range from 95 to 160 kcal/kg per day. Aside from growth, the factors of greatest quantitative importance are the activity state of the infant and the environmental conditions under which it is nursed. For most LBW infants, an energy intake of 120 kcal/kg per day is adequate.

## PROTEIN

The common practice of feeding LBW infants human milk was largely abandoned 40 to 50 years ago after Gordon et al. showed that higher protein intakes resulted in a greater rate of weight gain.[51] However, the formulas used in this study also contained more electrolytes and minerals than human milk, and some suggested that the greater weight gain was related to water retention secondary to the greater electrolyte/mineral intake rather than to the greater protein intake. Indeed, subsequent studies demonstrated that both total body water and extracellular fluid of infants fed high-protein, high-solute intakes were greater than those observed in infants fed low-solute formulas.[52] Nonetheless, a direct relationship exists between protein intake and weight gain.[52–54]

In general, a protein intake of approximately 3 g/kg per day, perhaps somewhat less, appears to be adequate for the LBW infant.[55] On the other hand, higher intakes appear to be well tolerated metabolically and these higher intakes also support a greater rate of weight gain.[54,55] The protein, of course, must be of such quality as to provide sufficient amounts of all essential amino acids, including, for the LBW infant, histidine,[56] tyrosine,[57] and cysteine.[57,58] In this regard, current LBW infant formulas contain "humanized" bovine milk protein (60% whey proteins and 40% caseins). However, despite a higher cyst(e)ine content, little evidence exists that this protein is more efficacious than unmodified bovine milk protein (18% whey protein and 82% caseins), particularly with respect to growth.[59] Of theoretic interest is the fact that plasma threonine concentrations of infants fed "humanized" bovine milk formulas are approximately double those observed in infants fed unmodified bovine milk protein, whereas plasma tyrosine concentrations are higher in infants fed unmodified bovine milk formulas.[59–61]

## FAT

Although fat accounts for about one half of the nonprotein energy content of human milk and most infant formulas, including those designed for LBW infants, the only known requirement for fat in human nutrition is to provide essential fatty acids. Until recently, it was thought that this requirement could be met by provision of 2 to 4% of the total energy intake as linoleic acid, but it is clear that some linolenic acid also is required.[62] In addition, the LBW infant, and perhaps the term infant as well, may not effectively convert linoleic and linolenic acids, respectively, to the longer chain, more unsaturated fatty acids of ω-6 and ω-3 fatty acid families.[63] Because these latter fatty acids rather than linoleic and linolenic acids accumulate in the central nervous system during development,[64,65] the longer chain, polyunsaturated fatty acids may be particularly important nutrients for the LBW infant. No formula now available contains the long-chain polyunsaturated fatty acids of either the ω-6 or the ω-3 fatty acid series, but recent studies suggest they may have beneficial effects.[66,67]

## CARBOHYDRATE

The central nervous system and the hematopoietic tissue depend to a large extent on glucose as a metabolic fuel. However, glucose can be produced from either exogenously administered protein or endogenous protein stores (i.e., gluconeogenesis). Thus, in contrast to requirements for specific amino acids and fatty acids, there appears to be no absolute requirement for carbohydrate. On the other hand, the various gluconeogenic mechanisms of LBW infants are not well developed[68]; thus, exogenous glucose is necessary to prevent hypoglycemia, particularly during the immediate neonatal period.

Carbohydrates, like fat, constitute about one half of the nonprotein energy content of human milk and infant formulas, including those designed for LBW infants. Although the predominant carbohydrate of most natural milks is lactose, LBW infant formulas usually contain a mixture of lactose and glucose polymer (see Table 46–7). Despite the fact that development of intestinal lactase activity lags behind development of other disaccharidases,[69] most viable infants tolerate lactose. In fact, satisfactory clinical progress has been observed with formulas that contain only lactose, only sucrose, only glucose, only glucose polymers, and mixtures of these sugars.

## FLUIDS

Several bases of reference have been suggested for estimating maintenance fluid requirements, e.g., body weight, body surface area, and energy expenditure. Energy expenditure, which focuses attention on the physiologic and nonphysiologic factors most likely to modify fluid requirements (e.g., body temperature, ambient temperature, ambient humidity, activity, and respiratory rate), seems most relevant. In the nongrowing older infant, the maintenance fluid requirement is approximately 1 ml/kcal expended.[70] This allotment replaces insensible water losses through the lungs and skin as well as obligatory renal and gastrointestinal losses.

Insensible water loss varies considerably in all infants, particularly LBW infants. Moreover, both pulmonary and cutaneous components of insensible water loss are related inversely to ambient humidity. Under usual nursery conditions, the insensible water loss of term infants is approximately 30 ml/100 kcal. In the small infant with altered skin permeability to water, cutaneous losses may be considerably greater,[71] although nursing the infant in relatively high humidity probably tends to decrease both this component of insensible fluid loss and pulmonary losses. Phototherapy, used commonly in LBW infants with hyperbilirubinemia, also increases insensible water losses.[72] Thus, the insensible water losses of LBW infants usually are at least twofold greater than those of the term infant.

Obligatory renal losses of LBW infants also are variable. Although even immature infants can regulate the volume of urine excreted according to the solute load and the available water, both renal concentrating and diluting mechanisms are somewhat limited.[73] In general, allowance for a urinary volume of 50 to 60 ml/100 kcal permits excretion of the usual range of solute loads at urine concentrations of 150 to 450 mOsm/L, which are achieved easily, even by an immature kidney.

In unfed infants, fluid losses through the gastrointestinal tract are minimal. If the infant is fed, however, approximately 10% of the fluid intake is lost in stool. Infants receiving phototherapy experience even greater stool losses of water.[72]

The fluid requirement for growth is a function of both the rate of growth and the water content of the newly synthesized tissue. The water content of tissue deposited during the last trimester of gestation is approximately 70% (see Table 46–5), whereas the water content of the tissue deposited by the term infant between birth and 4 months of age is 40 to 45%.[50] An estimate of 50 to 60% for the growing LBW infant seems reasonable.

The water requirements for insensible (30 to 60 ml/100 kcal) and obligatory losses (50 to 60 ml/100 kcal) as well as for growth (10 to 20 ml/100 kcal) are reduced by the endogenously produced water of oxidation, i.e., approximately 12 ml/100 kcal. Thus, the LBW infant, like the term infant, seems to have a minimum water requirement of 1 ml/kcal. The fasting infant, therefore, requires at least 65 to 75 ml/kg per day, whereas the growing infant requires at least 120 ml/kg per day; the immature infant and the infant undergoing phototherapy may require more. In general, a fluid intake of 140 ml/kg per day is well tolerated by most infants after the first few days of life; intakes above this amount are associated with an increased likelihood of developing patent ductus arteriosus.[74]

## ELECTROLYTES

The estimated daily obligatory electrolyte losses of the term infant after the first several days of life are approximately 0.5 mEq/kg of both sodium and chloride and approximately 0.75 mEq/kg of potassium. Because renal reabsorption mechanisms are not fully developed in the LBW infant, their renal losses are likely to be greater. Electrolyte losses probably are greater also in infants with increased fluid losses.

The electrolytes required for tissue synthesis depend on the rate of growth. Assuming continuation of the intrauterine growth rate (see Table 46–5), the daily requirements of these nutrients for tissue synthesis are approximately the amounts that accumulate during the last trimester of gestation, i.e., 1.0 to 1.5 mEq/kg of sodium and 0.5 to 1.0 mEq/kg of both potassium and chloride. If the rate of weight gain is more or less than the intrauterine rate, or if the composition of weight gain is different, the requirements obviously change proportionally.

The minimal daily sodium, potassium, and chloride requirements of the LBW infant receiving adequate protein and energy intakes and growing at the intrauterine rate are, respectively, 1.5 to 2.0 mEq/kg, 1.25 to 1.75 mEq/kg, and 1.0 to 1.5 mEq/kg. The quantities of potassium and chloride present in the volumes of both human milk and commonly used formulas usually ingested are sufficient to provide these requirements. However, the sodium content of human milk (approximately 1.2 mEq/100 kcal), even if completely absorbed, may be insufficient. On the other hand, the growth rate of LBW infants fed human milk is somewhat less than the intrauterine rate; therefore, their sodium requirement for growth probably is less than 1.5 mEq/kg per day. The intakes recommended by the Committee on Nutrition of the American Academy of Pediatrics are considerably greater than these minimal intakes (see Table 46–6).

## MINERALS

Early studies of calcium and phosphorus needs were directed toward defining the intake necessary to prevent hypocalcemia. Because this condition develops more commonly in infants fed formulas with a high content of phosphorus relative to calcium (i.e., a low calcium to phosphorus ratio), emphasis, until recently, was placed on the ratio of calcium to phosphorus intake rather than on absolute amounts of either mineral. Experience has shown that a ratio of roughly 1.5 to 2.0 is satisfactory.

The amount of calcium retained during the latter part of normal intrauterine growth is approximately 2.5 to 3.0 mmol/kg per day. The calcium content of human milk is sufficient to provide less than 1.0 mmol/kg per day, and this amount is not completely absorbed. Thus. if the calcium requirement of the LBW infant is assumed to be the amount necessary to allow continuation of the rate of accumulation that occurs in utero, human milk obviously contains inadequate calcium. The phosphorus content of human milk also is low. Moreover, LBW infants fed human milk have less dense skeletons radiographically than those fed formulas containing large amounts of calcium; many, in fact, develop rickets and/or fractures.[75] Thus, LBW infants fed human milk, including those fed their own mother's milk, require supplemental calcium and phosphorus for optimal skeletal mineralization.

Iron requirements depend on the existing body stores and the rate of growth. The LBW infant obviously has more limited stores of iron than the term infant and, therefore, is more susceptible to the development of iron deficiency, especially during periods of rapid growth. It has been estimated that the endogenous iron stores of the LBW infant, in the absence of exogenous intake, will be depleted sometime during the second or third month of life rather than during the fourth or fifth month of life as occurs in the term infant. However, most LBW infants experience further depletion of iron stores secondary to blood losses incident to biochemical monitoring during periods of clinical instability. Thus, the LBW infant should receive iron supplements or iron-fortified formulas as early as possible. Such supplements, however, may increase the infant's susceptibility to vitamin E deficiency,[76] especially when formulas high in polyunsaturated fatty acids are used (see subsequent section). In addition, the bactericidal properties of the iron-binding proteins of human milk (i.e., lactoferrin and lactoglobulin) are abolished if saturated with iron.[77] In light of these considerations, formulas that contain moderate amounts of polyunsaturated fats and ample vitamin E perhaps should be supplemented with only 1 mg of iron/100 kcal.[78] Current LBW infant formulas contain 0.37 to 1.88 mg/100 kcal (see Table 46–7).

Little information is available concerning the requirements of LBW infants for other trace minerals. In general, the recommended intakes of these minerals are based on either the amounts provided by human milk or the amounts recommended for term infants.

The American Academy of Pediatrics Committee on Nutrition recommends that formulas for term infants contain 0.5 mg of zinc/100 kcal.[79] This level of zinc intake, assuming 50% absorption from the gastrointestinal tract, should allow accumulation of zinc at the intrauterine rate. The concentration of zinc in human milk is approximately 3 to 5 mg/L; thus, it provides minimally adequate zinc to allow accumulation at the intrauterine rate. On the other hand, the zinc content of human milk is absorbed more efficiently than that of bovine milk.[80]

The iodine content of formulas for term infants recommended by the American Academy of Pediatrics Committee on Nutrition is 5 μg/100 kcal,[79] the iodine content of human milk. Because the uptake of radioiodine by the thyroid of LBW infants is in the same range as that of term infants, older children, and adults, this recommended intake is probably adequate.[81]

The recommended copper content of infant formulas is 60 μg/100 kcal.[79] Although this intake might not allow accumulation of copper at the intrauterine rate, it is approximately the amount present in human milk. Although some recommend a higher copper intake for

LBW infants, such intakes probably are not necessary because of the large hepatic stores of copper.

## VITAMINS

Specific recommendations concerning either requirements or advisable allowances of vitamins for LBW infants are not available; thus, it is usually suggested that the RDA for term infants be given. Infants fed sufficient amounts of either human milk or artificial formulas to produce adequate growth usually receive sufficient amounts of all vitamins, although human milk may be deficient in vitamin D. Nonetheless, because the consumption of sufficient volumes of formula to satisfy vitamin requirements may not be attained for several weeks, use of a supplement containing vitamins A, C, and D is recommended. In addition, the LBW infant may have special needs for vitamin E and folic acid.

Vitamin E functions as an antioxidant to prevent peroxidation of polyunsaturated fatty acids in various cell membranes. Thus, inadequate vitamin E intake not surprisingly results in erythrocyte hemolysis.[82] Because the polyunsaturated fatty acid content of all membranes is related to intake of these fatty acids, infant formulas containing vegetable oils of high polyunsaturated fatty acid content impose a greater vitamin E requirement. Such formulas, therefore, should have a higher vitamin E content. In general, the aim should be to provide at least 1 IU of vitamin E per gram of polyunsaturated fatty acids, i.e., a vitamin E to polyunsaturated fatty acid ratio of 1.

LBW infants fed formulas containing polyunsaturated fats and given therapeutic doses of iron also have a greater incidence of erythrocyte hemolysis and lower serum vitamin E levels than infants fed formulas containing less iron and polyunsaturated fats.[83] Thus, the relationship between the vitamin E and iron contents of the formula as well as the relationship between the vitamin E and polyunsaturated fat contents of the formula are important. For this reason, vitamin E intake warrants careful attention if iron supplements are given.

Large doses of vitamin E have been recommended to prevent both retrolental fibroplasia[84] and bronchopulmonary dysplasia.[85] However, these recommendations may not be warranted, particularly considering the potential toxicity of such large doses.

Folic acid functions as a coenzyme in many metabolic reactions including the synthesis of purines and pyrimidines; thus, it is essential for production of new cells. Studies of folate metabolism in preterm infants show that serum concentrations fall from approximately normal adult levels at birth to levels below this range by a few weeks of age, remain low until around 3 months of age, and then rise again to normal adult values. Although this decrease in serum folate concentration can be prevented by daily oral supplements of 50 μg, neither growth nor hemoglobin concentration of supplemented infants differs from that of unsupplemented infants.[86] Unsupplemented infants, however, have more hypersegmented neutrophils and lower erythrocyte folate levels. Thus, the recommendation that LBW infants receive supplemental folic acid (50 μg daily) is endorsed.[87]

## DELIVERY OF NUTRIENT REQUIREMENTS

For most LBW infants, the foregoing discussion of nutrient requirements is largely academic. Underlying illnesses as well as neurophysiologic deficiencies (e.g., poor or unsustained suck, uncoordinated sucking and swallowing mechanisms, delayed gastric emptying, and poor intestinal motility) make delivery of enteral nutrition virtually impossible, particularly during the early neonatal period. During this time, a nutritional regimen that prevents catabolism and allows some increment in lean body mass probably is satisfactory. This more realistic goal for the first several days of life can be achieved in sick LBW infants with a parenteral regimen that provides as few as 60 kcal/kg per day, an amino acid intake of 2.0 to 2.5 g/kg per day, and necessary electrolytes, minerals, and vitamins.[88] A similar regimen delivered enterally should be equally efficacious, provided intestinal absorption is not severely compromised.

Various methods of delivering nutrients intravenously (total parenteral nutrition) as well as methods of delivering feedings by the gastrointestinal tract (e.g., continuous nasogastric or transpyloric infusions) have been proposed as alternatives to more conventional feeding techniques. Although no one method is likely to be ideal for all situations, use of a combination of these methods of nutrient delivery, allowing the particular clinical problems of an individual infant to dictate the method of delivery, should improve nutritional management. In many infants, a combination of conventional as well as these less conventional methods of feeding permits delivery of sufficient nutrients to support "normal" growth by 1 to 2 weeks of age.

Within reason, every infant should have a trial of conventional feeding, i.e., tolerated nipple or gavage feedings of either human milk or a standard preterm infant formula, plus intravenous supplementation with 5 to 10% glucose solutions. If adequate nutrients cannot be delivered in this way, a trial of continuous nasogastric or transpyloric feedings is warranted. Tolerated enteral feedings delivered conventionally or by continuous infusion also can be supplemented by intravenous infusions of appropriate mixtures of glucose, amino acids, and/or lipid. In the event that enteral feedings are not tolerated, parenteral administration of a balanced nutritional mixture is indicated. A regimen that provides 75 kcal/kg per day plus amino acids, electrolytes, minerals, and vitamins can be delivered by peripheral vein infusion without imposing an unreasonable fluid load. Such a regimen almost certainly maintains existing body composition and, hence, is particularly applicable for infants who are likely to tolerate enteral intake within a brief period of time. Use of a central vein catheter allows delivery of a more concentrated nutrient mixture and is particularly useful in situations associated with prolonged intolerance of enteral feedings.

### ROLE OF HUMAN MILK IN FEEDING

Although many advocate human milk for feeding the LBW infant, evidence that it is nutritionally superior for this population is lacking. In fact, the growth rate of LBW infants fed human milk, even that of infants fed their own mother's milk, which has an approximately 20% higher protein concentration than term human milk,[89] is lower than that of infants fed LBW formulas.[90] Moreover, plasma albumin and transthyretin concentrations often fall to frankly low values.[91] In addition, the low amounts of calcium and phosphorus do not support adequate skeletal mineralization.

In contrast to the nutritional disadvantages of human milk for the LBW infant, its immunologic properties may be a distinct advantage. These properties (i.e., cellular as well as humoral components) theoretically confer passive immunity and/or enhance immunologic maturation, thereby providing some protection against infections and, perhaps, necrotizing enterocolitis. Recent studies show that the incidence of both infection[44] and necrotizing enterocolitis[40] are lower in infants fed either banked human milk or their own mother's milk. If confirmed, these advantages of human milk may far outweigh its nutritional disadvantages.

The steps involved in collection, storage, and dispensing of expressed human milk make inadvertent contamination likely. Thus, stringent hygienic techniques and bacterial screening are mandatory to ensure bacteriologic safety. Viral contamination also is a major concern. For example, cytomegalovirus (CMV) excretion in the milk of seropositive women is relatively common,[92] and CMV infection has been reported in infants fed CMV-positive milk.[93] Moreover, one case of human immunodeficiency virus (HIV) infection transmitted by human milk has been reported.[94] Herpes and rubella viruses and hepatitis B surface antigen also have been detected in human milk, but transmission of these viruses by milk has not been demonstrated.

More research is necessary to elucidate the role of human milk, provided by either the mother or a donor (or donors), in feeding the LBW infant. This research should be well underway before enormous expense and effort are spent in establishing milk banks to supply safe human milk for routine feeding of LBW infants. On the other hand, if an individual mother wishes to provide milk for her infant, the potential psychologic benefits of her involvement in the infant's care as well as the benefits with respect to eventual success in breast-feedings are strong reasons for encouraging milk expression until the infant can be breast-fed. Moreover, two commercial preparations for supplementing human milk with protein, calcium, phosphorus, sodium, and vitamins are available, and use of these supplements appears to overcome the nutritional inadequacies of human milk.

## REFERENCES


1. Food and Nutrition Board, National Research Council: Recommended Dietary allowances. 10th Ed. Washington, D.C., National Academy Press, 1989.
2. Holt, L.E., Jr., Snyderman, S.E.: JAMA, *175:*100–103, 1961.
3. Fomon, S.J., Thomas, L.N., Filer, L.J., et al.: Acta Pediatr. Scand., *62:*33–45, 1973.
4. Räihä, N.C.R.: Pediatrics, *75:*136–141, 1985.
5. Holliday, M.A.: Do dietary factors in the 6 to 12 month period of life affect blood pressure later in life? *In* Nutritional Needs of the Six to Twelve Month Old Infant. Edited by W.C. Heird. New York, Raven Press, 1991.
6. American Academy of Pediatrics Committee on Nutrition: Pediatrics, *58:*765–768, 1976.
7. Lakdewala, D.R., Widdowson, E.M.: Lancet, *1:*167–168, 1977.
8. Committee on Nutrition, American Academy of Pediatrics: Pediatrics, *65:*657–658, 1980.
9. Minton, S.D., Steichen, J.J., Tsang, R.C.: J. Pediatr., *95:*1037–1042, 1979.
10. Cunningham, A.J.: Morbidity in breast-fed and artificially fed infants. J. Pediatr., *90:*726–729, 1977.
11. Heird, W.C.: Nutritional Needs of the Six to Twelve-Month-Old Infant. New York, Raven Press, 1991.
12. Whitehead, R.G., Paul, A.A.: Dietary energy needs from 6 to 12 months of age. *In* Nutritional Needs of the Six to Twelve-Month-Old Infant. Edited by W.C. Heird. New York, Raven Press, 1991.
13. Montgomery, R.K.: Functional development of the gastrointestinal tract the small intestine. *In* Nutritional Needs of the Six to Twelve-Month-Old Infant. Edited by W.C. Heird. New York, Raven Press, 1991.
14. Mandel, I.D.: The nutritional impact on dental caries. *In* Nutritional Needs of the Six to Twelve-Month-Old Infant. Edited by W.C. Heird. New York, Raven Press, 1991.
15. Purvis, G.A., Bartholmey, S.J.: Infant feeding practices: Commercially prepared baby foods. *In* Nutrition During Infancy. Edited by R. Tsang, B. Nichols. Philadelphia, Hanley & Belfus, 1988.
16. American Academy of Pediatrics, Committee on Nutrition: Pediatrics, *72:*253–255, 1983.
17. Ryan, A.S., Martinez, G.A., Kreiger, F.W.: Am. J. Phys. Anthropol., *73:*539–548, 1987.
18. Martinez, G.A., Ryan, A.S., Malec, D.J.: Am. J. Dis. Child., *139:*1010–1018, 1985.
19. Crawford, M.A., Stassam, A.G., Stevens, P.A.: Prog. Lipid Res., *20:*31–40, 1981.

20. Davis, C.M.: Am. J. Dis. Child., *36:*651–679, 1928.
21. Birch, L.I., Johnson, S.I., Andersen, G., et al.: N. Engl. J. Med., *324:*232–235, 1991.
22. Weidman, W., Kwiterovich, P. Jr., Jesse, M.J., et al.: Circulation, *67:*1411A–1414A, 1983.
23. Wynder, E.L., Berenson, G.S., Epstein, F.H., et al.: Prev. Med., *12:*728–740, 1983.
24. Consensus Development Panel: JAMA, *253:*2080–2086, 1985.
25. American Academy of Pediatrics Committee on Nutrition: Pediatrics, *78:*521–525, 1986.
26. Ross, R., Glomset, J.A.: N. Engl. J. Med. (Part I), *295:*369–377, 1976; (Part II) *295:*420–425, 1976.
27. Small, D.M.: N. Engl. J. Med. (Part I) *297:*873–877, 1977; (Part II) *297:*924–929, 1977.
28. McNamara, J.J., Molot, M.A., Stremple, J.F., et al.: JAMA, *216:*1185–1187, 1971.
29. Enos, W.F., Holmes, R.H., Beyer, J.: JAMA, *152:*1090–1093, 1953.
30. Health United States 1984: U.S. Department of Health and Human Services Publication No. 851232. Washington, D.C., Government Printing Office, 1984.
31. Ziegler, E.E., O'Donnell, A.M., Nelson, S.E., et al.: Growth, *40:*329–340, 1976.
32. Heird, W.C.: Nutritional support of the pediatric patient including the low birth weight infant. *In* Nutritional Support of the Seriously Ill Patient. Edited by R.W. Winters and H.C. Greene. New York, Academic Press, 1983.
33. Fish, I., Winick, M.: Exp. Neurol., *25:*534–570, 1969.
34. Winick, M., Rosso, P.: Pediatr. Res., *3:*181–184, 1969.
35. Winick, M., Rosso, P., Waterlow, J.: Exp. Neurol., *26:*293–300, 1970.
36. Grantham-McGregor, S.M., Powell, C.A., Walker, S.P., et al.: Lancet, *338:*1–5, 1991.
37. Ross, G., Lipper, E.G., Auld, P.A.M.: Pediatrics, *76:*885–891, 1985.
38. American Academy of Pediatrics Committee on Nutrition: Pediatrics, *75:*976–986, 1985.
39. Lucas, A., Gore, S.M., Cole, T.J., et al.: Arch. Dis. Child., *59:*722–730, 1984.
40. Lucas, A., Cole, T.J.: Lancet, *336:*1519–1523, 1990.
41. Lucas, A.: Personal communication, 1991.
42. Lucas, A., Morley, R., Cole, T.J.: Lancet, *335:*1477–1481, 1990.
43. Lucas, A., Brooke, O.G., Baker, B.A., et al.: Arch. Dis. Child., *64:*902–909, 1989.
44. Heird, W.C.: Parenteral feeding. *In* Effective Care of the Newborn Infant. Edited by J.C. Sinclair, J.F. Lacey. Oxford, Oxford University Press. In press.
45. Whyte, R.K., Haslam, R., Vlainic, L., et al.: Pediatr. Res., *17:*891–898, 1983.
46. Reichman, B.L., Chessex, P., Putet, G., et al.: Pediatrics, *69:*446–451, 1982.
47. Schulze, K.F., Stefanski, M., Masterson, J., et al.: J. Pediatr., *110:*753–759, 1987.
48. Van Aerde, J., Sauer, P., Heim, T., et al.: Pediatr. Res., *13:*215–220, 1985.
49. Brooke, O.G., Alvear, J., Arnold, M.: Pediatr. Res., *13:*215–220, 1969.
50. Fomon, S.J.: Pediatrics, *40:*863–870, 1967.
51. Gordon, H.H., Levine, S.Z., McNamara, H.: Am. J. Dis. Child., *73:*442–452, 1947.
52. Kagan, B.M., Stanicova, V., Felix, N.S., et al.: Am. J. Clin. Nutr., *25:*1153–1167, 1972.
53. Davidson, M., Levine, S.Z., Bauer, C.H., et al.: J. Pediatr., *70:*694–713, 1967.
54. Kashyap, S., Forsyth, M., Zucker, C., et al.: J. Pediatr., *108:*955–963, 1986.
55. Kashyap, S., Schulze, K.F., Forsyth, M., et al.: J. Pediatr., *113:*713–721, 1988.
56. Snyderman, S.E., Boyer, A., Rothman, E., et al.: Pediatrics, *31:*786–801, 1963.
57. Snyderman, S.E.: The protein and amino acid requirements of the premature infant. *In* Metabolic Processes in the Fetus and Newborn Infant. Edited by J.H.P. Jonxis, H.K.A. Visser, J.A. Troelstra. Leiden, Steinfert Kruesse, 1971.
58. Sturman, J.A., Gaull, G.E., Räihä, N.C.R.: Science, *169:*74–76, 1970.
59. Kashyap, S., Okamoto, E., Kanaya, S., et al.: Pediatrics, *79:*748–755, 1987.
60. Rassin, D.K., Gaull, G.E., Heinonen, K., et al.: Pediatrics, *59:*407–422, 1977.
61. Rassin, D.K., Gaull, G.E., Räihä, N.C.R., et al.: J. Pediatr., *90:*356–360, 1977.
62. Holman, R.T., Johnson, S.B., Hateh, T.F.: Am. J. Clin. Nutr., *35:*617–623, 1982.
63. Carlson, S.E., Rhodes, P.G., Ferguson, M.G.: Am. J. Clin. Nutr., *44:*798–804, 1986.
64. Clandinin, M.T., Chappell, J.E., Leong, S., et al.: Early Hum. Dev., *4:*121–129, 1980.
65. Clandinin, M.T., Chappell, J.E., Leong, S., et al.: Early Hum. Dev., *4:*131–138, 1980.
66. Uauy, R.D., Birch, D.G., Birch, E.E., et al.: Pediatr. Res., *28:*485–492, 1990.
67. Carlson, S.E., Cooke, R.J., Rhodes, P.G., et al.: Pediatr. Res., *30:*404–412, 1991.
68. Williams, P.R., Fiser, R.H., Sperling, M.A., et al.: N. Engl. J. Med., *292:*612–614, 1975.
69. Boellner, S.W., Beard, A.G., Panos, T.C.: Pediatrics, *36:*542–550, 1965.
70. Wallace, W.M.: Am. J. Clin. Pathol., *23:*1133–1141, 1953.
71. Hammerlund, K., Nilsson, G.E., Oberg, P.A., et al.: Acta Pediatr. Scand., *72:*721–728, 1973.
72. Oh, W., Kareoki, H.: Am. J. Dis. Child., *124:*130–132, 1972.
73. Aperia, A., Broberger, O., Herin, P., et al.: Acta Pediatr. Scand. (Suppl.), *305:*61–65, 1983.
74. Stevenson, J.G.: J. Pediatr., *90:*257–261, 1977.
75. Steichen, J.J., Gratton, T.L., Tsang, R.C.: J. Pediatr., *96:*528–534, 1980.
76. Melborn, D.K., Gross, S.: J. Pediatr., *79:*569–580, 1971.
77. Bullen, J.J., Rogers, H.J., Leigh, L.: Br. Med. J., *1:*69–75, 1972.
78. Lundstrom, U., Siimes, M.D., Dallman, P.R.: J. Pediatr., *91:*878–883, 1977.
79. American Academy of Pediatrics Committee on Nutrition: Pediatrics, *57:*278–289, 1976.
80. Sanstrom, B., Cedeblad, A., Lonnerdal, B.: Am. J. Dis. Child., *137:*726–729, 1983.
81. Martmer, E.E., Corrigan, K.E., Charbeneau, H.P., et al.: Pediatrics, *17:*1956.
82. Oski, F.A., Barness, L.A.: J. Pediatr., *70:*211–220, 1967.
83. Williams, M.L., Shoot, R.J., O'Neal, P.L., et al.: N. Engl. J. Med., *292:*887–890, 1975.
84. Mintz-Hittner, H., Godio, L.B., Rudolph, A.J., et al.: N. Engl. J. Med., *305:*1366–1371, 1981.
85. Ehrenkranz, R.A., Bonta, B.W., Ablow, R.C., Warshaw, J.B.: N. Engl. J. Med., *299:*564–569, 1978.

**86.** Burland, W.L., Simpson, K., Lord, J.: Arch. Dis. Child., *46:*189–194, 1971.
**87.** Dallman, P.R.: J. Pediatr., *85:*742–752, 1974.
**88.** Anderson, T.L., Muttart, C.R., Bieber, M.A., et al.: J. Pediatr., *94:*947–951, 1979.
**89.** Atkinson, S.A., Anderson, G.H., Bryan, M.H.: Am. J. Clin. Nutr., *33:*811–815, 1980.
**90.** Gross, S.J.: N. Engl. J. Med., *308:*237–241, 1983.
**91.** Kashyap, S., Schulze, K.F., Forsyth, M., et al.: Am. J. Clin. Nutr., *52:*254–262, 1990.
**92.** Stagno, S., Reynolds, D.W., Pass, R.F., et al.: N. Engl. J. Med., *302:*1073–1076, 1980.
**93.** Ballard, R.A., Drew, W.L., Hufnagle, K.G., et al.: Am. J. Dis. Child. *133:*482–485, 1979.
**94.** Ziegler, J.R., Cooper, D.A., Johnson, R.O., et al.: Lancet, *1:*896–897, 1985.

CHAPTER 47

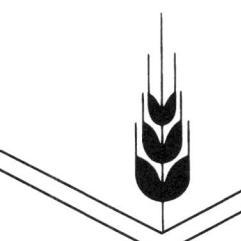

# Diet, Nutrition, and Adolescence

**Elizabeth J. Gong and Felix P. Heald**



The nutritional requirements of adolescents are influenced primarily by the normal events of puberty and the simultaneous spurt of growth. Puberty is an intensely anabolic period, with increases in height and weight, alterations in body composition resulting from increased lean body mass and changes in the quantity and distribution of fat, and enlargement of many organ systems. Adolescence is a unique period of development of physiologic, psychosocial, and cognitive levels, all of which impact on the nutritional needs of the adolescent. The teenager is a rapidly changing biologic organism, and so the nutritional management of adolescents must consider the rapid growth, maturation, and psychosocial changes of each individual. Three aspects of growth must be emphasized: the intensity and extent of the pubertal growth spurt; the sexual differences in the timing of growth, as well as the nature of change of body composition; and individual variation in the timing of the pubertal growth spurt.

The velocity of growth exerts a major influence on nutrient requirements. Adolescence is the only time in extrauterine life when growth velocity increases. The average American female experiences her most rapid spurt in linear growth between ages 10 and 13 years; the growth spurt of the average American male occurs about 2 years later, between 12 and 15 years. This time is frequently termed the period of maximum growth, and for both height and weight, it is greatest in girls in the year preceding menarche. The linear spurt during adolescence contributes about 15% to final adult height; its contribution to the adult weight is approximately 50%. Therefore, nutrition clearly plays a significant role in the doubling of body mass during pubescence. Because nutritional requirements are closely related to the rapid increase in body mass, it is of little surprise that peak nutritional requirements appear to occur during the year of maximum growth.

Although both adolescent males and females gain significant weight, gender-related differences exist with respect to the rate, quantity, composition, and distribution of tissues. During adolescence, boys tend to gain more weight at a faster rate, and their skeletal growth continues for a longer period of time than that of adolescent girls. Girls deposit relatively more total body fat; boys deposit more muscle mass. Patterns of body composition and distribution diverge during adolescence. Boys become leaner and paradoxically increase the number of actual adipose tissue cells while decreasing the percentage contribution of fat to total body mass. Girls have a steep rate of increase in actual fat deposition as well as an increase in the percentage of fat to total body mass and an increase in lean body mass. As a result of pubertal changes, males have a larger lean body mass, a larger skeleton, and less adipose tissue as total body mass than females. As lean body mass has more active metabolic function than adipose tissue, sex differences in body composition produce sex differences in the nutritional requirements of adolescents.[1,2]

The large individual variance in the time at which the growth spurt begins, as well as the intensity of growth, makes chronologic age a poor index of nutritional requirements. Physiologic growth, or maturational age, is a better indicator for establishing requirements or evaluating intakes. Figure 47–1 illustrates three normal males and three normal females in prepubertal, midpubertal, and postpubertal stages of development.[3] Al-

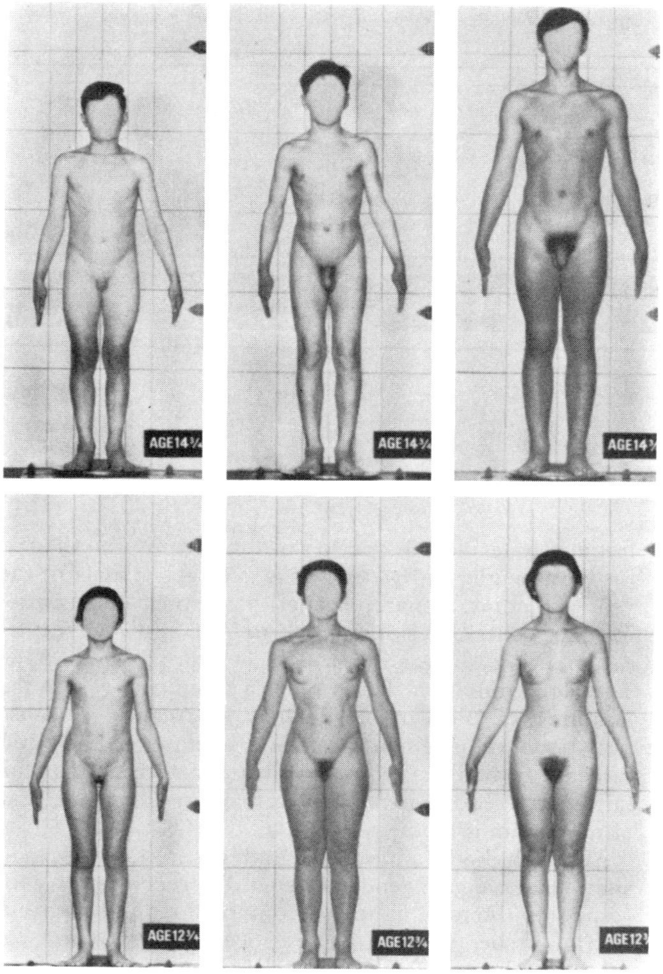
AGE 14¼
AGE 14¼
AGE 14¼
AGE 12¾
AGE 12¾
AGE 12¾

**FIGURE 47–1.** Differing degrees of adolescence at the same chronologic age. Top, Three boys all aged 14.25 years. Bottom, Three girls all aged 12.75 years. (From Tanner, J.M.: Growth and endocrinology of the adolescent. *In* Endocrine and Genetic Diseases of Children and Adolescents. 2nd Ed. Edited by L.I. Gardner. Philadelphia, W.B. Saunders, 1975.)

though each group is at the same chronologic age, each individual is at different physiologic age; each adolescent has a different rate of growth and different body composition, both important determinants of nutrient needs. Standards for assessing physiologic age have been developed. Tanner's Sexual Maturity Ratings are used widely clinically and are helpful in describing the stage of development of individual adolescents.[4]

## NUTRITIONAL REQUIREMENTS

Few actual data from adolescents are available on which to base the recommendations for their nutrient needs. Most recommendations are based on estimates of intakes associated with good health and growth, extrapolations from animal research, or interpolation from studies on children and adults. The most recent recommended dietary allowances (RDA) of the Food and Nutrition Board of the National Research Council for adolescents are given in terms of weight, sex, and age (4-year intervals, except for the age group 19 to 24 years; this age class has been extended in the 1989 RDA because peak bone mass probably is not attained before the age of 25 years).[5]

### ENERGY

The caloric requirements for the growing adolescent have not been studied enough to give an accurate expression of the energy needs of individual teenagers.

Some of the best data come from a study done by Wait, Blair, and Roberts.[6] Energy intake data from bomb calorimetry determinations support the thesis that the relationship of total calories to height or calories per unit of height per age were the preferred indices for determining caloric needs. From these observations, as well as supporting findings of Widdowson,[7] it appears that increments in height during adolescence may best represent the anabolic effect of this growth period.

The practical application of determining individual requirements using the kilocalorie per centimeter has been described. The RDA calculated on kilocalorie per centimeter of height for males and females are shown in Table 47–1.

In a group of normally growing teenagers followed longitudinally, Beal noted that for some teens, actual energy intake fell outside the range of the RDA.[8] Thus, even when using the parameter for calculating calories best supported by data (kcal/cm height), the margin of error is considerable. Nevertheless, kilocalorie per centimeter height may represent the best way of calculating individual energy requirements of adolescents at the present time.

A review of studies of energy intake of children and adolescents in the United States shows that girls appear to consume their peak caloric intake, about 2550 kcal, at the time of menarche (around 12 years). This peak demand is followed by a slow decline. In boys, the caloric intake appears to parallel the adolescent growth spurt, increasing until age 16 years to approximately 3400 kcal and then decreasing by 500 kcal by age 19 years.[9]

The most accepted way of assessing adequacy of energy intake is to evaluate growth and body composition. The normal variability of pubertal growth patterns makes ideal weight during puberty an untenable concept. A common practice is to plot height and weight on the National Center for Health Statistics (NCHS) growth chart with the percentiles for each age group.[10] This plot tells us the relative position of that teenager to the NCHS sample.[11] The growth data gathered in the NCHS survey published in 1973 form the basis for the growth charts currently used in the United States[11] (see Appendix Tables A–12d and A–12e). If multiple measurements over time are available, any significant changes in rates of linear growth or body mass can be detected by percentile shifts. However, the teenager in the 90th percentile for height may or may not be appropriately in the 90th percentile for weight. For example, a male at the 90th percentile weight for height with a triceps skinfold in the lower percentiles would be muscular. Another teenager in the 90th percentile weight for height with a triceps skinfold in the 75th percentile would be classified as obese (survey data summarized in Appendix Tables A–14a-1 to A–14a-4).

To determine appropriate weight-for-height for an adolescent and assess whether he or she has an excess or deficiency in energy intake, the Height and Weight of Youths 12–17 Years, United States[11] tables (Appendix Tables A–12f-1 to A–12f-6) are often used clinically. The data are problematic (such as sample size, lack of references to sexual maturity, ethnic differences, etc.), although the tables separate the percentiles of weight by age, sex, and height, providing a range of weights for a particular height and age. With the additional information gained from triceps percentiles (Appendix Tables A–14a-1 to A–14a-4), an assessment of obesity (triceps skinfold> 75th percentile) or underweight (triceps skinfold <25th percentile) can be made.

The National Center for Health data have been analyzed in such a sophisticated way that accurate assessment of growth and simple measures of body composition are available to measure the impact of energy excess or scarcity on the growing teenager. We must be aware, however, that the effects of marginal energy deficits have a subtle effect on growth. The work of Dreizen et al.[12] is one of the few studies in the United States describing the long-term effect of chronic mild malnutrition on growth. The net effect over time was to diminish the rate of growth during late childhood and adolescence and delay puberty by 2 years, but ultimately this group of malnourished youths in southeastern United States reached similar heights and weights as those of a comparison group. Keeping in mind the great variation in timing and intensity of growth seen in adolescents, we must empha-

**TABLE 47–1.** RECOMMENDED ENERGY INTAKES FOR ADOLESCENTS

| AGE (years) | AVERAGE ALLOWANCE (kcal/cm height)* | AVERAGE ALLOWANCE (kcal/day) |
|---|---|---|
| Males | | |
| 11–14 | 15.9 | 2500 |
| 15–18 | 17.0 | 3000 |
| 19–24 | 16.4 | 2900 |
| Females | | |
| 11–14 | 14.0 | 2200 |
| 15–18 | 13.5 | 2200 |
| 19–24 | 13.4 | 2200 |

*Average energy allowance (kilo-calories) and median height (cm) for the age group (Recommended Dietary Allowances, 1989).[5]

size the large variation in caloric intake in this group. Physical activity also contributes significantly to the total energy requirement of an individual, as does previous growth and nutritional status. When considering the energy requirements of adolescents, the importance of individual variation from one adolescent to another must be recognized in making nutritional recommendations. Table 47–2 presents energy expenditure, expressed in three different body weights, for different activities.[13] The different activities have highly variable energy costs and can be used to guide dietary advice or weight management. (Appendix Table A–8c compares calculated average energy expenditure and observed intakes in comparison with the WHO Committee for adolescents.)

## PROTEIN

As in energy recommendations, protein needs for an adolescent can be more useful when physiologic age is considered over chronologic age. Using the RDA for protein as it is related to height is probably the most useful method for determining protein needs for adolescents.[5] For adolescent males, the daily protein recommendation is 0.29, 0.34, and 0.33 g/cm height for the age groups 11 to 14, 15 to 18, and 19 to 24 years, respectively. For adolescent females, the daily recommendation is 0.29. 0.27, and 0.28 g/cm height for the age groups 11 to 14, 15 to 18, and 19 to 24 years, respectively. The requirement for protein is determined by the amount needed for maintenance plus that needed for growth of new tissue, which during adolescence may represent a substantial portion of the total need. Unfortunately, data on either of these determinants of requirements are lacking in adolescents and have been interpolated from results of studies involving infants and adults.[5,14]

The RDA for daily protein intake for adolescents ranges from 44 to 59 g.[5] Peak intakes of protein coincide with the peak in energy intake. The proportion of total energy intake represented by protein remains fairly constant, between 12 and 14%, throughout childhood and adolescence.[9]

Results of studies show that average intakes of protein in adolescents are above the recommended levels.[9,15,16] Although it appears most adolescents in the United States have sufficient intake of protein, some teenagers who restrict food intake because of a desire to lose weight, eating disorders such as anorexia nervosa and bulimia, or socioeconomic problems, may be at risk of poor protein intake. Without adequate caloric intake, protein is in gluconeogenesis and is unavailable for tissue synthesis. Heald and Hunt demonstrated that in the rapidly growing adolescent, protein metabolism is particularly sensitive to caloric restriction.[17]

Anthropometric measurements generally are simple to perform in order to assess protein status. Height, weight, and midarm circumference measurements (used to assess lean body mass) can be used as indicators of growth. Midarm circumference measurements and arm muscle area between the 25th and 75th percentiles probably represent good nutritional status.[18]

Biochemical assessments of protein nutriture include creatinine/height index and serum concentrations of certain proteins: albumin, transferrin, prealbumin, and retinol binding protein.[19–22] Determinations of prealbumin and retinol-binding protein are the most sensitive indicators of changes in diet that may indicate subclinical malnutrition.[22–25] A detailed evaluation of assessment procedures is given in Chapter 51.

## MINERALS

Because of the adolescent growth spurt, the need for three minerals is of particular importance: calcium to sustain increased skeletal mass, iron to aid expansion of

**TABLE 47–2.** ENERGY EXPENDITURE OF SELECTED ACTIVITIES (CALORIES EXPENDED/MINUTE ACTIVITY)

| ACTIVITY | kcal/min/kg | 45 kg | 55 kg | 65 kg |
|---|---|---|---|---|
| Basketball | 0.138 | 6.2 | 7.6 | 9.0 |
| Cycling 5.5 mph | 0.064 | 2.9 | 3.5 | 4.2 |
| 9.4 mph | 0.100 | 4.5 | 5.5 | 6.5 |
| Dancing (twist) | 0.168 | 7.6 | 9.2 | 10.9 |
| Football | 0.132 | 5.9 | 7.3 | 8.6 |
| Running 11.5 min./mile | 0.135 | 6.1 | 7.4 | 8.8 |
| 8 min./mile | 0.208 | 9.4 | 11.4 | 13.6 |
| Sitting quietly | 0.021 | 0.9 | 1.2 | 1.4 |
| Walking, normal pace | 0.080 | 3.6 | 4.4 | 5.2 |
| Writing, sitting | 0.029 | 1.3 | 1.6 | 1.9 |
| Vacuuming females | 0.045 | 2.0 | 2.5 | 2.9 |
| males | 0.048 | 2.2 | 2.6 | 3.1 |
| Ironing females | 0.033 | 1.5 | 1.8 | 2.1 |
| males | 0.064 | 2.9 | 3.5 | 4.2 |

(Adapted from McArdle, W.D., Katch, F.I., Katch, V.L.: Exercise Physiology: Energy, Nutrition, and Human Performance. Philadelphia, Lea & Febiger, 1981.)

red cell and muscle mass, and zinc to generate new skeletal and muscle tissues. In addition to significant increases in need, intake of these nutrients has been shown to be below the recommended levels for adolescents.[15,16,26–28]

The calcium intake of boys is higher than that for girls and is closer to achieving the recommended intakes.[29] Daily iron intakes as reported by the Ten State Nutrition Survey were relatively lower. Most (80%) of the girls 10 to 16 years of age were below the recommended 18 mg iron per day.[15] Some evidence shows an association between low concentrations of zinc in hair and poor growth. An analysis of food intake suggests poor eating habits.[30] The full extent of zinc deficiency and its adverse effect on puberty needs more inquiry.

### *CALCIUM*

With approximately 99% of the total body calcium in the skeleton,[31] the adolescent growth spurt associated with increased skeletal length and mass obviously has a significant impact on dietary requirements for calcium. Skeletal growth during adolescence accounts for approximately 45% of the adult skeletal mass. Because the absolute amount of calcium in the skeleton of a boy in the 95th percentile for height compared to that for another boy in the 5th percentile for height will differ by 36%, the calcium needs of these two boys will differ sharply because of the difference in skeletal size. The problem is compounded further by the normal differences in pubertal development, making age and sex alone poor predictors of individual calcium needs. Lastly, growth of the skeletal mass and gains in height and muscle mass continue after adolescence until the third decade of life.[32,33] Table 47–3 shows the average increments of body calcium for adolescence, as compared to the amount of daily increments of body calcium at the peak of the growth spurt.[34] At the peak of growth, the daily deposition of calcium is approximately double that for the average increment during the adolescent period. The daily peak increment of calcium during the growth spurt is greater, occurs later, and lasts longer in boys than in girls.[31]

**TABLE 47–3.** DAILY INCREMENTS IN BODY CONTENT DUE TO GROWTH

| | | AVERAGE FOR PERIOD 10–20 YR (mg) | AT PEAK OF GROWTH SPURT (mg) |
|---|---|---|---|
| Calcium | M | 210 | 400 |
| | F | 110 | 240 |
| Iron | M | 0.57 | 1.1 |
| | F | 0.23 | 0.9 |
| Nitrogen | M | 320 | 610 (3.8 g protein) |
| | F | 160 | 360 (2.2 g protein) |
| Zinc | M | 0.27 | 0.50 |
| | F | 0.18 | 0.31 |
| Magnesium | M | 4.4 | 8.4 |
| | F | 2.3 | 5.0 |

(From Forbes, G.B.: Nutritional requirements in adolescence. *In* Textbook of Pediatric Nutrition. Edition by R.M. Suskind. New York, Raven Press, 1981, by permission of Raven Press.)

The amount of calcium absorbed from different dietary sources varies. During peak periods of growth in adolescence, the average calcium retention is approximately 300 mg per day. Because the lower range of absorption is approximately 30%, a minimum of 900 mg calcium per day would be necessary during active skeletal growth.[35]

A wide difference exists in the daily allowances of calcium recommended by two expert committees. The World Health Organization recommends intakes of 600 to 700 mg per day for 11- to 15-year-old adolescents and 500 to 600 mg per day for 16- to 19-year-old adolescents.[36] In contrast, the National Research Council (NRC) recommends 1200 mg per day for these age groups.[5] The most recent RDA have extended the 1200 mg per day allowance through age 24 years to promote full mineral deposition.[5] It is apparent from these differences in recommended intakes that the amount of dietary calcium needed to sustain growth, as well as to provide maintenance, requires further study.

Establishing requirements for the teenage group is difficult because of the ability of many individuals to achieve equilibrium on a wide range of dietary intakes; the large error likely to occur in calculating calcium balance because of errors in measuring intakes and excretions; differences among individuals in rate of biologic maturation; and effects on calcium metabolism of protein, vitamin D, phosphorus, fiber,[34] caffeine, and sucrose.[35]

Surveys in the United States reveal that adolescent girls are less likely to meet the recommended levels of calcium than are teenage boys.[15,16,26] In addition, preliminary evidence suggests that adolescent females may need greater calcium in order to reach optimal bone mass. In a recent study, 1500 mg calcium per day was needed for maximal calcium retention in a small group of 14-year-old girls.[36]

Data from retrospective studies indicate that low calcium intakes during adolescence are associated with lower bone densities in women.[37,38] Decreased bone density may increase the risk of osteoporosis in later life.[39,40] Teen mothers who breast-feed may also be at risk for poor calcium balance. Lactating adolescents who consumed about 900 mg of calcium per day had a 10% decline in bone mineral content. Lactating teen mothers who consumed 1600 mg of calcium remained in calcium balance.[41]

### *IRON*

Iron deficiency is found in all races, both sexes, and all socioeconomic groups. Teenagers require additional amounts of iron to synthesize substantial amounts of new myoglobin and hemoglobin. As puberty is initiated, boys accumulate more lean body mass than girls. In fact, at the end of puberty, boys have twice the lean body mass of girls. Thus, Hepner calculated that for each additional kilogram of added tissue, males require 42 mg iron/kg body weight compared to 31 mg iron/kg body weight for girls.[42] In addition to the described sex differences, the normal biologic differences in body size make a tremendous difference in iron requirements. For example, a boy in the 97th percentile for body weight would require twice as much iron as a boy in the 3rd percentile.

The dietary intake of iron must be sufficient to account for the losses in feces, urine, skin, and menstruation, as well as to provide for expansion of red cell volume and for tissue growth in adolescence. The NRC recommends an additional 2 mg per day for males during the pubertal growth spurt (between ages 10 and 17 years), for a total of 12 mg of iron per day.[5] With menarche, the adolescent girl has additional iron loss from menstruation.[5] The NRC recommends an additional 5 mg per day for females starting with the pubertal growth spurt and menstruation, which begins approximately in the 11- to 14-year range. The iron recommendation for adolescent females is 15 mg per day.[5]

Unfortunately, few studies of iron requirements of adolescents have been performed. In a comprehensive review of iron requirements, Bowering et al. could find only one report on a controlled study with adolescents.[43] In the iron balance study of six adolescent girls, Schlaphoff and Johnson found that 0.62 to 1.82 mg per day (mean 1.0 mg per day) was retained, which included iron required to replace menstrual losses.[44] Assuming a rate of 10% absorption, they recommended a daily intake of 12 to 13 mg iron. Similar balance data are not available for boys. Finally, the amount of iron available in the American diet is estimated at 6 mg/1000 calories. Therefore, teenage girls whose caloric intake varies between 2000 and 2400 calories may find it difficult to ingest 15 mg of iron from dietary sources alone.

In the Ten State Nutrition Survey, between 5 and 10% of the teenagers had hemoglobin or hematocrit levels below normal.[15] Analysis of data from the Health and Nutrition Examination Survey II showed the highest prevalence of impaired iron status (ferritin model) was in teenagers—14.2% of the 15- to 19-year-old females and 12.1% of the 11- to 14-year-old males.[45] The results of other studies vary,[46,47] generally reporting more iron deficiency than iron deficiency anemia of the adolescents.

Results of several large surveys—the Ten State Nutrition Survey,[48] the Health and Nutrition Examination Survey I (HANES I),[47] and the Health and Nutrition Examination Survey II (HANES II)[49]—have shown a racial difference in hemoglobin level in adolescents. Blacks have approximately 1 g less hemoglobin than whites, which apparently is unrelated to socioeconomic level, education, diet, or obesity.[50] These differences have led many authors to recommend race-specific standards in screening for anemia.[51–56] Although use of different standards for hemoglobin concentration has been proposed, the biochemical basis for the racial difference of hemoglobin is unknown. The factors affecting hemoglobin differences, including genetic, socioeconomic, and dietary, are complex. At the present time, no data indicate that iron needs of black and white adolescents are different. Clearly, the standards for normal values used in any study will determine the amount of iron deficiency in any population. The prevalence of iron deficiency anemia will vary, depending on the standards for normal values and criteria for diagnosis used in the study. Measurements of hematocrit and hemoglobin, the most widely used screening procedures for anemia, are relatively insensitive indicators. The diagnosis of iron deficiency can be made by using the serum ferritin level, which provides the most accurate assessment of iron stores. Until more sophisticated studies are available, the true nature of iron deficiency anemia in adolescents awaits clarification.

Adolescent athletes may be at risk of iron deficiency caused by red blood cell destruction, increased need for red blood cell and tissue synthesis during puberty, or poor dietary intake.[54,55] Many (34 to 44%) teenage female runners have been found to be iron deficient, as assessed by low iron stores.[54,55] This deficiency is associated with abnormal gastrointestinal bleeding.[55]

Sports anemia may also be common; increased destruction of erythrocytes and a transient drop in hemoglobin concentration in the adolescent athlete results from an acute stress-response to exercise training. However, because the causes and treatments of sports anemia remain controversial, no basis currently exists for recommending iron supplementation for this transient condition.[56,57]

### *ZINC*

Zinc affects protein synthesis and is essential for the growth process. Zinc is particularly important in adolescence because of the rapid rate of growth and sexual maturation. Table 47–3 reveals that with the adolescent growth spurt comes greatly increased retention of zinc in both males and females, as compared to the average for the adolescent period. This striking increase in zinc retention is related to the increase of lean body mass observed during this period.[58]

In the tenth edition of the RDA[5] recommended daily zinc intake is reduced to 12 mg for adolescent females on the basis of their lower body weight. The recommendation for males remains at 15 mg per day.

Zinc deficiency has been associated with growth retardation and hypogonadism in adolescents.[59,60] Zinc supplementation resulted in accelerated growth and sexual maturation.[59,61] Poor dietary zinc sources and inhibition of zinc absorption from phytates in high-cereal diets contributed to the evolution of zinc deficiency and were major factors responsible for growth retardation and delayed sexual maturation.[60]

Evidence that adolescents undergoing rapid growth may be highly susceptible to inadequate dietary zinc is provided by Butrimovitz and Purdy.[62] These investigators found low plasma zinc concentrations during infancy and puberty, both periods of rapid growth. For adolescent girls and boys, plasma zinc levels were lowest at the ages when puberty was expected to occur.

Mild zinc deficiency has been reported in the United States. Hambidge et al. studied zinc status in apparently healthy children in Denver and found an association of low growth percentiles, diminished taste acuity, and low hair zinc levels.[63] Apparently, marginal zinc status may be a health problem in American children.

Adolescents undergoing rapid growth are at high risk of inadequate zinc levels. Young pregnant teenagers may be particularly susceptible to zinc deficiency, because of the rapid cell division and growth of the developing fetus as well as continued growth of the biologically immature teenager. These teenagers should be encouraged to include zinc-rich foods in their daily intake, such as poultry, lean meats, lowfat and nonfat dairy products, legumes, and grain products, particularly whole grains.[64]

### VITAMINS

Data on vitamin requirements for adolescents are even more limited than those for mineral requirements. The vitamin requirements for youth are interpolated from data on infant and adult allowances; Few data are derived directly from studies on adolescents. Emphasis should be placed on those vitamins necessary for the additional nutrient requirements of the pubertal growth spurt.

Vitamin A is required for vision, growth, cellular differentiation and proliferation, reproduction, and immune system integrity. Vitamin A levels and vitamin A intake in adolescents are considerably below the recommended amount.[15,16,65,66] Vitamin D is involved in maintaining homeostasis of calcium and phosphorus in the mineralization of bone. No controlled studies exist on vitamin D requirements for adolescents.

Vitamin C is essential for collagen synthesis. Vitamin C intakes in adolescents are often below the recommended levels.[67,68] Added to the unknown demands of growth, and changes in vitamin C status because of smoking[69,70] and oral contraceptive use,[71] some teenagers may have problems in vitamin C adequacy.

Because of its role in DNA synthesis, folate is important during periods of increased cell replication and growth. Folate status may be at risk in some adolescents, particularly those from low income populations[72] and pregnant teenagers.[73] The recent association of folate deficiency with neurotubal defects emphasizes the importance of adequate folate intake in teenage girls.[74] And yet, as assessed by dietary intakes and serum folate levels, poor folate status has been found in adolescent girls[75-77] and boys.[77]

Adolescents appear to have increased need for vitamin $B_{12}$, which is required for rapid cell growth, particularly during the growth spurt. Vitamin $B_6$ is involved in a large number of enzyme systems associated with nitrogen metabolism. The rapid growth of muscle mass, particularly in boys, makes vitamin $B_6$ adequacy important during puberty. Riboflavin, niacin, and thiamin are involved in energy metabolism and therefore also are important during puberty.

## SPECIAL NUTRITIONAL PROBLEMS

### OBESITY

Regulation of the amount of body fat in children and teenagers has been the subject of discussion and misunderstanding. Only in the last decade has a clearer picture of regulation of fat storage in the juvenile period emerged. In the past, obesity was thought to be a pure eating disorder and tinkering with the diet was a cure-all. As any health-care worker knows, juvenile obesity is particularly difficult to treat successfully over a long time.

A better understanding of the anatomy now reveals the complexities of regulating the size of the adipose tissue organ. The estimated number of adipocytes at birth is 5 billion. Primarily as a result of hyperplasia, but also influenced by some hypertrophy, the adipose tissue organ enlarges during growth until this number increases to an estimated 30 billion adipocytes in young adult life. The crucial issue in excessive adipose tissue development in teenagers is the nature versus nurture issue. Is excessive eating for whatever reason the cause of obesity? Or is the response of the child or teenager to food genetically modified to result in obesity? Our best information comes from studies of monozygotic and dizygotic twins. Using the Swedish twin registry, Borjorsen[78] and Stunkard[79] showed powerful genetic control over adiposity in children and adolescents. Confirmation in a population of twins in the United States has been reported.[80] That environment may play a facilitating role is likely. Thus, in juvenile-onset obesity, genetic background must be considered in assessment.

The long-term results of treatment of juvenile obesity with dietary counseling, anorectic drugs, and semistarvation have been dismal. The work of Brownell and co-workers gives some promise for the future.[81] Using the schools and involving the mothers, a well-structured behavioral modification program led to significant and long-term weight loss. Mellin et al.[82] used a variety of techniques with obese teens in nonschool sites and found significant improvement of relative body weight and weight-related behavior. The implications for these programs are important and suggest, if their work can be replicated, methods for incorporating practical public health programs for adiposity control in the community.

### EATING DISORDERS

Two major eating disorders, anorexia nervosa and bulimia (or bulimia nervosa), may pose major problems in adolescence.[83,84] Because of some of the psychologic changes in adolescence, it may be difficult to distinguish an adolescent with "normal" eating habits from one with an eating disorder. Adolescents may use food as a means of experimenting, gaining control, or establishing themselves as individuals. Dissatisfaction with body weight, fear of obesity resulting in unhealthy eating behavior, and preoccupation with dieting are common among today's youth, particularly adolescent girls.[85–87]

## HYPERTENSION

The prevalence of hypertension related to secondary causes is higher in adolescents than in adults.[88] Three elevated blood pressure readings (above the 95th percentile for age and sex, obtained on separate occasions) should be considered abnormal.[89] A blood pressure measurement of 140 mm Hg systolic and 90 mm Hg diastolic during adolescence is often used as the cut-off point for hypertension.[89,90] Dietary intervention should be part of the treatment of the adolescent with moderate or mild hypertension. Adolescents with severe hypertension should use dietary methods as an adjunct to pharmacologic therapy. Because many foods popular with teenagers are high in sodium and saturated fat,[91–93] education and behavior changes are important.

## PREGNANCY

The nutritional care of the pregnant adolescent must consider the health of both mother and infant. Knowledge of the role of nutrients is vital as is consideration of the principles of adolescent growth and development. Physiologically, the adolescent is at risk if she has not completed her growth.[94,95] Individual variability is great, but the majority of growth occurs before menarche. Linear growth in the adolescent female typically is not completed until approximately 4 years after the onset of menarche. Although the rate of growth after menarche has decelerated considerably, growth allowances should still be considered.

Gynecologic age (the difference between chronologic age and age at menarche) can give some indication of the physiologic maturity and growth potential. A young adolescent (with gynecologic age of 2 years or less) who becomes pregnant may still be growing. Her own needs for growth and development, along with the extra demands of fetal growth, increase the nutrient requirements of this young teen, as compared to those of a pregnant adult.[94,96]

The few studies that have focused on the energy needs of pregnant teenagers generally report that the teenagers frequently do not achieve the caloric intake recommended by the National Research Council.[5] Naeye raised the hypothesis that optimal weight gains for fetal survival may be higher in young teenagers, because both mother and infant compete for nutrients.[97] Results of further studies[98,99] also suggest that optimal weight gains for adolescents during pregnancy, particularly for those girls who are biologically immature, are greater than the adult recommendations of 25 to 35 pounds. Young adolescents (less than 2 years postmenarche) may deliver smaller infants for a given weight gain than do older women.[100,101] Inadequate weight gain during pregnancy has been associated with low-birth-weight infants.[102] Teenagers who smoke may be at increased risk of low prenatal weight gain and reduced infant birth weight.[103]

Preliminary data from our research using anthropometric measurements as predictors or low-birth-weight outcome in pregnant teenagers suggest that mothers of low-birth-weight infants tended to demonstrate a prenatal depletion of fat reserves (estimated from triceps skinfold measurements and from calculating arm fat area) as compared to the mothers of normal-birth-weight infants who accumulated fat.[104] In addition, prenatal protein stores of mothers of low-birth-weight infants changed little, whereas mothers delivering normal-birth-weight infants gained protein stores (estimated from midarm circumference measurements and arm muscle area calculations). Estimates of energy requirements indicate that sedentary adolescents needed at least 2400 to 2600 kcal per day. Physically active or rapidly growing adolescents needed additional energy, perhaps 50 kcal/kg of pregnant body weight per day.[105]

The issue of protein requirements for the pregnant adolescent is complex. Using careful nitrogen balance studies on pregnant teenagers, King et al. presented the best experimental data on which to base protein recommendations.[106] Their data suggested that nitrogen retention was greater than previously reported. In addition, maternal lean tissue of these adolescents increased during pregnancy, particularly during the last half of pregnancy.

Zinc metabolism is an important consideration during pregnancy. Data from a study of a small group of teenagers[107] are consistent with results of studies in adults, indicating that prenatal iron supplementation impairs zinc retention. However, these adolescents did not show a depression of serum zinc concentration during the second and third trimesters, as observed in adults, implying differences in zinc metabolism between adolescent and adult pregnancy.[107] Prenatal zinc supplementation in low-income teenagers has been associated with improved pregnancy outcome, reducing the number of premature births, as compared to a placebo group.[108]

On the basis of recent data, it appears pregnant teenagers, particularly those who may still be in their own growth phase, do have increased needs for nutrients during pregnancy. The pregnant adolescent needs an additional 300 calories and 10 to 16 more grams of protein each day, which can be supplied with the addition of foods such as those shown on Table 47–4.[109]

## VEGETARIAN DIETS

During a time of increased independence and decision-making, and greater influence by peers and role models, adolescents may use food as part of the process of

**TABLE 47–4.** FOODS TO INCREASE CALORIES AND PROTEIN FOR THE PREGNANT ADOLESCENT

| FOOD | CALORIES |
|---|---|
| Cereal (1 c), lowfat milk (8 oz), banana | 330 |
| Peanut butter (2 tbsp) sandwich | 320 |
| Cheese (2.5 oz) and 4 saltine crackers | 320 |
| Cheeseburger (regular) | 300 |
| Pizza, cheese (1/8 of 15″ pizza) | 290 |
| | PROTEIN (g) |
| Baked or refried beans (1 c) | 16 |
| Meat or poultry (2 oz) | 15 |
| Peanut butter (2 tbsp) sandwich | 15 |
| Pizza, cheese (1/8 of 15″ pizza) | 15 |
| Spaghetti with meat sauce (1 c) | 12 |
| Milk (12 oz) | 12 |
| Macaroni and cheese (3/4 c) | 11 |

(From Pennington, J.A.T.: Bowes and Church's Food Values of Portions Commonly Used. 15th Ed. New York, Harper & Row, 1989.)

individuation. Because the nutritional needs are high, vegetarian teenagers may be particularly at risk for nutritional deficiencies, especially at the time of the growth spurt.

Growing adolescents who are vegetarians may have problems in meeting their energy requirements because of the high-bulk content of vegetarian food patterns. In addition, many vegetarian diets are low in fat content.[110,111] Without sufficient energy intake, protein is used as an energy source and thus is unavailable for tissue synthesis and growth. Hence, the protein quality, protein quantity, and the energy intake of the individual must be assessed. Other nutrients of concern for the teenage vegetarian, particularly the strict vegetarian (who excludes all foods of animal origin), include calcium, iron, zinc, vitamins D, $B_{12}$, and $B_6$.[110–112]

Conscious effort and careful planning are necessary to ensure adequacy of these nutrients. Supplements may be necessary to meet the recommended allowances. The vegetarian should carefully plan a diet from a variety of foods. Protein complementation (the combining of different plant foods so that low essential amino acids of one protein source are complemented by the essential amino acids of another protein source, resulting in a complete protein) can ensure that the qualitative aspects of protein adequacy are met. An evaluation of the quantitative aspects of protein adequacy of the vegetarian is also necessary. The RDA for total protein intake during adolescence ranges from 44 to 56 g per day,[5] providing energy requirements are met.

Vegetarian food guides for adolescents are available in such sources as reports by Marino and King[113] and Smith[114] and the University of California's *Creative Eater's Handbook.*[115]

## REFERENCES


1. Marshall, W.A., Tanner, J.M.: Arch. Dis. Child., *44:*291–304, 1969.
2. Marshall, W.A., Tanner, J.M.: Arch. Dis. Child., *45:*13–24, 1970.
3. Tanner, J.M.: Growth and endocrinology of the adolescent. *In* Endocrine and Genetic Diseases of Children and Adolescents. 2nd Ed. Edited by L.I., Gardner. Philadelphia, W.B. Saunders, 1975.
4. Tanner, J.M.: Growth and Adolescence. 2nd Ed. Oxford, Blackwell Scientific, 1952.
5. Food and Nutrition Board, National Research Council: Recommended Dietary Allowances. 10th Ed. Washington, D.C., National Academy Press, 1989.
6. Wait, B., Blair, R., Roberts, L.: Am. J. Clin. Nutr., *22:*1383–1396, 1969.
7. Widdowson, E.M.: Medical Research Council Special Report Series No. 257. London, His Majesty Stationery Office, 1947.
8. Beal, V.A.: Nutritional intake. *In* Human Growth and Development. Edited by R.W. McCammon. Springfield, IL, Charles C Thomas, 1970.
9. Heald, F.P., Remmell, P.S., Mayer, J.: Caloric, protein and fat intake in children and adolescents. *In* Adolescent Nutrition and Growth. Edited by F.P. Heald. New York, Appleton-Century-Crofts, 1969.
10. National Center for Health Statistics: NCHS Growth Charts, 1976. Monthly Vital Statistics Report 25(3) Suppl. (HRA) 76-1120. Rockville, MD, National Center for Health, 1976.
11. National Center for Health Statistics: Height and weight of youths, 12-17 years, United States. *In* Vital and Health Statistics, Series 11, No. 124, Health Services and Mental Health Administration. Washington, D.C., U.S. Government Printing Office, 1973.
12. Dreizen, S., Spirakis, C.N., Stove, R.E.: J. Pediatr., *70:*256–263, 1967.
13. McArdle, W.D., Katch, F.I., Katch, V.L.: Exercise Physiology. Energy, Nutrition, and Human Performance. Philadelphia, Lea & Febiger, 1981.
14. Johnson, J.A.: Ann. N.Y. Acad. Sci., *69:*881–901, 1958.
15. Center for Disease Control: Ten State Nutrition Survey in the United States, 1968–1970. Atlanta, Health Services and Mental Health Administration, 1972.
16. National Center for Health Statistics: Caloric and Selected Nutrient Values for Persons 1–74 Years of Age. First Health and Examination Survey, 1971–1974, DHEW Publication (PHS) 79-1657. Hyattsville, MD, National Center for Health, 1979.
17. Heald, F.P., Hunt, S.M.: J. Pediatr., *66:*1035–1041, 1965.
18. Frisancho, A.R.: Am. J. Clin. Nutr., *27:*1052–1058, 1974.
19. Jensen, T.G., Englert, D., Dudrick, S.J.: Nutritional Assessment. A Manual for Practitioners. Norwalk, CT, Appleton-Century-Crofts, 1983.

20. Ingenbleek, Y., Van Den Schrieck, H., DeNayer, P.H., et al.: Clin. Chim. Acta, *63*:61–67, 1975.
21. Ingenbleek, Y., Devisscher, M., DeNayer, P.H., et al.: Lancet, *2*:106–108, 1972.
22. Shetty, P.S., Watrasiewicz, K.E., Jung, R.T., et al.: Lancet, *2*:230–232, 1979.
23. Hodges, R.E., Krehl, W.A.: Am. J. Clin. Nutr., *17*:200–210, 1965.
24. Hampton, M.C., Huenemann, R.L., Shapiro, L.R., et al.: J. Am. Diet. Assoc., *50*:385–396, 1967.
25. Wharton, M.A.: J. Am. Diet. Assoc., *24*:306–310, 1953.
26. Irwin, M.I., Kienholz, E.W.: J. Nutr., *103*:1019–1095, 1973.
27. Henkin, R.I.: Trace Elements in Nutrition. New York, Marcel Dekker, 1971.
28. Committee on Nutrition: American Academy of Pediatrics. Pediatrics, *62*:826–834, 1978.
29. Garn, S.M., Wagner, B.: The adolescent growth of the skeletal mass and its implications to mineral requirements. *In* Adolescent Nutrition and Growth. Edited by F.P. Heald. New York, Appleton-Century-Crofts, 1969.
30. Roche, A.F., Roberts, J., Hamill, P.V.: Vital Health Stat. [11], *167*:1–98, 1978.
31. Forbes, G.B.: Nutritional requirements in adolescence. *In* Textbook of Pediatric Nutrition. Edited by R.M. Suskind. New York, Raven Press, 1981.
32. Creenwood, C.T., Richardson, D.P.: World Rev. Nutr. Diet., *33*:1–41, 1979.
33. World Health Organization: Handbook on Human Nutritional Requirements. Monograph Series No. 61. Geneva, WHO, 1974.
34. Schuette, S.A., Linksweiler, H.M.: Calcium. *In* Present Knowledge of Nutrition. Fifth Ed. Washington, D.C., Nutrition Foundation, 1984.
35. Hollinbery, P.W., Massey, L.K.: Fed. Proc., *45*:375 (Abstract [@]1280), 1986.
36. Matkovic, V., Fontana, D., Tominac, C., et al. J. Bone Miner. Res., *1(Suppl. 1)*:Abstract 168, 1986.
37. Sandler, R.B., Slemenda, C.W., LaPorte, R.E., et al.: Am. J. Clin. Nutr., *42*:270–274, 1985.
38. Anderson, J.J.B., Tylavsky, F.A., Lacey, J., et al.: Fed. Proc., *46*:632 (Abstract 1841), 1987.
39. Heaney, R.P., Gallagher, J.C., Johnston, C.C., et al.: Am. J. Clin. Nutr., *36(Suppl.)*:986–1013, 1982.
*40. Allen, L.H.: Nutr. Today, *21*:6–10, 1986.
41. Chan, G.M., McNurry, M., Westover, K., et al.: Am. J. Clin. Nutr., *46*:319–323, 1987.
42. Hepner, R.E.: Nutrient Requirements in Adolescence. Cambridge. MIT Press, 1976.
43. Bowering, J., Sanchez, A.M., Irwin, M.I.: J. Nutr., *106*:985–1074, 1976.
44. Schlaphoff, D., Johnson, F.A.: J. Nutr., *39*:67–82, 1949.
45. Expert Scientific Working Group: Summary of a Report on the Iron Status of the United States Population. Am. J. Clin. Nutr., *42*:1318–1330, 1985.
46. National Academy of Sciences. Food and Nutrition Board: Iron Nutriture in Adolescence. DHEW Publications No. (HSA) 77-5100. Washington, D.C., U.S. Department of Health, Education and Welfare, 1976.
47. Johnson, C.L., Abraham, S.: Hemoglobin and Selected Iron-Related Findings of Persons 1-74 Years of Age: United States, 1971–74. DHEW Publication No. 46. Washington, D.C., U.S. Department of Health, Education and Welfare, 1979.
48. Garn, S.M., Smith, N.I., Clark, D.C.: J. Natl. Med. Assoc., *67*:91–96, 1975.
49. Yip, R., Johnson, C., Dallman, P.R.: Am. J. Clin. Nutr., *39*:427–436, 1984.
50. Dallman, P.R, Barr, G.D., Allen, C.M., et al.: Am. J. Clin. Nutr., *31*:377–380, 1978.
51. Garn, S.M., Smith, N.J., Clark, D.C.: Am. J. Clin. Nutr., *28*:563–568, 1975.
52. Owen, G.M., Yanochik, A.: Am. J. Public Health, *67*:865–866, 1977.
53. Daniel, W.A., Jr.: Nutritional requirements of adolescents. *In* Adolescent Nutrition. Edited by M. Winick. New York, John Wiley & Sons, 1982.
54. Brown, R.T., Mcintosh, S.M., Seabolt, V.R., et al.: J. Adolesc. Health Care, *6*:349–352, 1985.
55. Nickerson, H.J., Holubets, M.C., Weiller, B.R., et al.: J. Pediatr., *114*:657–663, 1989.
56. Sports and Cardiovascular Nutritionists (SCAN) Dietetic Practice Group: Sports Nutrition. A Guide for the Professional Working with Active People. Edited by J.B. Marcus Chicago, The American Dietetic Association, 1986.
57. Position of the American Dietetic Association: J. Am. Diet. Assoc., *87*:933–939, 1987.
58. Sandstead, H.H.: Am. J. Clin. Nutr., *26*:1251–1260, 1973.
59. Prasad, A.S., Schulert, A.R., Miale, A. Jr., et al.: J. Lab. Clin. Med., *61*:537–549, 1963.
60. Sandstead, H.H., Prasad, A.S., Schulert, A.R. et al.: Am. J. Clin. Nutr., *20*:422–442, 1967.
61. Prasad, A.S., Halsted, J.A., Nadimi, M.: Am. J. Med., *31*:532–545, 1961.
62. Butrimovitz, G.P., Purdy, C.: Am. J. Clin. Nutr., *31*:1409–1412, 1978.
63. Hambidge, K.M., Hambidge, C., Jacobs, M., et al.: Pediatr. Res, *6*:868–876, 1972.
64. Moser-Veillon, P.B.: J. Am. Diet. Assoc., *90*:1089–1093, 1990.
65. Canada National Survey: Nutrition. A National Priority. Ottawa, Department of National Health and Welfare, 1973.
66. Schor, B.C., Sanjur, D., Erikson, E.C.: J. Am. Diet. Assoc., *61*:415–420, 1972.
67. Huenemann, R.L., Shapiro, L., Hampton, M.C., et al.: J. Am. Diet. Assoc., *53*:17–24, 1968.
68. Nelson, M.: Dietary practices of adolescents. *In* Adolescent Nutrition. Edited by M. Winick. New York, John Wiley & Sons, 1982.
69. Pelletier, O.: Am. J. Clin. Nutr., *23*:520–524, 1970.
70. Schectman, G., Byrd, J.C., Gruchow, H.W.: Am. J. Public Health, *79*:158–162, 1989.
71. Rivers, J.M.: Am. J. Clin. Nutr., *28*:550–554, 1975.
72. Daniel, W.A., Gaines, E.G., Bennett, D.L.: Am. J. Clin. Nutr., *28*:363–370, 1975.
73. Vande Mark, M.S., Wright, A.C.: J. Am. Diet. Assoc., *61*:511—516, 1972.
74. Morbidity and Mortality Weekly Report, *40*:513–16, 1991.
75. Kirksey, A., Keaton, K., Abernathy, R.P., et al.: Am. J. Clin. Nutr., *31*:946–954, 1978.
76. Reiter, L.A., Boylan, L.M., Driskel, J., et al.: J. Am. Diet. Assoc., *87*:1065–1067, 1987.
77. Clark, A.J., Mossholder, S., Gates, R.: Am. J. Clin. Nutr., *46*:302–306, 1987.
78. Borjeson, M.: Acta Paediatr. Scand., *65*:279–287, 1976.
79. Stunkard, A.J., Harris, J.R., Pedersen, N.L., et al.: N. Engl. J. Med., *322*:1483–1487, 1990.
80. Bodurtha, J.N., Mosteller, M., Hewitt, J.K, et al.: Pediatr. Res., *28*:1–4, 1990.
81. Brownell, K.D., Kelman, J.H., Stunkard, A.J.: Pediatrics, *71*:515–523, 1983.

82. Mellin, L.M., Slinkard, L.A., Irwin, C.E., Jr.: J. Am. Diet. Assoc., *87:*333–338, 1987.
83. Committee on Diet and Health, Food and Nutrition Board, National Research Council: Diet and Health. Implications For Reducing Chronic Disease Risk. Washington, D.C., National Academy Press, 1989.
*84. Adams, L.B., Shafer, M.A.B.: J. Nutr. Ed., *20:*307–313, 1988.
85. Moore, D.C.: Arch. Dis. Child., *142:*1114–1118, 1988.
86. Moses, N., Banilivy, M.M., Lifshitz, F.: Pediatrics, *83:*393–398, 1989.
87. Casper, R.C., Offer, D.: Am. J. Clin. Nutr., *49(Suppl.):*1128–1129 (Abstract 6), 1989.
88. Neinstein, L.S.: Adolescent Health Care. A Practical Guide. Baltimore, Urban & Schwarzenberg, 1984.
89. Recommendations of the Task Force on Blood Pressure Control in Children. Pediatrics, *5(Suppl.):*797–820, 1977.
*90. Loggie, J.M.H., Rauh, L.W.: Med. Clin. North Am., *59:*1371–1383, 1975.
91. Morgan, K.J., Bundy, K.T.: Cereal Foods World, *26:*69–72, 1981.
92. Consumer Reports, September 1979, pp. 508–513.
93. Jacobson, M., Liebman, B.F., Moyer, G.: Salt. The Brand Name Guide to Sodium Content. New York, Workman Publishing, 1983.
94. Jacobson, M.S., Heald, F.P.: Nutritional risks of adolescent pregnancy and their management. *In* Premature Adolescent Pregnancy and Parenthood. Edited by E.R. McAnarney. New York. Grune & Stratton, 1983.
95. Rees, J.M. Worthington-Roberts, B.: Adolescence, nutrition, and pregnancy interrelationships. *In* Nutrition in Adolescence. Edited by L.K. Mahan, J.M. Rees. St. Louis, Times Mirror/Mosby College Publishing, 1984.
*96. Gong, E.J.: Weight issues and management. *In* Nutrition Management of the Pregnant Adolescent. A Practical Reference Guide. March of Dimes Birth Defects Foundation. Edited by M. Story. Washington, D.C., U.S. Department of Health and Human Services, U.S. Department of Agriculture, 1990.
97. Naeye, R.L.: Pediatrics, *67:*146–150, 1981.
98. Frisancho, A.R., Matos. J., Flegel P.: Am. J. Clin. Nutr., *38:*739–746, 1983.
99. Meserole, L.P., Worthington-Roberts, B.S.. Rees, J.M., et al.: J. Adolesc. Health Care, *5:*21–27, 1984.
100. Committee to Study the Prevention of Low Birthweight, Division of Health Promotion and Disease Prevention. Institute of Medicine. Preventing Low Birthweight. Washington, D.C., National Academy Press, 1985.
101. Subcommittee on Nutritional Status and Weight Gain During Pregnancy, Food and Nutrition Board. Institute of Medicine. National Academy of Sciences: Summary. Nutrition During Pregnancy. Part I. Weight Gain. Washington, D.C., National Academy Press, 1990.
102. Eastman, N.J., Jackson, E.: Obstet. Gynecol. *23:*1003–1025, 1968.
103. Muscati, S.K., Mackey, M.A., Newsom, B.: J. Nutr. Ed., *20:*299–306, 1988.
104. Maso, M., Gong, E.J., Jacobson, M.S., et al.: J. Adolesc. Health Care, *9:*188–193, 1988.
105. Blackburn, M.L., Calloway, D.H.: J. Am. Diet. Assoc., *65:*24–30, 1974.
106. King, J.C., Calloway, D.H., Margen, S.: J. Nutr., *103:*772–775, 1973.
107. Dawson, E.B., Albers, J., McGanity, W.J.: Am. J. Clin. Nutr., *50:*848–852, 1989.
108. Cherry, F.F., Sandstead, H.H., Rojas, P., et al.: Am. J. Clin. Nutr., *50:*945–954, 1989.
109. Pennington, J.A.T.: Bowes and Church's Food Values or Portions Commonly Used. 15th Ed. New York, Harper & Row, 1989.
110. Raper, N.R., Hill, M.M.: Nutr. Rev., *32(Suppl.):* 29–33, 1974.
*111. MacLean, W.C., Graham, G.G.: Am. J. Dis. Child., *134:*513–519, 1980.
112. Carruth, B.R.: J. Curr. Adolesc. Med., *2:*44–47, 1980.
*113. Marino, D.D., King, J.C.: Pediatr. Clin. North Am., *27:*125–139, 1980.
114. Smith, E.B.: J. Nutr. Ed., *7:*109–111, 1975.
115. University of California: The Creative Eater's Handbook. Better Nutrition Through Vegetarian Eating. Berkeley, University Student Health Service, 1982.


---

*Review article.

This work is supported in part by Maternal and Child Health Grant MCJ OQ0980, United States Department of Health and Human Services.

CHAPTER 48

# Nutrition in the Elderly

Lynne M. Ausman and Robert M. Russell



Currently, 25 million Americans are over the age of 65; by the year 2030, 57 million will be 65 or older. The increasing numbers of elderly and aged, especially in Western societies, presents challenges to those concerned with their physical and emotional well-being. An understanding of the role of both early and later nutrition in slowing or modulating the aging process and providing adequate nutriture for the elderly is important. Further, nutrient needs may change with aging, and the interaction of drugs and nutrients may play a major role in the nutrient needs of some elderly persons. A thorough and comprehensive review of all aspects of nutrition, aging, and the elderly can be found in the work of Munro and Danford.[1]

## THEORIES OF AGING

Aging is a gradual process taking place over many decades. Most theories of aging relate to impairment of DNA replication and loss of viability of the cell and hence the body's organs. The most common theories of aging relate to one or more of the following: immunologic breakdown, cellular proliferation, basal metabolic rate, rate of DNA repair, free radical damage, and/or the rate of protein synthesis and catabolism. One classification of general theories of aging is shown in Table 48–1.

### DIETARY RESTRICTION EXPERIMENTS WITH ANIMAL MODELS

Animal studies yield the strongest evidence that diet plays a major role in longevity and the aging process.[2–5] The most consistent finding from experimental rodent studies is that moderate dietary restriction markedly extends the lifespan of the experimental animals studied as compared to control animals fed ad libitum. Dietary restriction also decreases the incidence of several chronic

**TABLE 48–1.** SELECTED THEORIES OF AGING

| |
|---|
| Cellular |
| Free radical damage |
| Glycosylation and other cross-links |
| Changes in DNA or chromatin |
| Decreases in the accuracy or quantity of protein synthesis |
| Limited cell division capacity ("Hayflick limit") |
| Decrease in DNA repair activity |
| Organ Systems |
| Role of immune phenomena |
| Role of neuroendocrine phenomena |
| Population |
| Theories associating aging with differentiation or growth cessation |
| Rate of living |
| Theories based on the evolution of life span in mammals |

(Adapted from Weindruch, R.H., Walford, R.L.: The Retardation of Aging and Disease by Dietary Restriction. Springfield, IL, Charles C Thomas, 1988.)

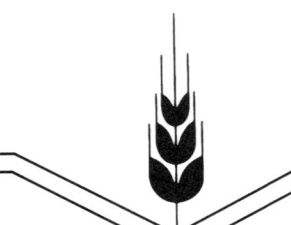

diseases such as glomerulonephritis, atherosclerosis, and tumors.

Dietary restriction by selective removal of individual macronutrients (fat, carbohydrate, or protein) has also been carried out. However, without a concomitant decrease in energy intake, little extension of life span has been found. Specific effects of protein or fat excess, however, can be shown to (1) increase the incidence of tumors and certain organ pathologies and (2) shorten the time of appearance of several physical, biochemical, and immunologic indices of early maturational development and aging.

The severity, age of initiation, and duration of the dietary perturbation play an important role in determining the eventual response to the dietary restriction. Many other factors including the species and strain of laboratory animal used are important variables in determining the outcome of these experiments. Individual micronutrients also have effects on life span and modulate the mechanisms of aging, at least to some extent. For example, increased levels of dietary antioxidants (ascorbic acid, α-tocopherol, carotenoids) may partially decrease cellular free-radical concentrations.[6,7] It is yet unclear whether any of these changes are related to the mechanism of aging.

## FACTORS AFFECTING NUTRITIONAL STATUS

The elderly are a more diverse population than any other age group; each individual has widely varying capabilities and levels of functioning. On the whole, elderly persons are more likely than younger adults to be in marginal nutritional health and thus be at higher risk for frank nutritional deficiency in times of stress or health-care problems. Physical, social, and emotional problems may interfere with appetite or may affect the ability to purchase, prepare, and consume an adequate diet.[8] These factors include whether or not a person lives alone, how many daily meals are eaten, who does the cooking and shopping and any physical impediments that would make this impossible, problems in chewing and denture use, adequate income to purchase appropriate foods, and alcohol and medication use.

## NUTRITIONAL REQUIREMENTS

A decline in organ function normally accompanies the aging process, especially in the older elderly (i.e., those more than 80 years old). Many of these changes in "normal" function might reasonably be expected to influence nutrient needs of the individual[9–11] (Table 48–2).

### ENERGY

Several studies have documented a decrease in the energy needs of the elderly. In the Baltimore Longitudinal Study of Aging, energy intakes of a sample of males decreased from 11.3 MJ (2700 kcal) per day at age 30 years to 8.8 MJ (2100 kcal) per day for those around 80 years. Two thirds of this reduction was attributable to a decrease in physical activity, and the remainder to a decrease in basal metabolism.[12] These findings have generally been supported by other studies. In NHANES II, young men and women, aged 24 to 34, were shown to consume 11.3 and 6.7 MJ (2700 and 1600 kcal) per day, whereas older individuals, aged 65 to 74, consumed 7.5 and 5.4 MJ (1800 and 1300 kcal) per day, respectively. The recommended energy intake from the 1989 Recommended Dietary Allowances (RDA) is 9.6 MJ (2300 kcal) for the reference 77-kg elderly male and 7.9 MJ (1900 kcal) for the reference 65-kg female 51 years of age and older.[13] In both cases, the 1989 RDA for energy is 125 kJ/kg (30 kcal/kg) per day, reduced from an earlier RDA of 138 kJ/kg (33 to 34 kcal/kg) per day. Variability of the measuring techniques may account for the wide range of apparent energy needs. A new laboratory method using excretion of administered $^{2}H_2{}^{18}O$ may be useful in estimating actual normal energy consumption of healthy elderly persons[14] (see Chapter 5).

### PROTEIN

High-protein diets may be less well digested and absorbed in the elderly as judged by a minor increase in fecal nitrogen content in response to a protein load.[15] However, little quantitative information is available regarding absorptive changes in the elderly for amino acids and peptides in more usual amounts.

The RDA currently recommends 0.8 g protein/kg body weight per day; this amount is adequate for the elderly when excessive energy intakes are observed (i.e., ≥167 kJ (= 40 kcal/kg) per day).[16] However, studies show that when an energy intake more usual for the elderly is used (e.g., 125 kJ (30 kcal/kg) per day), nitrogen balance is not attained in more than half the elderly subjects.[17,18] Another study suggests that the degree of adaptation of the individual to the lower energy or lower protein intake before the actual experimental trial began may account for many of the discrepancies in nitrogen needs reported in the literature.[19] The average protein consumption among the free-living elderly in Boston according to one study was 1.05 g/kg per day with no evidence that lower intakes were correlated with protein-energy malnutrition.[20] On the whole, a daily intake of 1 g/kg (and probably less) will meet the needs of this population.[1]

### CARBOHYDRATE

Carbohydrate absorption (mannitol, xylose, 3-O-methyl glucose) may be slightly impaired with advanced aging, although decreased renal function may interfere with interpretation of "absorption" test results when such results are based on urinary excretion.[21–23] In one

**TABLE 48–2.** CHANGES IN ORGAN FUNCTION WITH AGING THAT MAY INFLUENCE NUTRIENT STATUS*

| ORGAN FUNCTION | PHYSICAL CHANGE | IMPORTANCE TO NUTRITION |
|---|---|---|
| Taste and smell | Decreased taste buds and papilla on tongue<br>Decrease in taste and olfactory nerve endings<br>Change in taste and smell threshold | Loss of ability to detect salt and sweet<br>Decreased palatability causing poor food intake |
| Saliva secretion | Saliva flow may be reduced | Doubtful clinical significance |
| Esophageal function and swallowing | Minor changes including disordered contractions | Doubtful clinical significance |
| Gastric function and emptying | Decreased secretion of hydrochloric acid, intrinsic factor, and pepsin in 20% of healthy population > 60 years of age (atrophic gastritis); rapid rate of emptying of liquids, increased proximal small bowel pH, bacterial overgrowth in bowel | Decreased bioavailability of mineral, vitamins, and proteins; decreased absorption of protein bound vitamin $B_{12}$ and folate; increase in bacterial folate synthesis to counteract malabsorption |
| Liver and biliary function | Decreased size and blood flow; minor structural and biochemical changes; activity of drug metabolizing enzymes reduced | Rate of albumin synthesis may be decreased; drug dosages may need to be lower |
| Pancreatic secretion | Slightly lower bicarbonate and enzyme outputs | Doubtful clinical significance |
| Intestinal morphology and function | Insignificant changes in small bowel morphology | Doubtful clinical significance |
| Intestinal microflora | Bacterial overgrowth in proximal small bowel in atrophic gastritis | Functional significance unknown; influences supply of water-soluble vitamins and vitamin K |

(From Rosenberg, I.H., Russell, R.M., Bowman, B.B.: Aging and the digestive system. *In* Nutrition, Aging, and the Elderly. Edited by H.N. Munro and D.E. Danford. New York, Plenum Press, 1989.)

study in elderly persons 65 to 89 years of age, breath hydrogen was measured in response to a 100- to 200-g carbohydrate challenge to estimate carbohydrate malabsorption.[24] At the highest carbohydrate load, only 20% of the elderly had normal breath hydrogen results. However, interpretation of these results is uncertain because the increased breath hydrogen found in the elderly could be interpreted as carbohydrate malabsorption with age, increased bacterial enzyme activity in the small bowel, or both. Lactase activity decreases with age (especially in early life) but other brush border hydrolase activities appear to remain fairly constant.[25,26] The diminished lactase activity with age may create only a minor problem because most lactose-intolerant individuals can tolerate the lactose in a glass of milk (12.5 g).[27] Furthermore, in a double-blind study of healthy elderly persons given both lactose-containing and lactose-free products, about 30% of both groups showed bloating and discomfort associated with lactose intolerance. Although the elderly tend to avoid consumption of milk products (which are excellent sources of riboflavin, vitamin D, and calcium), the perceived bloating and discomfort may not be due to lactose intolerance. Therefore, accurate figures for the prevalence of lactose intolerance in the elderly are difficult to define.

There is no RDA for dietary carbohydrate. However, the United States Department of Agriculture (USDA), American Heart Association, and American Cancer Society, among others, recommend a dietary carbohydrate component of 55 to 60% of calories with an increase in the proportion of complex carbohydrates to simple sugars.

## FAT

Fat digestion and absorption in the elderly is equivalent to that of young adults when measured at normal consumption levels (100 g).[23,28] A study showed that at still higher dietary levels (120 g per day), the elderly showed slightly less fat absorption than the young adults did,[15] and another study reported that the institutionalized elderly showed even less.[29] Although not too common, fat malabsorption in the elderly, when found, is most often due to bacterial overgrowth of the small intestine, causing deconjugation of the bile salts. Gastric atrophy per se rarely causes fat malabsorption. Chylomicron appearance in blood after a 100-g fat meal is somewhat slower in the elderly as compared to young adults. However, an observed difference in gastric emptying times may have been responsible for this apparent slower lipid hydrolysis and uptake.[30]

There is no RDA for total fat. However, it is widely felt that a prudent diet with 30% or less of calories as fat (less than 10% saturated, 10 to 15% monounsaturated, and no more than 10% polyunsaturated fatty acids) may be just as important in the elderly as in young adults for preventing or ameliorating chronic diseases such as heart disease or cancer. At the same time, these amounts of polyunsaturated fat are consistent with a diet providing adequate amounts of essential fatty acids (linoleic and linolenic acid).[13]

## FLUID

Fluid balance is as important in the elderly as in other age groups. Nevertheless, it deserves particular attention because dehydration often goes unrecognized in the elderly. Poor fluid balance may be due to both inadequate (lower then normal) intake and excessive losses.[31] Chronically ill, immobilized, or demented patients and those with bladder control problems often fail to drink sufficient fluids. On the other hand, several clinical conditions such as fever, diarrhea, malabsorption, vomiting, and hemorrhage lead to excessive losses. Therapy with certain diuretics and laxative or hypertonic intravenous solutions also contribute to the problem. In the absence of severe clinical problems, consumption of 30 ml/kg per day is probably sufficient for the elderly.

## VITAMINS

Low to inadequate dietary intakes may account for much of the poor vitamin nutriture observed in the elderly.[32] In addition, physiologic changes associated with the aging gut may increase or decrease vitamin absorption, thereby influencing total dietary vitamin requirements. Table 48–3 lists the major water- and fat-soluble vitamins, the current RDA or Safe and Adequate Daily Dietary Intake, and an assessment of whether or not the current recommendation is appropriate for the elderly. A discussion of the individual vitamins follows below.

**Thiamin.** The 1989 RDA for the elderly for thiamin is 1.2 mg per day for males and 1.0 mg per day for females. When corrected for caloric consumption, intake should not decrease below 0.5 mg/1000 kcal. The NHANES I and II data indicated that the mean intake for the 65 to 75 year old age group was above this amount. Aging appears to be associated with an increased erythrocyte transketolase-activation coefficient in a small percentage of normal, free-living elderly persons.[33] It is not known whether this increase is normal for aging or represents nutritional inadequacy. There are no consistent changes in absorption of thiamin with age.[34,35] Thiamin deficiency in the elderly is due in large part to alcoholism accompanied by low thiamin intake. For most well elderly persons, however, the RDA for thiamin appears to be covering their needs.

**Riboflavin.** The 1989 RDA for riboflavin for the elderly is 1.4 and 1.2 mg per day for males and females, respec-

**TABLE 48–3.** ESTIMATE OF ADEQUACY OF 1989 RDA FOR VITAMINS FOR THE ELDERLY

| VITAMIN | CURRENT RDA FOR AGE 51+* | ADEQUACY OF RDA FOR ELDERLY | PHYSIOLOGIC REASON FOR CHANGE |
|---|---|---|---|
| Vitamin A | 800–1000 μg RE | May be too high | Change in unstirred water layer may lead to increased absorption in elderly. Decreased uptake by the liver of newly absorbed vitamin A. |
| Vitamin D | 5 μg | May be too low | Lack of sun exposure, reduced vitamin $D_3$ synthesis in skin and impaired renal 1-α hydroxylation suggest that the dietary requirement might be higher. |
| Vitamin E | 8–10 mg | I/C data† | — |
| Vitamin K | 65–80 μg | I/C data† | — |
| Thiamin | 1–1.2 mg | Adequate | — |
| Riboflavin | 1.2–1.4 mg | Adequate | — |
| Niacin | 13–15 mg | I/C data† | — |
| Vitamin $B_6$ | 1.6–2.0 mg | May be too low | Poor response to $B_6$ supplements in normal range suggests altered absorption or metabolism. |
| Folate | 180–200 μg | Adequate | — |
| Vitamin $B_{12}$ | 2.0 μg | May be too low | Atrophic gastritis and competition from bacterial overgrowth reduce availability of $B_{12}$. |
| Ascorbate | 60 mg | Adequate | — |
| Biotin | 30–100 μg‡ | I/C data† | — |
| Pantothenic | 4–7 mg‡ | I/C data† | — |

*RDA for female or male elderly 51+ years of age.
†Insufficient or conflicting data.
‡Safe and adequate daily dietary intake.
(From Suter, P.M., Russell, R.M.: Am. J. Clin. Nutr., *45*:501–512, 1987.)

tively. Deficiency of the vitamin as diagnosed by an increase in erythrocyte glutathione reductase activity coefficient[36,37] or a decrease in urinary riboflavin excretion[32] has been most often associated with low dietary intakes of riboflavin. Little evidence exists for altered absorption of the vitamin[38] or for altered tissue concentration with age;[39] therefore, current RDAs are expected to cover the elderly.

**Ascorbic Acid.** The current 1989 RDA for vitamin C is 60 mg per day for both sexes. Although the vitamin is widely abundant in many foods, levels of intake in the elderly vary widely. Factors such as smoking, medications, and emotional and environmental stress all adversely affect vitamin C nutriture.[40,41] Leukocyte and plasma vitamin C levels decline with age, although the significance of this is unclear.[42–44] Maintenance of the plasma level at 1.0 mg/dl would require, by extrapolation, 75 mg per day for females and 150 mg per day for males[45]; however, there is no evidence that saturating the body pool is optimal for this age group. Changes in tissue concentration with age are not consistent and there is little evidence that vitamin C absorption changes with aging.[42,43,46] Therefore, there is no evidence that vitamin C requirements per se change with aging.

**Niacin.** The 1989 RDA for niacin is 15 mg per day for male and 13 mg per day for female elderly persons, the same as for young adults. Individuals with low excretion of urinary N-methyl nicotinamide usually have a poor niacin intake or are very sick or very old (86 to 99 years);[37] in this latter case, decreased renal function should be considered. There is little if any evidence to indicate that niacin requirements change with age.[32]

**Vitamin $B_6$.** Because the vitamin $B_6$ content of many foods is not known, dietary intakes as calculated from food composition tables vary widely and may be low. Nevertheless, serum and plasma $B_6$ levels in the elderly show a decreasing trend with age. Studies indicating poor $B_6$ nutriture based on activity coefficient tests (response of whole blood $B_6$ enzymes to exogenous $B_6$ supplementation) show that with moderate oral supplementation, activity coefficients in some elderly persons still do not return to normal. The current RDA for vitamin $B_6$ in the elderly is 2.0 mg per day for men and 1.6 mg per day for women. However, it has been recently shown that the *average* requirement (without addition of 2 S.D. to ensure adequacy for most of the population) in both male and female elderly persons is about 2.0 mg per day.[47] Therefore, the RDA for vitamin $B_6$ should be considerably higher in the elderly.

**Folate.** Despite low folate intake levels, only 3 to 7% of persons in NHANES I[48] or in free-living elderly persons have low serum folate levels (i.e., <3.0 ng/ml). In a Swedish study of 35 elderly subjects,[49] intake of only 100 to 200 μg per day normalized whole-blood folate concentrations. Furthermore, although atrophic gastritis with aging causes malabsorption of folic acid due to a rise in pH of the proximal gastrointestinal tract, this is more than offset by the production and subsequent absorption of folate synthesized by bacteria overgrowth in the proximal small bowel.[50] The current RDA in the elderly is 200 μg per day for men and 180 μg per day for women. The reliability of the data on food folate content, however, has been questioned by Beecher and Matthews, who stress a need for the development of alternative methods in the measurement of folate in foods.[51]

**Vitamin $B_{12}$.** Serum or plasma vitamin $B_{12}$ levels in the elderly are often found to be low.[52–55] A low intake, especially among the poor elderly, and impaired absorption of vitamin $B_{12}$ may be important factors. A decreased digestive release of vitamin $B_{12}$ from food and bacterial overgrowth in the small bowel (as found in atrophic gastritis) leading to competition for vitamin $B_{12}$ seem to be important factors reducing absorption.[56,57] There is no evidence that atrophic gastritis per se is associated with decreased production of intrinsic factor. The current RDA of 2.0 μg per day is sufficient for most elderly persons, but may be too low for those with atrophic gastritis.

**Vitamin A.** Although vitamin A is not distributed widely in foods, excess daily amounts can be stored in the liver. Most individuals consume food rich in vitamin A 1 or 2 times per week. Estimates of vitamin A intakes derived from 24-hour recalls overestimate the number of individuals having low intakes.

Vitamin A tolerance curves show higher retinyl ester values in the elderly as compared to young adults.[58] This was recently shown to be due to reduced clearance of the lipid-rich lipoproteins carrying the retinyl esters in the elderly.[59] A change in character of the luminal epithelium or a decrease in the thickness or character of the unstirred water layer as demonstrated in elderly rats would suggest increased absorption. In addition, carotenes, the vitamin A precursors derived from plant pigments, are also a source of vitamin A activity, and these compounds may have a special beneficial effect in terms of cancer prevention. Therefore, although the need for preformed vitamin A for the elderly may be lower, it would be prudent to obtain a large fraction of the vitamin A requirement from the carotene-containing fruits and vegetables.

**Vitamin D.** Because vitamin D is found only in a few foods, which include sea food and fortified milk products, it is not surprising that over three-quarters of the elderly have vitamin D intakes less than two thirds of the RDA. The contribution of sunlight to the vitamin D status of the elderly is also reduced, because the elderly receive less sun exposure and have a decreased efficiency of vitamin D synthesis in the skin.[60] In institutionalized subjects with little access to sunlight exposure, the diet may not provide sufficient vitamin D.[61] Thus, the dietary need for vitamin D may be greater in the elderly than in individuals with sunlight exposure. Supplementation with 10 μg (400 IU per day), which is two times the RDA) is recommended for the homebound elderly or those in nursing homes.

In one study, although serum 25-OH D levels were not decreased in elderly subjects, average 1,25-$(OH)_2$-D levels were significantly lower in elderly osteoporotic females versus younger females,[62] suggesting impairment of renal conversion (renal 1-α-hydroxylase enzyme) of vitamin D to its active form. There was also a significant correlation between 1,25-$(OH)_2$-D levels and intestinal calcium absorption.

**Vitamin E.** As for vitamin C, the antioxidative properties of vitamin E (tocopherol) may play a role in retarding the aging process. The 1989 RDA for the elderly is 10 mg per day for males and 8 mg per day for females. Most populations consume adequate amounts although in one study 40% of a free-living population consumed <75% of the RDA from the diet alone.[63] Of note, one-third of this population took vitamin E supplements. Because the plasma α-tocopherol is carried passively in the lipid-rich lipoproteins (very low-density lipoproteins, or VLDL, and low-density lipoproteins, or LDL),[64,65] it is most accurate to express the vitamin E concentration in relation to blood lipid content.[66] When this is done, there is no relation between plasma vitamin E–lipid ratio and age.[67] The data examining tissue concentrations (platelets, liver, adrenal glands, heart) of vitamin E with age are inconsistent, and there is no evidence of increased vitamin E needs with age according to the erythrocyte hemolysis test.[32] Finally, there is no evidence for altered vitamin E absorption with aging.[65]

**Vitamin K.** With a new method to measure vitamin K metabolites in plasma, it has been possible to show that serum phylloquinone levels vary as a function of gender, age, and serum lipid levels.[68] One study showed that when expressed per millimole of triglyceride, plasma phylloquinone concentrations in the young subjects were $0.82 \times 10^{-6}$ mmol and in the elderly $0.62 \times 10^{-6}$ mmol.[69] The nutritional significance of this decrease in the elderly is not yet understood. The 1989 RDA for vitamin K for the elderly is an intake of 80 μg per day for men and 65 μg per day for women.

## MINERALS

**Calcium.** Calcium intake throughout one's lifetime appears to be a factor in the rate of occurrence of osteoporosis in the elderly. In both men and women the absorption of calcium decreases with age.[62,70] Calcium absorption may also decrease with the achlorhydria observed in some elderly persons.[71] In one study, calcium absorption was measured in 94 normal volunteers (aged 30 to 90) and 52 untreated women with postmenopausal osteoporosis.[62] Although fractional calcium absorption decreased with age, it was not correlated with calcium intake. It also appears that the elderly are less able to adapt to a low-calcium diet than young adults are.[72] Poor vitamin D nutriture and activity in the elderly is widely thought to be partially responsible for the decreased calcium absorption. In the NHANES I and II studies, average calcium intakes for women were about 500 mg per day, below the 1989 RDA of 800 mg per day. In studies in Yugoslavia, metacarpal cortical thickness was greater in a population that routinely consumed 1100 mg calcium per day as compared to a population with a typically low-calcium intake (500 mg per day).[73] Bone loss progressed with age in both districts, but the rate of hip fracture was higher in the population with the low calcium intake, suggesting lower calcium reserves before osteoporosis became apparent. In another study spinal bone loss in healthy postmenopausal elderly patients was decreased in women consuming more than 777 mg calcium per day as compared to those consuming less than 405 mg per day. Although calcium supplementation may be necessary for individuals with low intakes, supplementation exceeding total daily intake of 800 mg per day appears unnecessary.[75]

**Iron.** The iron deficiency seen in the elderly is due to inadequate iron intake, blood loss due to chronic disease, and/or reduced nonheme iron absorption secondary to the hypohydria or achlorhydria of atrophic gastritis.[76] Iron absorption per se does not appear to decline significantly with age,[77] although one study showed that red cell uptake of absorbed intestinal iron was reduced by about one-third.[78] In the NHANES I and II studies average iron intakes were 14 mg per day for men and 10 mg per day for women.[79] In these studies, a 4% prevalence of anemia in men was attributable more often to chronic disease and not to iron deficiency; iron-deficiency anemia without apparent disease was rare for women. Similarly, iron overload is rarely seen in the elderly. Therefore, it seems that the RDA for the elderly of 10 mg per day is adequate.

**Zinc.** Several studies indicate that zinc intakes of the elderly, 10 mg for males and 7 mg for females, are well below the 1989 RDA of 15 mg per day for men and 12 mg per day for women.[63,80] Zinc absorption as measured by isotopic studies decreases with age, although zinc balance remains intact.[81] There are conflicting data in the literature indicating normal or decreased plasma zinc concentrations in the elderly.[82,83] The significance of any decrease in plasma levels is difficult to ascertain, however, because diagnosis of zinc deficiency is problematic.

**Copper.** As determined by isotope studies, copper absorption in the elderly is similar to that in young adults.[84] The absorption of copper is affected by the presence of other trace minerals and factors in the diet that inhibit or enhance cation absorption (e.g., phytates, zinc, oxalates). A recent study in elderly males suggests that only 1.1 mg of copper is necessary for copper balance, an amount below the usual intake of 2 to 3 mg (also the RDA) observed in the elderly.[85]

**Other Trace Minerals.** The nutritional status and requirement of selenium, manganese, molybdenum, and chromium in relation to aging have been reviewed by Yunice and Hsu.[86]

## NUTRITIONAL STATUS

### DIETARY INTAKE

Dietary intakes and nutritional status of the elderly have been examined in several studies over the last 20 years. These range from the large nationwide NHANES I for 1971 to 1974[87] and NHANES II for 1976 to 1980,[88] to several smaller studies of specific populations of free-living and institutionalized elderly persons.[89–95] The sample population studied, the type of dietary instrument used, and the standards used for interpretation of the actual intake data influence the results of the study.

#### *METHODOLOGY OF DIET HISTORY*

Three instruments are currently in use: dietary food records, food recall, and food frequency. The food record requires an individual to record current food intake for 3 to 7 days. The recall method is done for consumption during the previous 24-hour period but may be particularly inappropriate for older persons with short-term memory problems. Finally, food frequency methods cover usual food consumption patterns for a 12-month period including all seasonal variations. Each of these methods incorporates questions on the use of dietary supplements and alcohol. The various advantages and disadvantages of each method have been reviewed[96–98] (see also Chap. 52). Many of these methods tend to underestimate food intake.[99] For some nutrients, especially vitamin $B_6$, folate, and zinc, actual content in foods is not well established.

#### *DIETARY INTAKE STANDARDS*

Standards used for interpretation of dietary data in the elderly range from the RDA in use at the time of the survey or a special standard set up especially for a particular study, such as two thirds of the RDA. Since the RDA of 1974, there have been separate categories for individuals 51 years of age or older.

### NUTRITIONAL EVALUATION

#### *BIOCHEMICAL STANDARDS*

The biochemical standards recommended for use for the elderly are currently the same as for adults.[100] Although some studies had speculated that serum albumin concentrations declined with aging, a recent study of 1066 healthy elderly persons found only minimal decreases in albumin with age.[101]

#### *HEMATOLOGIC STANDARDS*

Standards for the elderly for interpretation of hematologic data (e.g., red blood cells, white blood cells, hemoglobin) are slightly lower than those for young and middle-aged adults.[102] By convention, values that are lower than the tenth percentile for NHANES II are considered "at risk." There are as yet no reliable standards to indicate significant ethnic differences in the elderly.

#### *ANTHROPOMETRIC STANDARDS*

**Body Weight.** The correlation of obesity with increased morbidity and mortality is well known.[103–107] The pattern of distribution of the body fat (higher risk with increased waist to hip girth) may also be a factor in the excess morbidity and mortality.[108–111] However, the determination of obesity in the elderly is problematic, because few body weight standards specifically for the elderly are currently in use. One of the earliest standards is based on the accumulated body weight data of 5600 elderly men and women (65 to 94 years of age) who reported on an ambulatory basis to their doctor.[112] Data on the elderly up through age 74 are also available from the NHANES I and II studies. Using these data, Frisancho[113] has established body weight standards for persons 25 to 54 and 55 to 74 years of age for sex, age, height, and an estimation of frame size using elbow breadth[114] (see Appendix Tables A–11g and A–13). These standards are in close agreement with data from the Baltimore Longitudinal Aging Study.[115,116] Because body mass index, or BMI in the NHANES I and II studies and in several other studies was approximately 22.5 kg/m$^2$ for both sexes, the summary tables of Frisancho[113] have been prepared in weight ranges according to height and age but not gender.

The Metropolitan Life Tables[106] (see Appendix Tables A–11c to A–11e) are based on people aged 25 to 59 and do not account for possible changes in body weight and height with age; thus, they are probably not useful for the elderly. Furthermore, because these tables represent the experience of the insurance industry, they are certainly not an unbiased sample of the general population. Because the Build Study[105] of BMI versus mortality indicated minimal mortality for the elderly at a BMI greater than that calculated from the Metropolitan Life Tables, it appears that the Metropolitan Life Tables are not accurate or desirable for use in persons over the age of 54.

#### *OTHER ANTHROPOMETRIC STANDARDS*

Anthropometric data such as triceps skinfold have also been used to assess nutritional status of populations,[117,118] as well as to monitor responses to treatment of patients in a hospital setting.[119] Lean body mass declines with aging whereas body fat stores increase with aging.[120] The increased body fat is stored intra-abdominally and intramuscularly in the elderly as compared to subcutaneously in the young.[121] Thus, triceps skinfold thickness and measures derived from it (e.g., mid-arm muscle area) cannot accurately be used in the elderly to predict body fat content.

### REVIEW OF STUDIES OF INSTITUTIONAL AND FREE-LIVING ELDERLY POPULATIONS

A review of 28 dietary surveys that included data from elderly persons concluded that the mean calorie intake was most often found to be below the standard used.[122] In several large surveys of note,[63,87,88,94,95] mean energy intakes (kcal/kg per day) averaged 1792 to 2171 for males and 1168 to 1770 for females, generally lower than the 1989 RDA of 2300 for males and 1900 kcal per day for females. Calorie intakes of sedentary elderly may indeed be lower than current estimates. The low intakes may also be attributable to the tendency of many methods to underestimate food intake. Indeed, when the doubly labeled water method was used on an elderly population, total energy expenditure was greater than that estimated from food intake (Dr. Susan Roberts, unpublished data).

Nutritional status of elderly with respect to protein has been assessed by dietary intake and accompanying biochemical parameters. The average protein intakes in NHANES I and II as well as in other surveys of institutional and free-living elderly were above the 1989 RDA. Thus, protein nutriture, in the absence of chronic disease, appears adequate. In some studies, certain serum proteins (albumin, transferrin, prealbumin, retinol-binding protein) appear to decline with age.[95,123,124] A lower serum albumin level, when it occurs, is often not correlated with protein intake and may represent normal decreases for the elderly.[1,19,20] A recent study of serum albumin levels in healthy elderly appears to show minimal decreases with age.[101]

The nutritional status of the elderly with respect to several vitamins and minerals has been assessed. Based on both dietary intake and/or biochemical measures in the NHANES I and II studies as well as other studies,[61,94,95] the evidence for low intakes of calcium and vitamin D appears to be the most substantial and is attributable to the low intake of dairy products among certain groups of this population.

The situation with respect to vitamin $B_6$ nutriture is complex. Several studies show that vitamin $B_6$ intakes appear to be well below the RDA and that up to 28% of individuals showed abnormal erythrocyte aspartate aminotransferase stimulation tests.[94,95,125] However, it is thought that reported vitamin $B_6$ intakes would be somewhat higher if the food table values for vitamin $B_6$ (as well as for zinc, folate, and vitamin $B_{12}$) were more complete. As for any nutrient, it may be that current standards for biochemical tests of nutrient status for vitamin $B_6$ are inappropriate for the elderly. In addition, inferences of deficiency based on a single screening should be tempered by the fact that the intraindividual variance in biochemical measures is large enough to account for a portion of the "deficiency" at any one measurement time.[126]

Mean intakes of most other vitamins and minerals (with an adequate data base) appear adequate, although in a few studies, biochemical tests indicate that levels may be low in 5 to 20% of elderly people for thiamin, riboflavin, iron, and folate.[127]

#### *SUPPLEMENT USE BY THE ELDERLY*

In a study of a Meals on Wheels program, 14 of 33 subjects were considered at risk for protein-energy malnutrition. Supplementation with a liquid polymeric supplement for 4 months increased weight in a majority of subjects; the weight gain was associated with increases in serum albumin, total iron-binding capacity, folate, vitamin C, and vitamin $B_{12}$, thus providing evidence of an improved nutritional status.[128]

Supplement use was also examined as part of the nutritional status survey of free-living elderly in Boston.[129] Daily vitamin and mineral use was reported by about half of the elderly; vitamin C and E use were most common. Supplement use markedly decreased the number of individuals whose total daily intake (diet plus supplement) of vitamins $B_6$, $B_{12}$, and D and folate and calcium would be considered low. Of concern, both males and females were observed to consume excessive levels (at least 10 times the RDA) of vitamin A. These results are consistent with other studies of supplementation in the elderly.[130] However, an even greater prevalence of supplementation (72%) was observed in a survey of an affluent community of "health conscious" residents.[131]

## DRUG-NUTRIENT INTERACTION

Nutrients can affect drug action by altering the digestion, absorption, distribution, metabolism, and/or excretion of the drug (see Chap. 78). Less often recognized is that for all age groups, drugs may have an influence on the nutritional status of the individual. Drugs may exhibit their effects on nutritional status through several avenues: effects on food intake, alteration of nutrient absorption, alteration of nutrient metabolism, and alteration in nutrient excretion.[132–134] This is particularly important to consider in the elderly who often have multiple chronic diseases and are taking several medications or drugs concurrently. Risk of adverse side effects increases with number of drugs taken simultaneously and with the duration of exposure to the drugs.

## ALCOHOL AND NUTRITIONAL STATUS IN THE ELDERLY

Alcohol is the most common drug used by the population at large. In large amounts taken chronically, it is known to adversely affect nutritional status at all levels including reducing appetite and impairing nutrient absorption, nutrient metabolism, and nutrient excretion. It is also associated with several serious medical and social problems such as hepatic cirrhosis, adenocarcinoma of the gastrointestinal tract (particularly mouth, pharynx, larynx, and esophagus) and liver, and impaired driving. The majority of elderly individuals consuming alcohol do so in small amounts.[135] In another survey of 554 nonalcoholic subjects who had participated in a nutritional status assessment of the elderly in the Boston area, alcohol use was classified as <5 g per day, 5 to 14 g per day, or 15+ g per day.[136] Alcohol use was related to the nutritional, biochemical, and physical parameters of these individuals. Plasma retinol, ferritin and high-density lipid cholesterol concentrations were significantly increased, and serum copper, zinc, and potassium were significantly decreased in the 15+ g alcohol group as compared to the <5 g alcohol group. The statistically significant effects were small, however, and therefore of questionable biologic significance; the effects of alcohol on potassium and copper were observed only in patients using diuretics.

## REFERENCES


1. Munro H.N., Danford, D.E. (eds.): Nutrition, Aging, and the Elderly. New York, Plenum Press, 1989.
2. Weindruch, R.H., Walford, R.L.: The Retardation of Aging and Disease by Dietary Restriction. Springfield, IL, Charles C Thomas, 1988.
3. Masoro, E.J.: J. Nutr., *115:*842–848, 1985.
4. Snyder, D.L. (ed.): Dietary Restriction and Aging. (Prog. Clin. Biol. Res., *298*.) New York, Alan R. Liss, 1989.
5. McCay, C.M., Crowell, M.F., Maynard, L.A.,: J. Nutr., *10:*63–79, 1935.
6. Harman, D.: Free radical theory of aging: role of free radicals in the origination and evolution of life, aging, and disease processes. *In* Free Radicals, Aging, and Degenerative Diseases. Edited by J.E. Johnson, R.L. Walford, and D. Harman. New York, Alan R. Liss, 1986, p. 3.
7. Harman, D.: Proc. Natl. Acad. Sci. U.S.A., *78:*7124–7128, 1981.
8. Russell, R.M., Sahyoun, N.R.: The elderly. *In* Clinical Nutrition. 2nd Ed. Edited by E.M. Paige. Washington, D.C., C.V. Mosby, 1988, p. 110.
9. Bowman, B.B., Rosenberg, I.H.: Am. J. Clin. Nutr., *35:*1142–1151, 1982.
10. Thompson, A.B.R., Keelan, M.: Can. J. Physiol. Pharmacol., *64:*30–38, 1986.
11. Rosenberg, I.H., Russell, R.M., Bowman, B.B.: Aging and the digestive system. *In* Nutrition, Aging, and the Elderly. Edited by H.N. Munro and D.E. Danford. New York, Plenum Press, 1989.
12. McGandy, R.B., Barrows, C.H., Spanias, A., et al.: J. Gerontol., *21:*581–587, 1966.
13. Food and Nutrition Board, National Research Council: Recommended Dietary Allowances. 10th Ed. Washington, D.C., National Academy Press, 1989.
14. Prentice, A.M., Coward, W.A., Davies, H.L., et al.: Lancet, *1:*1419–1422, 1985.
15. Werner, I., Hambraeus, L.: The digestive capacity of elderly people. *In* Nutrition in Old Age. Edited by L.A. Carlson. Uppsala, Almquist and Wiksell, 1972, p. 55.
16. Cheng, A.H.R., Gomez, A., Gergan, J.G., et al.: Am. J. Clin. Nutr., *31:*12–22, 1978.
17. Uauy, R., Scrimshaw, N.S., Rand, W.M., et al.: Am. J. Clin. Nutr., *31:*779–785, 1978.
18. Gersovitz, M., Motil, D., Munro, H.N., et al.: Am. J. Clin. Nutr., *35:*6–14, 1982.
19. Munro, H.N., Suter, P.M., Russell, R.M.: Annu. Rev. Nutr., *7:*23–49, 1987.
20. Munro, H.N., McGandy, R.B., Hartz, S.C., et al.: Am. J. Clin. Nutr., *46:*586–592, 1987.
21. Beaumont, D.M., Cobden, I., Sheldon, W.L., Laker, M.F., James, O.F.W.: Age Ageing, *16:*294–300, 1987.
22. Guth, P.H.: Am. J. Dig. Dis., *13:*565–571, 1968.
23. Arora, S., Kassarjian, Z., Krasinski, S.D., et al.: Gastroenterology, *96:*1560–1565, 1989.
24. Feibusch, J.M., Holt, P.R.: Dig. Dis. Sci., *27:*1095–1100, 1982.
25. Welsh, J.D., Russell, L.C., Walker, A.W. Jr.: Gerontology, *66:*993–997, 1974.
26. Welsh, J.D., Poley, J.R., Bhatia, M., et al.: Gastroenterology, *75:*847–855, 1978.
27. Debongnie, J.C., Newcomer, A.D., Mcgill, D.B., Philips, F.S.: Dig. Dis. Sci., *24:*225–231, 1979.
28. Southgate, D.A.T., Durnin, J.V.G.A.: Br. J. Nutr., *24:*517–535, 1970.
29. Pelz, K.S., Goffried, S.P., Sooes, E.: Geriatrics, *23:*149–153, 1968.
30. Webster, S.G.P., Wilkinson, E.M., Gowland, E.: Age Ageing, *6:*113–117, 1977.
31. Rowe, J.W.: Renal and lower urinary tract diseases in the elderly. *In* The Practice of Geriatrics. Edited by E. Calkins, P.J. Davis, and A.B. Ford. Philadelphia, W.B. Saunders, 1986.
32. Suter, P.M., Russell, R.M.: Am. J. Clin. Nutr., *45:*501–512, 1987.
33. Iber, F.L., Blass, J.P., Brin, M., et al.: Am. J. Clin. Nutr., *36:*1067–1082, 1982.
34. Thomson, A.D.: Gerontol. Clin., *8:*345–361, 1966.
35. Breen, K.J., Buttigier, R., Iossifidis, S., et al.,: Am. J. Clin. Nutr., *42:*121–126, 1985.
36. Chen, L.H., Fan Chiang, W.L.: Int. J. Vitamin Nutr. Res., *51:*232–238, 1981.
37. Harrill, I., Cervone, N.: Am. J. Clin. Nutr., *30:*431–440, 1977.
38. Said, H.M., Hollander, D.: Life Sci., *36:*69–73, 1985.
39. Schaus, R., Kirk, J.E.: J. Gerontol., *11:*147–150, 1957.

40. Pelletier, O.: N. Y. Acad. Sci., *258:*156–168, 1975.
41. Sahud, M.A., Cohen, R.J.: Lancet, *1:*937–938, 1971.
42. Kirk, J.E., Chieffi, M.,: J. Gerontol., *8:*301–304, 1953.
43. Kirk, J.E., Chieffi, M.,: J. Gerontol., *8:*305–311, 1953.
44. Loh, H.S.: Int. J. Vitamin Nutr. Res., *42:*80–85, 1972.
45. Garry, P.J., Goodwin, J.S., Hunt, W.C., et al.: Am. J. Clin. Nutr., *36:*332–339, 1982.
46. Cheng, L., Cohen, M., Bhagavan, H.N.: Vitamin C and the elderly. *In* Handbook of nutrition in the aged. Edited by R.R. Watson. Boca Raton, FL, CRC Press, 1985, p. 157.
47. Ribaya-Mercado, J.D., Russell, R.M., Sahyoun, N., et al.: J. Nutr., *121:*1062–1074, 1991.
48. Senti, F.R., Pilch, S.M. (eds.): Assessment of the Folate Nutritional Status of the U.S. Population Based on Data Collected in the Second National Health and Nutrition Examination Survey, 1976–1980. Bethesda, MD, Federation of American Societies for Experimental Biology, 1984.
49. Jagerstad, M., Westesson, A.K.: Scand. J. Gastroenterol., *14 (Suppl. 52):*196–202, 1979.
50. Russell, R.M., Krasinski, S.D., Samloff, I.M., et al.: Gastroenterology, *91:*1476–1482, 1986.
51. Beecher, G.R., Matthews, R.H.: Nutrient composition of foods. *In* Present Knowledge in Nutrition. 6th Ed. Edited by L.M. Brown. Washington, D.C., International Life Sciences Institute, 1990, pp. 430–443.
52. Elwood, P.C., Shinton, N.K., Wilson, C.I.D., et al.: Br. J. Haematol., *21:*557–563, 1971.
53. Garry, P.J., Goodwin, J.S., Hunt, W.C.: J. Am. Geriatric Soc., *32:*719–726, 1984.
54. Magnus, E.M., Bache-Wiig, J.E., Aanderson, T.R., et al.: Scand. J. Haematol., *28:*360–366, 1982.
55. Bailey, L.B., Wagner, P.A., Christakis, G.J., et al.: J. Am. Gerentol. Soc., *28:*276–278, 1980.
56. Russell, R.M.: Implications of gastric atrophy for vitamin and mineral nutriture. *In* Nutrition and Aging. Edited by M.L. Hutchinson and H.N. Munro. New York, Academic Press, 1986, p. 59.
57. Suter, P.M., Golner B.B., Goldin, B.R., et al.: Gastroenterology, *101:*1039–1045, 1991.
58. Krasinski, S., Russell, R.M., Otradovec, C.L., et al.: Am. J. Clin. Nutr., *49:*112–120, 1989.
59. Krasinski, S.D., Cohn, J.S., Schaefer, E.J.: J. Clin. Invest., *85:*883–891, 1990.
60. MacLaughlin, J., Holick, M.F.: J. Clin. Invest., *76:*1536–1538, 1985.
61. Webb, A.R., Pilbeam, C., Hanafin, N., et al.: Am. J. Clin. Nutr., *51:*1075–1081, 1990.
62. Gallagher, J.C., Riggs, B.L., Eisman, J., et al.: J. Clin. Invest., *64:*729–736, 1979.
63. Garry, P.J., Goodwin, J.S., Hunt, W.C., et al.: Am. J. Clin. Nutr., *36:*319–331, 1982.
64. Horwitt, M.K., Harvey, C.C., Dahm, C.J. Jr.: N. Y. Acad. Sci., *203:*223–236, 1972.
65. Kelleher, J., Losowsky, M.S.: Vitamin E in the elderly. *In* Tocopherol, Oxygen and Biomembranes. Edited by C. DeDuve and O. Hayaishi. Amsterdam, Elsevier/North Holland Biomedical Press, 1978, p. 311.
66. Davies, E., Kelleher, J., Losowhy, M.S.: Clin. Chim. Acta, *24:*431–436, 1969.
67. Vatassery, G.T., Johnson, G.J., Johnson, G.J., et al.: J. Am. Coll. Nutr., *4:*369–375, 1983.
68. Haroon, Y., Bacon, D.S., Sadowski, J.A.: J. Chromatography, *384:*383–389, 1987.
69. Sadowski, J.A., Hood, S.J., Dallal, G.E., et al.: Am. J. Clin. Nutr., *50:*100–108, 1989.
70. Bullamore, J.R., Wilkinson, R., Gallagher, J.C., et al.: Lancet, *2:*535–537, 1970.
71. Krasinski, S.D., Russell, R.M., Samloff, I.M., et al.: J. Am. Geriatr. Soc., *34:*800–806, 1986.
72. Ireland, P., Fordtran, J.S.: J. Clin. Invest., *52:*2672–2681, 1973.
73. Matkovic, V., Kostial, K., Simonovic, I., et al.: Am. J. Clin. Nutr., *32:*540–549, 1979.
74. Dawson-Hughes, B., Jacques, P., Shipp, C.: Am. J. Clin. Nutr., *46:*685–687, 1987.
75. Dawson-Hughes B., Dallal G.E., Krall, E.A., et al.: N. Engl. J. Med., *323:*878–883, 1990.
76. Lynch, S.R., Finch, C.A., Monsen, E.R., et al.: Am. J. Clin. Nutr., *36:*1032–1045, 1982.
77. Bunker, V.W., Lawson, M.S., Clayton, B.E.: J. Clin. Pathol., *37:*1353–1357, 1984.
78. Marx, J.J.M.: Blood, *53:*204–211, 1979.
79. Pilch, S.M., Senti, F.R. (eds.): Assessment of the Iron Nutritional Status of the U.S. Population Based on Data Collected in the Second National Health and Nutrition Examination Survey, 1976–1980. Bethesda, MD, Federation of American Societies for Experimental Biology, 1984.
80. Pilch, S.M., Senti, F.R. (eds.): Assessment of the Zinc Nutritional Status of the U.S. Population Based on Data Collected in the Second National Health and Nutrition Examination Survey, 1976–1980. Bethesda, MD, Federation of the American Societies for Experimental Biology, 1984.
81. Turnlund, J.R., Durkin, N., Costa, F., et al.: J. Nutr., *116:*1239–1247, 1986.
82. Jacob, R.A., Russell, R.M., Sandstead, H.H.: Zinc and copper nutrition and aging. *In* Handbook of Nutrition in the Aged. Edited by R. Watson. Boca Raton, FL, CRC Press, 1985, p. 77.
83. Sandstead, H.D., Henriksen, L.K., Gerger, J.L., et al.: Am. J. Clin. Nutr., *36:*1046–1059, 1982.
84. Turnlund, J.R., Michel, M.C., Keyes, W.R.,: Am. J. Clin. Nutr., *36:*587–591, 1982.
85. Gibson, R.S., Martinez, O.B., MacDonald, C.: J. Gerontol., *40:*296–302, 1985.
86. Yunice, A.A., Hsu, J.M.: Homeostasis of trace elements in the aged. *In* Metabolism of Trace Metals in Man. Edited by O.M. Rennert and N.Y. Chan. Boca Raton, FL, CRC Press, 1984, pp. 99–127.
87. Lowenstein, F.W.: J. Am. College Nutr., *1:*165–177, 1982.
88. National Center for Health Statistics, Carroll, MD, Abraham, S, Dresser, CM: Vital and Health Statistics. Series 11, No. 231. DHHS Pub. No. (PHS) 83–1681. Public Health Service. Washington, D.C., U.S. Government Printing Office, 1983.
89. Attwood, E.C., Robey, E., Kramer, J.J., et al.: Age Ageing, *7:*46–56, 1978.
90. Stiedemann, M., Jansen, C., Harrill, I.: J. Am. Diet. Assoc., *73:*132–139, 1978.
91. Prothro, J., Mickles, M., Tolbert, B.: Am. J. Clin. Nutr., *29:*94–104, 1976.
92. Barr, S.I., Chrysomilides, S.A., Willis, E.J., Beattie, B.L.: Nutr. Res., *3:*417–431, 1983.
93. Kohrs, M.B., O'Neal, R., Preston, A., et al.: Am. J. Clin. Nutr., *31:*2186–2197, 1978.
94. McGandy, R.B., Russell, R.M., Hartz, S.C., et al.: Nutr. Res., *6:*785–798, 1986.

95. Sahyoun, N.R., Otradovec, C.L., Hartz, S.C., et al.: Am. J. Clin. Nutr., *47:*524–533, 1988.
96. Marr, J.W.: World Rev. Nutr. Diet., *13:*105–164, 1971.
97. Campbell, V.A., Dodds, M.L.: J. Am. Diet. Assoc., *51:*29–33, 1967.
98. Block, G.: Am. J. Epidemiol., *115:*492–505, 1982.
99. Russell, R.M., McGandy, R.B., Jelliffe, D.: Am. J. Med., *76:*767–769, 1984.
100. Morrow, F.D.: Clin. Nutr., *5:*112–120, 1986.
101. Campion, E.W., DeLabry, L.O., Glynn, R.J.: J. Gerontol., *43:*M18–M20, 1988.
102. National Center for Health Statistics, Fulwood, R., Johnson, C.L., et al.: Vital and Health Statistics. Series 11, No. 232. DHHS Pub. No. (PHS) 83–1682. Public Health Service. Washington, D.C., U.S. Government Printing Office, 1982.
103. Manson, J.E., Stampfer, M.J., Hennekens, C.H., et al.: JAMA, *257:*353–358, 1987.
104. Simopoulos, A.P., Van Itallie, T.B.: Ann. Intern. Med., *100:*285–295, 1984.
105. Chicago Society of Actuaries: Build Study, 1979. Chicago, Society of Actuaries and Association of Life Insurance Medical Directors of America, 1980.
106. Metropolitan Height and Weight Tables: New York, Metropolitan Insurance Company, 1983.
107. Garrison, R.J., Feinleib, M., Castelli, W.P., et al.: JAMA, *249:*2199–2203, 1983.
108. Kissebah, A.H., Vydelingum, N., Murray, R., et al.: J. Clin. Endocrinol. Metab., *54:*254–260, 1982.
109. Krotkiewski, M., Björntorp, P., Sjöström, L., et al.: J. Clin. Invest., *72:*1150–1162, 1983.
110. Lapidus, L., Bengtsson, C., Larsson, B., et al.: Br. Med. J., *289:*1257–1261, 1984.
111. Larsson, B., Svärdsudd, K., Welin, L., et al.: Br. Med. J., *288:*1401–1404, 1984.
112. Master, A.M., Lasser, R.P.: JAMA, *172:*658–662, 1960.
113. Frisancho, A.R.: Am. J. Clin. Nutr., *84:*808–819, 1984.
114. Frisancho, A.R., Flegel, P.N.: Am. J. Clin. Nutr., *37:*311–314, 1983.
115. Andres, R., Elahi, D., Tobin, J.D., et al: Ann. Intern. Med., *103:*1030–1033, 1985.
116. Andres, R.: Principles of Geriatric Medicine. New York, McGraw-Hill, 1985, p. 311.
117. National Center for Health Statistics, Najjar, M.F., Rowland, M.: Vital and Health Statistics. Series 11, No. 238. DHHS Pub. No. (PHS) 87–1688. Public Health Service. Washington, D.C., U.S. Government Printing Office, 1987.
118. Vir, S.C., Love, A.H.G.: Am. J. Clin. Nutr., *32:*1934–1947, 1979.
119. Blackburn, G.L., Thornton, P.A.: Med. Clin. North Am., *63:*1103–1115, 1979.
120. Forbes, G.B.: Hum. Biol., *48:*161–173, 1976.
121. Cohn, S.H., Ellis, K.J., Sawitsky, A., et al.: Am. J. Clin. Nutr., *34:*2839–2847, 1981.
122. O'Hanlon, P., Kohrs, M.B.: Am. J. Clin. Nutr., *31:*1257–1269, 1978.
123. Yearick, E.S., Wang, M.-S.L., Pisias, S.J.: J. Gerontol., *35:*663–671, 1980.
124. Jansen, C., Harrill, I.: Am. J. Clin. Nutr., *30:*1414–1422, 1977.
125. Smith, J.L., Wickiser, A.A., Korth, L.L., et al.: J. Am. Coll. Nutr., *3:*13–25, 1984.
126. Garry, P.J., Hunt, W.C., VanderJagt, D., et al.: Am. J. Clin. Nutr., *50:*1219–1230, 1989.
127. Garry, P.J., Goodwin, J.S., Hunt, W.C.: Am. J. Clin. Nutr., *36:*902–909, 1982.
128. Lipschitz, D.A., Mitchell, C.O., Steele, R.W., et al.: J. Parenter. Enter. Nutr., *9:*343–347, 1985.
129. Hartz, S.C., Otradovec, C.L., McGandy, R.B.,: J. Am. Coll. Nutr., *7:*119–128, 1988.
130. Hale, W.E., Stewart, R.B., Cerda, J.J., et al.: J. Am. Geriatr. Soc., *30:*401–403, 1982.
131. Gray, G.E., Paganini-Hill, A., Ross, R.K.: Am. J. Clin. Nutr., *38:*122–128, 1983.
132. Blumberg, J.B.: Trans. Pharmacol. Sci., *7:*33–35, 1986.
133. Blumberg, J.B.: Drug Nutr. Interact., *4:*99–106, 1985.
134. Roe, D.A. (ed.): Drugs and Nutrition in the Geriatric Patient. New York, Churchill Livingstone, 1984.
135. Russell, R.M.: Drug Nutr. Interact., *4:*165–170, 1985.
136. Jacques, P.F., Hartz, S.C., Russell, R.M.: FASEB J., *2:*A1613, 1988.


## SELECTED READINGS


Ausman, L.M., Russell, R.M.: Nutrition and the elderly. *In* Nutritional Biochemistry and Metabolism. Edited by Maria C. Linder. New York, Elsevier, 1991.

Hutchinson, M.L., Munro, H.N. (eds.): Nutrition and Aging. New York, Academic Press, 1986.

Morley, J.E., Glick, Z., Rubenstein, L.Z. (eds.): Geriatric Nutrition: A Comprehensive Review. New York, Raven Press, 1990.

Munro H.N., Danford, D.E. (eds.): Nutrition, Aging, and the Elderly. New York, Plenum Press, 1989.

CHAPTER 49

# Body Composition: Influence of Nutrition, Disease, Growth, and Aging

Gilbert B. Forbes



*Der sehr fettarme Muskel eines verhungerten Tiers kann nicht ohne weiteres dem fettreichen bei normaler Ernährung gegenübergestellt werden. Zülassig ist nur der Vergleich fettfrei berechneter Organe.*
—Adolph Magnus-Levy[1]*

The promulgation of Magnus-Levy's concept of fat-free tissue at the turn of the century paved the way for the development of techniques for estimating body composition in vivo. Physiologists of that era spoke of the existence of an "active protoplasmic mass," to which various metabolic phenomena could be related. The labors of the nineteenth century Continental chemists had established with some precision the composition of blood and tissue; now the twentieth century investigators were to supply the concept of volume, first with blood and later with other body fluid compartments, and to conceive the idea of metabolic balance. Soon after the discovery of deuterium Georg von Hevesy used this isotope to estimate total body water, and later Francis Moore introduced the concept of total exchangeable potassium and sodium. By applying Archimedes' principle, Albert Behnke showed us how to estimate the relative proportions of lean and fat in the human body. Rudolph Sievert found that the human body contained enough $^{40}K$ (a natural isotope) to be easily detectable, and thus opened the way for the use of this technique to estimate lean and fat in a noninvasive manner.[2] More recent years have seen the use of neutron activation, of special radiographic procedures (the latest being the computed tomography, or CT scan), of electrical conductivity and bioimpedance, and of nuclear magnetic resonance. Conceptualization and technical development both have played a role in this historical development, the one powerless without the other, to the point where we now possess a great deal of information on certain

*"The fat-poor muscle of a starved animal cannot be compared directly to one normally nourished and rich in fat. It is permitted only to compare organs on a fat-free basis."

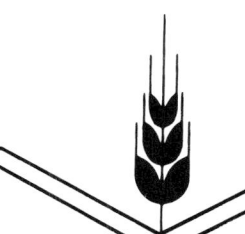

aspects of body composition throughout the age span of man.

## BODY WEIGHT AND HEIGHT

Body weight and height measurements are easily done and are of great use in assessing growth and nutritional status. For the infant and child growth velocity is truly a bioassay for energy balance and for certain hormonal functions; in the adult a change in weight suggests an abnormal process, nutritional or otherwise. See the Appendix for height-weight standards for fetal weight for gestational age and for infants, children, and adults (Appendix Tables A–11a to A–11g and A–12a to A–12e).

Normative values, despite what the adjective implies, cannot necessarily be construed as optimum. This is particularly apt to be true for a country such as the United States where there is an abundant supply of high-quality food, where a sizable fraction of the population is clearly overweight, and where it is the usual practice for adults to gain weight after they reach their maximum stature at 18 to 20 years for women and 21 to 25 years for men. In an attempt to define optimum, tables of "desirable weight" for height have been developed from actuarial data gathered by the Metropolitan Life Insurance Company; for their history see Appendix Tables A–11a to A–11g. These tables list such "desirable weights" for adults 25 years of age and older. Although no provision is made for age, adults are categorized by body frame size, which is determined by inspection or by elbow width; and the lack of precision in defining what is "desirable" is manifested by the range of values given for each frame and height category. These ranges vary progressively from 2.7 kg for the shortest "small frame" category to 11.8 kg for the tallest "large frame" category of persons.

### BODY MASS INDEX

Body mass index (BMI) is body weight divided by a power of height, usually (height),[2] which is said to be independent of stature. Calculations based on values for ideal body weight suggest that BMI for normal men and women should be in the range of 19 to 27 kg/m$^2$. Indeed, this range roughly corresponds to 25th to 75th percentile values recorded from adult individuals who participated in the 1971 to 1974 National Health and Nutrition Survey.[3] In the case of infants and children, average BMI values change with age,[3,4] beginning at 13 kg/m$^2$ at birth, reaching a peak of 18 at about 1 year, and then dropping to a nadir of 15 kg/m$^2$ at about age 6 years, to be followed by a rise to adult values during adolescence. Individuals with high indices are classified as overweight, even obese, and those with subnormal indices as undernourished. Although such classifications cannot be applied, for instance, to short muscular men, or to tall asthenic women, the BMI has found usefulness in evaluating groups of individuals.

However, the BMI is not always an accurate index of body composition. This is evident from the fact that despite the difference in body fat the average index is about the same for both sexes during the adolescent and young adult years.

Andres has analyzed the relationship between BMI and mortality in adults.[5] The curve is U-shaped: the lowest mortality rate is at a BMI of about 20 kg/m$^2$ for individuals 20 to 29 years old, and the nadir progressively moves upward with age to reach a value of about 27 kg/m$^2$ for those 60 to 69 years old. Based on morbidity, the lowest rate for Japanese men and women aged 30 to 59 years is at a BMI of 22 kg/m$^2$.[133] Of interest is the lack of a sex difference for this ideal body mass index. Because males generally have more lean body mass (LBM) and less fat than females at any given BMI, LBM size is a factor in health risk as well as body fat.

### CONSTANCY OF BODY WEIGHT

Support for the hypothesis that body weight is homeostatically controlled comes from the observation that many adults maintain their weight within narrow limits over long periods, and that many children maintain their relative weight status as they grow. The coefficients of variation for successive daily weights in adults is 0.4 to 0.8%.[6] Indeed, there is a tendency for overweight individuals following a period of weight loss to return to their previous weight. Parizkova's study of Olympic gymnasts showed that the gain in LBM and loss of body fat occasioned by training were completely reversed in time once the contests were finished.[7] Individuals who gain LBM and lose body fat in response to anabolic steroids tend to revert in time to their previous body composition status and weight when the drugs are stopped.[8,9] Short-term fluctuations in weight can result from changes in water balance, or changes in liver and muscle glycogen induced by diet or physical activity. Episodes of infection, serious trauma, enforced bed rest, malignancy, and nutritional inadequacy and surfeit lead to weight change; many women state that they gain weight towards the end of the menstrual cycle.

The fluctuations noted above indicate that homeostatic control is not perfect; nevertheless the absence of long-term change in healthy individuals suggests that energy balance oscillates around a mean of zero and that appetite (which controls intake) is geared in some mysterious manner to metabolic rate (which determines expenditure). When these homeostatic mechanisms fail, body weight will change significantly, and the result is obesity or anorexia nervosa.

### INFLUENCE OF HEREDITY

Garn,[10] Tanner et al.,[11] and Wingerd et al.[12] have offered charts and tables showing the effect of parental stature on the height of children, and there can be no doubt that a significant influence on children's height is the height of their parents. Family resemblances in relative weight and in body build are readily appreciated, as is the tendency towards obesity. Monozygotic twins are more concordant for body size, even if reared apart, than are dizygotic twins.[13] A genetic influence on metacarpal cortex thickness,[14] bone density,[15] and skinfold thickness,[16] body fat, lean body mass, BMI, and body fat distribution has been demonstrated.[17,18] Although family life-style and feeding practices may modulate the amount of body fat, both studies of adopted children and animal models provide additional evidence for the role of heredity.

Racial differences in stature are well known: generally speaking Asian adults are shorter than Caucasians and have a smaller LBM, and southern Europeans are shorter than northern Europeans. North American blacks exhibit higher values for total body K and Ca than whites do.[19] The average Pygmy male is 144 cm tall, the female 137 cm, and average birth weight is 2600 g.; each of these is roughly 80% of the respective Caucasian value.

### SECULAR CHANGES

Today's children are taller and heavier, and have an earlier puberty, than those of previous generations, a phenomenon that has occurred in all countries in which it has been studied. Although the reason for this change is not known, it is likely that improved nutrition is a prime factor.

### AGING

Once middle age is reached, there is a progressive decline in stature, the result of thoracic kyphosis, compression of intervertebral disks, and change in angulation of the femoral neck. Borkan et al. report a loss of 7.3 cm in males between age 22 and 82 years; and they estimate that 3.0 cm (41%) of the total change is secular in origin, and that 4.3 cm is due to aging.[20] The longitudinal data of Flynn et al. show a decline of 0.3 cm per decade in young adult males and 0.8 cm in females, with a gradual increase to 1.4 cm and 3.3 cm per decade, respectively, in those over 60 years of age.[21]

## BODY COMPOSITION

Body weight is the sum total of its parts. Modern techniques have made it possible to partition the body into several components, to carry out a "bloodless dissection."

### BODY FLUID VOLUMES

The various techniques used for measuring body fluid volumes are all based on the dilution principle: a known amount of material is injected intravenously, or in certain instances given by mouth, and after an interval for equilibration, a sample of blood or urine or saliva is obtained for analysis (in the case of metabolizable substances, several such samples are required, with subsequent extrapolation to time zero). When urinary losses are appreciable, a correction is made for these; however, losses into the lumen of the gastrointestinal tract are usually neglected.

The general equation, V being volume and C concentration, is

$$V_2 = \frac{C_1V_1}{C_2}$$

where $C_1V_1$ is the quantity of material administered, $C_2$ is the concentration in body fluid at equilibrium, and $V_2$ is body fluid volume.

Because the body is not a static system, true equilibrium may never be achieved, particularly so in the central nervous system and in bone, and there is always some question as to whether the apparent volume of distribution of the administered material coincides with that of the compartment in question. Intracellular fluid (ICF) volume cannot be determined directly, only by the difference between total body water and extracellular fluid (ECF) volume, and the value for the latter varies with the material used for its determination.

Plasma volume can be estimated with Evans blue dye (T-1824) or $^{131}$I-labeled albumin, and total red cell mass with red blood cells (RBCs) tagged with $^{32}$P, $^{51}$Cr, $^{55}$Fe, or $^{59}$Fe, or by carbon monoxide uptake. Materials for extracellular fluid volume are inulin, $^{35}S_2O_3^-$, $^{35}SO_4^{2-}$, $SCN^-$, $Br^-$, and $^{82}Br^-$. Cohn et al. have used the ratio of total body Cl (by neutron activation) to serum Cl for this purpose.[22] The first two materials in this list yield smaller values for ECF volume than the others do. Appropriate corrections for serum water must be made, and in the case of ionized injectates, corrections for the Donnan equilibrium.

Total body water is estimated by deuterium or tritium dilution, or by dilution of urea, alcohol, or N-acetyl-4-aminopyrine. Water labeled with oxygen-18 is now being used to estimate total body water.[23] Administered deuterium and tritium undergo some exchange with nonaqueous hydrogen, and hence overestimate total body water by 4 to 5%; such is not the case for oxygen-18. Bromide and $SCN^-$ both overestimate ECF volume by about 10% because of penetration of erythrocytes.

Some of these materials can be given by mouth, others must be given intravenously; some readily penetrate the cerebrospinal fluid, others do so very slowly; however, all appear in gastrointestinal secretions. This latter phenomenon poses a problem in animals with a large gastrointestinal tract.

Repeat determinations in normal subjects show that the total error (i.e., biologic variation plus technical error) ranges from 2 to 9% for the various assay methods. It should be remembered that body weight, which can be measured accurately, varies by at least 1% during the course of a 24-hour day, and that individuals tend to be 1 to 2 cm shorter in the evening than in the morning.

## TOTAL BODY CONTENT

The body content of a number of elements can now be assayed, by several methods. The technique of isotopic dilution can be applied to Na, K, and Cl as well as to water, by using the following equation:

$$Q = \frac{Q^* \text{ admin.} - Q^* \text{ excreted}}{Q^*/Q \text{ (serum, urine, saliva)}}$$

where Q is body content (g, mEq) and Q* is the isotope ($^{24}Na$, $^{22}Na$, $^{42}K$, $^{43}K$, $^{82}Br$, stable Br). Br is used because there is no convenient isotope of Cl. The result is expressed as total exchangeable content ($Na_e$, $K_e$, $Cl_e$), because this procedure underestimates total body content of both K and Na. Total exchangeable K is 90 to 95% of total body K, because of incomplete exchange with erythrocytes and brain. Total exchangeable Na is only 70 to 80% of total body Na, because of incomplete exchange with bone. However, Br dilution appears to be a good reflection of total body Cl.

Shizgal et al. have devised a method for estimating total exchangeable K ($K_e$) without the need to use the short-lived and inconvenient $^{42}K$ (t½ is 12 hours).[24] Total body water and total exchangeable Na ($Na_e$) are measured together with Na, K, and $H_2O$ in a sample of whole blood. Then,

$$K_e = \left[\frac{Na+K}{H_2O} \text{(blood)} \times \text{body } H_2O\right] - Na_e.$$

The correlation between measured $K_e$ and $K_e$ as estimated by this method is high. Because $Na_e$ is measured with long-lived $^{22}Na$, this method may not be suitable for children.

Francis Moore and his associates developed the concept of body cell mass (BCM), defined as "the working, energy-metabolizing portion of the human body in relation to its supporting structures."[25] It consists of the cellular components of muscle, viscera, blood, and brain; its size is estimated from total body K content, either as total exchangeable K from isotopic dilution or from $^{40}K$ counting. The BCM concept is useful because it encompasses those lean tissues most likely to be affected by nutrition, disease, or physical activity over relatively short periods. In normal subjects BCM would be expected to be about 57% of LBM.

Neutron activation has been used to estimate total body Na, Cl, N, Ca, and P.[26,27] The subject is irradiated with neutrons, and the induced radioactivity determined by suitable γ-ray detectors. The dose of radiation to the subject is about 30 millirads. However, the facilities required are expensive and highly sophisticated, so only a few are in existence.

The possibility exists of determining total body Mg, H, C, O, and individual organ content of I and Cd. Details can be found in reviews by Cohn.[27,28]

## $^{40}K$ COUNTING

The body contains enough of this naturally occurring isotope (t½ is $1.3 \times 10^9$ years, body content $3.7 \times 10^3$ Bq (0.1 μCi)) to permit its detection and quantitation by low background scintillation counters. From the known abundance of $^{40}K$ (0.012%) one can then calculate total body K content. This technique has the advantage of being noninvasive and requiring little cooperation by the subject.

There are two types of detectors: one or more sodium iodide crystals activated with thalium, and large plastic or liquid scintillation chambers, both in heavily shielded rooms. The former provide excellent resolution so that contaminating radioisotopes can be detected, but low efficiency; the latter have poor resolution, but high efficiency because the detector can be made large enough to completely surround the subject.* The former have a low background rate, of the order of one-third the net $^{40}K$ activity in adults, whereas the latter have, by virtue of their large size, a high background rate, amounting to 3 to 4 times the net $^{40}K$ activity. There are two factors that demand careful calibration of each instrument: the inverse square law of radiation, and the attenuation of $^{40}K$ γ rays by body tissues, especially the subcutaneous fat layer, which has a low K content. Instrument calibration is usually achieved by administering a known amount of $^{42}K$ (a short-lived isotope whose γ-ray energy is similar to that of $^{40}K$) to the subject and adding a like amount to a known quantity of KCl. From the ratio of $^{42}K$ to $^{40}K$ in the standard and the amount of $^{42}K$ in the subject's body one can calculate the quantity of $^{40}K$ in the subject, and so derive a calibration factor.

## BODY DENSITY

Archimedes is credited with the discovery that one can estimate the relative proportions of a two-component mixture, each of known density, by measuring the density of the whole system. Hence from a measurement of body density the relative proportions of lean (D = 1.100 g/cm³) and fat (D = 0.900 g/cm³) can be calculated. Let Wf represent weight of fat, Wl weight of lean, and Wb weight of body, and Vf, Vl, and Vb their respective volumes. Because density (D) = W/V, the relationship Vb = Vf + Vl can be written as

$$\frac{Wb}{Db} = \frac{Wf}{Df} + \frac{Wl}{Dl}$$

*During the 1960s the body burden of $^{137}Cs$ (a fallout product) was sufficient to cause interference with $^{40}K$ counts in low-resolution counters; however, today this is much less of a problem.

and because Wl = Wb − Wf, it follows that

$$\frac{Wb}{Db} - \frac{Wb}{Dl} = \frac{Wf}{Df} - \frac{Wf}{Dl}$$

whence

$$Wb\left(\frac{1}{Db} - \frac{1}{Dl}\right) = Wf\left(\frac{1}{Df} - \frac{1}{Dl}\right).$$

Dividing Wf by Wb yields the following (letting $\frac{1}{Df} - \frac{1}{Dl} = \frac{1}{a}$):

$$\frac{Wf}{Wb} = \frac{a}{Db} - \frac{a}{Dl}$$

Because Dl is known (letting $\frac{a}{Dl} = a'$),

$$\text{fraction fat } \frac{Wf}{Wb} = \frac{a}{Db} - a', \text{ and}$$

$$\text{fraction lean} = 1 - \frac{Wf}{Wb}.$$

Using the values for Df and Dl as noted, a = 4.95 and a′= 4.50. Brozek et al. suggest values of 4.570 and 4.142, respectively, based on calculations derived from induced weight losses and gains and compositional differences between lean and obese young men.[29] Body density can be measured by underwater weighing:

$$Db = \frac{W\ (\text{air})}{W\ (\text{air}) - W\ (\text{water})}$$

with appropriate corrections for the densities of water and air and for the volume of air in the lungs (gastrointestinal air is either neglected or assumed to be 100 ml). Body volume can also be estimated by water displacement, by helium dilution, application of Boyle's law, and even by special photographic and acoustic techniques, whence density is simply W/V. The underwater weighing technique is the only one in common use.

## TOTAL BODY ELECTRICAL CONDUCTIVITY (TOBEC)

The subject is placed in a hollow cylinder containing a solenoid coil driven by a 2.5 to 5 MHz oscillating radiofrequency current. The perturbation of the electromagnetic field by the subject is an index of electrical conductivity, which is a property of lean tissue. The second generation instrument requires the subject to be moved slowly through the cylinder; the use of Fourier analysis permits a better assessment of total body water and LBM.[30,31] The instrument has been validated against carcass analysis of rabbits and pigs.[32,33] Studies of both static subjects[34] and those losing weight[35] give evidence of the usefulness of this instrument. The energy delivered to the subject is so small (7 $mW/cm^2$) as to pose no hazard.

## BIOELECTRICAL IMPEDANCE

Electrodes are attached to the wrist and ankle; a weak alternating current (800 μA, 50 kHz) is applied and the voltage drop is detected by electrodes placed proximal to those carrying the current. The hypothesis is that the resistance (impedance) to the electrical current is directly proportional to the length (L) of the conductor (which is lean tissue) and inversely proportional to its cross-sectional area (A), so $R = pL/A$, where $p$ is volume resistivity. Multiplying the right hand side by L/L, $R = pL^2/V$, or in terms of height (H), volume $= pH^2/R$ (for some unexplained reason, standing height is used instead of total length between the electrodes).

The problems are that the body is far from a perfect cylinder, that $p$ undoubtedly varies from tissue to tissue, and that the arms and legs contribute almost all of the resistance of the body.[36] Reactance, a measure of cell membrane capitance, can also be recorded by the instrument; however, it is small in comparison to resistance and is usually neglected. Settle et al. provide a discussion of the principles of the technique.[37]

There are conflicting reports about the validity of this technique. Some report excellent correlations between impedance estimates of lean weight and density, total body water, and/or $^{40}K$ counting,[34,38,39] whereas others are of the opinion that this technique lacks sufficient precision.[36,40,41] A disturbing finding is the failure of the BIA technique to accurately predict body composition change during diet-induced weight loss.[42,43]

Many investigators have discovered that the precision of impedance estimates of lean weight is improved by adding weight, sex, and age to the basic $H^2/R$ parameter. Several prediction equations have been devised. The inclusion of height and weight in the final calculation is destined to improve predictability for the simple reason that lean weight is related to both of these parameters.

A note is in order about the conceptual basis for the techniques mentioned thus far. A large number of individual tissues have actually been analyzed for $H_2O$, K, N, and density; taken together with organ size these provide a basis for estimation of LBM in vivo. The TOBEC and bioimpedance techniques, on the other hand, can be evaluated only by comparison to other techniques, which are themselves subject to technical error.

## ANTHROPOMETRY

This technique includes *skinfold thickness*—really a double layer of skin and subcutaneous tissue, measured with special calipers—and various body circumferences. The usual sites for skinfold measurements are the midtriceps region, at the inferior tip of the scapula, and just above the iliac crest. Because human skin is only 0.5 to 2 mm thick, subcutaneous fat contributes the bulk of the measured value. One grasps the tissue between thumb and forefinger, shaking it gently to (it is hoped) exclude underlying muscle, and stretching it just far enough to permit the jaws of the spring-activated caliper to impinge on the tissue. Because the jaws compress the tissue, the caliper reading diminishes for a few seconds, and then the dial is read.* In subjects with moderately firm, rather thin subcutaneous tissue the measurement is easy to make, but those with flabby, easily compressible tissue and those with very firm tissue not easily deformable present a real problem. A recent comparison between caliper measurements and CT scans of the midarm region showed that the former progressively underestimated subcutaneous tissue thickness as thickness increased.[44]

The assumptions underlying this method are first, that the thickness of the subcutaneous fat mantle reflects total body fat, and second, that the sites chosen for the measurement, either singly or in combination, represent the average thickness of the entire mantle. Neither assumption has been proven true.

Cross-sectional area of the muscle-bone (M + B) and fat components of the arm can be calculated from arm circumference and skinfold thickness at the midpoint, as follows (T is triceps skinfold, B is biceps):

$$(\text{M} + \text{B})\ \text{area} = \frac{1}{4\pi}\left[\text{circ.} - \frac{\pi}{2}(\text{T} + \text{BSF})\right]^2,$$

and by subtraction from total area (circ.$^2/4\pi$) arm fat area. Data on arm (M + B) area and arm fat area for 6- to 17-year-old children have been published by the National Center for Health Statistics.[45†]

Extensive studies by many investigators have established relationships between various anthropometric measurements and LBM or body fat, and although the correlations are often not high, the simplicity of the techniques means that they can be readily applied to large numbers of individuals in the field. It is obvious that such measurements as skinfold thickness and abdominal and buttocks circumferences will bear some relationship to body fat, and that biacromial, wrist, and knee diameters will vary with LBM. The quantitative relationships between anthropometric measurements and body composition vary somewhat with age and sex, and indeed among various investigators; furthermore, there have been problems in applying the results to individuals other than those from whom the observations were made. For recent data, see Appendix Tables A–15a to A–15c.

Durnin and Womersley measured skinfold thickness and body density in a large number of men and women, and proceeded to develop relationships between density and the logarithm of the sum of four skinfolds (biceps, triceps, subscapular, and suprailiac).[46] They present a table from which the percentage of body fat for various age and sex groups can be read from the sum of skinfold values (see Appendix Table A–15a). Pollock et al. have constructed a similar table from which the percentage of fat can be read from the sum of skinfold measurements (triceps, iliac, thigh for women; chest, abdomen, thigh for men)[47] (see Appendix Table A–15b).

Although these tables have been widely used, there are some problems. Durnin and Womersley's table gives rather high estimates of the percentage of fat for subjects with low values for skinfold thickness.[46] Their estimates, as well as those of others employing different anthropometric formulations, do not provide satisfactory answers for subjects who are ill or who have lost considerable amounts of weight. The subcutaneous tissues in the elderly are easily compressed by the caliper jaws, which leads to falsely low readings.

Because LBM accounts for 70 to 90% of body weight in normal children and adults, it is obvious that LBM and weight will be related; in subjects of widely varying fat content one can anticipate that body fat and weight will also be related (Fig. 49–1). As will be noted later, LBM is a function of stature at all ages. It was the failure of weight-height functions for individuals whose excess weight consisted of muscle that led Albert Behnke to develop the specific gravity technique.

## FAT DISTRIBUTION

There is now considerable interest in body fat distribution as a possible factor in adult health. Lapidus et al.[48] and Larsson et al.[49] have shown in long-term studies that men and women with high ratios of abdomen circumference to hip circumference (the "apple" configuration) have a higher mortality from cardiovascular disease and stroke than those with low ratios (the "pear" configuration). There is evidence that the amount of visceral fat is related to the abdomen-to-hip ratio.[50]

Figure 49–1 shows a plot of abdomen-to-hip ratio against age for normal individuals studied in my laboratory. This ratio varies with age, and a definite sex difference develops by about age 12 years.

Tokunaga et al.[52] and Kvist et al.[53] have made CT scans of many regions of the body, from which they determined body fat volumes in both subcutaneous and internal sites. Of the total fat volume in women, it turns out that a large proportion is located in the pelvic, thigh, and hip regions.

*Satisfactory calipers are: Harpenden Caliper, H.E. Morse Co., Holland, Michigan; Holtain-Harpenden Caliper, Holtain Ltd., Brynberian, Crymmych, Pembrokeshire, Wales; and Lange Caliper, Cambridge Scientific Industries, Inc., Cambridge, Maryland.

†These values were calculated from arm circumference and triceps skinfold only, whence the formula becomes

$$(\text{M} + \text{B})\ \text{area} = \frac{1}{4\pi}[\text{circ.} - \pi\text{TSF}]^2.$$

The problem here is that triceps skinfold often differs from the biceps skinfold, and hence is not representative of the entire subcutaneous mantle of the arm.

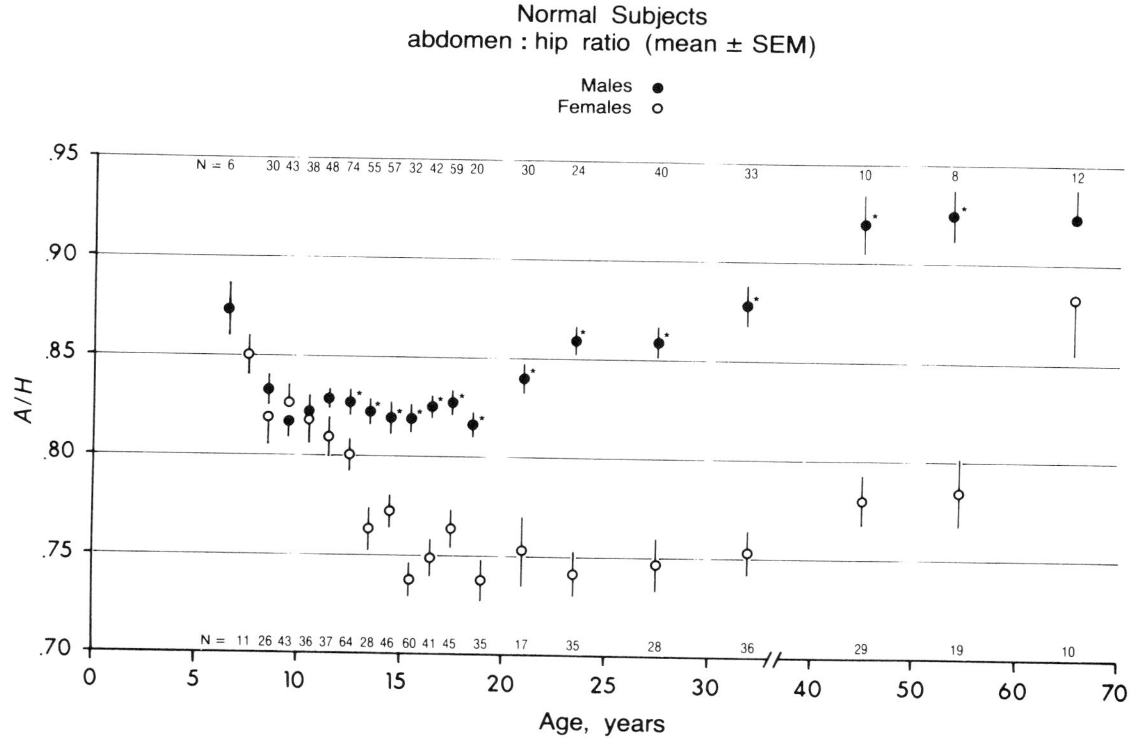
Normal Subjects
abdomen : hip ratio (mean ± SEM)
Males ●
Females ○
A/H
.95
.90
.85
.80
.75
.70
N = 6 30 43 38 48 74 55 57 32 42 59 20 30 24 40 33 10 8 12
N = 11 26 43 36 37 64 28 46 60 41 45 35 17 35 28 36 29 19 10
0 5 10 15 20 25 30 40 50 60 70
Age, years

**FIGURE 49–1.** Normative data for abdomen:hip ratio derived from 661 normal males and 646 normal females. Abdominal circumference was measured at the level of the umbilicus and hip circumference was measured at the maximum protuberance of the buttocks. Vertical bars are ± SEM. The asterisks represent a significant sex difference. (From Forbes, G.B.: The abdomen:hip ratio: normative data and observations on selected patients. Int. J. Obes., *14*:149–157, 1990.)

## URINARY CREATININE EXCRETION

The assumption that urinary creatinine (Cr) excretion is an index of muscle mass is supported by the work of Schutte et al. in dogs.[54] They found a good correlation between urinary Cr excretion and dissectable muscle mass in this species, and furthermore that there was a good correlation between Cr excretion and total plasma Cr (plasma Cr concentration times plasma volume). Urine collections must be timed accurately and the excretion rate can be affected by diet. Studies of subjects of widely varying body size have also shown a good relationship between Cr excretion and lean weight.[55] For subjects on ad libitum intake, this relationship is

$$\text{LBM (kg)} = 3.288 \text{ mmol/d Cr} (= 0.0291 \text{ mg/d Cr}) + 7.38 \quad r^2 = 0.97.$$[55]

For those on meat-free diets it is

$$\text{LBM (kg)} = 2.723 \text{ mmol/d Cr} (= 0.0241 \text{ mg/d Cr}) + 20.7 \quad r^2 = 0.91.$$[63]

Data from humans and animals show that fat-free skeletal muscle on average makes up 49% of total fat-free weight; thus, muscle mass can be easily calculated from the foregoing equation. The positive intercepts on the ordinate axis mean that the ratio of LBM, and of muscle mass to Cr excretion declines as Cr excretion increases. Notwithstanding the finding of positive ordinate intercepts by many investigators,[55] Schutte et al.[54] and Cheek[56] give single values of 17.9 kg and 20 kg muscle per gram urinary Cr excreted per day, respectively.

## METABOLIC BALANCE

The metabolic balance technique can detect small changes in body content and body composition. Sodium and chloride balance reflect changes in ECF, potassium and nitrogen changes in cell mass. For example, a change in body N content of 1.14 mol (16 g), equivalent to 0.5 kg LBM, is easily detected, whereas such a change is well within the error of body composition techniques. However, it cannot provide data on actual body content, and it is actually rather expensive when one adds up the cost of running a metabolic ward and supporting laboratory facilities.

The usual procedure is to subtract urine and fecal excretions from intake, and to neglect cutaneous losses since these are difficult to measure. If balance is strongly positive or negative the error in so doing is small, but it becomes appreciable as balance approaches zero. Cutaneous losses of N and K increase as their respective intakes rise. Many authors automatically subtract 0.36 to 0.57 mmol N (5 or 8 mg N)/kg per day. Another problem is the nonrandom nature of the intake and excretion variables, the result being that positive balances tend to be overestimated and negative balances underestimated, never the reverse. Corrections must be made for element content of blood samples and for menstrual losses. For those elements whose main route of excretion is fecal (such as Ca, Fe, and Pb) the balance periods must be long enough to account for day-to-day variations, and to include intestinal transit time.

Table 49–1 lists the advantages and disadvantages of the various techniques. Some are inexpensive, easy to use, and suitable for individuals in the field; others require a laboratory and expensive equipment; yet others are so sophisticated that few are actually in operation. Before proceeding, the investigator should determine the reliability and precision of the technique

**TABLE 49–1.** BODY COMPOSITION TECHNIQUES: ADVANTAGES AND DISADVANTAGES

| TECHNIQUE | ADVANTAGES | DISADVANTAGES |
|---|---|---|
| Density | Apparatus inexpensive<br>Estimates LBM and fat simultaneously<br>Nonhazardous<br>Can be repeated frequently | Subject cooperation necessary for underwater weighing technique<br>Unsuitable for young children, elderly<br>Error from intestinal gas |
| Dilution methods | Estimates body fluid volumes<br>Inexpensive<br>Great variety: Na, K, Cl (Br), $H_2O$ | Radiation exposure (some materials)<br>Blood samples needed (some materials)<br>Incomplete equilibration Na, K; overestimation by $D_2O$, THO; value for ECF depends on method used; $^{18}O_2$ assay requires elaborate equipment |
| $^{40}K$ counting | No hazard<br>Minimal subject cooperation<br>Can be repeated frequently | Instrument expensive<br>Proper calibration necessary<br>Problem in interpretation in subjects with K deficiency |
| Metabolic balance | No hazard<br>Suitable for many elements<br>Can detect small changes in body content (<1%) | Measures only *change* in body composition<br>Meticulous subject cooperation<br>Metabolic ward expensive<br>Error from unmeasured skin losses<br>Many laboratory analyses needed |
| Creatinine excretion | No hazard<br>Estimate of muscle mass | Meticulous subject cooperation<br>Influenced by diet, collection time critical<br>Day-to-day variation (c.v. 5–10%) |
| Anthropometry (skinfold thickness, circumferences) | Cheap<br>Direct estimate of body fat, regional muscle | Poor precision in obese subjects, and in those with firm subcutaneous tissue<br>Regional variation in subcutaneous fat layer; uncertainty ratio subcutaneous fat/total fat |
| CT scan | Organ size; fat distribution; bone | Instrument expensive<br>Radiation exposure |
| Electrical conductivity (TOBEC, EMME) | No hazard<br>Estimate of LBM | Apparatus expensive |
| Bioelectrical impedance | Apparatus inexpensive<br>No hazard<br>Estimate of LBM, $H_2O$ | Precision now under investigation* |
| Neutron activation | Minimal subject cooperation<br>Body content Ca, P, N, Na, Cl | Apparatus expensive<br>Calibration difficult<br>Radiation exposure |
| Nuclear magnetic resonance | Organ size, muscle, fat; fat distribution; total body water | Apparatus expensive |
| Dual photon absorptiometry | Bone mineral, total and regional; body fat, soft tissue lean | Expensive<br>Radiation exposure |
| Plain radiographs of extremities | Muscle, fat, bone cortex, cortex widths | Radiation exposure† |

*Although impedance measurement combined with height and weight can estimate LBM in static individuals, it alone is a relatively poor predictor of LBM change during weight gain and loss.[42,43]

†The cross-sectional area of the second metacarpal cortex has been used by Garn as an index of skeletal size.[57]

to be used. This is especially important in evaluating changes in body composition that result from nutrition or disease.

## OTHER TECHNIQUES

Some other techniques, which are listed below, are not in common use because of expense, the need for special diet precautions, or lack of advantage over other techniques.

1. Uptake of fat-soluble gases (cyclopropane, xenon, radiokrypton) provides a direct estimate of total body fat.[58]
2. Subcutaneous fat thickness by ultrasonography, infrared interactance.[59]
3. Urinary excretion of 3-methylhistidine as an index of muscle mass; a prerequisite is 3 days of a meat-free diet
4. Energy balance together with change in body weight yields a satisfactory estimate of body fat loss during weight reduction, according to Garrow;[60] the formula is

$$\Delta \text{ fat (kg)} = [\Delta E \text{ (Mcal)} - \Delta W \text{ (kg)}] /8,$$

which assumes energy equivalents of fat and lean as 9 and 1 kcal/g, respectively.

5. Estimates of body volume by special photographic techniques,[61] and by acoustic plethysmography;[62] density then is W/V

The estimation of lean weight and total body fat from measurements of body density, total body K, N, and $H_2O$, and from electrical conductivity and bioimpedance all carry the assumption that the composition of the LBM does not vary among normal adult individuals. The water, K, and N contents of the LBM do vary somewhat as determined by carcass analysis.[33,63] Of these, potassium exhibits the greatest variability, water the least. Bone has a low water content and a low K content but a high density in comparison to soft tissue; hence one must assume that bone-to-soft tissue ratios do not vary greatly among individuals. In their neutron activation studies Ellis and Cohn found that the whole body Ca/K ratio is related to stature, and so is a little lower in men than in women;[64,65] nonetheless, the limited variability of this ratio indicates that the bone-to-soft tissue ratio does not vary much among normal individuals.

Assessment of individuals with massive obesity presents a problem. They are unable to cooperate with the underwater weighing procedure, proper calibration of $^{40}K$ counters is difficult, skinfold measurements are imprecise, and the thickness may exceed the maximum jaw width of the usual calipers. Some patients have mild to moderate edema. Dilution methods and urinary Cr excretion should be satisfactory, however.

Another consideration stems from the fact that the ratio of ECF to total water varies somewhat with age, being higher in neonates than in young adults and then rising again in the elderly.[63] Hence neither the K, N, or $H_2O$ contents of the LBM, nor its density, can be considered to be constant throughout the age span of man. In dealing with diseased subjects or those who are losing weight, it must be remembered that the K/N ratio varies among body tissues, from a high of 0.336 (molar ratio) in erythrocytes to 0.070 in brain, 0.039 in skeletal muscle, 0.035 in viscera, to a low of 0.006 in plasma and skin (in terms of mmol K/g N, these values are 24, 5.0, 2.8, 2.5 and 0.45, respectively).[67] Hence the ratio of change in body K to change in body N resulting from a change in weight will depend on the particular tissue components involved. In states of underhydration or overhydration the density of the LBM will be altered, and in states of K deficiency the K content of the LBM will be subnormal.

Several investigators have used two or more techniques in the same subjects. Some report a reasonable correspondence between densitometric, body water, and $^{40}K$ techniques.[68,69] Cohn et al. found rather small coefficients of variation for body N/K and body $K/H_2O$ ratios in normal adults.[70] The results of $^{40}K$ and densitometric assays were comparable in a series of women with varying degrees of obesity,[71] and body K was closely related to body N in a group of adult men and women.[72]

The values for K, $H_2O$, and N contents of the LBM listed in Table 49–2 are based on cadaver analyses,[73] with the K/LBM ratio being altered for females on the basis of the reported sex difference in the $K_e/H_2O$ ratio.[74] Some investigators prefer to derive values for LBM composition from a comparison of in vivo assays. Cohn et al. have chosen values of 64.5 and 58 mmol K/kg LBM for males and females respectively,[70] whereas Womersley et al. suggest that these values should be 66.4 and 59.7.[75] Lukaski et al. derived a value of 62.6 mEq K/kg LBM for males.[69] They also offer a value of 746 ml $H_2O$/kg LBM; however, their values of 2.29 mol (32.1 g) N and 2.33 mmol (32.7 g) N/kg LBM are close to the value derived from cadaver analysis.

Values for total body K/N ratios have been reported: on a molar basis, these are 0.0263 to 0.0273 for males and 0.0234 to 0.0249 for females (1.88 to 1.95 mmol K/g N, and 1.67 to 1.78 mmol K/g N, respectively). Total body K/N ratios tend to be lower in older adults.[70] The average value from cadaver analysis is 0.0280 (2 mmol K/g N).

The variations noted previously reflect the criteria used to assess LBM and differences in analytical technique, or even biologic variability. There is a distinct tendency among investigators to use the densitometric technique as the "standard" to which the results of other techniques should be compared. Although densitometry has the advantage of being subject to less technical error than the other techniques, it is obviously impossible to determine its accuracy for living subjects, and it is likely

**TABLE 49–2.** CALCULATION OF LEAN BODY MASS AND FAT IN ADULTS (W = LBM + FAT)(KG)

| METHOD | FORMULA | REFERENCES AND COMMENTS |
|---|---|---|
| Density | Fraction fat = $\frac{4.95}{D} - 4.50$; $\frac{4.570}{D} - 4.142$ | Siri[6]; Brozek et al.[29] |
| Total body water | LBM = liters $H_2O$/0.73 | Multiply by 0.95 to correct for $^2H$ and $^3H$ exchange with nonaqueous hydrogen; no correction for $^{18}O_2$ |
| $^{40}K$ counting | LBM = mmol K/68.1 (M), 64.2 (F)<br>BCM = mmol K × 0.00833 | Multiply by 1.1 when $^{42}K$ dilution is used |
| Creatinine excretion | LBM = 3.288 Cr (mmol/d) (0.029 Cr mg/per day), + 7.38 | Ordinary diet |
| Neutron activation | LBM = mol N/2.36 | Change in LBM can be estimated from N balance |
| Anthropometry | Numerous formulas | |
| Density—total water | Fraction fat = $\frac{2.1366}{D} - 0.78\frac{H_2O}{W} - 1.394$ | Siri[6] |
| Neutron activation—total water—$^{40}K$ | LBM = 6.25 N + $H_2O$ + $\frac{Ca}{0.34}$ | Cohn et al.[22] |
| | LBM = BCM + ECF + $\frac{Ca}{0.017}$ | Cohn et al.[70] |
| Electrical conductivity (TOBEC) | Several formulas | |
| Bioimpedance | Numerous formulas | |

that the density of the LBM (upon which the test implicitly depends) varies with age (it does change with growth), and perhaps with sex. There would seem to be no a priori reason for choosing any one technique as the standard to which others must be compared.

## EFFECT OF AGE ON COMPOSITION OF THE LBM

The values listed in Table 49–2 pertain to young and middle-aged adults. Composition is different for the fetus and newborn, and changes occur with aging. Some of those changes are given in condensed form in Table 49–3. Water content falls progressively during early life, as does the ratio of ECF volume to total body water; this ratio rises again in old age. Potassium and nitrogen contents rise, as does calculated density. With aging, total body K declines a little faster than does total body N, so the K/N ratio falls.

## PRECISION OF VARIOUS TECHNIQUES

Two factors must be considered: technical error per se, and biologic variability. These include such phenomena as the random nature of radioactive isotope emissions and the day-to-day fluctuations in urinary Cr excretion. For isotope dilution procedures, for instance, four measurements are necessary, each subject to error: composition of the injectate and its volume, and assay of the equilibrium sample of body fluid for tracer and stable isotope. Densitometry entails measurement of residual pulmonary air volume as well as body weight both in air and submerged, together with an assumed value for intestinal air. Neutron activation requires that the neutron dose be known as well as the amount of induced radioactivity. Body weight exhibits diurnal and day-to-day variations, and it is safe to assume that certain features of body composition also exhibit some variability. An instructive exercise is to calculate the effect of adding or subtracting 500 ml $H_2O$ from an adult subject:

**TABLE 49–3.** COMPOSITION OF LEAN BODY MASS

| AGE | $H_2O$ (%) | ECF/ICF RATIO | K (mmol/kg) | N (mol/kg) | DENSITY (g/ml) |
|---|---|---|---|---|---|
| Fetus, 24 weeks | 89 | 1.9 | 40 | 1(1.4%) | |
| Birth | 81 | 1.5 | 49 | 1.7(2.4%) | 1.063 |
| Adult | 73 | 0.70 | 68 (64)* | 2.36(3.3%) | 1.10 |
| Elderly | | 0.85 | | | |

*Number in parentheses shows value for females.
Fomon et al. provide estimates for ages birth to 10 years.[77]

this will change the density and the K and N and $H_2O$ contents of the LBM slightly, as well as the ratio of element metabolic balance to weight change. It is the *total* error—technical plus biologic—that must be taken into account, and this can only be evaluated by replicate assays on individuals, a procedure not always feasible with assays involving radiation exposure.

The magnitude of the observed error will depend on the method used to express the results. When LBM is measured, fat is determined by subtraction, so in subjects where LBM exceeds 50% of body weight, the relative error for fat will be greater than that for LBM; the same is true for densitometry. The existence of rare individuals with estimated body fat contents of 1%, or even a negative value, is proof that error can occur.

Published data show coefficients of variation (c.v.) of 2 to 4% for $^{40}K$ counting, 2.5 to 6.1% for total exchangeable K, 5.5% for body Ca, 3.5% for total body N, and 5 to 10% for urinary Cr excretion. Densitometry appears to be the most reproducible technique (c.v. 1.2%); skinfold thickness is the worst, with recorded c.v. of 6 to 24%.[63] The c.v. for bioimpedance ranges from 1.3 to 7%,[30] and the c.v. for the TOBEC assay is said to be about 1%.[35] Errors can be reduced somewhat by making two or more assays at the start of an experimental procedure (e.g., induced weight loss) and again at the end.

## CHANGES IN BODY COMPOSITION WITH GROWTH AND AGING

Table 49–4 lists many of the elements to be found in the body of a male adult, the so-called "reference man" as determined by the International Committee on Radiation Protection.[76] Because the LBM of the average woman is about two thirds that of the average man, her body content will be, with the exception of $O_2$, C, and $H_2$, which are present in fat, two thirds to three fourths of the amounts listed. Hence I have added some values for the average woman as estimated from body composition assays of living subjects; the male values for Ca and P were also derived in this manner.

The values listed are averages; for some, such as F and Fe, the quantities depend on diet.

Average organ weights for an adult man are listed in Table 49–5, and are compared to those for the newborn infant. The adult weighing 20 times the newborn has 33 times as much muscle and 23 times as much skeleton, 19 times as much heart, and 10 times as much skin, liver, and kidney; however, the brain is only about 3 times as large. Please note that one third of the newborn skeleton consists of cartilage, and that relative organ size is different in the neonate: at this age muscle accounts for 22% of body weight, brain for 10%, and liver for 4%,

**TABLE 49–4.** REFERENCE MAN AND WOMAN: TOTAL BODY CONTENT

| SUBSTANCE* | AMOUNT IN GRAMS (mol) MALE | FEMALE |
|---|---|---|
| Water | 45,000 (2500 mol) | 31,000 (1700 mol) |
| Hydrogen, nonaqueous | 2,000 (1000 mol) | |
| Oxygen, nonaqueous | 2,900 (90 mol) | |
| Carbon | 16,000 (1333 mol) | |
| Nitrogen | 1,800 (64 mol) | 1,300 (46 mol) |
| Calcium | 1,100 (27 mol) | 830 (21 mol) |
| Phosphorus | 500 (16 mol) | 400 (13 mol) |
| Potassium | 140 (3600 mmol) | 100 (2560 mmol) |
| Sodium | 100 (4350 mmol) | 77 (3350 mmol) |
| Chlorine | 95 (2680 mmol) | 70 (2000 mmol) |
| Sulfur | 140 (4400 mmol) | |
| Magnesium | 19 (780 mmol) | |
| Silicon | 18 (640 mmol) | |
| Iron | 4.2 (75 mmol) | |
| Fluorine | 2.6 (140 mmol) | |
| Zinc | 2.3 (35 mmol) | |
| Copper | 0.07 (1.1 mmol) | |
| Manganese | 0.01 (180 μmol) | |
| Iodine | 0.01 (79 μmol) | |

*Seventeen additional elements (all less than 330 mg) are listed in reference 76. For many the body content is a function of diet. The body also contains a number of radioactive elements: uranium ($10^{-4}$ g), radium ($10^{-11}$ g), $^{90}$strontium, and $^{137}$cesium. The last two are fallout products from nuclear explosions; both are present in food and water, and both have long physical half-lives (28 and 27 years, respectively). The current body burden of $^{137}Cs$ is about 2nCi, which is considerably less than it was in the 1960s; it emits γ-rays, so the body content can be assayed in the whole body counter. Such measurements have been used during the past three decades to monitor fallout from the atomic bomb and from nuclear disasters.

**TABLE 49–5.** REFERENCE MAN AND NEONATE: GROSS ORGAN SIZE (g)

| | ADULT | NEWBORN |
|---|---|---|
| Weight | 70,000 | 3,400 |
| Skeletal muscle | 28,000 | 850 |
| Adipose tissue | 15,000 | |
| (fat 12,000) | | 500 |
| Skeleton | 10,000 | 440 |
| (cortical bone 4000, trabecular bone 1000 marrow 3000, cartilage 1100, periarticular tissue 900) | | (cartilage 140) |
| Skin | 4,900 | 510 |
| Liver | 1,800 | 170 |
| Brain | 1,400 | 440 |
| Heart | 330 | 17 |
| Kidneys | 310 | 34 |

(Data on the adult from International Committee on Radiation Protection: Report of the Task Group on Reference Man for Purposes of Radiation Protection. Oxford, Pergamon Press, 1975; data on the newborn from Widdowson, E., Dickerson, J.W.T.: Chemical composition of the body. *In* Mineral Metabolism. Edited by C.L. Comar and F. Bronner. New York, Academic Press, 1964.)

compared to 40%, 2%, and 2.6%, respectively, in the adult.

## LBM AND WEIGHT VARIABILITY COMPARED

Among individuals of the same age and sex body fat exhibits much more variability than LBM does. This is shown in Figure 49–2, which is based on my $^{40}$K assays of 164 women aged 14 to 50 years and 156 to 170 cm in stature. It is evident that body fat accounts for most of the variability in body weight. It should be emphasized, however, that LBM and fat are not completely independent entities. As shown later, a change in body weight that is the result of changes in energy balance usually involves both body components.

In women the maximum LBM is about 70 kg, in men about 100 kg. Perhaps there is a limit to LBM size, as there is for stature, whereas body fat can increase enormously (Fig. 49–2).

### *AGE AND SEX*

Figures 49–3 and 49–4 show average values for LBM and fat from midgestation through the eighth decade, as compiled from several sources. Note that the abscissa scale for Figure 49–3 is in postconception years. The fetus does not acquire appreciable amounts of body fat until the last trimester of gestation, and it turns out that the human neonate has a larger percentage of body fat (14%) than other mammals at birth. Relative body fat continues to increase during the first 6 months of postnatal life to a maximum of 25%, then falls to a nadir of about 13% in boys and 16% in girls in late childhood.

It is of interest that sexual dimorphism in body composition is present in early life, well in advance of mature gonadal function. Once adolescence is under way the sex difference becomes pronounced, the male spurt in LBM being much more rapid whereas females acquire more fat. Between the ages of 10 and 20 years the average increment in LBM is 33 kg in boys but only 16 kg in girls, and by age 20 years the male-to-female ratio is 1.45:1. This can be compared to a weight ratio of 1.25:1 and a height ratio of 1.08:1 at age 20 (Table 49–6). During the male adolescent spurt, the peak velocity for LBM coincides with peak height velocity.[7] It is likely that the sex difference in the magnitude of the adolescent spurt in LBM is due to the fact that the testosterone production rate in males is about 6 times that of females.

Based on cross-sectional data, the adult years are characterized by a slow fall in LBM; this fall takes place somewhat more rapidly in males, and from the data at hand it would appear that female LBM is preserved until the age of menopause. By age 75 years, LBM in males is roughly equivalent to that of the average 14 year old, and in females to that of the average 13 year old. So it appears that much of the LBM increment acquired during the adolescent growth spurt is dissipated by the aging process.

The studies of Cohn and associates show that there is a progressive decline in total body K, N, and Ca during the adult years.[22] Between ages 25 and 75 years body K declines by about 4.5% per decade and body N by about 3.5% per decade in both sexes; however, the decline in body Ca is 5.4% per decade in women, compared to 2% per decade in men. This last observation is in keeping

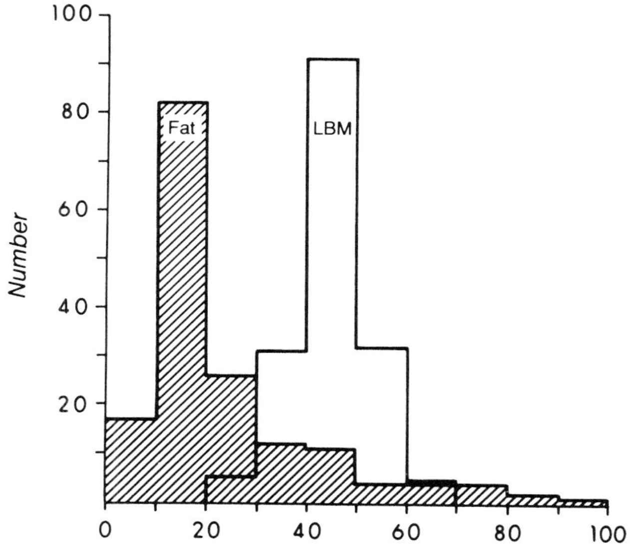
100
80
60
40
20
Number
Fat
LBM
0
20
40
60
80
100
Kilograms

**FIGURE 49–2.** Frequency distribution of lean body mass (LBM) and body fat for 164 females aged 14 to 50 years and 156 to 170 cm in height. Included are patients with anorexia nervosa and obesity as well as normal subjects.

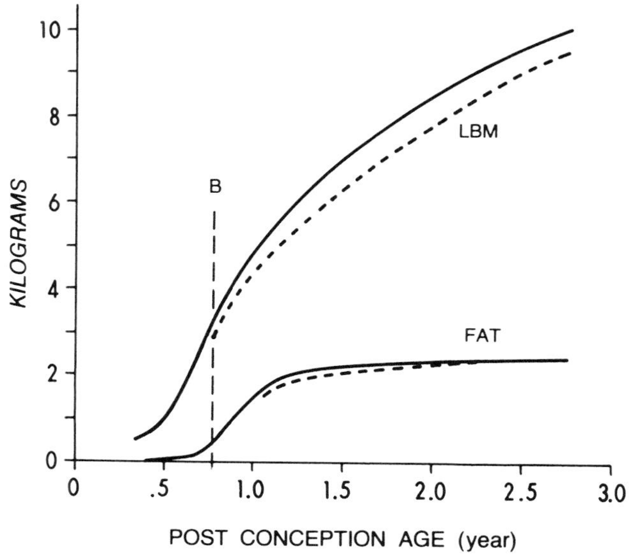
10
8
6
4
2
0
KILOGRAMS
B
LBM
FAT
0
.5
1.0
1.5
2.0
2.5
3.0
POST CONCEPTION AGE (year)

**FIGURE 49–3.** Average value for lean body mass (LBM) and fat in fetus and infant. Age is in postconception years. Boys, solid lines; girls, broken lines. (From Forbes, G.B.: Human Body Composition: Growth, Aging, Nutrition, and Activity. New York, Springer-Verlag, 1987.)

with observations on the decrease in density of the spine and appendicular skeleton, especially in women, with advancing years. However, it should be remembered that all of these values are derived from cross-sectional data.

A few investigators have managed to make repeated assays on adults over extended periods, and it should be noted that such longitudinal observations tend to show a somewhat smaller age decline than do the cross-sectional data. Steen et al. did repeated assays of total body water and body K in men and women from age 70 to age 81.[78] An analysis of the individual data, which were kindly provided by Dr. Bertil Steen, showed that those who lost significant amounts of weight lost more total body water and K than those who had minimal weight loss or some weight gain. On average the former group lost about 5 kg LBM per decade, the latter only 2 kg LBM per decade. Flynn et al. did repeated $^{40}$K assays on a large group of adults over an 18-year period.[21] Those individuals less than 51 years of age at the initial assay and who gained weight tended to gain LBM, and those who lost weight tended to lose LBM. On the other hand, older individuals tended to lose LBM regardless of body weight change; the average loss was about 4 kg per decade for both sexes.

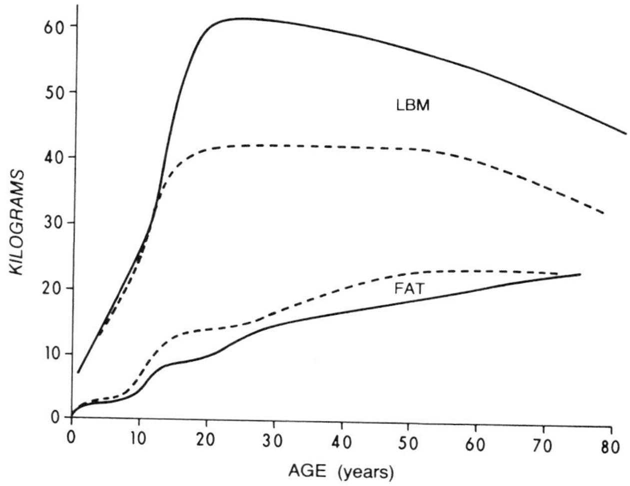
60
50
40
30
20
10
0
KILOGRAMS
LBM
FAT
0
10
20
30
40
50
60
70
80
AGE (years)

**FIGURE 49–4.** Average values for lean body mass (LBM) and fat in child and adult. Males, solid lines; females, broken lines. (Data from Forbes, G.B.: Human Body Composition: Growth, Aging, Nutrition, and Activity. New York, Springer-Verlag, 1987.)

Of three middle-aged males studied over periods of 26 to 31 years two showed an LBM decline of 1.6 kg per decade, whereas the third lost only 0.25 kg per decade.[63] This last subject tended to put on weight while the others did not; this observation taken in conjunction with those noted previously makes it necessary to consider body weight change in the evaluation of the age decline in lean body mass.

Longitudinal changes in thickness of the second metacarpal cortex, amounting to about 2% per decade, have been recorded by Fox et al. for normal male adults.[79]

As shown in Figures 49–3 and 49–4, girls have slightly more body fat than boys from an early age; once adolescence is under way girls acquire much more body fat than boys, and this sex difference persists throughout the adult years. These changes are reflected in triceps

**TABLE 49–6.** THE REFERENCE PERSON

| | NEWBORN | 10-YEAR-OLD BOY | 10-YEAR-OLD GIRL | ADULT MAN | ADULT WOMAN |
|---|---|---|---|---|---|
| Weight (kg) | 3.4 | 31 | 32 | 72 | 58 |
| LBM (kg) | 2.9 | 27 | 26 | 61 | 42 |
| % Fat | 14 | 13 | 19 | 15 | 28 |

skinfold thickness (Fig. 49–5). The great variability in this measurement is clearly evident.

*STATURE*

At all ages studied LBM is a function of height. On average the regression slope is 0.69 kg/cm in adult males and 0.29 kg/cm in adult females.[81] Skeletal size is also a function of height,[82] and Ellis and Cohn's data show that the same is true for total body Ca, the regression slope being 0.5 mol (20 g) Ca per centimeter.[64,65] According to their findings, a 186-cm male would be expected to have about 34 mol Ca (1370 g) in his body, a 154-cm female only 18 mol Ca (730 g). Data such as these mean that comparisons of LBM and total body Ca among individuals are valid only if height, as well as age and sex, is controlled.

Many athletes are taller than average, which is one reason why they tend to have a greater LBM. An analysis of the data compiled from several sources on male and female athletes showed that for most groups the regression slope of LBM on height was steeper than that for nonathletes.[63] Exceptions were basketball players, who have a lower LBM-to-height ratio, and weight lifters and body builders, who have a higher ratio than the others.

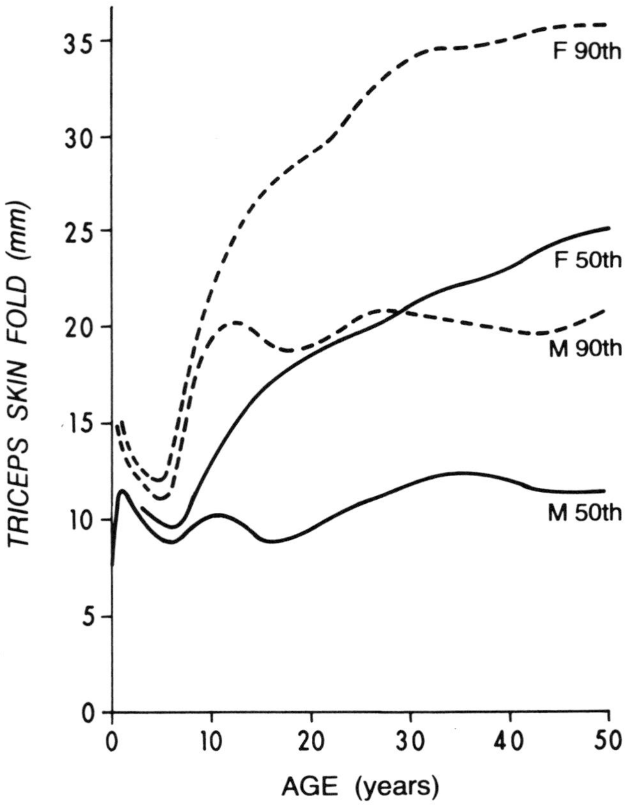
TRICEPS SKIN FOLD (mm)
35
30
25
20
15
10
5
0
10
20
30
40
50
AGE (years)
F 90th
F 50th
M 90th
M 50th

**FIGURE 49–5.** Fiftieth and ninetieth percentiles for triceps skinfold thickness. (Data on infants and children younger than 6 years from Tanner, J.M., Whitehouse, R.H.: Arch. Dis. Child., *50*:142–145, 1975; other data from Cronk, C.E., Roche, A.F.: Am. J. Clin. Nutr., *35*:351–354, 1982.)

*PREGNANCY*

Of the total weight gain during pregnancy, some 12 to 13 kg on average, the fetus, placenta, and amniotic fluid together account for about 4.2 kg. The remaining 8 kg is maternal tissue per se. All components of body water increase—plasma volume, extracellular and intracellular fluid volume—as well as total red cell mass; because the ratio of body water to body K increases, the increase in ECF volume is proportionately greater than that of ICF volume, which is in keeping with the observation that many pregnant women have mild edema. A portion of the weight gain—variously estimated at 2 to 4 kg—consists of fat.[63] Prentice et al. found no change in the BMR/LBM ratio during the course of pregnancy.[83]

*SOME CORRELATES OF BODY COMPOSITION*

Because the adult female has on average only about 70% the amount of LBM possessed by the average male, it is obvious that the requirements for energy and protein are correspondingly less. The Recommended Dietary Allowances (RDA) of the National Research Council reflect this sex difference. Both basal metabolic rate and blood volume are more closely related to LBM than to body weight; so it is to be expected that based on body weight they would be lower in the obese than in the nonobese.

It would seem prudent to adjust the dose of various drugs on the basis of LBM rather than body weight. Some of the adult decline in such metabolic parameters as glucose tolerance, adrenocorticoid hormone excretion, and maximal oxygen consumption may reflect the age-associated decline in LBM.

In considering studies done on individuals consuming protein-free diets (refs. in ref. 63), a linear relationship is seen between endogenous urinary nitrogen excretion and body cell mass. Dietary protein requirement is thus a function of BCM, and hence of LBM rather than body weight with its variable component of fat. On this basis, the need for protein—and perhaps for other dietary nutrients as well—should be less in the elderly than in the young adult, and less in women than in men.

## INFLUENCE OF NUTRITION

### ENERGY DEFICIT

Maintenance of body weight in the adult, and satisfactory growth rate in the child, depend on an adequate supply of energy. Subnormal intakes lead to a decline in growth velocity, and in the adult to a fall in body weight; generally speaking the rate of weight loss is a function of the magnitude of the energy deficit. After the first few days, fasting results in a loss of about 0.5 kg per day in the obese,[84] and about 0.35 kg per day in the nonobese.[85] Mathematical analysis shows that the weight loss during fasting is exponential,[86] which suggests that the loss rate is proportional to weight itself and so tends to diminish with time. The fractional loss rate is less in the obese than in the nonobese (0.34% per day versus 0.56% per day).

Smaller energy deficits produce slower rates of weight loss. Using data obtained during controlled observations on adults over periods of at least 5 weeks, it appears that 1400 to 1900-kcal diets produce a loss of 0.13 to 0.15 kg per day in nonobese males,[87,88] 0.16 to 0.20 kg per day in obese males, and 0.08 to 0.12 kg per day in obese females.[89]

### ENERGY EXCESS

Consumption of energy in excess of maintenance needs produces an increase in body weight; when subjects are under close observation it turns out that the increase is roughly proportional to the total excess energy consumed during the overfeeding period.[90] Indeed, a reevaluation of Neumann's and Gulick's classic studies on themselves showed that they always gained weight when they took excess food, and that they always lost when they ate less.[91]

The energy cost of the weight gain has been computed for several types of human subjects. On average this turns out to be 5.0 kcal/g gain for infants recovering from malnutrition,[92] 4.0 kcal/g gain for growing prematurely born infants,[93] 4.7 kcal/g for adolescent girls recovering from anorexia nervosa,[94] and 8.0 kcal/g for normal adults who are deliberately overfed;[90] the energy cost is about the same for women as it is for men. As will be shown later, the energy cost varies according to the composition of the tissue gained.

### EFFECT ON BODY COMPOSITION

Nutrition can affect lean weight as well as body fat. When compared to normal individuals of the same stature, age, and sex, undernourished subjects have a reduced LBM as well as less fat, and the obese have an increase in both.[63,95] Indeed, Keys and Brozek spoke of "obesity tissue" as consisting of protein and body fluid as well as fat.[96]

Careful studies of underfed subjects, employing either nitrogen balance or body composition techniques, have shown that significant weight reduction involves a loss of both LBM and fat. The relative contribution of each of these components to the total weight loss depends on two principal factors: the initial body fat content and the magnitude of the energy deficit.

During a fast thin individuals lose twice as much body N per unit weight loss as do obese individuals;[97] thin individuals consuming 1400 to 1900-kcal diets have a greater relative loss of LBM ($\Delta$LBM/$\Delta$W ratio) than do the obese.[63] The obese preferentially burn fat and so tend to conserve lean.

The second factor is equally important: for all categories of initial body fat content studied to date, the $\Delta$LBM/$\Delta$W loss ratio is directly related to the energy deficit. As Benedict et al. showed many years ago, even modest energy deficits lead to some loss of body N,[88] and densitometric techniques have confirmed the loss of LBM. One searches in vain for well-controlled studies showing that body N and LBM can be preserved on low-energy diets. Nitrogen losses do tend to diminish with time, however, both on low-energy diets and during fasting.[98,99] Indeed, in the latter situation it turns out that the N loss is exponential and that the fractional N loss is greater in the nonobese than in the obese.[97] This may partly account for the greater tolerance of the obese for fasting.

The combined influence of initial body fat content and energy deficit on the composition of the weight lost during weight reduction is shown in Table 49–7. Included are data on 70 men and 179 women who had body composition assays (total body water or densitometry or $^{40}$K counting) both prior to and after at least 4 weeks on a weight-reduction diet. Except for those given 300 kcal or less daily, all had adequate protein intakes. The values for the proportion of weight loss represented by LBM ($\Delta$LBM/$\Delta$W ratio) are grouped in categories according to initial body fat content and energy intake. The $\Delta$LBM/$\Delta$W ratio is seen to fall progressively for all energy intake categories as initial body fat increases; for any given value for the latter, the ratio progressively falls with increasing energy intakes (and hence decreasing energy deficits).

It is obvious that the amount of weight lost in response to a given energy deficit will vary with the composition of the weight loss. The energy value of fat is 9.4 kcal/g, and that of lean is about 1.1 kcal/g (protein has a value of 5.6 kcal/g, and LBM is 20% protein). Hence, in general, the obese will lose less weight for a given energy deficit

**TABLE 49–7.** EFFECT OF ENERGY DEFICIT (ΔLBM/ΔW RATIO)*

| INTAKE (kcal/day) | INITIAL BODY FAT (kg) 5–10 | 11–20 | 21–30 | 31–40 | 41–50 | 51–60 | 60+ |
|---|---|---|---|---|---|---|---|
| 0–300 | | | | .56(4) | .53(3) | | .40(7) |
| 450–900 | | | .51(7) | .38(35) | .31(17) | .26(10) | .21(17) |
| 1,100–1,400 | | | .26(21) | .13(31) | .14(17) | | |
| 1,600–1,900 | .69(18) | .49(14) | .21(45) | | | .15(3) | |

*Compilation of data from 19 reports (see reference 63). Values represent means; unfortunately, many of the data were presented in such a way as to preclude calculation of a standard deviation or a range. The number of subjects is given in parentheses.

than the nonobese because the former lose proportionately more fat. However, the entire process is confounded by the associated fall in basal metabolic rate (BMR), variability in physical activity, and lack of information on the actual energy deficit, so precise estimates are difficult to make.

Obese patients subjected to intestinal bypass or gastric stapling operations also lose LBM as they lose weight. In various studies 15 to 40% of the weight lost by these patients has consisted of LBM.[63]

The only animal known to preserve LBM during weight reduction is the hibernating bear, though migrating birds come close to this goal. In the absence of food and water this remarkable animal has been observed to lose 17 kg (13% of initial weight) during 60 days of hibernation without a change in LBM. However, when bears are fasted (but not thirsted) in summer, they behave as do other mammals in losing LBM as well as fat.

When undernourished individuals are induced to gain weight, LBM and fat both increase,[92,94,100] and it is obvious that the same is true for growing infants and children. There is also an increase in both components when normal adults are deliberately overfed. For such subjects the energy cost of the weight gain averages 8 kcal/g, and 38% of the gain consists of LBM.[90] In experiments involving rather modest degrees of overfeeding, Butterfield and Calloway found that 1 to 2 mg N was retained per kilocalorie of added energy (~ 45 mg LBM/kcal).[101] From their study of overfed twins Bouchard et al. concluded that genetic factors influenced the magnitude of the response.[102]

These data were collected from experiments lasting only a few weeks, the longest being 100 days. Because there are no controlled studies of longer duration in man, the situation over the long term is unknown.

The importance of adequate protein intake cannot be overemphasized. Although undernourished men can gain weight on low-protein diets, some LBM is lost at the same time that body fat is gained.[100] When Miller and Mumford gave excess food low in protein to normal individuals, they lost LBM (as judged by body K content) as they gained weight, whereas excess food high in protein produced a gain in LBM and a greater total gain per excess calorie consumed.[103] Hence low-protein diets are inefficient, even hazardous.

## BODY COMPOSITION IN OBESITY

Human obesity can occur only in the face of a positive energy balance, so in this sense it is a nutritional disease. It is fruitless to argue whether decreased physical activity or increased food intake is the prime factor: obesity results from a failure of those homeostatic mechanisms which in normal people serve to balance energy intake and outgo. Studies of obese children, adolescents, and young adults show that a portion (10 to 30%) of their excess weight consists of LBM; however, a few obese persons have normal LBM values.[95]* Such data force one to the conclusion that most obese individuals are overnourished, and that the foods eaten are nutritious. Autopsy observations show that the obese have larger hearts, kidneys, and livers.[105] Basal metabolic rate is increased,[106] as are blood hemoglobin levels[107] and metacarpal cortex thickness.[108] However, Shizgal et al. found that the ratios of ECF to total body water, and total exchangeable sodium to potassium, were much the same in the obese and nonobese.[109]

## BODY COMPOSITION IN UNDERNUTRITION

Examples to be considered here are individuals with more or less chronic energy deficits uncomplicated by significant infection or disease. They usually have normal or only slightly reduced serum protein levels, and are not incapacitated.

Patients with anorexia nervosa have very thin subcutaneous tissue, small heart and liver volumes, a reduced blood volume, and even some reduction in renal function.[110] There is a reduction in both LBM and body fat.[94]

*The situation is very different in animals rendered obese by experimentally produced hypothalamic lesions, for they tend to have a smaller LBM than controls do. Children and adolescents with the Prader-Willi syndrome (obesity, hypogonadism, muscle hypotonia, mild mental retardation) also have a subnormal LBM in the face of a supranormal body fat content.[104]

The same is true of undernourished male laborers; ECF volume, however was not reduced in these subjects, so the ratio of ECF volume to ICF volume is supranormal.[111]

## INFLUENCE OF PHYSICAL ACTIVITY

### EXERCISE

The phenomenon of work hypertrophy is well known; and this is nicely illustrated by the finding that the dominant arm of professional tennis players has larger muscles and thicker bones. However, the subcutaneous tissue thickness is about the same.[112]

Generally speaking, athletes of both sexes have a greater LBM than their nonathletic peers, and many have less body fat. The enlarged LBM is particularly true of weight lifters, "body builders," discus throwers, shot putters, and football players.

The question is whether the larger LBM is the result of training and exercise or is merely an inherent feature of the athletic individual. Studies have been done on individuals who have engaged in training and exercise programs of various types and who have presumably not taken androgenic-anabolic steroids. Although these studies show a tendency for LBM to rise and for body fat to fall, the documented changes have not been very great. Wilmore's review of 55 such studies shows that LBM increased in 22 (maximum 3.1 kg), decreased in 7, and was unchanged in 26.[113] Parizkova studied gymnasts in training for the Olympics.[7] LBM increased by an average of 1.8 kg in the males and 1.2 kg in the females, and there was an equivalent loss of body fat. Once the contests were finished, body composition reverted in time to its pretraining status.

The experiments described by Oscai et al. are of interest in this regard: when rats were forced to swim daily for many weeks (about 20% of their life span) they acquired more LBM (+5%) and less fat (−16%) than their *paired-weight sedentary* controls; skeletal muscle accounted for one third of the LBM increase.[114] However, when the exercised animals were compared to sedentary controls fed ad libitum the results were very different. Now the exercised animals weighed less than controls, and had a *smaller* LBM (by 14%) as well as less fat. The explanation is that the exercised animals ate less food and expended more energy, and so incurred an energy deficit.

The finding in experimental animals that exercise-induced increases in LBM depends on an adequate intake of food has been confirmed in humans. An analysis of Wilmore's compilation of body composition changes induced by exercise[113] shows that those subject groups who either maintained their weight or gained a little had a modest increase in LBM, whereas those who lost weight lost LBM as well as body fat.[115] This phenomenon has recently been confirmed by an analysis of individual subjects, including athletes and sedentary individuals, who engaged in exercise programs.[115] An additional finding was that body fat content influenced the body composition response to exercise and training: those individuals (of both sexes) with body fat burdens of 25 kg or more were able to sustain a greater weight loss without incurring a loss of LBM than those who were thin.[115] Bouchard et al. studied a group of males kept on a constant diet for 100 days while exercising vigorously.[116] Their estimated energy deficit was 353 MJ (84,370 kcal); average weight loss was 7.9 kg, of which 1.3 kg represented LBM.

Exercise and training cannot sustain lean weight, much less increase it, in the face of an appreciable energy deficit. Athletes who of necessity have high energy expenditures must eat well if they want to augment or even sustain their lean weight.

### IMMOBILIZATION AND SPACE TRAVEL

The decrease in muscle mass and bone density in immobilized or paralyzed limbs is a well-known phenomenon. Healthy young men placed in plaster spicas from the waist down for several weeks lost some nitrogen, calcium, and phosphorus, and had a reduction in blood volume, although body weight did not change.[117] Ordinary bed rest also results in negative balance of Ca, K, and P.[118] These authors found that exercise in the supine position was of no help in this respect. Studies of astronauts have included estimates of LBM. The loss of LBM during an 84-day flight varied according to the method used: 3.4 kg by $^{42}K$ dilution, 1.2 kg by densitometry, 2.6 kg by N balance, and 1.1 kg by total body water. The average is 2.1 kg LBM loss in the face of a 2.8 kg weight loss.[119] Blood volume declined by 10%.[120] The interpretation of these results is difficult because of the occurrence of mild hyponatremia, suggesting a change in body fluid osmolality, the strong positive N balance prior to the flight, and the fact that body weight was rapidly regained on returning to earth. Pitts and co-workers found an 8% drop in fat-free weight, a drop in total body Ca, and an increase in body fat in rats who had spent 18 days in space (see also Chap. 43).[121]

Thus the maintenance of normal body composition depends on gravity and normal physical activity as well as muscle innervation.

## IMPORTANCE OF BODY FAT

Data are now sufficient to show that relative changes in body composition are influenced by the amount of body fat. It has long been known that obese animals tolerate starvation better than thin ones, and the same is true of humans. Not only do the obese possess greater energy stores, but they also lose proportionally less lean tissue. Observations on individuals fed low-energy diets show that the relative contribution of LBM to the total weight loss is an inverse function of body fat content.[63,134] Animals are known to increase their body fat stores prior to hibernation.

When weight is gained in response to nutritional surfeit thin individuals tend to put on relatively more LBM than the obese do.

The body composition response to exercise is also influenced by body fat: those with generous fat burdens tend to lose less LBM and more fat when weight is lost during exercise than do those who are thin.[115] The limited data on migrating birds suggest that fatter species conserve LBM better than thinner ones in the face of what surely must be vigorous exercise.[63]

## INFLUENCE OF HORMONES*

Large doses of adrenal corticosteroids act to decrease muscle and bone mass; hence individuals with Cushing's syndrome have subnormal total body K and Ca and an increased Na/K ratio,[122] and total body K increases with treatment. Excessive amounts of parathyroid and thyroid hormones result in negative Ca balance, and the latter in loss of body N as well. Growth hormone treatment of children with hypopituitarism is associated with an increase in LBM and a decrease in body fat.[123] Individuals with acromegaly have increased body K, N, Na, and Ca and an increase in ECF volume.[124]

In normal individuals (including the elderly) growth hormone causes an increase in LBM and a loss of body fat,[125] and in cattle the effect on N balance is dose-related.[126]

Striking effects are produced by the androgenic-anabolic steroids: N balance becomes positive and animal studies have shown an increase in amino acid uptake in muscle and an increase in muscle size. Large doses enhance muscle protein synthesis[127] and produce a significant increase in LBM and a fall in body fat in man[63]; this effect is dose-related. These effects are apparently perceived by athletes, among whom the use of such steroids is said to be widespread.

Insulin has both anabolic and lipotropic activity, so deficiency of this hormone leads to negative N balance and fat dissolution. Normal pregnancy is associated with an increase in maternal LBM and fat, changes that are facilitated by the increased levels of testosterone, prolactin, progesterone, estrogen, and insulin that are known to occur, as well as the increase in food intake.

## INFLUENCE OF DISEASE

Cuthbertson showed many years ago that severe trauma to the limbs was accompanied by a significant loss of body N; the negative balance in his patients was as high as 9.8 mol (137 g), equivalent to a loss of 4 kg LBM.[128] Earlier Shaffer and Coleman had found that N losses occurred during the course of typhoid fever, and further that the addition of energy in the form of carbohydrate could minimize the N loss in such patients.[129] Beisel et al. recorded significant N losses in other types of infections, and showed that these losses exceeded those due to the decreased food intake that often accompanies infection.[130] They also recorded losses of K, Na, P, and Mg in their subjects. It is now common practice to provide extra nutrients—often by the parenteral route—to patients with severe trauma or infection, or who have had major surgery. Another feature of the metabolic response to surgery is an increase in the $Na_e/K_e$ ratio.[25]

Neuromuscular disease has a profound effect. Serial studies of boys with the Duchenne type of muscular dystrophy show a progressive departure from the normal total body K as they get older.[63]

Individuals with cirrhosis as well as those with cardiac failure have an increase in the ratio of Na space to total body water.[25]

As expected, individuals with osteoporosis have reduced total body Ca.[64] The loss of weight in patients with cancer involves LBM as well as fat.[110,131]

Severe malnutrition is associated with an increase in the ECF/ICF ratio, an increase in the $Na_e/K_e$ ratio,[131] an increase in intracellular Na in muscle, and a decrease in K. In such states it appears that ECF volume is better preserved than cell mass is, the shrunken cells retaining their fluid covering. Picou and co-workers evaluated the relative amounts of collagen and noncollagen protein in the bodies of malnourished infants.[132] Although the latter was reduced to about half the expected value, the former had not changed significantly. Skin and bone account for about 70% of the total body collagen.

The observations of Picou et al. help to explain the difference in calculated changes in body composition produced by different techniques. Tendon has a higher density and a lower K concentration than muscle does, so an increase in the ratio of collagen to noncollagen protein during weight loss would be expected to increase the density and to decrease the K content of the LBM. Hence the use of standard values for each will result in a slight underestimation of the LBM contribution to the weight loss by densitometry and an overestimation by $^{40}K$ counting. The finding of a smaller contribution of LBM to total weight loss by density than by $^{40}K$ counting during weight reduction by Garrow[60] and during space flight by Leonard et al.[119] is in keeping with this hypothesis. Such inconsistencies serve as a reminder that body composition techniques may not always yield precise results.

In conclusion, it is instructive to look at the relationship between the changes in LBM and the changes in body fat that have been recorded in various situations. In some instances the induced changes in LBM and fat are in the same direction: thus they act as *companions*, a decrease in one being accompanied by a decrease in the

*Although calcitriol is now considered a hormone, its action on body tissues will be presented in the chapter on vitamin D.

other, though usually not in the same proportion; the same is true for an increase. Under other circumstances LBM and fat behave as *strangers;* an increase in one is associated with a decrease in the other, and vice versa.

Figure 49–6 depicts in general terms the types of change in LBM and fat recorded for adult human subjects under various circumstances. Information on the hibernating bear and on animals with hypothalamic injury is included because these findings represent interesting departures.

When the stimulus is nutritional, a change in body weight is seen to involve both LBM and fat, and in the same direction. Despite a marked decrease in metabolic rate and in body temperature small hibernating mammals lose both LBM and fat. Established states that have evolved from nutritional excesses (obesity) or from nutritional deficits (anorexia nervosa) also exhibit concordant changes in LBM and fat. The hibernating bear is an interesting exception, for its weight loss consists entirely of fat.

The best example of discordant changes in LBM and fat is provided by the effect of androgen administration. Large doses of anabolic-androgenic steroids act to increase LBM (a proportion of which is muscle) and to decrease body fat, changes that are welcomed by athletes. Similar changes occur with the administration of growth hormone, both in normal and hypopituitary subjects. Obese patients with the Prader-Willi syndrome have a subnormal LBM despite their large burden of body fat, and the same is true for animals with experimental lesions of the hypothalamus. Hence these are not appropriate models for the usual type of human obesity.

Exercise and physical training can lead to a modest gain in LBM and a fall in body fat provided body weight does not change very much; however, if more than a few kilograms of weight are lost, LBM usually declines. Bed rest and zero gravity cause a modest reduction in LBM.

Modern techniques have thus defined a constellation of body composition changes in humans that are the result of various stimuli. Inferences derived from work on animals can now be tested in man, and the investigator is freed from the constraints of the metabolic balance method in now being able to assess body content at any point in time as well as changes that occur over long periods. A new dimension has been added to the phenomena of growth and aging.

| CHANGE OF LBM \ CHANGE OF FAT | + | 0 | – |
|---|---|---|---|
| + | OVERFEED<br>OBESITY<br>PREGNANCY<br>PUBERTY (F) | | ANDROGENS<br>GROWTH HORMONE<br>PUBERTY (M)<br>exercise |
| 0 | | STEADY STATE | HIBERNATION (bears) |
| – | AGEING<br>CNS INJURY<br>P-W SYNDROME<br>zero gravity<br>bedrest | | UNDERFEED<br>ANOREXIA<br>MALNUTRITION<br>HIBERNATION |

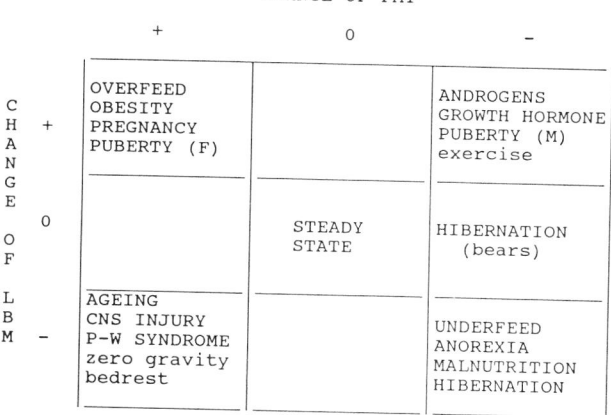

**FIGURE 49–6.** Classification of changes in lean body mass (LBM) and fat observed in various situations. Modest changes in lower case letters. P-W, Prader-Willi syndrome, an unusual and rare form of obesity associated with hypotonia and hypogonadism.

## REFERENCES


1. Magnus-Levy, A.: Physiologie des Stoffwechsels. *In* Handbuch der Pathologie des Stoffwechsels. Edited by C. von Noorden. Berlin, Hirschwald, 1906.
2. Forbes, G.B., Gallup, J., Hursh, J.B.: Science, *133:*101–102, 1961.
3. Cronk, C.E., Roche, A.F.: Am. J. Clin. Nutr., *35:*351–354, 1982.
4. van Wieringen, J.C.: Secular Changes in Growth. Leiden, Netherlands, Inst. Prev. Med., 1972.
5. Andres, R.: Ann. Intern. Med., *103:*1030–1033, 1985.
6. Khosla, T., Billewicz, W.Z.: Br. J. Nutr., *18:*227–239, 1964.
7. Parizkova, J.: Body Fat and Fitness. The Hague, Martinus Nijhoff b.v., 1977.
8. Forbes, G.B.: Some influences on lean body mass: exercise, androgens, pregnancy, and food. *In* Diet & Exercise: Synergism in Health Maintenance. Edited by P.L. White and T. Mondeika. Chicago, American Medical Association, 1982.
9. Forbes, G.B., Porta, C.R., Herr, B.E., et al.: JAMA, *267:*397–399, 1992.
10. Garn, S.M., Rohmann, C.C.: Pediatr. Clin. North Am., *13:*353–379, 1966.
11. Tanner, J.M., Goldstein, H., Whitehouse, R.H.: Arch. Dis. Child., *45:*755–762, 1970.
12. Wingerd, J., Salomon, I.L., Schoen, E.J.: Pediatrics, *52:*555–566, 1973.
13. Foch, T.T., McClearn, G.E.: Genetics, body weight, and obesity. *In* Obesity. Edited by A.J. Stunkard. Philadelphia, W.B. Saunders, 1980.
14. Smith, D.M., Nance, W.E., Kang, K.W., et al.: J. Clin. Invest., *52:*2800–2808, 1973.
15. Lutz, J., Tesar, R.: Am. J. Clin. Nutr., *52:*872–877, 1990.
16. Brook, C.G.D., Huntley, R.M.C., Slack, J.: Br. Med. J., *2:*719–721, 1975.
17. Bouchard, C., Savard, R., Després, J.-P., et al.: Hum. Biol., *57:*61–75, 1985.
18. Stunkard, A.J., Harris, J.R., Pedersen, N.L., et al.: N. Engl. J. Med., *322:*1483–1487, 1990.
19. Cohn, S.H., Abesamis, C., Zanzi, I., et al.: Am. J. Physiol., *232:*E419–E422, 1977.

20. Borkan, G.A., Hults, D.E., Glynn, R.J.: Hum. Biol., *55:*629–641, 1983.
21. Flynn, M.A., Nolph, G.B., Baker, A.S., et al.: Am. J. Clin. Nutr., *50:*713–717, 1989.
22. Cohn, S.H., Vaswani, A.N., Yasumura, S., et al.: Am. J. Clin. Nutr., *40:*255–259, 1984.
23. Schoeller, D.A., Van Sauten, D.W., Peterson, D.W., et al.: Am. J. Clin. Nutr., *33:*2686–2693, 1980.
24. Shizgal, H.M., Spanier, A.H., Humes, J., et al.: Am. J. Physiol., *233:*F253–F259, 1977.
25. Moore, F.D., Olesen, K.H., McMurray, J.D., et al.: The Body Cell Mass and Its Supporting Environment. Philadelphia, W.B. Saunders, 1963.
26. Cohn, S.H., Dombrowski, C.S.: J. Nucl. Med., *12:*499–505, 1971.
27. Cohn, S.H.: Med. Phys., *8:*145–154, 1981.
28. Cohn, S.H. (ed.): Non-invasive Measurements of Bone Mass and Their Clinical Application. Boca Raton, FL, CRC Press, 1981.
29. Brozek, J., Grande, F., Anderson, T., et al.: Ann. N. Y. Acad. Sci., *110:*113–140, 1963.
30. Van Loan, M., Mayclin, P.: Am. J. Clin. Nutr., *45:*131–137, 1987.
31. Fiarotto, M.L.: Measurements of total body electrical conductivity for the estimation of fat and fat-free mass. *In* New Techniques in Nutritional Research. Edited by R.G. Whitehead and A. Prentice. New York, Academic Press, 1991, pp. 281–301.
32. Klish, W.J., Forbes, G., Gordon, A., et al.: J. Pediatr. Gastroenterol. Nutr., *3:*199–204, 1984.
33. Keim, N.L., Mayclin, P.L., Taylor, S.J., et al.: Am. J. Clin. Nutr., *47:*180–185, 1988.
34. Segal, K.R., Gutin, B., Presta, E., et al.: J. Appl. Physiol., *58:*1565–1571, 1985.
35. Van Loan, M.D., Belko, A.Z., Mayclin, P.L., et al.: Am. J. Clin. Nutr., *46:*5–8, 1987.
36. Baumgartner, R.N., Chumlea, W.C., Roche, A.F.: Am. J. Clin. Nutr., *50:*221–226, 1989.
37. Settle, R.G., Foster, K.R., Epstein, B.R., et al.: Nutr. Cancer, *2:*72–80, 1980.
38. Lukaski, H.C., Bolonchuk, W.W., Hall, C.B., et al.: J. Appl. Physiol., *60:*1327–1332, 1986.
39. Kushner, R.F., Schoeller, D.A.: Am. J. Clin. Nutr., *44:*417–424, 1986.
40. Roche, A.F. (ed.): Hum. Biol., *59:*209–335, 1987.
41. Jackson, A.S., Pollock, M.L., Graves, J.E., et al.: J. Appl. Physiol., *64:*529–534, 1988.
42. Deurenberg, P., Weststrate, I.A., Hautvast, J.G.A.J.: Am. J. Clin. Nutr., *49:*33–36, 1989.
43. Forbes, G.B., Simon, W., Amatruda, J.M.: Am. J. Clin. Nutr., *56:*4–6, 1992.
44. Forbes, G.B., Brown, M.R., Griffiths, H.J.L.: Am. J. Clin. Nutr., *47:*929–931, 1988.
45. National Center for Health Statistics: DHEW Pub. No. (HRA) 74–614, Series 11, No. 132, 1974.
46. Durnin, J.V.G.A., Womersley, J.: Br. J. Nutr., *32:*77–97, 1974.
47. Pollock, M.L., Wilmore, J.H., Fox, S.M. III: Exercise in Health and Disease. Philadelphia, W.B. Saunders, 1984.
48. Lapidus, L., Bengtsson, C., Larsson, B., et al.: Br. Med. J., *289:*1257–1261, 1984.
49. Larsson, B., Svärdsudd, K., Welin, L., et al.: Br. Med. J., *288:*1401–1404, 1984.
50. Ashwell, M., Cole, T.J., Dixon, A.K.: Br. Med. J., *290:*1692–1694, 1985.
51. Forbes, G.B.: Int. J. Obes., *14:*149–157, 1990.
52. Tokunaga, K., Matsuzawa, Y., Ishikawa, K., et al.: Int. J. Obes., *7:*437–445, 1983.
53. Kvist, H., Sjöström, L., Tylén, U.: Int. J. Obes., *10:*53–67, 1986.
54. Schutte, J.E., Longhurst, J.C., Gaffney, F.A., et al.: J. Appl. Physiol., *51:*762–766, 1981.
55. Forbes, G.B., Bruining, G.J.: Am. J. Clin. Nutr., *29:*1359–1366, 1976.
56. Cheek, D.B.: Human Growth. Philadelphia, Lea & Febiger, 1968.
57. Garn, S.M.: The Earlier Gain and the Later Loss of Cortical Bone in Nutritional Perspective. Springfield, IL, Charles C Thomas, 1970.
58. Lesser, G.T., Perl, W., Steele, J.M.: J. Clin. Invest., *39:*1791–1806, 1960.
59. Conway, J.M., Norris, K.H., Bodwell, C.E.: Am. J. Clin. Nutr., *40:*1123–1130, 1984.
60. Garrow, J.S.: Treat Obesity Seriously. London, Churchill Livingstone, 1981.
61. Whipple, H.E., Silverzweig, S., Brozek, J. (eds.): Body Composition. Ann. N. Y. Acad. Sci., *110:*1–1018, 1963.
62. Sheng, H.-P., Adolph, A.L., Smith, E.O., et al.: Pediatr. Res., *24:*85–89, 1988.
63. Forbes, G.B.: Human Body Composition: Growth, Aging, Nutrition, and Activity. New York, Springer-Verlag, 1987.
64. Ellis, K.J., Cohn, S.H.: J. Appl. Physiol., *38:*455–460, 1975.
65. Cohn, S.H.: Personal communication.
66. Siri, W.E.: Body composition from fluid spaces and density: Analysis of methods. *In* Techniques for Measuring Body Composition. Edited by J. Brozek and A. Henschel. Washington, D.C., National Academy of Sciences, 1961.
67. Widdowson, E., Dickerson, J.W.T.: Chemical composition of the body. *In* Mineral Metabolism. Edited by C.L. Comar and F. Bronner. New York, Academic Press, 1964.
68. Krzywicki, H.J., Ward, G.M., Rahman, D.P., et al.: Am. J. Clin. Nutr., *27:*1380–1385, 1974.
69. Lukaski, H.C., Mendez, J., Buskirk, E.R., et al.: Am. J. Physiol., *240:*E302–E307, 1981; Metabolism, *30:*777–782, 1981.
70. Cohn, S.H., Vartsky, D., Yasumura, S., et al.: Am. J. Physiol., *239:*E524–E530, 1980.
71. Halliday, D., Hesp, R., Stalley, S.F., et al.: Int. J. Obes., *3:*1–6, 1979.
72. Morgan, D.B., Burkinshaw, L.: Clin. Sci., *65:*407–414, 1983.
73. Forbes, G.B.: Pediatrics, *29:*477–494, 1962.
74. Forbes, G.B., Schultz, F., Cafarelli, C., et al.: Health Phys., *15:*435–442, 1968.
75. Womersley, J., Boddy, K., King, P.C., et al.: Clin. Sci., *43:*469–475, 1972.
76. International Committee on Radiation Protection: Report of the Task Group on Reference Man for Purposes of Radiation Protection. Oxford, Pergamon Press, 1975.
77. Fomon, S.J., Haschke, F., Ziegler, E.E., et al.: Am. J. Clin. Nutr., *35:*1169–1175, 1982.
78. Steen, B.: Nutr. Rev., *46:*45–51, 1988.
79. Fox, K.M., Tobin, J.D., Plato, C.C.: Calcif. Tissue Res., *39:*218–224, 1986.
80. Tanner, J.M., Whitehouse, R.H.: Arch. Dis. Child., *50:*142–145, 1975.
81. Forbes, G.B.: Am. J. Clin. Nutr., *27:*595–602, 1974.
82. Borisov, B.K., Marei, A.N.: Health Phys., *27:*224–229, 1974.
83. Prentice, A.M., Goldberg, G.R., Davies, H.L., et al.: Br. J. Nutr., *62:*5–22, 1989.

84. Drenick, E.J., Swendseid, M.E., Blahd, W.H., et al.: JAMA, *187:*100–105, 1964.
85. Benedict, F.G.: A Study of Prolonged Fasting. Washington, D.C., Carnegie Institute, 1915.
86. Forbes, G.B.: Am. J. Clin. Nutr., *23:*1212–1219, 1970.
87. Keys, A., Brožek, J., Henschel, A., et al.: The Biology of Human Starvation. Minneapolis, University of Minnesota, 1950.
88. Benedict, F.G., Miles, W.R., Roth, P., et al.: Human Vitality and Efficiency under Prolonged Restricted Diet. Washington, D.C., Carnegie Institute, 1919.
89. Young, C.M., Scanlon, S.S., Im, H.S., et al.: Am. J. Clin. Nutr., *24:*290–296, 1971.
90. Forbes, G.B., Brown, M.R., Welle, S.L., et al.: Br. J. Nutr., *56:*1–9, 1986.
91. Forbes, G.B.: Am. J. Clin. Nutr., *39:*349–350, 1984.
92. Spady, D.W., Payne, P.R., Picou, D., et al.: Am. J. Clin. Nutr., *29:*1073–1088, 1976.
93. Reichman, B., Chessex, P., Putet, G., et al.: N. Engl. J. Med., *305:*1495–1500, 1981.
94. Forbes, G.B., Kreipe, R.E., Lipinski, B.A., et al.: Am. J. Clin. Nutr., *40:*1137–1145, 1984.
95. Forbes, G.B., Welle, S.L.: Int. J. Obes., *7:*99–108, 1983.
96. Keys, A., Brozek, J.: Physiol. Rev., *33:*245–345, 1953.
97. Forbes, G.B., Drenick, E.J.: Am. J. Clin. Nutr., *32:*1570–1574, 1979.
98. Fisler, J.S., Drenick, E.J., Blumfield, D.E., et al.: Am. J. Clin. Nutr., *35:*471–486, 1982.
99. Owen, O.E., Felig, P., Morgan, A.P., et al.: J. Clin. Invest., *48:*574–583, 1969.
100. Barac-Nieto, M., Spurr, G.B., Lotero, H., et al.: Am. J. Clin. Nutr., *32:*981–991, 1979.
101. Butterfield, G.E., Calloway, D.H.: Br. J. Nutr., *51:*171–184, 1984.
102. Bouchard, C., Tremblay, A., Després, J.-P., et al.: N. Engl. J. Med., *322:*1477–1482, 1990.
103. Miller, D.S., Mumford, P.: Am. J. Clin. Nutr., *20:*1212–1222, 1223–1229, 1967.
104. Schoeller, D.A., Levitsky, L.L., Bandini, L.G., et al.: Metabolism, *37:*115–120, 1988.
105. Naeye, R.L., Roode, P.: Am. J. Clin. Pathol., *54:*251–253, 1970.
106. James, W.P.T., Bailes, J., Davies, H.L., et al.: Lancet, *1:*1122–1125, 1978.
107. Garn, S.M., Ryan, A.S.: Am. J. Clin. Nutr., *36:*189–191, 1982.
108. Dalén, N., Hallberg, D., Lamke, B.: Acta Med. Scand., *197:*353–355, 1975.
109. Shizgal, H.M., Forse, R.A., Spanier, A.H., et al.: Surgery, *86:*60–68, 1979.
110. Heymsfield, S.B., McManus, C.B.: Cancer, *55:*238–249, 1985.
111. Barac-Nieto, M., Spurr, G.B., Lotero, H., et al.: Am. J. Clin. Nutr., *31:*23–40, 1978.
112. Buskirk, E.R., Anderson, K.L., Brozek, J.: Res. Q., *27:*127–131, 1956.
113. Wilmore, J.H.: Med. Sci. Sports, *15:*21–31, 1983.
114. Oscai, L.B., Holloszy, J.O.: J. Clin. Invest., *48:*2124–2128, 1969.
115. Forbes, G.B.: J. Appl. Physiol., *70:*994–997, 1991.
116. Bouchard, C., Tremblay, A., Nadeau, A.: Int. J. Obes., *14:*57–73, 1990.
117. Deitrick, J.E., Whedon, G.D., Shorr, E.: Am. J. Med., *4:*3–36, 1948.
118. Greanleaf, J.E., Bernauer, E.M., Juhos, L.T., et al.: J. Appl. Physiol., *43:*126–132, 1977.
119. Leonard, J.I., Leach, C.S., Rambaut, P.C.: Am. J. Clin. Nutr., *38:*667–679, 1983.
120. Rambaut, P.C., Smith, M.C. Jr., Leach C.S., et al.: Fed. Proc., *36:*1678–1682, 1977.
121. Pitts, G.C., Ushakov, A.S., Pace, N., et al.: Am. J. Physiol., *244:*R332–R337, 1983.
122. Aloia, J.F., Roginsky, M., Ellis, K., et al.: J. Clin. Endocrinol. Metab., *38:*981–985, 1974.
123. Collipp, P.J., Curti, V., Thomas, J., et al.: Metabolism, *22:*589–595, 1973.
124. Aloia, J.F., Roginsky, M.S., Jowsey, J., et al.: J. Clin. Endocrinol. Metab., *35:*543–551, 1972.
125. Rudman, D., Feller, A.G., Nagraj, H.S., et al.: N. Engl. J. Med., *323:*1–6, 1990.
126. Crooker, B.A., McGuire, M.A., Cohick, W.S., et al.: J. Nutr., *120:*1256–1263, 1990.
127. Griggs, R.C., Kingston, W., Jozefowicz, R.F., et al.: J. Appl. Physiol., *66:*498–503, 1989.
128. Cuthbertson, D.P.: Q. J. Med., *1:*233–246, 1932.
129. Shaffer, P.A., Coleman, W.: Arch. Intern. Med., *4:*538–600, 1909.
130. Beisel, W.R., Sawyer, W.D., Ryll, E.D., et al.: Ann. Intern. Med., *67:*744–779, 1967.
131. Shizgal, H.M.: Cancer, *55:*250–253, 1985.
132. Picou, D., Halliday, D., Garrow, J.S.: Clin. Sci., *30:*345–351, 1966.
133. Tokunaga, K., Matsuzawa, Y., Kotani, K., et al.: Int. J. Obes., *15:*1–6, 1991.
134. Prentice, A.M., Goldberg, G.R., Jebb, S.A., et al.: Proc. Nutr. Soc., *50:*441–458, 1991.

## SELECTED READINGS

Cheek, D.B.: Human Growth. Philadelphia, Lea & Febiger, 1968.
Cohn, S.H.: Measurement of total body calcium, sodium, chlorine, nitrogen and phosphorus in man by in vivo neutron activation analysis. Med. Phys., *8:*145–154, 1981.
Cohn, S.H. (ed.): Non-invasive Measurements of Bone Mass and Their Clinical Application. Boca Raton, FL, CRC Press, 1981.
Forbes, G.B.: Human Body Composition. New York, Springer-Verlag, 1987.
Keys, A., Brozek, J.: Body fat in adult man. Physiol. Rev., *33:*245–345, 1953.
Lukaski, H.C.: Methods for the assessment of human body composition: Traditional and new. Am. J. Clin. Nutr., *46:*537–556, 1987.
Moore, F.D., Olesen, K.H., McMurray, J.D., et al.: The Body Cell Mass and Its Supporting Environment. Philadelphia, W.B. Saunders, 1963.
Shephard, R.J.: Body Composition in Biological Anthropology. New York, Cambridge University Press, 1991.
Widdowson, E.M., Dickerson, J.W.T.: Chemical composition of the body. *In* Mineral Metabolism. Vol. 2, Part A. Edited by C.L. Comar and F. Bronner. New York, Academic Press, 1964, pp. 2–247.

PART III

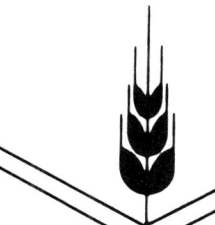

# Dietary and Nutritional Assessment of the Individual

CHAPTER **50**

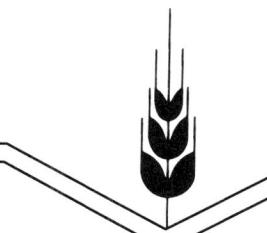

# Clinical and Functional Assessments

Khursheed N. Jeejeebhoy



Intake of a diet sufficient to meet or exceed the needs of an individual will keep the composition and function of an otherwise healthy individual within the normal range. This equilibrium is disturbed by (1) decreased intake, (2) increased requirements, and (3) altered utilization. When disequilibrium occurs, metabolism is altered, function is impaired, and finally loss of body tissue ensues. Metabolic changes in relation to energy and protein deficit occur within hours or days[1] of reducing nutrient intake (depending upon the severity of deficit), long before demonstrable anthropometric changes. Functional changes have predicted the occurrence of surgical complications better than anthropometric parameters,[2,3] specifically by showing that a reduction in muscle power is a better predictor of such complications than is weight loss or arm muscle circumference. Thus, malnutrition and its adverse consequences are recognized by inadequate intake, biochemical and functional changes, and eventually anthropometric effects. A detailed nutritional history and physical examination permit a global assessment of malnutrition and its risks and also allows identification of specific deficiencies.

## HISTORY AND PHYSICAL EXAMINATION

### HISTORY

Malnutrition is caused by an imbalance between intake and requirements. In addition, intake may be limited by impediments to eating and/or absorbing. The patient's history should therefore encompass information on the following:

**Weight changes.** Has the patient had recent and progressive weight changes? If so, in what direction? If weight has been lost, has this been voluntary (dieting) or involuntary?

**Altered intake of food or lack of specific food groups.** The patient should be questioned about his or her habitual diet and any change in the diet pattern with respect to the number of meals, the size of meals, and their contents in relation to the different food groups both prior to and during the current illness. The objective is to determine whether the diet is balanced and adequate in its nutrient content or is restricted and, if the latter, to what extent.

**Food supplements.** Details of nutrient supplements should be obtained. The use of potentially toxic levels of certain vitamins (especially A) should be determined. The reason for such supplements should be ascertained. Was it on medical advice? For example, iron is often prescribed for chronic anemia; if so, it is desirable to know what investigations, if any, had been done prior to receiving the advice.

**Ability to chew, swallow, and eat a normal diet.** Is the patient able to chew? Does he or she suffer from dental and oral problems that impede intake of food or the chewing of foods such as meat? Is there difficulty in eating because of a sore mouth or throat? Does swallowing cause pain (odynophagia)? Can the patient swallow?

If not, is the dysphagia for solids, liquids, or both? Can the obstruction to solids be overcome by swallowing liquids? If so, the patient has a motility disorder. If the food cannot progress and is regurgitated, then it is due to a mechanical problem such as a stricture.

**Satiety, discomfort, and appetite.** What happens when the food is eaten? Does the individual have a desire to eat? Is this desire normal, as compared to the premorbid state? After starting a meal, does early satiety prevent him or her from finishing the usual meal? Is the intake limited because of pain, postcibal discomfort, or diarrhea? Is the discomfort different with solids than with liquids?

**Vomiting.** Does the patient vomit? Is it copious and with ingested food? Is there a history of vomiting food eaten days before? Is pain in the abdomen relieved by vomiting?

**Change in bowel habits.** Is there a change in bowel habits? Does diarrhea occur, especially after eating? Is it watery or is it voluminous, foul-smelling, and yellow? Do the stools float on water, with difficulty in flushing the stool (steatorrhea)? Is pain relieved by bowel movements? Alternatively, does the patient suffer from constipation and bloating?

**Neuromuscular changes.** Is there tingling or numbness of the extremities or around the mouth, or spasms of the hands and/or toes?

**Presence of symptoms or signs suggestive of vitamin deficiency.** These include glossitis, stomatitis, and conjunctivitis. Is there a history of night blindness? Does the patient have petechial skin rashes?

**Presence of symptoms suggestive of trace element deficiency.** Has the patient been having excessive menses or chronic bleeding elsewhere? Is there swelling in the front of the neck? Is there a history of skin rashes or chronic infections suggestive of zinc deficiency? Chronic anemia may, on rare occasion, occur in patients with copper as well as iron deficiency, and diabetes can occur rarely in patients with chromium deficiency who are undergoing long-term total parenteral nutrition (TPN) without chromium.

**Previous medical history.** What is the patient's history with regard to previous or current illnesses, previous surgical procedures, medications, familial diseases, and socioeconomic status?

## PHYSICAL EXAMINATION

The physical examination corroborates and adds to the findings obtained by history.

**Weight and height.** The weight and height should be recorded at the start of the physical examination. The recorded values should be compared to records obtained earlier in the office or clinic or supplied by the patient. An assessment of the extent and rate of weight loss is important.

**General muscle and fat mass.** The presence of significant fat loss should be assessed by observations of the usual areas where adipose tissue is normally present. This includes an assessment of general loss of adipose tissue as judged by clearly defined bony, muscular, and venous outlines. A fold of skin is pinched to see whether any adipose tissue is present between the examining finger and thumb. Are the cheeks hollow (loss of fat) or filled out? Are the outlines of upper limb muscles and veins obscured or clearly defined (loss of fat)? Similarly, are the buttocks and perianal areas filled out or atrophic? The obvious loss of adipose tissue indicates severe energy deficit.

The wasting of muscle is judged by the hollowing of the temples (wasting of the temporalis), squaring of the shoulders (loss of deltoid), and wasting of the quadriceps. The latter is judged by observing difficulty in arising from a sitting position or from squatting, as well as difficulty in climbing stairs.

**Edema.** The presence of pitting edema on the lower limbs and over the sacrum may indicate hypoproteinemia or problems resulting in salt retention.

**Signs of Bone disease.** Bone tenderness, kyphosis, and thickening at the costochondral junction may be observed in patients with vitamin D deficiency. Kyphosis and tenderness over vertebral spines may indicate osteoporosis with collapse of vertebrae. Bone pain is one sign of hypervitaminosis A.

**Skin lesions.** Petechial and subcutaneous hemorrhages may be seen in vitamin C and K deficiencies. Perifollicular keratosis (thickening) may be seen in vitamin A deficiency. A scaly rash is observed with niacin/tryptophan deficiency. A red scaly rash around the mouth and the nasolabial folds and over the prominences of the joints may be seen in zinc deficiency. In zinc deficiency, hair loss may be observed. Protein-calorie deficiency is associated with thin, mosaic-patterned skin.

**Head and neck.** Patients with vitamin A deficiency have wrinkling and dryness of the conjunctiva observed best when the patient gazes laterally. In more severe cases, white plaques appear on the conjunctiva, just lateral to the cornea (Bitot's spots). Ophthalmoplegia may occur in advanced thiamin deficiency. Deficiency of vitamins of the B complex results in cheilosis (red scaly epithelium at the line of closure of lips), angular stomatitis (sodden epithelium with fissures radiating from the angle of the mouth), and glossitis (red denuded tongue); recall that these are also nonspecific changes and need investigation.

**Cardiorespiratory system.** Heart failure with dyspnea, peripheral edema, tachycardia, and a wide pulse pressure (high systolic and low diastolic pressure) may be a sign of thiamin deficiency. Patients with thiamin deficiency may have rapid respirations due to severe acidosis.

**Nervous system.** Ophthalmoplegia occurs in thiamin deficiency as part of the Wernicke-Korsakoff syndrome. In this condition, peripheral neuropathy with tingling, numbness of legs and hands, glove and stocking anesthesia, and weakness may also occur. Vitamin E deficiency causes myelopathy with ataxia, loss of position sense in the legs, and retinopathy with blindness. Classically, vitamin $B_{12}$ deficiency causes subacute combined degeneration of the spinal cord with loss of vibration and position sense, ataxia, and spastic paralysis of the lower limbs. Hypomagnesemia with hypocalcemia and hypokalemia are associated with circumoral and peripheral paresthesias and spasm of fingers and toes. Vertigo, blurred vision, and headache occur with long-term excessive intake of vitamin A.

## CLINICAL ASSESSMENT BASED ON A SUBJECTIVE GLOBAL ASSESSMENT OF THE PATIENT

The multiple manifestations of undernutrition emphasize the importance for the clinical assessment of nutritional status encompassing a variety of historical, symptomatic, and physical parameters, rather than relying heavily on anthropometric measurements and restricted laboratory test data. The clinical assessment should also be predictive of the adverse consequences of malnutrition, namely, to identify patients likely to develop nutritionally mediated complications. This approach has been termed subjective global assessment (SGA).[4–7]

### THEORETIC BASIS OF SUBJECTIVE GLOBAL ASSESSMENT

The basis of this assessment is, first, to determine whether there has been a true restriction of food intake and/or digestion and absorption and, second, to see whether associated effects on function and body composition have occurred.[7] It was hypothesized that (1) restoration of food intake can rapidly reduce the risk of malnutrition, and (2) if nutrient intake is restored to an optimal level to meet requirements, then the risk of complications is low even though the patient is still wasted and underweight.

### ASSESSMENT AND SCORING PROCEDURES

Details of the method have been published by me in collaboration with others, [7] and they are reviewed here with slight modification.

The specific features of the history and physical examination in the SGA method are listed in Table 50–1. Five features of the history are elicited. The first is weight loss in the previous 6 months, expressed both in kilograms and as proportional loss. My colleagues and I consider less than 5% a "small" loss, between 5 and 10% a "potentially significant" loss, and more than 10% a "definitely significant" loss. We also consider the rate of weight loss and its pattern. For example, if a patient has lost 10% of his or her weight in the period 6 months to 1 month prior to admission but has regained 3% of that weight in the subsequent month, resulting in a net loss of 7% for the entire period, he or she is considered to be better nourished than a patient who has lost 7% of his or her weight in the previous 6 months and continues to lose weight. Thus, it is possible for patients to suffer a net weight loss of significant proportions but still be considered well nourished if "true" weight (i.e., without edema) has recently stabilized or increased. The second feature of the history is dietary intake in relation to a patient's usual pattern. Patients are classified first as having normal or abnormal intake. The type, duration, and degree of abnormal intake are also noted (starvation, hypocaloric liquids, full liquid diet, suboptimal solid diet). The third feature of the history is the presence of significant gastrointestinal symptoms (anorexia, nausea, vomiting, diarrhea). By significant, my colleagues and I mean that these symptoms have persisted on virtually a daily basis for more than 2 weeks. Short-duration diarrhea or intermittent vomiting is not considered significant. Daily or twice-daily vomiting secondary to obstruction is considered significant. The fourth feature of the history is the patient's functional capacity or energy level (bedridden or full capacity). The last feature of the history concerns the metabolic demands of the patient's underlying disease state. An example of a high-stress disease is a severe flare of ulcerative colitis in which the patient has suffered a large volume of bloody diarrhea on a daily basis. A low-stress disease might be a smoldering infection or limited malignant tumor.

The features of the physical examination are noted as normal (0), mild (1+), moderate (2+), or severe (3+). The first is the loss of subcutaneous fat measured in the triceps region and the midaxillary line at the level of the lower ribs. These measurements are not precise, but are merely a subjective impression of the degree of subcutaneous tissue loss. The second feature is muscle wasting in the temporal areas and in the deltoids and quadriceps, as determined by loss of bulk and tone detectable by palpation. Obviously, a neurologic deficit will interfere with this assessment. The presence of edema in both the ankles and the sacral region and the presences of ascites are noted. Again, a co-existing disease such as congestive heart failure will modify the weight placed on the finding

**TABLE 50–1.** FEATURES OF SUBJECTIVE GLOBAL ASSESSMENT (SGA)

SELECT APPROPRIATE CATEGORY WITH A CHECKMARK, OR ENTER NUMERICAL VALUE WHERE INDICATED BY A "#")

A. History

1. Weight change and height
   Overall loss in past 6 months: Amt. = #__________kg; %loss = #__________ Height= #__________cm
   Change in past 2 weeks: __________ increase, __________ no change, __________ decrease.
2. Dietary intake change (relative to normal)
   __________No change.
   __________Change __________duration = #__________ weeks.
   Type: __________ suboptimal solid diet, __________ full liquid diet,
   __________ hypocaloric liquids __________, starvation.
   Supplement: (circle) nil, vitamin, minerals, #__________ frequency/week.
3. Gastrointestinal symptoms (that persisted for >2 weeks)
   __________none, __________nausea, __________vomiting, __________diarrhea, __________anorexia.
4. Functional capacity
   __________No dysfunction (e.g., full capacity).
   __________Dysfunction: duration #__________weeks.
   type: __________working suboptimally, __________ambulatory,__________
   __________bedridden.
5. Disease and its relation to nutritional requirements
   Primary diagnosis (specify)__________
   Metabolic demand (stress): __________no stress, __________low stress, __________moderate stress,
   __________high stress.

B. Physical (for each trait specify: 0 = normal, 1+ = mild, 2+ = moderate, 3+ = severe)

| | |
|---|---|
| #__________Loss of subcutaneous fat (triceps, chest) | #__________Ascites |
| #__________Muscle wasting (quadriceps, deltoids, temporalis) | #__________Mucosal lesions |
| #__________Ankle edema | #__________Cutaneous lesions |
| #__________Sacral edema | #__________Hair change |

C. SGA rating (select one)
   __________Well nourished.
   __________Moderately (or suspected of being) malnourished.
   __________Severely malnourished.

(Adapted from Detsky, A. S., McLaughlin, J. R., Baker, J. P., et al.: JPEN J. Parenter. Enteral Nutr., *11*:8–13, 1987.)

of edema. Mucosal and cutaneous lesions are recorded, as are color and appearance of the patient's hair.

On the basis of these features of the history and physical examination, clinicians identify an SGA rank that indicates the patient's nutritional status. These categories are: (1) well nourished, (2) moderate or suspected malnutrition, and (3) severe malnutrition. To arrive at an SGA rank, my colleagues and I do not use an explicit numeric weighting scheme. Rather, a rank is assigned on the basis of *subjective weighting*. Most of the judgment is based on the variables of weight loss, poor dietary intake, loss of subcutaneous tissue, and muscle wasting. For example, a patient could be assigned a B rank if he or she had at least a 5% weight loss in the few weeks prior to admission without stabilization or weight gain, definite reduction in dietary intake, and mild subcutaneous tissue loss. If the patient had considerable edema, ascites, or tumor mass, less influence would be given to the amount of weight loss. The other historical features are meant to help confirm the patient's self-report of weight loss and dietary change, but are given less weight. If the patient had a recent weight gain that did not appear to be merely fluid retention, an A rank would be assigned even if the net loss was between 5 and 10% and the patient had mild loss of subcutaneous tissue, especially if the patient had noted an improvement in the other historical features of the SGA (e.g., improvement in appetite). To receive a C rank, the patient would have to demonstrate obvious physical signs of malnutrition (severe loss of subcutaneous tissue, muscle wasting, and often some edema) in the presence of a clear and convincing pattern of ongoing weight loss. Such patients usually have had a net loss of at least 10% of their normal weight, in addition to many of the other historical features.

The assignment of rank should be based on unequivocal information. For example, if the data tending to a B rank (as opposed to an A rank) assignment are doubtful, then an A rank is appropriate. A C rank implies definite findings of severe malnutrition.

## ILLUSTRATIVE CASES

**Case A.** This 60-year-old woman admitted for elective resection of a colon carcinoma had lost 10% of her initial weight over 8 months prior to admission. Recently on supplements, however, she had gained some weight. She had been working and otherwise was active. On examination, there was no loss of muscle or fat and no edema. She was classified as A.

**Case B.** This 40-year-old man with acute Crohn's disease had lost 10% of his body weight within the past 2 weeks and was living mainly on liquids to avoid discomfort. He was ambulatory but was not at work. On examination, he had slight loss of subcutaneous tissue because of a reduced buccal fat pad and loose skin folds over the arms. No edema was present. He was assessed as B.

**Case C.** This patient was a 67-year-old man with esophageal cancer who had been unable to eat for 3 months. He had lost 15% of his body weight over the past 4 months and was continuing to lose weight. He had marked weakness and was able to move around the house but could no longer enjoy walking outdoors. On examination, he lacked subcutaneous tissue on palpation. Other features were hollow temples, squared shoulders, and mild pitting edema. He was assessed as C.

### PREDICTION OF NUTRITIONALLY ASSOCIATED COMPLICATIONS

Controlled studies by Baker et al. and Detsky et al. showed that SGA gave reproducible results when two blinded observers assessed the same patient.[4–7] In two studies, the two observers agreed in 81.4 and 91% of patients, respectively.[4,6] In addition, the first study noted a significant increase in septic complications and in the use of antibiotics, with a change in SGA from A to C grade.[4]

In a larger study,[6] the likelihood ratios of complications, both septic and nonseptic, increased from 0.66 in patients with an SGA of A to 4.44 in those with an SGA of C. Thus, an SGA of C increased the likelihood of complications by 7 times. Still another study showed that clinical judgment was superior to single objective parameters in predicting the development of nutritionally associated complications based on a careful evaluation of conditional probabilities and the sensitivity and specificity of the various clinical and objective parameters.[5]

The superiority of clinical judgment has been confirmed by Ottow et al.,[8] who showed that clinical judgment was superior to measurement of delayed cutaneous hypersensitivity (DCH) in predicting postoperative infection. Pettigrew and Hill confirmed that clinical assessment identified the risk of complications as effectively as the best plasma protein indicators.[9] The ultimate test of the ability of SGA to identify patients at risk was shown by a controlled trial of preoperative nutritional support.[10] In this trial, SGA predicted those patients who would show a reduction of complications by preoperative nutritional support.

In summary, the SGA provides a composite of criteria allowing informed clinical judgment based on estimates of (1) past nutritional intake, (2) the nature of the disease process and surgical or other treatments likely to affect future intake, (3) the extent of the catabolic effects of the disease, and (4) current physical status related to certain signs affected by nutritional status. Such an assessment not only provides an estimate of degree of undernutrition (if any), but also suggests pathophysiologic factors and differential diagnoses and allows one to estimate the likelihood of complications. Obviously, confirmation of the nature and extent of pathophysiologic factors and the severity of depletion of specific nutrients will require appropriate testing.

## FUNCTIONAL TESTS OF MALNUTRITION

SGA identifies patients at risk of complications by clinically assessing changes in intake of food, in body composition, and in function. It does not necessarily identify specific functional impairment or the amount of nutritional repletion needed to restore functional integrity. Functional impairment in malnutrition has been previously studied by examining changes in immune function,[11] in ability to perform work in an ergometer,[12] and in heart rate during maximal exercise.[13]

Immune competence as measured by DCH is reduced in malnutrition; however, several diseases[14] and drugs influence this measurement, making it a poor predictor of malnutrition in sick patients. The following factors nonspecifically alter DCH in the absence of malnutrition: (1) infections (viral, bacterial, and granulomatous); (2) uremia, cirrhosis, hepatitis, trauma, burns, and hemorrhage; (3) steroids, immunosupressants, cimetidine, warfarin, and perhaps aspirin; and (4) general anesthesia and surgical procedures. Hence in the critically sick patient, many factors can alter DCH and render it valueless in assessing the state of nutrition. Meakins et al. have shown that simply draining an abscess can reverse anergy.[15] Immunity therefore is neither a specific indicator of malnutrition nor easily studied.[11]

The use of exercise tolerance by ergometers and the measurement of heart rate are useful for population studies but difficult for sick patients with cardiorespiratory impairment and for patients under intensive care. These methods also depend upon the previous exercise status of the individual. An early study showing the role of impaired function in predicting postoperative complications was by Klidjian et al.[2] and Webb et al.[16] These investigators showed that the strength of the hand grip was predictive of the development of postoperative complications.

The direct relationship of effects of nutritional manipulations on changes in function was shown by Russell et al.[17] To study critically ill patients, it was necessary to develop a method that did not require the cooperation of the patient and where the effects of sepsis, drugs, trauma, surgical intervention, and anesthesia could be controlled. To do this, my colleagues and I selected a method developed by Edwards and used to study muscle fatigue.[18] It consisted of measuring the contraction of the adductor pollicis muscle in response to an electrical stimulus of the ulnar nerve at the wrist with unidirectional square wave pulses lasting only 50 to 70 microseconds at a range of frequencies from 10 to 50 Hz. There is a progressive increase in force with a maximal attained at 50 Hz. The plotted results constitute a force-frequency curve. In addition, when the nerve is stimulated at 20 Hz for 2 seconds and the stimulus is then switched off, the muscle relaxes after the initial contraction and the rate of this relaxation can be measured. Furthermore, if the stimulus at 20 Hz is continued, any loss of power represents fatigue of an objective nature (i.e., not due to voluntary relaxation). By studying the starving obese subject and the anorexic patient being refed, we showed that starvation caused the ratio of the force at 10 Hz/50 to 100 Hz to double and the relaxation rate to slow from a mean of about 10% of maximal force lost/10 milliseconds to 5 to 6%. In addition, we documented the development of fatigue in the muscle in starvation and that refeeding corrected these changes before there was any gain in body nitrogen.[17,19–22]

In other studies, Lenmarken et al. considered the relaxation rate to be a good index of the nutritional status.[23] More importantly Zeiderman and McMahon demonstrated that, in a group of preoperative surgical patients, the combination of an abnormal force-frequency curve and slow relaxation rate was the most specific and sensitive predictor of nutritionally associated complications when compared with other parameters of nutritional status such as hand grip strength, arm muscle circumference, and albumin and transferrin levels.[3] Windsor and Hill showed that muscle function, including hand grip, respiratory muscle strength, and relaxation rate of the adductor pollicis, were indicators of surgical complications rather than of weight loss.[24] In a study of patients with inflammatory bowel disease, Christie and Hill[25] confirmed our earlier observation,[19–22] with early restoration of muscle function preceding any significant increase in body protein. Furthermore, Chan et al. found that intravenous feeding rapidly restored muscle function in preoperative malnourished patients.[26]

Such findings are good evidence that muscle function is an index of nutritional changes and a predictor of the risks of complications in the sick individual. Preliminary studies suggest that muscle function changes rapidly on feeding; however, it is not clear whether the restoration of function is associated with an improvement in outcome. Studies by Hill and his colleagues suggest that grip strength, respiratory muscle strength, and function by electrical stimulation all demonstrate changes with nutrition.[24,25] Which one or ones are most useful should for assessment? The studies by Ziederman and McMahon suggest that electrical stimulation has greater predictive power than grip strength.[3] Moreover, respiratory muscle strength needs elaborate instrumentation in a pulmonary function laboratory, good cardiorespiratory status, and cooperation. My colleagues and I are of the opinion that the relaxation rate of single twitches may be a simple, minimally invasive, and reproducible way of studying muscle function in sick patients.

The term malnutrition implies a continuum that starts when the patient fails to eat enough to meet needs and progresses through a series of functional changes that precede any changes in body composition; these are related to the duration of reduced intake and its severity. To base the definition of malnutrition on any one of these changes is inappropriate. Only by recognizing the different facets of malnutrition can we define its various manifestations in relation to our clinical objectives. SGA provides a simple and effective clinical method of meeting these objectives, and muscle function analysis may be useful in determining optimal nutrient intake.

## REFERENCES


1. Owen, O.E., Reichard, G.A., Patel, M.S.: Adv. Exp. Med. Biol., *111*:119–188, 1979.
2. Klidjian, A.M., Foster, K.J., Kammerling, R.M., et al.: Br. Med. J., *2*:899–901, 1980.
3. Zeiderman, M.R., McMahon, M.J.: Clin. Nutr., *8*:161–166, 1989.
4. Baker, J.P., Detsky, A.S., Wesson, D.E., et al.: N. Engl. J. Med., *306*:969–972, 1982.
5. Detsky, A.S., Baker, J.P., Mendelson, R.A., et al.: J. Parenter. Enteral Nutr., *8*:153–159, 1984.
6. Detsky, A.S., Baker, J.P., O'Rourke, K., et al.: JPEN J. Parenter. Enteral Nutr., *11*:440–446, 1987.
7. Detsky, A.S., McLaughlin, J.R., Baker, J.P., et al.: JPEN J. Parenter. Enteral Nutr., *11*:8–13, 1987.
8. Ottow, R.T., Bruining, H.A., Jeekel, J.: Surg. Gynecol. Obstet., *159*:475–477, 1984.
9. Pettigrew, R.A., Hill, G.L.: Br. J. Surg., *73*:47–51, 1986.
10. Veterans Affairs Total Parenteral Nutrition Cooperative Study Group: N. Engl. J. Med., *325*:525–532, 1991.
11. Dominioni, L., Diogini, R.: JPEN J. Parenter. Enteral Nutr., *11*:*Suppl. 5*:70S–72S, 1987.
12. Desai, I.D., Garcia Tavares, M.L., Dutra de Oliveira, B.S., et al.: Am. J. Clin. Nutr., *34*:1925–1934, 1981.
13. Spurr, G.B., Barac-Nieto, M., Maksud, M.G.: Am. J. Clin. Nutr., *32*:767–778, 1979.
14. Dowd, P.S., Heatley, R.V.: Clin. Sci. Mol. Med., *66*:241–248, 1984.
15. Meakins, J.L., Christou, N.V., Shizgal, H.M., et al.: Ann. Surg., *190*:286–296, 1979.
16. Webb, A.R., Newman, L.A., Taylor, M., et al.: JPEN J. Parenter. Enteral Nutr., *13*:30–33, 1989.
17. Russell, D.McR., Pendergast, P.J., Darby, P.L., et al.: Am. J. Clin. Nutr., *38*:229–237, 1983.
18. Edwards, R.H.T.: Clin. Sci. Mol. Med., *54*:463–470, 1978.

**19.** Russell, D.McR., Leiter, L.A., Whitwell, J., et al.: Am. J. Clin. Nutr., *37:*133–138, 1983.
**20.** Russell, D.McR., Atwood, H.L., Whittaker, J., et al.: Clin. Sci., *67:*185–194, 1984.
**21.** Russell, D.McR., Walker, P.M., Leiter, L.A., et al.: Am. J. Clin. Nutr., *39:*503–513, 1984.
**22.** Brough, W., Horne, G., Blount, A., et al.: Br. Med. J., *293:*983–988, 1986.
**23.** Lenmarken, C., Sandstedt, S., Schenck, H.V., et al.: Clin. Nutr., *5:*99–103, 1986.
**24.** Windsor, J.A., Hill, G.L.: Ann. Surg., *207:*290–296, 1988.
**25.** Christie, P.M., Hill, G.L.: Gastroenterology, *99:*730–736, 1990.
**26.** Chan, S.T.F., McLaughlin, S.J., Ponting, G.A., et al.: Br. Med. J., *293:*1055–1056, 1986.

CHAPTER 51

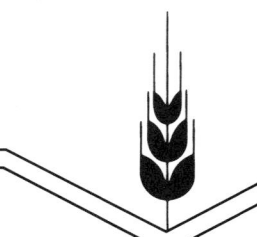

# Nutritional Assessment by Anthropometric and Biochemical Methods

**Steven B. Heymsfield, Ann Tighe, and Zi-Mian Wang**



Depletion of body nutrient stores and, ultimately, loss of specific cellular functions are common to many acute and chronic diseases. A hypothetic chronic illness of long duration is shown in Figure 51–1.[1] Progressive loss of fat-free body mass (FFM) is associated with the evolution of various complications, including loss of cell-mediated immunity, infections, bedsores, and, ultimately, death. A series of linkages implicit in Figure 51–1 is central to the nutritional assessment examination:

food intake < nutrient losses → negative protein balance → depletion of FFM → loss of protein-mediated cellular functions → clinical complications.

With nutritional therapy, loss of nutrients can be prevented or reversed and, ultimately, the risk of clinical complications can be minimized or eliminated. The aim of this chapter is to explore these relations further, specifically, to give a general overview of three components of the nutritional assessment examination—anthropometric measurements, nitrogen balance, and serum biochemical markers—that can be used in the evaluation of acutely and chronically ill malnourished patients.

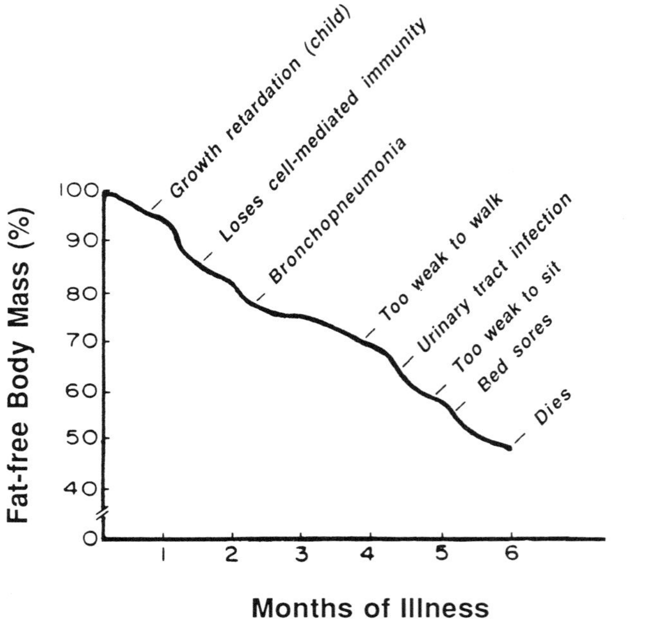

Growth retardation (child)
Loses cell-mediated immunity
Bronchopneumonia
Too weak to walk
Urinary tract infection
Too weak to sit
Bed sores
Dies
Fat-free Body Mass (%)
100
90
80
70
60
50
40
0
1
2
3
4
5
6
Months of Illness


**FIGURE 51–1.** The natural history of protein-energy malnutrition in a patient with chronic wasting illness. (Modified from Heymsfield, S.B., Bethel, R.A., Ansley, J.D., et al.: Ann. Intern. Med., *90*:63–71, 1979.)

## ASSESSMENT COMPONENTS

Maintaining optimum health requires adequate tissue levels of essential nutrients and a source of energy. More than 40 syndromes develop if tissue levels of these components are either too low or too high.[2] The emphasis in this chapter is on protein and energy because the large majority of patients seen for clinical evaluation have a disorder of protein-energy nutriture.[3,4]

### STEADY-STATE RELATIONS

The sequence of changes in progressive protein-energy malnutrition involves negative nutrient balance, loss of cellular functions, and, ultimately, clinical complications. This section gives an overview of the steady-state relations that exist among energy exchange, body weight, and body composition in health and describes how these relations are altered in pathologic states that cause negative nutrient balance.

Body weight is a fundamental component of nutritional assessment because it is an indirect marker of protein mass and energy stores. The relationships among body weight, protein mass, and body energy content are shown in Figure 51–2.[2]

A major portion of tissue function can be attributed to proteins that are activated by energy derived from metabolism of organic fuels.[5] As an organic compound, protein is also a metabolic fuel and, under conditions of weight stability, oxidation of amino acids provides about 15% of daily energy requirements.[6] The energy-producing reactions take this general form:

$$\text{Fuel}+O_2 \rightarrow \text{high energy intermediate} \rightarrow O_2+H_2O+\text{heat}+\text{urea}. \quad (1)$$

Urea is not metabolized further and is excreted unchanged in urine. During periods of nutritional deprivation, approximately half the total body protein mass can be used as metabolic fuel.[7] A greater loss of protein is incompatible with survival. Therefore, when food intake is less than nutrient losses, amino acids from proteins are oxidized to provide energy, various tissue functions are altered, and, ultimately, protracted negative protein balance results in death (see Chap. 56 on starvation).

The main sources of nonprotein energy are glycogen and fat or triglyceride. Glycogen is distributed primarily in liver and skeletal muscle.[8] Glycogen stores are small (~400 g), and carbohydrate oxidation on a usual diet in the United States accounts for about 50% of daily energy production.[6]

Fat is found almost entirely within adipocytes or fat cells.[9] Fat stores vary widely in humans, with fatty acid oxidation representing about 35% of energy production in the average American diet.[6] Both glycogen and fat are oxidized in reactions similar to that for protein (Equation 1), except urea is produced only with amino acid oxidation.

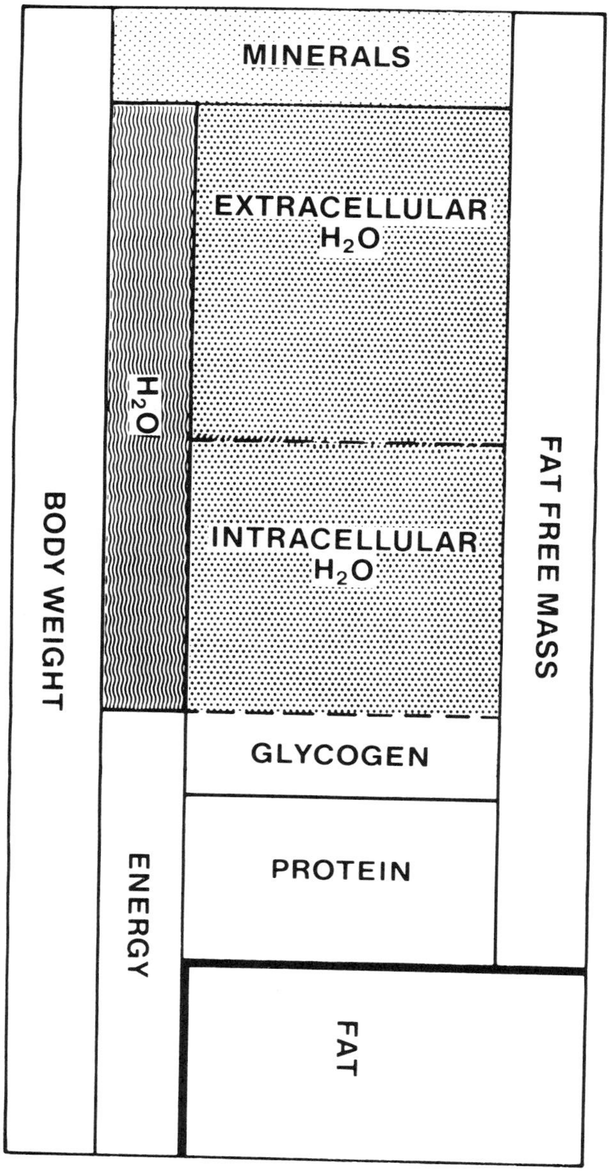
MINERALS
EXTRACELLULAR
H₂O
H₂O
INTRACELLULAR
H₂O
BODY WEIGHT
FAT FREE MASS
GLYCOGEN
PROTEIN
ENERGY
FAT

**FIGURE 51–2.** The major chemical determinants of body weight and how they relate to total body energy content.

The sum of protein, glycogen, and fat constitutes total body energy content (Fig. 51–2). These fuels account for over 90% of the nonaqueous portion of body weight.[10] Generalizations can be made on how body weight, protein, glycogen, fat, and energy stores relate to each other. Glycogen and protein are both solubilized by water and electrolytes. About 2 to 4 g water bind to 1 g of either glycogen or protein.[11] Changes in glycogen or protein balance are thus associated with greater changes in body weight than can be attributed to loss of the actual chemical component. For example, oxidation and loss of 100 g glycogen would result in approximately a 0.5-kg reduction in body weight.

The main remaining chemical components exclusive of fat are minerals, found primarily in the skeleton.[9,10] The total fat-free portion of body weight thus consists of protein, glycogen, water, and minerals. In health, the steady-state fractional contribution of each of these four components to total (FFM) is reasonably constant: 0.195, 0.01 to 0.02, 0.725, and 0.08, respectively. With long-term weight loss, the change in FFM is approximately the same as the relative reduction in protein.[2] Sharp changes in body weight and FFM may also reflect alterations in glycogen and fluid balance.

Fat maintains a relatively constant, although more complex relation to fat-free components (Fig. 51–3). Figure 51–3 shows a plot of total body fat/height(Ht)$^2$ versus body weight/Ht$^2$ in women. Fat was measured in the women by dual photon absorptiometry systems. The ratio body weight/Ht$^2$, referred to as body mass index (BMI, kg/m$^2$), is discussed later in more detail. Two important points are related to this figure. First, the intercept for zero total body fat is a BMI of ~13. This extrapolated value represents a theoretic female subject without any fat, a condition incompatible with survival. Second, the slope of the regression line (i.e., the change in fat adjusted for stature/the change in body weight adjusted for stature) of ~0.75 indicates that body weight added above a BMI of 13 is about three fourths fat and one fourth FFM. Webster and colleagues refer to the weight above a BMI of 13 as "excess weight" and suggest that weight gain or loss should approximate this composition.[12] The composition of "excess weight" may differ between men and women and between young and old subjects. A more complex analysis of the relations among body weight, protein, and fat is presented by Forbes.[13]

These associations among body weight, total body protein mass and energy content, and fluid are formulated into an important concept: that body weight under most conditions is an indirect marker of protein mass and energy stores. A loss or gain in body weight is usually assumed to reflect changes in protein mass and/or energy content.

Thus, body weight, total body protein mass and energy content, and chemical compartments exist in association with each other according to relatively simple rules. How these rules change in disease is important in nutritional assessment, as described in later sections of this chapter.

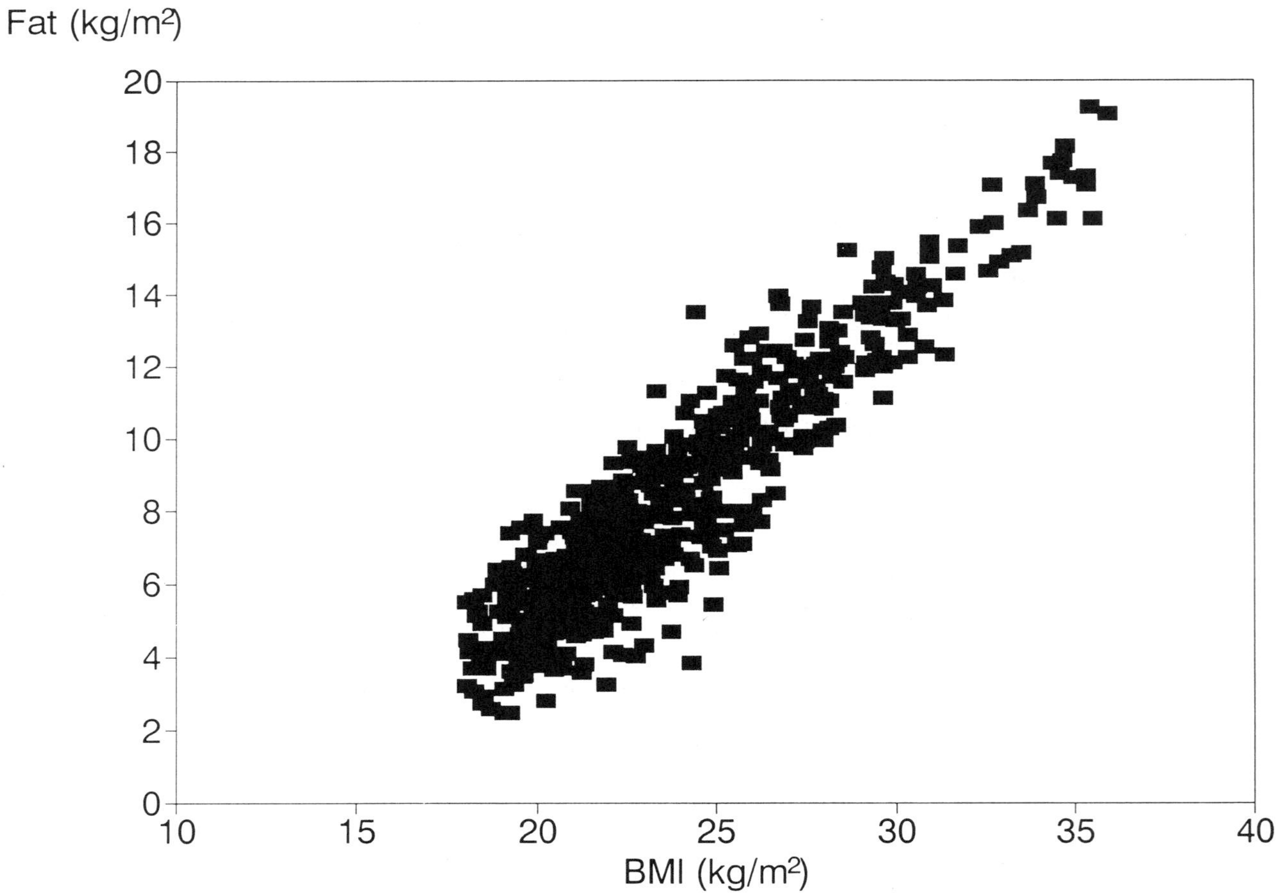
Fat (kg/m2)
20
18
16
14
12
10
8
6
4
2
0
10
15
20
25
30
35
40
BMI (kg/m2)

**FIGURE 51–3.** Relationship between total body fat (measured by dual-photon absorptiometry systems) adjusted for stature and body mass index (BMI) in 530 healthy women.

## BALANCE

Body composition is in a dynamic state throughout the day. Both total body protein mass and energy content decline between meals as a result of obligatory amino acid oxidation and metabolism of other fuels.[8,14] The result is negative protein and energy balance. With food intake, balance becomes positive, and total body protein and energy content increase. Over a typical day, net protein and energy balance are zero and body weight remains constant. These relations are depicted in Figure 51–4,[2] which presents a hypothetic healthy subject at point A. Body weight is stable and long-term balances of energy, protein, and water are zero. Figure 51–4 presents protein as nitrogen (N) as the two are related by a "constant" [protein = 16% N = 6.25 × N].

If the individual at point A develops an acute or chronic illness, then food intake may be inadequate to replace nutrient losses. The result is that net energy and nitrogen balance become negative and body weight is lost. If the condition persists and balance remains negative, the subject ultimately approaches the point at which survival is no longer possible ($B_u$ in Fig. 51–4). As mentioned earlier, the limits of survival with long-term underfeeding are a 50% loss in total body protein and a BMI of about 13. Loss of functional proteins and other essential nutrients results in the clinical complications described at the beginning of this chapter (see Fig. 51–1) and shown in Figure 51–4 as $C_u$. Clinically significant abnormalities in physiologic function and loss of total body protein are seen in most hospitalized patients who lose more than 20% of their preillness body weight.[15] The dynamics of protein metabolism differ in an acute catabolic illness, and this is discussed further in the section of this chapter on biochemical markers of nutritional status.

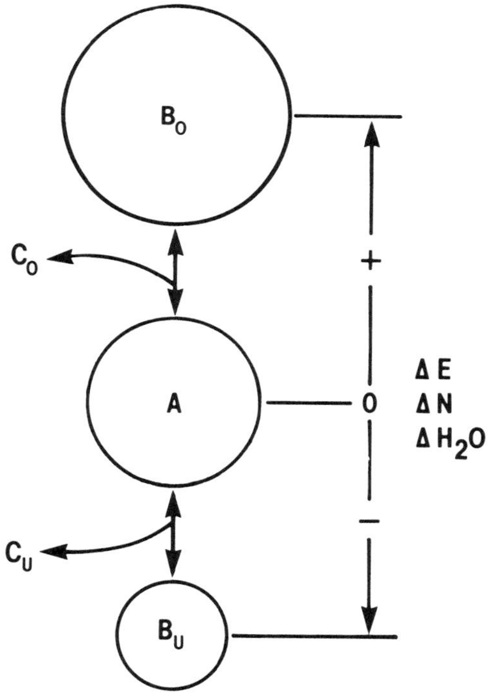

$B_O$
$C_O$
+
A
0
$\Delta$E
$\Delta$N
$\Delta H_2O$
−
$C_U$
$B_U$


**FIGURE 51–4.** Model depicting changes in metabolic balance and body composition in protein-energy malnutrition and obesity. Point A is the range of body composition and tissue function found in health. Weight is stable, and balances of energy, nitrogen (N), and water are zero. Disease causes negative metabolic balance, weight loss, and changes in body composition and tissue function. Point $B_u$ is the minimal range of body composition and tissue function that is compatible with survival. The course of a patient moving between points A and $B_u$ may be interrupted by a complication related to malnutrition, and this is indicated by point $C_u$. Positive balance leads to obesity, and a similar set of end points, $B_o$ and $C_o$, are designated.

Overeating relative to nutrient losses results in positive balance and, if sustained, the individual gains weight (Fig. 51–4). The maximum survivable body weight is approximately 500 kg or a body BMI of ~150. As with undernutrition, obesity is associated with complications ($C_O$ in Fig. 51–4). The proposed mechanisms that lead to these complications are described in Chapter 59.

Thus, some hypothetic optimal state of health exists (point A in Fig. 51–4) in which long-term balance is zero and health risks are at a minimum. Weight loss or gain is secondary to a change in energy and nitrogen balance and ultimately increases the individual's risk of developing various medical complications.

Figure 51–4 embodies the main components of nutritional assessment: to define the patient's status between points A, B, and C. These aims can be formulated into four specific questions:

1. What is the patient's body weight and body composition status relative to an arbitrarily defined healthy range?
2. If the patient is under- or overnourished, what are the mechanisms leading to either negative or positive nutrient balance?
3. Is the patient at risk of developing a complication related to altered nutritional status?
4. With nutritional treatment, is balance altered, and over time is the patient's weight and body composition moving towards the healthy range?

Question 2 is examined in other chapters and is not discussed further here. The focus in this review is on undernutrition, and Chapter 59 describes the evaluation of obese patients.

## FUNCTION

An important assumption of nutritional assessment is that body composition is an indirect measure of cellular function. Body composition estimates are usually highly correlated with specific functional tests. For example, anthropometric midarm muscle area is strongly correlated with forearm grip strength.[16] Body composition should not be assumed equivalent to tissue function, however: the two are different types of biologic measurements that serve different purposes but can, under certain conditions, be used in exchange for one another. An example of where mass and function can dissociate is the case of a patient with cardiomyopathy. Massive enlargement of the heart muscle is possible, yet the capacity of the myocardium to generate force and eject blood into the systemic circulation is severely impaired. The distinction between body composition estimates and cellular function indices should be kept in mind when evaluating the results of a patient's anthropometric and biochemical evaluations.

## ANTHROPOMETRY

### HISTORY

Anthropometry, a technique developed in the late nineteenth century by anthropologists, uses simple measuring devices to quantify differences in human form. The potential of anthropometric methods in assessing nutritional status was first realized in the late nineteenth century by Richer, who used skinfold thickness as an index of fatness.[17] The modern era of nutritional anthropometry began with the studies of Matiegka during World War I.[18] Matiegka's interest in the physical efficiency of soldiers led him to develop methods of anthropometrically subdividing the human body into muscle, fat, and bone. Anthropometric techniques are now widely used in many areas of human biologic research, and two important multiauthor books on the subject were prepared within the last decade.[19,20]

### FIVE-LEVEL MODEL

The purpose of anthropometric measurements is to quantify the major compositional determinants of body weight. A full appreciation of anthropometric measurements requires an understanding of human body composition and its organizational levels. According to Wang et al.,[9] human body composition can be studied at five levels: I, atomic; II, molecular; III, cellular; IV, tissue-system; and V, whole body. The five levels and their major compartments are shown in Figure 51–5.

**Atomic.** The first level of body composition consists of major elements that comprise body weight such as oxygen, hydrogen, carbon, nitrogen, calcium and so on. Whole-body measurements at this level are usually made by research techniques such as in vivo neutron activation analysis[21] (see Chap. 49). Elemental measurements are important in the study of body composition as they are used either directly (e.g., nitrogen balance as a measure of protein change) or to estimate compartments at other levels (e.g., total body calcium→ total bone mineral).[21] Anthropometric methods are available for estimating total body nitrogen, calcium, and potassium at the atomic level.[22]

**Molecular.** The second level of body composition consists of the major molecular compartments that comprise body weight such as water, protein, glycogen, mineral (osseous and nonosseous), and fat (see Fig. 51–2). Water and osseous minerals can now be measured directly, although no practical techniques are available for quantifying fat, protein, glycogen, or nonosseous minerals.[21,23]

The chemical compartments that cannot be measured directly can be estimated by indirect techniques. For example, total body protein can be estimated from total body nitrogen (an atomic level compartment).[21] This calculation assumes that most total body nitrogen is incorporated into protein and that the nitrogen content of protein is known and constant at 16%. Another important example is the indirect estimation of fat using a two-compartment model in which the molecular level is simplified to body weight = fat + FFM (see Fig. 51–2). Several two-compartment methods are used to estimate fat, such as underwater weighing, total body potassium, and total body water (TBW).[23] Each method relies on one or more assumptions that relate measurable aspects of body composition to the unknown compartment of interest. An example is the TBW-two-compartment method, which is formulated on the assumption that FFM has an average hydration of 73% (i.e., TBW/FFM = 0.73 or FFM = TBW/0.73). FFM and fat (i.e., body weight − FFM) can thus be estimated from TBW. Anthropometric methods of estimating total body fat are usually developed using one of these indirect techniques as the reference standard for quantifying fat.

The second level of body composition is important in nutritional assessment because fat and FFM are the major compartments in which energy stores are distributed (see Fig. 51–2), and FFM contains all the functional components of body weight. Fat has an energy density of 9.4 kcal/g, and all but 1 to 2 kg is metabolically available during periods of protracted negative energy balance. Protein and glycogen have respective energy densities of 5.65 and 4.1 kcal/g. Assuming that hydration is relatively normal, the metabolically available energy from FFM is 1.02 kcal/g.[24,25] Accordingly,

$$\text{Total body kcal} = [9.4 \times \text{total fat(g)}] + [1.02 \times \text{FFM(g)}]. \qquad (2)$$

Half of the energy contained within FFM can usually be used as fuel during long-term semistarvation.[25] Evaluation of fat and FFM thus allows the investigator or clinician to estimate total body energy content, available energy stores, and changes in energy balance over time.

FFM, the metabolically active compartment at the molecular level of body composition, is generally accepted as an index of protein nutriture. Changes in FFM

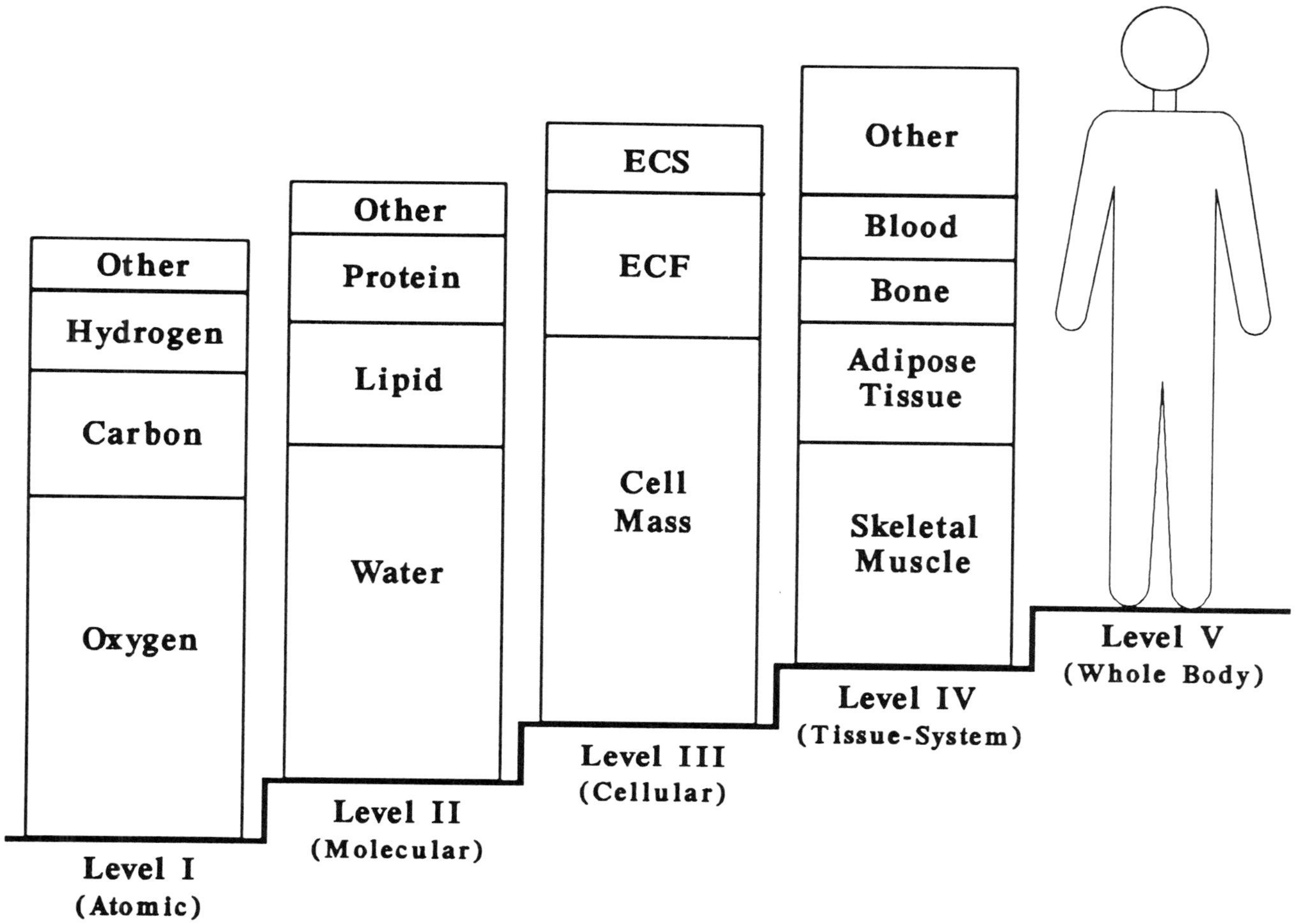
Other
Hydrogen
Carbon
Oxygen
Level I
(Atomic)
Other
Protein
Lipid
Water
Level II
(Molecular)
ECS
ECF
Cell Mass
Level III
(Cellular)
Other
Blood
Bone
Adipose Tissue
Skeletal Muscle
Level IV
(Tissue-System)
Level V
(Whole Body)

**FIGURE 51–5.** The five-level model of body composition. ECF and ECS, Extracellular fluid and solids. (From Wang, ZM., Pierson, R.N., Heymsfield, S.B.: Am. J. Clin. Nutr., *56*:19–28, 1992, with permission of the American Journal of Clinical Nutrition.)

over time are assumed to represent alterations in protein balance. Resting oxygen consumption, carbon dioxide production, and heat production (i.e., energy expenditure) are highly correlated with FFM (Fig. 51–6), and FFM accounts for most of the individual variation in energy expenditure.[26] Anthropometric methods are available for estimating TBW, FFM, and fat at the molecular level.[19,20,22,27]

**Cellular.** The cellular level of body composition consists of three main compartments: cells, extracellular fluid, and extracellular solids.[9] Measurement techniques are available for quantifying extracellular fluid and solids, although total cell weight or the weight of specific cell groups is difficult to quantify in vivo. A widely used model of body weight components at this level was suggested by Moore and his colleagues.[28] Cell mass was considered as two components: fat (a molecular level compartment) and fat-free cell mass. The fat-free cell mass was referred to by Moore et al. as "body cell mass

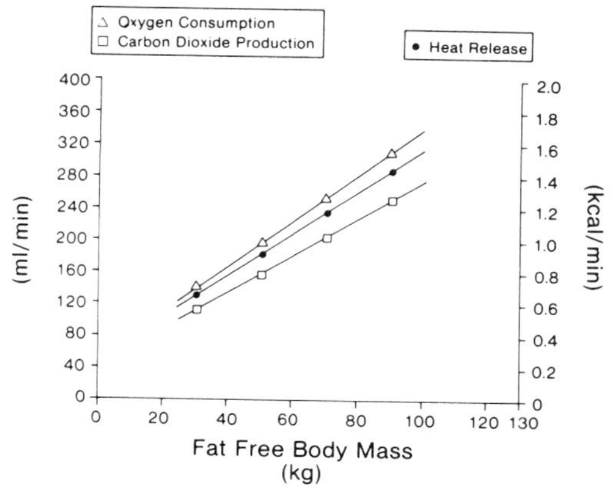
Oxygen Consumption
Carbon Dioxide Production
Heat Release
(ml/min)
(kcal/min)
Fat Free Body Mass
(kg)

**FIGURE 51–6.** Relationship between the fasting rate of oxygen consumption, carbon dioxide production, heat release in a gradient-layer calorimeter, and fat-free body mass (FFM). The healthy subjects were between the ages of 20 and 70 years and between 90 and 115% ideal body weight.

(BCM)," a compartment responsible for most of the body's metabolic processes. The investigators proposed that total body potassium or exchangeable potassium (both are atomic-level components that are approximately equivalent in amount) could be used to estimate BCM because the potassium concentration of intracellular fluid is relatively constant at 150 mmol/L and the ratio of intracellular fluid to solids is approximately 4:1 (i.e., intracellular fluid = body cell mass × 0.80). BCM could then be calculated using these relations combined with an estimate of either total body or exchangeable potassium (i.e., BCM = [TBK/150] × [1/0.80] or total body K × 0.0083). The equation for body weight according to Moore and his colleagues was thus equal to fat + body cell mass + extracellular fluids and solids.

The lack of more direct and specific methods of estimating cell mass is an important limitation in the field of body composition methodology.[9] This is because cells are the main functional compartments and their quantification would enable investigators to explore important physiologic and functional relations. At present, several anthropometric equations can be used to predict body cell mass at the cellular level[22,28,29] (see Appendix Tables A–15a, b, and c and Chap. 49).

**Tissue-System.** The tissue-system level of body composition consists of the major tissues and organs. The equation for body weight at this level is equal to adipose tissue + skeletal muscle + skeleton + residual (i.e., visceral organs, etc.).

Adipose tissue includes fat cells or adipocytes, blood vessels, and structural elements.[9] Adipose tissue is the primary site of fat storage, and in healthy adults the chemical composition of adipose tissue averages 80% fat, 18% water, and 2% protein.[10]

Adipose tissue is distributed mainly into the subcutaneous and internal or visceral compartments.[2] The proportions of total adipose tissue in the subcutaneous and visceral compartments are not constant. Distribution of adipose tissue is under hormonal and genetic control, with metabolic properties of adipose tissue varying among different anatomic locations.[30] Men, the elderly, and obese subjects tend to have a higher percentage of total adipose tissue in the visceral compartment than women, young, and lean subjects, respectively.[2,30] Weight gain or loss is associated with different relative rates of adipose tissue change in the subcutaneous and visceral compartments and from different subcutaneous sites.[31] This differential loss of adipose tissue is important when interpreting anthropometric measurements. A strong positive correlation exists between the amount of visceral adipose tissue and the health risks of obesity (see Chap. 59).

Skeletal muscle is the largest compartment within the adipose tissue-free body compartment, accounting for approximately half its weight in healthy adults.[9,10] Skeletal muscle consists of muscle tissue, nerves, tendons, and interstitial adipose tissue. Approximately 20% of fat-free skeletal muscle is protein, and muscle is the largest tissue reservoir of amino acids.[7] Depletion of up to 75% of skeletal muscle mass is possible during prolonged semistarvation.[7]

The response of visceral organs to semistarvation is variable. Organs decrease in weight at different rates during uncomplicated semistarvation. For example, liver mass decreases rapidly in rodents with underfeeding, whereas heart weight decreases at about the same rate as body weight.[31] The pattern of visceral organ changes in protein-energy malnutrition associated with physiologic stress may differ from that of uncomplicated underfeeding. An example is the severe weight loss that often accompanies metastatic malignant disease. Cancer cachexia in both animals and humans is accompanied by preservation of some visceral organs despite loss of body weight and atrophy of skeletal muscles.[32] The preservation of visceral organs with physiologic stress may represent an adaptive response to injury or infection that is the anatomic counterpart to increased synthesis of serum acute-phase reactants. The metabolic response to injury is described in a later section of this chapter.

Magnetic resonance imaging and computed tomography are used by investigators to quantify total body and regional adipose tissue and skeletal muscle.[23] Imaging and ultrasonic techniques can also be used to estimate visceral organ and skeletal weights. Skeletal muscle and adipose tissue are important compartments in nutritional assessment because they are readily measured by indirect anthropometric techniques. At present, many anthropometric equations can be used to predict total adipose tissue, skeletal muscle, and bone mass at the tissue-system level.[33,34]

**Whole Body.** The whole body level of body composition includes the main anthropometric dimensions such as body weight, stature, circumferences, breadths, and skinfold thicknesses. Other whole body estimates include total body density, volume, resistance, and reactance (see also Chap. 49).

**Features of the Model.** The five-level model has several important features. First, the model is consistent as a whole and each compartment is distinct.[9] Connections between compartments are important in relation to anthropometric methods, however. An example is a group of related compartments at levels I to IV, calcium, bone mineral, extracellular solids, skeleton, and bone breadths. Each of these compartments is distinct, and yet all five are linked because they are different constituents or dimensions of the human skeleton.[9]

Second, steady-state relations exist between many compartments at the same or different levels.[9] Steady state as defined here means a stable relation between compartments over a specified time interval, usually months or years. Some steady-state relations were described earlier, such as the hydration of FFM (0.73) and intracellular potassium concentration (150 mmol/L). These quantitative associations are important in developing body composition models that relate a direct measurement to an unmeasurable compartment of interest. For example, TBW can be measured directly and FFM then calculated as TBW/0.73.[23] The steady-state relations are particularly important in the field of anthropometry because all anthropometric measurements are at the whole body level and yet they are used primarily to infer information about levels I to IV. These steady-state relations allow us to establish the connections between level V and the other levels. Additionally, the steady-state relations are often altered with disease and thus change the quantitative associations established between anthropometric dimensions and other body compartments.

The following is a summary of anthropometric methods in the context of the five-level model.

## MEASUREMENTS

The anthropometric measurements in general use include body weight, stature, skinfolds, circumferences, and bone breadths. These whole body measurements either are used directly in nutritional assessment or they are used to estimate by indirect means compartments at the other five levels (Table 51–1). The following discussion groups the various anthropometric measurements and techniques into three categories: (1) body weight and stature; (2) estimates of fatness and energy stores; and (3) lean tissue indices, protein mass, and functional compartments.

**Body Weight and Stature.** Body weight is the sum of all compartments at each level of body composition. As described earlier, body weight is a rough measure of total body energy stores, and changes in weight parallel energy and protein balance. A significant correlation exists ($r = 0.6$, $p < 0.05$) between loss of body weight and change in total body protein in seriously ill adults.[15]

Body weight usually varies less than ± 0.1 kg per day in healthy adults.[2] A loss in weight of more than 0.5 kg per day either indicates negative energy or water balance or a combination of the two. Clinically significant weight loss is considered a relative decrease in weight of more than 10% over a time interval of less than 6 months.[2]

The severity of weight loss in an individual is determined by two factors: the rate of weight change over time and the total reduction in weight. The rate of weight loss in total starvation is approximately 0.4 kg per day, and survival is sustained to about 70% of desirable (i.e., ideal) body weight.[2] Semistarvation, the more typical cause of negative energy balance in patients, results in a more gradual loss in weight compared to that in total starvation. In extreme cases of chronic disease, the weight change may occur over years or decades. The minimal survivable body weight in humans is between 48 and 55% of desirable body weight or a BMI of between 13 and 15 (i.e., point $B_u$ in Fig. 51–4). Body weight at this point consists of less than 5% fat.[2] Exhaustion of the remaining metabolically usable fat mass results in rapid depletion of lean tissue and death.

The absolute body weight and rate of change in weight have prognostic value, and two aspects are recognized. The first is that an absolute body weight of less than 55 to 60% of desirable places the subject at or near the survival limits of semistarvation.[2] Further negative balance could not be tolerated for long. The second aspect is that a significant reduction in body weight from preillness weight (>10 to 20%) over a time interval of less than about 6 months places the patient at risk of developing functional impairment of multiple organ systems and an adverse clinical outcome.

Studley was among the first to associate weight loss with disease outcome.[35] In 1936, this pioneering investigator made the classic observation that marked weight loss prior to surgical procedures for peptic ulcer resulted in a higher postoperative mortality rate relative to that in weight-stable patients. Modern workers have identified weight loss as a major determinant of prognosis in many disease states and conditions, such as survival time in patients with carcinoma of the colon[36] and

**TABLE 51–1.** SOME CHARACTERISTIC COMPARTMENTS AT LEVELS I TO IV AND RELATED ANTHROPOMETRIC DIMENSIONS AT LEVEL V

| CHARACTERISTIC COMPARTMENTS | | | | ANTHROPOMETRIC DIMENSIONS (LEVEL V) | | | | |
|---|---|---|---|---|---|---|---|---|
| Level I | Level II | Level III | Level IV | BW | Stature | Circumferences | Skinfolds | Breadths |
| TBC | fat | fat cells | adipose tissue | X | | X | X | |
| | FFM | BCM +ECS +ECF | ATFW | X | | X | X | |
| TBCa, TBP | Mo | ECS | bone, skeleton | X | X | | | X |
| TBN, TBK | Pro, water, Ms | BCM | muscle + viscera | X | X | X | X | |
| TBNa, TBCl | Ms, water | ECF | blood + ISF | X | X | | | |

ATFW, Adipose tissue-free body weight; BCM, body cell mass; BW, body weight; ECF, extracellular fluid; ECS, extracellular solids; FFM, fat-free body mass; ISF, interstitial fluid; Levels I to V: atomic, molecular, cellular, tissue-system, and whole body levels of body composition, respectively; Mo, bone mineral; Ms, soft tissue mineral; Pro, protein; TBC, TBCa, TBCl, TBK, TBN, TBNa, TBP, total body carbon, calcium, chloride, potassium, nitrogen, sodium and phosphorus, respectively.

chronic obstructive lung disease.[37] Seltzer and his colleagues found a 19-fold increase in mortality in adult patients undergoing elective surgery who lost more than 10 lb body weight preoperatively compared to patients with no or small weight loss.[38]

An important study by Windsor and Hill refined Studley's classic observation by demonstrating that the postoperative patients with weight loss who are at the highest risk of complications are those who also have clinically obvious impairment in organ function.[39] Postoperative patients with clinically apparent organ impairment in this study also had significant abnormalities of a variety of measured physiologic functions and a reduced weight of total body protein. Summarizing this and other studies from his laboratory, Hill concluded that a weight loss of <10% of preillness body weight is usually not associated with functional abnormalities; a weight loss of between 10 and 20% of preillness body weight is accompanied by functional abnormalities in some patients; and a weight loss >20% of preillness body weight is associated with protein-energy malnutrition and multiple functional abnormalities in almost all patients.[15] Weight loss is thus an important indirect index of multiple physiologic functions and a guide to a patient's prognosis.

Body weight is measured longitudinally to establish the effectiveness of nutritional therapy. A change in weight reflects energy, protein, and water balance.

*Measurement.* In the hospital, body weight should be measured within ± 0.1 kg on a calibrated physician's scale. Special scales should be used in bedridden or wheelchair-bound patients. Edema, if present, should be recorded with the weight. The general procedure is to obtain a morning weight following evacuation of the bladder. The weight of the hospital gown can be subtracted from the total weight if the desired goal is nude weight. When comparing the patient's weight with standard values, the attire is usually presented in a footnote on the table. Serial weights should be measured on the same or a carefully calibrated scale. Intake and output records may be useful in interpreting the significance of changes in weight.

Reference tables provide a standard weight for height, and in some cases an adjustment is made for frame size (see Appendix Tables A–11c, d, and g). Height is usually measured by a sliding bar attached to the physician's scale, although more accurate techniques are used for research purposes. Height can be estimated in bedridden patients using knee-length prediction equations[40] (Table 51–2). The body weight reference table will usually specify the technique used to estimate frame size.

*Interpretation.* In four conditions, interpretation of body weight as an index of available energy supply must be used with caution:

1. Edema and ascites cause a relative increase in extracellular fluid and may mask loss in chemical or cellular components.
2. Massive tumor growth or organomegaly can mask loss in fat or lean tissues such as skeletal muscle.
3. Lean tissue and cellular atrophy are partially masked by residual fat and connective tissue in obese patients undergoing rapid or severe weight loss. Patients may still be overweight and yet suffer severe protein-energy malnutrition and also be at increased risk of adverse health outcomes secondary to semistarvation.
4. Large changes in energy intake cause corresponding changes in glycogen mass and bound water over several days. Similarly, large changes in sodium intake are associated with brief periods of fluid readjustment and body weight change.

For these reasons, and also to provide a more complete characterization of body composition, anthropometric methods are used to further compartmentalize body weight. These methods are described under two general headings as they relate to nutritional assessment: measures of fat stores and measures of lean tissues.

**TABLE 51–2.** PREDICTION OF ADULT STATURE FROM KNEE HEIGHT

This dimension is measured in centimeters using a broad-blade caliper, similar to the type of instrument used to measure an infant's length. The subject lies supine and bends the knee at a 90° angle. One blade of the caliper is placed over the anterior surface of the left thigh, above the condyles of the femur and just proximal to the patella. The caliper shaft is held parallel to the shaft of the tibia. Pressure is applied, and two readings should agree within ±0.5 cm. height (in cm) is then calculated from the following two prediction equations:

Height (men) = 64.19 − (0.4 × age) + (2.02 × knee height)
Height (women) = 84.88 − (0.24 × age) + (1.83 × knee height)

(Adapted from Chumlea, W.C., Roche, A.F., Steinbaugh, M.L.: Anthropometric approaches to the nutritional assessment of the elderly. *In* Nutrition, Aging, and the Elderly. Edited by H.N. Munro and D.E. Danford. New York, Plenum, 1989, pp. 335–361.)

**Fat.** Although fat refers specifically to a chemical component at the molecular level of body composition, this section as a whole relates to the following five-level sequence: I, carbon; II, fat; III, fat cells; IV, adipose tissue; and V, anthropometric dimensions (e.g., skinfolds/circumferences) (see Table 51–1). Anthropometric measurements are well suited for quantifying fatness because of the easy access provided by the subcutaneous adipose depot. Although more accurate and reproducible methods of estimating fatness exist, anthropometric methods are the simplest, safest, most practical, and least costly of the available techniques.

The amount of fat in healthy subjects varies greatly, with relatively small amounts in some highly trained athletes and relatively large amounts during the later stages of pregnancy. During protracted undernutrition, all but a small amount of total body fat can be utilized as metabolic fuel.[2] Two factors determine the adequacy of fat: the amount of total body triglyceride present and energy balance. Very little fat is sufficient if the individual is healthy and in zero energy balance. In contrast, a small amount of fat in the presence of marked negative energy balance implies a limited survival time. The usual practice is to compare fat values from an individual patient with reference standards and also to follow trends over time. During nutritional therapy, the measurement of fat provides an indirect guide to energy balance.

**TABLE 51–3** SKINFOLD MEASUREMENT SITES

1. **Biceps skinfold thickness.** Lift the skinfold on the anterior aspect of the upper arm, directly above the center of the cubital fossa, at the same level as the triceps skinfold and midarm circumference. The arm hangs relaxed at the patient's side, and the crest of the fold should run parallel to the long axis of the arm.
2. **Triceps skinfold thickness.** Grasp the skin and subcutaneous tissue 1 cm above the midpoint between the tip of the acromial process of the scapula and the olecranon process of the ulna. The fold runs parallel to the long axis of the arm. Care should be taken to ensure that the measurement is made in the midline posteriorly and that the arm hangs relaxed and vertical.
3. **Subscapular skinfold.** The skin is lifted 1 cm under the inferior angle of the scapula with the patient's shoulder and arm relaxed. The fold should run parallel to the natural cleavage lines of the skin; this is usually a line about 45° from the horizontal extending medially upwards.
4. **Suprailiac skinfold.** Pick up this skinfold 2 cm above the iliac crest in the midaxillary line. The crest of this fold should run horizontally.
5. **Thigh skinfold.** The skin is picked up on the posterior aspect at the same level as the thigh circumference. The crest of the skinfold should run parallel to the leg.
6. **Calf skinfold.** This skinfold is picked up on the posterior aspect of the calf at the same level as the calf circumference. The crest of the skinfold should run parallel to the leg.

*Measurement and Interpretation.* Three methods of assessing fatness are available: (1) the single skinfold method; (2) the limb fat area method; and (3) total body fat (or adipose tissue) calculated from multiple anthropometric measurements. The measurements common to all three techniques are now briefly reviewed, and the interested reader should consult additional references for added details.[19,20]

Measuring body fat requires two instruments: a skinfold caliper and a tape measure. The caliper should be a rugged and light instrument, and jaw pressure should be maintained at 10 g/mm$^2$ throughout the skinfold range. The contact surface area of the jaws can vary between 30 and 100 mm$^2$, and the jaws on some calipers remain parallel as they are opened wider. A calibration block is usually supplied with the instrument.

The tape measure should be durable, resist stretching, and have an accuracy of ± 0.1 cm. Plastic and fiberglass tapes meet these criteria, and calibration should be checked periodically against a meter stick.

Two types of measurement are usually made: skinfold thicknesses and limb or trunk circumferences. The location of six widely used skinfold sites and circumferences is described in Tables 51–3 and 51–4.[2] Skinfolds represent a double layer of subcutaneous tissue, including a small and relatively constant amount of skin and variable amounts of adipose tissue. Components at all five levels of body composition are thus represented by a skinfold measurement. For arm measurements, the most important aspect is to make repeated measurements using the same arm. Some workers recommend evaluating the nondominant arm; when comparing the patient's measurements with standard values, consult the arm selected in the reference table. Measuring techniques and methods of optimizing precision are presented in reference 19 and in Tables 51–5 and 51–6. Skinfold measurements are not accurate in massively obese patients.

**TABLE 51–4.** CIRCUMFERENTIAL MEASUREMENT SITES

1. **Mid-upper arm.** This circumference is taken at the midpoint between the acromial and olecranon processes of the scapula and the ulna, respectively. The arm should hang relaxed at the patient's side.
2. **Midthigh.** The subject stands with feet slightly apart and with weight evenly distributed on both feet. The tape is placed around the thigh horizontally at the midpoint between the lower extent of the gluteal fold and the crease immediately posterior to the patella.
3. **Midcalf.** With the subject standing in the same position as for the thigh circumference, the measurement is made with the tape horizontal at the maximal circumference of the calf.

**TABLE 51–5** METHODS OF MEASURING SKINFOLDS AND CIRCUMFERENCES

SKINFOLDS

1. Arrive at the anatomic site as defined in Tables 51–3 and 51–4
2. Lift the skin and fat layer from the underlying tissue by grasping the tissue with the thumb and forefinger.
3. Apply calipers about 1 cm distal from the thumb and forefinger, midway between the apex and base of the skinfold.
4. Continue to support the skinfold with the thumb and forefinger for the duration of the measurement.
5. After 2 to 3 seconds of caliper application, read skinfold to the nearest 0.5 mm.
6. Measurements are then made in triplicate until readings agree within ± 1.0 mm; results are then averaged.

CIRCUMFERENCES

1. The tape should be maintained in a horizontal position touching the skin and following the contours of the limb, but not compressing underlying tissue.
2. Measurements should be made to the nearest millimeter, in triplicate, as previously described for skinfolds.

**TABLE 51–6.** METHODS FOR OPTIMIZING PRECISION

1. Train observers by skilled professionals.
2. Use one rather than multiple observers for the same subject over time.
3. Mark the anatomic site of the skinfold and circumferential measurement with indelible ink when repeatedly measuring the same patient over a short time span.
4. Learn the anatomic landmarks, how to grasp the skinfold, how long to compress the skinfold site, and how to properly read the caliper scale.
5. Periodically assess interobserver and between-day measurement differences of the staff.

The absolute skinfold thickness can be used directly for comparison with reference tables and for longitudinal follow-up (see Appendix Table A–14). The limitation of evaluating one skinfold thickness is that a single measurement is a relatively poor predictor of the absolute amount and rate of change in total body fat because (1) large interindividual differences exist in fat distribution, (2) as total body fat changes, each skinfold site responds differently relative to changes in total body fat, and (3) the relationship between skinfold thickness and total body fat is complex (e.g., an exponential relationship exists between subcutaneous skinfold thickness and total body fat and between subcutaneous fat and internal fat.[2,33] Other factors that limit a single skinfold thickness as a measure of fatness include changes in the composition of adipose tissue with age and nutritional status; variation in skinfold distribution and compressibility with age; and the inclusion of a small amount of nonadipose tissues (e.g., skin) in the measurement.[2,20,33]

The final consideration is that the day-to-day variability in measuring the same skinfold is large, even when the rigorous procedures outlined in Table 51–6 are followed. Measuring skinfold thickness should therefore be considered a qualitative measure of the amount and rate of change in total body fat. The advantages are ease and rapidity of measurement, especially in bedridden patients.

Combining a limb skinfold thickness with a corresponding circumference allows calculation of limb fat areas (Table 51–7). Most of the problems related to a single skinfold measurement also occur with the limb fat area. The advantage generally ascribed to area calculations is that the result includes the contribution of limb circumference; two limbs with equal skinfolds but unequal circumferences will have different amounts of fat.

Many prediction equations are available for calculating total body fat from measured skinfold thicknesses, circumferences, and body weight. The most widely applied equation in current use was developed by Durnin and Womersley (Table 51–8). Subtracting total body fat from body weight provides a value for FFM. The advantages of calculating total body fat are: (1) more than one skinfold site is usually included in the calculation; and (2) the result (in kilograms) can be used directly to calculate energy reserves as fat. The latter values can then be integrated with estimates of energy balance calculations, thus providing a more physiologic description of the patient's nutritional state. A cautionary note is that, as with all prediction equations, results are most accurate on populations upon which the equation was derived. The accuracy of the Durnin-Womersley equation is unknown in patients with severe weight loss, and the technique should not be applied when a gross distortion in body habitus or obvious fluid accumulation is present. As emphasized by Damon and Goldman,

**TABLE 51–7** EQUATIONS FOR CALCULATING LIMB FAT AREAS

| EXTREMITY | EQUATION | COMMENTS |
|---|---|---|
| upper arm | arm fat area (cm$^2$) $= \left[\frac{MAC \times TSF}{2}\right] - \left[\frac{\pi \times (TSF)^2}{4}\right]$ | This general equation assumes a circular limb and muscle compartment and a symmetrically distributed fat rim. The accuracy of this equation in predicting mid-upper arm fat area is unknown. TSF, triceps skinfold (cm); MAC, midarm circumference (cm) |
| thigh | thigh fat area (cm$^2$) $= \left[\frac{MTC\ THSF}{2}\right] - \left[\frac{\pi\ (THSF)^2}{4}\right]$ | THSF, thigh skinfold (cm); MTC, midthigh circumference (cm) |
| calf | calf fat area (cm$^2$) $= \left[\frac{MCC\ CSF}{2}\right] - \left[\frac{\pi \times (CSF)^2}{4}\right]$ | CSF, calf skinfold (cm); MCC, midcalf circumference (cm) |

**TABLE 51–8.** CALCULATION OF FAT AND FAT-FREE BODY MASS ACCORDING TO THE METHOD OF DURNIN AND WOMERSLEY

**1.** Determine the patient's age and weight (kg).
**2.** Measure the following skinfolds in mm: biceps, triceps, subscapular, and suprailiac (Table 51–3 and 51–5).
**3.** Compute $\Sigma$ by adding the four skinfolds.
**4.** Compute the logarithm of $\Sigma$.
**5.** Apply one of the following age- and sex-adjusted equations to compute body density (D, g/ml)

Equations for men:

| Age range | |
|---|---|
| 17–19 | $D = 1.1620 - 0.0630 \times (\log \Sigma)$ |
| 20–29 | $D = 1.1631 - 0.0632 \times (\log \Sigma)$ |
| 30–39 | $D = 1.1422 - 0.0544 \times (\log \Sigma)$ |
| 40–49 | $D = 1.1620 - 0.0700 \times (\log \Sigma)$ |
| 50+ | $D = 1.1715 - 0.0779 \times (\log \Sigma)$ |

Equations for women:

| Age range | |
|---|---|
| 17–19 | $D = 1.1549 - 0.0678 \times (\log \Sigma)$ |
| 20–29 | $D = 1.1599 - 0.0717 \times (\log \Sigma)$ |
| 30–39 | $D = 1.1423 - 0.0632 \times (\log \Sigma)$ |
| 40–49 | $D = 1.1333 - 0.0612 \times (\log \Sigma)$ |
| 50+ | $D = 1.1339 - 0.0645 \times (\log \Sigma)$ |

**6.** Fat mass is then calculated as: fat mass (kg) = body weight (kg) $\times \left[\frac{4.95}{D} - 4.5\right]$
**7.** Fat-free body mass is then calculated as: FFM (kg) = body weight (kg) − fat mass (kg)

(Adapted from the data of Durnin, J.V.G.A., Womersley, J. and reprinted from Wright, R.A., Heymsfield, S.B. (eds.) Nutritional Assessment. Blackwell Scientific, 1984.)

skinfold measurements describe, but do not predict, total body fat.[41] More accurate methods of measuring fat are therefore usually applied in research studies of body composition.

It is customary to express total body fat estimates as a percentage of body weight. A problem in interpreting this approach is that, as an individual gains or loses weight, both fat and FFM change. Additionally, the relationship between total body fat and body weight has a nonzero intercept (see Fig. 51–3). The result is that a curvilinear relationship exists between total body fat,[12] expressed as a percentage of body weight, and body weight or BMI (Fig. 51–7). The complex relationship between percentage of fat and body weight can result in some confusing situations. A severely obese patient could lose a relatively large amount of weight and yet have a relatively small change in percentage of fat. A highly trained athlete and a severely malnourished patient might have an equivalent percentage of body weight as fat. To overcome these difficulties, VanItallie and colleagues suggest calculating a fat (or FFM)-stature index similar to BMI as: fat/Ht$^2$.[42] A low or high "fat mass index" would then represent a reduced or increased actual fat mass adjusted for stature, respectively. For example, fat mass index in a malnourished patient would be lower than in a highly trained athlete, even though both had an equivalent percentage of body weight as fat. This is because the athlete with a similar percentage of body weight as fat would have a larger absolute fat mass and also a larger FFM and greater body weight than the malnourished patient.

**Lean Tissues.** Lean tissues refer in general to the following sequence of compartments at the five levels of body composition: I, nitrogen, potassium, and calcium; II, FFM, water, and protein; III, body cell mass; IV, skeletal muscle, skeleton, and visceral organs, V, anthropometric measurements (e.g., skinfolds/circumferences) (see Table 51–1). These various compartments are associated with the major portion of whole body metabolic activity and biologic functions.

*Semistarvation.* Semistarvation results in negative balances of energy, protein, water, and minerals, a reduction in FFM and body cell mass, and atrophy of tissues and organs.[2,40] Not all lean compartments change at the same rate during periods of negative balance. At the molecular level, cellular proteins are depleted rapidly and connective tissue proteins are lost at a slower rate.[2] Similarly, at the cellular level, rapid changes can occur in body cell mass, whereas extracellular fluid is lost more slowly or may even increase in volume.[43] Organs and tissues also differ in their rate of weight loss during semistarvation. Liver mass decreases rapidly and brain weight changes very little if at all in uncomplicated semistarvation; liver and other visceral organs may be preserved in chronic catabolic conditions such as metastatic malignant diseases.[31] Skeletal muscle is a

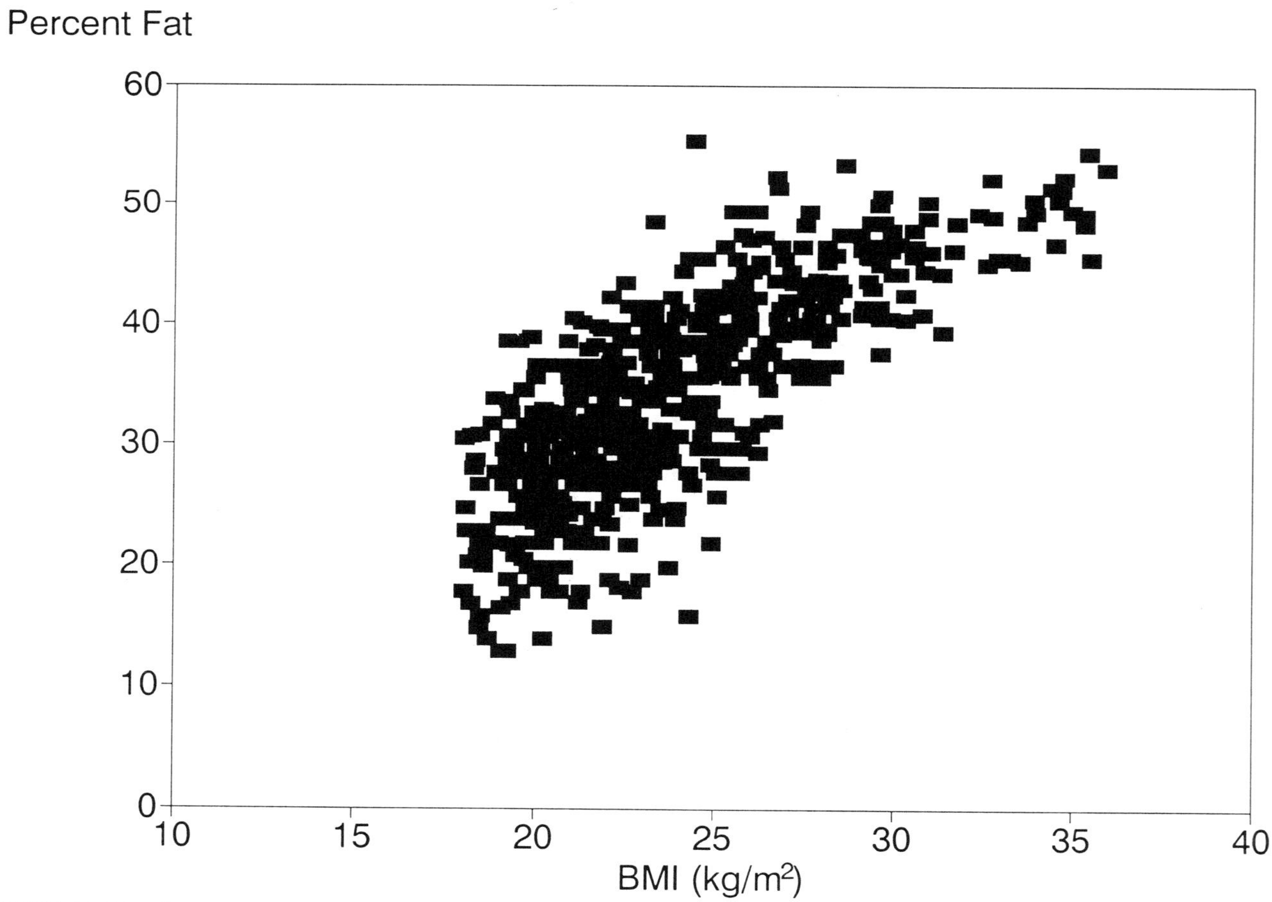
Percent Fat
60
50
40
30
20
10
0
10
15
20
25
30
35
40
BMI (kg/m²)

**FIGURE 51–7.** Percentage of body weight as fat in 530 women versus body mass index (BMI). Fat was measured by dual-photon absorptiometry systems.

major reservoir of amino acids for acute-phase protein synthesis and can decrease by up to 75% in weight during protein-energy malnutrition.[7,31] The malnourished patient with a reduced body weight therefore has a different composition at each of the five levels compared with his or her normally nourished counterpart. This explains why anthropometric equations developed in normal subjects may not predict a specific compartment with equal accuracy in an undernourished seriously ill patient.

In anthropometrically assessing the severity of malnutrition, an important goal is to define the amount and rate of change in total body or skeletal muscle protein.[7,31] The main anthropometric indices used for this assessment are FFM (level II) and limb muscle areas (level IV). As lower limits compatible with survival are known for both types of measurement,[2] the severity of protein-energy malnutrition is usually judged as the patient's value relative to the normal range on the one hand and the minimal range on the other. In terms of prognostic value, these measurements will provide some index of potential survival time; given the patient's anthropometric FFM or muscle index and nitrogen balance, progression towards or away from potentially lethal starvation can be established. During nutritional therapy and follow-up, the anthropometric FFM indices are used as measures of nitrogen balance, and specific details regarding interpretation are presented in the following paragraphs.

*Measurement and Interpretation.* Measuring FFM is accomplished by the skinfold methods, such as those described earlier in the section on fat (Table 51–8). The same cautions in measurement technique and selection of patients noted in the earlier discussion of fat also apply to FFM. With regard to interpretation, in theory multiplying FFM (in grams) by 0.195 and 1.02 provides the amount of total body protein in grams and metabolizable energy in kilocalories. Of the metabolizable energy in the healthy subject, about half of that in FFM is available during prolonged periods of semistarvation.[2] When combined with balance data and information on total body fat, these bedside calculations often provide an interesting insight into a patient's course. Unfortunately, the information needed for accurate prediction of total body protein cannot be derived from anthropometric FFM because of the changes in body hydration and variability of skinfold measurements described earlier. A large tumor burden or organomegaly of any cause may also add mass (as water, protein, and mineral) to FFM that is metabolically unavailable. In patients without serious derangements in body composition, FFM can be used to calculate resting metabolic rate (RMR) as [44]:

$$\text{RMR (kcal/d)} = 21.6 \times \text{FFM (kg)} + 370. \qquad (3)$$

This calculation, useful as energy expenditure adjusted for FFM, is largely independent of sex and age.[26,44]

Calculating the amount of limb muscle tissue from anthropometric data requires only two measurements: the limb circumference and the corresponding skinfold thickness. The midportion of the upper limb is usually studied, and little additional information is gathered by also measuring thigh and calf muscle areas.[31] Calf muscle measurement would, of course, be useful in subjects whose upper extremities are burned, amputated, edematous, or immobilized by casts or traction devices. The upper arm muscles tend to atrophy slightly more rapidly during semistarvation than the muscles of the thigh or calf, but the differences are not large.[31] The equations for calculating the limb muscle indices are provided in Table 51–9.

The primary application of limb muscle measurements is to obtain a measure of the amount and rate of change in skeletal muscle protein. The following three factors should therefore be considered[2]:

1. The mass of a skeletal muscle represents a three-dimensional measurement (i.e., volume), whereas limb muscle area and circumference are two- and one-dimensional indices, respectively.[2,31] As the muscle changes volume, the corresponding proportional changes in muscle area and circumference will be smaller than the change in volume. For example, a 50% decrease in muscle volume will correspond to a theoretic decrease in muscle area and circumference of 37 and 21%, respectively. As a rule, the relative change in muscle area will be larger than the change in muscle circumference. Therefore, although limb muscle area and circumference will be highly correlated with one another, the area measurement will provide a more realistic estimate of the relative change in muscle mass.

2. The equations for calculating limb muscle indices are based upon simple theoretic assumptions regarding arm geometry.[2,31] Actually, the calculated arm muscle area overestimates the amount of skeletal muscle by 15 to 25% in relatively young, nonobese subjects. Half of this overestimate is due to the inclusion of bone in the calculated area, and the remainder is due to errors in the assumptions and the inclusion of nonmuscle tissue (e.g., neurovascular bundle) in the result. Two methods of correcting this overestimate of muscle area are available. The first is to express results as a percentage of standard, because the standard value will also contain these "nonskeletal muscle" components. The second approach is to calculate a value for bone-free arm muscle area, as described in Table 51–9. Studies by Forbes and Baumgartner et al. suggest that arm muscle area assumptions are also inaccurate in obese and elderly subjects, respectively.[45,46] Further studies are therefore needed to improve our understanding of the relationship between anthropometric muscle estimates at level V of body composition and actual skeletal muscle mass at level IV.

3. Atrophic skeletal muscle differs in chemical composition from normal tissue. Per gram of muscle, the

**TABLE 51–9.** ANTHROPOMETRIC EQUATIONS FOR CALCULATING MUSCLE MASS

| EQUATION | COMMENT |
|---|---|
| **(1)** Calf muscle area $(cm)^2 = \frac{[MCC - \pi \times CSF]^2}{4\pi}$ | Includes bone area; assumes circular limb and muscle compartment and symmetric fat rim. Abbreviations as in Table 51–7. |
| **(2)** Thigh muscle area $(cm^2) = \frac{[MTC - \pi \times THSF]^2}{4\pi}$ | Bone corrections are available. |
| **(3)** Arm muscle circumference (cm) $= MAC - \pi \times TSF$ | Same assumption as for Equations 1 and 2; includes bone. Note that as muscle loses mass or volume in protein-energy malnutrition, circumferential measurements will change proportionately less than area measurements. The latter therefore more realistically depicts severity of muscle atropy. |
| **(4)** Arm muscle area $(cm^2) = \frac{[MAC - \pi \times TSF]^2}{4\pi}$ | Same assumption as Equations 1 and 2; includes bone. Equation overestimates actual muscle area; by expressing absolute value as a percentage of standard, the error is partially corrected. |
| **(5)** Arm muscle area $(cm^2) = \frac{[MAC - \pi \times TSF]^2}{4\pi} - 10$ (men)<br>Arm muscle area $(cm^2) = \frac{[MAC - \pi \times TSF]^2}{4\pi} - 6.5$ (women) | Same assumptions as Equations 1 and 2; the overestimate in Equation 4 is corrected, and the average value for bone area is also subtracted. Resulting value is therefore bone-free arm muscle area. As for all muscle derivatives on this table, the resulting value remains an approximation (± 8%) of actual muscle area. Arm muscle area estimates may be particularly inaccurate in obese and elderly subjects. |
| **(6)** Total body skeletal muscle mass (g) $= STAT \times (0.0553 \times CTG^2 + 0.0987 \times FG^2 + 0.0331 \times CCG^2) - 2445$ | Based on cadaver studies.[34] STAT, stature (cm); CTG, thigh circumference corrected for the front thigh skinfold thickness (cm); FG, uncorrected forearm circumference (cm); CCG, calf circumference corrected for the medial calf skinfold thickness (cm). |

amounts of water, total lipid, and collagen are increased, whereas the noncollagen proteins are reduced (Fig. 51–8). Thus, the concentration of functional proteins per unit arm muscle area or circumference is relatively lower in the atrophied muscle. Another chemical consideration is that muscle size can abruptly change by ± 5 to 10% in response to rapid changes in muscle glycogen as a result of the water-binding properties of glycogen.[31]

Thus, both anthropometric FFM and muscle indices are truly indirect markers of the active protein component of body weight. The two lean tissue indices should be considered approximate bedside guides to the amount of total body protein. Despite their approximate nature, anthropometric muscle estimates correlate with more complex methods of estimating skeletal muscle (e.g., urinary creatinine excretion) over the broad biologic range of muscle mass in humans (Fig. 51–9).

Small changes in total body protein cannot be detected by anthropometry, and nitrogen balance and other techniques must be used for this assessment. An example of the limitation of anthropometry is shown in Figure 51–10, where short-term changes in anthropometric arm muscle area with nutrition support are shown not to correlate with nitrogen balance.

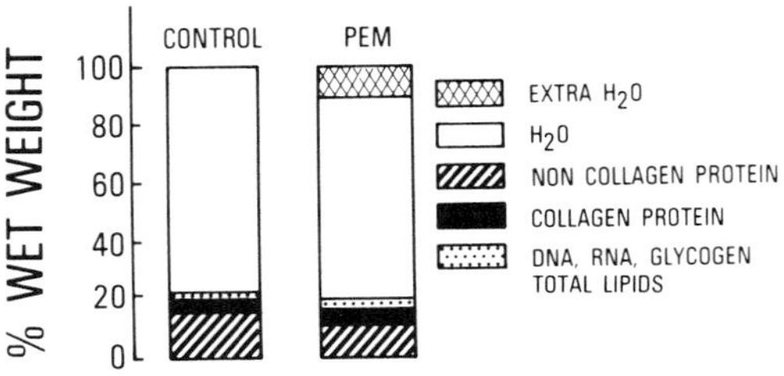
CONTROL
PEM
% WET WEIGHT
100
80
60
40
20
0
EXTRA H2O
H2O
NON COLLAGEN PROTEIN
COLLAGEN PROTEIN
DNA, RNA, GLYCOGEN
TOTAL LIPIDS

**FIGURE 51–8.** Muscle composition per gram of wet muscle weight in control subjects and in protein-energy malnourished (PEM) humans. Muscle specimens were collected at autopsy. Undernourished patients had relatively more water (including extra water), collagen proteins, and total lipids compared with controls. The extra water was calculated by assuming that muscle dry weight is normally 21% of wet weight. (From Heymsfield, S.B., Stevens, V., Noel, R., et al.: Am. J. Clin. Nutr., *36*:131–142, 1982; with permission of the American Journal of Clinical Nutrition.)

## REFERENCE VALUES

**Body Weight.** The patient's body weight is evaluated using two reference sources. The first reference values are those of the patient, and these include a "usual weight" by history or previous measured weight. This is

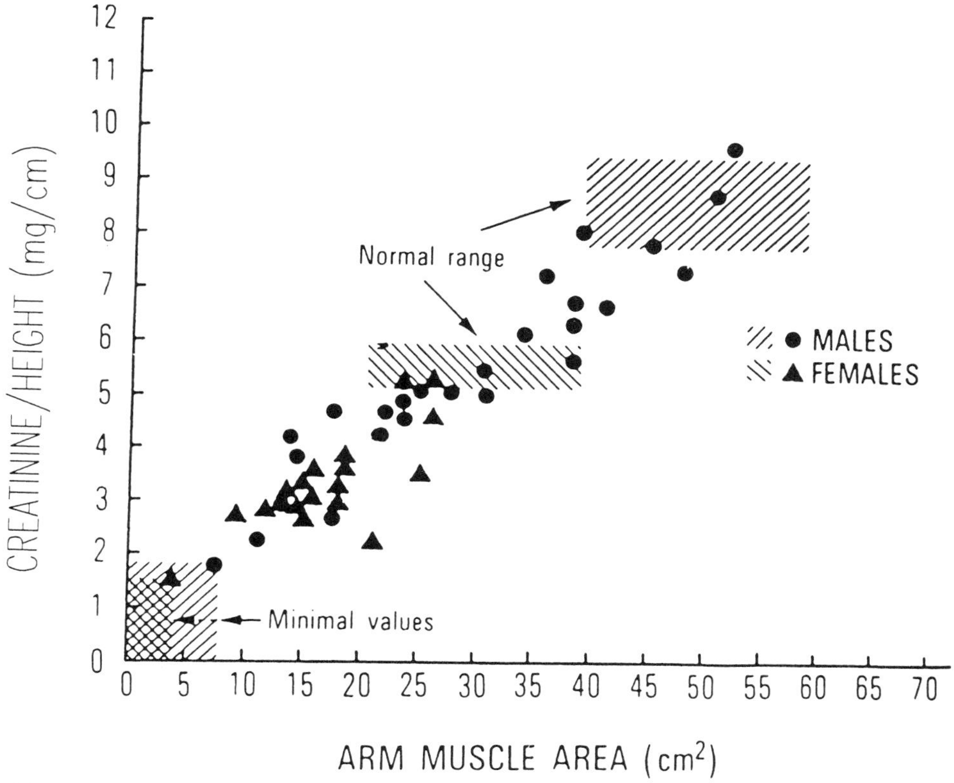
CREATININE/HEIGHT (mg/cm)
0
1
2
3
4
5
6
7
8
9
10
11
12
Normal range
Minimal values
MALES
FEMALES
0 5 10 15 20 25 30 35 40 45 50 55 60 65 70
ARM MUSCLE AREA (cm2)

**FIGURE 51–9.** Correlation between muscle indices creatinine/height and arm muscle area in healthy and undernourished subjects. The normal range and minimal values compatible with survival are indicated for males and females. (From Heymsfield, S.B., Casper, K.: JPEN J. Parenter. Enteral Nutr., *11*:36S–41S, 1987.)

important because many obese patients who lose weight during an illness and are thus potentially malnourished will still be overweight by conventional standards. The second reference source is the healthy population. In this approach, the individual's actual body weight is compared to that of a gender-, stature-, and age-appropriate reference or desirable body weight (see Appendix Tables A–11, A–12, and A–13). The subject's actual body weight is expressed as a percentage of desirable. The normal range for desirable body weight varies among different sources, but it usually is set between 90 and 120%. A body weight below or above these levels is consistent with undernutrition and obesity, respectively. A historical review of the development of reference body weight tables is provided in Appendix Table A–11a.

Another method of comparing the patient's weight with that of a reference population is to calculate a body weight (BW)-stature (S) index.[47] Most weight-stature indices in present use take the form $W/S^p$.[45] The term p indicates how stature is to be scaled. The main assumptions of weight-stature indices are that they are independent of height, represent an indirect index of body composition, mainly fatness, correlate with health outcomes, and can be generalized across different populations.

At present, the use of BMI, calculated as $BW/Ht^2$, is gaining acceptance as a weight-stature index for use in diagnosing both protein-energy malnutrition and obesity.[48,49] Most of the assumptions of weight-stature indices are fulfilled by BMI, although several limitations should be noted. First, although the correlation between BMI and total body fat is relatively strong ($r = 0.5 - 0.8$), individual variation is large and some subjects can be misclassified as undernourished or obese.[47] For example, some athletic subjects have a large skeletal muscle mass and a high BMI but are not obese. Another example, reported by Smalley and colleagues, is that a man with a BMI of 27 can have total body fat ranging from 10 to 31% of body weight.[50] Last, BMI may have a small stature dependence because individuals with short legs for their height have higher BMI values independent of fatness.[47,49]

Although no consistent BMI ranges are accepted by all investigators, a useful set of guidelines is presented in Table 51–10. The table gives a normal range (BMI $\geqq 18.5 < 25$) and three grades of both chronic protein-energy malnutrition and obesity. The investigators proposing these guidelines based their criteria on extensive reviews of functional measurements and health outcomes at various levels of BMI.[49,51] The diagnosis of protein-

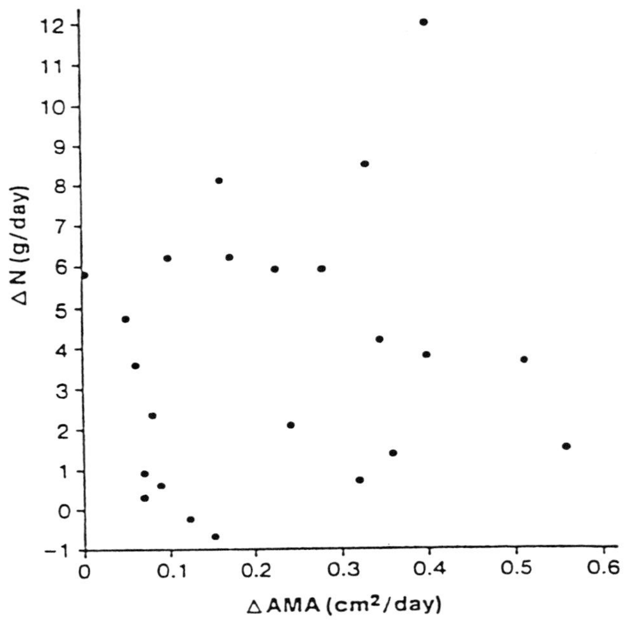
ΔN (g/day)
ΔAMA (cm²/day)

**FIGURE 51–10.** Nitrogen balance (N) measured on a metabolic ward versus change in arm muscle area (AMA) in subjects undergoing 1-week balance studies. (From Heymsfield, S.B., Casper, K.: JPEN J. Parenter. Enteral Nutr., *11*:36S–41S, 1987.)

**TABLE 51–10** BODY MASS INDEX AND GRADES OF CHRONIC PROTEIN-ENERGY MALNUTRITION AND OBESITY

| GRADE | BODY MASS INDEX |
|---|---|
| Obesity | |
| III | >40 |
| II | 30–40 |
| I | 25–29.9 |
| Normal | ≥18.5–<25 |
| Protein-energy malnutrition | |
| I | 17.0–18.4 |
| II | 16.0–16.9 |
| III | <16 |

(Adapted from James, W.P.T., Ferro-Luzzi, A., Waterlow, J.C.: Eur. J. Clin. Nutr., *42*:969–981; and McLaren, D.S.: A fresh look at anthropometric classification schemes in protein-energy malnutrition. *In* Anthropometric Assessment of Nutritional Status. Edited by J.H. Himes. New York, Wiley-Liss, 1991, pp. 273–286.)

energy malnutrition or obesity and their associated risks is often multifactorial and may require additional estimates including body composition, energy expenditure, organ/tissue function, and biochemical markers.

**Fat and Lean.** Two methods are used to process anthropometric data other than body weight. The first method is to express the individual's values relative to a healthy reference population. This method provides the anthropometric component used to assess whether and to what extent the patient is malnourished. The anthropometric reference tables present the results of large surveys and usually describe the general population. Appendix Tables A–12 to A–14 provide reference values for the United States population as a whole.

The reference tables usually present data in three forms: (1) as a mean ($\bar{x}$) value; (2) as $\bar{x}$ and standard deviation (SD); and (3) as percentiles. Describing a population in terms of $\bar{x}$ and SD assumes the measurement under study is symmetrically (normally) distributed. If data fit this model, then the $\bar{x} \pm 2SD$ includes 95% of the population. An abnormal value is more than 2 SD above or below the $\bar{x}$. Some tables provide only an $\bar{x}$, and the patient's value is then expressed as a percentage of the standard or reference value. A weakness of this approach is that tables of this type do not provide the observer with a method of determining whether the result is within the normal range. The second type of table includes the SD, or 95% range of the healthy population, thus indicating whether and to what degree the patient is abnormal. The third mode of expression is in terms of percentiles (e.g., Appendix Tables A–12 and A–13). The advantage of expressing results as a percentile rather than as a percentage of standard is that the reference population need not be symmetrically distributed. Often anthropometric surveys of populations produce "skewed" distributions, and therefore the easiest option is to present results in percentiles.[52] In this approach, the values of the subject exactly in the middle of the group are at the 50th percentile. If the patient's value is between the 5th and 95th percentile, the result is considered normal; below or above these respective values is abnormal.

No simple method of judging the severity or potential morbidity of protein-energy malnutrition from anthropometric data is available. Studies in adults have not yet clearly defined the "risk" of a subnormal anthropometric index, especially for results falling just below the normal range. Combining anthropometric data with the results of other components of the nutritional assessment provides some measure of potential morbidity.[53]

The second method of expressing anthropometric data is in terms of the individual's total body energy content, fat, and FFM. When estimated energy and nitrogen balance are combined with these body composition data, a whole spectrum of potential calculations is possible. Of course, these are approximations, but their application in teaching and solving simple clinical questions often proves useful.

## CLINICAL APPLICATIONS

Suggested applications of anthropometry are the following:

1. Weight and height should be recorded in the chart of every hospitalized patient. Weight indices, such as recent weight loss, should be added to the data base

for all patients who have a history of weight change. The weight of all patients undergoing short-term nutritional support should be measured daily.

2. The recommended uses of one skinfold measurement, limb fat area, and limb muscle area are:
   a. When body weight is an invalid index of energy reserves because of edema or massive tumor burden. The upper limb is usually not affected by dependent edema.
   b. When body weight is unmeasurable because of immobilizing devices, such as a cast or respirator.
   c. When patients are seen for nutritional consultation or are seen at rounds removed from the bedside. Anthropometric estimates provide a quantitative description of what is usually visible at the bedside. Although weight alone is useful in this regard, two patients of the same height and weight may differ in body composition.
   d. During the initial evaluation of hospitalized patients who are prescribed short-term nutritional support. Although changes in fat and lean tissue will most likely not be detected over a 1- to 2-week period, the baseline anthropometric data will become a permanent component of the nutritional data base. This information will then be available if a future re-evaluation is needed.
3. Total body fat and FFM are useful indices:
   a. In patients who are undergoing long-term nutritional follow-up over months or years. Limb muscle area measurements, preferably of the upper arm, should also be included in this group, to complete the body composition data base.
   b. In groups of subjects forming the basis of nutritional studies, when a more critical assessment of body composition is often useful and more accurate techniques of evaluating body composition are not available.
   c. In estimating resting metabolic rate based upon FFM.
   d. For teaching purposes, when the interrelation of metabolic balance, body composition, and nutritional therapy are the subject of discussion.

### AGING AND ANTHROPOMETRIC INDICES

Body composition changes throughout the adult life span, and this must be considered when evaluating anthropometric indices. Height declines and, assuming body weight remains unchanged, there is more fat and less FFM in an elderly subject than in a younger individual of the same sex.[40,54] Most of the loss in FFM can be accounted for by a decrease in skeletal muscle mass. A summary of how body composition changes with age and how anthropometric measures are affected is presented in Table 51–11.

A difficult problem in the elderly is estimation of height, especially in the wheelchair-bound, bedridden, or kyphotic subject. A useful approach is to measure knee height (see Table 51–2) to predict adult stature. Knee height undergoes little change with age in adults and provides an indirect estimate of stature that is difficult to obtain by conventional methods. Another approach is to estimate stature as twice the distance between the sternal notch and finger tips. The estimated value for height can then be used in calculating other assessment indices and for comparison of these results to height-adjusted reference values.

## NITROGEN BALANCE

### PHYSIOLOGY

Nitrogen balance, a measure of net change in total body protein mass, is based on the assumption that almost all total body nitrogen is incorporated into protein.[21,55] Nitrogen is approximately 16% of protein by weight: nitrogen (g) = protein (g) × 6.25. For example, a nitrogen balance of −1 g per day equals a 6.25-g reduction in total body protein. The overall nitrogen balance equation has six components:

$$\text{Nitrogen balance} = \text{N intake} - (\text{urinary N} + \text{fecal N} + \text{integumental N} + \Delta\ \text{nonprotein N} + \text{body fluid N losses}). \quad (4)$$

Nitrogen intake is the total amount of nitrogen supplied orally or parenterally to an individual. The value for nitrogen intake is most accurately determined by chemically measuring nitrogen in the nutrients provided. The micro-Kjeldahl technique, known for its accuracy, is the method usually used. Newer validated techniques, such as chemiluminescence,[56] are also available and may eventually replace the more complex Kjeldahl method. Less accurate but more practical is estimating nitrogen from product labels and nutrient data bases and handbooks.

The largest loss of nitrogen is in urine (Fig. 51–11). Urinary nitrogen losses for individuals on a general diet are: urea nitrogen, 80%; ammonia nitrogen, 7.4%; creatinine nitrogen, 6.4%; uric acid nitrogen, 2 to 3%; and other minor nitrogenous compounds, 1 to 2%.[57] Urea is synthesized in hepatic tissue by the enzyme pathway known as the Krebs-Henseleit cycle. Urea is a water-soluble end product of protein metabolism, which is distributed throughout the total body water. Most urea is excreted by the kidneys, with minor losses through sweat and other body secretions. In the intestinal tract, bacterial urease hydrolyzes urea to ammonia and carbon dioxide.[58] The ammonia is completely reabsorbed in healthy individuals, and only a negligible amount of urea can be detected in feces. Fecal urea increases in certain pathologic states.

Although urea usually constitutes 80% of total urinary nitrogen, this proportion varies with the amount and quality of proteins ingested. For example, Allison and Bird found that urea constituted 61.7% of total urinary

**TABLE 51–11.** EFFECTS OF AGING ON BODY COMPOSITION AND ANTHROPOMETRIC MEASUREMENTS

| ANTHROPOMETRIC MEASUREMENT | COMMENT |
|---|---|
| Weight | The average population value increases until the fifth decade and then plateaus or declines. |
| Height | Height decreases by 1 to 3 cm/20 years after maturity. The rate in height decline is race and sex dependent. |
| Fat | Fat increases as a percentage of body weight; redistribution occurs from subcutaneous to internal fat and between different subcutaneous sites. |
| Skinfold | The compressibility of skinfolds changes with age. There is a loss in the elastic recoil of skin and an increase in viscoelastic recovery time. Skinfolds in the elderly are often pendulous and difficult to measure. |
| Fat-free body mass | Fat-free body mass decreases as a percentage of body weight mainly because of a loss in skeleton and skeletal muscle mass. The mass of visceral organs remains unchanged or decreases only slightly with age. Skeletal muscle undergoes compositional changes, which include a relative increase in connective tissue and fat and relative loss in myofibrillar proteins. |

(From Wright, R.A., Heymsfield, S.B. (Eds.): Nutritional Assessment. Boston, Blackwell Scientific 1984.)

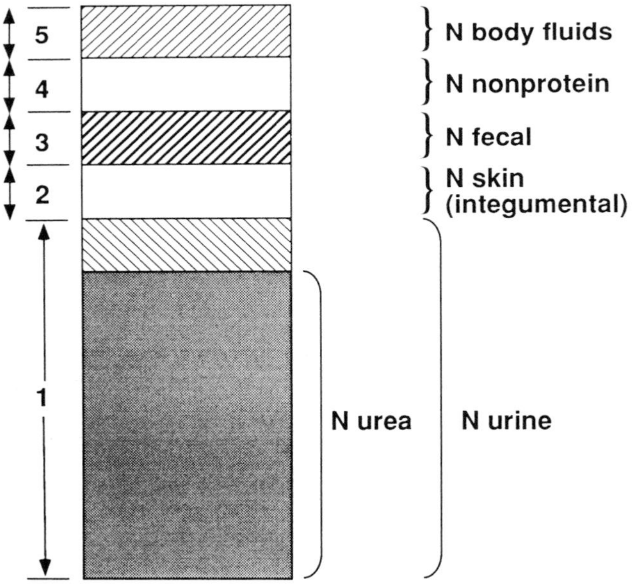
5
4
3
2
1
N body fluids
N nonprotein
N fecal
N skin (integumental)
N urea
N urine

**FIGURE 51–11.** Five forms of nitrogen (N) loss in hospitalized patients. (From Heymsfield, S.B., Tochilin, N., McManus, C.B., et al.: Clin. Consultations Nutr. Support, *4*:6–10, 1984.)

protein with a low-protein diet and 87.5% with a high-protein diet.[59] Some amino acids (e.g., arginine and glutamine) are effective in stimulating urea production;[58] a diet comprising low-quality proteins increases urea excretion more than does a diet comprising high-quality proteins.

In contrast to the situation for total urinary nitrogen, automated methods can be rapidly and easily used to measure urea nitrogen in most clinical laboratories. A common practice is to measure urinary urea nitrogen and then estimate total urinary nitrogen by dividing the urea nitrogen value by 0.8. Although this method provides a reasonable estimate of total urinary nitrogen, the actual fraction of total urinary nitrogen as urea varies. The average results of 7-day balance studies for patients with and without a history of malabsorption are presented in Table 51–12. Four diet categories are used: general, elemental 1 (free amino acids, 2% fat), elemental 2 (predigested protein formula, 2% fat), and polymeric (intact protein, 40% fat). The proportion of total nitrogen as urea ranged from 0.75 in the malabsorption patients on a polymeric diet to 0.87 in normal subjects on an elemental diet. The causes of these differences are unknown, but likely explanations include differences in the amount and quality of protein ingested, impaired protein absorption in the malabsorption patients, and reduced hydrolysis of urea in the intestine, an increase in

**TABLE 51–12.** AVERAGE RESULTS OF NITROGEN BALANCE STUDIES UNDER DIFFERING DIETARY CONDITIONS IN PATIENTS WITHOUT AND WITH MALABSORPTION

| PATIENTS/DIET | N | INTAKE | | UUN/TUN (A1) | APPARENT DIGESTIBILITY (A2) | TOTAL N LOSSES–UUN* G/DAY (A3) |
|---|---|---|---|---|---|---|
| | | % Fat | Protein (g) | | | |
| Nonmalabsorption | | | | | | |
| GHD (General hospital diet) | 10 | 40 | 16.5 | 0.80 | 0.88 | 4.1 |
| Enteral Formulas | | | | | | |
| $E_1$: Elemental, free amino acid | 22 | 2 | 15.8 | 0.87 | 0.96 | 2.6 |
| $E_2$: Elemental, predigested protein | 30 | 2 | 16.2 | 0.83 | 0.91 | 3.3 |
| P: Polymeric, intact protein | 33 | 40 | 15.5 | 0.85 | 0.90 | 3.4 |
| Formulas $E_1$ + $E_2$ + P | 85 | — | 15.3 | 0.85 | 0.92 | 3.1 |
| Malabsorption | | | | | | |
| GHD (General hospital diet) | 4 | 40 | 14.8 | 0.83 | 0.77 | 6.4 |
| Enteral Formulas | | | | | | |
| $E_1$: Elemental, free amino acid | 6 | 2 | 14.4 | 0.87 | 0.88 | 3.4 |
| $E_2$: Elemental, predigested protein | 6 | 2 | 14.9 | 0.78 | 0.82 | 4.9 |
| P: Polymeric, intact protein | 6 | 40 | 13.7 | 0.75 | 0.88 | 4.3 |
| Formulas $E_1$ + $E_2$ + P | 16 | — | 14.4 | 0.81 | 0.86 | 4.2 |

*Includes integumental N at 7 mg/kg for men and 8 mg/kg for women.
TUN, Total urine nitrogen; UUN, urine urea nitrogen.
(Modified from Heymsfield, S.B., Tochilin, N., McManus, C.B., et al.: Clin. Consultations Nutr. Support, *4*:6–10, 1984.)

fecal urea, and a reciprocal decrease in urinary urea in the malabsorption patients.

The percentage of urinary total nitrogen as amino acids or ammonia also varies in pathologic states. For example, metabolic alkalosis and acidosis, respectively, decrease and increase urinary excretion of ammonia. In cases of inborn errors of metabolism, such as 5-oxoprolinuria (pyroglutamic aciduria), α-amino nitrogen can be 30 to 50% of total urinary nitrogen.[57]

Fecal nitrogen comes from a mixture of desquamated epithelial cells, bacteria, and unabsorbed dietary protein. For a diet containing 100 g of protein, 70 g of endogenous digestive proteins mixes with food in the intestinal tract, and a total of 160 g of protein is then absorbed. Fecal protein content is 10 g per day, or 1 to 2 g of nitrogen. The apparent digestibility of protein (%) is calculated as

$$[(\text{Intake} - \text{stool losses})/\text{intake}] \times 100. \quad (5)$$

In this example, protein digestibility was 90%.

Apparent digestibility of protein varies with the amount of protein ingested; approximately 0.4 g of nitrogen per day remains in the stool when protein intake is zero. Thus the apparent digestibility of protein is low when protein intake is low. Prediction equations for calculating fecal nitrogen as a function of protein intake are available, but these are specific for the protein source on which the equations are based.[60] Apparent digestibility was 77 to 99% (mean 88%) in our subjects without a history of intestinal disease who were on a general diet; values were 59 to 94% (mean 77%) for malabsorption patients. Thus, in patients with malabsorption, fecal nitrogen can be as much as 41% of intake. Abnormal losses also occur in conditions such as protein-losing enteropathy.

Skin desquamation, sweat, nasal secretions, hair and nail clippings, menstrual flow, blood withdrawal for diagnostic studies, and seminal discharge all account for small integumental and miscellaneous nitrogen losses. In normal subjects, ambient temperature and protein intake influence integumental nitrogen; losses are abnormally large in exfoliative diseases and burns. A typical estimate of skin nitrogen loss per day for individuals consuming a general diet is 5 mg/kg of body weight; values decrease to 3 mg/kg with a protein-free diet.[61] The remaining miscellaneous nitrogen losses are estimated to be 2 and 3 mg/kg for men and women, respectively.[61] The average 70-kg man and 55-kg woman have an integumental daily nitrogen loss of 0.49 and 0.44 g, respectively. Nitrogen loss from skin can be measured only on a metabolic ward, and special techniques are required.

Most total body nitrogen occurs in protein, but there are also small amounts of nonprotein nitrogen. For nitrogen balance studies, the most important nonprotein-nitrogen considerations involve changes in total body urea nitrogen. An increase in blood urea nitrogen (BUN, in grams per deciliter) implies an increase in total body urea, which must then be subtracted from nitrogen intake to allow a true estimate of changes in total body protein. Because urea is distributed in total body water, the following equation proposed by Harvey et al. and Kopple is usually applied[62,63]:

$$\text{Nonprotein N (g/day)} = [(BUN_f - BUN_i) \times 0.6 \times BW_i + (BW_f - BW_i) \times BUN_f]/(day_f - day_i) \quad (6)$$

where i and f are the initial and final values for the balance period, and BW (in kilograms) is body weight. The value for nonprotein nitrogen can be either positive or negative. The equation is based on the assumption that water is 60% of body weight and that changes in weight are due to changes in total body water. For lean patients and patients with edema, the value 0.6 is too low; for obese individuals and for very young children, this value is too high. No simple corrections are available yet for these groups. Bioimpedance analysis may be useful in estimating initial total body water in these patients (see Chap. 49).

Finally, the nitrogen content of body fluid drainage, such as paracentesis or nasogastric aspirates, must be considered. The micro-Kjeldahl or chemiluminescence methods can be used to analyze total nitrogen in these fluids.

## INTERPRETATION

Interpretation of nitrogen balance studies is often difficult, even under rigorous metabolic-ward conditions. Overall nitrogen balance often is unexplainably high.[64] Wallace suggested that a cause for high values might be a tendency to overestimate intake (the patient consumes less food than is provided) and to underestimate nitrogen losses (specimens are inadequately collected).[65] An overestimate in intake occurs for patients not eating all the food on their plates and utensils or by receiving unrecorded nitrogen containing solutions such as blood; an underestimate in nitrogen losses occurs because of the many sources of unmeasured losses and incomplete urine and fecal collections. Forbes hypothesized that any changes in nitrogen intake require long periods for readjusting to a new nitrogen balance steady state.[66] Balance studies are usually too short for this to happen. Although the exact length of the required equilibrium period is not known, most researchers agree that at least 2 to 12 days are needed. The length of the readjustment period is related to the relative change in protein intake. Kurzer proposed that unmeasured losses, such as in nitrates and gaseous nitrogen, would falsely increase nitrogen balance;[67] however, questions remain regarding the size of these losses.[63,68]

Classic methods exist for confirming nitrogen balance results. For example, combinations of calcium phosphorus, and potassium balances can be used to calculate an "expected" or "theoretic" nitrogen balance. The theoretic nitrogen balance result can then be used to establish the validity of observed nitrogen balance.[63] This approach can be used on a metabolic ward to check the accuracy of nitrogen balance results.

Daily variation in a patient's nitrogen excretion must also be considered. On a metabolic ward, meticulous daily collection of urine resulted in a coefficient of variation of 2 to 8%, which was based on urinary creatinine output. Variability in nitrogen values is much greater for patients treated in a clinical service unless urine collections are strictly timed. Rand et al. noted that the intraindividual variation for nitrogen excretion was greater than that for creatinine.[68] These investigators concluded that nitrogen balance could be measured with a variability of 10% if the balance study took place during the last 5 days of a 15-day study.

## CLINICAL CALCULATION

For nitrogen balance studies, long equilibrium periods, accurate and multiple urine collections, and the ability to analyze diet, urine, and stool for total nitrogen are desirable features. Unfortunately, these conditions are rarely found in a clinical service, and thus the results of nitrogen balance studies must be interpreted cautiously.

Nitrogen intake is usually estimated from protein intake. With specialized nutrition support formulas, the amino acids present may not be 16% nitrogen, so caution should be used when interconverting between nitrogen and protein. Several alternatives exist for estimating or measuring the five nitrogen-loss factors (Fig. 51–11). Total urinary nitrogen is measured in 24-hour urine specimens and the results are averaged. Large errors can arise if short urine collections (<12 to 18 hours) are extrapolated to 24 hours.[63] In a recent study, Candio and colleagues observed that a 12-hour urinary urea nitrogen measurement was approximately equal to half the 24-hour urinary urea nitrogen.[69] The patients in this study, however, were critically ill but clinically stable and receiving constant infusions of nutrition-support solution. If only urea nitrogen can be measured by the clinical laboratory,[70] then total urine nitrogen can be approximated by

$$\text{Urinary N (g/day)} = \text{urea N (g/day)}/A1 \quad (7)$$

where A1 is approximation 1 in Table 51–12. A1 is diet dependent, so for inexact clinical purposes, the average value (for enteral formulas) of 0.85 is reasonable. We have no reason to believe that this value differs markedly for parenteral formulas. For the amount of protein supplied to most hospitalized patients, urinary nitrogen (grams per day) is approximately equal to urea nitrogen plus 1.5 to 2.0 g.[55]

The use of urinary urea nitrogen to estimate total urinary nitrogen was recently challenged by Konstantinides and colleagues,[71] who observed a ratio of urea nitrogen to total nitrogen that ranged from 0.12 to 1.12 in general surgical trauma patients. The conclusions of this study were critiqued by Flatt et al.,[72] who argued that most of the time (~95%) urinary urea nitrogen is a good surrogate (±1.8 g) for total urinary nitrogen.

Fecal nitrogen varies greatly even in patients without malabsorption and ranges from 0.2 to 3.5 g per day; patients without malabsorption receiving the free amino acid formula have the lowest values, and patients consuming solid food have the highest values. Average values for representative enteral formulas are between 0.6 and 1.9 g per day. One way to calculate fecal nitrogen is to multiply nitrogen intake by 1.0 minus approximation 2 (A2, the apparent digestibility of protein; Table 51–12). The average A2 value for the enteral formulas is 0.92 (i.e., 92%). For parenteral feeding, fecal nitrogen loss for patients without intestinal disease is 0.3 to 0.5 g/day.[55]

Integumental nitrogen loss (skin plus miscellaneous) is not clinically measurable, but a reasonable approximation is 7 mg/kg of body weight for men and 8 mg/kg for women.[61,73,74] These values were derived from data from healthy subjects who ingested a formula diet.

To estimate nonprotein nitrogen, body weight and BUN must be measured at the beginning and the end of urine collection. Equation 6, proposed by Harvey et al.,[62] is again used to calculate nonprotein nitrogen changes, which are usually small under clinical conditions.

Nitrogen is rarely measured in body drainage fluids. An estimated value can be acquired by determining the total protein concentration of the fluid (e.g., ascites) and calculating the amount of nitrogen removed.

Nitrogen balance can be calculated in several ways. If urea nitrogen is the only measurable nitrogen loss, then the following equation, which summarizes earlier suggestions, can be used to calculate nitrogen balance:

$$\text{Nitrogen balance (g/day)} = \text{N intake} - [(\text{urea N/A1}) + (1.0 - \text{A2})\ \text{N intake} + (\text{integumental N, nonprotein N, body fluid N})]. \quad (8)$$

The calculations are usually simplified by adding the approximate value for remaining nitrogen losses (A3) to urea nitrogen. For a nitrogen intake of 15 to 16 g per day, A3 is 2.6 to 4.1 g per day (mean 3.1 g per day) for enteral diets.[75] With parenteral feeding, the value is slightly lower, closer to the 2.5 to 3 g observed for elemental diets with free amino acids. This simplified calculation is as follows:

$$\text{Nitrogen balance (g/day)} = \text{N intake} - (\text{urea N} + \text{A3}). \quad (9)$$

Table 51–12 provides average values for A1, A2, and A3 for patients with malabsorption, but because the individual variability in fecal nitrogen losses is so large, a nitrogen balance study in this group should include a measurement of fecal nitrogen for a timed specimen.

## CASE STUDY

A 55-year-old woman with a 3-month history of chemically induced hepatitis was admitted to the hospital. Symptoms on admission included nausea, vomiting, fatigue, and anorexia. She was 67 in. (170 cm) tall and she weighed 104 lb (47.3 kg), which was 78 to 80% of both her usual and ideal weight.

A general diet was prescribed on admission, but a calorie count revealed the patient had poor oral intake. She continued to lose weight, and a nitrogen balance determination, calculated from average protein intake and daily urinary urea nitrogen measurement for 3 days, was negative (−7 g per day).

A polymeric formula that provided 1800 kcal and 61 g of protein per day was infused through a nasojejunal tube. Oral intake provided an additional 400 kcal and 15 g of protein per day. The patient's weight increased to 108 lb (49.1 kg). A repeat 3-day urinary urea nitrogen measurement averaged 7.7 g per day, her BUN value rose from 7 to 9 g/dl during the 3-day period, and her weight increased by 1 lb (0.4 kg). The therapeutic regimen was maintained for the remainder of her hospitalization.

The daily nitrogen balance for this patient was determined as follows:

$$\text{N intake (g)} = \text{dietary protein (g)}/6.25 = 76/6.25 = 12.2$$
$$\text{Urinary N (g)} = \text{urinary urea N (g)/A1} = 7.7/0.85 = 9.1$$
$$\text{Fecal N (g)} = (1.0 - \text{A2})\ \text{N intake} = (0.1)(12.2) = 1.2$$
$$\text{Integumental N (g)} = (\text{body weight at midbalance}) \times 0.0008 = 0.4$$
$$\text{Nonprotein N (g/day)} = [\text{BUN}_f - \text{BUN}_i) \times 0.6 \times \text{BW}_i + (\text{BW}_f - \text{BW}_i) \times \text{BUN}_f]/(\text{day}_f - \text{day}_i = [(0.09 - 0.07) \times 0.6 \times 49.1 + (49.5 - 49.1) \times 0.09]/3 = 0.2$$
$$\text{Body fluid N (g)} = 0.0$$

Thus, nitrogen balance = 12.2 g − 10.9 g = 1.3 g. If the simplified approach (Equation 9) is used, the sum of urea N losses (7.7 g) plus 3.4 g (A3 for a polymeric formula) is subtracted from N intake (12.2 g), and the N balance result is 1.1 g.

Calculated nitrogen balance can be used to estimate accretion of FFM, if constant composition of tissue is assumed, by converting the nitrogen to protein and assuming constant hydration. For example, of the 400 g gained by the patient in 3 days, approximately 24.4 g was protein and 125.1 g was FFM. FFM was calculated by assuming that 19.5% of lean tissue mass is protein. Cellular hydration is variable, however, and this type of analysis should be used for teaching purposes only.

## CLINICAL APPLICATIONS

During the nutritional treatment of severely ill, undernourished patients, a question may arise as to whether energy and nitrogen are adequate for maintenance or for new tissue growth. Several assessment indices are available for this determination, but each is beset with methodologic or interpretational problems similar to those for nitrogen balance. Until more sensitive and specific methods are available, nitrogen balance determination should be included as an assessment index.

Urinary urea nitrogen, under most circumstances, can be used in hospitalized patients to estimate total nitrogen losses. A suggestion is to estimate the patient's balance prior to treatment and thus establish good conditions for carrying out nitrogen balance studies. Measurements during treatment can then be compared to these initial results.[63] Results should be interpreted in the context of other assessment indices and clinical findings. An anabolic level of nitrogen balance is usually considered +2 to 4 g per day. If measurement conditions are optimized and results are conservatively interpreted, nitrogen balance should provide an early index of therapeutic efficacy.

## SERUM BIOCHEMICAL MARKERS

Serum biochemical markers are primarily proteins used in establishing the nutritional status of patients for determining whether they are at risk of complications and in monitoring nutritional treatment. Serum proteins are readily sampled by venipuncture, and, in most cases, measurement is simple and accurate; however, selecting a protein for analysis and proper interpretation of results requires a thorough understanding of three questions:

1. How does the concentration of the selected serum protein correlate with the total body amount and rate of change in the protein?
2. How does the serum protein relate to the amount and rate of change in total body protein?
3. Does an association exist between the serum protein concentration and the patient's outcome?

### SERUM ALBUMIN LEVELS

These three questions will be examined using the classic marker of nutritional status, serum albumin.

**Determinants of Serum Levels.** Review of the first question requires an understanding of the determinants of serum protein concentration. The concentration of albumin in serum is normally determined by three independent factors: (1) the rate of biosynthesis; (2) the volume and characteristics of the distribution space; and (3) the rate of breakdown or catabolism.[2,76,77] Two additional factors in diseased patients are the presence of abnormally large albumin losses and derangements in fluid status.[2,76,77]

Albumin synthesis consumes about 6% of daily nitrogen intake. Hepatocytes within the human liver synthesize albumin at a daily rate of 120 to 270 mg/kg body weight.[76–78] The biosynthetic rate of albumin is determined by dietary protein intake, ambient temperature, and plasma colloidal oncotic pressure near the biosynthetic site.[2] The rate of albumin synthesis is low in the presence of hypothyroidism, excessive levels of serum cortisol, physiologic stress, and hepatic parenchymal disease.[76,77] The rate of albumin synthesis is therefore multifactorial.

Once the albumin molecule is synthesized, it enters the circulation and then distributes in the intravascular and extravascular spaces. The total body albumin pool is normally between 3 and 5 g/kg body weight, and 30 to 40% of this is in the intravascular space.[2] Extravascular albumin is found in all lean tissues and approximately half of the total occurs in skin.[2,76,77] A shift of intravascular to extravascular albumin occurs in patients following surgery or thermal injury.[79,80] The opposite occurs in semistarvation, with a movement of albumin from the extravascular to the intravascular space.[2] The rate of rate albumin transfer between compartments is more rapid in tissues with discontinuous capillaries (e.g., liver, spleen, and gut) compared with organs and tissues that have a continuous capillary network (e.g., skin and skeletal muscle).[76,77,80]

The major catabolic sites of albumin are the intestinal tract and vascular endothelium, and approximately 6 to 10% of the pool is catabolized per day.[17,32] The half-life of albumin ranges between 14 and 20 days, with an equal probability of destruction for new and old molecules. The rate of albumin catabolism is increased by physiologic stress, by hypermetabolism, and by the presence of Cushing's syndrome and some malignant tumors.[2] The rate of albumin catabolism is lowered by semistarvation and hypometabolism. Multiple factors therefore determine albumin distribution and rate of catabolism.

Abnormally large losses of albumin occur in burns, nephrotic syndrome, and protein-losing enteropathy.[79,80] Finally, over- and underhydration cause a reduction and increase in the serum concentration of albumin, respectively.

To summarize these determinants of serum albumin concentration, the measured value of albumin in serum is determined by the rate of synthesis, the volume and nature of the distribution space, the rate of catabolism, the presence of abnormally large losses, and the state of hydration. A summary of albumin metabolism in several common disease states and conditions is provided in Table 51–13. The aim of Table 51–13 is to demonstrate the multiple determinants of albumin metabolism and serum albumin levels in a diversity of clinical conditions; it is not intended to be comprehensive in scope.

**Kinetics in Semistarvation.** How does the concentration of albumin in serum correspond to changes in total body albumin in the presence of uncomplicated protein-energy malnutrition? A general sequence of events can be recreated from animal and human studies.[2,78,80,81] The earliest change in albumin kinetics in response to dietary manipulation is an alteration in the rate of synthesis. With low protein-energy intake, the rate of synthesis falls rapidly and the result is negative albumin balance. If intake remains low, then the catabolic rate of albumin slows, thereby reducing the rate of whole body albumin loss. This tends to preserve serum levels, along with a second major adaptation, a shift of albumin from the extravascular to the intravascular space. These two adaptations preserve serum albumin levels, even though

**TABLE 51–13.** ALBUMIN METABOLISM IN SPECIFIC DISEASE STATES AND CONDITIONS

| DISEASE-CONDITION | COMMENTS |
|---|---|
| Nutritional | |
| Chronic semistarvation with balanced nutrient intake | Unchanged serum albumin level with decreased pool size, extravascular to intravascular albumin shift, and reduced albumin synthesis and breakdown[2,78,81] |
| Inadequate protein intake but adequate or excess intake of total calories | Reduced serum level from decreased albumin synthesis[80] |
| Endocrine | |
| Hypothyroidism | Decreased serum level secondary to reduced synthesis and breakdown with shift to extravascular space[76,77,80] |
| Hyperthyroidism | Unchanged serum level and pool size with both increased synthesis and catabolism[76,77,80] |
| Corticosteroid excess | Pool size unchanged with increased synthesis balanced by increased renal losses[76,77] |
| Carcinoid syndrome | Decreased synthesis from inadequate tryptophan[76,77] |
| Hepatic | |
| Severe liver failure | Decreased serum levels from reduced hepatic synthesis and extravascular losses (e.g., ascites); in some case, acute-phase response contributes to lowering of serum albumin levels[2,76,77] |
| Cirrhosis/chronic hepatitis | In addition to liver failure, possible presence of antialbumin antibodies[76,77] |
| Alcoholic liver disease | Ethanol-induced depression of synthesis and cellular release of albumin[76,77] |
| Gastrointestinal | Ileus and other gastrointestinal lesions possible causes of albumin sequestration in bowel and increased losses from protein-losing enteropathy; impaired amino acid uptake by gastrointestinal mucosa in some conditions[76,77,80] |
| Renal | |
| Chronic renal failure | Maintenance of serum levels if increased losses balanced by extravascular to intravascular shift of albumin[76,77] |
| Glomerular disease | Increased losses from albuminuria |
| Nephrotic syndrome | Increased losses due to albumin catabolism by renal tubular cells and albuminuria. |
| Dialysis (peritoneal) | Albumin losses ~ 8 g/day; increase with peritonitis |
| Uremia | Decreased synthesis secondary to disaggregation of hepatic polysomes |
| Cardiac | |
| Congesitive heart failure | Reduced serum levels from hemodilution; possible contribution of impaired hepatic and renal function[76,77] |
| Malignant Diseases | Tumor and radiation therapy both increase albumin catabolism |
| Thermal injury | Increased losses of extravascular albumin through skin, plus metabolic effects of physiologic stress[76,77] |
| Acute Physiologic Stress | Reduced serum levels with intravascular to extravascular shift of alumbin combined in some cases with lower synthesis and increased breakdown[80,83] |
| Aging | Reduced serum levels observed in subjects older than 70 years; mechanism unknown, but possibly underlying disease or influence of medications[84,85] |

the synthesis rate of albumin is reduced. A reasonable conclusion is that the relative decrease in whole body albumin will be greater than the lowering of serum albumin.

Although the reduction in serum albumin is small in uncomplicated protein-energy malnutrition, severe hypoalbuminemia is observed in association with some forms of malnutrition, and the specific causes of this finding are not entirely clear.[2,17] Explanations include: (1) maintenance of the individual on an intake low in protein but that provides an adequate or even excess amount of nonprotein energy; (2) the presence of other ongoing processes, such as an infection or one of the conditions listed in Table 51–13; (3) depletion of extravascular albumin, indicating severe protein-energy malnutrition; (4) fatty infiltration of the liver, resulting in disturbed hepatocyte function and albumin synthesis; and (5) severe muscle atrophy, leading to depletion of amino acid precursors for albumin synthesis. Whatever the mechanisms, the finding of hypoalbuminemia in children or adults with protein-energy malnutrition usually signals other serious metabolic derangements and an adverse prognosis. The relation of serum albumin levels to prognosis is described in a following section.

**Changes with Physiologic Stress.** Protein-energy malnutrition in hospitalized patients is often complicated by the presence of an injury or infection. During the acute catabolic phase of an injury or infection, the patient usually has a fever, a rise in plasma cortisol, leukocytosis, and a rapid (~7 to 8 hours) increase in synthesis and rise in serum levels of acute-phase reactants such as fibrinogen, haptoglobin, $\alpha_1$-glycoprotein, and C-reactive protein.[80,86] The synthesis and concentration of other serum proteins, including albumin, prealbumin, and transferrin, decrease. Interleukin-1 $\alpha$ and $\beta$, tumor necrosis factor/cachectin, and interleukin-6, which are synthesized by monocytic and phagocytic cells lining the hepatic and splenic vascular endothelium, are the major classes of monokines that regulate acute-phase protein synthesis following severe injury or elective surgery.[87–89] Counterregulatory hormones, including glucagon, epinephrine, and cortisol, also mediate the overall injury response and influence substrate availability and whole body protein metabolism.[90] The rise in acute-phase proteins is proportional to the severity of tissue injury in elective surgical and trauma patients.[80,86,91]

The hypoalbuminemia of injury, mediated by monokines and counterregulatory hormones, is caused by several independent mechanisms: a reduction in albumin synthesis secondary to anorexia with a decrease in dietary amino acid precursors; a reduction in albumin synthesis caused by direct downregulation of albumin gene expression and translation;[92] a rise in albumin catabolism;[79,83] and an increase in microvascular permeability and extravascular sequestration of albumin.[79,80,93] When semistarvation is combined with injury, the usual adaptive movement of albumin into the intravascular compartment is reversed; vascular permeability is increased, albumin is transferred into the extravascular space, and serum levels are not maintained as they are in the absence of physiologic stress.

The changes in albumin metabolism persist throughout the acute phase of an injury or catabolic illness. Serum albumin concentration thus remains low during the stress period, even when seemingly adequate levels of nutritional support are provided. The nadir in serum albumin levels is usually reached about 5 to 7 days following moderate trauma,[80,94] and the reduction in serum albumin concentration is about 0.5 g/dl following elective surgery.[76]

The serum level of albumin is therefore a poor index to the rate of albumin synthesis, whole body albumin mass, albumin balance, total body protein mass, and whole body nitrogen balance during the acute phase of a catabolic illness.[80,95] Serum levels of acute-phase proteins (e.g., C-reactive protein) can be used to establish the presence of physiologic stress and thus give insight into the validity of albumin and other serum proteins (Table 51–13) as nutritional markers.[80]

**Relation to Total Body Protein.** The second question is how does serum albumin relate to other proteins within FFM? Several studies show a strong correlation between serum albumin and body cell mass, and limited information suggests that relative changes in serum albumin and total body protein are about equal;[96] however, striking deviations from these generalizations occur. For example, a patient with anorexia nervosa may show severe muscle and liver atrophy, and yet serum albumin levels may be normal or near normal.[2] As indicated in the previous section, serum albumin levels following an acute injury or catabolic illness are largely independent of the amount and rate of change in total body albumin and protein mass.

**Relation to Outcome.** Is there an association between serum levels of albumin and the patient's outcome? Numerous studies spanning two decades link low serum levels of albumin with an increase in morbidity and mortality.[2,95] An example is the recent study of Hermann and colleagues in which 15,511 consecutive patients over the age of 40 years had serum albumin levels measured within 48 hours of hospital admission.[97] Normal serum albumin levels were defined by the investigators as $\geqq$3.4 g/dl, and hypoalbuminemia was present in 21% of the sample. Hermann and colleagues found that patients with hypoalbuminemia on admission stayed in the hospital longer, had an increased risk of dying during hospitalization, and were more likely to be readmitted than patients with normal serum albumin levels. All these differences in outcome were statistically significant when compared to findings in patients with normal levels of serum albumin. For example, mortality was 14% among the 3241 hypoalbuminemic patients and 4% among the 12,270 patients with normal serum albumin levels ($p < 0.0001$).

In another recent study, Hirsch and colleagues found that serum albumin levels were significantly ($p < 0.05$) higher in patients who survived complications following elective gastrointestinal surgery than in those with complications who did not survive.[98] The prognostic value of serum albumin levels extends beyond that of diseases or conditions observed within an acute-care setting. Phillips and colleagues prospectively studied 7735 British men as part of a regional heart study.[99] These investigators observed a marked increase in mortality rate with decreasing serum albumin levels, even following adjustments for age, cigarette smoking, social class, and other biochemical or functional indices.

Many mechanisms have been proposed to explain the association between serum albumin levels and the patient's outcome. A brief listing includes the following: inadequate protein intake with its associated functional consequences;[95,100] an acute-phase response of albumin in proportion to injury or disease severity;[80,91,95] a correlation between low serum albumin levels and poor wound healing[15,95] and impaired function of the immune system[15,95,96] and other organs and tissues;[15] and a link between serum albumin levels and other physiologic processes related to outcome such as drug or free-fatty acid binding by albumin,[101] suppression of inflammatory mediators from activated or damaged cells by albumin,[80] antioxidant capacity of albumin,[102,103] effects of albumin on platelet reactivity,[104] and influence of albumin on siderophore-mediated iron acquisition and malignant transformation.[102,103]

**Clinical Applications.** Serum albumin as a prognostic marker in many conditions is thus firmly established, but is it reasonable to also consider albumin a nutritional marker? This central and controversial question is best examined with the use of a diagram that integrates the complex interrelations among protein-energy malnutrition, clinical conditions, organ and tissue function, clinical outcome, and albumin metabolism (Fig. 51–12). Figure 51–12 shows that three interrelated processes may be present in an individual patient: protein-energy malnutrition, physiologic stress, and one or more of the conditions listed in Table 51–13 that directly influence albumin metabolism. These three processes in combination, mediated through effects on albumin synthesis, catabolism, distribution, abnormal losses, and hydration, all influence serum albumin levels. Acting through direct and indirect pathophysiologic effects, these three processes also affect organ/tissue function, immunocompetence, and body composition. Additionally, serum levels of albumin have direct functional effects on drug binding, platelet aggregability, and other processes. Serum albumin levels are thus multidetermined and relate both directly and indirectly to physiologic function, body composition, and, ultimately, to clinical outcome (Fig. 51–12). These complex but highly associated interrelations clearly show why low serum albumin levels are so closely linked with a patient's morbidity and mortality.

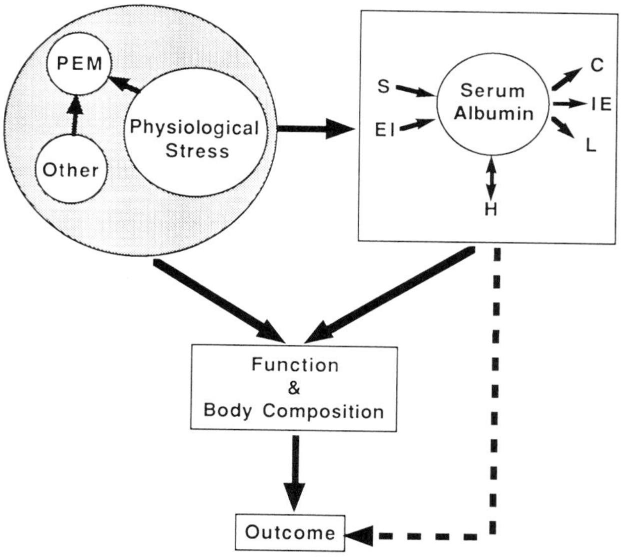
PEM
Other
Physiological Stress
S
EI
Serum Albumin
C
IE
L
H
Function & Body Composition
Outcome

**FIGURE 51–12.** The relationships among serum albumin levels, clinical conditions, body composition and various physiologic functions, and the patient's outcome. The dashed line represents the indirect link between serum albumin levels and clinical outcome. C, Rate of albumin catabolism; EI, rate of extravascular to intravascular transfer of albumin; H, changes in intravascular hydration; IE, rate of intravascular to extravascular transfer of albumin; L, rate of abnormal albumin losses; PEM, protein-energy malnutrition; S, rate of albumin synthesis.

On the other hand, it is clear that serum albumin levels are not solely determined by nutritional status, and therefore serum albumin levels do not, under most clinical circumstances, represent the direct effects of protein-energy malnutrition on the functional status of organs and tissues and on a patient's prognosis. Albumin and other similar serum proteins are valid nutritional markers only in the absence of clinical factors that influence nonacute-phase protein synthesis by the liver.

What role should we therefore assign to serum albumin in nutritional assessment? According to Bistrian, hypoalbuminemia is a reliable indicator of patients who are at increased risk and who are thus most likely to benefit from intensive nutritional evaluation and treatment.[105] Monitoring serum albumin levels during hospitalization might also provide an overall index of the patient's nutritional status, disease, hydration status, and potential for recovery. We emphasize, however, that serum levels of albumin and other similar proteins synthesized and exported by the liver cannot be used in hospitalized patients as discrete markers of protein nutriture unless other clinical factors that influence metabolism and serum levels are absent.

**Role in Classification of Protein-Energy Malnutrition.** Few concepts are more confusing to the practitioner than classification of different forms of protein-energy malnutrition in hospitalized patients. Early investigators, with minimal knowledge of underlying mechanisms, described two forms of protein-energy malnutrition, marasmus and kwashiorkor. These syndromes, which occur mainly in childhood, are amply described in Chapter 57. Severe depletion of fat and fat-free tissues, a small relative increase in extracellular fluid, a low energy expenditure, and normal or slightly reduced levels of serum albumin are characteristic of the marasmic form of protein-energy malnutrition. In contrast, in kwashiorkor fat stores are usually preserved whereas fat-free tissues are depleted, a large relative increase in extracellular fluid occurs, hypermetabolism may be present, fatty infiltration of the liver and hypoalbuminemia are severe, and functional derangements, such as immunoincompetence, are evident. Early descriptions of malnourished hospitalized patients often reported patients as suffering from "marasmus" or "kwashiorkor" because their laboratory and clinical findings resembled those reported in children from developing nations who had protein-energy malnutrition. Some investigators continue to use the terms marasmus and kwashiorkor to describe malnourished hospitalized patients, particularly those with normal or subnormal serum albumin levels, respectively. A more recent trend is to classify patients as malnourished with or without hypoalbuminemia. The criteria for diagnosing malnutrition are often unclear, however.

An example of the inappropriate use of serum albumin in nutritional assessment and diagnosis is the study of McClave and colleagues.[100] The investigators studied 180 patients receiving total parenteral nutrition and selected a subgroup of 68 with "hypoalbuminemic protein-calorie malnutrition" based on low levels of 3 "visceral proteins," including serum albumin. The patients with hypoalbuminemic malnutrition were found to have longer hospitalizations and generally poorer outcome measures than observed in the remaining patients. A criticism of this study is that serum albumin levels, and those of the other proteins analyzed, reflect mainly physiologic stress and other related pathologic processes (Table 51–13) and would therefore predictably correlate with outcome (dashed line in Fig. 51–12). The use of serum levels of albumin and other similar serum proteins in this context gives little information on protein-energy nutriture, and additional information would be required to establish a clear diagnosis of "protein-energy malnutrition."

A priority, which is beyond the scope of this chapter, is to clearly establish definitions, diagnostic criteria, and appropriate treatment for the different types of protein-energy malnutrition observed in hospitalized patients.

## OTHER BIOCHEMICAL MARKERS

The nonspecific and slow response of serum albumin levels to nutritional factors has led to the investigation of other serum proteins. In general, relative to albumin, these proteins have lower absolute biosynthetic rates, smaller total body pools, shorter half-lives, and lower serum levels. The key aspects of each of these proteins are summarized in Table 51–14. Under ideal conditions, these proteins are more sensitive indices of dietary protein and energy intake than serum albumin.[95] Synthesis rates and plasma levels change rapidly in response to dietary intake. For example, in a malnourished patient serum levels of albumin, transferrin, and prealbumin may normalize with appropriate nutrition support in 20 to 30 days, 7 days, and 3 days, respectively. The serum concentration of these proteins also responds to many of the same non-nutritional factors described earlier for albumin.[80] Interpretation must therefore be cautious.

In conclusion, anthropometry, nitrogen balance, and serum biochemical markers each have specific applications in the nutritional assessment of patients with acute or chronic illnesses. Their use should be integrated with the clinical, dietary, functional, and immunologic components of nutritional assessment described in other chapters. Taken collectively, these methods allow for a comprehensive analysis of each patient's nutritional status.

**TABLE 51–14.** SERUM PROTEINS USED IN NUTRITIONAL ASSESSMENT

| SERUM PROTEIN | APPROXIMATE MOLECULAR WEIGHT (DALTONS) | BIOSYNTHETIC SITE | NORMAL VALUE $\bar{x} \pm$ SD OR (RANGE)† | HALF-LIFE | FUNCTION | COMMENTS* |
|---|---|---|---|---|---|---|
| Albumin | 66,460 | Hepatocyte | 45 (35–50) | 18–20 days | Maintains plasma oncotic pressure; carrier for small molecules | Serum levels are determined by the processes described in the text |
| Transferrin | 79,550 | Hepatocyte | 2.3 (2.6–4.3) | 8–9 days | Binds $Fe^{++}$ in plasma and transports to bone marrow | Iron deficiency increases hepatic synthesis and plasma levels; increases during pregnancy, during estrogen therapy, and acute hepatitis; reduced in protein-losing enteropathy and nephropathy, chronic infections, uremia, and acute catabolic states; often measured indirectly by total iron-binding capacity; equations for indirect prediction should be developed locally |
| Prealbumin | 54,980 | Hepatocyte | 0.30 (0.2–0.4) | 2–3 days | Binds T3 and to a lesser extent T4; carrier for retinol-binding protein | Increased in patients with chronic renal failure on dialysis due to decreased renal catabolism; reduced in acute catabolic states, after surgery, in hyperthyroidism, in protein-losing enteropathy; increased in some cases of nephrotic syndrome; serum level determined by overall energy balance as well as nitrogen balance |
| Retinol-binding protein (RBP) | 20,960 | Hepatocyte | 0.372 ± 0.0073‡ | 12 hours | Transports vitamin A in plasma; binds noncovalently to prealbumin | Catabolized in renal proximal tubular cell; with renal disease RBP increases and half-life is prolonged; low in vitamin A deficiency, acute catabolic states, after surgery, and in hyperthyroidism |
| Insulin-like growth factor-1 (IGF-1) | 7,400 | Hepatocyte | 0.83 IU/ml (0.55–1.4) | 2–6 hours | One of a family of insulin-like peptides that have anabolic actions on fat, muscle, cartilage, and cultured cells | Referred to earlier as somatomedin-C; levels fall rapidly with fasting and quickly recover during refeeding; low values in hypothyroid patients, with estrogen administration, and possibly in obesity; may be a valid nutritional marker during acute-phase response |
| Fibronectin | 440,000 | Hepatocyte and other tissues | Plasma: 2.92 ± 0.2 Serum: 1.82 ± 0.16 | 4–24 hours | A glycoprotein found in many tissues; a soluble form appears in blood and behaves as an opsonic glycoprotein; may exert chemotactic activity and be involved in wound healing | Plasma fibronectin deficiency may contribute to host defense suppression with malnutrition; may be a sensitive marker during nutritional depletion and repletion; levels may be influenced by acute-phase response; more clinical studies needed; reference ranges not well studied |

*All the listed proteins are influenced by hydration and the presence of hepatocellular dysfunction.
†Units are gl/L. Normal range varies among centers; check local values.
‡Normal values are age and sex dependent. Table value is for pooled subjects.

## REFERENCES


1. Heymsfield, S.B., Bethel, R.A., Ansley, J.D., et al.: Ann. Intern. Med., *90*:63–71, 1979.
2. Heymsfield, S.B., Williams, P.J.: Nutritional assessment by clinical and biochemical methods. *In* Modern Nutrition in Health and Disease. 7th Ed. Edited by M.E. Shils and V.R. Young. Philadelphia, Lea & Febiger, 1988, pp. 817–860.
3. Bistrian, B.R., Blackburn, G.L., Vitale J., et al.: JAMA, *235*:1567–1570, 1976.
4. Bistrian, B.R., Blackburn, G.L., Hallowell, E.: JAMA, *230*:858, 1974.
5. Munro, H.N., Crim, M.C.: The proteins and amino acids. *In* Modern Nutrition in Health and Disease. 7th Ed. Edited by M.E. Shils and V.R. Young. Philadelphia, Lea & Febiger, 1988 pp. 1–37.
6. Garrow, J.S.: Their Composition, Measurement and Control: Energy Balance and Obesity in Man. Amsterdam, North Holland, 1974.
7. Heymsfield, S.B., McManus, C., Smith, J.: Am. J. Clin. Nutr., *35*:1192–1199, 1982.
8. Lehninger, A.L.: Organ interrelationships in the metabolism of mammals. *In* Biochemistry. 2nd Ed. Edited by A.L. Lehninger. New York, Worth, 1975, pp. 829–852.
9. Wang, Z.M., Pierson, R.N., Heymsfield, S.B.: Am. J. Clin. Nutr., *56*:19–28, 1992.
10. International Commission on Radiologic Protection: Report of the Task Group on Reference Man: Adopted by the Commission in October. New York, Pergamon, 1974.
11. Heymsfield, S.B., Stevens, V., Noel, R.: Am. J. Clin. Nutr., *36*:131–142, 1982.
12. Webster, J.D., Hesp, R., Garrow, J.S.: Human Nutr: Clin. Nutr., *38*:299–306, 1984.
13. Forbes, G.B.: Nutr. Rev., *45*:225–231, 1987.
14. Heymsfield, S.B., Casper, K., Funfar, J.: Am. J. Cardiol., *60*:75G–81G, 1987.
15. Hill, G.J.: JPEN J. Parenter. Enteral. Nutr., *16*:197–218, 1992.
16. Klidjian, A.M., Foster, K.J., Kammerling, R.M.: Br. Med. J., *281*:899–901, 1980.
17. Richer, P.: Nouv. Inconogr. Salpetriere, *3*:20–26, 1890.
18. Metiegka, J.: Am. J. Phys. Anthropol., *3*:223–230, 1921.
19. Lohman, T.G., Roche, A.F., Martorell, R. (Eds.): Anthropometric Standardization Reference Manual. Champaign, IL, Human Kinetics Books, 1988.
20. Himes, J.H. (Ed.): Anthropometric Assessment of Nutritional Status. New York, Wiley-Liss, 1991.
21. Heymsfield, S.B., Waki, M., Kehayias, J., et al.: Am. J. Physiol., *261*:E190–E198, 1991.
22. Ellis, K.J., Yasumura, S., Vartsky, D., et al.: J. Lab. Clin. Med., *99*:917, 1982.
23. Heymsfield, S.B., Waki, M.: Nutr. Rev., *49*:97–108, 1991.
24. Merrill, A.L., Watt, B.K.: Energy Value of Foods. Washington, D.C., United States Government Printing Office, 1973.
25. Heymsfield, S.B., Casper, K.: JPEN J. Parenter. Enteral Nutr., *11*:36S–41S, 1987.
26. Ravussin, E., Bogardus, C.: Am. J. Clin. Nutr., *49*:968–975, 1989.
27. Durnin, J.V.G.A., Womersley, J.: Br. J. Nutr., *32*:77–97, 1974.
28. Moore, F.D., Olesen, K.H., McMurray, J.D., et al.: The Body Cell Mass and Its Supporting Environment. Philadelphia, W.B. Saunders, 1963.
29. Burmeister, W., Bingert, A.: Klin. Wochenschr., *45*:409–416, 1967.
30. Kissebah, A.H., Freedman, D.S., Peiris, A.N.: Med. Clin. North Am., *73*:111–138, 1989.
31. Heymsfield, S.B., McManus, C.B., III, Seitz, S.B., et al.: Anthropometric assessment of adult protein-energy malnutrition. *In* Nutritional Assessment. Edited by R.A. Wright and S. Heymsfield. Boston, Blackwell Scientific Publications, 1984, pp. 27–82.
32. Heymsfield, S.B., McManus, C.B.: Cancer, *55*:238–243, 1985.
33. Sjöström, L.: Int. J. Obes., *15*:19–30, 1991.
34. Martin, A.D., Spenst, L.F., Drinkwater, D.T., et al.: Med. Sci. Sports Exerc., *22*:729–733, 1990.
35. Studley, H.O.: JAMA, *106*:458–460, 1936.
36. Nixon, D.W., Heymsfield, S.B., Cohen, A.B., et al.: Am. J. Med., *68*:683–690, 1980.
37. Vandenbergh, E., Van de Woestijne, K.P., Gyselen, A.: Am. Rev. Respir. Dis., *195*:556–566, 1967.
38. Seltzer, M.H., Slocum, B.A., Cataldi-Betcher, M.L.: JPEN J. Parenter. Enteral Nutr., *6*:218, 1982.
39. Windsor, J.A., Hill, G.: Ann. Surg., *207*:290–296, 1988.
40. Chumlea, W.C., Roche, A.F., Steinbaugh, M.L.: Anthropometric approaches to the nutritional assessment of the elderly. *In* Nutrition, Aging, and the Elderly. Edited by H.N. Munro and D.E. Danford. New York, Plenum, 1989, pp. 335–361.
41. Damon, A., Goldman, R.F.: Hum. Biol., *36*:32–44, 1964.
42. VanItallie, T.B., Yang, M.-U., Heymsfield S.B., et al.: Am. J. Clin. Nutr., *52*:953–959, 1990.
43. Keys, A., Brozek, J., Henschel, A., et al.: The Biology of Human Starvation. Vols. I and II. Minneapolis, University of Minnesota Press, 1950.
44. Cunningham, J.J.: Am. J. Clin. Nutr., *54*:963–969, 1991.
45. Forbes, G.B., Brown, M.R., Griffiths, H.J.L.: Am. J. Clin. Nutr., *47*:929–931, 1988.
46. Baumgartner, R.N., Rhyne, R.L., Garry, P.J., et al.: J. Nutr. In press.
47. Cole, T.J.: Weight–stature indices to measure underweight, overweight, and obesity. *In* Anthropometric Assessment of Nutritional Status. Edited by J.H. Himes. New York, Wiley-Liss, 1991.
48. Garn, S.M., Leonard, W.R., Hawthorne, V.M.: Am. J. Clin. Nutr., *44*:996–997, 1986.
49. James, W.P.T., Ferro-Luzzi, A., Waterlow, J.C.: Eur. J. Clin. Nutr., *42*:969–981, 1988.
50. Smalley, K.J., Knerr, A.K., Kendrick, Z.V., et al.: Am. J. Clin. Nutr., *52*:405, 1990.
51. McLaren, D.S.: A fresh look at anthropometric classification schemes in protein-energy malnutrition. *In* Anthropometric Assessment of Nutritional Status. Edited by J.H. Himes. New York, Wiley-Liss, 1991, pp. 273–286.
52. Galen, R.S., Gambino, S.R.: Beyond Normality: The Predictive Value and Efficiency of Medical Diagnoses. New York, John Wiley & Sons, 1975.
53. Jeejeebhoy, K.N., Detsky, A.S., Baker, J.P.: JPEN J. Parenter. Enteral Nutr., *14*:193S–196S, 1990.
54. Forbes, G.: Human Body Composition: Growth, Aging, Nutrition, and Activity. New York, Springer-Verlag, 1987.
55. Heymsfield, S.B., Tochilin, N., McManus, C.B., et al.: Clin. Consultations Nutr. Support, *4*:6–10, 1984.

56. Grimble, G.K., West, M.F.B., Acuti, A.B.C., et al.: JPEN J. Parenter. Enteral Nutr., *12:*100–106, 1988.
57. Lentner, C. (Ed.): Geigy Scientific Tables. Vol. 1. Basel, Ciba-Geigy, 1981, p. 63.
58. Walser, M.: Urea metabolism: regulation and sources of nitrogen. In: Amino Acids Metabolism and Medical Applications. Edited by G.L. Blackburn, G.P. Grant, and V.R. Young. Boston, John Wright-PSG, 1983.
59. Allison, J.B., Bird, JWC.: Elimination of nitrogen from the body. *In* Mammalian Protein Metabolism. Vol. I. Edited by H.N. Munro and J.B. Allison. Chicago, American Medical Association, 1977, pp. 141–146.
60. Cheng, A.H.R., Gomez, A., Bergan, J.G., et al.: Am. J. Clin. Nutr., *31:*12–22, 1978.
61. Calloway, D.H., Odell, A.C.F., Margen, S.: J. Nutr., *101:*775–786, 1971.
62. Harvey, K.B., Blumenkrantz, M.J., Levine, S.E., et al.: Am. J. Clin. Nutr., *33:*1586–1597, 1980.
63. Kopple, J.D.: JPEN J. Parenter. Enteral Nutr., *11:*79S–85S, 1987.
64. Hegsted, D.M.: J. Nutr., *106:*307–311, 1976.
65. Wallace, W.M.: Fed. Proc., *18:*1125–1130, 1959.
66. Forbes, G.B.: Nutr. Rev., *31:*297–300, 1973.
67. Kurzer, M.S.: Am. J. Clin. Nutr., *34:*1305–1313, 1981.
68. Rand, W.M., Scrimshaw, N.S., Young, V.R.: Conventional ("long-term") nitrogen balance studies for protein quality evaluation in adults: rationale and limitations. *In* Protein Quality in Humans: Assessment and in vitro Estimation. Edited by C.E. Bodwel, J.S. Adkins, and D.T. Hopkins. Westport, CT, AVI, 1981.
69. Candio, J.A., Hoffman, M.J., et al.: JPEN J. Parenter. Enteral Nutr., *15:*148–151, 1991.
70. Eckfeldt, J., Levine, A.S., Geiner, C., et al.: Clin. Chem., *28:*1500–1502, 1982.
71. Konstantinides, F.N., Konstantinides, N.N., et al.: JPEN J. Parenter. Enteral Nutr., *15:*189–193, 1991.
72. Flatt, J.P., Blackburn, G.L., Bistrian, B.R.: JPEN J. Parenter. Enteral Nutr., *16:*191–192, 1992.
73. Calloway, D.H., Margen, S.: J. Nutr., *101:*205–216, 1971.
74. Munro, H.N., Crim, M.: The proteins and amino acids. *In* Modern Nutrition in Health and Disease. 6th Ed. Edited by R.S. Goodhart and M.E. Shils. Philadelphia, Lea & Febiger, 1980, pp. 51–98.
75. Mackenzie, T.A., Blackburn, G.L., Flatt, J.P.: Fed. Proc., *33:*683, 1974.
76. Doweiko, J.P., Nompleggi, D.J.: JPEN J. Parenter. Enteral Nutr., *15:*476–483, 1991.
77. Doweiko, J.P., Nompleggi, D.J.: JPEN J. Parenter. Enteral Nutr., *15:*207–211, 1991.
78. James, W.P., Hay, A.M.: J. Clin. Invest., *47:*1958–1972, 1968.
79. Fleck, A., Raines, G., Hawker, F., et al.: Lancet, *1:*781–784, 1985.
80. Fleck, A., Path, F.R.C.: Nutrition, *4:*109–117, 1988.
81. Moore, F.D., Langohr, J.L., Ingebretson, M., et al.: Ann. Surg., *132:*1–19, 1950.
82. Soeters, P.B., Von Meyenfeldt, M.F., Meijerink, W.J.H., et al.: Lancet, *335:*348, 1990.
83. Dahn, M.S., Jacobs, L.A., Smith, S., et al.: Am. Surg., *6:*340–343, 1985.
84. Cooper, J.K., Gardner, C.: J. Am. Geriatr. Soc., *37:*1039–1042, 1989.
85. Greenblatt, D.J.: J. Am. Geriatr. Soc., *125:*20–22, 1979.
86. Stahl, W.M.: Crit. Care Med., *15:*545–550, 1987.
87. Pomposelli, J.J., Flores, E.A., Bistrian, B.R.: JPEN J. Parenter. Enteral Nutr., *12:*212–218, 1988.
88. Grimble, R.: Lancet, *335:*350, 1990.
89. Moldawer, L.L.: Nutrition, *4:*176–177, 1988.
90. Watters, J.M., Bessey, P.Q., Dinarello, C.A., et al.: Arch. Surg., *121:*179–190, 1986.
91. Boosalis, M.G., Ott, L., Levine, A.S., et al.: Crit. Care Med., *17:*741–747, 1989.
92. Perlmutter, D.H., Dinarello, C.A., Punsal, P.I., et al.: J. Clin. Invest., *78:*1349–1354, 1986.
93. Gosling, P., Beevers, D.G., Goode, G.E., et al.: Lancet, *335:*349–350, 1990.
94. Peterson, V.M., Moore, E.E., Jones, T.N., et al.: Surgery, *104:*199–207, 1988.
95. McMahon, M.M., Bistrian, B.: Dis. Mon., *36:*372–417, 1990.
96. Forse, R.A., Shizgal, H.M.: JPEN J. Parenter. Enteral Nutr., *4:*450–454, 1980.
97. Herrmann, F.R., Safran, C., Levkoff, S.E., et al.: Arch. Intern. Med., *152:*125–130, 1992.
98. Hirsch, S., Obaldia, N.D., Petermann, M., et al.: J. Am. Coll. Nutr., *11:*21–24, 1992.
99. Phillips, A., Shaper, A.G., Whincup, P.H.: Lancet, *2:*1434–1436, 1989.
100. McClave, S.A., Mitoraj, T.E., Thielmeier, K.A., et al.: JPEN J. Parenter. Enteral Nutr., *16:*337–342, 1992.
101. Williams, W.R., Pawlowicz, A., Davies, B.: Lancet, *335:*348–349, 1990.
102. Stevens, R.G.: Med. Oncol. Tumor Pharmacother., *7:*177–181, 1990.
103. Stevens, R.G., Blumberg, B.S.: Lancet, *335:*351, 1990.
104. Lorgeril, M.D., Guidollet, J., Renaud, S.: Lancet, *335:*339, 1990.
105. Bistrian, B.R.: Nutrition, *4:*175, 1988.

Partial support for the studies described in this chapter was provided by National Institutes of Health Grant P01-DK42818.

CHAPTER 52

# Dietary Assessment

Johanna T. Dwyer



Dietary assessment began in ancient times, but only in the twentieth century has it been possible to link it to nutrient intakes.[1,2] A major breakthrough in the early 1980s was the development of semiquantitative food frequency questionnaires derived from population-based dietary surveys. Their availability in a form that could be analyzed readily with computerized dietary analysis software made it possible to include dietary assessment in many studies.[3,4] Other developments include software programs available on microcomputers that permit direct data entry during interviews, and the availability of more complete computerized nutrient data bases and of rapid automated data processing techniques for analyzing dietary data.[5] Progress in our knowledge of food composition[6–9] and the advent of biochemical measures permitting partial validation of dietary methods with objective techniques has been good.[10] Finally, greater understanding of the statistical considerations involved in dietary assessment and in the interpretation of the health implications of findings have advanced the field.[11–13]

Dietary assessment and dietary status are important parts of the larger picture of characteristics that, taken together, describe the relationships between diet, health, and disease. This chapter aims to help readers make appropriate choices of dietary methods for their purposes.

## BASIC QUESTIONS TO ANSWER WHEN SELECTING A DIETARY ASSESSMENT METHOD

**Why Is the Study Being Done?** The purpose of the study must be determined because it influences the type of data that must be collected, the number of observations necessary, and the best methods to use. Some of the common reasons include screening assessment and evaluation of food and nutritional status, food safety and quality studies, and national food and nutrition planning. Excellent references are available to help guide choices for specific applications.[4,10,12,14–20]

**What Is Being Assessed?** The characteristics of interest may include nutrients or other food constituents, foods, food groups, dietary patterns, and characteristics. Table 52–1 ranks these in descending order according to the complexity of the methods that are required for their collection and analysis. If the focus is on nutrient intakes or other constituents that are widely dispersed in the food supply, information on the entire diet is usually needed. Information on total diet is also important because the absorption, use, and health effects of single

**TABLE 52–1.** TYPES OF DIETARY INFORMATION OF INTEREST

| FOCUS OF STUDY | TYPE OF INFORMATION NEEDED |
|---|---|
| Entire diet | Single or many nutrients or food constituents |
| | Interrelationships between these |
| Foods | Intake frequency of a single food or foods |
| | Form of food (such as retentiveness of sugar-containing foods in studies of dental caries) |
| | Type of food (animal, plant) |
| | Cooking or preparation method |
| | Food diversity |
| | Source of foods (feeding or meal program) |
| Food groups | Intake frequency of food groups |
| | Conformity with a good guidance system |
| Basic four food groups | Basic food exchange lists or some other food guidance system |
| Dietary patterns and characteristics | Typical meals |
| | Meal frequency |
| | Temporal patterns (time of mealing, snacking, drinking, breakfast eating) |
| | Location of eating (home or away from home) |
| | Use of vitamin-mineral supplements |
| | Other patterns (binging, spells of illness, fasting, dieting) |
| | Conformance with some recommended pattern (introduction of solids or weaning) |
| | Source of meals |
| | Associations of consumption with some other characteristic (such as mood or time in menstrual cycle) |
| | Type of feeding (breast, mixed, bottle) |

nutrients are frequently influenced by others. Also, intakes of many rather than a single nutrient are needed for most clinical and epidemiologic nutritional purposes.

Collection of data focused mainly on food frequencies or food groups is somewhat less time-consuming and complex to analyze, and may also be useful for some purposes, such as screening.[22] However, if food groups are used for assessing nutrient intakes, additional assumptions must be made that may limit their accuracy.

Most dietary studies include some additional information on food consumption patterns or dietary characteristics that are helpful for descriptive purposes, even if they are not necessary for the major purpose of the analysis. For specific purposes, combinations of information may be needed.[23,24]

**Who Is the Target Group?** The target group selected is important for three reasons: capabilities that influence choice of most appropriate assessment methods, generalizability of results, and period of observation likely to be necessary. Table 52–2 provides details on respondent characteristics that impose limitations on the choice of methods. Population sampling techniques must be employed if subjects are to be representative of a larger population. The target group's characteristics also influence how long the group must be studied.

**What Time Frame Is Important?** The purpose of dietary assessment is to provide a picture of intakes, usually typical intakes, because for most nutritional purposes, only these are likely to have significance. If only a day's intakes are needed, the task is greatly simplified.

**What Is the Focus of Analysis?** Table 52–3 describes the appropriate focus of analysis for several common types of studies. Methods differ in their validity and reliability for assessing individual intakes.[16,70] If the focus of analysis is individuals, more observations are usually needed than if the focus is on groups.[71] Statistical methods for analysis of dietary data have been well described.[72–76]

**How Great Is Respondent Burden?** Time involved varies from a few minutes to several hours, depending on the method chosen. Psychological burdens include the added work of remembering or recording food intake and the reporting of intakes that may be of a sensitive nature. Respondent burdens must be appropriate, and trade-offs often must be made between the investigator's desire to collect information that could conceivably be of interest and respondents' willingness to give it.

**What Are the Costs?** Objectives and costs entailed must be matched to resources before the study begins if it is to be successfully concluded. Some costs are immediately apparent, such as the need for forms and food models, and the time of the respondent and interviewer. There are also hidden costs such as the considerable amounts of

**TABLE 52–2.** IMPORTANT CONSIDERATIONS IN CHOOSING DIETARY ASSESSMENT METHODS IN PARTICULAR TARGET GROUPS

| TARGET GROUP AND REFERENCES | SPECIAL PROBLEMS |
|---|---|
| Pregnant women[25–30] | Intakes change over the course of pregnancy, so usual intakes must be assessed at specific points in time during pregnancy<br>Distortion of intakes owing to fear of noncompliance may be an issue<br>Intakes of certain substances such as alcohol and supplements may be of particular concern |
| Lactating women[31–33] | Maternal intakes and breast-feeding practices vary over the course of lactation and by individual<br>Maternal intakes are affected by extent to which infant is breast-feeding<br>Infant intakes may be supplemented with nutrients or foods<br>Composition of breast milk varies |
| Infants[34–37] | Intakes of breast milk must be assessed using special techniques such as test weighing or indirect estimates from doubly-labeled water studies<br>Mixed feedings (breast and other food) complicate assessment<br>Surrogate respondents must be used<br>Eating patterns and intakes vary greatly from month to month, hampering retrospective reporting methods<br>Special foods (formulas, baby and weaning foods) and portions commonly used must be included in food tables |
| Preschool children[38–45] | Surrogate respondents must be used (often several, because no one person is aware of child's entire intake)<br>Intakes vary greatly from day to day |
| School children [46–56] | Recall is limited; surrogate respondents or records may be needed to supplement recall<br>Literacy may be limited<br>Vocabulary and ability to describe foods may be limited<br>Reports may be of what was served, or what parent believes should have been provided, not what was eaten<br>Children have limited attention spans<br>Intakes may differ greatly between school days and other days |
| Adolescents[57–61] | Intakes change rapidly, especially during pubertal growth spurt, and may be more highly associated with physical maturation than age<br>Unusual patterns, including frequent meal skipping, snacks at unusual times of day, dieting fasting, bulimia, self-induced vomiting, laxative abuse, and sports training regimes may be present and not immediately apparent<br>Recall of food habits in childhood of interest may be unknown (e.g., duration of breast-feeding, weaning patterns) |
| Elderly[62–67] | Recall may be limited<br>Disabilities in hearing, sight, or attention may complicate assessment<br>Intakes may vary greatly from day to day if chronic illnesses affecting food intake are present |
| Illiterate individuals | Methods using printed information, instructions, or records cannot be used |
| The ill[20] | Reporting may be biased because of fears that noncompliance will be punished<br>Intakes may vary greatly from day to day with exacerbations in illness<br>Recall may be distorted by disease or by recollection of "usual" diet when well<br>Ability to pay attention, read, write, or hear may be affected by illness<br>"Net" intake may be affected by such conditions as fasting, vomiting, and diarrhea<br>Special dietary supplements or foods may be consumed in large amounts |
| Groups with unusual life styles[68,69] | "Usual" intakes may be difficult to describe; athletes and dancers may have special regimens while training or during competition or performance |

time needed for developing protocols, interview training, checking, coding, calculating and interpreting intakes. These are usually much greater than one imagines.[77]

**What Other Constraints Are Present?** Other constraints that need to be taken into account in choosing an assessment method include the skill and training of the interviewers in dietary assessment techniques, limitations imposed by the setting in which the interviews are being done, and the time and facilities available for analyzing the data.[14,78]

**How Accurately Must the Characteristic Be Measured?** Differences between actual and measured diets in assessment studies are influenced by representativeness and the many factors that affect the accuracy of measure-

**TABLE 52–3.** EXAMPLES OF TYPES OF INFORMATION DESIRED

| FOCUS OF INTEREST | EXAMPLES |
|---|---|
| Individuals | |
| Description of intake | Mean intake of group of individuals |
| Adequacy of intake | Absolute magnitude (means) of usual intakes of individual<br>Mean and distribution of intakes in a group to determine percentage at risk due to low intakes |
| Relationship of diet to nutritional status or development of disease | Relative magnitude (ranks) of individual's intakes within distribution of intakes for determining associations with nutritional status or disease |
| Case control or prospective analytic epidemiology studies | Categorization of intakes of individuals into exposed or unexposed groups |
| Cross-sectional studies of relationships between diet and nutritional status or behavior | |
| Groups | |
| Description of intakes at baseline or after intervention | Mean of group |
| Exploratory studies of Relationship of diet to health or disease | Mean of group |

(Adapted from Bingham, S.A., Nelson, M., Paul, A.A., et al.: Methods for data collection at an individual level. *In* Manual on Methodology for Food Consumption Studies. Edited by M.E. Cameron and W.A. Van Staveren. Oxford, Oxford University Press, 1988.)

ments. Accuracy depends on validity and reproducibility. The strengths and weaknesses of each method in these respects is discussed later.

## METHODS FOR OBTAINING INFORMATION ABOUT FOOD INTAKE

Table 52–4 summarizes methods for obtaining information about food intake. The major methods are retrospective, prospective, and combinations of the two. Table 52–5 summarizes the advantages and disadvantages of the various methods. Contrasts between methods for estimating specific nutrients and additional details are reviewed elsewhere.[14,16,79,80]

### RETROSPECTIVE METHODS

These include the 24-hour recall, food frequency recalls, semiquantitative food frequency recalls, and dietary histories. All of them rely heavily on the individual's memory and motivation to recall diets eaten in the near or more distant past. With probing they usually give higher estimates of intakes than do prospective methods.[73]

Accuracy of recall is related to interview setting, characteristics of the interviewer, effects of instruction, respondent variables such as commitment, memory, sex, age, education, recent health status, and diet, characteristics of the respondent's diet such as its stability over time, and a number of other factors.[81–83]

Given the proper incentives and training, there is abundant evidence that most adults can recollect what they ate over the past day or week well enough to place them reliably in tertiles or sextiles.[84] Recalls of actual food consumption during the previous 24- to 48-hour period are the most reliable, with the maximum period thought to be a month.[85] However, usual or customary habits and relative rankings going back much farther in time are probably also recalled.[17,86]

For epidemiologic purposes it is often sufficient if stable, semiquantitative, relative rankings for groups of respondents can be obtained. For such purposes the accuracy of long-term recall data is better.[79] For example one recent study showed that correlations between 7-day weighed dietary records collected at four occasions over a year and a semiquantitative food frequency questionnaire were good at the group level, but not at the individual level.[87] However, questions remain about whether the technique is valid enough for uses in some epidemiologic studies focusing on individuals. The reliability of recall after 1 or 2 years is

**TABLE 52–4.** DIETARY ASSESSMENT METHODS

| METHOD | DESCRIPTION |
|---|---|
| Retrospective methods | |
| 24-Hour recall | Interviewer prompts a respondent to recall and describe all foods and beverages he consumed over the past 24 hours, usually starting with the meal immediately preceding the interview<br>Food models, measuring cups and spoons, and other tools are used to get a rough estimate of portion sizes; may be face-to-face or by telephone |
| Food frequency questionnaire | Respondent records or describes usual intakes of a list of different foods and the frequency of consumption per day, week, or month, over a period of several months or a year; the number and type of food items vary, depending on the purpose of the assessment<br>Nutrient analyses are usually not possible |
| Semiquantitative food frequency questionnaire | Similar to a food frequency questionnaire; portion sizes are specified as standardized portion size or choice (of a range of sizes); foods are chosen to encompass the most frequently consumed foods as well as the most common sources of nutrients; the major sources of nutrients for a given population should be included for questionnaire to be valid |
| Burke-type dietary history | Respondent orally reports all foods and beverages consumed on a usual day, then the interview progresses to questions about the frequency and amount of consumption of these foods; often, the respondent provides additional documentation of several days' intakes in the form of food diaries; food models, cross-checks on food consumption, careful probing, and other techniques are also used |
| Prospective methods | |
| Weighed food record | With a food record, the individual weighs all food and drink consumed on a small scale rather than simply estimating portion sizes; all is recorded as eaten |
| Food record | The individual records everything he eats or drinks in the food diary, including estimated portion sizes at the time of consumption for several days or only at specified times |
| Telephone record | Instead of personal face-to-face interviews, telephones are used to report food intakes as soon as they have occurred |
| Photographic or videotape records | Individual photographs or videotapes of all foods to be eaten, at standardized distance |
| Electronic records (food recording electronic device, or FRED) | Respondent records foods intake on a specially programmed electronic recording device on which the subject can record his food intake |
| Portable electronic set of recording scales (PETRA) | Respondent records intake on an electronic weighing scale recording device and with a built-in memory; it operates by pressing a single button, weighing the foods to be eaten; weights are automatically recorded, then the description of the food is dictated on a microphone connected to the tape recorder and weighing scale |
| Duplicate portion analysis | A duplicate portion of the foods and beverages consumed by an individual is collected; foods are then chemically analyzed to obtain a direct nutrient analysis |
| Intakes and outputs | Applicable to confined individuals, usually in institutions; all foods entering and leaving the room are measured; the difference is assumed to be what the respondent ate |
| Direct observation: by video recording | Video cameras are used to monitor the individual's food intake over a certain period; Videotapes may then be reviewed and intakes recorded accordingly |
| Direct observation: by trained observers | In controlled or highly supervised environments intakes may be directly watched by trained observers who use any of the methods mentioned above; sometimes this observation is covert |

insufficient to classify individuals into tertiles or quantiles of exposure by their nutrient intakes, although it may be possible to do so for groups.[88] Another problem with long-term recall is that it is biased by current diet; these errors may affect patients differently than controls in epidemiologic studies.[20,88–90] If individuals cannot be categorized reliably with respect to differences in timing, dose, frequency, or duration of exposures on diet in case control or other studies then the associations between diet and later disease or mortality are difficult to study.

### *24-HOUR RECALLS*

Twenty-four-hour recalls cannot identify with precision those individuals whose intakes are likely to be high or low in the population. Group mean intakes may be reliable, however; those who report very high intakes on a given day are balanced out by those who report very low intakes. However, these individuals will not necessarily maintain their rankings on a second occasion; even though group means may be constant, their values usually exhibit regression toward

**TABLE 52–5.** ADVANTAGES AND DISADVANTAGES OF DIFFERENT DIETARY ASSESSMENT METHODS

| METHODS AND ADVANTAGES | DISADVANTAGES |
|---|---|
| Retrospective | |
| 24-hour recall | |
| Easy to administer | Does not provide adequate quantitative data on nutrient intakes |
| Time required to administer is short | Individual diets vary daily, so that a single day's intake may not be representative |
| Inexpensive | An experienced interviewer is required |
| Respondent burden is low | Relies heavily on memory, making it unsuitable for certain groups, such as the elderly |
| Useful in clinical settings | Selective forgetting of foods such as liquids, high-calorie snacks, alcohol, and fat occurs |
| More objective than diet history | Reported intake may not be actual intake, but rather what the interviewer wants to hear |
| Serial 24-hour recalls can provide estimates of usual intakes on individuals | Does not reflect differences in intake for weekday vs. weekend, season to season, or shift to shift |
| Data obtained can be repeated with reasonable accuracy | Data may not accurately reflect nutrient intakes for populations because of variations in food consumption from day to day |
| Good reliability between interviewers | May be a tendency to over-report intake at low levels and under-report intake at high levels of consumption, leading to "flat slope syndrome" with reports of group intakes |
| Food frequency questionnaire | |
| May be either self-administered or interviewer-administered | Response rates may be lower if questionnaire is self-administered |
| Inexpensive | Incomplete responses may be given |
| Quick to administer | Lists compiled for the general population are not useful for obtaining information on groups with different eating patterns (foods inappropriate) |
| Good at describing food intake patterns for diet and meal planning | Total consumption is difficult to obtain because not all foods can be included in lists; underestimation can occur |
| No observer bias | Respondent burden rises as the number of food items queried increases |
| Can be used for large population studies | Analysis is difficult without use of computers and special programs |
| Useful when purpose is to study association of a specific food or a small number of foods and disease such as alcohol and birth defects | Reliability is lower for individual foods than for food groups |
| Specific information about nutrients can be obtained if food sources of nutrients are confined to a few sources | Foods differ in extent to which they are over- and under-reported (errors are not random) |
| Can be analyzed rapidly for nutrients or food groups using a computer | Each questionnaire needs validation |
| Foods can be ranked in relation to intakes of certain food items or groups of foods | Translation of food groups to nutrient intakes requires that many assumptions be made |
| | For assessing single nutrients, short lists are acceptable |

the mean.[11,12] Thus quantitative estimates of intakes from single 24-hour recall data are highly suspect for individuals, but with several 24-hour recalls accuracy improves.

Single 24-hour recalls should not be used in surveys to report the number of individuals below some cut-off point for dietary adequacy. They will overestimate those whose intakes are truly low compared with dietary assessment measures that better reflect typical or usual intakes such as semiquantitative food frequencies, multiple days of records, or diet histories. In comparison to longer observation periods, distributions of nutrient intake obtained from single 24-hour recalls are more spread out, with more very high and very low values. Simply adding to groups size will not compensate for this.[11,12]

Twenty-four-hour recalls are also inappropriate to use in studies involving investigations of associations between intakes and biochemical or other health indices. With measures of diet on a single day, intraindividual variation in the dietary measure may be so great that it obscures these relationships, and correlations with biochemical parameters may be low or nonexistent even if a relatively strong association actually exists.

Errors of estimates of usual intake and their relative reliabilities vary from one nutrient to the next, and will also be influenced by how many observations are done.

### *FOOD FREQUENCY RECALLS*

Food frequency recalls are good for describing groups but have serious limitations for making statements

**TABLE 52–5.** ADVANTAGES AND DISADVANTAGES OF DIFFERENT DIETARY ASSESSMENT METHODS continued

| METHODS AND ADVANTAGES | DISADVANTAGES |
|---|---|
| Semiquantitative food frequency questionnaires | |
| Inexpensive<br>May be self-administered<br>Rapid<br>Usual diets are not altered<br>Can rank or categorize individuals by rank of nutrient intakes rather than measuring group means<br>Precoding and direct data entry to computer available to speed up analysis on some versions<br>Correlations between this and other methods are satisfactory for food items and targeted nutrients when groups are the focus of the analysis<br>Sufficiently simple to obtain dietary information in large epidemiologic studies that would not be possible with other methods<br>Can provide useful information on intake of a wide variety of nutrients<br>Validation studies are proceeding rapidly<br>Respondent burden varies | Good only for the general population, but not necessarily for specific groups<br>Culture-specific—i.e., assessment of intake in a culturally distinct group requires the creation and validation of another instrument<br>Unvalidated for individual dietary assessments<br>Needs to be constantly updated<br>Questionnaires available for adults cannot be used for children<br>Specific nutrients are measured, not all nutrients or food constituents<br>Not yet validated for those who eat modified or unusual diets (frequency and amount of intake from food groups may differ)<br>Ability to monitor short-term changes in food intake (weeks or months) is not known<br>Correlations for individual nutrient intakes obtained with semiquantitative food frequency questionnaires are poor compared to those obtained with diet histories and food records in household measures<br>May be reliable but invalid in some cases<br>Default codes with estimated variables may influence results unduly<br>May only reflect "core diets" of a week's duration |
| Burke-type dietary history | |
| Produces a more complete and detailed description of both qualitative and quantitative aspects of food intake than do food records, 24-hour recalls, or food frequency questionnaires<br>Eliminates individual day-to-day variations<br>Takes into consideration seasonal variations<br>Good for longitudinal studies<br>Provides good description of usual intake<br>Provides some data on previous diet before beginning prospective studies | Highly-trained nutritionists are required to administer dietary histories<br>Difficult to standardize because of considerable variability among and within interviewers<br>Depends on subject's memory<br>Time-consuming (takes about 1 to 2 hours to administer)<br>Diet histories overestimate intakes compared to food records collected over the same period because of bigger portion sizes and greater frequencies reported; also does not account for missed meals or sick days<br>Time frame actually used by subject for reporting intake history is uncertain, probably no longer than a few weeks<br>Costs of analysis are high because records must be checked, coded, and entered appropriately |
| Food diary | |
| What is eaten is recorded (or should be recorded at time of consumption)<br>Recording error can be minimized if subjects are given proper directions<br>Does not rely heavily on memory, and thus may be good for the elderly<br>Can be obtrusive | Food intake may be altered<br>Respondent burden is great<br>Individual must be literate and physically able to write<br>Respondent may not record intakes on assigned days<br>Difficult to estimate portion sizes<br>Food models or pictures may help<br>Underreporting is common<br>Number of sampled days must be sufficient to provide usual intake<br>Records must be checked and coded in standardized way<br>Measured food intakes are more valid than records above<br>Costs of coding and analysis are high<br>Sex difference exists—i.e., women are more competent than men in recording<br>Number of days surveyed depends on the nutrient being studied<br>The very act of recording may change what is eaten |

**TABLE 52–5.** ADVANTAGES AND DISADVANTAGES OF DIFFERENT DIETARY ASSESSMENT METHODS *continued*

| METHODS AND ADVANTAGES | DISADVANTAGES |
|---|---|
| Weighed food diary | |
| Increased accuracy of portion sizes over food diaries (where errors are substantial—up to 40% for foods and 25% for nutrients) | Respondent burden great, and may increase dropout rates<br>Consumption may be altered during recording days<br>Expensive<br>May restrict choice of food<br>Subjects must be highly motivated<br>Other disadvantages similar to those of food diary<br>Not highly portable<br>Obtrusive<br>Time-consuming<br>Scales may break |
| Telephone interviews | |
| Some anonymity is maintained<br>Respondent burden is low<br>Validity is good<br>Respondent acceptance is good<br>Effect of forgetting is minimum<br>Outreach is greater<br>May be easier to carry out after a face-to-face interview and instruction | Makes assumptions that portion sizes reported are actually eaten<br>Validation studies are incomplete |
| Records for monitoring specific foods or nutrients | |
| Immediate feedback<br>Easy, rapid way to monitor specific or nutrients for monitoring and adherence purposes in patients | Inaccurate for research<br>All food sources of nutrients not included |
| Special records | |
| Can be correlated with other measures such as hunger, blood sugar, mood | Time-consuming<br>Difficult to analyze |
| Photographic records | |
| Validity is good | Problems result with estimating portion sizes and identifying some foods from photographs<br>Food waste may not be taken into consideration, leading to overestimation<br>Necessary details may be lacking<br>Obtrusive<br>Respondent burden is high |
| Duplicate portion collection and analysis | |
| Highly accurate in metabolic research<br>Duplicate portion permits direct chemical analysis<br>Helpful for validating other methods for constituents on which food composition data are incomplete<br>Good for individuals consuming unusual foods | Intakes may be altered<br>High respondent burden<br>Expensive<br>Time-consuming and messy<br>Differences between duplicate portions and weighed records are large (7% for energy, larger for other nutrients) |

about the absolute magnitude of individual nutrient intakes of individuals.[14,16]

If only a single nutrient is of interest, lists are now available of about 100 foods that, by virtue of their composition, portion size, and the frequency with which they are eaten contribute the most to intakes of that nutrient in national surveys of representative samples of Americans.[91,92]

### *SEMIQUANTITATIVE FOOD FREQUENCY QUESTIONNAIRES*

The first food frequency questionnaires were used chiefly in abbreviated versions based on food groups in clinical situations and for special studies. Now questionnaires are available that are based on longer lists of the most common food and vitamin-mineral supplement

**TABLE 52–5.** ADVANTAGES AND DISADVANTAGES OF DIFFERENT DIETARY ASSESSMENT METHODS continued

| METHODS AND ADVANTAGES | DISADVANTAGES |
|---|---|
| Electronic records (food recording electronic device, or FRED) | |
| Preliminary validations are good | Requires considerable instructions and training |
| Decreased respondent burden | Special food groups must be constructed for population to be studied |
| Eliminates time for coding and data entry, as well as associated errors occurring at those stages | Portion size estimates often are imprecise |
| Can be used for patients who cannot write | |
| Measured intakes and outputs | |
| Low respondent burden | Others in the room may have eaten the food |
| Assessment can be accomplished without individual knowing about it | Individual may hide or throw away food (e.g., anorexics) |
| Good for individuals incapable of writing or remembering | Staff may forget to deliver or collect the food |
| Portable electronic set of tape recording scales (PETRA) | |
| Useful for patients who cannot write | Expensive |
| Cumulative weight is automatically recorded | Does not take plate waste into consideration |
| Records cannot be altered once entered | |
| Measures actual and habitual food intake | |
| Has been initially validated | |
| Time saved for coding and data entry | |
| Eliminates errors occurring during coding and data entry | |
| Direct observation by video recording | |
| Low respondent burden | High initial cost |
| Measures usual and habitual food intake | Not good for large studies |
| Highly accurate | May have technical problems (e.g., angle of camera, low-quality picture detail) |
| Details may be observed | Intakes may be altered if individual is aware of observation |
| Individual may or may not know he is being observed | Obtrusive |
| Direct observation by trained observers | |
| Low respondent burden | Expensive and time-consuming for observer |
| Overt or covert observation is possible | Not ideal for large studies |
| Precise measurements may be obtained | Intakes may be altered, especially if person is aware of observation |
| | Details may be overlooked |

sources of nutrients in representative sample of the American population. These are useful for providing semiquantitative estimates of nutrient intakes of groups.

The two semiquantitative food frequency questionnaires presently in widespread use that have been tested most extensively are the instrument developed by Willett et al. at Harvard University[87,93,94] and that developed by Block and co-workers at the National Cancer Institute.[95–98] They differ from each other in their method of construction, the reference populations used to select foods, the extent to which they have been validated, the reference portion sizes used, the number of foods they contain, the nutrient intakes they are designed to assess, the extent to which they account for overall intakes of these nutrients and of other constituents, the questions they ask on vitamin, mineral, and other dietary constituents, the nutrient data bases that have been used for translating findings from them into nutrient intakes, and probably in other respects. Specific questionnaires for key population groups are also available.[29,99–100]

The population-based questionnaires are good tools for providing estimates of the nutrient intakes of groups. However, they are now being widely and sometimes incorrectly used to provide quantitative estimates of dietary intakes of individuals. The basic problem that makes this procedure invalid is that the nutrient values for each food category on the questionnaire are derived from weighted averages or medians (based on group estimates) for each food of frequency × portion size × number of servings per occasion for each food in the category among the population used for validating it. Thus nutrient intakes for each food category are derived from weighted group estimates and reflect population, not individual, values. Individuals then provide their frequency of consumption of each food group category, with some estimate of portion and servings, and from these individual intake profiles are derived. However, overall nutrient intakes for the individual do not reflect their own individual weighted averages of food consumption frequency within each category. Rather, they are rough estimates of intakes of food groups, whose nutrient contents are assumed to be similar to that of the reference population at a given point in time, introducing a strong group effect. True differences between individuals may therefore be impossible to ascertain unless replicates are used.

Single food frequency, semiquantitative food frequency, and dietary history questionnaires are sometimes employed to minimize intraindividual variation because they purport to report typical or usual intakes. However, they are error-prone, and several repeated measures may be needed if they are used for these purposes. Their within-individual variation is often unknown, and threats to validity due to forgetting, unequal estimation errors, and different periods used as the interval for reporting introduce errors. In one study the precision of a self-administered semiquantitative food frequency questionnaire was assessed on nurses a year after the first questionnaire was distributed. After adjusting for energy intakes, intraclass correlation coefficients ranged from 0.5 for vitamin A intakes without supplements to 0.7 for sucrose; most energy-providing nutrients had correlation coefficients of about 0.5 to 0.6.[94] These low correlations present problems when data on usual intakes of individuals are required for correlation with biochemical or clinical parameters; unless very large numbers of subjects are available, significant correlations may be masked.[73,101]

When the focus of the study is to describe intakes of individuals, the number of observations necessary and the size of the group are larger than when groups are of interest.

#### *BURKE-TYPE DIETARY HISTORY*

This dietary history method is only infrequently used today because it takes so long, requires a trained, highly skilled nutritionist, and the results are difficult to code and process. It is less directive than list-based methods and for some purposes it may be appropriate, because it gives a complete profile of individual diet. Its project uses have been well described.[102]

### PROSPECTIVE METHODS

Table 52–4 describes the many prospective methods for obtaining food records at the time the food is eaten or shortly thereafter. These include collection of duplicate portions of all food eaten, records of weighed intakes using scales, food diaries, precoded lists for monitoring frequency of intake of specific foods and calculating intake of a nutrient of interest, other special records, telephone interviews on current intake, and photographic, videotaped, and electronic microcomputer records of consumption. Other techniques that are applicable in some situations are observations of intakes and food waste (as in intake and output studies in hospitals) and constant observation by trained observers.

The methods' strengths and limitations are presented in Table 52–5. They are all less affected by forgetting than retrospective methods. However, the very act of recording intake may inadvertently stimulate a greater consciousness about intake or otherwise lead the respondent to alter intakes during recording periods. Additional information for those who wish to use prospective methods in research studies is presented elsewhere.[4,14,16,17,103,104]

### COMBINATIONS OF METHODS

Often dietary assessment studies for research purposes employ several methods simultaneously to increase accuracy. For example, the United States Department of Agriculture (USDA) National Food Consumption Survey used a 24-hour recall combined with either 2- or 3-day written records, and the Department of Health and Human Service's Health and Nutrition Examination Survey used a 24-hour recall and food frequency information.[105] The monumental year-long diet study conducted by the USDA also used a variety of methods.[71] Newer national surveys are using telephone recalls and interactive computer recalls in addition to food records.[105]

## DESIGN CONSIDERATIONS IN DIET ASSESSMENT STUDIES

### REPRESENTATIVENESS, VALIDITY, RELIABILITY

Dietary assessment methods differ in the ease with which representative samples can be obtained as well as in their validity and reliability, and thus in the uses to which they should be put.[10,14,16,106]

Representativeness of the study population, the period under study, and the heterogeneity of food habits in the population are important considerations to take into account in drawing samples for study.

Validity is the degree to which a method measures what it claims to be measuring. It is difficult to assess the absolute validity of dietary methods because diet is constantly changing and the very act of observing often alters intakes. The major sources of error that affect validity are random response errors and bias (systematic errors), which in turn is due to either systematic errors in response or otherwise imperfect information. Therefore it is important to get estimates of validity so that suitable corrections in analysis can be made to account for errors.[18,70,97]

The most common validation technique used is concurrent validity; evaluation of the test dietary method against a "gold standard" reference method that is thought to be particularly accurate and precise.[79,106] Some underestimation of concurrent validity with records and recalls often occurs because of the use of small and possibly unrepresentative numbers of days, whereas there may be an overestimation with dietary histories and other such instruments.[101,107] After correcting for the variability of food records, correlations with diet records are about r = 0.5 to 0.7 for most nutrients.[70]

In actuality, because subjective response errors and bias are likely to be present in both methods, concurrent validity really only measures apparent validity; it does not provide information about whether the assessment method is producing the correct answer, only that it is producing the same answer. Lately efforts have been made to obtain estimates of true validity that eliminate this subjective element. One method is surreptitious weighing or observation of food intakes done at the same time that the individual keeps records. Biochemical markers for validation of intakes of some nutrients are now available. These include doubly-labeled water, which provides an estimate of energy intake.[108–111] Calculations of predicted versus actual energy intake and weight gain or loss are also helpful.[112,113] Urinary nitrogen appearance is used as a proxy for protein intakes.[113,114] All of these validation methods reveal that real underestimates of actual energy intakes are common when diaries or records are used. Some of the errors that lead to misclassification can be corrected for by using sample size formulas that take misclassification into account and increase the number of subjects accordingly.[75,115] Other formulas are available for adjusting the size of the confidence intervals.[73]

Reproducibility (also referred to as reliability or precision) is the degree to which the method gives the same results when it is used again and again in the same situation. It is affected most seriously by random response errors. These include random response errors and variation within an individual's food intake. Observer training and standardized techniques can reduce it.[70] Test-retest reliability is commonly used to measure it.[106] Larger numbers of observations can improve accuracy.[116]

### APPROPRIATE FOCUS FOR ANALYSIS

**Groups.** For descriptive clinical and epidemiologic purposes, group means from data collected using any method at a single time point may suffice. If means and distributions of food intakes within a group are desired, repeated assessments using 24-hour recalls or food records covering several days, semiquantitative food frequencies, or dietary histories may be helpful.[14] But most etiologic and analytic epidemiology studies, both case-control and prospective, involve the categorization of individuals into exposed and unexposed groups, and not simply the study of groups. They require data on individual intakes. If individuals' intakes cannot be categorized reliably into the distribution of intakes, the variability will be so great that it will be impossible to answer the questions posed.[18]

**Individuals.** For many purposes analysis focuses on individuals.[16,18,117] A single day's intake is usually inadequate to characterize an individual's usual intake correctly for placement into some range of nutrient distributions, such as quantiles. Thus multiple repeated records, recalls, or food frequency questionnaires totaling a much greater number of measurements than for groups are required to relate the absolute or relative magnitude of individuals' food consumption with morbidity or mortality. Data on the individual's usual or habitual diet are also required to identify those individuals in the larger population who need special attention, or to describe links between diet and nutritional status, morbidity, or mortality.

When the absolute magnitude of an individual's intake is needed (such as grams per day of fat or alcohol), the within-person variation in intakes is usually so large for most of the energy-yielding nutrients that 2 to 3 weeks' worth of weighed intakes would be required to obtain a precision of 10% in most (i.e., 90%) of the population.[118–119] Design considerations may make it impossible to study some nutrients because the number of dietary observations necessary to obtain accurate data are far more than subjects are willing to tolerate; thus multiple recalls may be a better choice.[10,16]

## CAUSES AND CONTROL OF VARIATION BETWEEN ACTUAL AND MEASURED DIETS

Table 52–6 summarizes the major sources of error that account for the differences between actual and measured diets, and likely vulnerabilities of each dietary assessment method. These problems and some ways to control them are described in greater depth elsewhere.[14,16,17,103]

### POPULATION SAMPLING ERRORS AND BIAS

*Lack of representativeness* causes differences between actual and measured diets in assessments. The three major sources of error involving representativeness are erroneous selection of the subjects to study, choice of an atypical period of observation, and heterogeneity of food intakes in the population. All are partially amenable to control with good study design.

*Population sampling error* is controlled by an appropriate sampling design that selects individuals who are representative of the larger population. Additional attention to appropriate substitutions for those who fail to volunteer, who drop out, or are uncooperative is also essential. If sampling is disregarded the actual population studied may not be representative of the reference population, and may be biased in physical, environmental, or other significant ways, threatening inference. Sampling errors may either underestimate or overestimate variability between individuals in the actual pop-

**TABLE 52–6.** SOURCES OF ERROR IN DIETARY ASSESSMENT METHODS

| METHOD | DUPLICATE PORTION | WEIGHED RECORD | ESTIMATED RECORD | 24-HOUR RECALL | DIET HISTORY | FOOD FREQUENCY | SQFF* |
|---|---|---|---|---|---|---|---|
| **Population** | | | | | | | |
| **Sampling error and bias** | + | + | + | + | + | + | + |
| **Response bias** | ? | ? | ? | ? | ? | ? | ? |
| **Response errors** | | | | | | | |
| Omitting foods | − | ? | ? | + | + | + | + |
| Adding foods | − | − | − | + | + | + | + |
| Estimate of weight of foods | − | − | + | + | + | + | + |
| Estimation of servings | − | − | − | − | + | + | + |
| Estimate of food consumption frequency | − | − | − | − | + | + | + |
| Day-to-day variation | + | + | + | + | − | − | − |
| Changes in diet | + | + | ? | − | − | − | − |
| **Coding errors** | − | + | + | + | + | + | + |
| **Errors in conversion of Foods to nutrients** | | | | | | | |
| Food sampling errors | + | − | − | − | − | − | − |
| Direct analysis | + | − | − | − | − | − | − |
| Food composition tables | − | + | + | + | + | + | + |
| Nutrient data base values used for groups of foods | − | − | − | − | − | + | + |
| Dietary analysis computational errors | + | + | + | + | + | + | + |

(Adapted from Bingham, S.A.: Dietary assessment of individuals: methods, accuracy, new techniques and recommendations. Nutr. Abstracts Rev., *57*:709, 1987; and Bingham, S.A., Nelson, M., Paul, A.A., et al.: Methods for data collection at the individual level. *In* Manual on Methodology for Food Consumption Studies. Edited by M.E. Cameron and W.A. Van Staveren. Oxford, Oxford University Press, 1988, p. 98.)

*Semiquantitative food frequency

ulation. Methods for survey sampling to avoid these problems are well described elsewhere.[78,120–122]

Some *random error* associated with time is always present in estimating dietary intake, because in affluent Western countries, peoples' intakes vary considerably and more or less randomly from day to day. Because they do, a single day's intakes, which may be particularly high or low, rarely suffices to describe the usual intakes of individuals. A large true variation in the person's current food intake (biologic within-person variation) decreases reproducibility. Its size depends on the food patterns of the individual being studied, as well as on the food constituent being assessed, the time frame of interest, and the dietary assessment technique used.

*Variation within individuals* in their food intake consists of day-to-day variations that are not accounted for in the design of the study, and on other random measurement errors that cannot be disentangled from true individual biologic variation. When within-person variation is high, reproducibility (precision) decreases. Within-individual variation is usually much greater than is the variation between individuals.[123] Data are available that provide some information on the scope of these variations in studies of adults,[118] young infants,[124] and other special populations.[125–126]

*Systematic errors* within individuals may also be present. Intakes may vary from weekday to weekend and season to season. Failure to obtain a representative sample of these days causes sampling bias. In clinical trials, intakes on reporting days often differ in important ways from typical diets. To avoid sampling bias and to select a valid sample, typical intake patterns must be identified. Then a suitable sampling design and weighting system can be developed so that each major source of time-related variability is represented appropriately. The stability of estimates of usual intake can also be enhanced by using more recalls or records for those nutrients having a great within-person variability.[101]

*Between-person variation* is that existing between people in their habitual food pattern. It varies for each nutrient. It increases as heterogeneity of the group being studied becomes greater. Within some populations systematic but unrecognized alterations in food intake may be unique to certain subgroups or individuals. These include dieting, binging, or periodic low intakes due to lack of money or illness. Large between-person variation in habitual food intake increases the difficulty of achieving representativeness in drawing samples from the population, increases the sample size needed, and makes inference difficult if it goes unrecognized. The identification of the sources of variation and their control in sample selection and later analysis is important because it can reduce between-person variation. When between-person variability is identified and controlled, either by selecting a homogeneous group or by selecting individuals in very heterogeneous strata in terms of their food intake, it can increase the ability to find differences.

## DURATION OF DATA COLLECTION

The number of days needed to assess nutrient intakes with sufficient accuracy to describe usual intakes and to provide a definitive test to show that differences exist depends on intra- and inter-individual variation in intakes for each nutrient.[10,16] If these are known, the measurement period necessary can be calculated. The number of individuals or groups who will be studied also influences the number of days that must be collected to get satisfactory accuracy.

A single day's intake almost always gives erroneous estimates of usual intakes because diets and nutrient intakes vary greatly from day to day. Several days' worth of intakes are usually necessary to characterize usual diets reliably. When the aim is to classify the nutrient intakes of individuals into tertiles, a week's worth of records is enough for some nutrients, but for vitamin A, riboflavin, iron, and cholesterol with very large intraindividual variations, a longer time will be needed. The practical significance is that so many days of observation may be needed and respondent burden may be so excessive that the study cannot be done. Estimates of how long data must be collected that are gleaned from the literature may be helpful in preliminary planning. However, empirical evidence on the actual population to be measured is also necessary because within-individual variation is not fixed; it varies from one study to another.[75,76]

## RESPONSE ERRORS

Most people are only vaguely aware of what they eat. Without training, food records and recalls collected from people will lack sufficient detail to be useful for most purposes. The quality of reporting and dietary data obtained can be greatly improved by training respondents, but retraining is needed after about a month.[82,127]

Response biases constitute serious threats to validity. With prospective record keeping the individual may consciously or unconsciously eat differently on reporting days either to make recording easier or to conform to what he perceives is an appropriate food intake. This bias is common in clinical trials among dietary intervention groups; the individual "eats to the study objectives" on recording days. Some individuals in both prospective and retrospective studies also report deliberately distorted diets that are not what they actually ate. In retrospective studies recalls of previous diet are also often inaccurate. Because current diet exerts a strong influence on recollection of past diet, faulty memory may be involved.[81] Alternatively, the respondent may wish to provide intakes he regarded as "good" eating habits that will please the observer.[127]

Reporting errors of a random type are common. They include failures of memory that lead to omissions and additions of foods. Recalls of past diet tend to be simple and stereotypical. Moreover, errors in estimating the portion size or weight of foods when they are not actually weighed are very large—as high as 50% for foods and 20% for nutrients.[16] Mistakes in the food consumption frequency also contribute.

Random reporting errors arise from the assessment method employed, the ability of the respondent, and the skill of the interviewer. They threaten accuracy because they decrease reproducibility. The use of probes, memory aids, and cross checks on reports of intakes minimizes these errors.[82]

Frequency of consumption[128] and portion size errors[129] also are common.

## CODING ERRORS

Coding dietary records validly and reliably is difficult but possible with coder training. When respondents describe foods vaguely many plausible coding alternatives exist. Errors can be large if each coder interprets the description differently.

The best practice is to obtain adequate information to begin with by training those who will administer dietary assessments and subjects so that the record obtained is complete and high in quality to begin with. Checking of records prior to and during coding can clear up remaining ambiguities. This is particularly important for food records, diaries, and recalls and for foods such as different fats and oils that are commonly added to foods.[130] In one recent study of fat intakes, for example, 15% of total fat intakes were of an unknown type, and about half of this could be identified with further probing.[131] The use of specialized data bases with complete values is helpful.[132] Whenever possible additional information needed on portion sizes, brands, and the like should be obtained from the respondent himself, the cook, or someone else who is familiar with the eating habits of the respondent. Information from restaurants or manufacturers may also be helpful for key items that are likely to be high in a nutrient of interest. Precoded interview schedules such as food frequency and semiquantitative food frequency questionnaires also need to be screened and checked to make sure that the respondent did not code incorrectly because of misunderstanding instructions.

Even when high-quality records have been received, well standardized decision rules and coding methods for handling unknowns and ambiguous items are necessary.

Simply omitting these items or allowing the coder to use his own discretion will introduce error.

## CONVERTING FOODS INTO NUTRIENTS OR OTHER CONSTITUENTS

All dietary assessment methods involve conversion of foods into nutrients or other constituents either by using values from direct chemical analysis of foods eaten or by using a food composition table or data base.[133] The process involves many problems and assumptions that can lead to substantial errors in estimating intakes.[7,8]

## ERRORS IN SAMPLING FOODS

Food composition values are not absolute and immutable quantities; rather, they are approximations. Technical errors relating to food composition include true random variability of composition of the individual food item, and biased food composition data owing to inadequate sampling. The best way to avoid these errors is to use a nutrient data base or food table that is as representative of the food supply as possible, and to recognize that some error is inevitable.

The nutrient composition of food is inherently variable. Samples of similar foods differ in their composition due to inherent biologic variability. In addition to genetics, environmental factors such as the soil in which food plants are grown, the feed consumed by livestock, post harvest or slaughter handling, time or circumstances of storage, and the effects of light, heat, humidity, and other conditions may alter nutrient composition. Food processing may introduce additional differences. The variability introduced by these factors differs from one food constituent to another.

For calculations of nutrient intakes to be valid, they must be based on foods that are representative samples of the food supply. The USDA has the largest and most comprehensive program for collection of food composition data in the world. The USDA uses methods that attempt to develop average values representative of the nutrient composition of foods available in this country. Efforts are constantly being made to upgrade the quality, quantity, completeness of information, and documentation provided.[6,134] Information on food composition is best when it is based on samples drawn for representativeness (as is done in the USDA program) rather than for convenience. The information in some other food composition data bases may include samples of convenience or lack documentation for values provided, making the data of uncertain quality. Content and comprehensiveness also differ. Errors may also occur in compiling nutrient values from several sources or laboratories to develop single representative values used in the food tables.

## ERRORS IN DIRECT CHEMICAL ANALYSIS

In some instances direct chemical analysis of duplicate samples of foods eaten is necessary to provide information on the presence of food constituents that are unavailable in standard tables. The errors involved here include both sampling errors in assuming that the foods chosen for analysis are representative of the entire food supply, and laboratory errors in the chemical analyses or biologic assays themselves. For most nutrients, comparisons between calculated and chemically analyzed values for total diets are closer than for individual foods.

### *CALCULATED VERSUS CHEMICALLY ANALYZED VALUES*

Calculated and chemically analyzed values rarely agree perfectly because of all the differences in food composition that have been discussed. In general, calculated and analyzed values for protein are closest. Values for total calories, carbohydrate, and fat are also fairly reliable, although the fat content of meat itself and cooking and eating practices vary a good deal and may increase errors. In contrast, the vitamin and mineral content of foods, especially that of the trace elements, is subject to much greater environmentally determined variation, and the differences between calculated and analyzed values are likely to be much greater.[9]

## FOOD COMPOSITION TABLES

Calculations of nutrient intakes must be based not only on representative samples of the food supply but on foods as actually eaten. Once the food is purchased, food preparation, trimming, and cooking techniques may further alter nutrient content to varying degrees. The use of food composition data bases that contain specific values for foods that differ in these respects can further improve the validity of nutrient intake estimates.[8]

Many different food composition tables and data bases are in use in the United States today. They vary in the timeliness, number, completeness, and specificity of the information they provide on food constituents. The major source of data on food composition in all of them is that compiled by the USDA and other government agencies. However, USDA data are frequently not identified as to source or brand name in the case of prepared foods, some proprietary food manufacturer data is not included, reports of additional research on food composition since publication of the tables may not be included, not all constituents of possible interest are necessarily covered, and availability of data is limited to published tables of food composition or data tapes. For these reasons other food tables that provide information on these issues have come into common use for many purposes.

Some data bases are in the public domain (e.g., USDA data bases).[135,136] Others are proprietary and available only for sale commercially. Publications of the National Nutrient Data Base Conferences usually provide information on these newer systems. The advantages of the proprietary data bases are that they often are produced in microcomputer-usable versions, are easier to use, provide additional values for special foods, brands of foods, and vitamin-mineral supplements, and include computer programs for manipulating and presenting values in a variety of ways. However, these data bases differ in the criteria used for assessing quality of composition data for acceptance, number of items or nutrients included, timeliness of data updates, descriptions of the source of the data, and ease of use, as well as in many other respects. Therefore it is important to study their characteristics before selecting them.

Food composition information on foods eaten in other countries is available from the International Network of Food and Data Systems (INFOODS), which has recently produced an international directory of food composition tables.[8] Differences exist between values obtained from nutrient data bases among different industrialized countries and even within countries at different times.[133] Some of these are real, and others are due to methodologic differences.[7] Therefore, caution is indicated when information from various food tables is combined. Although the completeness of information on food composition leaves much to be desired in the United States, in developing countries, the information available on food composition is considerably more fragmentary and incomplete.

The number of foods has increased at least five times in USDA tables of food composition over the past three decades, and the number of nutrients for which values are available have nearly doubled. The food composition tables must be up to date, especially if they are to be used for research.

As the food supply, formulation, and processing techniques change, new analyses are required to provide updated values on nutrient composition. One recent example is the closer trimming of fat from beef and pork cuts in the past few years, which has only recently been reflected in updates to relevant sections of the USDA food composition tables.

Methods for determining many nutrients and other constituents in foods are still being developed, and data are still sparse for many items of interest, such as dietary fiber and specific fatty acids.

A major difficulty with food tables for diet assessment purposes is missing values, especially for certain nutrients, naturally occurring compounds such as fiber or carotenoids, toxicants, environmental contaminants, and intentional food additives. New food products are being developed so rapidly that it is difficult to keep the ratio of the number of foods analyzed to the number of foods consumed constant or to increase it. Similarly, the number of food components of potential interest is immense; few analyses are available for many components, and for others, food analytic methods are not yet developed.[8] Thus complete information on each component of each food consumed in this country is unlikely to ever be available.

When data are lacking, imputed values, or "best estimates," of nutrients in similar foods can be used, but these are only approximations, introducing additional assumptions and errors. Good estimates can minimize errors. Pennington has developed tables of imputed values for many nutrients.[137] The estimation of values for other food constituents is more difficult. Consensus on standard protocols for imputation will facilitate comparisons between studies. Finally, the quality and quantity of the food composition data available may be so inadequate for many of the less-studied food constituents such as biotin or vitamin K that accurate calculations of their intakes are impossible, and only rough estimates can be obtained.

## ERRORS IN NUTRIENT DATA BASES USED FOR GROUPS OF FOODS

The computerized nutrient data bases used to analyze semiquantitative food frequency questionnaires usually consist of average values for different categories or groups of foods derived from a reference population.[87,95,138] Alternatively, foods contributing to variation among individuals are used to generate the lists.[139] They are vulnerable to errors due to changes in frequency of consumption (which is especially important), changes in the nutrient composition of individual foods, and changes in portion size of various foods within the food groups or categories. Portion size errors, although present, are smaller than those caused by mistaken frequency of consumption.[128,129] Because the food supply and consumption patterns are constantly changing even within categories, errors will arise if these questionnaires are not periodically updated. Before they are used in large-scale studies, validation is necessary. Finally, defaults and imputations may be incorrect or invalid.

## COMPUTATIONAL ERRORS WITH NUTRIENT ANALYSIS SYSTEMS

The calculation of nutrient intakes for large groups imposes a daunting burden unless computerized methods are used. Computerized nutrient analysis systems are available to minimize this onerous task and reduce inadvertent computational errors.[140] However, nutrient analysis systems only approximate actual consumption. All systems available presently have many limitations. It is sometimes wrongly assumed that computerized dietary analysis systems "cope with" all of the problems associated with dietary assessment. They are actually computational aids, not panaceas. Computerized systems cannot compensate for careless data collection, coding, or interpretation of results. Moreover, assumptions are made in some programs that may introduce errors and influence results. The way to minimize these errors is to study them closely before programs are adopted. This will help to avoid drawing invalid or grossly misleading conclusions from their outputs.[141]

Errors in some nutrient analysis systems may be so large that they obscure the effects of treatments or changes in intakes. Differences between systems exist in calculated intakes even when the same records are analyzed.[142–144] Comparisons across studies is facilitated by standardization.[145] Not only the disparate nutrient data bases but assumptions made in making calculations give rise to these errors. Assumptions include differences in portion sizes and weight/portion equivalence, factors for conversion from raw to prepared foods, listings of ingredients in recipe foods, values provided for nutrient-fortified foods, estimates of bioavailability of nutrients, and the defaults or imputed values used. A systematic method for reviewing nutrient data base capabilities has been devised.[5,146–148] It should be used to test programs before a choice is made on a dietary analysis system. Other reviews may also be helpful.[149]

## OTHER ISSUES

### DIFFERENCES BETWEEN CALCULATED AND BIOLOGICALLY AVAILABLE VALUES

Regardless of assessment method nutrient intakes calculated from food composition data bases do not necessarily represent food actually absorbed from the gut.[150] Most data bases do include adjustments to account for usual net absorption and utilization for the energy-providing nutrients, so that their biologically available intakes can be calculated directly. However, if disease or other causes of malabsorption are present these assumptions may need adjustment. For minerals and vitamins, estimates of net bioavailability are not incorporated in food tables because so many constituents of foods may promote or inhibit absorption. When bioavailability of their intakes is desired, it involves separate calculations.

### ERRORS IN INFERENCE FROM DIETARY INTAKE DATA TO NUTRITIONAL STATUS

Finally, incorrect inferences about nutritional status may be made from intake data.[13,20,151,152] No indicator provides definitive diagnosis of all forms of malnutrition and also supplies the information needed for shaping dietary interventions in individual cases.[10,13] Additional data are also required to get a complete picture of nutritional status.

In summary, all dietary assessment methods are imperfect. Their validity and reliability depend heavily on the skill of the interviewer, the instruction, training, and cooperation of the subject, and a valid and reliable nutrient data base or other system of analysis. The "best" method depends on the purpose of the investigation. In estimating individual nutritional status and designing treatments, a combination of dietary, biochemical, clinical, and anthropometric methods will continue to be the "gold standard" for most purposes.

## REFERENCES


1. Grivetti, L.E.: Nutr. Today, *26:*13–24, 1991.
2. Medlin, C., Skinner, J.D.: J. Am. Diet. Assoc., *88:*1250–1257, 1988.
3. Block, G., Hartman, A.M., Dresser, C.M., et al.: Am. J. Epidemiol., *124:*453, 1986.
4. Willett, W.: Nutritional Epidemiology. New York, Oxford University Press, 1990.
5. Hoover, L.W., Perloff, B.P.: Model for Review of Nutrient Data Base Capabilities. Columbia, Missouri, University of Missouri, 1981.
6. Hepburn, F.N.: Am. J. Clin. Nutr., *35:*1297–1301, 1982.
7. Rand, W.M.: J. Am. Diet. Assoc., *85:*1081–1083, 1985.
8. Rand, W.M., Windham, C.T., Wyse, B.W., et al. (eds.): Food Composition Data: A User's Perspective. Tokyo, The United Nations University, 1987.
9. Beecher, G.R., Khachik, R.: Analysis of micronutrients in foods. *In* Nutrition and Cancer Prevention. Edited by T.E. Moon and M.S. Miccozi. New York and Basel, Marcel Dekker, 1989, pp. 103–158.
10. Gibson, R.S.: Principles of Nutritional Assessment. New York, Oxford University Press, 1990.
11. Anderson, S.A. (ed.): Guidelines for Use of Dietary Intake Data. Bethesda, MD, Life Sciences Research Office, Federation of American Societies for Experimental Biology, 1986.
12. Food and Nutrition Board, National Research Council: Nutrient Adequacy. Assessment using Food Consumption Surveys. Subcommittee on Criteria for Dietary Evaluation, Coordinating Committee on Evaluation of Food Consumption Surveys. Washington, D.C., National Academy Press, 1986.
13. Beaton, G.H.: Nutr. Rev., *44:*349–358, 1986.
14. Cameron, M.E., Van Staveren, W.A. (eds.): Manual on Methodology for Food Consumption Studies. Oxford, Oxford University Press, 1988.
15. Pao, E.M., Cypel, Y.S.: Estimation of dietary intake. *In* Present Knowledge in Nutrition. Edited by M.L. Brown. Washington, D.C., International Life Sciences Institute, 1990. pp. 399–406.
16. Bingham, S: Nutr. Abst. Rev., *57:*707–742, 1987.
17. Mackerras, D: Interpreting Dietary Data. Sydney Department of Public Health, University of Sydney, 1990.

18. Block, G., Hartman, A.M.: Dietary Methods. *In* Nutrition and Cancer Prevention. Edited by T.E. Moon and M.S. Micozzi. New York and Basel, Marcel Dekker, 1989, pp. 159–181.
19. Pao, E.M., Sykes, K.E., Cypel, Y.S.: USDA Methodological Research for Large Scale Dietary Intake Surveys, 1975–88. Home Economics Research Report No. 49. Washington, D.C., United States Department of Agriculture, Human Nutrition Information Service, 1989.
20. Dwyer, J.T.: Assessment of dietary intake. *In* Modern Nutrition In Health and Disease. 7th Ed. Edited by M.E. Shils and V.R. Young. Philadelphia, 1988, pp. 887–902.
21. This reference has been deleted.
22. Russell-Briefel, R., Caggiula, A.W., Kuller, L.H.: Am. J. Epidemiol., *122*:628-636, 1985.
23. Barker, M.E., McClean, S.I., Thompson, K.A., et al.: Br. J. Nutr., *64*:319–329, 1990.
24. Randall, E., Marshall, J.R., Graham, S., et al.: Am. J. Clin. Nutr., *52*:739–745, 1990.
25. Rush, D., Kristal, A.R.: Am. J. Clin. Nutr., *35* (*Suppl. 5*):1259–1268, 1982.
26. Doyle, W., Crawford, M.A., Laurance, B.M., et al.: Hum. Nutr. Appl. Nutr., *36*:95–106, 1982.
27. Endres, J., Dunning, S., Poon, S.W., et al.: J. Am. Diet. Assoc., *87*:1011–1016, 1019, 1987.
28. Rush, D.: *In* The National WIC Evaluation: An Evaluation of the Special Supplemental Food Program for Women, Infants, and Children, Vol. III. Chapel Hill, Technical Research Triangle Institute and New York State Research Foundation for Mental Hygiene, 1987, pp. V:3–32, VI:4–VI:45.
29. Suitor, C.J.W., Gardner, J., Willett, W.C.: J. Am. Diet. Assoc., *889*:1786–1794, 1989.
30. Subcommittee on Nutritional Status and Weight Gain During Pregnancy: Dietary intake during pregnancy. *In* Institute of Medicine, Subcommittee on Nutritional Status and Weight Gain During Pregnancy Nutrition During Pregnancy. Washington, D.C., National Academy Press, 1990, pp. 258–271.
31. Stuff, J.E., Garza, C., Smith, E.O., et al.: Am. J. Clin. Nutr., *37*:300–306, 1983.
32. Jones, P.J., Winthrop, A.L., Schoeller, D.A., et al.: Pediatr. Res., *21*:242–246, 1987.
33. Subcommittee on Nutrition During Lactation: Nutrition during Lactation. Washington, D.C., National Academy Press, 1991.
34. Vobecky, J.S., Vobecky, J., Shapcott, D., et al.: Am. J. Clin. Nutr., *38*:730–738, 1983.
35. Eaton-Evans, J., Dugdale, A.E.: Hum. Nutr. Appl. Nutr., *40*:171–175, 1986.
36. Horst, C.H., Obermann De Boer, G.L., Kromhout, D.: Int. J. Epidemiol., *17*:217–221, 1988.
37. Quandt, S.A.; Am. J. Phys. Anthropol., *73*:515–523, 1987.
38. Morgan, J.: J. Hum. Nutr., *34*:376–381, 1980.
39. Leung, M., Yeung, D.L., Pennell, M.D., et al.: J. Am. Diet. Assoc., *84*:551–554, 1984.
40. Persson, L.A., Carlgren, G.: Int. J. Epidemiol., *13*:506–517, 1984.
41. Treiber, F.A., Leonard, S.B., Frank, G., et al.: J. Am. Diet. Assoc., *90*:814–820, 1990.
42. Walker, S.P., Powell, C.A., Grantham-McGregor, S.M.: Eur. J. Clin. Nutr., *44*:527–534, 1990.
43. Basch, C.E., Shea, S., Arliss, R., et al.: Am. J. Public Health, *80*:1314–1317, 1990.
44. Miller, J.Z, Kimes, T., Hui, S., et al.: J. Nutr., *121*:265–274, 1991.
45. Widdowson, E.M.: A study of Individual Childrens' Diets. MRC Special Report Series, No. 257. London, His Majesty's Stationery Office, 1947.
46. Hanes, S., Vermeersch, J., Gale, S.: Am. J. Clin. Nutr., *40*:390–413, 1984.
47. Frank, G.C., Berenson, G.S., Schilling, P.E., et al.: J. Am. Diet. Assoc., *71*:26–31, 1977.
48. Blom, L., Lundmark, K., Dahlquist, G., et al.: Acta Paediatr. Scand., *78*:858–864, 1989.
49. Rasanen, L.: Am. J. Clin. Nutr., *32*:2560–2567, 1979.
50. Eck, L.H., Klesges, R.C., Hanson, C.L.: J. Am. Diet. Assoc., *89*:784–789, 1989.
51. McPherson, R.S., Nichaman, M.Z., Kohl, H.W., et al.: Pediatrics, *86*:520–526, 1990.
52. Subcommittee on Nutritional Surveillance, Committee on Medical Aspect of Food Policy: Rep. Health Soc. Subj. (Lond.), *36*:1–293, 1989.
53. Knuiman, J.T., Rasanen, L., Ahola, M., et al.: J. Am. Diet. Assoc., *87*:303–307, 1987.
54. Baranowski, T., Dworkin, R., Henske, J.C., et al.: J. Am. Diet. Assoc., *86*:1381–1385, 1986.
55. Daniels, L.A.: Hum. Nutr. Appl. Nutr., *38*:110–118, 1984.
56. Hackett, A.F., Rugg Gunn, A.J., Appleton, D.R.: Hum. Nutr. Appl. Nutr., *37*:293–300, 1983.
57. Jenner, D.A., Neylon, K., Croft, S., et al.: Eur. J. Clin. Nutr., *43*:663–673, 1989.
58. Hackett, A.F., RuggGunn, A.J., Appleton, D.R., et al.: Hum. Nutr. Appl. Nutr., *40*:176–184, 1986.
59. Witschi, J.C., Capper, A.L, Ellison, R.C.: J. Am. Diet. Assoc., *90*:1429–1431, 1990.
60. Darke, S.J., Disselduff, M.M., Try, G.P.: Br. J. Nutr., *44*:237–241, 1980.
61. Skinner, J.D., Salvetti, N.N., Ezell, J.M., et al.: J. Am. Diet. Assoc., *85*:1093–1099, 1985.
62. Scythes, C.A., Zimmerman, S.A., Pennell, M.D., et al.: J. Nutr. Elderly, *8*:47–66, 1989.
63. Osler, M., Schrool, M.: Dan. Med. Bull., *37*:462–466, 1990.
64. McAvay, G., Rodin, J.: Appetite, *11*:97–110, 1988.
65. Davies, L, Holdsworth, M.D.: Hum. Nutr. Appl. Nutr., *39*:315–332, 1985.
66. Block, G.: Prev. Med., *18*:653–660, 1989.
67. Posner, B.E., Smigelski, C.G., Krachenfels, M.M.: J. Am. Diet. Assoc., *87*:452–456, 1987.
68. Lamar-Hildebrand, N., Saldanha, L., Endres, J.: J. Am. Diet. Assoc., *89*:1308–1310, 1989.
69. Bazzarre, T.L., Klwiner, S.M., Litchford, M.D.: J. Am. Coll. Nutr., *9*:136–142, 1990.
70. Block, G., Hartman, A.M.: Am. J. Clin. Nutr., *50*:1133–1138, 1989.
71. Basiotis, P.P., Thomas, R.G., Kelsay, J.L., et al.: Am. J. Clin. Nutr., *50*:448–453, 1989.
72. Borelli, R.: Br. J. Nutr., *63*:411–417, 1990.
73. Borelli, R., Cole, T.J., Di Biase, G., et al.: Eur. J. Clin. Nutr., *43*:453–463, 1989.
74. Marr, J.W., Heady, J.A.: Hum. Nutr. Appl. Nutr., *40*:347–364, 1986.
75. Liu, K., Stamler, J., Dwyer, A., et al.: J. Chronic Dis., *31*:399–418, 1978.
76. Liu, K.: Am. J. Epidemiol., *12*:864–874, 1988.

77. Black, A.E.: Appl. Nutr., *36A:*85–94, 1982.
78. Burk, M.C., Pao, E.M.: Home Economics Research Report No. 40. Washington, D.C., United States Department of Agriculture, 1976.
79. Block, G.: Am. J. Epidemiol., *115:*492–505, 1982.
80. Bull, N.L., Wheeler, E.F.: Hum. Nutr. Appl. Nutr., *40:*60–66, 1986.
81. Dwyer, J.T., Krall, E.A., Coleman, K.A.: J. Am. Diet. Assoc., *87:*1509–1512, 1987.
82. Krall, E.A., Dwyer, J.T., Coleman, K.A.: Nutr. Res., *8:*829–841, 1988.
83. Rohan, T., Potter, J.D.: Am. J. Epidemiol., *120:*876, 1984.
84. Wu, M.L., Whittemore, A.S., Jung, D.L.: Am. J. Epidemiol., *124:*326–335, 1986.
85. Van Staveren, W.A., West, C.E., Hoffmans, M.D., et al.: Am. J. Epidemiol., *123:*884–893, 1986.
86. Wu, M.L., Whittemore, A.S., Jung, D.L.: Am. J. Epidemiol., *128:*1137–1145, 1988.
87. Willett, W.C., Reynolds, R.D., Cottrell-Hoehner, S., et al.: J. Am. Diet. Assoc., *87:*43–47, 1987.
88. Dwyer, J.T., Gardner, J., Halvorsen, K., et al.: Am. J. Epidemiol., *130:*1033–1046, 1989.
89. Van Staveren, W.A., De Boer, J.O., Burema, J.: Am. J. Clin. Nutr., *42:*554–559, 1985.
90. Bakkum, A., Bloemberg, B., Van Staveren, W.A., et al.: Nutr. Cancer, *11:*41–53, 1988.
91. Block, G., Dresser, C.M., Hartman, A.M., et al.: Am. J. Epidemiol., *122:*13–40, 1985.
92. Pao, E.M., Flemming, K.H., Guenther, D.M., et al.: Human Nutrition Information Service Home Economics Research Report 49. Washington, D.C., United States Department of Agriculture, 1982.
93. Willett, W.C., Stampfer, M.J., Underwood, B.A., et al.: Am. J. Clin. Nutr., *38:*631–639, 1983.
94. Willett, W.C., Sampson, L., Stampfer, M.J., et al.: Am. J. Epidemiol., *122:*51–65, 1985.
95. Block, G., Hartman, A.M., Dresser, C.M., et al.: Am. J. Epidemiol., *124:*453–469, 1986.
96. National Cancer Institute Division of Cancer Prevention and Control: Health Habits and History Questionnaire. Bethesda, MD, National Institutes of Health, 1985.
97. Block, G., Hartman, A.M., Naughton, D.: Epidemiology, *1:*58–64, 1990.
98. Block, G., Woods, M., Potosky, A., et al.: J. Clin. Epidemiol., *43:*1327–1335, 1990.
99. Hankin, J.H.: Am. J. Clin. Nutr., *50:*1121–1127, 1989.
100. Hankin, J.H., Kolonel, L.N., Hinds, W.W.: J. Natl. Cancer Inst., *73:*1417–1422, 1984.
101. Potosky, A.L., Block, G., Hartman, A.M.: J. Am. Diet. Assoc., *90:*810–813, 1990.
102. Jain, M.: J. Am. Diet. Assoc., *89:*1647–1652, 1989.
103. Black, A.E.: Pitfalls in dietary assessment. *In* Recent Advances in Clinical Nutrition. Edited by A.N. Howard and I.M. Baird. London, John Libbey, 1981.
104. Fehily, A.M.: Hum. Nutr. Appl. Nutr., *37:*419–425, 1983.
105. Gable, C.B.: Am. J. Epidemiol., *121:*381–394, 1990.
106. Lee, H.H., Mcguire, V., Boyd, N.F.: J. Clin. Epidemiol., *42:*269–279, 1989.
107. Harlan, L., Block, G.: Epidemiology, *1:*224–231, 1990.
108. Livingstone, M.B.E., Prentice, A.M., Strain, J.J., et al.: Br. Med. J., *300:*708–712, 1990.
109. Klein, P.D., James, W.P., Wong, W.W., et al.: Hum. Nutr. Clin. Nutr., *38:*95–106, 1984.
110. Schoeller, D.A.: Nutr. Rev., *48:*373–379, 1990.
111. Harris, T., Woteki, C., Breifel, R.R., et al.: Am. J. Clin. Nutr., *50:*1145–1149, 1989.
112. Mertz, W., Tsui, J.C., Judd, J.T., et al.: Am. J. Clin. Nutr., *54:*291–295, 1991.
113. Bingham, S.A., Cummings, J.H.: Am. J. Clin. Nutr., *42:*1276–1289, 1985.
114. Hulten, B., Bengtsson, C., Isaksson, B.: Dur. J. Clin. Nutr., *44:*169–174, 1990.
115. Walker, A.M., Blettner, M.: Am. J. Epidemiol., *121:*783–900, 1985.
116. El Lozy, M.: J. Chronic Dis., *36:*237–249, 1983.
117. Van Beresteyln, E.C., Van't Hof, M.A., Van der Heiden-Winkeldermaat, H.J., et al.: J. Chronic Dis., *40:*1051–1058, 1987.
118. Basiotis, P.P., Wesh, S.O., Cronin, F.J., et al.: J. Nutr., *117:*1638–1641, 1987.
119. James, W.P.T., Bingham, S.A., Cole, T.J.: Nutr. Cancer, *2:*203–212, 1980.
120. Woteki, C.E.: Nutr. Rev., *44:*204–213, 1986.
121. Yetley, E., Johnson, C.: Annu. Rev. Nutr., *7:*441–463, 1987.
122. Johnson, S.R.: Cereal Foods World, *32:*186–190, 1987.
123. Sempos, C.T., Johnson, N.E., Smith, E.L., et al.: Am. J. Epidemiol., *12:*120, 1985.
124. Black, A.E., Cole, T.J., Wiles, S.J., et al.: Hum. Nutr. Appl. Nutr., *37:*448–458, 1983.
125. De Boer, J.O., Knuiman, J.T., West, C.E., et al.: Hum. Nutr. Appl. Nutr., *41:*225–232, 1987.
126. Nelson, M., Black, A.E., Morris, J.A., et al.: Am. J. Clin. Nutr., *5:*155–167, 1989.
127. Dwyer, J.T.: Assessing and monitoring dietary behaviors. *In* Nutrition Counseling Skills: Assessment, Treatment and Evaluation. Edited by L.G. Snetselaar. Rockville, MD, ASPEN Press, 1989, pp. 91–122.
128. Flegal, K.M., Larkin, F.A.: Am. J. Epidemiol., *131:*1046–1058, 1990.
129. Cohen, N.L., Laus, M.J.: The Contribution of Portion Data to Estimates of Nutrient Intake by Food Frequency. Res. Bull. No. 73. Amherst, MA, Massachusetts Agricultural Experiment Station, College of Food and Natural Resources, University of Massachusetts, 1990.
130. Broadhurst, A.J., Stockley, L., Wharf, S.G., et al.: Hum. Nutr. Appl. Nutr., *41:*101–106, 1987.
131. Milner, J.P., McGuire, V.M., Little, J.A.: Am. J. Clin. Nutr., *38:*964–970, 1983.
132. Dennis, B., Ernst, N., Hjortland, M., et al.: J. Am. Diet. Assoc., *77:*641–647, 1980.
133. Black, A.E., Ravenscroft, C., Paul, A.A.: Hum. Nutr. Appl. Nutr., *390:*9–18, 1985.
134. Stewart, K.K.: Food Nutr. Bull., *5:*54–65, 1983.
135. Consumer and Food Economics Institute, U.S. Department of Agriculture Composition of Foods: Raw, Processed, Prepared. Agricultural Handbook No. 8–1 to 8–15. Washington, D.C., United States Department of Agriculture, 1989 to 1991.
136. Pennington, J.A.T., Church, H.N.: Bowes and Church's Food Values of Portions Commonly used. 14th Ed. Philadelphia, J.B. Lippincott, 1985.
137. Pennington, J.A.T.: Dietary Nutrient Guide. Westport, CT, AVI Publishing, 1976.
138. Borrud, L.G., McPerson, R.S., Nichaman, M.Z., et al.: Nutr. Cancer, *12:*201–211, 1989.

**139.** Haile, R.W.C., Hunt, I.F., Buchecy, S., et al.: J. Am. Diet. Assoc., *86:*611–616, 1986.
**140.** Thompson, J.K., Dwyer, J.T.: Clin. Nutr., *6:*185–191, 1987.
**141.** Dwyer, J.T., Suitor, C.W.: J. Am. Diet. Assoc., *84:*302–312, 1984.
**142.** Adelman, M.O., Dwyer, J.T., Woods, M., et al.: J. Am. Diet. Assoc., *83:*421–428, 1983.
**143.** Frank, G.C., Farris, R.P., Berenson, G.S.: J. Am. Diet. Assoc., *84:*818–821, 1984.
**144.** Feskanich, D., Buzzard, I.M., Welch, B.T., et al.: J. Am. Diet. Assoc., *88:*1263–1267, 1988.
**145.** Tillotson, J.L., Gorder, D.D., DuChene, A.G., et al.: Clin. Trials, *7* (*Suppl. 3*):66S–90S, 1986.
**146.** Hoover, L.W.: J. Am. Diet. Assoc., *82:*501–505, 1983.
**147.** Hoover, L.W., Perloff, B.P.: J. Am. Diet. Assoc., *82:*506–508, 1983.
**148.** Hoover, L.W., Dowdy, R.P., Hughes, K.V.: J. Am. Diet. Assoc., *85:*297–304, 307, 1985.
**149.** Windham, C.T., Helm, A.A., Wyse, B.W.: Crit. Rev. Food Sci. Nutr., *29:*149–166, 1990.
**150.** Janghorbani, M., Young, V.R.: Am. J. Clin. Nutr., *30:*2021–2030, 1980.
**151.** Guthrie, H.A.: Nutr. Rev. *47:*33–38, 1989.
**152.** Dwyer, J.T.: Concept of nutritional status and its measurement. *In* Anthropometric Assessment of Nutritional Status. Edited by J.V. Himes. New York, Alan Liss, 1991, pp. 5–28.

## SELECTED READINGS

Bingham, S.A.: The dietary assessment of individuals: methods, accuracy, new techniques and recommendations. Nutr. Abstr. Rev. *57:*705–742, 1987.
Cameron, M.E., Van Staveren, W.A.: Manual on Methodology for Food Consumption Studies. Oxford, Oxford University Press, 1988.
Gibson, R.S.: Principles of Nutritional Assessment. New York, Oxford University Press, 1990.
Willett, W.: Nutritional Epidemiology. New York, Oxford University Press, 1990.
Partial Support for the preparation of this manuscript was furnished by grant MCJ 9120 from the Maternal and Child Health Service, United States Department of Health and Human Services, and through subcontracts to New England Medical Center, on grant 5R25-CA49612-02 from the National Cancer Institute, and grant U01HL47098 from the National Heart, Lung, and Blood Institute, National Institutes of Health. This paper has been funded at least in part from federal funds from the United States Department of Agriculture (USDA), Agricultural Research Service, under contract 533K065-10. The contents of this publication do not necessarily reflect the views or policies of USDA.

CHAPTER 53

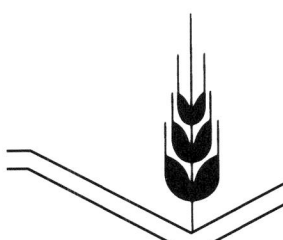

# Radiologic Findings in Nutritional Disturbances

**Robin C. Watson, Herman Grossman, and Morton A. Meyers**



The roentgenographic findings in nutritional disorders are somewhat varied. They may be distinctive, as in scurvy or rickets, but they are often nonspecific, as in osteoporosis and osteomalacia, and the diagnosis may depend upon secondary manifestations.[1–3] In addition, any radiographic abnormality occurs only in the face of prolonged deficiency or excessive intake. In all probability, the most striking changes are seen today as the result of malabsorption rather than deficient intake. However, particularly in underdeveloped areas, the latter is still a dominant factor. Generally, the earliest and most specific findings are seen in the child and adolescent, rather than in the adult, although with gastrointestinal abnormalities this tendency probably is reversed.

## OSTEOPOROSIS

Over the years the meaning of "osteoporosis" has blurred and it has become a vague, all-embracing word.[4,5]

In the normal subject there is a balance between osteoporosis and osteolysis and an adequate degree of bone mineralization. Osteoporosis represents a breakdown in this mechanism; osteogenesis is defective while osteolysis proceeds at the normal rate and the process of bone mineralization is unimpaired. The result is an overall loss of bone mass with respect to the volume of bone present. The bone elements, therefore, become sparse and brittle.

Radiographically the cortical bone thins, with an overall loss of bone density. The distance between the normally mineralized longitudinal, but thin, trabeculae increases (hence the term *porotic*), while there is a concomitant loss of transverse trabeculae.[6] These changes are usually first apparent in the spine; however, in advanced cases, the process may be seen to involve all bones. Fractures resulting from brittle quality of the bone are common and deformities may result. Most often seen are crush fractures of the spine with collapse of the vertebral end-plates and anterior wedging of the bodies, resulting in increased lordotic curves. Pseudofractures are not seen in this condition.

Osteoporosis may be seen in relation to:

1. senile and postmenopausal patients
2. malnutrition
3. hypovitaminosis C
4. endocrine disorders, such as Cushing's disease, acromegaly, hypothyroidism, and hyperthyroidism
5. the congenital defect of osteoporosis imperfecta
6. idiopathic conditions.

Interpretation is difficult because loss of the mass of bone must be extensive before this condition becomes radiographically apparent. Furthermore, the findings are nonspecific and there is no way of differentiating postmenopausal osteoporosis, for example, from that found in multiple myeloma.

Osteoporosis is, perhaps, most often seen in elderly patients, often in reduced circumstances, who have an associated dietary insufficiency, including that of vitamin C. Although there are perhaps fewer of these individuals than in the past, they exist in both rural and urban areas.

## SCURVY

Abnormalities in the skeleton in infantile scurvy have been studied by Park.[7] A disturbance of endochondral bone growth occurs, with subperiosteal hemorrhagic manifestations occurring without associated trauma. The bone changes occur symmetrically throughout the skeleton and are more widely distributed than are gross subperiosteal or intramedullary hemorrhages. As are the changes in rickets, those of scurvy are most marked where growth in length is normally most rapid: at the sternal end of the middle ribs, the lower end of the femur, the upper end of the humerus, both ends of the tibia and fibula, and the lower end of the radius and ulna, in approximately the order given.

The columns of cartilage cells in the proliferative cartilage in infantile scurvy tend to be irregular rather than linear. Whether this change represents a purely scorbutic process or whether it depends in part on an associated or antecedent rickets is not entirely certain. Scurvy interferes with the mechanism for removal of calcified cartilage matrix. It suppresses the formation of new trabeculae and, wherever there is bone already formed, resorption proceeds. These changes, morphologically important in themselves, affect the structure of bone also from a functional point of view by diminishing its capacity to withstand mechanical stress.

Roentgenographic changes are often diagnostic or suggestive. The costochondral junctions of the ribs are wide (Fig. 53–1*A* and *B*). The abrupt bony swelling culminates in a ridge where bone and cartilage meet. The sternochondral plate may be displaced posteriorly by atmospheric pressure where the cartilage has been pushed backward at the line of its separation from the bony shaft.

In the early stages, the changes in the bone are nonspecific, presenting poorly discernible trabeculae and thin cortices. As the disease progresses, a thick white line at the metaphysis develops (Figs. 53–2 and 53–3). Spurs develop at the cartilage shaft junction, and subepiphyseal atrophy casts a transverse line or band of diminished density[8] (Fig. 53–2). This zone of rarefaction is a linear break in the bone proximal and parallel to the white line. Peripheral metaphyseal clefts, the so-called corner sign, are characteristic of scurvy[7] (Fig. 53–3). Ossification centers have central rarefaction with heavy ring shadows (Fig. 53–2) on the margins. Epiphyseal separation may occur along the line of destruction, with linear displacement or compression of the epiphysis against the shaft.

Subperiosteal hemorrhages often appear on the larger long bones[8,9] (Fig. 53–4*A* and *B*). During healing the elevated periosteum becomes calcified (Fig. 53–4*B*), creating a heavy shell of subperiosteal bone. This shell of bone gradually shrinks and forms a new cortex. Subperichondrial hemorrhages over the epiphysis are said not to occur in scurvy.

## OSTEOMALACIA

In most countries osteomalacia is now considered to be the adult form of rickets. It represents an abnormality of the mineralizing process, whereas both osteogenesis and osteolysis proceed at a normal rate.[10] The result of the mineral deficiency is that the bone becomes soft and

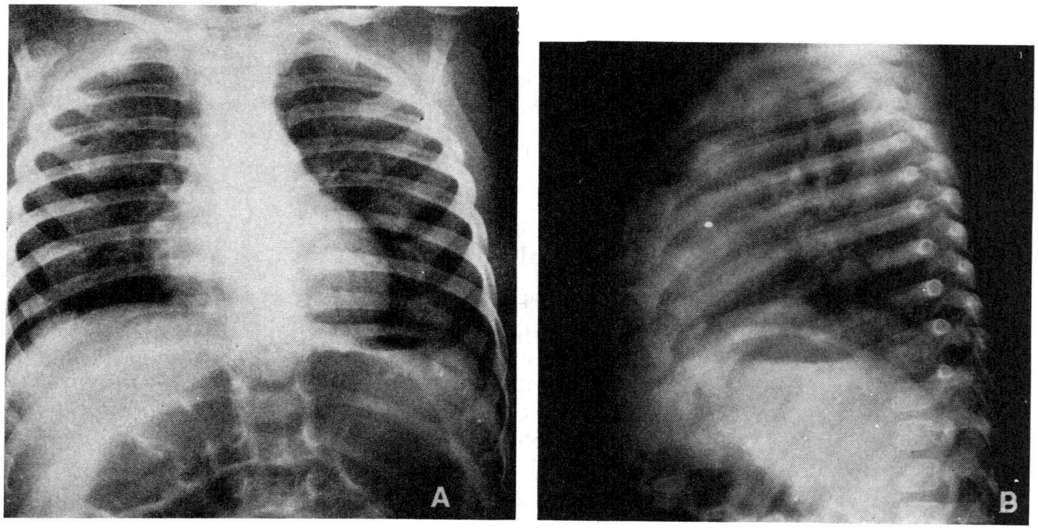
A
B

**FIGURE 53–1.** A 27-month-old boy with scurvy. Frontal *(A)* and lateral *(B)* chest roentgenograms demonstrate bony swelling at the costochondral junctions of the ribs.

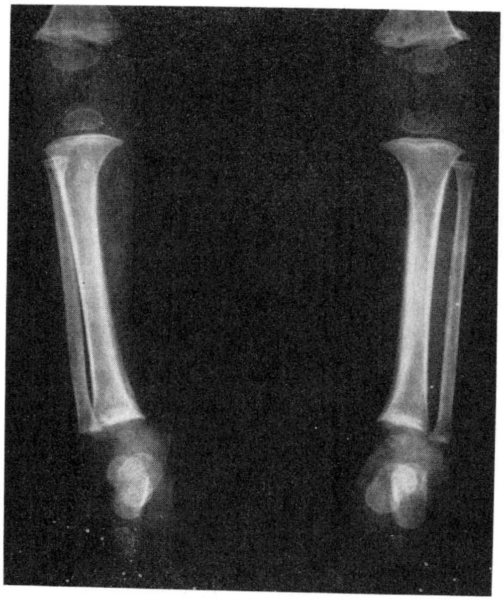

**FIGURE 53–2.** A 10-month-old boy with scurvy. A thick white line occurs at the metaphyses of the long bones of the knees. Linear breaks are present in the bones proximal and parallel to the white lines of the distal femur. Spurs are present and best seen at the ends of the femurs and medial aspect of the right tibia. The ossification centers have central rarefaction with heavy ring shadows on the margins. Periosteal new bone is along the medial aspects of the tibias

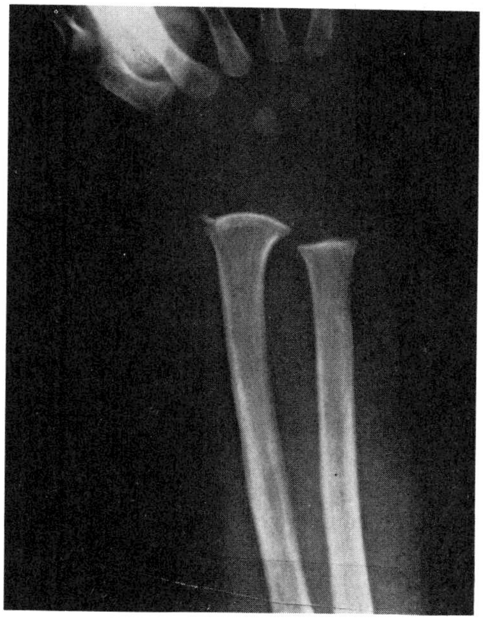

**FIGURE 53–3.** An 8-month-old girl with scurvy. Dense white lines and rarefaction are present at the distal ends of the radius and ulna. The "corner sign" of scurvy, noted at the distal lateral aspect of the radius, is the result of a defect at the angle between the provisional zone of calcification and the cortex.

pliable. Whereas in osteoporosis the thin and brittle bones fracture easily, in osteomalacia there is more likely to be bending of the bony structures. The bone mass is still of normal volume, but a loss of bone density occurs.[11]

Most often osteomalacia is related to malabsorption as a result of a variety of conditions: sprue, steatorrhea, pancreatic insufficiency, Crohn's disease, gastric or small bowel resections, fistulas, or chronic ulcerative colitis. Radiographically the bone density is decreased; however, this may be hard to recognize. The trabeculae are poorly defined and coarse, with widening of the intertrabecular spaces. The most striking feature is that, in areas of stress, pseudofractures appear as thin radiolucent lines extending across the cortex at right angles to the long axis of the bone.[12] These fractures are most often symmetrical and bilateral. With treatment, the margins become sclerotic, but angulation often occurs at the site. One theory is that the fractures are related to pulsating periosteal blood vessels; however, this relationship seems unlikely. In partially treated or untreated cases, these zones of lucency remain for considerable periods. The bones most commonly affected are the first or lower ribs, the pubic rami, the transverse processes of the lumbar vertebrae, the lateral scapular borders, the tibiae and fibulae and the shafts of the femoral necks. In chronic and untreated cases, gross skeletal deformities may result.

## RICKETS

Rickets, a disease of infancy and childhood, is a metabolic disorder of bone characterized by formation of normal collagen, matrix, and osteoid with a disturbance in calcium and phosphorus metabolism that prevents the normal deposition of calcium salts in the growing parts of the skeleton. The skeleton becomes weak, is unable to withstand the stress and strain to which it is ordinarily subjected, and yields and deforms. For the development of ordinary rickets, a deficiency must exist both in the short ultraviolet radiations of the sun and in the vitamin D present in certain foods. Osteomalacia is merely deficiency rickets occurring after endochondral growth has ended.

The roentgenograms give the most accurate information regarding rickets. The costochondral junctions, the most actively growing bones, are not accessible for clear radiographic study early in the course of rickets. The lower end of the femur is too thick and the junction of the epiphysis with the diaphysis is too uneven for slight changes to show distinctly. The lower ends of the radius and ulna are most useful for the study of rickets by x-ray pictures because of their small size and convenient location. Significant changes are often visible in the ulna when the radius appears to be normal.

The changes at the cartilage shaft junction are characterized by total or partial lack of calcification of the terminal segment of the shaft. This "invisible" provisional zone of calcification is seen only in rickets

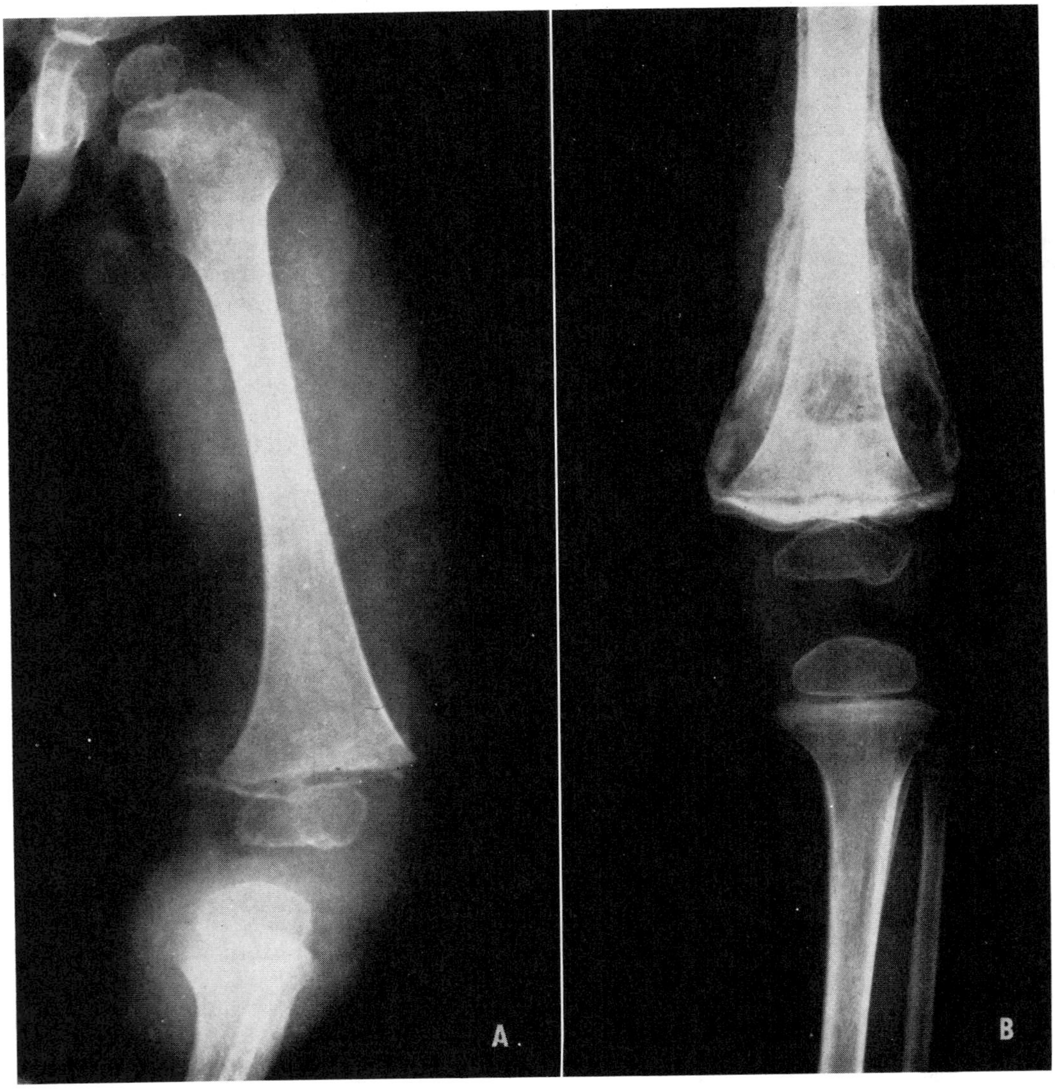
A
B

**FIGURE 53–4.** A 12-month-old boy with healing scurvy. *A*, Fracture of the provisional zone of calcification of the distal femur with early calcification is apparent. Displacement of the soft tissues is due to hematoma, which has not begun to calcify. *B*, Extensive calcification of elevated periosteum occurs after two weeks of vitamin C therapy.

(Fig. 53–5*A*). Cupping, spreading, cortical spurs, and fraying at the ends of bones are also seen in rickets, but not one of these changes itself is characteristic of this disease. Each may be seen in other conditions such as congenital syphilis or scurvy.

Cupping may not be evident until treatment is begun because of the lack of lime salts in the organic tissue that forms the cup (Fig. 53–5*B* and *C*). Cupping may be seen in scurvy, to a slight degree, in the ulnae of young, especially premature, infants whose bones are growing rapidly.

Cortical spurs are linear shadows that extend as prolongations of the shadows of the cortex along the sides of the proliferative cartilage[13] (Fig. 53–5*B*). They are not always in the direct line of the cortex but are external to it, since they lie in the perichondrial-periosteal layer that envelops the cortex. Such shadows may be found on one or both sides; they may be straight and in line of the cortex or they may arch outward. The shape and direction of the spurs are determined by the configuration of the proliferative cartilage. X-ray films often show the spurs lying external to the cortex, overlapping, and seeming to splint the cartilage shaft junction. This represents a new cortical layer forming outside the old. Spur formation also occurs in congenital syphilis.

Fraying consists of thread-like calcified shadows extending from the end of the shaft into the transparent cartilage[14] (Fig. 53–5*B*). These frayed densities are

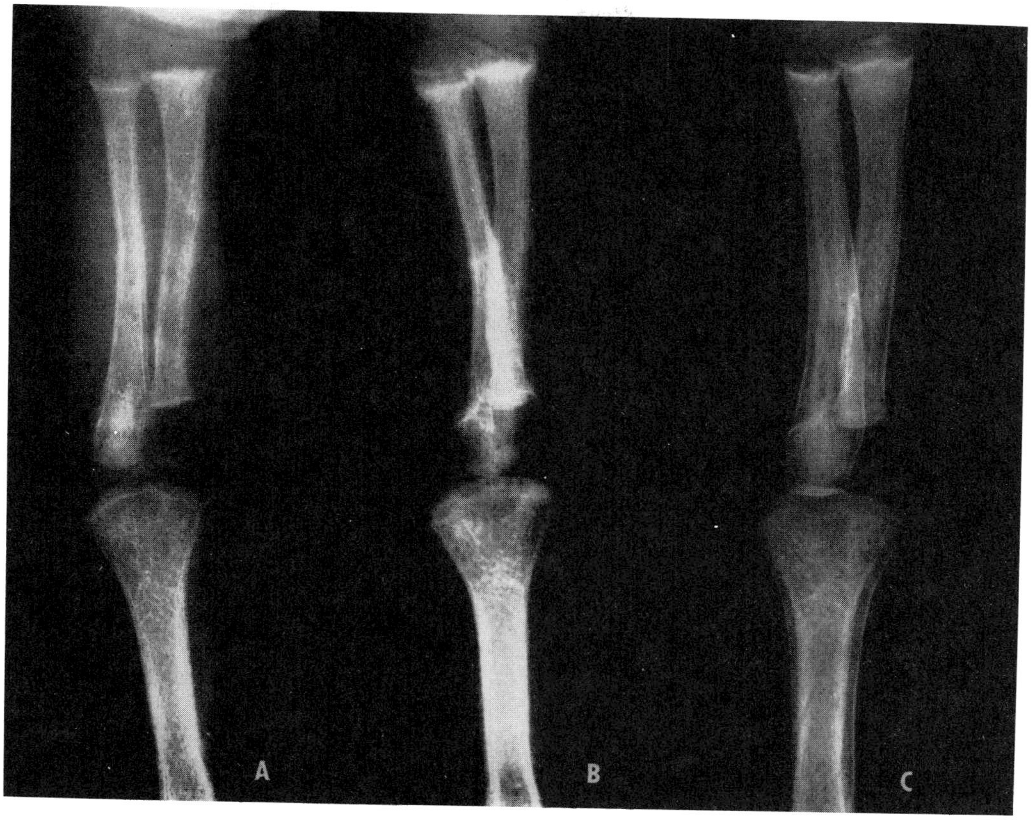
A
B
C

**FIGURE 53–5.** A 10-month-old boy during various stages of rickets. *A*, Noncalcified provisional zone, and fraying of the distal humerus are evident. Strands of calcified osteoid project from the sides of the bone. *B*, Cupping, spread metaphysis, fraying, and cortical spurs occur. Transverse linear recalcified density develops in rachitic metaphysis. A fracture is present in the midshaft of the radius. Greenstick fractures are common in the long bones. *C*, Metaphyseal spongiosum recalcifies and fuses with that of the provisional zone of calcification. Diffuse layer of recalcified cortex is present.

neither straight nor parallel but extend in various directions, exactly as would be expected from the disorder in the underlying pathologic condition.

In severe rickets, the shaft of the bone shows a diffuse rarefaction caused by the loss of lime. The cortex may be thin and, in places, invisible. Strands of osteoid may extend from the poorly defined cortex to the almost invisible periosteum, which contains enough lime salts to cast hair-like shadows sticking out from the sides of the bones (Fig. 53–5*A*). Other changes in the shaft that may be visible are complete or partial fracture, callus formation, curvature of the shaft, with great thickening on the concave side, or displacement of the epiphysis on the diaphysis.

Healing rickets is first observed in the provisional zone of calcification. A transverse linear recalcified density develops in the rachitic metaphysis beyond the visible end of the shaft and at a level the epiphyseal plate would have reached in the absence of rickets (Fig. 53–5*B*). As healing continues, the new provisional zone of calcification thickens. The metaphyseal spongiosum also recalcifies and fuses with that of the provisional zone of calcification. The cortex heals more slowly and is less conspicuous roentgenographically. However, when layers of osteoid have been deposited under the periosteum, recalcification of this osteoid discloses a diffuse layer or cortex, which may be of uniform density or lamellated (Fig. 53–5*C*).

Complete healing can be achieved in deficiency rickets. Distortion and sclerosis in the bone remain visible in the same level of the shaft for years, and cortical thickening on the concave surfaces of curvature deformities may also remain. Most bowing and angulation deformities result from displacement of the epiphyseal cartilage. Angulation deformities may also be secondary to pathologic fractures.

Rickets may be distinguished from scurvy by the tenderness and pain present with scurvy, which exceeds anything found in rickets. The various hemorrhagic phenomena seen with scurvy do not occur in rickets. Difficulty may be encountered in distinguishing the enlargement of the costochondral junctions found in scurvy from that found in rickets. Differentiation may be impossible.

Vitamin D and C deficiencies occur commonly together, since both vitamins must be given as accessories to the diet. If one is not given, it often happens that the other is omitted also. The association is thus due to chance, not to any chemical interrelationship between the two vitamins. However, a deficiency in one vitamin may prevent deficiency in the other from expressing itself by characteristic symptoms and signs. If vitamin D deficiency is sufficiently severe and prolonged, the lattice of calcified matrix framework, which is a characteristic feature of scurvy, cannot form at all or forms imperfectly. In scurvy the collapse of the brittle lattice framework is responsible for the fractures and the development of subperiosteal hemorrhage—and probably the pain and tenderness. Thus, as a result of suppressing the development of the lattice, vitamin D deficiency may prevent or modify important symptoms of scurvy, typical roentgenographic signs, and characteristic histology.

## IRON DEFICIENCY ANEMIA

Roentgenographic changes in the skeleton in association with congenital hemolytic anemia result from increased proliferation of hematopoietic tissue in the bone marrow.

In 1936 Sheldon first described a child with changes in the skull in association with iron deficiency anemia.[15] In the 1960s many other reports described such changes.[16–20] Lanzkowsky[21] reported several children with iron deficiency anemia who had changes in the metacarpals as well as in the skull.

The degree of change in the roentgenograms of the skull and metacarpals is variable. Children with marked changes are similar to those seen with severe congenital hemolytic anemias. The diploic space of the skull is widened in a nonuniform manner. The squama occipitalis is usually not wide, a result of normally deficient marrow in this portion of the skull. The trabeculae may be perpendicular to the inner table, presenting a radial pattern that may have a "hair-on-end" appearance (Figs. 53–6*A* and *B* and 53–7).

## HYPERVITAMINOSIS A

Early roentgenographic findings of chronic vitamin A poisoning may be limited to widened sutures in the skull and a bulging anterior fontanelle (Fig. 53–8*A* and *B*). The long bones (Figs. 53–9*A* and 53–10) may be normal at this stage of the disease. The 2-year-old patient represented in Figures 53–8 to 53–10 was seen for anorexia and vomiting. Because her fontanelle was full, a skull x-ray film was taken and demonstrated sutural diastasis. The dense line at the metaphyses of all long bones suggested lead poisoning. The history of a "poor eater" raised the possibility of pica, but careful questioning revealed that "extra" cod liver oil had been given, 100,000 units of vitamin A and 15,000 units of vitamin D, one to three times a day, intermittently during the previous 6 months. Serum vitamin A level was elevated. The dense line was considered to be caused by excess vitamin D. Two weeks after the diagnosis and the

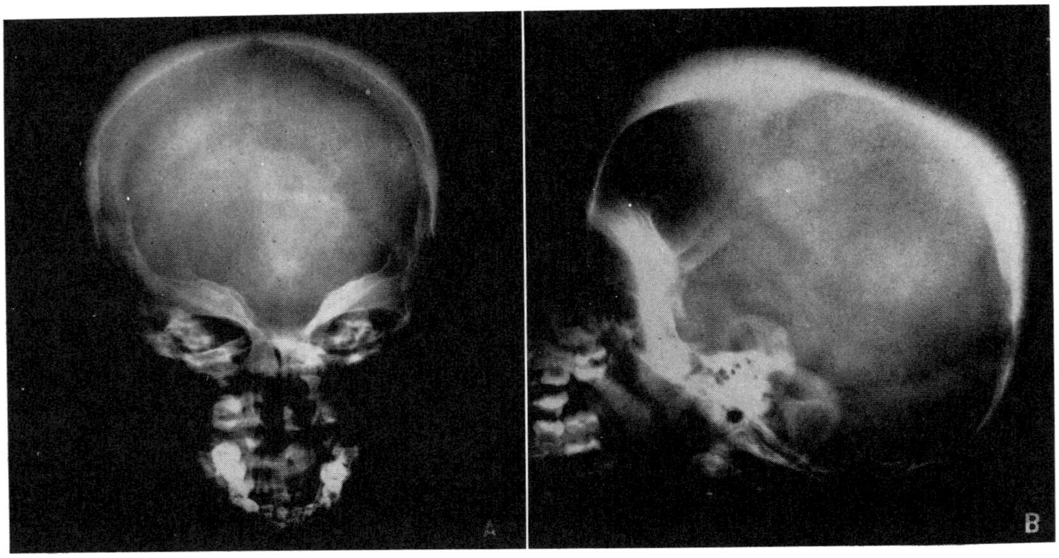
A
B

**FIGURE 53–6.** Frontal *(A)* and lateral *(B)* views of the skull in a young child with iron deficiency anemia demonstrating nonuniform widening of the diploic space with a "hair-on-end" appearance. (Courtesy of Dr. Philip Lanzkowsky.)

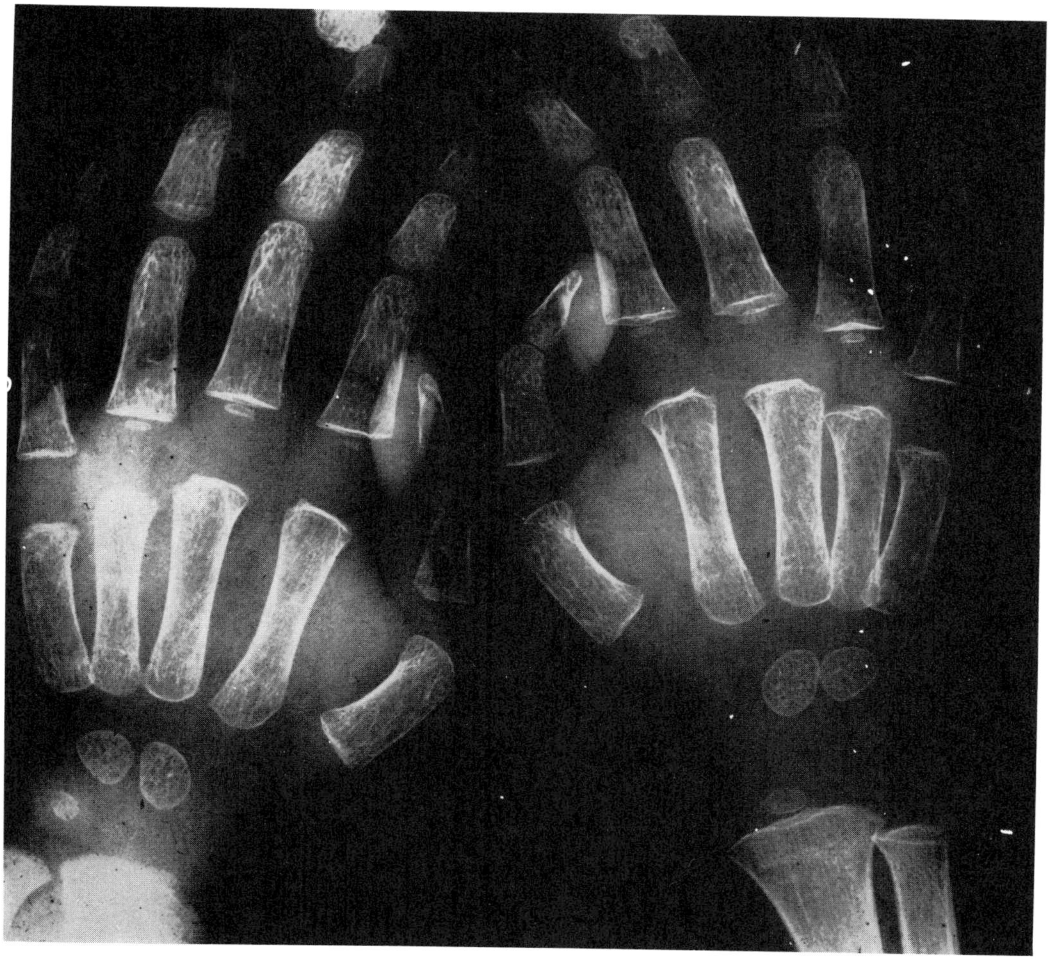

**FIGURE 53–7.** The hands of a child with iron deficiency anemia. Widening of the metacarpals, prominent trabeculae of the bones of the hands, and thin cortices are evident. (Courtesy of Dr. Philip Lanzkowsky.)

cessation of vitamin A, cortical hyperostosis was present on the ulnae (Fig. 53–9*B*) and the fibulae. The bone changes are usually symmetrical. Three weeks after admission of the child to the hospital, the serum vitamin A became normal but the hyperostosis continued.

When soft tissue swellings are noted in association with clinical symptoms of vitamin A toxicity (e.g., anorexia, pruritus, alopecia, desquamation of the skin), cortical thickening of long bones is present (Fig. 53–11*A*). Although vitamin A then is eliminated from the diet, the changes in the bones continue. The subperiosteal new bone continues to thicken (Fig. 53–11*B*). These cortical thickenings usually stop short of the ends of the shafts. In some patients metaphyseal cupping, splaying of the affected end of the shaft, hypertrophy of the contiguous epiphyseal ossification center, and premature fusion of this center with the shaft are found (Fig. 53–11*B* and *C*). Premature fusion of the center with its shafts is most often seen at the distal ends of the femurs and results in arrested growth, with permanent shortening of the affected bones. Although these changes at the metaphyses and epiphyses were demonstrated in experimental animals,[23,24] it was not until Pease[25] reported seven patients in 1962 that this complication of vitamin poisoning was universally accepted. Cortical hyperostosis of ribs also occurs with vitamin A poisoning (Fig. 53–12).

Caffey reviewed the many diseases that cause cupping of the metaphyses.[26] He believes that the basic defect is a reduced growth in the arterial segment of the epiphyseal plate. The "walls" of the cup are dependent on the periosteal and metaphyseal arteries, not on the epiphyseal arteries. Therefore, the peripheral zones of the bones continue to grow. Caffey suggests that in vitamin A poisoning, spontaneous immobilization is caused by exquisite pain and hyperesthesia. Immobilization causes slowing and stagnation of the blood, which lead to thrombosis of the arteries of the epiphyseal plate.

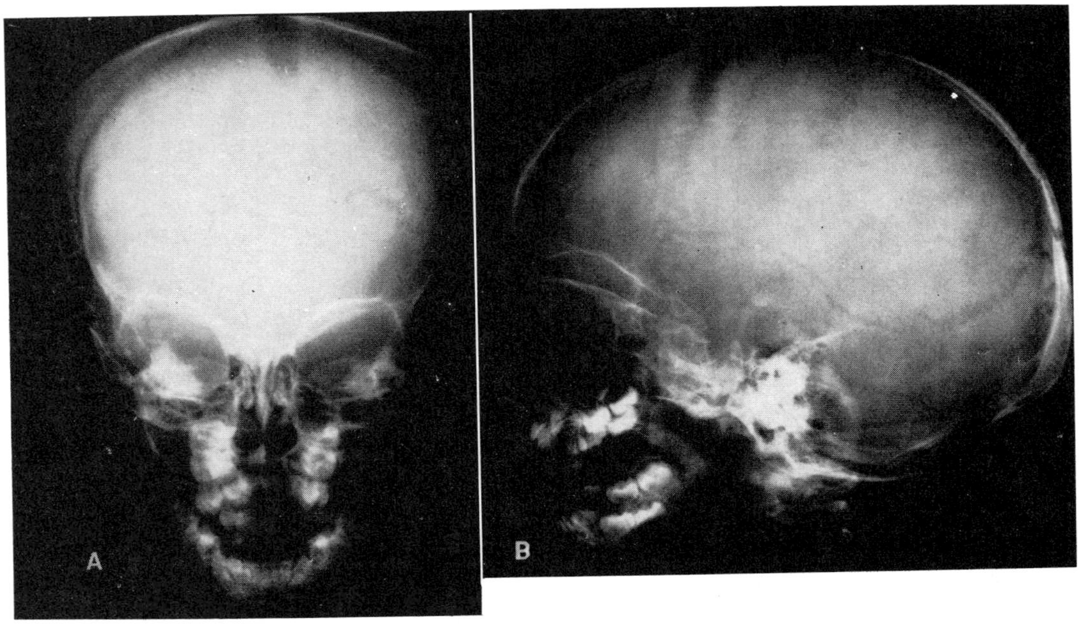
A
B

**FIGURE 53–8.** *A* and *B*. Skull of a 2-year-old girl, in frontal and lateral projections, with hypervitaminosis A showing wide sagittal and coronal sutures.

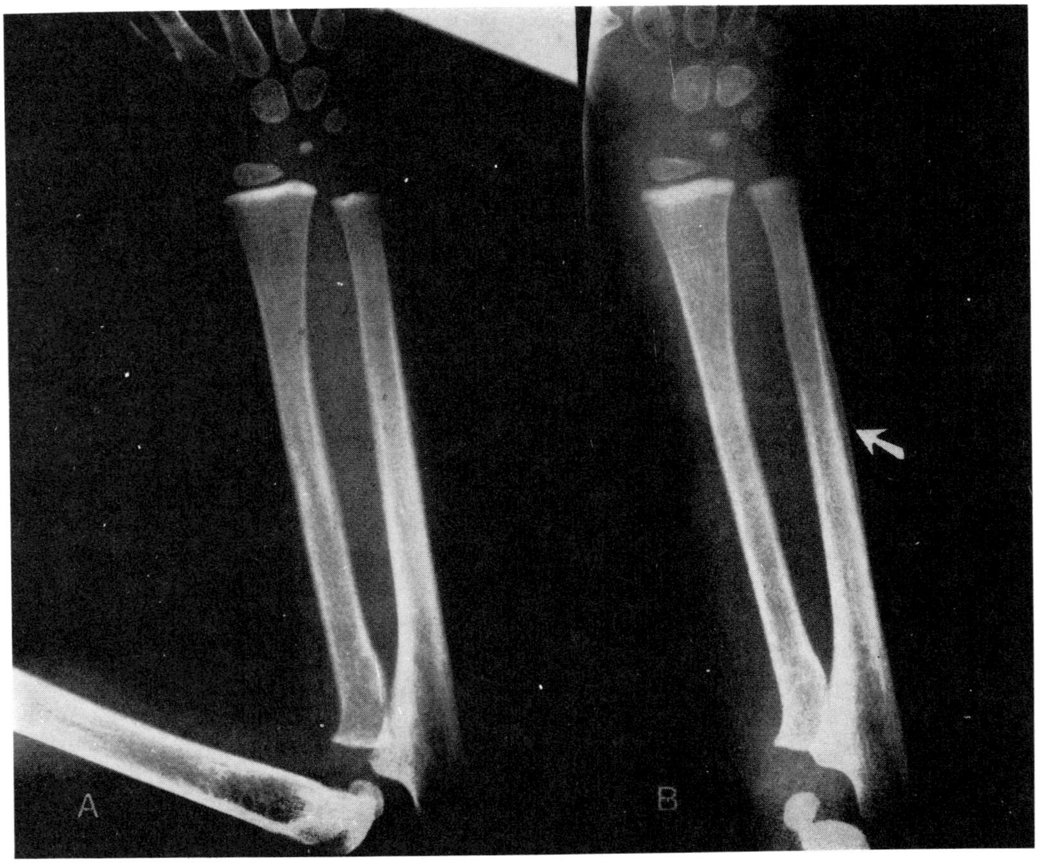
A
B

**FIGURE 53–9.** Same patient as in Figure 53–8. *A*, Dense line occurs at the distal end of radius and ulna. No subperiosteal new bone is present. *B*, Three weeks later periosteal new bone is seen on the lateral aspect of the ulna.

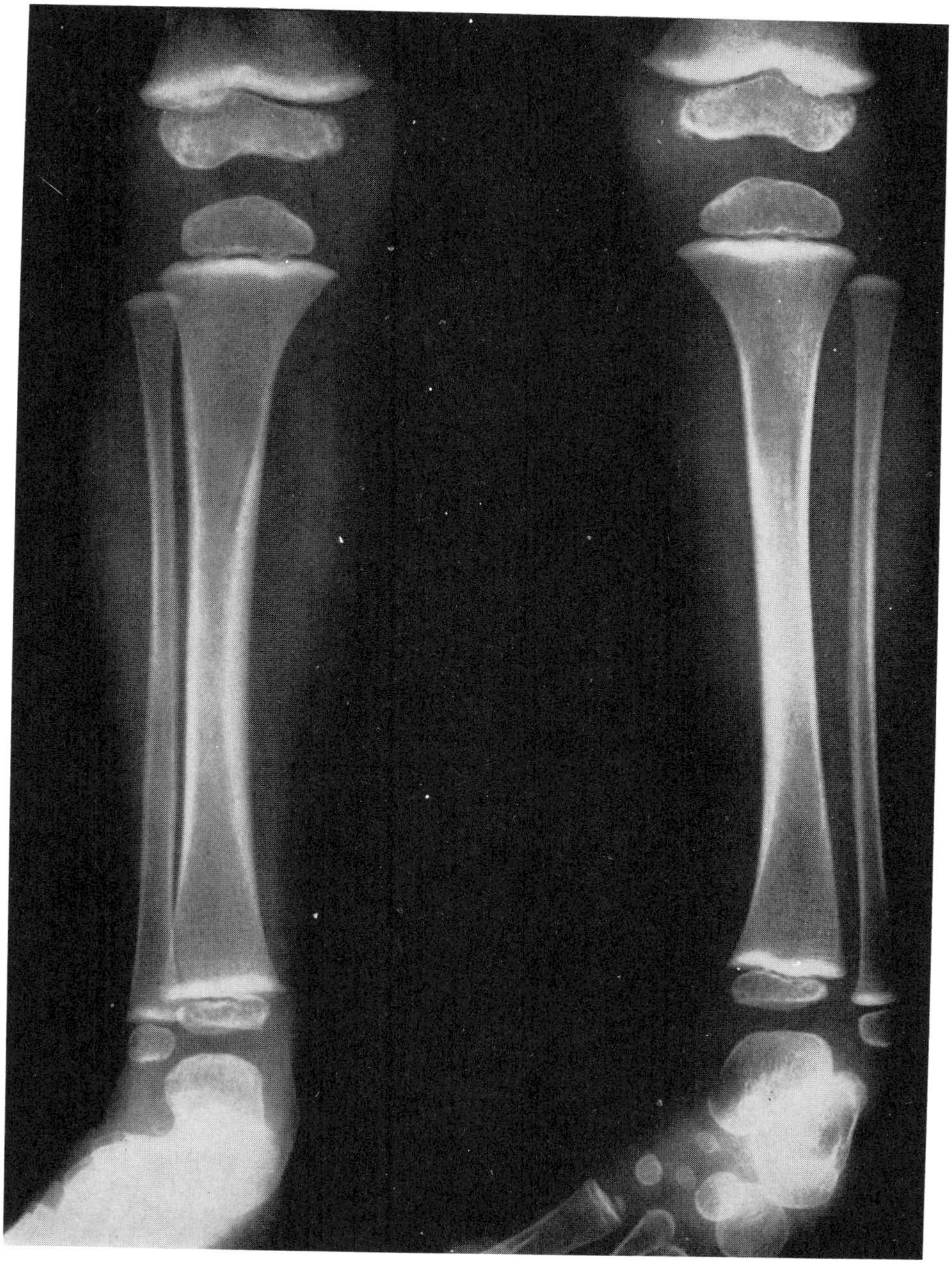

**FIGURE 53–10.** Same patient as in Figure 53–8. Initial roentgenograms of the metaphyses at the knees and ankles demonstrate dense lines. No periosteal new bone is present.

## HYPERVITAMINOSIS D

In the presence of an excess of vitamin D, an increased mobilization of mineral occurs with secondary hypercalcemia and phosphatemia.[27] Calcific deposits occur in the renal tubules with secondary renal failure, and sometimes death results. In the growing child, the zone of provisional calcification becomes relatively dense in comparison to the adjacent metaphyseal region. In addition, extensive periarticular and vessel calcification may be present with, in some cases, premature vascular calcification.[28,29] When the calcium intake is correspondingly high, thickening of the bony cortex may result so that, instead of decreased density, the bones may in fact be more dense. Distinguishing between this entity,

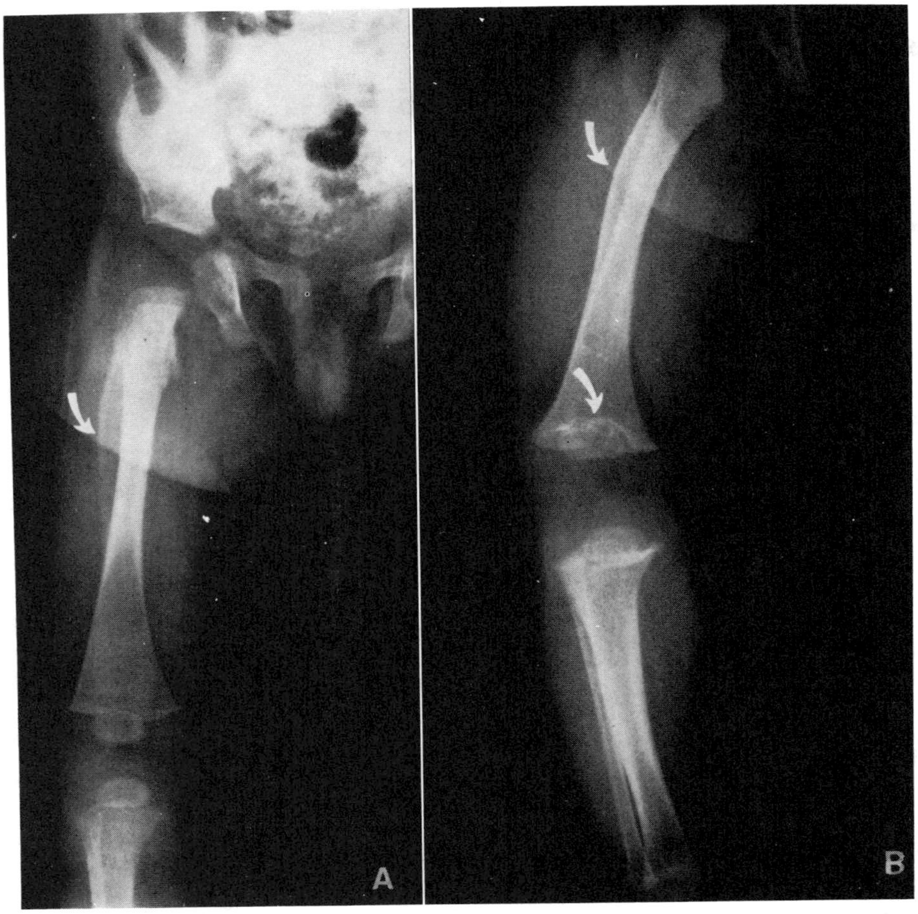
A
B

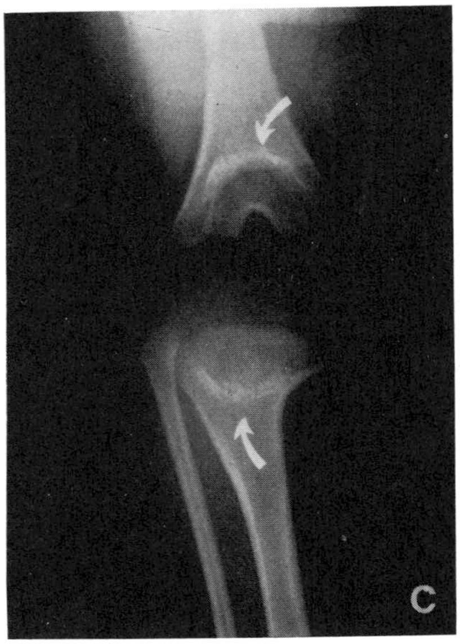
C

**FIGURE 53–11.** Frontal view of the right lower extremity of an 18-month-old child who had received 50,000 to 250,000 U vitamin A since 3 months of age. *A*, Cortical hyperostosis of the femur is evident. *B*, The cortical thickening is more dense and there is metaphyseal cupping of the femur and tibia 4 months after initial diagnosis. The distal end of the tibia is not affected. *C*, Nine months after the initial roentgenograms the cartilage plates are narrow, and the epiphyseal ossification centers and their respective shafts are fusing in the central segments of the cartilage plates. The ossification centers are buried into the metaphyseal cups. The joint spaces are increased. The defects were bilateral and symmetric. (Courtesy of Dr. A. Geffin.)

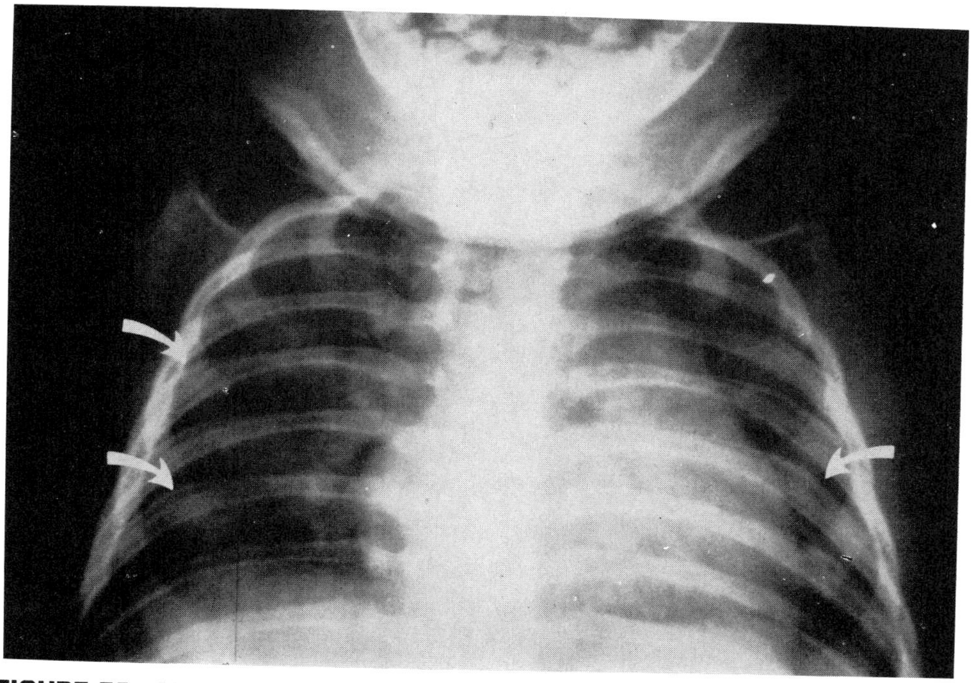

**FIGURE 53–12.** Same patient as in Figure 53–11. Chest roentgenogram shows cortical hyperostosis of many ribs caused by vitamin A poisoning.

hypercalcemia, and hypovitaminosis D can be difficult radiographically.

## SUTURAL DIASTASIS FOLLOWING RAPID WEIGHT GAIN

Sutural diastasis has been considered a sign of acute raised intracranial pressure in children, especially those under the age of 10 years. Capitanio and Kirkpatrick described three children with nutritional deprivation who developed increased head circumference and cranial sutures following the correction of malnutrition.[30] In 1970, two other reports added nine more children with these changes related to nutrition.[31,32] The increased head circumference and separation of the cranial sutures (Fig. 53–13*A* and *B*) are caused by cellular growth of the brain when nutrition is improved in previously malnourished young children.[33] Although the sutural diastasis simulates increased intracranial pressure, there are no abnormal neurologic signs or symptoms. No increased intracranial pressure has been noted and, in the one patient who had a pneumoencephalogram, the lateral ventricles were normal.

Distention of the stomach may be apparent on abdominal roentgenogram in nutritional deprivation. One patient had a small bowel study done as part of the workup for "failure to thrive." Thickened valvulae conniventes and separation of loops, noted on an early examination (Fig. 53–14*A*), were normal on an examination 1 month later (Fig. 53–14*B*). The pathogenesis of the gastrointestinal changes is not known, but it was thought that these findings were the result of edema, although the serum albumin was normal.

## MILK-ALKALI SYNDROME

With excessive ingestion of milk and alkali, usually related to peptic ulcer disease, insoluble calcium and phosphate precipitates may occur,[34] resulting in a renal tubular deposition of calcium with visible demonstration of nephrocalcinosis. To a certain extent, the condition can be relieved by limiting the intake of calcium. Soft tissue calcification, usually periarticular in nature, is also a feature of this syndrome; however, the most common finding is that of calculi within the upper urinary tracts.[35]

## FLUOROSIS

When fluorine is used to excess, probably above levels of 4 million ppm in water, or in the treatment of osteoporosis, multiple myeloma, or Paget's disease, certain side effects may be demonstrated.[36] Arguments persist as to the exact mechanism by which fluorine exerts its effects, but in all probability it acts by

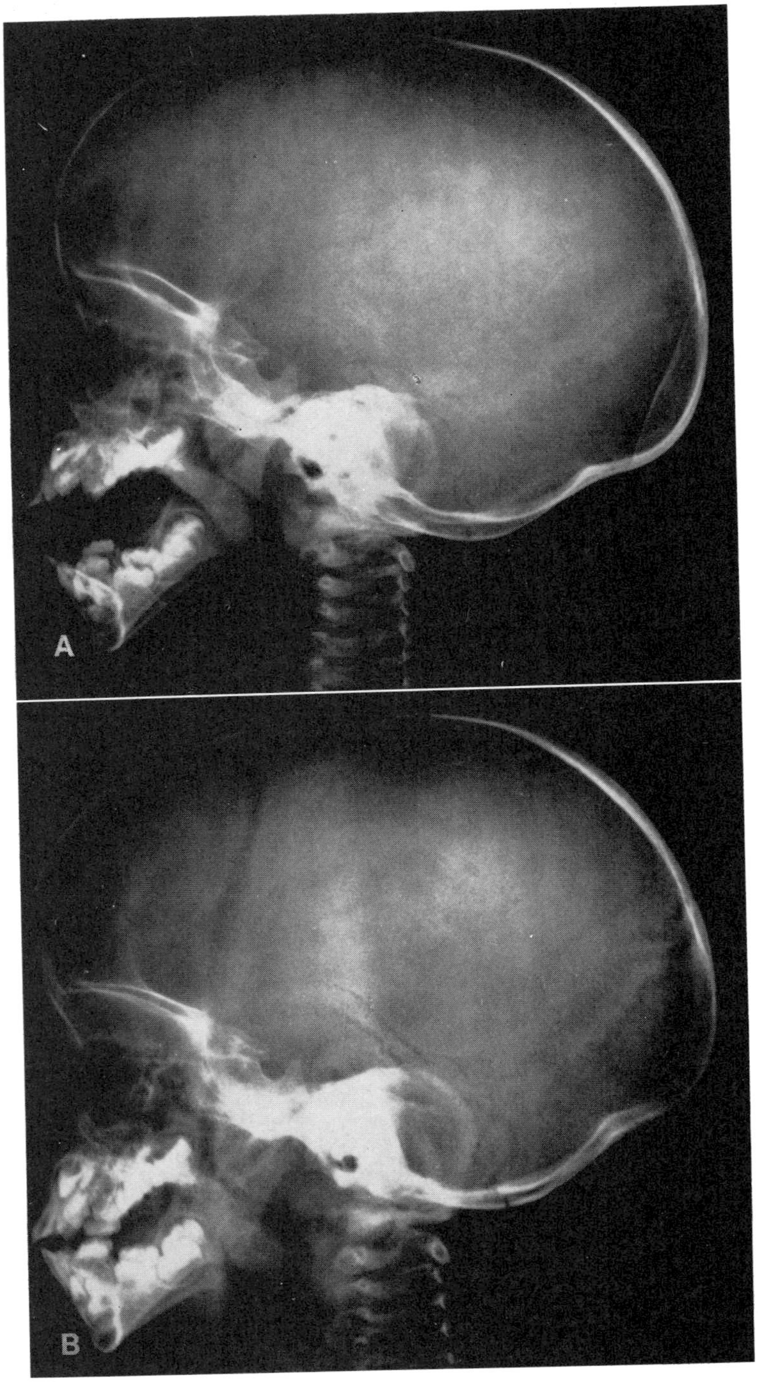
A
B

**FIGURE 53–13.** A 30-month-old boy hospitalized for failure to thrive. *A*, Lateral skull roentgenogram at time of admission is normal. *B*, Two months later, when the child had gained weight and was well, the lateral skull roentgenogram demonstrates wide coronal and lambdoid sutures.

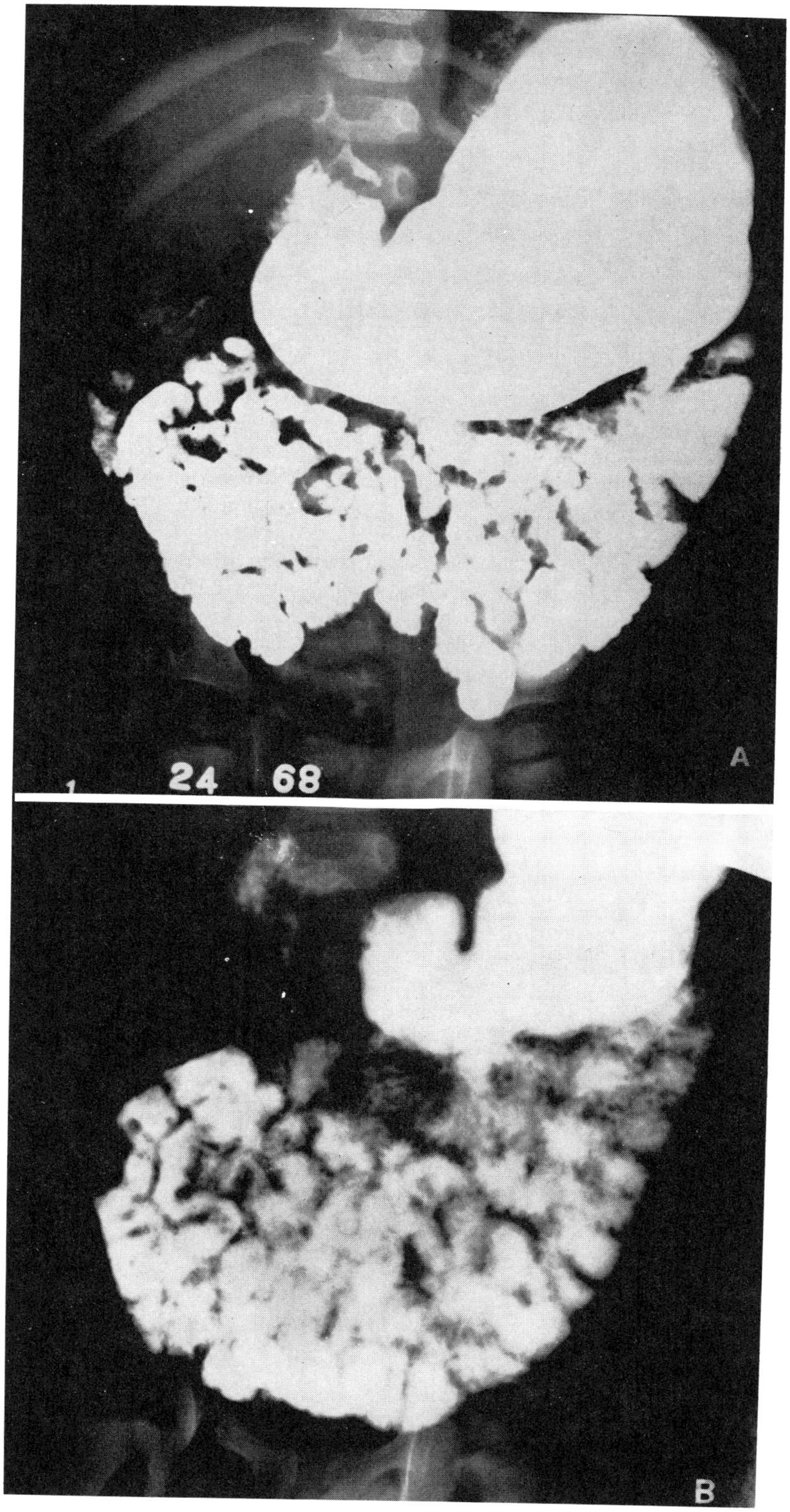
24 68
A
B

**FIGURE 53–14.** *A*, Gastrointestinal series 2 weeks after admission demonstrates a large stomach and separated loops of small intestine with thickened valvulae conniventes. *B*, Four weeks after the original study, when the patient was well, repeated intestinal studies show the small intestine to be normal.

decreasing the solubility of bone salts, thus impairing the process of osteolysis. Radiographically, thickening and coarsening of the trabeculae and similar changes in the cortex are seen. The overall result is one of increased density of the bony structure, although the underlying abnormality is sometimes difficult to visualize. Similar changes, of course, are seen in cases of myelosclerosis and myelofibrosis.

## LEAD AND BISMUTH POISONING

Both these heavy metals have an affinity for bone and act by replacing calcium. In these days the effects of bismuth are rarely seen, as it is seldom used for the treatment of syphilis in the growing child except when the mother has been treated during pregnancy. However, cases of lead poisoning still occur where eating lead paint has been the causative factor. In the growing child, deposition of heavy metals is principally seen in the region of the metaphyses of long bones, particularly where there is accelerated growth, i.e., the knee, ankle, and wrist. Intoxication makes itself evident by zones of increased density in this region. Confirmation may be obtained by the visualization of heavy metal content in the GI tract, together with widening of the skull sutures, indicating increased intracranial pressure.

## GASTROINTESTINAL DISTURBANCES

Although the clinical presentation of gastrointestinal abnormalities that may lead to nutritional disturbances is often nonspecific, gastrointestinal contrast studies may be crucial in making the correct initial diagnosis, in outlining the site and extent of disease, or in indicating the likely underlying entities requiring further investigation. In many of these conditions, x-ray interpretation relies upon subtle but characteristic findings. It must be emphasized that x-ray abnormalities may reflect pathologic anatomic changes or physiologic disturbances.

### MALABSORPTION SYNDROMES

**Sprue.** This group of diseases includes celiac diseases of children, nontropical sprue (gluten-induced enteropathy, idiopathic steatorrhea), and tropical sprue. Characteristic radiologic changes in the small intestine are present in almost all patients during the active phase of the disease.[37,38] The essential elements of this deficiency state include: (1) dilatation of small bowel loop, either diffusely or more markedly in the middle and distal jejunum, and (2) hypersecretion, shown by dilution of the barium suspension, often with striking flocculation and segmentation (Fig. 53–15*A* and *B*).

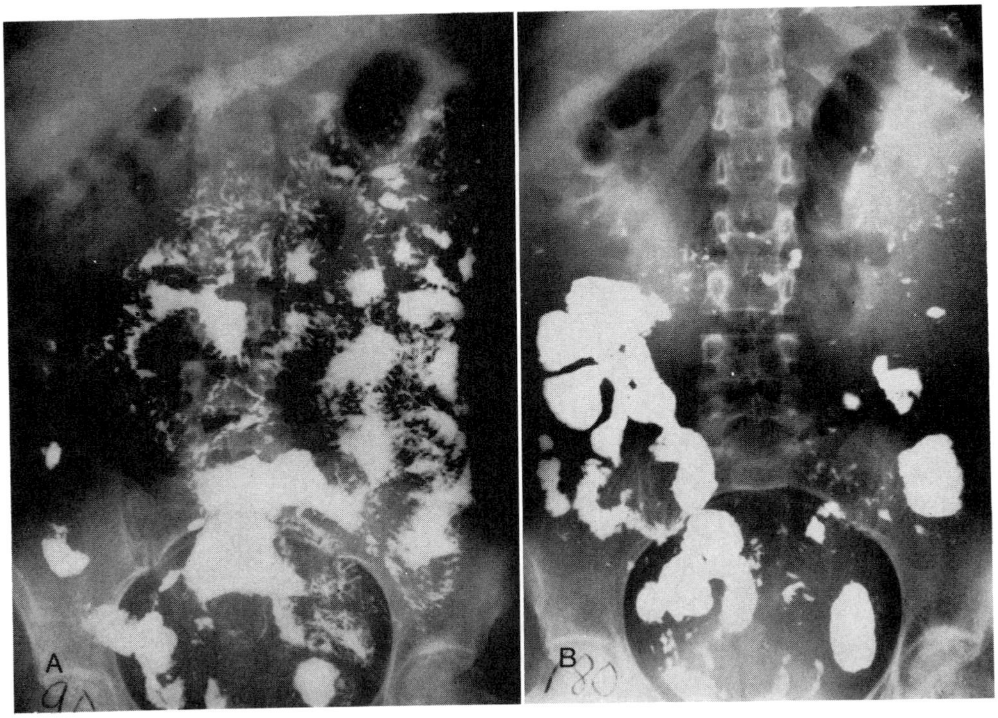
A
90
B
180

**FIGURE 53–15.** Nontropical sprue. *A*, At 90 minutes, conspicuous fragmentation and flocculation of the barium suspension are seen. Disordered motor activity is apparent. *B*, At 180 minutes, segmentation of the contrast within ileal loops, further reflecting hypersecretion.

Frazier et al. have shown that the classic "deficiency pattern" of segmentation within the small bowel is not necessarily associated with disordered motor function of the intestinal wall but is dependent upon the quality of the contents of the intestinal lumen.[39] The loops are flaccid and contract poorly, so that the transit time through the small bowel may be delayed. Little intrinsic change occurs in the mucosal folds. Their appearance is dependent upon the amount of secretions and peristaltic disorder. Short nonobstructive intussusceptions may transiently occur.[40]

The peculiar relationship of sprue and lymphosarcoma of the bowel[41] must be kept in mind. Not only may lymphoma demonstrate sprue-like malabsorption,[42] but the incidence of lymphoma complicating well-documented chronic cases of adult celiac disease is about 7%.[43] Roentgenographic study may be helpful in the distinction.[38]

Malabsorption and a sprue-like radiologic pattern may result from vascular insufficiency of the small bowel.[44,45] This condition must be suspected clinically if malabsorption appears in middle or later life, particularly if accompanied by abdominal angina or manifestations of atherosclerotic occlusive disease elsewhere. Abdominal aortography and selective arteriography may be crucial in establishing the diagnosis. Revascularization procedures have been shown to reverse the steatorrhea.[45]

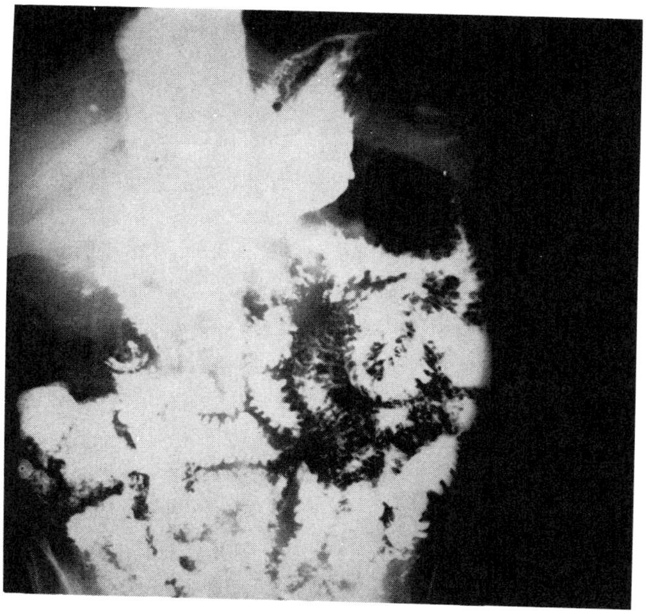

**FIGURE 53–16.** Whipple's disease. Markedly prominent valvulae conniventes without hypersecretion or dilatation are present.

**Whipple's Disease (Intestinal Lipodystrophy).** Although the multisystem involvement of this disease is shown by the major clinical manifestations of diarrhea, steatorrhea, arthralgias, increased skin pigmentation, lymphadenopathy, and serous effusions, the intestinal symptoms are usually predominant by the time the diagnosis is established.

Small intestinal series demonstrate definite thickening of the mucosal folds in the jejunum and duodenum and only occasionally in the ileum (Fig. 53–16). The coarsened folds are frequently wild and redundant in outline and may present slightly nodular contours. No significant hypersecretion or dilatation is shown; any flocculation or segmentation is minimal. There is normal peristaltic activity, and transit time from stomach to cecum is within normal limits.[46,47]

The diagnosis can be established by intestinal mucosal or lymph node biopsy. The small bowel villi are swollen and the lamina propria is infiltrated with macrophages containing PAS-positive bodies. These have been shown to be bacteria.[48] Improvement in the radiologic picture may parallel the clinical remission on long-term antibiotic therapy.[47]

**Scleroderma (Diffuse Systemic Sclerosis).** The hallmarks of sclerodermatous involvement of the alimentary tract are dilatation and a marked diminution in peristaltic activity. These symptoms reflect the underlying pathologic changes of collagen replacement of the muscular layers. Bacterial overgrowth in the intestinal lumen is now recognized as a major cause for steatorrhea in patients with scleroderma.

The esophagus is most commonly involved and presents hypomotility and some dilatation. Poor drainage results. Characteristic roentgenographic findings include failure of the esophagus to empty on prone films and stasis even in the erect position, with air-fluid levels (Fig. 53–17*A*).

In the intestines, large flaccid loops are seen without hypersecretion. The dilatation may appear most striking in the descending duodenum (Fig. 53–17*B*). Transit time is often markedly prolonged. Colonic dilatation and hypotonicity may also be present, with characteristic secondary pseudosacculations projecting from the antimesenteric border of the transverse colon (Fig. 53–17*C*).

**Amyloidosis.** The presence of malabsorption in some patients with amyloidosis has been well established.[49] In a report from the Mayo Clinic, Herskovic et al. reviewed 103 patients with amyloidosis and found 6 with documented steatorrhea.[50] With known gastrointestinal involvement, the incidence of malabsorption may approach 50%.[51] Radiologically, markedly diminished motility, conspicuous valvulae conniventes and, rarely, tumor-like deposits scattered throughout the intestinal tract may be present.[51]

**Disaccharidase Deficiency.** This condition is probably the most common abnormality of the small bowel in man, the only known mammal in whom lactase activity in the small intestine is maintained after weaning.

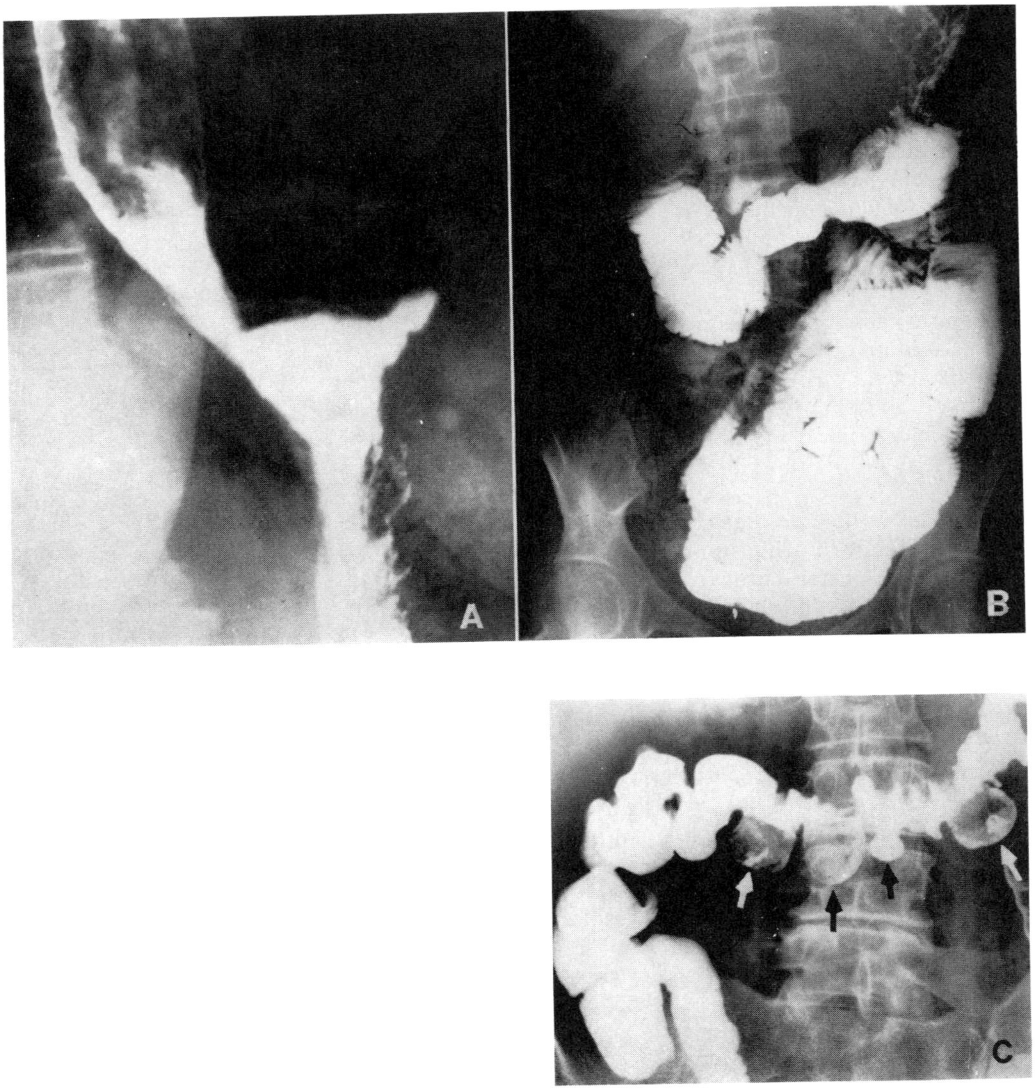
A
B
C

**FIGURE 53–17.** Scleroderma. *A*, Despite a nonobstructed lumen, differential fluid levels persist in the esophagus and stomach in the upright position. *B*, Diffuse involvement of the small bowel results in gross dilatation, most evident in the descending duodenum and jejunum. *C*, Asymmetric involvement of the colon is shown by large wide-mounted pseudosacculation (arrows).

Diarrhea, cramps, and flatulence after milk ingestion clinically indicate the disorder, which can be easily confirmed roentgenologically.[52,53] When 50 g of lactose are added to the usual barium mixture, characteristic changes occur in the small bowel series. These changes include dilution of the barium, particularly noticeable in the ileum and colon, and dilatation of the small bowel (Fig. 53–18). These effects are secondary to the ingress of water into the bowel lumen in response to the osmotic forces of the disaccharide. Rapid intestinal motility accompanies the dilatation.

Intestinal lactase deficiency occurs on a genetic basis and is also common in a variety of intestinal disorders. This radiologic technique is the most valuable screening aid for it. The addition of lactose to the barium sulfate mixture does not interfere with the examination of the small bowel in patients without disaccharidase deficiency. When a lactase deficiency is discovered, a conventional small bowel examination with barium alone is indicated to identify any morphologic abnormality.[53]

**Small Bowel Resection.** The severity of malabsorption after small bowel resection generally depends on the extent and site of resection, presence of the ileocecal valve, and the condition of the remaining small bowel

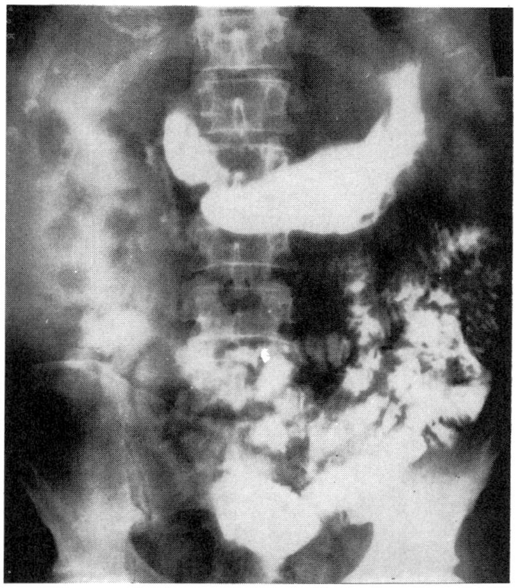

**FIGURE 53–18.** Lactase deficiency. A barium-lactose mixture results in progressive dilution and hypermotility.

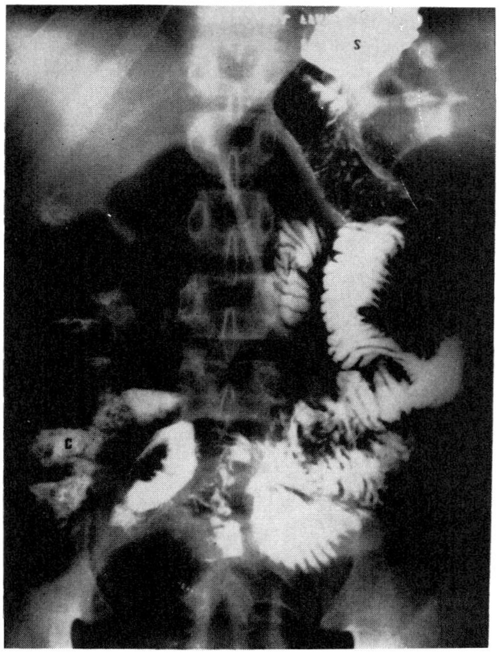
S
C

**FIGURE 53–19.** Massive small bowel resection for volvulus following gastrojejunostomy. Few small bowel loops, primarily jejunal as shown by their mucosal pattern, remain between the stomach pouch (S) and the cecum (C).

and other digestive organs.[54] These parameters of the "short-gut syndrome" can be evaluated by roentgenographic study (Fig. 53–19). On occasion, the exact extent of resection performed in the past is not known when malabsorption becomes a serious problem of management. Since the normal length of small intestine is variable, more important than knowledge of the length of bowel *removed* is an accurate appraisal of the length in the *remaining* functioning loops. Measurements derived from x-ray study after the passage of an opaque tube obviate the inaccuracy inherent in measuring the continuity of superimposed barium-filled loops.

Enteric fistulas and inadvertent gastroileostomy[55] result in a similar condition by bypassing the absorptive mechanisms of the small bowel (Fig. 53–20*A* and *B*).

**Diverticula, Blind Loops, and Strictures.** Common to all these conditions, which may result in malabsorption, is stasis of intestinal contents and bacterial overgrowth. Normally, the small bowel flora consists of predominantly gram-positive and anaerobic organisms. The ileocecal valve serves to separate two distinct groups of organisms: above, mainly streptococci, lactobacilli and fungi; below, coliforms, bacteroides, and anaerobic lactobacilli.[56] In a variety of disease states, an overgrowth of bacteria—especially the anaerobic bacteroides, lactobacilli, and clostridia—may occur and cause steatorrhea by deconjugating and/or dehydroxylating primary bile salts in the intestinal lumen.[57]

Diverticulosis of the small bowel is readily recognized as multiple outpouchings without gross intrinsic contractility from the mesenteric borders of the loops. Blind loops may be a result of (side-to-side) intestinal anastomoses, an obstructed postoperative loop, as in the afferent-loop syndrome following a Billroth II gastrojejunostomy (Fig. 53–21), multiple strictures of the intestine, as in the stenotic phase of regional enteritis,[38] or postradiation changes (Fig. 53–22). In radiation enteritis, lymphatic dilatation, bowel thickening, and avascularity may also contribute to the malabsorption.[58]

**Parasitic Diseases.** The enteritis caused by infestation with *Giardia lamblia*[59] or *Strongyloides stercoralis*[60] is reflected by roentgenographic alterations, which may first draw the attention of the clinician to the diagnosis.

**Dysgammaglobulinemia.** Hypogammaglobulinemia may underlie a clinical pattern of repeated infections and chronic or intermittent diarrhea and mild steatorrhea. In 1966, Hermans and his co-workers noted the association of nodular lymphoid hyperplasia of the small intestine, with or without giardiasis, in cases of dysgammaglobulinemia with a disproportionate deficiency of the IgA and IgM components.[61] These nodular hyperplastic lymphoid follicles in the lamina propria can be recognized as tiny, 1- to 3-mm filling defects, primarily in the duodenum and jejunum[62] (Fig. 53–23*A* and *B*). Their recognition may be an important clue in directing the clinician to evaluation of the gamma globulins and to intestinal biopsy for information necessary in management.

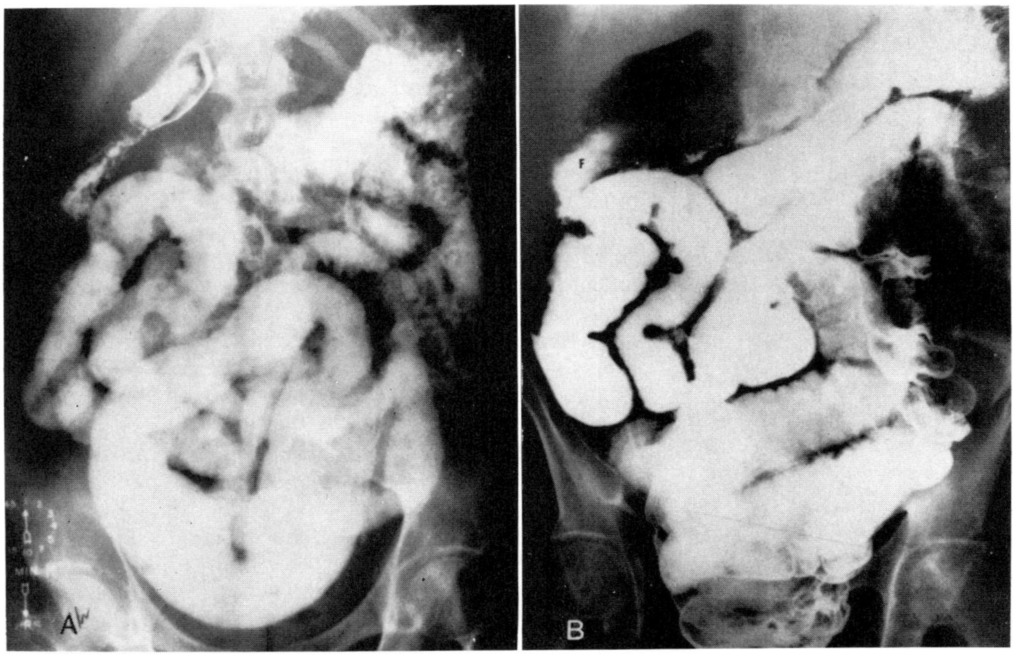
A
F
B

**FIGURE 53–20.** Enteric fistula producing malabsorption following ileotransversostomy. *A*, Dilatation and hypersecretion of small bowel loops. Although there is no flocculation or segmentation, these changes constitute a sprue-like pattern. *B*, During another examination, the fistula (F) between the distal ileum and descending duodenum is demonstrated.

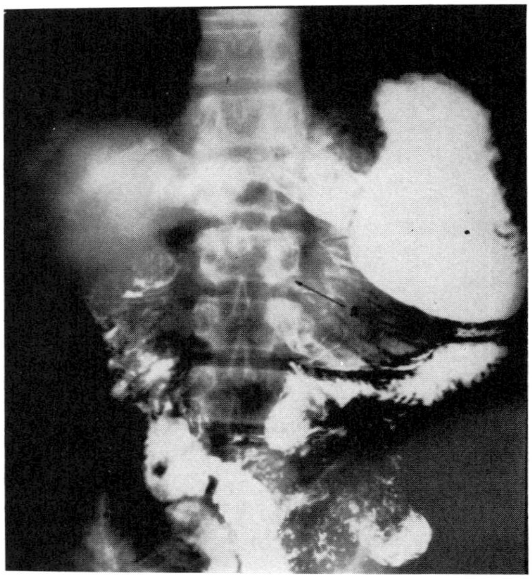

**FIGURE 53–21.** Afferent loop syndrome. The massively distended, obstructed afferent loop following a Billroth II gastrojejunostomy constitutes a blind loop leading to malabsorption.

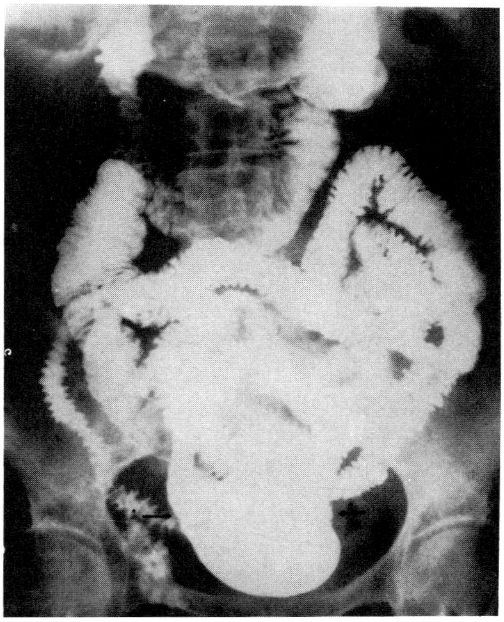

**FIGURE 53–22.** Blind loop secondary to radiation effects. Stasis within a fixed, distended loop occurs as a consequence of multiple strictures.

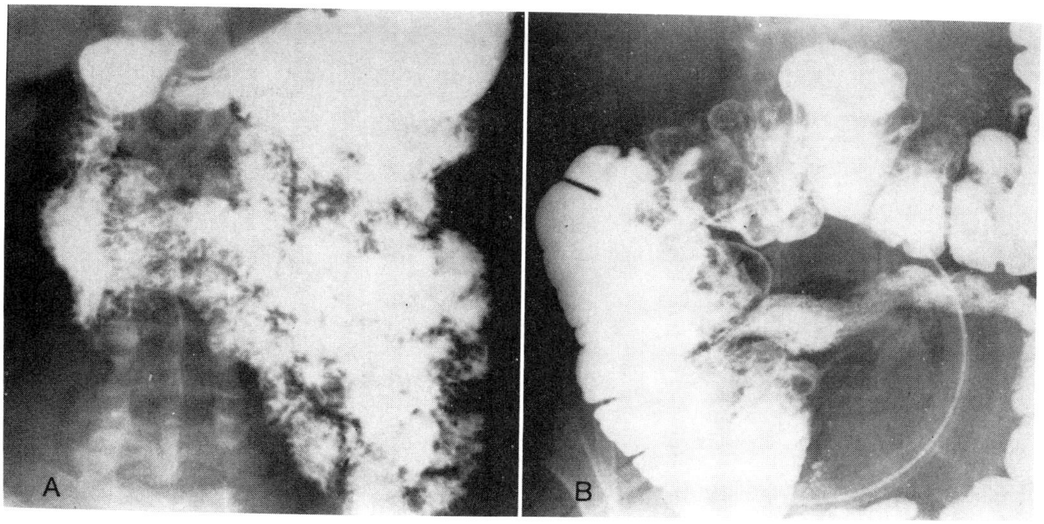
A
B

**FIGURE 53–23.** Nodular lymphoid hyperplasia of the small intestine associated with hypogammaglobulinemia. Two different cases illustrate multiple punctate to nodular submucosal filling defects in the jejunum *(A)* and terminal ileum *(B)*.

**Uncommon Constitutional Disorders.** In recent years, a number of uncommon systemic diseases in which malabsorption may be a significant complication have been recognized. Radiologic abnormalities in the gastrointestinal tract have been noted or are a conspicuous feature in the Canada-Cronkhite syndrome,[63] mastocytosis,[64] Degos' disease,[65] abetalipoproteinemia (Bassen-Kornzweig syndrome),[66] and Waldenström's macroglobulinemia.[67]

## PROTEIN-LOSING ENTEROPATHY

There is now widespread recognition that excessive gastrointestinal protein loss is a major cause of hypoproteinemia seen in association with a wide variety of disorders. Loss of protein secondary to exudation through an inflamed or ulcerated mucosa (as in regional enteritis or ulcerative colitis) or secondary to obstructed outflow of the gastrointestinal lymphatics (as in lymphoma or Whipple's disease) is well known. In an excellent review, Waldmann has compiled over 40 such gastrointestinal disorders and emphasizes that, in many of these patients with clearly defined gastrointestinal tract diseases, hypoproteinemia and edema may be the only clinical manifestations.[68]

**Giant Hypertrophy of the Gastric Mucosa (Menetrier's disease).** Massively enlarged gastric rugae may be the site of loss of plasma proteins, particularly albumin, into the lumen.[69] They characteristically are more prominent along the greater curvature and usually do not extend to involve the gastric antrum. The hypertrophied folds maintain pliability and are not nodular or ulcerated (Fig. 53–24).

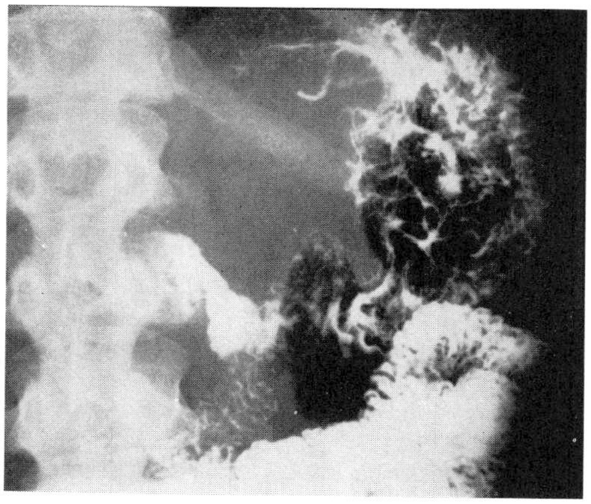

**FIGURE 53–24.** Menetrier's disease. Markedly enlarged gastric folds are particularly prominent in the upper two thirds of the stomach.

**Intestinal Lymphangiectasia.** This syndrome reflects a generalized disorder of the development of lymphatic channels. First defined by Waldmann in 1961, it is characterized by excessive loss of serum protein into the intestine with massive edema (often asymmetrical), chylous effusions, hypoalbuminemia, and hypogammaglobulinemia. The dilated lymphatic vessels invariably present in the intestinal wall may leak protein through an intact epithelium or may rupture and discharge their contents into the lumen of the gut. Isotopic studies are helpful in documenting the serum protein loss into the intestine.

The condition is being recognized with increased frequency, and x-ray study plays an important role in its

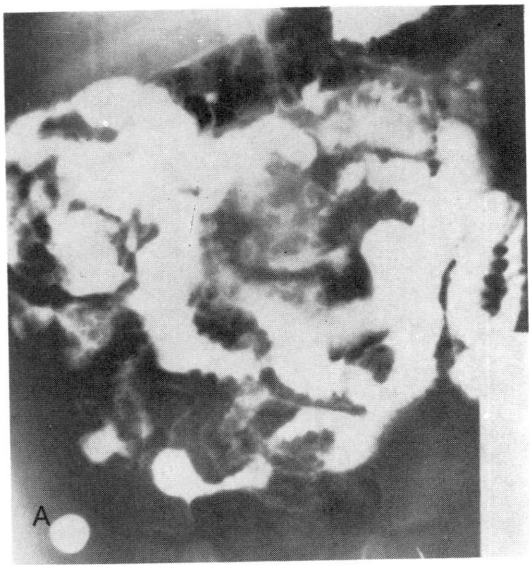
A

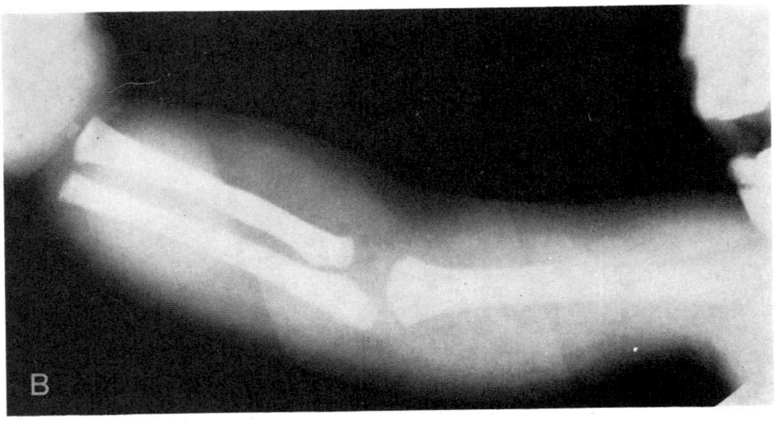
B

**FIGURE 53–25.** Intestinal lymphangiectasia in a 3-year-old child with severe protein-losing enteropathy. *A*, Prominent mucosal folds occur within mildly dilated small bowel loops containing increased secretions. *B*, Edematous involvement of the right upper extremity is apparent.

diagnosis. The characteristic appearance in the small bowel series consists of enlargement of the valvulae conniventes of both jejunum and ileum, increased secretions, and minimal or absent dilatation of the bowel (Fig. 53–25*A* and *B*). The fold enlargement may assume a "cobblestone" pattern. Punctate filling defects occasionally seen may represent the enormously enlarged villi secondary to dilated submucosal lymphatics.[70]

Hypoalbuminemia itself, below a level of 2.5g/dl resulting from other causes (e.g., nephrosis or hepatic cirrhosis), may result in edema of the bowel with diffusely thickened intestinal folds,[71] but usually does not exhibit increased intraluminal secretions.

Lymphangiographic findings support the concept that this disease is a systemic lymphatic dysplasia.[70,72] In the lower extremities, either hypoplasia of lymph vessels or dilated varicose lymphatics are present. In the abdomen, hypoplasia of lymph nodes or moderate contrast reflux into mesenteric lymphatics, associated with possible obstruction of the cisterna chyli and enlarged nodes, has been demonstrated.

**Villous Adenoma of the Colon.** Among the neoplasms of the gastrointestinal tract that may produce excess secretion of mucus to result in severe protein loss, villous adenoma of the colon is one of the most prominent. It is most common in the rectum where, because of its usual soft consistency, it may be easily missed on digital palpation. On barium enema examination, it is revealed by its characteristically irregular polypoid or flame-shaped contours as the contrast agent fills in the interstices between its frond-like projections (Fig. 53–26).

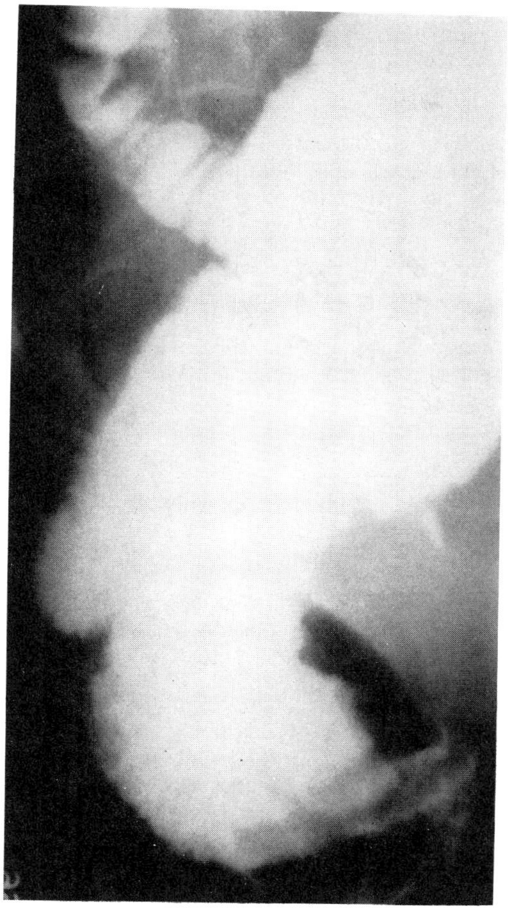

**FIGURE 53–26.** Villous adenoma of the rectum. Large circumferential mucosal mass with diffusely irregular contours is present.

## REFERENCES


1. Gould, D.M.: Am. J. Med. Sci., *223*:569, 1952.
2. Barnett, E., Nordin, B.E.C.: Br. J. Radiol., *34*:683, 1961.
3. Shapiro, R.: Clin. Radiol. *13*:238, 1962.
4. Harrison, M., Fraser, R., Mullan, B.: Lancet, *1*:1015, 1961.
5. Park, E.A.: Pediatrics, *33 (Suppl.)*:815, 1964.
6. Steinbach, H.L.: Radiol. Clin. North Am., *2*:191, 1964.
7. Park. E.A., Guild, H.G., Jackson, D., et al.: Arch. Dis. Child., *10*:265, 1935.
8. McLean, S., McIntosh, R.: Am. J. Dis. Child., *36*:875, 1928.
9. Kato, K.: Radiology, *18*:1096, 1932.
10. Albright, F., Burnett, C.H., Parson, W., et al.: Medicine, *25*:399, 1946.
11. Lasser, E.C.: Dynamic Factors in Roentgen Diagnosis, Baltimore. Williams & Wilkins, 1967.
12. Milkman, L.A.: A.J.R., *32*:622, 1934.
13. Park, E.A.: Harvey Lect., *34*:157, 1938–1939.
14. Park, E.A., Jackson, D.A.: J. Pediatr., *13*:748, 1938.
15. Sheldon, W.: Proc. R. Soc. Med., *29*:743, 1936.
16. Shahidi, N.T., Diamond, L.K.: N. Engl. J. Med., *262*:137, 1960.
17. Britton, H.A., Canby, J.P., Kohler, C.M.: Pediatrics, *25*:621, 1960.
18. Moseley, J.E.: J. Mt. Sinai Hosp., *29*:109, 1962.
19. Burko, J., Mellins, H.Z., Watson, J.: A.J.R., *86*:447, 1961.
20. Ryan, B.: Med. J. Aust., *1*:844, 1962.
21. Lanzkowsky, P.: Am. J. Dis. Child., *116*:16, 1968.
22. Holt, J.F., Hodges, F.J.: Year Book of Radiol., 1958–1959 Series. Chicago, Year Book Medical Publishers, 1958, p. 51.
23. Wolbach, S.B.: J. Bone Joint Surg., *45*:171, 1947.
24. Maddock, C.L., Wolbach, S.B., Maddock, S.: J. Nutr., *39*:117, 1949.
25. Pease, C.N.: J.A.M.A., *182*:980, 1962.
26. Caffey, J.: A.J.R. *108*:451, 1970.
27. Christiansen, W.R., Liebman, C., Sosman, M.: A.J.R., *65*:27, 1951.
28. Bauer, J.M., Freyberg, R.H.: J.A.M.A., *130*:1208, 1946.

29. Danowski, T.S., Winkler, A.W., Peters, J.P.: Ann. Intern. Med., *23:*22, 1945.
30. Capitanio, M.A., Kirkpatrick, J.A.: Radiology, *92:*53, 1969.
31. Sondheimer, F.K., Grossman, H., Winchester, P.: Arch. Neurol., *23:*314, 1970.
32. DeLevie, M., Nogrady, M.B.: J. Pediatr., *76:*523, 1970.
33. Wincik, M., Rosso, P.: J. Pediatr., *14:*774, 1969.
34. Wenger, J., Kersner, J.B., Palmer, W.L.: Am. J. Med., *24:*161, 1958.
35. Burnett, C.H., Commons, R.R., Albright, F., et al.: N. Engl. J. Med., *240:*787, 1949.
36. Leone, N.C., Stevenson, C.A., Hilbish, T.F., et al.: A.J.R., *74:*874, 1955.
37. Laws, J.W., Booth, C.C., Shawdon, H., et al.: Br. Med. J., *1:*1311, 1963.
38. Marshak, R.H., Lindner, A.E.: Semin. Roentgenol, *1:*138, 1966.
39. Frazier, A.C., French, J.M., Thompson, M.D.: Br. J. Radiol., *22:*123, 1949.
40. Ruoff, M., Lindner, A.E., Marshak, R.H.: A.J.R., *104:*525, 1968.
41. Sherlock, P., Winawer, S.J., Goldstein, M.J., et al.: Progress in Gastroenterology. Vol. II. New York, Grune & Stratton, 1970, pp. 367–391.
42. Sleisenger, M.H., Almy, T.P., Barr, D.P.: Am. J. Med., *15:*66, 1953.
43. Harris, O.E., Cooke, W.T., Thompson, H., et al.: Am. J. Med., *42:*899, 1967.
44. Shaw, R.S., Mayard, E.P.: N. Engl. J. Med., *258:*874, 1958.
45. Watt, J.K., Watson, W.C., Haase, S.: Br. Med. J., *3:*199, 1967.
46. Clemett, A.R., Marshak, R.H.: Radiol. Clin. North Am., *7:*105, 1969.
47. Rice, R.P., Roufail, W.N., Reeves, R.J.: Radiology, *88:*295, 1967.
48. Trier, J.S., Phelps, P.C., Edelman, S., et al.: Gastroenterology, *48:*684, 1965.
49. Gilat, T., Spiro, H.M.: Am. J. Dig. Dis., *13:*619, 1968.
50. Herskovic, T., Bartholomew, L.G., Green, P.A.: Arch. Intern. Med., *114:*629, 1964.
51. Legge, D.A., Carlson, H.C., Wollaeger, E.E.: A.J.R., *110:*406, 1970.
52. Laws, J.W., Neale, G.: Lancet, *2:*139, 1966.
53. Preger, L., Amberg, J.R.: A.J.R., *101:*287, 1967.
54. Winawer, S.J., Broitman, S.A., Wolochow, D.A., et al.: N. Engl. J. Med., *274:*72, 1966.
55. Katz, I, Karp, F.L.: A.J.R., *99:*162, 1967.
56. Gorbach, S.L., Plaut, A.G., Nahas, L., et al.: Gastroenterology, *53:*856, 1967.
57. Rosenberg, I.H., Hardison, W.G., Bull, D.M.: N. Engl. J. Med., *276:*1391, 1967.
58. Tankel, H.I., Clark, D.H., Lee, F.D.: Gut, *6:*560, 1965.
59. Marshak, R.H., Ruoff, M., Lindner, A.E.: A.J.R., *104:*557, 1968.
60. Louisy, C.L., Barton, C.L.: Radiology, *98:*535, 1971.
61. Hermans, P.E., Huizenga, K.A., Hoffman, H.N., et al.: Am. J. Med., *40:*78, 1966.
62. Hodgson, J.R., Hoffman, H.N., Huizenga, K.A.: Radiology, *88:*883, 1967.
63. Orimo, H., Fujita, T., Yoshikawa, M., et al.: Am. J. Med., *47:*445, 1969.
64. Clemett, A.R., Fishbone, G., Levine, R.J., et al.: A.J.R., *103:*405, 1968.
65. Strole, W.E., Clark, W.H., Isselbacher, K.G.: N. Engl. J. Med., *276:*195, 1967.
66. Stacy, G.S., Loop, J.W.: A.J.R., *92:*1072, 1964.
67. Khilnani, M.T., Keller, R.J., Cuttner, J.: Radiol. Clin. North Am., *7:*43, 1969.
68. Waldmann, T.A.: Gastroenterology, *50:*422, 1966.
69. Reese, D.F., Hodgson, J.R., Dockerty, M.B.: A.J.R., *88:*619, 1962.
70. Shimkin, P.M., Waldmann, T.A., Krugman, R.L.: A.J.R., *110:*827, 1970.
71. Marshak, R., Khilnani, M.T., Eliasoph, J., et al.: A.J.R., *101:*379, 1967.
72. Bookstein, J.J., French, A.B., Pollard, H.M.: Am. J. Dig. Dis., *10:*573, 1965.

CHAPTER 54

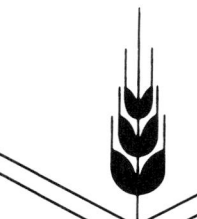

# Morphology and Dynamics of Bone: Nutritional Interactions

Michael D. Fallon†



Technical advances have permitted the more precise assessment of bone structure. These include the development of biochemical methods for the measurement of circulating hormones and vitamins that influence bone, and noninvasive radiologic methods allowing quantitative determination of bone mass, such as single and dual photon absorptiometry and computed tomography. The last enhances the detection of changes in skeletal mass previously unrecognized by routine radiographs. These diagnostic tools, however, are indirect markers of skeletal structure. Consequently, the procedure for a simplified bone biopsy technique and the ability to prepare undecalcified histologic sections of bone have permitted the direct examination of skeletal tissue. Examination of the microstructure of bone offers the advantage of determining not only the state of skeletal mineralization but also the level of bone remodeling activity.

†Deceased

## BONE AND NUTRITION

One of the major functions of the skeleton is related to nutrition. Bone is a dynamic organ that plays a role in calcium and mineral homeostasis. To understand how skeletal abnormalities occur as a result of nutritional disorders, it is necessary to understand the relationships between normal mineral homeostasis, bone structure, and bone cell physiology.

## HISTOLOGIC FEATURES OF BONE

Bone is a specialized connective tissue of mineralized extracellular collagenous matrix. The skeleton functions not only to provide mechanical support and protection, but also to serve as a mineral reservoir for calcium homeostasis.

Cortical bone, also called compact bone, is located in the diaphyses of the long tubular bones and provides structural support (Fig. 54–1). Trabecular or cancellous bone consists of spicules of bone, known as trabeculae, that transverse the marrow spaces. Although trabecular bone constitutes only 20% of the skeleton, the three-dimensional arrangement of the cancellous network provides an enormous surface area (see Fig. 54–1).

There are three main types of bone cells (Fig. 54–2). Bone matrix is synthesized by *osteoblasts,* the cuboidal mononuclear cells found along bone surfaces. *Osteocytes* represent osteoblasts that have been incorporated into

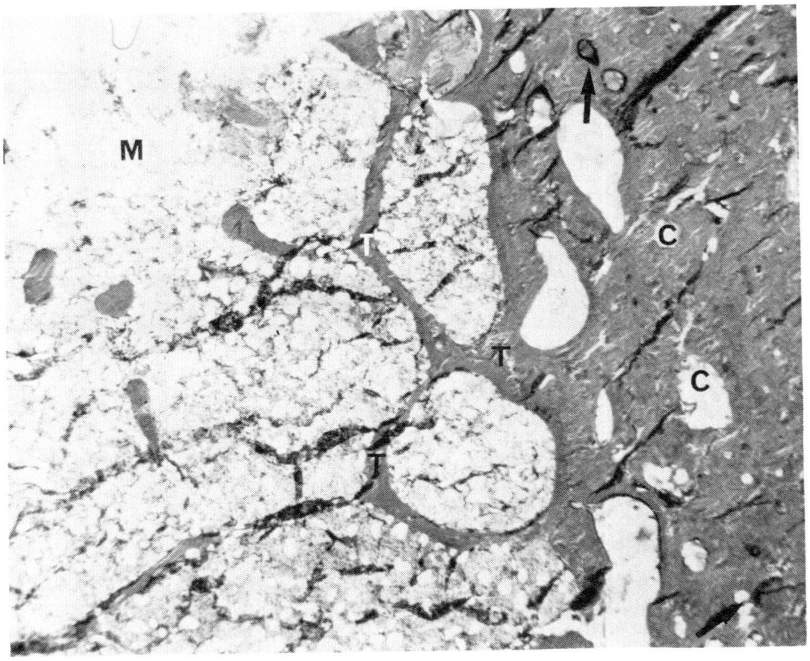
M
T
T
T
C
C

**FIGURE 54–1.** Transcortical core biopsy of normal iliac bone. Cortical bone (C) is of normal thickness and contains haversian canals (arrow). Trabecular bone (T) forms interconnecting plates or ribbons of bone. M, Marrow (undecalcified section, Masson trichrome stain; original magnification × 25).

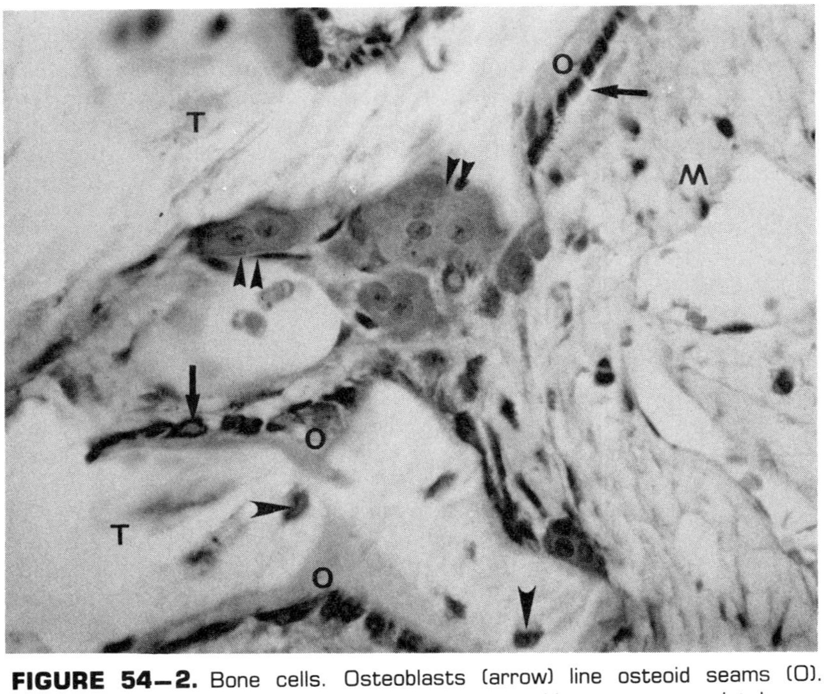
O
T
M
O
T
O

**FIGURE 54–2.** Bone cells. Osteoblasts (arrow) line osteoid seams (O). Osteocytes (single arrowhead) are entrapped osteoblasts, now completely surrounded by matrix of the trabecular bone (T). Large multinucleated osteoclasts (double arrowhead) resorb bone. M, Marrow (toluidine blue; original magnification × 340).

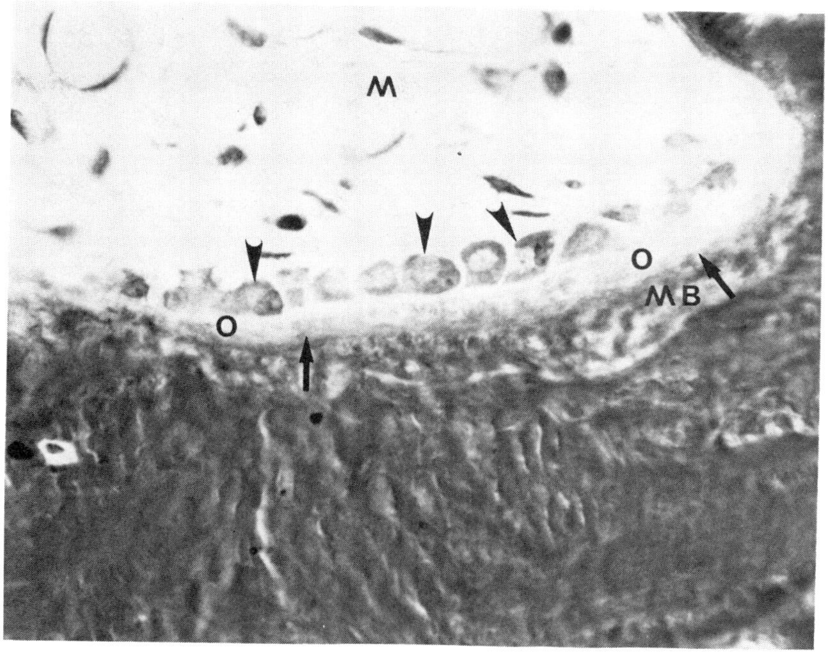
M
O
MB
O

**FIGURE 54–3.** Bone matrix synthesized by active, plump osteoblasts (arrowheads) forming an osteoid seam (O). Mineralization occurs at the junction between the mineralized bone (MB) and osteoid seam (arrows with O). M, Marrow (Masson trichrome stain; original magnification × 120).

the previously synthesized bone matrix. *Osteoclasts* are large multinucleated cells responsible for bone resorption.

Bone collagen is secreted in a highly organized manner, resulting in the formation of layers of bone matrix called lamellae. Bone matrix is composed of collagen and other noncollagenous proteins, which in the newly deposited unmineralized state are termed osteoid (Fig. 54–3). The osteoid layer found along trabecular bone surfaces is termed an osteoid seam. Mineralization of osteoid is an orderly process that begins with the deposition of amorphous calcium phosphate at the interface between the osteoid seam and mineralized bone (i.e., the mineralization front). These nascent mineral deposits subsequently "mature" into hydroxyapatite crystals, the mineral phase characteristic of adult bone.

The binding affinity of autofluorescent tetracycline antibiotics for immature mineral deposits, but not the mature crystal, enables the identification of calcification foci and subsequently permits the determination of the rate of bone mineralization.

### TETRACYCLINE AS AN IN VIVO BONE MARKER

Tetracycline antibiotics are utilized as biologic markers of mineralization.[1] During the first labeling course, tetracycline (dimethylchlortetracycline, oxytetracycline, or demeclocycline (1 g/day in divided doses) is administered for 3 days. After a 14-day, drug-free hiatus, a second course of tetracycline is given over a 3-day interval. The bone biopsy is obtained 3 to 4 days after the last dose of tetracycline.

Tetracycline fluorescence is evaluated on unstained nondecalcified tissue sections by ultraviolet light. The first course of tetracycline appears as a discrete fluorescent band within the mineralized bone (Fig. 54–4). The second, more recently administered, course of tetracycline is located at the current mineralization front. The distance between the two bands represents the amount of new bone synthesized and mineralized over the drug-free interval.

## GROWTH AND REMODELING

Growth refers to a net increase in skeletal mass occurring prior to epiphyseal plate closure. Modeling is the shaping process responsible for maintaining the characteristic morphology of the growing bone. Both growth and modeling require that bone formation (osteoblast activity) and resorption (osteoclast activity) occur at anatomically separate sites.

### COUPLING

Despite the fact that the skeleton is composed predominantly of inorganic extracellular matrix, bone is a dynamic organ, the microarchitecture of which is con-

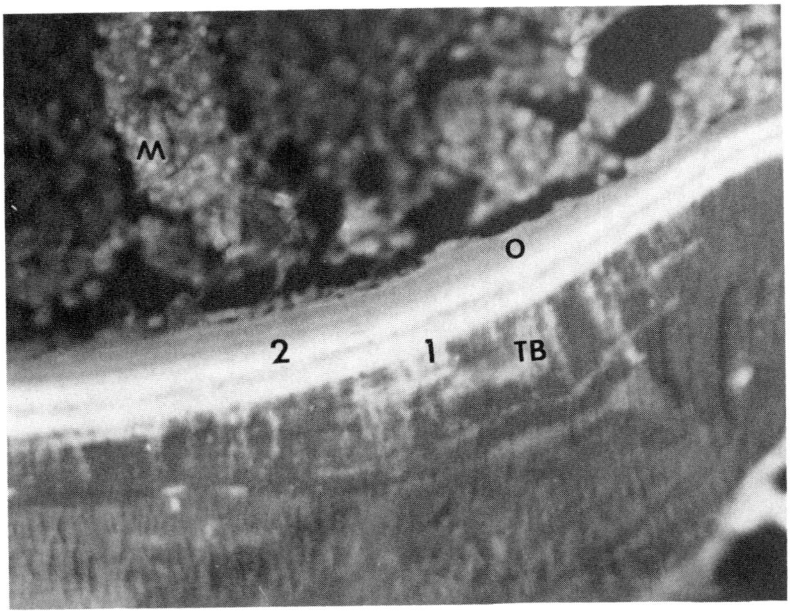
M
O
2
1
TB

**FIGURE 54–4.** Similar field as in Figure 54–3, as viewed by fluorescent light to reveal the dual tetracycline labels. The first course of tetracycline (1) is buried in the mineralized trabecular bone (TB). The second course of tetracycline (2) marks the recent mineralization fronts at the osteoid seam interface (O). M, Marrow.

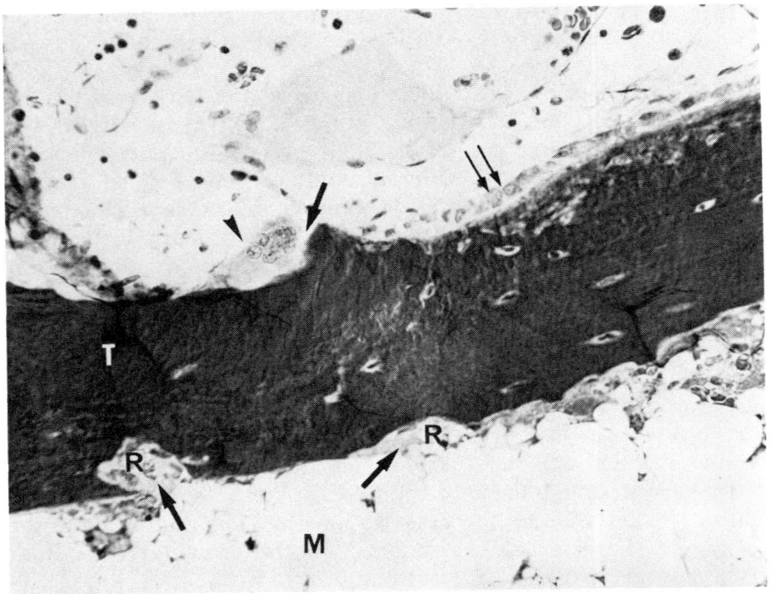
T
R
R
M

**FIGURE 54–5.** The normal remodeling cycle. An osteoclast (arrowhead) resorbs a packet of bone, i.e., Howship's lacuna (arrows). A reversal phase (R) denotes the transition phase between osteoclast activity and subsequent appearance of osteoblasts (double arrows). T, Trabecular bone; M, marrow (Masson trichrome stain; original magnification × 98).

stantly being modified by two groups of hormonally responsive bone cells: osteoblasts and osteoclasts. The linked activation of osteoclasts and osteoblasts, termed coupling, is the basis of bone turnover or remodeling, the continuous skeletal activity related to the maintenance of mineral homeostasis. In contrast to the structural modification associated with modeling, remodeling is characterized by the anatomic and sequential coupling of osteoclast and osteoblast activity (Fig. 54–5). Remodeling units are initiated by the appearance of osteoclasts that resorb a packet of bone, creating a scalloped resorption bay or Howship's lacuna. Following osteoclastic activity, a reversal phase of varying duration ensues. A densely staining metachromatic line, the cement line, is formed at the limits of the resorption focus. The appearance of osteoblasts marks the end of the reversal phase as lamellar bone matrix is deposited in an appositional fashion, filling in the resorptive defect.

## METABOLIC BONE DISEASES: DEFINITIONS OF OSTEOPENIA, OSTEOPOROSIS, AND OSTEOMALACIA

The ability of the skeleton to provide structural support depends upon the skeletal mass, i.e., the amount of bone tissue, as well as the quality of that tissue, i.e., the degree of mineralization (Fig. 54–6). The amount of bone tissue is determined primarily by the location and extent of bone removal and formation during the remodeling cycle. Because the mineralization process and the level of bone remodeling are influenced by several systemic factors, disorders of these activities result in generalized skeletal disease. When the bone mass can no longer sustain normal forces, skeletal fracture may ensue, leading to pain and deformity. Thus, a metabolic bone disease is defined as any generalized disorder of the skeleton, regardless of cause. Most metabolic bone diseases are due to either an imbalance in remodeling activity or a disorder of matrix mineralization (see Fig. 54–6).

Osteopenia is the generic term used to denote this generalized reduction in bone mass. By radiographic examination, the skeleton appears "washed out," or "demineralized." Osteoporosis and osteomalacia are the two major osteopenic syndromes. Osteoporosis is a group of diseases characterized by quantitatively low bone mass, but the composition of the remaining bone is chemically normal and, therefore, implies no assumption as to the pathogenesis. Osteomalacia, on the other hand, is a group of diseases characterized by bone that is qualitatively abnormal owing to an impaired state of mineralization. Defective mineralization of cartilage at the epiphyseal plate of growing bones is termed rickets.

### THE BONE BIOPSY

For any systemic skeletal disorder, a small sample of bone obtained from any skeletal site should be representative of the entire disease process. The iliac crest region is a readily accessible standardized biopsy site and reflects changes that may be occurring at more clinically relevant sites, such as the spine or long bones. By examination of this representative bone tissue, the level of bone remodeling activity and the rate of bone mineralization may be determined. The bone biopsy procedure

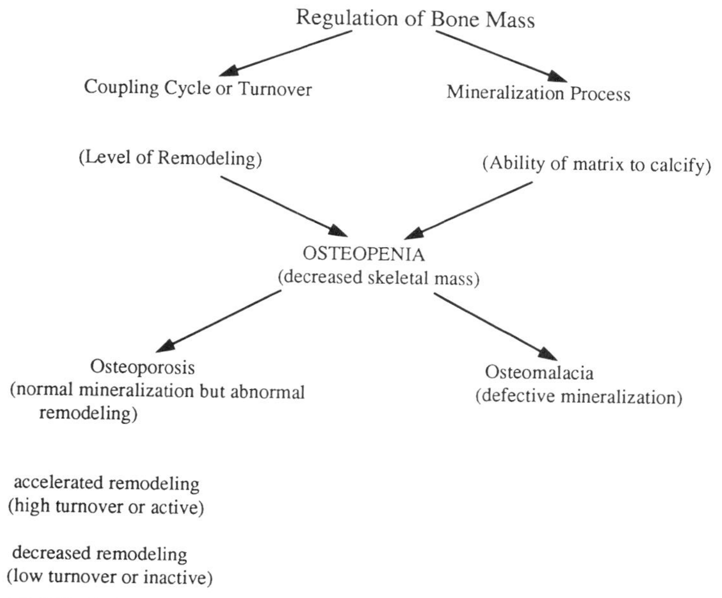
Regulation of Bone Mass
Coupling Cycle or Turnover
Mineralization Process
(Level of Remodeling)
(Ability of matrix to calcify)
OSTEOPENIA
(decreased skeletal mass)
Osteoporosis
(normal mineralization but abnormal remodeling)
Osteomalacia
(defective mineralization)
accelerated remodeling
(high turnover or active)
decreased remodeling
(low turnover or inactive)

**FIGURE 54–6.** Regulation of bone mass.

and the direct examination of bone tissue have become important tools in the differential diagnosis of metabolic bone diseases.

Trocars ranging from 5 to 8 mm in diameter are commercially available. A biopsy of the anterior iliac crest may be performed transcutaneously under local anesthesia, as shown in Figure 54–7, to produce a core or cylinder of bone. The actual biopsy procedure is described in detail elsewhere.[2]

**Processing Bone Biopsy Specimens.** Because the differentiation between the two major metabolic bone diseases, osteoporosis and osteomalacia, is based in part upon the quantity and quality of bone mineral, the ability to distinguish between calcified bone matrix and uncalcified bone matrix (osteoid) is critical. The traditional procedures for processing bone, acid decalcification and paraffin embedding, require the removal of inorganic matrix to facilitate histologic sectioning and, therefore, prevent the subsequent determination of the degree of skeletal mineralization.

In nondecalcified bone sections, osteomalacia is usually characterized by the accumulation of osteoid caused by a defect in the mineralization process. It must be recognized, however, that excess quantities of osteoid may result not only from a decreased rate of mineralization, but also from an accelerated rate of bone matrix synthesis. In routine nondecalcified bone sections, these two forms of osteoid excess appear identical (Fig. 54–8). Differentiation between these states is based upon the determination of mineralization rates, using tetracycline as an in vivo bone marker.

The mean distance between the midpoints of the double tetracycline labels is measured with a linear reticle. This distance divided by the number of days between the two courses of tetracycline is the *mineral appositional rate* and normally ranges from 0.4 to 0.9 μm per day (mean 0.65 μm per day).

As the bone apposition rate increases, the distance between the labels grows wider (Fig. 54–9). In contrast, with a reduced mineralization rate, the parallel bands become narrow and may fuse to produce single labels.

Abnormal patterns of fluorescent label deposition are the hallmark of osteomalacia, and represent the morpho-logic expression of defective mineralization.[3] The amount of tetracycline fluorescence is proportional to the amount of the immature amorphous calcium phosphate deposits in the mineralizing foci of the osteoid seam.

A common abnormal tetracycline pattern characteristic of osteomalacia is diffuse irregular fluorescence of an entire osteoid seam. Accumulation of immature bone mineral is thought to reflect a failure of maturation of amorphous calcium phosphate into hydroxyapatite crystals, thus permitting excessive tetracycline binding (Fig. 54–10). In some cases, osteoid seams are deficient in mineral and, therefore, osteoid is incapable of binding tetracycline, leading to an absence of fluorescence. As a

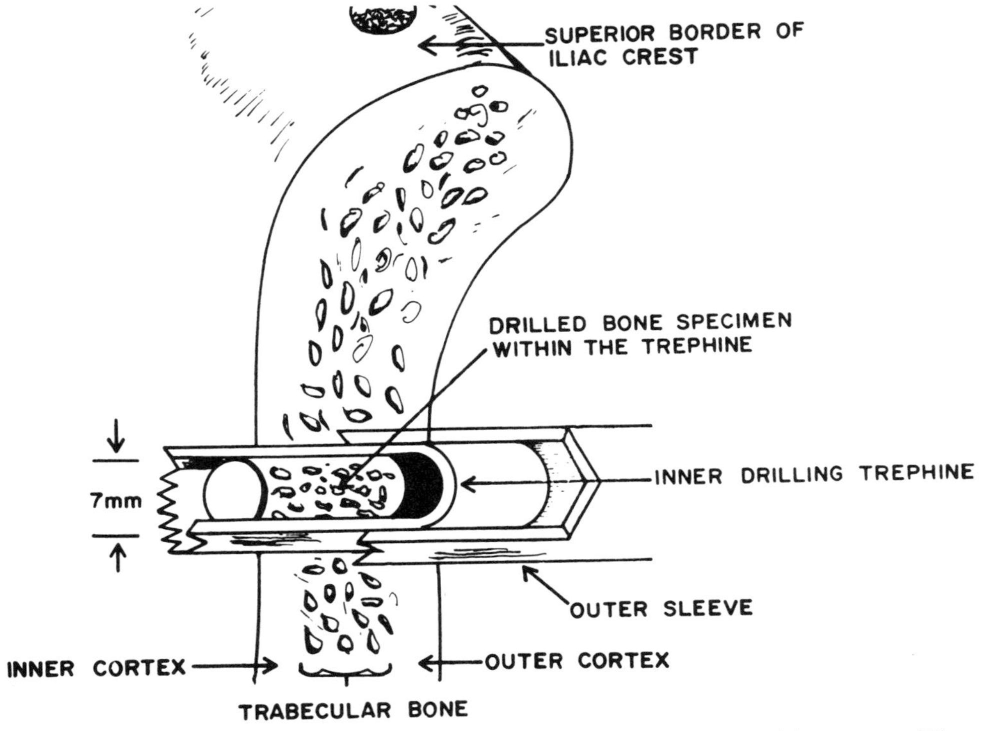
SUPERIOR BORDER OF ILIAC CREST
DRILLED BONE SPECIMEN WITHIN THE TREPHINE
INNER DRILLING TREPHINE
7mm
OUTER SLEEVE
INNER CORTEX
OUTER CORTEX
TRABECULAR BONE

**FIGURE 54–7.** Diagram showing the standard biopsy procedure for obtaining a core of iliac bone.

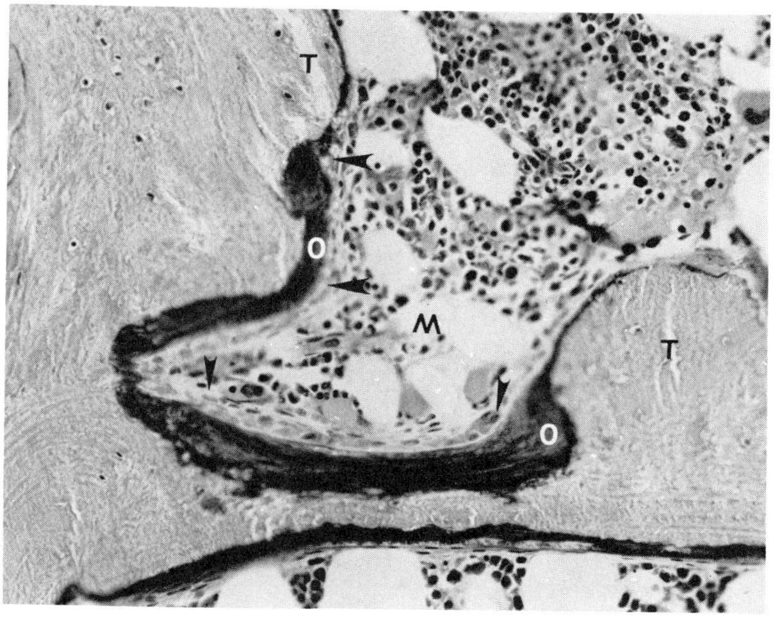
T
O
M
T
O

**FIGURE 54–8.** Increased quantity of osteoid (O). Increased thickness of the osteoid seam may be due to accelerated matrix synthesis by osteoblasts (arrowheads) stemming from an abnormally high remodeling condition, or it may result from defective mineralization secondary to an osteomalacic disorder. T, Trabecular bone; M, marrow (Goldner trichrome stain, original magnification × 250).

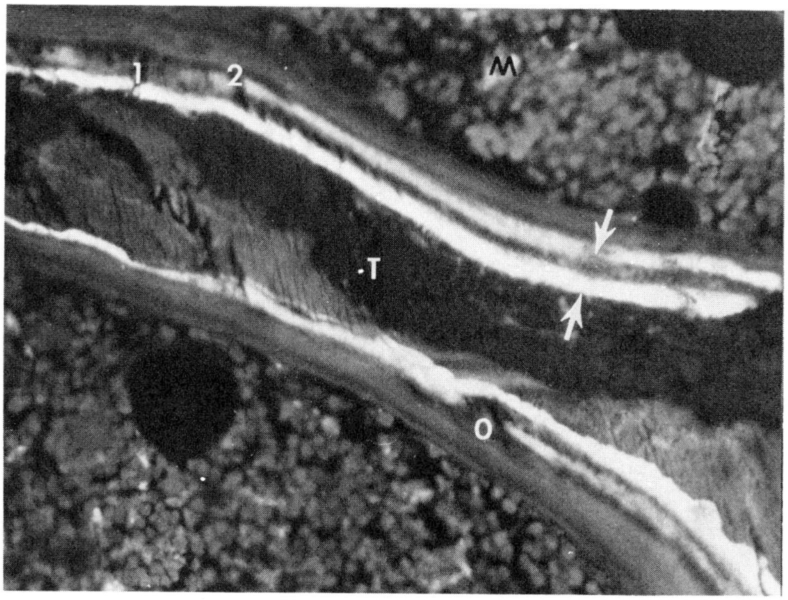
1
2
M
T
O

**FIGURE 54–9.** The increased quantity of osteoid in Figure 54–8 was proven to reflect active bone remodeling, and not osteomalacia as revealed by the widely spaced dual tetracycline labels (arrows). Compare label distance to that of normal tissue in Figure 54–4. T, Trabecular bone; M, marrow; O, osteoid; 1, first course of tetracycline; 2, second course of tetracycline.

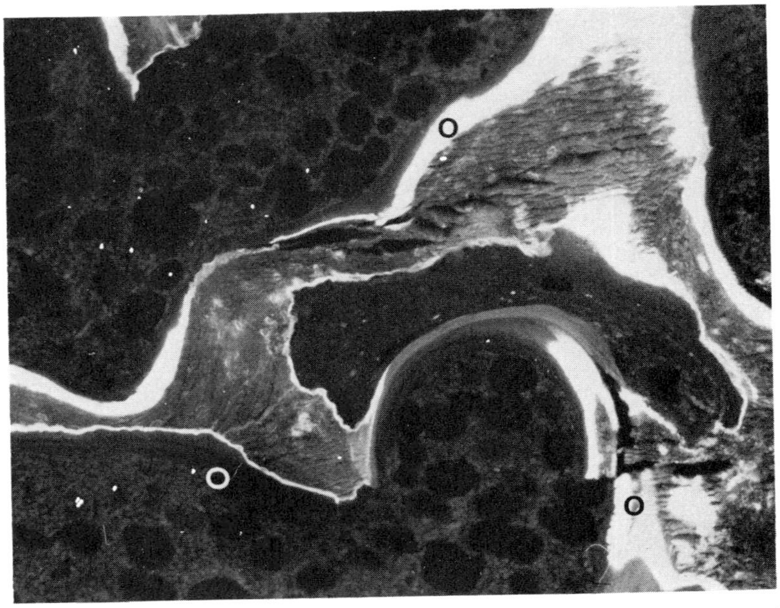
O
O
O

**FIGURE 54–10.** Abnormal tetracycline fluorescent pattern diagnostic of osteomalacia. Defective mineralization in this instance is revealed by wide, diffuse uptake of tetracycline at the broad osteoid seams (O) (unstained, fluorescent micrograph; original magnification × 60).

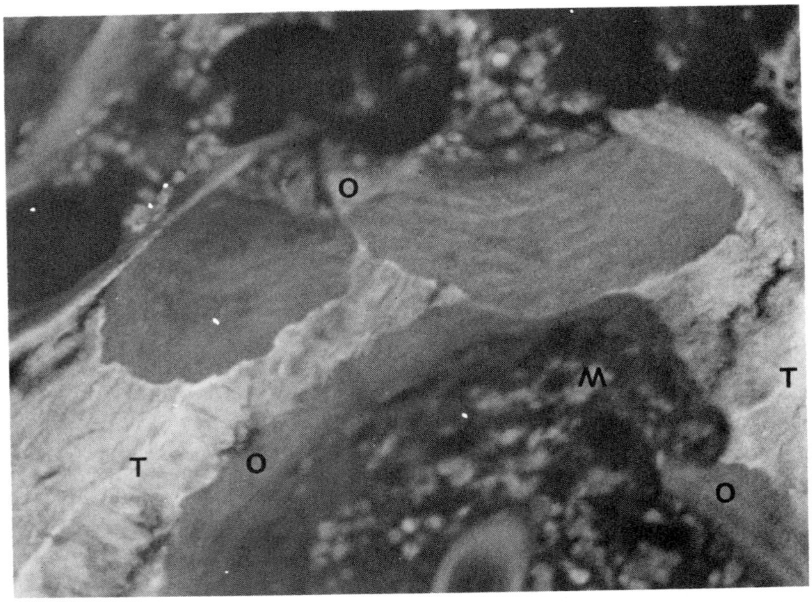
O
M
T
T
O
O

**FIGURE 54–11.** A second common abnormal tetracycline in vivo reaction diagnostic of osteomalacia. Defective mineralization in this instance is characterized by an absence of tetracycline uptake, with failure of the osteoid seams (O) to fluoresce. T, Trabecular bone; M, marrow; O, osteoid (unstained section; original magnification × 340).

result, the *mineralization front activity* (percentage of osteoid seams bearing normal tetracycline labels) is reduced (Fig. 54–11). It must be stressed that osteomalacia may occur with a normal quantity of osteoid (Fig. 54–12). Defective mineralization can only reliably be determined by kinetic tetracycline labeling.

The histologic techniques designed for the demonstration of bone mineral and tetracycline markers require

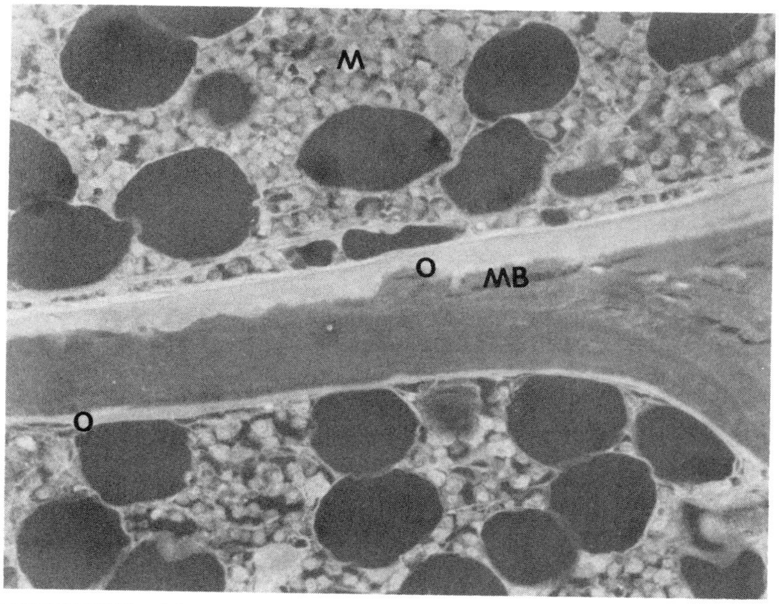
M
O
MB
O

**FIGURE 54–12.** This micrograph stresses the importance of performing in vivo tetracycline labeling prior to the biopsy. Despite a normal quantity of osteoid (O), the presence of a mineralization defect is demonstrated by the absence of tetracycline uptake at the mineralization fronts, i.e., the junction between the osteoid seams (O) and the mineralized bone interface (MB). Compare to Figures 54–8 and 54–9. M, Marrow (unstained section; original magnification × 250).

the examination of nondecalcified tissue. Thus, specialized embedding and sectioning procedures have been developed.

To obtain nondecalcified tissue sections, bone is embedded without prior demineralization in methyl methacrylate (MM) plastic and sectioned on a heavy-duty, sledge microtome equipped with a carbide-tungsten-tipped steel blade.[4] This technique is laborious and requires rigorous tissue dehydration, careful attention to resin preparation, polymerization, and specialized equipment, thereby limiting ready application. Alternative simplified procedures utilize less expensive and more commonly available equipment.[5] The routine histologic evaluation of bone has been made possible by sectioning glycol methacrylate (GMA)-embedded tissue on glass knives.

**Bone Histomorphometry.** Bone histomorphometry is the quantitative analysis of undecalcified bone in which the skeletal remodeling parameters are expressed in terms of volumes, surfaces, and cell numbers[6] (Fig. 54–13)(Table 54–1).

To obtain this information from the two-dimensional format, principles of stereology are used to reconstruct the third dimension. This principle, described by the French mineralogist Delesse in 1848, simply states that if measurements are made at random on infinitely thin sections, the ratio of areas is equal to the ratio of volumes. Areas are measured by counting the number of cross-marks or "hits" formed by an array of points in the grid (see Fig. 54–13). The points are projected onto the field from a grid in the microscope eyepiece. The average number of cross-marks or hits that fall on the histologic feature of interest (as a fraction of the total number of possible hits) is equal to the volume of that component within the total unit volume. Measurements of bone surfaces or perimeter lengths are obtained by counting the number of intersections between the bone perimeter and equidistant parallel grid lines. Distance between two items of interest, such as the distance between two tetracycline labels, is measured by a calibrated linear reticle.

**Bone Remodeling and Mineralization: Determinants of Bone Mass.** The level of bone remodeling activity is determined by a variety of calcium-regulating hormones (see Chaps. 7 and 17). During states of calcium deficiency, parathyroid hormone is secreted, which stimulates osteoclastic bone resorption and liberates calcium and phosphate from apatite crystals. At the same time, renal tubular reabsorption of calcium is stimulated and urinary excretion of phosphate is enhanced. Elevated PTH is also a stimulus for increased 1,25 dihydroxyvitamin D production by the kidney. Parent vitamin D, either produced in the skin by photoactivation or obtained by dietary sources, circulates in the blood and is converted to 25 hydroxyvitamin D by hepatic hydroxylase enzymes; 25 (OH) vitamin D serves as the renal substrate

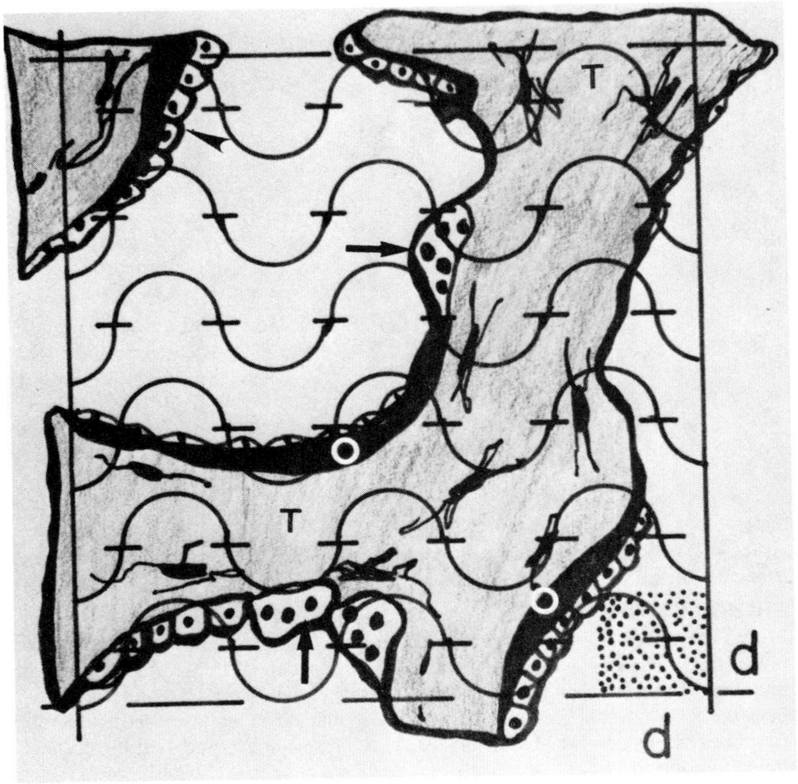
T
T
d
d

**FIGURE 54–13.** Histomorphometry. A Merz-Schenk grid in the microscope eyepiece is shown projected onto a field of mineralized bone (light shading), osteoid (dark shading), and marrow (no shading). Of the cross-marks or hits in the grid, 13 are superimposed on mineralized bone, 3 on osteoid, 16 on marrow, 2 on osteoclasts, and 2 on osteoblasts. Therefore, 44.4% of the field is bone. Because 3 of the 16 hits on bone fall on osteoid, the relative osteoid volume is 18.8%. The absolute area occupied by the grid is 36 times the square of the distance (d) between the hits (area = 36d$^2$). When viewed at 250 × magnification, "d" is measured by a calibrated ocular micrometer (the grid covers 0.155 mm$^2$). Approximately 200 fields (30 mm$^2$) should be measured for statistically valid results. The 6 semicircular parallel lines help compensate for nonrandomly oriented trabeculae, and the distance between the lines (d) is the same as that between hits. There are 18 intersections with the trabecular perimeter. Seven intersections are at osteoid surfaces, 5 are at resting mineralized surfaces, and 4 are at osteoclast-filled Howship's lacunae. Therefore, the osteoid surface is 38.9%, the resting surface 27.8%, and the active resorption surface 22.2% of the total number of intersections with the bone perimeter. O, Osteoid; T, trabecular bone; arrow, osteoclast; arrowheads, osteoblasts lining osteoid seam.

for further hydroxylation. This active dihydroxylated vitamin D stimulates intestinal absorption of calcium and, at supraphysiologic levels, stimulates osteoclastic activity.

Mineralization of osteoid matrix is promoted by optimum ambient calcium and phosphate levels maintained by the aforementioned hormones. Mineralization is facilitated by the enzyme alkaline phosphatase, which may remove endogenous crystallization inhibitors such as pyrophosphates. Other exogenous agents such as the diphosphonates, utilized in the treatment of Paget's disease of bone, and sodium fluoride, an experimental agent utilized in osteoporosis therapy, may inhibit further crystal accumulation and may induce osteomalacia. It is unclear whether vitamin D metabolites play a direct role in osteoid maturation and mineralization, or whether they promote mineralization secondarily by maintaining serum calcium and phosphorus levels (see section on vitamin D deficiency states).

Bone cell activity is influenced by physical forces, endocrine-hormone levels, and nutritional-metabolic factors, all of which are summarized in Table 54–2. Normally bone resorption and formation are in balance (Figs. 54–14 and 54–15). A net loss of bone tissue may

**TABLE 54–1.** HISTOMORPHOMETRIC PARAMETERS

| SYMBOL | DETERMINATION | RANGE | DEFINITION |
|---|---|---|---|
| TBV | trabecular bone volume | 15–25% | Percentage biopsy tissue occupied by mineralized and unmineralized bone tissue. |
| ROV | relative osteoid volume | 0.6–4.0% | Percentage trabecular bone volume composed of osteoid. |
| TOS | total osteoid surface | 4–20% | Percentage trabecular bone surface covered by osteoid seams. A function of the number of osteoblasts. |
| MOSW | mean osteoid seam width | 8–16 μm | Thickness of osteoid seams. A function of osteoblast cell activity. |
| OB | osteoblastic osteoid | 35–40% of osteoid or 1–8% of total trabecular surface | Percentage trabecular surface covered by osteoid lined by cuboidal osteoblasts. (Function of cell recruitment or number of osteoblasts.) |
| ARS | active resorptive surface | <0.5% | Percentage trabecular surface covered with osteoclasts. A function of the bone surface engaged in resorption. |
| OC | osteoclast number | 0.1–0.3/mm$^2$ | Number of osteoclasts per square millimeter of trabecular bone. |
| FIB | peritrabecular fibrosis | 0% | Percentage trabecular surface covered by fibrous tissue. |
| LEBF | linear extent of bone formation or fractional labeled surface | 10–17% | Extent of tetracycline labeled surface, as a fraction of the total trabecular surface. A function of the number of active cells. |
| MF | mineralization front activity | 60–80% | Percentage mineralized bone-osteoid seam interfaces labeled with tetracycline. |
| AR, CR | appositional rate, calcification rate | .4–.9 μm/day | Average amount of new matrix deposited and mineralized over the tetracycline labeling period. A function of cell activity. |
| MLT | mineralization lag time | 11–23 days | Derived by dividing the mean osteoid seam width by the appositional rate. An index of the length of time that osteoid once synthesized becomes mineralized. |
| BFR | bone formation rate | 0.3–0.8 μm/day | Amount of bone made per day. Derived from the LEBF multiplied by the AR. A function, therefore, of cell activity and cell number. |

occur from excessive bone resorption or deficient bone formation, or a combination of both, during the coupling cycle.

Bone remodeling activity may be categorized as either accelerated or reduced. Both of these high- and low-turnover states may result in a reduction of bone mass. Accelerated bone turnover is usually the result of an absolute increase in bone resorption. At the cellular level, osteoclast activity is enhanced such that a greater volume of bone is removed at a given remodeling site. These unusually deep Howship's lacunae cannot be filled by normal osteoblast activity (see Fig. 54–14, $B_1$ and $B_2$). At the tissue level (see Fig. 54–15, $B_1$ and $B_2$) there may be a recruitment of new bone remodeling units such that the number of active resorbing sites increases. Given the normal coupling of bone formation to resorption, accelerated bone turnover is often accompanied by an increase in bone formation. Despite this compensatory increase in bone formation at the cell and tissue level, a

**TABLE 54–2.** DETERMINANTS OF BONE TURNOVER

| | RESORPTION | FORMATION |
|---|---|---|
| Parathyroid hormone | ↑ | ↑ |
| Thyroxine | ↑ | ↑ |
| Calcitonin | ↓ | — |
| Estrogen | ↓ | — |
| Calcium | ↓ | — |
| Phosphate | ↓ | ↑ |
| 1.25 $(OH)_2$ vitamin D | ↑ | ↑ |
| Corticosteroids | ↓ or ↑ | |
| Growth hormone | ↑ | ↑ |

Determinants of Bone Mineralization
Promoters: Calcium, phosphate, vitamin D, alkaline phosphatase
Inhibitors: pyrophosphates, fluoride

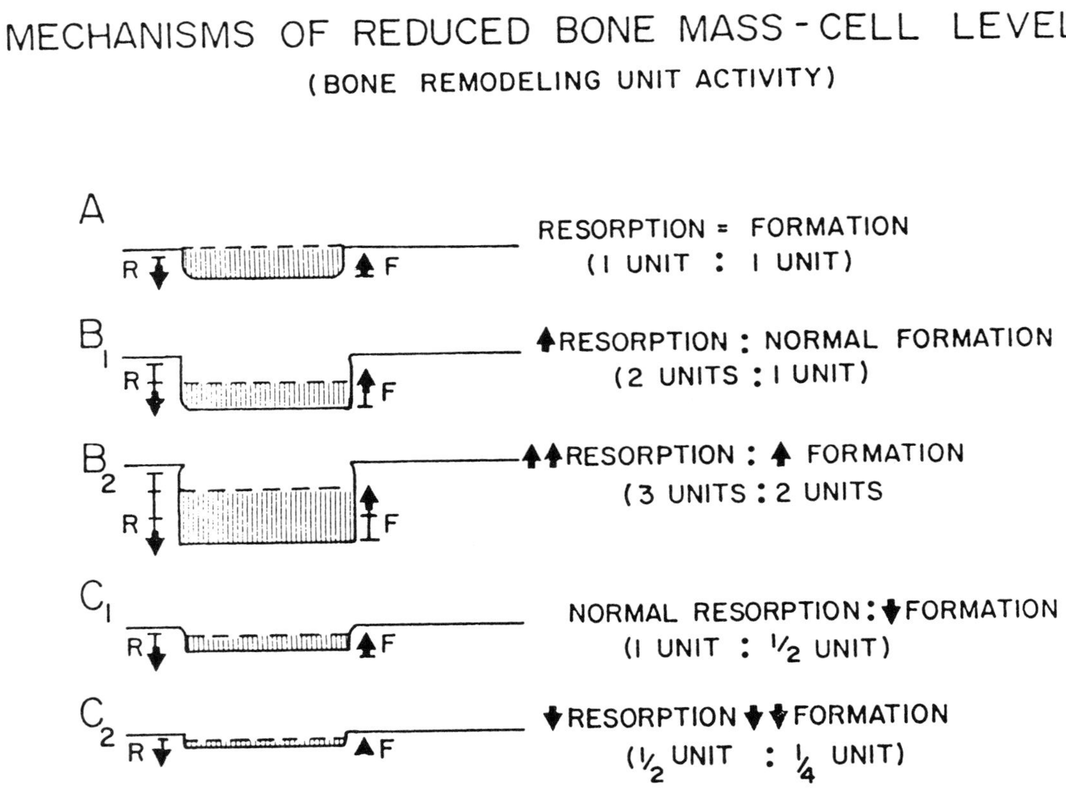
MECHANISMS OF REDUCED BONE MASS - CELL LEVEL
(BONE REMODELING UNIT ACTIVITY)
A
R
F
RESORPTION = FORMATION
(1 UNIT : 1 UNIT)
B1
R
F
↑RESORPTION : NORMAL FORMATION
(2 UNITS : 1 UNIT)
B2
R
F
↑↑RESORPTION : ↑ FORMATION
(3 UNITS : 2 UNITS
C1
R
F
NORMAL RESORPTION : ↓FORMATION
(1 UNIT : 1/2 UNIT)
C2
R
F
↓RESORPTION ↓↓FORMATION
(1/2 UNIT : 1/4 UNIT)

**FIGURE 54–14.** Mechanisms of reduced bone mass at the cell level. A depicts skeletal balance (R = F); $B_1$ and $B_2$ depict negative balance (R>F) with high turnover; $C_1$ and $C_2$ depict negative balance (R>F) with low turnover (see text).

net loss of bone ensues, owing to overriding bone resorptive activity (see Fig. 54–15, $B_2$).

Low bone remodeling states are often associated with a relative increase in bone resorption, such that the actual rate and extent of bone formation are reduced (see Figs. 54–14 and 54–15, $C_1$ and $C_2$). Even if bone resorption is reduced, there is often a greater reduction in osteoblast function, resulting in a lower level of turnover, that nonetheless produces a steady loss of bone mass.

## HISTOPATHOLOGIC APPEARANCE OF METABOLIC BONE DISEASES

Histologically, metabolic bone diseases appear as disorders of either increased remodeling activity, decreased remodeling activity, or defective mineralization (osteomalacia).

**Increased Bone Remodeling Activity (Accelerated Bone Turnover).** States of high turnover (see Fig. 54–15) are characterized by evidence of increased bone formation and increased resorption (Figs. 54–16 to 54–18). Histologic correlates of increased formation include: increased quantities of osteoid, increased osteoid surfaces, moderately increased osteoid seam thickness, and increased osteoblastic surfaces (Table 54–3). Tetracycline fluorescence may show an increase in the fraction of trabecular bone surfaces bearing double labels, indicating an increase in the linear extent of bone formation (Fig. 54–18*B*). The linear extent parameter is a function of the activation of additional osteoblasts. The mineralization rate (the distance between the double labels) may be increased, reflecting an augmentation of individual cell activity. Increased resorptive activity is manifested by an increase in the number of osteoclasts, and by the fraction of bone surfaces engaged in bone resorption resulting in Howship's lacunae complete with osteoclasts. Peritrabecular fibrous tissue deposition indicating osteitis fibrosa is a manifestation of general increased mesenchymal cell activity. This feature is not peculiar to hyperparathyroidism, but may be associated with any condition resulting in accelerated tissue turnover (Fig. 54–19).

**Decreased Bone Remodeling Activity (Reduced Bone Turnover).** These states show little evidence of either bone formation or resorption (Table 54–4). Consequently,osteoid seams are thin and scanty, osteoblasts are flattened, and osteoclasts are reduced in number (Fig. 54–20*A*). Few tetracycline labels are apparent, consis-

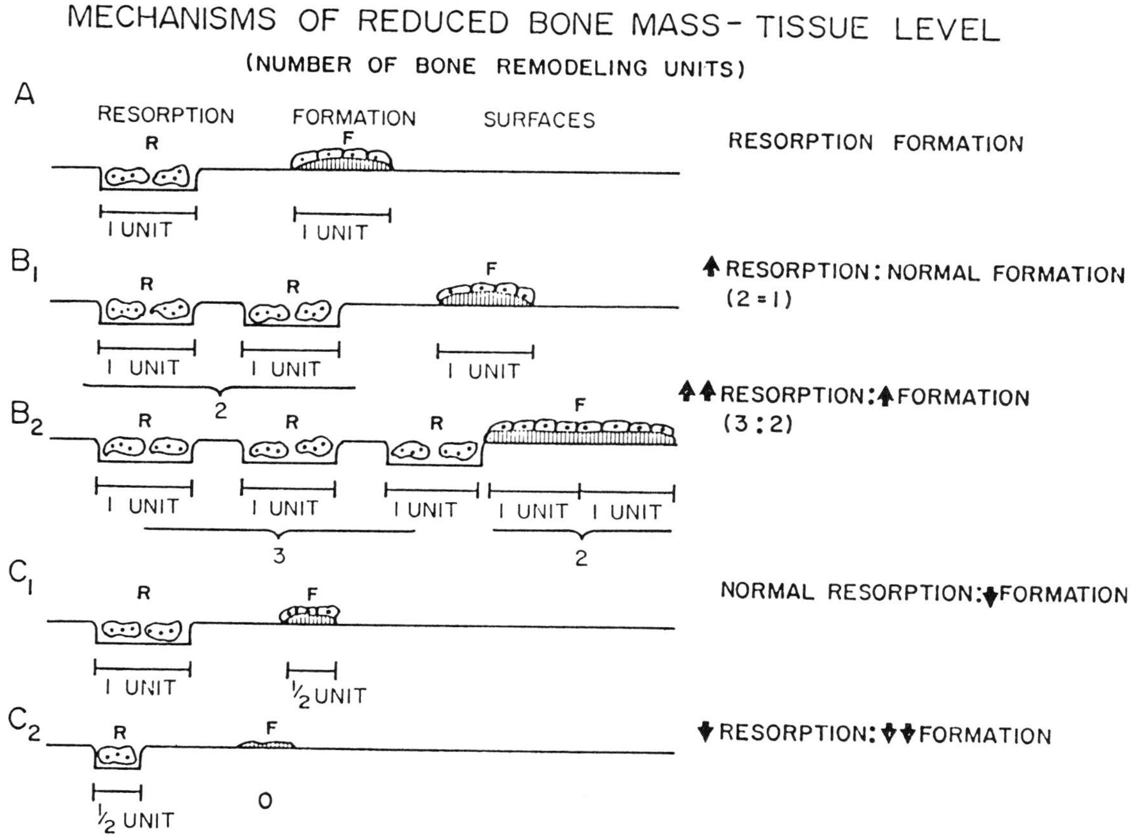
MECHANISMS OF REDUCED BONE MASS - TISSUE LEVEL
(NUMBER OF BONE REMODELING UNITS)
A
RESORPTION
R
FORMATION
F
SURFACES
RESORPTION FORMATION
I UNIT
I UNIT
B1
R
R
F
↑RESORPTION: NORMAL FORMATION
(2 = 1)
I UNIT
I UNIT
I UNIT
2
B2
R
R
R
F
↑↑RESORPTION: ↑FORMATION
(3 : 2)
I UNIT
I UNIT
I UNIT
I UNIT
I UNIT
3
2
C1
R
F
NORMAL RESORPTION: ↓FORMATION
I UNIT
½ UNIT
C2
R
F
↓RESORPTION: ↓↓FORMATION
½ UNIT
0

**FIGURE 54–15.** Mechanisms of reduced bone mass at the tissue level. A depicts skeletal balance (R surface = F surface); $B_1$ and $B_2$ depict negative balance (R surface > F surface) with high turnover; $C_1$ and $C_2$ depict negative balance (R surface > F surface) with low turnover (see text).

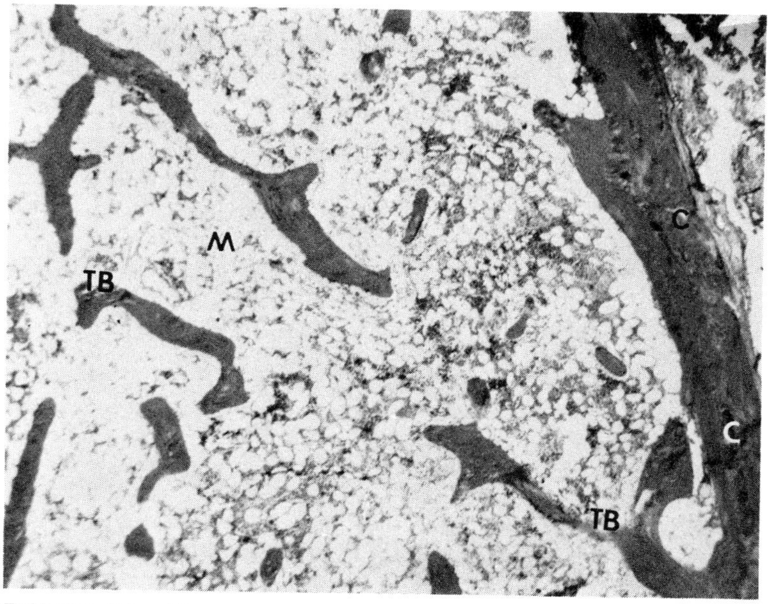
M
TB
TB
C
C

**FIGURE 54–16.** Osteoporosis. Low-power photomicrograph shows a reduction in cortical width (C) and a loss of trabecular bone spicules (TB). Compare to Figure 54–1. M, Marrow (Masson trichrome stain; original magnification × 25).

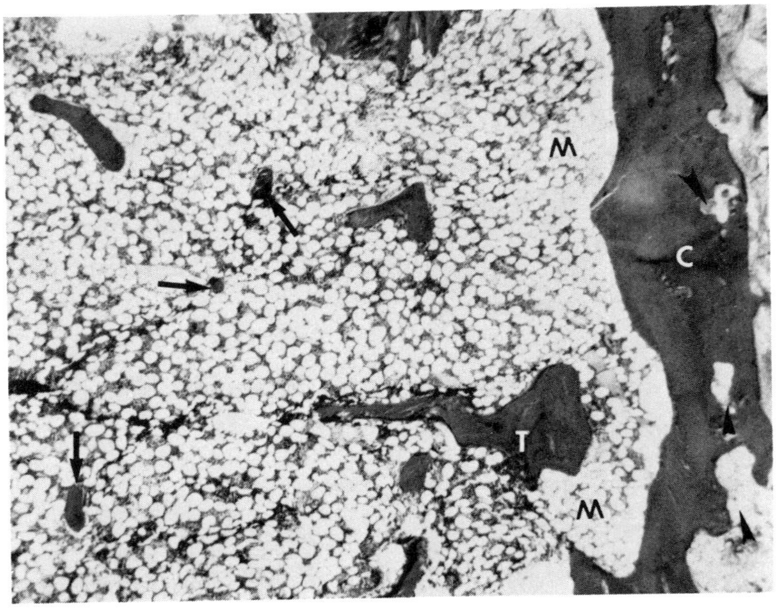
M
C
T
M

**FIGURE 54–17.** Osteoporosis. Low-power photomicrograph illustrates a further progression of the osteopenic state. Trabecular bone is now reduced to islands and thin spicules (arrows) of bone, instead of intact struts or bars. Compare to Figure 54–1. Note the reduction in cortical thickness, and an increase in cortical porosity (arrowheads) due to resorption of bone by activated osteoclasts within haversian cutting cones. C, Cortical bone; T, trabecular bone; M, marrow (Masson trichrome stain; original magnification× 25).

tent with the amount of osteoid seen by light microscopy. As a result, the *mineralization front activity* (fraction of tetracycline-labeled osteoid surface) is preserved, but is associated with a reduction in the linear extent of bone formation (fraction of labeled trabecular bone surfaces). Single fluorescent labels predominate (Fig. 54–20*B*), because the rate of bone matrix deposition is low enough to prevent spatial separation of the two courses of tetracycline.

**Osteomalacia.** Osteomalacia is usually characterized by excessive quantities of osteoid due to a failure of matrix calcification, despite continued matrix synthesis by osteoblasts (Table 54–5). Marked increases in the thickness of osteoid seams are characteristic, but osteomalacia may be associated with normal or even reduced quantities of osteoid.[7] The static and dynamic parameters that characterize osteomalacia include an increase in the amount of osteoid, and a reciprocal decrease in the rate of mineralization, respectively. These two components allow one to distinguish osteomalacia from other disorders of bone remodeling activity manifesting abnormal quantities of osteoid. In low-turnover states, for example, the mineralization rate may be low, but the quantity of osteoid is appropriately reduced. If the mineralization rate is not low, the presence of a mineralization defect is unlikely, despite the presence of excess amounts of osteoid, as seen in high-turnover states when matrix synthesis is accelerated.

Although osteomalacia is usually associated with low bone remodeling activity, features of osteoblast activation, osteoclast proliferation, and peritrabecular fibrosis, all indicative of accelerated turnover, may be present. Osteomalacia is, therefore, often seen in the context of a mixed bone lesion, coexisting with osteitis fibrosa. Examples of osteomalacia are shown in Figures 54–21*A* and *B*.

## SKELETAL MANIFESTATIONS OF NUTRITIONAL DISEASES

Bone plays a major role in calcium and mineral homeostasis and, as a result, the skeleton is sensitive to metabolic and hormonal imbalances. It is, therefore, not surprising that a wide variety of abnormalities of nutrition influence the skeleton (Table 54–6). Nutritional disorders either may result in defective mineralization producing osteomalacia or may manifest as osteoporosis. The osteoporotic conditions may result from either accelerated remodeling or reduced remodeling.

The skeleton is limited in the manner in which the tissue and cells respond to injury. The histologic differential diagnosis of metabolic diseases is, therefore, broad because various metabolic, endocrine, or nutritional disorders may produce similar morphologic changes in the skeleton.

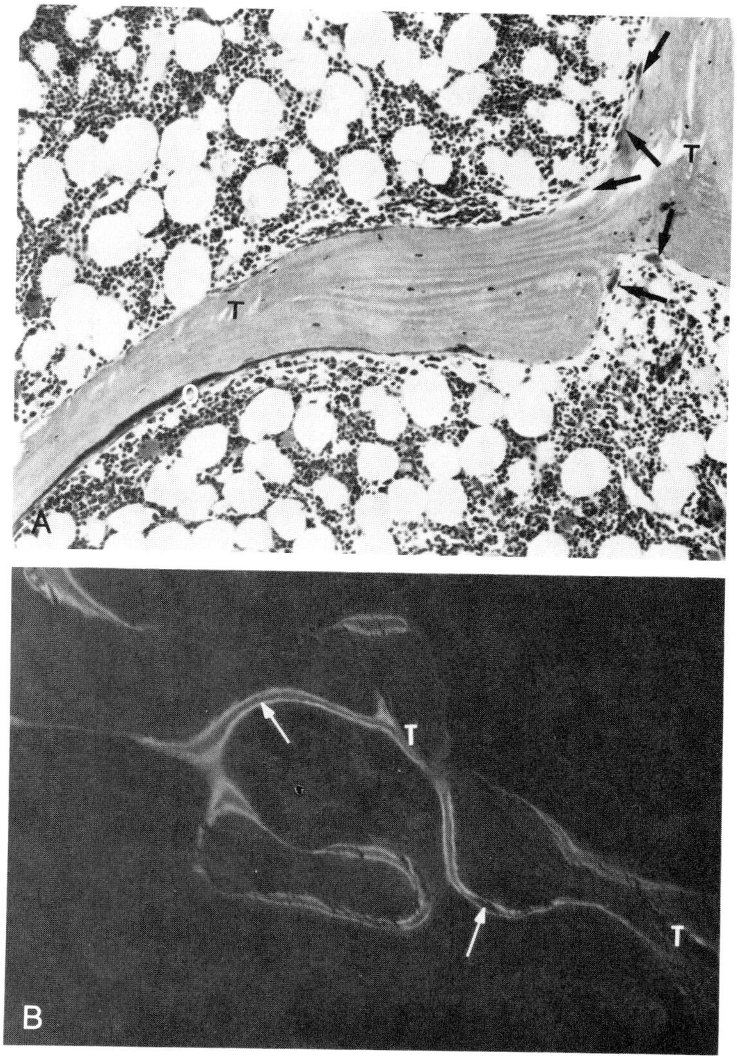
T
T
O
A
T
T
B

**FIGURE 54–18.** *A*, Active remodeling osteoporosis. Notice the increased total osteoid surface (O) and the increased number of osteoclasts (arrows) along the trabecular bone (T). This biopsy was taken from a patient with postgastrectomy osteoporosis (Masson trichrome stain; original magnification × 160). *B*, Corresponding fluorescent photomicrograph showing an increase in the linear extent of bone formation as revealed by the extensive double tetracycline-labeled surfaces (arrows). T, Trabecular bone (unstained section; original magnification × 98).

The primary role of the bone biopsy procedure, therefore, is not to provide a diagnosis of a specific disease, but rather to establish the level of bone turnover and to confirm or to exclude the presence of a mineralization defect. In this manner, a list of diagnostic possibilities is obtained, and the differential diagnosis is narrowed by a multidisciplinary approach involving clinical, laboratory, and radiologic findings.

## IDIOPATHIC OSTEOPOROSIS

Idiopathic or primary osteoporosis is subdivided by the age at presentation and sex of the individual (e.g., postmenopausal or senile). The age-related or involutional bone loss for both sexes is well characterized, such that there is a progressive loss of cortical and trabecular bone (see Figs. 54–16 and 54–17) with age in men and

**TABLE 54–3.** HISTOLOGIC FEATURES OF INCREASED BONE REMODELING ACTIVITY (ACCELERATED TURNOVER)

| |
|---|
| Bone Formation Parameters |
| Increased osteoid volume |
| Increased osteoid surface |
| Normal to increased osteoid seam width |
| Increased osteoblastic surface |
| Tetracycline Kinetic Parameters |
| Increased linear extent of bone formation |
| Double fluorescent labels predominate |
| Normal to increased appositional rate |
| Mineralization front activity maximal |
| Increased bone formation rate |
| Normal or decreased mineralization lag time |
| Bone Resorption Parameters |
| Increased osteoclast number |
| Increased active resorbing surface |
| Subperiosteal resorption |
| Other |
| Increased cortical porosity |
| Active cutting cones in cortex |
| Decreased cortical width |
| Osteitis fibrosa (peritrabecular fibrous tissue) |
| Woven bone |

women, with a transient accelerated phase of loss that occurs in women after the menopause. Although involutional osteoporosis is heterogeneous and the etiology complex, bone loss is thought to be due to a variety of age-related factors including osteoblast senescence with reduced bone formation, decreased calcium absorption with decreased production of 1,25 $(OH)_2$ vitamin D and gastrointestinal resistance to its action, mild secondary hyperparathyroidism, calcitonin deficiency, and estrogen withdrawal. When calcium absorption from the diet is insufficient to offset fecal and urinary calcium losses, calcium must be withdrawn from the bone. The minimum daily requirement is currently set at 800 mg per day. The middle-aged and elderly may have actual daily intakes far less than this amount. Although normal adults adapt to decreased calcium intake by increasing the fraction of absorbed dietary calcium, this compensatory mechanism is blunted by aging. Thus, the calcium requirement for postmenopausal women has been estimated to be as high as 1,500 mg per day to prevent negative calcium balance.

Although the importance of an adequate intake of calcium to promote growth is well known, the role of calcium intake in preventing osteoporosis is controversial.[8,9] Additional studies are required before final conclusions can be made.[10] In the meantime, prevention of osteoporosis should be directed at correcting low dietary calcium intakes (800 mg per day for adults and 1200 mg per day for adolescents are recommended daily allowances). The National Institutes of Health Consensus Conference on Osteoporosis recommended a daily calcium intake of 1000 to 1500 mg for all postmenopausal women (see Chap. 89).[11]

Histologically, postmenopausal osteoporosis is a heterogeneous disorder. Bone remodeling activity may be accelerated, normal, or decreased.[12] Serum and urine biochemical tests fail to separate these groups. This heterogeneity of osteoporosis may be partly responsible for the current disappointing results of drug therapy trials. It has been postulated, based upon bone biopsy-derived tetracycline dynamics and the identification of active and inactive groups, that different therapies may be required. For example, calcium is known to inhibit osteoclast activity. Patients with inactive osteoporosis who are treated with vitamin D and calcium may undergo further depression of an already low bone remodeling status, such that the restoration of bone mass is unlikely.[13] The treatment of osteoporosis is described in detail elsewhere and in Chapter 89.[10]

## CALCIUM DEFICIENCY, CHRONIC

The circulating calcium concentration is tightly regulated by a variety of hormones. The skeleton is the major reservoir for calcium, and during states of calcium deprivation, calcium homeostasis is maintained at the expense of the skeleton, even to the point of producing severe bone disease. The major response to hypocalcemia is the compensatory increase in parathyroid hormone secretion. Parathyroid hormone acts to increase bone resorption, and thereby to accelerate bone remodeling activity. Chronic hypocalcemia conditions such as chronic renal failure, vitamin D deficiency states, and mineral malabsorption secondary to gastrointestinal disease may exhibit evidence of increased bone turnover.

**Calcium Deficiency in Children.** Although calcium deficiency usually leads to secondary hyperparathyroidism with increased bone resorption, low dietary calcium intake in children may result in rickets and osteomalacia.[14] Defective mineralization is expressed more readily

**TABLE 54–4.** HISTOLOGIC FEATURES OF DECREASED BONE REMODELING ACTIVITY (REDUCED TURNOVER)

| |
|---|
| Bone Formation Parameters |
| Normal to decreased osteoid volume |
| Decreased osteoid surface |
| Normal to decreased osteoid seam width |
| Reduced osteoblastic surface |
| Tetracycline Kinetic Parameters |
| Decreased linear extent of bone formation |
| Single labels predominate |
| Normal to reduced appositional rate |
| Mineralization front activity low to normal |
| Low bone formation rate |
| Normal mineralization lag time |
| Bone Resorption Parameters |
| Decreased osteoclast number |
| Decreased active resorption surface |

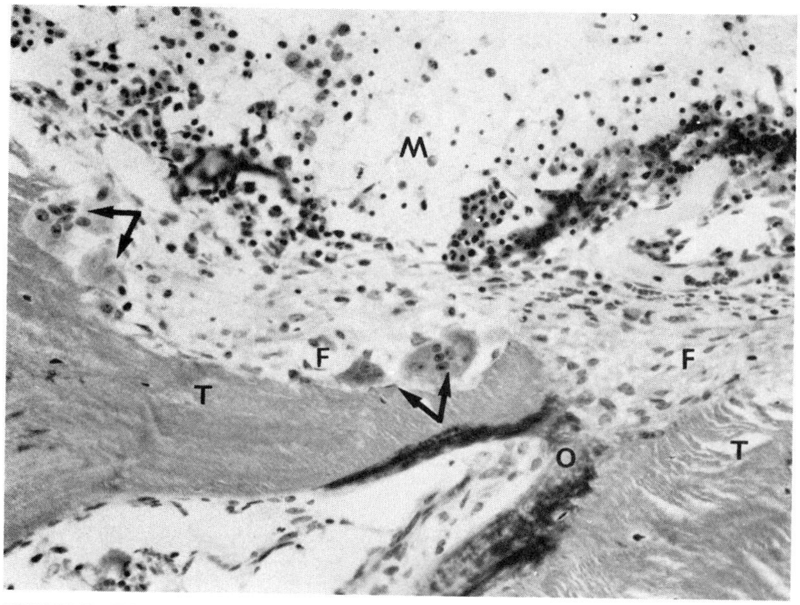
M
F
F
T
T
O

**FIGURE 54–19.** Osteitis fibrosa, a manifestation of accelerated bone turnover, characterized by increased numbers of osteoclasts (arrows) and peritrabecular fibrosis (F). This biopsy was obtained from an osteoporotic patient with mineral malabsorption due to small intestinal disease with subsequent hypocalcemia and secondary hyperparathyroidism. T, Trabecular bone; O, osteoid, M, marrow (Goldner trichrome stain; original magnification × 250).

in this younger group than in adults because of the increased calcium demands required during skeletal growth.

## HYPOPHOSPHATEMIA

Mineralization of skeletal tissue requires phosphorus as well as calcium in the deposition of amorphous calcium phosphate and in the formation of hydroxyapatite crystals. Various clinical disorders are associated with hypophosphatemia. The skeletal disease consists of rickets in children and osteomalacia in adults. Histologically, osteomalacia exists in a pure form, i.e., low-turnover osteomalacia without evidence of osteitis fibrosa.

**X-Linked Hypophosphatemia (XLH).** XLH, also known as vitamin D-resistant rickets, familial hypophosphatemia, and phosphate diabetes, is the most common form of hereditary rickets and osteomalacia. XLH is characterized by a primary defect in renal transport of phosphorus resulting in hypophosphatemia. Histologically, osteoid excess is usually marked, with extremely widened osteoid seams covering virtually all bone surfaces, resulting in osteosclerosis. In addition, hypomineralized zones surround the osteocytes, producing a ring of osteoid (Fig. 54–22). This "halo" effect is thought to represent a mineralization defect around newly formed osteocytes, and a characteristic feature of this disorder.[15]

**Sporadic Hypophosphatemia.** Renal phosphorus wasting may also occur without a family history and may be present any time from infancy to adulthood.

**Oncogenic Osteomalacia** Oncogenic osteomalacia is caused by a secreted tumor product that inhibits renal tubular reabsorption of phosphorus and the 1-hydroxylation of 25-hydroxyvitamin D, resulting in hypophosphatemia and inappropriately low levels of 1,25 $(OH)_2$ vitamin D. This form of secondary hypophosphatemic osteomalacia has been described with a variety of bone and soft tissue mesenchymal tumors and prostatic adenocarcinoma.[16] The bone disease remits after complete resection of the coexisting neoplasm.

**Antacid-Induced Osteomalacia.** Chronic consumption of phosphate-binding antacids can cause hypophosphatemic osteomalacia.[17] Phosphorus depletion is accompanied by hypophosphatemia with hypophosphaturia, hypercalciuria, and nephrolithiasis.

## PRIMARY VITAMIN D DEFICIENCY

Adequate serum calcium and phosphorus levels are required for normal matrix mineralization. It remains unclear, however, whether vitamin D metabolites affect the mineralization process by a direct effect on the osteoblast, or by indirect mechanisms through augmentation of intestinal calcium and phosphorus absorption. Experimental studies utilizing vitamin D-deficient rats

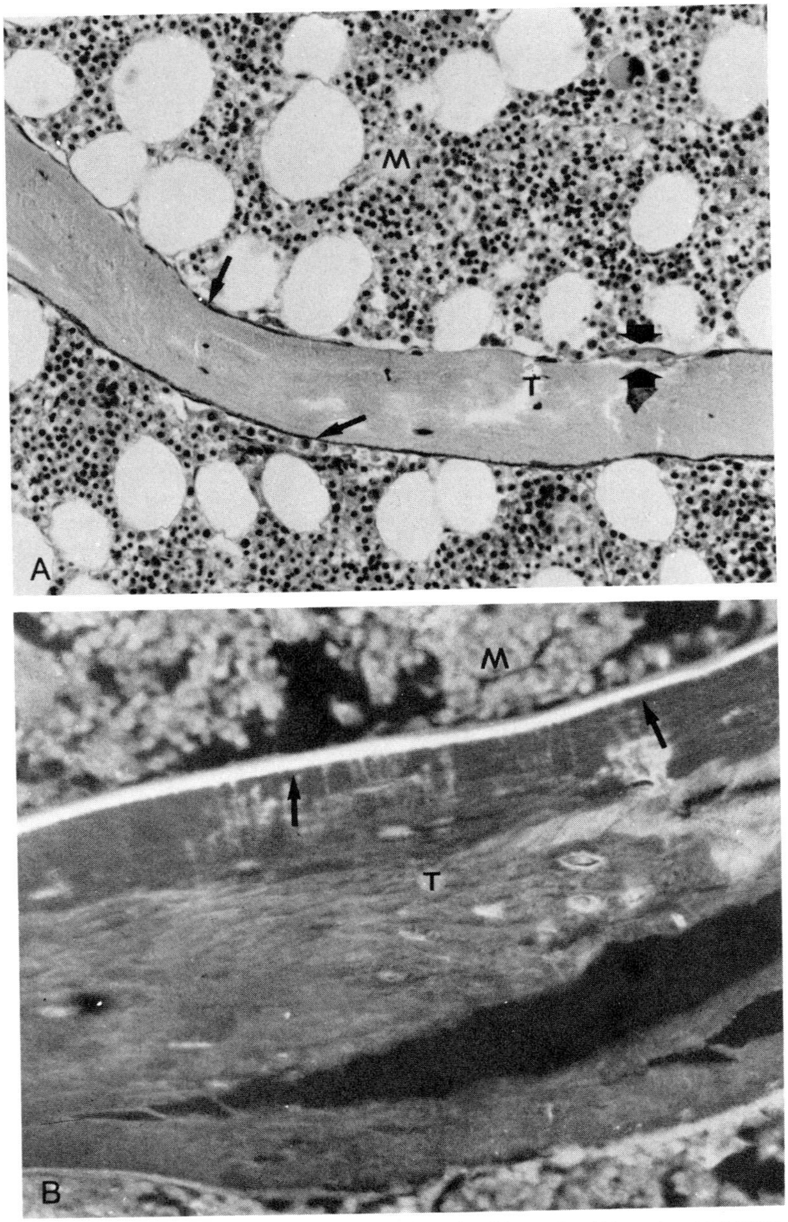
M
T
A
M
T
B

**FIGURE 54–20.** *A*, Inactive osteoporosis. Note the thin, almost nonexistent osteoid seams (arrows) and a single osteoclast (arrowheads). This biopsy is from a patient with anorexia nervosa and osteopenia. T, Trabecular bone; M, marrow (Goldner trichrome stain; original magnification × 160). *B*, Corresponding fluorescent micrograph showing superimposed single linear tetracycline labels (arrows). Because the rate of bone turnover is so low, not enough matrix was synthesized over the 2-week labeling period to allow spatial separation of the two fluorescent bands. T, Trabecular bone; M, marrow.

infused with calcium and phosphorus provided histomorphometric evidence that vitamin D was not essential for mineralization in growing rats.[18]

Because of the routine fortification of foodstuffs with vitamin D, dietary deficiency of this vitamin is now uncommon. Vitamin D deficiency, however, may still be encountered in certain clinical settings. Elderly individuals and institutionalized patients with poor diets and inadequate exposure to sunlight, food faddists, and alcoholics are prone to vitamin D deficiency. In addition to dietary restriction, vitamin D deficiency may occur following inadequate solar exposure.[19] Osteomalacia

**TABLE 54–5.** HISTOLOGIC FEATURES OF OSTEOMALACIA

| Bone Formation Parameters | Bone Remodeling Activity Status | |
|---|---|---|
| Osteoid excess common: | | |
| Increased osteoid volume | | |
| Increased osteoid surface | | |
| Markedly increased osteoid seam thickness | | |
| Subperiosteal osteoid | | |
| Cortical bone osteoid deposits | | |
| | Pure osteomalacia (low remodeling state): | Mixed osteomalacia osteitis fibrosa (high remodeling state): |
| Osteoblastic surface | Reduced | Normal to increased |
| Osteoblast number | Normal to decreased | Normal to increased |
| Active resorption surface | Normal to decreased | Normal to increased |
| Linear extent of bone formation | Reduced (may be 0) | May be reduced |
| Appositional rate | Reduced (often 0) | Reduced |
| Tetracycline labels | Predominantly abnormal<br>Diffuse, unlabeled | Predominantly abnormal<br>Diffuse, unlabeled |
| Mineralization front activity | Approaches 0 | Reduced |
| Bone formation rate | Reduced | Variable |
| Mineralization lag time | Increased | Increased |
| Peritrabecular fibrosis | Absent | Usually present |
| Subperiosteal resorption | Absent | May be present |

and rickets have been described in Asian immigrants who avoid exposure to sunlight.

Vitamin D functions to facilitate calcium absorption from the intestinal tract. Classic biochemical findings in vitamin D deficiency include near-normal serum calcium and a low serum phosphorus, reflecting bone resorption and the renal phosphaturic effect of parathyroid hormone. In the face of a falling serum calcium concentration, homeostatic mechanisms attempt to preserve the normal extracellular calcium level, at the expense of the mineral-deficient skeleton. The histologic appearance of bone reflects this combination of osteomalacia and osteitis fibrosa.[20] The histologic changes may be variable, and may reflect the degree and duration of vitamin D deficiency (see Fig. 54–21*A* and *B*). Milder forms of vitamin D deficiency may present as active bone remodeling disease resulting in osteoporosis, but not osteomalacia, because the mineralization may be ameliorated by compensatory secondary hyperparathyroidism.

## HEPATOBILIARY DISEASE

Vitamin D deficiency, despite adequate intake, may result from impaired vitamin D metabolism. Hepatic disease may decrease production of 25-OH vitamin D, owing to inadequate microsomal hydroxylase activity.

**Alcohol-Associated Liver Disease.** Fractures in alcoholics are generally due to trauma. Chronic alcoholism may also alter calcium homeostasis and may predispose the skeleton to fracture. Several studies have shown a reduction in trabecular bone mass in alcoholics. Furthermore, drinking alcoholic beverages has been implicated as a risk factor for primary osteoporosis. Two histologic studies of bone from alcoholics found evidence of osteomalacia (increased osteoid volume), although the kinetics of bone remodeling using double tetracycline labeling were not reported.[20,21] A study of eight males with a 10-year history of alcohol abuse showed a reduction in vertebral trabecular bone mass, with preservation of appendicular cortical bone. Histologically, a reduction in active bone formation and resorption was seen without evidence of osteomalacia.[22] Several explanations could account for a reduction in bone mass in the alcoholic, including nutritional deficiencies of calcium and vitamin D, malabsorption of calcium and vitamin D secondary to pancreatic or liver disease, abnormal metabolism of vitamin D due to cirrhosis of the liver, abnormal parathyroid secretion, and a direct toxic effect of ethanol on calcium absorption.

**Cholestatic Liver Disease.** *The metabolic bone disease most commonly associated with cholestatic liver disease is osteoporosis.*[23] It is manifested by bone pain, fractures, and reduced bone volume. Even in the two series of patients that reported a high incidence of osteomalacia,[21,24] 50% or more of the patients with cholestasis who had radiographic evidence of osteopenia proved histologically to have a *reduction* in both mineralized bone and osteoid.

In one histologic study, accelerated remodeling features were seen in iliac crest biopsy specimens from patients with primary biliary cirrhosis.[25] Despite find-

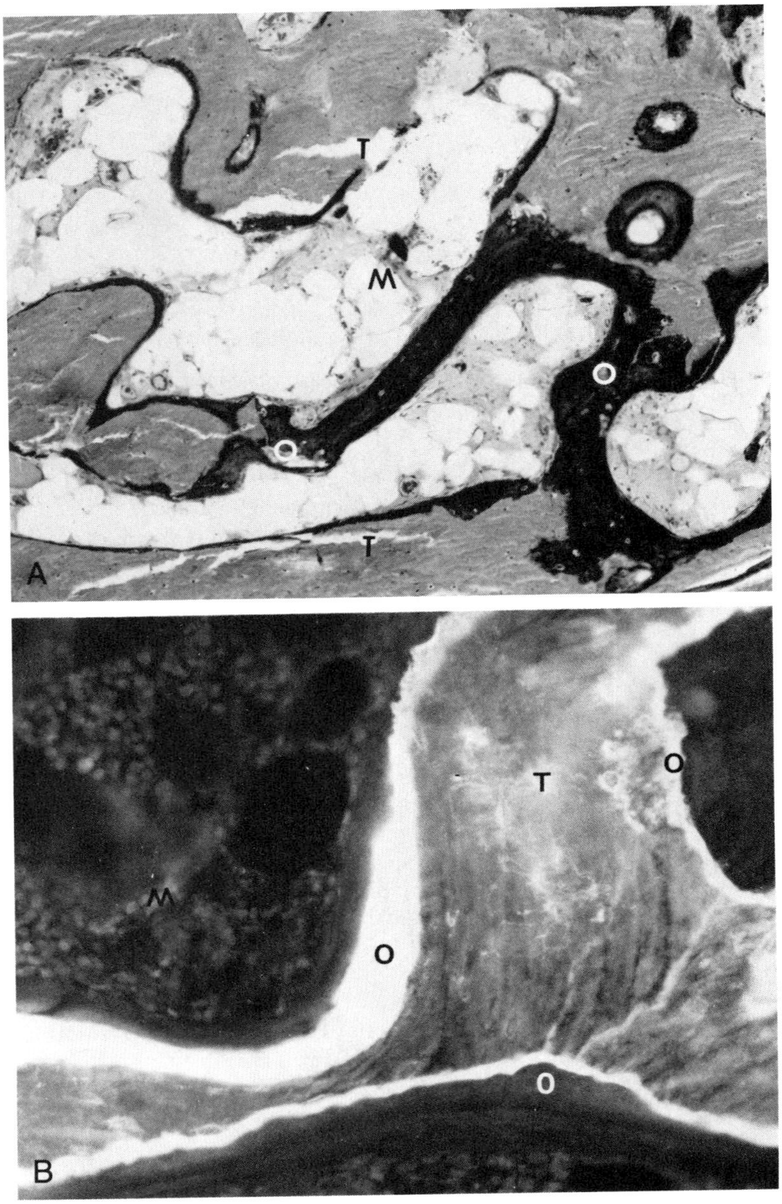
T
M
O
O
T
A
T
O
M
O
O
B

**FIGURE 54–21.** *A*, Osteomalacia due to vitamin D deficiency. The mineralization defect is manifested by marked increases in the quantity of osteoid (O). The relative osteoid volume is increased as a result of an increase in the osteoid surface as well as an augmentation of the mean osteoid seam width. M, Marrow; T, trabecular bone (Goldner trichrome stain; original magnification × 120). *B*, Corresponding fluorescent micrograph confirming the presence of a severe mineralization defect, as shown by the abnormal diffuse fluorescent tetracycline uptake at the osteoid seams (O). T, Trabecular bone; M, marrow.

ings of low circulating levels of 25-hydroxyvitamin D, histomorphometric analysis of bone failed to reveal evidence of osteomalacia. Hyperosteoidosis was absent, as measured by fractional osteoid surface, osteoid volume, or fractional osteoid volume. In addition, mineral appositional rates and calculated bone formation rate were normal. These findings suggest that vitamin D deficiency (hyperosteoidosis) does not contribute significantly to hepatic osteodystrophy observed in patients with primary biliary cirrhosis.

**TABLE 54–6.** BONE HISTOPATHOLOGY ASSOCIATED WITH SPECIFIC NUTRITIONAL DISORDERS

| | |
|---|---|
| I. Accelerated Remodeling States (high-turnover or active osteoporosis) | Idiopathic Osteoporosis: involutional (postmenopausal; senile). Secondary Osteoporosis: calcium deficiency states; chronic (secondary hyperparathyroidism); small intestinal disease (early, compensated mineral malabsorption); postgastrectomy (mineral malabsorption). |
| II. Reduced Remodeling States (low-turnover or inactive osteoporosis) | Idiopathic osteoporosis: involutional (postmenopausal; senile). Secondary osteoporosis: hepatic disease (cholestatic liver disease, biliary cirrhosis; alcohol-associated); severe systemic disease, starvation, inanition, anorexia nervosa; total parenteral nutrition. |
| III. Osteomalacia—Pure | X-linked hypophosphatemia (vitamin D-resistant rickets); sporadic hypophosphatemia; antacid-induced osteomalacia; oncogenic osteomalacia; primary vitamin D deficiency; chronic pancreatitis; metabolic acidosis; renal osteodystrophy (aluminum-associated osteomalacia). |
| IV. Osteomalacia—Mixed (Osteomalacia/Osteitis Fibrosa) | Primary vitamin D deficiency (nutritional, lack of solar exposure); small intestinal disease (vitamin D and calcium malabsorption); postgastrectomy (vitamin D and calcium malabsorption); renal osteodystrophy (mixed osteomalacia-osteitis fibrosa); calcium deficiency of children. |

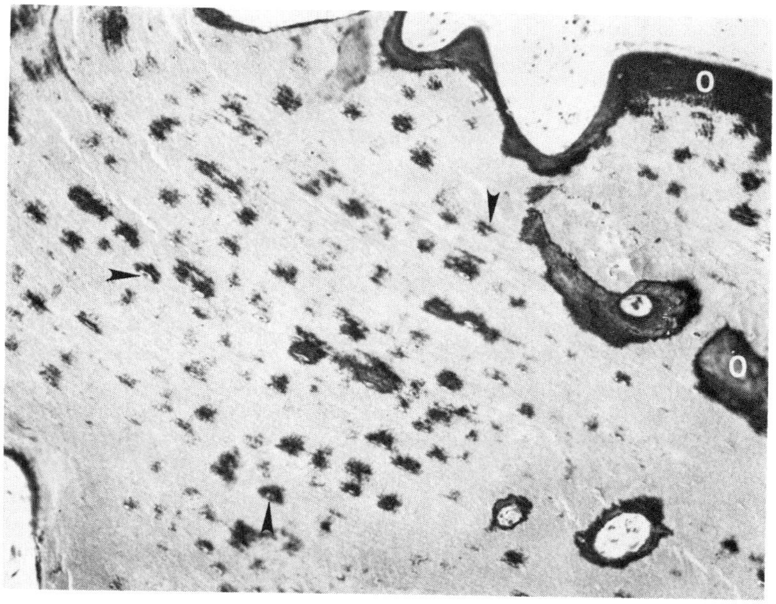
O
O

**FIGURE 54–22.** Osteomalacia of x-linked hypophosphatemia (vitamin D-resistant rickets). Hypophosphatemia promoted osteomalacia as shown histologically by the increased volume of osteoid (O) and presence of osteoid around osteocytes creating a "halo sign" (arrowheads). This periosteocytic mineralization defect is typical of XLH (Goldner trichrome stain; original magnification × 120).

## PARTIAL GASTRECTOMY

Dietary deficiency, impaired absorption of calcium, and malabsorption of vitamin D with steatorrhea may be seen in gastrectomy patients. The skeletal lesion may, therefore, be variable, depending upon the relative contribution by malabsorption of minerals versus vitamin D. In contrast to those with small bowel resection, most patients following partial gastrectomy develop osteoporosis rather than osteomalacia (see Fig. 54–18*A* and *B*). High-turnover features usually predominate in bone biopsy specimens.

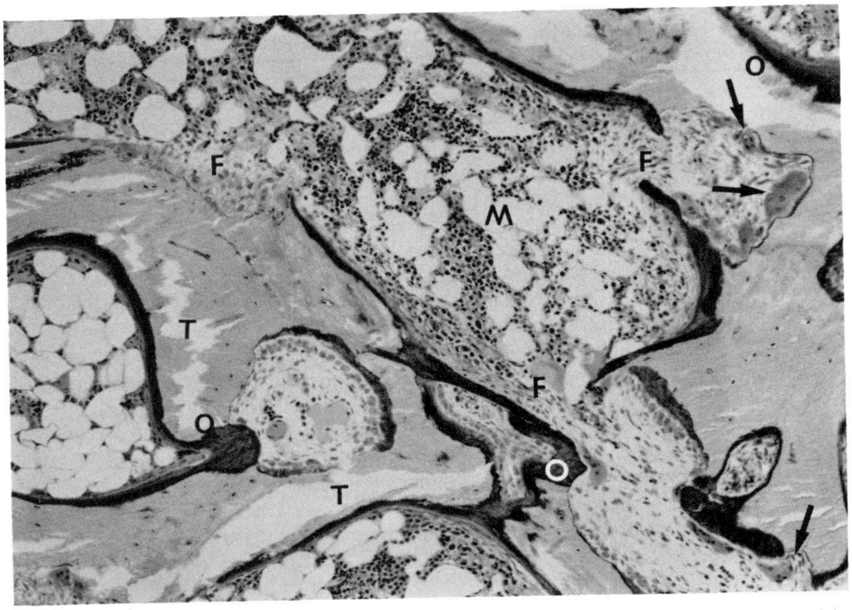
O
F
F
M
T
O
T
F
O

**FIGURE 54–23.** Renal osteodystrophy mixed with osteomalacia and osteitis fibrosa. Osteomalacia is suggested by the presence of a marked increased in the total osteoid surface (O), and was confirmed by abnormal tetracycline fluorescent patterns. Parathyroid hormone effect on the skeleton is evident by the presence of extensive peritrabecular fibrosis (F) and increased numbers of osteoclasts (arrows). T, Trabecular bone; M, marrow (Goldner trichrome stain; original magnification × 98).

## SMALL BOWEL DISEASE

Currently, osteomalacia in adulthood is frequently associated with intestinal malabsorption.[26] Chronic inflammatory disease of the small intestine, such as gluten-sensitive enteropathy and regional enteritis, often result in malabsorption of vitamin D and minerals. Anatomic defects, such as small bowel resections and small bowel bypass operations, may also produce these functional disorders. Malabsorption of vitamin D and calcium may be selective and may not be reflected by the degree of steatorrhea or necessarily by the extent, severity, and duration of small bowel disease. Malabsorption states may present with a reduction in bone mass without marked increases in osteoid (i.e., osteoporosis). Because symptomatic osteomalacia in patients with gastrointestinal disease may occur with a paucity of clinical and laboratory clues, the bone biopsy procedure has become the most reliable method for establishing the type and severity of the skeletal disease.

## TOTAL PARENTERAL NUTRITION (HYPERALIMENTATION)

Patients receiving total parenteral nutrition (TPN) have multiple derangements in mineral metabolism. Frequently, they have osteopenia, which may antedate their nutritional therapy. Rickets and osteomalacia have been associated with TPN.[27] This syndrome is characterized by bone pain, fractures, hypercalciuria, intermittent hypercalcemia, normal 25-OH vitamin D, reduced $1,25(OH)_2$ vitamin D, and normal parathyroid hormone concentrations. The pathogenesis of the bone changes remains unknown. Factors postulated include recognized trace metal deficiency and excess or altered vitamin D metabolism.[28] Aluminum plays a pathogenetic role in the development of the osteomalacia in patients receiving casein hydrolysates contaminated with aluminum.[29] Patients who are exposed to parenteral aluminum appear to develop a low-formation bone lesion that leads to symptoms and fractures. Total parenteral nutrition solutions should be carefully monitored to avoid aluminum contamination.

In one study of 13 home TPN patients, bone histomorphometry showed reduced bone volume and reduced osteoid with normal resorption and calcification rates.[30] These abnormalities were associated with hypercalciuria, but the plasma levels of $1,25(OH)_2D$ were normal. Abnormalities in bone metabolism in these patients suggest a fundamental decrease in bone matrix formation rather than a mineralization defect as the underlying mechanism.

## CHRONIC RENAL FAILURE

Renal osteodystrophy comprises the spectrum of skeletal and mineral alterations that attend chronic renal failure. The pattern of bone involvement may be catego-

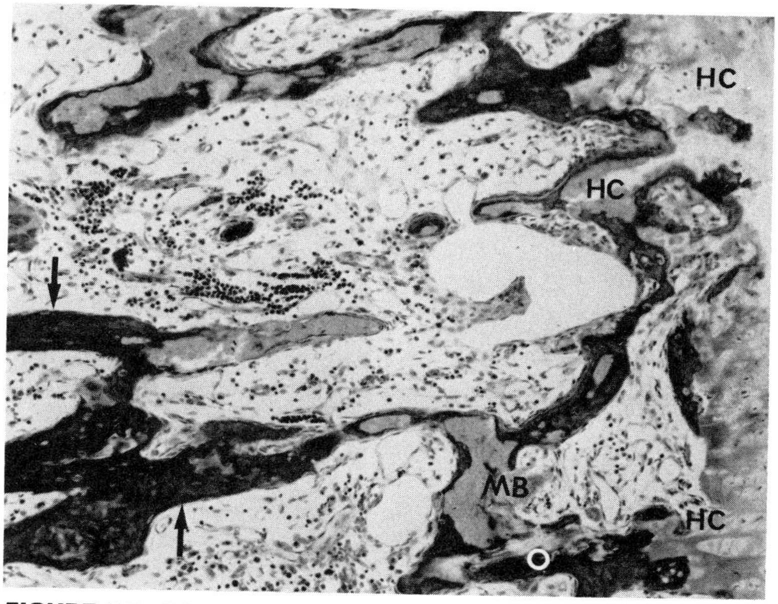
HC
HC
MB
HC
O

**FIGURE 54–24.** Rickets and osteomalacia in a child with chronic renal insufficiency. The mineralization defect of the cartilage, characteristic of rickets, consists of irregular tongues of poorly calcified hypertrophic chondrocytes (HC). Defective mineralization of the metaphyseal bone represents osteomalacia, with marked increases in osteoid (O). In some instances entire trabeculae consist of unmineralized matrix (arrows). Rickets and osteomalacia, from primary vitamin D deficiency, may also exhibit a similar histologic appearance, although of variable severity. MB, Metaphyseal bone (Goldner trichrome stain; original magnification × 250).

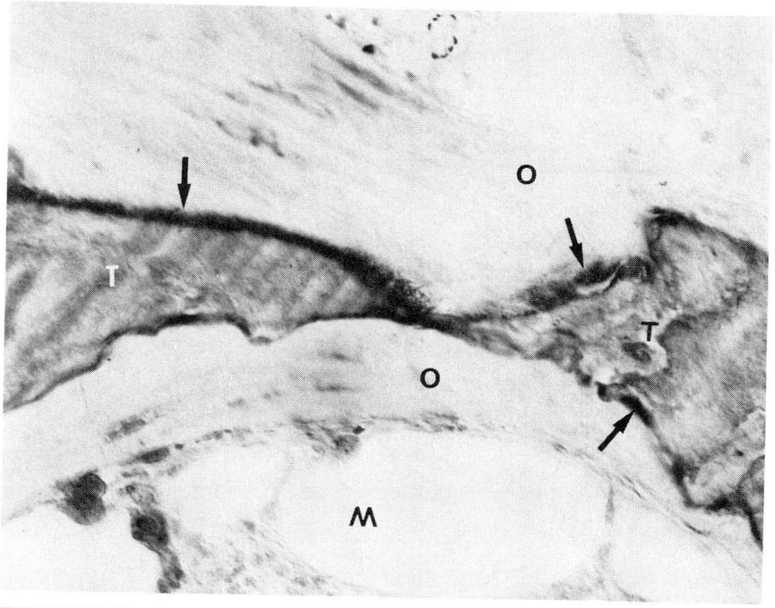
O
T
T
O
M

**FIGURE 54–25.** Positive aluminum histochemical stain, in a biopsy from a patient with renal osteodystrophy exhibiting pure osteomalacia. Reaction product (arrows) lines the mineralization fronts. O, Osteoid accumulation; T, trabecular bone; M, marrow (aluminum stain, no counterstain; original magnification × 250).

rized by histologic examination of tissue into three major groups: pure osteomalacia, mixed osteomalacia/osteitis fibrosis, and predominance of osteitis fibrosis. Mixed bone lesions and osteitis fibrosis-predominant lesions result from aberrations of vitamin D metabolism, calcium deficiency, phosphorus retention, and secondary hyperparathyroidism. In general, biochemical values and biologic changes are approximate indicators of the underlying bone changes. The type of skeletal lesions can only reliably be determined by direct examination of bone tissue.[31] Renal osteodystrophy is a complex disorder that is histologically heterogeneous. Osteomalacia

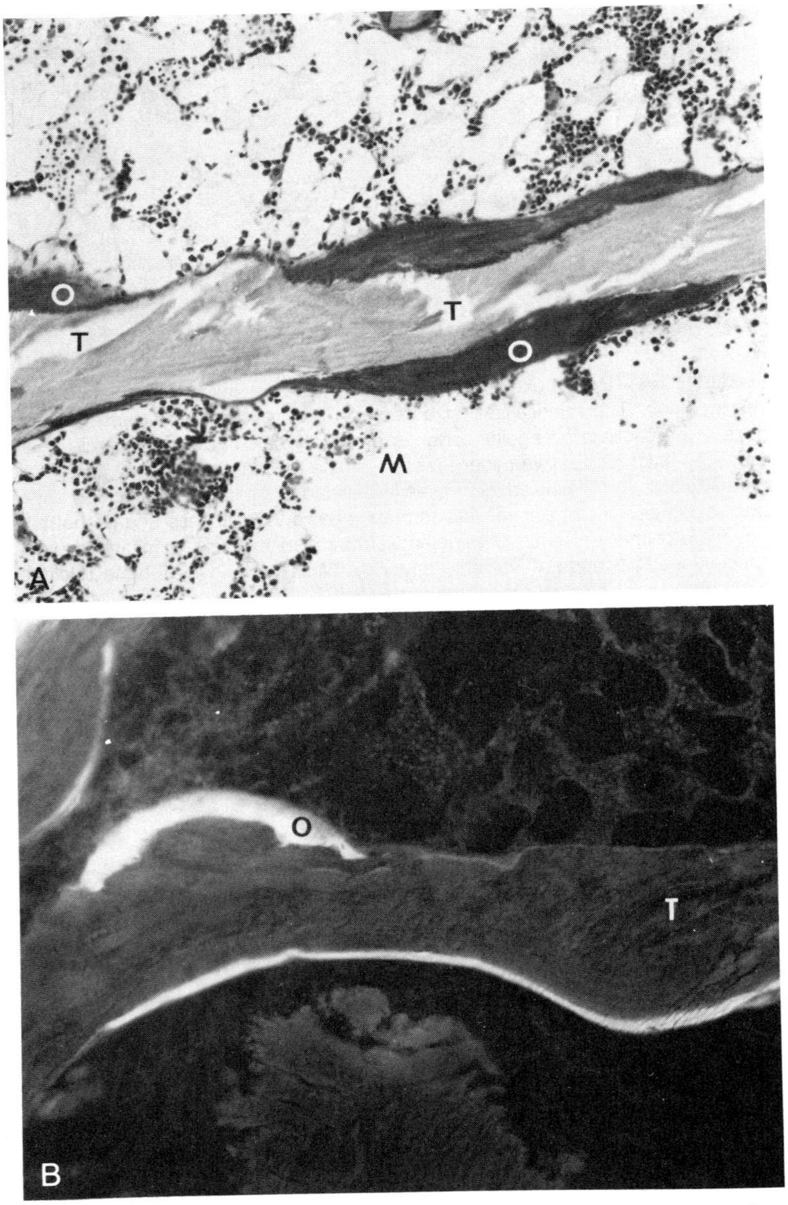
O
T
T
O
M
A
O
T
B

**FIGURE 54–26.** *A*, Osteomalacia caused by long-term, high-dose sodium fluoride therapy for osteoporosis. The pattern of fusiform osteoid accumulation (O) around several of the trabecular spicules (T) is characteristic of sodium fluoride-induced mineralization defect. M, Marrow (Goldner trichrome stain, original magnification × 250). *B*, By fluorescent microscopy, the unusual osteoid deposits seen by light microscopy exhibit diffuse tetracycline uptake. O, Osteoid; T, trabecular bone (unstained section; original magnification × 120).

may coexist with accelerated rate of mineralization in adjacent osteoid surfaces (Figs. 54–23 and 54–24). Therefore, the proportion of abnormally mineralizing osteoid seams can only be determined by evaluation of kinetic tetracycline markers.

The pure-osteomalacia form of renal bone disease has been associated with the accumulation of aluminum in bone (Fig. 54–25). The retention of aluminum due to the inability to excrete this metal in chronic renal insufficiency is associated with the deposition of this ion in bone tissue.[32]

## RENAL TUBULAR ACIDOSIS

Rickets or osteomalacia may occur in patients with chronic hyperchloremic acidosis due to renal tubular diseases.[33] A renal tubular defect results in impaired hydrogen ion excretion, promoting systemic acidosis. Calcium is lost from bone as the skeleton attempts to buffer the responses to chronic acidosis. The mechanism of osteomalacia is unknown, but may involve alterations in vitamin D metabolism. Alkali treatment alone has resulted in healing of the mineralization defect.

## STARVATION-INANITION

Bone formation may be affected not only at the level of mineralization but also during the earlier stage of organic matrix synthesis and secretion. General inhibition of cellular protein synthetic capacity may be associated with inanition, starvation, or chronic systemic disease. Anorexia nervosa has been associated with inactive or low-turnover osteoporosis.[34,35] (see Fig. 54–20).

## CRYSTAL POISONS, DRUG INDUCED

Osteomalacia may be produced by drugs that inhibit hydroxyapatite crystal growth. Sodium fluoride (an experimental agent used in the treatment of osteoporosis) (Fig. 54–26*A* and *B*) as well as diphosphonates (agents used to treat the skeletal lesions of Paget's disease of bone) may produce a mineralization defect if given for prolonged periods and in high doses.

## HYPOMAGNESEMIA

Hypocalcemia is a frequent complication of hypomagnesemia. Three factors have been implicated: altered PTH secretion, impaired PTH responsiveness, and impaired calcium-magnesium exchange in bone. Hypomagnesemia appears to produce a form of PTH resistance, with hypocalcemia and blunted osteoclastic bone resorption to exogenous PTH administration.[36] Histologic evaluation of bone from magnesium-deficient dogs shows features of reduced bone turnover consistent with a skeletal resistance to the actions of PTH.[37]

## REFERENCES


1. Frost, H.M.: Calcif. Tissue Res., *3*:211–237, 1969.
2. Rao, S.D., Matkovic, V., Duncan, H.: Henry Ford Hosp. Med. J., *28*:112–115, 1980.
3. Fallon, M.D., Teitelbaum, S.L.: Hum. Pathol., *13*:416–417, 1982.
4. Baron, R., Vignery, A., Neff, L., et al.: Processing undecalcified bone specimens for bone histomorphometry. *In* Bone Histomorphometry: Techniques and Interpretation. Edited by R.R. Recker. Boca Raton, FL, CRC Press, 1983, p. 13–35.
5. Fallon, M.D., Teitelbaum, S.L.: Calcif. Tissue Int., *33*:281–283, 1981.
6. Merz, W.A., Shenk, R.K.: Acta Anat., *75*:54–66, 1970.
7. Teitelbaum, S.L.: Clin. Endocrinol. Metab., *9*:43–62, 1980.
8. Thompson, D.L., Frame, B.: Ann. Intern. Med., *85*:789, 1976.
9. Gallagher, J.C., Riggs, B.L.: N. Engl. J. Med., *298*:1935, 1978.
10. Riggs, B.L., Melton, L.J.: N. Engl. J. Med., *314*:1676–1686, 1986.
11. Consensus Conference: Osteoporosis. JAMA, *252*:799–802, 1984.
12. Whyte, M.P., Bergfeld, M.A., Murphy, W.A., et al.: Am. J. Med., *72*:193–202, 1982.
13. Kleerekoper, M., Frame, B., Villanueva, A.R.: Treatment of osteoporosis with sodium fluoride alternating with calcium and vitamin D. *In* Osteoporosis: Recent Advances in Pathogenesis and Treatment. Edited by H.F. DeLuca, H.M. Frost, and W.S.S. Jee. Baltimore, University Park Press, 1981, pp. 441–448.
14. Marie, P.J., Pettifor, J.M., Ross, F.P., et al.: N. Engl. J. Med., *307*:584–588, 1982.
15. Choufoer, J.H., Steendijk, J.: Calcif. Tissue Int., *27*:101–104, 1979.
16. Taylor, H.C., Fallon, M.D., Valasco, M.E.: Ann. Intern. Med., *101*:786–788, 1984.
17. Carmichael, K.A., Fallon, M.D., Kaplan, F.S., et al.: Am. J. Med., *76*:1137–1139, 1984.
18. Weinstein, R.S., Underwood, J.L., Hutson, M.S., et al.: Am. J. Physiol., *246*:E499–505, 1984.
19. Kaplan, F.S., Soriano, S., Fallon, M.D., et al.: Clin. Orthop., *205*:216–221, 1986.
20. Verbanck, M., Verbanck, J., Bravman, J., et al.: Calcif. Tissue Res., *22(Suppl.)*:538, 1977.
21. Long, R.G., Meinhard, E., Skinner, R.K., et al.: Gut, *19*:85, 1978.

22. Bikle, D.D., Genant, H.K., Cann, C., et al.: Ann. Intern. Med., *103*:42–48, 1985.
23. Paterson, C.R., Losowski, M.S.: Scand. J. Gastroenterol., *2*:293–300, 1967.
24. Reed, J.S., Meredith, S.C., Nemchausky, B.A.: Gastroenterology, *78*:513–517, 1980.
25. Matloff, D.S., Kaplan, M.M., Neer, R.M., et al.: Gastroenterology, *83*:97–102, 1982.
26. Parfitt, A.M., Miller, M.J., Frame, B., et al.: Ann. Intern. Med., *89*:193–213, 1978.
27. Shike, M., Harrison, J.E., Strutridge, W.C., et al.: Ann. Intern. Med., *92*:343–350, 1980.
28. Shike, M., Strutridge, W.C., Tam. C.S., et al.: Ann. Intern. Med., *95*:560–568, 1981.
29. Ott, S.M., Maloney, N.A., Klein, G.L., et al.: Ann. Intern. Med., *99*:910–914, 1983.
30. Shike, M., Shils, M.E., Heller, A., et al.: Am. J. Clin. Nutr., *44*:89–98, 1986.
31. Hruska, K.A., Teitelbaum, S.L., Kopelman, R., et al.: Metab. Bone Dis. Relat. Res., *1*:39–44, 1978.
32. Ott, S.M., Maldrey, W.A., Coburn, J.W., et al.: N. Engl. J. Med., *307*:709–713, 1982.
33. Brenner, R.J., Spring, D.B., Sebastian, A., et al.: N. Engl. J. Med., *307*:217–221, 1982.
34. Rigotti, N.A., Nussbaum, S.R., Herzog, D.B., et al.: N. Engl. J. Med., *311*:1601–1606, 1984.
35. Kaplan, F.S.K., Pertschuk, M., Fallon, M., et al.: Clin. Orthop., *125*:64–68, 1986.
36. Breslau, N.A., Pak, C.Y.C.: Metabolism, *28*:1261–1276, 1979.
37. Freitag, J.J., Martin, K.J., Conrades, M.B., et al.: J. Clin. Invest., *64*:1238–1244, 1979.

CHAPTER **55**

# Clinical Manifestations of Human Vitamin and Mineral Disorders: A Resume

Donald S. McLaren



Nutritional disorders result from an imbalance between the body's requirements for nutrients and energy and the supply of these substrates of metabolism. This imbalance may take the form of either deficiency or excess and may be attributable either to an inappropriate intake or to defective utilization.

Despite the extensive understanding of human nutritional requirements, malnutrition continues to be one of the main causes or morbidity and mortality in developing regions of the world, especially in young children. In technologically advanced societies, primary undernutrition no longer constitutes a major hazard to health, but occurs in especially vulnerable groups in various ways. Some of these are related to the introduction and widespread use in recent years of techniques such as parenteral feeding and renal dialysis. Chronic alcoholism, drug abuse or even the medically supervised use of drugs, and food fadism may lead to deficiency disease states. Secondary undernutrition is the result of a variety of disease states is another matter of concern. The misuse of vitamins and elements can cause toxicity.

This chapter is confined to a consideration of nutritional disorders related to vitamins and essential elements. Disorders of protein and energy are considered elsewhere. A number of vitamin-dependency states have been identified in recent years. Their symptoms relate to the metabolic abnormalities produced by the respective apoenzyme disorders, and not to the vitamin per se, and they are considered under the appropriate vitamin.

The clinical manifestations of vitamin and essential element disorders consist of relevant symptoms elicited from the patient and signs observed on general physical examination.

## VITAMINS

### VITAMIN A (RETINOL)

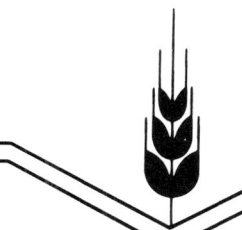

**Deficiency.** The symptoms and signs of vitamin A deficiency have been studied in greater detail than those of any other nutritional disorder.[1,2] The eye is primarily involved and the condition predominantly affects young children. Night blindness, an early feature, can be elicited by a careful history and some simple tests in a poorly illuminated room.[3] Color vision may also be affected. Dryness (xerosis) and unwettability of the bulbar conjunctiva follow. An advanced degree of this process is Bitot's spot, a heaping up of desquamated, keratinized epithelial cells (Fig. 55–1*A*). This condition usually occurs on the temporal aspect of the interpalpebral fissure near the corneal limbus, but less commonly also involves the nasal aspect and other parts of the bulbar conjunctiva. In older children and adults, Bitot's spots may be stigmata of earlier deficiency, or may be entirely unrelated to vitamin A deficiency. Corneal involvement, commencing as a superficial punctate keratopathy,[4] and proceeding to xerosis (Fig. 55–1*B*) and varying degrees of "ulceration" and liquefaction (keratomalacia) (Fig. 55–1*C*), frequently results in blindness. Punctate degenerative changes in the retina (xerophthalmic fundus) are a rare sign of chronic deficiency usually seen in older children.[5] Corneal scars may have many causes, but one of these is previous vitamin A deficiency. They may be fine nebulae or denser leucomata, or may consist of total scarring of a shrunken globe (phthisis bulbi) or corneal ectasia and anterior staphyloma.

Extraocular manifestations include perifollicular hyperkeratosis, a heaping up of hyperkeratinized skin epithelium around hair follicles. This condition is most commonly seen on the outer aspects of the upper arms and the thighs. It is also seen in starvation and has been attributed to B complex or essential fatty acid deficiency. Other changes, which include impaired taste, anorexia, vestibular disturbance, bone changes with pressure on cranial nerves, increased intracranial pressure, congenital malformations, and infertility, have been best demonstrated in animals.[6] More attention has been given recently to anemia that responds to vitamin A.[7]

**Toxicity.** Acute toxicity causes a rise in intracranial pressure, leading to drowsiness, irritability, headache, vomiting, and peeling of the skin. In infants the anterior fontanelle bulges (see Fig. 53–8).

Chronic poisoning produces a bizarre clinical picture that may be misdiagnosed if excessive intake is not suspected. It is characterized by anorexia, headache, blurred vision and diplopia, dry skin and pruritus, painful extremities due to periosteal thickening of the long bones (see Fig. 53–11), and hepatomegaly and splenomegaly.

Birth defects have been reported in the offspring of women receiving 13-*cis*-retinoic acid (isotretinoin) during pregnancy.[8]

**Hypercarotenosis.** This condition is caused by excessive intake of carotenoids. Yellow or orange discoloration of the skin (xanthosis cutis, carotenoderma) affects areas where sebum secretion is greatest (nasolabial folds, forehead, axillae, groins) and keratinized surfaces such as the palms and soles. The sclerae and buccal membranes are not affected.

## VITAMIN D (CALCIFEROL)

**Deficiency.** Vitamin D deficiency is manifested as rickets in children and as osteomalacia in adults. Those forms not due to primary nutrient deficiency also exhibit signs and symptoms of the underlying disease and of hypocalcemia.

*Rickets.* The rachitic infant is restless and sleeps poorly. Consequently, the occipital hair is denuded. Crainiotabes, softening of the bones of the skull and their ready depression on palpation, is often the earliest sign, but it must be present away from the suture lines to be diagnostic of rickets. Frontal bossing occurs and the fontanelles close late. Sitting, crawling, and walking are all delayed. If the disease is active when these activities occur, weight-bearing results in knock-knees or bowing of the arms or legs. Enlargement of the epiphyseal cartilages is most evident at the lower end of the radius and ulna and the upper ends of the tibia and fibula (see Fig. 53–5). The rachitic rosary, due to enlargement of the costochondral junctions of the ribs, is said to be smoother than that due to scurvy (see discussion of vitamin C). The chest may be deformed to give Harrison's sulcus or groove, which consists of a bilateral indentation of the lateral parts of the lower ribs. Other deformities of the chest, such as depression (funnel chest or pectus excavatum) and elevation (pigeon chest or pectus carinatum) of the sternum, are now considered to be congenital and not rachitic in origin.

*Osteomalacia.* The main features of this disease are bone pains and tenderness, skeletal deformity, and weakness of the proximal muscles. In severe cases all the bones are painful and tender, often sufficient to disturb sleep. Tenderness may be particularly marked over Looser's zones, usually occurring in the long bones, the pelvis, the ribs, and around the scapulae in a bilaterally symmetric pattern. Fractures of the softened bones are common. The proximal muscle weakness, the cause of which is uncertain, is more marked in some forms of osteomalacia than in others. Osteomalacia usually results in a waddling gait and difficulty in getting up and down stairs. In the elderly it may simulate paraplegia; in younger persons, it may simulate muscular dystrophy.

**Toxicity.** Some of the symptoms and signs are related to the hypercalcemia and are common to all causes of that condition. Anorexia, nausea, vomiting, and constipation are usually present. Weakness, hypotonia, stupor, and hypertension are less common. Polyuria and polydipsia are caused by hypercalciuria. Renal colic due to stone formation may result.

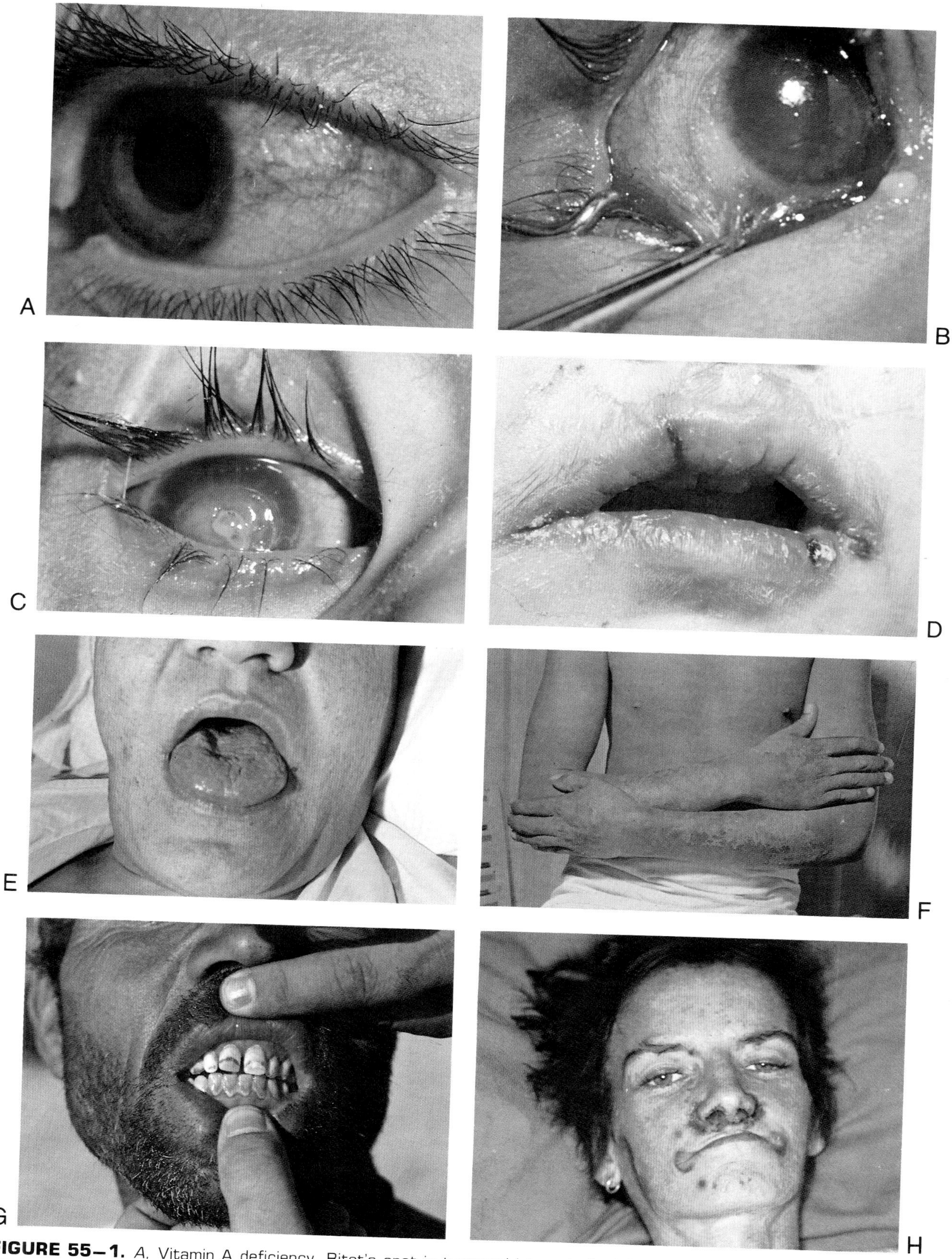
A
B
C
D
E
F
G
H

**FIGURE 55–1.** *A*, Vitamin A deficiency. Bitot's spot in temporal interpalpebral fissure. *B*, Vitamin A deficiency. Conjunctival and corneal xerosis. *C*, Vitamin A deficiency. Keratomalacia. *D*, Riboflavin deficiency. Cheilosis and angular stomatitis. *E*, Riboflavin deficiency. Magenta tongue. *F*, Niacin deficiency. Symmetric dermatosis of pellagra. *G*, Fluorosis. Early stage with brown mottling that is most marked on upper central incisors. *H*, Zinc deficiency. Typical dermatosis associated with alcoholic cirrhosis in this patient. (From Ilchyshyn, A., Mendelsohn, Z.: Br. Med. J., *284*:1676, 1982.)

Vitamin D excess has been reported to take two forms: mild and severe. In the mild form, the patient is usually 3 to 6 months of age, and the symptoms and signs are those already described. In the severe form, also seen in infants, in addition to the manifestations of hypercalcemia, there is mental retardation, stenosis of the aorta and the pulmonary arteries, and a characteristic facial appearance termed "elfin facies."[9]

## VITAMIN E (TOCOPHEROL)

**Deficiency.** In recent years clinical disease responsive to vitamin E has attracted considerable attention. Low-birth-weight infants are particularly susceptible, especially if fed formulas high in polyunsaturated fatty acids after hemolytic anemia made worse by iron supplements has occurred.[10,11] Defective vitamin E status of premature infants may also contribute to their greater susceptibility to platelet dysfunction, intraventricular hemorrhage, retinopathy of prematurity, and bronchopulmonary dysplasia. Lipofuscin deposition within muscle cells has been reported to account for the brown bowel syndrome.[12] The retinopathy of abeta- and hypolipoproteinemia is now considered to be mainly due to vitamin E deficiency.[13]

Of greatest importance at the present time are the neurologic syndromes that principally affect functions of the spinal cord posterior columns and the retina and that respond to vitamin E.[14] Among the underlying conditions reported have been cystic fibrosis, chronic pancreatitis, obstructive liver disease, abeta- or hypolipoproteinemia, short bowel syndrome, blind loop syndrome, and an unique inborn error of vitamin E metabolism.[15]

**Toxicity.** Low-birth-weight infants receiving prolonged pharmacologic doses of vitamin E are prone to a high incidence of sepsis and necrotizing enterocolitis.[16] Some years ago use of an intravenous vitamin E product that had not been approved by the United States Food and Drug Administration (FDA) led to pulmonary deterioration, thrombocytopenia, liver and renal failure, and a high mortality.[17]

## VITAMIN K

**Deficiency (Hypoprothrombinemia).** Hemorrhagic disease of the newborn may result in bleeding anywhere in the body, but the most common sites are the gut, producing melena neonatorum, cephalhematomas, and the umbilical stump. Bleeding may also result from circumcision. Generalized ecchymoses, often without petechiae, intracranial bleeding, and intramuscular hemorrhages are less common.

In the adult, bleeding from this cause is most common in chronic liver disease, obstructive jaundice, and in patients receiving anticoagulants, prolonged antibiotic therapy, or certain cephalosporin antibiotics, such as moxalactam disodium.

Rare instances of deficiency have been attributed to dietary restriction[18] or total parenteral nutrition[19] when inadequate amounts were added to the solutions or injected. Cases have been reported in the United States in 4- to 6-week-old infants, often with intracranial hemorrhage, who were exclusively breast-fed and did not receive vitamin K in the newborn period, usually because of home delivery.[20] Large doses of vitamin E may induce deficiency of vitamin K.[21]

**Toxicity.** Kernicterus (bilirubin encephalopathy) has occurred in low-birth-weight infants receiving large doses of menadione (75 mg) or its water-soluble derivatives. This has not occurred when vitamin K itself has been given. Lethargy, hypotonia, and loss of the sucking reflex are followed by opisthotonos, generalized spasticity, and frequently death from pulmonary complications. Survivors may develop the postkernicterus syndrome: high-frequency nerve deafness, athetoid cerebral palsy, and dental enamel dysplasia.

## THIAMIN (VITAMIN $B_1$)

**Deficiency.** Beriberi in the adult occurs in two distinct forms, wet and dry beriberi, in which the cardiovascular and the nervous systems, respectively, are affected. Both may be involved in the same patient but one or the other tends to predominate. Infantile beriberi is described separately.

Cardiovascular beriberi usually manifests as chronic high-output right and left-sided heart failure with tachycardia, rapid circulation time, elevated peripheral venous pressure, sodium retention, and edema.[22] A much less common acute fulminating form of heart failure (sometimes called "shoshin") is characterized by severe metabolic lactic acidosis, intense dyspnea, thirst, anxiety, and cardiovascular collapse. Signs also include stocking-glove cyanosis, extreme tachycardia, cardiomegaly and hepatomegaly, and neck vein distention. Edema is usually absent.[23] This highly fatal form is not uncommon as a cause of sudden death in young migrant laborers in the Orient subsisting on rice.

### Beriberi of the Nervous System[24]

*Cerebral Beriberi (Wernicke-Korsakoff Syndrome).* In its most severe form, mental confusion, accompanied by ophthalmoplegia due to paralysis of the 6th cranial nerve, leads to coma (Wernicke's encephalopathy).

Korsakoff's psychosis consists of loss of memory for distant events, inability to form new ones, and loss of insight and initiative. The patient is alert, able to converse, and can think and solve problems. Response to thiamin is complete in 25% of cases, partial in 50%. Ethanol is thought to have a direct part in neurotoxicity.[25,26]

*Peripheral neuropathy.* The most characteristic features are symmetric footdrop, associated with marked tenderness of the calf muscles, and a mild disturbance of sensation over the outer aspects of the legs and thighs and in patches over the abdomen, chest, and forearms. Ataxia with loss of position and vibration sense, burning paresthesias in the feet, and amblyopia are less common.

**Infantile Beriberi.** Early manifestations are anorexia, vomiting, pallor, restlessness, and insomnia. The disease progresses typically to (1) an acute, cardiac form in infants 2 to 4 months of age, (2) a subacute, aphonic form in those 5 to 7 months old, and (3) a chronic, pseudomeningeal form in those between 8 and 10 months of age. The acute form presents with dyspnea, cyanosis, a rapid, thready pulse, and other signs of acute heart failure. In the subacute form, aphonia or a characteristic hoarse cry, dysphagia, vomiting, and convulsions predominate. The chronic form is characterized by neck retraction, opisthotonos, edema, oliguria, constipation, and meteorism.[27]

**Subacute Necrotizing Encephalomyelopathy (SNE, Leigh's Disease).** This may be related to a defect in thiamin metabolism. About 100 cases have been reported.[28] Onset is usually before 1 year of age. Hypoventilation and apnea, cranial neuropathies, and hypotonia are the most common features.

**Toxicity.** Fatal anaphylactic shock and toxic reactions have occurred following large intravenous doses.[29]

## RIBOFLAVIN

**Deficiency.** The skin and mucous membranes are affected in what is known as the oroaculogenital syndrome. Areas of skin involved are usually those containing many sebaceous glands. These are mainly the nasolabial folds, alae nasi, external ears, eyelids, scrotum in the male, and labia majora in the female. They become reddened, scaly, greasy, painful, and pruritic. Plugs of inspissated sebum may accumulate in the hair follicles and give the appearance known as dyssebacea or sharkskin (Fig. 55–2).

At the angles of the mouth there are painful fissures known as angular stomatitis when active (see Fig. 55–1*D*). When chronic, these fissures give rise to one form of rhagades. Vertical fissures of the vermilion surface of the lips constitute cheilosis. These and the angular lesions may become infected with Candida albicans, giving rise to the appearance known as perlèche. The tongue may be painful and may have a magenta color (see Fig. 55–1*E*). These changes may also be seen in other nutrient deficiencies. Because deficiency is often multiple it is rarely possible in clinical practice to demonstrate the precise cause.

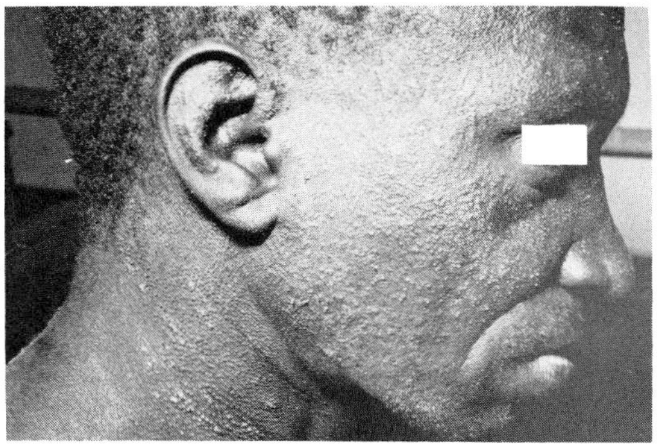

**FIGURE 55–2.** Dyssebacea associated with riboflavin deficiency.

Photophobia, lacrimation, and conjunctival injection are also often present. For unknown reasons, corneal neovascularization, so common in experimental animals, is rare in man.

## NIACIN

**Deficiency.** Pellagra affects primarily the skin, gastrointestinal tract, and nervous system.

Dermatosis is usually the earliest and most prominent manifestation. It is symmetric and appears on parts exposed to sunlight or trauma. Erythema progresses to keratosis and scaling with pigmentation (see Fig. 55–1*F*). The back of the hands, wrists, forearms, face, and neck (Casal's necklace) are typical affected areas. The skin and mucous membrane changes of riboflavin deficiency are also commonly present (see above).

The tongue often has a "raw beef" appearance, is bright red, swollen, and painful. Symptoms of gastritis, bouts of diarrhea, and signs of malabsorption suggest similar changes in the gastrointestinal tract.

Nervous system involvement is suggested in the early stages by periods of depression with insomnia, headaches, and dizziness. Later, tremulous movement or rigidity of the limbs occurs with loss of tendon reflexes, numbness, and paresis of the extremities, ultimately incapacitating the patient. In profound deficiency an encephalopathy has been described that resembles that of acute cerebral beriberi (see section on thiamin) but responds to some extent to niacin.

Mental disturbance is so prominent in some patients that there is a real danger that the true diagnosis may be missed and the patient could be incarcerated in a mental institution.

## PYRIDOXINE (VITAMIN $B_6$)

**Deficiency.** This is rarely severe enough to produce signs or symptoms. Volunteers receiving a deficiency diet and a pyridoxine antagonist became irritable and depressed.

Seborrheic dermatosis affected the nasolabial folds, cheeks, neck, and perineum. Several subjects also developed glossitis, cheilosis, angular stomatitis, blepharitis, and a peripheral neuropathy.

An uncommon form of sideroblastic anemia, often severe, has been reported to respond in some instances to pyridoxine, but most cases appear to be due to dependency rather than to deficiency.[30] Some years ago convulsions occurred in infants fed a milk formula in which the pyridoxine had been destroyed during processing.[31]

**Toxicity.** A sensory neuropathy has been attributed to the abuse of pyridoxine in megadoses.[32] Seven adults developed gradually progressive sensory ataxia and profound lower limb impairment of position and vibration sense. Touch, temperature, and pain perception were less affected. The motor and central nervous systems were unaffected. One review suggested that an impurity in the pharmacologic product might have been responsible.[33]

## BIOTIN

**Deficiency.** This deficiency has occasionally been induced in patients who have consumed large amounts of egg white over a prolonged period. Egg white contains avidin, which antagonizes the action of biotin. The skin of the face and hands becomes dry, shining, and scaling. The oral mucosa and tongue are swollen, magenta in color, and painful.

An infant with short-gut syndrome received total parenteral nutrition from 5 months of age. Five months later the infant lost all body hair and developed a waxy pallor, irritability, lethargy, mild hypotonia, and an erythematous rash. Biotin deficiency was confirmed biochemically, and all signs were reversed by supplementation.[34] Two adult patients receiving home parenteral nutrition after extensive gut resection developed severe hair loss that was reversed by 200 μg biotin given intravenously daily.[35]

## VITAMIN $B_{12}$ (COBALAMIN)

**Deficiency.** This may be primary or secondary, as in pernicious anemia.

*Pernicious anemia.* This condition usually manifests after middle age. There is a slight female preponderance. It may be associated with signs of other autoimmune diseases. The most common complaints—those associated with anemia—ordinarily do not arise until the anemia is well advanced. Neurologic changes may long precede the hematologic changes. The tongue may be red, smooth, shining, and painful. Anorexia, weight loss, indigestion, and episodic diarrhea are all usually present.

The typical patient has prematurely gray hair, blue eyes, and wide cheek bones. Mild jaundice gives the skin a lemon-yellow tint. A few patients have widespread pigmentation of a brownish color affecting nail beds and skin creases, but sparing the mucous membranes.

In advanced cases there is usually pyrexia, enlargement of the liver and spleen, and occasionally bruising due to thrombocytopenia. Older patients may present with congestive cardiac failure.

A distal sensory neuropathy with "glove and stocking" sensory loss, paresthesias, and areflexia may occur in isolation or more commonly together with a myelopathy known as subacute combined degeneration of the cord. In this condition the initial symptom is symmetric paresthesias of the feet or, occasionally, of the hands. There is increasing difficulty in walking due to a combination of weakness and loss of postural sense. Psychiatric disturbances, especially mild dementia, may be the presenting or only feature. Visual loss from optic atrophy is not uncommon.

Congenital lack of intrinsic factor presents before the age of 2 years with irritability, vomiting, diarrhea, weight loss, and anemia. It was reported that an infant exclusively breast-fed by a mother with a latent pernicious anemia developed megaloblastic anemia and neurologic abnormalities.[36]

**Primary Dietary Deficiency.** When dietary lack or malabsorption is the cause of deficiency, anemia is usually the most prominent feature, but glossitis, optic atrophy, and subacute combined degeneration of the cord have also been described. Megaloblastic anemia developed in an infant exclusively breast-fed by a vegan mother.[37]

## FOLIC ACID

**Deficiency.** The anemia has morphologic features similar to those of vitamin $B_{12}$ deficiency (see Chap. 25), but it develops much more rapidly. Subacute combined degeneration of the cord does not occur, but about 20% of patients may have peripheral neuropathy. The tongue may be red and painful in the acute stage. In chronic deficiency, the tongue papillae atrophy, leaving a shiny, smooth surface. Hyperpigmentation of the skin, similar to that seen occasionally in vitamin $B_{12}$ deficiency, has been reported.

Folic acid treatment before conception has been reported to prevent the occurrence of neural tube defects in infants of families in which these abnormalities have previously arisen.

Folate deficiency has been described in total parenteral nutrition with certain amino acid mixtures in the absence of supplementary folic acid.[37] A report shows that an infant exclusively breast-fed by a mother taking estrogen-progestogen contraceptive pills developed megaloblastic anemia responsive to folic acid.[39]

## PANTOTHENIC ACID

**Deficiency.** In adult volunteers on a deficient diet, researchers claimed that the "burning feet syndrome" resulted and that this condition responded to the vitamin. In clinical practice this distressing complaint has rarely responded to this treatment.

## VITAMIN C (ASCORBIC ACID)

**Deficiency.** Scurvy tends to affect either the very young or the elderly. The clinical picture differs in these two groups and requires separate consideration.

*Infantile Scurvy (Barlow's Disease).* The onset, usually in the second half of the first year of life, is preceded by a period of fretfulness, pallor, and loss of appetite. Localizing signs are tenderness and swelling, most marked at the knees or ankles. These signs result from characteristic bone changes demonstrable by radiograph (see Fig. 53–4*A*). Enlargement of the costochondral junctions produces the scorbutic rosary, which has a sharper feel than that due to rickets (see section on vitamin D). The infant often adopts the "pithed frog" position of maximum comfort, with the legs flexed at the knees and the hips partially flexed and externally rotated. The arms are less commonly involved. Hemorrhage and spongy changes in the gums are confined to the sites of teeth that have recently erupted or are about to do so. Bleeding may occur anywhere in the skin (the orbit is a not infrequent site) or from mucous membranes, including the renal tract. In infancy, intracranial hemorrhages are rapidly progressive if treatment is delayed, and death may occur. Petechiae and ecchymoses, usually found in the region of the bone lesions, are less common than in the adult. A microcytic hypochromic anemia is common. Older children may develop characteristic perifollicular hemorrhages and hair changes seen in the adult.

*Adult Scurvy.* Early symptoms are weakness, easy fatigue, and listlessness, followed by shortness of breath and aching bones, joints, and muscles, especially at night. These symptoms are followed by characteristic changes in the skin.[40] Acne, indistinguishable from that of adolescence, precedes defects in the hairs of the body. These defects consist of broken and coiled hairs and a "swan-neck" deformity resulting from their being flat instead of round in cross section. However, the true hallmark of scurvy in the adult is perifollicular hemorrhages and perifollicular hyperkeratosis, most common on the anterior aspect of the thorax, forearms, thighs, and legs and on the anterior abdominal wall (Fig. 55–3).

Frank bleeding is a late feature of scurvy. The classic gum changes are only associated with natural teeth or buried roots and are enhanced by poor dental hygiene and advanced caries. The interdental papillae become swollen and purple and bleed with trauma. In advanced scurvy the gums are spongy and friable, bleeding freely. Secondary infection leads to loosening of the teeth and to

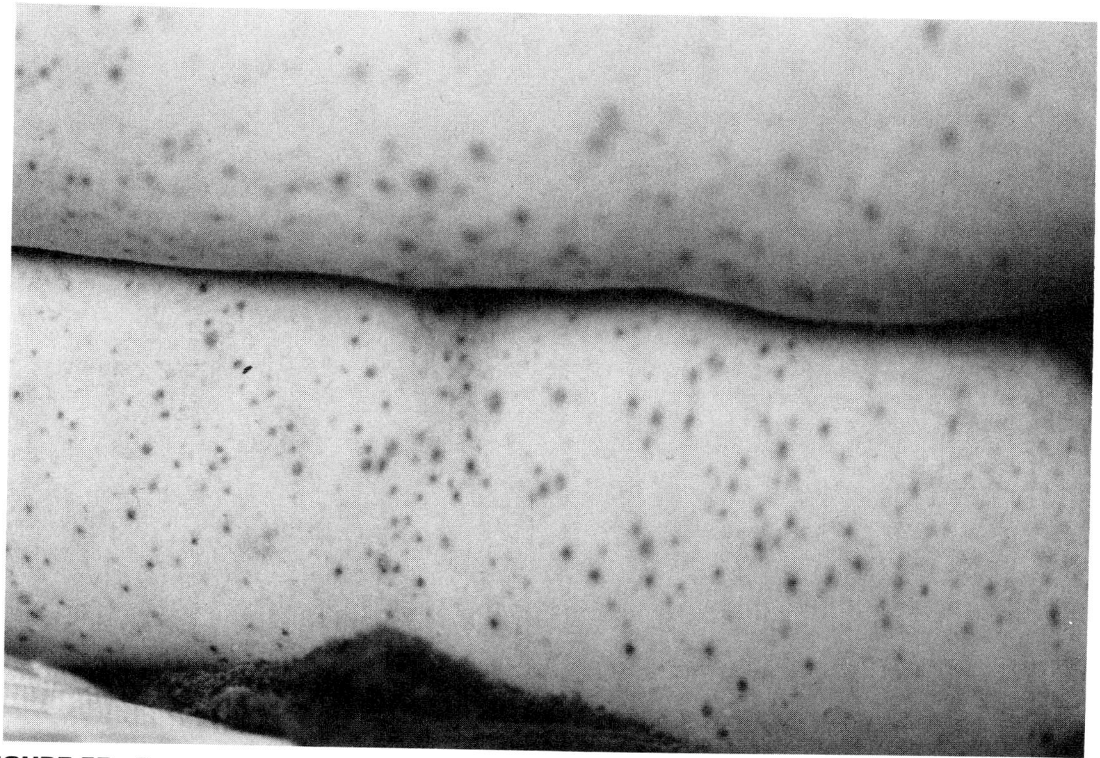

**FIGURE 55–3.** Perifollicular hemorrhages of the legs in adult scurvy.

gangrene (Fig. 55–4). Patients who are edentulous or whose teeth are in good repair have little or no evidence of scorbutic gingivitis. Hemorrhage commonly occurs deep in muscles and into joints. Multiple splinter hemorrhages may form a crescent near the distal ends of the nails. Old scars break down and new wounds fail to heal. Bleeding into viscera or the brain leads to convulsions and shock; death may occur abruptly.

### ESSENTIAL FATTY ACIDS

Although these are not vitamins it is convenient to consider the symptoms of deficiency of these fatty acids here.

**ω-6 Essential Fatty Acid Deficiency.** Growth retardation, sparse hair growth, a bran-like desquamation of the skin of the trunk, poor wound healing, and increased susceptibility to infection have been observed in infants receiving a formula deficient in essential fat or receiving long-term, lipid-free parenteral nutrition.

In adults reports have been associated with prolonged, usually lipid-free, total parenteral nutrition.[41] Sometimes there is only a dry, flaky skin, but more advanced deficiency results in scaling, eczematoid dermatosis, usually starting on the nasolabial folds and eyebrows and spreading across the face and neck (Fig. 55–5). Anemia and enlarged fatty liver have also been reported.

**ω-3 Essential Fatty Acid Deficiency.** The first human report was of a 7-year-old girl with extensive gut resection who received total parenteral nutrition rich in ω-6 but very low in ω-3 fatty acids. Neurologic changes included paresthesias, weakness, inability to walk, pain in the legs, and blurred vision.[42] These are reported to have responded to change of treatment, but it is possible that other deficiencies, including vitamin E, might have been responsible. Other possible cases have since been reported and the subject has been reviewed.[43] It now appears that the symptoms of the two kinds of fatty acid deficiency are distinct.

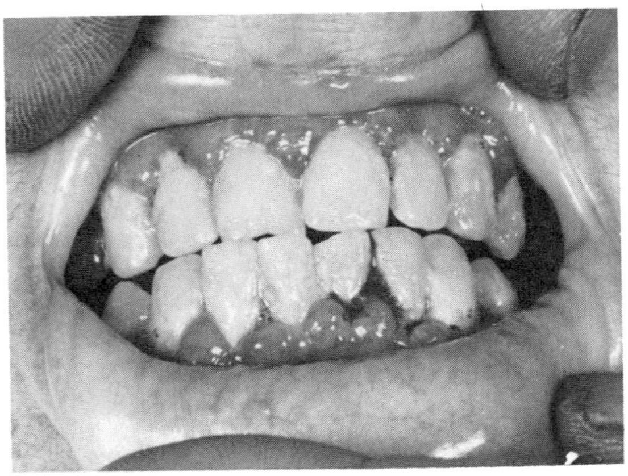

**FIGURE 55–4.** Gum changes of scurvy in food fadism. (From Sherlock, P., Rothschild, E.O.: JAMA, *199*:794–798, 1967.)

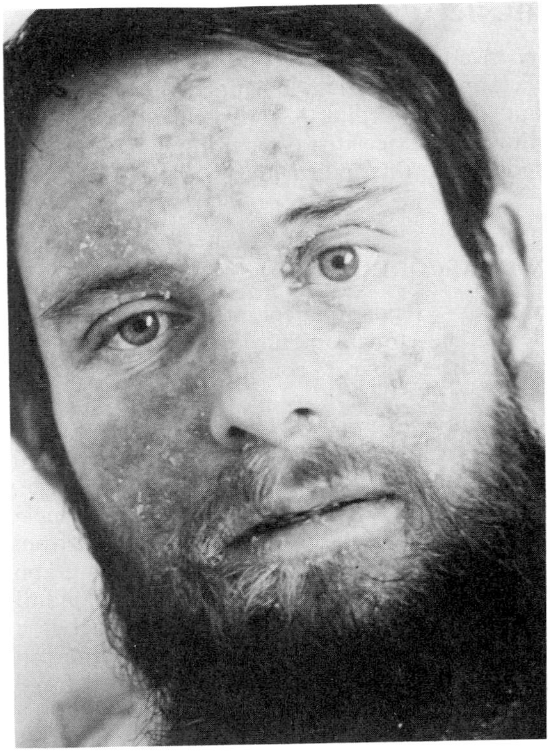

**FIGURE 55–5.** Dermatosis of essential fatty acid deficiency associated with total parenteral nutrition. (Courtesy of Dr. R.E. Hodges.)

## ESSENTIAL ELEMENTS

### *CALCIUM*

**Hypocalcemia.** Symptoms and signs of underlying disorders will be present. Hypocalcemia in clinical conditions is rarely caused by inadequate calcium ingestion but rather by disorders of calcium metabolism. The low blood calcium per se causes the nervous system to be affected. Depression and psychosis, progressing to dementia or encephalopathy, occur. The most characteristic syndrome is tetany, consisting of (1) paresthesias of the lips, tongue, fingers, and feet, (2) carpopedal spasm, resulting in "obstetrician's hand," a deformity that may be painful and prolonged, (3) generalized muscle aching, and (4) spasm of muscles of the face. At the earlier stage of latent tetany, the neuromuscular irritability may be elicited by provocative tests. Chvostek's sign is contraction of the facial muscles on light tapping of the facial nerve. Trousseau's sign is carpopedal spasm induced by restriction of the blood supply to a limb by a tourniquet applied for about 3 minutes. Cataract rarely is the earliest feature.

In the neonate and older infant tetany may manifest as rhythmic, focal myoclonic jerks, sometimes followed by convulsions, cyanosis, and heart failure. Muscular spasms and laryngismus stridulus may occur in young children.

**Osteoporosis.** Calcium deficiency plays an ill-defined part in this condition of loss of bone mass. It is common in the elderly, especially in postmenopausal white women. There is bone deformity, localized pain, and fracture. Osteomalacia may coexist. The most common deformity is loss of height due to vertebral collapse, which accounts for most of the pain. Fractures of the neck of the femur and Colles' fracture above the wrist are most commonly due to trauma, which may be trivial, in the elderly with osteoporosis.

**Calcium-Deficiency Rickets.** Reports from South Africa have suggested that true rickets can be produced by dietary calcium deficiency in the presence of normal vitamin D status.[44] The histologic changes of rickets were confirmed by biopsy and responded to calcium therapy alone.[45]

**Hypercalcemia.** This condition occurs from a variety of causes and produces a symptom complex that is, to some extent, characteristic of this state. Gastrointestinal symptoms include anorexia, nausea, vomiting, constipation, abdominal pain, and ileus. Renal system involvement produces polyuria, nocturia, polydipsia, stone formation, and sometimes hypertension and signs and symptoms of uremia. Muscle weakness and myopathy occur. More advanced disease, which causes psychosis, delerium, stupor, and coma, may prove fatal.

## POTASSIUM

**Deficiency.** This is usually due to excessive losses in urine or stool, less commonly to decreased intake as in starvation or failure to give potassium in intravenous solutions and losses in sweat as in cystic fibrosis.

Severe hypokalemia (serum K <3 mmol/L or <3 mEq/L) may cause muscle weakness leading to respiratory failure, paralytic ileus, hypotension, and tetany. Potassium nephropathy results in polyuria with secondary polydipsia. Cardiac effects are particularly prone to develop in patients receiving digitalis. The electrocardiogram (ECG) is characteristic with S-T segment depression, increased U wave amplitude, and T wave amplitude less than that of U wave in the same lead. Premature ventricular and atrial contractions and ventricular and atrial tachyarrhythmias occur.

**Toxicity (Hyperkalemia).** Acute oliguric states are often responsible, but excessive ingestion or infusion may produce symptoms even in the presence of normal renal function.

Cardiac toxicity, of serious import, starts with shortening of the Q-T interval of the ECG and tall, peaked T waves. Progressive toxicity with serum K >6.5 mmol/L (>6.5 mEq/L) causes nodal and ventricular arrhythmias, widening of the QRS complex, PR interval prolongation and disappearance of the P wave, and finally degeneration of the QRS complex with ventricular asystole or fibrillation and death.

## MAGNESIUM

**Deficiency.** In depletion studies in humans as well as in clinical practice, hypomagnesemia is accompanied by hypocalcemia and frequently hypokalemia.

The symptoms and signs in both experimental and clinical deficiency are primarily neuromuscular: Trousseau and Chvostek signs, muscle fasciculations, tremor, muscle spasm, personality changes, anorexia, nausea, and vomiting. Convulsions, with or without coma, seem to be more commonly seen in acute deficiency in infants than in adults. The clinical states with which magnesium depletion has been associated usually fall into the categories of malabsorptive syndromes, renal tubular abnormalities, endocrine dysfunction, and genetic and familial conditions.[46]

**Toxicity (Hypermagnesemia).** Elevated serum magnesium levels are not uncommon in renal failure patients receiving magnesium-containing drugs and in children with chronic constipation treated with magnesium sulfate enemas. With higher levels deep tendon reflexes disappear and ECG abnormalities appear. Hypertension, respiratory depression, narcosis, and ultimately cardiac arrest may occur with very high blood magnesium levels (see Chap. 8).

## PHOSPHORUS

**Hypophosphatemia.** This is defined as a lowered serum inorganic phosphate (<0.71 mmol, or 2.2 mg/dl) without any significant decrease in the total body phosphate in relation to total body nitrogen. This occurs usually in any situation stimulating anaerobic glycolysis, such as infusion of hypertonic glucose continuously without adequate phosphate replacement; this results in a shift of the serum inorganic phosphate into cells and a fall in the serum phosphate. The markedly depressed serum phosphate (usually <0.30 mmol, or 0.93 mg/dl) is associated in a matter of 3 to 4 days with circumoral and extremity paresthesias and red cell fragility and hemolysis among other dysfunctions.

**Deficiency.** Depletion of total body phosphate in relation to total body nitrogen occurs as the result of various diseases that lead to excess loss of phosphate in the stool (e.g., malabsorption, vitamin D deficiency) or in the urine (e.g., hyperparathyroidism, congenital or drug-induced renal tubular disorders, severe potassium depletion, diabetic ketoacidosis). In the management of advanced renal disease, administration of phosphate-binding gels intended to reduce phosphate absorption in association with restricted phosphate in the diet may lead to symptomatic phosphate deficiency[47,48] (Table 55–1).

## IODIDE (IODINE)

**Deficiency.** Enlargement of the thyroid gland is the most common clinical sign. When due to iodine lack this condition is termed simple, endemic, colloid, or euthyroid goiter. It is more common in women and is often noted at the onset of puberty, during pregnancy, or at the menopause. Early on the enlargement is soft, symmetric, and smooth, but later multiple nodules and cysts may appear. Most patients are euthyroid, a few have hyperthyroidism and, rarely, hypothyroidism occurs.

When endemic goiter is severe it is often accompanied by cretinism. Endemic cretinism occurs in two distinct forms, the myxedematous and the neurologic, which may coexist.[49] In most areas of the world the neurologic form is by far the more common. The clinical manifestations of the two conditions are shown in Table 55–2.

In recent years it has become evident that maternal iodine deficiency is an important cause in some parts of the world of fetal growth retardation, especially affecting development of the brain.

**Toxicity.** Prolonged excessive intake of iodine leads eventually to iodide-goiter and myxedema, especially in patients with preexisting Hashimoto's thyroiditis.

## IRON

**Deficiency.** This has its major impact, in common with other hematologic agents, on many systems through reduction in tissue oxygenation consequent upon decreased hemoglobin concentration. The clinical picture depends on the rapidity of the development of anemia, as well as on its severity.

Anemia of insidious onset manifests as increasing fatigue and slight pallor, best seen in the mucous membranes. Later, cardiorespiratory signs and symptoms include exertional dyspnea, tachycardia, palpitations, angina, claudication, night cramps, increased arterial and capillary pulsation, cardiac bruits, reversible cardiac enlargement and, if cardiac failure occurs, basal crepitations, peripheral edema, and ascites. Neuromuscular involvement is evidenced by headache, tinnitus, vertigo, cramps, faintness, increased cold sensitivity, and retinal hemorrhage. Gastrointestinal symptoms include anorexia, nausea, constipation, and diarrhea. Low-grade fever, menstrual irregularity, urinary frequency, and loss of libido may occur.

Iron deficiency per se has certain characteristics not usually associated with other forms of anemia. A nonspecific glossitis with almost complete loss of filiform papillae is common. Angular stomatitis is less frequent. Spoon-shaped nails (koilonychia) are characteristic of long-standing iron deficiency. The Patterson-Kelly (Plummer-Vinson) syndrome is the association of iron-deficiency anemia, glossitis, dysphagia, and achlorhydria, usually seen in middle-aged women, but more rarely than was formerly the case. In severe cases, postcricoid webs and malignant change in this region may occur. Signs of deficiency of some B group vitamins are often also present. Pica (geophagia) is an occasional feature. Even mild degrees of iron deficiency are considered to be an important factor in decreased work efficiency.[50] In infants certain aspects of intellectual function are impaired.

**TABLE 55–1.** MANIFESTATIONS OF PHOSPHATE DEPLETION AND/OR HYPOPHOSPHATEMIA

| ORGAN SYSTEM AFFECTED | MANIFESTATION |
|---|---|
| Constitutional | Anorexia, malaise, debility, lethargy |
| Neuropsychiatric | Altered sensorium, confusion, seizures, coma, decreased motor and sensory nerve conduction |
| Hematologic | Erythrocyte deformity, hemolysis, impaired phagocytosis, thrombocytopathia, hemorrhage |
| Metabolic | Insulin resistance and glucose intolerance |
| Gastrointestinal | Dysphagia, ileus, impaired liver function |
| Musculoskeletal | Rickets (osteomalacia), arthralgia, muscle weakness, rhabdomyolysis |
| Renal | Glycosuria, magnesuria, renal tubular acidosis |

(From Berner, Y.M., Shike, M.: Annu. Rev. Nutr., *8*:121–148, 1988.)

**TABLE 55–2.** COMPARATIVE CLINICAL FEATURES IN MYXOEDEMATOUS AND NEUROLOGIC CRETINISM

| FEATURE | MYXOEDEMATOUS CRETIN | NEUROLOGIC CRETIN |
|---|---|---|
| Mental retardation | Present, often severe | Present, often severe |
| Deaf-mutism | Absent | Usually present |
| Cerebral diplegia | Absent | Often present |
| Stature | Severe growth retardation | Usually normal, occasionally slight growth retardation |
| General features | Coarse dry skin, protuberant abdomen with umbilical hernia, large tongue | No physical signs of hypothyroidism |
| Reflexes | Delayed relaxation | Excessively brisk |
| ECG | Small voltage QRS complexes and other abnormalities of hypothyroidism | Normal |
| X-ray limbs | Epiphyseal dysgenesis | Normal |
| Effect of thyroid hormones | Improvement | No effect |

(From Hetzel, B.S., Hay, I.D.: Clin. Endocrinol., *11*:445–460, 1979.)

**Toxicity.** Acute poisoning causes vomiting, upper abdominal pain, pallor, cyanosis, diarrhea, drowsiness, and shock.

Chronic toxicity (hemochromatosis) or iron overload affects many tissues. Diabetes, often the presenting feature, eventually develops in about 80% of patients. The skin has a characteristic slate-gray coloration. The liver becomes enlarged and then cirrhotic, and hepatoma may develop. Cardiomyopathy leads to heart failure in about 15% of cases and is a common cause of death in younger people. Arthropathy develops in about 50% of patients. Pituitary failure may cause testicular atrophy and loss of libido. Focal hemosiderosis damages the lungs and kidneys.

## COPPER

**Deficiency.** The principle features are a hypochromic anemia unresponsive to iron therapy, neutropenia, and osteoporosis. Early radiologic findings are osteoporosis of the metaphyses and epiphyses and retarded bone age. Typical findings are increased density of the provisional zone of calcification and cupping with sickle-shaped spurs in the metaphyseal region. Other skeletal abnormalities include periosteal layering and submetaphyseal and rib fractures (Fig. 55–6).

Premature infants are especially vulnerable. In them the following signs have been observed: pallor, decreased pigmentation of skin and hair, prominent superficial veins, skin lesions resembling seborrheic dermatitis, failure to thrive, diarrhea, and hepatosplenomegaly. Some have shown features suggestive of central nervous system damage including hypotonia, apathy, psychomotor retardation, apparent lack of visual responses, and apneic episodes.

The most extreme form is seen in Menke's steely hair disease,[51] a complex X-linked disease of male infants in which there is both a failure to absorb copper and then to form functional cuproproteins. Interference with cross-linking of elastin and collagen can be blamed for many of the features: premature rupture of the membranes leading to premature birth, lax skin and joints, elongation and dilatation of major arteries leading to rupture and hemorrhage, subintimal thickening with partial occlusion of major arteries, hernias, and diverticulae of bladder and ureters causing recurrent infection or rupture. Osteoporosis, flaring of metaphyseal edges, and Wormian bones in cranial sutures may all be secondary to collagen abnormalities. Lack of pigmentation of skin and hair and abnormal spiral twisting (pili torti) and fragility of hair add to the characteristic appearance of affected babies. Neurologic development rarely progresses beyond 6 to 8 weeks and even these functions are lost during the ensuing months. Ataxia is striking in mild cases.

**Toxicity.** In Wilson's disease (hepatolenticular degeneration) accumulation of copper in the liver leads to cirrhosis and signs of liver failure. Deposits in the brain result in tremors, choreoathetoid movements, rigidity, dysarthria, and eventually dementia. Anemia and signs of renal failure are common. Characteristic changes in the eye are the Kayser-Fleischer ring, a brown or green ring near the limbus of the cornea, and a "sunflower" cataract.

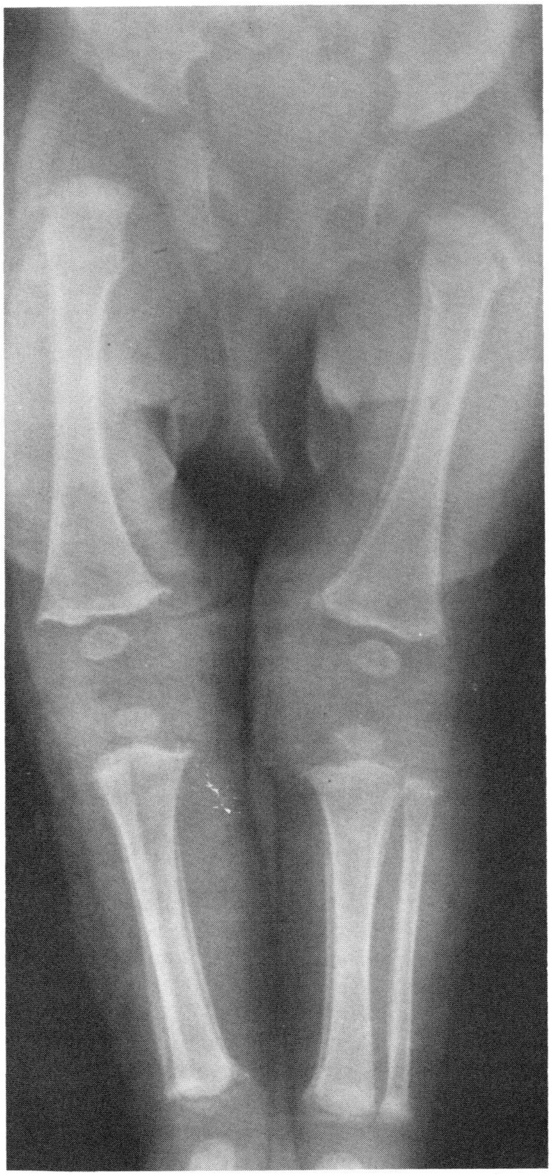

**FIGURE 55–6.** Bone changes due to copper deficiency. (From Bennani-Smires, C., Medina J., Young, L.W.: Am. J. Dis. Child., *134*:1155, 1980.)

Indian childhood cirrhosis is a common condition on the Indian subcontinent and has been reported in Indian children elsewhere.[52] It has been attributed to copper accumulation in the liver, probably as a result of the practice of feeding animal milk contaminated by boiling and storing in brass and copper pots.[53]

Acute poisoning has resulted from ingestion of solutions of copper salts or contaminated water supplies or dialysis fluid. In severe cases evidence of hepatic or renal failure (or both) is found.

## ZINC

**Deficiency.** In Iran a syndrome of dwarfism, hypogonadism, anemia, hepatosplenomegaly, rough dry skin, and lethargy associated with geophagia has been reported.[54] A similar syndrome associated with parasitism occurs in Egypt.[55] Hypogeusia (diminished taste) and growth retardation in otherwise healthy children have been found to respond to zinc supplementation in parts of North America.[56]

Some cases of night blindness and impaired dark adaptation, secondary to liver disease, malabsorption, or sickle cell anemia have responded to zinc therapy. Taste abnormalities and gonadal dysfunction in uremic males receiving renal dialysis have also improved with zinc. Wound healing is impaired.

Total parenteral nutrition with adequate zinc supplement has on occasion been responsible for an acute deficiency syndrome consisting of diarrhea, mental depression, alopecia, and dermatosis, usually around the orbits, nose, and mouth.[57]

Acrodermatitis enteropathica, an inherited disorder manifested in artificially fed infants, caused by a defect in zinc absorption, is characterized by extensive dermatitis, growth retardation, diarrhea, hair loss, and paronychia (see Chap. 10). The skin changes may resemble those seen in kwashiorkor, and a single report has claimed response to zinc.[58] The skin changes of zinc deficiency have a typical appearance: the distribution is often acro-orificial, commonly also involving the flexures and friction areas, and may become generalized. Exematoid, psoriaform, vesiculobullous, and pustular lesions may be present. The earliest skin lesions are bright reddish, nonscaly macules and patches.

**Toxicity.** Ingestion of the metal in large amounts, usually from an acid food or drink from a galvanized container, has caused vomiting and diarrhea. Excessive zinc intake, as in large daily doses (30 to 150 mg) for several weeks, interferes with copper absorption and leads to copper deficiency. Severe lethargy in dialysis patients has been attributed to excess zinc in dialysis fluids. Accidental intravenous administration of 1.5 g has proven fatal.

## FLUORINE (FLUORIDE)

**Deficiency.** Fluorine has not yet been proved to be an essential trace element for man, but areas with a low fluorine content of the water supply have high rates of dental caries. Fluoridation of the water, or use of supplemented tooth paste, has been associated with a significant fall in dental caries rates.

**Toxicity (Fluorosis).** This is associated with high levels (>10 ppm) in the drinking water. It is most evident in permanent teeth that develop during high fluorine intake. Deciduous teeth are affected only at very high levels. The earliest changes, chalky white, irregularly distributed patches on the surface of the enamel, become infiltrated by yellow or brown staining, giving rise to the characteristic "mottled" appearance (see Fig. 55–1*G*). Severe fluorosis weakens the enamel, resulting in surface pitting (Fig. 55–7).

Bone changes, consisting of deformity of the spine, and genu valgum, usually are seen only after prolonged high intake in adults.

## SELENIUM

**Deficiency.** It has been reported in China that an endemic disease, known as Keshan disease after its place of origin, and consisting of a highly fatal cardiomyopathy affecting mainly young children and women of the childbearing age, has responded to treatment with selenium.[59]

In the United States several patients have been reported to develop selenium deficiency on total parenteral nutrition.[60] Features have included fatal and responsive cardiomyopathy, muscle pain and tenderness, dyschromotrichia, white finger nail beds, and macrocytosis.

**Toxicity.** Endemic selenosis, long recognized in animals, has been suspected in some human communities. The most convincing evidence has been reported in China.[61] The most frequently observed signs were loss of hair and nails. Skin lesions and polyneuritis were less certainly attributed to selenium toxicity.

Alopecia and nail changes occurred in New York City from consumption of a "health store" supplement with excessive amounts of selenium.[62] In eight reported cases of acute poisoning, four were fatal.[63] Symptoms and signs were distinctive: metallic taste, odor of garlic due to methylation of selenium, mucosal irritation, gastroenteritis, paronychia, and red pigmentation of nails, hair, and teeth.

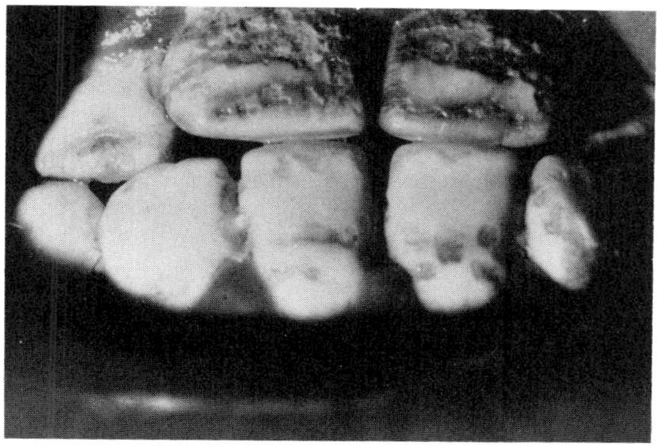

**FIGURE 55–7.** Pitting of enamel in severe fluorosis.

## CHROMIUM

**Deficiency.** A patient receiving total parenteral nutrition for more than 5 years unexpectedly developed 15% weight loss, a peripheral neuropathy, and glucose intolerance after $3\frac{1}{2}$ years of nutritional support.[64] These conditions were all reversed with chromium therapy. Two further cases have been reported, both with weight loss and hyperglycemia that responded to chromium.[65,66]

## COBALT

There is little evidence of a role for cobalt in human nutrition other than as a part of the vitamin $B_{12}$ molecule.

**Toxicity.** Cobalt had at one time been recommended for the treatment of anemia of nephritis and infection in addition to the usual hemopoietic agents. In this context it was reported to cause goiter, myxedema, and congestive heart failure in five patients.[67] A cardiomyopathy with a high mortality has been described after industrial exposure, during maintenance dialysis, and after drinking beer that was contaminated with cobalt during processing.[68]

## MOLYBDENUM

**Deficiency.** An autosomal recessive molybdenum cofactor deficiency, resulting in deficiencies of xanthine oxidase and sulfie oxidase, has been reported in more than 20 patients in the past decade.[69] There is severe brain damage, and the condition is fatal—about half the patients fail to survive beyond early infancy.

Only one case related to prolonged total parenteral nutrition has been reported to date.[70] Tachycardia, tachypnea, headache, night blindness, central scotomas, nausea, vomiting, lethargy, disorientation, and coma appeared to be reversed by 300 μg per day of molybdenum, and urinary excretion of abnormal metabolites was dramatically decreased.

**Toxicity.** Elevated blood levels of molybdenum were associated with a gout-like syndrome in Armenia in 1961.[71] Other symptoms and signs mentioned suggested some involvement of liver, gastrointestinal tract, and kidney. The pathogenesis was unclear.

## MANGANESE

One unsubstantiated case of human deficiency has been reported to have occurred when manganese was inadvertently omitted from an experimental diet fed to a volunteer. Clinical signs included weight loss, transient dermatitis, nausea and vomiting, changes in hair color, and slow growth of hair.[72]

**Toxicity.** This is usually limited to those who mine and refine ore. Prolonged exposure has caused neurologic changes resembling those of parkinsonism or Wilson's disease.

## REFERENCES


1. McLaren, D.S.: Nutritional Ophthalmology. New York, Academic Press, 1980.
2. Sommer, A.: Nutritional Blindness: Xerophthalmia and Keratomalacia. New York, Oxford University Press, 1982.
3. Sommer, A., Hussaini, G., Muhilal, et al.: Am. J. Clin. Nutr., *33:*887–891, 1980.
4. Sommer, A., Emran, N., Tamba, T.: Am. J. Ophthalmol., *87:*330–333, 1979.
5. Teng Khoen Hing: Ophthalmologica, *137:*81–85, 1959.
6. International Vitamin A Consultative Group: The Symptoms and Signs of Vitamin A Deficiency and their Relationship to Applied Nutrition. Washington, D.C., IVACG, 1981.
7. Mejia, L.A., Hodges, R.E., Arroyave, G., et al.: Am. J. Clin. Nutr., *30:*1175–1184, 1977.
8. Lammer, E.J., Chen, D.T., Hoar, R.M., et al.: N. Engl. J. Med., *313:*837–841, 1985.
9. Black, J.A., Bonham Carter, R.E.: Lancet, *2:*745–749, 1963.
10. Melhorn, D.K., Gross, S.: J. Pediatr., *79:*569–580, 1971.
11. Melhorn, D.K., Gross, S.: J. Pediatr., *79:*581–588, 1971.
12. Foster, C.S.: Histopathology, *3:*1–17, 1979.
13. Lloyd, J.K.: Disorders of lipid metabolism. *In* Textbook of Paediatric Nutrition. 2nd Ed. Edited by D.S. McLaren and D. Burman. Edinburgh, Churchill Livingstone, 1982.
14. Howard, L.J.: Nutr. Revs., *48:*169–177, 1990.
15. Sokol, R.J.: Ann. Rev. Nutr., *8:*351–373, 1988.
16. Johnson, L., Bowen, F.W. Jr., Abbasi, S., et al.: Pediatrics, *75:*619–638, 1985.
17. Lorch, V., Murphy, D., Hoersten, L.R., et al.: Pediatrics, *75:*598–602, 1985.
18. Kark, R., Lozner, E.L.: Lancet, *2:*1162–1163, 1939.
19. Berthoud, M., Bouvier, C.A., Krahenbuhl, B.: Schweiz Med. Wochenschr., *96:*1522–1524, 1966.
20. O'Connor, M.E., Livingstone, D.S., Hannah, J., et al.: Am. J. Dis. Child., *137:*601–602, 1983.
21. Corrigan, J.J., Marcus, F.I.: JAMA, *230:*1300–1301, 1974.
22. Campbell, C.H.: Lancet, *2:*446–449, 1984.
23. Jeffrey, F.E., Abelmann, W.H.: Am. J. Med., *50:*123–128, 1971.
24. Haas, R.H.: Annu. Rev. Nutr., *8:*483–515, 1988.
25. Editorial: Lancet, *2:*912–913, 1990.
26. Victor, M., Adams, R.D., Collins, G.H.: The Wernicke-Korsakoff Syndrome. Oxford, Blackwell, 1971.
27. Jelliffe, D.B.: Infant Nutrition in the Tropics and Subtropics. 2nd Ed. Geneva, WHO, 1968.
28. Pincus, J.H.: Dev. Med. Child. Neurol., *14:*87–101, 1972.
29. American Medical Association: Drug Evaluation. Chicago, AMA, 1980, p. 833.
30. Weintraub, L.R., Conrad, M.E., Crosby, W.H.: N. Engl. J. Med., *275:*169–176, 1966.
31. Coursin, D.B.: Vitam. Horm., *22:*756–786, 1964.
32. Schaumberg, H., Kaplan, J., Windebank, A., et al.: N. Engl. J. Med., *309:*445–448, 1983.
33. Rudman, D., Williams, P.J.: N. Engl. J. Med., *309:*488–489, 1983.
34. Mock, D.M., DeLorimer, A.A., Leberman, W.M., et al.: N. Engl. J. Med., *304:*820–823, 1981.
35. Innis, S.M., Allardyce, D.B.: Am. J. Clin. Nutr., *37:*185–187, 1983.
36. Johnson, P.R., Roloff, J.S.: J. Pediatr., *100:*917–919, 1982.
37. Higginbottom, M.C., Sweetman, K., Nyhan, W.L.: N. Engl. J. Med., *299:*317–320, 1978.
38. Anonymous: Nutr. Rev., *41:*51–53, 1983.
39. Mandel, H., Berant, M.: Arch. Dis. Child., *60:*971–972, 1985.
40. Hodges, R.E., Hood, J., Canham, J.E., et al.: Am. J. Clin. Nutr., *24:*432–443, 1971.
41. Fleming, C.R., Smith, L.M., Hodges, R.E.: Am. J. Clin. Nutr., *29:*976–983, 1976.
42. Holman, R.T., Johnson, S.B., Hatch, T.F.: Am. J. Clin. Nutr., *35:*617–623, 1982.
43. Anderson, G.J., Connor, W.E.: Am. J. Clin. Nutr., *49:*585–587, 1989.
44. Pettifor, J.M., Ross, P., Wang, J., et al.: J. Pediatr., *92:*320–324, 1978.
45. Marie, P.J., Pettifor, J.M., Ross, F.P., et al.: N. Engl. J. Med., *307:*584–588, 1982.
46. Shils, M.E.: Annu. Rev. Nutr., *8:*429–460, 1988.
47. Knochel, J.P.: N. Engl. J. Med., *313:*447–449, 1985.
48. Berner, Y.M., Shike, M.: Annu. Rev. Nutr., *8:*121–148, 1988.
49. Hetzel, B.S., Hay, I.D.: Clin. Endocrinol., *11:*445–460, 1979.
50. Andersen, H.T., Barkve, H.: Scand. J. Clin. Lab. Invest., *25*(Suppl.):*114:*1–62, 1970.
51. Danks, D.M.: Annu. Rev. Nutr., *8:*235–257, 1988.
52. Portmann, B., Tanner, M.S., Mowat, A.P., et al.: Lancet, *2:*1338–1340, 1978.
53. Tanner, M.S., Bhave, S.A., Kantarjian, A.H., et al.: Lancet, *2:*992–995, 1983.
54. Prasad, A.S., Halsted, J.A., Nadimi, M.: Am. J. Med., *31:*532–546, 1961.
55. Prasad, A.S., Miale, A. Jr., Farid, Z., et al.: Arch. Intern. Med., *111:*407–428, 1963.
56. Hambidge, K.M., Krebs, N.F., Walravens, P.A.: Nutr. Res., *1:*306–316, 1985.
57. Younaszai, H.D.: J. Parenter. Enter. Nutr., *7:*72–74, 1983.
58. Golden, M.H.N., Golden, B.E.: Am. J. Clin. Nutr., *34:*900–908, 1981.
59. Chen, X., Yang, G., Chen, J., et al.: Biol. Tr. El. Res., *2:*91–107, 1980.
60. Vinton, N.E., Dahlstrom, K.A., Strobel, C.T., et al.: J. Pediatr., *111:*711–717, 1987.
61. Yang, G., Wang, S., Zhou, R., et al.: Am. J. Clin. Nutr., *37:*872–881, 1983.
62. Centers for Disease Control: Morbid. Mortal. Wkly. Rep., *33:*157–158, 1984.
63. Ruta, D.A., Haider, S.: Br. Med. J., *299:*316–317, 1989.

**64.** Jeejeebhoy, K.N., Chu, R.C., Marliss, E.B., et al.: Am. J. Clin. Nutr., *30*:531–538, 1977.

**65.** Freund, H., Atamian, S., Fischer, J.E.: JAMA, *241*:496–498, 1979.

**66.** Brown, R.O., Forloines-Lynn, S., Cross, R.E., et al.: Dig. Dis. Sci., *31*:661–664, 1986.

**67.** Kriss, J.P., Carness, W.H., Gross, R.T.: JAMA, *157*:117–121, 1955.

**68.** Sullivan, J.F., Egan, J.D., George, R.P., et al.: J. Lab. Clin. Med., *68*:1022–1023, 1966.

**69.** Rajagopalan, K.V.: Annu. Rev. Nutr., *8*:401–427, 1988.

**70.** Abumrad, N.N., Schneider, A.J., Steel, D., et al.: Am. J. Clin. Nutr., *34*:2551–2559, 1981.

**71.** Kovalskii, V.V., Yatovaya, G.A., Shmavonyau, D.M.: Zh. Obshch. Biol., *22*:179, 1961.

**72.** Doisy, E.A., Jr.: Effects of deficiency in manganese upon plasma and cholesterol in man.: *In* Trace Element Metabolism in Animals. Vol. 2. Edited by W.G. Hoekstra, J.W. Suttie, H.E. Ganther, et al. Baltimore, University Park Press, 1974, pp. 668–670.

## SELECTED READING

McLaren, D.S.: A Colour Atlas and Text of Diet-Related Diseases. New Ed. London, Wolfe, 1992.

# Appendix

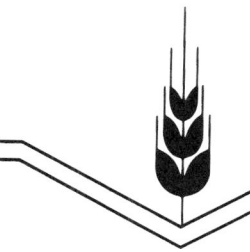

**Abby Stolper Bloch and Maurice E. Shils**

The Appendix for this edition has been appreciably revised and updated since the seventh edition. It has been divided into two segments. The first part provides basic reference data, various national and international recommendations, energy and nutrient requirements, and height and weight as well as body composition data. The second part is composed of tabular information on nutrient contents of various foods and diets for various disease entities. As always, such dietary prescriptions may require modification in accordance with the clinical status and reactions of the individual patient. An expanded section on supplemental exchange lists has been included in this edition. In addition, a listing of current commercially available nutrition formulations with manufacturer information is provided.

Past editions have included detailed formulations of commercially available dietary products for oral and tube-feeding purposes. Because such listings have been widely adopted and widely circulated by various companies and because revisions of such formulations are frequent, we have decided to eliminate such detailed data. Instead, Table A–37 simply lists the types and names of current formulas and provides the addresses and phone numbers where the latest information may be obtained.

In the following Appendix table of contents, section and subsection titles are given with designating numbers. The specific tables under these headings are designated by letter and/or number. In the text, each table has a designation specifying the section, subsection, and table.

# APPENDIX CONTENTS

## Table A–12 • PHYSICAL GROWTH STANDARDS



## Table A–13 • ADULT WEIGHT BY AGE AND SEX



## Table A–14 • WEIGHT AND SKINFOLD THICKNESS DATA

**TABLE A–1A.** CONVERSION FACTORS BETWEEN TRADITIONAL AND SI UNITS

Factors for converting nutrients expressed in metric or millequivalent units into International System (SI) units.

**1.** Definitions

**a.** Equivalent weight (EW) = atomic weight of element/valence of ionic form. Example with magnesium: atomic wt = 24, valence = 2+; therefore EW = 12

**b.** Quantity of an electrolyte in milliequivalents per liter (mEq/1) = mg of electrolyte/L/EW. Example: 48 mg of magnesium/L/12 = 4 mEq/L

**c.** Quantity of an electrolyte in mg/dl = (mEq/L × EW)/10

**d.** To convert mg/dl (= mg%) of an electrolyte to mEq/L mg/dl × 10/EW = mEq/L

**e.** 1 mol = 1 molecular or atomic weight of element or compound in grams (GMWt). In solutions this is usually expressed as moles per liter; i.e., 1 mol/L = 1 M; 1 mM (mmol) = 1 mol × $10^{-3}$; 1 μM (μmol) = 1 mol × $10^{-6}$; 1 nM (nmol) = 1 mol × $10^{-9}$

**f.**

**(1)** To convert mEq/L of an electrolyte or other ions in solution to mmol/L: mEq/L divided by valence = mmol/L; e.g., (a) 2 mEq/L of magnesium ($Mg^{2+}$) = 2/2 = 1 mmol/L; e.g., (b) 140 mEq $Na^{+}$/L = 140/L = 140 mmol/L

**(2)** To convert mg/dl to mmol/L: (mg/dl × 10/EW) divided by valence = mmol/L; e.g., 2 mg/dl of magnesium = (2 × 10/12) divided by 2 = 0.83 mmol/L

**(3)** For organic substances: mmol/L = wt in mg/L/MW (in mg)

**2.** SI units for expressing clinical laboratory data

These units are now widely used and are increasingly required for publication of scientific data in physical, biologic, and biomedical publications. Extensive SI conversion tables have been published together with an explanation of the rationale for their use and technical aspects of usage.[1–3]

**a.** The base units of interest in physical quantities used in clinical chemistry are:

| Quantity | Base Unit |
|---|---|
| mass | kilogram |
| time | second |
| amount | mole |
| length | meter |

A derived unit for energy is the kjoule(kJ) 4.18 kJ = 1 kcal
1 MJ = 239 kcal

**b.** Prefixes and symbols for decimal multiples and submultiples include:

| Factor | Prefix | Symbol | Factor | Prefix | Symbol |
|---|---|---|---|---|---|
| $10^{9}$ | giga | G | $10^{-3}$ | milli | m |
| $10^{6}$ | mega | M | $10^{-6}$ | micro | u |
| $10^{3}$ | kilo | k | $10^{-9}$ | nano | n |
| $10^{2}$ | hecto | h | $10^{-12}$ | pico | p |
| $10^{1}$ | deka | da | $10^{-15}$ | femto | f |
| $10^{-1}$ | deci | d | $10^{-18}$ | atto | a |
| $10^{-2}$ | centi | c | | | |

**3.** Conversion factors for selected compounds of nutrition interest*

| Component | (1) Present Unit | (2) Conversion Factor | (3) SI Unit Symbol | (4) Mass Conversion Factor |
|---|---|---|---|---|
| Albumin (s) | g/dl | 10 | g/L | — |
| Aluminum (s) | μg/L | 37.04 | nmol/L | μg/27 = mol |
| Amino acids | (see ref. 3, p. 119 for individual amino acids) | | | |
| Amino acid nitrogen (p) | mg/dl | 0.714 | mmol/L | mg/14 = mmol |
| Ascorbic acid (p) | mg/dl | 56.78 | μmol/L | mg/176 = mmol |
| Calcium (s) | mg/dl | 0.250 | mmol/L | mg/40 = mmol |
| Calcium (s) | mEq/dl | 0.500 | mmol/L | mEq/2 = mmol |
| β-Carotene† (s) | μ/dl | 0.0186 | μmol/L | ug/536.85 umol |
| Chloride (s) | mEq/L | 1.00 | mmol/L | mEq = mmol |
| Cholesterol (p) | mg/dl | 0.0259 | mmol/L | mg/386.6 = mmol |
| Copper (s) | μg/dl | 0.157 | μmol/L | μg/63.5 = umol |
| Cyanocobalamin ($B_{12}$) | pg/ml | 0.738 | pmol/L | pg/1355 = pmol |
| Ethanol (p) | mg/dl | 0.217 | mmol/L | mg/46 = mmol |
| Folic acid | ng/ml | 2.265 | nmol/L | ng/441.4 = nmol |
| Glucose (p) | mg/dl | 0.0555 | mmol/L | mg/180.2 = mmol |
| Iron (s) | μg/dl | 0.179 | μmol/L | μg/55.9 = umol |
| Phosphate (p) (as phosphorus) | mg/dl | 0.323 | mmol/L | mg/31 = mmol |
| Potassium (s) | mEq/L | 1.000 | mmol/L | mEq = mmol |
| Potassium | mg/dl | 0.256 | mmol/L | mg/39.1 = mmol |
| Magnesium (s) | mg/dl | 0.411 | mmol/L | mg/24.3 = mmol |
| Pyridoxal (B) | ng/ml | 5.981 | nmol/L | ng/167 = nmol |
| Retinol† (p,s) | μg/dl | 0.0349 | μmol/L | μg/286 = umol |
| Riboflavin (s) | μg/dl | 26.57 | nmol/L | μg/376 = nmol |
| Sodium (s) | mEq/L | 1.00 | mmol/L | mEq = mmol |
| Thiamin HCl (U) | μg/24 hr | 0.00298 | μmol/d | μg/337 = umol |
| α-Tocopherol (p) | mg/dl | 23.22 | μmol/L | μg/431 = umol |
| Vitamin $D_3$ | μg/dl | 26.01 | nmol/L | μg/384 = umol |
| Calcidiol | ng/ml | 2.498 | nmol/L | ng/400 = nmol |
| Zinc (s) | μg/dl | 0.153 | μmol/L | μg/65.4 = umol |

*To convert metric or equivalent unit per unit volume (column 1) to S.I. units per liter (column 3), multiply by the conversion factor in column 2. p = plasma; s = serum; B = blood; U = urine.

†See Appendix table A–1b for detailed conversion figures for retinol and carotene

## REFERENCES


1. Young, D.S.: Ann. Intern. Med., *106*:114, 1987.
2. Lundberg, G.D., Iberson, C., Radulescu, G.: JAMA, *255*: 2329, 1986.
3. Monsen, E.R.: J. Am. Diet. Assoc., *87*:356, 1987.

**TABLE A—1B.** FACTORS AND FORMULAS USED IN INTERCONVERTING UNITS OF VITAMIN A AND CAROTENOIDS

Factors
- 1 nmol retinol = 286.42 ng
- 1 nmol retinoic acid = 300.42 ng
- 1 nmol β-carotene = 536.85 ng

1 μg retinol equivalent (μg RE)
- = 1 μg all-*trans* retinol
- = 3.49 nmol all-*trans* retinol
- = 6 μg all-*trans* β-carotene
- = 11.18 nmol all-*trans* β-carotene
- = 12 μg other all-*trans* provitamin A carotenoids
- = 3.33 $IU_a$ (the international unit of all-*trans* retinol)
- = 10 $IU_c$ (the international unit of all-*trans* β-carotene)

1 $IU_a$
- = 0.3 μg all-*trans* retinol
- = 0.3 μg RE
- = 1.05 nmol all-*trans* retinol
- = 1.8 μg all-*trans* β-carotene
- = 3.35 nmol all-*trans* β-carotene
- = 3 $IU_c$
- = 3.6 μg other all-*trans* provitamin A carotenoids

1 $IU_c$
- = 0.6 μg all-*trans* β-carotene
- = 1.12 nmol all-*trans* β-carotene
- = 0.1 μg RE
- = 0.33 $IU_a$
- = 1.2 μg other all-*trans* provitamin A carotenoids

Formulas and Examples: All-*trans* configurations of retinol and carotenoids are assumed

1. μg RE = μg retinol + μg β-carotene/6
   A diet contains 500 μg retinol and 1800 μg β-carotene. Then,

   μg RE = 500 + 1800/6 = 800 μg RE

2. μg RE = $IU_a$/3.33 + $IU_c$/10
   A diet contains 1667 $IU_a$ of retinol and 3000 $IU_c$ of β-carotene. Then,

   μg RE = 1667/3.33 + 3000/10 = 800 μg RE

3. μg RE = μg β-carotene/6 + μg other provitamin A carotenoids/12
   A serving of sweet potato contains 2400 μg of β-carotene and 480 μg of other provitamin A carotenoids. Then,

   μg RE = 2400/6 + 480/12 = 440 μg RE

(continued)

**TABLE A–1B.** (continued)

4.

$$\% \ \mu g \text{ RE as retinol} = \left[1.5 - \frac{0.15 \text{ total IU}}{\text{total RE}}\right] \times 100$$

$$\% \ \mu g \text{ RE as carotenoids} = \left[\frac{0.15 \text{ total IU}}{\text{total RE}} - 0.5\right] \times 100$$

A 100-g portion of cheese contains a total of 300 μg RE and a total of 1200 IU, in which 1 $IU_a$ has been *assumed* to equal 1 $IU_c$. Then,

$$\% \text{ RE as retinol} = \left[1.5 - \frac{0.15 \times 1200}{300}\right] \times 100 = 90\%$$

$$\% \text{ RE as carotenoids} = \left[\frac{0.15 \times 1200}{300} - 0.5\right] \times 100 = 10\%$$

In this sample of cheese, therefore, 270 μg (270 μg RE) is present as retinol and 180 μg, or 30 μg RE, is present as β-carotene or its equivalent of other provitamin A carotenoids.

5.

$$IU_a = \frac{10 \ \mu g \text{ RE} - \text{total IU}}{2}$$

$$IU_c = \frac{3 \text{ total IU} - 10 \ \mu g \text{ RE}}{2}$$

In a cheese sample containing a total of 300 μg RE and a total of 1200 IU, in which 1 $IU_a$ is *assumed* to equal 1 $IU_c$,

$$IU_a = \frac{10 \times 300 - 1200}{2} = 900$$

$$IU_c = \frac{3 \times 1200 - 10 \times 300}{2} = 300$$

Note: Assumptions used from revised sections of the United States Department of Agriculture's *Handbook 8* (i.e., 8.1–8.10) are *(a)* that 1 $IU_a$ = 1 $IU_c$ and *(b)* that 1 RE = 1 μg of retinol = 6 μg of β-carotene = 12 μg of other provitamin A carotenoids.

In some cases, small negative values for $IU_c$ are obtained when the values for total IU and total RE are given for foods containing only preformed vitamin $A_1$ particularly in fortified foods like margarine. This aberrant calculation results from the rounding of analytic values. Similarly, small negative values for $IU_a$ may result for foods containing only carotenoids. In both cases, the negative values should be taken as zero.

Prepared by J.A. Olson. For further discussion of these interconversions, see Chapter 16.

**TABLE A–1C.** ATOMIC WEIGHTS (ALPHABETIC ORDER)

| ELEMENT | SYMBOL | ATOMIC NUMBER | ATOMIC WEIGHT | ELEMENT | SYMBOL | ATOMIC NUMBER | ATOMIC WEIGHT |
|---|---|---|---|---|---|---|---|
| Actinium | Ac | 89 | 227.0278* | Neodymium | Nd | 60 | 144.24 |
| Aluminum | Al | 13 | 26.981539 | Neon | Ne | 10 | 20.1797 |
| Americium | Am | 95 | 243.0614* | Neptunium | Np | 93 | 237.0482* |
| Antimony | Sb | 51 | 121.75 | Nickel | Ni | 28 | 58.69 |
| Argon | Ar | 18 | 39.948 | Niobium | Nb | 41 | 92.90638 |
| Arsenic | As | 33 | 74.92159 | Nitrogen | N | 7 | 14.00674 |
| Astatine | At | 85 | 209.9871* | Nobelium | No | 102 | 259.1009* |
| Barium | Ba | 56 | 137.327 | Osmium | Os | 76 | 190.2 |
| Berkelium | Bk | 97 | 247.0703* | Oxygen | O | 8 | 15.9994 |
| Beryllium | Be | 4 | 9.012182 | Palladium | Pd | 46 | 106.42 |
| Bismuth | Bi | 83 | 208.98037 | Phosphorus | P | 15 | 30.973762 |
| Boron | B | 5 | 10.811 | Platinum | Pt | 78 | 195.08 |
| Bromine | Br | 35 | 79.904 | Plutonium | Pu | 94 | 244.0642* |
| Cadmium | Cd | 48 | 112.411 | Polonium | Po | 84 | 208.9824* |
| Calcium | Ca | 20 | 40.078 | Potassium | K | 19 | 39.0983 |
| Californium | Cf | 98 | 251.0796* | Praseodymium | Pr | 59 | 140.90765 |
| Carbon | C | 6 | 12.011 | Promethium | Pm | 61 | 144.9127* |
| Cerium | Ce | 58 | 140.115 | Protactinium | Pa | 91 | 231.0359* |
| Cesium | Cs | 55 | 132.90543 | Radium | Ra | 88 | 226.0254* |
| Chlorine | Cl | 17 | 35.4527 | Radon | Rn | 86 | 222.0176* |
| Chromium | Cr | 24 | 51.9961 | Rhenium | Re | 75 | 186.207 |
| Cobalt | Co | 27 | 58.93320 | Rhodium | Rh | 45 | 102.90550 |
| Copper | Cu | 29 | 63.546 | Rubidium | Rb | 37 | 85.4678 |
| Curium | Cm | 96 | 247.0703* | Ruthenium | Ru | 44 | 101.07 |
| Dysprosium | Dy | 66 | 162.50 | Samarium | Sm | 62 | 150.36 |
| Einsteinium | Es | 99 | 252.083* | Scandium | Sc | 21 | 44.955910 |
| Erbium | Er | 68 | 167.26 | Selenium | Se | 34 | 78.96 |
| Europium | Eu | 63 | 151.965 | Silicon | Si | 14 | 28.0855 |
| Fermium | Fm | 100 | 257.0951* | Silver | Ag | 47 | 107.8682 |
| Fluorine | F | 9 | 18.9984032 | Sodium | Na | 11 | 22.989768 |
| Francium | Fr | 87 | 223.0197* | Strontium | Sr | 38 | 87.62 |
| Gadolinium | Gd | 64 | 157.25 | Sulfur | S | 16 | 32.066 |
| Gallium | Ga | 31 | 69.723 | Tantalum | Ta | 73 | 180.9479 |
| Germanium | Ge | 32 | 72.61 | Technetium | Tc | 43 | 97.9072* |
| Gold | Au | 79 | 196.96654 | Tellurium | Te | 52 | 127.60 |
| Hafnium | Hf | 72 | 178.49 | Terbium | Tb | 65 | 158.92534 |
| Helium | He | 2 | 4.002602 | Thallium | Tl | 81 | 204.3833 |
| Holmium | Ho | 67 | 164.93032 | Thorium | Th | 90 | 232.0381 |
| Hydrogen | H | 1 | 1.00794 | Thulium | Tm | 69 | 168.93421 |
| Indium | In | 49 | 114.82 | Tin | Sn | 50 | 118.710 |
| Iodine | I | 53 | 126.90447 | Titanium | Ti | 22 | 47.88 |
| Iridium | Ir | 77 | 192.22 | Tungsten | W | 74 | 183.85 |
| Iron | Fe | 26 | 55.847 | Unnilquadium | Unq | 104 | 261.11* |
| Krypton | Kr | 36 | 83.80 | Unnilpentium | Unp | 105 | 262.114* |
| Lanthanum | La | 57 | 138.9055 | Unnilhexium | Unh | 106 | 263.118* |
| Lawrencium | Lr | 103 | 262.11* | Unnilseptium | Uns | 107 | 262.12* |
| Lead | Pb | 82 | 207.2 | Uranium | U | 92 | 238.0289 |
| Lithium | Li | 3 | 6.941 | Vanadium | V | 23 | 50.9415 |
| Lutetium | Lu | 71 | 174.967 | Xenon | Xe | 54 | 131.29 |
| Magnesium | Mg | 12 | 24.3050 | Ytterbium | Yb | 70 | 173.04 |
| Manganese | Mn | 25 | 54.93805 | Yttrium | Y | 39 | 88.90585 |
| Mendelevium | Md | 101 | 258.10* | Zinc | Zn | 30 | 65.39 |
| Mercury | Hg | 80 | 200.59 | Zirconium | Zr | 40 | 91.224 |
| Molybdenum | Mo | 42 | 95.94 | | | | |

*Relative atomic mass of the isotope of that element with the longest known half-life.
(Based on 1987 IUPAC Table of Standard Atomic Weights of the Elements. *In* The Merck Index. 11th Ed. Rahway, NJ, Merck & Co., 1989.)

**TABLE A–1D.** WEIGHTS AND MEASURES

VOLUMES:

| Apothecaries' Measure | Metric | Household |
|---|---|---|
| 1 fluid dram (fl dr) | 4 milliliter (ml) | 1 teaspoon (tsp) |
| 2 fl dr | 8 ml | 1 dessert spoonful |
| ½ fluid ounce (fl oz) | 15 ml | 1 tablespoon (Tbsp) (3 tsp) |
| 1 fl oz. | 30 ml | 2 Tbsp (⅛ cup) |
| 1-½ fl oz | 45 ml | 1 jigger |
| 2 fl oz | 59 ml | 4 Tbsp (¼ cup) |
| 2-⅔ fl oz | 80 ml | 5-⅓ Tbsp (⅓ cup) |
| 4 fl oz | 118 ml | 8 Tbsp (½ cup) |
| 8 fl oz | 237 ml | 1 cup |
| 16 fl oz | 473 ml | 1 pint (pt) |
| 32 fl oz | 947 ml | 1 quart (qt) |
| 128 fl oz | 3,785 ml | 1 gallon (gal) |
| 3.38 fl oz | 1 deciliter (dl) (100 ml) | |
| 2.11 pt | 1 liter (L) (1,000 ml) | |

WEIGHTS:

| Avoirdupois | Metric |
|---|---|
| | 1 femtogram (fg) ($10^{-15}$ g) |
| | 1 picogram (pg) ($10^{-12}$ g) |
| | 1 nanogram (ng) ($10^{-9}$ g) |
| | 1 microgram ($\mu$g) ($10^{-6}$ g) |
| 1 grain (gr) | 0.065 g (65 mg) |
| 1 gram (0.035 oz) | 15.432 gr |
| 1 scruple (20 gr) | 1.296 g |
| 1 dram (dr) (= drachm) (27.3 gr) | 1.77 g |
| 1 oz (16 dr) | 28.35 g |
| 1 lb (16 oz) | 453.59 g |
| 1 ton (2,000 lb) | 0.91 metric tons |
| 1.015 gr | 1 milligram (mg) ($10^{-3}$ g) |
| | 1 centigram (cg) ($10^{-2}$ g) |
| | 1 decigram (dg) ($10^{-1}$ g) |
| 15.4 gr (0.035 oz) | 1 gram (g) |
| 2.2 lb | 1 kilogram (kg) ($10^{3}$ g) |

LENGTH/AREA:

| | Metric |
|---|---|
| 1 angstrom (A) | 10 millimeter (mm) |
| 1/2500 inch (in) | 1 micron ($\mu$) ($10^{-3}$ mm) = micrometer ($\mu$m) |
| 0.039 in | 1 mm |
| 0.39 in | 1 centimeter (cm) |
| 1 in | 2.54 cm |
| 1 foot (ft) (12 in) | 30.5 cm |
| 39.4 in | 1 meter (m) |
| 1 yard (yd) (3 ft) | 0.9 m |
| 1 rod (5.5 yd) | 4.95 m |
| 1093.6 yd (0.62 mile) | 1 kilometer (km) |
| 1 mile (mi) (5280 ft) | 1.61 km |
| 1 acre (160 square rods) | 0.4 hectare |

TEMPERATURE CONVERSIONS:

F to C: 5/9 (F − 32)

C to F: (9/5 × C) + 32

**TABLE A–1D.** WEIGHTS AND MEASURES

ELECTROLYTE DATA:

| Ion | | Atomic Wt (1) | Valence (2) | Equivalent Wt* 1 ÷ 2 |
|---|---|---|---|---|
| Bicarbonate | $HCO_3^-$ | 61.0 | 1 | 61.0 |
| Calcium | $Ca^{2+}$ | 40.1 | 2 | 20.0 |
| Chloride | $Cl^-$ | 35.5 | 1 | 35.5 |
| Magnesium | $Mg^{2+}$ | 24.3 | 2 | 12.2 |
| Phosphate† | $HPO_4^{2-}$ | 96.0 | 2 | 48.0† |
| Potassium | $K^+$ | 39.1 | 1 | 39.1 |
| Sodium | $Na^+$ | 23.0 | 1 | 23.0 |
| Sulfate | $SO_4^{2-}$ | 96.1 | 2 | 48.0 |

*Milliequivalent (mEq) = equivalent weight in milligrams (mg). To convert mg quantities of all electrolytes to mEq:

$$\frac{\text{mg of electrolyte}}{\text{equivalent weight in mg}} = \text{mEq}$$

To convert mEq quantities of all electrolytes to mg:

$$\text{mEq} \times \text{equivalent wt} = \text{mg}$$

To convert mg/dl to mEq/L:

$$\frac{\text{mg/dl} \times 10}{\text{equivalent wt in mg}} = \text{mEq/L}$$

To convert mEq/L to mg/dl: mEq/L × equivalent wt in mg × 0.1

†At the normal pH of plasma, 20% of the total inorganic phosphate radical is combined with one equivalent of base as $BH_2PO_4$, and 80% with two equivalents of base as $B_2HPO_4$. Under these conditions, base equivalence is therefore 0.2 + (0.8 × 2) = 1.8, and the equivalent weight of 53.3 is obtained by dividing the ionic weight by 1.8 instead of by 2. For phosphorus content of phosphate solutions, 1 mEq provides approximately 15 mg, and 1 mmol provides approximately 31 mg.

**TABLE A–2A.** MEDIAN HEIGHTS AND WEIGHTS AND RECOMMENDED ENERGY INTAKE IN THE UNITED STATES[a]

| CATEGORY | AGE (YEARS) OR CONDITION | WEIGHT (kg) | WEIGHT (lb) | HEIGHT (cm) | HEIGHT (in) | REE[b] (kcal/day) | AVERAGE ENERGY ALLOWANCE (kcal)[c] Multiples of REE | Per kg | Per day[d] |
|---|---|---|---|---|---|---|---|---|---|
| Infants | 0.0–0.5 | 6 | 13 | 60 | 24 | 320 | | 108 | 650 |
| | 0.5–1.0 | 9 | 20 | 71 | 28 | 500 | | 98 | 850 |
| Children | 1–3 | 13 | 29 | 90 | 35 | 740 | | 102 | 1,300 |
| | 4–6 | 20 | 44 | 112 | 44 | 950 | | 90 | 1,800 |
| | 7–10 | 28 | 62 | 132 | 52 | 1,130 | | 70 | 2,000 |
| Males | 11–14 | 45 | 99 | 157 | 62 | 1,440 | 1.70 | 55 | 2,500 |
| | 15–18 | 66 | 145 | 176 | 69 | 1,760 | 1.67 | 45 | 3,000 |
| | 19–24 | 72 | 160 | 177 | 70 | 1,780 | 1.67 | 40 | 2,900 |
| | 25–50 | 79 | 174 | 176 | 70 | 1,800 | 1.60 | 37 | 2,900 |
| | 51+ | 77 | 170 | 173 | 68 | 1,530 | 1.50 | 30 | 2,300 |
| Females | 11–14 | 46 | 101 | 157 | 62 | 1,310 | 1.67 | 47 | 2,200 |
| | 15–18 | 55 | 120 | 163 | 64 | 1,370 | 1.60 | 40 | 2,200 |
| | 19–24 | 58 | 128 | 164 | 65 | 1,350 | 1.60 | 38 | 2,200 |
| | 25–50 | 63 | 138 | 163 | 64 | 1,380 | 1.55 | 36 | 2,200 |
| | 51+ | 65 | 143 | 160 | 63 | 1,280 | 1.50 | 30 | 1,900 |
| Pregnant | 1st trimester | | | | | – | | | +0 |
| | 2nd trimester | | | | | | | | +300 |
| | 3rd trimester | | | | | | | | +300 |
| Lactating | 1st 6 months | | | | | | | | +500 |
| | 2nd 6 months | | | | | | | | +500 |

[a] Median Height/Weight used by the RDA are those which are the medians for the U.S. population of designated age as reported in NHANES II.
[b] Calculations based on WHO equation derived from BMR data (Table A–7a), then rounded.
[c] In the range of light to moderate activity, the coefficient of variation is ±20%.
[d] Figure is rounded.

(From Food and Nutrition Board, National Research Council: Recommended Dietary Allowances. 10th Ed. Washington, D.C., National Academy Press, 1989, p. 33.)

**TABLE A–2B.** RECOMMENDED DIETARY ALLOWANCES[a], REVISED 1989 (DESIGNED FOR THE MAINTENANCE OF GOOD NUTRITION OF PRACTICALLY ALL HEALTHY PEOPLE IN THE UNITED STATES)

| | | WEIGHT[b] | | HEIGHT[b] | | | FAT-SOLUBLE VITAMINS | | | |
|---|---|---|---|---|---|---|---|---|---|---|
| CATEGORY | AGE (YEARS) OR CONDITION | (kg) | (lb) | (cm) | (in) | PROTEIN (G) | Vitamin A (μg RE)[c] | Vitamin D (μg)[d] | Vitamin E (mg α-TE)[e] | Vitamin K (μg) |
| Infants | 0.0–0.5 | 6 | 13 | 60 | 24 | 13 | 375 | 7.5 | 3 | 5 |
| | 0.5–1.0 | 9 | 20 | 71 | 28 | 14 | 375 | 10 | 4 | 10 |
| Children | 1–3 | 13 | 29 | 90 | 35 | 16 | 400 | 10 | 6 | 15 |
| | 4–6 | 20 | 44 | 112 | 44 | 24 | 500 | 10 | 7 | 20 |
| | 7–10 | 28 | 62 | 132 | 52 | 28 | 700 | 10 | 7 | 30 |
| Males | 11–14 | 45 | 99 | 157 | 62 | 45 | 1,000 | 10 | 10 | 45 |
| | 15–18 | 66 | 145 | 176 | 69 | 59 | 1,000 | 10 | 10 | 65 |
| | 19–24 | 72 | 160 | 177 | 70 | 58 | 1,000 | 10 | 10 | 70 |
| | 25–50 | 79 | 174 | 176 | 70 | 63 | 1,000 | 5 | 10 | 80 |
| | 51+ | 77 | 170 | 173 | 68 | 63 | 1,000 | 5 | 10 | 80 |
| Females | 11–14 | 46 | 101 | 157 | 62 | 46 | 800 | 10 | 8 | 45 |
| | 15–18 | 55 | 120 | 163 | 64 | 44 | 800 | 10 | 8 | 55 |
| | 19–24 | 58 | 128 | 164 | 65 | 46 | 800 | 10 | 8 | 60 |
| | 25–50 | 63 | 138 | 163 | 64 | 50 | 800 | 5 | 8 | 65 |
| | 51+ | 65 | 143 | 160 | 63 | 50 | 800 | 5 | 8 | 65 |
| Pregnant | | | | | | 60 | 800 | 10 | 10 | 65 |
| Lactating | 1st 6 months | | | | | 65 | 1,300 | 10 | 12 | 65 |
| | 2nd 6 months | | | | | 62 | 1,200 | 10 | 11 | 65 |

[a]The allowances, expressed as average daily intakes over time, are intended to provide for individual variations among most normal persons as they live in the United States under usual environmental stresses. Diets should be based on a variety of common foods in order to provide other nutrients for which human requirements have been less well defined. See text for detailed discussion of allowances and of nutrients not tabulated.

[b]Weights and heights of reference adults are actual medians for the U.S. population of the designated age, as reported by NHANES II. The median weights and heights of those under 19 years of age were taken from Hamill et al. (1979). The use of these figures does not imply that the height-to-weight ratios are ideal.

[c]Retinol equivalents. 1 retinol equivalent = 1 μg retinol or 6 μg β-carotene. See text for calculation of vitamin A activity of diets as retinol equivalents.

[d]As cholecalciferol. 10 μg cholecalciferol = 400 IU of vitamin D.

[e]α-Tocopherol equivalents. 1 mg d-α tocopherol = 1 α-TE. See text for variation in allowances and calculation of vitamin E activity of the diet as α-tocopherol equivalents.

[f]1 NE (niacin equivalent) is equal to 1 mg of niacin or 60 mg of dietary tryptophan.

(From Food and Nutrition Board, National Research Council: Recommended Dietary Allowances. 10th Ed. Washington, D.C., National Academy Press, 1989.)

**TABLE A–2B.** (CONTINUED)

| WATER-SOLUBLE VITAMINS | | | | | | | MINERALS | | | | | | |
|---|---|---|---|---|---|---|---|---|---|---|---|---|---|
| Vitamin C (mg) | Thiamin (mg) | Riboflavin (mg) | Niacin (mg NE)[f] | Vitamin $B_6$ (mg) | Folate (μg) | Vitamin $B_{12}$ (μg) | Calcium (mg) | Phosphorus (mg) | Magnesium (mg) | Iron (mg) | Zinc (mg) | Iodine (μg) | Selenium (μg) |
| 30 | 0.3 | 0.4 | 5 | 0.3 | 25 | 0.3 | 400 | 300 | 40 | 6 | 5 | 40 | 10 |
| 35 | 0.4 | 0.5 | 6 | 0.6 | 35 | 0.5 | 600 | 500 | 60 | 10 | 5 | 50 | 15 |
| 40 | 0.7 | 0.8 | 9 | 1.0 | 50 | 0.7 | 800 | 800 | 80 | 10 | 10 | 70 | 20 |
| 45 | 0.9 | 1.1 | 12 | 1.1 | 75 | 1.0 | 800 | 800 | 120 | 10 | 10 | 90 | 20 |
| 45 | 1.0 | 1.2 | 13 | 1.4 | 100 | 1.4 | 800 | 800 | 170 | 10 | 10 | 120 | 30 |
| 50 | 1.3 | 1.5 | 17 | 1.7 | 150 | 2.0 | 1,200 | 1,200 | 270 | 12 | 15 | 150 | 40 |
| 60 | 1.5 | 1.8 | 20 | 2.0 | 200 | 2.0 | 1,200 | 1,200 | 400 | 12 | 15 | 150 | 50 |
| 60 | 1.5 | 1.7 | 19 | 2.0 | 200 | 2.0 | 1,200 | 1,200 | 350 | 10 | 15 | 150 | 70 |
| 60 | 1.5 | 1.7 | 19 | 2.0 | 200 | 2.0 | 800 | 800 | 350 | 10 | 15 | 150 | 70 |
| 60 | 1.2 | 1.4 | 15 | 2.0 | 200 | 2.0 | 800 | 800 | 350 | 10 | 15 | 150 | 70 |
| 50 | 1.1 | 1.3 | 15 | 1.4 | 150 | 2.0 | 1,200 | 1,200 | 280 | 15 | 12 | 150 | 45 |
| 60 | 1.1 | 1.3 | 15 | 1.5 | 180 | 2.0 | 1,200 | 1,200 | 300 | 15 | 12 | 150 | 50 |
| 60 | 1.1 | 1.3 | 15 | 1.6 | 180 | 2.0 | 1,200 | 1,200 | 280 | 15 | 12 | 150 | 55 |
| 60 | 1.1 | 1.3 | 15 | 1.6 | 180 | 2.0 | 800 | 800 | 280 | 15 | 12 | 150 | 55 |
| 60 | 1.0 | 1.2 | 13 | 1.6 | 180 | 2.0 | 800 | 800 | 280 | 10 | 12 | 150 | 55 |
| 70 | 1.5 | 1.6 | 17 | 2.2 | 400 | 2.2 | 1,200 | 1,200 | 320 | 30 | 15 | 175 | 65 |
| 95 | 1.6 | 1.8 | 20 | 2.1 | 280 | 2.6 | 1,200 | 1,200 | 355 | 15 | 19 | 200 | 75 |
| 90 | 1.6 | 1.7 | 20 | 2.1 | 260 | 2.6 | 1,200 | 1,200 | 340 | 15 | 16 | 200 | 75 |

**TABLE A–2C.** ESTIMATED SAFE AND ADEQUATE DAILY DIETARY INTAKES OF SELECTED VITAMINS AND MINERALS*

| CATEGORY | AGE (years) | VITAMINS: BIOTIN ($\mu g$) | VITAMINS: PANTOTHENIC ACID (mg) |
|---|---|---|---|
| Infants | 0–0.5 | 10 | 2 |
| | 0.5–1 | 15 | 3 |
| Children and adolescents | 1–3 | 20 | 3 |
| | 4–6 | 25 | 3–4 |
| | 7–10 | 30 | 4–5 |
| | 11+ | 30–100 | 4–7 |
| Adults | | 30–100 | 4–7 |

| CATEGORY | AGE (years) | TRACE ELEMENTS†: COPPER (mg) | MANGANESE (mg) | FLUORIDE (mg) | CHROMIUM ($\mu g$) | MOLYBDENUM ($\mu g$) |
|---|---|---|---|---|---|---|
| Infants | 0–0.5 | 0.4–0.6 | 0.3–0.6 | 0.1–0.5 | 10–40 | 15–30 |
| | 0.5–1 | 0.6–0.7 | 0.6–1.0 | 0.2–1.0 | 20–60 | 20–40 |
| Children and adolescents | 1–3 | 0.7–1.0 | 1.0–1.5 | 0.5–1.5 | 20–80 | 25–50 |
| | 4–6 | 1.0–1.5 | 1.5–2.0 | 1.0–2.5 | 30–120 | 30–75 |
| | 7–10 | 1.0–2.0 | 2.0–3.0 | 1.5–2.5 | 50–200 | 50–150 |
| | 11+ | 1.5–2.5 | 2.0–5.0 | 1.5–2.5 | 50–200 | 75–250 |
| Adults | | 1.5–3.0 | 2.0–5.0 | 1.5–4.0 | 50–200 | 75–250 |

*Because there is less information on which to base allowances, these figures are not given in the main table of RDA and are provided here in the form of ranges of recommended intakes.

†Because the toxic levels for many trace elements may be only several times usual intakes, the upper levels for the trace elements given in this table should not be habitually exceeded.

(From Food and Nutrition Board, National Research Council: Recommended Dietary Allowances. 10th Ed. Washington, D.C., National Academy Press, 1989, p. 284.)

**TABLE A–3A.** SUMMARY OF EXAMPLES OF RECOMMENDED NUTRIENTS BASED ON ENERGY EXPRESSED AS DAILY RATES, CANADA

| AGE | SEX | ENERGY (kcal) | THIAMIN (mg) | RIBOFLAVIN (mg) | NIACIN (ne[b]) | n-3 PUFA[a] (g) | n-6 PUFA (g) |
|---|---|---|---|---|---|---|---|
| Months | | | | | | | |
| 0–4 | Both | 600 | 0.3 | 0.3 | 4 | 0.5 | 3 |
| 5–12 | Both | 900 | 0.4 | 0.5 | 7 | 0.5 | 3 |
| Years | | | | | | | |
| 1 | Both | 1100 | 0.5 | 0.6 | 8 | 0.6 | 4 |
| 2–3 | Both | 1300 | 0.6 | 0.7 | 9 | 0.7 | 4 |
| 4–6 | Both | 1800 | 0.7 | 0.9 | 13 | 1.0 | 6 |
| 7–9 | M | 2200 | 0.9 | 1.1 | 16 | 1.2 | 7 |
| | F | 1900 | 0.8 | 1.0 | 14 | 1.0 | 6 |
| 10–12 | M | 2500 | 1.0 | 1.3 | 18 | 1.4 | 8 |
| | F | 2200 | 0.9 | 1.1 | 16 | 1.2 | 7 |
| 13–15 | M | 2800 | 1.1 | 1.4 | 20 | 1.5 | 9 |
| | F | 2200 | 0.9 | 1.1 | 16 | 1.2 | 7 |
| 16–18 | M | 3200 | 1.3 | 1.6 | 23 | 1.8 | 11 |
| | F | 2100 | 0.8 | 1.1 | 15 | 1.2 | 7 |
| 19–24 | M | 3000 | 1.2 | 1.5 | 22 | 1.6 | 10 |
| | F | 2100 | 0.8 | 1.1 | 15 | 1.2 | 7 |
| 25–49 | M | 2700 | 1.1 | 1.4 | 19 | 1.5 | 9 |
| | F | 1900 | 0.8[c] | 1.0[c] | 14[c] | 1.1[c] | 7[c] |
| 50–74 | M | 2300 | 0.9 | 1.2 | 16 | 1.3 | 8 |
| | F | 1800 | 0.8[c] | 1.0[c] | 14[c] | 1.1[c] | 7[c] |
| 75+ | M | 2000 | 0.8 | 1.0 | 14 | 1.1 | 7 |
| | F[d] | 1700 | 0.8[c] | 1.0[c] | 14[c] | 1.1[c] | 7[c] |
| Pregnancy (additional) | | | | | | | |
| 1st trimester | | 100 | 0.1 | 0.1 | 1 | 0.05 | 0.3 |
| 2nd trimester | | 300 | 0.1 | 0.3 | 2 | 0.16 | 0.9 |
| 3rd trimester | | 300 | 0.1 | 0.3 | 2 | 0.16 | 0.9 |
| Lactation (additional) | | 450 | 0.2 | 0.4 | 3 | 0.25 | 1.5 |

[a]PUFA, Polyunsaturated fatty acids.
[b]NE, Niacin equivalents.
[c]Level below which intake should not fall.
[d]Assumes moderate (more than average) physical activity.
(From Health and Welfare Canada: Nutrition Recommendations. The Report of the Scientific Review Committee. Ottawa; Supply and Services Canada, 1990. Reproduced with permission of the Minister of Supply and Services Canada 1992.)

**TABLE A–3B.** SUMMARY OF EXAMPLES OF RECOMMENDED NUTRIENT INTAKE BASED ON AGE AND BODY WEIGHT EXPRESSED AS DAILY RATES, CANADA

| AGE | SEX | WEIGHT (kg) | PROTEIN (g) | VIT. A (RE)[a] | VIT. D (μg) | VIT. E (mg) | VIT. C (mg) | FOLATE (μg) | VIT. $B_{12}$ (μg) | CALCIUM (mg) | PHOSPHORUS (mg) | MAGNESIUM (mg) | IRON (mg) | IODINE (μg) | ZINC (mg) |
|---|---|---|---|---|---|---|---|---|---|---|---|---|---|---|---|
| Months | | | | | | | | | | | | | | | |
| 0–4 | Both | 6.0 | 12[b] | 400 | 10 | 3 | 20 | 25 | 0.3 | 250[c] | 150 | 20 | 0.3[d] | 30 | 2[d] |
| 5–12 | Both | 9.0 | 12 | 400 | 10 | 3 | 20 | 40 | 0.4 | 400 | 200 | 32 | 7 | 40 | 3 |
| Years | | | | | | | | | | | | | | | |
| 1 | Both | 11 | 13 | 400 | 10 | 3 | 20 | 40 | 0.5 | 500 | 300 | 40 | 6 | 55 | 4 |
| 2–3 | Both | 14 | 16 | 400 | 5 | 4 | 20 | 50 | 0.6 | 550 | 350 | 50 | 6 | 65 | 4 |
| 4–6 | Both | 18 | 19 | 500 | 5 | 5 | 25 | 70 | 0.8 | 600 | 400 | 65 | 8 | 85 | 5 |
| 7–9 | M | 25 | 26 | 700 | 2.5 | 7 | 25 | 90 | 1.0 | 700 | 500 | 100 | 8 | 110 | 7 |
| | F | 25 | 26 | 700 | 2.5 | 6 | 25 | 90 | 1.0 | 700 | 500 | 100 | 8 | 95 | 7 |
| 10–12 | M | 34 | 34 | 800 | 2.5 | 8 | 25 | 120 | 1.0 | 900 | 700 | 130 | 8 | 125 | 9 |
| | F | 36 | 36 | 800 | 2.5 | 7 | 25 | 130 | 1.0 | 1100 | 800 | 135 | 8 | 110 | 9 |
| 13–15 | M | 50 | 49 | 900 | 2.5 | 9 | 30[e] | 175 | 1.0 | 1100 | 900 | 185 | 10 | 160 | 12 |
| | F | 48 | 46 | 800 | 2.5 | 7 | 30[e] | 170 | 1.0 | 1000 | 850 | 180 | 13 | 160 | 9 |
| 16–18 | M | 62 | 58 | 1000 | 2.5 | 10 | 40[e] | 220 | 1.0 | 900 | 1000 | 230 | 10 | 160 | 12 |
| | F | 53 | 47 | 800 | 2.5 | 7 | 30[e] | 190 | 1.0 | 700 | 850 | 200 | 12 | 160 | 9 |
| 19–24 | M | 71 | 61 | 1000 | 2.5 | 10 | 40[e] | 220 | 1.0 | 800 | 1000 | 240 | 9 | 160 | 12 |
| | F | 58 | 50 | 800 | 2.5 | 7 | 30[e] | 180 | 1.0 | 700 | 850 | 200 | 13 | 160 | 9 |
| 25–49 | M | 74 | 64 | 1000 | 2.5 | 9 | 40[e] | 230 | 1.0 | 800 | 1000 | 250 | 9 | 160 | 12 |
| | F | 59 | 51 | 800 | 2.5 | 6 | 30[e] | 185 | 1.0 | 700 | 850 | 200 | 13 | 160 | 9 |
| 50–74 | M | 73 | 63 | 1000 | 5 | 7 | 40[e] | 230 | 1.0 | 800 | 1000 | 250 | 9 | 160 | 12 |
| | F | 63 | 54 | 800 | 5 | 6 | 30[e] | 195 | 1.0 | 800 | 850 | 210 | 8 | 160 | 9 |
| 75+ | M | 69 | 59 | 1000 | 5 | 6 | 40[e] | 215 | 1.0 | 800 | 1000 | 230 | 9 | 160 | 12 |
| | F | 64 | 55 | 800 | 5 | 5 | 30[e] | 200 | 1.0 | 800 | 850 | 210 | 8 | 160 | 9 |
| Pregnancy (additional) | | | | | | | | | | | | | | | |
| 1st trimester | | | 5 | 0 | 2.5 | 2 | 0 | 200 | 0.2 | 500 | 200 | 15 | 0 | 25 | 6 |
| 2nd trimester | | | 20 | 0 | 2.5 | 2 | 10 | 200 | 0.2 | 500 | 200 | 45 | 5 | 25 | 6 |
| 3rd trimester | | | 24 | 0 | 2.5 | 2 | 10 | 200 | 0.2 | 500 | 200 | 45 | 10 | 25 | 6 |
| Lactation (additional) | | | 20 | 400 | 2.5 | 3 | 25 | 100 | 0.2 | 500 | 200 | 65 | 0 | 50 | 6 |

[a]Retinol Equivalents.
[b]Protein is assumed to be from breast milk and must be adjusted for infant formula.
[c]Infant formula with high phosphorus should contain 375 mg calcium.
[d]Breast milk is assumed to be the source of the mineral.
[e]Smokers should increase vitamin C by 50%.
(From Health and Welfare Canada: Nutrition Recommendations. The Report of the Scientific Review Committee. Ottawa, Supply and Services Canada, 1990. Reproduced with permission of the Minister of Supply and Services Canada 1992.)

**TABLE A–4A.** ESTIMATED AVERAGE REQUIREMENTS (EAR) FOR ENERGY, UNITED KINGDOM

| AGE | EAR MJ/D (KCAL/D) Males | Females |
|---|---|---|
| 0–3 months | 2.28 ( 545) | 2.16 ( 515) |
| 4–6 months | 2.89 ( 690) | 2.69 ( 645) |
| 7–9 months | 3.44 ( 825) | 3.20 ( 765) |
| 10–12 months | 3.85 ( 920) | 3.61 ( 865) |
| 1–3 years | 5.15 (1,230) | 4.86 (1,165) |
| 4–6 years | 7.16 (1,715) | 6.46 (1,545) |
| 7–10 years | 8.24 (1,970) | 7.28 (1,740) |
| 11–14 years | 9.27 (2,220) | 7.92 (1,845) |
| 15–18 years | 11.51 (2,755) | 8.83 (2,110) |
| 19–50 years | 10.60 (2,550) | 8.10 (1,940) |
| 51–59 years | 10.60 (2,550) | 8.00 (1,900) |
| 60–64 years | 9.93 (2,380) | 7.99 (1,900) |
| 65–74 years | 9.71 (2,330) | 7.96 (1,900) |
| 75+ years | 8.77 (2,100) | 7.61 (1,810) |
| Pregnancy | | +0.80*( 200) |
| Lactation: | | |
| 1 month | | +1.90 ( 450) |
| 2 months | | +2.20 ( 530) |
| 3 months | | +2.40 ( 570) |
| 4–6 months (Group 1) | | +2.00 ( 480) |
| 4–6 months (Group 2) | | +2.40 ( 570) |
| >6 months (Group 1) | | +1.00 ( 240) |
| >6 months (Group 2) | | +2.30 ( 550) |

*last trimester only

(From Report on Health and Social Subjects: Dietary Reference Values for Food and Energy and Nutrients for the United Kingdom. London, Her Majesty's Stationery Office, 1991.)

**TABLE A–4B.** REFERENCE NUTRIENT INTAKES FOR PROTEIN, UNITED KINGDOM

| AGE | REFERENCE NUTRIENT INTAKE[a] (g/d) | |
|---|---|---|
| 0–3 months | 12.5[b] | |
| 4–6 months | 12.7 | |
| 7–9 months | 13.7 | |
| 10–12 months | 14.9 | |
| 1–3 years | 14.5 | |
| 4–6 years | 19.7 | |
| 7–10 years | 28.3 | |
| Males | | |
| 11–14 years | 42.1 | |
| 15–18 years | 55.2 | |
| 19–50 years | 55.5 | |
| 50+ years | 53.3 | |
| Females | | |
| 11–14 years | 41.2 | |
| 15–18 years | 45.0 | |
| 19–50 years | 45.0 | |
| 50+ years | 46.5 | |
| Pregnancy[c] | | + 6 |
| Lactation[c] | | |
| 0–4 months | | +11 |
| 4+ months | | + 8 |

[a]These figures, based on egg and milk protein, assume complete digestibility.

[b]No values for infants 0 to 3 months are given by WHO. The reference nutrient intake is calculated from the recommendations of Committee on Medical Aspects of Food Policy (COMA).

[c]To be added to adult requirement through all stages of pregnancy and lactation.

(From Report on Health and Social Subjects: No. 41, Dietary Reference Values for Food Energy and Nutrients for the United Kingdom, Report of the Panel on Dietary Reference Values of the Committee on Medical Aspects of Food Policy. London, Her Majesty's Stationery Office, 1991.)

**TABLE A–4C.** REFERENCE NUTRIENT INTAKES FOR VITAMINS, UNITED KINGDOM

| AGE | THIAMIN (mg/d) | RIBOFLAVIN (mg/d) | NIACIN (NICOTINIC ACID EQUIVALENT) (mg/d) | VITAMIN $B_6$ (mg/d[a]) | VITAMIN $B_{12}$ (μg/d) | FOLATE (μg/d) | VITAMIN C (mg/d) | VITAMIN A (μg/d) | VITAMIN D (μg/d) |
|---|---|---|---|---|---|---|---|---|---|
| 0–3 months | 0.2 | 0.4 | 3 | 0.2 | 0.3 | 50 | 25 | 350 | 8.5 |
| 4–6 months | 0.2 | 0.4 | 3 | 0.2 | 0.3 | 50 | 25 | 350 | 8.5 |
| 7–9 months | 0.2 | 0.4 | 4 | 0.3 | 0.4 | 50 | 25 | 350 | 7 |
| 10–12 months | 0.3 | 0.4 | 5 | 0.4 | 0.4 | 50 | 25 | 350 | 7 |
| 1–3 years | 0.5 | 0.6 | 8 | 0.7 | 0.5 | 70 | 30 | 400 | 7 |
| 4–6 years | 0.7 | 0.8 | 11 | 0.9 | 0.8 | 100 | 30 | 500 | — |
| 7–10 years | 0.7 | 1.0 | 12 | 1.0 | 1.0 | 150 | 30 | 500 | — |
| Males | | | | | | | | | |
| 11–14 years | 0.9 | 1.2 | 15 | 1.2 | 1.2 | 200 | 35 | 600 | — |
| 15–18 years | 1.1 | 1.3 | 18 | 1.5 | 1.5 | 200 | 40 | 700 | — |
| 19–50 years | 1.0 | 1.3 | 17 | 1.4 | 1.5 | 200 | 40 | 700 | — |
| 50+ years | 0.9 | 1.3 | 16 | 1.4 | 1.5 | 200 | 40 | 700 | ** |
| Females | | | | | | | | | |
| 11–14 years | 0.7 | 1.1 | 12 | 1.0 | 1.2 | 200 | 35 | 600 | — |
| 15–18 years | 0.8 | 1.1 | 14 | 1.2 | 1.5 | 200 | 40 | 600 | — |
| 19–50 years | 0.8 | 1.1 | 13 | 1.2 | 1.5 | 200 | 40 | 600 | — |
| 50+ years | 0.8 | 1.1 | 12 | 1.2 | 1.5 | 200 | 40 | 600 | ** |
| Pregnancy | +0.1[b] | +0.3 | * | * | * | +100 | +10 | +100 | 10 |
| Lactation | | | | | | | | | |
| 0–4 months | +0.2 | +0.5 | +2 | * | +0.5 | + 60 | +30 | +350 | 10 |
| 4+ months | +0.2 | +0.5 | +2 | * | +0.5 | + 60 | +30 | +350 | 10 |

*No increment
**After age 65 the RNI is 10 μg/d for men and women
[a]Based on protein providing 14.7% of EAR for energy
[b]For last trimester only
(From Report on Health and Social Subjects: No. 41, Dietary Reference Values for Food Energy and Nutrients for the United Kingdom, Report of the Panel on Dietary Reference Values of the Committee on Medical Aspects of Food Policy. London, Her Majesty's Stationery Office, 1991.)

**TABLE A—4D.** REFERENCE NUTRIENT INTAKES FOR MINERALS, UNITED KINGDOM

| AGE | CALCIUM (mmol/d) | PHOSPHORUS[1] (mmol/d) | MAGNESIUM (mmol/d) | SODIUM (mmol/d[2]) | POTASSIUM (mmol/d[3]) | CHLORIDE[4] (mmol/d) | IRON (μmol/d) | ZINC (μmol/d) | COPPER (μmol/d) | SELENIUM (μmol/d) | IODINE (μmol/d) |
|---|---|---|---|---|---|---|---|---|---|---|---|
| 0–3 months | 13.1 | 13.1 | 2.2 | 9 | 20 | 9 | 30 | 60 | 5 | 0.1 | 0.4 |
| 4–6 months | 13.1 | 13.1 | 2.5 | 12 | 22 | 12 | 80 | 60 | 5 | 0.2 | 0.5 |
| 7–9 months | 13.1 | 13.1 | 3.2 | 14 | 18 | 14 | 140 | 75 | 5 | 0.1 | 0.5 |
| 10–12 months | 13.1 | 13.1 | 3.3 | 15 | 18 | 15 | 140 | 75 | 5 | 0.1 | 0.5 |
| 1–3 years | 8.8 | 8.8 | 3.5 | 22 | 20 | 22 | 120 | 75 | 6 | 0.2 | 0.6 |
| 4–6 years | 11.3 | 11.3 | 4.8 | 30 | 28 | 30 | 110 | 100 | 9 | 0.3 | 0.8 |
| 7–10 years | 13.8 | 13.8 | 8.0 | 50 | 50 | 50 | 160 | 110 | 11 | 0.4 | 0.9 |
| Males | | | | | | | | | | | |
| 11–14 years | 25.0 | 25.0 | 11.5 | 70 | 80 | 70 | 200 | 140 | 13 | 0.6 | 1.0 |
| 15–18 years | 25.0 | 25.0 | 12.3 | 70 | 90 | 70 | 200 | 145 | 16 | 0.9 | 1.0 |
| 19–50 years | 17.5 | 17.5 | 12.3 | 70 | 90 | 70 | 160 | 145 | 19 | 0.9 | 1.0 |
| 50+ years | 17.5 | 17.5 | 12.3 | 70 | 90 | 70 | 160 | 145 | 19 | 0.9 | 1.0 |
| Females | | | | | | | | | | | |
| 11–14 years | 20.0 | 10.0 | 11.5 | 70 | 80 | 70 | 260[5] | 140 | 13 | 0.6 | 1.0 |
| 15–18 years | 20.0 | 20.0 | 12.3 | 70 | 90 | 70 | 260[5] | 110 | 16 | 0.8 | 1.1 |
| 19–50 years | 17.5 | 17.5 | 10.9 | 70 | 90 | 70 | 260[5] | 110 | 19 | 0.8 | 1.1 |
| 50+ years | 17.5 | 17.5 | 10.9 | 70 | 90 | 70 | 160 | 110 | 19 | 0.8 | 1.1 |
| Pregnancy | * | * | * | * | * | * | * | * | * | * | * |
| Lactation | | | | | | | | | | | |
| 0–4 months | +14.3 | +14.3 | +2.1 | * | * | * | * | +90 | +5 | +0.2 | * |
| 4+ months | +14.3 | +14.3 | +2.1 | * | * | * | * | +40 | +5 | +0.2 | * |
| 0–3 months | 525 | 400 | 55 | 210 | 800 | 320 | 1.7 | 4.0 | 0.2 | 10 | 50 |
| 4–6 months | 525 | 400 | 60 | 280 | 850 | 400 | 4.3 | 4.0 | 0.3 | 13 | 60 |
| 7–9 months | 525 | 400 | 75 | 320 | 700 | 500 | 7.8 | 5.0 | 0.3 | 10 | 60 |
| 10–12 months | 525 | 400 | 80 | 350 | 700 | 500 | 7.8 | 5.0 | 0.3 | 10 | 60 |
| 1–3 years | 350 | 270 | 85 | 500 | 800 | 800 | 6.9 | 5.0 | 0.4 | 15 | 70 |
| 4–6 years | 450 | 350 | 120 | 700 | 1,100 | 1,100 | 6.1 | 6.5 | 0.6 | 20 | 100 |
| 7–10 years | 550 | 450 | 200 | 1,200 | 2,000 | 1,800 | 8.7 | 7.0 | 0.7 | 30 | 110 |
| Males | | | | | | | | | | | |
| 11–14 years | 1,000 | 775 | 280 | 1,600 | 3,100 | 2,500 | 11.3 | 9.0 | 0.8 | 45 | 130 |
| 15–18 years | 1,000 | 775 | 300 | 1,600 | 3,500 | 2,500 | 11.3 | 9.5 | 1.0 | 70 | 140 |
| 19–50 years | 700 | 550 | 300 | 1,600 | 3,500 | 2,500 | 8.7 | 9.5 | 1.2 | 75 | 140 |
| 50+ years | 700 | 550 | 300 | 1,600 | 3,500 | 2,500 | 8.7 | 9.5 | 1.2 | 75 | 140 |
| Females | | | | | | | | | | | |
| 11–14 years | 800 | 625 | 280 | 1,600 | 3,100 | 2,500 | 14.8[5] | 9.0 | 0.8 | 45 | 130 |
| 15–18 years | 800 | 625 | 300 | 1,600 | 3,500 | 2,500 | 14.8[5] | 7.0 | 1.0 | 60 | 140 |
| 19–50 years | 700 | 550 | 270 | 1,600 | 3,500 | 2,500 | 14.8[5] | 7.0 | 1.2 | 60 | 140 |
| 50+ years | 700 | 550 | 270 | 1,600 | 3,500 | 2,500 | 8.7 | 7.0 | 1.2 | 60 | 140 |
| Pregnancy | * | * | * | * | * | * | * | * | * | * | * |
| Lactation | | | | | | | | | | | |
| 0–4 months | +550 | +440 | + 50 | * | * | * | * | +6.0 | +0.3 | +15 | * |
| 4+ months | +550 | +440 | + 50 | * | * | * | * | +2.5 | +0.3 | +15 | * |

*No increment
[1]Phosphorus RNI is set equal to calcium in molar terms
[2]1 mmol sodium = 23 mg
[3]1 mmol potassium = 39 mg
[4]Corresponds to sodium 1 mmol = 35.5 mg
[5]Insufficient for women with high menstrual losses where the most practical way of meeting iron requirements is to take iron supplements

(From Report on Health and Social Subjects: No. 41, Dietary Reference Values for Food Energy and Nutrients for the United Kingdom, Report of the Panel on Dietary Reference Values of the Committee on Medical Aspects of Food Policy. London, Her Majesty's Stationery Office, 1991.)

**TABLE A—4E.** SAFE INTAKES, UNITED KINGDOM

| NUTRIENT | SAFE INTAKE |
|---|---|
| *Vitamins* | |
| Pantothenic acid | |
| adults | 3–7 mg/d |
| infants | 1.7 mg/d |
| Biotin | 10–200 μg/d |
| Vitamin E | |
| men | above 4 mg/d |
| women | above 3 mg/d |
| infants | 0.4 mg/g polyunsaturated fatty acids |
| Vitamin K | |
| adults | 1 μg/kg/d |
| infants | 10 μg/d |
| *Minerals* | |
| Manganese | |
| adults | 1.4 mg (26 μmol)/d |
| infants and children | 16 μg (0.3 μmol)/d |
| Molybdenum | |
| adults | 50–400 μg/d |
| infants, children, and adolescents | 0.5–1.5 μg/kg/d |
| Chromium | |
| adults | 25 μg (0.5 μmol)/d |
| children and adolescents | 0.1–1.0 μg (2–20 μmol)/kg/d |
| Fluoride (for infants only) | 0.05 mg (3 μmol)/kg/d |

For some nutrients, which are known to have important functions in humans, the Panel found insufficient reliable data on human requirements and were unable to set any dietary reference values for these. However, they decided on grounds of prudence to set a safe intake, particularly for infants and children. The safe intake was judged to be a level or range of intake at which there is no risk of deficiency and below a level where there is risk of undesirable effects. They are not therefore intended as a "toxic level," and although exceeding these safe intakes would not necessaily result in undesirable effects, equally there is no evidence for any benefits. The Panel agreed that the safe range of intakes set for the nutrients need not be exceeded.

(From Report on Health and Social Subjects: No. 41, Dietary Reference Values for Food Energy and Nutrients for the United Kingdom, Report of the Panel on Dietary Reference Values of the Committee on Medical Aspects of Food Policy. London, Her Majesty's Stationery Office, 1991.)

**TABLE A–5A.** RECOMMENDED DIETARY ALLOWANCES FOR PERSONS WITH LOW ACTIVITY, JAPAN

| AGE | ENERGY (kcal) M | ENERGY (kcal) F | PROTEIN (g) M | PROTEIN (g) F | FAT (%) | CALCIUM (g) M | CALCIUM (g) F | IRON (mg) M | IRON (mg) F | VITAMIN A (IU) M | VITAMIN A (IU) F | VITAMIN $B_1$ (mg) M | VITAMIN $B_1$ (mg) F | VITAMIN $B_2$ (mg) M | VITAMIN $B_2$ (mg) F | NIACIN (mg) M | NIACIN (mg) F | ASCORBIC ACID (mg) | VITAMIN D (IU) |
|---|---|---|---|---|---|---|---|---|---|---|---|---|---|---|---|---|---|---|---|
| 15~ | 2,350 | 2,000 | 85 | 70 | | 0.8 | | | | | | 0.9 | 0.8 | 1.3 | 1.1 | 16 | 13 | | |
| 16~ | 2,400 | 1,950 | 80 | 70 | | | | | | | | 1.0 | 0.8 | 1.3 | 1.1 | 16 | 13 | | |
| 17~ | 2,400 | 1,900 | 80 | 70 | 25~30 | | | 12 | 12 | | | 1.0 | 0.8 | 1.3 | 1.0 | 16 | 13 | | |
| 18~ | 2,350 | 1,850 | 75 | 65 | | 0.7 | | | | | | 0.9 | 0.7 | 1.3 | 1.0 | 16 | 12 | | |
| 19~ | 2,300 | 1,850 | 75 | 60 | | | | | | | | 0.9 | 0.7 | 1.3 | 1.0 | 15 | 12 | | |
| 20~29 | 2,250 | 1,800 | 70 | 60 | | | | | | | | 0.9 | 0.7 | 1.2 | 1.0 | 15 | 12 | | |
| 30~39 | 2,200 | 1,750 | 70 | 60 | | | | | | | | 0.9 | 0.7 | 1.2 | 1.0 | 15 | 12 | | |
| 40~49 | 2,150 | 1,700 | 70 | 60 | | | 0.6 | | 12 | 2,000 | 1,800 | 0.9 | 0.7 | 1.2 | 0.9 | 14 | 11 | 50 | 100 |
| 50~59 | 2,000 | 1,650 | 70 | 60 | | | | | | | | 0.8 | 0.7 | 1.1 | 0.9 | 13 | 11 | | |
| 60~64 | 1,850 | 1,550 | 70 | 60 | 20~25 | 0.6 | | 10 | | | | 0.7 | 0.6 | 1.0 | 0.9 | 12 | 10 | | |
| 65~69 | 1,800 | 1,500 | 70 | 60 | | | | | | | | 0.7 | 0.6 | 1.0 | 0.9 | 12 | 10 | | |
| 70~74 | 1,650 | 1,450 | 65 | 55 | | | | | 10† | | | 0.7 | 0.6 | 1.0 | 0.9 | 12 | 10 | | |
| 75~79 | 1,600 | 1,400 | 65 | 55 | | | | | | | | 0.7 | 0.6 | 1.0 | 0.9 | 12 | 10 | | |
| 80~ | 1,500 | 1,250 | 65 | 55 | | | | | | | | 0.7 | 0.6 | 1.0 | 0.9 | 12 | 10 | | |
| 1st Half Pregnancy* | | +150 | | +10 | | | +0.4 | | +3 | | +0 | | +0.1 | | +0.1 | | +1 | +10 | +300 |
| Last Half Pregnancy | | +350 | | +20 | 25~30 | | +0.4 | | +8 | | +200 | | +0.2 | | +0.2 | | +2 | +10 | +300 |
| Lactation | | +700 | | +20 | | | +0.5 | | +8 | | +1,400 | | +0.3 | | +0.4 | | +5 | +40 | +300 |

*Pregnancy increases are shown for convenience; however, values apply to each activity level.

†Decrease to 10 mg after menopause.

(From the Health Promotion and Nutrition Division, Health Policy Bureau, Ministry of Health and Welfare, Tokyo, Japan, 1991.)

**TABLE A–5B.** RECOMMENDED DIETARY ALLOWANCES FOR PERSONS WITH MEDIUM ACTIVITY OR GROWTH STAGES, JAPAN

| AGE | AVERAGE HEIGHT (CM) M | AVERAGE HEIGHT (CM) F | AVERAGE WEIGHT (kg) M | AVERAGE WEIGHT (kg) F | ENERGY (kcal) M | ENERGY (kcal) F | PROTEIN (g) M | PROTEIN (g) F | FAT (%) | CALCIUM (g) M | CALCIUM (g) F | IRON (mg) M | IRON (mg) F | VITAMIN A (IU) M | VITAMIN A (IU) F | VITAMIN $B_1$ (mg) M | VITAMIN $B_1$ (mg) F | VITAMIN $B_2$ (mg) M | VITAMIN $B_2$ (mg) F | NIACIN (mg) M | NIACIN (mg) F | ASCORBIC ACID (mg) | VITAMIN D (IU) |
|---|---|---|---|---|---|---|---|---|---|---|---|---|---|---|---|---|---|---|---|---|---|---|---|
| 0~mo | | | | | 120/kg | | 3.3/kg | | 45 | 0.4 | | 6 | | 1,300 | | 0.2 | | 0.3 | | 4 | | | |
| 2~mo | | | | | 110/kg | | 2.5/kg | | 45 | 0.4 | | 6 | | 1,300 | | 0.3 | | 0.4 | | 6 | | | |
| 6~mo | | | | | 100/kg | | 3.0/kg | | 30~40 | 0.4 | | 6 | | 1,000 | | 0.4 | | 0.5 | | 6 | | | |
| 1~yr | 80.7 | 79.6 | 10.95 | 10.35 | 960 | 910 | 30 | 30 | | | | | | | | 0.4 | 0.4 | 0.5 | 0.5 | 6 | 6 | | 400 |
| 2~ | 90.0 | 89.1 | 13.24 | 12.74 | 1,200 | 1,150 | 35 | 35 | | | | 7 | 7 | | | 0.5 | | 0.7 | 0.6 | 8 | 8 | | |
| 3~ | 97.3 | 96.6 | 15.04 | 14.70 | 1,400 | 1,350 | 40 | 40 | | | | | | 1,000 | 1,000 | | 0.5 | 0.8 | 0.7 | 9 | 9 | | |
| 4~ | 104.3 | 103.7 | 16.97 | 16.69 | 1,550 | 1,450 | 45 | 45 | | 0.4 | 0.4 | 8 | 8 | | | 0.6 | | | | 10 | | | |
| 5~ | 110.8 | 110.3 | 19.04 | 18.78 | 1,600 | 1,500 | 50 | 50 | | | | | | | | | 0.6 | 0.9 | 0.8 | | 10 | 40 | |
| 6~ | 117.0 | 116.5 | 21.35 | 21.04 | 1,700 | 1,600 | 55 | 50 | | | | | | | | 0.7 | | | | 11 | | | |
| 7~ | 122.7 | 122.2 | 23.85 | 23.44 | 1,800 | 1,650 | 60 | 55 | | | | 9 | 9 | 1,200 | 1,200 | | | | 0.9 | 12 | 11 | | |
| 8~ | 128.3 | 127.9 | 26.70 | 26.24 | 1,900 | 1,750 | 65 | 60 | | 0.5 | 0.5 | | | | | | 0.7 | 1.0 | | | | | |
| 9~ | 133.5 | 133.6 | 29.76 | 29.50 | 1,950 | 1,850 | 65 | 65 | | | 0.6 | | | | | 0.8 | | | 1.0 | 13 | 12 | | |
| 10~ | 138.8 | 139.8 | 33.21 | 33.54 | 2,050 | 1,950 | 70 | 70 | | 0.6 | | 10 | 10 | | | | | 1.1 | 1.1 | | 13 | | |
| 11~ | 144.6 | 146.5 | 37.26 | 38.46 | 2,150 | 2,100 | 75 | 75 | 25~30 | 0.7 | | | | 1,500 | 1,500 | | 0.8 | 1.2 | | 14 | 14 | | |
| 12~ | 151.4 | 151.9 | 42.29 | 43.31 | 2,350 | 2,250 | 80 | 80 | | 0.8 | 0.7 | | | | | 0.9 | | | 1.2 | 15 | | | |
| 13~ | 159.0 | 155.4 | 48.34 | 47.43 | 2,500 | 2,300 | 85 | 80 | | | | | | | | | | 1.3 | | 16 | | | |
| 14~ | 164.9 | 157.1 | 53.87 | 50.32 | 2,600 | 2,300 | 85 | 75 | | 0.9 | | | | | | 1.0 | | 1.4 | 1.3 | | | | |
| 15~ | 168.5 | 157.6 | 57.98 | 51.99 | 2,700 | 2,250 | 85 | 70 | | | | | | | | | 0.9 | | | 17 | 15 | | |
| 16~ | 169.9 | 158.0 | 60.21 | 52.87 | 2,700 | 2,200 | 80 | 70 | | 0.8 | | 12 | 12 | | | 1.1 | | 1.5 | 1.2 | | | | |
| 17~ | 170.8 | 158.1 | 61.55 | 52.92 | 2,700 | 2,150 | 80 | 70 | | | | | | | | | | | | 18 | | | 100 |
| 18~ | 171.3 | 158.1 | 62.18 | 52.52 | 2,650 | 2,100 | 75 | 65 | | 0.7 | | | | | | | | | | | | | |
| 19~ | 171.5 | 158.1 | 62.41 | 52.02 | 2,600 | 2,050 | 75 | 60 | | | | | | | | | | | | | 14 | | |
| 20~29 | 171.1 | 157.7 | 64.00 | 51.83 | 2,550 | 2,000 | 70 | 60 | | | | | | | | 1.0 | 0.8 | 1.4 | 1.1 | 17 | | 50 | |
| 30~39 | 169.8 | 156.7 | 65.48 | 54.09 | 2,500 | 2,000 | 70 | 60 | | | 0.6 | | | 2,000 | 1,800 | | | | | | | | |
| 40~49 | 167.8 | 154.6 | 65.10 | 55.14 | 2,400 | 1,950 | 70 | 60 | | | | | 12 | | | | | | | 16 | 13 | | |
| 50~59 | 164.2 | 151.9 | 61.93 | 54.13 | 2,250 | 1,850 | 70 | 60 | | | | | * | | | 0.9 | | 1.3 | | 15 | | | |
| 60~64 | 162.1 | 149.8 | 59.41 | 52.49 | 2,100 | 1,750 | 70 | 60 | 20~25 | 0.6 | | 10 | | | | | | | | | | | |
| 65~69 | 160.8 | 148.3 | 57.61 | 51.02 | 2,000 | 1,700 | 70 | 60 | | | | | | | | | | | 1.0 | | | | |
| 70~74 | 159.7 | 145.7 | 55.83 | 49.26 | 1,850 | 1,600 | 65 | 55 | | | | | 10 | | | 0.8 | 0.7 | 1.2 | | 14 | 12 | | |
| 75~79 | 158.7 | 145.0 | 54.07 | 47.22 | 1,750 | 1,550 | 65 | 55 | | | | | | | | | | | | | | | |
| 80~ | 157.6 | 142.4 | 52.38 | 44.53 | 1,650 | 1,400 | 65 | 55 | | | | | | | | | | | | | | | |

*Decrease to 10 mg after menopause.

(From the Health Promotion and Nutrition Division, Health Policy Bureau, Ministry of Health and Welfare, Tokyo, Japan, 1991.)

**TABLE A–5C.** RECOMMENDED DIETARY ALLOWANCES FOR PERSONS WITH MEDIUM-HIGH ACTIVITY, JAPAN

| AGE | ENERGY (kcal) M | ENERGY (kcal) F | PROTEIN (g) M | PROTEIN (g) F | FAT (%) | CALCIUM (g) M | CALCIUM (g) F | IRON (mg) M | IRON (mg) F | VITAMIN A (IU) M | VITAMIN A (IU) F | VITAMIN $B_1$ (mg) M | VITAMIN $B_1$ (mg) F | VITAMIN $B_2$ (mg) M | VITAMIN $B_2$ (mg) F | NIACIN (mg) M | NIACIN (mg) F | ASCORBIC ACID (mg) | VITAMIN D (IU) |
|---|---|---|---|---|---|---|---|---|---|---|---|---|---|---|---|---|---|---|---|
| 15~ | 3,200 | 2,650 | 100 | 85 | | 0.8 | | | | | | 1.3 | 1.1 | 1.8 | 1.5 | 21 | 17 | | |
| 16~ | 3,200 | 2,600 | 95 | 80 | | | | | | | | 1.3 | 1.0 | 1.8 | 1.4 | 21 | 17 | | |
| 17~ | 3,200 | 2,550 | 95 | 80 | | | | 12 | 12 | | | 1.3 | 1.0 | 1.8 | 1.4 | 21 | 17 | | |
| 18~ | 3,150 | 2,500 | 90 | 75 | | 0.7 | | | | | | 1.3 | 1.0 | 1.7 | 1.4 | 21 | 17 | | |
| 19~ | 3,100 | 2,450 | 90 | 70 | | | | | | | | 1.2 | 1.0 | 1.7 | 1.3 | 20 | 16 | | |
| 20~29 | 3,050 | 2,400 | 85 | 70 | 25~30 | | 0.6 | | | 2,000 | 1,800 | 1.2 | 1.0 | 1.7 | 1.3 | 20 | 16 | 50 | 100 |
| 30~39 | 2,950 | 2,350 | 85 | 70 | | | | | 12 | | | 1.2 | 0.9 | 1.6 | 1.3 | 19 | 16 | | |
| 40~49 | 2,850 | 2,300 | 85 | 70 | | | | | | | | 1.1 | 0.9 | 1.6 | 1.3 | 19 | 15 | | |
| 50~59 | 2,700 | 2,200 | 85 | 70 | | 0.6 | | 10 | * | | | 1.1 | 0.9 | 1.5 | 1.2 | 18 | 15 | | |
| 60~64 | 2,450 | 2,050 | 80 | 70 | | | | | | | | 1.0 | 0.8 | 1.3 | 1.1 | 16 | 14 | | |
| 65~69 | 2,350 | 2,000 | 80 | 70 | | | | | 10 | | | 1.0 | 0.8 | 1.3 | 1.1 | 16 | 14 | | |

*Decrease to 10 mg after menopause.
(From the Health Promotion and Nutrition Division, Health Policy Bureau, Ministry of Health and Welfare, Tokyo, Japan, 1991.)

**TABLE A–5D.** RECOMMENDED DIETARY ALLOWANCES FOR PERSONS WITH HIGH ACTIVITY, JAPAN

| AGE | ENERGY (kcal) M | ENERGY (kcal) F | PROTEIN (g) M | PROTEIN (g) F | FAT (%) | CALCIUM (g) M | CALCIUM (g) F | IRON (mg) M | IRON (mg) F | VITAMIN A (IU) M | VITAMIN A (IU) F | VITAMIN $B_1$ (mg) M | VITAMIN $B_1$ (mg) F | VITAMIN $B_2$ (mg) M | VITAMIN $B_2$ (mg) F | NIACIN (mg) M | NIACIN (mg) F | ASCORBIC ACID (mg) | VITAMIN D (IU) |
|---|---|---|---|---|---|---|---|---|---|---|---|---|---|---|---|---|---|---|---|
| 15~ | 3,750 | 3,100 | 115 | 95 | | 0.8 | | | | | | 1.5 | 1.2 | 2.1 | 1.7 | 25 | 20 | | |
| 16~ | 3,750 | 3,050 | 110 | 95 | | | | | | | | 1.5 | 1.2 | 2.1 | 1.7 | 25 | 20 | | |
| 17~ | 3,750 | 2,950 | 110 | 95 | | | | 12 | 12 | | | 1.5 | 1.2 | 2.1 | 1.6 | 25 | 19 | | |
| 18~ | 3,700 | 2,900 | 105 | 90 | | 0.7 | | | | | | 1.5 | 1.2 | 2.0 | 1.6 | 24 | 19 | | |
| 19~ | 3,700 | 2,850 | 105 | 85 | | | | | | | | 1.5 | 1.1 | 2.0 | 1.6 | 24 | 19 | | |
| 20~29 | 3,550 | 2,800 | 100 | 85 | 25~30 | | 0.6 | | | 2,000 | 1,800 | 1.4 | 1.1 | 2.0 | 1.5 | 23 | 18 | 50 | 100 |
| 30~39 | 3,450 | 2,750 | 100 | 85 | | | | | 12 | | | 1.4 | 1.1 | 1.9 | 1.5 | 23 | 18 | | |
| 40~49 | 3,350 | 2,700 | 100 | 85 | | 0.6 | | 10 | * | | | 1.3 | 1.1 | 1.8 | 1.5 | 22 | 18 | | |
| 50~59 | 3,150 | 2,600 | 100 | 85 | | | | | | | | 1.3 | 1.0 | 1.7 | 1.4 | 21 | 17 | | |
| 60~64 | 2,850 | 2,400 | 95 | 80 | | | | | | | | 1.1 | 1.0 | 1.6 | 1.3 | 19 | 16 | | |
| 65~69 | 2,750 | 2,300 | 95 | 80 | | | | | 10 | | | 1.1 | 1.0 | 1.6 | 1.3 | 19 | 16 | | |

*Decrease to 10 mg after menopause.
(From the Health Promotion and Nutrition Division, Health Policy Bureau, Ministry of Health and Welfare, Tokyo, Japan, 1991.)

Comments

1. These general guidelines are not for individual daily values. For individual nutrient requirements, other tables must be used.
2. An individual should take no more than 10 mg sodium daily.
3. Vitamin E: Males should have at least 8 mg, females should have at least 7 mg.
4. For those in the low activity category, more exercise is recommended. The values in Table A–5c represent the ideal intake for adults. These values are reflective of individuals who exercise accordingly.

**TABLE A–6.** RECOMMENDED DAILY DIETARY ALLOWANCES, KOREA*

| CATEGORY | AGE (years) | WEIGHT (kg) | HEIGHT (cm) | ENERGY (kcal) | PROTEIN (g) | VITAMIN A (re)† | Vitamin $B_1$ (mg) | VITAMIN $B_2$ (mg) | NIACIN (mg) | VITAMIN C (mg) | VITAMIN D (μg)‡ | CALCIUM (mg) | IRON (mg)§ |
|---|---|---|---|---|---|---|---|---|---|---|---|---|---|
| Infants | | | | | | | | | | | | | |
| | 0–3 mo | 5.5 | 58.5 | 800 | 25 | 350 | 0.40 | 0.48 | 6.4 | 35 | 10 | 400 | 10 |
| | 4–6 mo | 8.4 | 67.5 | 900 | 25 | 350 | 0.45 | 0.54 | 7.2 | 35 | 10 | 400 | 10 |
| | 7–9 mo | 9.5 | 76.0 | 1,000 | 30 | 350 | 0.50 | 0.60 | 8.0 | 35 | 10 | 400 | 15 |
| | 10–12 mo | 10.4 | 79.0 | 1,100 | 30 | 350 | 0.55 | 0.66 | 8.0 | 35 | 10 | 400 | 15 |
| Children | | | | | | | | | | | | | |
| | 1–3 | 12.6 | 87.0 | 1,200 | 35 | 350 | 0.60 | 0.72 | 8.0 | 40 | 10 | 500 | 15 |
| | 4–6 | 19.0 | 110.0 | 1,300 | 40 | 400 | 0.75 | 0.90 | 10.0 | 40 | 10 | 600 | 10 |
| | 7–9 | 26.0 | 130.0 | 1,800 | 50 | 500 | 0.90 | 1.08 | 12.0 | 40 | 10 | 700 | 10 |
| Males | | | | | | | | | | | | | |
| | 10–12 | 36.0 | 144.0 | 2,100 | 60 | 600 | 1.05 | 1.26 | 14.0 | 50 | 10 | 800 | 15 |
| | 13–15 | 51.0 | 161.0 | 2,600 | 80 | 700 | 1.30 | 1.36 | 17.0 | 50 | 10 | 800 | 18 |
| | 16–19 | 59.0 | 169.0 | 2,500 | 75 | 700 | 1.25 | 1.50 | 16.5 | 55 | 10 | 800 | 18 |
| | 20–29 | 64.0 | 170.5 | 2,500 | 70 | 700 | 1.25 | 1.50 | 16.5 | 55 | 5 | 600 | 10 |
| | 30–49 | 65.0 | 168.5 | 2,500 | 70 | 700 | 1.25 | 1.50 | 16.5 | 55 | 5 | 600 | 10 |
| | 50–64 | 63.0 | 168.0 | 2,200 | 70 | 700 | 1.10 | 1.32 | 14.5 | 55 | 5 | 600 | 10 |
| | 65 or older | 61.0 | 167.0 | 1,900 | 70 | 700 | 1.00 | 1.20 | 13.0 | 55 | 5 | 600 | 10 |
| Females | | | | | | | | | | | | | |
| | 10–12 | 37.0 | 145.0 | 2,000 | 60 | 600 | 1.00 | 1.20 | 13.0 | 50 | 10 | 800 | 18 |
| | 13–15 | 48.0 | 155.0 | 2,300 | 65 | 700 | 1.15 | 1.38 | 15.0 | 50 | 10 | 800 | 18 |
| | 16–19 | 52.0 | 158.0 | 2,200 | 60 | 700 | 1.10 | 1.32 | 14.5 | 55 | 10 | 700 | 18 |
| | 20–29 | 52.5 | 159.5 | 2,000 | 60 | 700 | 1.00 | 1.20 | 13.0 | 55 | 5 | 600 | 18 |
| | 30–49 | 55.0 | 158.0 | 2,000 | 60 | 700 | 1.00 | 1.20 | 13.0 | 55 | 5 | 600 | 18 |
| | 50–64 | 54.0 | 156.0 | 1,900 | 60 | 700 | 1.00 | 1.20 | 13.0 | 55 | 5 | 600 | 10 |
| | 65 or older | 53.0 | 156.0 | 1,600 | 60 | 700 | 1.00 | 1.20 | 13.0 | 55 | 5 | 600 | 10 |
| Pregnancy | | | | | | | | | | | | | |
| | | First half | | +150 | +30 | + 0 | +0.40 | +0.30 | +2.0 | +15 | +5 | +400 | +2 |
| | | Second half | | +350 | +30 | +100 | +0.40 | +0.30 | +2.0 | +15 | +5 | +400 | +2 |
| Lactation | | | | | | | | | | | | | |
| | | | | +700 | +30 | +300 | +0.60 | +0.50 | +6.0 | +35 | +5 | +500 | +2 |

*The allowances for energy are based on individuals of moderate activity. Data in this table are intended to provide only a standard figure under usual environment and given conditions.

†Retinol equivalent: 1 RE = 1 μg retinol = 6 μg β-carotene

‡Vitamin D : 10 μg = 400 IU.

§Supplemental iron should be taken to meet the increased requirement during pregnancy and lactation.

(From the Ministry of Health and Social Affairs, Kyonggi, Korea, 1989.)

**TABLE A–7A.** EQUATIONS FOR PREDICTING BASAL METABOLIC RATE FROM BODY WEIGHT (W)*

| AGE RANGE (years) | $KCAL_{th}$/DAY | CORRELATION COEFFICIENT | SD† | MJ/DAY | CORRELATION COEFFICIENT | SD |
|---|---|---|---|---|---|---|
| Males | | | | | | |
| 0–3 | 60.9 W − 54 | 0.97 | 53 | 0.255 W − 0.226 | 0.97 | 0.222 |
| 3–10 | 22.7 W + 495 | 0.86 | 62 | 0.0949 W + 2.07 | 0.86 | 0.259 |
| 10–18 | 17.5 W + 651 | 0.90 | 100 | 0.0732 W + 2.72 | 0.90 | 0.418 |
| 18–30 | 15.3 W + 679 | 0.65 | 151 | 0.0640 W + 2.84 | 0.65 | 0.632 |
| 30–60 | 11.6 W + 879 | 0.60 | 164 | 0.0485 W + 3.67 | 0.60 | 0.686 |
| > 60 | 13.5 W + 487 | 0.79 | 148 | 0.0565 W + 2.04 | 0.79 | 0.619 |
| Females | | | | | | |
| 0–3 | 61.0 W − 51 | 0.97 | 61 | 0.255 W − 0.214 | 0.97 | 0.255 |
| 3–10 | 22.5 W + 499 | 0.85 | 63 | 0.0941 W + 2.09 | 0.85 | 0.264 |
| 10–18 | 12.2 W + 746 | 0.75 | 117 | 0.0510 W + 3.12 | 0.75 | 0.489 |
| 18–30 | 14.7 W + 496 | 0.72 | 121 | 0.0615 W + 2.08 | 0.72 | 0.506 |
| 30–60 | 8.7 W + 829 | 0.70 | 108 | 0.0364 W + 3.47 | 0.70 | 0.452 |
| > 60 | 10.5 W + 596 | 0.74 | 108 | 0.0439 W + 2.49 | 0.74 | 0.452 |

*Since the present report was compiled, the data base for the equations contained in Schofield, W. N., et al.: Hum. Nutr. Clin. Nutr. *39(Suppl.)*, 1985 has been slightly expanded. They therefore differ from the equations shown in this table, but the differences are negligible.

†Standard deviation of differences between actual BMR and predicted estimates.

(From Energy and Protein Requirements: Report of a Joint FAO/WHO/UNU Expert Consultation. Technical Report Series No. 724. Geneva, World Health Organization, 1985, p. 71.)

**TABLE A–7B.** EXAMPLES OF PREDICTED BASAL METABOLIC RATE (BMR) IN SUBJECTS OF THE SAME HEIGHT BUT DIFFERENT WEIGHTS, PREDICTED FROM ACTUAL WEIGHT AND FROM MEDIAN ACCEPTABLE WEIGHT FOR HEIGHT

| | MAN, AGE 40, HEIGHT 1.8 M | | | WOMAN, AGE 25, HEIGHT 1.5 M | | |
|---|---|---|---|---|---|---|
| | Position in range* | | | Position in range* | | |
| | Upper | Median | Lower | Upper | Median | Lower |
| BMI† | 25 | 22 | 20 | 24 | 21 | 19 |
| Wt(kg) | 81.0 | 71.3 | 64.8 | 54.0 | 47.2 | 42.7 |
| BMR‡ from actual wt | | | | | | |
| $kcal_{th}$/day | 1,820 | 1,710 | 1,630 | 1,290 | 1,190 | 1,120 |
| MJ/day | 7.61 | 7.15 | 6.82 | 5.39 | 4.98 | 4.68 |
| BMR from median wt | | | | | | |
| $kcal_{th}$/day | 1,710 | 1,710 | 1,710 | 1,190 | 1,190 | 1,190 |
| MJ/day | 7.15 | 7.15 | 7.15 | 4.97 | 4.97 | 4.97 |

*Acceptable range of BMI (see Annex 2A in original reference).

†Body mass index = $wt(kg)/ht^2(m)$.

‡Predicted from equations in Table A–7a.

(From Energy and Protein Requirements: Report of a Joint FAO/WHO/UNU Expert Consultation. Technical Report Series No. 724, Geneva, World Health Organization, 1985, p. 72.)

**TABLE A–7C.** BASAL METABOLIC RATES OF ADOLESCENT BOYS AND GIRLS

| AGE (years) | HEIGHT* (cm) | WEIGHT† (kg) | BMR‡ Total ($kcal_{th}$/day) | BMR‡ Total (MJ/day) | BMR‡ per kg ($kcal_{th}$/day) | BMR‡ per kg (MJ/day) |
|---|---|---|---|---|---|---|
| Boys | | | | | | |
| 10–11 | 140 | 32.2 | 1215 | 5.08 | 37.7 | 0.16 |
| 11–12 | 147 | 37.0 | 1300 | 5.43 | 35.1 | 0.15 |
| 12–13 | 153 | 40.9 | 1370 | 5.73 | 33.4 | 0.14 |
| 13–14 | 160 | 47.0 | 1465 | 6.12 | 31.4 | 0.13 |
| 14–15 | 166 | 52.6 | 1570 | 6.57 | 29.9 | 0.12 |
| 15–16 | 171 | 58.0 | 1665 | 6.96 | 28.7 | 0.12 |
| 16–17 | 175 | 62.7 | 1750 | 7.32 | 27.9 | 0.12 |
| 17–18 | 177 | 65.0 | 1790 | 7.48 | 27.5 | 0.12 |
| Girls | | | | | | |
| 10–11 | 142 | 33.7 | 1160 | 4.85 | 34.3 | 0.14 |
| 11–12 | 148 | 38.7 | 1220 | 5.10 | 31.5 | 0.13 |
| 12–13 | 155 | 44.0 | 1280 | 5.38 | 29.1 | 0.12 |
| 13–14 | 159 | 48.8 | 1340 | 5.60 | 27.5 | 0.12 |
| 14–15 | 161 | 51.4 | 1375 | 5.75 | 26.7 | 0.11 |
| 15–16 | 162 | 53.0 | 1395 | 5.83 | 26.3 | 0.11 |
| 16–17 | 163 | 54.0 | 1405 | 5.87 | 26.0 | 0.11 |
| 17–18 | 164 | 54.4 | 1410 | 5.89 | 25.9 | 0.11 |

*Median height for age from NCHS standards.
†Median weight for height and age from Baldwin's standards (Annex 2(B) of original reference.
‡Boys: BMR = 17.5 W + 651 $kcal_{th}$/day (2.72 MJ/day). Girls: 12.2 W + 746 $kcal_{th}$/day (3.12 MJ/day).
(From Energy and Protein Requirements: Report of a joint FAO/WHO/UNU Expert Consultation. Technical Report Series No. 724. Geneva, World Health Organization, 1985, p. 72.)

**TABLE A–7D.** BASAL METABOLIC RATE IN ADULT MEN AND WOMEN IN RELATION TO HEIGHT AND MEDIAN ACCEPTABLE WEIGHT FOR HEIGHT* (VALUES GIVEN IN $KCAL_{TH}$ WITH MJ IN PARENTHESES)

| HEIGHT (m) | WEIGHT† (kg) | 18–30 YEARS Per kg per day | 18–30 YEARS Per day | 30–60 YEARS Per kg per day | 30–60 YEARS Per day | >60 YEARS Per kg per day | >60 YEARS Per day |
|---|---|---|---|---|---|---|---|
| Men | | | | | | | |
| 1.5 | 49.5 | 29.0 (121) | 1440 (6.03) | 29.4 (123) | 1450 (6.07) | 23.3 (98) | 1150 (4.81) |
| 1.6 | 56.5 | 27.4 (115) | 1540 (6.44) | 27.2 (114) | 1530 (6.40) | 22.2 (93) | 1250 (5.23) |
| 1.7 | 63.5 | 26.0 (109) | 1650 (6.90) | 25.4 (106) | 1620 (6.78) | 21.2 (89) | 1350 (5.65) |
| 1.8 | 71.5 | 24.8 (104) | 1770 (7.41) | 23.9 (99) | 1710 (7.15) | 20.3 (85) | 1450 (6.07) |
| 1.9 | 79.5 | 23.9 (100) | 1890 (7.91) | 22.7 (95) | 1800 (7.53) | 19.6 (82) | 1560 (6.53) |
| 2.0 | 88 | 23.0 (96) | 2030 (8.49) | 21.6 (90) | 1900 (7.95) | 19.0 (80) | 1670 (6.99) |
| Women | | | | | | | |
| 1.4 | 41 | 26.7 (112) | 1100 (4.60) | 28.8 (120) | 1190 (4.98) | 25.0 (105) | 1030 (4.31) |
| 1.5 | 47 | 25.2 (105) | 1190 (4.98) | 26.3 (110) | 1240 (5.19) | 23.1 (97) | 1090 (4.56) |
| 1.6 | 54 | 23.9 (100) | 1290 (5.40) | 24.1 (101) | 1300 (5.44) | 21.6 (90) | 1160 (4.85) |
| 1.7 | 61 | 22.9 (96) | 1390 (5.82) | 22.4 (94) | 1360 (5.69) | 20.3 (85) | 1230 (5.15) |
| 1.8 | 68 | 22.0 (92) | 1500 (6.28) | 20.9 (87) | 1420 (5.94) | 19.3 (81) | 1310 (5.48) |

*BMR from eqquations in Table A–7a rounded to 10 $kcal_{th}$.
†Weight taken as median acceptable weight for height: body mass index ($wt/ht^2$) = 22 in men, 21 in women.
(From Energy and Protein Requirements: Report of a joint FAO/WHO/UNU Expert Consultation. Technical Report Series No. 724. Geneva, World Health Organization, 1985, p. 72.)

**TABLE A–8A.** CALCULATED ENERGY REQUIREMENTS OF INFANTS FROM BIRTH TO 1 YEAR

| AGE (months) | INTAKE* (kcal$_{th}$/kg per day) | INTAKE* (kJ/kg per day) | CALCULATED ENERGY REQUIREMENT† (kcal$_{th}$/kg per day) | CALCULATED ENERGY REQUIREMENT† (kJ/kg per day) | MEDIAN BODY WEIGHT‡ Boys (kg) | MEDIAN BODY WEIGHT‡ Girls (kg) | TOTAL REQUIREMENT Boys (kcal$_{th}$/day) | TOTAL REQUIREMENT Boys (kJ/day) | TOTAL REQUIREMENT Girls (kcal$_{th}$/day) | TOTAL REQUIREMENT Girls (kJ/day) |
|---|---|---|---|---|---|---|---|---|---|---|
| 0.5 | 118 | 494 | 124 | 519 | 3.8 | 3.6 | 470 | 1,965 | 445 | 1,860 |
| 1–2 | 114 | 477 | 116 | 485 | 4.75 | 4.35 | 550 | 2,300 | 505 | 2,115 |
| 2–3 | 107 | 448 | 109 | 456 | 5.6 | 5.05 | 610 | 2,550 | 545 | 2,280 |
| 3–4 | 101 | 423 | 103 | 431 | 6.35 | 5.7 | 655 | 2,740 | 590 | 2,470 |
| 4–5 | 96 | 402 | 99 | 414 | 7.0 | 6.35 | 695 | 2,910 | 630 | 2,635 |
| 5–6 | 93 | 389 | 96.5 | 404 | 7.55 | 6.95 | 730 | 3,055 | 670 | 2,800 |
| 6–7 | 91 | 381 | 95 | 397 | 8.05 | 7.55 | 765 | 3,220 | 720 | 3,010 |
| 7–8 | 90 | 377 | 94.5 | 395 | 8.55 | 7.95 | 810 | 3,390 | 750 | 3,140 |
| 8–9 | 90 | 377 | 95 | 397 | 9.0 | 8.4 | 855 | 3,580 | 800 | 3,350 |
| 9–10 | 91 | 381 | 99 | 414 | 9.35 | 8.75 | 925 | 3,870 | 865 | 3,620 |
| 10–11 | 93 | 389 | 100 | 418 | 9.7 | 9.05 | 970 | 4,060 | 905 | 3,790 |
| 11–12 | 97 | 406 | 104.5 | 437 | 10.05 | 9.35 | 1,050 | 4,395 | 975 | 4,080 |
| 12 | 102 | 427 | | | | | | | | |

*Observed intakes at ages indicated, from data of sources given in original publication. Average intake predicted from equation (age in months): 1 (kcal$_{th}$/kg) = 123 − 8.9 age + 0.59 age. See original reference.

†Requirement over interval indicated, calculated as predicted intake + 5%. See original reference.

‡NCHS median weights at midpoint of month.

(From Energy and Protein Requirements: Report of a Joint FAO/WHO/UNU Expert Consultation. Technical Report Series No. 724. Geneva, World Health Organization, 1985, p. 91.)

**TABLE A–8B.** ESTIMATED AVERAGE DAILY ENERGY INTAKES AND REQUIREMENTS, AGES 1 TO 10 YEARS

| | BOYS | | | |
|---|---|---|---|---|
| | Intake* | | Requirement† | |
| Age (years) | (kcal$_{th}$/day) | (MJ/day) | (kcal$_{th}$/day) | (MJ/day) |
| 1–2 | 1,140 | 4.76 | 1,200 | 5.02 |
| 2–3 | 1,340 | 5.60 | 1,410 | 5.89 |
| 3–4 | 1,490 | 6.23 | 1,560 | 6.52 |
| 4–5 | 1,610 | 6.73 | 1,690 | 7.07 |
| 5–6 | 1,720 | 7.19 | 1,810 | 7.57 |
| 6–7 | 1,810 | 7.57 | 1,900 | 7.94 |
| 7–8 | 1,895 | 7.92 | 1,990 | 8.32 |
| 8–9 | 1,970 | 8.24 | 2,070 | 8.66 |
| 9–10 | 2,045 | 8.55 | 2,150 | 8.99 |

| | GIRLS | | | | REQUIREMENT BY WEIGHT‡ | | | |
|---|---|---|---|---|---|---|---|---|
| | Intake* | | Requirement† | | Boys | | Girls | |
| Age (years) | (kcal$_{th}$/day) | (MJ/day) | (kcal$_{th}$/day) | (MJ/day) | (kcal$_{th}$/kg per day) | (kJ/kg per day) | (kcal$_{th}$/kg per day) | (kJ/kg per day) |
| 1–2 | 1,090 | 4.56 | 1,140 | 4.76 | 104 | 435 | 108 | 452 |
| 2–3 | 1,250 | 5.23 | 1,310 | 5.48 | 104 | 410 | 102 | 427 |
| 3–4 | 1,370 | 5.73 | 1,440 | 6.02 | 99 | 414 | 95 | 397 |
| 4–5 | 1,465 | 6.12 | 1,540 | 6.44 | 95 | 397 | 92 | 385 |
| 5–6 | 1,550 | 6.48 | 1,630 | 6.81 | 92 | 385 | 88 | 368 |
| 6–7 | 1,620 | 6.77 | 1,700 | 7.11 | 88 | 368 | 83 | 347 |
| 7–8 | 1,685 | 7.05 | 1,770 | 7.40 | 83 | 347 | 76 | 318 |
| 8–9 | 1,740 | 7.28 | 1,830 | 7.65 | 77 | 322 | 69 | 268 |
| 9–10 | 1,795 | 7.51 | 1,880 | 7.86 | 72 | 301 | 62 | 259 |

*From data of Ferro-Luzzi and Durnin, Rome, FAO, 1981 (Document ESN: FAO/WHO/UNU/EPR/81/9).

†Intakes +5%. See original reference.

‡From NCHS median weights at midyear.

(From Energy and Protein Requirements: Report of a Joint FAO/WHO/UNU Expert consultation. Technical Report Series No. 724. Geneva, World Health Organization, 1985, pp. 94 and 95.)

**TABLE A–8C.** CALCULATED AVERAGE ENERGY EXPENDITURE AND OBSERVED INTAKES AND COMPARISON WITH RECOMMENDATIONS OF 1971 COMMITTEE FOR ADOLESCENTS AGED 10 TO 18 YEARS

| AGE (years) | EXPENDITURE (× BMR)* | EXPENDITURE (kcal$_{th}$/day) | (MJ/day) | INTAKE† (kcal$_{th}$/day) | (MJ/day) | 1971 COMMITTEE‡ RECOMMENDED REQUIREMENT (kcal$_{th}$/day) | (MJ/day) |
|---|---|---|---|---|---|---|---|
| Boys | | | | | | | |
| 10–11 | 1.76 | 2,140 | 8.95 | 2,110 | 8.82 | 2,500 | 10.46 |
| 11–12 | 1.73 | 2,240 | 9.37 | 2,170 | 9.07 | 2,600 | 10.87 |
| 12–13 | 1.69 | 2,310 | 9.66 | 2,200 | 9.20 | 2,700 | 11.29 |
| 13–14 | 1.67 | 2,440 | 10.20 | 2,280 | 9.53 | 2,800 | 11.71 |
| 14–15 | 1.65 | 2,590 | 10.83 | 2,340 | 9.79 | 2,900 | 12.13 |
| 15–16 | 1.62 | 2,700 | 11.29 | 2,390 | 9.99 | 3,000 | 12.55 |
| 16–17 | 1.60 | 2,800 | 11.71 | 2,440 | 10.20 | 3,050 | 12.76 |
| 17–18 | 1.60 | 2,870 | 12.0 | 2,490 | 10.41 | 3,100 | 12.97 |
| Girls | | | | | | | |
| 10–11 | 1.65 | 1,910 | 7.99 | 1,850 | 7.74 | 2,300 | 9.62 |
| 11–12 | 1.63 | 1,980 | 8.28 | 1,890 | 7.90 | 2,350 | 9.83 |
| 12–13 | 1.60 | 2,050 | 8.57 | 1,930 | 8.07 | 2,400 | 10.04 |
| 13–14 | 1.58 | 2,120 | 8.87 | 1,970 | 8.24 | 2,450 | 10.25 |
| 14–15 | 1.57 | 2,160 | 9.03 | 2,010 | 8.40 | 2,500 | 10.46 |
| 15–16 | 1.54 | 2,140 | 8.95 | 2,050 | 8.57 | 2,500 | 10.46 |
| 16–17 | 1.53 | 2,130 | 8.91 | 2,080 | 8.70 | 2,420 | 10.12 |
| 17–18 | 1.52 | 2,140 | 8.95 | 2,120 | 8.87 | 2,340 | 9.79 |

*Expenditure calculated as in original publication.
†Intakes from reference in original publication.
‡Reference in original 1971 publication. (cf ref. d)
(From Energy and Protein Requirements: Report of a Joint FAO/WHO/UNU Expert consultation. Technical Report Series No. 724. Geneva, World Health Organization, 1985, p. 98.)

**TABLE A–8D.** DERIVATION OF AVERAGE VALUES OF THE ENERGY COST OF THREE GRADES OF PHYSICAL ACTIVITY AT WORK FOR WOMEN AND MEN*

| | WOMEN† | | | | MEN‡ | | | |
|---|---|---|---|---|---|---|---|---|
| | Cost/min ($kcal_{th}$) | (kJ) | Average cost × BMR (gross) | (net) | Cost/min ($kcal_{th}$) | (kJ) | Average cost × BMR (gross) | (net) |
| Light work | | | | | | | | |
| 75% of time sitting or standing | 1.51 | 6.3 | | | 1.79 | 7.5 | | |
| 25% of time standing and moving | 1.70 | 7.1 | | | 2.51 | 10.5 | | |
| Average | 1.56 | 6.5 | 1.7 | 0.7 | 1.99 | 8.3 | 1.7 | 0.7 |
| Moderate work | | | | | | | | |
| 25% of time sitting or standing | 1.51 | 6.3 | | | 1.79 | 7.5 | | |
| 75% of time spent on specific occupational activity | 2.20 | 9.2 | | | 3.61 | 15.1 | | |
| Average | 2.03 | 8.5 | 2.2 | 1.2 | 3.16 | 13.2 | 2.7 | 1.7 |
| Heavy work | | | | | | | | |
| 40% of time sitting or standing | 1.51 | 6.3 | | | 1.79 | 7.5 | | |
| 60% of time spent on specific occupational activity | 3.21 | 13.4 | | | 6.22 | 26.0 | | |
| Average | 2.54 | 10.6 | 2.8 | 1.8 | 4.45 | 18.6 | 3.8 | 2.8 |

*Times and energy costs of sitting, standing, moving around, and work tasks are composite values derived from published and unpublished data (Annex 5) in original reference.

†Based on young adult females (18–30 years). Wt 55 kg, BMR 0.90 $kcal_{th}$(3.8) kJ)/min (Table A–7a.)

‡Based on young adult males (18–30 years). Wt 65 kg, BMR 1.16 $kcal_{th}$(4.9 kJ)/min (Table A–7a.)

(From Energy and Protein Requirements: Report of a Joint FAO/WHO/UNU Expert Consultation. Technical Report Series No. 724. Geneva, World Health Organization, 1985, p. 76.)

**TABLE A–8E.** AVERAGE DAILY ENERGY REQUIREMENT OF ADULTS WHOSE OCCUPATIONAL WORK IS CLASSIFIED AS LIGHT, MODERATE, OR HEAVY, EXPRESSED AS A MULTIPLE OF BASAL METABOLIC RATE

| | LIGHT | MODERATE | HEAVY |
|---|---|---|---|
| Men | 1.55 | 1.78 | 2.10 |
| Women | 1.56 | 1.64 | 1.82 |

(From Energy and Protein Requirements: Report of a Joint FAO/WHO/UNU Expert Consultation. Technical Report Series No. 724. Geneva, World Health Organization, 1985, p. 78.)

**TABLE A–8F.** NOMOGRAM FOR ESTIMATION OF CALORIC REQUIREMENTS

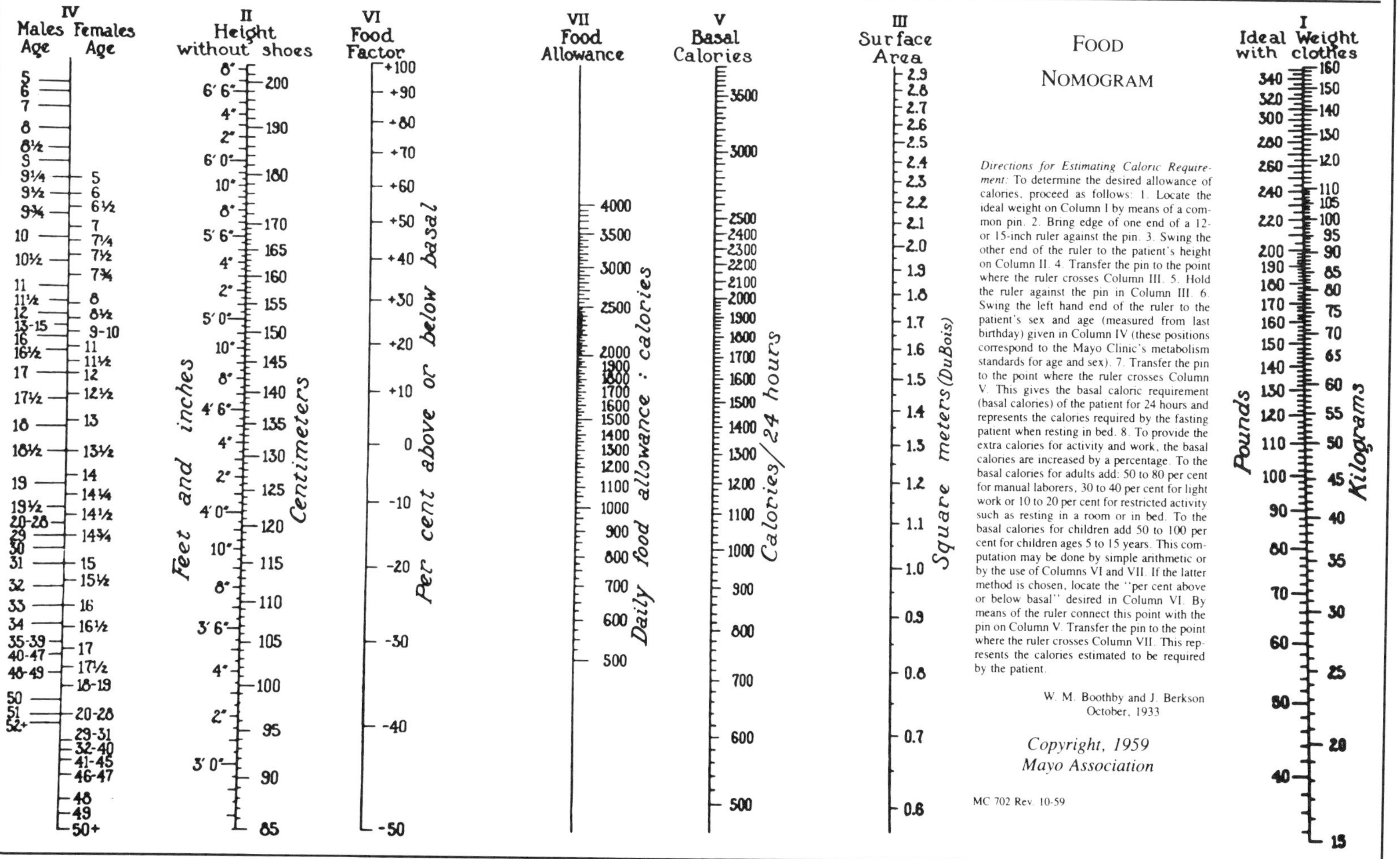
IV
Males Age / Females Age
Males: 5, 6, 7, 8, 8½, 9, 9¼, 9½, 9¾, 10, 10½, 11, 11½, 12, 13-15, 16, 16½, 17, 17½, 18, 18½, 19, 19½, 20-28, 29, 30, 31, 32, 33, 34, 35-39, 40-47, 48-49, 50, 51, 52+
Females: 5, 6, 6½, 7, 7¼, 7½, 7¾, 8, 8½, 9-10, 11, 11½, 12, 12½, 13, 13½, 14, 14¼, 14½, 14¾, 15, 15½, 16, 16½, 17, 17½, 18-19, 20-28, 29-31, 32-40, 41-45, 46-47, 48, 49, 50+
II
Height without shoes
Feet and inches
8", 6' 6", 4", 2", 6' 0", 10", 8", 5' 6", 4", 2", 5' 0", 10", 8", 4' 6", 4", 2", 4' 0", 10", 8", 3' 6", 4", 2", 3' 0"
Centimeters
200, 190, 180, 170, 165, 160, 155, 150, 145, 140, 135, 130, 125, 120, 115, 110, 105, 100, 95, 90, 85
VI
Food Factor
+100, +90, +80, +70, +60, +50, +40, +30, +20, +10, 0, -10, -20, -30, -40, -50
Per cent above or below basal
VII
Food Allowance
4000, 3500, 3000, 2500, 2000, 1900, 1800, 1700, 1600, 1500, 1400, 1300, 1200, 1100, 1000, 900, 800, 700, 600, 500
Daily food allowance : calories
V
Basal Calories
3500, 3000, 2500, 2400, 2300, 2200, 2100, 2000, 1900, 1800, 1700, 1600, 1500, 1400, 1300, 1200, 1100, 1000, 900, 800, 700, 600, 500
Calories/24 hours
III
Surface Area
2.9, 2.8, 2.7, 2.6, 2.5, 2.4, 2.3, 2.2, 2.1, 2.0, 1.9, 1.8, 1.7, 1.6, 1.5, 1.4, 1.3, 1.2, 1.1, 1.0, 0.9, 0.8, 0.7, 0.6
Square meters (DuBois)
FOOD
NOMOGRAM
Directions for Estimating Caloric Requirement: To determine the desired allowance of calories, proceed as follows: 1. Locate the ideal weight on Column I by means of a common pin. 2. Bring edge of one end of a 12- or 15-inch ruler against the pin. 3. Swing the other end of the ruler to the patient's height on Column II. 4. Transfer the pin to the point where the ruler crosses Column III. 5. Hold the ruler against the pin in Column III. 6. Swing the left hand end of the ruler to the patient's sex and age (measured from last birthday) given in Column IV (these positions correspond to the Mayo Clinic's metabolism standards for age and sex). 7. Transfer the pin to the point where the ruler crosses Column V. This gives the basal caloric requirement (basal calories) of the patient for 24 hours and represents the calories required by the fasting patient when resting in bed. 8. To provide the extra calories for activity and work, the basal calories are increased by a percentage. To the basal calories for adults add: 50 to 80 per cent for manual laborers, 30 to 40 per cent for light work or 10 to 20 per cent for restricted activity such as resting in a room or in bed. To the basal calories for children add 50 to 100 per cent for children ages 5 to 15 years. This computation may be done by simple arithmetic or by the use of Columns VI and VII. If the latter method is chosen, locate the "per cent above or below basal" desired in Column VI. By means of the ruler connect this point with the pin on Column V. Transfer the pin to the point where the ruler crosses Column VII. This represents the calories estimated to be required by the patient.
W. M. Boothby and J. Berkson
October, 1933
Copyright, 1959
Mayo Association
MC 702 Rev. 10-59
I
Ideal Weight with clothes
Pounds
340, 320, 300, 280, 260, 240, 220, 200, 190, 180, 170, 160, 150, 140, 130, 120, 110, 100, 90, 80, 70, 60, 50, 40
Kilograms
160, 150, 140, 130, 120, 110, 105, 100, 95, 90, 85, 80, 75, 70, 65, 60, 55, 50, 45, 40, 35, 30, 25, 20, 15

(From Pemberton, C.M., Gastineau, C.F.: Mayo Clinic Diet Manual. 5th Ed. Philadelphia, W.B. Saunders, 1981.)

**TABLE A–8G.** ESTIMATES OF ENERGY COST OF WEIGHT GAIN*

| SUBJECTS | | ENERGY COST ($kcal_{th}$/g) | (kJ/g) |
|---|---|---|---|
| Premature infants | | 4.9 | 20.5 |
| Premature infants | | 5.7 | 23.8 |
| Normal infants | | 5.6 | 23.4 |
| Infants recovering from malnutrition | | 5.55 | 23.2 |
| | | 4.6 | 19.2 |
| | | 3.5 | 14.6 |
| | | 4.4 | 18.4 |
| | | 7.1 | 29.7 |
| Adults, recovering from anorexia nervosa | | 6.4 | 26.7 |
| Adults, intentional overfeeding | | 8.2 | 34.3 |
| Pregnancy | Theoretic estimate† | 6.4 | 26.7 |

*See original references for data sources.

†Calculated as 80,000 $kcal_{th}$ (335 mJ) stored for 12.5 kg of weight gain.

(From Energy and Protein Requirements: Report of a Joint FAO/WHO/UNU Expert Consultation. Technical Report Series No. 724. Geneva, World Health Organization, 1985, p. 185.)

**TABLE A–9A.** VALUES FOR THE DIGESTIBILITY OF PROTEIN IN MAN*

| PROTEIN SOURCE | TRUE DIGESTIBILITY (mean ±SD) | | DIGESTIBILITY RELATIVE TO REFERENCE PROTEINS |
|---|---|---|---|
| Egg | 97 ± 3 | | |
| Milk, cheese | 95 ± 3 | 95 | 100 |
| Meat, fish | 94 ± 3 | | |
| Maize | 85 ± 6 | | 89 |
| Rice, polished | 88 ± 4 | | 93 |
| Wheat, whole | 86 ± 5 | | 90 |
| Wheat, refined | 96 ± 4 | | 101 |
| Oatmeal | 86 ± 7 | | 90 |
| Millet | 79 | | 83 |
| Peas, mature | 88 | | 93 |
| Peanut butter | 95 | | 100 |
| Soyflour | 86 ± 7 | | 90 |
| Beans | 78 | | 82 |
| Maize + beans | 78 | | 82 |
| Maize + beans + milk | 84 | | 88 |
| Indian rice diet | 77 | | 81 |
| Indian rice diet + milk | 87 | | 92 |
| Chinese mixed diet | 96 | | 98† |
| Brazilian mixed diet | 78 | | 82 |
| Filipino mixed diet | 88‡ | | 93 |
| American mixed diet | 96‡ | | 101 |
| Indian rice + bean diet | 78‡ | | 82 |

*See original reference for data sources.

†Relative to egg measured in the same study.

‡Recalculated from apparent digestibility, using $F_K$ = 12 mg N/kg (see original text).

(From Energy and Protein Requirements: Report of a Joint FAO/WHO/UNU Expert Consultation. Technical Report Series No. 724. Geneva, World Health Organization, 1985, p. 119.)

**TABLE A–9B-1.** DAILY AVERAGE (PER KG) ENERGY REQUIREMENTS AND SAFE LEVEL OF PROTEIN INTAKE FOR INFANTS AND CHILDREN AGED 3 MONTHS TO 10 YEARS (SEXES COMBINED UP TO 5 YEARS)

| AGE | MEDIAN WEIGHT (kg) | ENERGY REQUIREMENT ($kcal_{th}$/kg) | | ENERGY REQUIREMENT (kJ/kg) | | SAFE LEVEL OF PROTEIN INTAKE (g/kg)* |
|---|---|---|---|---|---|---|
| Months | | | | | | |
| 3–6 | 7.0 | 100 | | 418 | | 1.85 |
| 6–9 | 8.5 | 95 | | 397 | | 1.65 |
| 9–12 | 9.5 | 100 | | 418 | | 1.50 |
| Years | | | | | | |
| 1–2 | 11.0 | 105 | | 439 | | 1.20 |
| 2–3 | 13.5 | 100 | | 418 | | 1.15 |
| 3–5 | 16.5 | 95 | | 397 | | 1.10 |
| | | Boys | Girls | Boys | Girls | |
| 5–7 | 20.5 | 90 | 85 | 377 | 356 | 1.00 |
| 7–10 | 27.0 | 78 | 67 | 326 | 280 | 1.00 |

*Minimum level considered safe.

(From Diet, Nutrition and the Prevention of Chronic Diseases: Report of a WHO Study Group. Technical Report Series No. 797. Geneva, World Health Organization, 1990, pp. 167–168.

**TABLE A–9B-2.** DAILY AVERAGE ENERGY REQUIREMENTS AND SAFE LEVEL OF PROTEIN INTAKE FOR ADOLESCENTS AGED 10 TO 18 YEARS

| AGE (years) | MEDIAN WEIGHT (kg) | ENERGY REQUIREMENT ($kcal_{th}$) | ENERGY REQUIREMENT (kJ) | SAFE LEVEL OF PROTEIN INTAKE (g/kg)* |
|---|---|---|---|---|
| Boys | | | | |
| 10–12 | 34.5 | 2,200 | 9,200 | 1.00 |
| 12–14 | 44.0 | 2,400 | 10,000 | 1.00 |
| 14–16 | 55.5 | 2,650 | 11,100 | 0.95 |
| 16–18 | 64.0 | 2,850 | 11,900 | 0.90 |
| Girls | | | | |
| 10–12 | 36.0 | 1,950 | 8,200 | 1.00 |
| 12–14 | 46.5 | 2,100 | 8,800 | 0.95 |
| 14–16 | 52.0 | 2,150 | 9,000 | 0.90 |
| 16–18 | 54.0 | 2,150 | 9,000 | 0.80 |

*Minimum level considered safe.

(From Diet, Nutrition and the Prevention of Chronic Diseases: Report of a WHO Study Group. Technical Report Series No. 797. Geneva, World Health Organization, 1990, pp. 167–168.)

**TABLE A–9B-3.** DAILY AVERAGE ENERGY REQUIREMENTS AND SAFE LEVEL OF PROTEIN INTAKE FOR ADULTS*

| WEIGHT (kg) | ENERGY REQUIREMENT 18–30 years (kcal$_{th}$) | (kJ) | 30–60 years (kcal$_{th}$) | (kJ) | Over 60 years (kcal$_{th}$) | (kJ) | SAFE LEVEL OF PROTEIN INTAKE (g/day)† |
|---|---|---|---|---|---|---|---|
| Men | | | | | | | |
| 50 | 2,300 | 9,700 | 2,350 | 9,700 | 1,850 | 7,700 | 37.5 |
| 55 | 2,400 | 10,100 | 2,450 | 10,100 | 1,950 | 8,300 | 41.0 |
| 60 | 2,550 | 10,600 | 2,500 | 10,400 | 2,100 | 8,600 | 45.0 |
| 65 | 2,700 | 11,300 | 2,600 | 10,900 | 2,200 | 9,100 | 49.0 |
| 70 | 2,800 | 11,700 | 2,700 | 11,200 | 2,300 | 9,600 | 52.5 |
| 75 | 2,900 | 12,300 | 2,800 | 11,800 | 2,400 | 10,000 | 56.0 |
| 80 | 3,050 | 12,900 | 2,900 | 12,000 | 2,500 | 10,400 | 60.0 |
| Women | | | | | | | |
| 40 | 1,700 | 7,200 | 1,900 | 7,900 | 1,650 | 6,800 | 30.0 |
| 45 | 1,850 | 7,700 | 1,950 | 8,300 | 1,700 | 7,100 | 34.0 |
| 50 | 1,950 | 8,200 | 2,050 | 8,500 | 1,800 | 7,500 | 37.5 |
| 55 | 2,100 | 8,600 | 2,100 | 8,800 | 1,900 | 7,900 | 41.0 |
| 60 | 2,200 | 9,200 | 2,200 | 9,000 | 1,950 | 8,200 | 45.0 |
| 65 | 2,300 | 9,800 | 2,250 | 9,400 | 2,050 | 8,500 | 49.0 |
| 70 | 2,450 | 10,300 | 2,300 | 9,600 | 2,150 | 8,900 | 52.5 |
| 75 | 2,550 | 10,800 | 2,400 | 10,000 | 2,200 | 9,300 | 56.0 |

*For a basal metabolic rate factor of 1.6.

†Minimum level considered safe.

(From Diet, Nutrition and the Prevention of Chronic Diseases: Report of a WHO Study Group. Technical Report Series No. 797. Geneva, World Health Organization, 1990, pp. 167–168.)

**TABLE A–10.** RECOMMENDED DIETARY ALLOWANCES OF VITAMINS AND MINERALS

| AGE | VITAMIN A[a,b] SAFE LEVEL (μg retinol/day) | | FOLATE[a] (μg/day) | | VITAMIN $B_{12}$[a] (μg/day) | | VITAMIN C[c] (mg/day) | | VITAMIN D[c] (μg/day) | | IRON[a,d] ABSORBED (μg/kg per day) | | ZINC[e] (mg/day) | |
|---|---|---|---|---|---|---|---|---|---|---|---|---|---|---|
| | M | F | M | F | M | F | M | F | M | F | M | F | M | F |
| Infants (months) | | | | | | | | | | | | | | |
| 0–3 | 350 | | 16 | | 0.1 | | 20 | | 10 | | 120 | | 3.1 | |
| 4–6 | 350 | | 24 | | 0.1 | | 20 | | 10 | | 120 | | 3.1 | |
| 7–9 | 350 | | 32 | | 0.1 | | 20 | | 10 | | 120 | | 2.8 | |
| 10–12 | 350 | | 32 | | 0.1 | | 20 | | 10 | | 120 | | 2.8 | |
| Children and adults (years) | | | | | | | | | | | | | | |
| 1–2 | 400 | | 50 | | 1.0 | | 20 | | 10 | | 56 | | 4.0 | 3.9 |
| 3–4 | 400 | | 50 | | 1.0 | | 20 | | 10 | | 44 | | 4.0 | 3.9 |
| 5–6 | 400 | | 102 | | 1.0 | | 20 | | 10 | | 40 | | 4.0 | 3.9 |
| 7–10 | 400 | | 102 | | 1.0 | | 20 | | 2.5 | | 40 | | 4.0 | 3.9 |
| 11–12 | 500 | | 102 | | 1.0 | | 20 | | 2.5 | | 40 | | 7.0 | 6.6 |
| 13–14 | 600 | | 170 | | 1.0 | | 30 | | 2.5 | | 34 | 40 | 7.0 | 6.6 |
| 15–16 | 600 | 500 | 170 | | 1.0 | | 30 | | 2.5 | | 34 | 40 | 7.0 | 5.5 |
| 17–18 | 600 | 500 | 200 | 170 | 1.0 | | 30 | | 2.5 | | 34 | 40 | 7.0 | 5.5 |
| 19+ | 600 | 500 | 200 | 170 | 1.0 | | 30 | | 2.5 | | 18 | 43 | 5.5 | 5.5 |
| Pregnant women | | 600 | | 370 to 470 | | 1.4 | | 50 | | 10 | | [f] | | 6.4 to 7.5 |
| Lactating women | | 850 | | 270 | | 1.3 | | 50 | | 10 | | 24 | | 13.7 |
| Postmenopausal women | | 500 | | 170 | | 1.0 | | 30 | | 2.5 | | 18 | | 5.5 |

[a]Adapted from reference 1.
[b]Minimum level considered safe.
[c]Adapted from reference 2; 2.5 μg of cholecalciferol are equivalent to 100 IU of vitamin D.
[d]The amount of absorbed iron is a variable proportion of the intake, depending on the type of diet.
[e]Adapted from reference 3.
[f]Requirements during pregnancy depend on the woman's iron status before pregnancy.

## REFERENCES


1. FAO Food and Nutrition Series No. 23. Rome, Food and Agriculture Organization, 1988.
2. WHO Technical Report Series No. 452. Geneva, World Health Organization, 1970.
3. WHO Technical Report Series No. 532. Geneva, World Health Organization, 1973.


(From Diet, Nutrition and the Prevention of Chronic Diseases; Report of a WHO Study Group. Technical Report Series No. 797. Geneva, World Health Organization, 1990, p. 169.)

The Metropolitan Life Insurance Company presented their height and weight tables derived from data of the Build Study, 1979.[1] Metropolitan Life had previously utilized data from life insurance mortality studies compiled in the early 1900s and late 1950s to develop desirable weight tables in 1942,[2] 1943,[3] and 1959.[4] These studies reported the prevalence of mortality among insured persons according to variations in body build (height and weight) and also presented the average weight for height of persons by age. Such studies were designed to determine which groups (those underweight or overweight) showed a proportionately higher prevalence of mortality to yield information for underwriting purposes and for warranting changes in insurance policy premiums.

## AVERAGE WEIGHT BY HEIGHT TABLES AND AGE-GROUP

**Mortality Studies.** In the American life insurance industry, interest in build (height and weight) as factors that influence mortality dates back to 1885. In that year, the Union Mutual Life Insurance Company published a pamphlet containing the results of a study of the company's records on mortality in relation to build.[5] The first indepth study on the subject was presented in 1901 by a representative of the New York Life Insurance Company at the twelfth annual meeting of the Association of Life Insurance Medical Directors of America.[6] In this presentation it was pointed out that a certain amount of overweight had previously been looked on favorably. Nonetheless, the summary of this report noted that: "First among life insurance risks [is that] the [health] hazard increases in proportion to the degree of over- or underweight, second, whereas among overweights the mortality to be expected increases with [the] increased age of [the] applicant, among underweights the mortality decreases with advancing years."

**Height-Weight Tables.** The first height-weight table based on a considerable volume of statistics and taking age into account was the "Shepherd Table." This table was prepared in 1897 and was based on 74,162 male applicants accepted for life insurance in the United States and Canada.[7]

The basic study of height and weight based on life insurance statistics, however, was made as part of the Medico-Actuarial Mortality Investigation of 1912.[8] This study and the tables derived therefrom were the basis of the height-weight tables prepared for the general population. In addition to the study of the prevalence of mortality of certain groups of the insured population, the 1912 investigation included a study of the height and weight of a sample of persons insured from 1885 to 1900. The height and weight were recorded with the subjects wearing shoes and street clothes. A total of 221,819 men residing in the United States and Canada were included in this sample. At least 40% of the weights were estimated by the medical examiners. The data as tabulated were then smoothed to provide the figures for the height-weight age tables, and the adjusted tables became the basis for height-weight tables for males in the United States at this time.

Substantially the same procedure was employed to develop height-weight tables for women, but to secure enough cases for the preparation of tables it was necessary to add 126,504 policies issued after 1900 to the 10,000 included in the 1885 to 1900 sample.

In the Medical Impairment Study of 1929,[9] height-weight data were again collected on 667,000 men and 85,000 women. The average weights of both men and women in the 1929 study were not significantly different from those observed in the Medico-Actuarial Mortality Investigation. In fact, differences were so small that it was decided not to revise the standard height-weight tables except for those individuals younger than age 15.

## TABLES OF "IDEAL" OR "DESIRABLE" WEIGHTS

An article presented in 1920, "Is the 'Average' the Same as the 'Normal' for Weight and Blood Pressure?"[10] illustrates an important development in the preparation of height-weight tables. In this paper the "normal" weight group is defined as that having the lowest mortality rate. The article presented a table of "normal" weights, so defined, for medium-sized men averaging 68 inches in height, and several discussants added their tables of similarly defined normal weights for men of small, medium, and tall height. In 1922, complete height-weight tables were presented that showed this normal weight for each inch of height and for each age group.[11] In general, all such tables of normal weight indicated that the ideal weight in terms of mortality was the average weight for height at age 30.

## METROPOLITAN LIFE DEVELOPS "IDEAL" HEIGHT-WEIGHT TABLES

**Desirable Weight Tables, 1942 and 1943.** The concept of a "normal" weight, represented by the average weight of men at age 30, plus an awareness of the shortcomings of height and weight alone as complete indications of obesity, led to the development of "ideal" weight tables by the Metropolitan Life Insurance company.[2,3] Al-

(From Clinical Consultations in Nutrition Support, *3*:5–8, 1983. Reprinted with permission of Sidney Abraham and Clinical Consultants in Nutrition Support.)

though employed for many purposes, these tables were originally intended for use in health education. The basic data were derived from the standard height-weight tables of the Medico-Actuarial Study of 1912, using the average weight for each inch of height at age 30 for men and at age 25 for women. Arbitrary ranges were then developed, using the base figures as reference points. These ranges are approximately the standard deviation of average weights for a given height and include the lightest weight for persons with small frames to the heaviest weight for persons with large frames. The total was then arbitrarily divided into three overlapping ranges, and the resulting figures represented ideal weights for individuals of small, medium, and large frames. However, no definition of frame size was presented.

These tables were intended to aid people in achieving a weight below the average for their height. Before these tables were developed, only average weights for each inch of height by age and sex were available. The new approach represented a change in concept between average weight (assuming that the average value is optimal for health) and desirable weight (weight based on the criterion of longevity). The concept underlying these tables deemphasized the use of a single average at each height and refuted the popular notion that weight increments attendant with advancing age were normal and therefore not harmful.

**Desirable Weight Tables, 1959.** The next study of build in relation to mortality was made in conjunction with the Build and Blood Pressure Study of 1959.[4] This investigation was based on the combined experience of 26 life insurance companies in the United States and Canada from 1935 to 1954 and involved observation of nearly 5 million insured persons for periods up to 20 years. Only those insured persons ages 15 through 69 were included. The height and weight data were recorded with the subjects wearing street shoes and indoor clothing. More than 90% of the insured persons were reported to have been actually weighed and measured at the time of examination for life insurance. The study presented average weights for men and women for each inch of height, ranging from 62 to 76 inches for men and from 58 to 72 inches for women. To provide some indication of the sole effect of weight on mortality, persons with heart disease, cancer, or diabetes were excluded.

When the Build and Blood Pressure Study was completed, the "ideal weight" table, originally developed by the Metropolitan Life Insurance company in 1942 and 1943, was revised to conform to the latest data. The new table, called the "desirable weight" table (Table A–11b) was derived directly from weights associated with lowest mortality. Ranges of "desirable weight" for individuals 25 years and older with small, medium, and large frames were given, but again, no definition of frame size was included.

**1983 Metropolitan Height-Weight Tables.** Data published by the Society of Actuaries and the Association of Life Insurance Medical Directors of America in the Build Study, 1979,[1] are the source for the 1983 Metropolitan Life Insurance Height-Weight Tables (Table A–11c). The data are from 25 life insurance companies in the United States and Canada and show the prevalence of mortality from 1954 to 1972 of approximately 4.2 million insured men and women. Almost 90% of the recorded weights submitted for the study was obtained by actually weighing the applicants. As in the 1959 Build and Blood Pressure Study, applicants with major disease conditions at the time of policy issuance were excluded from the study. The terms "ideal body weight" and "desirable body weight," used in the earlier tables were not applied to the new height and weight tables because of the various misinterpretations of their meaning.

The findings from the Build Study, 1979, showed that the gap between the weights based on lowest mortality and average weights has narrowed considerably since the 1959 Build and Blood Pressure Study. Metropolitan Life considered this factor in developing the 1983 height-weight tables. Weight for height has increased in contrast to the 1959 tables, but the increased weights are still less than the average weights (see Table A–11f). Additionally, the increases in weight are not uniformly distributed throughout the 1983 height-weight tables. For each frame size, the weight increases for tall men or women were not as large as those for short men or women or for those of medium height.

In conjunction with investigations based on the life insurance data previously enumerated, long-term studies such as the Framingham Heart Study[12] and the Manitoba Study[13] all indicate that the weight associated with the greatest longevity tends to be below the average weight of the population under consideration and that "slimmer is better," provided that the underweight is not associated with a medical history of significant impairment.

## FRAME SIZE

The 1983 Metropolitan height-weight tables relate weight to body frame size. A distinction is made among persons with small, medium, and large frames. The previous Metropolitan height-weight tables also related weight to body frame size, but although the body frame sizes were statistically defined, no generally accepted method of measuring frame size was provided. Body frame size is an integral factor in considering variation in weight, assuming that persons with larger frames have larger lean body mass and therefore weigh more. In the 1983 tables, elbow breadth is now used to determine frame size in men and women (Table A–11d). The frame sizes were developed from elbow breadth measurements taken from the first National Health and Nutrition Examination Survey, 1971 to 1975,[14] and were distributed so that 50% of the population falls within the medium frame and 25% each falls within the small and large frames.

## SUMMARY

Major insurance mortality studies on insured populations in the United States and Canada conducted in 1912 by the Actuarial Society of America[8] and in 1959 and 1979 by the Society of Actuaries and the Association of Life Insurance Medical Directors of America[1,4] analyzed the mortality experience among insured persons according to variations of weight by height. The studies also presented data on the distribution of weight and height. The earliest study showed that the lowest mortality by build (weight for height) was found for those somewhat overweight at younger ages and among those underweight at older ages. In later mortality studies, it was generally found that insured persons whose weight was below the average lived longer than those whose weights were above average.

Since 1942, the Metropolitan Life Insurance Company has developed weight tables from data derived from each of the three major studies. The weights in each of the tables at given heights for men and women are classified according to frame size and refer to the weights associated with lowest mortality of policyholders. The weights were those obtained when the individual was originally insured. Because it is recognized that height and weight alone are incomplete indicators of excess weight, the weight tables also considered measurements of body build. In the tables issued in the 1940s,[2,3] 1959,[4] and 1983, three groups of frame size were identified. In each frame size, weight was given as a range rather than as a single value. However, no objective method was presented to estimate frame size in the earlier two tables. In the 1983 Metropolitan Height-Weight Tables, elbow breadth, unaffcted by degree of adiposity and closely representative of bony dimension, was suggested to estimate frame size in the three categories of body build.

The views herein are solely those of the author and do not necessarily represent those of the National Center for Health Statistics.

### REFERENCES

1. Build Study, 1979: Society of Actuaries and Association of Life Insurance Medical Directors of America. Philadelphia, Recording and Statistical Corporation, 1980.
2. Ideal Weight for Men: Stat. Bull. Metropol. Life Insur. Co., *23*:6, 1942.
3. Ideal weights for Woman: Stat. Bull. Metropol. Life Insur. Co., *24*:6, 1943.
4. New Weight Standards for Men and Women: Stat. Bull. Metropol. Life Insur. Co., *40*:1, 1959.
5. Grant, F. S.: Proc. Assoc. Life Insur. Med. Dir. Am., *2*:323–327, 1902.
6. Rogers, O. H.: Proc. Assoc. Life Insur. Med. Dir. Am., *1*:280–288, 1901.
7. Shepherd, G. R.: Proc. Assoc. Life Insur. Med. Dir. Am., *6*:46–58, 1912.
8. Medico-Actuarial Mortality Investigation. New York, Actuarial Society of America, 1912.
9. Medical Impairment Study, 1929. New York, The Association of Life Insurance Medical Directors of America and the Actuarial Society of America, 1931.
10. Hunter, A.: Trans. Actuar. Soc. Am., *21*:365–370, 1920.
11. Knight, A. S.: Proc. Assoc. Life Insur. Med. Dir. Am., *9*:193–199, 1922.
12. Hubert, H. B., Feinleib, M., McNamara, P. M., et al.: Circulation, *5*:968–977, 1983.
13. Rabkin, S. W., Mathewson, F. A. L., Hsu, P. H.: Am. J. Cardiol., *39*:452–458, 1977.
14. Public Use Data Tape, NHANES I—Anthropometry, goniometry, skeletal age, bone density, and cortical thickness, ages 1–74. Tape No. 4111, National Health and Nutrition Examination Survey, 1971–1975. Hyattsville, MD, National Center for Health Statistics.

**TABLE A–11B.** DESIRABLE WEIGHTS FOR MEN AND WOMEN AGED 25 AND OVER (IN POUNDS BY HEIGHT AND FRAME, IN INDOOR CLOTHING), 1959

MEN (IN SHOES, ONE-INCH HEELS)

| HEIGHT FEET | HEIGHT INCHES | SMALL FRAME | MEDIUM FRAME | LARGE FRAME |
|---|---|---|---|---|
| 5 | 2 | 112–120 | 118–129 | 126–141 |
| 5 | 3 | 115–123 | 121–133 | 129–144 |
| 5 | 4 | 118–126 | 124–136 | 132–148 |
| 5 | 5 | 121–129 | 127–139 | 135–152 |
| 5 | 6 | 124–133 | 130–143 | 138–156 |
| 5 | 7 | 128–137 | 134–147 | 142–161 |
| 5 | 8 | 132–141 | 138–152 | 147–166 |
| 5 | 9 | 136–145 | 142–156 | 151–170 |
| 5 | 10 | 140–150 | 146–160 | 155–174 |
| 5 | 11 | 144–154 | 150–165 | 159–179 |
| 6 | 0 | 148–158 | 154–170 | 164–184 |
| 6 | 1 | 152–162 | 158–175 | 168–189 |
| 6 | 2 | 156–167 | 162–180 | 173–194 |
| 6 | 3 | 160–171 | 167–185 | 178–199 |
| 6 | 4 | 164–175 | 172–190 | 182–204 |

WOMEN (IN SHOES, TWO-INCH HEELS)

| HEIGHT FEET | HEIGHT INCHES | SMALL FRAME | MEDIUM FRAME | LARGE FRAME |
|---|---|---|---|---|
| 4 | 10 | 92–98 | 96–107 | 104–119 |
| 4 | 11 | 94–101 | 98–110 | 106–122 |
| 5 | 0 | 96–104 | 101–113 | 109–125 |
| 5 | 1 | 99–107 | 104–116 | 112–128 |
| 5 | 2 | 102–110 | 107–119 | 115–131 |
| 5 | 3 | 105–113 | 110–122 | 118–134 |
| 5 | 4 | 108–116 | 113–126 | 121–138 |
| 5 | 5 | 111–119 | 116–130 | 125–142 |
| 5 | 6 | 114–123 | 120–135 | 129–146 |
| 5 | 7 | 118–127 | 124–139 | 133–150 |
| 5 | 8 | 122–131 | 128–143 | 137–154 |
| 5 | 9 | 126–135 | 132–147 | 141–158 |
| 5 | 10 | 130–140 | 136–151 | 145–163 |
| 5 | 11 | 134–144 | 140–155 | 149–168 |
| 6 | 0 | 138–148 | 144–159 | 153–173 |

(Data adapted from new weight standards for men and women. Stat. Bull. Metropol. Life Insur. Co., *40*:1, 1959.)

**TABLE A–11C.** HEIGHT-WEIGHT TABLES, 1983

MEN

| HEIGHT FEET | HEIGHT INCHES | SMALL FRAME | MEDIUM FRAME | LARGE FRAME |
|---|---|---|---|---|
| 5 | 2 | 128–134 | 131–141 | 138–150 |
| 5 | 3 | 130–136 | 133–143 | 140–153 |
| 5 | 4 | 132–138 | 135–145 | 142–156 |
| 5 | 5 | 134–140 | 137–148 | 144–160 |
| 5 | 6 | 136–142 | 139–151 | 146–164 |
| 5 | 7 | 138–145 | 142–154 | 149–168 |
| 5 | 8 | 140–148 | 145–157 | 152–172 |
| 5 | 9 | 142–151 | 148–160 | 155–176 |
| 5 | 10 | 144–154 | 151–163 | 158–180 |
| 5 | 11 | 146–157 | 154–166 | 161–184 |
| 6 | 0 | 149–160 | 157–170 | 164–188 |
| 6 | 1 | 152–164 | 160–174 | 168–192 |
| 6 | 2 | 155–168 | 164–178 | 172–197 |
| 6 | 3 | 158–172 | 167–182 | 176–202 |
| 6 | 4 | 162–176 | 171–187 | 181–207 |

WOMEN

| HEIGHT FEET | HEIGHT INCHES | SMALL FRAME | MEDIUM FRAME | LARGE FRAME |
|---|---|---|---|---|
| 4 | 10 | 102–111 | 109–121 | 118–131 |
| 4 | 11 | 103–113 | 111–123 | 120–134 |
| 5 | 0 | 104–115 | 113–126 | 122–137 |
| 5 | 1 | 106–118 | 115–129 | 125–140 |
| 5 | 2 | 108–121 | 118–132 | 128–143 |
| 5 | 3 | 111–124 | 121–135 | 131–147 |
| 5 | 4 | 114–127 | 124–138 | 134–151 |
| 5 | 5 | 117–130 | 127–141 | 137–155 |
| 5 | 6 | 120–133 | 130–144 | 140–159 |
| 5 | 7 | 123–136 | 133–147 | 143–163 |
| 5 | 8 | 126–139 | 136–150 | 146–167 |
| 5 | 9 | 129–142 | 139–153 | 149–170 |
| 5 | 10 | 132–145 | 142–156 | 152–173 |
| 5 | 11 | 135–148 | 145–159 | 155–176 |
| 6 | 0 | 138–151 | 148–162 | 158–179 |

Weight according to frame (ages 25 to 59) for men wearing indoor clothing weighing 5 lb, shoes with one-inch heels; for women, indoor clothing weighing 3 lb, shoes with one-inch heels.

Reprinted with permission from the Metropolitan Life Insurance Company, New York.)

| **TABLE A—11D.** HEIGHT AND ELBOW BREADTH FOR MEN AND WOMEN* | |
|---|---|
| HEIGHT IN ONE-INCH HEELS | ELBOW BREADTH |
| Men | |
| 5′2″–5′3″ | 2½″–2⅞″ |
| 5′4″–5′7″ | 2⅝″–2⅞″ |
| 5′8″–5′11″ | 2¾″–3″ |
| 6′0″–6′3″ | 2¾″–3⅛″ |
| 6′4″ | 2⅞″–3¼″ |
| Women | |
| 4′10″–4′11″ | 2¼″–2½″ |
| 5′0″–5′3″ | 2¼″–2½″ |
| 5′4″–5′7″ | 2⅜″–2⅝″ |
| 5′8″–5′11″ | 2⅜″–2⅝″ |
| 6′0″ | 2½″–2¾″ |

*See Table A–11f; see Table A–11g for data on frame size by elbow breadth from NHANES I and II.

Extend your arm and bend the forearm upward at a 90° angle. Keep fingers straight and turn the inside of your wrist toward your body. If you have a caliper, use it to measure the space between the two prominent bones on either side of your elbow. Without a caliper, place thumb and index finger of your other hand on these two bones. Measure the space between your fingers against a ruler or tape measure. Compare it with these tables that list elbow measurements for medium-frame men and women. Measurements lower than those listed indicate you have a small frame. Higher measurements indicate a larger frame.

(Reprinted with permission from Metropolitan Life Insurance Company, New York.)

**TABLE A—11E.** HEIGHT-WEIGHT TABLES (METRIC UNITS), 1983*

| | MEN | | | | WOMEN | | |
|---|---|---|---|---|---|---|---|
| HEIGHT (cm) | SMALL FRAME (kg) | MEDIUM FRAME (kg) | LARGE FRAME (kg) | HEIGHT (cm) | SMALL FRAME (kg) | MEDIUM FRAME (kg) | LARGE FRAME (kg) |
| 157.5 | 58.2–60.9 | 59.4–64.1 | 62.7–68.2 | 147.5 | 46.4–50.5 | 49.5–55.0 | 53.6–59.5 |
| 160 | 59.1–61.8 | 60.5–65.0 | 63.6–69.5 | 150 | 46.8–51.4 | 50.5–55.9 | 54.5–60.9 |
| 162.5 | 60.0–62.7 | 61.4–65.9 | 64.5–70.9 | 152.5 | 47.3–52.3 | 51.4–57.3 | 55.5–62.3 |
| 165 | 60.9–63.7 | 62.3–67.3 | 65.5–72.7 | 155 | 48.2–53.6 | 52.3–58.6 | 56.8–63.6 |
| 167.5 | 61.8–64.5 | 63.2–68.6 | 66.4–74.5 | 157.5 | 49.1–55.0 | 53.6–60.0 | 58.2–65.0 |
| 170 | 62.7–65.9 | 64.5–70.0 | 67.7–76.4 | 160 | 50.5–56.4 | 55.0–61.4 | 59.5–66.8 |
| 173 | 63.6–67.3 | 65.9–71.4 | 69.1–78.2 | 162.5 | 51.8–57.7 | 56.4–62.7 | 60.9–68.6 |
| 175 | 64.5–68.6 | 67.3–72.7 | 70.5–80.0 | 165 | 53.2–59.1 | 57.7–64.1 | 62.3–70.5 |
| 178 | 65.4–70.0 | 68.6–74.1 | 71.8–81.8 | 167.5 | 54.5–60.5 | 59.1–65.5 | 63.6–72.3 |
| 180 | 66.4–71.4 | 70.0–75.5 | 73.2–83.6 | 170 | 55.9–61.8 | 60.5–66.8 | 65.0–74.1 |
| 183 | 67.7–72.7 | 71.4–77.3 | 74.5–85.6 | 173 | 57.3–63.2 | 61.8–68.2 | 66.4–75.9 |
| 185.5 | 69.1–74.5 | 72.7–79.1 | 76.4–87.3 | 175 | 58.6–64.5 | 63.2–69.5 | 67.7–77.3 |
| 188 | 70.5–76.4 | 74.5–80.9 | 78.2–89.5 | 178 | 60.0–65.9 | 64.5–70.9 | 69.1–78.6 |
| 190.5 | 71.8–78.2 | 75.9–82.7 | 80.0–91.8 | 180 | 61.4–67.3 | 65.9–72.3 | 70.5–80.0 |
| 193 | 73.6–80.0 | 77.7–85.0 | 82.3–94.1 | 183 | 62.3–68.6 | 67.3–73.6 | 71.8–81.4 |

*The 1983 Metropolitan Height-Weight Tables are based on the 1979 Build Study.

The values are statistical computations from individuals ranging from 25 to 59 years of weights by height and body frame at which mortality has been found to be lowest or longevity the highest. Metropolitan Life does not advocate the use of the term "ideal," which has different meanings to various individuals, because the term was used originally in their 1942 to 1943 tables. If one wishes to use these tables in the sense that they are "ideal" in terms of lowest mortality, they are "appropriate" in that context. These tables do not provide weights related to minimizing illness, optimizing job performance, or creating the best appearance.

(Reprinted with permission from the Metropolitan Life Insurance Company, New York.)

**TABLE A–11F.** AVERAGE WEIGHTS BY HEIGHT AND AGE GROUP: 1959 AND 1979 BUILD AND BLOOD PRESSURE STUDIES

| | HEIGHT | | | | | | | | | | | | | | |
|---|---|---|---|---|---|---|---|---|---|---|---|---|---|---|---|
| MEN | 5′2″ | 5′3″ | 5′4″ | 5′5″ | 5′6″ | 5′7″ | 5′8″ | 5′9″ | 5′10″ | 5′11″ | 6′0″ | 6′1″ | 6′2″ | 6′3″ | 6′4″ |
| 15–16 Years* | | | | | | | | | | | | | | | |
| 1959 Study | 107 | 112 | 117 | 122 | 127 | 132 | 137 | 142 | 146 | 150 | 154 | 159 | 164 | 169 | † |
| 1979 Study | 112 | 116 | 121 | 127 | 133 | 137 | 143 | 148 | 153 | 159 | 162 | 168 | 173 | 178 | 184 |
| Weight Change | +5 | +4 | +4 | +5 | +6 | +5 | +6 | +6 | +7 | +9 | +8 | +9 | +9 | +9 | — |
| 17–19 Years | | | | | | | | | | | | | | | |
| 1959 Study | 119 | 123 | 127 | 131 | 135 | 139 | 143 | 147 | 151 | 155 | 160 | 164 | 168 | 172 | 176 |
| 1979 Study | 124 | 129 | 132 | 137 | 141 | 145 | 150 | 155 | 159 | 164 | 168 | 174 | 179 | 185 | 190 |
| Weight Change | +5 | +6 | +5 | +6 | +6 | +6 | +7 | +8 | +8 | +9 | +8 | +10 | +11 | +13 | +14 |
| 20–24 Years | | | | | | | | | | | | | | | |
| 1959 Study | 128 | 132 | 136 | 139 | 142 | 145 | 149 | 153 | 157 | 161 | 166 | 170 | 174 | 178 | 181 |
| 1979 Study | 130 | 136 | 139 | 143 | 148 | 153 | 157 | 163 | 167 | 171 | 176 | 182 | 187 | 193 | 198 |
| Weight Change | +2 | +4 | +3 | +4 | +6 | +8 | +8 | +10 | +10 | +10 | +10 | +12 | +13 | +15 | +17 |
| 25–29 Years | | | | | | | | | | | | | | | |
| 1959 Study | 134 | 138 | 141 | 144 | 148 | 151 | 155 | 159 | 163 | 167 | 172 | 177 | 182 | 186 | 190 |
| 1979 Study | 134 | 140 | 143 | 147 | 152 | 156 | 161 | 166 | 171 | 175 | 181 | 186 | 191 | 197 | 202 |
| Weight Change | +0 | +2 | +2 | +3 | +4 | +5 | +6 | +7 | +8 | +8 | +9 | +9 | +9 | +11 | +12 |
| 30–39 Years | | | | | | | | | | | | | | | |
| 1959 Study | 137 | 141 | 145 | 149 | 153 | 157 | 161 | 165 | 170 | 174 | 179 | 183 | 188 | 193 | 199 |
| 1979 Study | 138 | 143 | 147 | 151 | 156 | 160 | 165 | 170 | 174 | 179 | 184 | 190 | 195 | 201 | 206 |
| Weight Change | +1 | +2 | +2 | +2 | +3 | +3 | +4 | +5 | +4 | +5 | +5 | +7 | +7 | +8 | +7 |
| 40–49 Years | | | | | | | | | | | | | | | |
| 1959 Study | 140 | 144 | 148 | 152 | 156 | 161 | 165 | 169 | 174 | 178 | 183 | 187 | 192 | 197 | 203 |
| 1979 Study | 140 | 144 | 149 | 154 | 158 | 163 | 167 | 172 | 176 | 181 | 186 | 192 | 197 | 203 | 208 |
| Weight Change | +0 | +0 | +1 | +2 | +2 | +2 | +2 | +3 | +2 | +3 | +3 | +5 | +5 | +6 | +5 |
| 50–59 Years | | | | | | | | | | | | | | | |
| 1959 Study | 142 | 145 | 149 | 153 | 157 | 162 | 166 | 170 | 175 | 180 | 185 | 189 | 194 | 199 | 205 |
| 1979 Study | 141 | 145 | 150 | 155 | 159 | 164 | 168 | 173 | 177 | 182 | 187 | 193 | 198 | 204 | 209 |
| Weight Change | −1 | +0 | +1 | +2 | +2 | +2 | +2 | +3 | +2 | +2 | +2 | +4 | +4 | +5 | +4 |
| 60–69 Years | | | | | | | | | | | | | | | |
| 1959 Study | 139 | 142 | 146 | 150 | 154 | 159 | 163 | 168 | 173 | 178 | 183 | 188 | 193 | 198 | 204 |
| 1979 Study | 140 | 144 | 149 | 153 | 158 | 163 | 167 | 172 | 176 | 181 | 186 | 191 | 196 | 200 | 207 |
| Weight Change | +1 | +2 | +3 | +3 | +4 | +4 | +4 | +4 | +3 | +3 | +3 | +3 | +3 | +2 | +3 |

(Continued)

**TABLE A–11F.** (continued)

| WOMEN | HEIGHT | | | | | | | | | | | | | | |
|---|---|---|---|---|---|---|---|---|---|---|---|---|---|---|---|
| | 4'10" | 4'11" | 5'0" | 5'1" | 5'2" | 5'3" | 5'4" | 5'5" | 5'6" | 5'7" | 5'8" | 5'9" | 5'10" | 5'11" | 6'0" |
| 15–16 Years* | | | | | | | | | | | | | | | |
| 1959 Study | 97 | 100 | 103 | 107 | 111 | 114 | 117 | 121 | 125 | 128 | 132 | 136 | † | † | † |
| 1979 Study | 101 | 105 | 109 | 112 | 117 | 121 | 123 | 128 | 131 | 135 | 138 | 142 | 146 | 149 | 152 |
| Weight Change | +4 | +5 | +6 | +5 | +6 | +7 | +6 | +7 | +6 | +7 | +6 | +6 | — | — | — |
| 17–19 Years | | | | | | | | | | | | | | | |
| 1959 Study | 99 | 102 | 105 | 109 | 113 | 116 | 120 | 124 | 127 | 130 | 134 | 138 | 142 | 147 | 152 |
| 1979 Study | 103 | 108 | 111 | 115 | 119 | 123 | 126 | 129 | 132 | 136 | 140 | 145 | 148 | 150 | 154 |
| Weight Change | +4 | +6 | +6 | +6 | +6 | +7 | +6 | +5 | +5 | +6 | +6 | +7 | +6 | +3 | +2 |
| 20–24 Years | | | | | | | | | | | | | | | |
| 1959 Study | 102 | 105 | 108 | 112 | 115 | 118 | 121 | 125 | 129 | 132 | 136 | 140 | 144 | 149 | 154 |
| 1979 Study | 105 | 110 | 112 | 116 | 120 | 124 | 127 | 130 | 133 | 137 | 141 | 146 | 149 | 155 | 157 |
| Weight Change | +3 | +5 | +4 | +4 | +5 | +6 | +6 | +5 | +4 | +5 | +5 | +6 | +5 | +6 | +3 |
| 25–29 Years | | | | | | | | | | | | | | | |
| 1959 Study | 107 | 110 | 113 | 116 | 119 | 122 | 125 | 129 | 133 | 136 | 140 | 144 | 148 | 153 | 158 |
| 1979 Study | 110 | 112 | 114 | 119 | 121 | 125 | 128 | 132 | 134 | 138 | 142 | 148 | 150 | 156 | 159 |
| Weight Change | +3 | +2 | +1 | +3 | +2 | +3 | +3 | +3 | +1 | +2 | +2 | +4 | +2 | +3 | +1 |
| 30–39 Years | | | | | | | | | | | | | | | |
| 1959 Study | 115 | 117 | 120 | 123 | 126 | 129 | 132 | 135 | 139 | 142 | 146 | 150 | 154 | 159 | 164 |
| 1979 Study | 113 | 115 | 118 | 121 | 124 | 128 | 131 | 134 | 137 | 141 | 145 | 150 | 153 | 159 | 164 |
| Weight Change | −2 | −2 | −2 | −2 | −2 | −1 | −1 | −1 | −2 | −1 | −1 | 0 | −1 | 0 | 0 |
| 40–49 Years | | | | | | | | | | | | | | | |
| 1959 Study | 122 | 124 | 127 | 130 | 133 | 136 | 140 | 143 | 147 | 151 | 155 | 159 | 164 | 169 | 174 |
| 1979 Study | 118 | 121 | 123 | 127 | 129 | 133 | 136 | 139 | 143 | 147 | 150 | 155 | 158 | 162 | 168 |
| Weight Change | −4 | −3 | −4 | −3 | −4 | −3 | −4 | −4 | −4 | −4 | −5 | −4 | −6 | −7 | −6 |
| 50–59 Years | | | | | | | | | | | | | | | |
| 1959 Study | 125 | 127 | 130 | 133 | 136 | 140 | 144 | 148 | 152 | 156 | 160 | 164 | 169 | 174 | 180 |
| 1979 Study | 121 | 125 | 127 | 131 | 133 | 137 | 141 | 144 | 147 | 152 | 156 | 159 | 162 | 166 | 171 |
| Weight Change | −4 | −2 | −3 | −2 | −3 | −3 | −3 | −4 | −5 | −4 | −4 | −5 | −7 | −8 | −9 |
| 60–69 Years | | | | | | | | | | | | | | | |
| 1959 Study | 127 | 129 | 131 | 134 | 137 | 141 | 145 | 149 | 153 | 157 | 161 | 165 | † | † | † |
| 1979 Study | 123 | 127 | 130 | 133 | 136 | 140 | 143 | 147 | 150 | 155 | 158 | 161 | 163 | 167 | 172 |
| Weight Change | −4 | −2 | −1 | −1 | −1 | −1 | −2 | −2 | −3 | −2 | −3 | −4 | — | — | — |

*Height in shoes (feet and inches) and weight in indoor clothing (pounds).

†Average weights omitted in classes with too few cases for analysis.

(Data from Association of Life Insurance Medical Directors of America and Society of Actuaries. Compiled by Seltzer, F.: Dietetic Currents, *10*:17–22, 1983. Reprinted with permission of Ross Laboratories, Columbus, Ohio.)

**TABLE A–11G.** FRAME SIZE BY ELBOW BREADTH (cm) OF UNITED STATES MALE AND FEMALE ADULTS DERIVED FROM THE COMBINED NHANES I AND II DATA SETS*

| AGE (YEARS) | FRAME SIZE | | |
|---|---|---|---|
| | SMALL | MEDIUM | LARGE |
| MEN | | | |
| 18–24 | ≤6.6 | >6.6 AND <7.7 | ≥7.7 |
| 25–34 | ≤6.7 | >6.7 AND <7.9 | ≥7.9 |
| 35–44 | ≤6.7 | >6.7 AND <8.0 | ≥8.0 |
| 45–54 | ≤6.7 | >6.7 AND <8.1 | ≥8.1 |
| 55–64 | ≤6.7 | >6.7 AND <8.1 | ≥8.1 |
| 65–74 | ≤6.7 | >6.7 AND <8.1 | ≥8.1 |
| WOMEN | | | |
| 18–24 | ≤5.6 | >5.6 AND <6.5 | ≥6.5 |
| 25–34 | ≤5.7 | >5.7 AND <6.8 | ≥6.8 |
| 35–44 | ≤5.7 | >5.7 AND <7.1 | ≥7.1 |
| 45–54 | ≤5.7 | >5.7 AND <7.2 | ≥7.2 |
| 55–64 | ≤5.8 | >5.8 AND <7.2 | ≥7.2 |
| 65–74 | ≤5.8 | >5.8 AND <7.2 | ≥7.2 |

*The tenth and ninetieth percentiles, respectively, represent the predicted mean $\pm$1.282 times the SE. Similarly, the fifteenth and eighty-fifth percentiles are the predicted mean minus and plus, respectively, 1.036 times the SE of the regression equation. There were significant black-white population differences in weight and body composition when age and height were considered. However, when the comparisons were made with reference to age, height, and frame size, there were only minor interpopulation differences. For this reason, all races (white, black, and other) included in the NHANES I and II surveys were merged together for the purpose of calculating percentiles of anthropometric measurements.

(Combined NHANES I and II data sets from Frisancho, A.R.: Am, J. Clin. Nutr., *40*:808–819, 1984, with permission.)

**TABLE A–11H.** COMPARISON OF THE WEIGHT-FOR-HEIGHT TABLES FROM ACTUARIAL DATA (BUILD STUDY): NON-AGE-CORRECTED METROPOLITAN LIFE INSURANCE COMPANY AND AGE-SPECIFIC GERONTOLOGY RESEARCH CENTER RECOMMENDATIONS*

| | METROPOLITAN 1983 WEIGHTS FOR AGES 25–59† | | GERONTOLOGY RESEARCH CENTER WEIGHT RANGE FOR MEN AND WOMEN BY AGE (YEARS) | | | | |
|---|---|---|---|---|---|---|---|
| HEIGHT | MEN | WOMEN | 25 | 35 | 45 | 55 | 65 |
| ft-in | lb | | | | | | |
| 4–10 | — | 100–131 | 84–111 | 92–119 | 99–127 | 107–135 | 115–142 |
| 4–11 | — | 101–134 | 87–115 | 95–123 | 103–131 | 111–139 | 119–147 |
| 5–0 | — | 103–137 | 90–119 | 98–127 | 106–135 | 114–143 | 123–152 |
| 5–1 | 123–145 | 105–140 | 93–123 | 101–131 | 110–140 | 118–148 | 127–157 |
| 5–2 | 125–148 | 108–144 | 96–127 | 105–136 | 113–144 | 122–153 | 131–163 |
| 5–3 | 127–151 | 111–148 | 99–131 | 108–140 | 117–149 | 126–158 | 135–168 |
| 5–4 | 129–155 | 114–152 | 102–135 | 112–145 | 121–154 | 130–163 | 140–173 |
| 5–5 | 131–159 | 117–156 | 106–140 | 115–149 | 125–159 | 134–168 | 144–179 |
| 5–6 | 133–163 | 120–160 | 109–144 | 119–154 | 129–164 | 138–174 | 148–184 |
| 5–7 | 135–167 | 123–164 | 112–148 | 122–159 | 133–169 | 143–179 | 153–190 |
| 5–8 | 137–171 | 126–167 | 116–153 | 126–163 | 137–174 | 147–184 | 158–196 |
| 5–9 | 139–175 | 129–170 | 119–157 | 130–168 | 141–179 | 151–190 | 162–201 |
| 5–10 | 141–179 | 132–173 | 122–162 | 134–173 | 145–184 | 156–195 | 167–207 |
| 5–11 | 144–183 | 135–176 | 126–167 | 137–178 | 149–190 | 160–201 | 172–213 |
| 6–0 | 147–187 | — | 129–171 | 141–183 | 153–195 | 165–207 | 177–219 |
| 6–1 | 150–192 | — | 133–176 | 145–188 | 157–200 | 169–213 | 182–225 |
| 6–2 | 153–197 | — | 137–181 | 149–194 | 162–206 | 174–219 | 187–232 |
| 6–3 | 157–202 | — | 141–186 | 153–199 | 166–212 | 179–225 | 192–238 |
| 6–4 | — | — | 144–191 | 157–205 | 171–218 | 184–231 | 197–244 |

*Values in this table are for height without shoes and weight without clothes. To convert inches to centimeters, multiply by 2.54; to convert pounds to kilograms, multiply by 0.455.

†The weight range is the lower weight for small frame and the upper weight for large frame.

(Gerontology Research Center data from Andres, R.: Mortality and obesity: the rationale for age-specific height-weight tables. *In* Principles of Geriatric Medicine. Edited by R. Andres, E. Bierman, and W. R. Hazzard. New York, McGraw-Hill, 1985, pp. 311–318.)

**TABLE A–11I.** NOMOGRAPH FOR ESTIMATING BODY MASS INDEX (kg/m$^2$)*

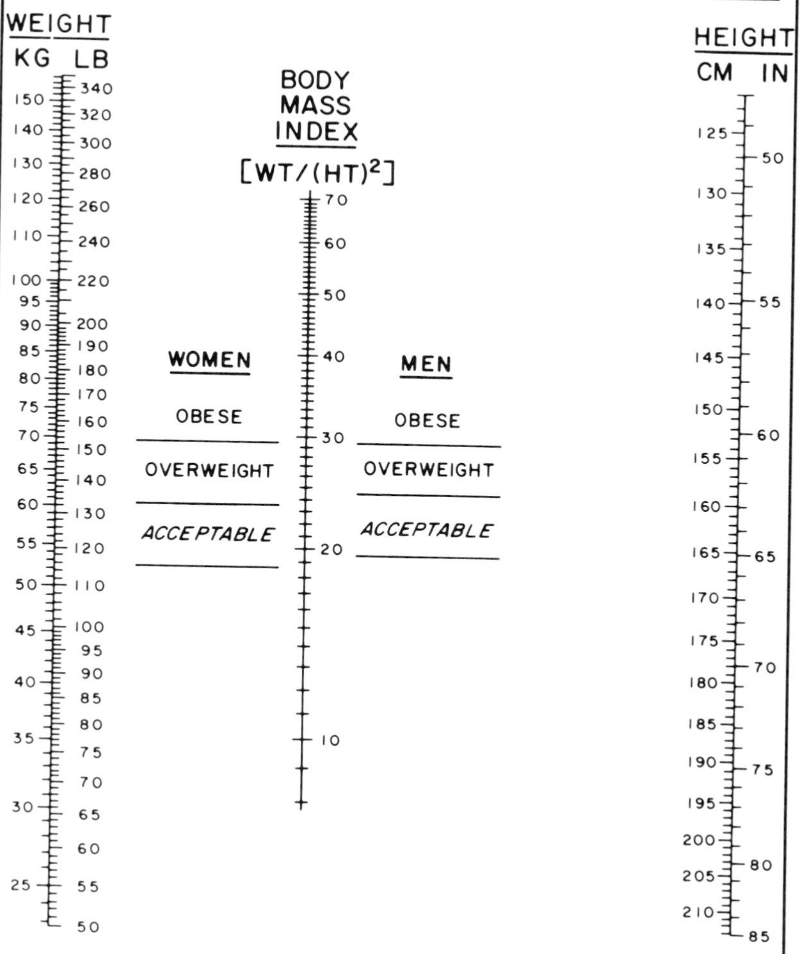
WEIGHT
KG LB
BODY MASS INDEX
[WT/(HT)$^2$]
WOMEN
OBESE
OVERWEIGHT
ACCEPTABLE
MEN
OBESE
OVERWEIGHT
ACCEPTABLE
HEIGHT
CM IN

*The ratio of weight/height$^2$ emerges from varied epidemiologic studies as the most generally useful index of relative body mass in adults. This nomograph facilitates use of this relationship in clinical situations. While showing the range of weight given as desirable in life insurance studies, the scale expresses relative weight as a continuous variable. This method encourages use of clinical judgment in interpreting "overweight" and "underweight" and in accounting for muscular and skeletal contributions to measured mass.

(From G. A. Bray, 1978.)

**TABLE A–11J.** DESIRABLE BODY MASS INDEX (BMI) IN RELATION TO AGE

| Age (years) | BMI (kg/m$^2$) |
|---|---|
| 19–24 | 19–24 |
| 25–34 | 20–25 |
| 35–44 | 21–26 |
| 45–54 | 22–27 |
| 55–65 | 23–28 |
| >65 | 24–29 |

(From Committee on Diet and Health, Food and Nutrition Board, National Research Council. Diet and Health: Implications for Reducing Chronic Disease Risk. Washington, D.C., National Academy Press, 1989, p. 564.)

**TABLE A—12A.** FETAL GROWTH STANDARDS: INTRAUTERINE WEIGHT* AND LENGTH† CHARTS

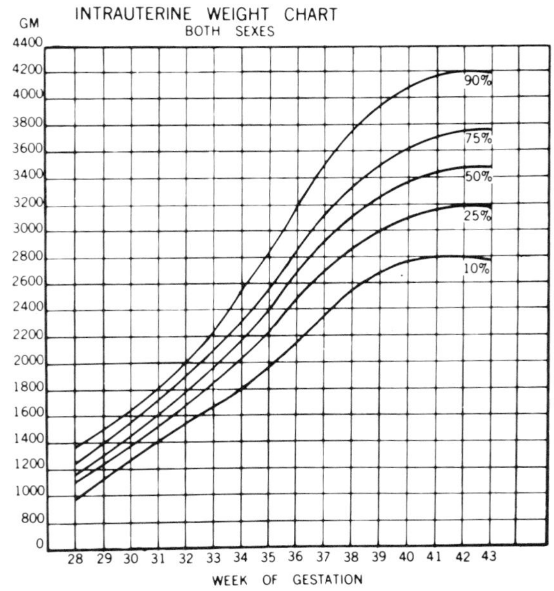
INTRAUTERINE WEIGHT CHART
BOTH SEXES
GM
4400
4200
4000
3800
3600
3400
3200
3000
2800
2600
2400
2200
2000
1800
1600
1400
1200
1000
800
0
90%
75%
50%
25%
10%
28 29 30 31 32 33 34 35 36 37 38 39 40 41 42 43
WEEK OF GESTATION

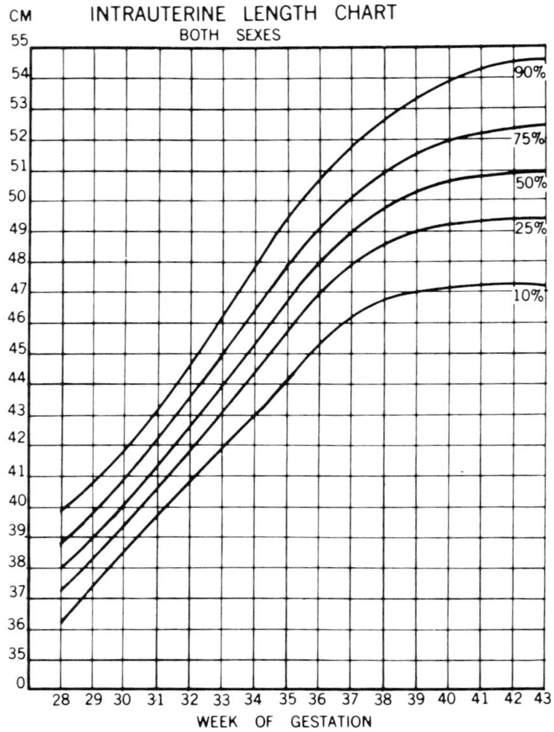
INTRAUTERINE LENGTH CHART
BOTH SEXES
CM
55
54
53
52
51
50
49
48
47
46
45
44
43
42
41
40
39
38
37
36
35
0
90%
75%
50%
25%
10%
28 29 30 31 32 33 34 35 36 37 38 39 40 41 42 43
WEEK OF GESTATION

*Fetal body weight percentiles from 28 to 43 weeks of gestation.
†Fetal body length percentiles from 28 to 43 weeks of gestation.
(From Naeye, R.L., Dixon J.B.: Pediatr. Res., *12*:989, 1978.)

**TABLE A–12B-1.** PHYSICAL GROWTH NCHS PERCENTILES: GIRLS FROM BIRTH TO 36 MONTHS

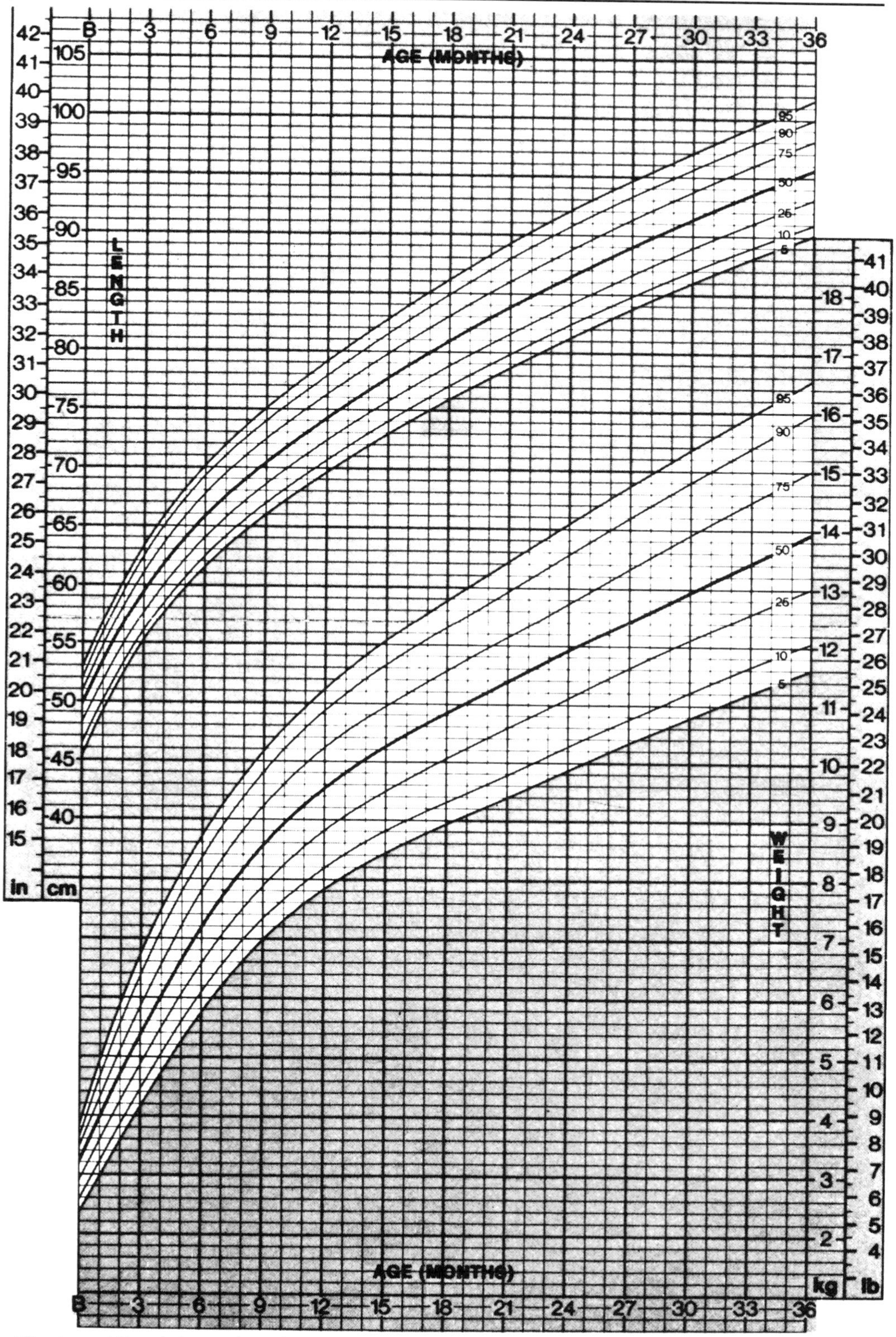
AGE (MONTHS)
LENGTH
WEIGHT
in
cm
kg
lb

(Courtesy of Ross Laboratories, who adapted the growth curves from the original data: National Center for Health Statistics, NCHS Growth Charts, 1976. Monthly Vital Statistics Report, Vol. 25, No. 3, Suppl. (HRA) 76–1120. Rockville, MD, Health Resources Administration, June, 1976. Data from The Fels Research Institute, Yellow Springs, Ohio.)

**TABLE A–12B-2.** PHYSICAL GROWTH NCHS PERCENTILES: BOYS FROM BIRTH TO 36 MONTHS

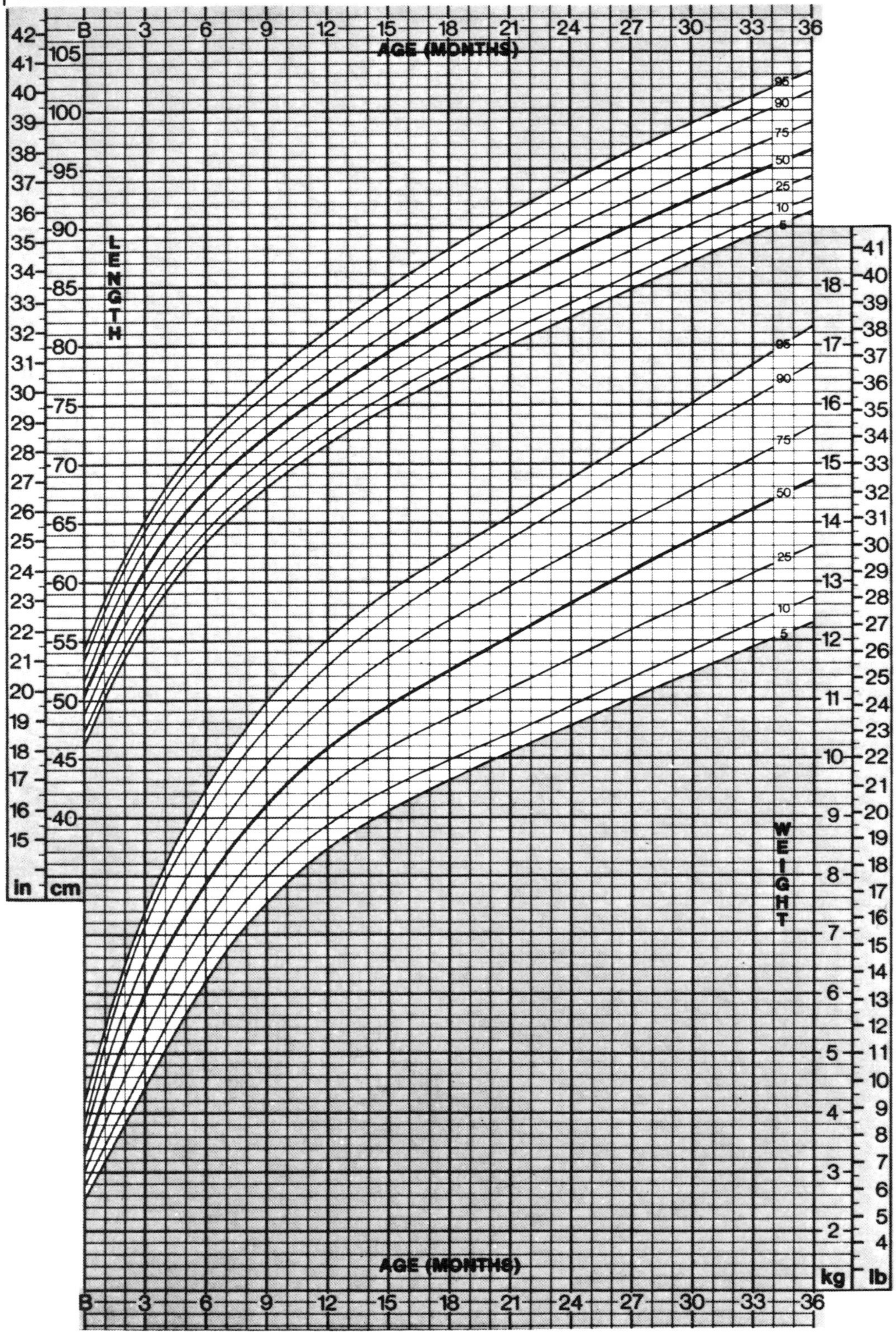
AGE (MONTHS)
B
3
6
9
12
15
18
21
24
27
30
33
36
LENGTH
WEIGHT
in
cm
kg
lb
95
90
75
50
25
10
5

(Courtesy of Ross Laboratories, who adapted the growth curves from the original data: National Center for Health Statistics, NCHS Growth Charts, 1976. Monthly Vital Statistics Report, Vol. 25, No. 3, Suppl. (HRA) 76–1120. Rockville, MD, Health Resources Administration, June, 1976. Data from The Fels Research Institute, Yellow Springs, Ohio.)

**TABLE A—12C-1.** PHYSICAL GROWTH NCHS PERCENTILES: GIRLS FROM 2 TO 18 YEARS

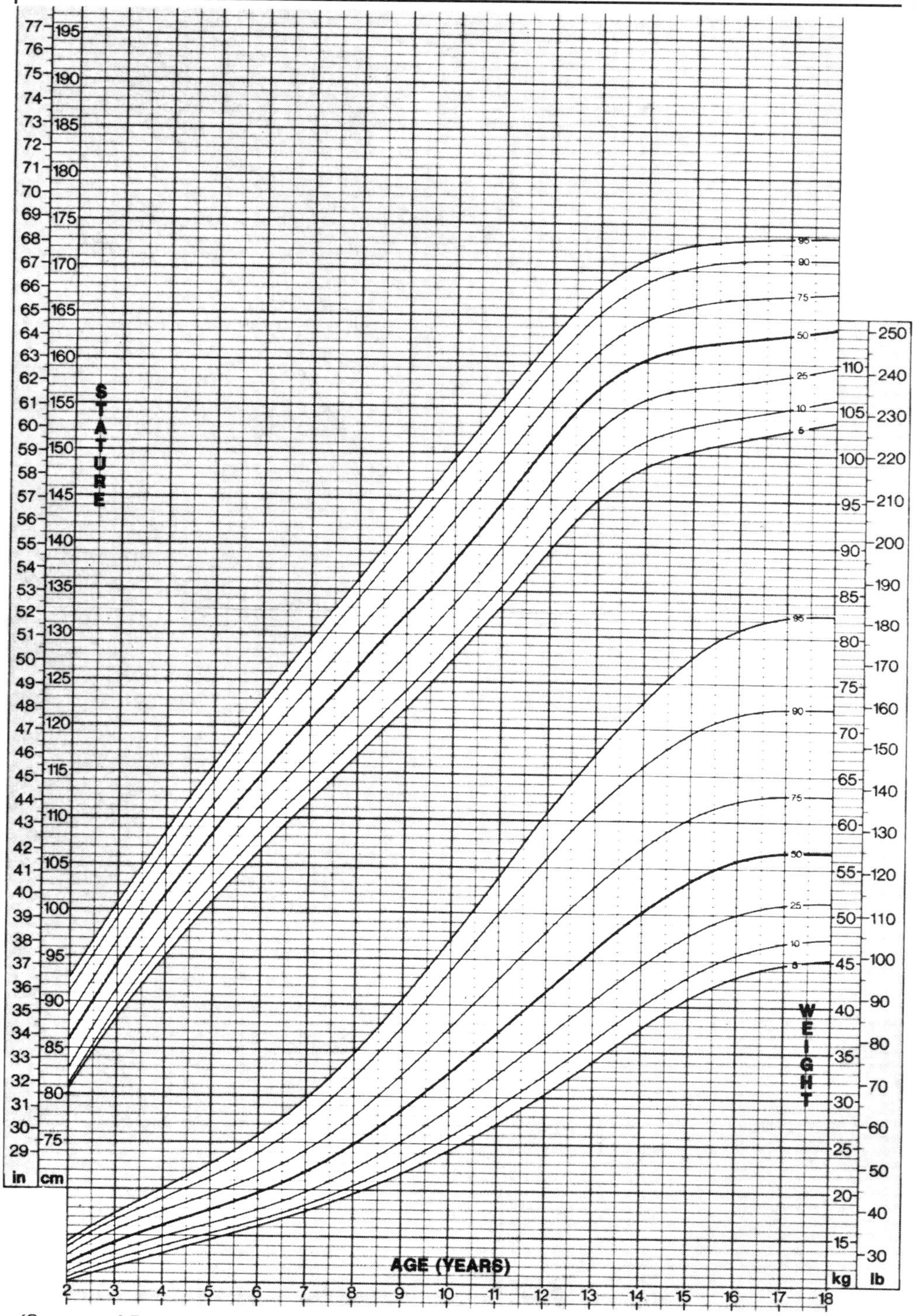

STATURE
WEIGHT
AGE (YEARS)
in
cm
kg
lb


(Courtesy of Ross Laboratories, who adapted the growth curves from the original data: National Center for Health Statistics, NCHS Growth Charts, 1976. Monthly Vital Statistics Report, Vol. 25, No. 3, Suppl. (HRA) 76—1120. Rockville, MD, Health Resources Administration, June, 1976. Data from The Fels Research Institute, Yellow Springs, Ohio.)

**TABLE A–12C-2.** PHYSICAL GROWTH NCHS PERCENTILES: BOYS FROM 2 TO 18 YEARS

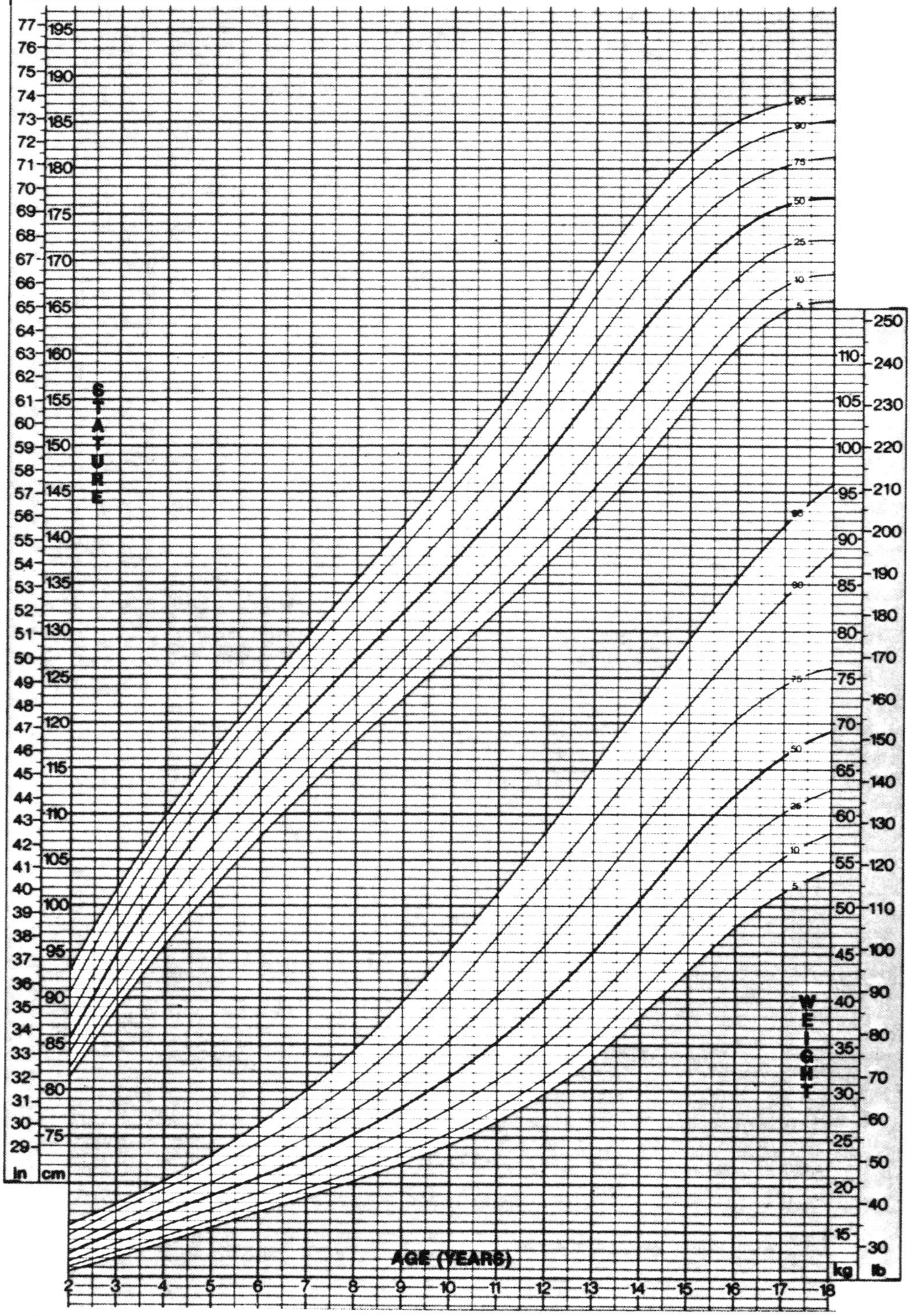

STATURE
WEIGHT
AGE (YEARS)
in
cm
kg
lb


(Courtesy of Ross Laboratories, who adapted the growth curves from the original data: National Center for Health Statistics, NCHS Growth Charts, 1976. Monthly Vital Statistics Report, Vol. 25, No. 3, Suppl. (HRA) 76–1120. Rockville, MD, Health Resources Administration, June, 1976. Data from The Fels Research Institute, Yellow Springs, Ohio.)

**TABLE A–12D.** HEIGHT IN CENTIMETERS FOR PERSONS 2 TO 19 YEARS OF AGE: NUMBER EXAMINED, MEAN, STANDARD DEVIATION, AND SELECTED PERCENTILES BY SEX AND AGE, UNITED STATES, 1976 TO 1980*

| SEX AND AGE (years) | NUMBER OF EXAMINED PERSONS | MEAN | STANDARD DEVIATION | PERCENTILE 5th | 10th | 15th | 25th | 50th | 75th | 85th | 90th | 95th |
|---|---|---|---|---|---|---|---|---|---|---|---|---|
| Male | | | | | | | | | | | | |
| 2 | 375 | 91.2 | 4.3 | 84.5 | 85.8 | 85.5 | 88.2 | 91.3 | 94.2 | 95.8 | 96.6 | 97.6 |
| 3 | 418 | 99.2 | 4.5 | 92.0 | 94.3 | 94.9 | 96.5 | 98.8 | 102.0 | 103.9 | 105.0 | 107.0 |
| 4 | 404 | 106.0 | 5.2 | 97.8 | 99.5 | 100.5 | 102.5 | 106.4 | 109.2 | 111.0 | 112.4 | 115.0 |
| 5 | 397 | 112.6 | 5.4 | 104.0 | 105.8 | 107.2 | 109.4 | 112.6 | 115.6 | 118.1 | 119.6 | 121.2 |
| 6 | 133 | 119.5 | 5.1 | 111.2 | 112.6 | 114.5 | 115.9 | 120.1 | 122.6 | 124.7 | 125.5 | 126.8 |
| 7 | 148 | 125.1 | 5.9 | 115.4 | 117.6 | 119.1 | 121.8 | 125.9 | 128.1 | 130.2 | 131.5 | 133.6 |
| 8 | 147 | 129.9 | 7.0 | 118.6 | 122.0 | 123.5 | 125.3 | 130.6 | 134.1 | 136.5 | 138.0 | 142.0 |
| 9 | 145 | 135.5 | 5.8 | 125.9 | 126.4 | 129.4 | 131.2 | 136.1 | 139.6 | 141.2 | 143.1 | 144.7 |
| 10 | 157 | 141.6 | 7.3 | 130.3 | 132.8 | 134.0 | 137.0 | 141.5 | 146.4 | 149.6 | 150.6 | 153.0 |
| 11 | 155 | 146.0 | 7.8 | 133.1 | 135.9 | 138.0 | 141.1 | 145.6 | 151.2 | 153.9 | 155.2 | 160.2 |
| 12 | 145 | 152.5 | 7.9 | 139.0 | 142.6 | 144.9 | 147.5 | 152.0 | 158.0 | 160.5 | 162.0 | 164.4 |
| 13 | 173 | 158.9 | 8.3 | 144.4 | 147.6 | 149.7 | 152.6 | 159.7 | 165.0 | 168.7 | 169.5 | 171.6 |
| 14 | 186 | 167.5 | 8.3 | 153.9 | 156.5 | 159.1 | 162.5 | 167.5 | 173.1 | 176.5 | 178.7 | 180.6 |
| 15 | 184 | 170.8 | 6.7 | 160.1 | 162.0 | 162.6 | 165.7 | 171.1 | 175.5 | 177.5 | 178.2 | 181.9 |
| 16 | 178 | 173.8 | 6.4 | 163.0 | 164.7 | 167.4 | 169.8 | 173.7 | 178.1 | 180.3 | 182.6 | 186.1 |
| 17 | 173 | 175.1 | 7.1 | 164.1 | 167.3 | 168.4 | 170.6 | 174.9 | 179.7 | 182.8 | 184.3 | 187.5 |
| 18 | 164 | 176.9 | 6.7 | 166.5 | 168.8 | 169.9 | 172.3 | 176.9 | 180.9 | 183.9 | 185.1 | 189.6 |
| 19 | 148 | 176.5 | 6.7 | 164.5 | 168.2 | 169.4 | 171.8 | 176.9 | 181.1 | 183.5 | 184.8 | 187.2 |
| Female | | | | | | | | | | | | |
| 2 | 336 | 89.7 | 4.2 | 83.1 | 84.4 | 85.5 | 86.7 | 89.8 | 92.2 | 93.6 | 94.9 | 97.2 |
| 3 | 366 | 97.5 | 4.8 | 89.6 | 91.1 | 92.5 | 94.5 | 97.6 | 100.8 | 102.5 | 103.4 | 104.5 |
| 4 | 396 | 104.6 | 5.0 | 96.1 | 98.2 | 99.5 | 101.5 | 104.5 | 108.2 | 109.8 | 110.7 | 112.4 |
| 5 | 364 | 111.6 | 5.3 | 103.0 | 105.1 | 106.4 | 108.1 | 111.6 | 115.2 | 116.5 | 118.8 | 120.3 |
| 6 | 135 | 118.4 | 6.1 | 109.9 | 111.1 | 111.5 | 113.3 | 118.5 | 122.2 | 124.5 | 126.5 | 128.7 |
| 7 | 157 | 123.7 | 6.7 | 113.3 | 116.6 | 117.4 | 119.6 | 124.1 | 128.1 | 130.1 | 132.2 | 134.7 |
| 8 | 123 | 130.2 | 5.7 | 120.8 | 123.4 | 124.4 | 125.8 | 130.6 | 133.2 | 135.4 | 137.5 | 140.5 |
| 9 | 149 | 134.4 | 7.6 | 124.0 | 126.4 | 127.8 | 129.0 | 134.8 | 139.0 | 140.7 | 142.6 | 147.1 |
| 10 | 136 | 141.9 | 6.5 | 131.6 | 133.6 | 135.1 | 137.6 | 141.6 | 146.3 | 148.1 | 150.4 | 153.8 |
| 11 | 140 | 147.9 | 7.8 | 134.7 | 139.3 | 140.6 | 142.2 | 147.9 | 152.2 | 154.7 | 156.9 | 162.7 |
| 12 | 147 | 154.4 | 7.2 | 143.9 | 145.7 | 146.7 | 149.2 | 154.8 | 158.6 | 161.9 | 164.7 | 165.9 |
| 13 | 162 | 158.9 | 6.6 | 149.0 | 150.3 | 152.7 | 155.3 | 159.0 | 163.0 | 164.5 | 166.9 | 170.3 |
| 14 | 178 | 160.8 | 6.4 | 151.0 | 152.7 | 154.5 | 156.7 | 160.9 | 165.1 | 166.9 | 168.2 | 172.3 |
| 15 | 145 | 163.2 | 6.2 | 153.0 | 155.2 | 157.1 | 159.1 | 163.1 | 167.1 | 170.2 | 172.4 | 173.5 |
| 16 | 170 | 162.9 | 6.1 | 152.0 | 154.5 | 157.2 | 159.1 | 163.2 | 166.4 | 169.4 | 171.4 | 173.3 |
| 17 | 134 | 163.5 | 5.7 | 153.8 | 156.8 | 158.5 | 160.4 | 163.1 | 166.7 | 169.7 | 170.7 | 172.2 |
| 18 | 170 | 162.4 | 6.8 | 150.7 | 154.2 | 155.6 | 158.0 | 162.7 | 166.2 | 169.1 | 171.5 | 174.0 |
| 19 | 158 | 163.5 | 5.6 | 153.8 | 156.8 | 157.7 | 159.7 | 163.7 | 167.2 | 169.5 | 170.4 | 172.1 |

*Height without shoes.

(From National Center for Health Statistics: Anthropometric Reference Data and Prevalence of Overweight, United States 1976–1980. DHHS Publication No. 87–1688. Hyattsville, MD, U.S. Department of Health and Human Services, Public Health Service, 1987.)

**TABLE A–12E.** WEIGHT IN KILOGRAMS FOR PERSONS 6 MONTHS TO 19 YEARS OF AGE: NUMBER EXAMINED, MEAN, STANDARD DEVIATION, AND SELECTED PERCENTILES BY SEX AND AGE, UNITED STATES, 1976 TO 1980*

| SEX AND AGE | NUMBER OF EXAMINED PERSONS | MEAN | STANDARD DEVIATION | PERCENTILE | | | | | | | | |
|---|---|---|---|---|---|---|---|---|---|---|---|---|
| | | | | 5th | 10th | 15th | 25th | 50th | 75th | 85th | 90th | 95th |
| Male | | | | | | | | | | | | |
| 6–11 months | 179 | 9.4 | 1.3 | 7.5 | 7.6 | 8.2 | 8.6 | 9.4 | 10.1 | 10.7 | 10.9 | 11.4 |
| 1 year | 370 | 11.8 | 1.9 | 9.6 | 10.0 | 10.3 | 10.8 | 11.7 | 12.6 | 13.1 | 13.6 | 14.4 |
| 2 years | 375 | 13.6 | 1.7 | 11.1 | 11.6 | 11.8 | 12.6 | 13.5 | 14.5 | 15.2 | 15.8 | 16.5 |
| 3 years | 418 | 15.7 | 2.0 | 12.9 | 13.5 | 13.9 | 14.4 | 15.4 | 16.8 | 17.4 | 17.9 | 19.1 |
| 4 years | 404 | 17.8 | 2.5 | 14.1 | 15.0 | 15.3 | 16.0 | 17.6 | 19.0 | 19.9 | 20.9 | 22.2 |
| 5 years | 397 | 19.8 | 3.0 | 16.0 | 16.8 | 17.1 | 17.7 | 19.4 | 21.3 | 22.9 | 23.7 | 25.4 |
| 6 years | 133 | 23.0 | 4.0 | 18.6 | 19.2 | 19.8 | 20.3 | 22.0 | 24.1 | 26.4 | 28.3 | 30.1 |
| 7 years | 148 | 25.1 | 3.9 | 19.7 | 20.8 | 21.2 | 22.2 | 24.8 | 26.9 | 28.2 | 29.6 | 33.9 |
| 8 years | 147 | 28.2 | 6.2 | 20.4 | 22.7 | 23.6 | 24.6 | 27.5 | 29.9 | 33.0 | 35.5 | 39.1 |
| 9 years | 145 | 31.1 | 6.3 | 24.0 | 25.6 | 26.0 | 27.1 | 30.2 | 33.0 | 35.4 | 38.6 | 43.1 |
| 10 yars | 157 | 36.4 | 7.7 | 27.2 | 28.2 | 29.6 | 31.4 | 34.8 | 39.2 | 43.5 | 46.3 | 53.4 |
| 11 years | 155 | 40.3 | 10.1 | 26.8 | 28.8 | 31.8 | 33.5 | 37.3 | 46.4 | 52.0 | 57.0 | 61.0 |
| 12 years | 145 | 44.2 | 10.1 | 30.7 | 32.5 | 35.4 | 37.8 | 42.5 | 48.8 | 52.6 | 58.9 | 67.5 |
| 13 years | 173 | 49.9 | 12.3 | 35.4 | 37.0 | 38.3 | 40.1 | 48.4 | 56.3 | 59.8 | 64.2 | 69.9 |
| 14 years | 186 | 57.1 | 11.0 | 41.0 | 44.5 | 46.4 | 49.8 | 56.4 | 63.3 | 66.1 | 68.9 | 77.0 |
| 15 years | 184 | 61.0 | 11.0 | 46.2 | 49.1 | 50.6 | 54.2 | 60.1 | 64.9 | 68.7 | 72.8 | 81.3 |
| 16 years | 178 | 67.1 | 12.4 | 51.4 | 54.3 | 56.1 | 58.7 | 64.4 | 73.6 | 78.1 | 82.2 | 91.2 |
| 17 years | 173 | 66.7 | 11.5 | 50.7 | 53.4 | 54.8 | 58.7 | 65.8 | 72.0 | 76.8 | 82.3 | 88.9 |
| 18 years | 164 | 71.1 | 12.7 | 54.1 | 56.6 | 60.3 | 61.9 | 70.4 | 76.6 | 80.0 | 83.5 | 95.3 |
| 19 years | 148 | 71.7 | 11.6 | 55.9 | 57.9 | 60.5 | 63.8 | 69.5 | 77.9 | 84.3 | 86.8 | 92.1 |
| Female | | | | | | | | | | | | |
| 6–11 months | 177 | 8.8 | 1.2 | 6.6 | 7.3 | 7.5 | 7.9 | 8.9 | 9.4 | 10.1 | 10.4 | 10.9 |
| 1 year | 336 | 10.8 | 1.4 | 8.8 | 9.1 | 9.4 | 9.9 | 10.7 | 11.7 | 12.4 | 12.7 | 13.4 |
| 2 years | 336 | 13.0 | 1.5 | 10.8 | 11.2 | 11.6 | 12.0 | 12.7 | 13.8 | 14.5 | 14.9 | 15.9 |
| 3 years | 366 | 14.9 | 2.1 | 11.7 | 12.3 | 12.9 | 13.4 | 14.7 | 16.1 | 17.0 | 17.4 | 18.4 |
| 4 years | 396 | 17.0 | 2.4 | 13.7 | 14.3 | 14.5 | 15.2 | 16.7 | 18.4 | 19.3 | 20.2 | 21.1 |
| 5 years | 364 | 19.6 | 3.3 | 15.3 | 16.1 | 16.7 | 17.2 | 19.0 | 21.2 | 22.8 | 24.7 | 26.6 |
| 6 years | 135 | 22.1 | 4.0 | 17.0 | 17.8 | 18.6 | 19.3 | 21.3 | 23.8 | 26.6 | 28.9 | 29.6 |
| 7 years | 157 | 24.7 | 5.0 | 19.2 | 19.5 | 19.8 | 21.4 | 23.8 | 27.1 | 28.7 | 30.3 | 34.0 |
| 8 years | 123 | 27.9 | 5.7 | 21.4 | 22.3 | 23.3 | 24.4 | 27.5 | 30.2 | 31.3 | 33.2 | 36.5 |
| 9 years | 149 | 31.9 | 8.4 | 22.9 | 25.0 | 25.8 | 27.0 | 29.7 | 33.6 | 39.3 | 43.3 | 48.4 |
| 10 years | 136 | 36.1 | 8.0 | 25.7 | 27.5 | 29.0 | 31.0 | 34.5 | 39.5 | 44.2 | 45.8 | 49.6 |
| 11 years | 140 | 41.8 | 10.9 | 29.8 | 30.3 | 31.3 | 33.9 | 40.3 | 45.8 | 51.0 | 56.6 | 60.0 |
| 12 years | 147 | 46.4 | 10.1 | 32.3 | 35.0 | 36.7 | 39.1 | 45.4 | 52.6 | 58.0 | 60.5 | 64.3 |
| 13 years | 162 | 50.9 | 11.8 | 35.4 | 39.0 | 40.3 | 44.1 | 49.0 | 55.2 | 60.9 | 66.4 | 76.3 |
| 14 years | 175 | 54.8 | 11.1 | 40.3 | 42.8 | 43.7 | 47.4 | 53.1 | 60.3 | 65.7 | 67.6 | 75.2 |
| 15 years | 145 | 55.1 | 9.8 | 44.0 | 45.1 | 46.5 | 48.2 | 53.3 | 59.6 | 62.2 | 65.5 | 76.6 |
| 16 years | 170 | 58.1 | 10.1 | 44.1 | 47.3 | 48.9 | 51.3 | 55.6 | 62.5 | 68.9 | 73.3 | 76.8 |
| 17 years | 134 | 59.6 | 11.4 | 44.5 | 48.9 | 50.5 | 52.2 | 58.4 | 63.4 | 68.4 | 71.6 | 81.8 |
| 18 years | 170 | 59.0 | 11.1 | 45.3 | 49.5 | 50.8 | 52.8 | 56.4 | 63.0 | 66.0 | 70.1 | 78.0 |
| 19 years | 158 | 60.2 | 11.0 | 48.5 | 49.7 | 51.7 | 53.9 | 57.1 | 64.4 | 70.7 | 74.8 | 78.1 |

*Includes clothing weight, estimated as ranging from 0.09 to 0.28 kilogram.

(From National Center for Health Statistics: Anthropometric Reference Data and Prevalence of Overweight, United States 1976–1980. DHHS Publication No. 87–1688. Hyattsville, MD, U.S. Department of Health and Human Services, Public Health Service, 1987.)

**TABLE A—12F-1.** WEIGHT IN KILOGRAMS OF YOUTHS AGED 12 YEARS AT LAST BIRTHDAY BY SEX AND HEIGHT GROUP IN CENTIMETERS: SAMPLE SIZE, ESTIMATED POPULATION SIZE, MEAN, STANDARD DEVIATION, STANDARD ERROR OF THE MEAN, AND SELECTED PERCENTILES, UNITED STATES, 1966 TO 1970

| SEX AND HEIGHT | *n* | *N* | $\bar{X}$ | *s* | $s_{\bar{x}}$ | PERCENTILE 5th | 10th | 25th | 50th | 75th | 90th | 95th |
|---|---|---|---|---|---|---|---|---|---|---|---|---|
| Male | | | | | | in kilograms | | | | | | |
| Under 130 | 5 | 15 | * | * | * | * | * | * | * | * | * | * |
| 130.0–134.9 | 4 | 8 | * | * | * | * | * | * | * | * | * | * |
| 135.0–139.9 | 34 | 111 | 32.50 | 3.741 | 0.727 | 26.6 | 27.6 | 30.2 | 31.6 | 34.7 | 37.7 | 39.4 |
| 140.0–144.9 | 80 | 241 | 34.28 | 3.635 | 0.601 | 28.1 | 30.0 | 31.8 | 34.1 | 36.5 | 38.6 | 40.7 |
| 145.0–149.9 | 123 | 386 | 39.27 | 6.243 | 0.615 | 32.1 | 33.2 | 35.7 | 38.2 | 40.9 | 46.1 | 52.5 |
| 150.0–154.9 | 156 | 513 | 42.90 | 6.314 | 0.480 | 34.9 | 36.1 | 38.2 | 42.1 | 46.0 | 51.6 | 56.3 |
| 155.0–159.9 | 135 | 432 | 47.35 | 7.551 | 0.769 | 38.3 | 39.4 | 41.9 | 46.2 | 50.5 | 57.4 | 61.9 |
| 160.0–164.9 | 65 | 201 | 50.82 | 8.735 | 1.388 | 42.1 | 42.7 | 44.9 | 48.4 | 56.0 | 61.1 | 67.1 |
| 165.0–169.9 | 29 | 88 | 55.75 | 8.811 | 2.031 | 43.3 | 46.4 | 49.0 | 54.4 | 59.9 | 68.3 | 76.6 |
| 170.0–174.9 | 8 | 21 | 62.37 | 4.503 | 1.993 | 54.0 | 58.1 | 60.1 | 61.0 | 66.0 | 69.1 | 69.5 |
| 175.0–179.9 | 3 | 10 | * | * | * | * | * | * | * | * | * | * |
| 180.0–184.9 | 1 | 2 | * | * | * | * | * | * | * | * | * | * |
| 185.0–189.9 | — | — | — | — | — | — | — | — | — | — | — | — |
| 190.0–194.9 | — | — | — | — | — | — | — | — | — | — | — | — |
| 195.0 and over | — | — | — | — | — | — | — | — | — | — | — | — |

**TABLE A—12F-1.** (continued)

| Sex and Height | *n* | *N* | $\bar{X}$ | *s* | $s_{\bar{x}}$ | PERCENTILE 5th | 10th | 25th | 50th | 75th | 90th | 95th |
|---|---|---|---|---|---|---|---|---|---|---|---|---|
| Female | | | | | | in kilograms | | | | | | |
| Under 130 | — | — | — | — | — | — | — | — | — | — | — | — |
| 130.0–134.9 | 3 | 10 | * | * | * | * | * | * | * | * | * | * |
| 135.0–139.9 | 12 | 44 | 29.41 | 3.372 | 0.914 | 25.0 | 25.0 | 26.4 | 28.9 | 32.1 | 34.1 | 34.2 |
| 140.0–144.9 | 32 | 116 | 38.30 | 7.314 | 1.194 | 28.8 | 30.6 | 33.3 | 36.8 | 41.4 | 49.2 | 55.1 |
| 145.0–149.9 | 72 | 258 | 39.78 | 6.205 | 0.975 | 31.8 | 32.8 | 35.5 | 38.5 | 42.8 | 48.3 | 50.6 |
| 150.0–154.9 | 147 | 517 | 44.00 | 7.421 | 0.677 | 34.4 | 35.8 | 38.9 | 42.8 | 47.4 | 52.9 | 57.4 |
| 155.0–159.9 | 144 | 525 | 48.74 | 8.369 | 0.714 | 37.9 | 39.2 | 43.0 | 46.8 | 53.8 | 60.7 | 63.5 |
| 160.0–164.9 | 95 | 336 | 53.06 | 8.010 | 0.658 | 42.5 | 43.9 | 47.2 | 51.1 | 57.2 | 65.6 | 69.6 |
| 165.0–169.9 | 31 | 117 | 54.89 | 7.022 | 1.384 | 43.9 | 47.1 | 50.4 | 53.1 | 59.7 | 64.5 | 71.3 |
| 170.0–174.9 | 11 | 42 | 63.66 | 14.501 | 6.214 | 48.7 | 50.1 | 50.8 | 56.7 | 82.2 | 86.0 | 86.1 |
| 175.0–179.9 | — | — | — | — | — | — | — | — | — | — | — | — |
| 180.0–184.9 | — | — | — | — | — | — | — | — | — | — | — | — |
| 185.0–189.9 | — | — | — | — | — | — | — | — | — | — | — | — |
| 190.0–194.9 | — | — | — | — | — | — | — | — | — | — | — | — |
| 195.0 and over | — | — | — | — | — | — | — | — | — | — | — | — |

*n*, Sample size; *N*, estimated number of youths in population in thousands; $\bar{X}$, mean; *s*, standard deviation; $s_{\bar{x}}$, standard error of the mean.

(From National Center for Health Statistics: Height and weight of youths 12–17 years, United States. *In* Vital and Health Statistics, Series 11, No. 124, Health Services and Mental Health Administration. Washington, D.C., U.S. Government Printing Office, 1973, pp. 282–288.)

**TABLE A—12F-2.** WEIGHT IN KILOGRAMS OF YOUTHS AGED 13 YEARS AT LAST BIRTHDAY BY SEX AND HEIGHT GROUP IN CENTIMETERS: SAMPLE SIZE, ESTIMATED POPULATION SIZE, MEAN, STANDARD DEVIATION, STANDARD ERROR OF THE MEAN, AND SELECTED PERCENTILES, UNITED STATES, 1966 TO 1970

| SEX AND HEIGHT | *n* | *N* | $\bar{X}$ | *s* | $s_{\bar{x}}$ | PERCENTILE 5th | 10th | 25th | 50th | 75th | 90th | 95th |
|---|---|---|---|---|---|---|---|---|---|---|---|---|
| Male | | | | | | in kilograms | | | | | | |
| Under 130 | — | — | — | — | — | — | — | — | — | — | — | — |
| 130.0–134.9 | 2 | 5 | * | * | * | * | * | * | * | * | * | * |
| 135.0–139.9 | 6 | 25 | 32.62 | 5.624 | 7.716 | 27.2 | 27.6 | 28.9 | 31.0 | 34.9 | 43.1 | 43.2 |
| 140.0–144.9 | 18 | 56 | 36.54 | 5.852 | 1.607 | 30.0 | 30.5 | 32.1 | 36.1 | 39.2 | 41.7 | 53.2 |
| 145.0–149.9 | 65 | 204 | 39.03 | 5.270 | 0.662 | 32.4 | 33.9 | 36.1 | 37.9 | 41.2 | 44.5 | 46.4 |
| 150.0–154.9 | 99 | 312 | 42.58 | 6.724 | 0.865 | 34.8 | 36.2 | 37.9 | 41.0 | 45.5 | 49.4 | 61.0 |
| 155.0–159.9 | 131 | 421 | 47.27 | 7.482 | 0.717 | 37.8 | 39.2 | 41.7 | 45.8 | 51.1 | 58.7 | 61.7 |
| 160.0–164.9 | 125 | 393 | 53.01 | 9.324 | 0.916 | 41.5 | 43.7 | 46.9 | 50.4 | 58.2 | 64.4 | 72.5 |
| 165.0–169.9 | 91 | 285 | 55.92 | 8.560 | 0.833 | 46.3 | 47.5 | 49.3 | 53.6 | 59.4 | 69.0 | 75.0 |
| 170.0–174.9 | 63 | 215 | 62.01 | 10.362 | 1.033 | 51.2 | 51.6 | 53.7 | 60.1 | 67.0 | 76.0 | 85.0 |
| 175.0–179.9 | 19 | 68 | 67.92 | 12.085 | 3.428 | 56.3 | 57.9 | 60.1 | 63.3 | 70.3 | 88.3 | 89.0 |
| 180.0–184.9 | 5 | 15 | * | * | * | * | * | * | * | * | * | * |
| 185.0–189.9 | — | — | — | — | — | — | — | — | — | — | — | — |
| 190.0–194.9 | — | — | — | — | — | — | — | — | — | — | — | — |
| 195.0 and over | — | — | — | — | — | — | — | — | — | — | — | — |
| Female | | | | | | | | | | | | |
| Under 130 | — | — | — | — | — | — | — | — | — | — | — | — |
| 130.0–134.9 | 1 | 3 | * | * | * | * | * | * | * | * | * | * |
| 135.0–139.9 | — | — | — | — | — | — | — | — | — | — | — | — |
| 140.0–144.9 | 15 | 51 | 37.13 | 7.317 | 2.259 | 26.6 | 27.5 | 30.5 | 36.7 | 40.1 | 44.5 | 56.1 |
| 145.0–149.9 | 47 | 165 | 42.23 | 6.880 | 0.888 | 34.7 | 35.6 | 38.2 | 40.5 | 44.2 | 53.6 | 57.6 |
| 150.0–154.9 | 98 | 329 | 44.32 | 7.029 | 0.787 | 35.6 | 36.5 | 39.2 | 42.9 | 47.3 | 53.7 | 57.9 |
| 155.0–159.9 | 152 | 499 | 49.75 | 8.757 | 0.699 | 39.1 | 39.9 | 43.8 | 48.4 | 53.8 | 61.0 | 65.9 |
| 160.0–164.9 | 156 | 515 | 53.16 | 8.399 | 0.522 | 41.2 | 43.9 | 47.7 | 52.2 | 57.0 | 63.8 | 68.5 |
| 165.0–169.9 | 86 | 284 | 58.17 | 9.125 | 0.921 | 46.2 | 47.4 | 52.2 | 58.1 | 61.5 | 69.3 | 76.2 |
| 170.0–174.9 | 24 | 87 | 58.11 | 13.209 | 2.343 | 46.2 | 47.1 | 48.4 | 52.9 | 65.3 | 68.6 | 96.8 |
| 175.0–179.9 | 3 | 10 | * | * | * | * | * | * | * | * | * | * |
| 180.0–184.9 | — | — | — | — | — | — | — | — | — | — | — | — |
| 185.0–189.9 | — | — | — | — | — | — | — | — | — | — | — | — |
| 190.0–194.9 | — | — | — | — | — | — | — | — | — | — | — | — |
| 195.0 and over | — | — | — | — | — | — | — | — | — | — | — | — |

*n*, Sample size; *N*, estimated number of youths in population in thousands; $\bar{X}$, mean; *s*, standard deviation; $s_{\bar{x}}$, standard error of the mean.

(From National Center for Health Statistics: Height and weight of youths 12–17 years, United States. *In* Vital and Health Statistics, Series 11, No. 124, Health Services and Mental Health Administration. Washington, D.C., U.S. Government Printing Office, 1973, pp. 282–288.)

**TABLE A—12F-3.** WEIGHT IN KILOGRAMS OF YOUTHS AGED 14 YEARS AT LAST BIRTHDAY BY SEX AND HEIGHT GROUP IN CENTIMETERS: SAMPLE SIZE, ESTIMATED POPULATION SIZE, MEAN, STANDARD DEVIATION, STANDARD ERROR OF THE MEAN, AND SELECTED PERCENTILES, UNITED STATES, 1966 TO 1970

| SEX AND HEIGHT | $n$ | $N$ | $\bar{X}$ | $s$ | $s_{\bar{s}}$ | PERCENTILE 5th | 10th | 25th | 50th | 75th | 90th | 95th |
|---|---|---|---|---|---|---|---|---|---|---|---|---|
| | | | | | | in kilograms | | | | | | |
| Male | | | | | | | | | | | | |
| Under 130 | — | — | — | — | — | — | — | — | — | — | — | — |
| 130.0–134.9 | — | — | — | — | — | — | — | — | — | — | — | — |
| 135.0–139.9 | 2 | 7 | * | * | * | * | * | * | * | * | * | * |
| 140.0–144.9 | 3 | 13 | * | * | * | * | * | * | * | * | * | * |
| 145.0–149.9 | 11 | 42 | 40.51 | 1.829 | 0.644 | 36.9 | 38.6 | 39.6 | 40.6 | 42.0 | 42.5 | 42.7 |
| 150.0–154.9 | 45 | 135 | 43.63 | 6.277 | 1.182 | 36.2 | 37.0 | 39.0 | 41.4 | 48.0 | 51.7 | 55.3 |
| 155.0–159.9 | 83 | 261 | 47.42 | 7.822 | 0.872 | 37.7 | 38.7 | 41.8 | 46.1 | 51.2 | 58.0 | 62.7 |
| 160.0–164.9 | 96 | 299 | 52.28 | 6.785 | 0.584 | 42.5 | 44.0 | 47.5 | 52.1 | 56.3 | 61.5 | 65.1 |
| 165.0–169.9 | 134 | 432 | 58.07 | 9.416 | 1.054 | 47.7 | 49.3 | 51.6 | 55.4 | 62.3 | 70.6 | 75.7 |
| 170.0–174.9 | 144 | 435 | 62.37 | 11.516 | 1.095 | 49.7 | 51.0 | 55.0 | 59.4 | 65.6 | 79.2 | 86.3 |
| 175.0–179.9 | 71 | 228 | 65.54 | 9.704 | 1.306 | 50.9 | 55.1 | 58.5 | 64.7 | 69.9 | 74.5 | 84.0 |
| 180.0–184.9 | 25 | 81 | 72.44 | 13.014 | 2.298 | 59.6 | 60.0 | 65.1 | 69.4 | 77.0 | 83.0 | 94.3 |
| 185.0–189.9 | 3 | 9 | * | * | * | * | * | * | * | * | * | * |
| 190.0–194.9 | 1 | 3 | * | * | * | * | * | * | * | * | * | * |
| 195.0 and over | — | — | — | — | — | — | — | — | — | — | — | — |
| Female | | | | | | | | | | | | |
| Under 130 | — | — | — | — | — | — | — | — | — | — | — | — |
| 130.0–134.9 | — | — | — | — | — | — | — | — | — | — | — | — |
| 135.0–139.9 | 1 | 2 | * | * | * | * | * | * | * | * | * | * |
| 140.0–144.9 | 2 | 6 | * | * | * | * | * | * | * | * | * | * |
| 145.0–149.9 | 17 | 52 | 42.00 | 5.879 | 1.683 | 32.0 | 35.3 | 36.3 | 42.3 | 47.5 | 49.5 | 51.1 |
| 150.0–154.9 | 64 | 196 | 48.26 | 6.797 | 0.926 | 37.7 | 39.2 | 42.5 | 47.9 | 53.3 | 55.9 | 58.8 |
| 155.0–159.9 | 157 | 508 | 51.35 | 7.705 | 0.520 | 41.2 | 43.4 | 46.3 | 49.6 | 55.6 | 62.2 | 64.3 |
| 160.0–164.9 | 186 | 603 | 54.59 | 8.810 | 0.707 | 43.0 | 45.0 | 48.4 | 53.0 | 59.7 | 66.7 | 70.7 |
| 165.0–169.9 | 114 | 372 | 58.46 | 10.185 | 0.955 | 45.9 | 47.5 | 52.1 | 56.8 | 61.8 | 70.5 | 76.4 |
| 170.0–174.9 | 36 | 121 | 64.37 | 15.821 | 2.814 | 49.2 | 52.1 | 56.2 | 59.8 | 70.5 | 72.9 | 99.4 |
| 175.0–179.9 | 7 | 28 | 61.33 | 5.496 | 2.620 | 51.7 | 52.0 | 57.7 | 59.8 | 64.6 | 70.2 | 70.6 |
| 180.0–184.9 | 2 | 7 | * | * | * | * | * | * | * | * | * | * |
| 185.0–189.9 | — | — | — | — | — | — | — | — | — | — | — | — |
| 190.0–194.9 | — | — | — | — | — | — | — | — | — | — | — | — |
| 195.0 and over | — | — | — | — | — | — | — | — | — | — | — | — |

*n*, Sample size; *N*, estimated number of youths in population in thousands; $\bar{X}$, mean; *s*, standard deviation; $s_{\bar{x}}$, standard error of the mean.
(From National Center for Health Statistics: Height and weight of youths 12–17 years, United States. *In* Vital and Health Statistics, Series 11, No. 124, Health Services and Mental Health Administration. Washington, D.C., U.S. Government Printing Office, 1973, pp. 282–288.)

**TABLE A—12F-4.** WEIGHT IN KILOGRAMS OF YOUTHS AGED 15 YEARS AT LAST BIRTHDAY BY SEX AND HEIGHT GROUP IN CENTIMETERS: SAMPLE SIZE, ESTIMATED POPULATION SIZE, MEAN, STANDARD DEVIATION, STANDARD ERROR OF THE MEAN, AND SELECTED PERCENTILES, UNITED STATES, 1966 TO 1970

| SEX AND HEIGHT | $n$ | $N$ | $\bar{X}$ | $s$ | $s_{\bar{x}}$ | PERCENTILE 5th | 10th | 25th | 50th | 75th | 90th | 95th |
|---|---|---|---|---|---|---|---|---|---|---|---|---|
| | | | | | | in kilograms | | | | | | |
| Male | | | | | | | | | | | | |
| Under 130 | — | — | — | — | — | — | — | — | — | — | — | — |
| 130.0–134.9 | — | — | — | — | — | — | — | — | — | — | — | — |
| 135.0–139.9 | — | — | — | — | — | — | — | — | — | — | — | — |
| 140.0–144.9 | — | — | — | — | — | — | — | — | — | — | — | — |
| 145.0–149.9 | 1 | 2 | * | * | * | * | * | * | * | * | * | * |
| 150.0–154.9 | 10 | 30 | 45.72 | 8.582 | 3.550 | 35.7 | 39.2 | 42.6 | 44.7 | 46.0 | 48.7 | 76.1 |
| 155.0–159.9 | 34 | 99 | 52.81 | 10.552 | 1.695 | 40.3 | 43.1 | 46.7 | 49.2 | 56.7 | 69.6 | 76.3 |
| 160.0–164.9 | 71 | 206 | 53.01 | 8.417 | 0.986 | 42.7 | 44.1 | 46.9 | 51.5 | 56.3 | 65.3 | 68.8 |
| 165.0–169.9 | 132 | 404 | 57.72 | 8.503 | 0.819 | 48.0 | 48.8 | 53.1 | 56.4 | 61.3 | 67.1 | 73.3 |
| 170.0–174.9 | 176 | 574 | 62.88 | 8.464 | 0.633 | 51.6 | 53.4 | 56.7 | 61.9 | 67.2 | 72.9 | 78.1 |
| 175.0–179.9 | 118 | 374 | 65.80 | 9.457 | 1.045 | 53.1 | 55.6 | 59.7 | 64.3 | 69.5 | 80.2 | 89.2 |
| 180.0–184.9 | 51 | 144 | 72.00 | 11.928 | 1.724 | 54.6 | 60.3 | 64.4 | 70.2 | 78.4 | 84.4 | 96.6 |
| 185.0–189.9 | 14 | 48 | 74.21 | 15.035 | 5.200 | 58.3 | 58.5 | 62.9 | 70.7 | 84.6 | 92.4 | 110.8 |
| 190.0–194.9 | 6 | 15 | 83.39 | 16.431 | 10.332 | 66.4 | 66.7 | 69.6 | 73.8 | 103.0 | 105.7 | 106.2 |
| 195.0 and over | — | — | — | — | — | — | — | — | — | — | — | — |
| Female | | | | | | | | | | | | |
| Under 130 | — | — | — | — | — | — | — | — | — | — | — | — |
| 130.0–134.9 | — | — | — | — | — | — | — | — | — | — | — | — |
| 135.0–139.9 | — | — | — | — | — | — | — | — | — | — | — | — |
| 140.0–144.9 | 2 | 5 | * | * | * | * | * | * | * | * | * | * |
| 145.0–149.9 | 15 | 51 | 47.91 | 7.875 | 3.623 | 36.0 | 39.4 | 42.1 | 45.4 | 52.7 | 55.7 | 66.3 |
| 150.0–154.9 | 69 | 242 | 49.69 | 8.895 | 1.190 | 39.1 | 40.6 | 44.3 | 48.1 | 52.8 | 60.5 | 68.3 |
| 155.0–159.9 | 111 | 400 | 51.52 | 8.473 | 0.934 | 41.4 | 43.5 | 46.3 | 50.8 | 55.1 | 59.8 | 65.2 |
| 160.0–164.9 | 137 | 509 | 57.03 | 10.828 | 0.875 | 45.1 | 47.3 | 50.2 | 55.0 | 60.2 | 71.7 | 77.7 |
| 165.0–169.9 | 109 | 398 | 60.71 | 10.357 | 1.053 | 47.5 | 49.3 | 55.1 | 58.4 | 65.7 | 74.1 | 81.0 |
| 170.0–174.9 | 49 | 188 | 65.27 | 10.730 | 1.880 | 49.7 | 53.6 | 57.2 | 61.2 | 71.6 | 85.3 | 86.4 |
| 175.0–179.9 | 7 | 23 | 63.30 | 8.872 | 4.807 | 49.7 | 49.9 | 53.8 | 62.4 | 71.1 | 71.9 | 79.2 |
| 180.0–184.9 | 3 | 26 | * | * | * | * | * | * | * | * | * | * |
| 185.0–189.9 | 1 | 3 | * | * | * | * | * | * | * | * | * | * |
| 190.0–194.9 | — | — | — | — | — | — | — | — | — | — | — | — |
| 195.0 and over | — | — | — | — | — | — | — | — | — | — | — | — |

$n$, Sample size; $N$, estimated number of youths in population in thousands; $\bar{X}$, mean; $s$, standard deviation; $s_{\bar{x}}$, standard error of the mean.
(From National Center for Health Statistics: Height and weight of youths 12–17 years, United States. *In* Vital and Health Statistics, Series 11, No. 124, Health Services and Mental Health Administration. Washington, D.C., U.S. Government Printing Office, 1973, pp. 282–288.)

**TABLE A—12F-5.** WEIGHT IN KILOGRAMS OF YOUTHS AGED 16 YEARS AT LAST BIRTHDAY BY SEX AND HEIGHT GROUP IN CENTIMETERS: SAMPLE SIZE, ESTIMATED POPULATION SIZE, MEAN, STANDARD DEVIATION, STANDARD ERROR OF THE MEAN, AND SELECTED PERCENTILES, UNITED STATES, 1966 TO 1970

| SEX AND HEIGHT | $n$ | $N$ | $\overline{X}$ | $s$ | $s_{\overline{x}}$ | PERCENTILE 5th | 10th | 25th | 50th | 75th | 90th | 95th |
|---|---|---|---|---|---|---|---|---|---|---|---|---|
| Male | | | | | | in kilograms | | | | | | |
| Under 130 | — | — | — | — | — | — | — | — | — | — | — | — |
| 130.0–134.9 | — | — | — | — | — | — | — | — | — | — | — | — |
| 135.0–139.9 | — | — | — | — | — | — | — | — | — | — | — | — |
| 140.0–144.9 | — | — | — | — | — | — | — | — | — | — | — | — |
| 145.0–149.9 | 1 | 1 | * | * | * | * | * | * | * | * | * | * |
| 150.0–154.9 | 4 | 12 | * | * | * | * | * | * | * | * | * | * |
| 155.0–159.9 | 11 | 33 | 49.89 | 7.323 | 3.572 | 42.0 | 42.2 | 44.7 | 46.8 | 54.4 | 59.8 | 67.2 |
| 160.0–164.9 | 32 | 108 | 53.09 | 6.459 | 1.273 | 44.2 | 44.9 | 48.2 | 51.4 | 58.0 | 60.9 | 66.1 |
| 165.0–169.9 | 87 | 275 | 59.39 | 9.178 | 0.981 | 48.5 | 49.8 | 52.7 | 58.0 | 63.9 | 69.3 | 75.9 |
| 170.0–174.9 | 166 | 552 | 62.66 | 7.556 | 0.629 | 51.6 | 53.8 | 57.5 | 61.6 | 67.1 | 73.1 | 78.0 |
| 175.0–179.9 | 149 | 511 | 67.33 | 9.018 | 0.856 | 56.3 | 58.2 | 61.0 | 65.4 | 72.5 | 80.1 | 83.8 |
| 180.0–184.9 | 72 | 227 | 72.38 | 12.485 | 1.993 | 58.3 | 59.3 | 64.4 | 68.9 | 76.5 | 90.2 | 96.9 |
| 185.0–189.9 | 29 | 95 | 81.06 | 14.268 | 3.265 | 63.7 | 66.6 | 69.7 | 78.4 | 90.3 | 97.0 | 111.4 |
| 190.0–194.9 | 3 | 10 | * | * | * | * | * | * | * | * | * | * |
| 195.0 and over | 2 | 7 | * | * | * | * | * | * | * | * | * | * |
| Female | | | | | | | | | | | | |
| Under 130 | — | — | — | — | — | — | — | — | — | — | — | — |
| 130.0–134.9 | — | — | — | — | — | — | — | — | — | — | — | — |
| 135.0–139.9 | — | — | — | — | — | — | — | — | — | — | — | — |
| 140.0–144.9 | 2 | 5 | * | * | * | * | * | * | * | * | * | * |
| 145.0–149.9 | 10 | 33 | 52.58 | 8.198 | 3.191 | 43.9 | 44.1 | 44.9 | 51.0 | 54.5 | 72.0 | 72.1 |
| 150.0–154.9 | 57 | 178 | 51.79 | 10.457 | 1.053 | 41.4 | 42.0 | 45.8 | 48.9 | 54.1 | 61.5 | 83.3 |
| 155.0–159.9 | 117 | 354 | 53.20 | 7.766 | 0.734 | 44.0 | 45.6 | 48.4 | 51.6 | 56.4 | 61.9 | 69.0 |
| 160.0–164.9 | 160 | 547 | 57.71 | 11.129 | 1.246 | 46.1 | 47.3 | 51.5 | 55.5 | 61.2 | 69.5 | 75.1 |
| 165.0–169.9 | 122 | 450 | 61.72 | 11.998 | 0.802 | 47.1 | 48.8 | 53.3 | 59.1 | 67.3 | 78.7 | 86.7 |
| 170.0–174.9 | 53 | 170 | 63.61 | 8.734 | 1.126 | 52.9 | 53.8 | 58.1 | 62.1 | 66.8 | 73.8 | 84.2 |
| 175.0–179.9 | 14 | 45 | 72.55 | 15.012 | 5.224 | 58.6 | 58.8 | 61.7 | 65.9 | 80.6 | 99.1 | 105.5 |
| 180.0–184.9 | 1 | 2 | * | * | * | * | * | * | * | * | * | * |
| 185.0–189.9 | — | — | — | — | — | — | — | — | — | — | — | — |
| 190.0–194.9 | — | — | — | — | — | — | — | — | — | — | — | — |
| 195.0 and over | — | — | — | — | — | — | — | — | — | — | — | — |

*n*, Sample size; *N*, estimated number of youths in population in thousands; $\overline{X}$, mean; *s*, standard deviation; $s_{\overline{x}}$, standard error of the mean.
(From National Center for Health Statistics: Height and weight of youths 12–17 years, United States. *In* Vital and Health Statistics, Series 11, No. 124, Health Services and Mental Health Administration. Washington, D.C., U.S. Government Printing Office, 1973, pp. 282–288.)

**TABLE A—12F-6.** WEIGHT IN KILOGRAMS OF YOUTHS AGED 17 YEARS AT LAST BIRTHDAY BY SEX AND HEIGHT GROUP IN CENTIMETERS: SAMPLE SIZE, ESTIMATED POPULATION SIZE, MEAN, STANDARD DEVIATION, STANDARD ERROR OF THE MEAN, AND SELECTED PERCENTILES, UNITED STATES, 1966 TO 1970

| SEX AND HEIGHT | *n* | *N* | $\bar{X}$ | *s* | $s_{\bar{x}}$ | PERCENTILE 5th | 10th | 25th | 50th | 75th | 90th | 95th |
|---|---|---|---|---|---|---|---|---|---|---|---|---|
| | | | | | | in kilograms | | | | | | |
| Male | | | | | | | | | | | | |
| Under 130 | — | — | — | — | — | — | — | — | — | — | — | — |
| 130.0–134.9 | — | — | — | — | — | — | — | — | — | — | — | — |
| 135.0–139.9 | — | — | — | — | — | — | — | — | — | — | — | — |
| 140.0–144.9 | — | — | — | — | — | — | — | — | — | — | — | — |
| 145.0–149.9 | — | — | — | — | — | — | — | — | — | — | — | — |
| 150.0–154.9 | 1 | 3 | * | * | * | * | * | * | * | * | * | * |
| 155.0–159.9 | 11 | 39 | 54.63 | 9.397 | 3.414 | 43.8 | 46.4 | 48.2 | 49.7 | 57.8 | 69.9 | 73.2 |
| 160.0–164.9 | 25 | 81 | 57.75 | 6.503 | 1.355 | 49.7 | 51.1 | 52.5 | 56.9 | 61.6 | 70.1 | 70.8 |
| 165.0–169.9 | 63 | 248 | 62.57 | 8.344 | 1.224 | 50.2 | 53.2 | 56.4 | 61.5 | 66.9 | 72.7 | 77.3 |
| 170.0–174.9 | 115 | 396 | 67.06 | 11.163 | 0.704 | 53.3 | 55.5 | 59.5 | 64.6 | 71.9 | 80.9 | 91.6 |
| 175.0–179.9 | 151 | 537 | 68.37 | 9.907 | 0.831 | 56.9 | 58.9 | 61.5 | 66.5 | 73.6 | 79.4 | 88.4 |
| 180.0–184.9 | 80 | 297 | 73.31 | 12.454 | 1.335 | 59.6 | 61.0 | 65.1 | 71.2 | 78.4 | 91.8 | 102.7 |
| 185.0–189.9 | 36 | 133 | 76.03 | 9.171 | 1.301 | 62.4 | 66.3 | 70.5 | 75.3 | 80.8 | 90.3 | 92.9 |
| 190.0–194.9 | 7 | 25 | 81.40 | 10.985 | 7.588 | 62.9 | 62.9 | 67.8 | 87.3 | 90.3 | 90.6 | 90.6 |
| 195.0 and over | — | — | — | — | — | — | — | — | — | — | — | — |
| Female | | | | | | | | | | | | |
| Under 130 | — | — | — | — | — | — | — | — | — | — | — | — |
| 130.0–134.9 | — | — | — | — | — | — | — | — | — | — | — | — |
| 135.0–139.9 | — | — | — | — | — | — | — | — | — | — | — | — |
| 140.0–144.9 | 2 | 5 | * | * | * | * | * | * | * | * | * | * |
| 145.0–149.9 | 8 | 26 | 43.49 | 3.939 | 1.604 | 38.6 | 38.8 | 40.1 | 45.1 | 45.7 | 51.1 | 51.2 |
| 150.0–154.9 | 43 | 151 | 49.96 | 6.508 | 0.827 | 41.6 | 42.3 | 44.6 | 48.9 | 53.5 | 59.2 | 64.1 |
| 155.0–159.9 | 103 | 385 | 54.71 | 9.903 | 0.775 | 44.4 | 45.5 | 48.7 | 53.2 | 57.7 | 61.6 | 76.2 |
| 160.0–164.9 | 133 | 506 | 57.79 | 10.620 | 1.028 | 46.8 | 48.0 | 50.2 | 55.4 | 61.5 | 72.3 | 82.3 |
| 165.0–169.9 | 116 | 433 | 60.63 | 10.117 | 1.182 | 47.9 | 50.3 | 55.1 | 59.3 | 65.1 | 69.4 | 71.6 |
| 170.0–174.9 | 51 | 186 | 62.18 | 9.132 | 1.407 | 50.6 | 52.9 | 55.5 | 60.2 | 65.7 | 76.1 | 82.7 |
| 175.0–179.9 | 12 | 47 | 65.76 | 8.405 | 2.229 | 54.9 | 56.7 | 60.1 | 61.7 | 75.2 | 75.9 | 83.0 |
| 180.0–184.9 | 1 | 2 | * | * | * | * | * | * | * | * | * | * |
| 185.0–189.9 | — | — | — | — | — | — | — | — | — | — | — | — |
| 190.0–194.9 | — | — | — | — | — | — | — | — | — | — | — | — |
| 195.0 and over | — | — | — | — | — | — | — | — | — | — | — | — |

*n*, Sample size; *N*, estimated number of youths in population in thousands; $\bar{X}$, mean; *s*, standard deviation; $s_{\bar{x}}$, standard error of the mean.
(From National Center for Health Statistics: Height and weight of youths 12–17 years, United States. *In* Vital and Health Statistics, Series 11, No. 124, Health Services and Mental Health Administration. Washington, D.C., U.S. Government Printing Office, 1973, pp. 282–288.)

**TABLE A–13A.** WEIGHT IN KILOGRAMS FOR WOMEN 18 TO 74 YEARS OF AGE: NUMBER EXAMINED, MEAN, STANDARD DEVIATION, AND SELECTED PERCENTILES BY RACE AND AGE, UNITED STATES, 1976 TO 1980*

| RACE AND AGE (years) | NUMBER OF EXAMINED PERSONS | MEAN | STANDARD DEVIATION | PERCENTILE | | | | | | | | |
|---|---|---|---|---|---|---|---|---|---|---|---|---|
| | | | | 5th | 10th | 15th | 25th | 50th | 75th | 85th | 90th | 95th |
| All races† | | | | | | | | | | | | |
| 18–74 | 6,588 | 65.4 | 14.6 | 47.7 | 50.3 | 52.2 | 55.4 | 62.4 | 72.1 | 79.2 | 84.4 | 93.1 |
| 18–24 | 1,066 | 60.6 | 11.9 | 46.6 | 49.1 | 50.6 | 53.2 | 58.0 | 65.0 | 70.4 | 75.3 | 82.9 |
| 25–34 | 1,170 | 64.2 | 15.0 | 47.4 | 49.6 | 51.4 | 54.3 | 60.9 | 69.6 | 78.4 | 84.1 | 93.5 |
| 35–44 | 844 | 67.1 | 15.2 | 49.2 | 52.0 | 53.3 | 56.9 | 63.4 | 73.9 | 81.7 | 87.5 | 98.9 |
| 45–54 | 763 | 68.0 | 15.3 | 48.5 | 51.3 | 53.3 | 57.3 | 65.5 | 75.7 | 82.1 | 87.6 | 96.0 |
| 55–64 | 1,329 | 67.9 | 14.7 | 48.6 | 51.3 | 54.1 | 57.3 | 65.2 | 75.3 | 82.3 | 87.5 | 95.1 |
| 65–74 | 1,416 | 66.6 | 13.8 | 47.1 | 50.8 | 53.2 | 57.4 | 64.8 | 73.8 | 79.8 | 84.4 | 91.3 |
| White | | | | | | | | | | | | |
| 18–74 | 5,686 | 64.8 | 14.1 | 47.7 | 50.3 | 52.2 | 55.2 | 62.1 | 71.1 | 77.9 | 83.3 | 91.5 |
| 18–24 | 892 | 60.4 | 11.6 | 47.3 | 49.5 | 50.8 | 53.3 | 57.9 | 64.8 | 69.7 | 74.3 | 82.4 |
| 25–34 | 1,000 | 63.6 | 14.5 | 47.3 | 49.5 | 51.3 | 54.0 | 60.6 | 68.9 | 76.3 | 81.5 | 89.7 |
| 35–44 | 726 | 66.1 | 14.5 | 49.3 | 51.8 | 52.9 | 56.3 | 62.4 | 71.9 | 79.7 | 85.8 | 94.9 |
| 45–54 | 647 | 67.3 | 14.4 | 48.6 | 51.3 | 53.4 | 57.0 | 65.0 | 74.8 | 81.1 | 85.6 | 94.5 |
| 55–64 | 1,176 | 67.2 | 14.4 | 48.5 | 50.7 | 53.7 | 57.1 | 64.7 | 74.5 | 81.8 | 86.2 | 92.8 |
| 65–74 | 1,245 | 66.2 | 13.7 | 47.2 | 50.7 | 52.9 | 57.2 | 64.3 | 72.9 | 79.2 | 84.3 | 91.2 |
| Black | | | | | | | | | | | | |
| 18–74 | 782 | 71.2 | 17.3 | 48.8 | 51.6 | 55.1 | 59.1 | 67.8 | 80.6 | 87.4 | 94.9 | 105.1 |
| 18–24 | 147 | 63.1 | 13.9 | 46.2 | 49.0 | 50.6 | 53.8 | 60.4 | 70.0 | 75.8 | 79.1 | 89.3 |
| 25–34 | 145 | 69.3 | 16.7 | 48.3 | 50.8 | 53.1 | 57.8 | 65.3 | 80.2 | 87.1 | 91.5 | 102.7 |
| 35–44 | 103 | 75.3 | 18.4 | 50.7 | 55.2 | 57.2 | 63.0 | 70.2 | 85.2 | 95.3 | 103.5 | 113.1 |
| 45–54 | 100 | 77.7 | 18.8 | 55.1 | 60.3 | 60.8 | 64.5 | 74.3 | 83.6 | 94.5 | 98.2 | 117.5 |
| 55–64 | 135 | 75.8 | 16.4 | 54.2 | 55.2 | 57.6 | 65.4 | 74.6 | 83.4 | 91.9 | 95.5 | 108.5 |
| 65–74 | 152 | 72.4 | 13.6 | 52.9 | 56.4 | 60.3 | 64.0 | 70.0 | 82.2 | 84.4 | 86.5 | 98.1 |

*Includes clothing weight, estimated as ranging from 0.09 to 0.28 kilogram.

†Includes all other races not shown as separate categories.

(From National Center for Health Statistics: Anthropometric Reference Data and Prevalence of Overweight, United States 1976–1980. DHHS Publication No. 87–1688. Hyattsville, MD, U.S. Department of Health and Human Services, Public Health Service, 1987.)

**TABLE A–13B.** WEIGHT IN KILOGRAMS FOR MEN 18 TO 74 YEARS OF AGE: NUMBER EXAMINED, MEAN, STANDARD DEVIATION, AND SELECTED PERCENTILES BY RACE AND AGE, UNITED STATES, 1976 TO 1980*

| RACE AND AGE (years) | NUMBER OF EXAMINED PERSONS | MEAN | STANDARD DEVIATION | PERCENTILE 5th | 10th | 15th | 25th | 50th | 75th | 85th | 90th | 95th |
|---|---|---|---|---|---|---|---|---|---|---|---|---|
| All races† | | | | | | | | | | | | |
| 18–74 | 5,916 | 78.1 | 13.5 | 58.6 | 62.3 | 64.9 | 68.7 | 76.9 | 85.6 | 91.3 | 95.7 | 102.7 |
| 18–24 | 988 | 73.8 | 12.7 | 56.8 | 60.4 | 61.9 | 64.8 | 72.0 | 80.3 | 85.1 | 90.4 | 99.5 |
| 25–34 | 1,067 | 78.7 | 13.7 | 59.5 | 62.9 | 65.4 | 69.3 | 77.5 | 85.6 | 91.1 | 95.1 | 102.7 |
| 35–44 | 745 | 80.9 | 13.4 | 59.7 | 65.1 | 67.7 | 72.1 | 79.9 | 88.1 | 94.8 | 98.8 | 104.3 |
| 45–54 | 690 | 80.9 | 13.6 | 60.8 | 65.2 | 67.2 | 71.7 | 79.0 | 89.4 | 94.5 | 99.5 | 105.3 |
| 55–64 | 1,227 | 78.8 | 12.8 | 59.9 | 63.8 | 66.4 | 70.2 | 77.7 | 85.6 | 90.5 | 94.7 | 102.3 |
| 65–74 | 1,199 | 74.8 | 12.8 | 54.4 | 58.5 | 61.2 | 66.1 | 74.2 | 82.7 | 87.9 | 91.2 | 96.6 |
| White | | | | | | | | | | | | |
| 18–74 | 5,148 | 78.5 | 13.1 | 59.3 | 62.8 | 65.5 | 69.4 | 77.3 | 85.6 | 91.4 | 95.5 | 102.3 |
| 18–24 | 846 | 74.2 | 12.8 | 56.8 | 60.5 | 62.0 | 65.0 | 72.4 | 80.6 | 85.5 | 91.0 | 100.0 |
| 25–34 | 901 | 79.0 | 13.1 | 59.9 | 63.7 | 65.9 | 69.8 | 78.0 | 85.6 | 91.3 | 95.3 | 102.7 |
| 35–44 | 653 | 81.4 | 12.8 | 62.3 | 66.6 | 68.8 | 72.9 | 80.1 | 88.2 | 94.6 | 98.7 | 104.1 |
| 45–54 | 617 | 81.0 | 13.4 | 62.0 | 66.1 | 67.3 | 71.9 | 79.0 | 89.4 | 94.2 | 99.0 | 104.5 |
| 55–64 | 1,086 | 78.9 | 12.4 | 60.5 | 64.5 | 66.6 | 70.6 | 78.2 | 85.6 | 90.4 | 94.5 | 101.7 |
| 65–74 | 1,045 | 75.4 | 12.4 | 55.5 | 59.5 | 62.5 | 67.0 | 74.7 | 83.0 | 87.9 | 91.2 | 96.0 |
| Black | | | | | | | | | | | | |
| 18–74 | 649 | 77.9 | 15.2 | 58.0 | 61.1 | 63.6 | 67.2 | 75.3 | 85.4 | 92.9 | 98.3 | 105.4 |
| 18–24 | 121 | 72.2 | 12.0 | 58.3 | 60.9 | 62.3 | 64.9 | 70.8 | 77.1 | 81.8 | 83.7 | 93.6 |
| 25–34 | 139 | 78.2 | 16.3 | 58.7 | 63.4 | 64.9 | 68.4 | 75.3 | 84.4 | 90.6 | 92.2 | 106.3 |
| 35–44 | 70 | 82.5 | 15.4 | * | 61.7 | 65.2 | 69.7 | 83.1 | 94.8 | 100.4 | 104.2 | * |
| 45–54 | 62 | 82.4 | 14.5 | * | 64.7 | 67.0 | 73.2 | 81.8 | 93.0 | 100.0 | 102.5 | * |
| 55–64 | 129 | 78.6 | 14.7 | 56.8 | 61.4 | 64.3 | 68.0 | 77.0 | 86.5 | 93.8 | 98.6 | 104.7 |
| 65–74 | 128 | 73.3 | 15.3 | 52.5 | 56.7 | 58.0 | 61.0 | 71.2 | 81.1 | 90.8 | 97.3 | 105.1 |

*Includes clothing weight, estimated as ranging from 0.09 to 0.28 kilogram.
†Includes all other races not shown as separate categories.
(From National Center for Health Statistics: Anthropometric Reference Data and Prevalence of Overweight, United States 1976–1980. DHHS Publication No. 87–1688. Hyattsville, MD, U.S. Department of Health and Human Services, Public Health Service, 1987.)

**TABLE A–13C.** HEIGHT IN CENTIMETERS FOR WOMEN 18 TO 74 YEARS OF AGE: NUMBER EXAMINED, MEAN, STANDARD DEVIATION, AND SELECTED PERCENTILES BY RACE AND AGE, UNITED STATES, 1976 TO 1980*

| RACE AND AGE (years) | NUMBER OF EXAMINED PERSONS | MEAN | STANDARD DEVIATION | PERCENTILE | | | | | | | | |
|---|---|---|---|---|---|---|---|---|---|---|---|---|
| | | | | 5th | 10th | 15th | 25th | 50th | 75th | 85th | 90th | 95th |
| All races[†] | | | | | | | | | | | | |
| 18–74 | 6,588 | 161.8 | 6.6 | 150.9 | 153.6 | 155.2 | 157.4 | 161.7 | 166.3 | 168.6 | 170.3 | 172.6 |
| 18–24 | 1,066 | 163.4 | 6.6 | 152.9 | 155.2 | 156.7 | 159.0 | 163.7 | 167.6 | 170.0 | 171.6 | 174.0 |
| 25–34 | 1,170 | 163.1 | 6.3 | 153.2 | 155.2 | 156.6 | 158.7 | 163.1 | 167.6 | 169.9 | 171.3 | 173.7 |
| 35–44 | 844 | 162.8 | 6.3 | 152.6 | 155.5 | 156.7 | 158.5 | 162.5 | 167.0 | 169.3 | 171.0 | 173.5 |
| 45–54 | 763 | 161.3 | 6.4 | 150.5 | 152.9 | 154.5 | 156.8 | 161.3 | 165.6 | 167.7 | 169.4 | 171.8 |
| 55–64 | 1,329 | 160.1 | 6.4 | 149.2 | 151.8 | 153.7 | 155.9 | 160.3 | 164.5 | 166.7 | 168.0 | 170.3 |
| 65–74 | 1,416 | 158.1 | 6.2 | 147.9 | 150.0 | 151.7 | 154.1 | 158.4 | 162.2 | 164.5 | 166.0 | 167.7 |
| White | | | | | | | | | | | | |
| 18–74 | 5,686 | 161.9 | 6.5 | 151.3 | 153.8 | 155.4 | 157.6 | 161.9 | 165.4 | 168.7 | 170.3 | 172.7 |
| 18–24 | 892 | 163.7 | 6.4 | 153.1 | 155.7 | 157.1 | 159.4 | 163.9 | 167.7 | 170.1 | 171.8 | 174.0 |
| 25–34 | 1,000 | 163.3 | 6.2 | 153.5 | 155.4 | 156.6 | 158.9 | 163.3 | 167.8 | 170.1 | 171.5 | 173.7 |
| 35–44 | 726 | 162.9 | 6.3 | 152.6 | 155.6 | 156.7 | 158.4 | 162.6 | 167.0 | 169.4 | 171.2 | 173.5 |
| 45–54 | 647 | 161.5 | 6.2 | 151.5 | 153.6 | 155.2 | 157.2 | 161.3 | 165.7 | 167.6 | 169.4 | 171.7 |
| 55–64 | 1,176 | 160.1 | 6.3 | 149.6 | 151.9 | 153.9 | 156.1 | 160.3 | 164.4 | 166.5 | 167.7 | 170.1 |
| 65–74 | 1,245 | 158.1 | 6.2 | 147.8 | 150.1 | 151.7 | 154.1 | 158.5 | 162.2 | 164.5 | 166.0 | 167.7 |
| Black | | | | | | | | | | | | |
| 18–74 | 782 | 162.1 | 6.7 | 150.6 | 154.2 | 155.2 | 157.6 | 162.2 | 166.6 | 168.9 | 170.4 | 173.0 |
| 18–24 | 147 | 163.2 | 6.9 | 152.8 | 155.1 | 156.4 | 158.6 | 163.0 | 168.1 | 170.2 | 171.1 | 174.8 |
| 25–34 | 145 | 162.3 | 6.3 | 151.3 | 154.8 | 156.3 | 158.1 | 162.5 | 166.2 | 168.6 | 170.4 | 174.1 |
| 35–44 | 103 | 163.3 | 5.5 | 155.2 | 156.9 | 157.3 | 159.7 | 162.5 | 167.0 | 168.7 | 170.1 | 171.7 |
| 45–54 | 100 | 161.7 | 6.9 | 150.4 | 152.6 | 154.4 | 155.2 | 162.1 | 167.5 | 169.3 | 170.5 | 171.9 |
| 55–64 | 135 | 161.0 | 7.4 | 148.7 | 149.2 | 153.4 | 155.8 | 161.8 | 166.5 | 169.1 | 171.0 | 174.5 |
| 65–74 | 152 | 158.8 | 6.2 | 148.2 | 150.4 | 152.6 | 155.6 | 159.1 | 163.0 | 164.7 | 166.4 | 169.4 |

*Height without shoes.

[†]Includes all other races not shown as separate categories.

(From National Center for Health Statistics: Anthropometric Reference Data and Prevalence of Overweight, United States 1976–1980. DHHS Publication No. 87–1688. Hyattsville, MD, U.S. Department of Health and Human Services, Public Health Service, 1987.)

**TABLE A–13D.** HEIGHT IN CENTIMETERS FOR MEN 18 TO 74 YEARS OF AGE: NUMBER EXAMINED, MEAN, STANDARD DEVIATION, AND SELECTED PERCENTILES BY RACE AND AGE, UNITED STATES, 1976 TO 1980*

| RACE AND AGE (years) | NUMBER OF EXAMINED PERSONS | MEAN | STANDARD DEVIATION | PERCENTILE 5th | 10th | 15th | 25th | 50th | 75th | 85th | 90th | 95th |
|---|---|---|---|---|---|---|---|---|---|---|---|---|
| All races† | | | | | | | | | | | | |
| 18–74 | 5,916 | 175.5 | 7.2 | 163.9 | 166.4 | 168.2 | 171.1 | 175.7 | 180.4 | 182.9 | 184.5 | 187.0 |
| 18–24 | 988 | 177.0 | 7.1 | 165.8 | 168.3 | 169.8 | 172.2 | 177.0 | 181.6 | 183.9 | 186.0 | 189.6 |
| 25–34 | 1,067 | 176.7 | 6.7 | 165.5 | 167.9 | 170.0 | 172.2 | 176.8 | 181.2 | 183.6 | 185.3 | 187.4 |
| 35–44 | 745 | 176.3 | 7.3 | 164.1 | 166.4 | 168.8 | 172.2 | 176.5 | 181.2 | 183.6 | 185.2 | 188.0 |
| 45–54 | 690 | 175.2 | 6.6 | 164.5 | 167.2 | 168.3 | 170.7 | 175.1 | 179.8 | 182.5 | 184.3 | 185.7 |
| 55–64 | 1,227 | 173.7 | 6.9 | 162.1 | 165.4 | 166.8 | 169.2 | 173.7 | 178.5 | 180.6 | 182.2 | 184.6 |
| 65–74 | 1,199 | 171.3 | 7.1 | 159.3 | 162.3 | 164.1 | 166.3 | 171.5 | 176.1 | 178.6 | 180.4 | 183.1 |
| White | | | | | | | | | | | | |
| 18–74 | 5,148 | 175.7 | 7.1 | 164.2 | 166.7 | 168.6 | 171.2 | 175.9 | 180.5 | 183.0 | 184.6 | 187.2 |
| 18–24 | 846 | 177.2 | 7.0 | 166.3 | 168.6 | 170.1 | 172.4 | 177.1 | 181.9 | 184.1 | 186.4 | 189.7 |
| 25–34 | 901 | 177.0 | 6.6 | 165.8 | 168.2 | 170.6 | 172.5 | 177.0 | 181.4 | 183.8 | 185.4 | 187.7 |
| 35–44 | 653 | 176.7 | 7.3 | 164.5 | 166.7 | 169.6 | 172.6 | 176.8 | 181.7 | 183.7 | 185.8 | 188.0 |
| 45–54 | 617 | 175.4 | 6.8 | 164.6 | 167.3 | 168.9 | 171.2 | 175.3 | 179.8 | 182.5 | 184.3 | 185.7 |
| 55–64 | 1,086 | 173.8 | 6.8 | 163.1 | 165.6 | 167.2 | 169.5 | 173.6 | 178.5 | 180.7 | 182.2 | 184.5 |
| 65–74 | 1,045 | 171.6 | 6.9 | 159.6 | 162.9 | 164.6 | 166.9 | 171.6 | 176.4 | 178.7 | 180.5 | 183.3 |
| Black | | | | | | | | | | | | |
| 18–74 | 649 | 175.5 | 7.0 | 164.3 | 166.5 | 168.1 | 171.1 | 175.7 | 180.3 | 183.0 | 184.5 | 186.5 |
| 18–24 | 121 | 176.7 | 7.0 | 165.1 | 167.6 | 169.9 | 172.5 | 177.9 | 181.0 | 183.8 | 185.0 | 186.4 |
| 25–34 | 139 | 176.7 | 6.9 | 165.5 | 168.5 | 169.6 | 172.4 | 177.1 | 181.8 | 183.2 | 184.7 | 187.1 |
| 35–44 | 70 | 176.5 | 6.4 | * | 167.6 | 170.7 | 172.8 | 175.2 | 179.9 | 181.9 | 185.1 | * |
| 45–54 | 62 | 174.2 | 6.7 | * | 167.6 | 167.7 | 169.1 | 172.8 | 178.4 | 183.2 | 184.5 | * |
| 55–64 | 129 | 174.2 | 6.9 | 162.7 | 165.3 | 166.8 | 168.6 | 174.6 | 178.8 | 180.7 | 182.8 | 186.8 |
| 65–74 | 128 | 171.2 | 6.5 | 161.2 | 162.6 | 163.8 | 165.9 | 171.6 | 175.3 | 177.7 | 180.8 | 182.2 |

*Height without shoes.

†Includes all other races not shown as separate categories.

(From National Center for Health Statistics: Anthropometric Reference Data and Prevalence of Overweight, United States 1976–1980. DHHS Publication No. 87–1688. Hyattsville, MD, U.S. Department of Health and Human Services, Public Health Service, 1987.)

**TABLE A–13E.** PROVISIONAL AGE- AND SEX-SPECIFIC REFERENCE VALUES FOR WEIGHT IN KILOGRAMS (POUNDS) IN ELDERLY SUBJECTS*,†

| AGE GROUP (YEARS) | 5% | 50% | 95% |
|---|---|---|---|
| Men | | | |
| 65 | 62.6 (138.0) | 79.5 (175.0) | 102.0 (224.9) |
| 70 | 59.7 (131.6) | 76.5 (168.7) | 99.1 (218.5) |
| 75 | 56.8 (125.2) | 73.6 (162.3) | 96.3 (212.3) |
| 80 | 53.9 (118.8) | 70.7 (155.9) | 93.4 (205.9) |
| 85 | 51.0 (112.4) | 67.8 (149.5) | 90.5 (199.5) |
| 90 | 48.1 (106.0) | 64.9 (143.1) | 87.6 (193.1) |
| Women | | | |
| 65 | 51.2 (112.9) | 66.8 (147.3) | 87.1 (192.0) |
| 70 | 49.0 (108.0) | 64.6 (142.4) | 84.9 (187.2) |
| 75 | 46.8 (103.2) | 62.4 (137.6) | 82.8 (182.5) |
| 80 | 44.7 (98.5) | 60.2 (132.7) | 80.6 (177.7) |
| 85 | 42.5 (93.7) | 58.0 (127.9) | 78.4 (172.8) |
| 90 | 40.3 (88.8) | 55.9 (123.2) | 76.2 (168.0) |

*Data from 119 men and 150 women. The subjects were all ambulatory.

†See Tables A–14b-1 through A–14b-6 for data compiled by Frisancho (Am. J. Clin. Nutr., *40*:808–819, 1984) from NHANES I and II.

(From Chumlea, W.C., Roche, A.F., Mukherjee, D.: Nutritional Assessment of the Elderly through Anthropometry. Ohio, Wright State University School of Medicine, 1984.)

**TABLE A–14A-1.** TRICEPS SKINFOLD THICKNESS: GIRLS, 1 TO 17 YEARS, UNITED STATES, 1971 TO 1974

| RACE AND AGE IN YEARS | NUMBER IN SAMPLE | ESTIMATED POPULATION IN THOUSANDS | MEAN[†] | STANDARD DEVIATION | PERCENTILE 5th | 10th | 15th | 25th | 50th | 75th | 85th | 90th | 95th |
|---|---|---|---|---|---|---|---|---|---|---|---|---|---|
| | | | | | Triceps Skinfold in Millimeters | | | | | | | | |
| All Races* | | | | | | | | | | | | | |
| 1 | 267 | 1,620 | 10.1 | 2.8 | 6.0 | 6.5 | 7.0 | 8.0 | 10.0 | 12.0 | 13.0 | 14.0 | 15.0 |
| 2 | 272 | 1,708 | 10.5 | 2.5 | 7.0 | 7.5 | 8.0 | 9.0 | 10.0 | 12.0 | 13.5 | 14.0 | 15.0 |
| 3 | 292 | 1,701 | 10.9 | 2.7 | 6.0 | 7.0 | 8.0 | 9.0 | 11.0 | 12.5 | 13.5 | 14.0 | 15.0 |
| 4 | 281 | 1,599 | 10.5 | 2.7 | 7.0 | 7.5 | 8.0 | 8.0 | 10.0 | 12.0 | 13.0 | 14.0 | 15.0 |
| 5 | 314 | 1,695 | 10.5 | 3.8 | 6.0 | 7.0 | 7.0 | 8.0 | 10.0 | 12.0 | 13.0 | 15.0 | 17.5 |
| 6 | 176 | 1,787 | 10.3 | 3.3 | 6.0 | 6.5 | 7.0 | 8.0 | 10.0 | 12.0 | 13.0 | 13.5 | 15.0 |
| 7 | 169 | 1,754 | 10.8 | 4.2 | 4.0 | 6.0 | 7.0 | 8.0 | 10.5 | 12.0 | 15.0 | 16.0 | 18.0 |
| 8 | 152 | 1,800 | 12.3 | 4.8 | 6.5 | 8.0 | 8.0 | 9.0 | 11.0 | 15.0 | 17.0 | 18.0 | 22.5 |
| 9 | 171 | 2,017 | 13.2 | 4.8 | 7.0 | 7.5 | 8.0 | 10.0 | 12.5 | 16.0 | 18.0 | 20.0 | 22.0 |
| 10 | 197 | 2,173 | 13.1 | 5.0 | 7.0 | 8.0 | 8.0 | 9.5 | 12.0 | 15.5 | 19.0 | 20.0 | 23.0 |
| 11 | 166 | 1,911 | 14.5 | 6.2 | 7.0 | 8.0 | 8.5 | 10.0 | 13.0 | 18.0 | 20.5 | 23.5 | 28.5 |
| 12 | 177 | 1,812 | 15.0 | 5.9 | 7.5 | 8.0 | 9.0 | 10.5 | 14.0 | 18.5 | 20.0 | 23.0 | 27.0 |
| 13 | 198 | 2,175 | 16.2 | 6.8 | 7.0 | 8.0 | 10.0 | 11.5 | 15.0 | 20.0 | 24.0 | 25.0 | 30.0 |
| 14 | 184 | 2,036 | 17.5 | 7.3 | 8.5 | 9.5 | 10.0 | 13.0 | 16.0 | 21.0 | 24.0 | 27.0 | 33.0 |
| 15 | 171 | 2,163 | 17.0 | 7.0 | 8.0 | 10.0 | 11.0 | 12.0 | 16.0 | 20.5 | 23.0 | 25.0 | 28.5 |
| 16 | 175 | 2,145 | 18.2 | 6.7 | 10.0 | 10.5 | 12.0 | 13.5 | 17.0 | 21.0 | 24.0 | 26.0 | 32.5 |
| 17 | 157 | 1,804 | 19.6 | 8.1 | 10.0 | 11.5 | 12.0 | 13.0 | 19.0 | 24.0 | 26.5 | 29.5 | 35.0 |
| White | | | | | | | | | | | | | |
| 1 | 189 | 1,328 | 10.2 | 2.8 | 6.0 | 7.0 | 7.0 | 8.0 | 10.0 | 12.0 | 13.0 | 13.5 | 15.5 |
| 2 | 203 | 1,434 | 10.6 | 2.6 | 7.0 | 7.5 | 8.0 | 9.0 | 10.0 | 12.0 | 13.5 | 14.0 | 15.0 |
| 3 | 211 | 1,438 | 11.1 | 2.6 | 7.0 | 8.0 | 8.5 | 9.0 | 11.0 | 13.0 | 13.5 | 14.0 | 15.0 |
| 4 | 204 | 1,339 | 10.8 | 2.6 | 7.5 | 8.0 | 8.0 | 9.0 | 10.5 | 12.0 | 13.0 | 14.5 | 16.0 |
| 5 | 224 | 1,416 | 10.7 | 3.7 | 6.0 | 7.0 | 8.0 | 8.5 | 10.0 | 12.0 | 13.0 | 15.0 | 17.5 |
| 6 | 125 | 1,445 | 10.6 | 3.3 | 6.5 | 7.0 | 7.5 | 8.0 | 10.5 | 12.0 | 13.0 | 14.0 | 16.0 |
| 7 | 122 | 1,507 | 10.9 | 4.2 | 4.0 | 6.0 | 7.0 | 8.0 | 11.0 | 12.0 | 15.0 | 15.5 | 17.5 |
| 8 | 117 | 1,507 | 12.4 | 4.7 | 7.0 | 8.0 | 8.0 | 9.0 | 11.5 | 15.0 | 16.5 | 18.0 | 22.0 |
| 9 | 129 | 1,751 | 13.6 | 4.6 | 7.5 | 8.0 | 9.0 | 10.0 | 13.0 | 16.0 | 18.0 | 20.0 | 22.0 |
| 10 | 148 | 1,855 | 13.4 | 4.8 | 7.5 | 8.0 | 8.5 | 10.0 | 12.5 | 15.5 | 19.0 | 20.0 | 23.0 |
| 11 | 122 | 1,569 | 14.9 | 6.1 | 8.0 | 8.5 | 9.0 | 10.0 | 13.0 | 17.5 | 20.5 | 24.5 | 28.5 |
| 12 | 128 | 1,506 | 15.2 | 5.6 | 8.0 | 9.0 | 10.0 | 11.0 | 14.0 | 18.5 | 20.0 | 23.0 | 26.0 |
| 13 | 153 | 1,886 | 16.2 | 6.8 | 7.0 | 8.0 | 10.0 | 11.5 | 15.0 | 20.0 | 24.0 | 25.0 | 28.5 |
| 14 | 132 | 1,731 | 17.8 | 7.3 | 9.0 | 9.5 | 10.5 | 13.0 | 16.7 | 21.0 | 24.0 | 28.5 | 33.0 |
| 15 | 125 | 1,752 | 17.7 | 6.7 | 9.0 | 10.5 | 11.0 | 13.0 | 17.0 | 21.0 | 24.0 | 25.0 | 28.5 |
| 16 | 141 | 1,933 | 18.2 | 6.6 | 10.0 | 10.5 | 12.5 | 14.0 | 17.0 | 21.0 | 24.0 | 26.0 | 32.1 |
| 17 | 117 | 1,549 | 19.8 | 8.0 | 10.0 | 12.0 | 12.5 | 13.5 | 19.0 | 24.0 | 26.5 | 29.5 | 35.0 |
| Black | | | | | | | | | | | | | |
| 1 | 73 | 257 | 10.0 | 3.0 | 5.5 | 5.5 | 7.0 | 8.0 | 10.0 | 12.0 | 13.0 | 14.0 | 15.0 |
| 2 | 66 | 261 | 10.0 | 2.3 | 7.0 | 8.0 | 8.0 | 8.0 | 10.0 | 11.0 | 12.0 | 14.0 | 15.5 |
| 3 | 78 | 245 | 9.7 | 2.9 | 6.0 | 7.0 | 7.0 | 8.0 | 10.0 | 11.0 | 12.0 | 13.0 | 14.0 |
| 4 | 73 | 246 | 8.8 | 2.7 | 5.0 | 6.0 | 7.0 | 7.0 | 8.0 | 10.5 | 12.0 | 13.0 | 14.0 |
| 5 | 88 | 265 | 9.4 | 3.9 | 5.0 | 5.0 | 6.5 | 7.0 | 8.0 | 10.0 | 12.0 | 13.5 | 17.0 |
| 6 | 50 | 336 | 9.0 | 3.1 | 5.5 | 6.0 | 6.0 | 8.0 | 8.0 | 10.0 | 11.5 | 12.0 | 13.0 |
| 7 | 46 | 241 | 10.1 | 4.0 | 5.0 | 6.0 | 7.0 | 7.5 | 9.0 | 11.0 | 17.5 | 18.0 | 18.0 |
| 8 | 35 | 293 | 11.5 | 5.1 | 5.0 | 6.5 | 7.0 | 8.0 | 10.0 | 13.5 | 18.0 | 18.0 | 23.0 |
| 9 | 41 | 247 | 10.2 | 5.1 | 5.5 | 6.0 | 6.0 | 6.5 | 8.0 | 12.0 | 18.0 | 18.0 | 20.0 |
| 10 | 48 | 303 | 11.7 | 5.6 | 6.5 | 6.5 | 7.0 | 7.5 | 10.0 | 16.0 | 18.0 | 19.0 | 24.0 |
| 11 | 42 | 315 | 12.7 | 6.4 | 4.0 | 5.0 | 6.5 | 7.5 | 10.0 | 18.0 | 22.0 | 23.0 | 23.0 |
| 12 | 47 | 284 | 13.6 | 7.6 | 5.5 | 6.0 | 6.0 | 7.5 | 12.0 | 17.0 | 22.0 | 25.0 | 30.0 |
| 13 | 44 | 287 | 16.1 | 7.0 | 7.0 | 8.5 | 10.0 | 11.0 | 14.0 | 18.0 | 24.0 | 24.0 | 33.5 |
| 14 | 50 | 265 | 15.9 | 6.7 | 8.0 | 8.0 | 9.0 | 10.5 | 14.0 | 20.5 | 24.0 | 24.5 | 24.5 |
| 15 | 46 | 411 | 14.0 | 7.6 | 6.5 | 6.5 | 8.0 | 10.0 | 12.5 | 16.0 | 16.5 | 20.0 | 32.8 |
| 16 | 33 | 203 | 18.9 | 8.0 | 8.0 | 8.0 | 10.0 | 12.0 | 19.0 | 24.0 | 24.5 | 33.0 | 33.1 |
| 17 | 39 | 239 | 16.9 | 6.6 | 7.5 | 9.0 | 11.0 | 12.0 | 14.5 | 20.0 | 24.0 | 28.0 | 31.0 |

*Includes data for races that are not shown separately.

[†]Measurements made in the right arm.

(From the National Center for Health Statistics, Department of Health and Human Services. See also Bishop, C.W., Bowen, P.E., Ritchey, S.J.: Am. J. Clin. Nutr., *34*:2530–2539, 1981.)

**TABLE A–14A-2.** SUBSCAPULAR SKINFOLD THICKNESS: GIRLS, 1 TO 17 YEARS, UNITED STATES, 1971 TO 1974

| RACE AND AGE IN YEARS | NUMBER IN SAMPLE | ESTIMATED POPULATION IN THOUSANDS | MEAN† | STANDARD DEVIATION | PERCENTILE | | | | | | | | |
|---|---|---|---|---|---|---|---|---|---|---|---|---|---|
| | | | | | 5th | 10th | 15th | 25th | 50th | 75th | 85th | 90th | 95th |
| All Races* | | | | | Subscapular Skinfold in Millimeters | | | | | | | | |
| 1 | 267 | 1,620 | 6.2 | 1.9 | 4.0 | 4.0 | 4.0 | 5.0 | 6.0 | 8.0 | 8.0 | 9.0 | 9.0 |
| 2 | 272 | 1,708 | 6.2 | 2.4 | 4.0 | 4.0 | 4.0 | 5.0 | 6.0 | 7.0 | 8.0 | 9.0 | 10.0 |
| 3 | 292 | 1,701 | 5.8 | 2.0 | 4.0 | 4.0 | 4.0 | 4.5 | 5.5 | 6.5 | 7.0 | 8.0 | 9.0 |
| 4 | 281 | 1,599 | 5.6 | 1.9 | 3.5 | 4.0 | 4.0 | 4.5 | 5.0 | 6.0 | 7.0 | 8.0 | 9.0 |
| 5 | 314 | 1,695 | 6.2 | 3.3 | 3.5 | 4.0 | 4.0 | 4.0 | 5.0 | 6.5 | 8.0 | 9.0 | 15.0 |
| 6 | 176 | 1,787 | 6.0 | 2.8 | 3.0 | 4.0 | 4.0 | 4.5 | 5.5 | 6.5 | 7.0 | 8.0 | 10.0 |
| 7 | 169 | 1,754 | 6.2 | 3.3 | 3.0 | 4.0 | 4.0 | 4.5 | 5.0 | 7.0 | 9.0 | 10.5 | 11.5 |
| 8 | 152 | 1,800 | 7.7 | 5.5 | 3.5 | 4.0 | 4.0 | 4.5 | 5.5 | 8.0 | 12.5 | 14.5 | 19.5 |
| 9 | 171 | 2,017 | 8.5 | 5.0 | 4.0 | 4.0 | 4.5 | 5.0 | 7.0 | 10.0 | 13.0 | 17.0 | 19.0 |
| 10 | 197 | 2,173 | 8.6 | 5.1 | 4.0 | 4.5 | 5.0 | 5.5 | 6.5 | 10.0 | 13.0 | 18.0 | 20.0 |
| 11 | 166 | 1,911 | 10.1 | 6.4 | 4.0 | 5.0 | 5.0 | 6.0 | 8.0 | 13.0 | 16.0 | 19.0 | 25.5 |
| 12 | 177 | 1,812 | 11.1 | 6.8 | 5.0 | 5.0 | 5.5 | 6.0 | 9.5 | 13.0 | 16.0 | 20.0 | 25.0 |
| 13 | 198 | 2,175 | 11.9 | 7.1 | 5.0 | 6.0 | 6.0 | 7.0 | 9.5 | 15.0 | 19.0 | 23.4 | 26.0 |
| 14 | 184 | 2,036 | 13.0 | 8.0 | 5.0 | 6.0 | 6.5 | 8.0 | 10.0 | 16.0 | 19.0 | 24.0 | 28.0 |
| 15 | 171 | 2,163 | 12.2 | 7.2 | 6.0 | 6.5 | 7.0 | 7.5 | 10.0 | 14.0 | 18.0 | 20.0 | 27.0 |
| 16 | 175 | 2,145 | 13.4 | 7.8 | 6.0 | 7.0 | 7.5 | 8.0 | 10.5 | 15.0 | 21.0 | 25.5 | 29.0 |
| 17 | 157 | 1,804 | 15.6 | 9.4 | 6.5 | 7.0 | 7.5 | 9.0 | 12.5 | 20.0 | 25.5 | 27.0 | 34.1 |
| White | | | | | | | | | | | | | |
| 1 | 189 | 1,328 | 6.3 | 1.9 | 3.5 | 4.0 | 4.0 | 5.0 | 6.0 | 8.0 | 8.0 | 9.0 | 9.5 |
| 2 | 203 | 1,434 | 6.0 | 2.1 | 4.0 | 4.0 | 4.0 | 5.0 | 6.0 | 7.0 | 8.0 | 8.5 | 10.0 |
| 3 | 211 | 1,438 | 5.8 | 1.9 | 4.0 | 4.0 | 4.0 | 5.0 | 5.5 | 6.5 | 7.0 | 8.0 | 9.0 |
| 4 | 204 | 1,339 | 5.7 | 1.9 | 3.5 | 4.0 | 4.0 | 4.5 | 5.0 | 6.0 | 7.0 | 8.0 | 9.0 |
| 5 | 224 | 1,416 | 6.2 | 3.2 | 3.5 | 4.0 | 4.0 | 4.5 | 5.5 | 6.5 | 8.0 | 10.0 | 15.0 |
| 6 | 125 | 1,445 | 6.0 | 2.7 | 3.0 | 3.5 | 4.0 | 4.5 | 6.0 | 6.5 | 7.0 | 8.0 | 10.0 |
| 7 | 122 | 1,507 | 6.2 | 3.4 | 3.0 | 3.5 | 4.0 | 4.5 | 5.0 | 7.0 | 8.5 | 10.0 | 12.5 |
| 8 | 117 | 1,507 | 7.6 | 5.6 | 3.5 | 4.0 | 4.0 | 4.5 | 6.0 | 8.0 | 10.0 | 13.0 | 21.0 |
| 9 | 129 | 1,751 | 8.5 | 4.7 | 4.0 | 4.5 | 5.0 | 5.0 | 7.0 | 10.0 | 13.0 | 16.0 | 18.0 |
| 10 | 148 | 1,855 | 8.8 | 5.1 | 4.0 | 4.5 | 5.0 | 5.5 | 7.0 | 10.0 | 13.0 | 18.0 | 20.0 |
| 11 | 122 | 1,569 | 10.3 | 6.7 | 4.0 | 5.0 | 5.0 | 6.0 | 8.0 | 13.0 | 16.5 | 20.5 | 25.5 |
| 12 | 128 | 1,506 | 11.1 | 6.4 | 5.0 | 5.0 | 6.0 | 6.5 | 9.5 | 13.5 | 17.0 | 20.0 | 22.0 |
| 13 | 153 | 1,886 | 11.6 | 6.9 | 5.0 | 5.5 | 6.0 | 7.0 | 9.0 | 15.0 | 19.0 | 21.0 | 25.0 |
| 14 | 132 | 1,731 | 13.2 | 8.2 | 5.0 | 6.0 | 6.5 | 8.0 | 10.5 | 16.0 | 20.0 | 24.0 | 30.0 |
| 15 | 125 | 1,752 | 12.4 | 6.9 | 6.0 | 7.0 | 7.0 | 8.0 | 10.0 | 14.5 | 18.0 | 20.0 | 27.0 |
| 16 | 141 | 1,933 | 12.9 | 7.3 | 6.0 | 7.0 | 7.5 | 8.0 | 10.0 | 15.0 | 20.5 | 25.0 | 28.5 |
| 17 | 117 | 1,549 | 15.2 | 9.3 | 6.0 | 7.0 | 7.5 | 8.0 | 12.5 | 18.0 | 25.0 | 26.5 | 34.0 |
| Black | | | | | | | | | | | | | |
| 1 | 73 | 257 | 6.1 | 2.0 | 4.0 | 4.0 | 4.0 | 5.0 | 5.5 | 8.0 | 8.5 | 9.0 | 9.0 |
| 2 | 66 | 261 | 6.8 | 3.3 | 4.0 | 4.0 | 4.5 | 5.0 | 6.0 | 7.5 | 9.5 | 12.0 | 15.5 |
| 3 | 78 | 245 | 5.5 | 2.0 | 4.0 | 4.0 | 4.0 | 4.5 | 5.0 | 6.0 | 7.0 | 7.0 | 8.0 |
| 4 | 73 | 246 | 5.2 | 1.7 | 3.0 | 3.5 | 4.0 | 4.0 | 5.0 | 6.0 | 6.0 | 8.0 | 8.5 |
| 5 | 88 | 265 | 5.8 | 3.5 | 4.0 | 4.0 | 4.0 | 4.0 | 5.0 | 6.0 | 6.5 | 7.0 | 13.0 |
| 6 | 50 | 336 | 6.0 | 3.3 | 3.0 | 4.0 | 4.0 | 4.5 | 5.0 | 7.0 | 7.5 | 7.5 | 10.0 |
| 7 | 46 | 241 | 6.4 | 2.6 | 3.0 | 4.0 | 4.0 | 5.0 | 5.5 | 8.0 | 11.0 | 11.0 | 11.0 |
| 8 | 35 | 293 | 8.2 | 5.2 | 4.0 | 4.0 | 4.0 | 4.5 | 5.0 | 14.0 | 15.0 | 16.0 | 17.5 |
| 9 | 41 | 247 | 8.3 | 6.4 | 4.0 | 4.0 | 4.0 | 4.5 | 5.5 | 7.5 | 14.5 | 24.0 | 24.0 |
| 10 | 48 | 303 | 8.1 | 5.5 | 4.0 | 4.0 | 4.5 | 5.0 | 6.0 | 8.0 | 12.5 | 14.3 | 22.0 |
| 11 | 42 | 315 | 9.2 | 4.5 | 4.0 | 5.0 | 5.0 | 5.5 | 8.0 | 11.0 | 14.5 | 14.5 | 15.5 |
| 12 | 47 | 284 | 10.7 | 8.6 | 4.5 | 5.0 | 5.0 | 5.5 | 7.0 | 11.5 | 16.0 | 28.0 | 31.0 |
| 13 | 44 | 287 | 13.9 | 8.1 | 6.0 | 6.0 | 6.5 | 8.0 | 12.0 | 15.0 | 26.0 | 26.0 | 28.4 |
| 14 | 50 | 265 | 12.5 | 7.3 | 6.0 | 6.0 | 6.5 | 7.0 | 10.0 | 16.5 | 23.0 | 23.0 | 25.0 |
| 15 | 46 | 411 | 11.2 | 8.4 | 5.5 | 5.5 | 6.0 | 6.5 | 7.5 | 10.5 | 19.0 | 20.0 | 33.4 |
| 16 | 33 | 203 | 17.8 | 10.7 | 6.0 | 7.0 | 8.0 | 10.5 | 15.0 | 24.5 | 31.0 | 38.0 | 38.0 |
| 17 | 39 | 239 | 16.4 | 8.4 | 7.0 | 7.5 | 8.0 | 9.0 | 12.5 | 23.5 | 27.0 | 28.0 | 30.0 |

*Includes data for races that are not shown separately.

†Measurements made in the right arm.

(From the National Center for Health Statistics, Department of Health and Human Services. See also Bishop, C.W., Bowen, P.E., Ritchey, S.J.: Am. J. Clin. Nutr., *34*:2530–2539, 1981.)

**TABLE A–14A-3.** TRICEPS SKINFOLD THICKNESS: BOYS, 1 TO 17 YEARS, UNITED STATES, 1971 TO 1974

| RACE AND AGE IN YEARS | NUMBER IN SAMPLE | ESTIMATED POPULATION IN THOUSANDS | MEAN† | STANDARD DEVIATION | PERCENTILE 5th | 10th | 15th | 25th | 50th | 75th | 85th | 90th | 95th |
|---|---|---|---|---|---|---|---|---|---|---|---|---|---|
| All Races* | | | | | Triceps Skinfold in Millimeters | | | | | | | | |
| 1 | 286 | 1,693 | 10.4 | 3.1 | 6.0 | 7.0 | 7.5 | 8.0 | 10.0 | 12.0 | 14.0 | 15.0 | 16.0 |
| 2 | 298 | 1,747 | 10.0 | 2.7 | 6.0 | 6.5 | 7.0 | 8.0 | 10.0 | 12.0 | 12.5 | 13.5 | 15.0 |
| 3 | 308 | 1,807 | 9.9 | 2.7 | 6.5 | 7.0 | 7.0 | 8.0 | 10.0 | 11.0 | 12.5 | 13.1 | 14.5 |
| 4 | 304 | 1,815 | 9.4 | 2.5 | 5.0 | 6.5 | 7.0 | 8.0 | 9.0 | 11.0 | 12.0 | 12.5 | 14.0 |
| 5 | 273 | 1,563 | 9.5 | 3.3 | 5.0 | 6.0 | 7.0 | 7.0 | 9.0 | 11.0 | 12.5 | 13.5 | 15.0 |
| 6 | 179 | 1,673 | 8.6 | 3.0 | 5.0 | 5.5 | 6.0 | 6.5 | 8.0 | 10.0 | 12.0 | 12.0 | 14.0 |
| 7 | 164 | 1,979 | 8.9 | 3.5 | 4.0 | 5.0 | 6.0 | 6.5 | 8.0 | 10.0 | 12.0 | 13.0 | 15.5 |
| 8 | 152 | 1,861 | 9.0 | 3.3 | 5.0 | 5.5 | 6.0 | 6.5 | 8.0 | 10.0 | 12.0 | 13.0 | 16.0 |
| 9 | 169 | 2,019 | 10.6 | 4.8 | 5.0 | 6.0 | 6.5 | 7.0 | 9.0 | 14.0 | 17.0 | 17.0 | 19.0 |
| 10 | 184 | 2,205 | 10.9 | 4.4 | 5.5 | 6.0 | 6.0 | 8.0 | 10.0 | 13.5 | 15.0 | 17.0 | 19.5 |
| 11 | 178 | 2,177 | 11.9 | 6.4 | 5.0 | 6.0 | 6.0 | 7.5 | 10.0 | 14.5 | 18.0 | 20.0 | 24.0 |
| 12 | 200 | 2,304 | 11.9 | 6.3 | 4.5 | 6.0 | 6.5 | 8.0 | 10.5 | 13.5 | 16.5 | 20.0 | 27.0 |
| 13 | 174 | 1,978 | 11.2 | 6.6 | 5.0 | 5.0 | 5.5 | 7.0 | 10.0 | 13.0 | 19.0 | 22.0 | 25.0 |
| 14 | 174 | 2,030 | 10.3 | 6.2 | 4.0 | 5.0 | 5.5 | 6.5 | 8.0 | 12.0 | 16.5 | 19.0 | 22.5 |
| 15 | 171 | 2,093 | 10.0 | 6.1 | 4.0 | 5.0 | 5.0 | 6.0 | 8.0 | 11.5 | 15.0 | 19.0 | 23.5 |
| 16 | 169 | 2,019 | 9.7 | 5.2 | 4.0 | 5.0 | 5.0 | 6.0 | 8.0 | 12.0 | 14.0 | 17.0 | 22.0 |
| 17 | 176 | 2,095 | 9.2 | 5.4 | 4.0 | 5.0 | 5.0 | 6.0 | 7.5 | 11.0 | 12.5 | 15.0 | 19.0 |
| White | | | | | | | | | | | | | |
| 1 | 211 | 1,402 | 10.7 | 3.0 | 7.0 | 7.0 | 7.5 | 8.0 | 10.0 | 12.0 | 14.0 | 15.0 | 16.5 |
| 2 | 217 | 1,461 | 9.9 | 2.6 | 6.0 | 6.5 | 7.0 | 8.0 | 10.0 | 12.0 | 12.5 | 13.0 | 14.7 |
| 3 | 226 | 1,536 | 9.9 | 2.6 | 6.5 | 7.0 | 7.0 | 8.0 | 10.0 | 11.0 | 12.5 | 13.5 | 14.5 |
| 4 | 229 | 1,547 | 9.6 | 2.4 | 6.0 | 7.0 | 7.0 | 8.0 | 10.0 | 11.0 | 12.0 | 12.5 | 14.0 |
| 5 | 207 | 1,319 | 9.8 | 3.2 | 6.0 | 6.5 | 7.0 | 7.5 | 9.0 | 11.0 | 12.5 | 13.5 | 15.0 |
| 6 | 126 | 1,343 | 8.9 | 3.1 | 5.5 | 5.6 | 6.0 | 7.0 | 9.0 | 10.0 | 12.0 | 12.5 | 14.0 |
| 7 | 125 | 1,718 | 9.1 | 3.5 | 5.0 | 6.0 | 6.0 | 7.0 | 8.0 | 10.5 | 12.0 | 13.5 | 17.0 |
| 8 | 116 | 1,644 | 9.1 | 3.3 | 5.0 | 5.5 | 6.0 | 7.0 | 8.5 | 10.5 | 12.0 | 13.0 | 16.0 |
| 9 | 117 | 1,636 | 11.1 | 4.8 | 5.5 | 6.5 | 6.5 | 7.5 | 10.0 | 14.0 | 17.0 | 17.0 | 19.0 |
| 10 | 148 | 1,909 | 11.1 | 4.2 | 5.5 | 6.0 | 7.0 | 8.0 | 10.0 | 14.0 | 15.5 | 17.0 | 19.5 |
| 11 | 132 | 1,823 | 12.5 | 6.5 | 6.0 | 6.0 | 7.0 | 8.0 | 10.0 | 15.0 | 19.0 | 20.5 | 24.5 |
| 12 | 152 | 1,970 | 12.4 | 6.1 | 6.0 | 6.0 | 7.0 | 8.5 | 11.0 | 14.0 | 18.0 | 21.0 | 27.0 |
| 13 | 129 | 1,697 | 11.7 | 6.7 | 5.0 | 5.0 | 6.0 | 7.0 | 10.0 | 14.0 | 19.0 | 22.0 | 25.5 |
| 14 | 134 | 1,730 | 10.9 | 6.4 | 4.0 | 5.0 | 6.0 | 7.0 | 9.0 | 13.0 | 18.0 | 20.0 | 24.0 |
| 15 | 124 | 1,728 | 10.2 | 6.1 | 4.0 | 5.0 | 6.0 | 6.0 | 8.0 | 12.0 | 15.0 | 19.0 | 24.0 |
| 16 | 128 | 1,752 | 10.1 | 5.2 | 4.0 | 5.0 | 5.0 | 6.5 | 9.0 | 12.5 | 15.0 | 17.0 | 22.0 |
| 17 | 139 | 1,831 | 9.3 | 5.4 | 4.5 | 5.0 | 5.5 | 6.0 | 7.5 | 11.0 | 13.0 | 15.0 | 19.0 |
| Black | | | | | | | | | | | | | |
| 1 | 72 | 280 | 9.4 | 3.4 | 4.5 | 6.0 | 7.0 | 8.0 | 8.0 | 11.0 | 12.0 | 13.0 | 15.0 |
| 2 | 77 | 267 | 10.1 | 3.2 | 4.5 | 6.0 | 6.5 | 8.0 | 10.0 | 12.0 | 14.0 | 15.0 | 15.0 |
| 3 | 72 | 212 | 9.1 | 2.6 | 6.0 | 6.5 | 6.5 | 7.0 | 9.0 | 10.5 | 12.0 | 12.0 | 13.0 |
| 4 | 74 | 260 | 8.0 | 2.6 | 5.0 | 5.0 | 5.0 | 6.5 | 7.0 | 9.0 | 10.0 | 10.5 | 15.0 |
| 5 | 64 | 226 | 7.7 | 3.4 | 4.5 | 5.0 | 5.0 | 5.0 | 7.0 | 9.0 | 10.0 | 12.0 | 15.5 |
| 6 | 52 | 321 | 7.1 | 1.8 | 4.0 | 4.0 | 5.0 | 6.0 | 7.0 | 8.0 | 9.0 | 9.0 | 9.0 |
| 7 | 38 | 253 | 7.5 | 3.2 | 4.0 | 4.0 | 4.0 | 5.0 | 6.5 | 9.0 | 11.5 | 13.0 | 15.0 |
| 8 | 33 | 203 | 7.8 | 3.4 | 4.0 | 5.0 | 5.0 | 6.0 | 6.5 | 10.0 | 11.0 | 11.0 | 12.5 |
| 9 | 52 | 383 | 8.2 | 3.9 | 3.5 | 4.0 | 4.5 | 6.0 | 7.0 | 8.0 | 12.0 | 13.0 | 18.0 |
| 10 | 33 | 251 | 9.1 | 5.3 | 5.0 | 5.0 | 6.0 | 6.0 | 7.5 | 10.0 | 13.0 | 15.0 | 20.0 |
| 11 | 43 | 313 | 8.0 | 5.0 | 4.0 | 4.0 | 5.0 | 5.0 | 6.0 | 8.5 | 11.0 | 12.0 | 15.0 |
| 12 | 47 | 316 | 9.4 | 7.0 | 4.0 | 4.0 | 4.5 | 6.0 | 7.5 | 10.7 | 11.0 | 15.0 | 24.0 |
| 13 | 45 | 281 | 8.2 | 4.4 | 4.0 | 5.0 | 5.0 | 5.0 | 7.0 | 8.5 | 11.0 | 19.0 | 19.0 |
| 14 | 39 | 282 | 6.6 | 2.6 | 3.5 | 3.5 | 3.5 | 5.0 | 6.5 | 7.0 | 8.0 | 9.0 | 12.0 |
| 15 | 43 | 310 | 8.9 | 6.1 | 4.0 | 4.5 | 5.0 | 5.0 | 6.5 | 9.0 | 10.0 | 21.0 | 21.0 |
| 16 | 41 | 267 | 7.2 | 4.8 | 4.0 | 4.0 | 4.0 | 5.0 | 6.0 | 7.5 | 8.0 | 11.0 | 15.0 |
| 17 | 35 | 235 | 8.7 | 5.8 | 3.5 | 3.5 | 5.0 | 5.0 | 7.0 | 10.5 | 12.0 | 12.0 | 23.2 |

*Includes data for races that are not shown separately.
†Measurements made in the right arm.
(From the National Center for Health Statistics, Department of Health and Human Services. See also Bishop, C.W., Bowen, P.E., Ritchey, S.J.: Am. J. Clin. Nutr., *34*:2530–2539, 1981.)

**TABLE A–14A-4.** SUBSCAPULAR SKINFOLD THICKNESS: BOYS, 1 TO 17 YEARS, UNITED STATES, 1971 TO 1974

| RACE AND AGE IN YEARS | NUMBER IN SAMPLE | ESTIMATED POPULATION IN THOUSANDS | MEAN† | STANDARD DEVIATION | PERCENTILE 5th | 10th | 15th | 25th | 50th | 75th | 85th | 90th | 95th |
|---|---|---|---|---|---|---|---|---|---|---|---|---|---|
| All Races* | | | | | Subscapular Skinfold in Millimeters | | | | | | | | |
| 1 | 286 | 1,693 | 6.2 | 1.9 | 4.0 | 4.0 | 4.0 | 5.0 | 6.0 | 7.0 | 8.0 | 8.5 | 10.0 |
| 2 | 298 | 1,747 | 5.7 | 2.0 | 3.0 | 4.0 | 4.0 | 4.5 | 5.0 | 6.5 | 7.0 | 8.0 | 10.0 |
| 3 | 308 | 1,807 | 5.4 | 2.0 | 3.5 | 4.0 | 4.0 | 4.0 | 5.0 | 6.0 | 6.8 | 7.0 | 9.5 |
| 4 | 304 | 1,815 | 5.1 | 1.7 | 3.0 | 3.5 | 4.0 | 4.0 | 5.0 | 6.0 | 6.0 | 7.0 | 7.0 |
| 5 | 273 | 1,563 | 5.3 | 2.7 | 3.0 | 3.5 | 4.0 | 4.0 | 5.0 | 6.0 | 7.0 | 7.0 | 8.0 |
| 6 | 179 | 1,673 | 5.1 | 2.4 | 3.0 | 3.0 | 3.5 | 4.0 | 4.5 | 5.0 | 6.0 | 7.0 | 9.0 |
| 7 | 164 | 1,979 | 5.5 | 3.0 | 3.0 | 3.0 | 3.5 | 4.0 | 4.5 | 6.0 | 7.0 | 9.0 | 11.0 |
| 8 | 152 | 1,861 | 5.1 | 2.3 | 3.0 | 3.0 | 3.5 | 4.0 | 4.5 | 6.0 | 6.0 | 7.5 | 9.0 |
| 9 | 169 | 2,019 | 7.1 | 5.1 | 3.5 | 3.5 | 4.0 | 4.0 | 5.0 | 8.0 | 11.0 | 14.0 | 14.0 |
| 10 | 184 | 2,205 | 6.8 | 4.5 | 3.5 | 4.0 | 4.0 | 4.0 | 5.5 | 7.0 | 10.0 | 12.0 | 18.0 |
| 11 | 178 | 2,177 | 8.0 | 6.2 | 4.0 | 4.0 | 4.0 | 4.5 | 6.0 | 8.5 | 13.0 | 15.0 | 19.0 |
| 12 | 200 | 2,304 | 8.0 | 6.0 | 3.5 | 4.0 | 4.5 | 5.0 | 6.0 | 9.0 | 11.0 | 14.0 | 20.5 |
| 13 | 174 | 1,978 | 8.8 | 6.9 | 3.5 | 4.0 | 4.5 | 5.0 | 6.5 | 9.0 | 13.5 | 17.0 | 26.0 |
| 14 | 174 | 2,030 | 8.5 | 6.1 | 4.0 | 4.5 | 5.0 | 5.0 | 6.5 | 9.0 | 13.0 | 16.0 | 20.0 |
| 15 | 171 | 2,093 | 9.1 | 6.5 | 4.0 | 5.0 | 5.0 | 5.5 | 7.0 | 10.0 | 13.0 | 15.5 | 23.0 |
| 16 | 169 | 2,019 | 9.8 | 6.2 | 5.0 | 5.5 | 6.0 | 6.5 | 8.0 | 10.5 | 13.5 | 16.5 | 23.5 |
| 17 | 176 | 2,095 | 9.7 | 5.9 | 5.0 | 5.5 | 6.0 | 7.0 | 8.0 | 10.0 | 13.0 | 16.0 | 23.0 |
| White | | | | | | | | | | | | | |
| 1 | 211 | 1,402 | 6.3 | 2.0 | 4.0 | 4.0 | 4.0 | 5.0 | 6.0 | 7.0 | 8.0 | 8.5 | 10.0 |
| 2 | 217 | 1,461 | 5.6 | 1.9 | 3.0 | 3.5 | 4.0 | 4.0 | 5.0 | 6.0 | 7.0 | 7.5 | 10.0 |
| 3 | 226 | 1,536 | 5.4 | 2.0 | 3.5 | 4.0 | 4.0 | 4.0 | 5.0 | 6.0 | 6.5 | 7.0 | 10.0 |
| 4 | 229 | 1,547 | 5.2 | 1.8 | 3.0 | 4.0 | 4.0 | 4.0 | 5.0 | 6.0 | 6.0 | 7.0 | 7.0 |
| 5 | 207 | 1,319 | 5.3 | 2.7 | 3.0 | 3.5 | 4.0 | 4.0 | 5.0 | 6.0 | 7.0 | 7.0 | 8.0 |
| 6 | 126 | 1,343 | 5.1 | 2.4 | 3.0 | 3.5 | 3.5 | 4.0 | 4.5 | 5.5 | 6.0 | 7.0 | 10.0 |
| 7 | 125 | 1,718 | 5.6 | 3.1 | 3.0 | 3.0 | 3.5 | 4.0 | 5.0 | 6.0 | 7.0 | 8.0 | 11.5 |
| 8 | 116 | 1,644 | 5.1 | 2.3 | 3.0 | 3.0 | 3.0 | 4.0 | 4.5 | 6.0 | 6.0 | 7.5 | 11.0 |
| 9 | 117 | 1,636 | 7.2 | 4.7 | 3.5 | 4.0 | 4.0 | 4.0 | 5.0 | 8.5 | 11.5 | 14.0 | 14.0 |
| 10 | 148 | 1,909 | 6.8 | 4.5 | 3.0 | 4.0 | 4.0 | 4.0 | 5.5 | 7.0 | 9.5 | 12.0 | 18.0 |
| 11 | 132 | 1,823 | 8.2 | 6.4 | 3.5 | 4.0 | 4.0 | 4.5 | 6.0 | 9.0 | 14.0 | 15.0 | 20.0 |
| 12 | 152 | 1,970 | 8.1 | 5.8 | 3.5 | 4.0 | 4.0 | 5.0 | 6.0 | 9.0 | 11.5 | 14.0 | 21.0 |
| 13 | 129 | 1,697 | 9.0 | 7.1 | 3.5 | 4.0 | 4.0 | 5.0 | 6.5 | 9.0 | 14.0 | 17.0 | 27.0 |
| 14 | 134 | 1,730 | 9.0 | 6.5 | 4.0 | 5.0 | 5.0 | 5.5 | 6.5 | 9.0 | 14.0 | 16.0 | 20.0 |
| 15 | 124 | 1,728 | 8.8 | 6.4 | 4.0 | 5.0 | 5.0 | 5.5 | 7.0 | 9.0 | 13.0 | 15.0 | 22.0 |
| 16 | 128 | 1,752 | 9.9 | 6.4 | 5.0 | 5.0 | 6.0 | 6.5 | 8.0 | 11.0 | 13.5 | 17.0 | 23.5 |
| 17 | 139 | 1,831 | 9.7 | 6.1 | 5.0 | 5.5 | 6.0 | 6.5 | 8.0 | 10.0 | 13.0 | 16.0 | 23.0 |
| Black | | | | | | | | | | | | | |
| 1 | 72 | 280 | 6.0 | 1.6 | 4.0 | 4.0 | 4.0 | 5.0 | 6.0 | 7.0 | 7.5 | 8.0 | 9.0 |
| 2 | 77 | 267 | 6.5 | 2.4 | 4.0 | 4.0 | 4.0 | 5.0 | 5.5 | 7.0 | 10.0 | 11.5 | 11.5 |
| 3 | 72 | 212 | 5.3 | 1.6 | 3.5 | 4.0 | 4.0 | 4.0 | 5.0 | 6.0 | 6.5 | 6.5 | 9.0 |
| 4 | 74 | 260 | 4.8 | 1.2 | 3.0 | 3.0 | 3.5 | 4.0 | 5.0 | 5.1 | 6.0 | 6.0 | 8.0 |
| 5 | 64 | 226 | 5.1 | 2.5 | 2.5 | 3.0 | 3.0 | 4.0 | 4.5 | 5.0 | 7.0 | 7.0 | 8.5 |
| 6 | 52 | 321 | 4.9 | 2.1 | 3.0 | 3.0 | 3.5 | 4.0 | 5.0 | 5.0 | 5.5 | 7.0 | 7.0 |
| 7 | 38 | 253 | 5.2 | 2.4 | 3.0 | 3.0 | 3.0 | 3.5 | 4.0 | 6.0 | 8.0 | 10.0 | 11.0 |
| 8 | 33 | 203 | 5.5 | 2.1 | 3.5 | 3.5 | 4.0 | 4.0 | 5.0 | 6.0 | 7.5 | 9.0 | 9.0 |
| 9 | 52 | 383 | 6.6 | 6.3 | 3.0 | 3.0 | 3.0 | 4.0 | 5.0 | 6.0 | 8.0 | 8.0 | 30.0 |
| 10 | 33 | 251 | 6.7 | 3.8 | 4.0 | 4.0 | 4.0 | 4.5 | 5.0 | 7.0 | 9.0 | 12.0 | 18.5 |
| 11 | 43 | 313 | 6.7 | 4.9 | 4.0 | 4.0 | 4.0 | 5.0 | 5.5 | 6.5 | 8.0 | 8.0 | 12.5 |
| 12 | 47 | 316 | 7.4 | 6.9 | 4.0 | 4.0 | 4.5 | 4.5 | 5.0 | 7.0 | 7.0 | 17.0 | 19.0 |
| 13 | 45 | 281 | 7.6 | 5.9 | 4.0 | 4.5 | 4.5 | 5.0 | 6.0 | 7.0 | 8.0 | 18.5 | 26.0 |
| 14 | 39 | 282 | 6.1 | 2.1 | 4.0 | 4.0 | 5.0 | 5.0 | 6.0 | 7.0 | 7.0 | 7.5 | 12.0 |
| 15 | 43 | 310 | 10.6 | 6.7 | 4.0 | 5.0 | 5.5 | 7.0 | 9.0 | 12.0 | 12.0 | 24.0 | 24.0 |
| 16 | 41 | 267 | 8.5 | 4.2 | 5.5 | 5.5 | 6.5 | 6.5 | 7.0 | 9.0 | 9.5 | 10.0 | 16.0 |
| 17 | 35 | 235 | 9.6 | 5.2 | 6.0 | 6.0 | 6.0 | 7.0 | 8.0 | 10.0 | 12.0 | 16.0 | 16.0 |

*Includes data for races that are not shown separately.

†Measurements made in the right arm.

(From the National Center for Health Statistics, Department of Health and Human Services. See also Bishop, C.W., Bowen, P.E., Ritchey, S.J.: Am. J. Clin. Nutr., *34*:2530–2539, 1981.)

**TABLE A–14B-1.** SELECTED PERCENTILES OF WEIGHT, TRICEPS AND SUBSCAPULAR SKINFOLDS, AND BONE-FREE UPPER ARM MUSCLE AREA (AMA) FOR UNITED STATES MEN AND WOMEN WITH SMALL FRAMES (25 TO 54 YEARS OLD)

| HT | | | WT (kg) | | | | | | | TRICEPS (mm) | | | | | | | SUBSCAPULAR (mm) | | | | | | | BONE-FREE AMA ($cm^2$) | | | | | | |
|---|---|---|---|---|---|---|---|---|---|---|---|---|---|---|---|---|---|---|---|---|---|---|---|---|---|---|---|---|---|---|
| in | cm | n | 5 | 10 | 15 | 50 | 85 | 90 | 95 | 5 | 10 | 15 | 50 | 85 | 90 | 95 | 5 | 10 | 15 | 50 | 85 | 90 | 95 | 5 | 10 | 15 | 50 | 85 | 90 | 95 |
| Men | | | | | | | | | | | | | | | | | | | | | | | | | | | | | | |
| 62 | 157 | 23 | 46* | 50* | 52* | 64 | 71* | 74* | 77* | | | | 11 | | | | | | | 16 | | | | | | | 52 | | | |
| 63 | 160 | 43 | 48* | 51* | 53 | 61 | 70 | 75* | 79* | | | 6 | 10 | 17 | | | | | 8 | 12 | 20 | | | | | 32 | 48 | 54 | | |
| 64 | 163 | 73 | 49* | 53 | 55 | 66 | 76 | 76 | 80* | | 5 | 5 | 10 | 16 | 18 | | | 7 | 7 | 15 | 25 | 29 | | | 37 | 38 | 49 | 58 | 63 | |
| 65 | 165 | 112 | 52 | 53 | 58 | 66 | 77 | 81 | 84 | 4 | 5 | 6 | 11 | 17 | 19 | 21 | 7 | 8 | 9 | 14 | 25 | 28 | 35 | 31 | 35 | 37 | 47 | 60 | 63 | 71 |
| 66 | 168 | 129 | 56 | 57 | 59 | 67 | 78 | 83 | 84 | 5 | 6 | 6 | 11 | 18 | 18 | 20 | 7 | 8 | 8 | 14 | 26 | 26 | 32 | 31 | 36 | 38 | 49 | 60 | 62 | 71 |
| 67 | 170 | 132 | 56 | 60 | 62 | 71 | 82 | 83 | 88 | 5 | 6 | 6 | 11 | 18 | 20 | 22 | 6 | 7 | 9 | 15 | 23 | 25 | 30 | 35 | 39 | 41 | 49 | 58 | 60 | 62 |
| 68 | 173 | 107 | 56 | 59 | 62 | 71 | 79 | 82 | 85 | 5 | 6 | 6 | 10 | 15 | 16 | 20 | 7 | 8 | 9 | 13 | 24 | 30 | 40 | 33 | 37 | 40 | 49 | 59 | 62 | 69 |
| 69 | 175 | 97 | 57* | 62 | 65 | 74 | 84 | 87 | 88* | | 6 | 6 | 11 | 17 | 20 | | | 7 | 7 | 13 | 24 | 26 | | | 36 | 40 | 58 | 61 | 63 | |
| 70 | 178 | 46 | 59* | 62* | 67 | 75 | 87 | 86* | 90* | | | 7 | 10 | 17 | | | | | 9 | 14 | 23 | | | | | 35 | 48 | 57 | | |
| 71 | 180 | 49 | 60* | 64* | 70 | 76 | 79 | 88* | 91* | | | 7 | 10 | 16 | | | | | 8 | 13 | 22 | | | | | 39 | 47 | 52 | | |
| 72 | 183 | 21 | 62* | 65* | 67* | 74 | 87* | 89* | 93* | | | | 10 | | | | | | | 14 | | | | | | | 45 | | | |
| 73 | 185 | 9 | 63* | 67* | 69* | 79* | 89* | 91* | 94* | | | | | | | | | | | | | | | | | | | | | |
| 74 | 188 | 6 | 65* | 68* | 71* | 80* | 90* | 92* | 96* | | | | | | | | | | | | | | | | | | | | | |
| Women | | | | | | | | | | | | | | | | | | | | | | | | | | | | | | |
| 58 | 147 | 53 | 37* | 43 | 43 | 52 | 58 | 62 | 66* | | 12 | 13 | 24 | 30 | 33 | | | 10 | 12 | 23 | 34 | 38 | | | 22 | 24 | 29 | 36 | 44 | |
| 59 | 150 | 108 | 42 | 43 | 44 | 53 | 63 | 69 | 72 | 8 | 11 | 14 | 21 | 29 | 36 | 37 | 6 | 9 | 10 | 17 | 29 | 32 | 34 | 17 | 20 | 22 | 28 | 38 | 39 | 43 |
| 60 | 152 | 142 | 42 | 44 | 45 | 53 | 63 | 65 | 70 | 8 | 11 | 12 | 21 | 28 | 29 | 33 | 6 | 7 | 8 | 18 | 27 | 32 | 39 | 19 | 21 | 22 | 28 | 36 | 40 | 44 |
| 61 | 155 | 218 | 44 | 46 | 47 | 54 | 64 | 66 | 72 | 11 | 12 | 14 | 21 | 28 | 31 | 34 | 7 | 8 | 9 | 16 | 28 | 32 | 36 | 20 | 21 | 23 | 28 | 38 | 39 | 42 |
| 62 | 157 | 255 | 44 | 47 | 48 | 55 | 63 | 64 | 70 | 10 | 12 | 14 | 20 | 28 | 31 | 34 | 6 | 7 | 8 | 14 | 22 | 27 | 32 | 20 | 21 | 21 | 27 | 33 | 35 | 37 |
| 63 | 160 | 239 | 46 | 48 | 49 | 55 | 65 | 68 | 79 | 10 | 11 | 13 | 20 | 27 | 30 | 36 | 6 | 7 | 7 | 14 | 27 | 29 | 31 | 20 | 21 | 22 | 27 | 33 | 35 | 38 |
| 64 | 163 | 146 | 49 | 50 | 51 | 57 | 67 | 68 | 74 | 10 | 13 | 13 | 20 | 28 | 30 | 34 | 6 | 7 | 8 | 13 | 24 | 27 | 34 | 22 | 23 | 23 | 28 | 34 | 38 | 42 |
| 65 | 165 | 113 | 50 | 52 | 53 | 60 | 70 | 72 | 80 | 12 | 13 | 14 | 22 | 29 | 31 | 34 | 7 | 8 | 8 | 15 | 26 | 30 | 33 | 21 | 22 | 23 | 28 | 37 | 39 | 47 |
| 66 | 168 | 47 | 46* | 49* | 54 | 58 | 65 | 71* | 74* | | | 12 | 19 | 30 | | | | | 9 | 12 | 25 | | | | | 23 | 27 | 35 | | |
| 67 | 170 | 18 | 47* | 50* | 52* | 59 | 70* | 72* | 76* | | | | 18 | | | | | | | 13 | | | | | | | 26 | | | |
| 68 | 173 | 18 | 48* | 51* | 53* | 62 | 71* | 73* | 77* | | | | 20 | | | | | | | 15 | | | | | | | 25 | | | |
| 69 | 175 | 5 | 49* | 52* | 54* | 63* | 72* | 74* | 78* | | | | | | | | | | | | | | | | | | | | | |
| 70 | 178 | 1 | 50* | 53* | 55* | 64* | 73* | 75* | 79* | | | | | | | | | | | | | | | | | | | | | |

*Value estimated through linear regression equation.

(From Frisancho, A. R.: Am. J. Clin. Nutr., *40*:808–819, 1984, with permission.)

**TABLE A–14B-2.** SELECTED PERCENTILES OF WEIGHT, TRICEPS AND SUBSCAPULAR SKINFOLDS, AND BONE-FREE UPPER ARM MUSCLE AREA (AMA) FOR UNITED STATES MEN AND WOMEN WITH MEDIUM FRAMES (25 TO 54 YEARS OLD)

| HT | | | WT (kg) | | | | | | | TRICEPS (mm) | | | | | | | SUBSCAPULAR (mm) | | | | | | | BONE-FREE AMA (cm$^2$) | | | | | | |
|---|---|---|---|---|---|---|---|---|---|---|---|---|---|---|---|---|---|---|---|---|---|---|---|---|---|---|---|---|---|---|
| in | cm | n | 5 | 10 | 15 | 50 | 85 | 90 | 95 | 5 | 10 | 15 | 50 | 85 | 90 | 95 | 5 | 10 | 15 | 50 | 85 | 90 | 95 | 5 | 10 | 15 | 50 | 85 | 90 | 95 |
| Men | | | | | | | | | | | | | | | | | | | | | | | | | | | | | | |
| 62 | 157 | 10 | 51* | 55* | 58* | 68 | 81* | 83* | 87* | | | | 15 | | | | | | | 13 | | | | | | | 58 | | | |
| 63 | 160 | 30 | 52* | 56* | 59* | 71 | 82* | 85* | 89* | | | | 11 | | | | | | | 18 | | | | | | | 55 | | | |
| 64 | 163 | 71 | 54* | 60 | 61 | 71 | 83 | 84 | 90* | | 6 | 6 | 12 | 18 | 20 | | | 7 | 9 | 17 | 30 | 32 | | | 43 | 47 | 56 | 67 | 71 | |
| 65 | 165 | 154 | 59 | 62 | 65 | 74 | 87 | 90 | 94 | 5 | 7 | 8 | 12 | 20 | 22 | 25 | 8 | 9 | 10 | 16 | 26 | 29 | 32 | 40 | 43 | 45 | 56 | 67 | 69 | 70 |
| 66 | 168 | 212 | 58 | 61 | 65 | 75 | 85 | 87 | 93 | 5 | 6 | 7 | 11 | 16 | 18 | 22 | 7 | 7 | 9 | 16 | 25 | 27 | 33 | 38 | 42 | 44 | 55 | 69 | 72 | 78 |
| 67 | 170 | 409 | 62 | 66 | 68 | 77 | 89 | 93 | 100 | 5 | 7 | 7 | 13 | 21 | 23 | 28 | 8 | 9 | 10 | 18 | 26 | 30 | 33 | 39 | 42 | 44 | 53 | 66 | 69 | 73 |
| 68 | 173 | 478 | 60 | 64 | 66 | 78 | 89 | 92 | 97 | 4 | 5 | 7 | 11 | 18 | 20 | 24 | 7 | 8 | 9 | 16 | 25 | 28 | 31 | 41 | 44 | 45 | 55 | 67 | 71 | 76 |
| 69 | 175 | 464 | 63 | 66 | 68 | 78 | 90 | 93 | 97 | 5 | 6 | 7 | 12 | 18 | 20 | 24 | 7 | 8 | 9 | 16 | 25 | 27 | 31 | 38 | 41 | 44 | 54 | 66 | 69 | 73 |
| 70 | 178 | 419 | 64 | 66 | 70 | 81 | 90 | 93 | 97 | 5 | 6 | 7 | 12 | 18 | 20 | 23 | 7 | 8 | 9 | 15 | 24 | 27 | 30 | 39 | 42 | 43 | 55 | 65 | 68 | 72 |
| 71 | 180 | 282 | 62 | 68 | 70 | 81 | 92 | 96 | 100 | 4 | 5 | 7 | 12 | 19 | 21 | 25 | 7 | 8 | 9 | 14 | 24 | 27 | 30 | 37 | 41 | 44 | 54 | 67 | 68 | 73 |
| 72 | 183 | 231 | 68 | 71 | 74 | 84 | 97 | 100 | 104 | 5 | 7 | 7 | 12 | 20 | 22 | 26 | 7 | 8 | 9 | 15 | 26 | 30 | 32 | 40 | 42 | 44 | 56 | 65 | 67 | 74 |
| 73 | 185 | 106 | 70 | 72 | 75 | 85 | 100 | 101 | 104 | 6 | 7 | 8 | 12 | 20 | 24 | 27 | 8 | 9 | 9 | 15 | 25 | 29 | 32 | 39 | 42 | 43 | 55 | 67 | 69 | 73 |
| 74 | 188 | 50 | 68* | 76 | 77 | 88 | 100 | 100 | 104* | | 6 | 9 | 13 | 21 | 23 | | | 7 | 9 | 14 | 25 | 30 | | | 43 | 43 | 55 | 62 | 63 | |
| Women | | | | | | | | | | | | | | | | | | | | | | | | | | | | | | |
| 58 | 147 | 40 | 41* | 46* | 50 | 63 | 77 | 75* | 79* | | | 20 | 25 | 40 | | | | | 15 | 23 | 38 | | | | | 24 | 35 | 42 | | |
| 59 | 150 | 104 | 47 | 50 | 52 | 66 | 76 | 79 | 85 | 15 | 19 | 21 | 30 | 37 | 40 | 40 | 10 | 12 | 13 | 29 | 38 | 39 | 43 | 23 | 24 | 26 | 33 | 43 | 45 | 49 |
| 60 | 152 | 208 | 47 | 50 | 52 | 60 | 77 | 79 | 85 | 14 | 15 | 17 | 26 | 35 | 37 | 41 | 8 | 10 | 11 | 22 | 35 | 37 | 41 | 22 | 25 | 25 | 32 | 42 | 45 | 49 |
| 61 | 155 | 465 | 47 | 49 | 51 | 61 | 73 | 78 | 86 | 11 | 14 | 15 | 25 | 34 | 36 | 42 | 7 | 9 | 10 | 19 | 32 | 36 | 42 | 21 | 24 | 25 | 31 | 42 | 45 | 51 |
| 62 | 157 | 644 | 49 | 50 | 52 | 61 | 73 | 77 | 83 | 12 | 14 | 16 | 24 | 34 | 36 | 40 | 7 | 9 | 10 | 18 | 33 | 37 | 40 | 21 | 23 | 25 | 31 | 40 | 43 | 48 |
| 63 | 160 | 685 | 49 | 51 | 53 | 62 | 77 | 80 | 88 | 12 | 13 | 15 | 24 | 33 | 35 | 38 | 7 | 8 | 10 | 18 | 31 | 34 | 38 | 22 | 23 | 25 | 32 | 41 | 43 | 50 |
| 64 | 163 | 722 | 50 | 52 | 54 | 62 | 76 | 82 | 87 | 11 | 14 | 15 | 23 | 33 | 36 | 40 | 7 | 7 | 8 | 16 | 31 | 35 | 38 | 21 | 23 | 24 | 31 | 40 | 43 | 48 |
| 65 | 165 | 628 | 52 | 54 | 55 | 63 | 75 | 80 | 89 | 12 | 14 | 15 | 22 | 31 | 34 | 38 | 7 | 8 | 8 | 15 | 29 | 33 | 38 | 21 | 23 | 24 | 31 | 40 | 43 | 49 |
| 66 | 168 | 428 | 52 | 54 | 55 | 63 | 75 | 78 | 83 | 11 | 13 | 14 | 22 | 31 | 33 | 37 | 7 | 8 | 9 | 14 | 28 | 30 | 35 | 21 | 23 | 24 | 30 | 39 | 41 | 44 |
| 67 | 170 | 257 | 54 | 56 | 57 | 65 | 79 | 82 | 88 | 12 | 13 | 15 | 21 | 29 | 30 | 35 | 7 | 8 | 8 | 15 | 28 | 32 | 37 | 22 | 24 | 25 | 30 | 40 | 43 | 48 |
| 68 | 173 | 119 | 58 | 59 | 60 | 67 | 77 | 85 | 87 | 10 | 14 | 15 | 22 | 31 | 32 | 36 | 8 | 8 | 9 | 15 | 29 | 33 | 35 | 22 | 24 | 25 | 30 | 37 | 38 | 39 |
| 69 | 175 | 59 | 49* | 58 | 60 | 68 | 79 | 82 | 87* | | 11 | 12 | 19 | 29 | 31 | | | 8 | 8 | 12 | 25 | 29 | | | 23 | 24 | 30 | 36 | 39 | |
| 70 | 178 | 15 | 50* | 54* | 57* | 70 | 80* | 83* | 87* | | | | 19 | | | | | | | 20 | | | | | | | 32 | | | |

*Value estimated through linear regression equation.

(From Frisancho, A. R.: Am. J. Clin. Nutr., *40*:808–819, 1984, with permission.)

**TABLE A–14B-3.** SELECTED PERCENTILES OF WEIGHT, TRICEPS AND SUBSCAPULAR SKINFOLDS, AND BONE-FREE UPPER ARM MUSCLE AREA (AMA) FOR UNITED STATES MEN AND WOMEN WITH LARGE FRAMES (25 TO 54 YEARS OLD)

| HT | | | WT (kg) | | | | | | | TRICEPS (mm) | | | | | | | SUBSCAPULAR (mm) | | | | | | | BONE-FREE AMA ($cm^2$) | | | | | | |
|---|---|---|---|---|---|---|---|---|---|---|---|---|---|---|---|---|---|---|---|---|---|---|---|---|---|---|---|---|---|---|
| in | cm | n | 5 | 10 | 15 | 50 | 85 | 90 | 95 | 5 | 10 | 15 | 50 | 85 | 90 | 95 | 5 | 10 | 15 | 50 | 85 | 90 | 95 | 5 | 10 | 15 | 50 | 85 | 90 | 95 |
| Men | | | | | | | | | | | | | | | | | | | | | | | | | | | | | | |
| 62 | 157 | 1 | 57* | 62* | 66* | 82* | 99* | 103* | 108* | | | | | | | | | | | | | | | | | | | | | |
| 63 | 160 | 1 | 58* | 63* | 67* | 83* | 100* | 104* | 109* | | | | | | | | | | | | | | | | | | | | | |
| 64 | 163 | 5 | 59* | 64* | 68* | 84* | 101* | 105* | 110* | | | | | | | | | | | | | | | | | | | | | |
| 65 | 165 | 15 | 60* | 65* | 69* | 79 | 102* | 106* | 111* | | | | 14 | | | | | | | 21 | | | | | | | 62 | | | |
| 66 | 168 | 37 | 60* | 65* | 75 | 84 | 103 | 106* | 112* | | | 9 | 14 | 30 | | | | | 13 | 22 | 36 | | | | | 48 | 58 | 76 | | |
| 67 | 170 | 54 | 62* | 70 | 71 | 84 | 102 | 111 | 113* | | 7 | 7 | 11 | 23 | 27 | | | 8 | 11 | 20 | 36 | 40 | | | 50 | 52 | 61 | 73 | 78 | |
| 68 | 173 | 84 | 63* | 74 | 76 | 86 | 101 | 104 | 114* | | 9 | 10 | 14 | 22 | 23 | | | 12 | 14 | 20 | 31 | 35 | | | 51 | 53 | 65 | 78 | 86 | |
| 69 | 175 | 126 | 68 | 71 | 74 | 89 | 103 | 105 | 114 | 6 | 7 | 8 | 15 | 25 | 29 | 31 | 9 | 10 | 11 | 18 | 31 | 32 | 38 | 46 | 48 | 49 | 61 | 73 | 78 | 83 |
| 70 | 178 | 150 | 68 | 72 | 74 | 87 | 106 | 112 | 114 | 7 | 7 | 7 | 14 | 23 | 25 | 30 | 7 | 10 | 11 | 17 | 31 | 35 | 38 | 43 | 47 | 50 | 61 | 75 | 77 | 86 |
| 71 | 180 | 123 | 73 | 78 | 82 | 91 | 113 | 116 | 123 | 6 | 8 | 10 | 15 | 25 | 27 | 31 | 9 | 11 | 11 | 20 | 35 | 40 | 46 | 47 | 48 | 50 | 62 | 75 | 81 | 83 |
| 72 | 183 | 114 | 73 | 76 | 78 | 91 | 109 | 112 | 121 | 5 | 6 | 7 | 12 | 20 | 22 | 25 | 8 | 9 | 9 | 19 | 28 | 30 | 36 | 45 | 48 | 50 | 61 | 77 | 80 | 86 |
| 73 | 185 | 109 | 72 | 77 | 79 | 93 | 106 | 107 | 116 | 5 | 6 | 7 | 13 | 19 | 22 | 31 | 7 | 9 | 9 | 18 | 27 | 28 | 30 | 47 | 49 | 51 | 66 | 79 | 83 | 86 |
| 74 | 188 | 37 | 69* | 74* | 82 | 92 | 105 | 115* | 120* | | | 8 | 12 | 19 | | | | | 9 | 18 | 32 | | | | | 53 | 66 | 78 | | |
| Women | | | | | | | | | | | | | | | | | | | | | | | | | | | | | | |
| 58 | 147 | 6 | 56* | 63* | 67* | 86* | 105* | 110* | 117* | | | | | | | | | | | | | | | | | | | | | |
| 59 | 150 | 19 | 56* | 62* | 67* | 78 | 105* | 109* | 116* | | | | 36 | | | | | | | 35 | | | | | | | 45 | | | |
| 60 | 152 | 32 | 55* | 62* | 66* | 87 | 104* | 109* | 116* | | | | 38 | | | | | | | 42 | | | | | | | 44 | | | |
| 61 | 155 | 92 | 54* | 64 | 66 | 81 | 105 | 117 | 115* | | 25 | 26 | 36 | 48 | 50 | | | 17 | 17 | 35 | 48 | 53 | | | 29 | 33 | 41 | 62 | 74 | |
| 62 | 157 | 135 | 59 | 61 | 65 | 81 | 103 | 107 | 113 | 16 | 19 | 22 | 34 | 48 | 48 | 50 | 13 | 16 | 18 | 32 | 48 | 51 | 55 | 26 | 28 | 31 | 44 | 56 | 63 | 72 |
| 63 | 160 | 162 | 58 | 63 | 67 | 83 | 105 | 109 | 119 | 18 | 20 | 22 | 34 | 46 | 48 | 51 | 11 | 14 | 16 | 32 | 44 | 48 | 50 | 27 | 30 | 32 | 43 | 60 | 65 | 77 |
| 64 | 163 | 196 | 59 | 62 | 63 | 79 | 102 | 104 | 112 | 16 | 20 | 21 | 32 | 43 | 45 | 49 | 10 | 12 | 15 | 28 | 42 | 46 | 50 | 26 | 28 | 29 | 39 | 50 | 55 | 63 |
| 65 | 165 | 242 | 59 | 61 | 63 | 81 | 103 | 109 | 114 | 17 | 20 | 21 | 31 | 43 | 46 | 48 | 10 | 12 | 14 | 29 | 42 | 48 | 52 | 27 | 28 | 29 | 39 | 56 | 59 | 67 |
| 66 | 168 | 166 | 55 | 58 | 62 | 75 | 95 | 100 | 107 | 13 | 17 | 18 | 27 | 40 | 43 | 45 | 8 | 9 | 11 | 25 | 36 | 40 | 45 | 23 | 24 | 27 | 35 | 49 | 53 | 69 |
| 67 | 170 | 144 | 58 | 60 | 65 | 80 | 100 | 108 | 114 | 13 | 16 | 17 | 30 | 41 | 43 | 49 | 7 | 10 | 11 | 25 | 41 | 46 | 55 | 25 | 28 | 30 | 37 | 50 | 53 | 55 |
| 68 | 173 | 81 | 51* | 66 | 66 | 76 | 104 | 105 | 111* | | 16 | 20 | 29 | 37 | 40 | | | 10 | 12 | 21 | 45 | 48 | | | 28 | 30 | 38 | 51 | 54 | |
| 69 | 175 | 39 | 50* | 57* | 68 | 79 | 105 | 104* | 111* | | | 21 | 30 | 42 | | | | | 11 | 20 | 43 | | | | | 27 | 35 | 49 | | |
| 70 | 178 | 17 | 50* | 56* | 61* | 76 | 99* | 104* | 110* | | | | 20 | | | | | | | 16 | | | | | | | 37 | | | |

*Value estimated through linear regression equation.

(From Frisancho, A. R.: Am. J. Clin. Nutr., *40*:808–819, 1984, with permission.)

**TABLE A–14B-4.** SELECTED PERCENTILES OF WEIGHT, TRICEPS AND SUBSCAPULAR SKINFOLDS, AND BONE-FREE UPPER ARM MUSCLE AREA (AMA) FOR UNITED STATES MEN AND WOMEN WITH SMALL FRAMES (55 TO 74 YEARS OLD)

| HT | | | WT (kg) | | | | | | | TRICEPS (mm) | | | | | | | SUBSCAPULAR (mm) | | | | | | | BONE-FREE AMA (cm$^2$) | | | | | | |
|---|---|---|---|---|---|---|---|---|---|---|---|---|---|---|---|---|---|---|---|---|---|---|---|---|---|---|---|---|---|---|
| in | cm | n | 5 | 10 | 15 | 50 | 85 | 90 | 95 | 5 | 10 | 15 | 50 | 85 | 90 | 95 | 5 | 10 | 15 | 50 | 85 | 90 | 95 | 5 | 10 | 15 | 50 | 85 | 90 | 95 |
| Men | | | | | | | | | | | | | | | | | | | | | | | | | | | | | | |
| 62 | 157 | 47 | 45* | 49* | 56 | 61 | 68 | 73* | 77* | | | 6 | 9 | 12 | | | | | 11 | 16 | 23 | | | | | 38 | 46 | 52 | | |
| 63 | 160 | 78 | 47* | 49 | 51 | 62 | 71 | 71 | 79* | | 5 | 5 | 10 | 16 | 17 | | | 6 | 6 | 12 | 21 | 22 | | | 34 | 35 | 43 | 54 | 55 | |
| 64 | 163 | 107 | 47 | 50 | 54 | 63 | 72 | 74 | 80 | 4 | 4 | 4 | 9 | 20 | 21 | 22 | 6 | 7 | 7 | 14 | 24 | 25 | 29 | 26 | 30 | 31 | 44 | 53 | 54 | 56 |
| 65 | 165 | 132 | 48 | 54 | 59 | 70 | 80 | 90 | 90 | 5 | 6 | 7 | 11 | 18 | 19 | 24 | 6 | 8 | 8 | 16 | 28 | 28 | 29 | 26 | 30 | 34 | 48 | 57 | 60 | 62 |
| 66 | 168 | 112 | 51 | 55 | 59 | 68 | 77 | 80 | 84 | 5 | 6 | 7 | 11 | 16 | 20 | 20 | 7 | 7 | 8 | 15 | 25 | 26 | 30 | 25 | 31 | 35 | 45 | 54 | 58 | 64 |
| 67 | 170 | 128 | 55 | 60 | 61 | 69 | 79 | 81 | 88 | 5 | 6 | 6 | 10 | 15 | 17 | 25 | 7 | 8 | 9 | 13 | 22 | 25 | 31 | 30 | 36 | 37 | 45 | 53 | 55 | 59 |
| 68 | 173 | 95 | 54* | 54 | 58 | 70 | 79 | 81 | 86* | | 5 | 5 | 10 | 15 | 17 | | | 7 | 7 | 13 | 21 | 22 | | | 35 | 35 | 43 | 55 | 60 | |
| 69 | 175 | 47 | 56* | 59* | 63 | 75 | 81 | 84* | 88* | | | 8 | 10 | 15 | | | | | 10 | 16 | 27 | | | | | 38 | 47 | 62 | | |
| 70 | 178 | 29 | 57* | 61* | 63* | 76 | 83* | 86* | 89* | | | | 11 | | | | | | | 13 | | | | | | | 48 | | | |
| 71 | 180 | 14 | 59* | 62* | 65* | 69 | 85* | 87* | 91* | | | | 9 | | | | | | | 10 | | | | | | | 43 | | | |
| 72 | 183 | 6 | 60* | 64* | 66* | 76* | 86* | 89* | 92* | | | | | | | | | | | | | | | | | | | | | |
| 73 | 185 | 1 | 62* | 65* | 68* | 78* | 88* | 90* | 94* | | | | | | | | | | | | | | | | | | | | | |
| 74 | 188 | 1 | 63* | 67* | 69* | 77* | 89* | 92* | 95* | | | | | | | | | | | | | | | | | | | | | |
| Women | | | | | | | | | | | | | | | | | | | | | | | | | | | | | | |
| 58 | 147 | 85 | 39* | 46 | 48 | 54 | 63 | 65 | 71* | | 14 | 16 | 21 | 31 | 34 | | | 8 | 9 | 18 | 32 | 33 | | | 22 | 23 | 29 | 40 | 42 | |
| 59 | 150 | 122 | 41 | 45 | 48 | 55 | 66 | 68 | 74 | 11 | 13 | 15 | 21 | 30 | 31 | 33 | 6 | 7 | 9 | 19 | 29 | 30 | 33 | 22 | 23 | 24 | 30 | 39 | 40 | 44 |
| 60 | 152 | 157 | 43 | 45 | 47 | 54 | 67 | 70 | 73 | 10 | 11 | 13 | 20 | 29 | 31 | 35 | 5 | 7 | 8 | 15 | 27 | 32 | 36 | 20 | 22 | 23 | 30 | 37 | 41 | 44 |
| 61 | 155 | 145 | 43 | 43 | 45 | 56 | 65 | 70 | 71 | 10 | 12 | 14 | 22 | 29 | 29 | 32 | 6 | 7 | 8 | 17 | 29 | 31 | 34 | 18 | 21 | 23 | 28 | 36 | 40 | 42 |
| 62 | 157 | 158 | 47 | 49 | 52 | 58 | 67 | 69 | 73 | 11 | 11 | 12 | 21 | 29 | 30 | 32 | 7 | 8 | 9 | 17 | 25 | 26 | 30 | 20 | 23 | 24 | 30 | 37 | 40 | 43 |
| 63 | 160 | 89 | 42* | 45 | 49 | 58 | 67 | 68 | 74* | | 12 | 13 | 20 | 29 | 30 | | | 6 | 7 | 14 | 25 | 27 | | | 19 | 20 | 27 | 35 | 36 | |
| 64 | 163 | 50 | 43* | 47 | 49 | 60 | 68 | 70 | 75* | | 12 | 13 | 21 | 27 | 29 | | | 6 | 7 | 18 | 24 | 25 | | | 21 | 21 | 28 | 37 | 42 | |
| 65 | 165 | 26 | 43* | 47* | 49* | 60 | 69* | 72* | 75* | | | | 18 | | | | | | | 13 | | | | | | | 28 | | | |
| 66 | 168 | 12 | 44* | 48* | 50* | 68 | 70* | 72* | 76* | | | | 23 | | | | | | | 13 | | | | | | | 33 | | | |
| 67 | 170 | 1 | 45* | 48* | 51* | 61* | 71* | 73* | 77* | | | | | | | | | | | | | | | | | | | | | |
| 68 | 173 | 1 | 45* | 49* | 51* | 61* | 71* | 74* | 77* | | | | | | | | | | | | | | | | | | | | | |
| 69 | 175 | 0 | 46* | 49* | 52* | 62* | 72* | 74* | 78* | | | | | | | | | | | | | | | | | | | | | |
| 70 | 178 | 0 | 47* | 50* | 52* | 63* | 73* | 75* | 79* | | | | | | | | | | | | | | | | | | | | | |

*Value estimated through linear regression equation.

(From Frisancho, A. R.: Am. J. Clin. Nutr., *40*:808–819, 1984, with permission.)

**TABLE A–14B-5.** SELECTED PERCENTILES OF WEIGHT, TRICEPS AND SUBSCAPULAR SKINFOLDS, AND BONE-FREE UPPER ARM MUSCLE AREA (AMA) FOR UNITED STATES MEN AND WOMEN WITH MEDIUM FRAMES (55 TO 74 YEARS OLD)

| HT | | | WT (kg) | | | | | | | TRICEPS (mm) | | | | | | | SUBSCAPULAR (mm) | | | | | | | BONE-FREE AMA (cm²) | | | | | | |
|---|---|---|---|---|---|---|---|---|---|---|---|---|---|---|---|---|---|---|---|---|---|---|---|---|---|---|---|---|---|---|
| in | cm | n | 5 | 10 | 15 | 50 | 85 | 90 | 95 | 5 | 10 | 15 | 50 | 85 | 90 | 95 | 5 | 10 | 15 | 50 | 85 | 90 | 95 | 5 | 10 | 15 | 50 | 85 | 90 | 95 |
| Men | | | | | | | | | | | | | | | | | | | | | | | | | | | | | | |
| 62 | 157 | 49 | 50* | 54* | 59 | 68 | 77 | 81* | 85* | | | 5 | 12 | 25 | | | | | 11 | 19 | 27 | | | | | 39 | 48 | 61 | | |
| 63 | 160 | 89 | 51* | 57 | 60 | 70 | 80 | 82 | 87* | | 7 | 7 | 11 | 20 | 23 | | | 8 | 10 | 15 | 26 | 28 | | | 36 | 38 | 50 | 60 | 63 | |
| 64 | 163 | 210 | 55 | 59 | 62 | 71 | 82 | 83 | 91 | 5 | 6 | 6 | 10 | 17 | 20 | 26 | 6 | 7 | 9 | 15 | 25 | 27 | 35 | 35 | 39 | 40 | 51 | 64 | 66 | 71 |
| 65 | 165 | 335 | 56 | 60 | 64 | 72 | 83 | 86 | 89 | 5 | 6 | 7 | 11 | 17 | 19 | 24 | 7 | 8 | 9 | 17 | 25 | 29 | 31 | 35 | 38 | 41 | 52 | 63 | 65 | 72 |
| 66 | 168 | 405 | 57 | 62 | 66 | 74 | 83 | 84 | 89 | 6 | 6 | 7 | 12 | 18 | 19 | 22 | 7 | 9 | 10 | 16 | 25 | 28 | 31 | 34 | 39 | 42 | 51 | 60 | 62 | 67 |
| 67 | 170 | 509 | 59 | 64 | 66 | 78 | 87 | 89 | 94 | 5 | 6 | 7 | 12 | 18 | 20 | 23 | 7 | 9 | 10 | 17 | 26 | 29 | 34 | 35 | 39 | 42 | 52 | 65 | 67 | 70 |
| 68 | 173 | 413 | 62 | 66 | 68 | 78 | 89 | 95 | 101 | 6 | 7 | 8 | 12 | 18 | 21 | 23 | 7 | 9 | 10 | 17 | 26 | 29 | 32 | 37 | 40 | 42 | 52 | 65 | 67 | 70 |
| 69 | 175 | 366 | 62 | 66 | 68 | 77 | 90 | 93 | 99 | 5 | 6 | 7 | 12 | 19 | 22 | 25 | 6 | 8 | 9 | 16 | 25 | 28 | 30 | 31 | 36 | 40 | 51 | 62 | 65 | 72 |
| 70 | 178 | 248 | 62 | 68 | 71 | 80 | 90 | 95 | 101 | 6 | 7 | 7 | 11 | 18 | 19 | 21 | 7 | 9 | 10 | 16 | 25 | 27 | 30 | 36 | 41 | 44 | 53 | 63 | 65 | 68 |
| 71 | 180 | 146 | 68 | 70 | 72 | 84 | 94 | 97 | 101 | 5 | 6 | 6 | 11 | 16 | 17 | 20 | 7 | 9 | 10 | 15 | 25 | 26 | 31 | 36 | 42 | 44 | 56 | 65 | 67 | 71 |
| 72 | 183 | 81 | 66* | 65 | 69 | 81 | 96 | 97 | 101* | | 6 | 8 | 11 | 19 | 20 | | | 8 | 10 | 16 | 28 | 30 | | | 27 | 39 | 50 | 58 | 59 | |
| 73 | 185 | 35 | 68* | 72* | 79 | 88 | 93 | 99* | 103* | | | 8 | 13 | 16 | | | | | 10 | 15 | 26 | | | | | 43 | 56 | 67 | | |
| 74 | 188 | 11 | 69* | 73* | 76* | 95 | 98* | 101* | 104* | | | | 11 | | | | | | | 18 | | | | | | | 56 | | | |
| Women | | | | | | | | | | | | | | | | | | | | | | | | | | | | | | |
| 58 | 147 | 105 | 40 | 44 | 49 | 57 | 72 | 82 | 85 | 5 | 13 | 17 | 28 | 40 | 40 | 41 | 3 | 7 | 10 | 25 | 37 | 43 | 48 | 21 | 23 | 25 | 32 | 46 | 47 | 51 |
| 59 | 150 | 198 | 47 | 49 | 52 | 62 | 74 | 78 | 86 | 12 | 15 | 18 | 26 | 34 | 38 | 41 | 8 | 9 | 11 | 23 | 32 | 36 | 43 | 24 | 26 | 27 | 35 | 44 | 48 | 48 |
| 60 | 152 | 358 | 47 | 50 | 52 | 65 | 76 | 79 | 86 | 13 | 17 | 18 | 25 | 33 | 34 | 38 | 8 | 10 | 12 | 22 | 34 | 36 | 40 | 21 | 24 | 26 | 35 | 45 | 49 | 57 |
| 61 | 155 | 543 | 49 | 51 | 54 | 64 | 78 | 81 | 86 | 13 | 16 | 18 | 25 | 35 | 37 | 42 | 8 | 10 | 10 | 20 | 33 | 36 | 42 | 22 | 24 | 26 | 34 | 44 | 49 | 52 |
| 62 | 157 | 576 | 49 | 53 | 54 | 64 | 78 | 82 | 88 | 13 | 15 | 17 | 24 | 33 | 36 | 39 | 7 | 8 | 10 | 20 | 33 | 36 | 38 | 24 | 25 | 26 | 35 | 45 | 47 | 54 |
| 63 | 160 | 551 | 52 | 54 | 55 | 65 | 79 | 83 | 89 | 12 | 14 | 16 | 24 | 32 | 35 | 38 | 8 | 8 | 10 | 18 | 32 | 37 | 41 | 24 | 26 | 27 | 35 | 44 | 45 | 51 |
| 64 | 163 | 406 | 51 | 54 | 57 | 66 | 78 | 81 | 87 | 12 | 14 | 16 | 25 | 33 | 34 | 37 | 7 | 9 | 10 | 17 | 30 | 33 | 38 | 21 | 24 | 26 | 33 | 44 | 46 | 49 |
| 65 | 165 | 307 | 54 | 56 | 59 | 67 | 78 | 84 | 88 | 14 | 16 | 17 | 24 | 33 | 35 | 39 | 7 | 8 | 9 | 17 | 30 | 35 | 37 | 24 | 25 | 27 | 34 | 44 | 45 | 50 |
| 66 | 168 | 119 | 54 | 57 | 57 | 66 | 79 | 85 | 88 | 12 | 13 | 16 | 24 | 33 | 33 | 36 | 6 | 7 | 8 | 16 | 30 | 31 | 34 | 24 | 26 | 27 | 33 | 41 | 43 | 49 |
| 67 | 170 | 63 | 51* | 59 | 61 | 72 | 82 | 85 | 89* | | 17 | 17 | 27 | 35 | 35 | | | 9 | 10 | 19 | 35 | 35 | | | 27 | 28 | 32 | 41 | 43 | |
| 68 | 173 | 28 | 52* | 56* | 59* | 70 | 83* | 86* | 90* | | | | 25 | | | | | | | 16 | | | | | | | 36 | | | |
| 69 | 175 | 5 | 53* | 57* | 60* | 72* | 84* | 87* | 91* | | | | | | | | | | | | | | | | | | | | | |
| 70 | 178 | 1 | 54* | 58* | 61* | 73* | 85* | 88* | 92* | | | | | | | | | | | | | | | | | | | | | |

*Value estimated through linear regression equation.
(From Frisancho, A. R.: Am. J. Clin. Nutr., *40*:808–819, 1984, with permission.)

**TABLE A–14B-6.** SELECTED PERCENTILES OF WEIGHT, TRICEPS AND SUBSCAPULAR SKINFOLDS, AND BONE-FREE UPPER ARM MUSCLE AREA (AMA) FOR UNITED STATES MEN AND WOMEN WITH LARGE FRAMES (55 TO 74 YEARS OLD)

| HT | | | WT (kg) | | | | | | | TRICEPS (mm) | | | | | | | SUBSCAPULAR (mm) | | | | | | | BONE-FREE AMA ($cm^2$) | | | | | | |
|---|---|---|---|---|---|---|---|---|---|---|---|---|---|---|---|---|---|---|---|---|---|---|---|---|---|---|---|---|---|---|
| in | cm | n | 5 | 10 | 15 | 50 | 85 | 90 | 95 | 5 | 10 | 15 | 50 | 85 | 90 | 95 | 5 | 10 | 15 | 50 | 85 | 90 | 95 | 5 | 10 | 15 | 50 | 85 | 90 | 95 |
| Men | | | | | | | | | | | | | | | | | | | | | | | | | | | | | | |
| 62 | 157 | 7 | 54* | 59* | 63* | 77* | 91* | 95* | 100* | | | | | | | | | | | | | | | | | | | | | |
| 63 | 160 | 12 | 55* | 60* | 64* | 80 | 92* | 96* | 101* | | | | 15 | | | | | | | 20 | | | | | | | 57 | | | |
| 64 | 163 | 20 | 57* | 62* | 65* | 77 | 94* | 97* | 102* | | | | 21 | | | | | | | 31 | | | | | | | 44 | | | |
| 65 | 165 | 36 | 58* | 63* | 73 | 79 | 89 | 98* | 103* | | | 11 | 14 | 22 | | | | | 14 | 19 | 27 | | | | | 44 | 59 | 66 | | |
| 66 | 168 | 58 | 59* | 67 | 73 | 80 | 101 | 102 | 105* | | 7 | 8 | 13 | 21 | 25 | | | 9 | 11 | 20 | 31 | 35 | | | 43 | 47 | 56 | 67 | 72 | |
| 67 | 170 | 114 | 65 | 71 | 73 | 85 | 103 | 108 | 112 | 6 | 8 | 9 | 16 | 21 | 25 | 27 | 8 | 11 | 12 | 20 | 35 | 35 | 38 | 41 | 43 | 44 | 56 | 71 | 73 | 79 |
| 68 | 173 | 128 | 67 | 71 | 73 | 83 | 95 | 98 | 111 | 6 | 7 | 8 | 13 | 20 | 21 | 23 | 8 | 10 | 11 | 18 | 27 | 30 | 32 | 41 | 43 | 46 | 57 | 69 | 70 | 74 |
| 69 | 175 | 131 | 65 | 70 | 74 | 84 | 96 | 98 | 105 | 6 | 7 | 8 | 12 | 18 | 20 | 23 | 7 | 11 | 11 | 19 | 27 | 30 | 33 | 40 | 45 | 45 | 58 | 70 | 72 | 79 |
| 70 | 178 | 144 | 68 | 73 | 77 | 87 | 102 | 104 | 117 | 5 | 6 | 8 | 14 | 22 | 25 | 31 | 9 | 11 | 13 | 20 | 30 | 33 | 37 | 43 | 48 | 50 | 59 | 70 | 71 | 87 |
| 71 | 180 | 95 | 65* | 70 | 70 | 84 | 102 | 109 | 111* | | 6 | 6 | 13 | 18 | 22 | | | 8 | 9 | 15 | 30 | 30 | | | 46 | 47 | 54 | 70 | 75 | |
| 72 | 183 | 72 | 67* | 76 | 81 | 90 | 108 | 112 | 112* | | 8 | 8 | 13 | 23 | 26 | | | 8 | 9 | 20 | 28 | 31 | | | 47 | 48 | 59 | 73 | 78 | |
| 73 | 185 | 23 | 68* | 73* | 76* | 88 | 105* | 108* | 113* | | | | 11 | | | | | | | 19 | | | | | | | 59 | | | |
| 74 | 188 | 15 | 69* | 74* | 78* | 89 | 106* | 109* | 114* | | | | 12 | | | | | | | 15 | | | | | | | 54 | | | |
| Women | | | | | | | | | | | | | | | | | | | | | | | | | | | | | | |
| 58 | 147 | 14 | 53* | 59* | 63* | 92 | 95* | 99* | 104* | | | | 45 | | | | | | | 44 | | | | | | | 50 | | | |
| 59 | 150 | 26 | 54* | 59* | 63* | 78 | 95* | 99* | 105* | | | | 36 | | | | | | | 31 | | | | | | | 49 | | | |
| 60 | 152 | 72 | 54* | 65 | 69 | 78 | 87 | 88 | 105* | | 25 | 26 | 35 | 44 | 45 | | | 19 | 21 | 31 | 42 | 45 | | | 28 | 33 | 41 | 58 | 60 | |
| 61 | 155 | 117 | 64 | 68 | 69 | 79 | 94 | 95 | 106 | 18 | 22 | 24 | 33 | 40 | 44 | 46 | 13 | 16 | 19 | 29 | 40 | 43 | 48 | 31 | 32 | 34 | 44 | 59 | 61 | 71 |
| 62 | 157 | 126 | 59 | 61 | 63 | 82 | 93 | 101 | 111 | 19 | 24 | 24 | 32 | 40 | 43 | 50 | 13 | 19 | 22 | 30 | 39 | 48 | 53 | 28 | 29 | 34 | 43 | 59 | 63 | 76 |
| 63 | 160 | 154 | 61 | 65 | 67 | 80 | 100 | 102 | 118 | 20 | 24 | 25 | 33 | 41 | 43 | 45 | 13 | 15 | 16 | 29 | 40 | 45 | 51 | 27 | 32 | 33 | 41 | 56 | 62 | 67 |
| 64 | 163 | 147 | 60 | 65 | 67 | 77 | 97 | 102 | 119 | 18 | 22 | 23 | 29 | 42 | 46 | 50 | 10 | 12 | 16 | 24 | 41 | 46 | 55 | 28 | 29 | 32 | 41 | 54 | 60 | 78 |
| 65 | 165 | 117 | 60 | 66 | 69 | 80 | 98 | 102 | 111 | 15 | 17 | 20 | 30 | 43 | 44 | 46 | 8 | 9 | 12 | 26 | 42 | 46 | 48 | 29 | 32 | 32 | 42 | 53 | 57 | 65 |
| 66 | 168 | 64 | 57* | 60 | 63 | 82 | 98 | 105 | 109* | | 18 | 18 | 27 | 35 | 40 | | | 9 | 12 | 26 | 34 | 36 | | | 31 | 31 | 40 | 57 | 58 | |
| 67 | 170 | 40 | 58* | 64* | 68 | 80 | 105 | 104* | 109* | | | 22 | 32 | 44 | | | | | 14 | 25 | 46 | | | | | 30 | 40 | 58 | | |
| 68 | 173 | 17 | 58* | 64* | 68* | 79 | 100* | 104* | 110* | | | | 26 | | | | | | | 21 | | | | | | | 48 | | | |
| 69 | 175 | 7 | 59* | 65* | 69* | 85* | 101* | 105* | 110* | | | | | | | | | | | | | | | | | | | | | |
| 70 | 178 | 2 | 60* | 65* | 69* | 85* | 101* | 105* | 111* | | | | | | | | | | | | | | | | | | | | | |

*Value estimated through linear regression equation.

(From Frisancho, A. R.: Am. J. Clin. Nutr., *40*:808–819, 1984, with permission.)

**TABLE A–14C-1.** MIDARM MUSCLE CIRCUMFERENCE IN ADULTS (18 TO 74 YEARS), UNITED STATES*†

| AGE GROUP (years) | SAMPLE SIZE | ESTIMATED POPULATION (millions) | MEAN (cm) | PERCENTILE | | | | | | |
|---|---|---|---|---|---|---|---|---|---|---|
| | | | | 5th | 10th | 25th | 50th | 75th | 90th | 95th |
| Men | | | | | | | | | | |
| 18–74 | 5,261 | 61.18 | 28.0 | 23.8 | 24.8 | 26.3 | 27.9 | 29.6 | 31.4 | 32.5 |
| 18–24 | 773 | 11.78 | 27.4 | 23.5 | 24.4 | 25.8 | 27.2 | 28.9 | 30.8 | 32.3 |
| 25–34 | 804 | 13.00 | 28.3 | 24.2 | 25.3 | 26.5 | 28.0 | 30.0 | 31.7 | 32.9 |
| 35–44 | 664 | 10.68 | 28.8 | 25.0 | 25.6 | 27.1 | 28.7 | 30.3 | 32.1 | 33.0 |
| 45–54 | 765 | 11.15 | 28.2 | 24.0 | 24.9 | 26.5 | 28.1 | 29.8 | 31.5 | 32.6 |
| 55–64 | 598 | 9.07 | 27.8 | 22.8 | 24.4 | 26.2 | 27.9 | 29.6 | 31.0 | 31.8 |
| 65–74 | 1,657 | 5.50 | 26.8 | 22.5 | 23.7 | 25.3 | 26.9 | 28.5 | 29.9 | 30.7 |
| Women | | | | | | | | | | |
| 18–74 | 8,410 | 67.84 | 22.2 | 18.4 | 19.0 | 20.2 | 21.8 | 23.6 | 25.8 | 27.4 |
| 18–24 | 1,523 | 12.89 | 20.9 | 17.7 | 18.5 | 19.4 | 20.6 | 22.1 | 23.6 | 24.9 |
| 25–34 | 1,896 | 13.93 | 21.7 | 18.3 | 18.9 | 20.0 | 21.4 | 22.9 | 24.9 | 26.6 |
| 35–44 | 1,664 | 11.59 | 22.5 | 18.5 | 19.2 | 20.6 | 22.0 | 24.0 | 26.1 | 27.4 |
| 45–54 | 836 | 12.16 | 22.7 | 18.8 | 19.5 | 20.7 | 22.2 | 24.3 | 26.6 | 27.8 |
| 55–64 | 669 | 9.98 | 22.8 | 18.6 | 19.5 | 20.8 | 22.6 | 24.4 | 26.3 | 28.1 |
| 65–74 | 1,822 | 7.28 | 22.8 | 18.6 | 19.5 | 20.8 | 22.5 | 24.4 | 26.5 | 28.1 |

*Measurements made in the right arm.
†See Tables A–14b-1 through A–14b-6 for data compiled by Frisancho (Am. J. Clin. Nutri., *40*:808–819, 1984) from NHANES I and II.
(From Bishop. C. W., Bowen, P.E., Ritchey, S.J.: Am. J. Clin. Nutr., *34*:2530–2539, 1981 [NHANES 1].)

**TABLE A–14C-2.** MIDARM MUSCLE AREA IN ADULTS (18 TO 74 YEARS), UNITED STATES*†

| AGE GROUP (years) | SAMPLE SIZE | ESTIMATED POPULATION (millions) | MEAN (cm) | PERCENTILE | | | | | | |
|---|---|---|---|---|---|---|---|---|---|---|
| | | | | 5th | 10th | 25th | 50th | 75th | 90th | 95th |
| Men | | | | | | | | | | |
| 18–74 | 5,261 | 61.18 | 62.4 | 45.1 | 49.0 | 55.1 | 62.0 | 69.8 | 78.5 | 84.1 |
| 18–24 | 773 | 11.78 | 59.8 | 44.0 | 47.4 | 53.0 | 58.9 | 66.5 | 75.5 | 83.1 |
| 25–34 | 804 | 13.00 | 63.8 | 46.6 | 51.0 | 55.9 | 62.4 | 71.7 | 80.0 | 86.2 |
| 35–44 | 664 | 10.68 | 66.0 | 49.8 | 52.2 | 58.5 | 65.6 | 73.1 | 82.0 | 86.7 |
| 45–54 | 765 | 11.15 | 63.3 | 45.9 | 49.4 | 55.9 | 62.9 | 70.7 | 79.0 | 84.6 |
| 55–64 | 598 | 9.07 | 61.5 | 41.4 | 47.4 | 54.7 | 62.0 | 69.8 | 76.5 | 80.5 |
| 65–74 | 1,657 | 5.50 | 57.2 | 40.3 | 44.7 | 51.0 | 57.6 | 64.7 | 71.2 | 75.0 |
| Women | | | | | | | | | | |
| 18–74 | 8,410 | 67.84 | 39.2 | 27.0 | 28.7 | 32.5 | 37.8 | 44.3 | 53.0 | 59.8 |
| 18–24 | 1,523 | 12.89 | 34.8 | 24.9 | 27.2 | 30.0 | 33.8 | 38.9 | 44.3 | 49.4 |
| 25–34 | 1,896 | 13.93 | 37.5 | 26.7 | 28.4 | 31.8 | 36.5 | 41.8 | 49.4 | 56.3 |
| 35–44 | 1,664 | 11.59 | 40.3 | 27.2 | 29.4 | 33.8 | 38.5 | 45.9 | 54.2 | 59.8 |
| 45–54 | 836 | 12.16 | 41.0 | 28.1 | 30.3 | 34.1 | 39.2 | 47.0 | 56.3 | 61.5 |
| 55–64 | 669 | 9.98 | 41.4 | 27.5 | 30.3 | 34.4 | 40.7 | 47.4 | 55.1 | 62.9 |
| 65–74 | 1,822 | 7.28 | 41.4 | 27.5 | 30.3 | 34.4 | 40.3 | 47.4 | 55.9 | 62.9 |

*Measurements made in the right arm.
†See Tables A–14b-1 through A–14b-6 for data compiled by Frisancho (Am. J. Clin. Nutri., *40*:808–819, 1984) from NHANES I and II.
(From Bishop. C. W., Bowen, P.E., Ritchey, S.J.: Am. J. Clin. Nutr., *34*:2530–2539, 1981 [NHANES 1].)

**TABLE A–14C-3.** AGE CORRECTION FOR ESTIMATES OF WEIGHT, TRICEPS AND SUBSCAPULAR SKINFOLD THICKNESSES, AND BONE-FREE UPPER ARM MUSCLE AREA (AMA)

| AGE GROUP: FRAME SIZE | MEDIAN AGE | WEIGHT | TRICEPS SKINFOLD | SUBSCAPULAR SKINFOLD | ARM MUSCLE AREA |
|---|---|---|---|---|---|
| Men | | | | | |
| 25–54 | | | | | |
| Small | 39 | 0.074 | 0.016 | 0.080 | 0.030 |
| Medium | 39 | 0.080 | 0.005 | 0.083 | 0.055 |
| Large | 40 | 0.000 | −0.024 | 0.049 | 0.026 |
| 55–74 | | | | | |
| Small | 66 | −0.329 | −0.036 | −0.115 | −0.407 |
| Medium | 67 | −0.435 | −0.040 | −0.125 | −0.521 |
| Large | 67 | −0.562 | −0.054 | −0.185 | −0.644 |
| Women | | | | | |
| 25–54 | | | | | |
| Small | 37 | 0.165 | 0.166 | 0.142 | 0.087 |
| Medium | 37 | 0.234 | 0.189 | 0.214 | 0.191 |
| Large | 37 | 0.284 | 0.191 | 0.233 | 0.270 |
| 55–74 | | | | | |
| Small | 67 | −0.027 | −0.072 | −0.013 | 0.036 |
| Medium | 66 | −0.196 | −0.210 | −0.221 | −0.033 |
| Large | 67 | −0.466 | −0.370 | −0.515 | −0.378 |

(From Frisancho, A.R.: Am. J. Clin. Nutr., *40*:808–819, 1984, with permission.)

**TABLE A–14D-1.** PROVISIONAL PERCENTILES FOR TRICEPS SKINFOLD THICKNESS IN THE ELDERLY*†

| AGE GROUP (Years) | PERCENTILE 5th | 50th | 95th |
|---|---|---|---|
| Men | | | |
| 65 | 8.6 | 13.8 | 27.0 |
| 70 | 7.7 | 12.9 | 26.1 |
| 75 | 6.8 | 12.0 | 25.2 |
| 80 | 6.0 | 11.2 | 24.3 |
| 85 | 5.1 | 10.3 | 23.4 |
| 90 | 4.2 | 9.4 | 22.6 |
| Women | | | |
| 65 | 13.5 | 21.6 | 33.0 |
| 70 | 12.5 | 20.6 | 32.0 |
| 75 | 11.5 | 19.6 | 31.0 |
| 80 | 10.5 | 18.6 | 30.0 |
| 85 | 9.5 | 17.6 | 29.0 |
| 90 | 8.5 | 16.6 | 28.0 |

*Data are from 119 men and 150 women. All subjects were ambulatory, and measurements were made in the recumbent position on the left side.

†See Tables A–14b-1 and A–14b-2 for data compiled by Frisancho (Am. J. Clin. Nutr., *40*:808–819, 1984) from NHANES I and II.

(From Chumlea, W.C., Roche, A.F., Mukherjee, D.: Nutritional Assessment of the Elderly Through Anthropometry. Ohio, Wright State University School of Medicine, 1984.)

**TABLE A–14D-2.** PROVISIONAL PERCENTILES FOR MIDARM MUSCLE AREA ($cm^2$) IN THE ELDERLY*†

| AGE GROUP (Years) | PERCENTILE 5th | 50th | 95th |
|---|---|---|---|
| Men | | | |
| 65 | 43.2 | 59.4 | 77.1 |
| 70 | 41.4 | 57.7 | 75.3 |
| 75 | 39.6 | 55.9 | 73.5 |
| 80 | 37.8 | 54.1 | 71.7 |
| 85 | 36.0 | 52.3 | 69.9 |
| 90 | 34.3 | 50.5 | 68.2 |
| Women | | | |
| 65 | 33.5 | 44.5 | 66.4 |
| 70 | 33.0 | 44.1 | 65.9 |
| 75 | 32.6 | 43.6 | 65.5 |
| 80 | 32.2 | 43.2 | 65.1 |
| 85 | 31.8 | 42.8 | 64.7 |
| 90 | 31.3 | 42.4 | 64.2 |

*Data are from 119 men and 150 women. All subjects were ambulatory, and measurements were made in the recumbent position on the left side.

†See Tables A–14b-1 and A–14b-2 for data compiled by Frisancho (Am. J. Clin. Nutr., *40*:808–819, 1984) from NHANES I and II.

(From Chumlea, W.C., Roche, A.F., Mukherjee, D.: Nutritional Assessment of the Elderly Through Anthropometry. Ohio, Wright State University School of Medicine, 1984.)

## TABLES A–15A TO C. BODY FAT ESTIMATIONS FROM SKINFOLD DATA

Various investigators have developed equations for predicting the proportions of body fat by anthropometric measures of specific regions. Durnin and Womersley used four different skinfolds (Table A–15-b). Pollock, Schmidt, and Jackson have prepared tables based on three sites, including thigh skinfolds (Tables A–13-b and A–15-c). Because some technicians have difficulty in obtaining consistent results with thigh skinfold measurements, data also are available based on other equations that do not use this skinfold. These data are included in the following sources:

Golding, L.A., Meyers, C.R., Sinning, W.E.: Y's Way to Physical Fitness: The Complete Guide to Fitness Testing and Instruction. 3rd Ed. Champaign, IL, Human Kinetics Publishers, 1989.

Pollock, M.L., Schmidt, D.H., Jackson, A.S.: Compr. Ther., *6*:12–27, 1980.

Jackson, A.S. and Pollock, M.L.: Phys. Sportsmed., *13*:76–90, 1985.

**TABLE A–15A.** EQUIVALENT FAT CONTENT, AS PERCENTAGE OF BODY WEIGHT, FOR A RANGE OF VALUES FOR THE SUM OF FOUR SKINFOLDS*

| SKINFOLDS (mm) | MEN (AGE IN YEARS) | | | | WOMEN (AGE IN YEARS) | | | |
|---|---|---|---|---|---|---|---|---|
| | 17–29 | 30–39 | 40–49 | 50+ | 16–29 | 30–39 | 40–49 | 50+ |
| 15 | 4.8 | | | | 10.5 | | | |
| 20 | 8.1 | 12.2 | 12.2 | 12.6 | 14.1 | 17.0 | 19.8 | 21.4 |
| 25 | 10.5 | 14.2 | 15.0 | 15.6 | 16.8 | 19.4 | 22.2 | 24.0 |
| 30 | 12.9 | 16.2 | 17.7 | 18.6 | 19.5 | 21.8 | 24.5 | 26.6 |
| 35 | 14.7 | 17.7 | 19.6 | 20.8 | 21.5 | 23.7 | 26.4 | 28.5 |
| 40 | 16.4 | 19.2 | 21.4 | 22.9 | 23.4 | 25.5 | 28.2 | 30.3 |
| 45 | 17.7 | 20.4 | 23.0 | 24.7 | 25.0 | 26.9 | 29.6 | 31.9 |
| 50 | 19.0 | 21.5 | 24.6 | 26.5 | 26.5 | 28.2 | 31.0 | 33.4 |
| 55 | 20.1 | 22.5 | 25.9 | 27.9 | 27.8 | 29.4 | 32.1 | 34.6 |
| 60 | 21.2 | 23.5 | 27.1 | 29.2 | 29.1 | 30.6 | 33.2 | 35.7 |
| 65 | 22.2 | 24.3 | 28.2 | 30.4 | 30.2 | 31.6 | 34.1 | 36.7 |
| 70 | 23.1 | 25.1 | 29.3 | 31.6 | 31.2 | 32.5 | 35.0 | 37.7 |
| 75 | 24.0 | 25.9 | 30.3 | 32.7 | 32.2 | 33.4 | 35.9 | 38.7 |
| 80 | 24.8 | 26.6 | 31.2 | 33.8 | 33.1 | 34.3 | 36.7 | 39.6 |
| 85 | 25.5 | 27.2 | 32.1 | 34.8 | 34.0 | 35.1 | 37.5 | 40.4 |
| 90 | 26.2 | 27.8 | 33.0 | 35.8 | 34.8 | 35.8 | 38.3 | 41.2 |
| 95 | 26.9 | 28.4 | 33.7 | 36.6 | 35.6 | 36.5 | 39.0 | 41.9 |
| 100 | 27.6 | 29.0 | 34.4 | 37.4 | 36.4 | 37.2 | 39.7 | 42.6 |
| 105 | 28.2 | 29.6 | 35.1 | 38.2 | 37.1 | 37.9 | 40.4 | 43.3 |
| 110 | 28.8 | 30.1 | 35.8 | 39.0 | 37.8 | 38.6 | 41.0 | 43.9 |
| 115 | 29.4 | 30.6 | 36.4 | 39.7 | 38.4 | 39.1 | 41.5 | 44.5 |
| 120 | 30.0 | 31.1 | 37.0 | 40.4 | 39.0 | 39.6 | 42.0 | 45.1 |
| 125 | 31.0 | 31.5 | 37.6 | 41.1 | 39.6 | 40.1 | 42.5 | 45.7 |
| 130 | 31.5 | 31.9 | 38.2 | 41.8 | 40.2 | 40.6 | 43.0 | 46.2 |
| 135 | 32.0 | 32.3 | 38.7 | 42.4 | 40.8 | 41.1 | 43.5 | 46.7 |
| 140 | 32.5 | 32.7 | 39.2 | 43.0 | 41.3 | 41.6 | 44.0 | 47.2 |
| 145 | 32.9 | 33.1 | 39.7 | 43.6 | 41.8 | 42.1 | 44.5 | 47.7 |
| 150 | 33.3 | 33.5 | 40.2 | 44.1 | 42.3 | 42.6 | 45.0 | 48.2 |
| 155 | 33.7 | 33.9 | 40.7 | 44.6 | 42.8 | 43.1 | 45.4 | 48.7 |
| 160 | 34.1 | 34.3 | 41.2 | 45.1 | 43.3 | 43.6 | 45.8 | 49.2 |
| 165 | 34.5 | 34.6 | 41.6 | 45.6 | 43.7 | 44.0 | 46.2 | 49.6 |
| 170 | 34.9 | 34.8 | 42.0 | 46.1 | 44.1 | 44.4 | 46.6 | 50.0 |
| 175 | 35.3 | | | | | 44.8 | 47.0 | 50.4 |
| 180 | 35.6 | | | | | 45.2 | 47.4 | 50.8 |
| 185 | 35.9 | | | | | 45.6 | 47.8 | 51.2 |
| 190 | | | | | | 45.9 | 48.2 | 51.6 |
| 195 | | | | | | 46.2 | 48.5 | 52.0 |
| 200 | | | | | | 46.5 | 48.8 | 52.4 |
| 205 | | | | | | | 49.1 | 52.7 |
| 210 | | | | | | | 49.4 | 53.0 |

*Biceps, triceps, subscapular, and suprailiac of men and women of different ages.
(From Durnin, J.V.G.A., Womersley, J.: Br. J. Nutr., *32*:77–97, 1974, with permission.)

**TABLE A–15B.** PERCENTAGE OF BODY FAT ESTIMATION FOR WOMEN FROM AGE AND TRICEPS, SUPRAILIUM, AND THIGH SKINFOLDS*

| SUM OF SKINFOLDS (mm) | AGE TO THE LAST YEAR | | | | | | | | |
|---|---|---|---|---|---|---|---|---|---|
| | Under 22 | 23 to 27 | 28 to 32 | 33 to 37 | 38 to 42 | 43 to 47 | 48 to 52 | 53 to 57 | Over 58 |
| 23–25 | 9.7 | 9.9 | 10.2 | 10.4 | 10.7 | 10.9 | 11.2 | 11.4 | 11.7 |
| 26–28 | 11.0 | 11.2 | 11.5 | 11.7 | 12.0 | 12.3 | 12.5 | 12.7 | 13.0 |
| 29–31 | 12.3 | 12.5 | 12.8 | 13.0 | 13.3 | 13.5 | 13.8 | 14.0 | 14.3 |
| 32–34 | 13.6 | 13.8 | 14.0 | 14.3 | 14.5 | 14.8 | 15.0 | 15.3 | 15.5 |
| 35–37 | 14.8 | 15.0 | 15.3 | 15.5 | 15.8 | 16.0 | 16.3 | 16.5 | 16.8 |
| 38–40 | 16.0 | 16.3 | 16.5 | 16.7 | 17.0 | 17.2 | 17.5 | 17.7 | 18.0 |
| 41–43 | 17.2 | 17.4 | 17.7 | 17.9 | 18.2 | 18.4 | 18.7 | 18.9 | 19.2 |
| 44–46 | 18.3 | 18.6 | 18.8 | 19.1 | 19.3 | 19.6 | 19.8 | 20.1 | 20.3 |
| 47–49 | 19.5 | 19.7 | 20.0 | 20.2 | 20.5 | 20.7 | 21.0 | 21.2 | 21.5 |
| 50–52 | 20.6 | 20.8 | 21.1 | 21.3 | 21.6 | 21.8 | 22.1 | 22.3 | 22.6 |
| 53–55 | 21.7 | 21.9 | 22.1 | 22.4 | 22.6 | 22.9 | 23.1 | 23.4 | 23.6 |
| 56–58 | 22.7 | 23.0 | 23.2 | 23.4 | 23.7 | 23.9 | 24.2 | 24.4 | 24.7 |
| 59–61 | 23.7 | 24.0 | 24.2 | 24.5 | 24.7 | 25.0 | 25.2 | 25.5 | 25.7 |
| 62–64 | 24.7 | 25.0 | 25.2 | 25.5 | 25.7 | 26.0 | 26.7 | 26.4 | 26.7 |
| 65–67 | 25.7 | 25.9 | 26.2 | 26.4 | 26.7 | 26.9 | 27.2 | 27.4 | 27.7 |
| 68–70 | 26.6 | 26.9 | 27.1 | 27.4 | 27.6 | 27.9 | 28.1 | 28.4 | 28.6 |
| 71–73 | 27.5 | 27.8 | 28.0 | 28.3 | 28.5 | 28.8 | 28.0 | 29.3 | 29.5 |
| 74–76 | 28.4 | 28.7 | 28.9 | 29.2 | 29.4 | 29.7 | 29.9 | 30.2 | 30.4 |
| 77–79 | 29.3 | 29.5 | 29.8 | 30.0 | 30.3 | 30.5 | 30.8 | 31.0 | 31.3 |
| 80–82 | 30.1 | 30.4 | 30.6 | 30.9 | 31.1 | 31.4 | 31.6 | 31.9 | 32.1 |
| 83–85 | 30.9 | 31.2 | 31.4 | 31.7 | 31.9 | 32.2 | 32.4 | 32.7 | 32.9 |
| 86–88 | 31.7 | 32.0 | 32.2 | 32.5 | 32.7 | 32.9 | 33.2 | 33.4 | 33.7 |
| 89–91 | 32.5 | 32.7 | 33.0 | 33.2 | 33.5 | 33.7 | 33.9 | 34.2 | 34.4 |
| 92–94 | 33.2 | 33.4 | 33.7 | 33.9 | 34.2 | 34.4 | 34.7 | 34.9 | 35.2 |
| 95–97 | 33.9 | 34.1 | 34.4 | 34.6 | 34.9 | 35.1 | 35.4 | 35.6 | 35.9 |
| 98–100 | 34.6 | 34.8 | 35.1 | 35.3 | 35.5 | 35.8 | 36.0 | 36.3 | 36.5 |
| 101–103 | 35.3 | 35.4 | 35.7 | 35.9 | 36.2 | 36.4 | 36.7 | 36.9 | 37.2 |
| 104–106 | 35.8 | 36.1 | 36.3 | 36.6 | 36.8 | 37.1 | 37.3 | 37.5 | 37.8 |
| 107–109 | 36.4 | 36.7 | 36.9 | 37.1 | 37.4 | 37.6 | 37.9 | 38.1 | 38.4 |
| 110–112 | 37.0 | 37.2 | 37.5 | 37.7 | 38.0 | 38.2 | 38.5 | 38.7 | 38.9 |
| 113–115 | 37.5 | 37.8 | 38.0 | 38.2 | 38.5 | 38.7 | 39.0 | 39.2 | 39.5 |
| 116–118 | 38.0 | 38.3 | 38.5 | 38.8 | 39.0 | 39.3 | 39.5 | 39.7 | 40.0 |
| 119–121 | 38.5 | 38.7 | 39.0 | 39.2 | 39.5 | 39.7 | 40.0 | 40.2 | 40.5 |
| 122–124 | 39.0 | 39.2 | 39.4 | 39.7 | 39.9 | 40.2 | 40.4 | 40.7 | 40.9 |
| 125–127 | 39.4 | 39.6 | 39.9 | 40.1 | 40.4 | 40.6 | 40.9 | 41.1 | 41.4 |
| 128–130 | 39.8 | 40.0 | 40.3 | 40.5 | 40.8 | 41.0 | 41.3 | 41.5 | 41.8 |

*Percentage of fat calculated by the formula of Siri: percentage of fat = $(4.95/D_b - 4.5) \times 100$, where $D_b$ = body density.

(Reprinted with permission from Pollock, M.L., Schmidt, D.H., and Jackson, A.S.: Measurement of cardiorespiratory fitness and body composition in the clinical setting. Compr. Ther., *6*:12–27, 1980.)

**TABLE A–15C.** PERCENTAGE OF BODY FAT ESTIMATION FOR MEN FROM AGE AND THE SUM OF CHEST, ABDOMINAL, AND THIGH SKINFOLDS*

| SUM OF SKINFOLDS (mm) | AGE TO THE LAST YEAR | | | | | | | | |
|---|---|---|---|---|---|---|---|---|---|
| | Under 22 | 23 to 27 | 28 to 32 | 33 to 37 | 38 to 42 | 43 to 47 | 48 to 52 | 53 to 57 | Over 58 |
| 23–25 | 9.7 | 9.9 | 10.2 | 10.4 | 10.7 | 10.9 | 11.2 | 11.4 | 11.7 |
| 26–28 | 11.0 | 11.2 | 11.5 | 11.7 | 12.0 | 12.3 | 12.5 | 12.7 | 13.0 |
| 29–31 | 12.3 | 12.5 | 12.8 | 13.0 | 13.3 | 13.5 | 13.8 | 14.0 | 14.3 |
| 32–34 | 13.6 | 13.8 | 14.0 | 14.3 | 14.5 | 14.8 | 15.0 | 15.3 | 15.5 |
| 35–37 | 14.8 | 15.0 | 15.3 | 15.5 | 15.8 | 16.0 | 16.3 | 16.5 | 16.8 |
| 38–40 | 16.0 | 16.3 | 16.5 | 16.7 | 17.0 | 17.2 | 17.5 | 17.7 | 18.0 |
| 41–43 | 17.2 | 17.4 | 17.7 | 17.9 | 18.2 | 18.4 | 18.7 | 18.9 | 19.2 |
| 44–46 | 18.3 | 18.6 | 18.8 | 19.1 | 19.3 | 19.6 | 19.8 | 20.1 | 20.3 |
| 47–49 | 19.5 | 19.7 | 20.0 | 20.2 | 20.5 | 20.7 | 21.0 | 21.2 | 21.5 |
| 50–52 | 20.6 | 20.8 | 21.1 | 21.3 | 21.6 | 21.8 | 22.1 | 22.3 | 22.6 |
| 53–55 | 21.7 | 21.9 | 22.1 | 22.4 | 22.6 | 22.9 | 23.1 | 23.4 | 23.6 |
| 56–58 | 22.7 | 23.0 | 23.2 | 23.4 | 23.7 | 23.9 | 24.2 | 24.4 | 24.7 |
| 59–61 | 23.7 | 24.0 | 24.2 | 24.5 | 24.7 | 25.0 | 25.2 | 25.5 | 25.7 |
| 62–64 | 24.7 | 25.0 | 25.2 | 25.5 | 25.7 | 26.0 | 26.7 | 26.4 | 26.7 |
| 65–67 | 25.7 | 25.9 | 26.2 | 26.4 | 26.7 | 26.9 | 27.2 | 27.4 | 27.7 |
| 68–70 | 26.6 | 26.9 | 27.1 | 27.4 | 27.6 | 27.9 | 28.1 | 28.4 | 28.6 |
| 71–73 | 27.5 | 27.8 | 28.0 | 28.3 | 28.5 | 28.8 | 29.0 | 29.3 | 29.5 |
| 74–76 | 28.4 | 28.7 | 28.9 | 29.2 | 29.4 | 29.7 | 29.9 | 30.2 | 30.4 |
| 77–79 | 29.3 | 29.5 | 29.8 | 30.0 | 30.3 | 30.5 | 30.8 | 31.0 | 31.3 |
| 80–82 | 30.1 | 30.4 | 30.6 | 30.9 | 31.1 | 31.4 | 31.6 | 31.9 | 32.1 |
| 83–85 | 30.9 | 31.2 | 31.4 | 31.7 | 31.9 | 32.2 | 32.4 | 32.7 | 32.9 |
| 86–88 | 31.7 | 32.0 | 32.2 | 32.5 | 32.7 | 32.9 | 33.2 | 33.4 | 33.7 |
| 89–91 | 32.5 | 32.7 | 33.0 | 33.2 | 33.5 | 33.7 | 33.9 | 34.2 | 34.4 |
| 92–94 | 33.2 | 33.4 | 33.7 | 33.9 | 34.2 | 34.4 | 34.7 | 34.9 | 35.2 |
| 95–97 | 33.9 | 34.1 | 34.4 | 34.6 | 34.9 | 35.1 | 35.4 | 35.6 | 35.9 |
| 98–100 | 34.6 | 34.8 | 35.1 | 35.3 | 35.5 | 35.8 | 36.0 | 36.3 | 36.5 |
| 101–103 | 35.3 | 35.4 | 35.7 | 35.9 | 36.2 | 36.4 | 36.7 | 36.9 | 37.2 |
| 104–106 | 35.8 | 36.1 | 36.3 | 36.6 | 36.8 | 37.1 | 37.3 | 37.5 | 37.8 |
| 107–109 | 36.4 | 36.7 | 36.9 | 37.1 | 37.4 | 37.6 | 37.9 | 38.1 | 38.4 |
| 110–112 | 37.0 | 37.2 | 37.5 | 37.7 | 38.0 | 38.2 | 38.5 | 38.7 | 38.9 |
| 113–115 | 37.5 | 37.8 | 38.0 | 38.2 | 38.5 | 38.7 | 39.0 | 39.2 | 39.5 |
| 116–118 | 38.0 | 38.3 | 38.5 | 38.8 | 39.0 | 39.3 | 39.5 | 39.7 | 40.0 |
| 119–121 | 38.5 | 38.7 | 39.0 | 39.2 | 39.5 | 39.7 | 40.0 | 40.2 | 40.5 |
| 122–124 | 39.0 | 39.2 | 39.4 | 39.7 | 39.9 | 40.2 | 40.4 | 40.7 | 40.9 |
| 125–127 | 39.4 | 39.6 | 39.9 | 40.1 | 40.4 | 40.6 | 40.9 | 41.1 | 41.4 |
| 128–130 | 39.8 | 40.0 | 40.3 | 40.5 | 40.8 | 41.0 | 41.3 | 41.5 | 41.8 |

*Percentage of fat calculated by the formula of Siri: percentage of fat = $(4.95/D_b - 4.5) \times 100$, where $D_b$ = body density.

(Reprinted with permission from Pollock, M.L., Schmidt, D.H., and Jackson, A.S.: Measurement of cardiorespiratory fitness and body composition in the clinical setting. Compr. Ther., *6*:12–27, 1980.)

**TABLE A–16A.** DIETARY RECOMMENDATIONS IN INDUSTRIALIZED AND DEVELOPING COUNTRIES, 1977 TO 1989*

| Country/region or Source of Recommendation | Target Group(s) | Maintain Appropriate Body Weight, Exercise | Limit or Reduce Total Fat (% Energy) | Reduce Saturated Fatty Acids (% Energy) |
|---|---|---|---|---|
| Australia 1983 | GP | Yes | Yes | NC |
| 1987, targets for 1995 | GP | Reduce obesity prevalence to 30% | 35% | NS |
| 1987, targets for 2000 | GP | To 25% | 33% | NS |
| Canada 1982 | GP | Yes | 35% | Yes |
| Czechoslovakia 1988 | GP | Yes, reduce by 10–15% | Yes, reduce by 15 g/day | Yes |
| France 1981 | GP | Yes | 30–35% | Yes |
| Germany, Federal Republic of, 1985 | GP | Yes | Yes | NS |
| Hungary 1988 | GP | Yes | Avoid too much | Use vegetable oil |
| India 1988 | HR (affluent people) | Yes | 15–20% | NC |
| Ireland 1984 | GP | Yes | ≤35% | Yes |
| Japan 1985 | GP | Yes | 20–25% | Yes |
| Latin America 1988 | GP | Yes | 20–25% | ≤8 |
| Netherlands 1983–1984 | GP | Yes | 30–35% | Yes |
| 1986 | GP | Yes | 30–35% | Yes |
| New Zealand 1982 | GP<br>HR | Yes | Yes | Yes |
| Norway 1981–1982 | GP | NC | <35% | Yes |
| Poland 1988 | GP | Yes | ≈30% | Yes |
| Sweden 1981 | GP | Yes | 25–35% | Yes |
| 1985 | GP | Yes | Reduce by 5% energy by 1990; to ≈30% by 2000 | NS |
| United Kingdom 1983 | GP | Yes | 30% | 10 |
| United States of America 1977 | GP | Yes | 27–33% | Yes |
| 1979 | GP | Yes | Yes | Yes |
| 1985 | GP | Yes | Yes | Yes |
| 1988 | GP<br>HR | Yes | Yes | Yes |
| 1989 | GP | Balance energy intake and expenditure | ≤30% | <10% for individuals, 7–8% population mean |
| WHO 1988 | | | | |
| Intermediate goals | GP | BMI | 35% | 15% |
| Ultimate goals | | 20–25 | 20–30% | 10–15% |

*BMI = Body-mass index; GP = General population; HR = High-risk groups; NC = No comment; NS = Not specified; P/S = Ratio of polyunsaturated to saturated fatty acids; RDA = Recommended dietary allowance.

(From Diet, Nutrition and the Prevention of Chronic Diseases. Report of a WHO Study Group. Technical Report Series No. 797. Geneva, WHO, 1990, pp. 180–181.)

**TABLE A–16A.** CONTINUED.

| Increase Polyunsaturated Fatty Acids (% Energy) | Limit Cholesterol (mg/day) | Limit Free Sugars (% Energy) | Increase Complex Carbohydrates (% Energy for Total Carbohydrates) |
|---|---|---|---|
| NC | NC | Yes | Yes |
| NS | NS | <14% | Indirectly |
| NS | NS | <12% | Indirectly |
| Yes | No | Yes | Yes |
| No | NS | Yes | Yes, more plant foods, vegetables, cereals, legumes |
| NS | NS | Yes | 50–55% |
| NS | NS | Avoid excess | Yes; fresh fruits and vegetables, whole-grain cereals |
| NS | NS | Yes | Yes, fresh vegetables, salads, whole-grains |
| Balance (*n*-3)/(*n*-6) ratio | NC | Yes | Yes; avoid refined and polished grains |
| NC | NC | Moderation; ≤7 g/day for weight reduction | Yes |
| Use vegetables and fish oils | NC | NC | NC |
| P/S ≈1.0 | <100 mg/1000 $kcal_{th}$ in children, up to 300 mg/day | Yes | Yes |
| Maximum 10% | Yes | Yes | NS |
| P/S = 1.0 | <30 mg/MJ | Mono- and disaccharides 15–25% | 45–55% |
| NS | NS | Yes | Yes |
| P/S = 0.5 | NS | <10% | Yes; 50–60% |
| NS | Yes, <300 mg | ≤10% | Yes |
| P/S = 0.5 | Yes | <10% | Yes; 50–60% |
| P/S = >0.5 | NS | Decrease by 3% energy by 1990 | Yes; increase starch to 45–50% energy by 2000 |
| NS | No | To 20 kg/year | Through whole grains, vegetables, cereals, fruits |
| Yes | 250–350 | Yes | Yes |
| NS | Yes | Yes | Yes |
| No | Yes | Yes | Adequate starch and fiber |
| No | Yes | Yes | Yes |
| Up to 10 for individuals and ≈7 population mean | <300 | Yes | ≥55%; ≥5 servings/day vegetables and fruits; ≥6 daily servings cereals, breads, and legumes |
| P/S ≥0.5 | <100 mg/1000 $kcal_{th}$ | 10% | >40% |
| P/S = 1.0 | | | 45–55% |

**TABLE A–16A.** CONTINUED.

| Increase Dietary Fiber (g/day) | Restrict Sodium Chloride (g/day) | Moderate Alcohol Intake (% energy) | Other Recommendations |
|---|---|---|---|
| Yes | Yes | Yes | Promote breast-feeding; variety |
| 25 | 130 mmol/day | <5% | Promote water fluoridation, increase prevalence of breast-feeding |
| 30 | 100 mmol/day | <5% | |
| Yes | Yes | Yes | Exercise |
| Yes | Yes | Yes | Increase vitamin C intake; more plant foods; nutrition education; variety |
| Yes | Yes | <10% | Water fluoridation |
| Yes | Yes | Yes | Variety; small, frequent meals, proper cooking; sufficient protein |
| Yes | Yes | Yes | Variety; focus on cooking methods; consume milk and cheese as skimmed-milk products; 4 or 5 even meals daily; food labelling |
| Include grains, leafy vegetables, and whole grains | Yes | NC | Breast-feeding; water fluoridation upper limit 1 mg/L; different recommendation for general, poorer population |
| To 20–35 | <9 | <5% | Reduce protein to 1 g/kg of body weight daily; more vegetable protein |
| NC | <10 | NC | Varied diet (at least 30 different foods daily); home cooking; pleasant eating environment |
| >8 g/1000 $\text{kcal}_{th}$ | ≤5; in profuse sweating, up to 10 | NC | Protein 10–12% energy; variety; dietary interactions; vitamin C with iron-containing foods; calcium intake |
| NC | NC | Yes | Variety |
| 3 g/MJ | Yes | <9 g/day | Variety |
| Yes | Yes | Yes | Variety; less animal protein; water fluoridation |
| Yes | NC | NC | Maintain adequate nutrient intake |
| Yes | ? | ? | ? |
| >30 | ≈7–8 | Yes | Varied diet, exercise, regular meals |
| Increase by 7–8 g/day by 1990 and to 30–35 g by 2000 | Reduce by 1–2 g/day by 1990 to 7–8 g by 2000 | Yes | Year 1990 and year 2000 goals |
| To 30 | Decrease by 3 g/day | <4% | Long-term proposals: food labeling; nutrition education; greater proportion of vegetable protein |
| Yes | <8 | Yes | Limit additives and processed foods |
| NS | Yes | Yes | More fish, poultry, legumes; less red meat |
| Yes | Yes | Yes | Variety in diet; consider high-risk groups |
| Yes | Yes | Yes | Fluoridation of water; adolescent girls and women increase intake of calcium-rich foods; children, adolescents, and women of child-bearing age increase intake of iron-rich foods |
| Indirectly through vegetables, fruits, and cereals | ≤6 with a goal of 4.5 | <30 g of ethanol or <2 drinks/day | Population and individual goals; avoid dietary supplements in excess of RDAs; drink fluoridated water; limit protein intake to less than twice the RDA; comments on future goals |
| >30 | 7–8 | Yes | Increase nutrient density of food; water fluoridation; iodine prophylaxis |
| | 5 | | |

**TABLE A–16B.** DIETARY RECOMMENDATIONS TO REDUCE CORONARY HEART DISEASE RISK IN INDUSTRIALIZED COUNTRIES*

| COUNTRY/REGION OR SOURCE OF RECOMMENDATION | TARGET GROUP(S) | BODY WEIGHT/EXERCISE | TOTAL FAT (% ENERGY) |
|---|---|---|---|
| Australia | | | |
| 1979 | HR | Avoid obesity | Reduce to 30–35 |
| Canada | | | |
| 1977 | GP | Maintain appropriate body weight | Reduce to 35 |
| 1988 | GP<br>HR | Adjust energy intake and expenditure | <30 |
| Europe | | | |
| 1987 | GP<br>HR | Control obesity; increase exercise | ≤30 |
| Finland | | | |
| 1987 | GP<br>HR | Avoid excess weight; exercise | <30 |
| Finland, Norway, Sweden | | | |
| 1968 | GP | Reduce energy intake to avoid obesity; exercise | Reduce to 25–35 |
| Germany, Federal Republic of | | | |
| 1975 | GP | NC | Reduce |
| Japan | | | |
| 1983 | GP | NC | 20–25 |
| Netherlands | | | |
| 1973 | GP | Maintain appropriate body weight | 33 |
| New Zealand | | | |
| 1976 | GP<br>HR | Maintain appropriate body weight | 35 |
| United Kingdom | | | |
| 1982 | GP | Avoid obesity; increase exercise | 30 |
| 1984 | GP | Avoid obesity; exercise | Reduce to 35 |
| United States of America | | | |
| 1984 | GP | Control obesity | <30 |
| 1985 | GP<br>HR | Maintain appropriate body weight | <30 |
| 1988 | GP | Maintain appropriate body weight | <30 |
| WHO | | | |
| 1982 | GP | Avoid obesity | Reduce to 20–30 |
| 1988 | HR | BMI 20–25, regular exercise | 20–30 |

*BMI = Body-mass index; GP = General population; HR = High-risk groups; NC = No comment; NS = Not specified; P:S = Ratio of polyunsaturated to saturated fatty acids.

(From Diet, Nutrition and the Prevention of Chronic Diseases. Report of a WHO Study Group. Technical Report Series No. 797. Geneva, WHO, 1990, pp. 182–183. With permission.)

**TABLE A–16B.** CONTINUED.

| SATURATED FAT (% ENERGY) | POLYUNSATURATED FAT (% ENERGY) | CHOLESTEROL (MG/DAY) | COMPLEX CARBOHYDRATES AND FIBER |
|---|---|---|---|
| P:S = 1.0 | P:S = 1.0 | Restrict | Eat enough |
| 10 | 10 | NC | Increase |
| <10 | <10 | Restrict through less meats and egg yolks; for HR <300 | Increase |
| <10 | Increase oleic and linoleic acids | <300 | Increase, especially vegetables, fruits, cereals, legumes |
| <10 | P:S >0.5 | Reduce | NC |
| Reduce | Increase | NC | Increase vegetables, fruits, potatoes |
| Reduce | Increase | Reduce | NC |
| NC | Cook with vegetable oil | NC | Increase |
| Restrict | 10–13 | 250–300 | Increase to make up energy need |
| Reduce especially for HR | HR should substitute for saturated fatty acids | Reduce | NC |
| <10 | NC | NC | Increase |
| Reduce to 15 | P/S≈0.45 | NS | Increase breads, cereals, vegetables, fruits |
| 8 | <10 | <250 | Increase to make up energy loss |
| 10 | Up to 10 | 250–300 | Endorsed earlier recommendations |
| <10 | Up to 10 | <300 | Increase, ≥50% energy from total carbohydrates |
| <10 | Up to 10 | <300 | Increase |
| 10 | Up to 10 P/S >1.0 | <100 mg/1000 $kcal_{th}$ | 45–55% energy >30 g fiber/day |

**TABLE A–16B.** CONTINUED.

| FREE SUGARS | SODIUM CHLORIDE (G/DAY) | ALCOHOL INTAKE | OTHER RECOMMENDATIONS |
|---|---|---|---|
| Use less | Restrict | Moderation | Focus on HR groups; food labelling; recommendations safe for GP |
| NC | Restrict | NC | Variety of foods |
| NC | Limit | Limit | Focus on HR groups; limit protein to 10–15 % energy |
| Reduce | Moderation | Moderation, <25–30 g/day | Nutrition education; collaboration among government and other groups; food labelling |
| NC | Reduce; for HR <5 | Moderation | Avoid trace element deficiencies; food labelling; focus on HR groups |
| Decrease | NC | NC | 10–12% of energy from protein; 30–50% of animal origin |
| NC | NC | NC | NC |
| Reduce | Limit to <10 | Avoid too much | Variety; eat enough protein, half from vegetables and half from animal sources; eat enough potassium, especially from green vegetables; eat lean meat and fish and fewer sweets |
| Use little | NC | NC | NC |
| Restrict to reduce weight | NC | Restrict to reduce weight | NC |
| NC | NC | NC | Special attention to children |
| Do not increase | Decrease | Avoid excess; <90 ml/day men; <65 ml/day women | Special recommendations for governments, professionals, industry |
| NC | 5 | NC | NC |
| | NC | NC | Guidelines for health professionals, industry, and public |
| NS | <3 (as sodium) | 30–50 g ethanol/day | Protein to make up remainder of energy; wide variety of foods |
| NC | <5 | Drink less | Emphasis on plant foods, fish, poultry, lean meats, low-fat dairy products, and fewer whole eggs |
| 10% energy | <5 | Limit | Increase nutrient density; water fluoridation 0.7–1.2 mg/L; iodine prophylaxis; intermediate and ultimate goals |

**TABLE A–16C.** DIETARY RECOMMENDATIONS TO REDUCE CANCER RISK IN INDUSTRIALIZED COUNTRIES*

| COUNTRY/ REGION | MAINTAIN APPROPRIATE BODY WEIGHT, EXERCISE | LIMIT OR REDUCE TOTAL FAT (% ENERGY) | MODIFY RATIO OF DIETARY FATS | PROMOTE FRUIT AND VEGETABLE INTAKE | INCREASE COMPLEX CARBOHYDRATE/ FIBER INTAKE |
|---|---|---|---|---|---|
| Canada 1985 | Yes | Reduce | Decrease saturated fatty acids and cholesterol | Yes | More fiber-containing foods |
| Europe 1986 | Yes | To ≈30 | NC | Yes | Yes |
| Japan 1983 | NC | Avoid excess | NC | Especially green/ yellow vegetables, oranges, carotene, and fungi | Unrefined cereal, seafood, fiber-rich legumes |
| United States of America 1982 | NC | To ≈30 | NC | Especially citrus fruits, green and yellow and cruciferous vegetables | Whole-grain products, vegetables, and fruits |
| 1984 | Yes | To ≈30 | NC | Especially vitamin A- and C-rich foods and cruciferous vegetables | High-fiber foods, whole-grain cereals |
| 1987 | Yes | To ≈30 | NC | Vitamin A-rich, green and yellow vegetables, citrus fruits | Whole-grain products, 20–30 g fiber/day |

*NC = No comment; NS = Not specified.

(From Diet, Nutrition and the Prevention of Chronic Diseases. Report of a WHO Study Group. Technical Report Series No. 797. Geneva, World Health Organization, 1990, pp. 184–185.)

**TABLE A–16C.** CONTINUED

| RESTRICT SODIUM CHLORIDE | FOOD PREPARATION METHODS | ALCOHOL INTAKE | OTHER RECOMMENDATIONS |
|---|---|---|---|
| NS | Minimize cured, pickled, and smoked foods | Two or fewer drinks per day, if any | NC |
| To <5 g/day | As above; avoid frying and high-temperature cooking | Drink less, if at all | Varied diet; no food supplements; recommendations to government, scientists, and industry |
| Yes | Avoid hot drinks and burned foods | Drink less, if at all | Varied diet; chew food well |
| Minimize cured and pickled foods | Minimize cured, pickled, and smoked foods | Drink less, if at all | Avoid food supplements; monitor and test mutagens and carcinogens; recommendations to government, scientists, and industry |
| NS | As above | As above | NC |
| NS | As above, avoid frying and high-temperature cooking | As above | Balanced diet; read labels |

**TABLE A–16D.** NATIONAL NUTRITION OBJECTIVES FOR THE YEAR 2000

**A.** *Health Status Objectives*

**1.** Reduce deaths from coronary heart disease to no more than 100 per 100,000 persons (age-adjusted baseline: 135 per 100,000 in 1987).

**2.** Reverse the rise in deaths from cancer to achieve a rate of no more than 130 per 100,000 persons (age-adjusted baseline: 133 per 100,000 in 1987).

**3.** Reduce the overweight population to no more than 20% among adults aged 20 years and older and no more than 15% among adolescents aged 12 through 19 years (baseline: 26% for adults aged 20 through 74 years in 1976 to 1980, 24% for men and 27% for women; 15% for adolescents aged 12 through 19 years in 1976 to 1980).

**4.** Reduce growth retardation among low-income children aged 5 years and younger to less than 10% (baseline: up to 16% among low-income children in 1988, depending on age and race/ethnicity).

**B.** *Risk Reduction Objectives*

**5.** Reduce dietary fat intake to an average of 30% of calories or less and reduce average saturated fat intake to less than 10% of calories among persons aged 2 years and older (baseline: 36% of calories from total fat and 13% from saturated fat for persons aged 20 through 74 years in 1976 to 1980; 36% and 13% for women aged 19 through 50 years in 1985).

**6.** Increase complex carbohydrates and fiber-containing foods in the diets of adults to 5 or more daily servings for vegetables (including legumes) and fruits, and to 6 or more daily servings for grain products (baseline: 2.5 servings of vegetables and fruits and 3 servings of grain products for women aged 19 through 50 years in 1985).

**7.** Increase to at least 50% the proportion of overweight persons aged 12 years and older who have adopted sound dietary practices combined with regular physical activity to attain an appropriate body weight (baseline: 30% of overweight women and 25% of overweight men for people aged 18 years and older in 1985).

**8.** Increase calcium intake so that at least 50% of youth aged 12 through 24 years and at least 50% of pregnant and lactating women are consuming 3 or more servings daily of foods rich in calcium, and at least 50% of adults aged 25 years and older are consuming 2 or more servings daily (baseline: 7% of women and 14% of men aged 19 through 24 years and 24% of pregnant and lactating women consumed 3 or more servings daily, and 15% of women and 23% of men aged 25 through 50 years consumed 2 or more servings daily in 1985 to 1986).

**9.** Decrease salt and sodium intake so that at least 65% of those who prepare home-cooked meals do so without adding salt, at least 80% of persons avoid using salt at the table, and at least 40% of adults regularly purchase foods modified or lower in sodium (baseline: 54% of women aged 19 through 50 years who prepared most of the meals did not use salt in food preparation, and 68% of women aged 19 through 50 years did not use salt at the table in 1985; 20% of all persons aged 18 years and older regularly purchased foods with reduced salt and sodium content in 1988).

**10.** Reduce iron deficiency to less than 3% among children aged 1 through 4 years and among women of childbearing age (baseline: 9% for children aged 1 through 2 years, 4% for children aged 3 through 4 years, and 5% for women aged 20 through 44 years in 1976 to 1980).

**11.** Increase to at least 75% the proportion of mothers who breast-feed their babies in the early postpartum period and to at least 50% the proportion who continue to breast-feed until their babies are 5 to 6 months old (baseline: 54% at discharge from birth site and 21% at 5 to 6 months in 1988).

**12.** Increase to at least 75% the proportion of parents and caregivers who use feeding practices that prevent baby-bottle tooth decay.

**13.** Increase to at least 85% the proportion of persons aged 18 years and older who use food labels to make nutritious food selections (baseline: 74% used labels to make food selections in 1988).

**C.** *Service and Protection Objectives*

**14.** Achieve useful and informative nutrition labeling for virtually all processed foods and for at least 40% of fresh meats, poultry, fish, fruits, vegetables, baked foods, and ready-to-eat carry-out foods (baseline: 60% of processed foods regulated by the Food and Drug Administration had nutrition labeling in 1988; baseline data on fresh and carry-out foods are unavailable).

**15.** Increase the available processed food products that are reduced in fat and saturated fat to at least 5000 brand items (baseline: 2500 brand items reduced in fat in 1986).

**16.** Increase to at least 90% the proportion of restaurants and institutional service operations than offer identifiable low-fat, low-calorie food choices, consistent with the nutrition principles in the *Dietary Guidelines for Americans.*

**17.** Increase to at least 90% the proportion of school lunch and breakfast services and child-care food services that offer menus consistent with the nutrition principles in the *Dietary Guidelines for Americans.*

**18.** Increase to at least 80% the receipt of home food services by people aged 65 years and older who cannot prepare their own meals or are otherwise in need of home-delivered meals.

**19.** Increase to at least 75% the proportion of schools in the United States that provide nutrition education from preschool through 12th grade, preferably as part of quality school health education.

**20.** Increase to at least 50% the proportion of worksites with 50 or more employees that offer nutrition education and/or weight management programs for employees (baseline: 17% offered nutrition education activities and 15% offered weight-control activities in 1985).

**21.** Increase to at least 75% the proportion of primary care providers who provide nutrition assessment and counseling and/or referral to qualified nutritionists or dietitians (baseline: physicians provided diet counseling for an estimated 40 to 50% of patients in 1988).

(From Nutrition in Healthy People 2000. *In* National Health Promotion and Disease Prevention Objectives. Washington, D.C., U.S. Government Printing Office, 1991.)

**TABLE A–16E.** RECOMMENDED DIET MODIFICATIONS TO LOWER BLOOD CHOLESTEROL

For Table A–16e, National Cholesterol Education Program (NCEP) Recommendations and Diets in the United States, see Table A–28, Recommendations for Phased Dietary Modification in the Prevention and Therapy of Hyperlipidemia (NCEP Step-One and Step-Two Diets).

**TABLE A–17.** BEVERAGES AND ALCOHOLIC DRINKS: CALORIES AND SELECTED ELECTROLYTES (PER 100 ML)*

| BEVERAGE | CALORIES | SODIUM (mg) | SODIUM (mEq) | POTASSIUM (mg) | POTASSIUM (mEq) | PHOSPHORUS (mg) |
|---|---|---|---|---|---|---|
| Cola (avg.) | 48.1–55.0† | 0.8–4.7 (mg)† | | 0–4.4 (mg)† | | 18.1–25† |
| Diet cola (avg.) | 0.1–0.5† | 0.8–13.0 (mg)† | | 0–33.2 (mg)† | | 8.5–17.6† |
| Patio grape/orange | 52 | 11.2 | 0.5 | 4.1 | 0.1 | — |
| Mountain Dew | 49 | 8.7 | 0.4 | 2.7 | 0.1 | — |
| Teem | 41 | 8.6 | 0.4 | — | — | — |
| Root beer | 45 | 1 | 0.1 | 3.9 | 0.1 | — |
| Club soda | 0 | 21.9 | 1.0 | — | — | 0 |
| Sprite | 48 | 15.4 | 0.7 | 0.4 | — | — |
| Fanta (avg.) | 53 | 6.4 | 0.3 | 0.6 | — | — |
| Fresca | 1 | 12.1 | 0.5 | — | — | — |
| Fanta ginger ale | 42 | 9.4 | 0.4 | — | — | — |
| Slice | 45 | 3 | 0.1 | 27.6 | 0.7 | — |
| Apricot nectar | 56 | 3 | 0.1 | 114 | 2.9 | 9 |
| Apple juice | 47 | 3 | 0.1 | 119 | 3 | 7 |
| Cranberry juice | 58 | 4 | 0.2 | 24 | 0.6 | 1 |
| Grape juice, canned | 61 | 3 | 0.1 | 132 | 3.4 | 11 |
| Grapefruit juice, unsweetened | 38 | trace | — | 153 | 3.9 | 11 |
| Orange juice, unsweetened or fresh | 45 | 1 | 0.1 | 200 | 5.1 | 17 |
| Pear nectar | 60 | 4 | 0.2 | 13 | 0.3 | 3 |
| Peach nectar | 54 | 7 | 0.3 | 40 | 1 | 6 |
| Pineapple juice, unsweetened | 56 | trace | — | 134 | 3.4 | 8 |
| Tomato juice | 20 | 200.7 | 8.7 | 227 | 5.8 | 16.5 |
| Fruit-flavored beverage | 45 | — | — | — | — | — |
| Beer, regular | 41 | 5.3 | 0.2 | 25 | 0.6 | 12.4 |
| Beer, light | 28 | 2.8 | 0.1 | 18.1 | 0.5 | 12.1 |
| Gin, rum, vodka, whiskey (86 proof) | 250 | trace | — | 3.6 | 0.1 | — |
| Table wine, 12.2% alcohol/vol. | 86 | 3.5 | 0.1 | 93.1 | 2.4 | 10.3 |
| Dessert wine, 18.5% alcohol/vol. | 137 | 3.3 | 0.1 | 76.7 | 2 | — |

Alcoholic beverages are customarily served in special glassware, the size of which tends to standardize the alcoholic content:

| | | | |
|---|---|---|---|
| 1 cordial glass | = 20 ml | 1 burgundy glass | = 120 ml |
| 1 brandy glass | = 30 ml | 1 champagne glass | = 150 ml |
| 1 jigger | = 45 ml | 1 tumbler | = 240–360 ml |
| 1 sherry glass | = 60 ml | 1 mixing glass | = 360 ml |
| 1 cocktail glass | = 90 ml | | |

*Brand name data supplied by the commercial producer of the product. Other data obtained from Composition of Foods, Fruits, and Fruit Juices: Raw, Processed, Prepared. Agriculture Handbook No. 8–9. Consumer Nutrition Center, Washington, U.S. Department of Agriculture, 1982.
†Range.

**TABLE A–18A.** DIETARY FIBER CONTENT OF SELECTED FOODS*,† (g/100 g EDIBLE PORTION)

| FOOD ITEM | MOISTURE | TOTAL DIETARY FIBER (AOAC)‡ |
|---|---|---|
| Breads, Crackers, and Cakes | | |
| Bagels, plain | 31.6 | 2.1 |
| Biscuits, made from refrigerated dough, baked | 28.7 | 1.5 |
| Bread | | |
| Bran | 37.7 | 8.5 |
| Cornbread mix, baked | 34.4 | 2.4 |
| Cracked-wheat | 35.9 | 5.3 |
| French | 33.9 | 2.7 |
| Hollywood-type, light | 37.8 | 4.8 |
| Italian | 34.1 | 3.1 |
| Mixed-grain | 38.2 | 7.1 |
| Oatmeal | 36.7 | 3.9 |
| Pita | | |
| White | 32.1 | 1.6 |
| Whole-wheat | 30.6 | 7.5 |
| Pumpernickel | 38.3 | 5.9 |
| Reduced-calorie, high-fiber | | |
| Wheat | 43.7 | 11.3 |
| White | 41.8 | 9.3 |
| Rye | 37.0 | 6.2 |
| Wheat | 37.0 | 4.3 |
| White | 37.1 | 2.3 |
| Whole-wheat | 38.3 | 6.9 |
| Bread crumbs, plain or seasoned | 5.7 | 4.2 |
| Bread stuffing, flavored, from dry mix | 65.1 | 2.9 |
| Cake mix | | |
| Chocolate, prepared | 33.3 | 2.2 |
| Yellow, prepared | 40.0 | 0.8 |
| Cakes | | |
| Boston cream pie | 47.6 | 1.3 |
| Coffeecake | | |
| Crumb topping | 22.3 | 3.3 |
| Fruit | 31.7 | 2.5 |
| Fruitcake, commercial | 22.0 | 3.5 |
| Gingerbread, from dry mix | 38.5 | 3.2 |
| Cheesecake | | |
| Commercial | 44.6 | 2.1 |
| From no-bake mix | 44.4 | 1.9 |
| Cookies | | |
| Brownies | 12.6 | 2.4 |
| Brownies with nuts | 12.6 | 2.6 |
| Butter | 4.7 | 2.4 |
| Chocolate chip | 4.0 | 2.7 |
| Chocolate sandwich | 2.2 | 3.0 |
| Fig bar | 16.7 | 4.6 |
| Fortune | 8.0 | 1.6 |
| Oatmeal | 5.7 | 3.1 |
| Oatmeal, soft-type | — | 2.7 |
| Peanut butter | 6.7 | 1.8 |
| Shortbread with pecans | 3.3 | 1.8 |
| Vanilla sandwich | 2.1 | 1.5 |
| Crackers | | |
| Cheese, sandwich with peanut butter filling | 4.0 | 1.1 |
| Crisp bread, rye | 6.1 | 16.2 |
| Graham | | |
| Regular | 4.1 | 2.7 |
| Honey | 4.1 | 2.7 |

**TABLE A–18A.** CONTINUED

| FOOD ITEM | MOISTURE | TOTAL DIETARY FIBER (AOAC)‡ |
|---|---|---|
| Matzoh | | |
| Plain | 6.1 | 3.0 |
| Egg/onion | 8.0 | 5.0 |
| Whole-wheat | 3.0 | 11.6 |
| Melba toast | | |
| Plain | 5.6 | 6.5 |
| Rye | 6.7 | 8.0 |
| Wheat | 6.1 | 7.4 |
| Rye | 7.2 | 15.8 |
| Saltines | — | 2.7 |
| Snack-type | 4.2 | 2.0 |
| Wheat | 3.2 | 5.5 |
| Whole-wheat | 2.7 | 10.4 |
| Croutons, plain or seasoned | 5.6 | 5.0 |
| Doughnuts | | |
| Cake | 19.7 | 1.7 |
| Yeast-leavened, glazed | 26.7 | 2.1 |
| English muffin, whole-wheat | 45.7 | 6.3 |
| French toast, commercial, ready-to-eat | 48.1 | 2.8 |
| Ice cream cones | | |
| Sugar, rolled-type | 3.0 | 4.6 |
| Wafer-type | 5.3 | 4.1 |
| Muffins, commercial | | |
| Blueberry | 37.3 | 3.6 |
| Oat bran | 35.0 | 7.5 |
| Pancake, waffle mix, prepared | 50.4 | 1.3 |
| Pastry, Danish | | |
| Fruit | 27.6 | 1.9 |
| Plain | 19.3 | 1.2 |
| Pies, commercial | | |
| Apple | 51.7 | 1.7 |
| Cherry | 46.2 | 0.8 |
| Chocolate, cream | 43.5 | 2.0 |
| Egg custard | 46.5 | 1.2 |
| Fruit and coconut | — | 0.9 |
| Lemon meringue | 41.7 | 1.2 |
| Pecan | 19.8 | 3.5 |
| Pumpkin | 58.1 | 2.7 |
| Rolls, dinner, egg | 30.4 | 3.8 |
| Taco shells | 6.0 | 8.1 |
| Toaster pastries | 8.9 | 1.0 |
| Tortillas | | |
| Corn | 43.6 | 5.2 |
| Flour, wheat | 26.2 | 3.1 |
| Waffles, commercial, frozen, ready-to-eat | 45.0 | 2.4 |
| <u>Breakfast Cereals, Ready-to-Eat</u> | | |
| Bran | | |
| High-fiber | 2.9 | 35.3 |
| Extra fiber | — | 45.9 |
| Bran flakes | 2.9 | 18.8 |
| Bran flakes with raisins | 8.3 | 13.4 |
| Corn flakes | | |
| Frosted or sugar-sparkled | 1.9 | 2.2 |
| Plain | 2.8 | 2.0 |
| Fiber cereal with fruit | — | 14.8 |
| Granola | 3.3 | 10.5 |
| Oat cereal | 5.0 | 10.6 |
| Oat flakes, fortified | 3.1 | 3.0 |
| Puffed wheat, sugar-coated | 1.5 | 1.5 |
| Rice, crispy | 2.4 | 1.2 |

**TABLE A—18A.** CONTINUED

| FOOD ITEM | MOISTURE | TOTAL DIETARY FIBER (AOAC)‡ |
|---|---|---|
| Wheat and malted barley | | |
| Flakes | 3.4 | 6.8 |
| Nuggets | 3.2 | 6.5 |
| with raisins | — | 6.0 |
| Wheat flakes | 4.3 | 9.0 |
| Cereal Grains | | |
| Barley | 9.4 | 17.3 |
| Bulgur, dry | 8.0 | 18.3 |
| Corn flour, whole-grain | 10.9 | 13.4 |
| Cornmeal | | |
| Degermed | 11.6 | 5.2 |
| Whole-grain | 10.3 | 11.0 |
| Cornstarch | 8.3 | 0.9 |
| Farina, regular or instant, cooked | 85.8 | 1.4 |
| Hominy, canned | 79.8 | 2.5 |
| Millet, hulled, raw | — | 8.5 |
| Oat bran, raw | 6.6 | 15.9 |
| Oat flour | 7.8 | 9.6 |
| Oats, rolled or oatmeal, dry | 8.8 | 10.3 |
| Rice, brown, long-grain, cooked | 73.1 | 1.7 |
| Rice, white | | |
| glutinous, raw | 10.0 | 2.8 |
| Long-grain | | |
| Parboiled, cooked | — | 0.5 |
| Precooked or instant, cooked | 76.4 | 0.8 |
| Rye flour, medium or light | 9.4 | 14.6 |
| Semolina | 12.7 | 3.9 |
| Tapioca, pearl, dry | 12.0 | 1.1 |
| Wheat bran, crude | 9.9 | 42.4 |
| Wheat flour | | |
| White, all-purpose | 11.8 | 2.7 |
| Whole-grain | 10.9 | 12.6 |
| Wheat germ, toasted | 2.9 | 12.9 |
| Wild rice, raw | 7.8 | 5.2 |
| Fruits and Fruit Products | | |
| Apples, raw: | | |
| With skin | 83.9 | 2.2 |
| Without skin | 84.5 | 1.9 |
| Apple juice, unsweetened | 87.9 | 0.1 |
| Applesauce, unsweetened | 88.4 | 1.5 |
| Apricots, dried | 31.1 | 7.8 |
| Apricot nectar | 84.9 | 0.6 |
| Bananas, raw | 74.3 | 1.6 |
| Blueberries, raw | 84.6 | 2.3 |
| Cantaloupe, raw | 89.8 | 0.8 |
| Figs, dried | 28.4 | 9.3 |
| Fruit cocktail, canned in heavy syrup, drained | — | 1.5 |
| Grapefruit, raw | 90.9 | 0.6 |
| Grapes, Thompson, seedless, raw | 81.3 | 0.7 |
| Kiwifruit, raw | 83.0 | 3.4 |
| Nectarines, raw | 86.3 | 1.6 |
| Olives | | |
| Green | — | 2.6 |
| ripe | — | 3.0 |
| Orange, raw | 86.8 | 2.4 |
| Orange juice, frozen concentrate, prepared | 88.1 | 0.2 |

**TABLE A–18A.** CONTINUED

| FOOD ITEM | MOISTURE | TOTAL DIETARY FIBER (AOAC)‡ |
|---|---|---|
| Peach | | |
| Canned in juice, drained | — | 1.0 |
| Dried | 31.8 | 8.2 |
| Raw | 87.7 | 1.6 |
| Pears, raw | 83.8 | 2.6 |
| Pineapple | | |
| Canned in heavy syrup, chunks, drained | 79.0 | 1.1 |
| Raw | 86.5 | 1.2 |
| Prune | | |
| Dried | 32.4 | 7.2 |
| Stewed | — | 6.6 |
| Prune juice | 81.2 | 1.0 |
| Raisins | 15.4 | 5.3 |
| Strawberries | 91.6 | 2.6 |
| Watermelon | 91.5 | 0.4 |
| Legumes, Nuts, and Seeds | | |
| Almonds, oil-roasted | 3.3 | 11.2 |
| Baked beans, canned | | |
| Barbecue-style | — | 5.8 |
| Sweet or tomato sauce, plain | 72.6 | 7.7 |
| Beans, Great Northern, canned, drained | 69.9 | 5.4 |
| Cashews, oil-roasted | 5.4 | 6.0 |
| Chickpeas, canned, drained | 68.2 | 5.8 |
| Coconut, raw | 47.0 | 9.0 |
| Cowpeas (black-eyed peas), cooked, drained | 70.0 | 9.6 |
| Hazelnuts, oil-roasted | 1.2 | 6.4 |
| Lima beans, cooked, drained | 69.8 | 7.2 |
| Miso | 47.4 | 5.4 |
| Mixed nuts, oil-roasted, with peanuts | — | 9.0 |
| Peanut | | |
| Dry-roasted | 1.6 | 8.0 |
| Oil-roasted | 2.0 | 8.8 |
| Peanut butter | | |
| Chunky | 1.1 | 6.6 |
| Smooth | 1.4 | 6.0 |
| Pecans, dried | 4.8 | 6.5 |
| Pistachio nuts | 3.9 | 10.8 |
| Sunflower seeds, oil-roasted | 2.6 | 6.8 |
| Tahini | 3.0 | 9.3 |
| Tofu | 84.6 | 1.2 |
| Walnuts, dried | | |
| Black | 4.4 | 5.0 |
| English | 3.6 | 4.8 |
| Pasta | | |
| Noodles, Chinese, chow mein | 0.7 | 3.9 |
| Noodles, egg, regular, cooked | 68.7 | 2.2 |
| Noodles, Japanese, dry | | |
| Somen | 9.2 | 4.3 |
| Udon | 8.7 | 5.4 |
| Spaghetti and macaroni, cooked | 64.7 | 1.6 |
| Spaghetti, dry | | |
| Spinach | 8.7 | 10.6 |
| Whole-wheat | 7.1 | 11.8 |
| Snacks | | |
| Banana chips | 4.3 | 7.7 |
| Corn cakes | 4.6 | 1.9 |

**TABLE A–18A.** CONTINUED

| FOOD ITEM | MOISTURE | TOTAL DIETARY FIBER (AOAC)‡ |
|---|---|---|
| Corn-based, extruded | | |
| Chips | | |
| Barbecue-flavor | 1.2 | 5.2 |
| Plain | 1.0 | 4.4 |
| Puffs or twists, cheese-flavor | 1.5 | 1.0 |
| CORNNUTS | | |
| Barbecue-flavor | 1.6 | 8.4 |
| Nacho-flavor | 2.1 | 8.0 |
| Plain | 1.3 | 6.9 |
| Crisped rice bar | | |
| Almond | 6.7 | 3.6 |
| Chocolate chip | 7.0 | 2.2 |
| Granola bars | | |
| Hard | | |
| Chocolate chip | 2.4 | 4.4 |
| Plain | 3.9 | 5.3 |
| Soft | | |
| Milk-chocolate–coated, chocolate chip | 3.6 | 3.4 |
| Uncoated | | |
| Chocolate chip | 5.4 | 4.8 |
| Chocolate chip, graham, and marshmallow | 6.0 | 4.0 |
| Nut and raisin | 6.1 | 5.6 |
| Peanut butter | 7.3 | 4.3 |
| Peanut butter and chocolate chip | 5.9 | 4.2 |
| Plain | 6.4 | 4.6 |
| Raisin | 6.4 | 4.3 |
| Popcorn | | |
| Air-popped | 4.1 | 15.1 |
| Caramel-coated | | |
| With peanuts | 3.3 | 3.8 |
| Without peanuts | 2.8 | 5.2 |
| Cheese-flavor | 2.5 | 9.9 |
| Oil-popped | 2.8 | 10.0 |
| Potato chips | | |
| Barbecue-flavor | 1.9 | 4.4 |
| Plain | 1.9 | 4.8 |
| Sour-cream-and-onion–flavor | 1.8 | 5.2 |
| Potato chips, made from dried potatoes, plain | 1.4 | 3.6 |
| Potato sticks | 2.2 | 3.4 |
| Pretzels, hard, plain | 3.3 | 2.8 |
| Rice cakes, brown rice | | |
| Buckwheat | 5.9 | 3.8 |
| Corn | 5.9 | 2.9 |
| Multigrain | 6.3 | 3.0 |
| Plain | 5.8 | 4.2 |
| Rye | 6.8 | 4.0 |
| Tortilla chips | | |
| Nacho-flavor | 1.7 | 5.3 |
| Plain | 1.8 | 6.5 |
| Sweets | | |
| Baking chocolate, unsweetened, squares | 1.3 | 15.4 |
| Candies | | |
| ALPINE WHITE Bar With Almonds | 1.1 | 5.4 |

**TABLE A—18A.** CONTINUED

| FOOD ITEM | MOISTURE | TOTAL DIETARY FIBER (AOAC)‡ |
|---|---|---|
| BABY RUTH Bar | 5.0 | 2.9 |
| BUTTERFINGER Bar | 5.6 | 2.7 |
| Caramels | 8.5 | 1.2 |
| CHUNKY Bar | 2.9 | 4.8 |
| Milk chocolate | 1.3 | 2.8 |
| Milk chocolate, with almonds | 1.5 | 6.2 |
| M&M's Plain Chocolate Candies | 1.4 | 3.1 |
| NESTLE CRUNCH Milk Chocolate With Crisp Rice | 1.7 | 2.6 |
| O'HENRY | 5.9 | 3.5 |
| Cocoa, dry powder, unsweetened | 3.0 | 29.8 |
| Jams and preserves | 34.5 | 1.2 |
| Jellies | 28.4 | 0.6 |
| Pie fillings, canned | | |
| Apple | 73.4 | 1.0 |
| Cherry | 69.7 | 0.6 |
| Vegetables and Vegetable Products | | |
| Artichokes, raw | 84.4 | 5.2 |
| Beans, snap | | |
| Canned, drained, solids | 93.3 | 1.3 |
| Raw | 90.3 | 1.8 |
| Beets, canned, drained, solids | 91.0 | 1.7 |
| Broccoli | | |
| Cooked | 90.2 | 2.6 |
| Raw | 90.7 | 2.8 |
| Brussel sprouts, boiled | 87.3 | 4.3 |
| Cabbage, Chinese | | |
| Cooked | 95.4 | 1.6 |
| Raw | 94.9 | 1.0 |
| Cabbage, red | | |
| Cooked | 93.6 | 2.0 |
| Raw | 91.6 | 2.0 |
| Cabbage, white, raw | 91.5 | 2.4 |
| Carrots | | |
| Canned, drained, solids | 93.0 | 1.5 |
| Raw | 87.8 | 3.2 |
| Cauliflower | | |
| Cooked | 92.5 | 2.2 |
| Raw | 92.3 | 2.4 |
| Celery, raw | 94.7 | 1.6 |
| Chives | 92.0 | 3.2 |
| Corn, sweet | | |
| Canned | | |
| Brine pack, drained, solids | 76.9 | 1.4 |
| Cream-style | 78.7 | 1.2 |
| Cooked | 69.6 | 3.7 |
| Cucumbers | | |
| Raw | 96.0 | 1.0 |
| Pared | — | 0.5 |
| Lettuce | | |
| Butterhead or iceberg | 95.7 | 1.0 |
| Romaine | 94.9 | 1.7 |
| Mushrooms | | |
| Boiled | 91.1 | 2.2 |
| Raw | 91.8 | 1.3 |
| Onions, raw | 90.1 | 1.6 |
| Parsley, raw | 88.3 | 4.4 |

**TABLE A–18A.** CONTINUED

| FOOD ITEM | MOISTURE | TOTAL DIETARY FIBER (AOAC)‡ |
|---|---|---|
| Peas, edible, podded | | |
| Cooked | 88.9 | 2.8 |
| Raw | 88.9 | 2.6 |
| Peas, sweet, canned, drained, solids | 81.7 | 3.4 |
| Peppers, sweet, raw | 92.8 | 1.6 |
| Pickles | | |
| Dill | 93.8 | 1.2 |
| Sweet | 68.9 | 1.1 |
| Potatoes | | |
| Baked | | |
| Flesh | 75.4 | 1.5 |
| Skin | 47.3 | 4.0 |
| Boiled | 77.0 | 1.5 |
| French-fried, home-prepared from frozen | 52.9 | 4.2 |
| Hashed brown | 56.1 | 2.0 |
| Spinach | | |
| Boiled | 91.2 | 2.2 |
| Raw | 91.6 | 2.6 |
| Squash | | |
| Summer, cooked | 93.7 | 1.4 |
| Winter, cooked | 89.0 | 2.8 |
| Sweet potatoes | | |
| Canned, drained, solids | 72.5 | 1.8 |
| Cooked | 72.8 | 3.0 |
| Tomato, raw | 94.0 | 1.3 |
| Tomato products | | |
| Catsup | — | 1.6 |
| Paste | 74.1 | 4.3 |
| Puree | 87.3 | 2.3 |
| Sauce | 89.1 | 1.5 |
| Turnip greens | | |
| Boiled | 93.2 | 3.1 |
| Raw | 91.1 | 2.4 |
| Turnips, boiled | 93.6 | 2.0 |
| Vegetables, mixed, frozen, cooked | 83.2 | 3.8 |
| Water chestnuts, canned, drained, solids | 87.9 | 2.2 |
| Watercress | 95.1 | 2.3 |

*Modified from the Provisional Table on the Dietary Fiber Content of Selected Foods, HNIS/PT-106, 1988 and from updated Appendix Tables 8–19, Aug. 1991, and 8–20, Oct. 1989.

†Appreciation is expressed to the U.S. Department of Agriculture, Human Nutrition Information Service, Nutrition Monitoring Division for assistance in obtaining these data.

‡The total dietary fiber in foods is measured by the enzymatic-gravimetric method (the Association of Official Analytical Chemists (AOAC) official method of analysis). Duplicate samples of dried foods, with fat extracted if containing >10% fat, are gelatinized with Termamyl (heat-stable α-amylase) and then enzymatically digested with protease and amyloglucosidase to remove protein and starch. (When analyzing mixed diets, fat is always extracted prior to determining total dietary fiber.) Four volumes of ethyl alcohol (EtOH) are added to precipitated soluble dietary fiber. Total residue is filtered and then washed with 78% EtOH, 95% EtOH, and acetone. After drying, residue is weighed. One duplicate is analyzed for protein; the other is incinerated at 525° and ash is determined.

$$\text{Total dietary fiber} = \text{weight residue} - \text{weight (protein + ash)}$$

**TABLE A–18B.** NONSTARCH POLYSACCHARIDE CONTENT OF SELECTED FOODS

| FOOD ITEM | TOTAL g/100g FRESH WEIGHT |
|---|---|
| Vegetables and Legumes | |
| Beans, baked, canned | 3.5 |
| Beans, French, cooked | 3.1 |
| Beans, red kidney, cooked | 6.7 |
| Cabbage, red, cooked | 3.3 |
| Carrots, raw | 2.4 |
| Lentils, red, cooked | 1.9 |
| Onion, cooked | 1.8 |
| Peas, garden, canned | 4.0 |
| Potato, boiled, fresh | 1.1 |
| Potato Crisps | 4.9 |
| Sprouts, Brussel, boiled | 4.8 |
| Fruits and Nuts | |
| Apple, Golden Delicious with skin | 1.7 |
| Apricots, fresh | 2.3 |
| Avocado, fresh | 4.4 |
| Canteloupe | 0.6 |
| Coconut, fresh | 7.3 |
| Figs, dried | 7.5 |
| Kiwi fruit, no skin | 1.7 |
| Peanuts, roasted | 6.2 |
| Raisins, dried | 2.1 |
| Cereal Products | |
| Bran flakes | 11.3 |
| Corn flakes | 0.9 |
| Oatmeal, coarse | 7.0 |
| Popcorn | 9.8 |
| Pumpernickel bread | 7.5 |
| Shredded wheat | 9.8 |
| Spaghetti, white, cooked | 1.7 |
| Spaghetti, whole-wheat, cooked | 3.5 |
| White bread | 1.6 |
| Wholemeal bread (average) | 5.0 |

(From references 23 and 24 in Chapter 4. Courtesy of Dr. Barbara Schneeman.)

**TABLE A–19A.** AVERAGE VALUES FOR TRIGLYCERIDES, FATTY ACIDS (FA), AND CHOLESTEROL IN SELECTED FOODS AND OILS (INCLUDING OMEGA-3 FA) (PER 100 g EDIBLE PORTION)

| | FAT (g) | SFA (g) | MFA (g) | PFA (g) | M18:1 (g) | P18:2 (g) | P18:3 (g) | P:S | CHOL (mg) | S14:0 (g) | S16:0 (g) | S18:0 (g) | P20:5 (g) | P22:5 (g) | P22:6 (g) |
|---|---|---|---|---|---|---|---|---|---|---|---|---|---|---|---|
| Meats | | | | | | | | | | | | | | | |
| Liver calf | 6.90 | 2.56 | 1.49 | 1.09 | 1.28 | .61 | 0.08 | 0.43 | 561.00 | 0.00 | 1.40 | 1.16 | 0.00 | 0.00 | 0.00 |
| Liver pork | 4.40 | 1.41 | 0.63 | 1.05 | 0.56 | 0.42 | 0.04 | 0.74 | 355.00 | 0.02 | 0.53 | 0.84 | 0.00 | 0.04 | 0.03 |
| Kidney, beef | 3.44 | 1.09 | 0.74 | 0.74 | 0.61 | 0.40 | 0.01 | 0.68 | 387.00 | 0.06 | 0.47 | 0.51 | 0.00 | 0.00 | 0.00 |
| Kidney pork | 4.70 | 1.51 | 1.55 | 0.38 | 1.40 | 0.25 | 0.01 | 0.25 | 480.00 | 0.05 | 0.85 | 0.60 | 0.00 | 0.00 | 0.00 |
| Brains, beef | 12.53 | 2.92 | 2.50 | 1.44 | 2.00 | 0.03 | 0.00 | 0.49 | 2054.00 | 0.06 | 1.51 | 1.27 | 0.00 | 0.30 | 0.67 |
| Brains, pork | 9.51 | 2.15 | 1.72 | 1.47 | 1.10 | 0.09 | 0.12 | 0.68 | 2552.00 | 0.04 | 1.06 | 1.03 | 0.00 | 0.22 | 0.46 |
| Beef, 5% fat, cooked | 4.90 | 1.68 | 1.90 | 0.22 | 1.75 | 0.17 | 0.02 | 0.13 | 84.00 | 0.11 | 1.02 | 0.54 | 0.00 | 0.00 | 0.00 |
| Beef, 26% fat, cooked | 25.98 | 10.52 | 11.16 | 0.90 | 10.04 | 0.61 | 0.27 | 0.09 | 84.00 | 0.85 | 6.45 | 3.07 | 0.00 | 0.00 | 0.00 |
| Lamb, 9% fat, cooked | 9.17 | 3.28 | 4.02 | 0.60 | 3.72 | 0.49 | 0.05 | 0.18 | 92.00 | 0.29 | 1.76 | 1.13 | 0.00 | 0.00 | 0.00 |
| Lamb, 36% fat, cooked | 36.00 | 16.80 | 14.68 | 2.10 | 13.80 | 1.36 | 0.68 | 0.13 | 98.00 | 1.45 | 8.28 | 6.18 | 0.00 | 0.00 | 0.00 |
| Veal, 6% fat, cooked | 5.81 | 2.31 | 2.16 | 0.43 | 1.87 | 0.32 | 0.04 | 0.19 | 109.00 | 0.21 | 1.23 | 0.77 | 0.00 | 0.00 | 0.00 |
| Veal, 25% fat, cooked | 21.20 | 9.21 | 9.24 | 1.30 | 7.82 | 0.87 | 0.33 | 0.14 | 101.00 | 0.94 | 4.84 | 3.19 | 0.00 | 0.00 | 0.00 |
| Chicken, light meat, unknown part, skin removed before cooking | 3.87 | 1.15 | 1.05 | 0.92 | 0.88 | 0.66 | 0.02 | 0.80 | 77.00 | 0.03 | 0.67 | 0.32 | 0.00 | 0.03 | 0.03 |
| Duck, domestic, skin removed before cooking | 11.94 | 4.37 | 4.02 | 1.49 | 3.56 | 1.34 | 0.15 | 0.34 | 92.50 | 0.05 | 2.53 | 1.34 | 0.00 | 0.00 | 0.00 |
| Ground beef, unknown % fat | 22.56 | 8.86 | 9.88 | 0.84 | 8.63 | 0.62 | 0.09 | 0.09 | 89.00 | 0.64 | 5.10 | 2.66 | 0.00 | 0.00 | 0.00 |
| Bologna, beef, regular | 28.49 | 12.07 | 13.80 | 1.09 | 12.16 | 0.85 | 0.24 | 0.09 | 58.00 | 0.87 | 6.64 | 4.05 | 0.00 | 0.00 | 0.00 |
| Pork, fresh, 25% fat, cooked | 25.13 | 9.08 | 11.52 | 2.84 | 10.59 | 2.29 | 0.45 | 0.31 | 82.00 | 0.32 | 5.60 | 2.94 | 0.00 | 0.00 | 0.00 |
| Frankfurter, all beef (Kosher), regular | 28.54 | 12.05 | 13.62 | 1.38 | 11.99 | 1.11 | 0.27 | 0.11 | 61.00 | 0.94 | 6.52 | 3.96 | 0.00 | 0.00 | 0.00 |
| Frankfurter, chicken | 17.70 | 5.89 | 5.58 | 5.00 | 5.30 | 6.46 | 0.36 | 0.85 | 107.00 | 0.30 | 3.62 | 1.83 | 0.00 | 0.00 | 0.00 |
| Frankfurter, regular, beef and pork | 29.15 | 10.76 | 13.67 | 2.73 | 12.36 | 2.34 | 0.39 | 0.25 | 50.00 | 0.53 | 6.45 | 3.65 | 0.00 | 0.00 | 0.00 |
| Pork, cured, 23% fat, cooked | 23.48 | 8.38 | 11.03 | 2.51 | 10.15 | 2.15 | 0.36 | 0.30 | 67.00 | 0.25 | 5.12 | 2.93 | 0.00 | 0.00 | 0.00 |
| Salami, pork | 33.72 | 11.89 | 16.00 | 3.74 | 14.67 | 3.27 | 0.28 | 0.31 | 79.00 | 0.52 | 7.64 | 3.56 | 0.00 | 0.00 | 0.00 |
| Bacon, regular cut | 49.24 | 17.42 | 23.69 | 5.81 | 21.96 | 4.89 | 0.79 | 0.33 | 85.00 | 0.62 | 10.98 | 5.67 | 0.00 | 0.00 | 0.00 |
| Fish | | | | | | | | | | | | | | | |
| Mussel, cooked from fresh or frozen | 1.95 | 0.19 | 0.17 | 0.55 | 0.07 | 0.03 | 0.01 | 2.89 | 67.00 | 0.03 | 0.12 | 0.04 | 0.14 | 0.10 | 0.15 |
| Fish, 0 to 2.9% fat | 1.53 | 0.36 | 0.31 | 0.63 | 0.15 | 0.01 | 0.02 | 1.75 | 68.00 | 0.06 | 0.23 | 0.05 | 0.24 | 0.05 | 0.26 |
| Fish, 3.0 to 6.9% fat | 4.31 | 0.83 | 1.33 | 1.54 | 0.79 | 0.32 | 0.15 | 1.86 | 73.00 | 0.09 | 0.49 | 0.17 | 0.18 | 0.13 | 0.55 |
| Fish, 7.0 to 10.9% fat | 7.54 | 1.39 | 2.61 | 2.20 | 1.52 | 0.32 | 0.24 | 1.58 | 49.00 | 0.35 | 0.79 | 0.24 | 0.41 | 0.27 | 0.62 |
| Fish, 11.0 to 14.9% fat | 12.14 | 4.50 | 3.31 | 1.46 | 0.75 | 0.05 | 0.00 | 0.32 | 64.00 | 0.21 | 0.95 | 0.35 | 0.13 | 0.11 | 0.03 |
| Herring, smoked/kippered, canned and drained | 12.37 | 2.79 | 5.11 | 2.92 | 2.07 | 0.18 | 0.14 | 1.05 | 82.00 | 0.76 | 1.85 | 0.15 | 0.97 | 0.07 | 1.18 |

| | | | | | | | | | | | | | | | |
|---|---|---|---|---|---|---|---|---|---|---|---|---|---|---|---|
| Salmon, canned, drained, with salt | 6.05 | 1.53 | 1.81 | 2.05 | 1.07 | 0.06 | 0.06 | 1.34 | 55.00 | 0.05 | 1.35 | 0.13 | 0.84 | 0.05 | 0.81 |
| Sardines, canned in oil, drained | 11.45 | 1.53 | 3.87 | 5.15 | 2.14 | 3.54 | 0.50 | 3.37 | 142.00 | 0.19 | 0.99 | 0.34 | 0.47 | 0.00 | 0.51 |
| Tuna, canned, oil pack, regular, drained | 8.21 | 1.53 | 2.95 | 2.88 | 2.84 | 2.68 | 0.07 | 1.88 | 18.00 | 0.03 | 1.41 | 0.09 | 0.03 | 0.00 | 0.10 |
| Tuna, canned, water pack, regular, drained, not rinsed | 0.50 | 0.16 | 0.14 | 0.13 | 0.07 | 0.00 | 0.00 | 0.81 | 18.00 | 0.03 | 0.11 | 0.02 | 0.04 | 0.01 | 0.07 |
| Clams, cooked from fresh or frozen | 1.95 | 0.19 | 0.17 | 0.55 | 0.07 | 0.03 | 0.01 | 2.89 | 67.00 | 0.03 | 0.12 | 0.04 | 0.14 | 0.10 | 0.15 |
| Crab, hardshell, Alaskan King | 1.77 | 0.23 | 0.28 | 0.68 | 0.15 | 0.03 | 0.02 | 2.96 | 100.00 | 0.02 | 0.14 | 0.06 | 0.24 | 0.05 | 0.23 |
| Lobster, cooked from fresh or frozen | 0.59 | 0.11 | 0.16 | 0.09 | 0.09 | 0.00 | 0.00 | 0.82 | 72.00 | 0.01 | 0.08 | 0.02 | 0.05 | 0.00 | 0.03 |
| Oyster, cooked from fresh or frozen, Pacific | 4.95 | 1.26 | 0.50 | 1.48 | 0.19 | 0.10 | 0.07 | 1.17 | 109.00 | 0.22 | 0.87 | 0.12 | 0.42 | 0.10 | 0.46 |
| Scallops | 1.40 | 0.15 | 0.07 | 0.48 | 0.03 | 0.01 | 0.00 | 3.20 | 31.81 | 0.02 | 0.10 | 0.02 | 0.17 | 0.03 | 0.20 |
| Shrimp, cooked from fresh or frozen | 1.08 | 0.29 | 0.20 | 0.44 | 0.11 | 0.02 | 0.01 | 1.52 | 195.00 | 0.02 | 0.14 | 0.10 | 0.17 | 0.02 | 0.14 |
| Caviar | 17.90 | 4.21 | 5.86 | 5.66 | 2.94 | 0.99 | 0.55 | 1.34 | 588.00 | 0.90 | 1.87 | 0.72 | 1.03 | 0.81 | 1.35 |
| <u>Eggs Dairy</u> | | | | | | | | | | | | | | | |
| Eggs, whole, cooked | 10.02 | 3.10 | 3.81 | 1.36 | 3.47 | 1.15 | 0.03 | 0.44 | 425.00 | 0.03 | 2.23 | 0.78 | 0.00 | 0.00 | 0.04 |
| Eggs, yolk only, cooked | 30.87 | 9.55 | 11.74 | 4.20 | 10.70 | 3.54 | 0.10 | 0.44 | 1281.00 | 0.10 | 6.86 | 2.42 | 0.01 | 0.00 | 0.11 |
| Eggs, white only, cooked | 0.00 | 0.00 | 0.00 | 0.00 | 0.00 | 0.00 | 0.00 | 0.00 | 0.00 | 0.00 | 0.00 | 0.00 | 0.00 | 0.00 | 0.00 |
| Cream, coffee creamer, liquid/frozen | 9.97 | 9.30 | 0.11 | 0.00 | 0.11 | 0.00 | 0.00 | 0.00 | 0.00 | 1.00 | 0.43 | 0.60 | 0.00 | 0.00 | 0.00 |
| Cream, coffee creamer, powder, regular | 35.48 | 32.52 | 0.97 | 0.01 | 0.97 | 0.00 | 0.01 | 0.00 | 0.00 | 5.99 | 3.75 | 6.34 | 0.00 | 0.00 | 0.00 |
| Cream, coffee creamer, liquid/frozen | 11.28 | 1.68 | 4.85 | 4.25 | 4.79 | 3.94 | 0.29 | 2.53 | 0.00 | 0.01 | 1.10 | 0.56 | 0.00 | 0.00 | 0.00 |
| Cream, half and half, 10 to 12% fat | 11.50 | 7.16 | 3.32 | 0.43 | 2.89 | 0.26 | 0.17 | 0.06 | 36.90 | 1.16 | 3.02 | 1.39 | 0.00 | 0.00 | 0.00 |
| Cream, light/coffee cream, 20% fat | 19.31 | 12.02 | 5.58 | 0.72 | 4.86 | 0.44 | 0.28 | 0.06 | 66.10 | 1.94 | 5.08 | 2.34 | 0.00 | 0.00 | 0.00 |
| Milk, buttermilk, 1% fat | 0.88 | 0.55 | 0.25 | 0.03 | 0.22 | 0.02 | 0.01 | 0.05 | 3.50 | 0.09 | 0.23 | 0.11 | 0.00 | 0.00 | 0.00 |
| Milk, skim | 0.18 | 0.12 | 0.05 | 0.01 | 0.04 | 0.00 | 0.00 | 0.08 | 1.80 | 0.02 | 0.05 | 0.02 | 0.00 | 0.00 | 0.00 |
| Milk, 1% fat | 1.06 | 0.66 | 0.31 | 0.04 | 0.27 | 0.02 | 0.01 | 0.06 | 4.00 | 0.11 | 0.28 | 0.13 | 0.00 | 0.00 | 0.00 |
| Milk, 2% fat | 1.92 | 1.19 | 0.55 | 0.07 | 0.48 | 0.04 | 0.03 | 0.06 | 7.50 | 0.19 | 0.50 | 0.23 | 0.00 | 0.00 | 0.00 |
| Milk, whole, 3.5 to 4% fat | 3.34 | 2.08 | 0.96 | 0.12 | 0.84 | 0.07 | 0.05 | 0.06 | 13.60 | 0.34 | 0.88 | 0.40 | 0.00 | 0.00 | 0.00 |
| Parmesan cheese, dry | 30.02 | 19.07 | 8.73 | 0.66 | 7.74 | 0.32 | 0.34 | 0.03 | 78.70 | 3.38 | 8.10 | 2.67 | 0.00 | 0.00 | 0.00 |
| American cheese, processed | 31.25 | 19.69 | 8.95 | 0.99 | 7.51 | 0.61 | 0.38 | 0.05 | 94.40 | 3.21 | 9.10 | 3.80 | 0.00 | 0.00 | 0.00 |
| Cottage cheese, lowfat, 2% fat | 1.93 | 1.22 | 0.55 | 0.06 | 0.45 | 0.04 | 0.02 | 0.05 | 8.40 | 0.20 | 0.58 | 0.22 | 0.00 | 0.00 | 0.00 |
| Cottage cheese, regular or creamed, 4% fat | 4.51 | 2.85 | 1.28 | 0.14 | 1.06 | 0.10 | 0.04 | 0.05 | 14.90 | 0.47 | 1.36 | 0.51 | 0.00 | 0.00 | 0.00 |
| Cream cheese, Neufchatel | 23.43 | 14.80 | 6.77 | 0.65 | 5.66 | 0.45 | 0.20 | 0.04 | 76.10 | 2.35 | 6.88 | 2.98 | 0.00 | 0.00 | 0.00 |
| Cheddar cheese, natural | 33.14 | 21.09 | 9.39 | 0.94 | 7.90 | 0.58 | 0.36 | 0.04 | 104.90 | 3.33 | 9.80 | 4.01 | 0.00 | 0.00 | 0.00 |
| Swiss cheese, natural | 27.45 | 17.78 | 7.27 | 0.97 | 6.02 | 0.62 | 0.35 | 0.05 | 91.70 | 3.06 | 7.79 | 3.25 | 0.00 | 0.00 | 0.00 |

**TABLE A–19A.** AVERAGE VALUES FOR TRIGLYCERIDES, FATTY ACIDS (FA), AND CHOLESTEROL IN SELECTED FOODS AND OILS (INCLUDING OMEGA-3 FA) (PER 100 g EDIBLE PORTION) (CONTINUED)

| | | | | | | | | | | | | | | | |
|---|---|---|---|---|---|---|---|---|---|---|---|---|---|---|---|
| Monterey Jack cheese, natural | 30.04 | 19.11 | 8.71 | 0.66 | 7.34 | 0.43 | 0.23 | 0.03 | 95.60 | 3.07 | 9.22 | 3.57 | 0.00 | 0.00 | 0.00 |
| Mozzarella cheese, part skim milk | 17.12 | 10.88 | 4.85 | 0.51 | 4.17 | 0.36 | 0.15 | 0.05 | 54.00 | 1.72 | 5.22 | 2.08 | 0.00 | 0.00 | 0.00 |
| Brie cheese | 24.26 | 15.26 | 7.02 | 0.72 | 5.75 | 0.45 | 0.27 | 0.05 | 72.00 | 2.69 | 7.23 | 2.52 | 0.00 | 0.00 | 0.00 |
| Cheese, Kraft Light N' Lively Singles, American flavor | 15.50 | 9.77 | 4.44 | 0.49 | 3.73 | 0.30 | 0.19 | 0.05 | 52.91 | 1.59 | 4.51 | 1.88 | 0.00 | 0.00 | 0.00 |
| Cheese, Borden Lite-Line Singles, American flavor | 8.20 | 4.99 | 2.34 | 0.26 | 1.94 | 0.19 | 0.07 | 0.05 | 45.00 | 0.82 | 2.47 | 0.88 | 0.00 | 0.00 | 0.00 |
| Yogurt, frozen, fruit or vanilla, whole milk, 3 to 4% fat | 3.24 | 2.10 | 0.90 | 0.09 | 0.75 | 0.06 | 0.03 | 0.04 | 9.74 | 0.33 | 0.87 | 0.30 | 0.00 | 0.00 | 0.00 |
| Yogurt, frozen, fruit or vanilla, low fat, 1 to 2% fat | 1.08 | 0.70 | 0.30 | 0.03 | 0.25 | 0.02 | 0.01 | 0.04 | 4.20 | 0.11 | 0.29 | 0.10 | 0.00 | 0.00 | 0.00 |
| Yogurt, plain, lowfat, 1 to 2% fat | 1.55 | 1.00 | 0.43 | 0.04 | 0.35 | 0.03 | 0.01 | 0.04 | 6.10 | 0.16 | 0.42 | 0.15 | 0.00 | 0.00 | 0.00 |
| Yogurt, fruit, nonfat, <1% fat | 0.20 | 0.12 | 0.05 | 0.01 | 0.00 | 0.00 | 0.00 | 0.08 | 2.00 | 0.00 | 0.00 | 0.00 | 0.00 | 0.00 | 0.00 |
| Yogurt, fruit, whole milk, 3 to 4% fat | 3.24 | 2.10 | 0.90 | 0.09 | 0.75 | 0.06 | 0.03 | 0.04 | 9.74 | 0.33 | 0.87 | 0.30 | 0.00 | 0.00 | 0.00 |
| Ice cream and frozen desserts, regular, 10% fat, other flavors include chocolate chip | 10.77 | 6.70 | 3.11 | 0.40 | 2.71 | 0.24 | 0.16 | 0.06 | 44.70 | 1.08 | 2.83 | 1.30 | 0.00 | 0.00 | 0.00 |
| Sherbet, plain | 1.98 | 1.23 | 0.57 | 0.07 | 0.50 | 0.04 | 0.03 | 0.06 | 7.30 | 0.20 | 0.52 | 0.24 | 0.00 | 0.00 | 0.00 |
| Ice cream and frozen desserts, regular 5% fat, other flavors include chocolate chip | 4.30 | 2.68 | 1.24 | 0.16 | 1.08 | 0.10 | 0.06 | 0.06 | 13.90 | 0.43 | 1.13 | 0.52 | 0.00 | 0.00 | 0.00 |
| Fats/Oils | | | | | | | | | | | | | | | |
| Oils, canola | 100.00 | 7.10 | 58.90 | 29.60 | 56.10 | 20.30 | 9.30 | 4.17 | 0.00 | 0.00 | 4.00 | 1.80 | 0.00 | 0.00 | 0.00 |
| Oils, corn | 100.00 | 12.70 | 24.20 | 58.70 | 24.20 | 58.00 | 0.00 | 4.62 | 0.00 | 0.00 | 10.90 | 1.80 | 0.00 | 0.00 | 0.00 |
| Oils, sunflower | 100.00 | 10.30 | 19.50 | 65.70 | 19.50 | 65.70 | 0.00 | 6.38 | 0.00 | 0.00 | 5.90 | 4.50 | 0.00 | 0.00 | 0.00 |
| Oils, cottonseed | 100.00 | 25.90 | 17.80 | 51.90 | 17.00 | 51.50 | 0.20 | 2.00 | 0.00 | 0.80 | 22.70 | 2.30 | 0.00 | 0.00 | 0.00 |
| Oils, safflower | 100.00 | 9.10 | 12.10 | 74.50 | 11.70 | 74.10 | 0.40 | 8.19 | 0.00 | 0.10 | 6.20 | 2.20 | 0.00 | 0.00 | 0.00 |
| Oils, sesame | 100.00 | 14.20 | 39.70 | 41.70 | 39.30 | 41.30 | 0.30 | 2.94 | 0.00 | 0.00 | 8.90 | 4.80 | 0.00 | 0.00 | 0.00 |
| Oils, soybean (partially hydrogenated) | 100.00 | 14.90 | 43.00 | 37.60 | 42.50 | 34.90 | 2.60 | 2.52 | 0.00 | 0.10 | 9.80 | 5.00 | 0.00 | 0.00 | 0.00 |
| Oils, olive | 100.00 | 13.50 | 73.70 | 8.40 | 72.50 | 7.90 | 0.60 | 0.62 | 0.00 | 0.00 | 11.00 | 2.20 | 0.00 | 0.00 | 0.00 |
| Oils, peanut | 100.00 | 16.90 | 46.20 | 32.00 | 44.80 | 32.00 | 0.00 | 1.89 | 0.00 | 0.10 | 9.50 | 2.20 | 0.00 | 0.00 | 0.00 |
| Oils, coconut | 100.00 | 86.50 | 5.80 | 1.80 | 5.80 | 1.80 | 0.00 | 0.02 | 0.00 | 16.80 | 8.20 | 2.80 | 0.00 | 0.00 | 0.00 |
| Oils, palm | 100.00 | 49.30 | 37.00 | 9.30 | 36.60 | 9.10 | 0.20 | 0.19 | 0.00 | 1.00 | 43.50 | 4.30 | 0.00 | 0.00 | 0.00 |

| | | | | | | | | | | | | | | | |
|---|---|---|---|---|---|---|---|---|---|---|---|---|---|---|---|
| Oils, palm kernel | 100.00 | 81.40 | 11.40 | 1.60 | 11.40 | 1.60 | 0.00 | 0.02 | 0.00 | 16.40 | 8.10 | 2.80 | 0.00 | 0.00 | 0.00 |
| Shortening, vegetable | 100.00 | 25.00 | 44.50 | 26.10 | 44.50 | 24.50 | 1.60 | 1.04 | 0.00 | 0.40 | 14.10 | 10.60 | 0.00 | 0.00 | 0.00 |
| Margarine, regular, stick, salted, corn oil | 80.50 | 19.85 | 36.48 | 18.62 | 36.48 | 18.62 | 0.00 | 0.94 | 0.00 | 1.08 | 11.54 | 7.23 | 0.00 | 0.00 | 0.00 |
| Lard | 100.00 | 39.20 | 45.10 | 11.20 | 41.20 | 10.20 | 1.00 | 0.29 | 95.00 | 1.30 | 23.80 | 13.50 | 0.00 | 0.00 | 0.00 |
| Butter, regular, salted | 81.11 | 50.49 | 23.43 | 3.01 | 20.40 | 1.83 | 1.18 | 0.06 | 218.90 | 8.16 | 21.33 | 9.83 | 0.00 | 0.00 | 0.00 |
| Oils, medium chain triglyceride | 100.00 | 94.50 | 0.00 | 0.00 | 0.00 | 0.00 | 0.00 | 0.00 | 0.00 | 0.00 | 0.00 | 0.00 | 0.00 | 0.00 | 0.00 |
| Mayonnaise/mayo-type dressing, real, regular, commercial | 79.40 | 11.80 | 22.70 | 41.30 | 22.50 | 37.10 | 4.20 | 3.50 | 59.00 | 0.10 | 8.50 | 3.10 | 0.00 | 0.00 | 0.00 |
| Oils, rapeseed | 100.00 | 6.80 | 55.50 | 33.30 | 53.80 | 22.10 | 11.10 | 4.90 | 0.00 | 0.00 | 4.80 | 1.60 | 0.00 | 0.00 | 0.00 |
| Miscellaneous | | | | | | | | | | | | | | | |
| Peanuts, peanut butter, with salt | 49.98 | 9.59 | 23.58 | 14.36 | 22.96 | 14.10 | 0.08 | 1.50 | 0.00 | 0.05 | 5.50 | 2.14 | 0.00 | 0.00 | 0.00 |
| Almonds, roasted, dry roasted, salted | 56.53 | 5.27 | 36.71 | 11.86 | 36.03 | 11.36 | 0.40 | 2.25 | 0.00 | 0.32 | 3.74 | 1.11 | 0.00 | 0.00 | 0.00 |
| Cashews, roasted, dry roasted, salted | 48.21 | 9.70 | 28.41 | 8.15 | 27.89 | 7.97 | 0.17 | 0.84 | 0.00 | 0.36 | 4.53 | 3.09 | 0.00 | 0.00 | 0.00 |
| Peanuts, roasted, dry roasted, salted | 49.30 | 6.84 | 24.46 | 15.58 | 23.79 | 15.58 | 0.00 | 2.28 | 0.00 | 0.02 | 5.16 | 1.10 | 0.00 | 0.00 | 0.00 |
| Walnuts | 61.87 | 5.59 | 14.17 | 39.13 | 13.30 | 31.76 | 6.81 | 7.00 | 0.00 | 0.19 | 4.24 | 1.08 | 0.00 | 0.00 | 0.00 |
| Olives, black | 10.68 | 1.41 | 7.89 | 0.91 | 7.77 | 0.85 | 0.06 | 0.65 | 0.00 | 0.00 | 1.18 | 0.24 | 0.00 | 0.00 | 0.00 |
| Candy, chocolate pieces, fudge, plain | 10.78 | 4.93 | 4.53 | 0.93 | 4.48 | 0.86 | 0.06 | 0.19 | 3.92 | 0.10 | 2.29 | 2.35 | 0.00 | 0.00 | 0.00 |
| Avocado, unknown type | 15.32 | 2.44 | 9.61 | 1.95 | 8.96 | 1.84 | 0.11 | 0.80 | 0.00 | 0.00 | 2.40 | 0.03 | 0.00 | 0.00 | 0.00 |
| Coconut, fresh | 33.49 | 29.70 | 1.42 | 0.37 | 1.42 | 0.37 | 0.00 | 0.01 | 0.00 | 5.87 | 2.84 | 1.73 | 0.00 | 0.00 | 0.00 |
| Soybeans, cooked from dried | 8.97 | 1.30 | 1.98 | 5.06 | 1.96 | 4.46 | 0.60 | 3.89 | 0.00 | 0.02 | 0.95 | 0.32 | 0.00 | 0.00 | 0.00 |
| Peas, black-eyed, cooked from dried | 0.53 | 0.14 | 0.04 | 0.22 | 0.04 | 0.14 | 0.08 | 1.57 | 0.00 | 0.00 | 0.11 | 0.02 | 0.00 | 0.00 | 0.00 |
| Split peas, yellow or green, cooked from dried | 0.39 | 0.05 | 0.08 | 0.16 | 0.08 | 0.14 | 0.03 | 3.20 | 0.00 | 0.00 | 0.04 | 0.01 | 0.00 | 0.00 | 0.00 |

SFA = saturated fatty acid, MFA = monounsaturated fatty acid, PFA = polyunsaturated fatty acid, M18:1 = oleic acid, P18:2 = linoleic acid, P18:3 = linolenic acid, S14:0 = myristic acid, S16:0 = palmitic acid, S18:0 = stearic acid, P20:5 = omega-3 (eicosapentaenoic acid), P22:5 = omega-3 (docosapentaenoic acid), P22:6 = omega-3 (docosahexaenoic acid).

(With appreciation to the Nutrition Coding Center, University of Minneapolis, Minneapolis, MN for the compilation and preparation of these tables. Data are based on Version 19 of the NCC Nutrient Data Base.)

**TABLE A–19B.** AVERAGE VALUES FOR TRIGLYCERIDES, FATTY ACIDS (FA), AND CHOLESTEROL OF MARINE FOODS AND OILS (INCLUDING OMEGA-3 FA)

| FISH (100 g) | FAT (g) | CHOL (mg) | SFA (g) | MFA (g) | PFA (g) | M18:1 (g) | P18:2 (g) | P18:3 (g) | P20:5 (g) | P22:5 (g) | P22:6 (g) |
|---|---|---|---|---|---|---|---|---|---|---|---|
| Anchovy, European, raw | 4.84 | — | 1.28 | 1.19 | 1.64 | 0.62 | 0.10 | — | 0.50 | — | 0.90 |
| Bass, striped, raw | 2.33 | 80.00 | 0.51 | 0.66 | 0.78 | 0.45 | 0.02 | 0.02 | 0.17 | — | 0.59 |
| Bluefish, raw | 4.24 | 58.82 | 0.92 | 1.79 | 1.06 | 0.68 | 0.06 | trace | 0.25 | 0.06 | 0.52 |
| Burbot, raw | 0.81 | 60.00 | 0.16 | 0.13 | 0.30 | 0.10 | 0.01 | — | 0.07 | 0.03 | 0.10 |
| Carp, raw | 5.60 | 65.88 | 1.08 | 2.33 | 1.44 | 1.15 | 0.52 | 0.27 | 0.24 | 0.08 | 0.11 |
| Catfish, wild, raw | 2.82 | 58.00 | 0.72 | 0.84 | 0.87 | 0.59 | 0.10 | 0.07 | 0.13 | 0.10 | 0.23 |
| Catfish, farmed, raw | 7.59 | 47.00 | 1.77 | 3.59 | 1.57 | 3.17 | 0.88 | 0.10 | 0.07 | 0.09 | 0.21 |
| Cod, Atlantic, raw | 0.67 | 43.53 | 0.13 | 0.09 | 0.23 | 0.06 | 0.01 | trace | 0.10 | — | 0.20 |
| Eel, all varieties, raw | 11.66 | 126.00 | 2.35 | 7.19 | 0.95 | 2.78 | 0.20 | 0.70 | 0.10 | — | 0.10 |
| Flounder, unspecified, raw | 1.00 | 46.00 | 0.20 | 0.30 | 0.30 | — | — | trace | 0.10 | — | 0.10 |
| Haddock, raw | 0.72 | 57.65 | 0.13 | 0.12 | 0.24 | 0.07 | 0.01 | trace | 0.10 | — | 0.10 |
| Halibut, raw | 2.29 | 31.77 | 0.33 | 0.65 | 0.84 | 0.36 | 0.03 | 0.07 | 0.07 | 0.09 | 0.29 |
| Herring, Atlantic, raw | 9.04 | 60.00 | 2.03 | 3.74 | 2.13 | 1.52 | 0.13 | 0.10 | 0.70 | — | 0.90 |
| Mackerel, Atlantic, raw | 13.87 | 70.07 | 3.26 | 4.06 | 4.76 | 2.28 | 0.22 | 0.16 | 0.90 | 0.21 | 1.40 |
| Mussel, blue, raw | 2.20 | 38.00 | 0.40 | 0.50 | 0.60 | trace | — | — | 0.20 | 1.03 | 0.37 |
| Octopus, raw | 1.01 | — | 0.30 | 0.10 | 0.30 | — | — | — | 0.10 | — | 0.10 |
| Oyster, Eastern, wild, raw | 2.46 | 53.00 | 0.77 | 0.31 | 0.97 | 0.12 | 0.06 | 0.05 | 0.27 | 0.06 | 0.29 |
| Oyster, Eastern, farmed, raw | 1.55 | 25.00 | 0.44 | 0.15 | 0.59 | 0.07 | 0.03 | 0.04 | 0.19 | — | 0.20 |
| Perch, all varieties, raw | 0.92 | 89.41 | 0.19 | 0.15 | 0.37 | 0.07 | 0.01 | 0.10 | 0.90 | — | 1.60 |
| Pike, walleye, raw | 1.21 | 85.88 | 0.25 | 0.29 | 0.45 | 0.20 | 0.03 | 0.01 | 0.09 | 0.04 | 0.23 |
| Pollock, Atlantic, raw | 0.98 | 71.06 | 0.14 | 0.11 | 0.48 | 0.07 | 0.01 | — | 0.07 | 0.02 | 0.35 |
| Sablefish, raw | 15.30 | 49.00 | 3.20 | 8.06 | 2.04 | 4.07 | 0.17 | 0.10 | 0.68 | 0.17 | 0.72 |
| Salmon, Chinook, raw | 10.45 | 65.88 | 2.51 | 4.48 | 2.08 | 2.80 | 0.11 | 0.09 | 0.79 | 0.23 | 0.57 |
| Salmon, coho, wild, raw | 5.93 | 45.00 | 1.26 | 2.13 | 1.99 | 1.20 | 0.21 | 0.16 | 0.43 | 0.23 | 0.66 |
| Salmon, coho, farmed, raw | 7.67 | 51.00 | 1.82 | 3.33 | 1.86 | 1.72 | 0.35 | 0.08 | 0.39 | — | 0.82 |
| Sea bass, all, raw | 2.00 | 41.18 | 0.51 | 0.42 | 0.74 | 0.29 | 0.02 | trace | 0.10 | — | 0.30 |
| Smelt, rainbow, raw | 2.58 | 75.00 | 0.48 | 0.68 | 0.94 | 0.43 | 0.05 | 0.10 | 0.30 | — | 0.40 |
| Squid, short, finned, raw | 1.50 | 0.40 | 0.42 | 0.09 | 0.52 | — | — | trace | 0.16 | 0.52 | 0.36 |
| Red snapper, raw | 1.34 | 37.06 | 0.29 | 0.25 | 0.46 | 0.17 | 0.02 | trace | trace | — | 0.20 |
| Sole, European, raw | 1.20 | 50.00 | 0.30 | 0.40 | 0.20 | — | 0.00 | trace | trace | — | 0.10 |
| Sturgeon, all, raw | 4.04 | — | 0.92 | 1.94 | 0.69 | 1.44 | 0.07 | 0.10 | 0.19 | 0.05 | 0.09 |
| Swordfish, raw | 4.01 | 38.82 | 1.10 | 1.54 | 0.92 | 1.09 | 0.03 | — | 0.10 | 0.00 | 0.10 |
| Trout, rainbow, wild, raw | 3.46 | 59.00 | 0.72 | 1.13 | 1.24 | 0.61 | 0.24 | 0.12 | 0.17 | 0.11 | 0.42 |
| Trout, rainbow, farmed, raw | 5.40 | 59.00 | 1.55 | 1.54 | 1.81 | 1.06 | 0.71 | 0.06 | 0.26 | — | 0.67 |
| Tuna, bluefin, fresh, raw | 4.91 | 37.65 | 1.26 | 1.37 | 1.67 | 0.92 | 0.05 | — | 0.40 | — | 1.20 |
| Whitefish, all, raw | 5.85 | 60.00 | 0.91 | 2.00 | 2.15 | 1.35 | 0.27 | 0.18 | 0.32 | 0.16 | 0.94 |
| Cod liver oil | 100.00 | 570.00 | 22.61 | 46.71 | 22.54 | 20.65 | 0.94 | 0.94 | 6.90 | 0.94 | 10.97 |
| Herring oil | 100.00 | 766.00 | 21.29 | 56.56 | 15.60 | 11.96 | 1.15 | 0.76 | 6.27 | 0.62 | 4.21 |
| Menhaden oil | 100.00 | 521.00 | 30.43 | 26.69 | 34.20 | 14.53 | 2.15 | 1.49 | 13.17 | 4.92 | 8.56 |
| Max EPA conc fish body oil | 100.00 | 600.00 | 25.40 | 28.30 | 41.10 | — | — | 0.00 | 17.80 | — | 11.60 |
| Salmon oil | 100.00 | 485.00 | 19.87 | 29.04 | 40.32 | 16.98 | 1.54 | 1.06 | 13.02 | 2.99 | 18.23 |

SFA = saturated fatty acid, MFA = monounsaturated fatty acid, PFA = polyunsaturated fatty acid, M18:1 = oleic acid, P18:2 = linoleic acid, P18:3 = linolenic acid, P20:5 = omega-3 (eicosapentaenoic acid), P22:5 = omega-3 (docosapentaenoic acid), P22:6 = omega-3 (docosahexaenoic acid).

(From Provisional Table on the Content of Omega-3 Fatty Acids and Other Fat Components in Selected Foods, U.S. Department of Agriculture, Human Nutrition Information Service, HNIS/PT-103, 1988. Other data obtained from Composition of Finfish and Shellfish Products, Agriculture Handbook No. 8-15, 1991 Supplement. Consumer Nutrition Center, Washington, U.S. Department of Agriculture, 1991.)

Trace is less than 0.05 g/100 g food.

— denotes Lack of reliable data for nutrient known to be present.

**TABLE A–20.** PROTEIN, SODIUM, POTASSIUM, CALCIUM, PHOSPHORUS, AND MAGNESIUM CONTENT OF SELECTED COMMON FOODS PER SERVING PORTION

| FOOD NAME | SERVING PORTION | Pro (g) | Na (mg) | K (mg) | Ca (mg) | $PO_4$ (mg) | Mg (mg) |
|---|---|---|---|---|---|---|---|
| Dairy Products | | | | | | | |
| Egg, whole, raw, large | 1.0 Item | 6.250 | 63.000 | 60.000 | 25.000 | 89.000 | 5.000 |
| Cheese, cottage, uncreamed | 1.0 Oz | 4.888 | 3.715 | 9.189 | 8.994 | 29.523 | 1.173 |
| Cream, coffee, table, light | 1.0 Tbsp | 0.405 | 5.937 | 18.250 | 14.437 | 12.000 | 1.312 |
| Cream, sour, cultured | 1.0 Tbsp | 0.454 | 7.687 | 20.687 | 16.750 | 12.187 | 1.625 |
| Milk, buttermilk, fluid | 1.0 Cup | 8.110 | 257.000 | 371.000 | 285.000 | 219.000 | 27.000 |
| Milk, whole, 3.3% fat, fluid | 1.0 Cup | 8.030 | 120.000 | 370.000 | 291.000 | 228.000 | 33.000 |
| Milk, nonfat/skim, fluid | 1.0 Cup | 8.350 | 126.000 | 406.000 | 302.000 | 247.000 | 28.000 |
| Milk, whole, low sodium | 1.0 Cup | 7.560 | 6.000 | 617.000 | 246.000 | 209.000 | 12.000 |
| Fats | | | | | | | |
| Butter, regular | 1.0 Tbsp | 0.119 | 116.000 | 3.640 | 3.360 | 3.220 | 0.280 |
| Vegetable oil, corn | 1.0 Tsp | 0.000 | 0.000 | 0.000 | 0.000 | 0.000 | 0.000 |
| Vegetable oil, olive | 1.0 Tsp | 0.000 | 0.002 | 0.000 | 0.008 | 0.055 | 0.000 |
| Shortening, veg, soybn/cottnsd | 1.0 Tsp | 0.000 | 0.000 | 0.000 | 0.000 | 0.000 | 0.000 |
| Margarine, reg, hard, unsalted | 1.0 Tsp | 0.000 | 0.100 | 1.160 | 0.820 | 0.630 | 0.070 |
| Mayonnaise, soy, commercial | 1.0 Tsp | 0.067 | 26.133 | 1.667 | 0.667 | 1.333 | 0.047 |
| Cereals | | | | | | | |
| Bran flakes, Kellogg's | 0.5 Cup | 2.455 | 152.000 | 124.000 | 9.550 | 96.000 | 35.500 |
| Corn flakes, Kellogg's | 0.5 Cup | 0.920 | 116.000 | 10.450 | 0.341 | 7.150 | 1.360 |
| Cream of rice, cooked | 1.0 Cup | 2.200 | 2.440 | 48.800 | 7.320 | 41.500 | 7.320 |
| Cream of wheat, instant | 1.0 Cup | 4.400 | 6.000 | 48.000 | 59.000 | 43.000 | 14.000 |
| Farina, cooked, enriched | 1.0 Cup | 3.260 | 0.000 | 30.300 | 4.660 | 28.000 | 4.660 |
| Oatmeal, cooked | 1.0 Cup | 6.080 | 2.340 | 131.000 | 18.700 | 178.000 | 56.200 |
| Wheat, puffed, plain | 0.5 Cup | 0.880 | 0.240 | 20.900 | 1.680 | 21.300 | 8.700 |
| Wheat, shredded, biscuit | 1.0 Item | 2.600 | 0.472 | 77.000 | 9.680 | 86.000 | 40.100 |
| Rice Krispies | 0.5 Cup | 0.965 | 170.000 | 14.750 | 1.990 | 17.200 | 5.100 |
| Breads, Cookies, Crackers | | | | | | | |
| Bread, white, soft | 1.0 Slice | 2.070 | 129.000 | 28.000 | 31.500 | 27.000 | 5.250 |
| Bread, whole-wheat, soft | 1.0 Slice | 2.690 | 178.000 | 49.300 | 20.200 | 72.800 | 26.000 |
| Crackers, graham, plain | 1.0 Item | 0.500 | 33.000 | 27.500 | 3.000 | 10.500 | 3.570 |
| Crackers, sodium free/whole wheat | 1.0 Serving | 1.000 | 1.000 | 35.000 | — | — | — |
| Crackers, saltines | 1.0 Item | 0.250 | 36.800 | 3.250 | 0.500 | 2.500 | 0.770 |
| Muffin, English, plain | 0.5 Item | 2.215 | 179.000 | 157.000 | 45.350 | 31.350 | 5.300 |
| Bread, Italian, enriched | 1.0 Slice | 3.000 | 152.000 | 22.000 | 5.000 | 23.000 | — |
| Roll, hard, enriched | 0.5 Item | 2.500 | 156.000 | 24.500 | 12.000 | 23.000 | 5.750 |
| Roll, hamburger/hotdog | 1.0 Item | 3.430 | 241.000 | 36.800 | 53.600 | 32.800 | 7.600 |
| Cookies, vanilla wafer | 5.0 Items | 1.000 | 50.000 | 14.500 | 8.000 | 12.500 | 3.400 |
| Meat, Fish | | | | | | | |
| Pot roast, arm, beef, cooked | 1.0 Oz | 9.355 | 18.711 | 81.931 | 2.551 | 75.978 | 6.804 |
| Hamburger patty, beef/lean | 1.0 Oz | 7.004 | 21.679 | 85.384 | 3.002 | 44.693 | 6.004 |
| Steak, sirloin, lean, broiled | 1.0 Oz | 8.606 | 18.731 | 114.000 | 3.119 | 69.356 | 9.062 |
| Chicken, leg, no skin, roasted | 1.0 Oz | 7.669 | 25.963 | 68.637 | 3.402 | 51.925 | 6.864 |
| Chicken, breast, roasted | 1.0 Oz | 8.447 | 19.961 | 69.429 | 4.050 | 60.750 | 7.811 |
| Lamb, all cuts, lean/fat, cooked | 1.0 Oz | 6.971 | 20.345 | 87.718 | 4.669 | 53.365 | 6.671 |
| Turkey, dark meat, no skin | 1.0 Oz | 8.100 | 22.275 | 82.215 | 9.113 | 57.915 | 6.885 |
| Turkey, light, no skin, roasted | 1.0 Oz | 8.485 | 18.023 | 86.265 | 5.468 | 62.168 | 7.898 |
| Veal, all cuts, lean, cooked | 1.0 Oz | 9.039 | 25.348 | 96.056 | 6.671 | 71.042 | 8.005 |
| Bluefish | 1.0 Oz | 5.689 | 17.010 | 105.000 | 1.890 | 64.449 | 9.450 |
| Flatfish, raw | 1.0 Oz | 5.336 | 23.014 | 102.000 | 5.003 | 52.031 | 9.005 |
| Cod, cooked, dry heat | 1.0 Oz | 6.473 | 22.050 | 69.143 | 3.969 | 39.060 | 11.970 |
| Halibut, broiled, dry | 1.0 Oz | 7.571 | 19.578 | 163.000 | 17.010 | 80.714 | 30.351 |
| Shrimp, raw, mixed species | 1.0 Oz | 5.751 | 42.525 | 52.650 | 15.188 | 58.725 | 10.125 |
| Tuna, can/oil, drained | 1.0 Oz | 8.272 | 100.000 | 58.701 | 3.702 | 88.052 | 8.805 |
| Tuna, diet, low sodium | 1.0 Oz | 7.656 | 11.380 | 73.670 | 1.418 | 62.390 | 9.074 |
| Sweets | | | | | | | |
| Honey, strained/extracted | 1.0 Tbsp | 0.000 | 1.000 | 11.000 | 1.000 | 1.000 | 0.630 |
| Ice milk, van, hard, 4.3% fat | 0.5 Cup | 2.580 | 52.500 | 133.000 | 88.000 | 64.500 | 9.500 |
| Ice cream, van, hard, 10% fat | 0.5 Cup | 2.400 | 58.000 | 129.000 | 88.000 | 67.000 | 9.000 |

**TABLE A–20.** CONTINUED

| FOOD NAME | SERVING PORTION | Pro (g) | Na (mg) | K (mg) | Ca (mg) | $PO_4$ (mg) | Mg (mg) |
|---|---|---|---|---|---|---|---|
| Sweets | | | | | | | |
| Ice cream, van, hard, 16% fat | 0.5 Cup | 2.065 | 54.000 | 111.000 | 75.500 | 57.500 | 8.000 |
| Jams/preserves, regular | 1.0 Tbsp | 0.000 | 2.000 | 18.000 | 4.000 | 2.000 | — |
| Sherbet, orange, 2% fat | 0.5 Cup | 1.080 | 44.000 | 99.000 | 51.500 | 37.000 | 7.500 |
| Sugar, brown, pressed down | 0.5 Cup | 0.000 | 33.000 | 379.000 | 93.500 | 21.000 | — |
| Sugar, white, granulated | 1.0 Tbsp | 0.000 | 0.120 | 0.000 | 0.000 | 0.000 | — |
| Juices | | | | | | | |
| Apple juice, can and bottle | 3.5 Fl ozs | 0.066 | 3.062 | 129.000 | 7.612 | 7.875 | 3.500 |
| Apricot nectar, can | 3.5 Fl ozs | 0.402 | 3.937 | 125.000 | 7.700 | 9.887 | 5.687 |
| Cranberry juice, bottle | 3.5 Fl ozs | 0.000 | 4.375 | 19.906 | 3.321 | 2.214 | 2.214 |
| Grape juice, can | 3.5 Fl ozs | 0.000 | 0.000 | 38.500 | 3.500 | 3.500 | — |
| Grapefruit juice, can, unsweetened | 3.5 Fl ozs | 0.560 | 1.081 | 165.000 | 7.569 | 11.900 | 10.806 |
| Lemon juice, can and bottle | 3.5 Fl ozs | 0.427 | 22.400 | 109.000 | 11.725 | 9.625 | 8.531 |
| Orange juice, can | 3.5 Fl ozs | 0.643 | 2.179 | 191.000 | 8.706 | 15.268 | 11.987 |
| Pear nectar, can | 3.5 Fl ozs | 0.120 | 4.375 | 14.219 | 5.469 | 3.281 | 3.281 |
| Pineapple juice, can | 3.5 Fl ozs | 0.350 | 1.094 | 147.000 | 18.593 | 8.750 | 14.219 |
| Prune juice, can and bottle | 3.5 Fl ozs | 0.682 | 4.462 | 309.000 | 13.431 | 28.000 | 15.662 |
| Tomato juice, can | 3.5 Fl ozs | 0.809 | 385.000 | 235.000 | 9.625 | 20.300 | 11.725 |
| Tomato juice, low sodium | 3.5 Fl ozs | 0.809 | 10.675 | 235.000 | 9.625 | 20.300 | 11.725 |
| Vegetables | | | | | | | |
| Asparagus, can, spears | 0.5 Cup | 2.590 | 472.000 | 208.000 | 19.350 | 52.000 | 12.100 |
| Asparagus, can, low sodium | 0.5 Cup | 2.195 | 425.000 | 187.000 | 17.100 | 46.350 | 11.000 |
| Beans, snap, green, can, cuts | 0.5 Cup | 0.775 | 170.000 | 73.500 | 17.550 | 12.850 | 8.800 |
| Beans, green, can, low sodium | 0.5 Cup | 0.780 | 1.360 | 74.000 | 16.000 | 13.000 | 9.000 |
| Beans, snap, wax, raw, boiled | 0.5 Cup | 1.180 | 1.875 | 187.000 | 28.750 | 24.000 | 15.650 |
| Beets, can, whole | 0.5 Cup | 1.025 | 324.000 | 175.000 | 17.200 | 19.700 | 19.700 |
| Beets, can, diet, low sodium | 0.5 Cup | 1.025 | 324.000 | 175.000 | 17.200 | 19.700 | 19.700 |
| Broccoli, raw, boiled, drained | 0.5 Cup | 2.310 | 20.150 | 227.000 | 35.650 | 45.750 | 18.600 |
| Cabbage, common, boiled, drained | 0.5 Cup | 0.695 | 13.800 | 149.000 | 23.950 | 18.150 | 10.900 |
| Carrots, can, sliced, drained | 0.5 Cup | 0.467 | 176.000 | 131.000 | 18.250 | 17.500 | 5.850 |
| Carrots, can, low sodium | 0.5 Cup | 0.750 | 47.950 | 213.000 | 30.750 | 24.600 | 11.050 |
| Carrot, raw, whole, scraped | 1.0 Item | 0.740 | 25.200 | 233.000 | 19.400 | 31.700 | 10.800 |
| Cauliflower, raw, boiled, drained | 0.5 Cup | 1.160 | 4.000 | 200.000 | 17.000 | 22.000 | 7.000 |
| Celery, Pascal, raw, stalk | 1.0 Item | 0.300 | 34.800 | 115.000 | 16.000 | 10.000 | 4.400 |
| Corn, sweet, can, drained | 0.5 Cup | 2.160 | 267.000 | 161.000 | 4.125 | 53.500 | 16.500 |
| Corn, sweet, can, low sodium | 0.5 Cup | 2.480 | 3.840 | 196.000 | 5.100 | 65.500 | 20.500 |
| Cucumber, raw, sliced | 0.5 Cup | 0.281 | 1.040 | 77.500 | 7.300 | 8.850 | 5.700 |
| Peas, green, can, drained | 0.5 Cup | 3.755 | 186.000 | 147.000 | 17.000 | 57.000 | 14.450 |
| Peas, green, can, low sodium | 0.5 Cup | 3.755 | 1.700 | 147.000 | 17.000 | 57.000 | 14.450 |
| Tomato, raw, red, ripe | 1.0 Item | 1.050 | 11.100 | 273.000 | 6.150 | 29.500 | 13.500 |
| Tomato, red, can, stewed | 0.5 Cup | 1.185 | 324.000 | 305.000 | 42.100 | 25.500 | 15.300 |
| Tomato, can, low sodium, diet | 0.5 Cup | 1.115 | 15.600 | 265.000 | 31.200 | 22.800 | 14.400 |
| Potato, boiled, peeled before cooked | 1.0 Item | 2.310 | 6.750 | 443.000 | 10.800 | 54.000 | 27.000 |
| Noodles, egg, enriched, cooked | 0.5 Cup | 3.500 | 1.500 | 35.000 | 8.000 | 47.000 | 21.600 |
| Rice, white, parboiled, cooked | 0.5 Cup | 2.005 | 2.625 | 32.400 | 16.650 | 36.750 | 10.500 |
| Fruits | | | | | | | |
| Apples, raw, unpeeled | 1.0 Item | 0.262 | 1.000 | 159.000 | 10.000 | 10.000 | 6.000 |
| Apples, raw, peeled | 1.0 Item | 0.190 | 0.000 | 144.000 | 5.000 | 9.000 | 4.000 |
| Applesauce, can, unsweetened | 0.5 Cup | 0.208 | 2.440 | 91.500 | 3.660 | 8.550 | 3.660 |
| Apricots, can, light syrup | 0.5 Cup | 0.675 | 5.000 | 175.000 | 13.900 | 17.000 | 10.500 |
| Bananas, raw, peeled | 1.0 Item | 1.170 | 1.140 | 451.000 | 6.840 | 22.000 | 33.000 |
| Blueberries, raw | 0.5 Cup | 0.486 | 4.350 | 64.500 | 4.350 | 7.250 | 3.625 |
| Cherries, sweet, can/juice | 0.5 Cup | 1.140 | 3.750 | 164.000 | 17.500 | 27.500 | 15.000 |
| Grapefruit, red/pnk/wht, raw | 0.5 Cup | 0.725 | 0.500 | 161.000 | 13.500 | 10.000 | 9.500 |
| Oranges, raw, all varieties | 1.0 Item | 1.230 | 0.000 | 237.000 | 52.400 | 18.300 | 13.100 |
| Peaches, raw, whole | 1.0 Item | 0.609 | 0.000 | 171.000 | 4.350 | 10.400 | 6.090 |
| Peaches, can, light syrup | 0.5 Cup | 0.565 | 6.500 | 122.000 | 4.500 | 13.500 | 6.000 |
| Pears, raw, bartlet, unpeeled | 1.0 Item | 0.647 | 0.000 | 208.000 | 18.300 | 18.300 | 9.960 |
| Pineapple, can/juice | 0.5 Cup | 0.525 | 2.000 | 153.000 | 17.500 | 7.500 | 17.500 |
| Strawberries, raw, whole | 0.5 Cup | 0.455 | 0.745 | 124.000 | 10.450 | 14.150 | 7.450 |

Pro = protein, Na = sodium, K = potassium, Ca = calcium, $PO_4$ = phosphorus, Mg = magnesium.

(Created on Nutritionist III, Version 7, N-Squared Computing, 1991. Data compiled from U.S. Department of Agriculture Handbook 8- Series, manufacturers' data, published journals, and industry sources. Appreciation expressed to Ms. Lori Cohen, M.S., R.D., for her assistance in preparing this table.)

**TABLE A–21A.** VITAMIN A, VITAMIN E, α-TOCOPHEROL (TOC), VITAMIN C, THIAMIN, RIBOFLAVIN, NIACIN, VITAMIN $B_6$, VITAMIN $B_{12}$, AND FOLATE CONTENT OF SELECTED COMMON FOODS PER SERVING PORTION

| FOOD NAME | SERVING PORTION | A* (RE) | E† (mg) | α-TOC (mg) | C (mg) | THIAMIN (mg) | RIBO (mg) | NIACIN (mg) | $B_6$ (mg) | $B_{12}$ (μg) | FOLATE (μg) |
|---|---|---|---|---|---|---|---|---|---|---|---|
| Dairy Products | | | | | | | | | | | |
| Egg, whole, raw, large | 1.0 Item | 95.200 | 0.700 | 0.350 | 0.000 | 0.031 | 0.254 | 0.037 | 0.070 | 0.500 | 23.000 |
| Cheese, cottage, uncreamed | 1.0 Oz | 2.581 | — | 0.181 | 0.000 | 0.007 | 0.040 | 0.044 | 0.023 | 0.235 | 4.106 |
| Cream, coffee, table, light | 1.0 Tbsp | 32.437 | 0.094 | — | 0.114 | 0.005 | 0.022 | 0.009 | 0.005 | 0.033 | 0.375 |
| Cream, sour, cultured | 1.0 Tbsp | 34.124 | — | — | 0.124 | 0.005 | 0.021 | 0.010 | 0.002 | 0.043 | 1.562 |
| Milk, buttermilk, fluid | 1.0 Cup | 24.300 | 0.980 | — | 2.400 | 0.083 | 0.377 | 0.142 | 0.083 | 0.537 | 12.300 |
| Milk, whole, 3.3% fat, fluid | 1.0 Cup | 92.200 | 0.220 | 0.146 | 2.290 | 0.093 | 0.395 | 0.205 | 0.102 | 0.871 | 12.000 |
| Milk, nonfat/skim, fluid | 1.0 Cup | 150.000 | 0.221 | 0.147 | 2.400 | 0.088 | 0.343 | 0.216 | 0.098 | 0.926 | 13.000 |
| Milk, whole, low sodium | 1.0 Cup | 95.200 | 0.220 | 0.146 | 2.290 | 0.049 | 0.256 | 0.105 | 0.083 | 0.876 | 12.200 |
| Fats | | | | | | | | | | | |
| Butter, regular | 1.0 Tbsp | 105.000 | 0.221 | 0.221 | 0.000 | 0.001 | 0.005 | 0.006 | 0.000 | 0.018 | 0.420 |
| Vegetable oil, corn | 1.0 Tsp | 0.000 | 3.771 | 0.650 | 0.000 | 0.000 | 0.000 | 0.000 | 0.000 | 0.000 | 0.000 |
| Vegetable oil, olive | 1.0 Tsp | 0.000 | 0.569 | 0.535 | 0.000 | 0.000 | 0.000 | 0.000 | 0.000 | 0.000 | 0.000 |
| Shortening, veg, soybn/cottnsd | 1.0 Tsp | 0.000 | 2.771 | 0.342 | 0.000 | 0.000 | 0.000 | 0.000 | 0.000 | 0.000 | 0.000 |
| Margarine, reg, hard, unsalted | 1.0 Tsp | 47.000 | 2.710 | 0.423 | 0.004 | 0.000 | 0.001 | 0.001 | 0.000 | 0.003 | 0.030 |
| Mayonnaise, soy, commercial | 1.0 Tsp | 3.900 | 2.667 | 0.967 | 0.000 | 0.000 | 0.000 | 0.000 | 0.027 | 0.012 | 0.360 |
| Cereals | | | | | | | | | | | |
| Bran flakes, Kellogg's | 0.5 Cup | 258.000 | 0.412 | 0.082 | 0.000 | 0.254 | 0.293 | 3.430 | 0.351 | 1.050 | 69.000 |
| Corn flakes, Kellogg's | 0.5 Cup | 150.000 | — | 0.012 | 6.000 | 0.148 | 0.171 | 2.000 | 0.205 | 0.000 | 40.050 |
| Cream of rice, cooked | 1.0 Cup | 0.000 | — | — | 0.000 | 0.000 | 0.000 | 0.976 | 0.066 | 0.000 | 7.320 |
| Cream of wheat, instant | 1.0 Cup | 0.000 | — | — | 0.000 | 0.200 | 0.100 | 1.800 | 0.029 | 0.000 | 11.000 |
| Farina, cooked, enriched | 1.0 Cup | — | 2.190 | — | — | 0.186 | 0.117 | 1.280 | 0.023 | 0.000 | 4.660 |
| Oatmeal, cooked | 1.0 Cup | 4.680 | 5.400 | 3.530 | — | 0.257 | 0.047 | 0.304 | 0.047 | 0.000 | 9.360 |
| Wheat, puffed, plain | 0.5 Cup | 0.000 | — | 0.040 | 0.000 | 0.012 | 0.014 | 0.650 | 0.010 | 0.000 | 1.920 |
| Wheat, shredded, biscuit | 1.0 Item | 0.000 | 0.508 | 0.085 | 0.000 | 0.070 | 0.060 | 1.080 | 0.060 | 0.000 | 12.000 |
| Rice Krispies | 0.5 Cup | 188.000 | 0.040 | 0.006 | 7.550 | 0.185 | 0.213 | 2.500 | 0.256 | 0.000 | 50.000 |
| Breads, Cookies, Crackers | | | | | | | | | | | |
| Bread, white, soft | 1.0 Slice | 0.000 | 0.298 | 0.030 | 0.000 | 0.118 | 0.078 | 0.938 | 0.009 | 0.000 | 8.750 |
| Bread, whole-wheat, soft | 1.0 Slice | 0.000 | 0.252 | 0.028 | 0.000 | 0.098 | 0.059 | 1.070 | 0.052 | 0.000 | 15.400 |
| Crackers, graham, plain | 1.0 Item | 0.000 | 0.128 | 0.026 | 0.000 | 0.010 | 0.040 | 0.250 | 0.006 | 0.000 | 0.910 |
| Crackers, sodium free/whole-wheat | 1.0 Serving | — | — | — | — | — | — | — | — | — | — |
| Crackers, saltines | 1.0 Item | 0.000 | 0.050 | 0.010 | 0.000 | 0.125 | 0.013 | 0.100 | 0.001 | 0.000 | 0.495 |
| Muffin, English, plain | 0.5 Item | 0.000 | — | — | 0.000 | 0.129 | 0.090 | 1.050 | 0.011 | 0.000 | 8.950 |
| Bread, Italian, enriched | 1.0 Slice | 0.000 | 0.357 | 0.036 | 0.000 | 0.120 | 0.070 | 1.000 | 0.016 | 0.000 | 10.500 |
| Roll, hard, enriched | 0.5 Item | 0.000 | 0.133 | 0.010 | 0.000 | 0.100 | 0.060 | 0.850 | 0.009 | 0.000 | 14.750 |
| Roll, hamburger/hotdog | 1.0 Item | 0.000 | 0.212 | 0.016 | 0.000 | 0.196 | 0.132 | 1.580 | 0.014 | — | 14.800 |
| Cookies, vanilla wafer | 5.0 Items | 5.000 | 1.090 | 0.515 | 0.000 | 0.050 | 0.045 | 0.400 | — | — | — |
| Meat, Fish | | | | | | | | | | | |
| Pot roast, arm, beef, cooked | 1.0 Oz | 0.000 | — | 0.040 | 0.000 | 0.023 | 0.082 | 1.055 | 0.094 | 0.964 | 3.118 |
| Hamburger patty, beef, lean | 1.0 Oz | 3.005 | 0.172 | 0.101 | 0.000 | 0.014 | 0.060 | 1.464 | 0.073 | 0.667 | 2.668 |
| Steak, sirloin, lean, broiled | 1.0 Oz | 1.519 | 0.156 | 0.037 | 0.000 | 0.036 | 0.084 | 1.215 | 0.128 | 0.810 | 2.835 |
| Chicken, leg, no skin, roasted | 1.0 Oz | 5.372 | 0.156 | 0.099 | 0.000 | 0.021 | 0.066 | 1.791 | 0.104 | 0.093 | 2.387 |

**TABLE A–21A.** CONTINUED

| FOOD NAME | SERVING PORTION | A* (RE) | E† (mg) | α-TOC (mg) | C (mg) | THIAMIN (mg) | RIBO (mg) | NIACIN (mg) | $B_6$ (mg) | $B_{12}$ (μg) | FOLATE (μg) |
|---|---|---|---|---|---|---|---|---|---|---|---|
| Meat, Fish | | | | | | | | | | | |
| Chicken, breast, roasted | 1.0 Oz | 7.912 | 0.156 | 0.099 | 0.000 | 0.019 | 0.034 | 3.602 | 0.156 | 0.093 | 0.868 |
| Lamb, all cuts, lean/fat, cooked | 1.0 Oz | — | — | — | — | 0.027 | 0.073 | 1.888 | 0.037 | 0.724 | 5.003 |
| Turkey, dark meat, no skin | 1.0 Oz | 0.000 | — | 0.181 | 0.000 | 0.018 | 0.070 | 1.035 | 0.101 | 0.105 | 2.552 |
| Turkey, light, no skin, roasted | 1.0 Oz | 0.000 | — | 0.026 | 0.000 | 0.017 | 0.037 | 1.938 | 0.152 | 0.105 | 1.620 |
| Veal, all cuts, lean, cooked | 1.0 Oz | — | — | — | — | 0.017 | 0.097 | 2.388 | 0.093 | 0.470 | 4.336 |
| Bluefish | 1.0 Oz | 33.831 | — | — | 0.016 | 0.016 | 0.023 | 1.688 | 0.114 | 1.529 | 0.454 |
| Flatfish, raw | 1.0 Oz | 2.668 | — | — | — | 0.025 | 0.022 | 0.820 | 0.059 | 0.430 | — |
| Cod, cooked, dry heat | 1.0 Oz | 3.969 | — | — | 0.283 | 0.025 | 0.022 | 0.712 | 0.080 | 0.298 | 2.300 |
| Halibut, broiled, dry | 1.0 Oz | 15.309 | — | — | 0.000 | 0.020 | 0.026 | 2.021 | 0.112 | 0.387 | 3.902 |
| Shrimp, raw, mixed species | 1.0 Oz | — | — | — | — | 0.008 | 0.012 | 0.725 | 0.028 | 0.328 | 0.810 |
| Tuna, can/oil, drained | 1.0 Oz | 6.537 | — | 0.474 | 0.000 | 0.011 | 0.034 | 3.502 | 0.031 | 0.624 | 1.504 |
| Tuna, diet, low sodium | 1.0 Oz | 6.898 | 0.799 | — | — | 0.009 | 0.014 | 3.514 | 0.105 | 0.397 | 0.000 |
| Sweets | | | | | | | | | | | |
| Honey, strained/extracted | 1.0 Tbsp | 0.000 | — | — | 0.000 | 0.000 | 0.010 | 0.100 | 0.004 | 0.000 | — |
| Ice milk, van, hard, 4.3% fat | 0.5 Cup | 26.000 | 0.230 | 0.040 | 0.380 | 0.038 | 0.174 | 0.059 | 0.043 | 0.438 | 1.500 |
| Ice cream, van, hard, 10% fat | 0.5 Cup | 66.500 | 0.233 | 0.040 | 0.350 | 0.026 | 0.165 | 0.067 | 0.031 | 0.313 | 1.500 |
| Ice cream, van, hard, 16% fat | 0.5 Cup | 104.000 | 0.259 | 0.045 | 0.305 | 0.022 | 0.142 | 0.058 | 0.027 | 0.269 | 1.000 |
| Jams/preserves, regular | 1.0 Tbsp | 0.000 | — | 0.018 | 0.000 | 0.000 | 0.010 | 0.000 | 0.004 | 0.000 | 1.600 |
| Sherbet, orange, 2% fat | 0.5 Cup | 19.500 | — | — | 1.930 | 0.016 | 0.045 | 0.066 | 0.013 | 0.079 | 7.000 |
| Sugar, brown, pressed down | 0.5 Cup | 0.000 | — | — | 0.000 | 0.010 | 0.035 | 0.200 | — | — | — |
| Sugar, white, granulated | 1.0 Tbsp | 0.000 | — | — | 0.000 | 0.000 | 0.000 | 0.000 | — | — | — |
| Juices | | | | | | | | | | | |
| Apple juice, can and bottle | 3.5 Fl ozs | 0.087 | — | 0.011 | 1.006 | 0.023 | 0.018 | 0.108 | 0.032 | 0.000 | 0.108 |
| Apricot nectar, can | 3.5 Fl ozs | 144.000 | — | — | 0.661 | 0.010 | 0.015 | 0.286 | — | 0.000 | 1.426 |
| Cranberry juice, bottle | 3.5 Fl ozs | 0.000 | — | — | 39.199 | 0.010 | 0.010 | 0.039 | 0.021 | 0.000 | 0.221 |
| Grape juice, can | 3.5 Fl ozs | 0.000 | — | — | 17.500 | 0.010 | 0.010 | 0.109 | 0.021 | 0.000 | 1.050 |
| Grapefruit juice, can, unsweetened | 3.5 Fl ozs | 0.787 | 0.195 | 0.043 | 31.543 | 0.045 | 0.021 | 0.250 | 0.021 | 0.000 | 11.244 |
| Lemon juice, can and bottle | 3.5 Fl ozs | 1.619 | — | — | 26.468 | 0.044 | 0.010 | 0.210 | 0.046 | 0.000 | 10.762 |
| Orange juice, can | 3.5 Fl ozs | 19.118 | 0.218 | 0.044 | 37.493 | 0.065 | 0.031 | 0.342 | 0.096 | 0.000 | 19.731 |
| Pear nectar, can | 3.5 Fl ozs | 0.044 | — | — | 1.203 | 0.002 | 0.014 | 0.140 | 0.015 | 0.000 | 1.312 |
| Pineapple juice, can | 3.5 Fl ozs | 0.525 | — | — | 11.725 | 0.060 | 0.024 | 0.281 | 0.105 | 0.000 | 25.287 |
| Prune juice, can and bottle | 3.5 Fl ozs | 0.394 | — | — | 4.594 | 0.018 | 0.078 | 0.879 | 0.244 | 0.000 | 0.446 |
| Tomato juice, can | 3.5 Fl ozs | 59.936 | 0.757 | 0.234 | 19.556 | 0.050 | 0.033 | 0.717 | 0.119 | 0.000 | 21.262 |
| Tomato juice, low sodium | 3.5 Fl ozs | 59.936 | 0.757 | 0.235 | 19.556 | 0.050 | 0.033 | 0.717 | 0.119 | 0.000 | 21.262 |
| Vegetables | | | | | | | | | | | |
| Asparagus, can, spears | 0.5 Cup | 64.000 | — | 0.460 | 22.250 | 0.074 | 0.121 | 1.155 | 0.133 | 0.000 | 116.000 |
| Asparagus, can, low sodium | 0.5 Cup | 57.500 | — | 0.464 | 20.000 | 0.066 | 0.109 | 1.040 | 0.120 | 0.000 | 104.000 |

**TABLE A–21A.** CONTINUED

| FOOD NAME | SERVING PORTION | A* (RE) | E† (mg) | α-TOC (mg) | C (mg) | THIAMIN (mg) | RIBO (mg) | NIACIN (mg) | $B_6$ (mg) | $B_{12}$ (μg) | FOLATE (μg) |
|---|---|---|---|---|---|---|---|---|---|---|---|
| Vegetables | | | | | | | | | | | |
| Beans, snap, green, can, cuts | 0.5 Cup | 23.650 | 0.034 | 0.021 | 3.240 | 0.010 | 0.038 | 0.135 | 0.025 | 0.000 | 21.450 |
| Beans, green, can, low sodium | 0.5 Cup | — | 0.034 | 0.021 | 3.200 | 0.010 | 0.038 | 0.137 | — | 0.000 | 21.600 |
| Beans, snap, wax, raw, boiled | 0.5 Cup | 41.900 | — | 0.182 | 6.050 | 0.047 | 0.061 | 0.384 | 0.035 | 0.000 | 20.800 |
| Beets, can, whole | 0.5 Cup | 1.238 | — | 0.037 | 4.795 | 0.013 | 0.047 | 0.186 | 0.068 | 0.000 | 35.650 |
| Beets, can, diet, low sodium | 0.5 Cup | 1.238 | — | 0.037 | 4.795 | 0.013 | 0.047 | 0.186 | 0.068 | 0.000 | 35.650 |
| Broccoli, raw, boiled, drained | 0.5 Cup | 108.000 | 0.496 | 0.357 | 58.000 | 0.043 | 0.088 | 0.445 | 0.111 | 0.000 | 38.750 |
| Cabbage, common, boiled drained | 0.5 Cup | 6.550 | 1.210 | 1.210 | 17.600 | 0.042 | 0.040 | 0.165 | 0.047 | 0.000 | 14.700 |
| Carrots, can, sliced, drained | 0.5 Cup | 1005.000 | 0.336 | 0.307 | 1.970 | 0.013 | 0.022 | 0.403 | 0.082 | 0.000 | 6.700 |
| Carrots, can, low sodium | 0.5 Cup | 1620.000 | 0.565 | 0.515 | 3.445 | 0.024 | 0.033 | 0.520 | 0.138 | 0.000 | 9.950 |
| Carrot, raw, whole, scraped | 1.0 Item | 2025.000 | 0.367 | 0.317 | 6.700 | 0.070 | 0.042 | 0.668 | 0.106 | 0.000 | 10.100 |
| Cauliflower, raw, boiled, drained | 0.5 Cup | 0.900 | 0.057 | 0.019 | 34.300 | 0.039 | 0.032 | 0.342 | 0.125 | 0.000 | 31.700 |
| Celery, Pascal, raw, stalk | 1.0 Item | 5.200 | 0.292 | 0.144 | 2.800 | 0.018 | 0.018 | 0.129 | 0.035 | 0.000 | 11.200 |
| Corn, sweet, can, drained | 0.5 Cup | 13.200 | 0.510 | 0.033 | 7.000 | 0.027 | 0.065 | 0.990 | 0.039 | 0.000 | 40.100 |
| Corn, sweet, can, low sodium | 0.5 Cup | 15.350 | 0.795 | 0.051 | 8.600 | 0.033 | 0.078 | 1.200 | 0.048 | 0.000 | 48.750 |
| Cucumber, raw, sliced | 0.5 Cup | 2.600 | 0.161 | 0.078 | 2.445 | 0.016 | 0.010 | 0.156 | 0.027 | 0.000 | 7.250 |
| Peas, green, can, drained | 0.5 Cup | 65.500 | 2.235 | 0.017 | 8.150 | 0.103 | 0.066 | 0.620 | 0.055 | 0.000 | 37.650 |
| Peas, green, can, low sodium | 0.5 Cup | 65.500 | 2.235 | 0.017 | 8.150 | 0.103 | 0.066 | 0.620 | 0.055 | 0.000 | 37.650 |
| Tomato, raw, red, ripe | 1.0 Item | 76.300 | 0.603 | 0.418 | 23.500 | 0.073 | 0.059 | 0.772 | 0.098 | 0.000 | 18.500 |
| Tomato, red, can, stewed | 0.5 Cup | 70.000 | 0.905 | 0.281 | 16.950 | 0.059 | 0.045 | 0.910 | 0.022 | 0.000 | 6.900 |
| Tomato, can, low sodium, diet | 0.5 Cup | 72.000 | — | 0.264 | 18.150 | 0.054 | 0.037 | 0.880 | 0.108 | 0.000 | 9.350 |

**TABLE A–21A.** CONTINUED

| FOOD NAME | SERVING PORTION | A* (RE) | E† (mg) | α-TOC (mg) | C (mg) | THIAMIN (mg) | RIBO (mg) | NIACIN (mg) | $B_6$ (mg) | $B_{12}$ (μg) | FOLATE (μg) |
|---|---|---|---|---|---|---|---|---|---|---|---|
| Vegetables | | | | | | | | | | | |
| Potato, boiled, peeled before cooked | 1.0 Item | 0.000 | 0.081 | 0.041 | 9.990 | 0.132 | 0.026 | 1.770 | 0.363 | 0.000 | 12.000 |
| Noodles, egg, enriched cooked | 0.5 Cup | 5.500 | — | — | 0.000 | 0.110 | 0.065 | 0.950 | 0.071 | 0.000 | 9.600 |
| Rice, white, parboiled, cooked | 0.5 Cup | 0.000 | 0.342 | 0.097 | 0.000 | 0.219 | 0.016 | 1.225 | 0.016 | 0.000 | 3.000 |
| Fruit | | | | | | | | | | | |
| Apple, raw, unpeeled | 1.0 Item | 7.400 | 0.911 | 0.814 | 7.800 | 0.023 | 0.019 | 0.106 | 0.066 | 0.000 | 3.900 |
| Apple, raw, peeled | 1.0 Item | 5.600 | 0.845 | 0.346 | 5.120 | 0.022 | 0.013 | 0.116 | 0.059 | 0.000 | 0.500 |
| Applesauce, can, unsweetened | 0.5 Cup | 3.500 | — | 0.110 | 1.465 | 0.016 | 0.031 | 0.230 | 0.032 | 0.000 | 0.730 |
| Apricots, can, light syrup | 0.5 Cup | 167.000 | — | 1.125 | 3.415 | 0.020 | 0.026 | 0.385 | 0.069 | 0.000 | 2.150 |
| Bananas, raw, peeled | 1.0 Item | 9.200 | 0.365 | 0.308 | 10.400 | 0.051 | 0.114 | 0.616 | 0.659 | 0.000 | 21.800 |
| Blueberries, raw | 0.5 Cup | 7.250 | — | — | 9.450 | 0.035 | 0.037 | 0.261 | 0.026 | 0.000 | 4.640 |
| Cherries, sweet, can/ juice | 0.5 Cup | 15.650 | — | — | 3.125 | 0.023 | 0.030 | 0.510 | 0.038 | 0.000 | 5.250 |
| Grapefruit, red/pnk/ wht, raw | 0.5 Cup | 14.500 | — | — | 39.550 | 0.042 | 0.023 | 0.288 | 0.049 | 0.000 | 11.700 |
| Oranges, raw, all varieties | 1.0 Item | 26.900 | 0.314 | 0.314 | 69.700 | 0.114 | 0.052 | 0.369 | 0.079 | 0.000 | 39.700 |
| Peaches, raw, whole | 1.0 Item | 46.500 | — | 0.087 | 5.740 | 0.015 | 0.036 | 0.861 | 0.016 | 0.000 | 2.960 |
| Peaches, can, light syrup | 0.5 Cup | 44.500 | — | — | 2.950 | 0.012 | 0.032 | 0.745 | 0.024 | 0.000 | 4.100 |
| Pears, raw, bartlet, unpeeled | 1.0 Item | 3.300 | — | 0.820 | 6.640 | 0.033 | 0.066 | 0.166 | 0.030 | 0.000 | 12.100 |
| Pineapple, can/juice | 0.5 Cup | 4.750 | 0.125 | 0.125 | 11.900 | 0.119 | 0.024 | 0.355 | 0.093 | 0.000 | 6.000 |
| Strawberries, raw, whole | 0.5 Cup | 2.050 | 0.194 | 0.090 | 42.250 | 0.015 | 0.049 | 0.172 | 0.044 | 0.000 | 13.200 |

*RE = μg retinol + μg β-carotene (0.167) + μg other carotenes (0.083)

1 RE = 3.33 IU from vitamin A (retinol)
10 IU from β-carotene

†mg of vitamin E represents mg of total tocopherol including α-tocopherol.

— denotes Lack of reliable data for nutrient to be present.

(Created on Nutritionist III, Version 7, N-Squared Computing, 1991. Data compiled from U.S. Department of Agriculture Handbook 8- Series, manufacturers' data, published journals, and industry sources. Appreciation expressed to Ms. Lori Cohen, M.S., R.D., for her assistance in preparing this table.)

**TABLE A–21B.** RETENTION OF NUTRIENTS IN COOKED VEGETABLES[1]

| | ASCORBIC ACID (%) | THIAMIN (%) | RIBOFLAVIN (%) | NIACIN (%) | PANTOTHENIC ACID[6] (%) | VITAMIN $B_6$ (%) | FOLACIN[7] (%) | VITAMIN A (%) |
|---|---|---|---|---|---|---|---|---|
| Potatoes | | | | | | | | |
| Prepared from raw | | | | | | | | |
| Baked in skin | 80 | 85 | 95 | 95 | 90 | 95 | 90 | —[8] |
| Boiled in skin | 75 | 80 | 95 | 95 | 90 | 95 | 90 | — |
| Boiled without skin | 75 | 80 | 95 | 95 | 90 | 95 | 75 | — |
| Fried | 80 | 80 | 95 | 95 | 90 | 95 | 75 | — |
| Hashed-brown[2] | 25 | 40 | 85 | 80 | — | — | 65 | — |
| Mashed | 75 | 80 | 95 | 95 | 90 | 95 | 75 | — |
| Scalloped and au gratin | 80 | 80 | 95 | 95 | 90 | 95 | 75 | — |
| Prepared from frozen | | | | | | | | |
| French fried, heated | 50 | 75 | 95 | 95 | 90 | 95 | 75 | — |
| Baked, stuffed, heated | 80 | 85 | 95 | 95 | 90 | 95 | 80 | — |
| Hashed-brown | 80 | 80 | 95 | 95 | 90 | 95 | 80 | — |
| Sweet Potatoes | | | | | | | | |
| Prepared from raw | | | | | | | | |
| Baked in skin | 80 | 85 | 95 | 95 | 90 | 95 | 90 | 90 |
| Boiled in skin | 75 | 80 | 95 | 95 | 90 | 95 | 90 | 85 |
| Prepared from frozen | | | | | | | | |
| Baked | 80 | 80 | 95 | 95 | 90 | 95 | 80 | 90 |
| Boiled | 75 | 80 | 95 | 95 | 90 | 95 | 80 | 85 |
| Tomatoes (prepared from raw, baked, boiled, or stewed) | 95 | 95 | 95 | 95 | 95 | 95 | 70 | 95 |
| Other Vegetables (cooked in small or moderate amount of water until tender) | | | | | | | | |
| Prepared from raw, drained | | | | | | | | |
| Greens, dark and leafy[3] | 60 | 85 | 95 | 90 | 95 | 90 | 65 | 95 |
| Roots, bulbs, other vegetables of high starch and/or sugar content[4] | 70 | 85 | 95 | 95 | 90 | 95 | 70 | 90 |
| Other[5] | 80 | 85 | 95 | 90 | 90 | 90 | 70 | 90 |
| Prepared from frozen, drained | | | | | | | | |
| Greens, dark and leafy[3] | 60 | 90 | 95 | 90 | 95 | 90 | 55 | 95 |
| Roots, bulbs, other vegetables of high starch and/or sugar content[4] | 70 | 90 | 95 | 95 | 90 | 95 | 70 | 90 |
| Other[5] | 80 | 90 | 95 | 90 | 90 | 90 | 70 | 90 |

[1] $\% \text{ True Retention} = \frac{\text{Nutrient content per g of cooked food} \times \text{g of food after cooking}}{\text{Nutrient content per g of raw food} \times \text{g of food before cooking}} \times 100$

[2] Potatoes were pared, boiled, and held overnight before hashed-browning.

[3] Vegetables such as beet greens, Chinese cabbage, collards, mustard greens, spinach, Swiss chard, turnip greens, and other wild greens.

[4] Vegetables such as beets, carrots, green peas, lima beans, onions, parsnips, rutabagas, salsify, turnips, summer and winter squash, and other immature seeds of the legume group.

[5] Vegetables such as asparagus, bean sprouts, broccoli, brussels sprouts, cabbage, cauliflower, eggplant, kohlrabi, okra, and sweet peppers.

[6] Because of limited data, values are based on nutrient retention data from other cooked plant products.

[7] Values are based on limited data.

[8] Dashes denote lack of reliable data.

(From Composition of Foods, Raw, Processed, Prepared. 1990 Supplement. Washington, D.C., U.S. Department of Agriculture, Human Nutrition Information Service, Agriculture Handbook No. 8.)

**TABLE A–22.** IRON, ZINC, COPPER, SELENIUM, AND MANGANESE CONTENT OF SELECTED FOODS, IN MG (100 g = 3½ oz)*

| FOOD NAME | Fe | Zn | Cu | Se | Mn |
|---|---|---|---|---|---|
| **Dairy Products** | | | | | |
| Egg, whole, raw, large | 1.440 | 1.100 | 0.014 | 0.044 | 0.024 |
| Cheese, cottage, uncreamed | 0.228 | 0.469 | 0.028 | 0.023 | 0.003 |
| Cream, coffee, table, light | 0.042 | 0.271 | 0.008 | 0.000 | 0.001 |
| Cream, sour, cultured | 0.061 | 0.270 | 0.019 | — | 0.003 |
| Milk, buttermilk, fluid | 0.049 | 0.420 | 0.011 | 0.001 | 0.002 |
| Milk, whole, 3.3% fat, fluid | 0.049 | 0.381 | 0.010 | 0.001 | 0.004 |
| Milk, nonfat/skim, fluid | 0.041 | 0.400 | 0.011 | 0.003 | 0.002 |
| Milk, whole, low sodium | 0.050 | 0.380 | 0.010 | 0.001 | 0.004 |
| **Fats** | | | | | |
| Butter, regular, tablespoon | 0.157 | 0.050 | 0.014 | 0.000 | 0.007 |
| Vegetable oil, corn | 0.000 | 0.000 | 0.000 | — | 0.000 |
| Vegetable oil, olive | 0.384 | 0.060 | 0.074 | — | — |
| Shortening, veg, soybn/cottnsd | 0.000 | 0.000 | 0.000 | — | 0.000 |
| Margarine, reg, hard, unsalted | 0.000 | 0.000 | — | 0.000 | — |
| Mayonnaise, soy, commercial | 0.714 | 0.143 | 0.243 | — | — |
| **Cereals** | | | | | |
| Bran flakes, Kellogg's | 63.590 | 13.205 | 0.741 | 0.010 | 4.333 |
| Corn flakes, Kellogg's | 6.300 | 0.282 | 0.066 | 0.004 | 0.084 |
| Cream of rice, cooked | 0.200 | 0.160 | 0.034 | — | 0.144 |
| Cream of wheat, instant | 4.979 | 0.170 | 0.038 | — | — |
| Farina, cooked, enriched | 0.502 | 0.070 | 0.011 | — | — |
| Oatmeal, cooked | 0.679 | 0.491 | 0.055 | 0.009 | 0.585 |
| Wheat, puffed, plain | 4.733 | 2.358 | 0.408 | — | 1.758 |
| Wheat, shredded, biscuit | 3.136 | 2.500 | 0.500 | — | 3.072 |
| Rice Krispies | 6.303 | 1.690 | 0.250 | 0.014 | 0.989 |
| **Breads, Cookies, Crackers** | | | | | |
| Bread, white, soft | 2.840 | 0.620 | 0.140 | 0.028 | 0.280 |
| Bread, whole-wheat, soft | 3.373 | 1.655 | 0.338 | 0.046 | — |
| Crackers, graham, plain | 3.571 | 0.757 | 0.857 | 0.014 | — |
| Crackers, sodium free/ whole-wheat | — | — | — | — | — |
| Crackers, saltines | 4.545 | 0.618 | 0.182 | 0.145 | — |
| Muffin, English, plain | 2.821 | 0.720 | 0.311 | 0.027 | — |
| Bread, Italian, enriched | 2.333 | — | — | 0.027 | — |
| Roll, hamburger/hotdog | 2.975 | 0.620 | 0.165 | 0.030 | — |
| Cookies, vanilla wafer | 1.500 | — | — | 0.000 | — |
| **Meat, Fish** | | | | | |
| Pot roast, arm, beef, cooked | 3.790 | 8.660 | 0.164 | 0.006 | 0.019 |
| Hamburger patty, beef/lean | 2.106 | 5.365 | 0.066 | 0.024 | 0.014 |
| Steak, sirloin, lean, broiled | 3.357 | 6.518 | 0.146 | 0.034 | 0.018 |
| Chicken, leg, no skin, roasted | 1.305 | 2.853 | 0.080 | 0.014 | 0.021 |
| Chicken, breast, roasted | 1.061 | 1.020 | 0.050 | 0.027 | 0.018 |
| Lamb, all cuts, lean/fat, cooked | 1.871 | 4.459 | 0.119 | — | 0.022 |
| Turkey, dark meat, no skin | 2.336 | 4.464 | 0.160 | 0.025 | 0.023 |
| Turkey, light, no skin, roasted | 1.343 | 2.036 | 0.042 | — | 0.020 |
| Veal, all cuts, lean, cooked | 1.165 | 5.094 | 0.120 | — | 0.038 |
| Bluefish | 0.480 | 0.807 | 0.053 | — | 0.021 |
| Flatfish, raw | 0.353 | 0.459 | 0.032 | — | 0.016 |
| Cod, cooked, dry heat | 0.490 | 0.578 | 0.036 | 0.045 | 0.020 |
| Halibut, broiled, dry | 1.071 | 0.529 | 0.035 | 0.060 | 0.020 |
| Shrimp, raw, mixed species | 2.400 | 1.114 | 0.271 | — | 0.057 |
| Tuna, can/oil, drained | 1.388 | 0.900 | 0.071 | 0.072 | 0.015 |
| Tuna, diet, low sodium | 1.201 | 0.500 | 0.060 | 0.116 | 0.039 |
| **Sweets** | | | | | |
| Honey, strained/extracted | 0.476 | 0.095 | 0.038 | 0.005 | 0.029 |
| Ice milk, van, hard, 4.3% fat | 0.137 | 0.420 | 0.023 | 0.002 | 0.009 |
| Ice cream, van, hard, 10% fat | 0.090 | 1.060 | 0.019 | 0.002 | 0.006 |
| Ice cream, van, hard, 16% fat | 0.068 | 0.818 | 0.019 | 0.002 | 0.006 |
| Jams/preserves, regular | 1.000 | — | 0.310 | 0.000 | — |
| Sherbet, orange, 2% fat | 0.161 | 0.689 | 0.030 | — | 0.011 |
| Sugar, brown, pressed down | 3.409 | — | 0.350 | 0.001 | — |
| Sugar, white, granulated | 0.000 | 0.050 | 0.017 | 0.000 | — |

**TABLE A–22.** CONTINUED

| FOOD NAME | Fe | Zn | Cu | Se | Mn |
|---|---|---|---|---|---|
| Juices | | | | | |
| Apple juice, can and bottle | 0.371 | 0.028 | 0.022 | 0.001 | 0.113 |
| Apricot nectar, can | 0.382 | 0.092 | 0.073 | — | 0.032 |
| Cranberry juice, bottle | 0.150 | 0.070 | 0.018 | 0.000 | 0.193 |
| Grape juice, can | 0.096 | — | — | — | — |
| Grapefruit juice, can, unsweetened | 0.200 | 0.090 | 0.038 | 0.000 | 0.020 |
| Lemon juice, can and bottle | 0.130 | 0.060 | 0.037 | 0.000 | 0.020 |
| Orange juice, can | 0.442 | 0.070 | 0.057 | 0.000 | 0.014 |
| Pear nectar, can | 0.260 | 0.070 | 0.067 | 0.000 | 0.030 |
| Pineapple juice, can | 0.260 | 0.110 | 0.090 | 0.001 | 0.992 |
| Prune juice, can and bottle | 1.180 | 0.210 | 0.068 | 0.000 | 0.151 |
| Tomato juice, can | 0.582 | 0.140 | 0.101 | 0.000 | 0.077 |
| Tomato juice, low sodium | 0.582 | 0.140 | 0.101 | 0.000 | 0.077 |
| Vegetables | | | | | |
| Asparagus, can, spears | 1.831 | 0.400 | 0.096 | 0.004 | 0.170 |
| Asparagus, can, low sodium | 0.582 | 0.471 | 0.107 | 0.001 | 0.152 |
| Beans, snap, green, can, cuts | 0.904 | 0.290 | 0.038 | 0.001 | 0.200 |
| Beans, green, can, low sodium | 0.897 | 0.294 | 0.038 | 0.001 | 0.200 |
| Beans, snap, wax, raw, boiled | 1.280 | 0.360 | 0.103 | 0.001 | 0.294 |
| Beets, can, whole | 0.671 | 0.230 | 0.097 | 0.000 | 0.241 |
| Beets, can, diet, low sodium | 0.671 | 0.230 | 0.097 | 0.001 | 0.241 |
| Broccoli, raw, boiled, drained | 0.839 | 0.380 | 0.043 | 0.002 | 0.218 |
| Cabbage, common, boiled, drained | 0.390 | 0.160 | 0.028 | 0.002 | 0.129 |
| Carrots, can, sliced, drained | 0.640 | 0.260 | 0.104 | 0.001 | 0.450 |
| Carrots, can, low sodium | 0.610 | 0.290 | 0.103 | 0.001 | 0.451 |
| Carrot, raw, whole, scrapd | 0.500 | 0.200 | 0.047 | 0.003 | 0.142 |
| Cauliflower, raw, boiled, drained | 0.419 | 0.242 | 0.090 | 0.001 | 0.177 |
| Celery, pascal, raw, stalk | 0.400 | 0.130 | 0.035 | 0.000 | 0.035 |
| Corn, sweet, can, drained | 0.861 | 0.390 | 0.058 | 0.001 | 0.173 |
| Corn, sweet, can, low sodium | 0.350 | 0.359 | 0.056 | 0.000 | 0.033 |
| Cucumber, raw, sliced | 0.280 | 0.230 | 0.040 | 0.001 | 0.061 |
| Peas, green, can, drained | 0.953 | 0.712 | 0.082 | 0.001 | 0.303 |
| Peas, green, can, low sodium | 0.953 | 0.712 | 0.082 | 0.001 | 0.303 |
| Tomato, raw, red, ripe | 0.450 | 0.089 | 0.074 | 0.001 | 0.105 |
| Tomato, red, can, stewed | 0.729 | 0.170 | 0.112 | 0.001 | 0.059 |
| Tomato, can, low sodium, diet | 0.608 | 0.160 | 0.110 | 0.001 | — |
| Potato, boiled, peeled before cooked | 0.310 | 0.270 | 0.167 | 0.001 | 0.140 |
| Noodles, egg, enriched, cooked | 0.875 | — | 0.169 | 0.059 | — |
| Rice, white, parboiled, cooked | 1.126 | 0.310 | 0.094 | 0.020 | 0.260 |
| Fruits | | | | | |
| Apples, raw, unpeeled | 0.181 | 0.036 | 0.041 | 0.001 | 0.045 |
| Apple, raw, peeled | 0.070 | 0.039 | 0.031 | 0.001 | 0.023 |
| Applesauce, can, unsweetened | 0.119 | 0.030 | 0.026 | 0.000 | 0.075 |
| Apricots, can, light syrup | 0.391 | 0.107 | 0.079 | 0.000 | 0.052 |
| Bananas, raw, peeled | 0.307 | 0.160 | 0.104 | 0.001 | 0.152 |
| Blueberries, raw | 0.170 | 0.110 | 0.061 | 0.001 | 0.282 |
| Cherries, sweet, can/juice | 0.580 | 0.100 | 0.073 | 0.000 | 0.061 |
| Grapefruit, red/pnk/wht, raw | 0.087 | 0.070 | 0.047 | — | 0.012 |
| Oranges, raw, all varieties | 0.100 | 0.069 | 0.045 | 0.002 | 0.025 |
| Peaches, raw, whole | 0.110 | 0.140 | 0.068 | 0.001 | 0.047 |
| Peaches, can, light syrup | 0.359 | 0.088 | 0.052 | — | 0.046 |
| Pears, raw, Bartlet, unpeeled | 0.250 | 0.120 | 0.113 | 0.001 | 0.076 |
| Pineapple, can/juice | 0.280 | 0.100 | 0.086 | 0.001 | 1.120 |
| Strawberries, raw, whole | 0.380 | 0.130 | 0.049 | 0.001 | 0.290 |

*Values for five trace elements have been provided in this table. Other trace elements have been analyzed and can be found in the following article by Hunt and Mullen: Concentration of boron and other elements in human foods and personal-care products, J. Am. Diet Assoc., *91*:558–568, 1991. These authors report the analyzed concentrations of boron and molybdenum, as well as of calcium, copper, iron, magnesium, and manganese in selected foods and personal-care products (analgesics, antibiotics, decongestants, antihistamines, dental hygiene products, gastric antacids, and laxatives). For those interested in obtaining data on these nutrients, this article may serve as a helpful reference.

Fe = iron, Zn = zinc, Cu = copper, Se = selenium, Mn = manganese.

— denotes Lack of reliable data for nutrient known to be present.

(Created on Nutritionist III, Version 7, N-Squared Computing, 1991. Data compiled from U.S. Department of Agriculture Handbook 8- Series, manufacturers' data, published journals, and industry sources. Appreciation expressed to Ms. Lori Cohen, M.S., R.D., for her assistance in preparing this table.)

**TABLE A–23A.** STANDARD EXCHANGE LISTS*,†

The reason for dividing food into six different groups is that foods vary in their carbohydrate, protein, fat, and calorie content. Each exchange list contains foods that are alike; each choice contains about the same amount of carbohydrate, protein, fat, and calories.

The following chart shows the amount of these nutrients in one serving from each exchange list.

| *Exchange List* | *Carbohydrate (g)* | *Protein (g)* | *Fat (g)* | *Calories* |
|---|---|---|---|---|
| Starch/bread | 15 | 3 | trace | 80 |
| Meat (lean) | — | 7 | 3 | 55 |
| (medium-fat) | — | 7 | 5 | 75 |
| (high-fat) | — | 7 | 8 | 100 |
| Vegetable | 5 | 2 | — | 25 |
| Fruit | 15 | — | — | 60 |
| Milk (skim) | 12 | 8 | trace | 90 |
| (low-fat) | 12 | 8 | 5 | 120 |
| (whole) | 12 | 8 | 8 | 150 |
| Fat | — | — | 5 | 45 |

As you read the exchange lists, you will notice that one choice often is a larger amount of food than another choice from the same list. Because foods are so different, each food is measured or weighed so the amount of carbohydrate, protein, fat, and calories is the same in each choice.

*The exchange lists are based on material in the *Exchange Lists for Meal Planning* prepared by Committees of the American Diabetes Association, Inc., and the American Dietetic Association in cooperation with the National Institute of Arthritis, Metabolism, and Digestive Diseases and the National Heart and Lung Institutes of Health, Public Health Service, U.S. Department of Health and Human Services.

†From the American Diabetes Assoc., 1986, with permission.

**TABLE A—23A.** CONTINUED

STARCH/BREAD LIST

Each item in this list contains about 15 g of carbohydrate, 3 g of protein, a trace of fat, and 80 calories.

Whole-grain products average about 2 g of fiber per serving. Some foods are higher in fiber. Those foods that contain 3 or more g of fiber per serving are identified with the fiber symbol.†

You can choose your starch servings from any of the items on this list. If you want to eat a starch food that is not on this list, the general rule is that:

- ½ cup of cereal, grain, or pasta is one serving
- 1 ounce of a bread product is one serving

| | |
|---|---|
| *Cereals/Grains/Pasta* | |
| Bran cereals†, flaked | ½ cup |
| Bran cereals†, concentrated (such as Bran Buds, All Bran | ⅓ cup |
| Puffed cereal | 1½ cup |
| Grapenuts | 3 Tbsp |
| Shredded wheat | ½ cup |
| Other ready-to-eat unsweetened cereals | ¾ cup |
| Cooked cereals | ½ cup |
| Bulgur (cooked) | ½ cup |
| Grits (cooked) | ½ cup |
| Pasta (cooked) | ½ cup |
| Rice, white or brown (cooked) | ⅓ cup |
| Cornmeal (dry) | 2½ Tbsp |
| Wheat germ† | 3 Tbsp |
| *Dried Beans, Peas/Lentils* | |
| Beans† and peas† (cooked), e.g., kidney, white, split, blackeye | ⅓ cup |
| Lentils† (cooked) | ⅓ cup |
| Baked beans† | ¼ cup |
| *Starchy Vegetables* | |
| Corn† | ½ cup |
| Corn on cob†, 6″ long | 1 |
| Lima beans† | ½ cup |
| Peas, green† (canned or frozen) | ½ cup |
| Plantain† | ½ cup |
| Potato, baked | 1 small (3 oz) |
| Potato, mashed | ½ cup |
| Squash, winter† (acorn, butternut) | ¾ cup |
| Yam, sweet potato, plain | ⅓ cup |
| *Bread* | |
| Whole wheat | 1 slice (1 oz) |
| Pita, 6″ across | ½ |
| Raisin, unfrosted | 1 slice (1 oz) |
| Rye†, pumpernickel† | 1 slice (1 oz) |
| White (including French, Italian) | 1 slice (1 oz) |
| Bagel | ½ (1 oz) |
| Bread sticks, crisp, 4″ long × ½″ | 2 (⅔ oz) |
| Croutons, low-fat | 1 cup |
| English muffin | ½ |
| Plain roll, small | 1 (1 oz) |
| Frankfurter or hamburger bun | ½ (1 oz) |
| Tortilla, 6″ across | 1 |
| *Crackers/ Snacks* | |
| Animal crackers | 8 |
| Graham crackers, 2½″ square | 3 |
| Matzoth | ¾ oz |
| Melba toast | 5 slices |
| Oyster crackers | 24 |
| Popcorn (popped, no fat added) | 3 cups |
| Pretzels | ¾ oz |
| Rye crisp, 2″ × 3½″ | 4 |
| Saltine-type crackers | 6 |
| Whole-wheat crackers, no fat added (crispbreads, such as Finn, Kavli, Wasa) | 2–4 slices (¾ oz) |
| *Starch Foods Prepared With Fat (Count as 1 starch/bread serving plus 1 fat serving)* | |
| Biscuit, 2½″ across | 1 |
| Chow mein noodles | ½ cup |
| Cornbread, 2″ cube | 1 (2 oz) |
| Cracker, round butter type | 6 |
| French fried potatoes, 2″ to 3½″ long | 10 (1½ oz) |
| Muffin, plain, small | 1 |
| Pancake, 4″ across | 2 |
| Waffle, 4½″ square | 1 |
| Stuffing, bread (prepared) | ¼ cup |
| Taco shell, 6″ across | 2 |
| Whole-wheat crackers, fat added (such as Triscuits) | 4–6 (1 oz) |

†3 g or more of fiber per serving.

**TABLE A—23A.** CONTINUED

MEAT LIST

Each serving of meat and substitutes on this list contains varying amounts of fat and calories. The list is divided into three parts based on the amount of fat and calories: lean meat, medium-fat meat, and high-fat meat. One ounce (one meat exchange) of each of these includes:

| | *Carbohydrate (g)* | *Protein (g)* | *Fat (g)* | *Calories* |
|---|---|---|---|---|
| Lean | 0 | 7 | 3 | 55 |
| Medium-fat | 0 | 7 | 5 | 75 |
| High-fat | 0 | 7 | 8 | 100 |

You are encouraged to use more lean and medium-fat meat, poultry, and fish in your meal plan. This will help decrease your fat intake, which may help decrease your risk for heart disease. The items from the high-fat group are high in saturated fat, cholesterol, and calories. You should limit your choices from the high-fat group to three (3) times per week. Meat and substitutes do not contribute any fiber to your meal plan. Meat and meat substitutes that have 400 mg or more of sodium are identified with a § symbol.

*Tips:*

1. Bake, roast, broil, grill, or boil these foods rather than frying them with added fat.
2. Use a nonstick pan spray or a nonstick pan to brown or fry these foods.
3. Trim off visible fat before and after cooking.
4. Do not add flour, bread crumbs, coating mixes, or fat to these foods when preparing them.
5. Weigh meat after removing bones and fat, and after cooking. Three ounces of cooked meat is about equal to 4 ounces of raw meat. Some examples of meat portions are:
   - 2 oz meat (2 meat exchanges) = 1 small chicken leg or thigh
     ½ cup cottage cheese or tuna
   - 3 oz meat (3 meat exchanges) = 1 medium pork chop
     1 small hamburger
     ½ chicken breast (1 side)
     1 unbreaded fish fillet
     cooked meat, about the size of a deck of cards
6. Restaurants usually serve prime cuts of meat, which are high in fat and calories.

*Lean Meat and Substitutes*

(One exchange is equal to any one of the following items)

| | | |
|---|---|---|
| Beef: | USDA Good or Choice grades of lean beef, such as round, sirloin, and flank steak, tenderloin, and chipped beef§ | 1 oz |
| Pork: | Lean pork, such as fresh ham; canned, cured, or boiled ham; Canadian bacon§, tenderloin | 1 oz |
| Veal: | All cuts are lean except for veal cutlets (ground or cubed). Examples of lean veal are chops and roasts. | 1 oz |
| Poultry: | Chicken, turkey, Cornish hen (without skin) | 1 oz |
| Fish: | All fresh and frozen fish | 1 oz |
| | Crab, lobster, scallops, shrimp, clams (fresh, or canned in water§) | 2 oz |
| | Oysters | 6 medium |
| | Tuna§ (canned in water) | ¼ cup |
| | Herring (uncreamed or smoked) | 1 oz |
| | Sardines (canned) | 2 medium |
| Wild Game: | Venison, rabbit, squirrel | 1 oz |
| | Pheasant, duck, goose (without skin) | 1 oz |
| Cheese: | Any cottage cheese | ¼ cup |
| | Grated Parmesan | 2 Tbsp |
| | Diet cheese§ with less than 55 calories per oz | 1 oz |
| Other: | 95% fat-free luncheon meat§ | 1 oz |
| | Egg whites | 3 whites |
| | Egg substitutes with less than 55 calories per ¼ cup | ¼ cup |

**TABLE A–23A.** CONTINUED

| | | |
|---|---|---|
| *Medium-Fat Meat and Substitutes* | | |
| (One exchange is equal to any one of the following items) | | |
| Beef: | Most beef products fall into this category. Examples are all ground beef, roast (rib, chuck, rump), steak (cubed, Porterhouse, T-bone), and meatloaf | 1 oz |
| Pork: | Most pork products fall into this category. Examples are chops, loin roast. Boston butt, cutlets | 1 oz |
| Lamb: | Most lamb products fall into this category. Examples are chops, leg, and roast | 1 oz |
| Veal: | Cutlet (ground or cubed, unbreaded) | 1 oz |
| Poultry: | Chicken (with skin), domestic duck or goose (well-drained of fat), ground turkey | 1 oz |
| Fish: | Tuna§ (canned in oil and drained), salmon§ (canned) | 1 oz |
| Cheese: | Skim or part-skim milk cheeses, such as | ¼ cup |
| | Ricotta | ¼ cup |
| | Mozzarella | 1 oz |
| | Diet cheeses§ with 56–80 calories per oz | 1 oz |
| Other: | 86% fat-free luncheon meat§ | 1 oz |
| | Egg (high in cholesterol, limit to 3 per week) | 1 |
| | Egg substitutes with 56–80 calories per ¼ cup | ¼ cup |
| | Tofu (2½″ × 2¾″ × 1″) | 4 oz |
| | Liver, heart, kidney, sweetbreads (high in cholesterol) | 1 oz |
| *High-Fat Meat and Substitutes* | | |
| Remember, these items are high in saturated fat, cholesterol, and calories, and should be used only three (3) times per week. | | |
| (One exchange is equal to any one of the following items) | | |
| Beef: | Most USDA Prime cuts of beef, such as ribs, corned beef§ | 1 oz |
| Pork: | Spareribs, ground pork, pork sausage§ (patty or link) | 1 oz |
| Lamb: | Patties (ground lamb) | 1 oz |
| Fish: | Any fried fish product | 1 oz |
| Cheese: | All regular cheese,§ such as American, Blue, Cheddar, Monterey, Swiss | 1 oz |
| Other: | Luncheon meat,§ such as bologna, salami, pimento loaf | 1 oz |
| | Sausage,§ such as Polish, Italian, knockwurst, smoked | 1 oz |
| | Bratwurst§ | 1 oz |
| | Frankfurter§ (turkey or chicken)†† | 1 frank (10/lb) |
| | Peanut butter (contains unsaturated fat) | 1 Tbsp |

§400 mg or more of sodium per exchange.
††Frankfurter (beef, pork or combination). Count as one high-fat meat plus one fat exchange: 1 frank (10/lb).

**TABLE A–23A.** CONTINUED

VEGETABLE LIST

Each vegetable serving on this list contains about 5 g of carbohydrate, 2 g of protein, and 25 calories. Vegetables contain 2–3 g of dietary fiber. Vegetables that contain 400 mg or more of sodium per serving are identified with a § symbol.

Vegetables are a good source of vitamins and minerals. Fresh and frozen vegetables have more vitamins and less added salt. Rinsing canned vegetables will remove much of the salt.

Unless otherwise noted, the serving size for vegetables is:

- ½ cup of cooked vegetables or vegetable juice
- 1 cup of raw vegetables

| | | |
|---|---|---|
| Artichoke (½ medium) | Eggplant | Rutabaga |
| Asparagus | Greens (collard, mustard, turnip) | Sauerkraut§ |
| Beans (green, wax, Italian) | Kohlrabi | Spinach, cooked |
| Bean sprouts | Leeks | Summer squash (crookneck) |
| Beets | Mushrooms, cooked | Tomato (1 large) |
| Broccoli | Okra | Tomato/vegetable juice§ |
| Brussels sprouts | Onions | Turnips |
| Cabbage, cooked | Pea pods | Water chestnuts |
| Carrots | Peppers (green) | Zucchini, cooked |
| Cauliflower | | |

Starchy vegetables, such as corn, peas, and potatoes, are found on the Starch/Bread list.

For free vegetables, see Free Food list.

FRUIT LIST

Each item on this list contains about 15 g of carbohydrate and 60 calories. Fresh, frozen, and dry fruits have about 2 g of fiber per serving. Fruits that have 3 g or more of fiber per serving have a † symbol. Fruit juices contain very little dietary fiber.

The carbohydrate and calorie contents for a fruit serving are based on the usual serving of the most commonly eaten fruits. Use fresh fruits, or fruits frozen or canned without sugar added. Whole fruit is more filling than fruit juice, and may be a better choice for those who are trying to lose weight. Unless otherwise noted, the serving size for fruit is:

- ½ cup of fresh fruit or fruit juice
- ¼ cup of dried fruit

*Fresh, frozen, and unsweetened canned fruit*

| | |
|---|---|
| Apple (raw, 2″ across) | 1 apple |
| Applesauce (unsweetened) | ½ cup |
| Apricots (medium, raw) | 4 apricots |
| Apricots (canned) | ½ cup, or 4 halves |
| Banana (9″ long) | ½ banana |
| †Blackberries (raw) | ¾ cup |
| †Blueberries (raw) | ¾ cup |
| Cantaloupe (5″ across) | ⅓ melon |
| (cubes) | 1 cup |
| Cherries (large, sweet, raw) | 12 cherries |
| Cherries (canned) | ½ cup |
| Figs (raw, 2″ across) | 2 figs |
| Fruit cocktail (canned) | ½ cup |
| Grapefruit (medium) | ½ grapefruit |
| Grapefruit (segments) | ¾ cup |
| Grapes (small) | 15 grapes |
| Honeydew melon (medium) | ⅛ melon |
| (cubes) | 1 cup |
| Kiwi (large) | 1 kiwi |
| Mandarin oranges | ¾ cup |
| Mango (small) | ½ mango |
| †Nectarine (1½″ across) | 1 nectarine |
| Orange (2½″ across) | 1 orange |
| Papaya | 1 cup |
| Peach (2¾″ across) | 1 peach, or ¾ cup |
| Peaches (canned) | ½ cup, or 2 halves |
| Pear | ½ large, 1 small |
| Pears (canned) | ½ cup, or 2 halves |
| Persimmon (medium, native) | 2 persimmons |
| Pineapple (raw) | ¾ cup |
| Pineapple (canned) | ⅓ cup |
| Plum (raw, 2″ across) | 2 plums |
| †Pomegranate | ½ pomegranate |
| †Raspberries (raw) | 1 cup |
| †Strawberries (raw, whole) | 1¼ cup |
| †Tangerine (2½″ across) | 2 tangerines |
| Watermelon (cubes) | 1¼ cup |

*Dried Fruit*

| | |
|---|---|
| †Apples | 4 rings |
| †Apricots | 7 halves |
| Dates | 2½ medium |
| †Figs | 1½ |
| †Prunes | 3 medium |
| Raisins | 2 Tbsp |

*Fruit Juice*

| | |
|---|---|
| Apple juice/cider | ½ cup |
| Cranberry juice cocktail | ⅓ cup |
| Grapefruit juice | ½ cup |
| Grape juice | ⅓ cup |
| Orange juice | ½ cup |
| Pineapple juice | ½ cup |
| Prune juice | ⅓ cup |

§400 mg or more of sodium per serving.
†3 g or more of fiber per serving.

**TABLE A—23A.** CONTINUED

MILK LIST

Each serving of milk or milk products on this list contains about 12 g of carbohydrate and 8 g of protein. The amount of fat in milk is measured in percent (%) of butterfat. The calories vary, depending on what kind of milk you choose. The list is divided into three parts based on the amount of fat and calories: skim/very low-fat milk, low-fat milk, and whole milk. One serving (one milk exchange) of each of these includes:

| | *Carbohydrate (g)* | *Protein (g)* | *Fat (g)* | *Calories* |
|---|---|---|---|---|
| Skim/Very low-fat | 12 | 8 | trace | 90 |
| Low-fat | 12 | 8 | 5 | 120 |
| Whole | 12 | 8 | 8 | 150 |

Milk is the body's main source of calcium, the mineral needed for growth and repair of bones. Yogurt is also a good source of calcium. Yogurt and many dry or powdered milk products have different amounts of fat. If you have questions about a particular item, read the label to find out the fat and calorie content.

Milk is good to drink, but it can also be added to cereal and to other foods. Many tasty dishes, such as sugar-free pudding, are made with milk (see the Combination Foods list). Plain yogurt is delicious with one of your fruit servings mixed with it.

*Skim and Very Low-fat Milk*

- 1 cup skim milk
- 1 cup ½% milk
- 1 cup 1% milk
- 1 cup low-fat buttermilk
- ½ cup evaporated skim milk
- ⅓ cup dry nonfat milk
- 8-oz carton plain nonfat yogurt

*Low-Fat Milk*

- 1 cup fluid 2% milk
- 8-oz carton plain low-fat yogurt (with added nonfat milk solids)

*Whole Milk*

The whole milk group has much more fat per serving than the skim and low-fat groups. Whole milk has more than 3¼% butterfat. Try to limit your choices from the whole milk group as much as possible.

- 1 cup whole milk
- ½ cup evaporated whole milk
- 8-oz carton whole plain yogurt

FAT LIST

Each serving on the fat list contains about 5 g of fat and 45 calories.

The foods on the fat list contain mostly fat, although some items may also contain a small amount of protein. All fats are high in calories and should be carefully measured. Everyone should modify their fat intake by eating unsaturated fats instead of saturated fats. The sodium content of these foods varies widely. Check the label for sodium information.

| *Unsaturated Fats* | |
|---|---|
| Avocado | ⅛ medium |
| Margarine | 1 tsp |
| Margarine, diet# | 1 Tbsp |
| Mayonnaise | 1 tsp |
| Mayonnaise, reduced-calorie# | 1 Tbsp |
| Nuts and seeds: | |
| Almonds, dry roasted | 6 whole |
| Cashews, dry roasted | 1 Tbsp |
| Pecans | 2 whole |
| Peanuts | 20 small, 10 large |
| Walnuts | 2 whole |
| Other nuts | 1 Tbsp |
| Seeds, pine nuts, sunflower (without shells) | 1 Tbsp |
| Pumpkin seeds | 2 tsp |
| Oil (corn, cottonseed, safflower, soybean, sunflower, olive, peanut) | 1 tsp |
| Olives# | 10 small, 5 large |
| Salad dressing, mayonnaise-type | 2 tsp |
| Salad dressing, mayonnaise-type, reduced-calorie | 1 Tbsp |
| Salad dressing (all varieties)# | 1 Tbsp |
| Salad dressing, reduced-calorie (2 Tbsp of low-calorie is a free food)§ | 2 Tbsp |

| *Saturated Fats* | |
|---|---|
| Butter | 1 tsp |
| Bacon | 1 slice |
| Chitterlings | ½ oz |
| Coconut, shredded | 2 Tbsp |
| Coffee whitener, liquid | 2 Tbsp |
| Coffee whitener, powder | 4 tsp |
| Cream (light, coffee, table) | 2 Tbsp |
| Cream, sour | 2 Tbsp |
| Cream (heavy, whipping) | 1 Tbsp |
| Cream cheese | 1 Tbsp |
| Salt pork | ¼ oz |

#If more than one or two servings are eaten, foods have 400 mg or more of sodium.
§400 mg or more of sodium per serving.

**TABLE A–23A.** CONTINUED

FREE FOODS

A free food is any food or drink that contains 20 calories or less per serving. You can eat as much as you want of those items that have no serving size specified. You may eat 2 or 3 servings per day of those items that have a specific serving size. Be sure to spread them out through the day.

*Drinks*
Bouillon§ or broth without fat†
Bouillon, low-sodium
Carbonated drinks, sugar-free
Carbonated water
Club soda
Cocoa powder, unsweetened (1 Tbsp)
Coffee/Tea
Drink mixes, sugar-free
Mineral water
Tonic water, sugar-free

*Nonstick pan spray*

*Fruit*
Cranberries, unsweetened (½ cup)
Rhubarb, unsweetened (½ cup)

*Vegetables (raw, 1 cup)*
Cabbage
Celery
Chinese cabbage†
Cucumber
Green onion
Hot peppers
Mushrooms
Radishes
Zucchini†
Salad greens
  Endive
  Escarole
  Lettuce
  Romaine
  Spinach

*Sweet Substitutes*
Candy, hard, sugar-free
Gelatin, sugar-free
Gum, sugar-free
Jam/jelly, sugar-free (2 tsp)
Pancake syrup, sugar-free (¼ cup)
Sugar substitutes (saccharin, Equal)
Whipped topping, low calorie

*Condiments*
Catsup (1 Tbsp)
Horseradish
Mustard
Pickles§, dill, unsweetened
Salad dressing, low-calorie (2 Tbsp)
Taco sauce (1 Tbsp)
Vinegar

Seasonings can be very helpful in making food taste better. Be careful of how much sodium you use. Read the label and choose those seasonings that do not contain sodium or salt.

Basil (fresh)
Celery seeds
Cinnamon
Chili powder
Chives
Curry
Dill
Flavoring extracts (e.g., vanilla, lemon, almond, walnut, peppermint, butter)
Garlic
Garlic powder
Herbs
Hot pepper sauce
Lemon
lemon juice
Lemon pepper
Lime
Lime juice
Mint
Onion powder
Oregano
Paprika
Pepper
Pimento
Spices
Soy sauce§
Soy sauce, low-sodium
Wine, used in cooking (¼ cup)
Worcestershire sauce

COMBINATION FOODS

Much of the food we eat is mixed together in various combinations. These combination foods do not fit into only one exchange list. It can be difficult to tell what is in a certain casserole dish or baked food item. This is a list of average values for some typical combination foods. This list will help you fit these foods into your meal plan. Ask your dietitian for information about any other foods you would like to eat. The *American Diabetes Association/American Dietetic Association Family Cookbooks* and the *American Diabetes Association Holiday Cookbook* have many recipes and further information about many foods, including combination foods. Check your library or local bookstore.

| *Food* | *Amount* | *Exchanges* |
|---|---|---|
| Casseroles, homemade | 1 cup (8 oz) | 2 starch, 2 medium-fat meat, 1 fat |
| Cheese pizza§ thin crust | ¼ of 15 oz or ¼ of 10″ | 2 starch, 1 medium-fat meat, 1 fat |
| Chili with beans†§ (commercial) | 1 cup (8 oz) | 2 starch, 2 medium-fat meat, 2 fat |
| Chow mein† (without noodles or rice) | 2 cups (16 oz) | 1 starch, 2 vegetable, 2 lean meat |
| Macaroni and cheese§ | 1 cup (8 oz) | 2 starch, 1 medium-fat meat, 2 fat |
| Soup | | |
| Bean† | 1 cup (8 oz) | 1 starch, 1 vegetable, 1 lean meat |
| Chunky, all varieties | 10¾ oz can | 1 starch, 1 vegetable, 1 medium-fat meat |
| Cream§ (made with water) | 1 cup (8 oz) | 1 starch, 1 fat |
| Vegetable§ or broth§ | 1 cup (8 oz) | 1 starch |
| Spaghetti and meatballs§ (canned) | 1 cup (8 oz) | 2 starch, 1 medium-fat meat, 1 fat |
| Sugar-free pudding (made with skim milk) | ½ cup | 1 starch |
| *If beans are used as a meat substitute:* | | |
| Dried beans,† peas,† lentils† | 1 cup (cooked) | 2 starch, 1 lean meat |

†3 g or more of fiber per serving.
§400 mg or more of sodium per serving.

**TABLE A–23A.** CONTINUED

FOODS FOR OCCASIONAL USE

Moderate amounts of some foods can be used in your meal plan, in spite of their sugar or fat content, as long as you can maintain blood glucose control. The following list includes average exchange values for some of these foods. Because they are concentrated sources of carbohydrate, you will notice that the portion sizes are very small. Check with your dietitian for advice on how often and when you can eat them.

| *Food* | *Amount* | *Exchanges* |
|---|---|---|
| Angel food cake | 1/12 cake | 2 starch |
| Cake, no icing | 1/12 cake, or a 3″ square | 2 starch, 2 fat |
| Cookies | 2 small (1 3/4″ across) | 1 starch, 1 fat |
| Frozen fruit yogurt | 1/3 cup | 1 starch |
| Gingersnaps | 3 | 1 starch |
| Granola | 1/4 cup | 1 starch, 1 fat |
| Granola bars | 1 small | 1 starch, 1 fat |
| Ice cream, any flavor | 1/2 cup | 1 starch, 2 fat |
| Ice milk, any flavor | 1/2 cup | 1 starch, 1 fat |
| Sherbet, any flavor | 1/4 cup | 1 starch |
| Snack chips,§ all varieties | 1 oz | 1 starch, 2 fat |
| Vanilla wafers | 6 small | 1 starch, 1 fat |

MANAGEMENT TIPS

Some food you buy uncooked will weigh less after you cook it. This is true of most meats. Starches often swell in cooking, so a small amount of uncooked starch will become a much larger amount of cooked food. The following table shows some of the changes:

| *Food (Starch Group)* | *Uncooked* | *Cooked* |
|---|---|---|
| Oatmeal | 3 level Tbsp | 1/2 cup |
| Cream of wheat | 2 level Tbsp | 1/2 cup |
| Grits | 3 level Tbsp | 1/2 cup |
| Rice | 2 level Tbsp | 1/3 cup |
| Spaghetti | 1/4 cup | 1/2 cup |
| Noodles | 1/3 cup | 1/2 cup |
| Macaroni | 1/4 cup | 1/2 cup |
| Dried beans | 3 Tbsp | 1/3 cup |
| Dried peas | 3 Tbsp | 1/3 cup |
| Lentils | 2 Tbsp | 1/3 cup |
| *Food (Meat Group)* | | |
| Hamburger | 4 oz | 3 oz |
| Chicken | 1 small drumstick | 1 oz |
| | 1/2 breast (1 side) | 3 oz |

- Read food labels. Remember—*dietetic* does not mean *diabetic!* When you see the word "dietetic" on a food label, it means that something has been changed or replaced. It may have less salt, less fat, or less sugar. It does not mean that the food is sugar-free or calorie-free. Some dietetic foods may be useful. Those that contain 20 calories or less per serving may be eaten as many as 3 times a day as free foods.
- Know your sweeteners. Two types of sweeteners are on the market: those with calories and those without calories. Sweeteners with calories, such as fructose, sorbitol, and mannitol, when used in large amounts, may cause cramping and diarrhea. Remember, these sweeteners do have calories that add up. Sweeteners without calories include saccharin and aspartame (Equal, Nutrasweet) and may be used in moderation.

§If more than one serving is eaten, these foods have 400 mg or more of sodium.

**TABLE A–23B.** DIABETIC EXCHANGES FOR AFRICAN-AMERICAN (SOUTHERN) COOKERY

| FOOD EXCHANGE GROUP | FOOD | PORTION | SODIUM CONTENT |
|---|---|---|---|
| Starch/Bread | | | |
| (80 calories per exchange) | Biscuit, 2″ diameter | 1 (add 2 fat) | 262 mg |
| | Cornbread, 2″ × 2″ × 1″ | 1 (add 1 fat) | 220 mg |
| | Corn muffin, 2″ diameter | 1 (add 1 fat) | 250 mg |
| | Crackling bread, 2″ × 2″ × 1″ | 1 (add 2 fat) | High |
| | CooCoo (cornmeal, okra, butter, salt, and water) | (equals 1 veg/1 fat) | High |
| | Cornmeal | 2 Tbsp | Low |
| | Black-eyed peas | ½ cup (add ½ lean meat) | 6 mg |
| | Pinto beans | ¼ cup (add ½ lean meat) | 2 mg |
| | Baked beans (no pork) | ¼ cup | 239 mg |
| | Grits (instant/cooked) | ½ cup | 385 mg |
| | Hoe cake, 2″ × 2″ × 1″ | 1 (add 2 fat) | Medium |
| | Hominy (canned) | ½ cup | 720 mg |
| | Hoppin john (frozen) | ½ cup (add 1 fat, ½ bread) | High |
| | Hush puppies | 2 small pieces (add 2 fats) | High |
| | Spoon bread | ½ cup (add 1 lean meat, 1 fat) | High |
| | Pound cake, 3½″ × 3″ × ½″ | 1 (add 2 fat) | Low |
| | Custard (baked) | ½ cup (add 1 lean meat, ½ fat) | Medium |
| Meat | | | |
| *Lean Meat* | Chicken gizzard | 1 oz | 19 mg |
| (55 calories per ounce) | Pork | | |
| | Hog maw, stomach | ⅓ cup | 30 mg |
| | Sousemeat | 3″ × 2″ × ¼″ | High |
| | Pig ear | 1 medium | Low |
| | Fish | | |
| | Catfish, 4″ × 2″ × ¼″ | 1 | Low |
| | Mullet, 4″ × 2″ × ¼″ | 1 | Low |
| | Perch, 4″ × 2″ × ¼″ | 1 | Low |
| | Snapper, 4″ × 2″ × ¼″ | 1 | Low |
| | Sardines | 3 drained | High |
| *Medium-Fat Meat* | Pork | | |
| (75 calories per ounce) | Chipped ham | 1 oz | High |
| | Fresh butt | 1 oz | High |
| | Neck bones | ½ cup | High |
| | Pork cubes (lean) | 1 oz | High |
| | Tongue | 1 oz | High |
| | Organ meats | | |
| | Heart (beef) | 1 oz | 35 mg |
| | Kidney | 1 oz | 71 mg |
| | Liver (pork) | 1 oz | 14 mg |
| | Sweetbreads | 1 oz | 32 mg |
| | Fish | | |
| | Eel, American (fresh) | 1 oz | 25 mg |
| | Mackerel (fresh) | 1 oz | 17 mg |
| *High-Fat Meat* | Barbecued ribs | 1 oz | High |
| (100 calories per ounce) | Country ham | 1 oz | High |
| | Devild ham (canned) | 1 oz | High |
| | Pork belly (fresh) | 1 oz | |
| | Hock (smoked) | 1 oz | |
| | Pig's feet | 1 (equals 2 exchanges) | |
| | Pork shank | 1 oz | |
| | Pork tail | 1 oz | |
| | Sausage (bulk, patties, link) | 1 oz | High |
| | Pig snout | 1 (equals 2 exchanges) | |

**TABLE A–23B.** CONTINUED

| FOOD EXCHANGE GROUP | FOOD | PORTION | SODIUM CONTENT |
|---|---|---|---|
| *Luncheon Meats* (100 calories per ounce) | Bologna | 1 oz | High |
| | Frankfurter (hot dogs) | 1 oz | High |
| | Sausage link (canned or frozen) | 1 oz (add 1 fat) | 215 mg |
| | Sausage links (brown and serve) | 1 oz (add 1 fat) | High |
| | Small Vienna sausage | 3 (add 1 fat) | High |
| | Spam | 1 oz | High |
| | Treat | 1 oz | High |
| | Scrapple | 1 oz | High |
| *Organ Meats* | Brains | ¼ cup | 70 mg |
| *Combination Meats* | Chicken and dumplings | 3 oz (equals 2 lean meat, 1 veg, 1 bread, 1 fat) | High |
| | Chili, 1 cup | (equals 2 medium-fat meat, 2 bread, 2 fat) | High |
| | Smothered chicken (no skin) | ¼ broiler (equals 4 lean meat, ½ bread) | High |
| | Steamed fish with butter | 3 oz (equals 4 lean meat, ½ fat) | Low |
| Vegetable (25 calories per exchange) | Collard (cooked without fat) | ½ cup | 25 mg |
| | Kale (cooked without fat) | ½ cup | 29 mg |
| | Mustard (cooked without fat) | ½ cup | 18 mg |
| | Turnip (cooked withou fat) | cup | 8.5 mg |
| | Poke salad (cooked without fat) | 1 cup | High |
| | Rape | ½ cup (add 2 fat) | High |
| | Greens (cooked with fat) | ½ cup | High |
| | Okra | 8-9 pods | High |
| | Chickory (raw) | 1 cup | 6 mg |
| | Cressie greens (raw) | 1 cup | 5 mg per 10 sprigs |
| Fruit (60 calories per exchange) | No additions | | |
| Milk (90 calories per exchange) | Buttermilk (skim milk) | 1 cup | 257 mg |
| | Buttermilk (whole milk) | 1 cup (omit 2 fat) | 250 mg |
| Fats (Saturated) (45 calories per teaspoon) | Bacon (thick sliced, crisp) | 1 strip | High |
| | Bacon (thin/medium sliced, crisp) | 1 strip | High |
| | Bacon grease | 1 tsp | High |
| | Chitterlings, fried | 2 Tbsp | High |
| | Crackling, pork | 1½ tsp | High |
| | Fat back | ¾″ cube | High |
| | Salt pork | ¾″ cube | High |
| | Slab of bacon, 1″ × 1″ × ¼″ | 1 slice | High |
| | Streak o'lean, 1″ × 1″ × ¼″ | 1 slice | High |

(Adapted with permission from The American Diabetes Association, Washington, D.C. Area Affiliate, Inc.: Exchange Lists for Meal Planning: Black American Cookery. 1987.)

**TABLE A–23C.** SUPPLEMENTARY EXCHANGE LISTS FOR CHINESE-AMERICAN FOODS

| FOOD EXCHANGE GROUP | FOOD | PORTION |
|---|---|---|
| Starch/Bread | Cellophane or mung bean noodles (cooked) | ¾ cup |
| | Ginkgo seeds | ½ cup |
| | Lotus root, ¼″-thick slice, 2½″ diameter | 10 slices |
| | Mung beans or green gram beans (cooked) | ⅓ cup |
| | Red beans (cooked) | ⅓ cup |
| | Rice congee or soup | ¾ cup |
| | Rice vermicelli or noodles (cooked) | ½ cup |
| | Taro (cooked) | ⅓ cup |
| Meat and Meat Substitutes | | |
| *Lean Meat* | Beef jerky, 3½″ × 1″* | ½ oz |
| | Dried scallop | 1 large |
| | Dried shrimp | 1 Tbsp or 10 medium shrimp |
| | Soybeans (cooked) | 3 Tbsp |
| | Squid | 2 oz |
| | Tripe (beef) | 2 oz |
| *Medium-fat Meat and Substitutes* | Beef tongue | 1 oz |
| | Tofu or soybean curd, 2½″ × 2¾″ × 1″† | 4 oz or ½ cup |
| *High-fat Meat* | Salted duck egg‡§ | 1 |
| | Thousand-year-old or preserved limed duck egg‡§ | 1 |
| *High-fat Meat + 1 Fat* | Chinese sausage (pork and spices and/or liver)*§ | 1 (2 oz) |
| Vegetables (½ cup cooked or 1 cup raw unless indicated otherwise) | Amaranth or Chinese spinach (cooked) | |
| | Arrowheads, or fresh corms (raw), 3½″ diameter | |
| | Baby corn (canned)* | |
| | Bamboo shoots | |
| | Bitter melon or bitter gourd | |
| | Chayote | |
| | Chinese celery | |
| | Chinese eggplant (white or purple) | |
| | Chinese or black mushroom (dried) | 2 medium |
| | Hairy melon or hairy cucumber | |
| | Leeks† | |
| | Luffa (angled or smooth) | |
| | Mung bean sprouts | |
| | Mustard greens† | |
| | Peapods or sugar peas† | |
| | Soybean sprouts (cooked or raw) | ½ cup |
| | Straw mushrooms | |
| | Turnip† | |
| | Water chestnuts (canned)† | ½ cup |
| | Winter melon or wax gourd | |
| | Yard-long beans | |
| Fruits | Carambola or star fruit (raw) | 2 medium |
| | Chinese banana (raw) | 1 dwarf |
| | Guava (raw) | 1 medium |
| | Kumquats (raw) | 5 medium |
| | Litchi or lychee (raw) | 10 |
| | Litchi or lychee (canned, drained) | ½ cup |
| | Longan (raw) | 30 |
| | Longan (canned, drained) | ¾ cup |
| | Mango (raw)† | ½ small |
| | Papaya (raw), 3½″ diameter, 5⅛″ hight† | ½ |
| | Persimmon, Japanese (soft type) (raw) | ½ |
| | Pummelo (raw) | ¾ cup |
| Milk | Soybean milk (unsweetened) | 1 cup |
| Fats | Coconut milk | 1 Tbsp |
| | Sesame paste | 1½ tsp |
| | Sesame seeds (whole, dried) | 1 Tbsp |

**TABLE A–23C.** CONTINUED

| FOOD EXCHANGE GROUP | FOOD | PORTION |
|---|---|---|
| Free Foods | Amaranth or Chinese spinach | |
| | Bok choy | |
| | Chili pepper (raw)† | 1 |
| | Chinese or Peking cabbage† | |
| | Choy sum or Chinese flowering cabbage | |
| | Coriander | |
| | Garland chrysanthemum | |
| | Ginger | ¼ cup |
| | Mustard greens (salted and soured) | 2 Tbsp |
| | Oriental radish or daikon | |
| | Watercress | |
| Combination | Mock duck or wheat gluten (canned) | ½ cup (equals ½ starch/ bread, 1 lean meat) |

*400 mg or more of sodium per serving.
†Foods are included in *Exchange Lists for Meal Planning,* 1986. © American Diabetes Association and The American Dietetic Association.
‡Probably 400 mg or more of sodium per serving, based on author's estimate.
§Limit high-fat meat choices to 3 times per week.
(From The American Dietetic Association and The American Diabetes Association, Inc.: Ethnic and Regional Food Practices: A Series. Chinese Food Practices, Customs and Holidays. 1990. With permission.)

**TABLE A–23D.** SUPPLEMENTARY EXCHANGE LISTS FOR HMONG-AMERICAN FOODS

| FOOD EXCHANGE GROUP | FOOD | PORTION |
|---|---|---|
| Starch/Bread | Cellophane or mung bean noodles (cooked) | 3/4 cup |
| | Rice vermicelli or noodles (cooked) | 1/2 cup |
| | Rice soup | 3/4 cup |
| Meat and Meat Substitutes | | |
| *Lean Meat* | Pheasant† | 1 oz |
| | Squirrel† | 1 oz |
| | Venison† | 1 oz |
| *Medium-fat Meat and Substitutes* | Pig's feet | 2½ oz (equals 2 exchanges) |
| | Tofu or soybean curd, 2½″ × 2¾″ × 1″ | 4 oz or ½ cup |
| *High-fat Meat* | Ground pork†‡ | 1 oz |
| Vegetables (½ cup cooked or 1 cup raw unless indicated otherwise) | Bamboo shoots | |
| | Bitter melon or bitter gourd | |
| | Chinese onion (leeks†) | |
| | Cucuzzi squash (spaghetti squash) | |
| | Luffa gourd/squash | |
| | Mustard greens† | |
| | Mung bean sprouts | |
| | Pumpkin | |
| | Sugar peas, snow peas, sweet peas, peapods† | |
| | Yard-long beans, pod and seeds | ½ cup |
| Fruits | Apple pear, Asian pear (raw), 2¼″ high, 2½″ diameter | 1 |
| | Guava (raw) | 1½ medium |
| | Jackfruit (raw) | ½ cup |
| | Mango (raw)† | ½ small |
| | Papaya (raw), 5⅛″ high, 3½″ diameter† | ½ or 1 cup |
| Fats | Beef fat | 1 tsp |
| | Chicken fat | 1 tsp |
| | Coconut cream or milk | 1 Tbsp |
| | Coconut (raw)† | 2 Tbsp |
| | Pork lard | 1 tsp |
| | Pork intestine, chitterlings† | ½ oz |
| Free Foods | Fish sauce* | |
| | Pumpkin or squash blossom | |
| | Soy sauce*† | |
| | Tender vines and leaves of pumpkin, squash, luffa gourd, and pea plants | |
| Occasional Foods | Condensed milk, sweetened | 1 oz (equals 1½ starch/bread) |

*400 mg or more of sodium per serving.
†Foods are included in *Exchange Lists for Meal Planning,* 1986. © American Diabetes Association and The American Dietetic Association.
‡Limit high-fat meat choice to 3 times per week.
(From The American Dietetic Association and The American Diabetes Association, Inc.: Ethnic and Regional Food Practices, a Series. Hmong Food Practices, Customs and Holidays. 1992. With permission.)

**TABLE A–23E.** DIABETIC EXCHANGES FOR AN INDIAN DIET

| FOOD EXCHANGE GROUP | FOOD | PORTION |
|---|---|---|
| Starch/Bread | Arrowroot flour (uncooked) | 2 Tbsp |
| | Barley (uncooked) | 1½ Tbsp |
| | Colacassia (cooked) | ¼ cup |
| | Indian breads* | |
| | Chapati, 5″–6″ diameter | 1 medium |
| | Dosa, 5″–6″ diameter | 1 medium |
| | Idli, 2½″–3″ diameter | 1 medium |
| | Puri, 5″ diameter | 1 large (omit 2½ fat) |
| | Phulka, 5″ to 6″ diameter | 1 medium |
| | Phoa (rice flakes, Indian style) (uncooked) | 3 Tbsp |
| | Plantain (raw) | ½ medium |
| | Rice flour (uncooked) | 2 Tbsp |
| | Sago (uncooked) | 1¼ Tbsp |
| | Suji (cream of wheat) (uncooked) | 2 Tbsp |
| | Upma (plain without vegetable) (cooked) | ½ cup |
| | Vermicelli (thinner than very thin spaghetti) (uncooked) | ½ cup |
| | Whole-wheat flour | 2½ Tbsp |
| Meat and Meat Substitutes | | |
| *Lean Meat and Substitutes* (omit 1 starch/bread for each) | Bengal gram dhal (Chana, whole, split) (uncooked) | 2 Tbsp |
| | Bengal gram dhal (roasted) (uncooked) | 3 Tbsp |
| | Black gram dhal (Urad dhal) (uncooked) | 2 Tbsp |
| | Green gram dhal (Mung dhal) (uncooked) | 2 Tbsp |
| | Masur dhal (uncooked) | 2 Tbsp |
| | Toordhal (uncooked) | 2 Tbsp |
| | Besan (chick pea flour) (uncooked) | 3 Tbsp |
| *High-Fat Meat and Substitute* | Pannir (cheese) made with whole milk | ¼ cup |
| Vegetables (½ cup cooked or 1 cup raw unless indicated otherwise) | Ashgourd (cooked) | |
| | Bitter gourd (cooked) | |
| | Bottle gourd (cooked) | 1⅓ cup |
| | Chow-chow (cooked) | |
| | Cluster beans (cooked) | |
| | Drumstick (cooked) | |
| | Fenugreek leaves (cooked) | |
| | Ladies fingers (cooked) (okra) | |
| | Ridge gourd (cooked) | |
| | White radish (cooked) | |
| Fruits | Guava (fresh) | ½ cup |
| Milk | Curds (yogurt) made from skim milk (plain) | 1 cup |
| Fats | Coconut (grated) (unsweetened) | 2 Tbsp |
| | Coconut chutney | 2 Tbsp |
| | Coconut oil | 1 tsp |
| | Ghee (clarified butter) | 1 tsp |
| | Mustard oil | 1 tsp |
| | Sesame oil | 1 tsp |

*Exchange values for Indian breads from *Diabetic Diet,* Dietetic Department, Christian Medical College and Hospital, Vellore, India.
(Adapted with permission from The American Diabetes Association, Washington, D.C. Area Affiliate, Inc.: Supplement to Exchange Lists for Meal Planning: Indian Cookery.)

**TABLE A–23F.** SUPPLEMENTARY EXCHANGE LISTS FOR EASTERN EUROPEAN (JEWISH) FOODS*

| FOOD EXCHANGE GROUP | FOOD | PORTION |
|---|---|---|
| Starch/Bread | Bagel† or bialy | ½ small, 1 oz |
| | Bulgur (cooked)† | ½ cup |
| | Bulke | ½ medium |
| | Farfel (dry) | ½ cup |
| | Hallah | 1 slice, 1 oz |
| | Kasha (cooked) | ½ cup |
| | Kasha (raw) | 2 Tbsp |
| | Lentils† | ⅓ cup |
| | Matzoh† | ¾ oz |
| | Matzoh meal | 2½ Tbsp |
| | Potato starch (flour) | 2 Tbsp |
| | Pumpernickel bread† | 1 slice, 1 oz |
| | Rye bread† | 1 slice, 1 oz |
| | Split peas† | ⅓ cup |
| Starch/Bread Prepared with Fat | Matzoh ball‡ | 3 balls, 1½ oz (equals 1 starch/bread + 1 fat) |
| | Potato pancake | ½ pancake (equals 1 starch/bread + 1 fat) |
| Meat | | |
| *Lean meat* | Flanken† | 1 oz |
| | Gefilte fish | 2 oz |
| | Herring† (smoked, uncreamed) | 1 oz |
| | Lox† | 1 oz |
| | Sardines† (canned, drained) | 2 medium |
| | Smelts | 1 oz |
| *Medium-fat meat* | Beef tongue | 1 oz |
| | Brisket | 1 oz |
| | Chopped liver§ | ¼ cup |
| | Corned beef† | 1 oz |
| | Sablefish (smoked) | 1 oz |
| | Salmon† (canned) | ¼ cup |
| *High-fat meat* | Pastrami | 1 oz |
| Vegetables | Borscht (no sugar or sour cream) | ½ cup |
| | Sorrel | ½ cup |
| Fats | Cream cheese† | 1 Tbsp |
| | Nondairy creamer† (liquid) | 2 Tbsp |
| | Nondairy creamer† (powder) | 4 tsp |
| | Schmaltz | 1 tsp |
| | Sour cream† | 2 Tbsp |
| Free Foods (in reasonable amounts) | Horseradish† | |
| | Pickles, dill† | |
| Occasional Foods | Sweet kosher wine | ½ cup (equals 2 fat) |

*Unless otherwise specified, all foods are 1 exchange.

†Foods are included on the American Diabetes Association and American Dietetic Association *Exchange Lists for Meal Planning.* 1986. © American Diabetes Association and The American Dietetic Association.

‡High in sodium.

§No additional salt in recipe.

(From The American Dietetic Association and The American Diabetes Association, Inc. Ethnic and Regional Food Practices, a Series. Jewish Food Practices, Customs and Holidays, 1989. With permission.)

**TABLE A–23G.** SUPPLEMENTARY EXCHANGE LISTS FOR MEXICAN-AMERICAN FOODS*

| FOOD EXCHANGE GROUP | FOOD | PORTION |
|---|---|---|
| Starch/Bread | Bolillo (French roll), 4½″ to 5″ long | ¼ |
| | Frijoles cocidos† (cooked beans) | ⅓ cup |
| | Frijoles cocidos | 1 cup (equals 2 starch/bread + 1 lean meat) |
| | Frijoles refritos (refried beans) (no fat added) | ⅓ cup |
| | Tortilla, corn, 7½″ across (ready to bake)‡ | 1 |
| | Tortilla, flour, 7″ across (ready to bake)‡ | 1 (equals 1½ starch/bread) |
| | Tortilla, flour, 9″ across (ready to bake)‡ | ⅓ |
| Starch/Bread Prepared with Fat | Frijoles refritos (fat added) | ⅓ cup (equals 1 starch/bread + 1 fat) |
| | Taco shell, 5″ across (ready to use) | 2 (equals 1 starch/bread + 1 fat) |
| | Tortilla, flour, 7″ across (fried with added fat) | 1 (equals 1½ starch/bread + 1 fat) |
| | Tortilla, corn, 7½″ across (fried with added fat) | 1 (equals 1 starch/bread + 1 fat) |
| | Tortilla, flour, 9″ across (fried with added fat) | 1 (equals 3 starch/bread + 2 fat) |
| Meat | | |
| *Lean meat* | Menudo (tripe soup) | ½ cup |
| *Medium-fat meat* | Queso fresco (cheese made with skim milk) | ¼ cup (2 oz) |
| *High-fat meat* | Chorizo (Mexican sausage) | 1 oz (equals 1 high-fat meat + 1 fat) |
| Vegetables | Chayote (squash) (cooked) | ½ cup |
| | Jícama (yambean root) (raw) | ½ cup |
| | Nopales (cactus) (raw) | ½ cup |
| Fruits | Mango† | ½ small |
| | Papaya† | 1 cup |
| Fats | Avocado† | ⅛ medium |
| Free Foods | Jalapeño chilis | |
| | Salsa de chile (chili/taco sauce) | |
| | Verdolagas (purslane) | |
| Occasional Foods | Pan dulce (sweet bread), 4½″ across | 1 (equals 4 starch/bread + 1 fat) |

*Unless otherwise specified, all foods are 1 exchange.
†Food and amount are same as in 1986 *Exchange Lists for Meal Planning.* © American Diabetes Association, Inc., The American Dietetic Association.
‡Food, amount, or both differ from 1986 *Exchange Lists for Meal Planning* because of new information.
(From The American Dietetic Association and The American Diabetes Association, Inc. Ethnic and Regional Food Practices, a Series. Mexican Food Practices, Customs and Holidays, 1989. With permission.)

**TABLE A–23H.** SUPPLEMENTARY EXCHANGE LISTS FOR TRADITIONAL NAVAJO FOODS*

| FOOD EXCHANGE GROUP | FOOD | PORTION |
|---|---|---|
| Starch/Bread | Blue corn mush | ¾ cup |
| | Flour tortilla, 8″ diameter | ¼ |
| | Steamed corn hominy (cooked) | ½ cup |
| Meat | | |
| *Lean meat* | Mutton, flesh (lean only) (cooked without added fat) | 1 oz |
| *High-fat meat* | Mutton, flesh (lean and fat) (cooked without added fat) | 1 oz |
| Fats | Piñon nuts | 1 Tbsp (about 25 nuts) |

*Nutrition practitioners who work with Navajo clients with noninsulin-dependent diabetes mellitus do not often use the Exchange system in client education sessions. This listing is presented for the few occasions when supplementary Exchange values may be needed.
(From The American Dietetic Association and The American Diabetes Association, Inc. Ethnic and Regional Food Practices, a Series. Navajo Food Practices, Customs and Holidays, 1991. With permission.)

**TABLE A–23I.** DIABETIC EXCHANGES FOR A GENERAL ASIAN-AMERICAN DIET

| FOOD EXCHANGE GROUP | FOOD | PORTION |
|---|---|---|
| Starch/Bread | Arrowroot | 3 small |
| | Arrowroot starch | 2 Tbsp |
| | Cellophane noodles (cooked) | ½ cup |
| | Chestnuts (shelled) | ¼ cup |
| | Chowmein noodles | ½ cup (omit 1 fat) |
| | Congee (rice soup)* | 1 cup |
| | Cornstarch* | 2 Tbsp |
| | Fungi (woodears) (dried) | 1 oz (omit 1 Fruit) |
| | Gingko seeds (dried) | 1½ oz |
| | Glutinous rice, (cooked)* | ¼ cup |
| | Glutinous rice flour* | 1 Tbsp |
| | Lanka (jackfruit) | ⅓ cup |
| | Lotus root | ⅔ segment |
| | Lotus seeds (dried) | 1 oz |
| | Millet | 1 oz (omit ½ Bread) |
| | Mung bean noodles | ½ cup |
| | Rice noodles (sticks) | |
| | Cooked | ½ cup |
| | Dry | 1 oz |
| | Tamarind | 1 oz |
| | Tapioca pearles (dry) | 1 Tbsp |
| | Taro (dasheen) | ¼ cup |
| Meat and Meat Substitutes | | |
| *Lean Meat and Substitutes* | Dried beans and peas (cooked) | ½ cup (omit 1 Bread) |
| | Black-eyed peas | |
| | Broad beans (horse beans) | |
| | Garbanzo | |
| | Kidney | |
| | Lentils | |
| | Lima | |
| | Mung | |
| | Navy | |
| | Pinto | |
| | Abalone | 1 oz |
| | Chicken wings | 1 wing |
| | Dried duck feet | ½ oz |
| | Gefilte fish | 1 oz |
| | Octopus | 1¾ oz |
| | Shrimp (dried) | ½ oz |
| | Squid (calamares) | 1¾ oz |
| *Medium-Fat Meat and Substitutes* | Bean curd cheese | 2 oz |
| | Fishmaw (fish stomach) | 2 oz |
| | Oxtail | 1 oz |
| | Soybeans (cooked) | ⅓ cup |
| | Tofu (soybean curd) 2½″ × 2¾″ × 1″ | 1 portion |
| *High-Fat Meat and Substitutes* | Anchovies | 10 |
| | Chinese sausage | 1 oz |
| | Eel | 1 oz |
| | Pork feet (fresh) | 2 oz (omit 1 Fat) |
| | Preserved duck egg | ⅔ egg |

**TABLE A–23I.** CONTINUED

| FOOD EXCHANGE GROUP | FOOD | PORTION |
|---|---|---|
| Vegetables | Bok choy (cooked) | 1 cup |
| | Bamboo shoots (canned, drained) | 3/4 cup |
| | Banana flower | 1/2 cup |
| | Bitter melon (balsam pear) | 1/2 cup |
| | Chinese radish (daikon) | 1 cup |
| | Dried Chinese mushrooms (soaked) | 1/2 cup |
| | Green beans (Chinese) | 1/2 cup |
| | Hairy cucumber | 1/2 cup |
| | Kohlrabi | 3/4 cup |
| | Leek (Chinese onion) | 1/2 cup |
| | Lotus seeds | 1 oz |
| | Mung bean sprouts | 1 cup |
| | Mustard green root | 1/2 cup |
| | Pear squash (chayote) | 1/2 medium |
| | Salted celery cabbage | Free |
| | Salted Chinese cabbage | 1/2 cup |
| | Scallions, 5″ × 1/2″ | 3 |
| | Seaweed (dried, soaked, drained) | 1/2 cup |
| | Snow peas | 1/2 cup |
| | Straw mushrooms | 1/2 cup |
| | Water chestnuts | 4 |
| | White eggplant (Chinese) | 1/2 cup |
| | Winter melon (Wax gourd) | 1 cup |
| Fruit | Carambola (star fruit) | 1 |
| | Dried red dates | 4 |
| | Guava (fresh) | 1/2 cup |
| | Kumquats (fresh) | 3 |
| | Litchis (dried or fresh) | 6 |
| | Longans (dried) | 5 |
| | Pomegranate | 1/2 |
| Milk | Coconut milk* | 1 cup (omit 12 fats) |
| | Soymilk | 1 cup (add 1/2 starch/bread) |
| Fats | Chicken fat or pork fat | 1 tsp |
| | Nuts | |
| | Cashew | 7 large (omit 1 Vegetable) |
| | Macadamia | 6 |
| | Pine | 1/3 oz |
| | Pistachio (shelled) | 1/3 oz |
| | Oils | 1 tsp |
| | Peanut | |
| | Safflower | |
| | Sesame | |
| | Soy (tou yo) | |
| | Seeds (dried) | |
| | Pumpkin | 1 Tbsp |
| | Sesame | 1 Tbsp |
| | Watermelon | 1/2 oz |
| | Sesame seed paste | 1 tsp |
| Miscellaneous Foods | | |
| *YES! YES! YES!* | Anise, curry powder, flower spice, ground ginger, mustard sauce, oyster sauce, parsley, soy sauce, tangerine peel, tea, vinegar, 5-spices powder. | |
| *NO! NO! NO!* | Brown sugar, hoisin sauce, molasses, moon cake, plum sauce, red preserved ginger, rock sugar, sweet buns, sweet coconut tarts, sweet mung bean soup. | |

*See Professional Guidelines, *In* American Diabetes Association, Washington, D.C. Area Affiliate, Inc.: Supplement to Exchange Lists for Meal Planning Oriental Cookery, 1979, p. 18.

(Adapted with permission from The American Diabetes Association, Washington, D.C. Area Affiliate, Inc.: Supplement to Exchange Lists for Meal Planning Oriental Cookery. 1979.)

**TABLE A—23J.** DIET EXCHANGES FOR A VEGETARIAN DIET*

| FOOD EXCHANGE GROUP | FOOD | PORTION |
|---|---|---|
| Starch/Bread | Brown rice (cooked) | ⅓ cup |
| | Buckwheat flour (dark) | 3 Tbsp |
| | Bulgur wheat | 2 Tbsp |
| | Millet (cooked) | ½ cup |
| | Miso | 3 Tbsp |
| | Oats (dry) | ¼ cup |
| | Pita (Syrian) bread | ½ of a 2½-oz loaf |
| | Rye flour | 3 Tbsp |
| | Wheat berries (cooked) | ⅓ cup |
| | Wild rice (cooked) | ½ cup |
| Meat and Meat Substitutes | | |
| *Lean Meat and Substitutes* | Dried beans and peas (cooked) | ½ cup |
| | (omit 1 bread for each listing) | |
| | Black-eyed peas | |
| | Broad beans | |
| | Garbanzo | |
| | Kidney | |
| | Lentils | |
| | Lima | |
| | Mung | |
| | Navy | |
| | Pinto | |
| | Soy flour | ¼ cup (omit ½ bread) |
| *Medium-fat Meat and Substitutes†* | Cheeses | |
| | Camembert | 1 oz |
| | Edam | 1 oz |
| | Liederkranz | 1 oz |
| | Soybeans | ⅓ cup |
| | Tofu, 2½″ × 2¾″ × 1″ | 1 portion |
| *High-fat Meat and Substitutes* | Cheeses | |
| | Blue, Roquefort | 1 oz |
| | Brick | 1 oz |
| | Gorgonzola | 1 oz |
| | Gouda | 1 oz |
| | Gruyère | 1 oz |
| | Limburger | 1 oz |
| | Muenster | 1 oz |
| | Parmesan | 1 oz |
| | Swiss | 1 oz |
| | Hummus | 4 Tbsp (omit 1 bread) |
| | Peanuts‡ | 4 Tbsp (omit ½ bread and 2 fat) |
| | Pignolia nuts‡ | 6 Tbsp (omit ½ vegetable and 1 fat) |
| | Pumpkin seeds‡ | 4 Tbsp (omit ½ bread and 1½ fat) |
| | Sesame seeds‡ | 4 Tbsp (omit ½ bread and 2 fat) |
| | Sunflower seeds‡ | 4 Tbsp (omit ½ bread and 2 fat) |
| Vegetables | Bamboo shoots | ¾ cup |
| | Bean sprouts (raw or cooked) | |
| | Alfalfa | 1 cup |
| | Mung | 1 cup |
| | Soy | 1 cup |
| | Water chestnuts | 4 |
| Fruit | Carrot juice | ½ cup |
| Milk | Kefir | 1 cup (omit 2 fats) |
| | Soy milk (fortified) | 1 cup (add ½ bread) |
| Fats | Tahini | 1 tsp |

**TABLE A–23J** CONTINUED

Food containing complementary proteins may be eaten together, thereby increasing protein quality. Examples of foods that may be complemented to yield high-quality protein are listed below.

| FOOD | COMPLEMENTARY PROTEIN |
|---|---|
| Grains | Combine rice with: cheese, legumes, sesame<br>Combine wheat with: legumes, peanuts and milk, sesame, and soybean<br>Combine corn with: legumes |
| Legumes | Combine beans with: wheat, corn<br>Combine soybeans with: rice and wheat, corn and milk, wheat and sesame, peanuts and sesame, peanuts and wheat and rice |
| Nuts and seeds | Combined sesame with: beans, peanuts and soybeans, soybeans and wheat<br>Combine peanuts with: sunflower seeds |

DIET PATTERNS

| Lacto-Ovovegetarian | Strict Vegetarian |
|---|---|
| Calories: 1,500 | Calories: 1,500 |
| $CH_2O$—190 g 50% | $CH_2O$—190 g 50% |
| Protein—75 g 20% | Protein—75 g 20% |
| Fat—47 g 30% | Fat—47 g 30% |
| Daily Food Allowance | Daily Food Allowance |
| 3 Skim Milk Exchanges | 3 Soybean Milk Exchanges (Note: Add ½ bread for each cup) |
| 2 Vegetable Exchanges | 2 Vegetable Exchanges |
| 4 Fruit Exchanges | 4 Fruit Exchanges |
| 7 Bread Exchanges | 7 Bread Exchanges |
| 4 Lean Meat Exchanges | 4 Lean Meat Exchanges |
| 1 Medium-fat Meat Exchange | 1 Medium-fat Meat Exchange |
| 6 Fat Exchanges | 6 Fat Exchanges |
| Meal Pattern | Meal Pattern |
| *Breakfast* | *Breakfast* |
| 1 Fruit Exchange | 1 Fruit Exchange |
| 2 Bread Exchanges | 2 Bread Exchanges |
| 1 Medium-fat Meat Exchange | 1 Medium-fat Meat Exchange |
| 2 Fat Exchanges | 2 Fat Exchanges |
| 1 Skim Milk Exchange | 1 Milk Exchange |
| *Lunch* | *Lunch* |
| 2 Lean Meat Exchanges | 2 Lean Meat Exchanges |
| 2 Bread Exchanges | 2 Bread Exchanges |
| 1 Vegetable Exchange | 1 Vegetable Exchange |
| 2 Fruit Exchanges | 2 Fruit Exchanges |
| 2 Fat Exchanges | 2 Fat Exchanges |
| *Dinner* | *Dinner* |
| 2 Lean Meat Exchanges | 2 Lean Meat Exchanges |
| 2 Bread Exchanges | 2 Bread Exchanges |
| 1 Vegetable Exchange | 1 Vegetable Exchange |
| 1 Fruit Exchange | 1 Fruit Exchange |
| 2 Fat Exchanges | 2 Fat Exchanges |
| 1 Skim Milk Exchange | 1 Milk Exchange |
| *Bedtime Snack* | *Bedtime Snack* |
| 1 Skim Milk Exchange | 1 Milk Exchange |
| 1 Bread Exchange | 1 Bread Exchange |

**TABLE A–23J.** CONTINUED

GUIDELINES FOR THE PROFESSIONAL

You may revise the patient's meal plan to allow more calories from carbohydrate (50 to 60%) because of the high consumption of complex carbohydrates by vegetarians.

Many vegetarians use butter instead of margarine because it is considered a natural food.

The commercial meat analogues are very high in sodium, ranging in values from 300 mg to 3,000 mg/100 g edible portion. Nutritional analyses of these products are available upon request from Loma Linda Foods, Riverside, California 92505, and Worthington Foods, Miles Laboratories, Worthington, Ohio 43085.

Some vegetarians use diet supplements, such as wheat germ and brewer's yeast. Include these in the diet as follows:

Brewer's yeast, powder: 1 level Tbsp = ½ Lean Meat Exchange
Wheat germ: ¼ cup = 1 Bread Exchange

Vegetarian diets, unless fortified, could be deficient in iron. Iron absorption is enhanced by the inclusion of a vitamin C–rich food at each meal.

Vegetarian diets excluding dairy products may be inadequate in riboflavin and calcium. Two cups daily of fortified soybean milk or appropriate supplements should prevent deficiency.

For the strict vegetarian, vitamin $B_{12}$ is also required as a vitamin supplement if 2 cups of fortified soybean milk are not consumed daily.

SUGGESTED READING FOR VEGETARIANS


1. Position of the American Dietetic Association: Vegetarian Diets, J. Am. Diet. Assoc., *88*:3, 351–355, 1988.
2. Lappe, F.M.: Diet for a Small Planet. New York, Ballantine Books, 1991.
3. Robertson, L., Flinders, C., Ruppenthal, B.: The New Laurel's Kitchen. Berkeley, CA, Ten Speed Press, 1986.
4. Hodgkin, G., Maloney, S.: Diet Manual Utilizing a Vegetarian Diet Plan. 7th Ed. Loma Linda, CA, The Seventh Day Adventist Dietetic Association, 1990.
5. Hinman, B., Snyder, N.: Lean and Luscious and Meatless. Prima Publications, Rocklin, CA, 1992.
6. Mangum, K.: Life's Simple Pleasures: Fine Vegetarian Cooking for Sharing and Celebration. Pacific Press Publications, Boise, ID, 1990.
7. Baird, P.: Quick Harvest: A Vegetarian's Guide to Microwave Cooking. New York, Prentice-Hall, 1991.


*Supplement to Exchange Lists for Meal Planning Vegetarian Cookery. American Diabetes Association, Washington, D.C. Area Affiliate, Inc., Food and Nutrition Committee, 1978. See Table A–23a for Standard Exchange lists.

†Meat analogs: Vegetable protein foods that closely duplicate the flavor, texture, and appearance of meat—"meatless" meats. See company information in the Guidelines for the Professional given above.

‡Seeds and nuts can be considered a "High-fat Meat" exchange and a complete protein only when they are complemented.

**TABLE A–24A.** GLYCEMIC INDEX VALUES OF SOME FOODS ADJUSTED SO THE GLYCEMIC INDEX OF WHITE BREAD IS 100*

| FOOD | MEAN | FOOD | MEAN |
|---|---|---|---|
| Breads | | Legumes | |
| Rye (crispbread) | 95 | Baked beans (canned) | 70 |
| Rye (wholemeal) | 89 | Bengal gram dal | 12 |
| Rye (whole grain, i.e., pumpernickel) | 68 | Butter beans | 46 |
| Wheat (white) | 100 | Chick peas (dried) | 47 |
| Wheat (wholemeal) | 100 | Chick peas (canned) | 60 |
| Pasta | | Green peas (canned) | 50 |
| Macaroni (white, boiled 5 min) | 64 | Green peas (dried) | 65 |
| Spaghetti (brown, boiled 15 min) | 61 | Garden peas (frozen) | 65 |
| Spaghetti (white, boiled 15 min) | 67 | Haricot beans (white, dried) | 54 |
| Star pasta (white, boiled 5 min) | 54 | Kidney beans (dried) | 43 |
| Cereal Grains | | Kidney beans (canned) | 74 |
| Barley (pearled) | 36 | Lentils (green, dried) | 36 |
| Buckwheat | 78 | Lentils (green, canned) | 74 |
| Bulgur | 65 | Lentils (red, dried) | 38 |
| Millet | 103 | Pinto beans (dried) | 60 |
| Rice (brown) | 81 | Pinto beans (canned) | 64 |
| Rice (instant, boiled 1 min) | 65 | Peanuts | 15 |
| Rice (polished, boiled 5 min) | 58 | Soya beans (dried) | 20 |
| Rice (polished, boiled 10-25 min) | 81 | Soya beans (canned) | 22 |
| Rice (parboiled, boiled 5 min) | 54 | Fruit | |
| Rice (parboiled, boiled 15 min) | 68 | Apple | 52 |
| Rye kernels | 47 | Apple juice | 45 |
| Sweet corn | 80 | Banana | 84 |
| Wheat kernels | 63 | Orange | 59 |
| Breakfast Cereals | | Orange juice | 71 |
| "All Bran" | 74 | Raisins | 93 |
| Cornflakes | 121 | Sugars | |
| Muesli | 96 | Fructose | 26 |
| Porridge oats | 89 | Glucose | 138 |
| Puffed rice | 132 | Honey | 126 |
| Puffed wheat | 110 | Lactose | 57 |
| Shredded wheat | 97 | Maltose | 152 |
| "Weetabix" | 109 | Sucrose | 83 |
| Cookies | | Dairy Products | |
| Digestive | 82 | Custard | 59 |
| Oatmeal | 78 | Ice cream | 69 |
| "Rich tea" | 80 | Skim milk | 46 |
| Plain crackers (water biscuits) | 100 | Whole milk | 44 |
| Shortbread cookies | 88 | Yogurt | 52 |
| Root Vegetables | | Snack Foods | |
| Potato (instant) | 120 | Corn chips | 99 |
| Potato (mashed) | 98 | Potato chips | 77 |
| Potato (new/white boiled) | 80 | | |
| Potato (Russett, baked) | 116 | | |
| Potato (sweet) | 70 | | |
| Yam | 74 | | |

*Glycemic index is defined as the blood glucose repsonse to a 50-g available carbohydrate portion of a food expressed as a percentage of the response to the same amount of carbohydrate from a standard food, in this case white bread (see Chap. 39). (From Wolever, T. M. S.: World Rev. Nutr. Diet., *62*:120–185, 1990.)

**TABLE A—24B.** DIETS FOR WEIGHT REDUCTION AND FOR DIABETIC PERSONS*

| | TOTAL DAILY INTAKE (kcal) | | | |
|---|---|---|---|---|
| NUTRIENT CLASS | 800 | 1,200 | 1,800 | 2,250 |
| Carbohydrate (g) | 109 (54%) | 154 (51%) | 249 (55%) | 309 (55%) |
| Protein | 54 (27%) | 60 (20%) | 84 (19%) | 107 (19%) |
| Fat (g) | 17 (19%) | 40 (29%) | 54 (27%) | 65 (26%) |
| FOOD GROUP | TOTAL EXCHANGES FOR ONE DAY (see Table A—23) | | | |
| Skim milk | 2 | 2 | 2 | 2 |
| Vegetable | 2 | 2 | 3 | 6 |
| Fruit | 3 | 4 | 5 | 7 |
| Bread† | 2 | 4 | 9 | 10 |
| Meat | 4‡ | 4 | 5 | 7 |
| Unsaturated Fat | 1 | 4 | 4 | 4 |
| MEAL | SAMPLE MEAL PATTERN (servings based on exchanges) | | | |
| Breakfast | | | | |
| Skim milk | ½ | 1 | 1 | 1 |
| Fruit | 1 | 1 | 1 | 1 + 1 midmeal |
| Bread | 1 | 1 | 2 | 2 + 1 midmeal |
| Meat | 0 | 0 | 0 | 1 |
| Unsaturated fat | 1 | 1 | 1 | 1 |
| Lunch | | | | |
| Skim milk | 1 | ½ | 0 | 0 |
| Vegetable | 0 | 1 | 1 | 2 + 2 midmeal |
| Fruit | 1 | 1 | 2 | 1 + 1 midmeal |
| Bread | ½ | 1 | 3 | 2 |
| Meat | 1 | 1 | 2 | 2 |
| Unsaturated fat | 0 | 1 | 1 | 1 |
| Dinner | | | | |
| Skim milk | ½ | 0 | 0 | 0 |
| Vegetable | 2 | 1 | 2 | 2 |
| Fruit | 1 | 1 | 1 | 2 |
| Bread | ½ | 1 | 2 | 3 |
| Meat | 3 | 3 | 3 | 4 |
| Unsaturated fat | 0 | 1 | 1 | 1 |
| Evening | | | | |
| Skim milk | 0 | ½ | 1 | 1 |
| Vegetable | 0 | 0 | 0 | 0 |
| Fruit | 0 | 1 | 1 | 1 |
| Bread | 0 | 1 | 2 | 2 |
| Meat | 0 | 0 | 0 | 0 |
| Unsaturated fat | 0 | 1 | 1 | 1 |

*This table, prepared by us with assistance from Ms. Lori Cohen, R.D., is based on the dietary recommendations in Nutrition Guide for Professionals: Diabetes Education and Meal Planning, Powers, M. (Ed.), American Diabetes Association, Inc., and The American Dietetic Association, 1988. See Table A—25 for nutrition guidelines.

†In Exchange lists, trace fat is listed for breads. For calculation purposes, 1 g fat can be used when amount of breads contribute significantly to diet (i.e., > 6 servings per day).

‡Lean meat exchanges are used to calculate the 800-kcal meal pattern. All other meal patterns are based on medium-fat meat exchange.

**TABLE A–25.** NUTRITION GUIDELINES FOR PERSONS WITH NONINSULIN-DEPENDENT DIABETES MELLITUS

| | LEAN PERSONS | OBESE PERSONS |
|---|---|---|
| Energy | Enough to maintain desirable body weight<br>Men and physically active women require 30 kcal/kg desirable body weight<br>Sedentary persons and persons older than 55 years require 28 kcal/kg desirable body weight | Enough to achieve reasonable body weight*<br>20 kcal/kg desirable body weight |
| Carbohydrate | Up to 55 to 60% of total energy | Same |
| Sucrose | Can be included with an individualized diet plan† | Low nutrient density; limit on low-calorie diets |
| Fiber | Up to 40 g/day, with emphasis on water-soluble fiber | 25 g/1,000 kcal |
| Protein | Recommended dietary allowance is 0.8 g/kg body weight | Minimum of 60 g when restricted to ≤1,200-kcal diet‡ |
| Fat | Ideally <30% of energy | Same |
| Polyunsaturated fats | Up to 10% of energy | |
| Saturated fats | <10% of energy | |
| Monounsaturated fats | 10 to 15% of energy | |
| Cholesterol | <300 mg/day | |
| Alternative Sweeteners | Use is acceptable | Same |
| Sodum | Not to exceed 3,000 mg/day | Same |
| Alcohol | Occasional or no use; limit to 1 to 2 alcohol equivalents 1 to 2 times per week | Same |
| Vitamins/Minerals | No evidence that diabetes causes increased need | |
| Snacks | Individualized on the basis of preferences and glucose patterns; snack should be coordinated with insulin schedule if on insulin | Not necessary; if desired, should be included in total day's meal plan. If on insulin, coordinate with insulin schedule or adjust insulin as needed. |

*Reasonable body weight is that which is achievable and maintainable for the patient, although it may not be in the range considered desirable. For example, a reasonable weight goal for a patient weighing 105 kg may be 95 kg, although desirable body weight may actually be closer to 84 kg. Losing 4.5 to 9 kg may dramatically improve a person's glucose intolerance and may be a maintainable weight loss. Individual weight goals should be discussed and set.

†Individualization should be based on nutritional adequacy, promotion of diet adherence, and glucose and lipid control. Postprandial glucose response to a high-sucrose snack or meal should be evaluated; use of food and glucose records is helpful.

‡For example, 12% of a 1,200-kcal diet is only 36 g protein, which is less than the Recommended Dietary Allowance (9) for a 163-cm-tall woman; 20% of a 1,200-kcal diet will provide the recommended 60 g protein.

(From Beebe, C. A., Pastors, J. G., Powers, M. A., et al.: Nutrition management for individuals with noninsulin-dependent diabetes mellitus in the 1990's: A review by the Diabetes Care and Education dietetic practice group. J. Am. Diet. Assoc., *91*:199, 1991. With permission.)

**TABLE 1–26A.** RENAL DIETS

*Purpose:* The diet for chronic renal insufficiency (CRI) is designed to slow the progression of kidney disease and possibly delay the need for maintenance dialysis. The diet for chronic renal failure (CRF) is designed to meet nutritional requirements, minimize uremic complications, and maintain acceptable blood chemistries, blood pressure, and fluid status in patients with impaired renal function.

*Use:* The CRI diet (often called the predialysis diet) is indicated for patients with chronic renal insufficiency who do not yet require dialysis. The CRF diet is used for patients requiring hemodialysis or peritoneal dialysis treatments.

*Modifications:* The CRI diet is restricted in two major areas—protein and phosphorus. Restrictions of sodium, potassium, fluid, and calories are based on individual needs.[1-5] Generally, the CRF diet reflects controlled intake of protein, potassium, sodium, phosphorus, and fluids. Additional modifications of fat, cholesterol, triglycerides, and fiber may be necessary based on individual requirements.[6,7] Certain underlying conditions may require the adjustment of kilocalories.

SUMMARY OF NUTRIENT RECOMMENDATIONS FOR ADULT PATIENTS WITH CRI, HEMODIALYSIS, AND PERITONEAL DIALYSIS[4-12]

| Nutrient | CRI | Hemodialysis | Peritoneal Dialysis |
|---|---|---|---|
| Protein | 0.6-0.8 g/kg ideal body weight | 1.1-1.4 g/kg ideal body weight; at least 60% high biologic value | 1.2-1.5 g/kg ideal body weight<br>1.2-1.3 maintenance<br>1.5 repletion<br>1.2 reduction or with diabetes |
| Energy | Normal weight: 35 kcal/kg ideal body weight<br>Obese: 20-30 kcal/kg ideal body weight<br>Underweight or catabolic: 45 kcal/kg ideal body weight | 30-35 kcal/kg ideal body weight | 20-50 kcal/kg ideal body weight<br>25-35 maintenance<br>35-50 repletion<br>20-25 reduction<br>35 with diabetes (for CAPD and CCPD, include dialysate calories)* |
| Phosphorus | 5-10 mg/kg ideal body weight (IBW) | < 17 mg/kg IBW or approximately 800-1,200 mg/day | < 17 mg/kg IBW or approximately 1,200 mg/day |
| Sodium | 1,000-3,000 mg/day if necessary; additional sodium may be required with salt-losing nephropathic conditions | 1,000-3,000 mg/day | Individualized based on blood pressure and weight; CAPD and CCPD, 3,000-4,000 mg/day; IPD, 2,000-3,000 mg/day* |
| Potassium | Generally not restricted unless potassium is elevated and urine output is < 1 L/d | 40 mg/kg ideal body weight or approximately 50-80 mEq/day | Generally unrestricted with CAPD and CCPD; IPD, 2,000-3,000 mg/day* |
| Fluid | Generally unrestricted; balance fluid intake with urine output in patients with edema or congestive heart failure | 500-750 ml/day plus urine output or approximately 750-1,500 ml/day | CAPD and CCPD, approximately 2,000-3,000 ml/day based on daily weight fluctuations and blood pressure; IPD, same as for hemodialysis* |
| Calcium | 1,200-1,600 mg/day | Approximately 1,000-1,800 mg/day supplement as needed to maintain normal serum level | Same as for hemodialysis |
| Fat | None | Limit cholesterol to < 300 mg/day; emphasize use of polyunsaturated fats | Same as for hemodialysis |

*Adequacy:* The CRI diet is deficient in calcium, iron, vitamin $B_{12}$, and zinc because of the low-phosphorus, low-protein intake. The need for vitamin and mineral supplementation should be assessed on an individual basis.[10] CRF diets containing less than 60 g of protein may be deficient in niacin, riboflavin, thiamin, and calcium for men and calcium and iron for women, according to the 1989 Recommended Dietary Allowances.

**REFERENCES**


1. Zeller, K.: N. Engl. J. Med., *324*:78–84, 1991.
2. Ihle, B. V.: N. Engl. J. Med., *321*:1773–1777, 1989.
3. Mitch, W. E.: *In* Nutrition and the Kidney. Edited by W. E. Mitch and S. Klahr. Boston, Little Brown, 1988.
4. Kopple, J. D.: *In* Modern Nutrition in Health and Disease. Edited by M. E. Shils and R. Young. Philadelphia, Lea & Febiger, 1988.
5. Blumen Krantz, M. J.: *In* Handbook of Dialysis. Edited by J. T. Daugirdas and T. S. Ing. Boston, Little Brown, 1988.
6. Alvestrand, A. S.: *In* Nutrition and the Kidney. Edited by W. E. Mitch and S. Klahr. Boston, Little Brown, 1988.
7. Diamond, S. M. Henrich, D. E.: *In* Nutrition and the Kidney. Edited by W. E. Mitch and S. Klahr. Boston, Little Brown, 1988.
8. Bergstrom, J.: Clin. Nephrol., *21*:29–35, 1984.
9. Hruska, A.: *In* Nutrition and the Kidney. Edited by W. E. Mitch and S. Klahr. Boston, Little Brown, 1988.
10. Wolkens, K., Schiro, K. (eds.): Suggested Guidelines for the Nutrition Care of Renal Patients. 2nd Ed. Chicago, The American Dietetic Association, 1992.
11. Renal Dietitians Dietetic Practice Group: National Renal Diet. Chicago, The American Dietetic Association, to be published.
12. Gillit, D., Stover, J., Spinozzi, N.S. (Eds.): A Clinical Guide to Nutrition Care in End-Stage Renal Disease. Chicago, American Dietetic Association, 1987.


*CAPD = continuous ambulatory peritoneal dialysis; CCPD = continuous cyclic peritoneal dialysis; IPD = intermittent peritoneal dialysis.
(Modified from The Manual of Clinical Dietetics. 4th Ed. Chicago, American Dietetic Association, 1992. With permission.)

**TABLE A–26B-1.** SAMPLE MENU FOR CHRONIC RENAL INSUFFICIENCY (70-kg man; 40 g protein, 2,000 kcal, 600 mg phosphorus)

| BREAKFAST | LUNCH | DINNER |
|---|---|---|
| Orange juice (½ cup) | Roast beef (1 oz) | Baked chicken thigh (1 oz) |
| Cinnamon applesauce (½ cup) | Bread (2 slices) | White rice (½ cup) |
| Cornflakes (1 cup) | Mayonnaise (1 Tbsp) | Green beans (½ cup) |
| Toast (1 slice) | Lettuce salad (1 cup) | Low-sodium vegetable soup (½ cup) |
| Margarine (1 tsp) | Vinegar and oil dressing (1 Tbsp) | Dinner roll (1 small) |
| Jelly or jam (1 tsp) | Sliced canned peaches (1 cup) | Margarine (2 tsp) |
| Liquid nondairy creamer (½ cup) | Graham crackers (2) | Jelly |
| Coffee or tea with sugar | Lemon-lime soda (1 cup) | Strawberries (1 cup) |
| | | Tea with sugar |
| | | Lemonade (½ cup) |
| | **SNACK** | |
| | Apple pie (1 slice) | |
| | Tea with sugar | |

APPROXIMATE NUTRIENT ANALYSIS

| | | | |
|---|---|---|---|
| Energy (kcal) | 2,057.2 | Sodium (mg) | 1,798.4 |
| Protein (g) (7.9% of kcal) | 40.6 | Zinc (mg) | 5.7 |
| Carbohydrate (g) (61.8% of kcal) | 317.6 | Vitamin A (μg RE) | 994.8 |
| Total fat (g) (32.4% of kcal) | 74.2 | Vitamin C (mg) | 180.2 |
| Saturated fatty acids (g) | 14.6 | Thiamin (mg) | 1.6 |
| Monounsaturated fatty acids (g) | 28.0 | Riboflavin (mg) | 1.4 |
| Polyunsaturated fatty acids (g) | 26.7 | Niacin (mg) | 19.1 |
| Cholesterol (mg) | 64.7 | Folate (μg) | 309.0 |
| Calcium (mg) | 258.1 | Vitamin $B_6$ (mg) | 1.3 |
| Iron (mg) | 12.5 | Vitamin $B_{12}$ (μg) | 1.0 |
| Magnesium (mg) | 172.9 | Dietary fiber (g) | 17.7 |
| Phosphorus (mg) | 549.3 | Water-insoluble fiber (g) | 11.4 |
| Potassium (mg) | 2,138.0 | | |

(From The Manual of Clinical Dietetics. 4th Ed. Chicago, American Dietetic Association, 1992. With permission.)

**TABLE A–26B-2.** SAMPLE MENU FOR HEMODIALYSIS (70-kg man; 85 g protein, 2 g sodium, 2 g potassium, 1,000 mg phosphorus, 1,000 ml fluid)

| BREAKFAST | LUNCH | DINNER |
|---|---|---|
| Cranberry juice (½ cup) | Low-sodium vegetable soup (½ cup) | Broiled chicken (3 oz) |
| Grapefruit (½) | Unsalted crackers (4) | White rice (½ cup) |
| Cornflakes (¾ cup) | Lean hamburger patty (3 oz) | Green beans (½ cup) |
| White toast (2 slices) | Hamburger bun (1) | Hard dinner roll (1) |
| Margarine (2 tsp) | Unsalted mayonnaise (1 Tbsp) | Margarine (2 tsp) |
| Jelly (1 tbsp) | Lettuce | Lettuce salad (1 cup) |
| Hard-boiled egg (1) | Canned pears (½ cup) | Salt-free vinegar and oil dressing (1 Tbsp) |
| Coffee (½ cup) | Graham crackers (4) | Baked apple with sugar (1) |
| Sugar (4 tsp) | Lemonade (½ cup) | 2% milk (½ cup) |
| Liquid nondairy creamer (½ cup) | | |
| | **SNACK THROUGHOUT DAY** | |
| | Hard candy (6 pieces) | |
| | Lollipop (1 small) | |
| | Ginger ale (1 cup) | |

APPROXIMATE NUTRIENT ANALYSIS

| | | | |
|---|---|---|---|
| Energy (kcal) | 2,618.4 | Sodium (mg) | 1,901.7 |
| Protein (g) (12.6% of kcal) | 82.2 | Zinc (mg) | 9.7 |
| Carbohydrate (g) (58.4% of kcal) | 382.3 | Vitamin A (μg RE) | 860.3 |
| Total fat (g) (30% of kcal) | 87.2 | Vitamin C (mg) | 132.0 |
| Saturated fatty acids (g) | 21.8 | Thiamin (mg) | 1.6 |
| Monounsaturated fatty acids (g) | 32.7 | Riboflavin (mg) | 1.7 |
| Polyunsaturated fatty acids (g) | 25.0 | Niacin (mg) | 26.4 |
| Cholesterol (mg) | 347.8 | Folate (μg) | 235.0 |
| Calcium (mg) | 458.0 | Vitamin $B_6$ (mg) | 1.8 |
| Iron (mg) | 15.4 | Vitamin $B_{12}$ (μg) | 3.0 |
| Magnesium (mg) | 196.5 | Dietary fiber (g) | 17.9 |
| Phosphorus (mg) | 946.4 | Water-insoluble fiber (g) | 11.9 |
| Potassium (mg) | 2,069.4 | | |

(From The Manual of Clinical Dietetics. 4th Ed. Chicago, American Dietetic Association, 1992. With permission.)

**TABLE A–26B-3.** SAMPLE MENU FOR PERITONEAL DIALYSIS (70-kg man; 105 g protein, 3 g sodium, 1.4 g phosphorus, 3–4 g potassium)

| BREAKFAST | LUNCH | DINNER |
|---|---|---|
| Cranberry juice (½ cup) | Low-sodium vegetable soup (1 cup) | Green salad (3½ oz) |
| Cornflakes (¾ cup) | Lean hamburger patty (3 oz) | Vinegar and oil dressing (1 Tbsp) |
| Banana (½) | Hamburger bun | Broiled chicken breast (4 oz) |
| White toast (2 slices) | Sliced tomato (2 oz) and lettuce | Herbed white rice (½ cup) |
| Margarine (2 tsp) | Fresh fruit salad (½ cup) | Broccoli spears (2) |
| Skim milk (½ cup) | Graham crackers (4) | Hard dinner roll (1) |
| Coffee/tea | Coffee/tea | Margarine (2 tsp) |
| | | Fresh strawberries (¾ cup) |
| | | Coffee/tea |
| | **SNACK** | |
| | Unsalted crackers (5) | |
| | Tuna salad (½ cup) | |
| | Orange (1 medium) | |

APPROXIMATE NUTRIENT ANALYSIS

| | | | |
|---|---|---|---|
| Energy (kcal) | 2,125.6 | Sodium (mg) | 1,964.8 |
| Protein (g) (20.2% of kcal) | 107.6 | Zinc (mg) | 10.2 |
| Carbohydrate (g) (46.8% of kcal) | 248.8 | Vitamin A (μg RE) | 1,077.0 |
| Total fat (g) (33.4% of kcal) | 78.8 | Vitamin C (mg) | 278.4 |
| Saturated fatty acids (g) | 19.3 | Thiamin (mg) | 1.9 |
| Monounsaturated fatty acids (g) | 28.2 | Riboflavin (mg) | 1.9 |
| Polyunsaturated fatty acids (g) | 24.3 | Niacin (mg) | 40.0 |
| Cholesterol (mg) | 193.6 | Folate (μg) | 340.3 |
| Calcium (mg) | 549.9 | Vitamin $B_6$ (mg) | 2.9 |
| Iron (mg) | 16.5 | Vitamin $B_{12}$ (μg) | 3.9 |
| Magnesium (mg) | 280.5 | Dietary fiber (g) | 18.7 |
| Phosphorus (mg) | 1,069.6 | Water-insoluble fiber (g) | 10.9 |
| Potassium (mg) | 3,170.0 | | |

*Note:* Calories provided may need to be adjusted based on calories absorbed from the dialysate exchanges.
(From The Manual of Clinical Dietetics. 4th Ed. Chicago, American Dietetic Association, 1992. With permission.)

**TABLE A–26C.** AVERAGE CALCULATION FIGURES FOR PLANNING CRI AND CRF DIETS*

| FOOD EXCHANGES | kcal | Pro (g) | Na (mg) | K (mg) | Phos (mg) |
|---|---|---|---|---|---|
| Milk | 120 | 4.0 | 80 | 185 | 110 |
| Milk substitutes† | 140 | 0.5 | 40 | 80 | 30 |
| Meat | 65 | 7.0 | 25 | 100 | 65 |
| Starches | 90 | 2.0 | 80 | 35 | 35 |
| Vegetables‡ | | | | | |
| Low K | 25 | 1.0 | 15 | 70 | 20 |
| Medium K | 25 | 1.0 | 15 | 150 | 20 |
| High K | 25 | 1.0 | 15 | 270 | 20 |
| Fruits | | | | | |
| Low K | 70 | 0.5 | Trace | 70 | 15 |
| Medium K | 70 | 0.5 | Trace | 150 | 15 |
| High K | 70 | 0.5 | Trace | 270 | 15 |
| Fats | 45 | Trace | 55 | 10 | 5 |
| High-calorie choices§ | 100 | Trace | 15 | 20 | 5 |
| Beverages | Varies | Varies | Varies | Varies | Varies |
| Salt choices | — | — | 250 | — | — |

*Serving sizes for each food choice are shown in the following renal exchange lists (Table A–26d).
†Milk substitute choices are nondairy products that can be used in lieu of milk and milk products.
‡Average sodium level values do not include canned vegetables. Add 250 mg sodium for canned vegetables with added salt.
§High-calorie choices are foods high in carbohydrates that contain only a trace of protein and minimal electrolytes. These should be used to raise calorie intake to the desired level.

**TABLE A–26D.** RENAL EXCHANGE LISTS

| | |
|---|---|
| **MILK EXCHANGES FOR CRI AND CRF PATIENTS** (Average per choice: 4 g protein, 120 kcal, 80 mg sodium, 185 mg potassium, 110 mg phosphorus) | |
| Milk (nonfat, low-fat, whole) | ½ cup |
| Alterna | 1 cup |
| Buttermilk, cultured | ½ cup |
| Chocolate milk | ½ cup |
| Light cream or half and half | ½ cup |
| Ice milk or ice cream | ½ cup |
| Yogurt, plain or fruit-flavored | ½ cup |
| Evaporated milk | ¼ cup |
| Cream cheese | 3 Tbsp |
| Sour cream | 4 Tbsp |
| Sherbet | 1 cup |
| Sweetened condensed milk | ¼ cup |
| **NONDAIRY MILK SUBSTITUTES FOR CRI AND CRF PATIENTS** (Average per choice: 0.5 g protein, 140 kcal, 40 mg sodium, 80 mg potassium, 30 mg phosphorus) | |
| Dessert, nondairy frozen | ½ cup |
| Dessert topping, nondairy frozen | ½ cup |
| Liquid nondairy creamer, polyunsaturated | ½ cup |
| **MEAT EXCHANGES FOR CRI AND CRF PATIENTS** (Average per ounce: 7 g protein, 65 kcal, 25 mg sodium, 100 mg potassium, 65 mg phosphorus) | |
| *Prepared without added salt* | |
| Beef | |
| Round, sirloin, flank, cubed, T-bone, and porterhouse steak; tenderloin, rib, chuck, and rump roast; ground beef or ground chuck | 1 oz |
| Pork | |
| Fresh ham, tenderloin, chops, loin roast, cutlets | 1 oz |
| Lamb | |
| Chops, leg, roasts | 1 oz |
| Veal | |
| Chops, roasts, cutlets | 1 oz |
| Poultry | |
| Chicken, turkey, Cornish hen, domestic duck, and goose | 1 oz |
| Fish | |
| All fresh and frozen fish | 1 oz |
| Lobster, scallops, shrimp, clams | 1 oz |
| Crab, oysters | 1½ oz |
| Canned tuna, canned salmon (unsalted) | 1 oz |
| Sardines (unsalted)* | 1 oz |
| Wild game | |
| Venison, rabbit, squirrel, pheasant, duck, goose | 1 oz |
| Egg | |
| Whole | 1 large |
| Egg white or yolk | 2 large |
| Low-cholesterol egg product | ¼ cup |
| Chitterlings | 2 oz |
| Organ meats* | 1 oz |
| *Prepared with added salt* | |
| Beef | |
| Deli-style roast beef† | 1 oz |
| Pork | |
| Boiled or deli-style ham† | 1 oz |
| Poultry | |
| Deli-style chicken or turkey† | 1 oz |
| Fish | |
| Canned tuna, canned salmon† | 1 oz |
| Sardines† | 1 oz |
| Cheese | |
| Cottage† | ¼ cup |
| *High in sodium, phosphorus, and/or saturated fat* (should be used in limited quantities) | |
| Bacon | |
| Frankfurters, bratwurst, Polish sausage | |
| Lunch meats, including bologna, braunschweiger, liverwurst, picnic loaf, salami, summer sausage | |
| All cheese except cottage cheese | |

**TABLE A–26D.** CONTINUED

| STARCH EXCHANGES FOR CRI AND CRF PATIENTS (Average per choice: 2 g protein, 90 kcal, 80 mg sodium, 35 mg potassium, 35 mg phosphorus) | |
|---|---|
| *Breads and rolls* | |
| Bread (French, Italian, raisin, light rye, sourdough white) | 1 slice (1 oz) |
| Bagel | ½ small (1 oz) |
| Bun, hamburger or hot dog | ½ |
| Danish pastry or sweet roll, no nuts | ½ small |
| Dinner roll or hard roll | 1 small |
| Doughnut | 1 small |
| English muffin | ½ |
| Muffin, no nuts, bran or whole-wheat | 1 small (1 oz) |
| Pancake‡§ | 1 small |
| Pita or pocket bread, 6″ | ½ |
| Tortilla, corn, 6″ | 2 |
| Tortilla, flour, 6″ | 1 |
| Waffle‡§ | 1 small (1 oz) |
| *Cereals and grains* | |
| Cereals, ready-to-eat, most brands§ | ¾ cup |
| Puffed rice | 2 cups |
| Puffed wheat | 1 cup |
| Cooked cereal | |
| Cream of rice or wheat, farina, Malt-O-Meal | ½ cup |
| Oat bran or oatmeal, Ralston | ⅓ cup |
| Corn meal, cooked | ¾ cup |
| Grits, cooked | ½ cup |
| Flour, all-purpose | 2½ Tbsp |
| Pasta (noodles, macaroni, spaghetti), cooked | ½ cup |
| Pasta made with egg (egg noodles), cooked | ⅓ cup |
| Rice, white or brown, cooked | ½ cup |
| *Crackers and snacks* | |
| Crackers (saltines, round butter) | 4 |
| Graham crackers | 3 squares |
| Melba toast | 3 oblong |
| RyKrisp§ | 3 |
| Popcorn, plain | 1½ cups popped |
| Tortilla chips | ¾ oz (9 chips) |
| Pretzels,§ sticks or rings | ¾ oz (10 sticks) |
| *Desserts* | |
| Cake, angelfood | 1/20 cake or 1 oz |
| Cake, 2″ × 2″ | 1 square or 1½ oz |
| Sandwich cookies‡§ | 4 |
| Shortbread cookies | 4 |
| Sugar cookies | 4 |
| Sugar wafers | 4 |
| Vanilla wafers | 10 |
| Fruit pie (apple, berry, cherry, peach) | ⅛ pie |
| Sweetened gelatin | ½ cup |
| *High in poor-quality protein and phosphorus* (should be used rarely and in limited quantities) | |
| Bran cereal or muffins, Grape-Nuts, granola cereal or bars | |
| Boxed, frozen, or canned meals, entrees, or side dishes | |
| Pumpernickel, dark rye, whole-wheat or oatmeal breads | |
| Whole-wheat crackers | |
| Whole-wheat cereals | |
| *Starchy vegetables for CRI PATIENTS* | |
| Corn | ⅓ cup or ½ ear |
| Green peas | ¼ cup |
| Potatoes, boiled, mashed | ½ cup |
| Potatoes, baked, white or sweet | 1 small (3 oz) |
| Potatoes, french fried | ½ cup or 10 small |
| Potatoes, hashed brown | ½ cup |
| Squash, butternut, mashed | ½ cup |
| Squash, winter, baked (all other varieties), cubed | 1 cup |

**TABLE A–26D.** CONTINUED

VEGETABLE EXCHANGES FOR CRI PATIENTS

(Average per choice: 1 g protein, 25 kcal, 15 mg sodium, 20 mg phosphorus. See Starch List for other vegetables. Prepared or canned without added salt.||)

*1 cup serving*
Alfalfa sprouts
Cabbage
Celery
Cucumber (or ½ whole)
Eggplant
Endive
Escarole
Lettuce, all varieties
Pepper, green, sweet
Radishes, sliced (or 15 small)
Turnips
Watercress

*½ cup serving*
Artichoke
Bamboo shoots
Bean sprouts
Beans, green or wax
Beets
Carrots (or 1 small)
Cauliflower
Chard
Chinese cabbage
Collard greens
Kale
Kohlrabi
Mushrooms, fresh (or 4 medium)
Onions
Parsnips¶
Pumpkin
Rutabagas¶
Squash, summer
Tomato (or 1 medium)
Tomato juice, unsalted
Tomato juice, regular#
Tomato puree
Turnip greens
Vegetable juice cocktail, unsalted
Vegetable juice cocktail, regular#

*¼ serving*
Asparagus (or 2 spears)
Avocado (¼ whole)
Beet greens
Broccoli
Brussels sprouts
Chili pepper
Mushrooms, cooked
Mustard greens
Okra
Snow peas
Spinach
Tomato sauce

VEGETABLE EXCHANGES FOR CRF PATIENTS

(Average per choice: 1 g protein, 25 kcal, 15 mg sodium, 20 mg phosphorus. ½ cup per choice unless otherwise indicated. Prepared or canned without added salt.||)

*Low potassium (0–100 mg)*
Alfalfa sprouts (1 cup)
Bamboo shoots, canned
Bean sprouts
Beans, green or wax
Cabbage, raw
Chard, raw
Chinese cabbage, raw
Cucumber, peeled
Endive
Lettuce, all varieties (1 cup)
Escarole
Pepper, green, sweet
Watercress
Water chestnuts, canned

*Medium potassium (101–200 mg)*
Artichoke
Broccoli
Cabbage, cooked
Carrots (1 small raw)
Cauliflower
Celery, raw (1 stalk)
Collards
Corn (or ½ ear)¶
Eggplant
Kale
Mushrooms, canned¶ or fresh
Mustard greens
Onions
Peas, green¶
Radishes
Snow peas¶
Spinach, raw
Squash, summer
Turnip greens
Turnips

*High potassium (201–350 mg)*
Asparagus¶ (5 spears)
Avocado (¼ whole)
Bamboo shoots,** fresh cooked
Beet greens** (¼ cup)
Beets
Brussels sprouts¶
Celery, cooked
Chard**
Kohlrabi
Mushrooms,¶ fresh cooked
Okra¶
Parsnips¶
Pepper, chili
Potato,** baked (½ medium)
Potato,¶ boiled or mashed
Potato,** hash browned
Potato chips** (1 oz or 14 chips)
Pumpkin
Rutabagas
Spinach, cooked¶**
Sweet potato¶**
Tomato (1 medium)
Tomato juice, unsalted
Tomato juice, regular#
Tomato paste¶ (2 Tbsp)
Winter squash¶ (¼ cup)

**TABLE A–26D.** CONTINUED

**FRUIT EXCHANGES FOR CRI PATIENTS**
(Average per choice: 0.5 g protein, 70 kcal, 15 mg phosphorus)

*1 cup serving*

Apple (1 medium)
Apple juice
Applesauce
Cranberries
Cranberry juice cocktail
Papaya nectar
Peach nectar
Pear nectar
Pear, canned or fresh (1 medium)
Tangerine (1 medium)

*½ cup serving*

Apricot nectar
Banana (½ small)
Blueberries
Figs, canned
Fruit cocktail
Grape juice
Grapefruit (½ medium)
Grapefruit juice
Grapes (15 small)
Gooseberries
Kiwifruit (½ medium)
Lemon (½ medium)
Lemon juice
Mango (½ medium)
Nectarine (½ medium)
Orange (½ medium)
Peach, canned or fresh (½ medium)
Pineapple
Plums, canned or fresh (1 medium)
Rhubarb
Strawberries
Watermelon

*¼ cup serving*

Apricots (2 halves)
Apricots, dried (2)
Blackberries
Cantaloupe (⅛ small)
Cherries
Dates (2 Tbsp)
Figs, dried (1 whole)
Honeydew melon (⅛ small)
Orange juice
Papaya (¼ medium)
Prune juice
Prunes, cooked (5)
Raisins (2 Tbsp)
Raspberries

**FRUIT EXCHANGES FOR CRF PATIENTS**
(Average per choice: 0.5 g protein, 70 kcal, 15 mg phosphorus, ½ cup per choice unless otherwise indicated)

*Low potassium (0–100 mg)*

Applesauce
Blueberries
Cranberries (1 cup)
Cranberry juice cocktail (1 cup)
Grape juice
Lemon (½)
Papaya nectar
Peach nectar
Pear nectar
Pears, canned

*Medium potassium (101–200 mg)*

Apple (1 small, 2½″ diameter)
Apple juice
Apricot nectar
Blackberries
Cherries, sour or sweet
Fruit cocktail
Gooseberries
Grapefruit (½ small)
Grapefruit juice
Grapes (15 small)
Lemon juice
Mango
Papaya
Peach, canned
Peach, fresh (1 small, 2″ diameter)
Pineapple, canned or fresh
Plums, canned or fresh (1 medium)
Raisins (2 Tbsp)
Raspberries
Rhubarb
Strawberries
Tangerine (2½″ diameter)
Watermelon (1 cup)

*High potassium (201–350 mg)*

Apricots, canned or fresh (2 halves)
Apricots, dried (5)
Banana** (½ medium)
Cantaloupe (⅛ small)
Dates (¼ cup)
Figs, dried (2 whole)
Honeydew melon (⅛ small)
Kiwifruit (½ medium)
Nectarine (1 small, 2″ diameter)
Orange (1 small, 2½″ diameter)
Orange juice
Pear, fresh (1 medium)
Prune juice**
Prunes,** dried or canned (5)

**TABLE A–26D.** CONTINUED

FAT EXCHANGES FOR CRI AND CRF PATIENTS

(Average per choice: trace protein, 45 kcal, 55 mg sodium, 10 mg potassium, 5 mg phosphorus)

| | |
|---|---|
| *Unsaturated fats* | |
| Margarine | 1 tsp |
| Reduced-calorie margarine | 1 Tbsp |
| Mayonnaise | 1 tsp |
| Low-calorie mayonnaise | 1 Tbsp |
| Oil | |
| Safflower, sunflower, corn, soybean, olive, peanut, canola | 1 tsp |
| Salad dressing, mayonnaise-type | 2 tsp |
| Salad dressing, oil-type | 1 Tbsp |
| Low-calorie salad dressing (mayonnaise-type)†† | 2 Tbsp |
| Low-calorie salad dressing†† (oil-type) | 2 Tbsp |
| Tartar sauce | 1½ tsp |
| *Saturated fats* | |
| Butter | 1 tsp |
| Coconut | 2 Tbsp |
| Powdered coffee whitener | 1 Tbsp |
| Solid shortening | 1 tsp |

HIGH CALORIE CHOICES FOR CRI AND CRF PATIENTS

(Average per choice: trace protein, 100 kcal, 15 mg sodium, 20 mg potassium, 5 mg phosphorus)

| | | | |
|---|---|---|---|
| *Beverages* (count within fluid allowance) | | Fruit-flavored drink | 1 cup |
| Carbonated beverages | 1 cup | Kool-Aid | 1 cup |
| Fruit flavors, root beer, colas,‡‡ or pepper type | | Limeade | 1 cup |
| Cranberry juice cocktail | 1 cup | Lemonade | 1 cup |
| *Frozen desserts* (count within fluid allowance) | | Tang | 1 cup |
| Fruit ice | ½ cup | Wine§§ | ½ cup |
| Juice bar (3 oz) | 1 bar | | |
| | | Popsicle (3 oz) | 1 bar |
| | | Sorbet | ½ cup |
| *Candy and sweets* | | | |
| Candy corn | 20 or 1 oz | Butter mints | 14 |
| Gumdrops | 15 small | Fruit chews | 4 |
| Hard candy | 4 pieces | Chewy fruit snacks | 1 pouch |
| Jellybeans | 10 | Fruit Roll-Ups | 2 |
| LifeSavers or cough drops | 12 | Cranberry sauce or relish | ¼ cup |
| Marshmallows | 5 large | | |
| Honey | 2 Tbsp | | |
| Sugar, brown or white | 2 Tbsp | | |
| Jam or jelly | 2 Tbsp | | |
| Sugar, powdered | 3 Tbsp | | |
| Marmalade | 2 Tbsp | | |
| Syrup | 2 Tbsp | | |
| *Special low-protein products for CRI PATIENTS* | | | |
| Low-protein gelled dessert | ½ cup | | |
| Low-protein bread | 1 slice | | |
| Low-protein cookies | 2 | | |
| Low-protein pasta | ½ cup | | |
| Low-protein rusk | 2 slices | | |

**TABLE A–26D.** CONTINUED

| SALT CHOICES FOR CRI AND CRF PATIENTS (Average per choice: 250 mg sodium) | |
|---|---|
| Salt | 1/8 tsp |
| Seasoned salts (onion, garlic) | 1/8 tsp |
| Accent | 1/4 tsp |
| Barbecue sauce | 2 Tbsp |
| Bouillon | 1/3 cup |
| Catsup | 1 1/2 Tbsp |
| Chili sauce | 1 1/2 Tbsp |
| Dill pickle | 1/6 large or 1/2 oz |
| Mustard | 4 tsp |
| Olives, green | 2 medium or 1/3 oz |
| Olives, black | 3 large or 1 oz |
| Soy sauce | 3/4 tsp |
| Steak sauce | 2 1/2 tsp |
| Sweet pickle relish | 2 1/2 Tbsp |
| Taco sauce | 2 Tbsp |
| Tamari sauce | 3/4 tsp |
| Teriyaki sauce | 1 1/4 tsp |
| Worcestershire sauce | 1 Tbsp |

BEVERAGE CHOICES FOR CRF PATIENTS

*The following beverages may be used as desired within daily fluid allowance.*
Carbonated beverages (except Moxie, colas, and pepper-type)
Ice
Lemonade
Limeade
Mineral water
Water
*The following beverages contain moderate amounts of potassium and/or phosphorus and should be used in limited quantities.*
Beer and wine§§
Coffee, regular or decaffeinated
Coffee substitute (cereal grain beverage)
Fruit-flavored drinks with added vitamin C
Tea
Thirst quencher beverages
*The following liquids are very high in sodium and/or potassium and should only be used as advised by a physician or dietitian.*
Bouillon
Broth
Consomme
Salt-free broth or bouillon containing potassium chloride (KCl)
*Remember:* anything *that is liquid* or melts at room temperature must also be counted in fluid allowance (for example, ice cream, Popsicles, sherbet, gelatin).

*High phosphorus—≥ 100 mg/serving.
†High sodium—each serving counts as 1 meat choice and 1 salt choice.
‡High phosphorus—≥ 70 mg/serving.
§High sodium—each serving counts as 1 starch choice and 1 salt choice.
||For vegetables canned with salt, add 250 mg sodium and count as 1 vegetable choice and 1 salt choice.
¶High phosphorus—≥ 40 mg/serving.
#Very high sodium—each serving counts as 1 vegetable choice and 2 salt choices.
**Very high potassium—≥ 300 mg/serving.
††High sodium—each serving counts as 1 fat choice and 1 salt choice.
‡‡High phosphorus—≥ 20 mg/serving.
§§Check with physician for recommendation regarding alcohol.

Alterna, Ross Laboratories; Malt-O-Meal, Malt-O-Meal Co; Ralston, RyKrisp, Ralston Purina Co; Grape-Nuts, Kool-Aid, Tang, General Foods Corp; Popsicle, Popsicle Industries Inc; LifeSavers, Nabisco Brands, Inc; Fruit Roll-Ups, General Mills, Inc; Accent, Pet Inc; Moxie, Monarch Co, Atlanta GA 30341.

(Modified from Renal Dietitians Dietetic Practice Group: National Renal Diet. Chicago, The American Dietetic Association. In press. With permission.)

**TABLE A–27A.** SODIUM-CONTROLLED DIETS

*Purpose:* The goal of sodium restriction is to manage hypertension in sodium-sensitive individuals and promote the loss of excess fluids in edema and ascites.

*General Rules*

**1.** Avoid the use of all salt, baking soda, and/or baking powder in cooking and for table use.
**2.** Avoid medicines, laxatives, and salt substitutes unless prescribed by a physician.
**3.** Read labels carefully for sodium or salt content of packaged foods.

*Modifications*

**1.** *3,000 mg sodium (130 mEq).* Eliminate high-sodium processed foods and beverages, such as fast foods; salad dressings; smoked, salted, and koshered meats; regular canned food; pickled vegetables; luncheon meats; and commercially softened water. Allow up to 0.25 tsp table salt in cooking or at the table.
**2.** *2,000 mg sodium (87 mEq).* Eliminate processed and prepared foods and beverages high in sodium. Do not allow any salt in the preparation of foods or at the table. Limit milk and milk products to 16 fl oz daily. Check labels of canned and instant grain products for high-sodium sources.
**3.** *1,000 mg sodium (45 mEq).* Eliminate processed and prepared foods and beverages high in sodium. Omit regular canned foods, many frozen foods, deli foods, fast foods, cheeses, margarines, and regular salad dressings. Limit regular breads to 2 servings per day. Limit milk and milk products to 16 fl oz daily. Do not allow any salt in food preparation or for table use.
**4.** *500 mg sodium (22 mEq).* Omit canned or processed foods containing salt. Do not use any salt in food preparation or at the table. Omit vegetables containing high amounts of natural sodium. Limit meat to 6 oz daily, and milk and milk products to 8 fl oz daily. Use low-sodium bread in place of regular, and distilled water for cooking and drinking. This meal plan is used on a short-term basis only.
**5.** *250 mg sodium (11 mEq).* Use this meal plan for short terms only. Include the same foods as those in the 500-mg sodium diet, but use low-sodium milk in place of regular milk.

*Adequacy:* Based on the individual's food choices, the diets are adequate in all nutrients according to the 1989 National Research Council's Recommended Dietary Allowances. Unless carefully planned, however, the 250-mg and the 500-mg sodium diets can be inadequate in some nutrients.

(From The Manual of Clinical Dietetics. 4th Ed. Chicago, American Dietetic Association, 1992. With permission.)

**TABLE A–27B-1.** SAMPLE MENU FOR 3,000-MG SODIUM DIET*

| BREAKFAST | LUNCH | DINNER |
|---|---|---|
| Orange juice (½ cup) | Low-sodium vegetable soup (1 cup) | Green salad (3½ oz) |
| Whole-grain cereal (¾ cup) | Unsalted crackers (4) | Vinegar and oil dressing (1 Tbsp) |
| Banana (½) | Lean beef patty (3 oz) | Broiled skinless chicken breast (3 oz) |
| Whole-wheat toast (2 slices) | Hamburger bun (1) | Herbed brown rice (½ cup) |
| Margarine (2 tsp) | Mustard (1 Tbsp) | Steamed broccoli (½ cup) |
| Jelly or jam (1 Tbsp) | Catsup (1 Tbsp) | Whole-grain roll (1) |
| 2% milk (1 cup) | Sliced tomato (2 oz) and lettuce | Margarine (2 tsp) |
| Coffee/tea | Fresh fruit salad (½ cup) | Low-fat frozen yogurt (½ cup) |
| | Graham crackers (4) | Medium apple (1) |
| | 2% milk (1 cup) | Coffee/tea |
| | Coffee/tea | |

APPROXIMATE NUTRIENT ANALYSIS

| | | | |
|---|---|---|---|
| Energy (kcal) | 2,144.7 | Sodium (mg) | 2,334.8 |
| Protein (g) (19.2% of kcal) | 103.1 | Zinc (mg) | 13.3 |
| Carbohydrate (g) (54.1% of kcal) | 290.2 | Vitamin A (μg RE) | 1,409.2 |
| Total fat (g) (29.2% of kcal) | 69.6 | Vitamin C (mg) | 167.1 |
| Saturated fatty acids (g) | 22.6 | Thiamin (mg) | 1.8 |
| Monounsaturated fatty acids (g) | 25.0 | Riboflavin (mg) | 2.4 |
| Polyunsaturated fatty acids (g) | 15.0 | Niacin (mg) | 31.1 |
| Cholesterol (mg) | 186.6 | Folate (μg) | 400.3 |
| Calcium (mg) | 1,147.8 | Vitamin $B_6$ (mg) | 2.9 |
| Iron (mg) | 16.9 | Vitamin $B_{12}$ (μg) | 4.3 |
| Magnesium (mg) | 459.8 | Dietary fiber (g) | 24.2 |
| Phosphorus (mg) | 1,604.3 | Water-insoluble fiber (g) | 17.2 |
| Potassium (mg) | 4,056.5 | | |

*May use up to ¼ tsp salt per day in cooking and at the table.

(From The Manual of Clinical Dietetics. 4th Ed. Chicago, American Dietetic Association, 1992. With permission.)

**TABLE A–27B-2.** SAMPLE MENU FOR 2,000-MG SODIUM DIET

| BREAKFAST | LUNCH | DINNER |
|---|---|---|
| Orange juice (½ cup) | Low-sodium vegetable soup (1 cup) | Green salad (3½ oz) |
| Whole-grain cereal (¾ cup) | Unsalted crackers (4) | Salt-free vinegar and oil dressing (1 Tbsp) |
| Banana (½) | Lean beef patty (3 oz) | Broiled skinless chicken breast (3 oz) |
| Whole-wheat toast (2 slices) | Hamburger bun (1) | Herbed brown rice (½ cup) |
| Margarine (2 tsp) | Mustard (1 Tbsp) | Steamed broccoli (½ cup) |
| Jelly or jam (1 Tbsp) | Low-sodium mayonnaise (1 Tbsp) | Whole-grain roll (1) |
| 2% milk (1 cup) | Sliced tomato (2 oz) and lettuce | Margarine (2 tsp) |
| Coffee/tea | Fresh fruit salad (½ cup) | Italian fruit ice (½ cup) |
| | Graham crackers (4) | Medium apple (1) |
| | 2% milk (1 cup) | Coffee/tea |
| | Coffee/tea | |

APPROXIMATE NUTRIENT ANALYSIS

| | | | |
|---|---|---|---|
| Energy (kcal) | 2,239.7 | Sodium (mg) | 1,749.0 |
| Protein (g) (17.5% of kcal) | 98.1 | Zinc (mg) | 12.3 |
| Carbohydrate (g) (53.2% of kcal) | 297.8 | Vitamin A (μg RE) | 1,393.9 |
| Total fat (g) (31.5% of kcal) | 78.5 | Vitamin C (mg) | 165.2 |
| Saturated fatty acids (g) | 22.9 | Thiamin (mg) | 1.8 |
| Monounsaturated fatty acids (g) | 27.8 | Riboflavin (mg) | 2.2 |
| Polyunsaturated fatty acids (g) | 20.8 | Niacin (mg) | 30.7 |
| Cholesterol (mg) | 190.9 | Folate (μg) | 388.9 |
| Calcium (mg) | 989.5 | Vitamin $B_6$ (mg) | 2.9 |
| Iron (mg) | 16.2 | Vitamin $B_{12}$ (μg) | 3.9 |
| Magnesium (mg) | 422.8 | Dietary fiber (g) | 23.3 |
| Phosphorus (mg) | 1,462.2 | Water-insoluble fiber (g) | 16.4 |
| Potassium (mg) | 3,751.4 | | |

(From The Manual of Clinical Dietetics. 4th Ed. Chicago, American Dietetic Association, 1992. With permission.)

**TABLE A–27B-3.** SAMPLE MENU FOR 1,000-MG SODIUM DIET

| BREAKFAST | LUNCH | DINNER |
|---|---|---|
| Orange juice (½ cup) | Low-sodium vegetable soup (1 cup) | Green salad (3½ oz) |
| Shredded wheat cereal (¾ cup) | Unsalted crackers (4) | Salt-free vinegar and oil dressing (1 Tbsp) |
| Banana (½) | Lean beef patty (3 oz) | Broiled skinless chicken breast (3 oz) |
| Low sodium whole-wheat toast (2 slices) | Low-sodium bread (2 sices) | Herbed brown rice (½ cup) |
| Unsalted margarine (2 tsp) | Low-sodium mayonnaise (1 Tbsp) | Steamed broccoli (½ cup) |
| Jelly or jam (1 Tbsp) | Sliced tomato (2 oz) and lettuce | Whole-grain roll (1) |
| 2% milk (1 cup) | Fresh fruit salad (½ cup) | Unsalted margarine (2 tsp) |
| Coffee/tea | Graham crackers (4) | Italian fruit ice (½ cup) |
| | 2% milk (1 cup) | Medium apple (1) |
| | Coffee/tea | Coffee/tea |

APPROXIMATE NUTRIENT ANALYSIS

| | | | |
|---|---|---|---|
| Energy (kcal) | 2,255.1 | Sodium (mg) | 1,040.7 |
| Protein (g) (17.9% of kcal) | 100.9 | Zinc (mg) | 13.4 |
| Carbohydrate (g) (54% of kcal) | 304.2 | Vitamin A (μg RE) | 1,111.9 |
| Total fat (g) (31.1% of kcal) | 78.0 | Vitamin C (mg) | 153.9 |
| Saturated fatty acids (g) | 22.7 | Thiamin (mg) | 1.5 |
| Monounsaturated fatty acids (g) | 27.5 | Riboflavin (mg) | 1.9 |
| Polyunsaturated fatty acids (g) | 20.8 | Niacin (mg) | 28.2 |
| Cholesterol (mg) | 191.1 | Folate (μg) | 336.4 |
| Calcium (mg) | 952.5 | Vitamin $B_6$ (mg) | 2.6 |
| Iron (mg) | 14.6 | Vitamin $B_{12}$ (μg) | 3.9 |
| Magnesium (mg) | 469.6 | Dietary fiber (g) | 26.7 |
| Phosphorus (mg) | 1,563.6 | Water-insoluble fiber (g) | 19.7 |
| Potassium (mg) | 3,863.0 | | |

(From The Manual of Clinical Dietetics. 4th Ed. Chicago, American Dietetic Association, 1992. With permission.)

**TABLE A–27B-4.** SAMPLE MENU FOR 500-MG SODIUM DIET

| BREAKFAST | LUNCH | DINNER |
|---|---|---|
| Orange juice (½ cup) | Low-sodium vegetable soup (1 cup) | Green salad (3½ oz) |
| Shredded wheat cereal (¾ cup) | Unsalted crackers (4) | Salt-free vinegar and oil dressing (1 Tbsp) |
| Banana (½) | Lean beef patty (3 oz) | Broiled skinless chicken breast (3 oz) |
| Low sodium whole-wheat toast (2 slices) | Low-sodium bread (2 sices) | Herbed brown rice (½ cup) |
| Unsalted margarine (2 tsp) | Low-sodium mayonnaise (1 Tbsp) | Steamed broccoli (½ cup) |
| Jelly or jam (1 Tbsp) | Sliced tomato (2 oz) and lettuce | Low-sodium bread (1 slice) |
| 2% milk (1 cup) | Unsalted pretzels (1 oz) | Unsalted margarine (2 tsp) |
| Coffee/tea | Fresh fruit salad (½ cup) | Italian fruit ice (½ cup) |
| | Fruit juice (1 cup) | Medium apple (1) |
| | Coffee/tea | Coffee/tea |

APPROXIMATE NUTRIENT ANALYSIS

| | | | |
|---|---|---|---|
| Energy (kcal) | 2,220.8 | Sodium (mg) | 594.7 |
| Protein (g) (17.3% of kcal) | 96.0 | Zinc (mg) | 12.3 |
| Carbohydrate (g) (57.2% of kcal) | 317.4 | Vitamin A (μg RE) | 1,109.7 |
| Total fat (g) (28.5% of kcal) | 70.3 | Vitamin C (mg) | 232.0 |
| Saturated fatty acids (g) | 18.6 | Thiamin (mg) | 1.6 |
| Monounsaturated fatty acids (g) | 24.8 | Riboflavin (mg) | 1.6 |
| Polyunsaturated fatty acids (g) | 20.2 | Niacin (mg) | 28.7 |
| Cholesterol (mg) | 170.3 | Folate (μg) | 347.2 |
| Calcium (mg) | 652.5 | Vitamin $B_6$ (mg) | 2.6 |
| Iron (mg) | 15.3 | Vitamin $B_{12}$ (μg) | 3.0 |
| Magnesium (mg) | 438.1 | Dietary fiber (g) | 26.6 |
| Phosphorus (mg) | 1,316.2 | Water-insoluble fiber (g) | 19.2 |
| Potassium (mg) | 3,552.3 | | |

(From The Manual of Clinical Dietetics. 4th Ed. Chicago, American Dietetic Association, 1992. With permission.)

**TABLE A–27C.** GUIDELINES FOR FOOD SELECTION

| FOOD CATEGORY | FOODS RECOMMENDED | FOODS EXCLUDED FOR 3,000-MG SODIUM DIET | ADDITIONAL FOODS EXCLUDED FOR 2,000-MG SODIUM DIET* | ADDITIONAL FOODS EXCLUDED FOR 1,000-MG SODIUM DIET* |
|---|---|---|---|---|
| Beverages | Milk<br>Eggnog<br>Buttermilk (limit to 1 cup per week)<br>Low-sodium or salt-free vegetable juices<br>Regular vegetable or tomato juice (limit to ½ cup per day) | Greater than ½ cup regular vegetable or tomato juice<br>Commercially softened water for drinking or cooking | Buttermilk (>½ cup), malted milk, chocolate milk, milkshake<br>Regular milk (>2 cups)<br>Regular vegetable or tomato juice | No additional restrictions |
| Vegetables (2–4 servings per day) | Fresh and frozen vegetables<br>Low-sodium canned, drained vegetables | Sauerkraut<br>Pickled vegetables and others prepared in brine<br>Vegetables seasoned with bacon, ham, or pork | Regular canned vegetables<br>Frozen vegetables prepared in sauce | Frozen peas, frozen lima beans, frozen mixed vegetables |
| Fruits (2 or more servings per day) | All fruits and fruit juices | No additional restrictions | Fruits processed with salt or sodium-containing compounds | No additional restrictions |
| Breads and cereals (4 or more servings per day) | Enriched white, wheat, rye, and pumpernickel<br>Most cereals, hard rolls, and dinner rolls<br>Crackers<br>Unsalted snack crackers<br>Breadsticks<br>Biscuits, muffins, cornbread, pancakes, and waffles | Breads and rolls with salted tops<br>Instant hot cereals | Quick breads<br>Instant hot cereals<br>Cooked dry cereals with added sodium<br>Crackers with salted tops<br>Self-rising flour and biscuit mixes<br>Regular bread crumbs or cracker crumbs<br>Commercial bread stuffing | Sweet rolls, crackers, and other products containing salt, baking powder, or self-rising flour<br>Dry cereals |
| Potato or substitute | White or sweet potatoes<br>Squash<br>Enriched rice, barley, noodles, spaghetti, macaroni, and other pastas<br>Homemade bread stuffing | Commercially prepared potato, rice, and pasta mixes<br>Commercial stuffing | No additional restrictions | Instant potatoes |

**TABLE A–27C.** CONTINUED

| FOOD CATEGORY | FOODS RECOMMENDED | FOODS EXCLUDED FOR 3,000-MG SODIUM DIET | ADDITIONAL FOODS EXCLUDED FOR 2,000-MG SODIUM DIET* | ADDITIONAL FOODS EXCLUDED FOR 1,000-MG SODIUM DIET* |
|---|---|---|---|---|
| Meat or substitute | Fresh or fresh-frozen meats (beef, lamb, pork, veal, and game)<br>Fresh or fresh-frozen poultry (chicken, turkey, Cornish hen, and others)<br>Fresh-water or fresh-frozen unbreaded fish<br>Most shellfish<br>Canned tuna, rinsed<br>Canned salmon, rinsed<br>Eggs and egg substitutes<br>Cheese in limited amounts<br>Low-sodium cheese as desired<br>Ricotta cheese and cream cheese (limit 2 oz per day)<br>Cottage cheese, drained<br>Regular yogurt<br>Regular peanut butter (3 times per week)<br>Dried peas and beans<br>Frozen dinners (<600 mg sodium) | Any meat, fish, or poultry that is smoked, cured, salted, koshered, or canned (bacon, chipped beef, coldcuts, ham, hot dogs, and sausages)<br>Sardines, anchovies, marinated herring, and pickled meats<br>Pickled eggs<br>Frozen breaded meats<br>Processed cheese, cheese spreads, and sauces<br>Salted nuts | Crab<br>Lobster<br>Regular hard and processed cheese<br>Regular peanut butter<br>Frozen dinner entrees (<500 mg sodium) | All shellfish<br>Egg substitutes |
| Fats | Butter or margarine<br>Vegetable oils<br>Low-sodium salad dressing as desired<br>Regular salad dressing in limited amounts<br>Light, sour, and heavy cream | Salad dressings containing bacon, bacon fat, bacon bits, and salt pork<br>Snack dips made with instant soup mixes and/or processed cheese | No additional restrictions | Nondairy cream ($\leq$1 fl oz allowed per day)<br>Salted butter or margarine<br>Regular mayonnaise |
| Soups | Commercial canned and dehydrated soups, broth, and bouillon<br>Homemade soups without added salt, made with allowed vegetables<br>Homemade broth<br>Low-sodium canned soups and broths | Excessive amounts of canned or dehydrated soups (>1 cup per week) | Regular canned or dehydrated commercial soups, broths, or bouillon | No additional restrictions |

**TABLE A—27C.** CONTINUED

| FOOD CATEGORY | FOODS RECOMMENDED | FOODS EXCLUDED FOR 3,000-MG SODIUM DIET | ADDITIONAL FOODS EXCLUDED FOR 2,000-MG SODIUM DIET* | ADDITIONAL FOODS EXCLUDED FOR 1,000-MG SODIUM DIET* |
|---|---|---|---|---|
| Sweets and desserts | Any sweets and desserts allowed | No additional restrictions | Desserts and sweets made with milk exceeding allowance | All candies made with sweet chocolate, nuts, or coconut<br>Desserts make with rennin, rennin tablets<br>Sherbets and flavored gelatin (>½ cup per day)<br>Salted bakery foods, homemade or commercial |
| Miscellaneous | Limit added salt to ¼ tsp per day used at the table or in cooking<br>Salt substitute with physician's approval<br>Pepper, herbs, and spices<br>Vinegar<br>Lemon or lime juice<br>Hot pepper sauce<br>Low-sodium soy sauce<br>Unsalted tortilla chips, pretzels, potato chips, popcorn | Any seasoning containing salt (garlic salt, celery salt, onion salt, and seasoned salt)<br>Sea salt, rock salt, and kosher salt<br>Any other seasoning containing salt and sodium compounds (meat tenderizers, monosodium glutamate [MSG: Accent])<br>Regular soy sauce<br>Teriyaki sauce<br>Most flavored vinegars<br>Regular snack chips | Regular catsup, chili sauce, mustard, pickles, relishes, olives, and horseradish<br>Barbecue, Worcestershire, and steak sauce<br>Canned gravies and mixes | No additional restrictions |

*Guidelines for food selection for 500-mg sodium diet.* Use the 1000-mg sodium diet guidelines with the following modifications:

- Use low sodium bread only.
- Omit sherbet and flavored gelatin.
- Limit meat to 6 oz per day. One egg may be used per day in place of 1 oz of meat.
- Omit the following vegetables: beets, beet greens, carrots, kale, spinach, celery, white turnips, rutabagas, mustard greens, chard, peas, and dandelion greens.
- Use distilled water.
- Limit milk and milk products to 8 oz per day.

*The foods listed under the 2 "Additional Foods Excluded" categories represent additions to the foods already excluded either in the preceding column (for 2,000-mg diet) or in the preceding 2 columns (for 1,000-mg diet).

(Adapted from The Manual of Clinical Dietetics. 4th ed. Chicago, American Dietetic Association, 1992. With permission.)

**TABLE A—28A.** RECOMMENDED DIET MODIFICATIONS TO LOWER BLOOD CHOLESTEROL

*Purpose:* The general aim of dietary therapy is to reduce elevated cholesterol levels while maintaining a nutritionally adequate eating pattern.

*Use:* Dietary therapy should occur in two steps, the Step-One and Step-Two Diets, that are designed to progressively reduce intakes of saturated fatty acids and cholesterol and to promote weight loss in patients who are overweight by eliminating excess total calories. The Step-One Diet should be prescribed and explained by the physician and his or her staff. This diet involves an intake of total fat less than 30% of calories, saturated fatty acids less than 10% of calories, and cholesterol less than 300 mg/day. The Step-Two Diet, used if the response to the Step-One Diet is insufficient, calls for a further reduction in saturated fatty acid intake to less than 7% of calories and in cholesterol to less than 200 mg/day. The Step-One Diet calls for the reduction of the major and obvious sources of saturated fatty acids and cholesterol in the diet; for many patients this can be achieved without a radical alteration in dietary habits. The Step-Two Diet requires careful attention to the whole diet to reduce intake of saturated fatty acids and cholesterol to a minimal level compatible with an acceptable and nutritious diet. Involvement of a registered dietitian is useful, particularly for intensive dietary therapy, such as the Step-Two Diet.

After starting the Step-One Diet, the total serum cholesterol level should be measured and adherence to the diet assessed at 4 to 6 weeks and at 3 months. If the total cholesterol monitoring goal is met, the LDL-cholesterol level should be measured to confirm that the LDL goal has been achieved. If this is the case, the patient enters a long-term monitoring program and is seen quarterly for the first year and twice yearly thereafter. At these visits total cholesterol level should be measured, and dietary and behavior modifications reinforced.

If the cholesterol goal has not been achieved with the Step-One Diet, the patient should generally be referred to a registered dietitian. With the aid of the dietitian, the patient should progress to the Step-Two Diet, or to another trial on the Step-One Diet (with progression to the Step-Two Diet if the response is still not satisfactory). On the Step-Two Diet, total cholesterol levels should again be measured and adherence to the diet assessed after 4 to 6 weeks and at 3 months of therapy. If the desired goal for total cholesterol (and for LDL-cholesterol) lowering has been attained, long-term monitoring can begin. If not, drug therapy should be considered. A minimum of 6 months of intensive dietary therapy and counseling should usually be carried out before initiating drug therapy; shorter periods can be considered in patients with severe elevations of LDL-cholesterol (> 225 mg/dl) or with definite coronary heart disease. Drug therapy should be added to, and not substituted for, dietary therapy.

*Adequacy:* Based on the individual's food choices, the diets are adequate in all nutrients according to the National Research Council's Recommended Dietary Allowances.

NATIONAL CHOLESTEROL EDUCATION PROGRAM: STEP-ONE AND STEP-TWO DIETS

| | RECOMMENDED INTAKE | |
|---|---|---|
| NUTRIENT | Step-One Diet | Step-Two Diet |
| Total fat | Less than 30% of total calories | |
| Saturated fatty acids | Less than 10% of total calories | Less than 7% of total calories |
| Polyunsaturated fatty acids | Up to 10% of total calories | |
| Monounsaturated fatty acids | 10% to 15% of total calories | |
| Carbohydrates | 50% to 60% of total calories | |
| Protein | 10% to 20% of total calories | |
| Cholesterol | Less than 300 mg/day | Less than 200 mg/day |
| Total calories | To achieve and maintain desirable weight | |

(With permission from The National Cholesterol Education Program, Report of the Expert Panel on Detection, Evaluation, and Treatment of High Blood Cholesterol in Adults. U.S. Department of Health and Human Services, Public Health Service National Institutes of Health Publication No. 89-2925, 1989.)

**TABLE A–28B.** STEP-ONE DIET

| FOOD CATEGORY | CHOOSE | DECREASE |
|---|---|---|
| Fish, chicken, turkey, and lean meat | Fish; poultry without skin; lean cuts of beef, lamb, pork or veal; shellfish | Fatty cuts of beef, lamb, pork; spare ribs; organ meats; regular cold cuts; sausage; hot dogs; bacon; sardines; roe |
| Skim and low-fat milk, cheese, yogurt, and dairy substitutes | Skim or 1% fat milk (liquid, powdered, evaporated); buttermilk | Whole milk (4% fat) (regular, evaporated, condensed); cream; half and half; 2% milk; imitation milk products; most nondairy creamers; whipped toppings |
| | Nonfat (0% fat) or low-fat yogurt | Whole-milk yogurt |
| | Low-fat cottage cheese (1% or 2% fat) | Whole-milk cottage cheese (4% fat) |
| | Low-fat, farmer, or pot cheeses (all of these should be labeled no more than 2 to 6 g fat/oz) | All natural cheeses (e.g., blue, roquefort, camembert, cheddar, swiss) |
| | Low-fat or "light" cream cheese, low-fat or "light" sour cream | Cream cheeses, sour cream |
| | Sherbet or sorbet | Ice cream |
| Eggs | Egg whites (2 whites = 1 whole egg in recipes), cholesterol-free egg substitutes | Egg yolks |
| Fruits and vegetables | Fresh, frozen, canned, or dried fruits and vegetables | Vegetables prepared in butter, cream, or other sauces |
| Breads and cereals | Homemade baked goods using unsaturated oils sparingly, angel food cake, low-fat crackers, low-fat cookies | Commercial baked goods: pies, cakes, doughnuts, croissants, pastries, muffins, biscuits, high-fat crackers, high-fat cookies |
| | Rice, pasta | Egg noodles |
| | Whole-grain breads and cereals (oatmeal, whole-wheat, rye, bran, multigrain, etc.) | Breads in which eggs are major ingredient |
| Fats and oils | Baking cocoa | Chocolate |
| | Unsaturated vegetable oils: corn, olive, rapeseed (canola oil), safflower, sesame, soybean, sunflower | Butter, coconut oil, palm oil, palm kernel oil, lard, bacon fat |
| | Margarine or shortening made from one of the unsaturated oils listed above | |
| | Diet margarine | |
| | Mayonnaise, salad dressings made with unsaturated oils listed above | Dressings made with egg yolk |
| | Low-fat dressings | |
| | Seeds and nuts | Coconut |

**TABLE A–28C-1.** SAMPLE MENU FOR STEP-ONE DIET

| BREAKFAST | LUNCH | DINNER |
|---|---|---|
| Orange juice (½ cup) | Vegetable soup (1 cup) | Green salad (3½ oz) |
| Whole-grain cereal (¾ cup) | Saltine crackers (4) | Vinegar and oil dressing (1 tbsp) |
| Banana (½) | Lean beef patty (3 oz) | Broiled skinless chicken breast (3 oz) |
| Whole-wheat toast (2 slices) | Hamburger bun (1) | Herbed brown rice (½ cup) |
| Diet margarine (2 tsp) | Mustard (1 tbsp) | Steamed broccoli (½ cup) |
| Jelly or jam (1 tbsp) | Low-fat mayonnaise (2 tsp) | Whole-grain roll (1) |
| 1% milk (1 cup) | Sliced tomato (2 oz) and lettuce | Diet margarine (2 tsp) |
| Coffee/tea | Fresh fruit salad (½ cup) | Low-fat frozen yogurt (½ cup) |
| | Graham crackers (4) | Medium apple (1) |
| | 1% milk (1 cup) | Coffee/tea |
| | Coffee/tea | |

APPROXIMATE NUTRIENT ANALYSIS

| | | | | | |
|---|---|---|---|---|---|
| Energy (kcal) | 2,054.7 | Iron (mg) | 16.5 | Thiamin (mg) | 1.8 |
| Protein (g) (19.9% of kcal) | 102.1 | Magnesium (mg) | 456.4 | Riboflavin (mg) | 2.4 |
| Carbohydrate (g) (55.5% of kcal) | 285.3 | Phosphorus (mg) | 1,610.8 | Niacin (mg) | 29.0 |
| Total fat (g) (27.1% of kcal) | 61.8 | Potassium (mg) | 3,978.0 | Folate (μg) | 400.6 |
| Saturated fatty acids (g) | 19.4 | Sodium (mg) | 3,190.1 | Vitamin $B_6$ (mg) | 2.8 |
| Monounsaturated fatty acids (g) | 21.1 | Zinc (mg) | 14.4 | Vitamin $B_{12}$ (μg) | 4.4 |
| Polyunsaturated fatty acids (g) | 14.8 | Vitamin A (μg RE) | 1,378.8 | Dietary fiber (g) | 24.1 |
| Cholesterol (mg) | 167.8 | Vitamin C (mg) | 165.2 | Water-insoluble fiber (g) | 17.0 |
| Calcium (mg) | 1,126.4 | | | | |

(From The Manual of Clinical Dietetics. Chicago, American Dietetic Association, 1992. With permission.)

**TABLE A–28C-2.** SAMPLE MENU FOR STEP-TWO DIET

| BREAKFAST | LUNCH | DINNER |
|---|---|---|
| Orange juice (½ cup) | Vegetable soup (1 cup) | Green salad (3½ oz) |
| Whole-grain cereal (¾ cup) | Saltine crackers (4) | Vinegar and oil dressing (1 tbsp) |
| Banana (½) | Sliced turkey (3 oz) | Broiled skinless chicken breast (3 oz) |
| Whole-wheat toast (2 slices) | Whole-wheat bread (2 slices) | Herbed brown rice (½ cup) |
| Diet margarine (2 tsp) | Mustard (1 tbsp) | Steamed broccoli (½ cup) |
| Jelly or jam (1 tbsp) | Low-fat mayonnaise (2 tsp) | Whole-grain roll (1) |
| Skim milk (1 cup) | Sliced tomato (2 oz) and lettuce | Diet margarine (2 tsp) |
| Coffee/tea | Fresh fruit salad (½ cup) | Low-fat frozen yogurt (½ cup) |
| | Graham crackers (4) | Medium apple (1) |
| | Skim milk (1 cup) | Coffee/tea |
| | Coffee/tea | |

APPROXIMATE NUTRIENT ANALYSIS

| | | | | | |
|---|---|---|---|---|---|
| Energy (kcal) | 1,892.5 | Iron (mg) | 15.6 | Thiamin (mg) | 1.7 |
| Protein (g) (21.6% of kcal) | 102.3 | Magnesium (mg) | 471.0 | Riboflavin (mg) | 2.1 |
| Carbohydrate (g) (61.2% of kcal) | 289.7 | Phosphorus (mg) | 1,734.4 | Niacin (mg) | 32.6 |
| Total fat (g) (20.4% of kcal) | 42.9 | Potassium (mg) | 4,024.4 | Folate (μg) | 413.5 |
| Saturated fatty acids (g) | 10.6 | Sodium (mg) | 3,565.7 | Vitamin $B_6$ (mg) | 2.8 |
| Monounsaturated fatty acids (g) | 13.3 | Zinc (mg) | 12.4 | Vitamin $B_{12}$ (μg) | 3.1 |
| Polyunsaturated fatty acids (g) | 14.7 | Vitamin A (μg RE) | 1,392.5 | Dietary fiber (g) | 25.3 |
| Cholesterol (mg) | 126.5 | Vitamin C (mg) | 165.3 | Water-insoluble fiber (g) | 18.0 |
| Calcium (mg) | 1,129.9 | | | | |

(From The Manual of Clinical Dietetics. Chicago, American Dietetic Association, 1992. With permission.)

**TABLE A–29A.** GUIDELINES FOR FOOD SELECTION FOR FAT-RESTRICTED DIET (25 g or 50 g of FAT)

| FOOD CATEGORY | RECOMMENDED | MAY CAUSE DISTRESS |
|---|---|---|
| Beverages | Skim milk; skim buttermilk; powdered and evaporated skim milk; coffee; tea; soda; other nondairy drinks | 1%, 2%, whole milks; buttermilk made with whole milk; chocolate milk; evaporated milk; cream |
| Breads and cereals | Whole-grain breads; enriched breads; saltines; soda crackers; cold and cooked cereals; whole-grain cereal except granola-type; unbuttered popcorn; plain corn or flour tortillas | Biscuits; breads containing egg or cheese; sweet rolls; pancakes; French toast; doughnuts; waffles; fritters; buttered popcorn; muffins; granola-type cereals and breads to which extra fat is added; popovers; snack crackers with added fat; snack chips; stuffing; fried tortillas |
| Desserts | Sherbet; fruit ice; gelatin; angel food cake; vanilla wafers; graham crackers; meringues; pudding made with skim milk; fat-free commercial baked products; nonfat ice cream and frozen yogurt | All other cakes, cookies, pies, and pastries; puddings made with whole milk or eggs; cream puffs |
| Fats<br>Amount listed equals 1 fat equivalent; 3 to 5 equivalents/day allowed for 50-g fat diet.<br>(Unsaturated fats are recommended. | *Unsaturated*<br>Margarine (1 tsp)<br>Diet margarine (1 Tbsp)<br>Mayonnaise<br>reduced-calorie (1 Tbsp)<br>regular (1 tsp)<br>Creamy salad dressings<br>reduced-calorie (1 Tbsp)<br>regular (2 tsp)<br>Other salad dressings<br>reduced-calorie (2 Tbsp)<br>regular (1 Tbsp)<br>Vegetable oils (1 tsp)<br>Nuts<br>almonds (6 whole)<br>cashews (1 Tbsp or 2 whole)<br>peanuts (20 small or 10 large)<br>peanut butter (2 tsp)<br>cashew butter (2 tsp)<br>walnuts (2 whole)<br>pistachios (18 whole)<br>other nuts (1 Tbsp)<br>Seeds<br>sesame (1 Tbsp)<br>sunflower (1 Tbsp)<br>pumpkin (2 tsp)<br>Olives (10 small or 5 large)<br>*Saturated*<br>Bacon (1 slice)<br>Bacon fat (1 tsp)<br>Butter (1 tsp)<br>Whipped butter (2 tsp)<br>Chitterlings (½ oz)<br>Shredded coconut (2 Tbsp)<br>Cream<br>light, coffee, table (2 Tbsp)<br>heavy whipping (1 Tbsp)<br>Sour cream (2 Tbsp)<br>Cream cheese (1 Tbsp)<br>Coffee whitener<br>liquid (2 Tbsp)<br>powder (4 tsp)<br>Lard (1 tsp)<br>Oil<br>coconut (1 tsp)<br>palm (1 tsp)<br>Shortening (1 tsp)<br>Sour cream (2 Tbsp)<br>Salt pork (¼ oz) | Any in excess of amounts prescribed on diets and all others |

**TABLE A—29A.** CONTINUED

| FOOD CATEGORY | RECOMMENDED | MAY CAUSE DISTRESS |
|---|---|---|
| Fruits | Fresh, frozen, canned, or dried fruit; fruit juices | Avocado |
| Meats and meat substitutes<br>For 50-g fat diet, 6 oz/day<br>For 25-g fat diet, 5 oz/day<br>(Recommended preparation methods are broiling, roasting, grilling, or boiling; weigh meat after cooking.) | Poultry<br>breast meat without skin<br>Veal<br>all cuts<br>Lean beef<br>USDA good or choice cuts (i.e., round, sirloin, flank steak, tenderloin, and chopped beef); roast (rib, chuck, rump); steak (cube, Porterhouse, T-bone); meatloaf made with ground beef (95% lean)<br>Lean pork<br>fresh, canned, cured, or boiled ham; Canadian bacon; tenderloin; chops; loin roast; Boston butt; cutlets<br>Lean lamb<br>chops, leg, or roast<br>Fish<br>all fresh, frozen, or canned in water: crab, lobster, scallops, shrimp, clams, oysters, tuna; herring (uncreamed or smoked); sardines (canned, drained); salmon (canned in water)<br>Luncheon meats<br>95% fat-free; lean ham, turkey, or beef<br>Legumes<br>cooked, canned, without added fat<br>Tofu, tempeh, natto<br>Cheese<br>skim-milk cheeses; cottage cheese; parmesan cheese<br>Low-fat yogurt; non-fat yogurt as desired<br>Eggs<br>poached; soft or hard cooked; scrambled, not fried in fat; count 1 egg as 1 oz of meat in daily meat allowance; egg substitutes as desired | Any fried, fatty, or heavily marbled meat, fish, or poultry<br>Poultry<br>duck, goose<br>Beef<br>most USDA prime cuts of beef, ribs, corned beef<br>Pork<br>spareribs; ground pork sausage (patty or link); ham hocks; pigs' feet; chitterlings<br>Lamb<br>patties (ground lamb)<br>Fish<br>tuna (packed in oil)<br>salmon (packed in oil)<br>Luncheon meats<br>most, including bologna, salami, pimento loaf<br>Sausage<br>Polish; Italian; knockwurst; smoked bratwurst; frankfurter<br>Legumes (cooked with added fat) |
| Potatoes and potato substitutes | Potatoes; rice; barley; noodles; spaghetti, macaroni, and other pastas | Fried potatoes; fried rice; potato chips; chow mein noodles |
| Soups | Fat-free broth; fat-free vegetable soup; cream soup made with skim milk and allowed fat; packaged dehydrated soups | All others |
| Sweets | Sugar; honey; jelly; jam; marmalade; molasses; maple syrup; sourballs; gumdrops; jelly beans; marshmallows; hard candy; cocoa powder | Butter, coconut, chocolate, and cream candies |
| Vegetables | All fresh, frozen, or canned vegetables prepared without fats, oil, or fat-containing sauces | Buttered, au gratin, creamed, or fried vegetables unless made with allowed fat allowance |
| Miscellaneous | Catsup; chili sauce; vinegar; pickles; vanilla; unbuttered popcorn; white sauce made with skim milk and allowed fat; mustard; all herbs and seasonings; apple butter | Olives and nuts in excess of specified portions; cream sauces; gravies; buttered popcorn |

(From The Manual of Clinical Dietetics. 4th Ed. Chicago, American Dietetic Association, 1992. With permission.)

**TABLE A–29B-1.** SAMPLE MENU FOR FAT-RESTRICTED DIET (25 g of FAT)

| BREAKFAST | LUNCH | DINNER |
|---|---|---|
| Orange juice (1 cup) | Fat-free vegetable soup (1 cup) | Green salad (3½ oz) |
| Whole-grain cereal (¾ cup) | Saltine crackers (4) | Fat-free dressing (1 Tbsp) |
| Banana (1) | Sliced turkey (2 oz) | Broiled skinless chicken breast (2 oz) |
| Whole-wheat toast (2 slices) | Whole-wheat bread (2 slices) | Herbed brown rice (½ cup) |
| Jelly or jam (2 Tbsp) | Mustard (1 Tbsp) | Steamed broccoli (½ cup) |
| Skim milk (1 cup) | Fat-free mayonnaise (1 Tbsp) | Whole-grain roll (1) |
| Coffee/tea | Sliced tomato (2 oz) and lettuce | Jelly or jam (1 Tbsp) |
| SNACK | Fresh fruit salad (½ cup) | Fruit ice or sorbet (½ cup) |
| Canned or fresh fruit (1 cup) | Graham crackers (4) | Medium apple (1) |
| Skim milk (½ cup) | Skim milk (1 cup) | Coffee/tea |
| | Coffee/tea | |

APPROXIMATE NUTRIENT ANALYSIS

| | | | |
|---|---|---|---|
| Energy (kcal) | 2,016.4 | Sodium (mg) | 3,259.9 |
| Protein (g) (18.8% of kcal) | 94.7 | Zinc (mg) | 11.6 |
| Carbohydrate (g) (75.6% of kcal) | 380.9 | Vitamin A (μg RE) | 1,261.1 |
| Total fat (g) (9.8% of kcal) | 22.0 | Vitamin C (mg) | 271.7 |
| Saturated fatty acids (g) | 6.8 | Thiamin (mg) | 1.8 |
| Monounsaturated fatty acids (g) | 6.4 | Riboflavin (mg) | 2.2 |
| Polyunsaturated fatty acids (g) | 5.2 | Niacin (mg) | 28.7 |
| Cholesterol (mg) | 110.7 | Folate (μg) | 493.2 |
| Calcium (mg) | 1,169.7 | Vitamin $B_6$ (mg) | 3.3 |
| Iron (mg) | 16.6 | Vitamin $B_{12}$ (μg) | 2.9 |
| Magnesium (mg) | 512.5 | Dietary fiber (g) | 29.3 |
| Phosphorus (mg) | 1,672.1 | Water-insoluble fiber (g) | 20.2 |
| Potassium (mg) | 4,681.4 | | |

(From The Manual of Clinical Dietetics. 4th Ed. Chicago, American Dietetic Association, 1992. With permission.)

**TABLE A–29B-2.** SAMPLE MENU FOR FAT-RESTRICTED DIET (50 g of FAT) )

| BREAKFAST | LUNCH | DINNER |
|---|---|---|
| Orange juice (½ cup) | Fat-free vegetable soup (1 cup) | Green salad (3½ oz) |
| Whole-grain cereal (¾ cup) | Saltine crackers (4) | Fat-free dressing (1 Tbsp) |
| Banana (½) | Lean beef patty (3 oz) | Broiled skinless chicken breast (3 oz) |
| Whole-wheat toast (2 slices) | Hamburger bun (1) | Herbed brown rice (½ cup) |
| Margarine (1 tsp) | Mustard (1 Tbsp) | Steamed broccoli (½ cup) |
| Jelly or jam (1 Tbsp) | Reduced-calorie mayonnaise (1 Tbsp) | Whole-grain roll (1) |
| Skim milk (1 cup) | Sliced tomato (2 oz) and lettuce | Margarine (1 tsp) |
| Coffee/tea | Fresh fruit salad (½ cup) | Fruit ice or sorbet (½ cup) |
| SNACK | Graham crackers (4) | Medium apple (1) |
| Canned peaches (½ cup) | Skim milk (1 cup) | Coffee/tea |
| Skim milk (½ cup) | Coffee/tea | |

APPROXIMATE NUTRIENT ANALYSIS

| | | | |
|---|---|---|---|
| Energy (kcal) | 2,053.2 | Sodium (mg) | 3,016.8 |
| Protein (g) (20.1% of kcal) | 103.3 | Zinc (mg) | 14.2 |
| Carbohydrate (g) (60.7% of kcal) | 311.7 | Vitamin A (μg RE) | 1,373.5 |
| Total fat (g) (21.6% of kcal) | 49.3 | Vitamin C (mg) | 171.7 |
| Saturated fatty acids (g) | 15.2 | Thiamin (mg) | 1.8 |
| Monounsaturated fatty acids (g) | 18.6 | Riboflavin (mg) | 2.3 |
| Polyunsaturated fatty acids (g) | 9.4 | Niacin (mg) | 29.7 |
| Cholesterol (mg) | 159.0 | Folate (μg) | 400.4 |
| Calcium (mg) | 1141.8 | Vitamin $B_6$ (mg) | 2.9 |
| Iron (mg) | 16.3 | Vitamin $B_{12}$ (μg) | 4.5 |
| Magnesium (mg) | 440.4 | Dietary fiber (g) | 24.4 |
| Phosphorus (mg) | 1,642.1 | Water-insoluble fiber (g) | 16.9 |
| Potassium (mg) | 4,170.9 | | |

(From The Manual of Clinical Dietetics. 4th Ed. Chicago, American Dietetic Association, 1992. With permission.)

**TABLE A–30A.** RESTRICTED-FIBER DIET

*Purpose:* The fiber- and residue-restricted diet is designed to prevent blockage of a stenosed gastrointestinal tract and to reduce the frequency and volume of fecal output while prolonging intestinal transit time.

*Suggested General Guidelines:*

1. Limit milk and milk products to 2 cups daily. If lactose intolerant, see lactose-controlled diet.
2. Limit fruits to the following: juices without pulp (excluding prune), canned fruit, and ripe bananas. Most raw fruits should be avoided, such as dates, figs, prunes, apples, blackberries, boysenberries, peaches, grapes, pears, pineapple, rhubarb, and fresh grapefruit and orange sections.
3. Limit vegetables to the following: vegetable juices without pulp, lettuce, and cooked/canned vegetables without seeds, such as asparagus, beets, green beans, seedless tomatoes, spinach, eggplant, and acorn squash.
4. Use only white or refined bread and cereal products, or baked products using refined flour. Cooked white and sweet potatoes without skin, white rice, and refined pasta are allowed.
5. Avoid tough fibrous meats with gristle: Allow ground or well-cooked tender beef, lamb, ham, veal, pork, poultry, fish, and organ meats. Eggs and cheese are acceptable.
6. Avoid peanuts, coconut, nuts, seeds, popcorn, dried beans, peas, legumes, and lentils.

*Modifications:* A low-fiber diet is not synonymous with a low-residue diet. The term residue refers to both the indigestible content of a food that acts as a laxative and the total postdigestive luminal contents that increase fecal output.[1,2] A low-fiber diet also can be a low-residue diet if milk and products that contain milk are limited to 2 cups or less per day, prune juice is omitted, and meat and shellfish with tough connective tissue are avoided. Milk, prune juice, and connective tissue from meats are low in fiber but may increase colonic residue and stool weight by mechanisms other than dietary fiber.[1]

*Adequacy:* Based on the individual's food choices, the diet is adequate in all nutrients according to the National Research Council's Recommended Dietary Allowances, 1989. Vitamin and mineral supplementation may be indicated, however, when illness results in suboptimal intakes and increased requirements. The benefit of long-term restriction of dietary fiber remains controversial. Strict reductions in milk products, vegetables, and fruit intake may necessitate calcium, ascorbic acid, and folate supplementation. Individual response, particularly in patients with ulcerative colitis and Crohn's disease, must be monitored to avoid an overly restrictive regimen and to determine continued indication for this diet.

*References*

1. Kramer, P.: The meaning of high and low residue diets. *Gastroenterology, 47*:649, 1964.
2. Connell, A.M.: The role of fibre in the gastrointestinal tract. *In* The Clinical Role of Fibre. Edited by P.E. Bowen, A.M. Connell, et al. Toronto, Ontario, Canada, Medical Education Services, 1985.

(From The Manual of Clinical Dietetics. 4th Ed. Chicago, American Dietetic Association, 1992. With permission.)

**TABLE A—30B.** HIGH-FIBER DIET

*Purpose:* The diet is designed to be high in dietary fiber. It is useful for decreasing intraluminal colonic pressure, increasing gastrointestinal motility and increasing the volume and weight of material that reaches the distal colon. Both soluble and insoluble fibers exert these physiologic effects, whereas only soluble fibers exert metabolic effects, such as delayed glucose absorption, increased sensitivity to insulin, altered intestinal enzyme activity, binding of bile acids, and decrease in serum cholesterol and triglyceride levels.

*General Guidelines*

1. The reported positive effects of fiber are derived from a diet high in fiber-rich foods. Increased fiber intake should come from a variety of food sources rather than dietary fiber supplements. This approach is more likely to ensure increased intake of minerals and other nutrients.
2. Consumption of adequate amounts of liquids (eight 8-fluid-ounce glasses per day) in conjunction with high-fiber intake is recommended.
3. Prior to recommending a twofold increase in dietary fiber consumption, an assessment of current fiber intake should be made. Estimates of fiber content of household portions of foods are shown in Table A—30c.
4. Advise gradual increase of dietary fiber intake to minimize potential side effects.

*Fiber Components and Food Sources*

*Water-soluble fibers* are hydrated, resulting in gel-like or viscous substances, and are fermented by colonic bacteria.

| Water-soluble fibers: | Foods containing water-soluble fibers include: |
|---|---|
| Gum<br>Mucilages<br>Pectin<br>Some hemicellulose | Fruits, vegetables, barley, legumes, oat, and oat bran |

*Water-insoluble fibers* remain essentially unchanged during digestion.

| Water-insoluble fibers: | Foods containing water-insoluble fibers include: |
|---|---|
| Cellulose<br>Lignin<br>Some hemicellulose | Fruits, vegetables, cereals, whole-wheat products, and wheat bran |

*Adequacy:* Depending on individual food selection, the high-fiber diet is adequate in all nutrients according to the National Research Council's Recommended Dietary Allowances, 1989.

The adequacy of the high-fiber diet may be questionable for individuals whose mineral intake is marginal because of poor dietary practices or for "at-risk" groups (children, pregnant or lactating women, elderly or chronically ill persons). Some studies indicate that excessive intakes of some dietary fiber sources may bind and interfere with the absorption of the following minerals: calcium, copper, iron, magnesium, selenium, and zinc.[1] It is hypothesized, however, that long-term high-fiber diet would not by itself cause mineral or nutrient imbalances in the general population.[2,3] Intake of adequate fluids is necessary because of hygroscopic nature of fiber.

The American Dietetic Association recommends a daily dietary fiber intake of 20 to 35 g from a variety of sources combined with a low-fat, high-carbohydrate diet.[4]

*References*


1. Walter, A.: Mineral metabolism. *In Dietary Fibre, Fibre-Depleted Foods and Disease.* Edited by H. Trowell, D. Burkitt, and K. Heaton. Orlando, Academic Press, 1985.
2. Gordon, D.T.: Total dietary fiber and mineral absorption. *In Dietary Fiber Chemistry, Physiology and Health Effects.* Edited by D. Kritchevsky, C. Bonfield, and J.W. Anderson. New York, Plenum Press, 1990.
3. Slavin, J.L.: Dietary fiber: classification, chemical analyses and food sources. J. Am. Diet. Assoc., *87*:1164, 1987.
4. Position of The American Dietetic Association: Health implications of dietary fiber. Technical support paper. J. Am. Diet. Assoc., *88*:216, 1988.


*Further Reading*


Anderson, J.W.: Fiber and health: an overview. *Am. J. Gastroenterol, 82*:892, 1986.

Judd, P., Truswell, S.: Dietary fibre and blood lipids in man. *In Dietary Fibre Perspectives, Reviews and Bibliography.* Edited by A. Leeds. London, John Libbey, 1985.

Klurfeld, D.M.: The role of dietary fiber in gastrointestinal disease. *J. Am. Diet. Assoc., 87*:1178, 1987.

Lanza, E., and Batrum, R.: A critical review of fiber analysis and data. *J. Am. Diet. Assoc., 86*:732, 1986.


(Modified from The Manual of Clinical Dietetics. 4th Ed. Chicago, American Dietetic Association, 1992. With permission.)

**TABLE A–30C.** DIETARY FIBER CONTENT OF FOODS IN COMMONLY SERVED PORTIONS

| FOOD GROUP | <1 g | 1–1.9 g | 2–2.9 g | 3–3.9 g | 4–4.9 g | 5–5.9 g | > 6 g |
|---|---|---|---|---|---|---|---|
| Breads (1 slice) | Bagel<br>White<br>French | Whole-wheat | Bran muffin (1) | NA* | NA | NA | NA |
| Cereals (1 oz) | Rice Krispies<br>Special K<br>Cornflakes | Oatmeal<br>Nutri-Grain<br>Cheerios | Wheaties<br>Shredded Wheat | Most<br>Honey Bran | Bran Chex<br>40% Bran Flakes<br>Raisin Bran | Corn Bran | All-Bran<br>Bran Buds<br>100% Bran |
| Pasta (1 cup) | NA | Macaroni<br>Spaghetti | NA | Whole-wheat spaghetti | NA | NA | NA |
| Rice (½ cup) | White | Brown | NA | NA | NA | NA | NA |
| Legumes (½ cup cooked) | NA | NA | NA | Lentils | Lima beans<br>Dried peas | NA | Kidney beans<br>Baked beans<br>Navy beans |
| Vegetables (½ cup unless otherwise stated | Cucumber<br>Lettuce (1 cup)<br>Green pepper | Asparagus<br>Green beans<br>Cabbage<br>Cauliflower<br>Potato without skin (1)<br>Celery | Broccoli<br>Brussels sprouts<br>Carrots<br>Corn<br>Potato with skin (1)<br>Spinach | Peas | NA | NA | NA |
| Fruits (1 medium unless other-wise stated) | Grapes (20)<br>Watermelon (1 cup) | Apricots (3)<br>Grapefruit (½)<br>Peach with skin<br>Pineapple (½ cup) | Apple, without skin<br>Banana<br>Orange | Apple, with skin<br>Pear, with skin<br>Raspberries (½ cup) | NA | NA | NA |

*Not applicable.

(Slavin, J.L.: Dietary fiber: Classification, chemical analyses, and food sources. J. Am. Diet. Assoc., *87*:1164, 1987. Reprinted with permission.)

**TABLE A–30D-1.** SAMPLE MENU FOR FIBER- AND RESIDUE-RESTRICTED DIET

| BREAKFAST | LUNCH | DINNER |
|---|---|---|
| Strained orange juice (½ cup) | Vegetable broth (1 cup) | Strained tomato juice (½ cup) |
| Puffed rice cereal (¾ cup) | Saltine crackers (4) | Broiled skinless chicken breast (3 oz) |
| Canned peaches (½ cup) | Lean beef patty (3 oz) | White rice (½ cup) |
| White bread toast (2 slices) | Hamburger bun without seeds (1) | Cooked spinach (½ cup) |
| Margarine (2 tsp) | Mustard (1 Tbsp) | White roll (1) |
| Jelly (1 Tbsp) | Catsup (1 Tbsp) | Margarine (2 tsp) |
| 2% milk (1 cup) | Canned fruit cocktail (½ cup) | Low-fat frozen yogurt (½ cup) |
| Coffee/tea | Vanilla wafer cookies (2) | Applesauce (½ cup) |
| | 2% milk (1 cup) | Coffee/tea |
| | Coffee/tea | |

APPROXIMATE NUTRIENT ANALYSIS

| | | | |
|---|---|---|---|
| Energy (kcal) | 1,857.2 | Sodium (mg) | 2,954.5 |
| Protein (g) (20.9% of kcal) | 97.0 | Zinc (mg) | 11.7 |
| Carbohydrate (g) (52.1% of kcal) | 241.9 | Vitamin A (μg RE) | 1,398.2 |
| Total fat (g) (27.6% of kcal) | 53.0 | Vitamin C (mg) | 132.1 |
| Saturated fatty acids (g) | 20.3 | Thiamin (mg) | 1.4 |
| Monounsaturated fatty acids (g) | 21.3 | Riboflavin (mg) | 2.0 |
| Polyunsaturated fatty acids (g) | 9.2 | Niacin (mg) | 25.4 |
| Cholesterol (mg) | 181.8 | Folate (μg) | 274.2 |
| Calcium (mg) | 1,138.7 | Vitamin $B_6$ (mg) | 1.7 |
| Iron (mg) | 13.2 | Vitamin $B_{12}$ (μg) | 4.2 |
| Magnesium (mg) | 346.5 | Dietary fiber (g) | 14.3 |
| Phosphorus (mg) | 1,315.6 | Water-insoluble fiber (g) | 9.0 |
| Potassium (mg) | 3,482.6 | | |

(From The Manual of Clinical Dietetics. 4th Ed. Chicago, American Dietetic Association, 1992. With permission.)

**TABLE A–30D-2.** SAMPLE MENU FOR HIGH-FIBER DIET*

| BREAKFAST | LUNCH | DINNER |
|---|---|---|
| Orange juice (½ cup) | Split pea soup (1 cup) | Green salad (3½ oz) |
| Whole-grain cereal (¾ cup) | Whole-wheat crackers (4) | Vinegar and oil dressing (1 Tbsp) |
| Raisins (2 Tbsp) | Lean beef patty (3 oz) | Broiled skinless chicken breast (3 oz) |
| Whole wheat toast (2 slices) | Hamburger bun (1) | Herbed brown rice (½ cup) |
| Margarine (2 tsp) | Mustard (1 Tbsp) | Steamed broccoli (½ cup) |
| Jelly or jam (1 Tbsp) | Catsup (1 Tbsp) | Whole-grain roll (1) |
| 2% milk (1 cup) | Sliced tomato (2 oz) and lettuce | Margarine (2 tsp) |
| Coffee/tea | Fresh fruit salad (½ cup) | Low-fat frozen yogurt (½ cup) |
| | Bran muffin (1) | Medium pear (1) |
| | 2% milk (1 cup) | Coffee/tea |
| | Coffee/tea | |

APPROXIMATE NUTRIENT ANALYSIS

| | | | |
|---|---|---|---|
| Energy (kcal) | 2,195.0 | Sodium (mg) | 3,175.6 |
| Protein (g) (19.4% of kcal) | 106.4 | Zinc (mg) | 14.4 |
| Carbohydrate (g) (54.0% of kcal) | 296.0 | Vitamin A (μg RE) | 1,381.1 |
| Total fat (g) (29.6% of kcal) | 72.1 | Vitamin C (mg) | 160.4 |
| Saturated fatty acids (g) | 23.0 | Thiamin (mg) | 1.8 |
| Monounsaturated fatty acids (g) | 25.7 | Riboflavin (mg) | 2.4 |
| Polyunsaturated fatty acids (g) | 16.0 | Niacin (mg) | 28.6 |
| Cholesterol (mg) | 190.9 | Folate (μg) | 425.4 |
| Calcium (mg) | 1,241.8 | Vitamin $B_6$ (mg) | 2.4 |
| Iron (mg) | 18.4 | Vitamin $B_{12}$ (μg) | 4.3 |
| Magnesium (mg) | 511.7 | Dietary fiber (g) | 30.8 |
| Phosphorus (mg) | 1,763.0 | Water-insoluble fiber (g) | 21.1 |
| Potassium (mg) | 4,328.5 | | |

*For further fat restriction, decrease servings of margarine and salad dressing. Use skimmed or 1% milk and milk products.
(From The Manual of Clinical Dietetics. 4th Ed. American Dietetic Association, 1992. With permission.)

**TABLE A—31A.** SOFT DIET

*Purpose:* The soft diet is designed for patients who are physically or neurologically unable to tolerate a general diet.
*Adequacy:* Based on the individual's food choice, the diet is adequate in all nutrients according to the National Research Council's Recommended Dietary Allowances, 1989.

**TABLE A—31B.** GUIDELINES FOR FOOD SELECTION FOR SOFT DIET

| FOOD CATEGORY | RECOMMENDED | MAY CAUSE DISTRESS |
|---|---|---|
| Beverages | Milk and milk products; all other beverages | Alcoholic beverages |
| Breads and cereals | White, refined-wheat, or light-rye enriched breads, soft rolls and crackers; cooked or ready-to-eat cereals | Coarse cereals (e.g., bran); whole-grain breads or crackers with seeds; bread or bread products with nuts or dried fruits |
| Desserts | Cakes, cookies, pies, pudding, custard, ice cream, sherbet, and gelatin made with allowed foods; fruit ice and frozen pops | All sweets and desserts containing nuts, coconut, or dried fruits not allowed; fried pastries (e.g., doughnuts) |
| Fats | Butter or fortified margarine; salad dressings; all fats and oils | Highly seasoned salad dressings |
| Fruits | All fruit juices; cooked or canned fruit; avocado, banana, grapefruit, and orange sections without membrane; soft fruits (e.g., melons, strawberries) | Other fresh and dried fruits |
| Meats and meat substitutes | All lean, tender meats, poultry, fish, and shellfish; crisp bacon; eggs; mild-flavored cheeses; creamy peanut butter; soybean and other meat substitutes; plain or flavored yogurt | Strong-smelling or highly seasoned meats, cheeses, or fish (e.g., luncheon meats, frankfurters, sausage); yogurt with nuts or dried fruits |
| Potato or substitute | Potatoes; enriched rice, barley, spaghetti, macaroni, and other pasta | Potato chips, fried potatoes |
| Soups | Soups made with allowed foods | Highly seasoned soups and soups made with gas-producing vegetables |
| Sweets | Sugar; syrup; honey; jelly and seedless jam; hard candies; plain chocolate candies; molasses; marshmallows | Any with nuts or coconut |
| Vegetables | All vegetable juices; cooked vegetables and lettuce as tolerated; salads made from allowed foods | Raw and fried vegetables; whole kernel corn; gas-producing vegetables (eg, broccoli, Brussels sprouts, cabbage, onions, leeks, cauliflower, cucumber, green pepper, rutabagas, turnips, sauerkraut, dried peas, dried beans) |
| Miscellaneous | Iodized salt; flavorings; mildly flavored gravies and sauces; pepper, herbs, spices, catsup, mustard, and vinegar in moderation | Strongly flavored seasonings and condiments (e.g., garlic, chili sauce, chili pepper, horseradish); pickles; popcorn; nuts and coconut |

(From The Manual of Clinical Dietetics. 4th Ed. Chicago, American Dietetic Association, 1992. With permission.)

**TABLE A–31C.** SAMPLE MENU FOR SOFT DIET

| BREAKFAST | LUNCH | DINNER |
|---|---|---|
| Orange juice (½ cup) | Vegetable soup (1 cup) | Tomato juice (6 oz) |
| Refined cold cereal (¾ cup) | Saltine crackers (4) | Broiled skinless chicken breast (3 oz) |
| Banana (½ cup) | Lean beef patty (3 oz) | Enriched rice (½ cup) |
| White toast (2 slices) | Hamburger bun (1) | Steamed green beans (½ cup) |
| Margarine (2 tsp) | Mustard (1 Tbsp) | Soft dinner roll (1) |
| Jelly or jam (1 Tbsp) | Mayonnaise (1 Tbsp) | Margarine (2 tsp) |
| 2% milk (1 cup) | Lettuce leaf | Low-fat frozen yogurt (½ cup) |
| Coffee/tea | Canned fruit cocktail (½ cup) | Applesauce (½ cup) |
| | Graham crackers (4) | Coffee/tea |
| | 2% milk (1 cup) | |
| | Coffee/tea | |

APPROXIMATE NUTRIENT ANALYSIS

| | | | |
|---|---|---|---|
| Energy (kcal) | 2,142.6 | Sodium (mg) | 3,581.9 |
| Protein (g) (17.9% of kcal) | 96.0 | Zinc (mg) | 12.5 |
| Carbohydrate (g) (57.1% of kcal) | 305.8 | Vitamin A (μg RE) | 944.5 |
| Total fat (g) (25.5% of kcal) | 60.8 | Vitamin C (mg) | 118.3 |
| Saturated fatty acids (g) | 21.8 | Thiamin (mg) | 2.0 |
| Monounsaturated fatty acids (g) | 23.0 | Riboflavin (mg) | 2.4 |
| Polyunsaturated fatty acids (g) | 9.9 | Niacin (mg) | 30.9 |
| Cholesterol (mg) | 185.9 | Folate (μg) | 327.2 |
| Calcium (mg) | 1,038.7 | Vitamin $B_6$ (mg) | 2.5 |
| Iron (mg) | 15.4 | Vitamin $B_{12}$ (μg) | 4.4 |
| Magnesium (mg) | 308.9 | Dietary fiber (g) | 16.5 |
| Phosphorus (mg) | 1,319.1 | Water-insoluble fiber (g) | 11.1 |
| Potassium (mg) | 3,389.7 | | |

(From The Manual of Clinical Dietetics. 4th Ed. Chicago, American Dietetic Association, 1992. With permission.)

**TABLE A—32.** DYSPHAGIA DIET

Stage I—Dysphagia puree, no liquids
Stage II—Dysphagia puree plus thick liquids
Stage III—Dysphagia puree plus thin liquids
Stage IV—Dysphagia mechanical soft foods, no liquids
Stage V—Dysphagia mechanical soft foods plus thick liquids
Stage VI—Dysphagia mechanical soft foods plus thin liquids

STAGE I—DYSPHAGIA PUREE, NO LIQUIDS

No liquids are provided unless specified by physician's order. Includes smooth, moist, and pureed foods that require little or no chewing but form a moist, cohesive bolus.

| Food Group | Foods Allowed | Foods Avoided |
|---|---|---|
| Milk products | Pudding, custard, ice cream, plain or flavored yogurt (without fruit) | All others |
| Meat, poultry, and eggs | Pureed meat, chicken, fish; soufflés, soft cooked or poached eggs | All others |
| Vegetables and fruits | Pureed vegetables, fruits; applesauce, frozen fruit juices | All others |
| Breads and cereals | Thick cooked cereals, mashed potato | All others |
| Fats | Butter, margarine, sour cream | All others |
| Miscellaneous | Salt, pepper, ketchup, mustard, jelly, gelatin dessert | None |

STAGE II—DYSPHAGIA PUREE PLUS THICK LIQUIDS

Includes all foods allowed in stage I with the addition of the following *thick liquids.*

| Food Group | Liquids Allowed | Liquids Avoided |
|---|---|---|
| Milk products | Thickened eggnog, Carnation Instant Breakfast, milk shakes | All others |
| Soups | Thick creamed soups | Broth |
| Fruits | Thinned pureed fruits, nectar, vegetable juice | All others |

STAGE III—DYSPHAGIA PUREE PLUS THIN LIQUIDS

Includes all foods allowed in stage II with the addition of the following *thin liquids.*

| Food Group | Liquids Allowed | Liquids Avoided |
|---|---|---|
| Milk products | Eggnog, Carnation Instant Breakfast, milk | None |
| Soup | Thin creamed soups, broth | None |
| Beverages | Coffee, tea, soda, fruit juices | None |

*Note:* Once a patient has mastered stage III, the diet can be either progressed in consistency (i.e., to stage V) or changed to puree.

STAGE IV—DYSPHAGIA MECHANICAL SOFT FOODS, NO LIQUIDS

No liquids are provided unless specified by physician's order. Includes minced and soft foods that require little or no chewing but form a soft, cohesive bolus.

| Food Group | Liquids Allowed | Liquids Avoided |
|---|---|---|
| Milk products | Pudding, custard, ice cream, cream pies; plain, flavored, fruited yogurt | All others |
| Cheeses | Small-curd cottage cheese, ricotta cheese, American cheese, grated cheese | All others |
| Eggs | Soft scrambled eggs, crustless quiche, soufflés, egg salad | All others |
| Meat, fish, and poultry | Ground meat or poultry with gravy; chicken or tuna salad (without celery); meat loaf; hamburger; baked or broiled fish; salmon loaf; pasta casseroles | |

**TABLE A–32.** CONTINUED

| Food Group | Foods Allowed | Foods Avoided |
|---|---|---|
| Vegetables | Cooked and diced carrots, beets, chopped or creamed spinach, butternut or acorn squash | Raw vegetables, other cooked vegetables |
| Potatoes, rice, and noodles | Mashed or baked (without skin) potatoes, macaroni and cheese, egg noodles, spaghetti with gravy or sauce | Rice, coarse grain (kasha, buckwheat, bran) |
| Fruit | Mashed banana, canned or cooked fruits cut into small pieces | Fruits with pits, raisins; all others |
| Breads and cereals | Bread, soft rolls, muffins, soft French toast, pancakes, cooked cereal, dry cereals soaked in milk, cakes without nuts | Dry crackers, breads with seeds, raisins, nuts |
| Fats | Butter, margarine, sour cream, gravy, mayonnaise | Nuts, seeds |

STAGE V—DYSPHAGIA MECHANICAL SOFT FOODS PLUS THICK LIQUIDS

Includes all food from stage IV with the addition of *thick liquids* as outlined in stage II.

STAGE VI—DYSPHAGIA MECHANICAL SOFT FOODS PLUS THIN LIQUIDS

Includes all food from stage IV with the addition of *thin liquids* as outlined in stage III.

*Note:* Once a patient has mastered stage VI, the diet can be either progressed in consistency (i.e., to regular) or changed to mechanical soft foods.

Patients at stages I and IV need to have fluid status monitored and fluid requirements met by alternate means.

Milk products may not be tolerated by individuals who are susceptible to increased mucus production probably secondary to casein, a milk protein. If this becomes a problem, substitutes should be found.

Suggestions for dietitians:

1. A member of the medical or nursing staff or dysphagia team should be present at the bedside when a patient initially receives a dysphagia diet or advances to a higher stage to evaluate the patient's tolerance of the stage.
2. The dietitian should work closely with medical and nursing staff for continued evaluation of the patient's diet tolerance and progression.
3. Calorie counts are indicated to evaluate adequacy of intake and to justify the need for supplementation or nutrition support.
4. The dietitian should work closely with the dysphagia team for physiologic evaluation of the patient's ability to chew and swallow to select the correct diet stage.
5. The dietitian should encourage small, frequent meals, particularly in the first stages of the diet.
6. As a guide, the following list gives a progression of food consistencies in order of increasing swallowing difficulty:
   - stiff jelled consistency
   - standard jelled consistency
   - thick purees
   - applesauce consistency
   - thick soup consistency
   - nectar consistency
   - standard thin liquids
   - chunk consistency (ground or diced)

Eating tips:

1. Food should be taken in small portions (½ tsp at a time).
2. The patient should sit upright with hips flexed at a 90° angle.
3. If possible, the neck should be at a 90° angle and flexed slightly forward.
4. The patient should sit up for 15 to 30 minutes both before and after meals.
5. Food should be placed on the unaffected side when possible.
6. Cold or hot foods may be better tolerated than foods at room temperature.

(From Antiaspiration-dysphagia Diet. *In* Diet Manual. New York, Memorial Sloan-Kettering Cancer Center, 1989. Reprinted by permission; and Bloch, A.S.: Nutrition Management of the Cancer Patient. Aspen, Rockville, MD, 1990. With permission.)

## TABLE A–33A. ANTIDUMPING (POSTGASTRECTOMY) DIET

*Purpose:* This diet is designed to provide adequate calories and nutrients to support tissue healing and prevent weight loss and dumping syndrome after gastric surgery.[1–6]

*Modifications:* The diet limits beverages and liquids at meals, limits the intake of simple carbohydrates, and is high in protein and moderate in fat. Small, frequent feedings should be provided daily.[1,2] If no complications occur, additional foods are added as tolerated. Some patients are able to advance to a general diet within 2 to 3 weeks.[1]

After surgery, the diet generally progresses as follows:[1,2]

1. Ice chips held in mouth or small sips of water. Some people tolerate warm water better than ice chips or cold water.
2. Low-carbohydrate, clear liquids, such as broth, bouillon, unsweetened gelatin, or diluted unsweetened fruit juices, are given next.
3. The postgastrectomy diet then begins, with gradual progression to a general diet as tolerated.

It is important to note that the stated guidelines must be tailored to each patient's surgery, food tolerances, and nutrition problems and deficiencies.

*General Guidelines*[1,2,4,5,7,8]

1. Liquids should be given 30 to 60 minutes after meals and limited to 0.5-to 1-cup servings. At least 6 cups of fluid, however, should be consumed daily to replace losses resulting from diarrhea. Carbonated beverages and milk are not recommended initially.
2. Small, frequent feedings should be provided. The number of feedings depends on the patient's tolerance to specific portions of food. Foods should be eaten slowly and chewed well.
3. The diet should be low in simple carbohydrates, high in complex carbohydrates and protein, and moderate in fat.
4. All food and drink should be moderate in temperature. Cold drinks tend to cause increased gastric motility.
5. If "dumping" is a problem, the patient should lie down 20 to 30 minutes after meals to retard transit to the small bowel.
6. Introduce small amounts of milk to determine tolerance. If milk intolerance is found to be caused by a lactase deficiency, a lactose-restricted diet may be necessary (see Table A–35).
7. If adequate caloric intake cannot be provided because of steatorrhea, use of medium-chain triglyceride products may be needed.
8. Pectin, a dietary fiber found in fruits and vegetables, may be helpful for treating dumping syndrome. Pectin delays gastric emptying, slows carbohydrate absorption, and reduces the glycemic response.

*Adequacy:* The adequacy of the diet depends on the extent of surgery, as well as on individual food tolerances. With careful selection, this diet is adequate in all nutrients. After gastric surgery some patients experience malabsorption, which may be specific for macronutrients (e.g., carbohydrates, proteins, and fats) or micronutrients (e.g., folate, vitamin $B_{12}$, iron, vitamin D, and calcium).[2] Vitamin and mineral supplementation may be necessary depending on the extent of surgery and on whether the symptoms of dumping syndrome persist.[1,2]

*References*


1. Zeman, F.J.: *Clinical Nutrition and Dietetics.* 2nd Ed. New York, Macmillan, 1991.
2. Desai, M. Jeejeebhoy, K.N. *In* Modern Nutrition in Health and Disease. 7th Ed. Edited by M.E. Shils and V.R. Young. Philadelphia, Lea & Febiger, 1988.
3. Braga, M., Zuliani, L., Foppa, L., et al.: Br. J. Surg., *75*:477, 1988
4. Jordan, P. *In* Hardy's Textbook of Surgery. 2nd Ed. Edited by J. Hardy. Philadelphia, J.B. Lippincott, 1988.
5. Williams, S.R.: Nutrition and Diet Therapy. 6th Ed. St. Louis, Times Mirror/Mosby College Publishing, 1989.
6. Meyer, J.H. *In* Gastrointestinal Disease: Pathophysiology, Diagnosis, and Management. 4th Ed. Edited by M.H. Sleisenger, J.S. Fordtran. Philadelphia, W.B. Saunders, 1989.
7. Sawyers, J.L.: Am. J. Surg., *159*:8–13, 1990.
8. Alpers, D., Crouse, R., Stenson, W.: Manual of Nutritional Therapeutics. 2nd Ed. Boston, Little Brown, 1988.

**TABLE A—33B.** GUIDELINES FOR FOOD SELECTION FOR ANTIDUMPING (POSTGASTRECTOMY) DIET

| FOOD CATEGORY | RECOMMENDED | MAY CAUSE DISTRESS* |
|---|---|---|
| Beverages† | Milk as tolerated; coffee; tea; unsweetened or diluted fruit drinks; unsweetened carbonated beverages | Alcohol; chocolate milk drinks; milkshakes; sweetened fruit drinks; sweetened carbonated beverages |
| Breads and cereals | Whole-grain or enriched breads and cereals; English muffins and bagels; unsweetened, cooked cereals | Breads made with dried fruits, nuts, and seeds; pastries; donuts; muffins |
| Cereals | Unsweetened dry and cooked cereals | Sugar-coated cereals, coarse cereals (e.g., bran) |
| Desserts | Plain cakes and cookies; sugar-free pudding, gelatin dessert, custard, yogurt, and frozen yogurt | All sweets and desserts made with chocolate or dried fruits; sweetened gelatin dessert; fried pastries; ice cream; ice milk; regular fruited or frozen yogurt |
| Fats | Butter; margarine; salad dressings; mayonnaise; vegetable oils; sour cream; cream cheese as tolerated | None |
| Fruits | Unsweetened canned fruits and fruit juice†; fresh fruits | All dried fruits; sweetened fruit juice; fruits canned in heavy syrup |
| Meats and meat substitutes | Lean tender meats; fish; poultry; shellfish; eggs; peanut butter; cottage cheese; mild cheeses; highly seasoned and spicy meats | Fried meats or eggs |
| Potato and potato substitutes | Potatoes; enriched rice; barley; noodles; spaghetti, macaroni, and other pastas | Any to which sugar has been added (e.g., candied sweet potatoes) |
| Soups | Soups made with allowed foods; spicy soups as tolerated | Soups prepared with heavy cream or high-fat ingredients |
| Sweets | Sugar substitutes and sweets made with sugar substitutes | Sugar; syrup; honey; jelly; jam; molasses; marshmallows |
| Vegetables | Cooked (fresh, frozen, canned) vegetables or vegetable juice†; raw vegetables as tolerated | Any to which sugar has been added |
| Miscellaneous | Iodized salt; pepper; mildly flavored sauces and gravies; strongly flavored seasonings as tolerated | None |

*If no adverse symptoms occur, these foods can be added as tolerated.
†All fluids should be consumed 30 to 60 minutes after meals and limited to ½- to 1-cup servings.
(From The Manual of Clinical Dietetics. 4th Ed. Chicago, American Dietetic Association, 1992. With permission.)

**TABLE A—33C.** SAMPLE MENU FOR ANTIDUMPING (POSTGASTRECTOMY) DIET*

| BREAKFAST | LUNCH | DINNER |
|---|---|---|
| Grapefruit (½) | Lean hamburger patty (2 oz) | Broiled skinless chicken breast (3 oz) |
| Oatmeal (½ cup) | Hamburger bun (1) | Herbed brown rice (½ cup) |
| Whole-wheat toast (1 slice) | Mayonnaise (1 Tbsp) | Steamed broccoli (½ cup) |
| Margarine (1 tsp) | Sliced tomato (2 oz) and lettuce | Margarine (2 tsp) |
| 2% milk† (½ cup) | Fresh fruit salad (½ cup) | Unsweetened applesauce (½ cup) |
| Coffee/tea† (½ cup) | 2% milk† (½ cup) | 2% milk† (½ cup) |
| | Coffee/tea† (½ cup) | Coffee/tea† (½ cup) |
| MIDMORNING SNACK | MIDAFTERNOON SNACK | BEDTIME SNACK |
| Cheese (1 oz) | Roast beef (1 oz) | Peanut butter (2 Tbsp) |
| Saltine crackers (4) | Bread (1 slice) | Graham crackers (4) |
| Banana (½) | Mustard (1 tsp) | 2% milk† (½ cup) |
| | Vegetable soup† (1 cup) | |

APPROXIMATE NUTRIENT ANALYSIS

| | | | |
|---|---|---|---|
| Energy (kcal) | 2,055.9 | Sodium (mg) | 3,016.3 |
| Protein (g) (20.9% of kcal) | 107.4 | Zinc (mg) | 14.1 |
| Carbohydrate (g) (41.7% of kcal) | 214.1 | Vitamin A (μg RE) | 823.3 |
| Total fat (g) (39.4% of kcal) | 90.0 | Vitamin C (mg) | 136.2 |
| Saturated fatty acids (g) | 29.8 | Thiamin (mg) | 1.4 |
| Monounsaturated fatty acids (g) | 33.5 | Riboflavin (mg) | 1.9 |
| Polyunsaturated fatty acids (g) | 19.3 | Niacin (mg) | 27.1 |
| Cholesterol (mg) | 215.2 | Folate (μg) | 240.5 |
| Calcium (mg) | 1,035.6 | Vitamin $B_6$ (mg) | 2.3 |
| Iron (mg) | 12.0 | Vitamin $B_{12}$ (μg) | 4.3 |
| Magnesium (mg) | 409.9 | Dietary fiber (g) | 21.6 |
| Phosphorus (mg) | 1,652.2 | Water-insoluble fiber (g) | 14.0 |
| Potassium (mg) | 3,270.6 | | |

*The sample menu incorporates six (6) meals per day. The number of feedings depends on the patient's tolerance to food portions and therefore should be adjusted accordingly.

†Liquid should be given 30 to 60 minutes after the meal and limited to ½ cup to 1 cup servings.

(From The Manual of Clinical Dietetics. 4th Ed. Chicago, American Dietetic Association, 1992. With permission.)

**TABLE A–34.** GLUTEN-RESTRICTED AND GLIADIN- AND PROLAMIN-FREE (Wheat-, Rye-, Oat, and Barley-Free) DIET INSTRUCTION

This menu pattern is designed to provide adequate nutrition while eliminating wheat, rye, oats, and barley from the diet. The fraction of gluten protein in wheat that injures the intestine of susceptible persons is gliadin. The equivalent toxic protein fractions in barley, rye, and oats are prolamins. When all sources of gliadin and prolamin are removed from the diet, the intestine is able to regenerate, and normal function is usually restored.

Gliadin and prolamin may be either present in foods as a basic ingredient (i.e., listed as wheat, rye, oats, or barley) or added as a derivative when a food is processed or prepared. Thus, *reading labels carefully is very important!* A great deal of confusion occurs about the presence of gliadin- and prolamin-containing additives in foods. This table includes lists of both nebulous ingredients and common additives.

Since flour and cereal products are quite often used in the preparation of foods, it is important to be aware of the methods of preparation used as well as the foods themselves. This is especially true when dining out.

| FOOD GROUP WITH SUGGESTED DAILY INTAKE | FOODS ALLOWED | FOODS TO AVOID |
|---|---|---|
| Milk (2 or more cups) | Fresh, dry, evaporated, or condensed milk; cream; sour cream;* whipping cream; yogurt* | Malted milk; some commercial chocolate drinks; some nondairy creamers.† |
| Meat, fish, poultry | All kinds of fresh meats, fish, other seafood, poultry; fish canned in oil, brine, or vegetable broth; some meat products, such as hot dogs and lunch meats† | Prepared meats containing wheat, rye, oats, or barley, such as some sausages,† hot dogs,† bologna†; luncheon meats†; ground beef and pork with oat bran added in the form of "Oatrim" or "LeanMaker"; chili con carne†; bread-containing products, such as swiss steak, meat loaf, and croquettes; tuna canned with hydrolyzed protein†; turkey with hydrolyzed vegetable protein (HVP) injected as part of the basting solution; "imitation Crab" containing wheat starch or other unacceptable filler. |
| Cheeses (Can be used for meat and milk groups) | All aged cheeses, such as cheddar, swiss, edam, parmesan; cottage cheese;* cream cheese;* pasteurized processed cheese*† | Any cheese product containing *oat gum* as an ingredient. |
| Eggs | Plain or in cooking. | Eggs in sauce made from wheat, rye, oat, or barley. Usually wheat flour is used in white sauce. |
| Potato or other starch | White and sweet potatoes; yams; hominy; rice; wild rice; special pasta made from rice, soy, or corn‡; some oriental rice and bean thread noodles. | Regular noodles; spaghetti or macaroni (semolina = wheat); most packaged rice mixes and frozen rice side dishes; frozen potato products with wheat starch or wheat flour added. |
| Vegetables (2 or more servings) | All plain, fresh, frozen, or canned; dried peas, beans, and lentils; some commercially prepared vegetables† | Creamed vegetables†; vegetables canned in sauce†; some canned baked beans†; commercially prepared vegetables and salads† |
| Fruits | All fresh, frozen, canned, or dried; all fruit juices; some canned pie fillings | Thickened or prepared fruits; some pie fillings† |
| Breads (3 or more servings) | Specially prepared breads using only allowed flours. Breads may be purchased ready-to-eat or as mixes to prepare at home. Recipes have been developed for home use and for use in automatic bread machines.‡ | Those containing wheat, rye, oats, and/or barley flours. Avoid those with buckwheat, millet, amaranth, quinoa, spelt, or teff.§ *Beware: wheat-free* does not always mean gliadin- and prolamin-free! Breads made from "carob-soy flour" may contain 80% wheat flour! |
| Cereals (1 or more servings) | *Hot cereals*<br>Corn meal<br>Cream of Rice<br>Hominy<br>Rice<br>*Cold cereals*<br>Puffed Rice<br>Corn Pops<br>Fruity and Choc. Pebbles<br>Kenmei<br>Sun Flakes (corn & rice)<br>Special cereals made without malt or malt flavoring. | Those containing wheat, rye, oats, barley, graham, wheat germ, malt or malt flavoring, kasha, bulgar, buckwheat,§ millet,§ amaranth,§ quinoa,§ spelt,§ teff.§<br>New products with "unusual" grains are constantly being introduced. Do not use them until you can clear them with a reliable source. |

**TABLE A–34.** CONTINUED

| FOOD GROUP WITH SUGGESTED DAILY INTAKE | FOODS ALLOWED | FOODS TO AVOID |
|---|---|---|
| Crackers and snack foods | Rice wafers; rice crackers; plain corn and potato chips; rice cakes†; pure cornmeal tortillas; popcorn; caramel corn† | Those with wheat, rye, barley, oats, or other questionable (grain-like) ingredients. *Read labels carefully.* Some coating mixes used on chips contain wheat flour! If the product shows "brown rice syrup," contact the manufacturer to check for "barley malt enzymes" used in processing. |
| Soups | Homemade broth and soup using allowed ingredients; a few canned soups;† specialty dry soup mixes‡ | Most canned soups† and soup mixes†; bouillon and bouillon cubes with hydrolyzed vegetable protein (HVP). HVP may appear as "flavoring" or "natural flavoring" ingredient. |
| Flours and thickening agents | Arrowroot starch (A)<br>Corn bean (B)<br>Corn flour‡ (B, C, D)<br>Corn germ (B)<br>Corn meal (B, C, D)<br>Potato flour (B, C, E)<br>Potato starch flour (B, C, E)<br>Rice bran (B)<br>Rice flours<br>Plain (B, C, D, E)<br>Brown (B, C, D, E)<br>Sweet (A, B, C, F)<br>Rice polish‡ (B, C, G)<br>Rice starch (A)<br>Soy flour‡ (B, C, G)<br>Tapioca starch (A) | Wheat starch<br>Wheat germ, bran<br>Wheat flour<br>Rye<br>Oats<br>Barley<br>Buckwheat§<br>Amaranth§<br>Quinoa§<br>Spelt§<br>Teff§<br>"Carob-soy" flour containing 80% wheat flour (made by Sterling Foods Co., Seattle) |
| A = good thickening agent; B = good combined with other flours; C = best combined with milk and eggs in baked products; D = grainy-textured products; E = drier product than with other flours; F = moister product than with other flours; G = adds distinct flavor to product, use with moderation. | | |
| Fats | Butter; margarine; vegetable oil; hydrogenated vegetable oil; nuts; peanut butter; some salad dressings†; mayonnaise† (mayonnaise made with cider or wine vinegar is found at Kosher delis) | Some commercial salad dressings†‖ |
| Desserts | Cakes; quick breads; pastries; puddings made with allowed ingredients; Cornstarch; tapioca; rice puddings; gelatin desserts; cook and serve puddings; "expensive" ice cream with a few simple ingredients; sorbet; frozen Yogurt†; sherbet† | Commercial cakes, cookies, pies, made with wheat, rye, oats, barley, millet, amaranth, buckwheat, quinoa, spelt, teff; Jello "instant" pudding; products containing brown rice syrup made with barley malt enzyme. |
| Beverages | Instant and ground coffee; instant tea; carbonated beverages†; pure cocoa powder; wines made in United States; rums; some root beers†; vodka distilled from grapes or potatoes. | Ovaltine; malted milk; ale; beer; gin; whiskeys‖; vodka distilled from grain; flavored coffees†; some herbal teas with barley or barley malt added† |
| Sweets | Jelly; jam; honey; brown and white sugar; molasses; most syrups†; some candy†; chocolate; pure cocoa; coconut; marshmallows† | Some commercial candies; foods with malt/malt flavoring or "natural flavoring"†; See's Molasses Chews; chocolate-coated nuts, which may be rolled in wheat flour†; brown rice syrup made with barley malt enzyme† |
| Miscellaneous | Spices (salt, pure pepper, cloves, ginger, nutmeg, cinnamon, allspice, etc.); herbs (oregano, rosemary, etc.); food coloring; alcohol-free extracts; yeast; baking soda; baking powder; cream of tartar; dry mustard; cider, rice and wine vinegars; olives; monosodium glutamate (MSG) made in United States | Condiments made with wheat-derived distilled white vinegar‖; alcohol-based extracts‖; some curry powders†; some dry seasoning mixes†; some gravy extracts†; some meat sauces†; most soy sauces†; some chewing gum†; communion wafers/bread# |

**TABLE A—34.** CONTINUED

*Check vegetable gum used.
†Consult label and contact manufacturer to clarify questionable ingredients.
‡See Special Products List for availability and ordering information.
§Additional information is needed before this product can be cleared.
||Distilled white vinegar uses grain as a starting material. Most often the grain mash includes wheat. Whiskies, including "corn whiskey," use wheat, rye, oats, or barley in their mash. According to chemistry professors consulted, in large-scale distillation processes, such as those used in the manufacture of whiskey and vinegar, it is possible that a very small amount of protein may be carried over into the distillate. The presence of such a small amount of gliadin and/or prolamin must be tested via immunoassay. Currently, we are advising gliadin- and prolamin-intolerant individuals to use cider, wine, or rice vinegar in such food preparation as making salad dressings, pickles, and in cooking. To be 100% safe, purchase or make condiments with cider, wine or rice vinegar. These condiments (ketchup, mustard, mayonnaise, pickles) are usually available in kosher delis. Foods with nongrain vinegars are produced for Passover.
#Contact the Gluten Intolerance Group of North America to obtain instructions for making communion wafers from acceptable ingredients. Note: In Catholic communion, host crumbs are often added to the wine before it is served. A workable solution is to arrange to use a goblet of your own.

| NEBULOUS INGREDIENT | INCLUDE | AVOID |
|---|---|---|
| "Hydrolyzed vegetable protein" or "hydrolyzed protein" | Those from soy, corn, or milk | Mixtures of wheat, corn, and soy* |
| "Flour" or "cereal products" | Rice flour, corn flour, corn meal, potato flour, soy flour | Wheat, rye, oats, barley, amaranth, quinoa, spelt, teff, millet, buckwheat |
| 'Vegetable protein" | Soy, corn | Wheat, rye, oats, barley |
| "Vegetable broth" | In the United States, this must contain two or more of the following: beans, cabbage, carrots, celery, garlic, onions, parsley, peas, potatoes, green bell pepper, red bell pepper, spinach, or tomatoes. It cannot contain any other ingredients. *It can be used.* | |
| "Malt" or "malt flavoring" | Those derived from corn. | Those derived from barley or barley malt syrup. |
| "Brown rice syrup" | Rice only. | Rice plus barley malt enzyme. |
| "Starch" | In the United States, it must be *cornstarch.* | |
| "Modified starch" or "modified food starch" | Arrowroot, corn, potato waxy maize, maize. | Wheat starch |
| "Vegetable gum" | Carob bean, locust bean, cellulose, guar, gum arabic, gum acacia, gum tragacanth, xanthan gum | Oat gum. |
| "Soy sauce" or "soy sauce solids" | Those that *do not* contain wheat *(soy only)* | Those brewed from wheat and soy. |
| "Mono-" and "diglycerides" | Those using *non*wheat-based carrier. | Those using a wheat starch carrier. |

These questionable ingredients must be cleared with the manufacturer before they are eaten. A sample letter requesting information on starting materials and packaging and processing ingredients is available at the end of this table.

*Hydrolyzed vegetable protein: A combination of wheat, corn, and soy is primarily used as starting material for hydrolyzed vegetable protein (HVP). When wheat protein is "hydrolyzed," its large amino acid chains are broken down into smaller chains. Some protein reseachers believe the same sequence of amino acids found in these smaller chains contain the same toxicity as the intact gliadin subfraction of the gluten protein. Thus, HVP made from wheat is not recommended for use on a gliadin-free diet.

ADDITIVES THAT ARE GLIADIN- AND PROLAMIN-FREE*

| | | |
|---|---|---|
| Adipic acid | Gums: acacia, arabic, carob bean, cellulose, guar, locust bean, tragacanth, xanthan | Riboflvin |
| Ascorbic acid | | |
| | | Sodium acid pyraphosphate |
| BHA | | Sodium ascorbate |
| BHT | Invert sugar | Sodium benzoate |
| Beta carotene | | Sodium caseinate |
| Biotin | Lactic acid | Sodium citrate |
| | Lactose | Sodium hexametaphosphate |
| Calcium chloride | Lecithin | Sodium nitrate |
| Calcium pantothenate | | Sodium silaco aluminate |
| Calcium phosphate | Magnesium hydroxide | Sorbitol—mannitol |
| Carboxymethylcellulose | Malic acid | Sucrose |
| Carrageenan | Microcrystallin cellulose | Sulfosuccinate |
| Citric acid | Monosodium glutamate (MSG) made in United States | |
| Corn sweetener | | Tartaric acid |
| Corn syrup solids | | Thiamine hydrochloride |
| | Niacin—niacinamide | Tri-calcium phosphate |
| Demineralized whey | | |
| Dextrimaltose | Polyglycerol | Vanillan |
| Dextrose—dextrins | Polysorbate 60; 80 | Vitamin A (palmitate) |
| Dioctyl sodium sulfosuccinate | Potassium citrate | Vitamins and minerals |
| | Potassium iodide | |
| Folic acid—folacin | Propylene glycol monostearate | |
| Fructose | Propylgallate | |
| Fumaric acid | Pyridoxine hydrochloride | |

*The above is not an exhaustive list.

**TABLE A—34.** CONTINUED

| MEDICATIONS | |
|---|---|
| All medications have fillers/dispersing agents added. These are usually lactose or corn starch. Wheat starch may also be used. *Before you take any medication, take the following precautions.*<br>*Over-the-Counter Drug:* Read the list of active and inactive ingredients carefully. Use the list of "Nebulous Ingredients" in this table to spot potential problems. Ask your pharmacist to "translate" the terms you do not know.<br>*Prescription Drug:* Inactive ingredients are *not* listed. Even your pharmacist must call the drug company to obtain this information! When the pharmaceutical company is contacted, they will need the lot number of the product so they can check the formulation of the batch you will be taking. A list of drug companies with addresses and phone numbers can be found in the Physicians' Desk Reference.<br>*Liquid Cold and Flu Medications:* These medications often contain alcohol. Check source. | |
| SPECIAL PRODUCTS LIST | |
| AlpineAire Foods<br>P.O. Box 926<br>Nevada City, CA 95959<br>916-272-1971 | Freeze-dried foods for backpacking. Vacuumed packed. No preservatives, no added sugar, no artificial flavors or colors. Note: The "vegetable pasta" in Pasta Roma and Vegetable Pasta Stew *contains wheat flour.*<br>Mail orders accepted. |
| Bickford Laboratories<br>282 S. Main Street<br>Akron, OH 44308<br>216-762-4666 | Forty-nine varieties of alcohol-free flavorings. Selection ranges from common flavorings, like vanilla and almond, to exotic.<br>Mail orders accepted. |
| DeBoles<br>Garden City Park, NY 11040 | Corn pasta products, including ribbon noodles, macaroni, and spaghetti. |
| Dietary Specialties<br>P.O. Box 227<br>Rochester, NY 14601<br>1-800-544-0099 | A wide assortment of mixes, crackers, cookies, and pasta. Many exclusive imported items.<br>Mail orders accepted. |
| Ener-G Foods, Inc.<br>P.O. Box 84487<br>Seattle, WA 98124-5787<br>1-800-331-5222 | Excellent assortment of flours and flour mixes. Will ship in bulk (20# boxes). Variety of baked products, dry soup mixes, flavorings.<br>Mail orders accepted. |
| Lundberg Family Farms<br>Box 369<br>Richvale, CA 95974<br>916-882-4551 | Interesting variety of combination rices. Brown rice cereals and rice cakes.<br>Note: Sweet Dreams Brown Rice Syrup is made using barley malt enzyme. Products made with this syrup should be avoided. Soups contain wheat-derived soy sauce.<br>Mail orders accepted. |
| Med-Diet Inc.<br>3050 Ranchview Lane<br>Plymouth, MN 55447<br>1-800-med-diet | Carries various brands of breads, crackers, cookies, cake and muffin mixes, and pasta.<br>Note: Their order blank is not designed for those who must eliminate gliadin and prolamin. Request their list of "wheat/gluten-free foods that contain no wheat starch" so you'll know what to order! |
| Red Mill Farms, Inc.<br>290 S. 5th Street<br>Brooklyn, NY 11211<br>718-384-2150 | Three suitable products that are also lactose free: Dutch Chocolate Cake, Banana-Nut Cake, and Coconut Macaroons. All vacuumed packed.<br>Mail orders accepted. |
| Tad Enterprizes<br>9356 Pleasant<br>Tinley Park, IL 60477<br>708-429-2101 | Carry a variety of flours for gliadin- and prolamin-free baking.<br>Mail orders accepted. |
| Van Brode's Milling<br>Clinton, MA 01510 | Carries some cold breakfast cereals (malt free). Write for complete product information. |

**TABLE A–34.** CONTINUED

| WRITING EFFECTIVE LETTERS TO FOOD MANUFACTURERS* |
|---|
| Clarifying questionable ingredients on product labels and in medications is essential for those following this diet. Manufacturers are usually courteous and prompt when answering questions regarding their products. The usefulness of their reply, however, often depends on how the question is posed. Use the following letter format when you need to contact a a manufacturer. |

Your Address
Date

Dear Sir/Madam:

I am on a gluten-restricted, gliadin- and prolamin-free diet for the treatment of celiac sprue (dermatitis herpetiformis). I must avoid the protein found in wheat, rye, oats, and barley, since they cause an immune response which damages the lining of my intestine.

Although I would like to use your product, (insert name), your ingredient listing does not give adequate information for me to determine if it would be suitable. Specifically, I need to know

examples would be:

the source of your "food starch modified"
whether your "soy sauce solids" are derived from wheat
what "natural flavorings" you use in this product
from what source your "vegetable gum" is derived
the inacive ingredients used in the medication, including those used in the coatings and capsules

Another likely source of gliadin and prolamin contamination is the incidental ingredients which are used in the packaging and processing of your product. Since these incidental ingredients are not listed on the packaging, I am relying on your thoroughness to clarify these substances.

If it would be possible, I would appreciate a copy of your response to be forwarded to: The Gluten Intolerance Group of North America
P.O. Box 23053
Seattle, WA 98102-0353

This will allow your efforts to be shared with others through our national organization which reaches health-care personnel as well as persons with celiac sprue and dermatitis herpetiformis. If you have questions regardiing these disorders and the required dietary restrictions, please direct them to our national office.

Thank you for your efforts on my behalf.

Sincerely,
Your Signature

*Additional information on celiac sprue and dermatitis herpetiformis may be obtained from The Gluten Intolerance Group of North America, P.O. Box 23053, Seattle WA 98102-0353.

## TABLE A–35A. LACTOSE-CONTROLLED DIET

*Purpose:* The lactose-controlled diet is designed to prevent or reduce bloating, flatulence, cramping, and diarrhea associated with ingesting lactose-containing products.

*Modifications:* The diet is a general one that restricts or eliminates lactose-containing foods and beverages. Since tolerance of lactose may vary, the diet is usually administered on a trial-and-error basis.[1] Individual tolerance determines the amount of lactose allowed; many patients may be able to tolerate 5 to 8 g of lactose at a given time, especially if they consume it with a meal.[2]

Labels should be read carefully, and foods containing milk, lactose, milk solids, whey, curds, skim milk powder, and skim milk solids should be avoided. In addition to dairy products, the following food categories may contain lactose: breads, candy and cookies; cold cuts, hot dogs, and bologna; commercial sauces and gravies; cream soups; dry cereals; frostings; frozen breaded fish and chicken; prepared and processed foods; salad dressings containing milk or cheese; sugar substitutes; and instant drink mixes. Moreover, some medications and vitamins may contain lactose as a carrier. Lactate, lactalbumin, lactulate, and calcium compounds are salts of lactic acid and do not contain lactose.

Patients should be encouraged to experiment with the lactose-reduced or lactose-free products currently available. In addition, lactase enzyme is available in droplet form for use with lactose-containing beverages and in tablet form for ingestion prior to consuming a lactose-containing meal. Lactobacillus acidophilus milk is not equivalent to lactase-treated milk.

Tolerance to lactose is variable; if a patient is asymptomatic, no restrictions are necessary. If the patient experiences adverse reactions to lactose, cessation of symptoms should occur within 3 to 5 days on a lactose-controlled diet. Further testing may be necessary if symptoms persist.[2] Small amounts of lactose-containing food (approximately 3 g) several times a day may be tolerated better than a large amount of lactose ingested at one time.[3] Studies have shown that yogurt is significantly better tolerated than milk because of its high lactase activity.[3,4] Different brands and processing methods, however, may affect tolerance to yogurt.

*Adequacy:* Depending on individual food choices, the diet can provide adequate amounts of all essential nutrients. Calcium, vitamin D, and riboflavin may be deficient if all dairy products are avoided. Use of lactose-hydrolyzed milk and milk products could satisfy these nutrient needs; otherwise, supplementation may be necessary.

*References*


**1.** Shils, M.E., Young, V.R. (Eds.): Modern Nutrition in Health and Disease. 7th Ed. Philadelphia, Lea & Febiger, 1988.
**2.** Martini, M. Savaiano, D.: Am. J. Clin. Nutr., *47*:57–60, 1988.
**3.** Onwulata, C.I., Rao, D.R., Vankineni, P.: Am. J. Clin. Nutr., *49*:1233–1237, 1989.
**4.** Wytock, D.H., DiPalma, J.A.: Am. J. Clin. Nutr., *47*:454–457, 1988.


*Further Reading*


Burlant, A.: Lactose-Free Cooking. Wayne, NJ, Lockley Publishing, 1990.
Dobler, M.L.: Lactose Intolerance. Chicago, The American Dietetic Association, 1991, catalog no. 0881.
Martens, R.A., Martens, S.: The Milk Sugar Dilemma. 2nd Ed. Lansing, Medi-Ed Press, 1987.
Zukin, J.: Dairy-Free Cookbook. Rocklin, CA, Prima Publishing and Communications, 1989.


*Special Product Information*

Lactaid can be purchased in tablets, drops, or as lactase-treated milk and cheese products.

Lactaid Hotline
800-257-8650
9 AM–4 PM Eastern time
Monday through Friday
In Canada: 800-387-5711

Lactaid, Inc.
P.O. Box 111
Pleasantville, NJ 08232

Lactase tablets are produced by:

Kremers-Urban Company
P.O. Box 2038
Milwaukee, WI 53201

Dairy Ease tablets and lactose-treated milk (skim, 1%, and 2% fat) are produced by:

Winthrop Consumer Products
Glenbrook Laboratories
Division of Sterling Drug, Inc.
90 Park Ave.
New York, NY 10016

(From The Manual of Clinical Dietetics. 4th Ed. Chicago, American Dietetic Association, 1992. With permission.)

**TABLE A–35B.** GUIDELINES FOR FOOD SELECTION FOR LACTOSE-CONTROLLED DIET*

| FOOD CATEGORY | RECOMMENDED | MAY CAUSE DISTRESS* |
|---|---|---|
| Beverages | All beverages with allowed ingredients; soybean milks; other lactose-free supplements; lactase-hydrolyzed milk | Milk, milk products, or acidophilus milk as tolerance dictates |
| Breads and cereals | Whole-grain or enriched breads and cereals | Depending on tolerance, some breads and cereals prepared with milk or milk products may need to be avoided |
| Desserts | Cakes, cookies, pies; flavored gelatin desserts; water ices made with allowed foods | Any prepared with milk or milk products (e.g., sherbet, ice cream, ice milk, custard, pudding, commercial desserts, and mixes) |
| Fats | Butter or margarine; salad dressings; nondairy creamer; all oils | Any prepared with lactose-containing ingredients |
| Fruits | All fruits and juices | None |
| Meats and meat substitutes | All meats, poultry, fish; eggs; peanut butter; dried peas and beans; hard, aged, and processed cheese, if tolerated; yogurt as tolerated | Cold cuts and frankfurters that contain lactose filler; cottage cheese |
| Potatoes and potato substitutes | Potatoes; enriched rice; barley; noodles, spaghetti, macaroni, and other pastas | Potatoes or substitutes prepared with milk or milk products; mixes prepared with lactose-containing ingredients |
| Soups | Broth; bouillon; soups made with allowed ingredients | Soups prepared with milk or milk products |
| Sweets | Sugar; corn syrup; pure maple syrup; honey; jellies; jams; pure sugar candies; marshmallows | Chocolate; caramels; any candies made with lactose-containing ingredients |
| Vegetables | All | Vegetables prepared with milk or milk products |
| Miscellaneous | All spices, seasonings, flavorings | Any prepared with milk or milk products |

*A lactose-free diet, from which virtually all known sources of lactose are eliminated, may be indicated for patients with severe intolerance or a congenital lactase deficiency.

(From The Manual of Clinical Dietetics. 4th Ed. American Dietetic Association, 1992. With permission.)

**TABLE A—35C.** SAMPLE MENU FOR LACTOSE-CONTROLLED DIET*

| BREAKFAST | LUNCH | DINNER |
|---|---|---|
| Orange juice (½ cup) | Vegetable soup (1 cup) | Green salad (3½ oz) |
| Whole-grain cereal (¾ cup) | Saltine crackers (4) | Oil and vinegar dressing (1 Tbsp) |
| Banana (½) | Lean beef patty (3 oz) | Broiled skinless chicken breast (3 oz) |
| Whole-wheat toast (2 slices) | Hamburger bun (1) | Herbed brown rice (½ cup) |
| Margarine (2 tsp) | Catsup (1 Tbsp) | Steamed broccoli (½ cup) |
| Jelly or jam (1 Tbsp) | Mustard (1 Tbsp) | Whole-grain roll (1) |
| Lactose-reduced 2% milk (1 cup) | Sliced tomato (2 oz) and lettuce | Margarine (2 tsp) |
| Coffee/tea | Fresh fruit salad (½ cup) | Fruit ice (½ cup) |
| | Graham crackers (4) | Medium apple (1) |
| | Lactose-reduced 2% milk (1 cup) | Coffee/tea |
| | Coffee/tea | |

APPROXIMATE NUTRIENT ANALYSIS

| | | | |
|---|---|---|---|
| Energy (kcal) | 2,157.2 | Sodium (mg) | 3,069.8 |
| Protein (g) (15.6% of kcal) | 83.9 | Zinc (mg) | 11.7 |
| Carbohydrate (g) (56.8% of kcal) | 306.3 | Vitamin A (µg RE) | 1,111.5 |
| Total fat (g) (30.1% of kcal) | 72.1 | Vitamin C (mg) | 256.8 |
| Saturated fatty acids (g) | 18.3 | Thiamin (mg) | 1.7 |
| Monounsaturated fatty acids (g) | 27.3 | Riboflavin (mg) | 1.4 |
| Polyunsaturated fatty acids (g) | 19.4 | Niacin (mg) | 29.0 |
| Cholesterol (mg) | 144.4 | Folate (µg) | 471.0 |
| Calcium (mg) | 1,413.5 | Vitamin $B_6$ (mg) | 2.5 |
| Iron (mg) | 16.1 | Vitamin $B_{12}$ (µg) | 2.2 |
| Magnesium (mg) | 380.2 | Dietary fiber (g) | 23.5 |
| Phosphorus (mg) | 1,121.7 | Water-insoluble fiber (g) | 16.4 |
| Potassium (mg) | 3,580.2 | | |

*If lactose-reduced milk is not tolerated, substitute ½ cup nondairy creamer at breakfast and fruit juice at lunch. A calcium supplement should also be provided.

(From The Manual of Clinical Dietetics. 4th Ed. Chicago, American Dietetic Association, 1992. With permission.)

**TABLE A–35D.** LACTOSE CONTENT OF SELECTED MILK, MILK PRODUCTS, AND SUBSTITUTES*

| PRODUCT | | LACTOSE (APPROX. g/UNIT) |
|---|---|---|
| Milk | 1 cup—244 g | 11 |
| Low-fat milk (2% fat) | 1 cup—244 g | 9–13 |
| Skim milk | 1 cup—244 g | 12–14 |
| Chocolate milk | 1 cup—244 g | 10–12 |
| Sweetened condensed whole milk | 1 cup—306 g | 35 |
| Dried whole milk | 1 cup—128 g | 48 |
| Nonfat dry milk, instant | 1½ cup—91 g | 46 |
| Buttermilk fluid | 1 cup—245 g | 9–11 |
| Whipped cream topping | 1 Tbsp—3 g | 0.4 |
| Light Cream | 1 Tbsp—15 g | 0.6 |
| Half and Half | 1 Tbsp—15 g | 0.6 |
| Low-fat yogurts† | 8 oz—227–258 g | 11–15 |
| Cheese: | | |
| Blue, cream, Parmesan, Colby | 1 oz—28 g | 0.7–0.8 |
| Camembert, Limburger | 1 oz—28 g | 0.1 |
| Cheddar, Gouda | 1 oz—28 g | 0.4–0.6 |
| Cheese, pasteurized, processed: | | |
| American | 1 oz—28 g | 0.5 |
| Pimento | 1 oz—28 g | 0.5–1.7 |
| Swiss | 1 oz—28 g | 0.4–0.6 |
| Cottage cheese | 1 cup—210 g | 5–6 |
| Cottage cheese, low-fat (2% fat) | 1 cup—226 g | 7–8 |
| Butter | 2 pats—10 g | 0.1 |
| Oleomargarine | 2 pats—10 g | 0 |
| Ice cream | | |
| Vanilla, regular | 1 cup—133 g | 9 |
| French, soft | 1 cup—173 g | 9 |
| Ice milk, vanilla | 1 cup—131 g | 10 |
| Sherbet, orange | 1 cup—193 g | 4 |
| Ice, orange | 100 g | 0 |

*Lactaid milk and other dairy products have lactose reduced by 70%. With further treatment, these products can be 100% lactose-free.

†Bacterial lactase in unpasteurized yogurt survives transit through the stomach, thus allowing digestion of the lactose present in yogurt. This process enables lactase-deficient individuals to consume these dairy products in moderate amounts (from ½ to 1 pint) with fewer or no symptoms. Data from Kolars, J.C., Levitt, M.D., Aouji, M., et al.: N. Engl. J. Med., *310*:1–3, 1984.

Lactase-deficient patients have been reported to experience no gastrointestinal distress after consuming pasteurized yogurt (500 g) even though the lactase activity is significantly destroyed by pasteurization. In contrast, cultured milk does result in gastrointestinal distress for lactose-intolerant individuals. Data from Savaiano, D.A., AbouElAnouar, A., Smith, D.E., et al.: Am. J. Clin. Nutr., *40*:1219–1223, 1984.

(From Walsh, J.D.: Am. J. Clin. Nutr., *31*:592–596, 1978. With permission of the author and publisher.)

**TABLE A–36.** OXALATE CONTENT OF SELECTED FOODS AND FOOD GROUPS

FOODS TO USE: THESE CONTAIN SMALL AMOUNTS OF OXALATE
0–2 mg OXALATE PER SERVING

| Vegetables | Fruits | Beverages | Miscellaneous |
|---|---|---|---|
| Broccoli | Avocados | Apple juice | Butter |
| Brussels sprouts | Bananas | Barley water | Cheese, cheddar |
| Cabbage | Cherries | Beer, bottled | Chicken noodle soup |
| Cauliflower | Grapes, Thompson seedless | Cider | Cornflakes |
| Chives | Mangoes | Coca-Cola | Eggs |
| Cucumbers | Melons | Grapefruit juice | Egg noodle (chow mein) |
| Lettuce | Nectarines | Lemon squash drink (lemonade) | Fish (except sardines) |
| Mushrooms | Peaches, canned | Lucozade, bottled | Jelly with allowed fruit |
| Onions | Hiley | Milk | Lemon juice |
| Peas | Stokes | Orange juice | Lime juice |
| Potatoes, white | Pineapples | Pepsi-Cola | Macaroni |
| Radishes | Plums, golden gage, green gage | Pineapple juice | Margarine |
| Rice | | Sherry, dry | Meats |
| Turnips | | Wine | Oatmeal, porridge |
| | | | Oxtail soup |
| | | | Poultry |
| | | | Red plum jam |
| | | | Sweets, boiled |

FOODS TO AVOID: THESE CONTAIN LARGE AMOUNTS OF OXALATE
>15 mg OXALATE PER SERVING

| Vegetables | Fruits | Beverages | Miscellaneous |
|---|---|---|---|
| Beans in tomato sauce | Blackberries | Beer, lager | Chocolate |
| Beets | Blueberries | Tuborg Pilsner | Cocoa |
| Celery | Currants, red | Ovaltine (24 mg/8 oz) | Grits (white corn) |
| Chard, Swiss | Gooseberries, green | Tea (132–181.2 mg/8 oz) | Peanuts |
| Collards | Grapes, Concord | | Pecans |
| Dandelion greens | Lemon peel | | Soybean crackers |
| Eggplant | Lime peel | | Wheat germ |
| Escarole | Raspberries, black | | |
| Leeks | Rhubarb | | |
| Okra | | | |
| Parsley | | | |
| Peppers, green | | | |
| Pokeweed | | | |
| Potatoes, sweet | | | |
| Rutabagas | | | |
| Spinach | | | |
| Squash, summer | | | |

LOW-OXALATE MEAL PLAN
(40–50 mg)

| Foods | Little or No Oxalate Content<br><2 mg Oxalate/Serving<br>Eat as Desired | Moderate Oxalate Content<br>2–10 mg Oxalate/Serving<br>Limit: 2 (½ cup) Servings/Day | High Oxalate Content<br>>10 mg Oxalate/Serving<br>Avoid Completely |
|---|---|---|---|
| Beverages/Juices | Apple juice | Coffee, any kind (8 oz serving) | Beer: draft |
| | Beer, bottled | Cranberry juice (4 oz) | Stout, Guinness Draft |
| | Coca-Cola (12 oz limit/day) | Grape juice (4 oz) | Lager, Tuborg Pilsner |
| | Distilled alcohol | Orange juice (4 oz) | Juices containing berries |
| | Grapefruit juice | Tomato juice (4 oz) | Ovaltine and other mixed beverage mixes |
| | Lemonade or limeade without peel | Nescafé powder | Tea, cocoa |
| | Wine, red, rosé | | |
| | Pepsi-Cola (12 oz limit/day) | | |
| | Pineapple juice | | |
| | Tap water (prefered for extra calcium) | | |
| Milk (2 or more cups) | Buttermilk | | |
| | Low-fat milk | | |
| | Low-fat yogurt with allowed fruit | | |
| | Skim milk | | |

**TABLE A–36.** CONTINUED

LOW-OXALATE MEAL PLAN
(40–50 mg)

| Foods | Little or No Oxalate Content<br><2 mg Oxalate/Serving<br>Eat as Desired | Moderate Oxalate Content<br>2–10 mg Oxalate/Serving<br>Limit: 2 (½ cup) Servings/Day | High Oxalate Content<br>>10 mg Oxalate/Serving<br>Avoid Completely |
|---|---|---|---|
| Meat Group | Eggs<br>Cheese, cheddar<br>Lean lamb, beef, or pork<br>Poultry<br>Seafood | Sardines | Baked beans canned in tomato sauce<br>Peanut butter<br>Soybean curd (Tofu) |
| Vegetables | Brussels sprouts<br>Cauliflower<br>Cabbage<br>Mushrooms<br>Onions<br>Peas, green<br>Potatoes (Irish)<br>Radishes | Asparagus<br>Broccoli<br>Carrots<br>Corn, sweet white, sweet yellow<br>Cucumbers, peeled<br>Green peas, canned<br>Lettuce, iceberg<br>Lima beans<br>Parsnips<br>Tomato, 1 small<br>Turnips | Beans, green, wax, dried<br>Beets, tops, root, greens<br>Celery<br>Chard, Swiss<br>Chives<br>Collards<br>Dandelion greens<br>Eggplant<br>Escarole<br>Kale<br>Leeks<br>Mustard greens<br>Okra<br>Parsley<br>Peppers, green<br>Pokeweed<br>Potatoes, sweet<br>Rutabagas<br>Spinach<br>Squash, summer<br>Watercress |
| Fruits | Avocados<br>Banana<br>Cherries, Bing<br>Grapefruit<br>Grapes, Thompson seedless<br>Mangoes<br>Melons<br>cantaloupe<br>casaba<br>honeydew<br>watermelon<br>Nectarines<br>Peaches, Hiley<br>Plums, green or Golden Age | Apples<br>Apricots<br>Cherries, edible portion<br>Currants, black<br>Oranges, edible portion<br>Peaches, Alberta<br>Pears<br>Pineapples<br>Plums, Damson<br>Prunes, Italian | Blackberries<br>Blueberries<br>Currants, red<br>Dewberries<br>Fruit cocktail<br>Gooseberries<br>Grapes, Concord<br>Lemon peel<br>Lime peel<br>Orange peel<br>Raspberries<br>Rhubarb<br>Strawberries<br>Tangerines |
| Bread Starches | Cornflakes<br>Macaroni<br>Noodles<br>Oatmeal<br>Rice<br>Spaghetti<br>White bread | Cornbread<br>Sponge cake<br>Spaghetti, canned in tomato sauce | Fruit cake<br>Grits, white corn<br>Soybean crackers<br>Wheat germ |
| Fats and Oils | Bacon<br>Mayonnaise<br>Salad dressing<br>Vegetable oils | | Peanuts<br>Pecans |
| Miscellaneous | Jelly or preserves (made with allowed fruits)<br>Lemon, lime juice<br>Salt, pepper (1 tsp/day)<br>Soups with ingredients allowed<br>Sugar | Chicken noodle soup, dehydrated | Chocolate, cocoa<br>Pepper (in excess of 1 tsp/day)<br>Vegetable soup<br>Tomato soup |

(From The Low Oxalate Diet Book, General Clinical Research Center, University of California at San Diego Medical Center and San Diego Chapter of National Foundation for Ileitis and Colitis, 1981. With permission.)

**TABLE A–37.** COMMERCIAL NUTRITION FORMULATIONS FOR ORAL AND TUBE FEEDING

The sixth and seventh editions included numerous tables providing detailed nutrient composition of a variety of available commercial formulas. In more recent years, the companies making these formulas have uniformly provided updated information in reprints that are widely distributed. These reprints often contain the composition of formulas produced by other companies as well as their own. Additionally, new and revised commercial preparations appear on the market in increasing numbers, whereas some older formulas have been removed. These commercial reference guides make the continued publication of detailed formulations unnecessary and actually undesirable in this volume. Thus, outdated information can be avoided.

A list is provided below of the companies currently producing and marketing such formulations. Address and telephone numbers are included to help the reader to obtain the most current information on a specific product. Each company also produces an enteral product reference list that provides nutrient analysis on each product, as well as other relevant information needed to make informed choices. They may be contacted for such publications or for other educational materials they provide. In addition, a list is included of the names of current formulations by dietary use characteristics.

COMPANY LISTS WITH IDENTIFICATION CODE

*CLINTEC Nutrition Company (C)*
Affiliated with Baxter Healthcare Corporation
and Nestles S.A.
Three Parkway North, Suite 500
P.O. Box 760
Deerfield, IL 60015-0760
1-800-422-2752

*KENDALL McGAW (K)*
2525 McGaw Avenue
P.O. Box 19791
Irvine, CA 92713
714-660-2000
1-800-854-6851 (Technical Assistance)

*MEAD JOHNSON ENTERAL NUTRITIONALS (M)*
Mead Johnson Nutrition Group
A Bristol Myers Squibb Company
Evansville, IN 47721
1-800-457-3550

*ELAN PHARMA (E)*
320 Charles Street
Cambridge, MA 02141
617-868-6400
1-800-237-3535

*ROSS LABORATORIES (R)*
Division of Abbott Laboratories
625 Cleveland Avenue
Columbus, OH 43215
614-227-3333
1-800-544-7495

*SANDOZ NUTRITION (S)*
5300 West 23rd Street
Minneapolis, MN 55416
1-800-999-9978

*SHERWOOD MEDICAL (SH)*
1915 Olive Street
St. Louis, MO 63103-1642
314-621-7788
1-800-428-4400

**TABLE A–37.** CONTINUED

CURRENT LIST OF FORMULATIONS FOR ORAL AND/OR ENTERAL FEEDING BY DIETARY USE CHARACTERISTICS

*Complete Diet Formulations Containing Some Natural Foods with Varying Residue*
Carnation Instant Breakfast (C)
Carnation Instant Breakfast, no sugar (C)
Compleat Regular (S)
Compleat Modified (S)
Meritene Powder (S)
Sustagen (M)
Vitaneed (SH)

*Complete Defined-formula Diets with Intact Purified Protein, Low Residue, and No Lactose*
Attain (SH)
CitriSource (S)
Citrotein (S)
Comply (SH)
Ensure (R)
Ensure HN (R)
Ensure Plus (R)
Ensure Plus HN (R)
Entrition 0.5 (C)
Entrition HN (C)
Fortical (SH)
Fortison (SH)
Fortison, L.S. (SH)
Introlan (E)
Introlite (R)
Isocal (M)
Isocal HCN (M)
Isocal HN (M)
Isolan (E)
Isosource (S)
Isosource HN (S)
Isotein HN (S)
Magnacal (SH)
Nitrolan (E)
Nutren 1.0 (C)
Nutren 1.5 (C)
Nutren 2.0 (C)
Nutrilan (E)
Osmolite (R)
Osmolite HN (R)
Portagen (M)
Pre-Attain (SH)
Pre-Fortison (SH)
Promote (R)
Replete Oral (C)
Resource Liquid (S)
Resource Plus Liquid (S)
Ross SLD (R)
Susta II (M)
Sustacal (M)
Sustacal HC (M)
Sustacal 8.8 (M)
Travasorb MCT (C)
Two Cal HN (R)
Ultralan (E)

**TABLE A–37.** CONTINUED

| |
|---|
| *Complete Defined Formula Diets with Intact Purified Protein, No Lactose-Containing Fiber* |
| Ensure with Fiber (R) |
| Fiberlan (E) |
| Fibersource (S) |
| Fibersource HN (S) |
| Jevity (R) |
| Nutren with Fiber (C) |
| Profiber (SH) |
| Replete with Fiber (C) |
| Sustacal with Fiber (M) |
| Ultracal (M) |
| *Defined Formula Diets with Hydrolyzed Protein or Amino Acids, Low Residue, and No Lactose* |
| Accupep HPF (SH) |
| Alitraq (R) |
| Criticare HN (M) |
| Peptamen (C) |
| Reabilan (E) |
| Reabilan HN (E) |
| Tolerex (S) |
| Travasorb HN (C) |
| Travasorb (C) |
| Vital HN (R) |
| Vivonex T.E.N. (S) |
| *Disease-Specific Formulations* |
| Alterna (R) |
| Aminess Essential Amino Acid Tablets (C) |
| Amin-Aid (K) |
| Glucerna (R) |
| Hepatic-Aid II (K) |
| Immun-Aid (K) |
| Impact (S) |
| Impact with Fiber (S) |
| Lipisorb (M) |
| Nepro (R) |
| Nutri Hep (C) |
| Nutrivent (C) |
| Perative (R) |
| Protain XL (SH) |
| Pulmocare (R) |
| Replena (R) |
| Replete (C) |
| Stresstein (S) |
| Suplena (R) |
| Traum-Aid HBC (K) |
| TraumaCal (M) |
| Travasorb Hepatic (C) |
| Travasorb Renal (C) |

( ) = Company identification, see preceding list.

*O'Brien KMI is now Elan Pharma. The Newtrition product line is now the Elan product line.

# INDEX

Page numbers in *italics* indicate figures; numbers followed by "t" indicate tables.